# *Surgical Diseases*
# *~ of the ~*
# *Pancreas*

THIRD EDITION

# *Surgical Diseases ~ of the ~ Pancreas*

THIRD EDITION

EDITED BY

*John M. Howard, MD, FACS, FRCS-Edinburgh (Hon), FCS-Brazil (Hon)*

*Professor of Surgery, Emeritus*
*Medical College of Ohio*
*Toledo, Ohio*

*Yasuo Idezuki, MD*

*Professor and Chairman*
*Department of Surgery*
*Saitama Medical Center, Saitama Medical School*
*Saitama, Japan*

*Ingemar Ihse, MD, PhD*

*Professor and Chairman*
*Department of Surgery*
*University Hospital*
*Lund, Sweden*

*Richard A. Prinz, MD*

*Helen Shedd Kieth Professor and Chairman*
*Department of General Surgery*
*Rush-Presbyterian-St. Luke's Medical Center*
*Chicago, Illinois*

Williams & Wilkins

A WAVERLY COMPANY

BALTIMORE • PHILADELPHIA • LONDON • PARIS • BANGKOK
BUENOS AIRES • HONG KONG • MUNICH • SYDNEY • TOKYO • WROCLAW

Editor: *Carroll C. Cann*
Managing Editor: *Joanne Husovsky*
Marketing Manager: *Diane M. Harnish*
Production Coordinator: *Peter J. Carley*
Project Editor: *Jeffrey S. Myers*
Designer: *Graphic World Publishing Services*
Illustration Planner: *Lorraine Wrzosek*
Cover Designer: *Graphic World Publishing Services*
Typesetter and Digitized Illustrations: *Graphic World, Inc.*
Printer/Binder: *Walsworth Publishing Co.*



351 West Camden Street
Baltimore, Maryland 21201-2436 USA

Rose Tree Corporate Center
1400 North Providence Road
Building II, Suite 5025
Media, Pennsylvania 19063-2043 USA



Accurate indications, adverse reactions and dosage schedules for drugs are provided in this book, but it is possible that they may change. The reader is urged to review the package information data of the manufacturers of the medications mentioned.

*Printed in the United States of America*

First Edition, 1976
Second Edition, 1987

**Library of Congress Cataloging-in-Publication Data**

Surgical diseases of the pancreas/edited by John Howard . . . [et al.].—2nd ed.
p. cm.
Rev. ed. of: Surgical diseases of the pancreas/John M. Howard, George L. Jordan, Jr., Howard A. Reber. 1987.
Includes bibliographical references and index.
ISBN 0-683-18019-3
1. Pancreas—Surgery. 2. Pancreas—Diseases. I. Howard, John M. (John Malone), 1919-
[DNLM: 1. Pancreas—surgery. 2. Pancreatic Diseases. WI 830 S962 1998]
RD546.H65 1998
617.5′57—dc21
DNLM/DLC
for Library of Congress

97-22075
CIP

The publishers have made every effort to trace the copyright holders for borrowed material. If they have inadvertently overlooked any, they will be pleased to make the necessary arrangements at the first opportunity.

To purchase additional copies of this book, call our customer service department at (800) 638-0672 or fax orders to (800) 447-8438. For other book services, including chapter reprints and large quantity sales, ask for the Special Sales department.

Canadian customers should call (800) 665-1148, or fax (800) 665-0103. For all other calls originating outside of the United States, please call (410) 528-4223 or fax us at (410) 528-8550.

Visit Williams and Wilkins on the Internet: http://www.wwilkins.com or contact our customer service department at custserv@wwilkins.com. Williams & Wilkins customer service representatives are available from 8:30 am to 6:00 pm, EST, Monday through Friday, for telephone access.

97 98 99 00
1 2 3 4 5 6 7 8 9 10

# *Dedication*

Dedicated to our beloved wives—Nina, Yuko, Maggan, and Lori.
Without their love, patience, and encouragement over the years,
it would not have been possible.

And to the late George L. Jordon, Jr., MD,
Distinguished Professor, Baylor University College of Medicine,
scholar, surgeon, and friend.

# Foreword

Jonathan E. Rhoads, MD

The pancreas is a complex organ. Situated as it is behind the duodenum, behind the stomach, extending to the hilum of the spleen, it is the last bastion to be attacked by modern surgery. Furthermore, the attacks on pancreatic disease, particularly adenocarcinoma of the pancreas, have had very limited success, so that pancreatic pathology remains a frontier on which many persons in many countries are endeavoring to advance. Much has been learned yet many problems remain to be solved. Had I been asked how many chapters it would take to cover the subject, I would have flunked the test. The present volume has over 80 chapters, each covering a different facet of pancreatic disease, diagnosis, and therapy.

When Dr. Howard wrote to ask if I would prepare a foreword for this third edition, I was very close to my 90th birthday and looked back on my own keen interest but very limited success in treating pancreatic disease. I had met and greatly admired Dr. Allen O. Whipple and in 1941 carried out a Whipple operation with the sudden death of the patient from a pulmonary embolus on the 10th postoperative day. There followed at fairly long intervals other efforts, some temporary successes, and experience with numerous serious complications, often related to leakage of activated pancreatic juice with autodigestion and hemorrhage. These experiences led us to try the technique of pancreatogastrostomy, which we learned from an article by Melbourne and which I still believe has certain significant advantages in reconnecting the duct of Wirsung with the GI tract (1). Later, with collaborators, I carried out laborious reviews of the literature of islet cell adenomas and had the opportunity to operate on some adenomas. Still later, I was called upon to write a chapter on the history of pancreatic surgery, in which I was joined by a niece, then a medical student. Intermingled with this personal background, it has been my privilege to follow the career of Dr. John M. Howard, the senior editor of this volume. A student at the School of Medicine of the University of Pennsylvania 1941–1944, he interned at its teaching hospital and took his residency training there with I.S. Ravdin during the years when I was an active member of the department. A few years after leaving the University of Pennsylvania and after serving as Director of the U.S. Army's Surgical Research Team in Korea, Dr. Howard was appointed Chairman of the Department of Surgery at Emory University, where he had the opportunity of studying numerous cases of pancreatitis at the municipal hospital in Atlanta. It was there that he and his resident, Dr. Joseph Owens, drew attention to the first correlation between alcoholism and calcification in the pancreas. In Chapters 19 and 30 of the present volume, he summarizes his observations on different types of pancreatitis. After moving to his present situation as a Professor of Surgery at the Medical College of Ohio, he reported a unique series of pancreatoduodenectomies (2), personally performed, which was subsequently extended (3) to over 70 consecutive operations without an intervening death. More recently, he has reported a series of over 70 cases of necrotizing pancreatitis with a mortality rate of less than 3% (4).

Thus, both pancreatic carcinoma and pancreatitis have been a lifelong study by the senior editor of this volume, and he is the personal author of chapters on each of these important segments of the whole story. Professor Yasuo Idezuki has recently been President of the Japan Surgical Association, President of the International Society of Surgery, and Vice-President of the International Federation of Surgical Colleges. This extremely able surgeon has been a key to the numerous valuable studies recently carried out by Japanese authors and published in the Japanese and English literature. Dr. Ingemar Ihse of the University of Lund has been an honorary member of the American Surgical Association where I have had the opportunity of becoming acquainted with him and with Dr. Richard Prinz, who enjoys an eminent place in American surgery as Keith Professor of Surgery at Rush in Chicago. Furthermore, it has been my pleasure to know a number of the other contributors of chapters. Knowing these individuals, I have the greatest confidence in the fidelity of the book in correctly representing the present state of knowledge. More perhaps than any recent monograph, it conveys a world view of the subject.

On a rough count of the various chapters, I find 47 authored from the United States, 14 from Japan, 4 from Canada, 11 from Sweden, 2 from Germany, 6 from England, 1 from Switzerland, 1 from Scotland, 3 from Belgium, 1 from France, and 1 from Australia. The final count may vary slightly from this, as some of the manuscripts have not yet been finalized. Much of the Western world has been poorly informed, if not blind to much of the important work going forward in Japan in recent years.

As has been already stated, there remains much to be accomplished in surgery of the pancreas. Even with modern equipment such as ultrasound, CT, angiography, MRI, and blood analyses for pancreatic enzymes, the diagnoses are often difficult and may be delayed. Therapy for neoplasms has progressed significantly, yet outcome studies remain discouraging in the experience of most clinics. Thus, one of the great contributions of the book is to define the frontiers of the subject so that future workers will know what has been accomplished and what problems remain unsolved. The editors and authors are to be congratulated on completion of this definitive study and its presentation to the medical public.

In addition to defining the frontiers of scientific knowledge, it affords the operating surgeon the most complete background so far available for the management of pancreatic disease.

1. Mackie JA, Rhoads JE, Park CD. Pancreato-gastrostomy: a further evaluation. Ann Surg 1975;181:541–545.
2. Howard JM. Benign and malignant disease of the pancreas. J R Coll Surg Edinb 1981;26:206–213.
3. Howard JM. Historical aspects and future of pancreatoduodenectomy. J Hepat Bil Pancr Surg 1996;*3*:149–153.
4. Howard JM. Studies of acute pancreatitis with retroperitoneal necrosis: ''the suet syndrome.'' Improvements in patient survival. J Hepat Bil Pancr Surg 1996;3:195–202.

# *Foreword*

Ryoichi Tsuchiya, MD
Nagasaki

The book *Surgical Diseases of the Pancreas,* edited by Drs. Howard and Jordan, was published 37 years ago. The first editor, Dr. John Malone Howard, was only 41 years old at that time, yet, it was the best guidebook for surgeons who were then interested in treating pancreatic diseases. During the following quarter of a century, tremendous developments including rapid progress in diagnostic methods for pancreatic diseases were made, and experiences with the diseases "piled up." The second book with the same title, published in 1987, was edited by Drs. Howard, Jordan, and Reber and made the greatest such contribution in the world. It was with great pleasure that I recently learned from Dr. Howard that a new book using the same title, edited by Drs. Howard, Idezuki, Ihse, and Prinz, was being launched and that an effort is being made to better incorporate the tremendous work being done in Japan with that of the Western countries. I have been highly honored to be asked to write a foreword for this new book.

The work done in the past 15 years in Japan has been mainly concerned with carcinoma of the pancreas. In 1982, the Japanese Pancreatic Society published "General Rules for Surgical and Pathological Studies on Carcinoma of the Pancreas," which provided guidelines to standardize definitions of surgical practice and pathology and was used as the basis for reporting all cases of pancreatic cancer to the Japanese Pancreatic Cancer Registry. Using the general rules, the Japanese Pancreatic Society has been able to collect and analyze a considerable database annually since 1981. The results have shown high resectability rates with a low mortality rate and have indicated an important survival benefit for patients with small pancreatic cancers (1).

Most general surgeons in the Western countries are pessimistic when they deal with a patient with carcinoma of the pancreas, since even the most extensive and aggressive operation such as regional pancreatectomy could not improve the operative results. On the contrary, most surgeons in Japan were resolved to cure the disease by surgery and had started performing more aggressive resectional procedures in 1975. Although their long-term postoperative survival rates have not been improved, their high rate of resectability and their low postoperative mortality rate reflect great improvement in surgical techniques. Their contributions have also included an elucidation of our knowledge of the pathology of carcinoma of the pancreas regarding its patterns of invasion and lymph node metastases. One reason why most Japanese surgeons have taken a resectional policy for pancreatic cancer and why a more aggressive approach could have been taken, may be due to our National Health Care Insurance System in Japan, which was established in 1960. The Japanese people have not had to worry about any excessive economic burden, even when they were hospitalized and underwent operation, and surgeons did not necessarily consider the cost-effectiveness of their operations.

Looking far to the past, the first use of the word "pancreas" is found in Aristotle's *Historia Animalium.* In the 11th line of column B on page 514 of Becker's edition, there is a line saying "another to the *so-called* pancreas." It is said that Aristotle (384–322 BC) wrote this treatise during his wandering years from 347 BC to 335 BC (3). Herophilus of Chalcedon (330/320–260/250 BC) was the first to dissect both human and animal bodies and was called the Father of Anatomy by posterity. It is said that he described many organs, including the pancreas, and defined and named the duodenum and the prostate (4). According to Staden, 11 works are explicitly ascribed to Herophilus by ancient sources. Of these, six works, *On Anatomy*, *On Pulses*, *Midwifery*, *Therapeutics*, *Dialectics*, and *Against Common Opinions*, seem to be of indisputable authenticity. From his treatise *On Anatomy*, three texts are preserved, one each from Book II on the liver, Book III on the female reproductive organ, and Book IV on veins. (There is, therefore, no evidence in the remaining fragments that Herophilus referred to the pancreas). However, in his treatise *De Semine*, Galen (129–199 AD) referred to some glands suggestive of the pancreas, and he mentioned that these glands had been actively investigated by Herophilus and his younger contemporary Eudemus (6). Rufus of Ephesus (about AD 100) wrote of the pancreas in his treatise *On the names of the parts of the body*, using only 14 Greek words (7). The words mean "the, lying and being attached to the primary portion of the intestine, adipose and glandular flesh, pancreas." Thus, unlike Aristotle who wrote of the "so-called pancreas," Rufus wrote of the "pancreas." Apparently the existence of the gland had gained professional acceptance. Galen refers to the pancreas in the 11th paragraph of the fourth book of the treatise *On the usefulness of the parts of the body (De Usu Partium):* "it is for this reason, I suppose, that the omentum is attached to the spleen and the part called pancreas" (8). Also in the second paragraph of the fifth book there is the following sentence: "Nature, realizing this, created a glandular body called the pancreas" (9). Galen noted another name for the organ in his treatise *De venarium arteriarumque diffectione*, that is, "the pancreas which some other people name 'Kallikreas' (beautiful flesh)" (10). He never indicated who "some other people" were, but I believe that some people, at least in the medical field, were fascinated with the "pancreas" even in the time of antiquity.

This third edition of *Surgical Diseases of the Pancreas* is the fruit of endeavors of representative pancreatologists in the 20th century, and it will become the root and trunk toward efflorescence in the 21st century.

1. Tsuchiya R, Tusunoda T, Ishida T, Saitoh Y. Resection for cancer of the pancreas—the Japanese experience. Bailliere's Clin Gastroenterol 1990;4:931–939.
2. Academia Regia Borusiza, Aristotelis Opera. (The works of Aristotle) Revised: Bekker I., 1831:514.
3. Hotta A, Aristoteles. Shimizu Shoin Tokyo 1979:49–52 (in Japanese).
4. Major RH. A history of medicine. Springfield, IL: Charles C Thomas, 1954:143.
5. Hiatt JR, Hiatt N. Galen—a father of medicine. J Am Coll Surg 1994;178:110–116. (According to Garrison FH (Introduction to the history of medicine. Philadelphia: WB Saunders, 1929:112) the dates for Galen are 131–201 AD, and C Singer refers to AD 129–199 (A short history of anatomy from the Greeks to Harvey. New York: Dover 1957:46).)
6. von Staden H. Herophilus. New York: Cambridge University Press, 1989:153–209.
7. Fitzgerald PJ, Morrison AB. The pancreas. Baltimore: Williams & Wilkins, 1980:2.
8. May MT. Galen, On the usefulness of the parts of the body. New York: Cornell University Press, 1968:220.
9. May MT. Galen, On the usefulness of the parts of the body. New York: Cornell University Press, 1968:246.
10. Kühn CG. Clavdii Galeni Opera Omnia (The Complete Works of Claudius Galen) Hildesheim, Germany: Georg Olms, 1964; 2:781.

# Foreword

Kenneth W. Warren, MD, FACS

Except for the brain and the liver, the pancreas is the most complex organ in the body. It is a deep, dark, defiant organ, long regarded as bête noire of even the most intrepid surgeon. Reluctant to betray its myriad secrets, this organ has engaged the attention of anatomists, physiologists, chemists, other basic scientists, and clinicians for centuries. Despite the complexity of the organ and the mysteries surrounding it, the pancreas is not essential to life. Signal research efforts have made it possible to live without a pancreas.

Most of the current knowledge regarding the pancreas, including the means of diagnosing and treating its diverse pathologic conditions, has occurred during the 20th century. The avalanche of new information and innovative techniques in this field during the last 50 years is reflected in this textbook.

The third edition of this book, edited by Drs. Howard, Idezuki, Ihse, and Prinz contains 86 chapters authored by surgeons, gastroenterologists, pathologists, and radiologists, with especial expertise and experience in their respective disciplines, gives comprehensive and authoritative coverage to the surgical diseases of the pancreas. The editors have selected authors of the various chapters to reflect the geographic interest in and knowledge of the subject; thus, a balanced view of the European, Asian, South Pacific, and American experience is achieved.

A careful review of the contents of this textbook defies the experienced pancreatic surgeon to suggest a subject that is not adequately addressed. In this rapidly changing area, the contributors emphasize that a basic understanding of the anatomy, physiology, and pathology of the pancreas is fundamental to continued progress in this field.

Dr. Howard has a long sustained interest in the pancreas, reflected in his numerous authoritative contributions to the literature and his lively participation in national and international conferences regarding this subject.

Dr. Ihse is an admirable choice to represent the distinguished contributors from Europe. Dr. Prinz is a recognized authority in pancreatic surgery. Professor Idezuki is a worthy ambassador of the Japanese and South Pacific contingent.

This book recognizes the major contributions of the nonsurgical specialists whose application of new diagnostic and therapeutic techniques and interventions have changed the treatment of pancreatic disease.

The cooperation and interdependence that now exist among surgeons and the related disciplines have established a common bond among specialties that has been beneficial to us and, most of all, to the patient.

In this third edition, one sees the relentless advancement of the frontiers of knowledge, the development of new techniques, and the refinement of old ones. Taken together, they have reduced morbidity and saved numerous lives.

# Preface

John M. Howard, MD
Yasuo Idezuki, MD
Ingemar Ihse, MD
Richard A. Prinz, MD

Entirely new fields of science related to diseases of the pancreas have recently emerged: invasive radiology, laparoscopic and endoscopic surgery, advanced imagery, molecular biology, immunology as related to pancreatic transplantation, and advances in immunohistochemistry. As a result, knowledge of pancreatic disease is progressing so rapidly, involving so many disciplines, that surgery of the pancreas is changing as it responds to challenges on many frontiers.

The overriding goal in the development of this edition of *Surgical Diseases of the Pancreas* has been the mobilization of information relative to the science and skills of pancreatic surgery from around the world, incorporating with Europe, North America, and Australia the tremendous energy and expertise that have emerged during recent years from Japan. Within the fields of surgery, especially surgery of the pancreas, there has been little or no previous effort to merge or integrate the clinical and scientific streams flowing from East and West.

This book is oriented toward clinicians, including clinical investigators in the field of pancreatic diseases.

Detailed data from the animal laboratories have been largely omitted to present a factual background on the best available observations from studies of man. A limited duplication of material from chapter to chapter will be noted and is not an oversight, as we thought it desirable, to permit each chapter to be better understood without the need to refer to other sections for supplementary information. It also allows presentation of different perspectives by different authors. Where operative techniques are of vital importance, such as pancreatic resection for cancer, especially where these techniques are advancing beyond the standards of the past decade, such techniques have been illustrated.

Cigarette smoking has been clearly demonstrated to be a major hazard, perhaps the major hazard, leading to pancreatic cancer. The ever-increasing incidence of pancreatic cancer may for the first time be diminishing in one or two countries of the world where this etiologic relationship has been recognized by the population. This information is either unknown or has failed to influence the population of much of the world.

Centers of excellence in the field of pancreatic surgery have been created on several continents and in numerous countries. The rate of collection of information has therefore rapidly increased. In Japan, in a collaborative effort between many institutions, over 30,000 patients with pancreatic cancer have been entered into an ongoing central registry. Pancreatoduodenectomy is now being safely performed in multiple centers with a postoperative mortality rate well below 5%. The operation has been developed to such an extent that it can now, with reasonable safety, be evaluated as a *palliative* procedure for pancreatic cancer in experienced centers, a result all too often obtained from "curative" resections. Multimodal protocols for adjuvant therapy of pancreatic cancer are being evaluated throughout Japan, North America, and Europe. Numerous surgical centers throughout the world, particularly in Japan, have extended the scope of pancreatic resection and its associated lymphadenectomy with results that suggest increasing survivals.

Knowledge of the multiple etiologies and natural histories of acute as well as chronic pancreatitis has continued to expand. At present, approximately 200 etiological factors have been suggested or proven to cause acute pancreatitis in the many climates and cultures around the world. Knowledge and experience gained in the treatment of severe acute pancreatitis with massive necrosis of peripancreatic tissues have resulted in mortality rates that are now beginning to fall below 5%.

Pancreatic transplantation is reaching new heights of practicality. The world of pancreatic surgery is enlarging in scientific and geographic scope; yet in a sense, diminishing, as barriers to communication fall. It is the purpose of the new edition of *Surgical Diseases of the Pancreas* to present the principles and frontiers of clinical surgery from around the world, while contributing to the bridging of the barriers of communication. Each has required diligence by the authors, editors, and publishers.

# Acknowledgments

We acknowledge our gratitude to our distinguished colleagues who have contributed knowledge and expertise to the many chapters of this book. Let us also note what a wonderful resource for the expansion of international culture and the joys of camaraderie that our colleagues around the world have provided us. They have enriched our lives.

In addition we wish to acknowledge our professional debts to our clinical colleagues at home; past and present: our residents, students, fellows, and peers with whom we have had the privilege to work and from whom we continue to learn. Dr. Jonathan E. Rhoads, Dr. Ryoichi Tsuchiya, and Dr. Kenneth W. Warren, surgical teachers and statesmen, who through a lifetime of surgery have taught us more by scholarship and example than they will ever know.

We are individually indebted to our secretaries, Paula Williams, Patricia O'Connor, and Sheryl Orok of Toledo, Mrs. Monica Lundin Hansson of Lund, and Mrs. Linda Wahrer of Chicago.

In addition, we wish to express our appreciation to the staff of our respective libraries and to Mr. Roy Schneider, artist of the Medical College of Ohio.

Finally, we are indebted to Joanne Husovski, Carroll Cann, and Grant Lashbrook of Williams & Wilkins.

# Contributors

***Afaf G.E. Absood, PhD***
Visiting Research Scientist
Department of Surgery
Yale University
New Haven, Connecticut

***Bo Ahrén, MD, PhD***
Department of Medicine
Malmo University Hospital
Malmo, Sweden

***Måns Åkerman, MD, PhD, FIAC***
Assistant Professor
Department of Pathology and Cytology
University Hospital
Lund, Sweden

***David C. Allison, MD, PhD***
Professor of Surgery
Director of Surgical Research
Department of Surgery
Medical College of Ohio
Toledo, Ohio

***Dana K. Andersen, MD***
Professor and Vice-chairman, Department of Surgery
Chief, Section of Surgical Gastroenterology,
Yale University School of Medicine
Chief, General Surgery Service, Yale-New Haven Hospital
New Haven, Connecticut

***Roland Andersson, MD, PhD***
Associate Professor
Department of Surgery
University Hospital
Lund, Sweden

***Åke Andrén-Sandberg, MD***
Associate Professor
Department of Surgery
University Hospital
Lund, Sweden

***Stanley W. Ashley, MD***
Associate Professor of Surgery, Harvard Medical School
Senior Surgeon, Brigham and Women's Hospital
Department of Surgery
Brigham & Women's Hospital
Boston, Massachusetts

***Yutaka Atomi, MD***
Professor
Department of Surgery
Kyorin Medical School
Tokyo, Japan

***Jan Axelson, MD, PhD***
Department of Surgery
University Hospital
Lund, Sweden

***Pia Lena Bäckman, MD***
Department of Surgery
University Hospital
Lund, Sweden

***Yasutsugu Bandai, MD***
Surgeon in Chief
Department of Surgery
Central Hospital of Social Health Insurance
Tokyo, Japan

***Jeffrey L. Barnett, MD***
Associate Professor of Internal Medicine
Gastroenterology Division
The University of Michigan Medical Center
Ann Arbor, Michigan

***John Barrett, MD, FRCS (I), FACS***
Chairman, Department of Trauma
Director of Trauma Services
Department of Trauma
Cook County Hospital
Chicago, Illinois

***Claudio Bassi, MD***
Surgical Department Pancreatic Unit
Borgo Roma University Hospital
University of Verona
Verona, Italy

***Joyce A. Battle, MD***
Assistant Professor of Radiation Therapy
Vice Chief of Service
Medical College of Ohio
Toledo, Ohio

***James M. Becker, MD***
James Utley Professor and Chairman, Department of Surgery, Boston University School of Medicine
Surgeon-in-Chief, Boston Medical Center
Department of Surgery
Boston University Medical Center
Boston, Massachusetts

***Hans G. Beger, MD, FACS***
Professor and Head
Department of General Surgery
University Hospital of Surgery
University of Ulm
Ulm, Germany

***Richard H. Bell, Jr., MD***
Professor and Vice-Chairman, Department of Surgery, University of Washington School of Medicine
Chief, Surgical Service, Veterans Affairs Puget Sound Health Care System
Department of Surgery
VA Puget Sound Health Care System
Seattle, Washington

***Leslie H. Blumgart, MD, FRCS, FACS***
Chief, Hepatobiliary Service,
Memorial Sloan-Kettering Cancer Center
Professor of Surgery, Cornell University Medical College
Department of Surgery
Memorial Sloan-Kettering Cancer Center
New York, New York

***Peter Boyle, PhD***
Director
Division of Epidemiology and Biostatistics
European Institute of Oncology
Milan, Italy

***John W. Braasch, MD, PhD***
Assistant Clinical Professor of Surgery,
Harvard Medical School
Senior Consultant in Surgery, Former Chairman,
Department of General Surgery, Lahey Hitchcock Medical Center
Department of General Surgery
Lahey Hitchcock Clinic
Burlington, Massachusetts

***Edward L. Bradley III, MD***
Professor and Vice-Chairman, Department of Surgery,
State University of New York at Buffalo
Chief of Surgery, Buffalo General Hospital
Department of Surgery
State University of New York at Buffalo
Buffalo, New York

***Murray F. Brennan, MD, MCh, FACS, FRACS***
Chairman
Department of Surgery
Memorial Sloan-Kettering Cancer Center
New York, New York

***Markus W. Büchler, MD***
Professor and Chairman
Department of Visceral and Transplantation Surgery
University of Bern, Inselspital
Bern, Switzerland

***Peter C. Buetow, Major, MC USA***
Associate Professor of Radiology, F. Edward Hebert School of Medicine, Uniformed Services
University of the Health Sciences, Bethesda, Maryland
Chief, Gastrointestinal Radiology,
Department of Radiologic Pathology,
Armed Forces Institute of Pathology, Washington, DC
Washington, DC

***Harvey L. Bumpers, MD***
Assistant Professor of Surgery
Department of Surgery
State University of New York at Buffalo
School of Medicine and Biomedical Sciences
Buffalo, New York

***Guillaume Cadiot, MD, PhD***
Associate Professor of Medicine
Department of Hepato-Gastroenterology
Hopital Bichat-Claude Bernard
Paris, France

***John L. Cameron, MD***
Professor and Chairman
Department of Surgery
The Johns Hopkins University School of Medicine
Baltimore, Maryland

***Sir David C. Carter, MD, FRCS, FACS***
Professor of Surgery
The University of Edinburgh
Edinburgh, Scotland, UK

***Arnold G. Coran, MD***
Pediatric Surgery Associate
Section of Pediatric Surgery
University of Michigan Medical Center
Ann Arbor, Michigan

***Alfred Cuschieri, MD***
Professor of Surgery
Department of Surgery
University of Dundee
Ninewells Hospital and Medical School
Dundee, Scotland

***Sigmund Dawiskiba, MD***
Department of Pathology and Cytology
Division of Cytology
University Hospital
Lund, Sweden

***Romano Delcore, MD***
Department of Surgery
University of Kansas Medical Center
Kansas City, Missouri

***Daniel J. Deziel, MD***
Associate Professor of Surgery, Rush Medical College
Attending Surgeon, Rush-Presbyterian-St. Luke's Medical Center
Rush Medical College
Rush-Presbyterian-St. Luke's Medical Center
Chicago, Illinois

***Ralph R. Dobelbower, MD, PhD, FACR***
Professor
Department of Radiation Therapy
Medical College of Ohio
Toledo, Ohio

***Jean Michel Dubernard, MD***
Urology-Transplantation
Edouard Herriot Hospital
Lyon, France

***Scott Engum, MD***
Assistant Professor, Pediatric Surgery
Pediatric Surgery
James Whitcomb Riley Hospital for Children,
Indiana University School of Medicine
Indianapolis, Indiana

***Toshifumi Eto, MD***
Director
Department of Surgery
Eto Hospital
Isahaya City, Japan

***Massimo Falconi, MD***
Researcher of Senior Assistant of the Surgical Department
Surgical Department Pancreatic Unit
Borgo Roma University Hospital
University of Verona
Verona, Italy

***David R. Fletcher, MBBS, MD, FRACS***
Professor of Surgery and Head
Department of Surgery
University of Western Australia
Fremantle Hospital
Fremantle, Western Australia

***Yuman Fong, MD***
Assistant Attending Surgeon
Department of Surgery
Memorial Sloan-Kettering Cancer Center
New York, New York

***Stanley R. Friesen, MD, PhD***
Professor Emeritus
Departments of Surgery and History and Philosophy of Medicine
University of Kansas School of Medicine
Kansas University Medical Center
Prairie Village, Kansas

***David Fromm, MD***
Penberthy Professor and Chairman,
Department of Surgery, Wayne State University
Surgeon in Chief, Detroit Medical Center Department of Surgery
Department of Surgery
University Health Center
Detroit, Michigan

***Louis M. Gianakakis, MS***
Medical student
Department of General Surgery
Rush-Presbyterian-St. Luke's Medical Center
Chicago, Illinois

***Vay Liang W. Go, MD***
Editor-in-Chief
Pancreas, Official Journal of the American Pancreatic Association and the Japan Pancreas Society
Los Angeles, California

***Constantine V. Godellas, MD***
Surgical Oncology Fellow
Department of Surgery
Memorial Sloan-Kettering Cancer Center
New York, New York

***Jay L. Grosfeld, MD***
Professor and Chairman, Department of Surgery,
Indiana University School of Medicine
Surgeon-in-Chief, J.W. Riley Hospital for Children
Department of Surgery
Indianapolis, Indiana

***Mustafa Guvendi, MD, FACS***
Associate Professor of Clinical Surgery
Medical College of Ohio
Toledo, Ohio

***Carroll M. Harmon, MD, PhD***
Assistant Professor of Surgery
Section of Pediatric Surgery
University of Michigan Medical Center
Ann Arbor, Michigan

***Marquis Hart, MD***
Assistant Professor
Department of Surgery
University of California, San Diego Medical Center
San Diego, California

***Takehisa Hiraoka, MD***
Associate Professor
First Department of Surgery
Kumamoto University School of Medicine
Kumamoto, Honjo, Japan

***John M. Howard, MD, FACS, FRCS-Edinburgh (Hon), FCS Brazil (Hon.)***
Professor of Surgery, Emeritus
Medical College of Ohio
Toledo, Ohio

***Yasuo Idezuki, MD***
Professor and Chairman
Department of Surgery
Saitama Medical Center, Saitama Medical School
Saitama, Japan

***Ingemar Ihse, MD, PhD***
Professor and Chairman
Department of Surgery
University Hospital
Lund, Sweden

***Clem W. Imrie, MD***
Consultant Surgeon, Pancreato-Biliary Team
AA and Honorary Professor of Surgery
Department of Surgery
Royal Infirmary
Glasgow, Scotland, UK

***Lee Jenkins, MD***
Department of General Surgery
Rush-Presbyterian-St. Luke's Medical Center
Chicago, Illinois

***Raymond J. Joehl, MD***
James R. Hines Professor of Surgery
Chief, Division of General Surgery
Department of Surgery
Northwestern University Medical School
Chicago, Illinois

***Leon G. Josephs, MD***
Department of Surgery
Boston University Medical Center
Boston, Massachusetts

***Keiichiro Kanemitsu, MD***
Associate
First Department of Surgery
Kumamoto University School of Medicine
Kumamoto, Japan

***Kogoro Kasahara, MD, PhD***
Professor
Department of Surgery
Jichi Medical School
Tochigi, Japan

***Yoshifumi Kawarada, MD, FACS***
Professor and Chairman
First Department of Surgery, School of Medicine
Mie University School of Medicine
Tsu, Mie, Japan

***Roger G. Keith, MD, FRCSC, FRCS, FACS***
Fred H. Wigmore Professor of Surgery and Chairman,
Department of Surgery, University of Saskatchewan
Chief of Surgery, Royal University Hospital
Department of Surgery
Saskatoon, Saskatchewan, Canada

***Günter Klöppel, MD***
Professor and Head
Department of Pathology
University of Kiel
Kiel, Germany

***Tomoo Kosuge, MD***
Head, Hepatopancreatiobiliary Unit, Department of Surgery, National Cancer Center Hospital
Invited Lecturer, Second Department of Surgery, Faculty of Medicine, University of Tokyo
HPB unit, Department of Surgery
National Cancer Center Hospital
Tokyo, Japan

***Keiichi Kubota, MD, PhD***
Assistant Professor
Second Department of Surgery, Faculty of Medicine
University of Tokyo
Tokyo, Japan

***R. Kunz, MD***
Department of General Surgery
University of Ulm
Ulm, Germany

***Akira Kuroda, MD***
Vice Director and Head, Department of Surgery
Department of Surgery
Hospital of the Imperial Household
Tokyo, Japan

***Jörgen Larsson, MD***
Professor of Surgery
Department of Surgery
Huddinge General Hospital
Huddinge, Sweden

***Gregory LaValle, MD***
Assistant Professor of Surgery
Department of Surgery; Division of Surgical Oncology
Ohio State University Hospitals
Columbus, Ohio

***Thomas L. Lawson, MD***
Professor and Chairman
Department of Radiology
Loyola University Stritch School of Medicine
Maywood, Illinois

**Peter Layer, MD**
Professor of Medicine
Division of Gastroenterology
University of Essen
Department of Medicine/Gastroenterology
Essen, Germany

**Glen A. Lehman, MD**
Professor of Medicine
Division of Gastroenterology/Hepatology
Department of Medicine
Indiana University Medical Center
Indianapolis, Indiana

**Nicholas R. Lemoine, MD, PhD, MRCPath**
Professor of Molecular Pathology and ICRF Consultant
Clinical Scientist
ICRF Oncology Unit
Royal PostGraduate Medical School,
Hammersmith Hospital
London, UK

**Kenneth A. Leslie, MD**
Department of Surgery
London Health Sciences Center
University of Western Ontario
London, Ontario

**Keith D. Lillemoe, MD**
Professor
Department of Surgery
Johns Hopkins Hospital
Baltimore, Maryland

**Qiang Liu, MD**
Department of General Surgery
Rush-Presbyterian-St. Luke's Medical Center
Chicago, Illinois

**Albert B. Lowenfels, MD**
Professor of Surgery and Community
and Preventive Medicine
Department of Surgery
New York Medical College
Valhalla, New York

**Patrick Maisonneuve, Ing.**
Deputy Director
Division of Epidemiology and Biostatistics
European Institute of Oncology
Milan, Italy

**Masatoshi Makuuchi, MD, PhD**
Professor and Chairman
Second Department of Surgery, Faculty of Medicine
University of Tokyo
Bunkyo-ku, Tokyo, Japan

**Xavier Martin, MD**
Professor of Urology
Service d'Urologie et Chirurgie de la Transplantation
Hopital Edouard Herriot
Lyon, France

**Deborah Martinez, MD**
Surgical Oncology Fellow
Department of Surgery; Division of Surgical Oncology
Ohio State University Hospitals
Columbus, Ohio

**Lawrence P. McChesney, MD**
Servico d'Urologie et Chirurgie de la Transplantation
Hopital Edouard Herriot
Lyon, France

**C. S. Frances McCormick, MB BCh, MSc, MRCPath**
Clinical Research Fellow
Departments of Histopathology and Clinical Oncology
ICRF Oncology Unit
Royal PostGraduate Medical School,
Hammersmith Hospital
London, UK

**Louis T. Merriam, MD**
Resident in General Surgery and Research Fellow
Department of Surgery
Northwestern University Medical School
Chicago, Illinois

**Michel Mignon, MD**
Professor of Medicine, University of Paris VII
Department Head, Department of Hepato-Gastroenterology, Hopital Bichat-Claude Bernard,
Hopitaux de Paris
Hopital Bichat-Claude Bernard
Paris, France

**Alexander R. Miller, MD**
Chief Resident in Surgery
Department of Surgery, Division of Gastroenterologic
and General Surgery
Mayo Medical School and Mayo Foundation
Rochester, Minnesota

**Donald L. Miller, MD**
Chief, Vascular/Interventional Radiology, National Naval
Medical Center, Bethesda
Professor of Radiology, Department of Radiology
and Nuclear Medicine
F. Edward Hebert School of Medicine
Uniformed Services University of the Health Sciences
Bethesda National Naval Medical Center
Rockville, Maryland

**Itsuo Miyazaki, MD**
Professor and Chairman
Second Department of Surgery, Faculty of Medicine
Kanazawa University
Kanazawa, Japan

**A. R. Moossa, MD**
Professor and Chairman
Department of Surgery
University of California San Diego Medical Center
San Diego, California

***Toshiyuki Mori, MD, PhD***
Associate Professor of Surgery
Kyorin University
Tokyo, Japan

***Hideo Nagai, MD, PhD***
Associate Professor
Department of Surgery
Jichi Medical School
Minami-Kawachi-machi
Tochigi, Japan

***Takukazu Nagakawa, MD***
Professor and Chairman of Surgery
Department of Health Science
Kanazawa University
Kanazawa, Japan

***Kimberly K. Nagy, MD***
Assistant Professor of General Surgery,
Rush Medical College
Chair, Division of Research and Education,
Cook County Hospital
Department of Trauma
Chicago, Illinois

***John P. Neoptolemos, MA, MB, BChir, MD, FRCS***
Professor and Deparment Head
Department of Surgery
University of Liverpool
Royal Liverpool Hospital
Liverpool, UK

***Isto H. Nordback, MD***
Department of Surgery
Tampere University Hospital
Tampere, Finland

***Jeffrey A. Norton, MD***
Professor of Surgery, Washington University School of Medicine
Chief of Endocrine and Oncologic Surgery,
Barnes-Jewish Hospital
Department of Surgery
St. Louis, Missouri

***Thomas O'Dorisio, MD***
Ohio State University College of Medicine
Columbus, Ohio

***Mary C. Olson, MD***
Associate Professor of Radiology
Director, Computed Tomography
Department of Radiology
Loyola University Medical Center
Maywood, Illinois

***Chung Owyang, MD***
Professor of Internal Medicine
H. Marvin Pollard Collegiate Professor and Chief
Division of Gastroenterology
The University of Michigan
Ann Arbor, Michigan

***Paolo Pederzoli, MD***
Professor of Surgery
Surgical Department Pancreatic Unit
Borgo Roma University Hospital
University of Verona
Verona, Italy

***Gary R. Peplinski, MD***
Resident in Surgery, Barnes-Jewish Hospital, Washington University School of Medicine
Department of Surgery
Washington University School of Medicine
Barnes-Jewish Hospital
St. Louis, Missouri

***C.S. Pitchumoni, MD, FRCP(C), FACP***
Professor of Medicine and Professor of Community and Preventive Medicine
New York Medical College
Director of Medicine, Our Lady of Mercy Medical Center
Department of Medicine
Bronx, New York

***Henry A. Pitt, MD***
Johns Hopkins Hospital
Baltimore, Maryland

***Harold V. Posniak, MD***
Associate Professor of Radiology
Department of Radiology
Loyola University Medical Center
Stritch School of Medicine
Maywood, Illinois

***Parviz M. Pour, MD***
Eppley Institute; University of Nebraska Medical Center
Omaha, Nebraska

***Richard A. Prinz, MD***
Helen Shedd Keith Professor and Chairman
Department of General Surgery
Rush-Presbyterian-St. Luke's Medical Center
Chicago, Illinois

***Ib Rasmussen, MD***
University Department of Surgery
Royal Infirmary
Edinburgh, Scotland

***Howard A. Reber, MD***
UCLA School of Medicine
Center for Health Sciences
Los Angeles, California

***Finn P. Reinholt, MD, PhD***
Associate Professor of Pathology
Department of Immunology,
Microbiology, Pathology, and Infectious Disease
Huddinge Hospital, Karolinska Institutet
Huddinge, Sweden

***Harry Richter, III, MD***
Assistant Professor of Surgery, University of Illinois
College of Medicine
Chairman, Theoretical Surgery, Cook County Hospital
Department of Surgery
Cook County Hospital
Chicago, Illinois

***Thomas Rösch, MD***
Director of GI Endoscopy
Assistant Professor of Medicine
Department of Internal Medicine II
Technical University of Munich
Klinikum rechts der Isar
Munchen, Germany

***Lawrence Rosenberg, MD, PhD, FRCSC, FACS***
Director, Centre for Pancreatic Diseases,
Montreal General Hospital
Professor of Surgery and Medicine,
McGill University
Montreal General Hospital
Montreal, Quebec, Canada

***Michael Rünzi, MD***
Assistant Professor of Medicine
Division of Gastroenterology
Department of Medicine
University of Essen
Essen, Germany

***R. C. G. Russell, MS, FRCS***
Consultant Surgeon
Department of Surgery
University College Hospitals London
London, UK

***Michael S. Sabel, MD***
Instructor
Department of General Surgery
Rush-Presbyterian-St. Luke's Medical Center
Chicago, Illinois

***Michael G. Sarr, MD***
Professor of Surgery,
Mayo Medical School
Chair, Division of Gastroenterologic and General Surgery,
Mayo Clinic
Department of Surgery
Division of Gastroenterologic and General Surgery
Mayo Clinic
Rochester, Minnesota

***Katsusuke Satake, MD***
Associate Professor
First Department of Surgery
Osaka City University Medical School
Osaka, Japan

***M. H. Schoenberg, MD***
Department of General Surgery
University of Ulm
Ulm, Germany

***Stuart Sherman, MD***
Associate Professor of Medicine and Radiology
Division of Gastroenterology/Hepatology
Department of Medicine
Indiana University Medical Center
Indianapolis, Indiana

***Kazuaki Shimada, MD***
HPB Unit
Department of Surgery
National Cancer Center Hospital
Tokyo, Japan

***Kazuyuki Shimomura, MD***
Assistant Professor
Department of Surgery
Saitama Medical Center
Saitama Medical School
Saitama, Japan

***Michael A. Skinner, MD***
Assistant Professor of Surgery, Division of Pediatric
Surgery, Department of Surgery, Washington University
School of Medicine, St. Louis Children's Hospital
Department of Surgery
St. Louis Children's Hospital
St. Louis, Missouri

***William H. Smith-Mensah, MD***
Department of Surgery
Medical College of Ohio
Toledo, Ohio

***Seth A. Spector, MD***
Resident in General Surgery and Post-Doctoral
Research Fellow
Department of Surgery
Yale University School of Medicine
New Haven, Connecticut

***Edgar D. Staren, MD, PhD***
Department of General Surgery
Rush-Presbyterian-St. Luke's Medical Center
Chicago, Illinois

***Hans Stridbeck, MD, PhD***
Associate Professor of Diagnostic Radiology
Department of Diagnostic Radiology
University Hospital
Lund, Sweden

***Mark T. Toyama, MD***
Department of Surgery
UCLA School of Medicine
Los Angeles, California

***Gregory G. Tsiotos, MD***
Gastrointestinal Surgery Scholar
Department of Surgery
Mayo Clinic
Rochester, Minnesota

***Tsukasa Tsunoda, MD, DMedSc***
Professor and Chairman
Department of Gastroenterologic Surgery
Kawasaki Medical School
Kurashiki City, Okayama, Japan

***Waldemar Uhl, MD***
Professor
Department of Visceral and Transplantation Surgery
University Hospital of Bern
Inselspital, Switzerland

***Jonathan A. van Heerden, MD, MB, FRCS(C), FACS, FRCS(Edin), FRCPS (Glas)***
Professor of Surgery, Mayo Medical School
Fred C. Andersen Professor, Mayo Foundation
Mayo Clinic
Department of Surgery
Division of Gastroenterologic and General Surgery
Mayo Clinic
Rochester, Minnesota

***Mathew Varughese, MD, FRCS***
Emeritus Professor of Surgery, University of Kerala
Retired Professor and Director, Department of Surgery,
Medical College Hospital
Department of Surgery
University of Kerala
Kerala, India

***John Webber, MD***
National Institute of Health Research Fellow
Department of Surgery
Wayne State University
University Health Center
Detroit, Michigan

***Robin C. N. Williamson, MA, MD***
Professor and Director of Surgery
Department of Surgery
Royal Postgraduate Medical School
Hammersmith Hospital
London, UK

***Paul G. Wilson, MB, ChB, MRCP***
University Research Fellow
Department of Medicine
University of Birmingham
Queen Elizabeth Hospital
Brimingham, UK

***Junji Yamamoto, MD***
Department of Surgery
National Cancer Center Hospital
Tokyo, Japan

***Charles J. Yeo, MD***
Professor
Department of Surgery
The Johns Hopkins University School of Medicine
Baltimore, Maryland

***Toru Yusa, MD***
Department of Surgery
University Hospital
Lund, Sweden

***Kaspar Z'graggen, MD***
Department of Visceral and Transplantation Surgery
University of Bern
Inselspital, Switzerland

# Contents

## SECTION VI
### CHRONIC PANCREATITIS



## SECTION VII
### SPECIAL CONSIDERATIONS



## SECTION VIII
### PANCREATIC PSEUDOCYSTS



## SECTION IX
### TUMORS OF THE EXOCRINE PANCREAS

## SECTION X
### Clinical Management of Carcinoma of the Exocrine Pancreas



## SECTION XI
### Other Pancreatic Tumors, Clinical Management



## SECTION XII
### Adjacent Tumors Requiring Pancreatic Resection



## SECTION XIII
### True Cysts and Cystic Tumors of the Pancreas



## SECTION XIV
### The Endocrine Pancreas

## SECTION XV
### SPECIAL PROBLEMS

SECTION I

FOUNDATIONS OF CLINICAL PRACTICE

# 1

# *Embryology and Congenital Anomalies of the Pancreas*

Carroll M. Harmon and Arnold G. Coran

## EMBRYOLOGY

The end result of pancreatic embryogenesis is a complex, self-organized, adaptive organ consisting of ductal, acinar, islet, and interstitial cells that must interact with great precision to carry out its normal physiologic function. Despite the fact that the pancreas is a single organ, it houses two quite different types of glandular tissue: the exocrine cells that secrete enzymes into the intestine and the endocrine cells that secrete hormones into the blood stream. Recently, there has been renewed interest in studying the embryogenesis of the pancreas. A better understanding of the ontogeny of specific cell populations may yield more effective treatment of diseases of pancreatic cellular dysfunction such as diabetic mellitus, idiopathic hyperinsulinemic hypoglycemia of infancy, cystic fibrosis, and pancreatic exocrine insufficiency, as well as pancreatic tumors of exocrine or endocrine origin.

### Morphologic Development of the Pancreas

The human pancreas develops during the 4th to 7th weeks of fetal life, arising from dorsal and ventral epithelial evaginations of foregut endoderm into the surrounding splanchnic mesoderm. This description was first made in the human embryo by Phisalix in 1888 (1). The ventral anlage of the pancreas arises directly from the liver diverticulum, which grows from the ventral side of the foregut into the transverse septum during the 4th to 5th week. The ventral bud of the pancreas may be paired transiently, forming right and left lobes with small ducts that open into the hepatic diverticulum (2). The left ventral bud later regresses completely (2). The dorsal pancreatic diverticulum arises slightly before the ventral bud and develops from the duodenum, almost opposite the liver primordium. In the human embryo, by the 6th week, the dorsal primordium, growing faster than the ventral anlage, has extended into the dorsal mesentery. During this time, the ventral primordium has been carried away from the duodenum by the elongation of the proximal part of the liver diverticulum, from which it arises. As the duodenum grows and rotates to the right, the ventral bud and hepaticopancreatic orifice move around until they come in contact with the dorsal pancreatic bud (Fig. 1.1). The tip of the ventral bud comes to lie behind the superior mesenteric vein and the root of the portal vein (3).

During the 7th week, the smaller ventral primordium fuses with the proximal part of the dorsal pancreas, so that the ventral component creates the uncinate process and the posteroinferior part of the pancreatic head. The dorsal structure forms the remainder of the head, body, and tail. The ductal system of the pancreas develops as the two pancreatic buds grow rapidly and form new protrusions leading to a highly branched structure. At the ultrastructural level, this process is seen as highly folded epithelial sheets with apical and basal surfaces in continuity with those of the gut tube (4). Following fusion of the two pancreatic primordia, the two ductal systems anastomose. The main pancreatic duct, or duct of Wirsung, is created by the fusion of the persisting duct of the ventral anlage and the distal portion of the duct of the dorsal anlage. The proximal, cephalic portion of the dorsal duct may regress or persist as a functioning route opening to the minor papilla as the accessory pancreatic duct, or the duct of Santorini (Fig. 1.2). Under normal circumstances, by the end of the 7th week, little gross evidence remains of the double origin of the pancreas.

Acinar cells are histologically apparent during the 3rd month along the lateral wall and at the end of the ducts. During the 4th month, zymogen granules appear in the cytoplasm of the acinar cells. Endocrine cells appear earlier in development and are initially visible as scattered individual cells embedded in the ducts during the 10th to 14th week. Later they are visible in clusters and, toward the end of gestation, as typical islets.

The origin of the endocrine and exocrine cells of the pancreas has been a topic of controversy. Despite their functional differences, observational studies strongly suggest that both endocrine and exocrine cells arise from the same endodermal rudiment, making the pancreas an integrated organ from a biologic point of view. For many years, the pancreatic endocrine cells were believed to be a component of the APUD neuroendocrine system derived from the neural crest. This theory was disproven by experiments that created a chimera using quail neuroectoderm and chick endomesoderm. Endocrine cells of the pancreas as well as endocrine cells of gut epithelium, had the chick-type markers (5). This, and other studies, support the notion that endocrine cells arise from endodermal epithelium. More recent experimental data suggest that acinar and islet cells differentiate from lineage-specific primitive ductlike cells (3). It is not certain, however, whether these terminally differentiated cells arise from monoclonal precursor cells or are continuously recruited from ductal or other undifferentiated epithelium. Extensive investigation has been conducted to determine the details of normal pancreatic embryogenesis with particular interest focused on the islet cells. If, as some investigators believe, the postnatal pancreas retains the capacity to regenerate new functional islet cells, and if this process reiterates the normal ontogeny of islet cell development, then a clear understanding of normal pancreatic embryogenesis could lead to more effective treatment of the 30 million people worldwide with diabetes mellitus (6).

### Cellular and Molecular Development of the Pancreas

The cellular and molecular events that lead to and regulate the development of the pancreas are quite complex, and to date, the way in which endocrine, acinar, and ductal cell lineages are generated from the embryonic foregut has not been determined. Historically, the pancreas has long been considered an organ whose development was determined by specific epitheliomesenchymal interactions, in which undifferentiated epithelium in the duodenal anlage is stimulated by the overlying mesenchyme to grow and differentiate into mature pancreas. The search for a "mesenchymal factor" located in the region of the budding pancreatic epithelium has been under way for over 30 years. In 1962, Golosow and Grobstein found that isolated mouse pancreas epithelium would not differentiate in the absence of mesenchyme and suggested that there was a soluble growth factor secreted by mesenchymal cells that was required by the epithelium (7). By 1973, a pancreatic mitogen in chick embryo was partially purified by Ronzio and Rutter; however, the definitive identification of this factor, or factors, has remained elusive (8). Using an embryonic mouse model, Gittes et al. have shown that mesenchyme *is* necessary for normal acinar development but not for formation of islet cells, which appear to arise from an early pancreatic precursor cell (9). Recent experimental work has identified a variety of soluble factors, such as cytokines, which are released from mesenchymal cells and act in a paracrine fashion to at least influence pancreatic cell growth. For instance, in vitro experiments in rats have demonstrated that epidermal growth factor (EGF) promotes the development of pancreatic duct tissue; transforming growth factor-beta (TGF-ß) promotes the development of endocrine cells while inhibiting the growth of acini (10). In addition, interferon-γ, nerve growth hormone, insulin-like growth factor II, and transforming growth factor-alpha have all been implicated in islet cell growth and differentiation.

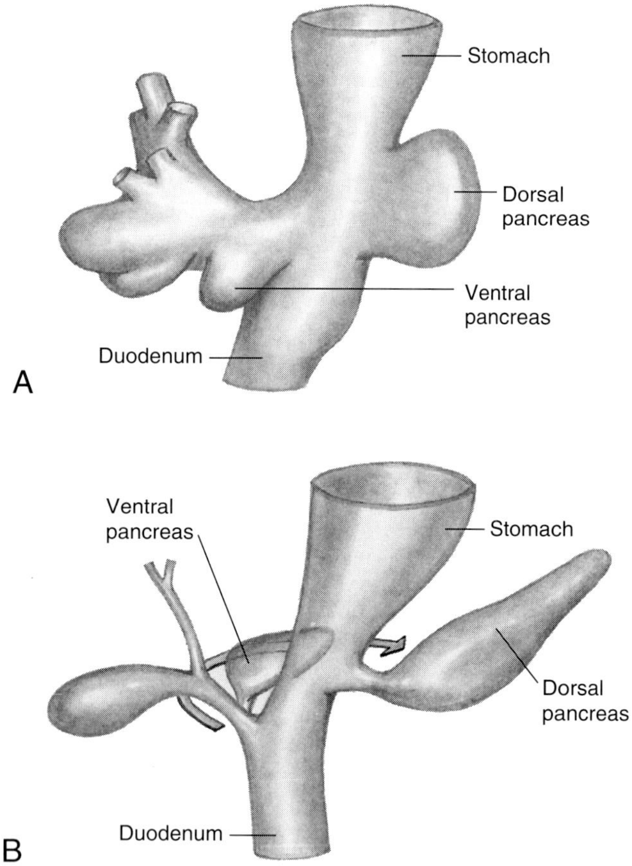


**FIG. 1.1.** Embryology of the pancreas. **A.** In the 5-week embryo, the ventral pancreatic bud lies caudal to the dorsal pancreatic bud. The common bile duct and the duct of the ventral pancreas drain into the duodenum through the major papilla, and the dorsal pancreatic duct drains through the accessory papilla. Persistence of this anatomy results in pancreas divisum. **B.** At 6 weeks' gestation, the dorsal and ventral pancreas fuse. The duct of Wirsung (to the ampulla of Vater) becomes the main pancreatic drainage duct, although the accessory papilla may persist. (Redrawn from Greenfield LJ, et al. Surgery: scientific principles and practice. Philadelphia: JB Lippincott, 1993.)

Despite the significant influence of the mesenchyme on pancreatic growth and differentiation, there appears to be growing support for inherent endodermal cell determination of pancreatic embryogenesis. There must be a region within the endoderm of the foregut that is committed to form the pancreas at some stage *before* the appearance of the pancreatic buds or the expression of terminal differentiation products such as digestive enzymes and hormones. This region would presumably consist of a set of cells committed to become the pancreas because of the activation of a certain set of genes. These presumptive genes have been referred to as the "epigenetic code" for the pancreas and most likely code for a particular combination of transcription factors that regulate subsequent gene expression (11). One important component of the pancreatic epigenetic code is likely to be the homeobox gene, insulin-promotor factor-1 (IPF-1), also called PDX-1. This gene is expressed in the entire early pancreatic rudiment and part of the surrounding gut tube. When the IPF-1 gene is removed from mice by targeted mutagenesis, the embryos completely lack a pancreas (11); this is due to a direct alteration in the pancreatic epithelium and not the surrounding mesenchyme (12).

One experimental approach to studying the early events in pancreatic embryogenesis has been the identification of molecular markers of individual pancreatic cell types. For example, use of protein immunostaining techniques show that insulin and glucagon appear in the mouse about 9.5 days after conception, whereas cells containing amylase are detected from about 14.5 days, and those expressing somatostatin and pancreatic polypeptide appear later (11).

With the advent of molecular biologic techniques that allow evaluation of cell-specific gene expression, additional information is available regarding the timing and regulation of specific pancreatic cell differentiation. Gittes and Rutter have used the reverse-transcriptase polymerase chain reaction (RT-PCR) to examine mRNA levels of cellular pancreatic terminal differentiation products in the wall of the duodenum, at the site from which the pancreas will develop, and in the early pancreatic bud epithelium (13). Endocrine cell products such as somatostatin, insulin, and glucagon gene transcripts were detected in the foregut wall before bud evagination (8.5–9.5 days) (13). Exocrine cell gene products such as amylase were identified later in development (12.5 days) but prior to discrete acinar structure

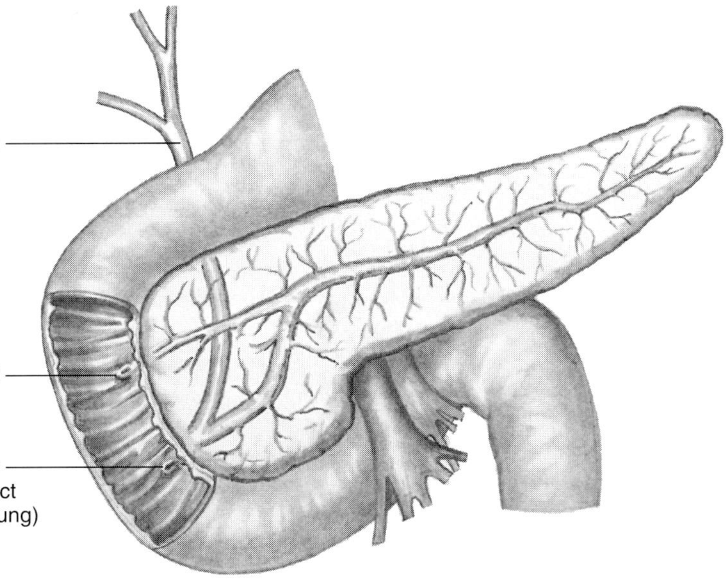


**FIG. 1.2.** Normal pancreatic ductal anatomy.

formation (13). The detection of primitive undifferentiated pancreatic epithelial cells that are capable of gene and protein expression typical of differentiated, mature cell types suggests that these precursor cell are committed to a specific cell lineage. However, cells within one lineage are capable of turning genes on and off at different times, so that there is no guarantee, for example, that cells expressing insulin at 11.5 days are precursors of mature ß cells (3). The complex issue of whether differentiated terminal cells such as mature acinar cells or islet cells arise from individual monoclonal progenitors or whether they both arise from a multipotential cell associated with the ductal epithelium will continue to be debated and studied. In the future, the ability to modify tissue and cells by use of transgenesis and targeted mutagenesis in the mouse model should provide powerful data regarding pancreatic cell lineage development.

## CONGENITAL ANOMALIES OF THE PANCREAS

### Agenesis, Aplasia, and Hypoplasia of the Pancreas

**Agenesis of the Pancreas.** Complete agenesis of the total pancreas in a living newborn is extremely rare and fatal. As of 1994, only five cases of complete pancreatic agenesis had been reported in the literature (14). All five infants exhibited moderate-to-severe intrauterine growth retardation (IUGR), hyperglycemia, and viscous meconium; four of five had other associated congenital anomalies. In addition to pancreatic agenesis, two of the cases were also associated with agenesis of the gallbladder. One infant also had a ventricular septal defect and a congenital diaphragmatic hernia, and another infant also had a truncus arteriosus communis. All infants developed hyperglycemia and ketonemia or lactic acidosis and died within 2 weeks of birth (14).

**Aplasia of a Pancreatic Anlage.** Aplasia of part of the pancreas is also a relatively rare anomaly. Pancreatic aplasia, or failure of development of either the ventral or dorsal anlage, occurs most often in the dorsal anlage. There appears to be some confusion in the literature regarding true aplasia of the dorsal pancreas. With the advent of more sophisticated imaging modalities such as ultrasound, computerized tomography (CT) scan, and magnetic resonance imaging (MRI), more case reports of the absence of the body and tail of the pancreas are being published. These reports may represent at least four anatomic or pathologic processes: *(a)* true aplasia of the dorsal pancreatic anlagen, *(b)* hypoplasia of the excretory tissue of the dorsal pancreas, *(c)* defective development in a part of the dorsal pancreatic primordium, or *(d)* secondary obliteration of the body and tail, after fibrotic degeneration (as after acute pancreatitis) or lipomatous atrophy. The etiology of true dorsal pancreatic aplasia is unknown. A recent report of a woman and her two sons who all had "agenesis" of the dorsal pancreas diagnosed by imaging studies and endoscopic retrograde pancreatography may suggest an hereditary mechanism in the pathogenesis of this anomaly (15).

**Hypoplasia of the Pancreas.** The term *hypoplasia* has been used in the past to describe cases of absence of the body and tail of the pancreas, since this term refers to partial development. In this situation, "hypoplasia" suggests that the head of the pancreas, which develops from a portion of the dorsal pancreatic primordium, is intact. Hypoplasia more accurately signifies incomplete development of the cells in the pancreas. Hypoplasia is typically of the exocrine acinar cells, which has also been referred to as acinar aplasia, again creating some terminology confusion. This condition may be a component of Schwachman's syndrome (pancreatic insufficiency, bone marrow dysfunction, metaphyseal dysplasia, and other anomalies) (16).

### Annular Pancreas

An annular pancreas is a rare malformation in which a band of pancreatic tissue surrounds the descending portion of the duodenum with smooth continuation to the head of the pancreas. The pancreatic tissue of the annulus is histologically normal, containing both acini and islets. A number of theories have developed to explain formation of the annular pancreas. The most widely accepted theory is that described by Lecco in 1910 (17). This theory states that there is fixation of the tip of the ventral pancreatic primordium to the duodenal wall before rotation during the 5th week. With subsequent growth, this results in fusion of this ventral tip with the dorsal primordium on the far side, thus encircling the duodenum. In this case the duct within the ring of the annulus would pass dorsally to the right and enter the fused main pancreatic duct. In a recent review of 61 cases with adequate documentation of ductal anatomy this type of ductal anatomy was identified in 42 (69%) (18). Other anatomic descriptions of annular pancreas have resulted in additional theories of the embryogenesis of this anomaly. Baldwin, also in 1910, proposed that annular pancreas resulted from the failure of the involution of the left ventral pancreatic bud, with ventral extension of this anlage creating the annulus (19). A third theory proposes that the pancreatic ring forms from primitive differentiating pancreatic tissue in the region of the duodenum early in development and results in several ducts opening directly from the annular pancreas into the duodenum (20) (Fig. 1.3).

More recent immunohistochemical studies on annular pancreas have confirmed that the tissue of the annular pancreas arises from the ventral primordium. The islets are irregular in shape, and there is a very high proportion of (pancreatic polypeptide) PP cells similar to what is seen in the ventral pancreatic primordium and in the uncinate process of the normal pancreas (21).

The incidence of annular pancreas is reported as 3 in 20,000 autopsies (18). Some 75% of infants with annular pancreas have other anomalies. Duodenal stenosis or atresia is present at the site of the annulus in about 40%, and trisomy 21 (Down's syndrome) is present in about 16%. Intestinal malrotation, tracheoesophageal fistula, and congenital heart defects are also not uncommon. There are case reports of annular pancreas in association with duodenal obstruction and partial situs inversus referred to as *m*ultiple *o*rgan *m*alrotation *s*yndrome (MOMS) (22). Recently England et al. reported two cases of annular pancreas associated with pancreas divisum and reviewed the literature (18). There are also rare reports of annular pancreas associated with congenital absence of the gallbladder, and a recent report describes primary extrahepatic biliary obstruction secondary to a constricting pancreatic annulus (23, 24). A family with two individuals in two successive generations who were affected by annular pancreas and duodenal obstruction suggests autosomal dominant transmission for this anomaly (25).

Though annular pancreas is of congenital origin, symptoms may arise at any age. Furthermore, it has been estimated that two-thirds of those with this anomaly remain asymptomatic for life (26). Infants who are symptomatic from annular pancreas often present in the first days of life with duodenal obstruction. However, partial obstruction of the duodenum related to stenosis associated with annular pancreas may present later in childhood. Infants or children with associated malrotation can also present with symptoms of acute duodenal or intestinal obstruction related to volvulus and not directly to the annular pancreas. Beyond infancy, there is a peak incidence of symptomatic annular pancreas in adulthood during the 4th decade, and males are more prone to symptoms than females (18). Presenting symptoms in adults with annular pancreas are most frequently pain (69%), nausea with or without intermittent vomiting (60%), gastric or duodenal ulceration (26–48%), and pancreatitis (15–50%) (18). As mentioned above, symptoms of extrahepatic biliary obstruction such as jaundice have also been reported (24, 27, 28).

The diagnosis of annular pancreas has traditionally been made at the time of surgical exploration for duodenal obstruction with or without a preoperative upper gastrointestinal contrast study. Recently, radiographic imaging has played a more prominent role in suggesting the diagnosis of annular pancreas. There are now several reports of the role of sonography in the diagnosis of annular pancreas and associated duodenal obstruction in the fetus and infant (29–31). In older children and adults, CT and MRI have proven helpful in the diagnosis of annular pancreas, particular in association with pancreatitis (32, 33). The definitive diagnosis of annular pancreas is being more commonly made by the use of endoscopic retrograde cholangiopancreatography (ERCP), particularly in adults. Endoscopic ultrasound may prove more useful for making the diagnosis in a less invasive manner.

The treatment of annular pancreas is dictated by symptoms. No therapy is warranted in the two-thirds of patients without symptoms. The most common indication for operative therapy in infants and children with annular pancreas is associated duodenal stenosis or obstruction. A variety of operations has been used in the treatment of duodenal obstruction related to annular pancreas. Division of the constricting ring of pancreatic tissue is tempting; however, there are substantial complications related to this procedure, including *(a)* failure to relieve the duodenal obstruction, which typically is related to intrinsic stenosis or atresia, and *(b)* division of the annular pancreatic ductal system, resulting in pancreatic fistula. Gastrojejunostomy has also been

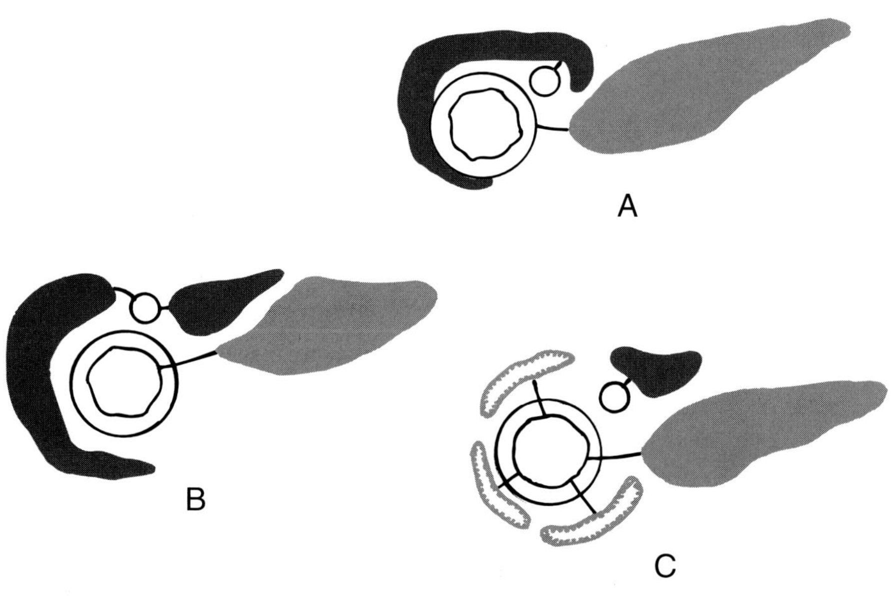


**FIG. 1.3.** Theories of the embryogenesis of the annular pancreas. **A.** Fixation of the distal tip of the ventral primordium to the duodenal wall prior to rotation. **B.** Failure of the involution of the left ventral pancreatic bud with ventral extension. **C.** Fusion of aberrant pancreatic tissue in the region of the duodenum.

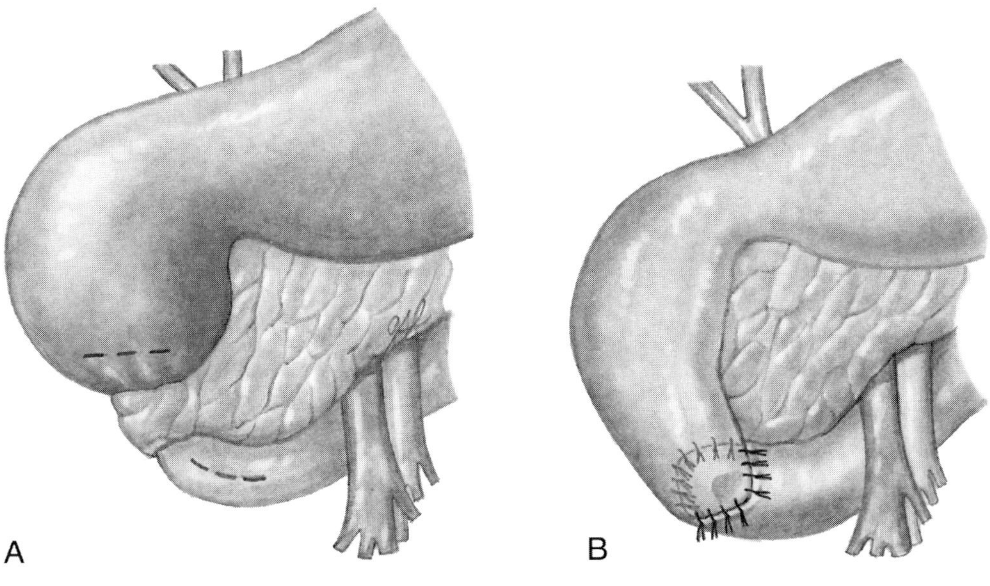

**FIG. 1.4. A.** Duodenoduodenostomy is performed by making a transverse duodenotomy in the proximal dilated duodenum and a longitudinal duodenotomy of the same length in the distal segment. It is important that the proximal transverse duodenotomy is some distance from the annular pancreas to avoid an injury to the pancreatic or biliary ductal system. **B.** A single layer of interrupted sutures with posterior knots tied on the inside of the lumen is performed creating a "diamond shaped" anastomosis.

used and is a relatively simple procedure; however, ulceration at the anastomosis and poor drainage of the afferent limb are serious postoperative complications. Bypass of the obstructing lesion has also been treated by duodenojejunostomy. The operation of choice for duodenal obstruction associated with annular pancreas is duodenoduodenostomy as described by Weitzman and Brennan in 1974 (33). This procedure bypasses the obstructing lesion by creating an anastomosis between the side of the dilated proximal duodenum and the side of the decompressed distal duodenum (Fig. 1.4). In cases of massive dilation of the proximal duodenum and stomach, a tube gastrostomy is also advocated by some surgeons.

Annular pancreas is also associated with acute and chronic pancreatitis, particularly in adults (18). The diagnosis of annular pancreas in the setting of pancreatitis is typically made by abdominal CT scan and ERCP. Management of patients with pancreatitis associated with annular pancreas should initially be nonoperative, as is the approach in most cases of typical pancreatitis. However, a variety of surgical procedures has been used in treating pancreatitis associated with annular pancreas, including sphincterotomy, sphincteroplasty, and endoscopic pancreatic stent placement (28). Pancreaticojejunostomy, with or without duodenoduodenostomy, has also been used with success in the treatment of chronic pancreatitis associated with annular pancreas (18). In select cases, pancreaticoduodenectomy has been successful in treating chronic pancreatitis associated with annular pancreas (34).

### Pancreas Divisum

Pancreas divisum (PD) was originally described by Opie in 1903 (35). Historically, the term *pancreas divisum* signified a very rare congenital anomaly in which the parenchyma of the ventral and dorsal pancreas is separated as a double pancreas (2). Recently, the term has been widely used to describe anatomic variations that result when the dorsal and ventral pancreatic ducts do not fuse normally. The presence of two completely separate pancreatic ducts, referred to as type 1 pancreatic divisum by Warshaw et al., is not unusual and is reported to occur in 4–14% of autopsy studies and in 2–7% of patients undergoing ERCP (36). In addition, a substantial number of patients with "pancreas divisum" (5–23%) have only a dorsal duct with no evidence of a ventral duct of Wirsung. This anatomic variant has been referred to as type 2 divisum. Another variation is a dominant dorsal duct with only a small, narrow filamentous connection between the dorsal and ventral ducts (type 3). Common to all variants of PD is that all or most pancreatic secretion flows through the accessory papilla (Fig. 1.5).

The anatomic variant of PD is not necessarily abnormal. The clinical relevance of PD has been, and continues to be, very controversial (36–43). No clinical study has definitively proven a statistically significant, independent association of PD and pancreatitis. However, a growing body of evidence suggests that PD plays a direct role in pancreatitis.

Three groups of patients have been considered to have symptoms related to PD, those with *(a)* acute recurrent pancreatitis, *(b)* chronic pancreatitis, and *(c)* chronic upper abdominal pain. In patients with acute recurrent pancreatitis, the incidence of PD rises to 12–25%, suggesting an association between the two conditions (44). In a group of patients undergoing ERCP specifically for the evaluation of pancreatitis, compared with other indications, a statistically significant difference was noted between the number of patients with pancreatitis and PD and the number without pancreatitis but with PD (41). In another review involving 1825 consecutive ERCPs, the 137 patients with PD had a significantly higher incidence of acute recurrent idiopathic pancreatitis (50%) than either control patients who underwent ERCP or the general population (45).

Pancreatitis associated with PD is believed to be secondary to the finding that the accessory papilla, through which the bulk of pancreatic flow occurs in PD, is narrower than the normal main pancreatic duct of the ventral pancreas. The dorsal duct in cases of PD and pancreatitis has a mean orifice size of 0.6 mm, compared with 3 mm in normal adults (46). Asymptomatic patients with PD frequently have a dorsal duct orifice that is readily cannulated by a 1-mm cannula (46). If the orifice of the accessory papilla is stenotic or too small to handle the flow of pancreatic juice, obstructive pancreatitis or pancreatic pain can result. The obstruction of the dorsal duct is typically neither complete nor permanent, accounting for the intermittent nature of attacks of pancreatitis or pain. Stenosis of the lesser papilla is

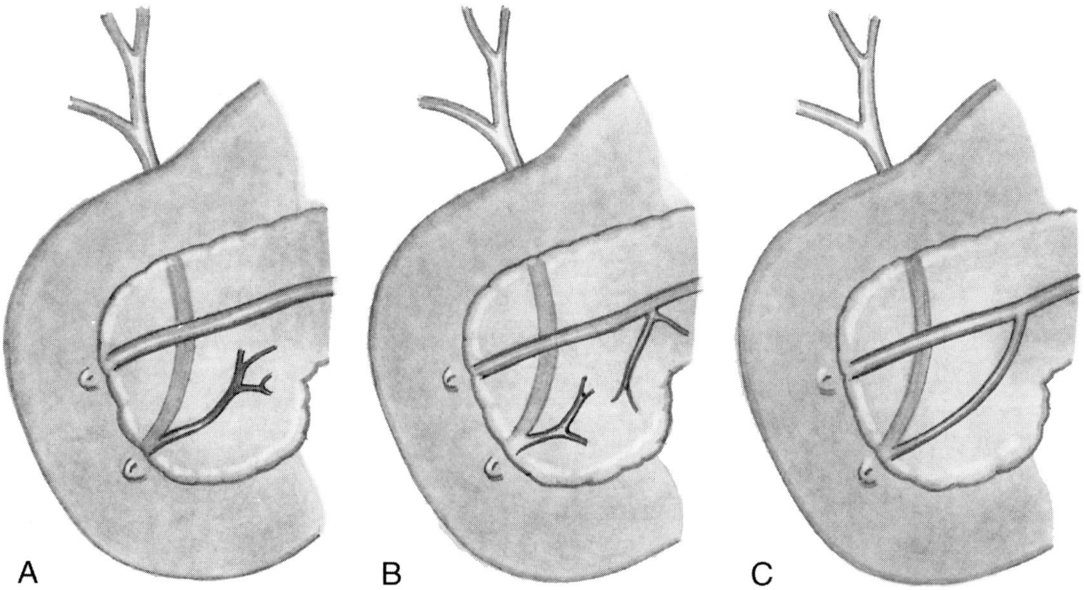


**FIG. 1.5.** Anatomic variation of PD. **A.** Two completely separate pancreatic ducts, with the main duct being much smaller than the accessory duct. **B.** Absent or diminutive main pancreatic duct with a prominent dorsal accessory duct. **C.** A small narrow connection between the large dorsal and diminutive ventral duct.

probably developmental, because there is usually a diminutive orifice without evidence of inflammation.

ERCP is necessary to establish the diagnosis of PD. Visualization of both major and minor papillae and two separate ductal systems, or as mentioned, a complete absence of the duct of Wirsung is required for the definitive diagnosis of PD. The physiologic relevance of PD may be determined by using intravenous secretin stimulation of pancreatic secretions while performing real-time ultrasound imaging of the pancreatic ducts. A functional stenosis of the accessory papilla with secretion-induced proximal ductal dilation is thought to be characteristic of clinically important PD. The secretin stimulation test is controversial; Warshaw et al. reported a 78% sensitivity for the test when judged against intraoperative accessory papilla orifice diameter, while other authors have not agreed about the usefulness of the test (36, 46).

All other causes of pancreatitis must be excluded before surgical or endoscopic intervention for symptomatic PD. Several recent studies have evaluated the efficacy of endoscopic dorsal duct stenting and/or sphincterotomy in treating patients with acute recurrent pancreatitis, chronic pancreatitis, and chronic abdominal pain syndrome in association with PD. Most studies have shown short-term improvement of symptoms in treating patients with acute recurrent pancreatitis; however, complication rates have been relatively high (15%), and the long-term success of stenting has not been satisfactory (46–50).

Operative dorsal duct sphincterotomy, with or without sphincteroplasty, is the preferred surgical treatment for patients with PD and recurrent attacks of acute pancreatitis with documented hyperamylasemia. The operation is performed through a transverse duodenotomy opposite the ampulla of Vater. The accessory papilla is identified and dilated, and a sphincterotomy of the accessory sphincter is performed to the level of the junction of the dorsal pancreatic duct and the circular fibers of the duodenal muscularis. Some surgeons prefer to perform a sphincteroplasty as well; however, because of the more direct route of the dorsal duct from the pancreas into the duodenal wall, this addition may not be necessary (46). Concomitant cholecystectomy and sphincteroplasty of the ampulla of Vater and the orifice of the ventral pancreatic duct are also advocated by some surgeons (51). In the unusual case of chronic pancreatitis attributed to PD, a longitudinal pancreaticojejunostomy should be constructed to the dilated dorsal pancreatic duct.

Endoscopic stenting of the dorsal pancreatic duct should be considered as a predictive study in patients with PD and chronic abdominal pain syndrome. Consistent relief of pain during an extended period of dorsal duct intubation without pancreatitis can be considered an indication for operative sphincterotomy.

### Congenital Pancreatic Cysts

Except for posttraumatic pseudocysts, cysts arising from the pancreas are rare in children. Congenital cysts may be unilocular or multilocular and are frequently associated with cysts in other organs. An example is the cysts seen in von Hippel-Lindau disease, which is characterized by hereditary cerebellar cysts, hemangiomas of the retina, and cysts of the pancreas and other organs. Congenital cysts are lined by epithelium and acinar tissue and are most commonly seen in the body and tail of the pancreas. They are usually asymptomatic unless they cause extrinsic pressure on adjacent viscera such as the stomach and the transverse colon. Treatment of congenital cysts consists of either total excision or internal drainage into the stomach or jejunum.

### Persistent Hyperinsulinemic Hypoglycemia of Infancy (Nesidioblastosis)

Persistent hyperinsulinemic hypoglycemia of infancy (PHHI) should be considered a congenital pancreatic anomaly. PHHI, historically referred to as nesidioblastosis or islet cell dysplasia, is an autosomal recessive disorder characterized by unregulated secretion of insulin and hypoglycemia. Hypoglycemia of infancy and childhood also has several extrapancreatic causes. These include panhypopituitarism, isolated growth hormone deficiency, adrenal insufficiency, hypothyroidism, congenital adrenal hyperplasia (adrenogenital syndrome), the Beckwith-Wiedemann syndrome, inborn errors of gluconeogenesis (e.g., fructose-1,6-diphosphatase deficiency), leucine sensitivity, and others. One must recognize and consider these possibilities with appropriate diagnostic tests. These causes are all rare, and most infants with refractory hypoglycemia have PHHI.

The precise pathophysiology of PHHI is uncertain; however, most studies suggest that there is a defect in glucose-regulated insulin secretion in pancreatic islet ß cells. As implied in the terms nesidioblastosis and islet cell dysplasia, histologic examination of an affected pancreas often suggests ß cell and islet hyperplasia. Using linkage analysis, the PHHI gene has been localized to chromosome 11p14-15.1 (52). More recently, a mutation in the sulfonylurea receptor (SUR) gene has been implicated as the cause of familial PHHI (53). The SUR is a subunit of the ß cell ATP-sensitive potassium channel, which modulates insulin secretion, and a truncation of this receptor would allow unregulated insulin secretion (53).

Infants with PHHI present with symptomatic hypoglycemia. Frank seizures or other neurologic symptoms are typical. PHHI is suspected clinically if Whipple's triad is demonstrated: *(a)* mental status changes or dizziness are precipitated by fasting or exercise; *(b)* fasting blood glucose concentrations are below 40–50 mg/dL; and *(c)* symptoms are relieved by oral or intravenous administration of glucose. An insulin/glucose ratio (insulin in IU/mL divided by glucose in mg/dL) above 0.5 with fasting is highly suggestive of this disease. In infants and children, the absolute ratio of insulin to glucose is not so important as in adults, but an insulin level above 5 IU/mL in the presence of hypoglycemia is diagnostic. Low serum levels of ß-hydroxybutyrate have been considered an important diagnostic feature of PHHI in infants and children. There have recently been reports of the prenatal diagnosis of familial PHHI in susceptible infants by measuring high levels of insulin and C-peptide and low levels of glucose in amniotic fluid (54).

Infants with PHHI are initially managed medically, with maintenance of blood glucose levels above 40 mg/dL. This is best carried out by infusing hypertonic glucose solutions through a permanent central venous catheter. In addition, diazoxide (15 mg/kg/day) may be administered to counteract the effects of insulin and raise plasma glucose levels. The somatostatin analogue octreotide has also been used to treat PHHI in the short, as well as long, term. In one study, octreotide stabilized glucose levels and reduced the glucose infusion in 16 neonates with PHHI who did not respond to diazoxide; however, glucose control was inadequate to avoid subtotal pancreatectomy (55). Another series of eight infants treated long term with octreotide reported good results without the need for surgical intervention (56).

Despite the occasional reports of successful long-term medical management, at present, most infants with PHHI should be considered for a 95–99% pancreatectomy early in the course of the disease, because of the risk of serious permanent neurologic impairment with ineffective medical therapy. Pancreatectomy (95–99%) has been considered effective in the past by reducing the number of ß cells considered to be excessive in "nesidioblastosis." With the recent identification of a specific islet ß cell protein mutation resulting in excessive insulin secretion (i.e. a functional ß cell abnormality), 95–99% pancreatectomy would not be expected to result in normal insulin secretion and glucose metabolism, though it may effectively treat the patient. In fact, recent evidence suggests that children with PHHI have impaired insulin response to glucose and lack suppressibility of endogenous insulin secretion years after clinical remission, whether treated medically or by near total pancreatectomy (57).

The operation is conducted through a long upper abdominal transverse incision, and the lesser omentum is opened to expose the entire pancreas. If an islet cell adenoma is found, it should be removed without further resection of the pancreas. If no adenoma is found, the patient is assumed to have PHHI. Intraoperative ultrasound examination of the pancreas may be useful in this evaluation. The next step in the surgical algorithm is a 95% pancreatectomy with preservation of the spleen. The entire pancreas from the tail to the head is resected, including the uncinate process, leaving a small rim of pancreatic tissue within the C loop of the duodenum. If a child remains hypoglycemic after 95% pancreatectomy, a 99% or near-total pancreatectomy with preservation of the duodenum is required (Fig. 1.6). This procedure involves removal of pancreatic tissue from the distal common bile duct and the region of the duodenal arterial arcade. The entire common bile duct is exposed but should remain undamaged during the dissection.

After a 95% or 99% pancreatectomy, a child tends to be hyperglycemic for some time. In the case of 95% pancreatectomy, the patient often returns to euglycemia. In contrast, with the 99% pancreatectomy, diabetes mellitus may result, and insulin therapy may be required. An 80% (subtotal) pancreatectomy has no place in the management of PHHI in infancy and childhood.

### Heterotopic Pancreas

Pancreatic heterotopia occurs during human embryonic development and has been found in 1–2% of people examined post

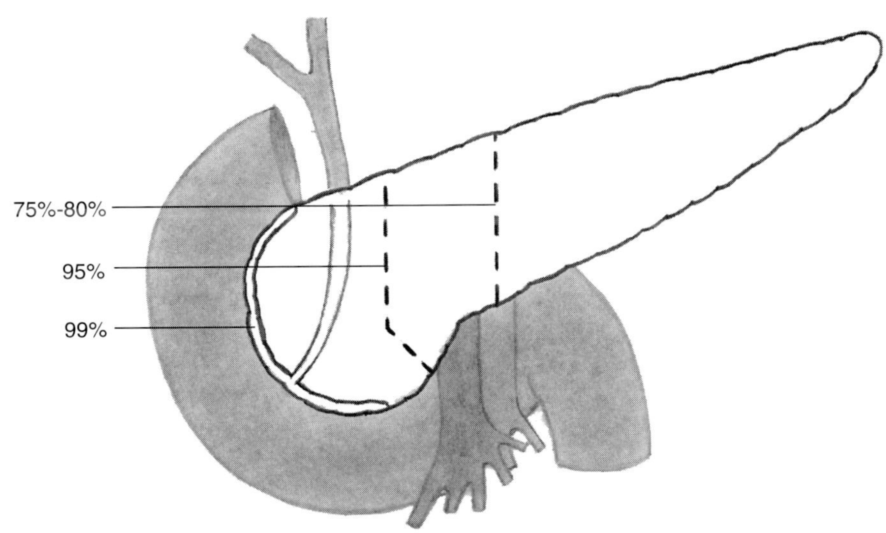


**FIG. 1.6.** Schematic illustration of various degrees of pancreatic resection.

mortem. It is most common in the stomach, duodenum, and Meckel's diverticulum. More unusual intestinal locations include esophagus, jejunum, ileum, colon, rectum, and appendix (58–62). Also reported are pancreatic rests located in the hepatobiliary tree, anomalous bronchoesophageal fistulae, omentum, mesentery, mediastinal cysts, and the skin of the abdominal wall (58, 63–66).

There are two theories of embryogenesis of pancreatic heterotopia: metaplasia and transplantation. The metaplasia theory appears to have the most support and includes *(a)* abnormal differentiation of multipotential endodermal cells in situ and *(b)* differentiation of mature gastric or intestinal epithelial cells during adult life, as the result of inflammation (58). Based on the concept of the development of the pancreas from a region of endoderm containing an epigenetic code, it is reasonable to assume that other structures that develop from the foregut region such as the stomach, duodenum, and biliary tree may well contain a very similar epigenetic code. Activation of one or a few genes in these regions may allow development of heterotopic pancreas (3). In addition, the finding that most heterotopic patches of pancreas have ductal openings into the lumen of the gut strongly suggests in situ differentiation rather than migration from elsewhere (3). In addition, there is immunohistochemical support for both acinar and islet cells developing from primitive duct cells in heterotopic pancreas as has been discussed previously for normal pancreatic development (67). The theory of transplantation explains heterotopia as the adhesion of embryonic pancreatic cells to neighboring structures during rotation of pancreatic primordia (58).

Most patients with heterotopic pancreas exhibit no symptoms. When symptoms develop, they are related to the location of the aberrant pancreatic mass. When located in the stomach or duodenum, the symptoms can be similar to those of peptic ulcer disease, such as pain or vomiting. Intestinal bleeding or symptoms of intussusception or peritonitis are typical of pancreatic rests in the appendix, small intestine, or Meckel's diverticulum. Malignant degeneration has been reported in several heterotopic pancreatic locations, including the esophagogastric junction, the duodenum, and the jejunum (60, 68, 69). Symptoms of biliary obstruction, hydrops of the gallbladder, and pancreatitis in the ectopic pancreatic mass, have been reported (58, 66, 70). There is also one case report of nesidioblastosis arising from heterotopic pancreas (71).

The treatment of heterotopic pancreas is surgical, with the procedure depending on the site of heterotopia. Local excision, with or without frozen section diagnosis, is appropriate when heterotopic pancreas is a coincidental finding at exploration (60, 72). Typical procedures for symptomatic heterotopic pancreas include limited bowel resection for obstructive, inflammatory, or bleeding symptoms or more extensive resection for malignancy (i.e., pancreaticoduodenectomy for duodenal lesions) (60).

## REFERENCES


1. Phisalix C. Etude d'yn embryon humain de 10 millimetres. Arch Zool Exp Gen Hist Nat Morph Histol Evol Animaux 1888;6:279.
2. Kozu T, Suda K, Tokiu F. Pancreatic development and anatomical variation. Gastrointest Clin North Am 1995;5:1–30.
3. Slack JMW. Developmental biology of the pancreas. Development 1995;121:1569–1580.
4. Pietet R, Routter WJ. Development of the embryonic endocrine pancreas. In: Steiner DF, Frenkel N, eds. Handbook of physiology, sect 7, vol 1, American Physiology Society. Washington, DC: Williams & Wilkins, 1972:25–66.
5. Andrew A. An experimental investigation into the possible neural crest origin of pancreatic APUD (islet) cells. J Embryol Exp Morphol 1976;35:577–593.
6. Rosenberg L. In vivo cell transformation; neogenesis of beta cells from a pancreatic ductal cells. Cell Transplant 1995;4:371–383.
7. Golosow N, Grobstein C. Epitheliomesenchymal interaction in pancreatic morphogenesis. Dev Biol 1962;4:242–255.
8. Ronzio RA, Rutter WJ. Effects of a partially purified factor from chick embryos on macromolecular synthesis of embryonic pancreatic epithelia. Dev Biol 1973;30:307–320.
9. Gittes GK, Galante PE, Hanahan D, Rutter WJ, Debase HT. Lineage-specific morphogenesis in the developing pancreas: role of mesenchymal factors. Development 1996;122(2):439–447.
10. Sanvito F, Herrea PL, Huarte J, et al. TGF-beta 1 influences the relative development of the exocrine and endocrine pancreas in vitro. Development 1994;120:3451–3462.
11. Jonsson J, Carlsson L, Edlund T, Edlund H. Insulin-promoter-factor 1 is required for pancreas development in mice. Nature 1994; 371:606–609.
12. Ahlgren U, Jonsson J, Edlund H. The morphogenesis of the pancreatic mesenchyme is uncoupled from that of the pancreatic epithelium in IPF1/PDX1-deficient mice. Development 1996; 122(5):1409–1416.
13. Gittes G, Rutter WJ. Onset of cell-specific gene expression in the developing mouse pancreas. Proc Natl Acad Sci USA 1992;89: 1128–1132.
14. Voldsgaard P, Kryger-Baggesen N, Lisse I. Agenesis of pancreas. Acta Paediatr 1994;83:791–793.
15. Wilding R, Schnedl WJ, Reisinger EC, et al. Agenesis of the dorsal pancreas in a women with diabetes mellitus and in both her sons. Gastroenterology 1993;104:1182–1186.
16. Zairat'iants OV, Miagkova LP, Podymova SA, Mel'nichenko GA, Burmakin IA. Congenital hypoplasia of the pancreas with lipomatosis and bone marrow dysfunction (Schwachman syndrome). Arkh Patol 1991;53:71–74.
17. Lecco TM. Zur Morphologie des Pankreas annulare. Sitzungsber Wien Akad Wissen Math Naturw Kl 1910;119:391–406.
18. England RE, Newcomer MK, Leung JW, Cotton PB. Case report: annular pancreas divisum—a report of two cases and review of the literature. Br J Radiol 1995;68:324–328.
19. Baldwin WM. Specimen of annular pancreas. Anat Rec 1910;4: 299–304.
20. Erimoglu C. A case of pancreas annulare. Proc K Ned Akad Wet (Biol Med) 1952;55:18.
21. Suda K. Immunohistochemical and gross dissection studies of the annular pancreas. Acta Pathol Jpn 1990;40:505–508.
22. Adeyemi SD. Combination of annular pancreas and partial situs inversus: a multiple organ malrotation syndrome associated with duodenal obstruction. J Pediatr Surg 1988;23:188–191.
23. Heij HA, Niessen GJ. Annular pancreas associated with congenital absence of the gallbladder. J Pediatr Surg 1987;22:1033.
24. Baggott BB, Long WB. Annular pancreas as a cause of extrahepatic biliary obstruction. Am J Gastroenterol 1991;86:224–226.
25. Hendricks SK, Sybert VP. Association of annular pancreas and duodenal obstruction—evidence for Mendelian inheritance? Clin Genet 1991;39:383–385.
26. Bickford B, Williamson JCFL. Annular pancreas. Br J Surg 1952;39: 49–52.
27. Lloyd-Jones W, Mountain JC, Warren KW. Annular pancreas in the adult. Ann Surg 1972;176:163–170.
28. Urayama S, Kozarek R, Ball T, et al. Presentation and treatment of annular pancreas in adult population. Am J Gastroenterol 1995;90:995–999.
29. Pahci A, Maggi E, Giancotti A, Torcia F, De Prosperi V. Ultasound diagnosis of fetal annular pancreas. J Perinat Med 1989;17: 361–364.
30. Orr LA, Powell RW, Melhem RE. Sonographic demonstration of annular pancreas in the newborn. J Ultrasound Med 1992;11: 373–375.
31. Norton KI, Tenreiro R, Rabinowitz JG. Sonographic demonstration of annular pancreas and distal duodenal obstruction in a newborn. Pediatr Radiol 1992;22:66–67.
32. Nguyen K, Pace R, Groll A. CT appearance of annular pancreas: a case report. J Can Assoc Radiol 1989;40:322–323.
33. Weitzman JJ, Brennan LP. An improved technique for the correction of duodenal obstruction in the neonate. J Pediatr Surg 1974;9:385–386.
34. Dowsett JF, Rode J, Russell RC. Annular pancreas: a clinical, endoscopic and immunohistochemical study. Gut 1989;30: 130–135.

35. Opie EL. The anatomy of the pancreas. Johns Hopkins Bull 1903;14:229–232.
36. Warshaw AL, Simeone JF, Scharpiro RH, Flavin-Warshaw B. Evaluation and treatment of the dominant dorsal duct syndrome (pancreas divisum redefined). Am J Surg 1990;159:59–64.
37. Sugawa C, Walt AJ, Nunez DC, et al. Pancreas divisum: is it normal anatomic varient? Am J Surg 1987;153:62–67.
38. Thompson MH, Williamson RCN, Salmon PR. The clinical relevance of isolated ventral pancreas. Br J Surg 1981;68:101–104.
39. Delhaye M, Engelholm L, Cremer M. Pancreas divisum: controversial clinical significance. Dig Dis 1988;6:30–39.
40. Delhaye M, Cremer M. Clinical significance of pancreas divisum. Acta Gastroenterol Belg 1992;55:306–313.
41. Brenner P, Duncombe V, Ham JM. Pancreatitis and pancreas divisum: aetiological and surgical considerations. Aust NZ J Surg 1990;60:899–903.
42. Kozarek RA, Ball TJ, Patterson DJ, Brandabur JJ, Raltz SL. Endoscopic approach to pancreas divisum. Dig Dis Sci 1995;40:1974–1981.
43. Burtin P, Person B, Charneau J, Boyer J. Pancreas divisum and pancreatitis: a coincidental association? Endoscopy 1991;23:55–58.
44. Leese T, Chiche L, Bismuth H. Pancreatitis caused by congenital anomalies of the pancreatic ducts. Surgery 1989;105:125–130.
45. Bernard JP, Sahel J, Giovannini M, Sarles H. Pancreas divisum is a probable cause of acute pancreatitis: a report of 137 cases. Pancreas 1990;5:248–254.
46. Keith R. Surgery for pancreas divisum. Gastrointest Clin North Am 1995;5(1):171–181.
47. Coleman SD, Eisen GM, Troughton AB, Cotton PB. Endoscopic treatment in pancreas divisum. Am J Gastroenterol 1994;89:1152–1155.
48. Lans JI, Geenen JE, Johanson JF, Hogan WJ. Endoscopic therapy in patients with pancreas divisum and acute pancreatitis: a prospective, randomized, controlled clinical trial. Gastrointest Endosc 1992;38:430–434.
49. Siegel JH, Ben-Zvi JS, Pullano W, Cooperman A. Effectiveness of endoscopic drainage for pancreas divisum: endoscopic and surgical results in 31 patients. Endoscopy 1990;22:129–133.
50. Lehman GA, Sherman S, Nisi R, Hawes RH. Pancreas divisum: results of minor papilla sphincterotomy. Gastrointest Endosc 1993;39:1–8.
51. Adzick NS, Shamberger RC, Winters HS, Hendren WH. Surgical treatment of pancreas divisum causing pancreatitis in children. J Pediatr Surg 1989;24:54–58.
52. Thomas PM, Cote GJ, Hallman DM, Mathew PM. Homozygosity mapping, to chromosome 11p, of the gene for familial persistent hyperinsulinemic of infancy. Am J Hum Genet 1995;56(2):416–421.
53. Thomas PM, Cote GJ, Wohllk N, et al. Mutations in the sulfonylurea receptor gene in familial persistent hyperinsulinemic hypoglycemia of infancy. Science 1995;268(5209):426–429.
54. Aparicio L, Carpenter MW, Schwartz R, Gruppuso PA. Prenatal diagnosis of familial neonatal hyperinsulinemia. Acta Paediatr 1993;82(8):683–686.
55. Thornton PS, Alter CA, Katz LE, Baker L, Stanley CA. Short- and long-term use of octreotide in the treatment of congenital hyperinsulinism. J Pediatr 1993;123(4):637–643.
56. Glaser B, Hirsch HJ, Landau H. Persistent hyperinsulinemic hypoglycemia of infancy: long-term octreotide treatment without pancreatectomy. J Pediatr 1993;123(4):644–650.
57. Leibowitz G, Glaser B, Higazi AA, Salameh M, Cerasi E, Landau H. Hyperinsulinemic hypoglycemia of infancy (nesidioblastosis) in clinical remission; high incidence of diabetes mellitus and persistent beta-cell dysfunction at long-term follow-up. J Clin Endocrinol Metab 1995;80(2):386–392.
58. Skandalakis JE, Gray SW, Ricketts R, Skandalakis LJ. The pancreas. In: Skandalakis JE, Gray SW. Embryology for Surgeons. 2nd ed. Baltimore: Williams & Wilkins, 1994.
59. Tanigawa K, Yamashita S, Tezuka H, Morita S, Ohtsubo T, Maeda R. Diagnostic difficulty in a case of heterotopic pancreatic tissue of the ileum. Am J Gastroenterol 1993;88(3):451–453.
60. Tanaka K, Tsunoda T, Eto T, et al. Diagnosis and management of heterotopic pancreas. Int Surg 1993;78(1):32–35.
61. Noffsinger AE, Hyams DM, Fenoglio-Preiser CM. Esophageal heterotopic pancreas presenting as an inflammatory mass. Dig Dis Sci 1995;40(11):2373–2379.
62. Gugulski A, Regula J, Orlowska J, Butruk E. Heterotopic pancreas in the rectum (Letter). Endoscopy 1994;26(4):372.
63. Terada T, Nakanuma Y, Kakita A. Pathologic observations of intrahepatic peribiliary glands in 1000 consecutive autopsy livers. Heterotopic pancreas in the liver. Gastroenterology 1990;98(5 pt 1):1333–1337.
64. Anagnostopoulos D, Lappas E, Kasselas V, Sfougaris D. The heterotopic pancreas in children. Apropos of 4 new cases. Chir Pediatr 1990;31(3):164–166.
65. Shim YT, Kim SY. Heterotopic gastric mucosa and pancreatic tissue in the skin of the abdominal wall. J Pediatr Surg 1992;27(12):1539–1540.
66. Tsunoda T, Eto T, Yamada M, et al. Heterotopic pancreas: a rare cause of bile duct dilatation—report of a case and review of the literature. Jpn J Surg 1990;20(2):217–220.
67. Yamagiwa H, Onishi N, Nishii M. Heterotopic pancreas of the stomach. Histogenesis and immunohistochemistry. Acta Pathol Jpn 1992;42(4):249–254.
68. Guillou L, Nordback P, Gerber C, Schneider RP. Ductal adenocarcinoma arising in a heterotopic pancreas situated in a hiatal hernia. Arch Pathol Lab Med 1994;118(5):568–571.
69. Jeng KS, Yang KC, Kuo SH. Malignant degeneration of heterotopic pancreas. Gastrointest Endosc 1991;37(2):196–198.
70. Inceoglu R, Dosluoglu HH, Kullu S, Ahiskali R, Doslu FA. An unusual cause of hydropic gallbladder and biliary colic—heterotopic pancreatic tissue in the cystic duct: report of a case and review of the literature. Surg Today 1993;23(6):532–534.
71. Risaliti A, Pizzolitto S. Nesidioblastosis arising from heterotopic pancreas and presenting with hypertension. A clinical, immunohistochemical and ultrastructural study. Ann Chir 1989;43(6):459–464.
72. Farrar WB, Scott M, PJ O'Dwyer. Heterotopic pancreas. Ir J Med Sci 1990;159(1):19–20.

# 2

# *Surgical Anatomy of the Pancreas*

Akira Kuroda and Hideo Nagai

## MACROSCOPY AND TOPOGRAPHY

The pancreas is a soft, pale-yellow, coarsely lobulated organ 12–20 cm long, 3–5 cm wide, and 1–3 cm thick, weighing 60–125 g in adults (1–3). The topography of the pancreas is shown in Figure 2.1. It lies relatively fixed in the retroperitoneum behind the peritoneal floor of the lesser sac, extending from the medial margin of the duodenum to the hilum of the spleen, in an oblique position, higher on the left at about the L1-L2 level.

Anatomically, the pancreas is divided into four portions: the head (the portion to the right of the superior mesenteric vein), the neck (the portion lying over the superior mesenteric vessels), the body, and the tail (the portion to the left of these vessels). The border of the latter two portions is not clearly defined. According to the classification of pancreatic cancer proposed by the Japan Pancreas Society in 1996, the head of the gland is the portion to the right of the left border of the superior mesenteric and portal vein, and the remaining gland is bisected into the body (the right half) and the tail (the left half) (4).

The width and thickness of the pancreas are greatest at the head and taper through the body to the tail. The anterior surface of the pancreas is covered by the peritoneum, but the posterior surface has no peritoneal covering except in the tail.

### Head

The head is intimately surrounded by the duodenal loop. The connection of both organs is generally loose enough for blunt dissection except for the area of the accessory papilla, in which the pancreatic tissue occasionally invades the submucosal or muscular layer of the duodenum (5). Anteriorly, the head is covered by the pylorus above and transverse colon below and is traversed by the attachment of the transverse mesocolon, which may be quite short here. The posterior surface of the head is separated by the avascular fusion fascia of Treitz from the hilum and vessels of the right kidney, the inferior vena cava, the left renal vein, and the aorta.

There are three major patterns of the relationship of the common bile duct to the head of the pancreas: partial coverage of the duct by pancreatic tissue from behind (51.5%), total coverage of the duct passing through the pancreas (30%), and the duct running externally in a groove on the posterior aspect of the gland (16.5%) (6) (Fig. 2.2).

### Uncinate Process

The uncinate process is a projection from the inferior left margin of the head, passing behind the portal vein and the superior mesenteric vessels and anterior to the vena cava, the aorta, and the left renal vein (Fig. 2.3). The uncinate process may be absent *(A)*, but usually extends posterior to the superior mesenteric vein *(B)*. It may rarely extend over the left margin of the superior mesenteric artery *(C)* or even encircle the mesenteric vessels.

### Neck

The neck is a narrow portion of the pancreas overlying the superior mesenteric vessels. Its posterior surface is grooved by the portal vein, which is formed by the confluence of the superior mesenteric and splenic veins. Anteriorly, the neck is covered by the pylorus and the lesser sac, and superiorly, it is related to the celiac trunk and the root of its tributaries.

## BODY AND TAIL

The body and tail extend to the left, paralleling the splenic vessels in general. Anteriorly, these portions are covered by the stomach, the gastrocolic ligament, and the transverse colon. The transverse mesocolon attaches to the inferior aspect of the body and tail of the pancreas. Inferiorly, the body lies adjacent to the fourth portion of the duodenum and the ligament of Treitz. The tail may or may not reach the hilum of the spleen.

The posterior surfaces of the body and tail, together with the splenic vessels, are separated by the avascular fusion fascia of Toldt from the aorta, the left adrenal gland, the left renal vessels, and the upper third of the left kidney.

### Retroperitoneal Fasciae and Spaces Relevant to the Pancreas

Abdominal organs and their mesenteric structures undergo complex rotation and fixation during the fetal period (Fig. 2.4*A*). The visceral peritoneum overlying the pancreas, duodenum, ascending colon, and descending colon together with their mesenteries confronts the posterior parietal peritoneum. The two opposing peritoneal layers often become fused during gestation to form a fibrous membrane referred to as "fusion fascia" (7). The fusion fasciae behind the head of the pancreas and behind the body and tail are named after Treitz and Toldt, respectively (Fig. 2.4, *A* and *B*).

With its fixation onto the posterior parietal peritoneum, the pancreas now is included in the retroperitoneal space, which is bounded anteriorly by the peritoneum and posteriorly by the transversalis fascia. Meyers (8) divided the retroperitoneal spaces into three compartments based on their demarcation by the anterior and posterior layers of the renal fascia (Gerota's fascia) (Fig. 2.4*B*). The anterior pararenal space is ventral to the anterior renal fascia and contains the pancreas, the major peripancreatic vessels, the extraperitoneal segments of the ascending and descending colon, and the duodenum. The perirenal space includes the kidney, adrenal gland and perirenal fat and

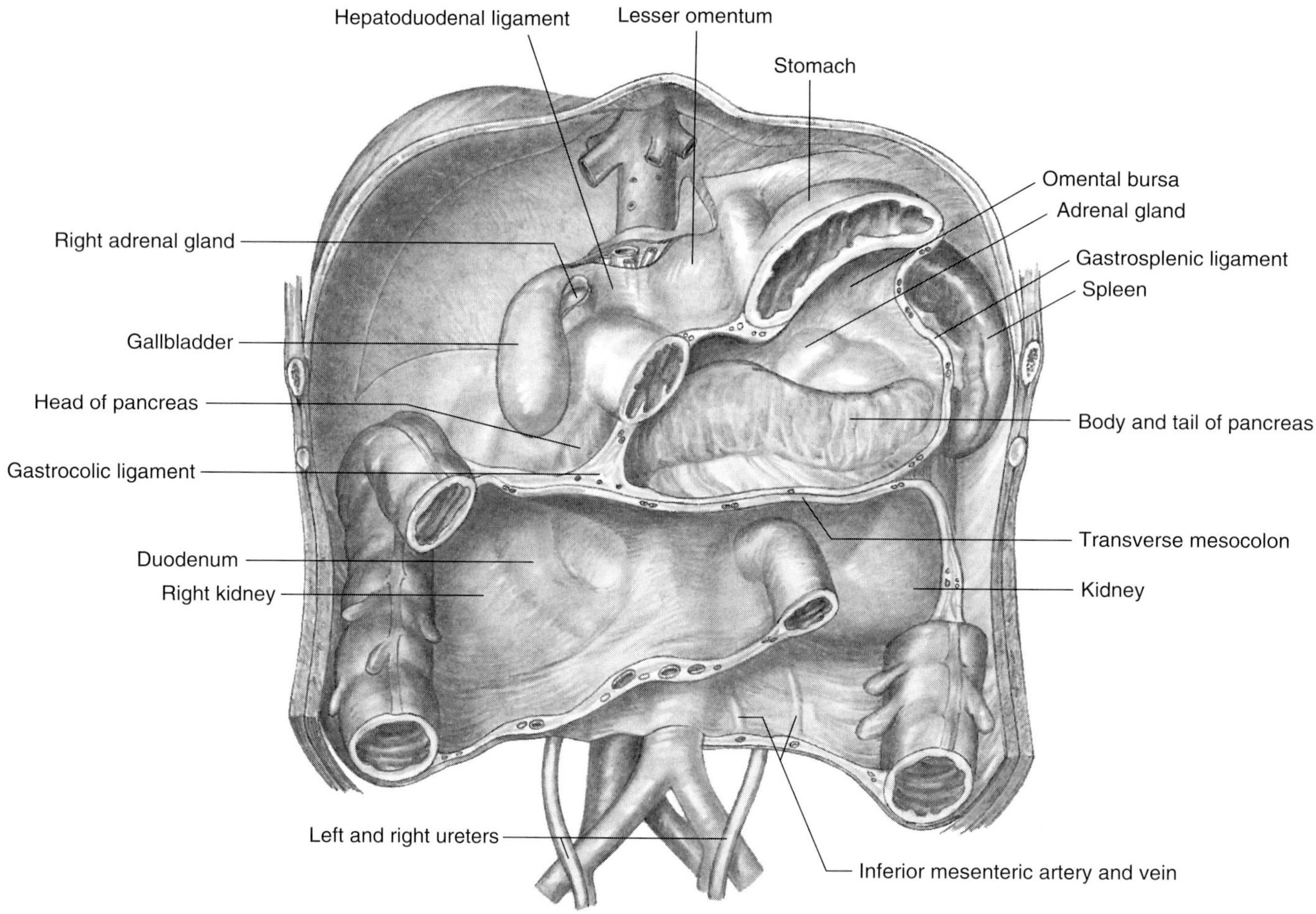


**FIG. 2.1.** Anatomic relationship between the pancreas and neighboring organs, with special emphasis on peritoneal reflections.

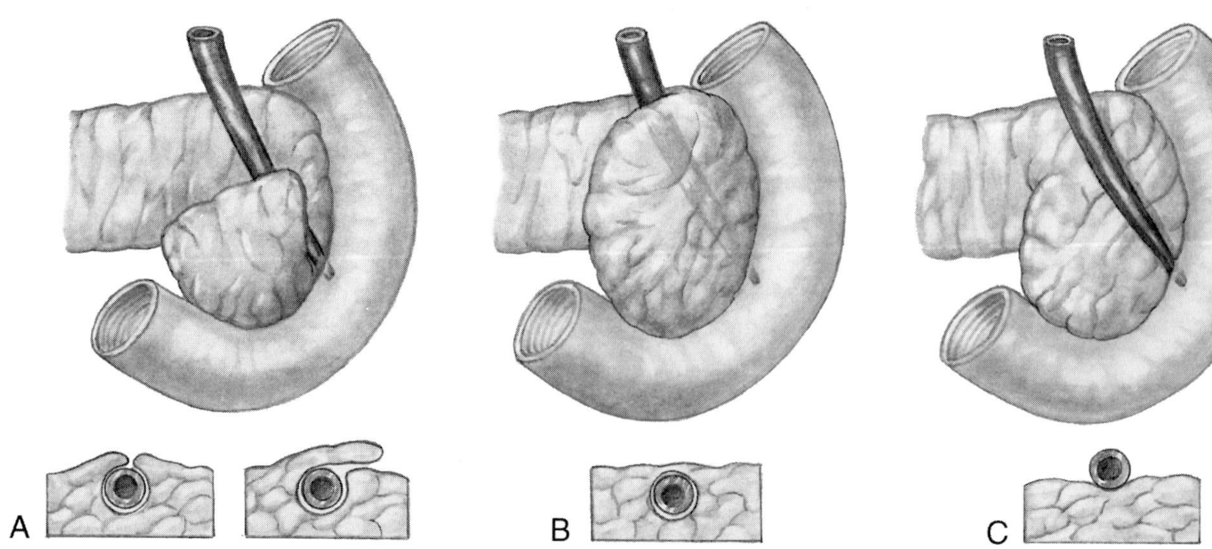


**FIG. 2.2.** Relationship of the common bile duct to the posterior aspect of the pancreatic head. **A.** Partially covered. **B.** Completely covered. **C.** Uncovered.

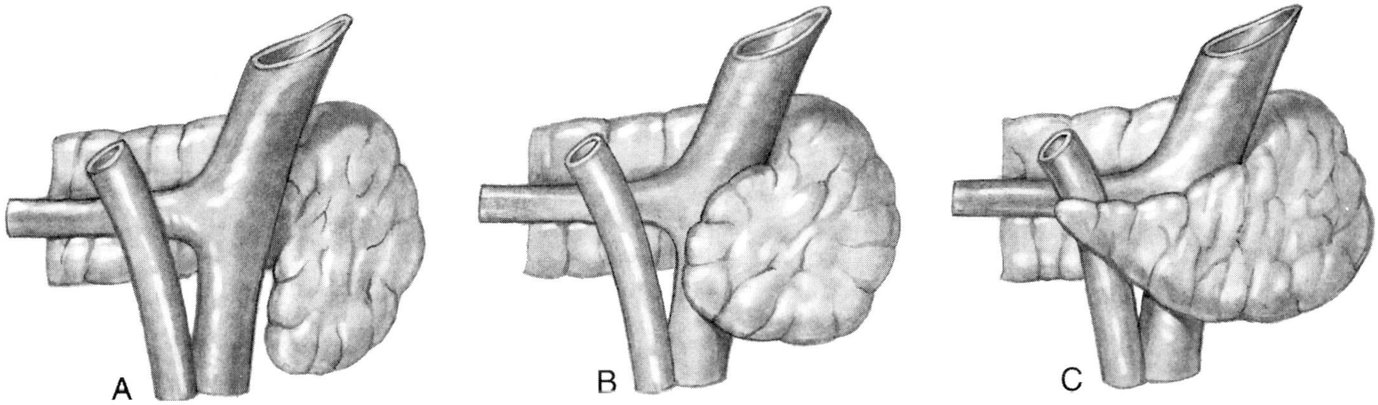


**FIG. 2.3.** Extension of the uncinate process. Three different variations are shown (A, B, C).

is enclosed by the anterior and posterior renal fascia. The posterior pararenal space is dorsal to the perirenal space and includes pararenal fat but no organs.

## PANCREATIC DUCTAL SYSTEM

The pancreas develops from both the ventral and the dorsal pancreatic anlages, which arise from the endodermal epithelium of the duodenum. Both anlages and their ducts usually fuse during the 7th embryonic week. The duct of the ventral anlage and of the dorsal anlage distal to the junction of both ducts serves as the main pancreatic duct (duct of Wirsung). The duct of the dorsal anlage proximal to the junction becomes the accessory pancreatic duct (duct of Santorini) (9).

The main pancreatic duct begins at the terminus of the tail of the gland. It runs midway between the superior and inferior margins through the body and closer to the posterior surface at the neck, to reach the head region. In the head, the main duct inclines caudally and dorsally and passes to the left caudal side of the intrapancreatic portion of the common bile duct, with which it usually unites to form the common channel before opening into the duodenum at the major duodenal papilla (the papilla of Vater). The dorsocaudal portion of the head is drained by the main pancreatic duct.

The accessory pancreatic duct usually begins near the neck of the gland at its junction with the main duct. It runs superior to the main duct and anterior to the common bile duct, to open into the duodenum at the minor duodenal papilla, about 2 cm anteriosuperior to the major papilla (2). The cephalad and ventrocaudal portions of the head are drained by the accessory duct.

Besides the usual pattern of conjunction of both the main and accessory pancreatic ducts (Fig. 2.5*A*), there are variations, including hypoplasia and aplasia of the accessory duct (Fig. 2.5, *A–B, –C*) as well as nonunion of the ducts (Fig. 2.5, *A–D*). The accessory duct may carry most of the pancreatic secretion with or without conjunction with the main duct (Fig. 2.5, *A–E, –F*). The last pattern is termed pancreas divisum (10).

Communication of the main and accessory ducts is present in 90% of persons, and patency of the accessory duct orifice is reported in 33–60% (11). Some 60% of the ducts are in the usual configuration (Fig. 2.5*A*), 30% have suppression of the accessory duct (Fig. 2.5, *A–B, –C, –D*), and 10% have suppression of the main duct (Fig. 2.5, *A–E, –F*) (12). On extremely rare occasions, the accessory duct drains all of the pancreatic secretion through the minor papilla, and no pancreatic duct opens into the major duodenal papilla.

Both the main duct and the accessory duct have numerous tributaries radiating chiefly at right angles from the stem duct. Some 20–30 branches join the main duct in the body of the pancreas (13). The head of the pancreas has a rather complicated ramification caused by fusion of the ventral and dorsal anlages. Its caudal part, including the uncinate process, is characterized by descending branches (rami capitis inferiores) from both the main and the accessory ducts.

## TERMINATION OF THE COMMON BILE DUCT AND THE MAIN PANCREATIC DUCT

The main pancreatic and common bile ducts unite in the duodenal wall in 85% of cases to form a common channel that has been termed the ampulla of Vater (11). The common channel, 1–14 mm long, opens on the major duodenal papilla with a single opening (Fig. 2.6*A*). Rare types in the termination of both ducts are shown in Figure 2.6, *B* and *C*. Both ducts open on the major duodenal papilla via separate orifices (Fig. 2.6*B*) or open into the duodenum at separate points (Fig. 2.6*C*).

## ARTERIAL ANATOMY

The pancreas receives its blood supply from branches of the celiac axis and the superior mesenteric artery. A typical pattern of branch configuration is shown in Figure 2.7 (2, 9). Nonetheless, normal variations are not rare.

### Head

The gastroduodenal artery, which is typically the first major branch of the common hepatic artery arising from the celiac axis (Fig. 2.7), gives off a pair (posterior and anterior, in this order) of the superior pancreaticoduodenal arteries. The superior pancreaticoduodenal arteries descend on the posterior and anterior surfaces of the head of the pancreas to anastomose with a pair (posterior and anterior) of the inferior pancreaticoduodenal arteries, forming the posterior and anterior pancreatic arcades. The anterior and posterior superior pancreaticoduodenal arteries are almost always constant in origin, while the anterior and posterior inferior pancreaticoduodenal arteries arise separately or have a common trunk from the superior mesenteric artery (14). The separate branch or the common trunk of the inferior pancreaticoduodenal arteries often shares the same branch from the superior mesenteric artery with the first jejunal artery.

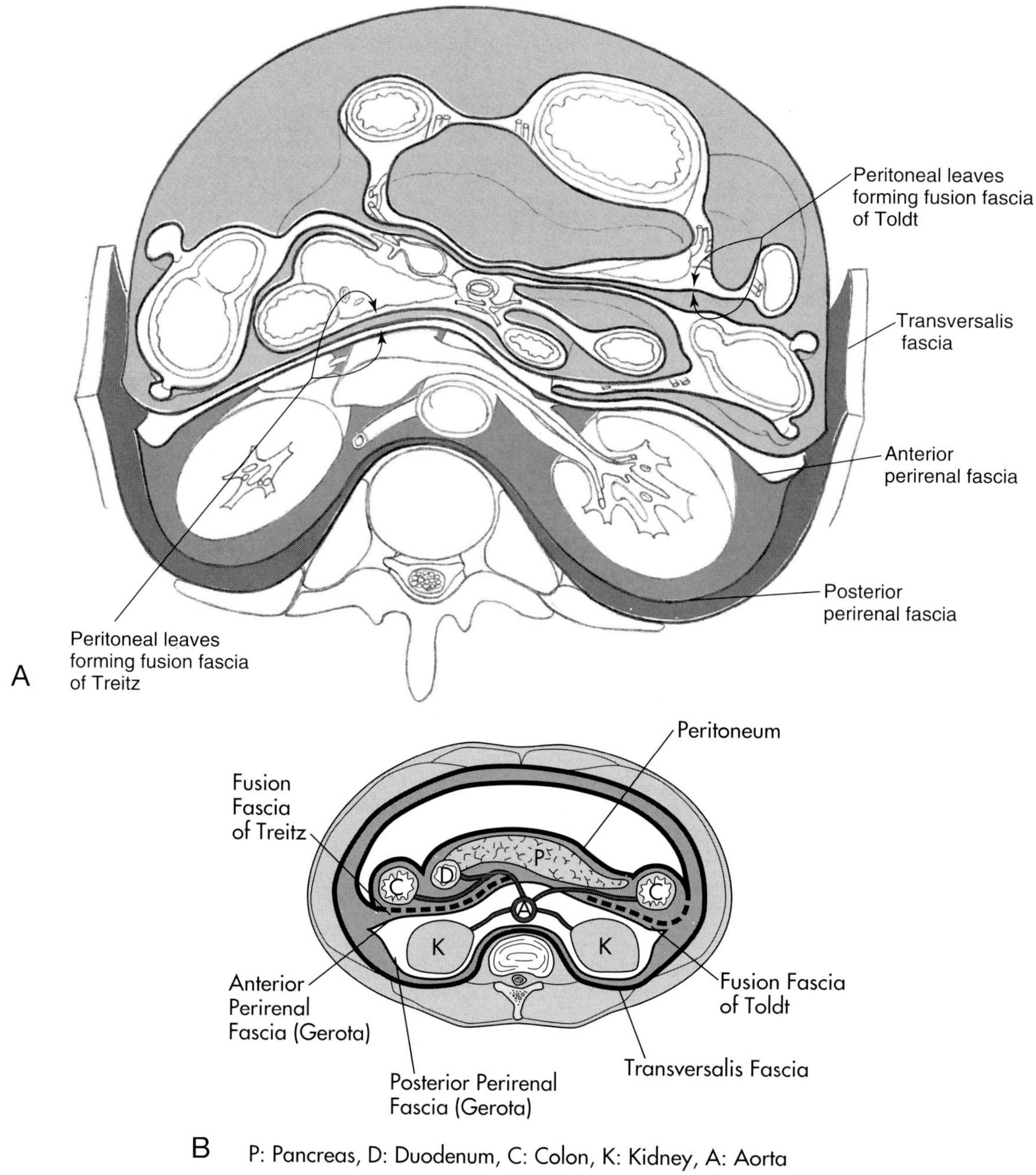


**FIG. 2.4.** **A.** Anteroinferior view of peritoneal reflections and fasciae relevant to the pancreas in a primordial state before formation of fusion fasciae. **B.** Three compartments of the retroperitoneal space. *Light gray color:* anterior pararenal space derived from fixation of the primordially intraperitoneal organs. *Medium gray color:* perirenal space surrounded by Gerota's renal fascia. *Dark gray color:* posterior pararenal space demarcated postrolaterally by the transversalis fascia and anteromedially by Gerota's renal fascia. *P,* pancreas; *D,* duodenum; *C,* colon; *K,* kidney; *A,* aorta.

The head of the pancreas and the duodenum are supplied with blood mainly from these arcades. When considering the duodenum-preserving pancreatic head resection (DPPHR), now performed in selected cases of benign or low-grade malignant tumor of the head of the pancreas (15), one should recognize the vascular anatomy of the pancreaticoduodenal arcades in more detail (5, 16, 17).

The posterior arcade arising from the gastroduodenal artery generally runs in front of the retroduodenal choledochus and then behind the pancreatic head. The posterior arcade passes within the fusion fascia of Treitz, which is easily detachable from the pancreatic parenchyma.

The anterior arcade, a terminal branch of the gastroduodenal artery, runs toward a point 1.5 cm below the papilla of Vater and frequently turns to the posterior aspect of the pancreatic head, which overhangs the anterior surface of the duodenal wall (5, 16, 17) (Fig. 2.8).

The superior portion of the anterior arcade lies partly embedded in the pancreatic parenchyma, while its inferior portion has a relatively loose attachment to the pancreatic parenchyma. Therefore, separation of the posterior arcade from the pancreas by dividing the pancreatic branches and sparing the duodenal tributaries is rather easy, whereas complete preservation of the entire anterior arcade seems difficult. Another difference be-

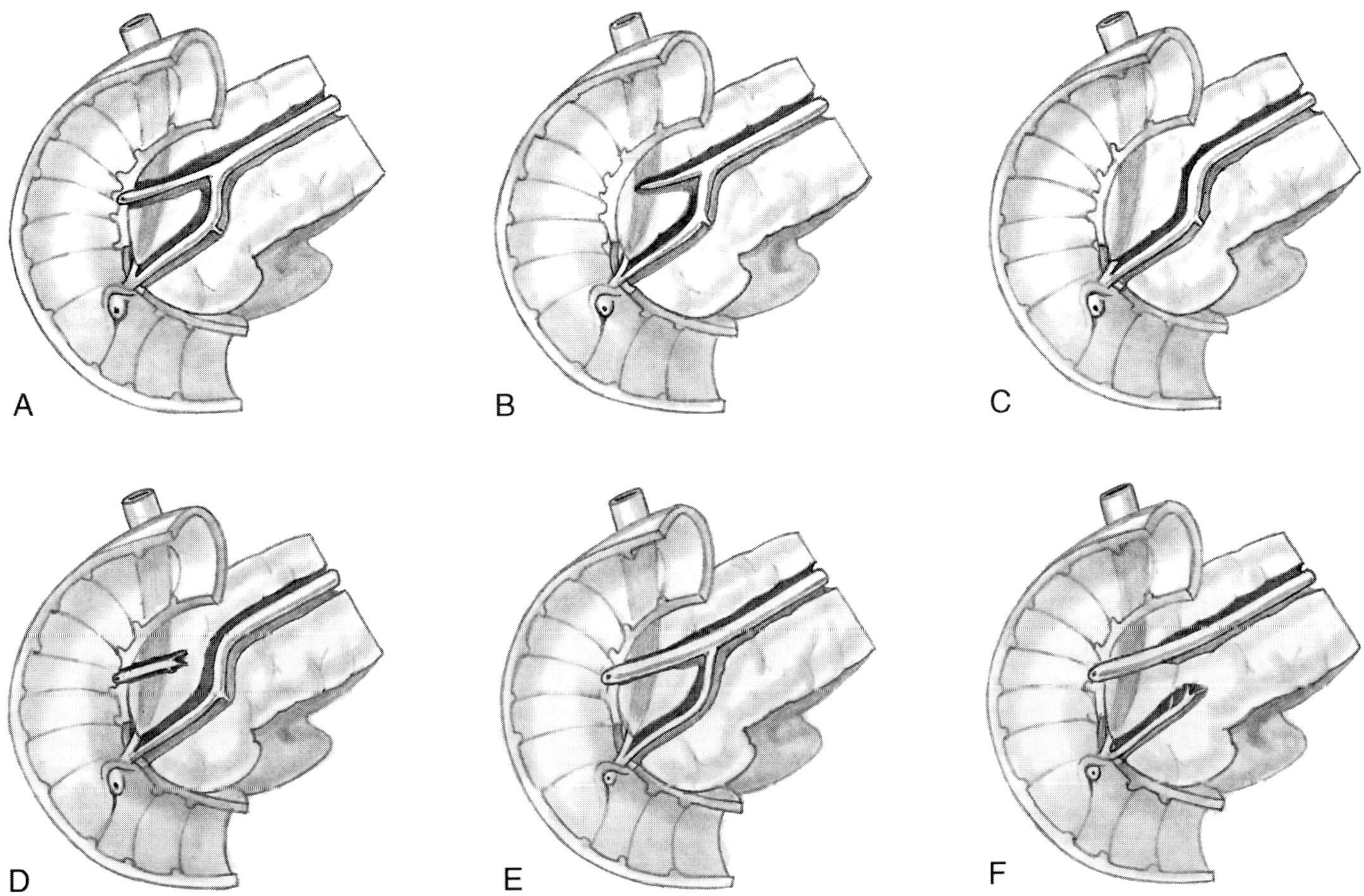


**FIG. 2.5.** Variations of course and termination of the pancreatic ducts (A-F). See the text for description. (With permission from Kuroda A, Nagai H. Gross anatomy of the pancreas. In: Pour PM, Konishi G, Kloppel G, Longnecker DS, eds. Atlas of exocrine pancreatic tumors: morphology, biology, and diagnosis with an international guide for tumor classification. Tokyo: Springer-Verlag, 1994:1–15.)

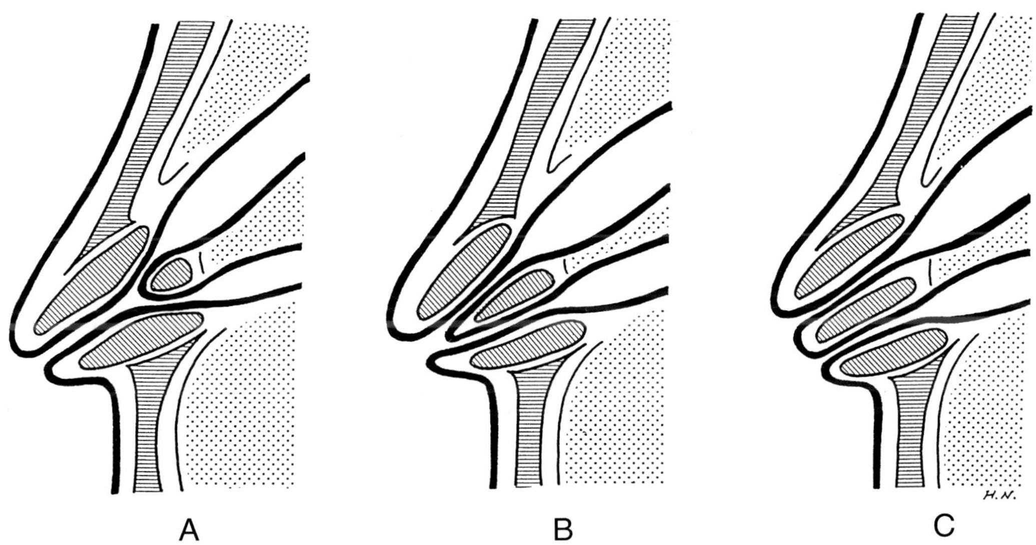


**FIG. 2.6.** Variations in termination of the common bile duct and the main pancreatic duct at the major duodenal papilla (A-C). (With permission from Kuroda A, Nagai H. Gross anatomy of the pancreas. In: Pour PM, Konishi G, Kloppel G, Longnecker DS, eds. Atlas of exocrine pancreatic tumors: morphology, biology, and diagnosis with an international guide for tumor classification. Tokyo: Springer-Verlag, 1994:1–15.)

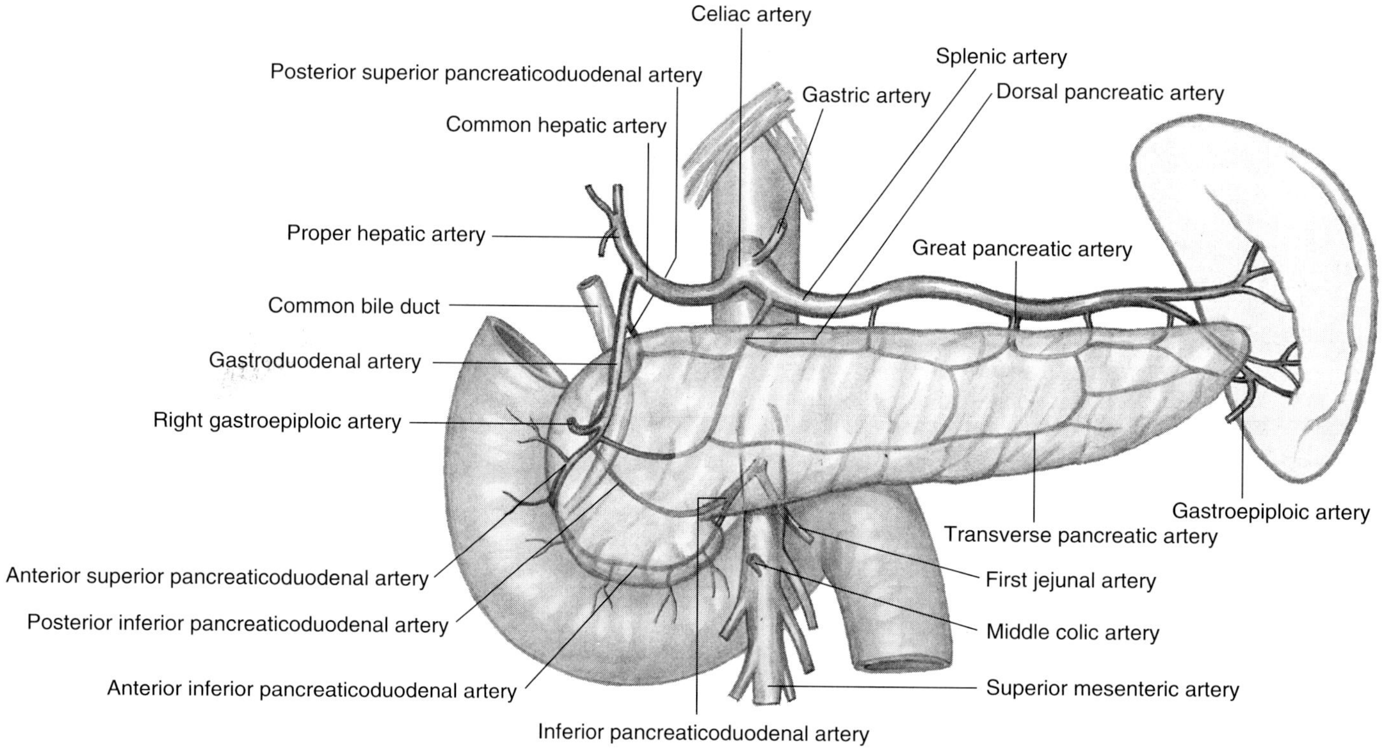


**FIG. 2.7.** Arterial blood supply to the pancreas. (With permission from Kuroda A, Nagai H. Gross anatomy of the pancreas. In: Pour PM, Konishi G, Kloppel G, Longnecker DS, eds. Atlas of exocrine pancreatic tumors: morphology, biology, and diagnosis with an international guide for tumor classification. Tokyo: Springer-Verlag, 1994:1–15.)

tween the posterior and anterior arcades is their course in relation to the duodenum: the posterior arcade passes farther from the duodenum and in a more cephalad position than does its anterior counterpart.

The blood supply to the distal part of the common bile duct and the duodenal papilla of Vater is mainly provided by the branches from the posterior superior pancreaticoduodenal artery.

Most of the arterial anomalies related to pancreatic surgery involve the common hepatic artery and its branches. An aberrant common hepatic artery and right hepatic artery arising from the superior mesenteric artery occur in 4.5% and 25% of subjects, respectively (18). Both of these anomalous vessels usually run just behind the pancreatic head and uncinate process and can communicate with the posterior pancreaticoduodenal arcade.

### Body and Tail

The dorsal pancreatic artery lies behind the neck of the gland, arising from the splenic (40%), the celiac (22%), the superior mesenteric (14%), or the common hepatic artery (12%) (19). It runs downward to the lower border of the pancreas and divides into left and right branches. To the left, it gives off the transverse (inferior) pancreatic artery, and to the right, it sends branches to the head and the uncinate process to anastomose with the superior pancreaticoduodenal or the gastroduodenal artery.

The dorsal pancreatic artery provides the main blood supply to the neck and body of the pancreas. The transverse (inferior) pancreatic artery is the left branch of the dorsal pancreatic artery in 90% of cases and may arise from the gastroduodenal, the right gastroepiploic, or the superior pancreaticoduodenal artery. It runs along the inferior margin of the pancreas to anastomose with the great pancreatic and the caudal pancreatic arteries.

The great pancreatic (pancreatica magna) artery is the largest artery among the 2–10 pancreatic branches of the splenic artery, which courses along the superior margin of the body and tail of the gland. It usually arises around the border between the body and tail of the gland and divides into left and right branches to anastomose with the transverse pancreatic, the dorsal pancreatic, and the caudal pancreatic arteries.

The caudal pancreatic arteries are small branches of the splenic or the left gastroepiploic artery. The transverse pancreatic, the great pancreatic, and the caudal pancreatic arteries supply blood to the body and tail of the pancreas.

## VENOUS ANATOMY

The venous blood of the pancreas (Fig. 2.9) drains into the portal system around the gland: the splenic, the superior mesenteric, the inferior mesenteric, and the portal veins (2, 9, 11).

The splenic vein, running inferior to the splenic artery along the posterior aspect of the body and tail of the pancreas, joins the superior mesenteric vein, which passes anterior to the inferomedial aspect of the uncinate process to form the portal vein behind the neck of the pancreas. The inferior mesenteric vein drains into the splenic (60%) or the superior mesenteric vein (9).

In general, the pancreatic veins parallel the arteries. The head of the pancreas is drained by the anterior and posterior, superior, and inferior pancreaticoduodenal veins. The posterior superior pancreaticoduodenal vein is almost always present, crosses the choledochus posteriorly (sometimes anteriorly), and terminates in the right posterior wall of the portal vein. The posterior and anterior inferior pancreaticoduodenal veins drain, as a common trunk or separately, into the first jejunal vein after passing behind the superior mesenteric vein.

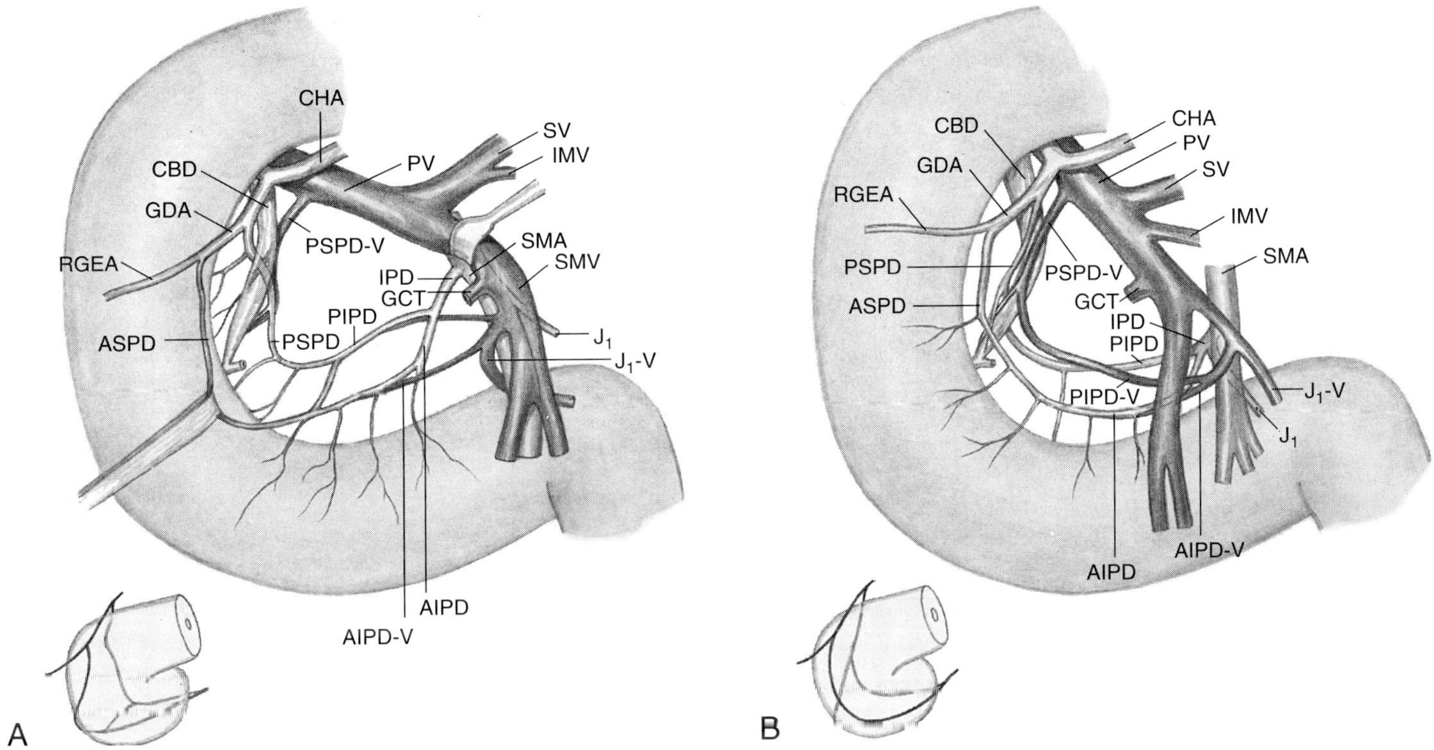


**FIG. 2.8.** Vascular anatomy of the pancreatic head crucial for duodenum-preserving pancreatic head resection. **A.** A rather common distribution of the vessels in that the anterior inferior pancreaticoduodenal artery *(AIPD)* usually runs mostly behind the lower portion of the pancreatic head, and the posterior superior pancreaticoduodenal vein *(PSPD-V)* courses posterior to the common bile duct *(CBD)*, and in that the first jejunal vein *($J_1$-V)* turns behind the superior mesenteric artery *(SMA)* and the inferior mesenteric vein *(IMV)* flows into the splenic vein *(SV)*. **B.** A less common distribution of the vessels with different courses, in that the *PSPD-V* runs anterior to the *CBD* and the inferior pancreaticoduodenal vein flows into the *$J_1$-V* coursing in front of the *SMA*. *AIPD-V,* anterior inferior pancreaticoduodenal vein; *ASPD,* anterior superior pancreaticoduodenal artery; *CHA,* common hepatic artery; *GCT,* gastrocolic trunk; *GDA,* gastroduodenal artery; *IPD,* inferior pancreaticoduodenal artery; *$J_1$,* first jejunal artery; *PIPD,* posterior inferior pancreaticoduodenal artery; *PSPD,* posterior superior pancreaticoduodenal artery; *PV,* portal vein; *RGEA,* right gastroepiploic artery; *SMV,* superior mesenteric vein. (Modified from Nagai H, Ohki J, Kondo Y, et al. Duodenal-sparing resection of the pancreatic head with preservation of duodenal vascular arcades (in Japanese). Geka (Surgery) 1995;57:816–825.)

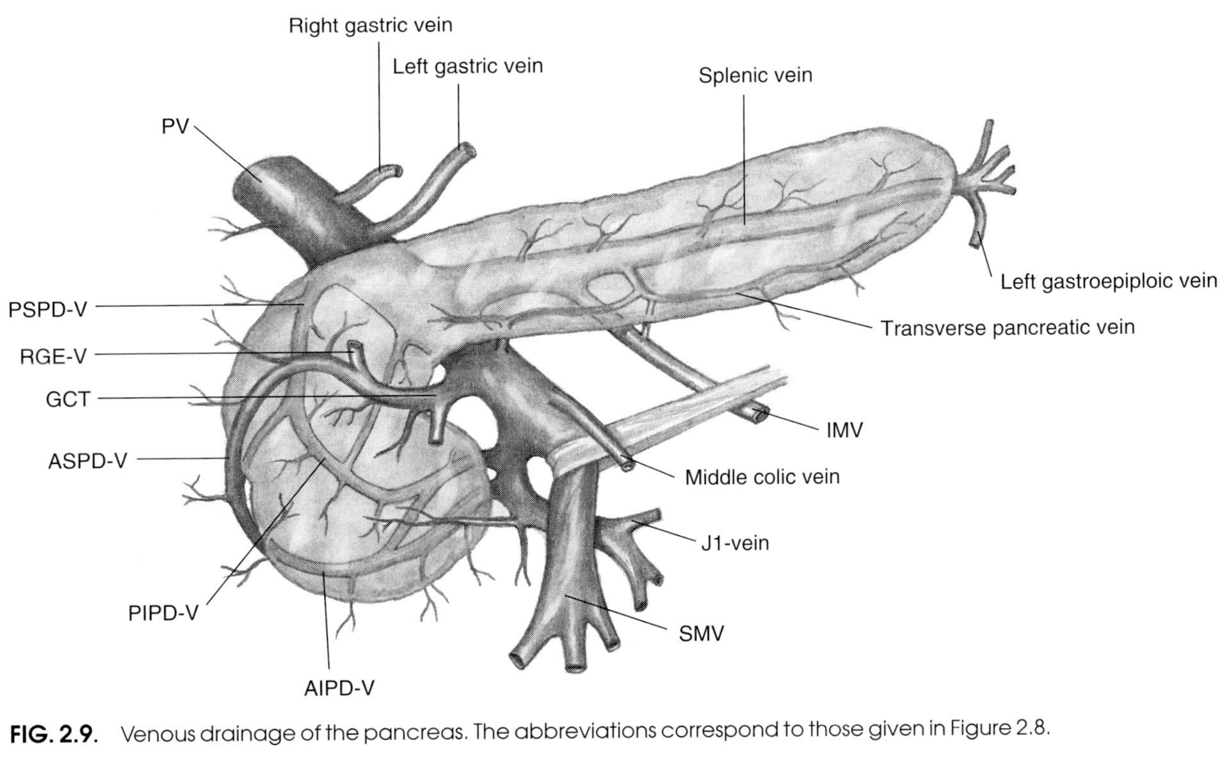


**FIG. 2.9.** Venous drainage of the pancreas. The abbreviations correspond to those given in Figure 2.8.

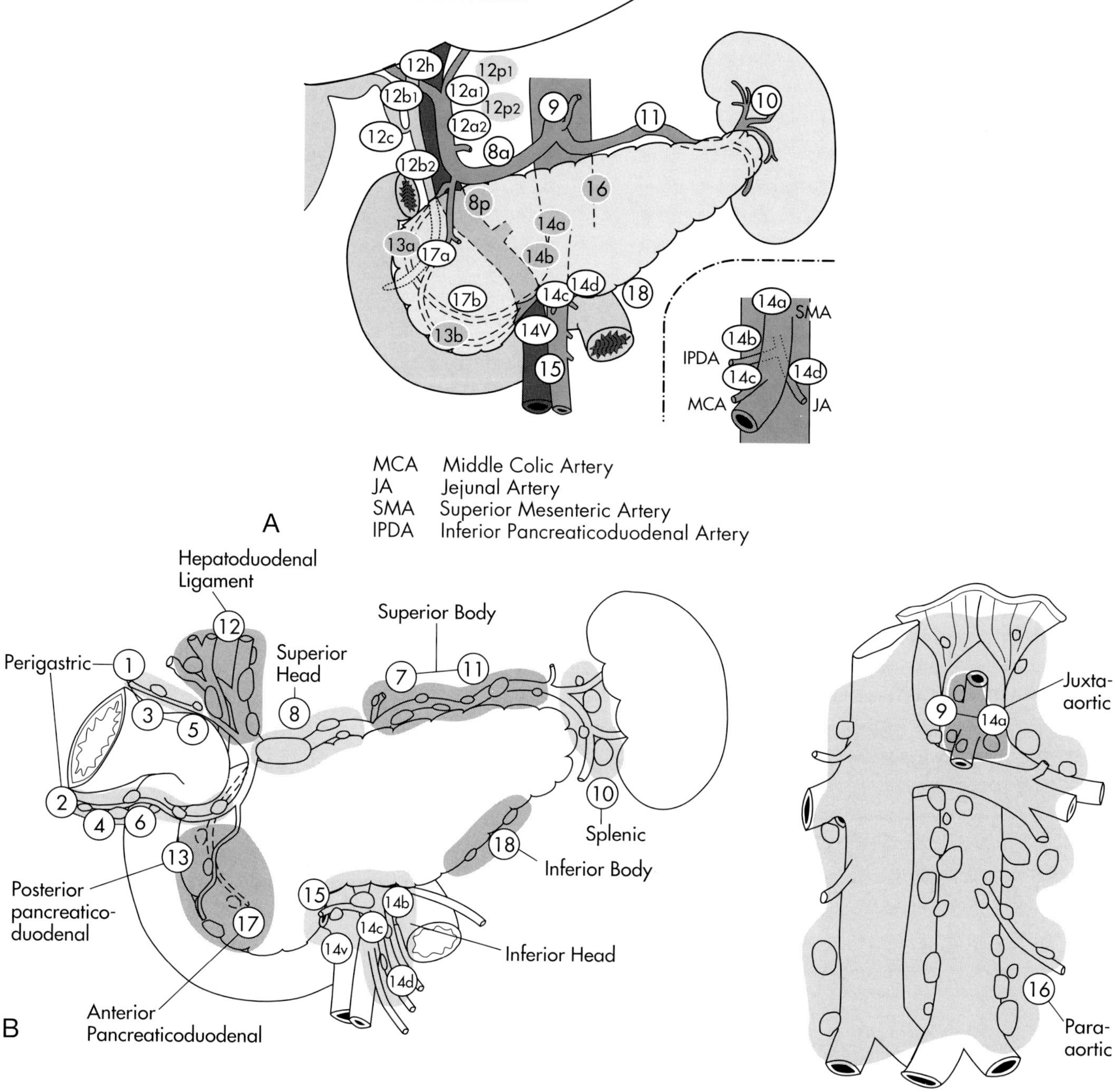


**FIG. 2.10.** Classifications of the regional lymph nodes of the pancreas. **A.** Stations and their nomenclature of the lymph nodes proposed by the Japan Pancreas Society. Lymph node stations: *1,* right cardial lymph nodes; *2,* left cardial lymph nodes; *3,* lymph nodes along the lesser curvature of the stomach; *4,* lymph nodes along the greater curvature of the stomach; *5,* suprapyloric lymph nodes; *6,* infrapyloric lymph nodes; *7,* lymph nodes along the left gastric artery; *8,* lymph nodes along the common hepatic artery; *8a,* anterosuperior nodes; *8p,* posterior nodes; *9,* lymph nodes around the celiac artery; *10,* lymph nodes at the splenic hilum; *11,* lymph nodes along the splenic artery; *12,* lymph nodes in the hepatoduodenal ligament; *12h,* lymph nodes of the hepatic hilum (porta hepatis); *12a,* lymph nodes along the hepatic artery; $12a_1$, superior nodes; $12a_2$, inferior nodes; *12p,* lymph nodes posterior to the portal vein; $12p_1$, superior nodes; $12p_2$, inferior nodes; *12b,* lymph nodes along the bile duct; $12b_1$, superior nodes; $12b_2$, inferior nodes; *12c,* lymph nodes around the cystic duct; *13,* lymph nodes on the posterior surface of the head of the pancreas; *13a,* superior nodes; *13b,* inferior nodes; *14,* lymph nodes at the root of the mesentery; *14A,* lymph nodes along the superior mesenteric artery; *14a,* lymph nodes at the origin of the superior mesenteric artery; *14b,* lymph nodes at the origin of the inferior pancreaticoduodenal artery; *14c,* lymph nodes at the origin of the middle colic artery; *14d,* lymph nodes along the first jejunal branch; *14V,* lymph nodes along the superior mesenteric vein; *15,* lymph nodes along the middle colic vessels; *16,* lymph nodes around the abdominal aorta; $16a_1$, lymph nodes around the aortic hiatus of the diaphragm; $16a_2$, lymph nodes around the abdominal aorta (from the superior margin of the celiac trunk to the inferior margin of the left renal vein); $16b_1$, lymph nodes around the abdominal aorta (from the inferior margin of the left renal vein to the superior margin of the inferior mesenteric artery); $16b_2$, lymph nodes around the abdominal aorta (from the superior margin of the inferior mesenteric artery to the aortic bifurcation); *17,* lymph nodes on the anterior surface of the head of the pancreas; *17a,* superior nodes; *17b,* inferior nodes; *18,* lymph nodes along the inferior margin of the body and tail of the pancreas. **B.** The authors' simplified version of the Japan Pancreas Society's classification. The numbers indicate the lymph node station numbers proposed by the Japan Pancreas Society. (With permission from Nagai H, Kuroda A, Morioka Y. Lymphatic and local spread of T1 and T2 pancreatic cancer: a study of autopsy material. Ann Surg 1986;204:65–71.)

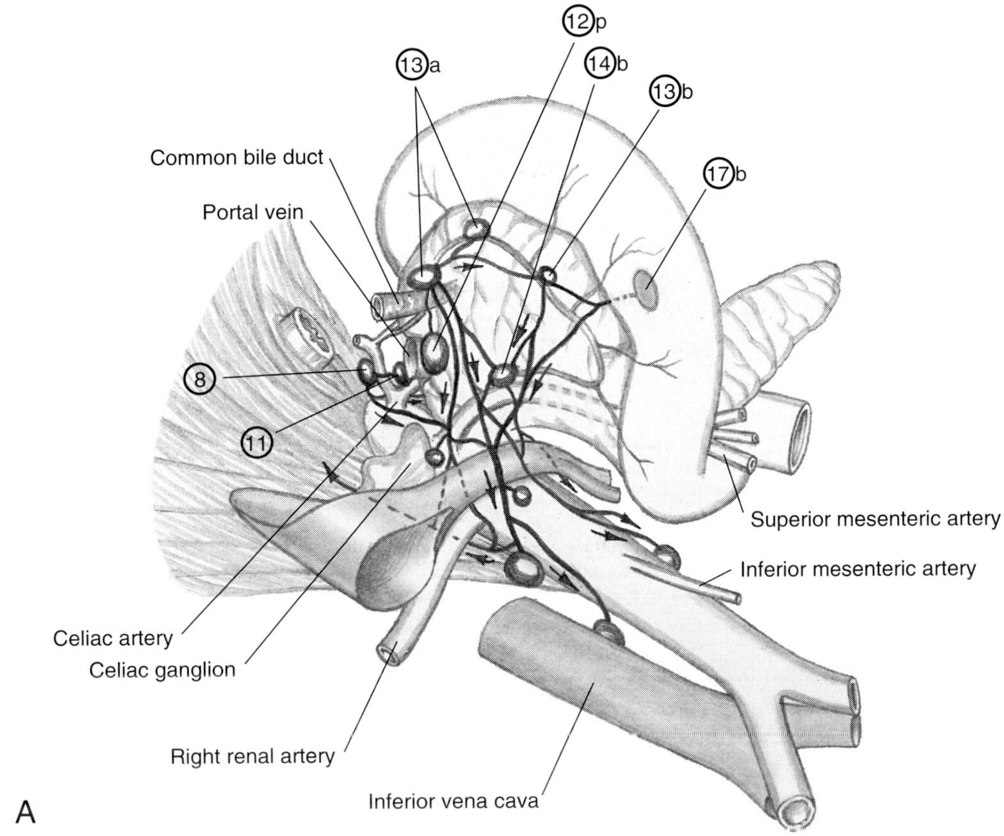


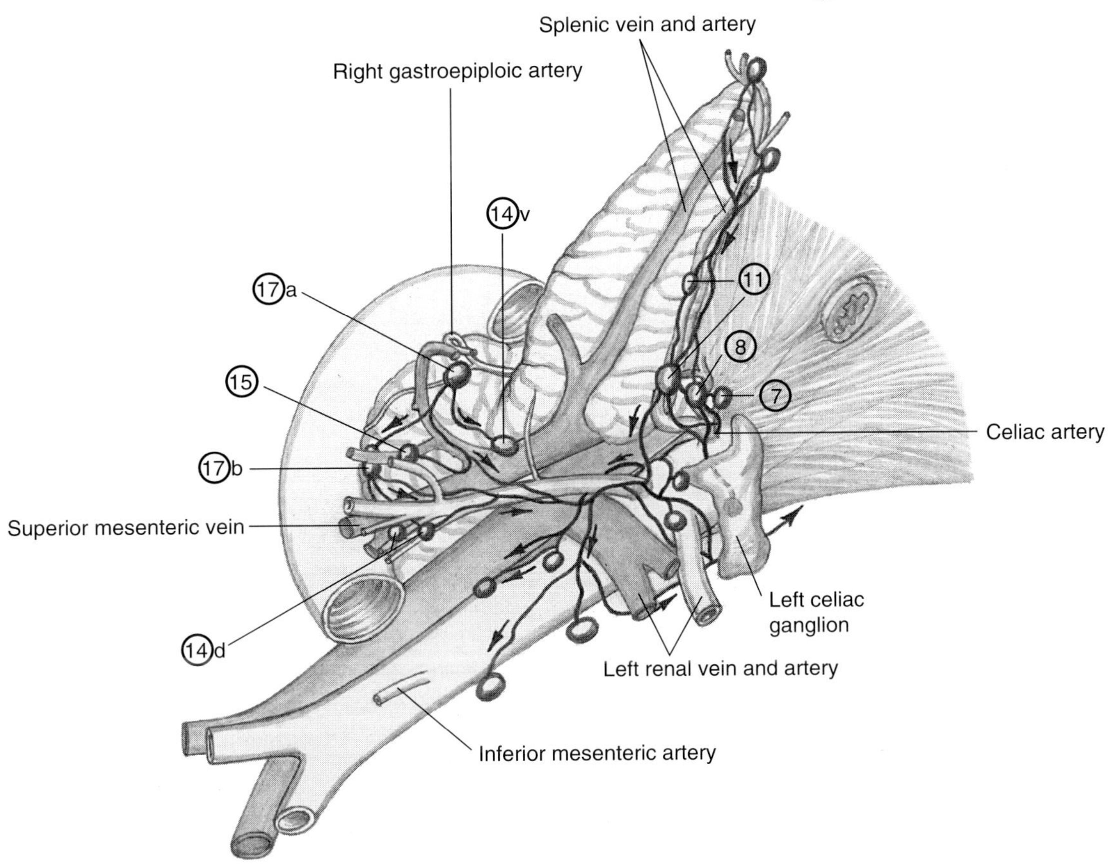


**FIG. 2.11.** Lymphatic drainage from the pancreas. The numbers indicate the numerical grouping of the peripancreatic nodes proposed by the Japan Pancreas Society. **A.** Drainage from the posterior aspect of the pancreatic head. **B.** Lymph flow from the anterior surface of the pancreatic head and from the body and tail of the pancreas. (With permission from Nagai H. An anatomical and pathological study of autopsy material on metastasis of pancreatic cancer to para-aortic lymph nodes (in Japanese). J Jpn Surg Soc (Nihon Geka Gakkai Zasshi) 1987;88:308–317.)

The anterior superior pancreaticoduodenal vein terminates in the superior mesenteric vein via the gastrocolic trunk, a vessel formed by the confluence of the right gastroepiploic and colic veins.

The body and tail of the pancreas are drained by the splenic vein above and the transverse pancreatic vein below. The splenic vein receives 3–13 short pancreatic venous branches. The transverse pancreatic vein terminates in the superior mesenteric vein, or occasionally, the splenic vein or the gastrocolic trunk.

## LYMPHATIC ANATOMY

The intralobular tissue of the pancreas is devoid of lymphatics, and lymph capillaries of the gland arise in the interlobular tissue. Lymph capillaries are collected by anastomosing networks to form large lymph ducts that reach the surface of the pancreas, usually along blood vessels.

The lymphatics from the pancreas empty into the regional lymph nodes. Various classifications of the regional nodes of the pancreas have been proposed by several authors. The Japan Pancreas Society's classification and its simplified version by the authors are shown in Figure 2.10, *A* and *B* (4, 18).

**Lymph Drainage from the Head of the Pancreas (Fig. 2.11).** The main lymphatic flow from the head of the pancreas reaches the anterior *(17)* and posterior *(13)* pancreaticoduodenal nodes. Some lymphatics from the head of the pancreas skip the pancreaticoduodenal nodes to flow directly into the inferior head *(14b, c, d, v)*, juxtaaortic *(9, 14a)*, or paraaortic nodes *(16)*.

The efferent lmphatics from the anterior pancreaticoduodenal nodes *(17)* reach the inferior head *(14b, c, d, v)* lymph nodes or flow directly into the intestinal lymph trunks that terminate in the juxtaaortic *(9, 14a)* and paraaortic *(16)* nodes. Most of the efferent lymphatics from the posterior pancreaticoduodenal nodes course down toward the juxtaaortic *(9, 14a)* and paraaortic *(16)* nodes.

The paraaortic lymph nodes *(16)* receiving the direct or indirect lymphatic flow from the pancreas are mainly located on the bilateral and anterior aspects of the aorta, ranging from the celiac axis to the origin of the inferior mesenteric artery (21, 22). Some of the lymphatics from the pancreas flow directly into the following collecting lymphatic trunks: lumbar lymphatic trunks, cisterna chyli, and thoracic duct.

### Lymph Drainage from the Body and Tail of the Pancreas (Fig. 2.11)

Most lymphatics from the body and tail of the pancreas empty into the splenic *(10)* and superior body *(11)* lymph nodes. Some lymphatics flow into the inferior head *(14b, c, d, v)*, inferior body *(18)*, juxtaaortic *(9, 14a)*, or paraaortic nodes *(16)*.

Efferent lymphatics from the splenic *(10)*, superior body *(11)*, inferior body *(18)*, and inferior head *(14b, c, d, v)* nodes proceed to the juxtaaortic *(9, 14a)* and paraaortic *(16)* nodes (21, 23).

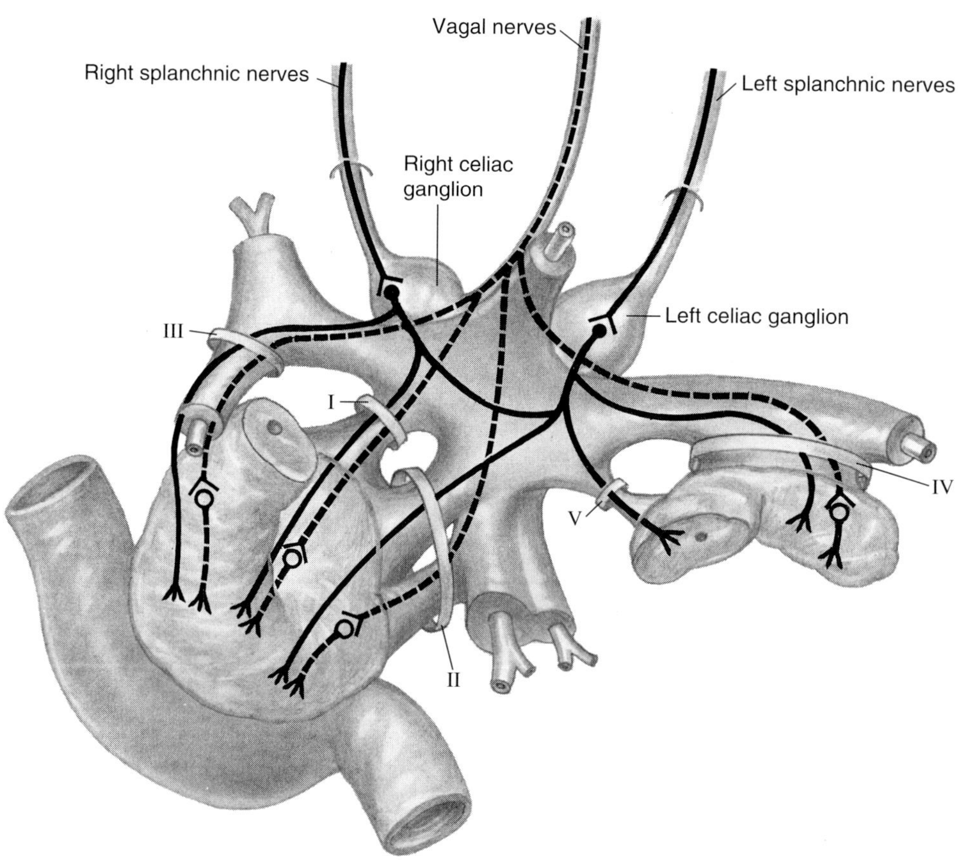


**FIG. 2.12.** The anatomy of the nerves of the pancreas. Only efferent fibers are shown. *I*, plexus pancreaticus capitalis I; *II*, plexus pancreaticus capitalis II; *III*, plexus along the gastroduodenal artery; *IV*, plexus from around the splenic artery; *V*, plexus from the left celiac ganglion and the celiac plexus. (With permission from Kuroda A, Nagai H. Gross anatomy of the pancreas. In: Pour PM, Konishi G, Kloppel G, Longnecker DS, eds. Atlas of exocrine pancreatic tumors: morphology, biology, and diagnosis with an international guide for tumor classification. Tokyo: Springer-Verlag, 1994:1–15.)

## ANATOMY OF THE NERVES

Like other abdominal organs, the pancreas is innervated by sympathetic and parasympathetic nerves. The sympathetic nerves of the pancreas mainly originate from the greater and lesser splanchnic nerves. The greater splanchnic nerve is usually formed by branches from T4-T10 sympathetic ganglia, and the lesser splanchnic nerve consists of the nerve fibers from T9-L2 sympathetic ganglia. The splanchnic nerves pass through the diaphragmatic crura to enter the celiac plexus and ganglia, and make synaptic connections with neurons in the ganglia.

The parasympathetic innervation of the pancreas originates from the vagus nerve. Although most of the vagal nerve fibers related to the pancreas pass through the celiac ganglia without synapsing, some reach the pancreas directly via the hepatic and gastric rami of the vagus nerve.

The main routes of both the sympathetic and parasympathetic nerves from the celiac plexus and ganglia to the pancreas are as follows:

1. The direct route from the celiac ganglion to the posterior surface of the head of the pancreas ("plexus pancreaticus capitalis I") (23) (Fig. 2.12)
2. The route from the bilateral celiac ganglion to the left margin of the uncinate process via the plexus around the superior mesenteric artery ("plexus pancreaticus capitalis II") (24) (Fig. 2.12)
3. The route from the plexus around the common hepatic artery to the anterior region of the head of the pancreas, coursing along the gastroduodenal artery and its tributaries
4. The route from the left celiac ganglia to the body and tail of the pancreas via the plexus around the splenic artery and its tributaries
5. The direct route from the left celiac ganglion and the celiac plexus to the posterior region of the pancreatic body

Via these routes, numerous extrinsic nerve fibers enter the gland through the capsule, often following the course of the vascular supply.

The postganglionic sympathetic fibers directly innervate blood vessels and islets, while the parasympathetic fibers terminate in intrapancreatic ganglia, and the postganglionic fibers are distributed to acini and ducts. In addition, the pancreas is richly innervated by intrinsic peptidergic nerves (25).

The nerve plexuses of the pancreas, especially the plexus pancreaticus capitalis I and II, serve as the main routes of perineural extrapancreatic spread of cancer of the head (20, 26).

## REFERENCES


1. Cubilla LA, Fitzgerald PJ. Tumors of the exocrine pancreas: gross anatomy. In: Hartmann WH, Sobin LH, eds. Atlas of tumor pathology, 2nd series. Fascicle 19. Washington, DC: Armed Forces Institute of Pathology.
2. Quinlan RM. Anatomy and embryology of the pancreas. In: Zuidema GD, ed. Shackelford's surgery of the alimentary tract, vol III. 3rd ed. Philadelphia: WB Saunders, 1991:3–18.
3. Friedman AC, Birns MT. The pancreas: embryology, anatomy, histology, and physiology. In: Friedman AC, ed. Radiology of the liver, biliary tract, pancreas, and spleen. Baltimore: Williams & Wilkins, 1987:619–642.
4. Japan Pancreas Society. Japanese classification of pancreatic carcinoma: the first English edition. Tokyo: Kanehara, 1996.
5. Kimura W, Nagai H. Study of surgical anatomy for duodenum-preserving resection of the head of the pancreas. Ann Surg 1995;221:359–363.
6. Smanio T. Varying relations of the common bile duct with the posterior face of the pancreatic head in Negroes and white persons. J Int Coll Surg 1954;22:150–172.
7. Tobin CE. The renal fascia and its relation to the transversalis fascia. Anat Rec 1944;89:295–311.
8. Meyers MA. Acute extraperitoneal infection. Semin Roentgenol 1973;8:445–464.
9. Freeny PC, Lawson TL. Radiology of the pancreas. Berlin: Springer-Verlag, 1982.
10. Kuroda A, Nagai H. Gross anatomy of the pancreas. In: Pour PM, Konishi G, Kloppel G, Longnecker DS, eds. Atlas of exocrine pancreatic tumors. Morphology, biology, and diagnosis with an international guide for tumor classification. Tokyo: Springer-Verlag, 1994:1–15.
11. Skandalakis JE, Gray SW, Skandalakis LJ. Surgical anatomy of the pancreas. In: Howard JM, Jordan JR, Reber HA, eds. Surgical diseases of the pancreas. Philadelphia: Lea & Febiger, 1987: 11–36.
12. Gray SW, Skandalakis JE, Skandalakis LJ. Embryology and congenital anomalies of the pancreas. In: Howard JM, Jordan JR, Reber HA, eds. Surgical diseases of the pancreas. Philadelphia: Lea & Febiger, 1987:37–45.
13. Ansel HJ. The normal pancreatic duct. In: Silvis SE, Rohrmann CA Jr, Ansel HJ, eds. Text and atlas of endoscopic retrograde cholangio-pancreatography. Tokyo: Igaku-Shoin, 1995:311–335.
14. Nebesar RA, Kornblith PL, Pollard JJ, Michels NA. Celiac and superior mesenteric arteries: a correlation of angiograms and dissections. Boston: Little, Brown, and Co., 1969.
15. Takada T, Yasuda K, Uchiyama K, Hasegawa H. Duodenum-preserving pancreatoduodenectomy: a new technique for complete excision of the head of the pancreas with preservation of biliary and alimentary integrity. Hepatogastroenterology 1993;40: 356–359
16. Nagai H, Ohki J, Kondo Y, et al. Duodenal-sparing resection of the pancreatic head with preservation of duodenal vascular arcades (in Japanese). Geka (Surgery) 1995;57:816–825.
17. Bertelli E, Di Gregorio F, Bertelli L, et al. The arterial blood supply of the pancreas: a review. I. The superior pancreaticoduodenal and the anterior pancreaticoduodenal arteries: an anatomical and radiological study. Surg Radiol Anat 1995;17:97–106.
18. Trede M. Embryology and surgical anatomy of the pancreas. In: Trede M, Carter DC, eds. Surgery of the pancreas. Edinburgh: Churchill Livingstone, 1993:17–27.
19. Marzoli GP, Vesentini S, Mangiante G. Elements of surgical anatomy of the pancreas. In: Scuro LA, Dragradi A, eds. Topics in acute and chronic pancreatitis. Berlin: Springer-Verlag, 1981: 11–22.
20. Nagai H, Kuroda A, Morioka Y. Lymphatic and local spread of T1 and T2 pancreatic cancer: a study of autopsy material. Ann Surg 1986;204:65–71.
21. Nagai H. An anatomical and pathological study of autopsy material on metastasis of pancreatic cancer to para-aortic lymph nodes (in Japanese). J Jpn Surg Soc (Nihon Geka Gakkai Zasshi) 1987;88:308–317.
22. Nagakawa T, Kobayashi H, Ueno K, et al. Clinical study of lymphatic flow to the paraaortic lymph nodes in carcinoma of the head of the pancreas. Cancer 1994;73:1155–1162.
23. Donatini B, Hidden G. Routes of lymphatic drainage from the pancreas: a suggested segmentation. Surg Radiol Anat 1992;14: 35–42.
24. Yoshioka H, Wakabayashi T. The pancreatic neurotomy on the head of the pancreas for relief of pain due to chronic pancreatitis: a new technical procedure and its results. Arch Surg 1958;76:546–554.
25. Holst JJ. Neural regulation of pancreatic exocrine function. In: Go VLW, Gardner JD, Brooks FP, Lebenthal E, DiMagno EP, Scheele GA, eds. The exocrine pancreas: biology, pathology and diseases. New York: Raven, 1986:287–300.
26. Nagakawa T, Mori K, Kayahara M, et al. Three-dimensional studies on the structure of the tissue surrounding the superior mesenteric artery. Int J Pancreatol 1994;15:129–138.

# 3

# Physiologic Basis for the Surgical Management of the Exocrine Pancreas

Lawrence Rosenberg

The objective of this chapter is to provide the reader with the physiologic background that is required to understand and manage diseases of the exocrine pancreas. The discussion does not address issues related to the endocrine pancreas because this subject is dealt with elsewhere.

The chapter first reviews the basic physiology of the exocrine pancreas to provide the framework for understanding the pathophysiology of disease. These physiologic principles are then applied to a number of selected clinical situations to demonstrate that an understanding of basic physiology can be used to design strategies for the management of patients with pancreatic disease.

The pancreas is divided both functionally and structurally into an exocrine portion (acinar and duct cells) and an endocrine portion (the islets of Langerhans). The exocrine component secretes into the intestine a pancreatic juice that is the product of two distinct types of secretory process: enzyme secretion and electrolyte secretion. Pancreatic enzymes constitute the most significant mechanism for food digestion. They are secreted by a complex process involving synthesis, intracellular transport, modification, condensation and eventual discharge by exocytosis. In the intestine, the initially inactive enzymes are converted to their active form in a cascade fashion. Enterokinase present on the intestinal brush border converts trypsinogen to trypsin, which in turn activates most of the remaining pancreatic enzymes (proteases, lipases, phospholipases, and others). Amylase does not require activation and is secreted in an enzymatically active form.

By contrast, the process of electrolyte secretion involves the selective, coordinated transport of ions across the basolateral and apical membranes of the secretory cells, which, because of the osmotic imbalance created, are followed by water in isotonic proportions. The bicarbonate neutralizes gastric acid and maintains the intraluminal pH above 6.0 in all but the most proximal 15 cm of small intestine. Maintaining the pH above this level is important for three reasons: *(a)* it prevents damage of the duodenal mucosa by gastric acid and pepsin, *(b)* it provides an optimal biochemical environment for the action of pancreatic and brush border digestive enzymes, and *(c)* it is required to keep certain bile salts in a soluble, dissociated form.

The normal pancreas is rather robust; it has a large reserve of exocrine capacity. Malabsorption of fat or protein does not usually occur until exocrine secretion is reduced to less than 10% of normal. This degree of major impairment requires the destruction of most of the exocrine pancreas, as typically occurs late in the clinical course of chronic pancreatitis.

## BASIC PHYSIOLOGY OF THE EXOCRINE PANCREAS

### Anatomic and Functional Basis for Secretion

While pancreatic secretion is a function of the synthetic and transport functions of acinar and ductular cells, these processes are ultimately dependent on and influenced by an adequate blood supply and innervation. Therefore, before examining the mechanisms and control of pancreatic secretion, the functional and anatomic bases for secretion are briefly reviewed.

**Blood Supply.** The pancreas receives its blood supply from branches of both the celiac and superior mesenteric arteries. Once these have penetrated the substance of the pancreas, the vessels anastomose freely, forming an interconnected network that renders the pancreas relatively resistant to ischemia.

At the microvascular level, the blood supply to the islets and acinar tissue is in the form of a portal system. While arterioles supply both the islets and the exocrine elements, the capillary system of the islets enters into vessels that also supply the exocrine tissue (1–3). Approximately 10–25% of total pancreatic blood goes to the islets (4); therefore, these cells, which constitute 1–2% of the pancreatic mass (5), are perfused at 10–20 times the rate of exocrine tissue. The physiologic significance of this vascular organization lies in the potential effects of high concentrations of islet hormones on exocrine pancreatic function (6, 7).

The factors that regulate pancreatic blood flow have been reviewed by Solomon (8). Intestinal perfusion with hydrochloric acid (HCl) increases pancreatic bicarbonate secretion, but only large amounts of HCl will cause a concomitant increase in pancreatic blood flow (9). The effects of protein and fat and their digestion products have not been studied. Under certain conditions, various hormones and neurotransmitters also influence pancreatic blood flow. Secretin (10), vasoactive intestinal polypeptide (VIP) (11), glucagon (12), cholecystokinin (CCK) or its analogues (13), α- and β-adrenergic agonists (10, 14), low-dose dopamine (15), cortisone (10), histamine, vagal stimulation and acetylcholine (16), and prostaglandins (12) have been reported to increase flow. Conflicting results, however, have been obtained in other studies (14–16). The physiologic importance of these multiple agents, as well as their mechanism of action on blood flow, remain to be more fully characterized.

The two major hormonal stimulants of pancreatic enzyme secretion, CCK and secretin, when administered by continuous intravenous infusion, stimulate pancreatic secretion but have no or only transient effects on pancreatic blood flow (9, 17). Even when given by bolus injection, secretin stimulates pancreatic bicarbonate secretion at doses far lower than those required to increase blood flow (18). Therefore, in his review of pancreatic blood flow, Solomon (8) concluded there was no evidence that pancreatic blood flow increases in response to stimulation of secretion. This implies that exocrine pancreatic secretion is not blood flow–limited under normal conditions.

**Neuroanatomy and Physiology.** The pancreas receives its extrinsic innervation from branches of the vagus and splanchnic nerves that carry both efferent secretory and vasomotor fibers and afferent sensory fibers. The intrinsic innervation of the pancreas, the nerve fibers in the substance of the gland, consists of postganglionic adrenergic fibers, pre- and postganglionic cholinergic fibers, and their associated ganglia, peptidergic neurons, and sensory (afferent) fibers.

The noradrenaline-secreting adrenergic nerve fibers innervate primarily the pancreatic vasculature (19), with some innervation of the islets. These fibers do not appear to contribute to the innervation of the exocrine tissue.

The acetylcholine-secreting postganglionic cholinergic fibers supply both acinar and islet cells (20). There are also peptidergic fibers in the pancreas that contain VIP, calcitonin gene–related peptide (CGRP), substance P, enkephalins, and bombesin-like peptides (21–23) as well as dopamine- and serotonin-containing fibers (24, 25). Their target tissues and specific functions are unknown, and their roles in the regulation of exocrine pancreatic secretion are presently being elucidated.

There are no specialized efferent nerve endings in the pancreas (8). Instead, efferent nerve fibers secrete their transmitters along the length of their axons. The transmitters then diffuse to target cells as a form of paracrine interaction. Acetylcholine released by cholinergic postganglionic fibers directly stimulates digestive enzyme secretion by acinar cells, acts synergistically with secretin on fluid and bicarbonate secretion by duct cells, and modulates islet hormone secretion in response to a meal by stimulating the release of pancreatic polypeptide (PP). Adrenergic postganglionic fibers release noradrenaline, which acts to decrease blood flow by producing arteriolar constriction and decreases secretion rates of digestive enzymes, fluid, and bicarbonate.

**Structure-Function Correlates.** The exocrine cells of the pancreas constitute about 85% of the mass of the gland (5), with the vast majority being acinar cells. Ductal epithelium comprises only about 11% of the gland by volume.

The pancreas is classically described as a compound acinar gland, with acini being terminal elements. Their enzymes are secreted into terminal ductules, which drain into larger and larger intralobular and interlobular ducts (26). This concept has been challenged in recent years by Bockman et al. (27), who have postulated the existence of multiple interconnecting small ducts composed of acinar cells. This new concept is based on three-dimensional reconstructions that indicate a syncytial network of ducts whose walls contain specialized areas with acinar cells.

Acinar cells are arranged in acini, spheroid clusters of 15–20 or more pyramidal cells oriented with their apical membranes abutting a common lumen (28). Each acinar cell is equipped with the ultrastructural elements associated with high rates of protein synthesis, processing, storage, and secretion—an abundant rough endoplasmic reticulum, transitional vesicles, a well developed Golgi apparatus, and apically located zymogen granules. Duct cells appear to be far less specialized, being typical cuboidal or columnar secretory epithelial cells (28).

## Composition of Exocrine Pancreatic Secretions

Pancreatic juice is a mixture of two distinctly different fluids. One of these is a high-volume solution of sodium bicarbonate. The other is a solution of sodium chloride that contains high concentrations of digestive enzymes and other substances. The composite solution is an alkaline, enzyme-rich juice that serves to neutralize gastric acid and digest food.

**Water and Electrolytes.** Humans secrete pancreatic juice with a maximal bicarbonate concentration of 130–150 mM, and the concentrations of bicarbonate and the other major anion, chloride, depend on flow rate (29) and are a function of two separate processes. One process is the admixture of two fluids, one high in bicarbonate (from duct cells), the other low (from acinar cells), which are secreted at varying rates (Fig. 3.1). The other process is the passive diffusion of bicarbonate from the duct lumen to the interstitial space, with chloride diffusing in the opposite direction to maintain electrochemical neutrality (Fig. 3.2). This process is flow rate–dependent; the slower the rate of flow, the greater is the time of contact between duct fluid and interstitial fluid through the diffusional barrier of the duct cells. At a slow rate, most of the bicarbonate present above its concentration in the interstitial space diffuses out of the duct system and is replaced by chloride. As flow rates increase, a smaller proportion of bicarbonate is lost, until at high flow rates, the proportion of bicarbonate lost by diffusion is low.

At basal levels of flow, bicarbonate concentration is low (30–60 mM), while chloride concentration is high (Fig. 3.2). As the flow rate increases, bicarbonate concentration increases until it reaches maximum value at about half the maximal rate of flow. Chloride concentration decreases, so that the sum of bicarbonate and chloride concentrations is a constant value. The maximal flow rate in humans is about 4–5 mL/min. Interestingly, Solomon points out that the bicarbonate output (moles/unit time) increases exponentially with flow to reach a value about equal to the maximal rate of $H^+$ output in humans (8).

The major cations in pancreatic juice, sodium and potassium, are present in concentrations that approximate those in plasma; neither one shows a change in concentration as a function of the flow rate of pancreatic juice. Other ionic constituents are present, but in very low concentrations.

**Digestive Enzymes.** Pancreatic acinar cells synthesize and secrete at least 10 different hydrolases, which are the major enzymes responsible for intraluminal digestion of macronutrients to forms that can be absorbed. Several of the hydrolases have two or more isozymes (enzymes with minor structural differences but similar actions), and with the two other peptide secretory products—(pro)colipase and trypsin inhibitor—the total number of secretory products in pancreatic juice is more than 20 (Table 3.1).

Digestive enzymes are either proteases, lipases, amylases, or nucleases. Proteases represent approximately 70% of the total digestive enzyme pool in humans (30). Amylase and lipase, the other major enzymes, are present in small amounts, but they all have very high enzymatic activities (30).

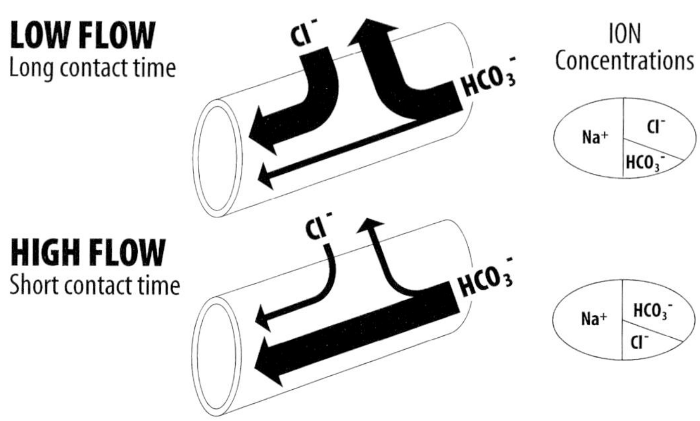


**FIG. 3.1.** Concentrations of anions in pancreatic juice are a function of the flow rate (process I). Back-diffusion of bicarbonate is time dependent.

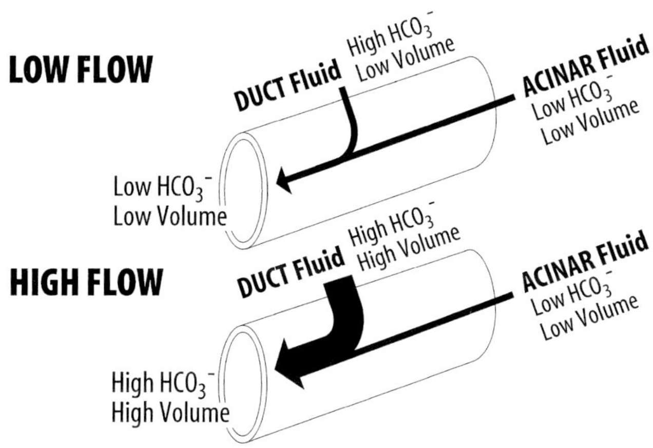


**FIG. 3.2.** Concentrations of anions in pancreatic juice are a function of the flow rate (process II). Admixture of two fluids with different concentrations of bicarbonate.

**TABLE 3.1. Human Pancreatic Enzymes and Proenzymes**

| |
|---|
| Proteolytic enzymes |
| Trypsinogen 1 |
| Trypsinogen 2 |
| Trypsinogen 3 |
| (Pro)carboxypeptidase A |
| (Pro)carboxypeptidase B |
| (Pro)elastase 2 |
| (Pro)protease E |
| Kallikreinogen |
| Amylolytic enzyme |
| Amylase |
| Lipolytic enzymes |
| Lipase |
| (Pro)phospholipase $A_2$ |
| (Pro)colipase I, II |
| Carboxyl ester hydrolase |
| Nucleases |
| Deoxyribonuclease I |
| Ribonuclease |
| Others |
| Secretory trypsin inhibitor |

Besides their function in normal digestion, pancreatic enzymes have been implicated in the pathophysiology of human disease. Intrapancreatic protease activation appears to play an important role in the initiation of acute pancreatitis, and the activities of lipase and phospholipase may contribute to the systemic complications seen in the more severe form of the disease.

Several digestive enzymes are potentially damaging to pancreatic cell membranes. However, these enzymes are synthesized and secreted as inactive precursor forms, or zymogens. Zymogens require activation in the intestinal lumen before they become enzymatically active (Fig. 3.3).

Trypsinogen, the precursor form of trypsin, is activated by the brush border enzyme enterokinase in the small intestine (Fig. 3.3). Trypsin can also catalyze the activation of trypsinogen, but this is much slower than activation by enterokinase. All other zymogens can be activated only by trypsin (Fig. 3.4), making it a central enzyme that controls the activity of all other enzymes.

Why doesn't the pancreas digest itself? All digestive enzymes are segregated from the cytoplasm of the acinar cell within membranes. Those enzymes that can digest membranes are synthesized and secreted as inactive zymogens, and the activation of these zymogens normally occurs only after they have been secreted into the intestine (Figs. 3.3 and 3.4). The acinar cell also synthesizes a trypsin inhibitor that blocks any trypsin that is inadvertently present in the acinar cell. When these protective mechanisms fail, acute pancreatitis may result.

If reflux of duodenal contents into the pancreatic duct occurs, it is possible that the colocalization of enterokinase and trypsin in the ductal system may also lead to the intrapancreatic activation of trypsinogen and other zymogens. In addition, trypsinogen may autocatalyze its own activation in the pancreas, although this is a very slow process. Finally, the lysosomal acid hydrolase, cathepsin $B_1$, can also convert trypsinogen to trypsin. Colocalization of trypsinogen and cathepsin $B_1$ is thought to be an early event in the initiation of acute pancreatitis.

**Mucin.** Goblet cells are present in appreciable numbers in the main and interlobular ducts of the exocrine pancreas and in glands in the periductal stroma (31–34). Mucins have been purified from human pancreatic juice and appear to be similar in biochemical characteristics to intestinal mucins (35). It has been suggested that pancreatic mucins form a protective barrier against backflux of bicarbonate ions and degradation of the duct epithelium by digestive enzymes (36), but these suppositions remain to be tested.

## Mechanisms of Secretion

**Water and Electrolytes.** Recent interest in pancreatic duct secretory mechanisms has been sparked by the recognition that the duct system is intimately involved in several pathologic disturbances of pancreatic function including those associated with pancreatitis, cystic fibrosis, and pancreatic neoplasms. Therefore, it is important to review the basic physiology of duct cell function, as this helps to provide some insight into the pathophysiology of the pancreatic duct system and hence a framework for planning intervention strategies.

The secretion of the bicarbonate-poor fluid of the acinar cell and the bicarbonate-rich fluid of the duct cell appears to be the result of two different cellular mechanisms. Fluid secretion by acinar cells is strongly dependent on extracellular $Ca^{2+}$, whereas duct cell secretion is not (37). Duct cell secretion is strictly dependent on the presence of bicarbonate or other weak acid conjugates, whereas acinar secretion is not (37, 38). Finally, duct cell secretion requires the active transport of bicarbonate (or $H^+$ or $OH^-$), but acinar secretion does not.

What is the cellular mechanism by which bicarbonate secretion occurs? Current evidence suggests that the secretion of bicarbonate by duct cells is an active, energy-requiring (Fig. 3.5) process, because bicarbonate is secreted against both concentration and electrochemical gradients (26, 39). This is borne out by the demonstration that specific inhibitors of Na,K-ATPase (40), which is located predominantly in the basolateral region of the duct cell (41), decrease pancreatic bicarbonate secretion. Pan-

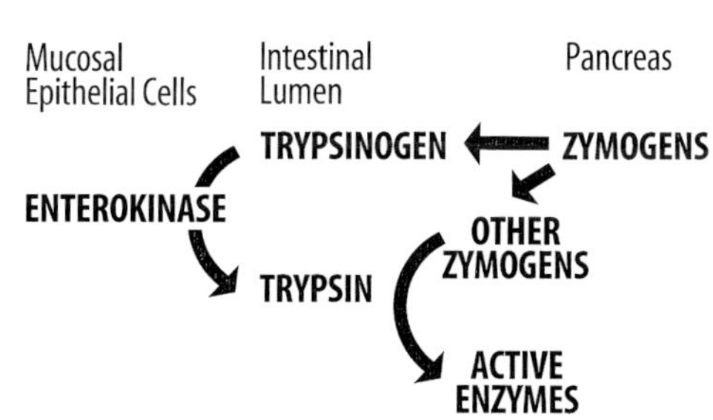


**FIG. 3.3.** Pancreatic enzyme activation begins in the intestine with the activation of trypsinogen by the brush border enzyme enterokinase.

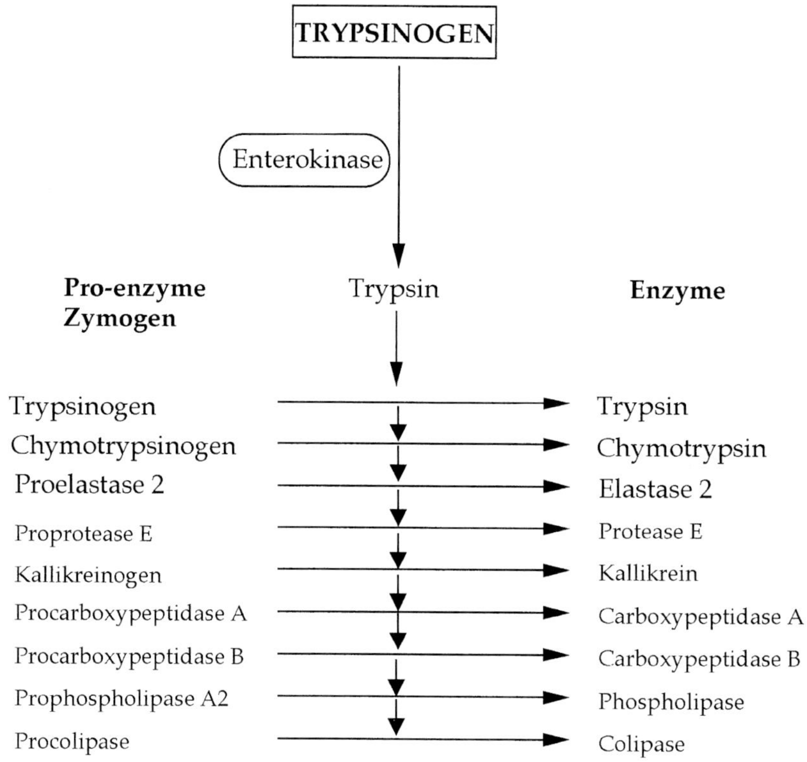


**FIG. 3.4.** The cascade of pancreatic zymogen activation by trypsin.

creatic bicarbonate secretion is also decreased by specific inhibitors of carbonic anhydrase (42), which has been localized to duct cells, although the exact location—cytoplasm or luminal or basolateral membrane—remains to be determined.

Secretion of a bicarbonate-rich fluid by the duct cell may occur in two possible ways: active transport of $HCO_3^-$ (or $OH^-$) from intracellular space to duct lumen or active transport of $H^+$ from the intracellular or intraluminal space to the interstitial space. Regardless of the precise mechanism, however, the end result is the same. These mechanisms of secretion have been examined by Solomon (8). In the active $HCO_3^-$ transport model, carbonic anhydrase acts intracellularly to catalyze the formation of carbonic acid from $CO_2$ and $H_2O$; most of the $CO_2$ that forms $HCO_3^-$ comes from plasma and not duct cell metabolism (38). Carbonic acid dissociates rapidly into $HCO_3^-$ and $H^+$. $HCO_3^-$ is then assumed to be transported across the apical (i.e., luminal) membrane of the duct cell. In the second model, $H^+$ is transported either from the intraluminal space to the duct cell or from the duct cell to the interstitial space. The $H^+$ comes from carbonic acid, the production of which is catalyzed by carbonic anhydrase. In this model, the energy required for active transport of $H^+$ is assumed to come from coupling to the Na,K-ATPase, with $Na^+$ moving down the gradient established by the sodium pump. The other major ions of pancreatic juice—$Cl^-$, $Na^+$, $K^+$—are presumed to diffuse passively into pancreatic juice. Thus the dependence of bicarbonate secretion on active sodium transport appears to be due to the important but general role of the sodium pump in maintaining the intracellular milieu, as well as to a possible contribution of this pump to the sodium gradient required for active $H^+$ transport (8).

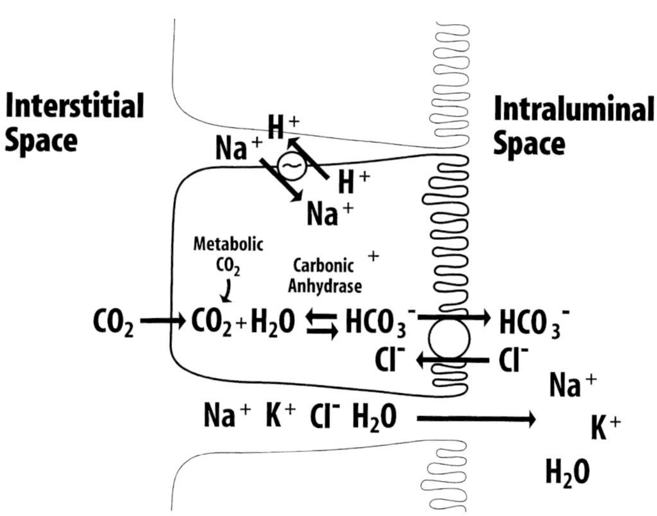


**FIG. 3.5.** The secretion of bicarbonate by duct cells is an active, energy-requiring process.

The cellular control mechanisms for fluid secretion by duct cells are still being characterized, as are the membrane receptors on duct cells. This is because, until recently, it was difficult to purify enough functionally intact duct cells from the pancreas, where they comprise a small proportion of the total cell population. While there are reports of rodent and guinea pig studies using microdissected ducts and cells dispersed by collagenase digestion, very few data are available on the function of the human duct cell.

**Mucin.** The goblet cell is a specialized pancreatic duct cell that synthesizes mucin. Very little is known of the mechanisms that regulate pancreatic mucus secretion (43). Carbachol, VIP, and bombesin, but not secretin or CCK, cause goblet cell degranulation in an in vitro guinea pig model (34). Since acetylcholine, VIP, and gastrin-releasing peptide (the mammalian analogue of bombesin) are all found in intrapancreatic nerves (44, 45), these observations implicate neural rather than hormonal regulation of duct mucus secretion. The signal transduction pathways that mediate exocytosis of mucus-containing granules in goblet cells remain to be determined.

Many questions remain about the normal regulation of pancreatic duct cell function and about the pathophysiology of disease states such as cystic fibrosis, chronic pancreatitis, and pancreatic cancer. It is clear that not all potential regulators of bicarbonate and mucus secretion have been identified. Several peptidergic neurotransmitters including VIP, substance P, enkephalins, neuropeptide Y, calcitonin–gene related peptide, and gastrin-releasing peptide have been localized histochemically to nerve terminals within the periductal connective tissue (44, 45). The intracellular mechanisms by which these candidate regulatory molecules direct duct fluid and goblet cell secretion, and their importance as modulators of duct cell function, remain to be determined. Further, Hootman indicates that virtually nothing is known of the interaction of these potential regulators at the subcellular level—how the signaling pathways that they activate interact and at what points they impinge on one another to modulate either bicarbonate or mucus secretion (43). Obviously, much work remains to be done in this area.

**Digestive Enzymes.** The synthesis, packaging, intracellular transport, and secretion of digestive enzymes by the pancreatic acinar cell is an extremely complex topic, and only an overview is offered here.

Protein synthesis begins with the active transport of amino acids into the acinar cell, a process probably linked to the movement of $Na^+$ down its electrochemical gradient (46). Digestive proteins are then synthesized on ribosomes attached to membrane-bound cisternae of the endoplasmic reticulum. Most if not all newly synthesized proteins, including the digestive enzymes, include a signal peptide at their amino-terminal end, composed of relatively lipophilic amino acids (47). This signal peptide is necessary for penetrating the cisternal membrane, after which the signal peptide is cleaved by endopeptidases. The remaining protein moiety is then transported to the Golgi complex where further processing (i.e., glycosylation, proteolytic processing) occurs (48). Finally, the processed peptides are packaged into membrane-bound zymogen granules and stored in the apical domain of the cell (48). Secretion of the enzyme contents of zymogen granules occurs by exocytosis, when fusion between the zymogen granule membrane and the apical plasma membrane of the acinar cell occurs. Prevailing evidence suggests that enzyme synthesis and intracellular transport is an extraordinarily dynamic and flexible system that responds quickly to increased demand for additional secretion (49). In addition, the rate and pattern of enzyme synthesis are modulated by CCK and acetylcholine (50).

Stimulation of secretion at the cellular level has been reviewed in detail by Solomon (8). Acinar cells from rat and guinea pig possess specific membrane receptors for CCK, acetylcholine, bombesin, substance P, secretin, and VIP, epidermal growth factor (EGF), and insulin-like growth factor-1 (IGF-1). Activation of these receptors by the appropriate regulatory molecule leads to a cascade of intracellular events that includes depolarization of plasma membrane potential, increased cytoplasmic levels of cyclic AMP and cyclic GMP, increased cytoplasmic levels of $Ca^{2+}$, breakdown of phosphatidylinositol, and phosphorylation of specific proteins; the end result is protein secretion. The two earliest events appear to be increased cyclic nucleotide and $Ca^{2+}$ levels. Both secretin and VIP increase cyclic AMP levels in acinar cells but not $Ca^{2+}$ levels, and they do not alter the effects of other stimulants on intracellular events (51). A second group of stimulants—CCK, bombesin, acetylcholine, and substance P—increases cyclic GMP and $Ca^{2+}$ levels in acinar cells. The cyclic GMP increase does not appear to be directly related to initiation of enzyme secretion (52), but the increase in intracellular $Ca^{2+}$ is an absolute requirement. Unfortunately, the receptors on the human acinar cell have not yet been fully characterized.

### Control of Pancreatic Secretion

**Secretion in the Interdigestive Period.** The secretion of pancreatic juice in the period between meals is generally quite low. Basal secretion of digestive enzymes occurs at a level that is 5–10% of the maximal enzyme secretory response to exogenous CCK (53, 54), while bicarbonate secretion is only 1 or 2% of the maximal response to secretin (53, 55). In humans, pancreatic secretion in the interdigestive period occurs in a cyclic fashion (56), but the phenomenon has been best studied in a canine model (56, 57). Enzyme and bicarbonate secretion increase every 1–2 hours, beginning several hours after the last meal, and lasts for 15–20 minutes (56, 57). While the cause of the cyclic nature of basal pancreatic secretion is unknown, available evidence suggests that a neurohumoral factor is involved. Two hormones, motilin and PP, have been implicated in the regulation of pancreatic secretion in dogs (58, 59). Motilin induces cyclic increases in secretion (59), while PP plays an inhibitory role (60). The release of the two hormones is dependent on cholinergic tone; thus, atropine blocks their cyclic increase in the circulation (59). Atropine also dramatically reduces the secretion of enzymes in the interdigestive period (61), an action that appears to be mediated by completely blocking the action of motilin on the exocrine pancreas (59).

**Pancreatic Secretion in Response to a Meal.** The primary function of the exocrine pancreas is to secrete enzymes and bicarbonate in response to a meal. Traditionally, this secretory response has been divided into three phases on the basis of the sites of action of the mediators involved.

**Cephalic Phase.** At the start of a meal, the smell, taste, chewing, and swallowing of food, without the entry of acid or chyme into the duodenum, induce significant increases in pancreatic secretion of fluid, bicarbonate, and digestive enzymes (61–65). The enzyme secretory response in humans amounts to about 50% of the maximal response to exogenous CCK (8). This phenomenon has been attributed to increased vagal tone, which results in increased intrapancreatic postganglionic cholinergic input, thereby stimulating secretion of both enzymes and bicarbonate. However, the effect of vagotomy on such pancreatic secretory responses has not been studied. These neurons in the pancreas are activated by central input during the cephalic phase and by vasovagal reflexes initiated later by the stimulation of the gastric and intestinal phases. The activation of these fibers may thus release not only a classic neurotransmitter, acetylcholine, but also neuropeptides, such as VIP (21) and gastrin-releasing peptide (GRP) (22). Peptides may coexist with nonpeptide transmitters in autonomic nerves, and activation of such fibers may thus release both acetylcholine and VIP (21). Thus, peptidergic neurons in the exocrine pancreas appear to play important roles in the regulation of the exocrine pancreas.

**Gastric Phase.** The stomach indirectly influences pancreatic secretion by determining the amount and timing of entry of pancreatic stimulants into the duodenum. Gastric distension, however, can directly stimulate pancreatic secretion, although the increases are small compared with the maximal responses to secretin or CCK (66, 67). The effect of distension does not depend on entrance of gastric acid into the duodenum (67), and the pancreatic response to gastric distension can be blocked by atropine and vagotomy.

**Intestinal Phase.** Intestinal phase mechanisms are probably responsible for most of the pancreatic response to a meal. There are three major intestinal phase stimulants of pancreatic secretion.

Peptides and amino acids in the intestine initiate pancreatic enzyme secretion (68). The maximal attainable pancreatic response to intestinal amino acids is significantly less than the maximal response to exogenous CCK (53).

Intact triglycerides in the intestinal lumen do not stimulate pancreatic secretion, in contrast to fatty acids and monoglycerides, which are strong stimulants (69–71). The maximal enzyme secretory response, in fact, can be nearly equal to that provoked by exogenous CCK (69). Fatty acids and monoglycerides also stimulate more bicarbonate secretion than do amino acids (71).

The third major intestinal phase stimulant of pancreatic secretion, gastric acid, has been reviewed by Solomon (8). In the basal state, unbuffered HCl at low pH is delivered into the duodenum; however, the load is small. A meal of mixed composition is a strong stimulant of gastric acid secretion. The protein component of the meal is a strong buffer of acid, however; therefore, the concentration of free unbuffered $H^+$ in gastric contents is lower than it would be if no buffering occurred. The pH of chyme, which is emptied during a solid meal, is still low, however, and has been measured as low as pH 2.0–2.5 (72). Acid in the intestine can itself act as a stimulant of pancreatic fluid and bicarbonate secretion, although large amounts of acid can stimulate a small enzyme secretory response.

Another characteristic of pancreatic stimulation by acid in the intestine is that there is a pH threshold for the stimulation of secretion of pancreatic bicarbonate. No matter how much acid is infused into the intestine at pH values above this threshold, no stimulation of secretion occurs. In humans, pH values below 3.0 are required to cause an increase in plasma secretin and duodenal neutralization of infused acid (73). The magnitude of the pancreatic bicarbonate response to acid is correlated with the length of proximal small bowel that is acidified (74). The intraluminal pH of the duodenum distal to the ampulla of Vater does not drop below 5.0–6.0 in either the fasting or fed state (75). Therefore, only in the first stage and proximal second stage of the duodenum is the intraluminal pH sufficiently low to stimulate pancreatic secretion. Finally, while the mucosal receptors for acid are activated at pH values below 4.5, the actual pancreatic secretory response is then determined by the number of receptors that are activated. In other words, the stimulation of pancreatic bicarbonate secretion is a function of the absolute amount of titratable acid present in the duodenum, not its pH (8).

Calcium and bile are among other factors that have been implicated in the intestinal phase of pancreatic secretion. While intestinal perfusion with calcium has been demonstrated to stimulate pancreatic enzyme secretion (76), the reported effects of bile and bile salts on secretion have been contradictory (8). Clearly, although many of the complexities of the intestinal phase of pancreatic secretion have been elaborated, more investigation is required before all the factors involved have been identified and their interactions delineated fully.

**Hormonal Regulation of Postprandial Pancreatic Secretion.** Hormones or peptides that influence pancreatic secretion include secretin (16, 77), CCK (17, 78), neurotensin (9, 79), insulin (18, 80), pancreatic polypeptide (PP) (19, 81), peptide YY (81), glucagon (20, 82), somatostatin (SMS) (21, 83), pancreastatin (22, 84), thyrotropin-releasing hormone (TRH) (23, 85), and CGRP (24, 86).

The importance of secretin and CCK in the regulation of postprandial pancreatic stimulation has been well established during the past decade (77, 78), although much of the evidence comes from studies in dogs (87, 88) and rats (89). The human evidence for the role of secretin has been summarized by Solomon (8) as follows: *(a)* fasting plasma levels of secretin are low in nonanesthetized subjects, and small but sustained increases in plasma secretin after food can be detected; *(b)* a reduction of basal or meal-induced gastric acid secretion also reduces plasma secretin levels; *(c)* the pH threshold for stimulation of pancreatic bicarbonate secretion and secretin release are identical, and the degree of secretin release is correlated with the duodenal load of $H^+$ and titratable acid; *(d)* the intravenous administration of secretin in doses that reproduce meal-induced plasma levels stimulates pancreatic bicarbonate secretion; and finally, *(e)* strong evidence for a central role of secretin in mediating postprandial pancreatic bicarbonate secretion comes from studies in which the administration of antiserum directed against secretin reduced bicarbonate secretion by more than 80% (87).

Pancreatic bicarbonate secretion in response to secretin is potentiated by vagal stimulation in cats (90), and atropine causes a profound inhibition of pancreatic bicarbonate secretion stimulated by a physiologic dose of secretin in humans (91). During the postprandial period, the interaction between secretin and intrinsic cholinergic nerve fibers may play an important role in pancreatic secretion. In humans, atropine abolished the potentiation between secretin and CCK-8 for bicarbonate secretion (92). These observations strongly suggest that the action of secretin on the exocrine pancreas depends heavily on intrinsic cholinergic input.

Uncertainty persists, however, with respect to the role played by CCK in the human pancreas. Basal plasma concentrations of CCK are low (93–95) but may be increased significantly by a meal or intraduodenal fat (94, 95). The issue that remains to be clarified, however, is whether the plasma levels of CCK measured after a meal are the cause of any part of the pancreatic secretory response.

Truncal vagotomy or the administration of atropine dramatically decreases the pancreatic bicarbonate and enzyme secretory responses to intravenous CCK-octapeptide or to intraduodenal fat, protein, and acid (92, 96–99). This has been attributed to a blockade of a classic vagovagal reflex from the intestine to the pancreas, and it suggests that cholinergic input in the pancreas is needed for the action of endogenous CCK. Receptors for acetylcholine have in fact been identified on pancreatic acinar cells, and their activation produces maximal stimulation of enzyme secretion (100). Therefore it appears that this entero-pancreatic reflex is the mediator for most of the pancreatic enzyme response to a meal.

A number of peptides inhibit pancreatic secretion stimulated by secretin and/or CCK; they are PP (81), peptide YY (81), glucagon (82), somatostatin (83), pancreastatin (84), galanin (30), TRH (85), and CGRP (86). Among them, PP (60) and somatostatin (101) are the recognized inhibitory hormones that appear to play important physiologic roles in pancreatic secretion.

**Negative Feedback Regulation.** For bicarbonate secretion, negative feedback regulation is controlled by the pH of the duodenal luminal contents. As acid enters the duodenum, pH decreases. Intestinal mechanisms initiate pancreatic bicarbonate secretion, which in turn neutralizes acid and raises the pH. This decreases the drive for bicarbonate secretion. Evidence for an inhibitory feedback mechanism regulating pancreatic enzyme secretion is far more controversial.

Diversion of pancreaticobiliary juice from the proximal intestine in the rat causes a marked increase in pancreatic enzyme secretion. Trypsin, chymotrypsin, or pancreaticobiliary juice infused into the duodenum suppresses pancreatic enzyme secretion (102). Pancreatic proteases in the upper small intestine suppress pancreatic exocrine secretion in several species, including humans, where pancreatic secretion in only the intestinal phase of pancreatic secretion is suppressed by pancreatic proteases (103, 104).

The suppressive effect of proteases on pancreatic secretion

has been attributed to the inhibition of the release of secretin and CCK, because suppression was reversed by intravenous administration of these two hormones in physiologic doses (105). Although the release of CCK has been shown to be suppressed by pancreatic proteases, it has not been determined whether the release of secretin is also subject to the same feedback regulation.

Release of CCK (106, 107) and secretin (53, 108) in rats is mediated by releasing peptides secreted from the intestinal mucosa into the duodenal lumen. These observations indicate that luminally secreted peptides signal gut endocrine cells, such as secretin and/or CCK cells, for their release into the circulation. These releasing peptides are inactivated in the upper small intestine lumen by pancreatic proteases. Thus, when the proteases are inactivated, the release of both secretin and CCK is enhanced, leading to increased pancreatic secretion of both bicarbonate and enzymes. Thus, pancreatic proteases play an important role in the negative feedback regulation of pancreatic exocrine secretion.

The issue of whether or not a similar mechanism exists in man has engendered much debate. Ihse et al. (108) reported that when bile and pancreatic flow from the duodenum was completely obstructed by a carcinoma of the ampulla of Vater, infusion of active pancreaticobiliary juice or trypsin into the duodenum caused a rapid fall in pancreatic secretion. Conversely, intraduodenal infusion of pancreatic juice treated with soybean trypsin inhibitor failed to suppress pancreatic secretion. These observations strongly suggest that feedback regulation of pancreatic enzyme secretion occurs in man. Finally, Owyang et al. (103) demonstrated that intraduodenal infusion of trypsin inhibited phenyalanine-stimulated pancreatic enzyme secretion in association with a decrease in plasma CCK levels to basal values, thereby demonstrating that feedback regulation of pancreatic enzyme secretion occurs in man and that it is, at least in part, mediated by release of CCK.

Even though plasma CCK levels dropped to basal values during intraduodenal perfusion of phenylalanine and trypsin, there still remained a significant increase in pancreatic enzyme secretion. This suggests that pancreatic secretion is regulated by more than one mechanism. It is conceivable that trypsin in the duodenum inhibits pancreatic enzyme secretion through suppression of CCK release but has no effect on other stimulatory factors, such as the enteropancreatic cholinergic reflexes that also play an important role in the intestinal phase of pancreatic enzyme secretion. The enteropancreatic reflex can also be activated by distension or administration of hyperosmolar solutions in the duodenum, eliciting pancreatic enzyme secretion without raising the plasma CCK levels. This effect is inhibited by atropine, suggesting that it is cholinergically mediated. Pancreatic response to duodenal volume or osmolarity is not suppressed by trypsin, indicating that the reflex is not affected by intraluminal proteases. Secretion of PP is under cholinergic control, and this peptide acts by interfering with cholinergic transmission, making it an ideal candidate to modulate pancreatic secretion by the vagal cholinergic pathway (109).

**Role of the Endocrine Pancreas on the Regulation of the Exocrine Pancreas.** It was demonstrated many years ago (110) that insulin potentiates CCK-stimulated pancreatic amylase secretion in rats. Conversely, the elimination of circulating insulin by a specific antiinsulin antibody resulted in a complete suppression of postprandial pancreatic secretion (80). Data obtained from a perfused pancreas model suggest that the effect of insulin on pancreatic secretion is, in part, mediated by its paracrine action (111). Moreover, the insulin action on the exocrine pancreas is thought to result, in part, from suppression of the local release of somatostatin. Whether these mechanisms are operative in the human pancreas remains to be determined.

## PHYSIOLOGIC BASIS FOR THE SURGICAL MANAGEMENT OF THE EXOCRINE PANCREAS

This section demonstrates how an understanding of basic pancreatic physiology can be applied in the management of clinical situations that are commonly encountered in surgical practice. A series of clinical scenarios is presented to highlight a physiologic approach to pancreatic disease. This discussion serves merely to introduce these topics, each of which is addressed in far greater detail in other chapters.

### Pancreatic Surgery, Acute Pancreatitis, and Nutritional Support

**Problem: How Do I "Rest" the Pancreas and Feed My Patient?** Conservative patient management after pancreatic surgery or following an attack of acute pancreatitis attempts to minimize pancreatic stimulation by discontinuing oral intake and reducing gastric acid secretion. Patients in both situations are frequently starved, often for extended periods, and are thus prone to malnutrition (112).

Intravenous hyperalimentation (also called total parenteral nutrition, or TPN) is one way in which this problem can be addressed. However, TPN is expensive and has a defined morbidity. Fortunately, many of these patients have an intact gastrointestinal (GI) tract that can be used for feeding. It is beyond the scope of this chapter to discuss the relative merits of enteral feeding and intravenous feeding, but feeding into the GI tract is generally to be preferred when possible.

In the settings under discussion, elemental diets are theoretically attractive in the management of such patients. Based on the underlying physiology reviewed above, an attenuated pancreatic secretory response might be expected with elemental nutrients, since less digestion is necessary. This assumption, though, is only partially valid. As discussed above, important stimulants to pancreatic secretion include gastric and duodenal acidity (which stimulate secretin-induced volume and bicarbonate secretion), ingested intraluminal fatty acids and amino acids (which cause CCK-induced enzyme secretion), and gastrin.

Intraduodenal infusion of corn oil or amino acids in dogs (113, 114), and intrajejunal amino acid infusion in humans (115) produced significant increases in pancreatic enzyme output. With an intraduodenal, hyperosmolar, elemental diet with a high carbohydrate and amino acid composition at neutral pH, much less enzyme was secreted than with pure acidic amino acids (116).

Numerous dog studies have compared the pancreatic secretory response after elemental diets and whole or blenderized food and studied differences between oral and intraintestinal administration (117–120). Generally, an intrajejunal or intraduodenal elemental diet causes little or no pancreatic secretory response (117), although this opinion is by no means universally accepted (120). But despite some apparent pancreatic stimulation, elemental diets can improve nitrogen balance without worsening symptoms in severe pancreatitis (121).

### Finding the Pancreatic Duct Orifice in the Operating Room

**Problem: How to Locate the Pancreatic Duct Intraoperatively?** This is really a trivial annoyance, more than anything. Many surgeons have found themselves in the operating room staring at the inside of the duodenum unable to identify the orifice of the papilla of Vater. This can be easily accomplished if the common bile duct is opened and a probe passed down into the duodenum. However, if the pancreatic duct empties independently of the bile duct or if one is trying to localize the minor papilla of Santorini, then the intravenous administration of secretin, because of its stimulatory effect on the exocrine pancreas (as discussed above) will usually allow localization of the papilla because pancreatic juice appears to squirt rather abruptly into the duodenum.

### Pancreatic Surgery, Trauma, Fistulae, and Pancreatic Ascites

**Problem: What to Do with a Leaking Pancreatic Ductal System?** A leak from the pancreatic duct system is potentially one of the most devastating complications following pancreatic surgery, trauma, and acute pancreatitis, and it can lead to substantial morbidity and sometimes death. Not only may one or more fluid collections form about the pancreas and elsewhere in the peritoneal cavity, but these may become secondarily infected and develop into abscesses. This sets the stage for necrosis, systemic sepsis, and possibly death. Many, if not most, of these problems could be obviated if there was an effective means to shut off pancreatic secretion. For the sake of this discussion, I will limit my remarks to the reduction of perioperative complications following pancreatic surgery.

Though the mortality rate following pancreatic resection has improved considerably in recent years, it remains between 3 and 10% (122). Complications, including medical and surgical morbidity, occur in 30–40% of patients (122). Major complications after pancreatic resection (fistula, abscess, and sepsis) are chiefly associated with exocrine pancreatic secretion.

Inhibiting exocrine pancreatic secretion to prevent postoperative complications is an appealing concept that is based solely on the physiology of exocrine secretion. First reported in 1979 (123), a continuous intravenous infusion of somatostatin was administered to patients perioperatively after Whipple's resection, and a reduced complication rate was found.

While native somatostatin strongly inhibits basal and stimulated exocrine pancreatic secretion, it is of limited clinical use because of its extremely short half-life. The synthetic somatostatin analogue octreotide is more potent in inhibiting pancreatic exocrine secretion and has a much longer half-life than the native hormone. In two large randomized controlled trials, octreotide significantly reduced complications in patients undergoing elective pancreatic surgery (122, 124). The use of octreotide for the treatment of established pancreatic fistulae and pancreatic ascites has also been reported (125–128).

### Chronic Pancreatitis: Pain, Exocrine Insufficiency, and Diabetes

**Problem: Is There a Role for Surgical Intervention—When and How?** Intractable pain in patients with large-duct pancreatitis is generally considered to be the prime indication for a longitudinal pancreaticojejunostomy (129). Some 85% (74/87) of patients operated on experienced pain relief, including 58 patients with a dilated main pancreatic duct (MPD) and elevated MPD pressure, compared with 2% (1/56) of nonoperated patients. In contrast, nine patients with normal pressure did not profit from decompression (130). Nealon and Thompson have suggested that this procedure may also retard the progressive loss of exocrine and endocrine function that is part of the chronic pancreatitis syndrome. As a result, they have suggested that preservation of function should also be considered an indication for the procedure (130, 131).

These observations support the hypothesis that elevated tissue pressure contributes to the pain in this disorder and that early operative drainage performed before the appearance of irreversible functional impairment may be beneficial in patients with chronic pancreatitis (132).

### Chronic Pancreatitis and Pain: Medical Therapy

**Problem: If Surgery Isn't Appropriate—Then What?** Pain in chronic pancreatitis may be related to elevated pancreatic tissue pressures and activation of secretory pathways. Theoretically, the intraluminal delivery of pancreatic proteases would act via a negative feedback loop to reduce the CCK- or cholinergic-mediated pancreatic secretion, thereby reducing pain (133).

The existence of feedback regulation of pancreatic enzyme secretion in man may have important clinical implications. It is conceivable that in patients with chronic pancreatitis, decreased pancreatic enzyme secretion may potentially result in elevated plasma CCK levels. This may reflect a failure in the feedback modulation of CCK release secondary to a deficiency of pancreatic enzyme secretion. This, in turn, may cause hyperstimulation of the pancreas and produce pain. Thus, effective enzyme replacement therapy should reduce stimulation, decrease intraductal pressure, and diminish pain. Is there evidence to support this thesis?

Serine proteases (trypsin, chymotrypsin, and elastase) contained within pancreatic enzyme preparations exert a controlling influence on pancreatic secretion when they are delivered to the duodenum. The relief of abdominal pain following oral administration of pancreatic enzymes is based upon this feedback concept. When employed appropriately, this therapy affords considerable pain relief to selected patients with chronic pancreatitis and often is the only successful treatment in such patients (134).

Feedback control of pancreatic secretion by serine proteases in humans has been established (103). The mechanism appears to involve a reduction in the secretion of pancreatic enzymes mediated by the presence of ingested enzymes in the duodenum. As discussed above in the section on negative feedback regulation, the ability of ingested enzymes to initiate changes in pancreatic exocrine secretion, and thereby possibly modify pain, involves a peptide in the mucosa of the small intestine, called CCK-releasing peptide (CCK-RP), which releases CCK into the circulation.

In the fasting state, basal pancreatic secretion supplies just enough enzymes in the duodenum to denature CCK-RP and thus limits the steady-state release of CCK to only small amounts. In chronic pancreatitis, trypsin output is diminished. As a result, CCK-RP is not denatured and is available to release excessive amounts of CCK. The pancreas remains under strong stimulation from this hormone. This stimulation is thought to cause pancreatic pain, but the mechanism remains to be elucidated. Support for this theory comes from studies of chronic pancreatitis patients with elevated CCK blood levels, who demonstrated a decrease in CCK levels when the duodenum was perfused with proteases or when pancreatic enzymes were given orally (135).

Oral enzyme therapy provides increased trypsin within the duodenum. Trypsin denatures CCK-RP, thereby reducing CCK release. The result is a decrease in pancreatic stimulation and less pain. Oral enzyme therapy also reduces CCK release in response to food (106, 136, 137). Therefore, the use of exogenous pancreatic enzymes for the treatment of pain in chronic pancreatitis has a firm physiologic basis.

Another approach to this problem, again based on a physiologic understanding of the function of the exocrine pancreas, involves the use of the long-acting somatostatin analogue octreotide (138, 139). Somatostatin acts directly on the pancreas to inhibit secretion by the acinar cells by preventing secretin-induced cyclic AMP production and also indirectly, by decreasing circulating levels of CCK (140). Thus octreotide may complement the effects of pancreatic enzyme supplementation in the treatment of chronic pancreatic pain by further suppressing pancreatic secretion (141).

### Exocrine Insufficiency in Chronic Pancreatitis and after Pancreatic Resection

**Problem: Can It Be Managed, and What Are the Pitfalls?** The pancreas normally secretes a large excess of digestive enzymes, therefore clinically evident pancreatic insufficiency requires a substantial loss of pancreatic function; at least 90% of the normal secretory response to intestinal stimulants must be lost before evident pancreatic insufficiency occurs (142).

Decreased lipase secretion in chronic pancreatitis results in a marked reduction in the hydrolysis of dietary triglycerides and vitamin A esters. Calorie deficiency, steatorrhea, and diarrhea commonly occur (Fig. 3.6).

The basic physiology of pancreatic enzyme activation, as described in the first part of this chapter, would predict that treatment of the digestive enzyme deficit in chronic pancreatitis by orally administered enzymes may fail because *(a)* low intragastric pH produces irreversible inactivation of pancreatic enzymes and *(b)* decreased pancreatic bicarbonate secretion leads to a low intraduodenal pH unsuitable for optimal activity of administered enzyme supplements. These problems can be overcome either by increasing the intragastric pH or by coating the orally administered enzymes to increase effective concentrations of enzymes in the intestine (143).

## Endoscopic Retrograde Cholangiopancreatography (ERCP) and Pancreatitis

**Problem: Can Procedure-Related Pancreatitis Be Prevented?** ERCP is associated with a certain incidence of acute pancreatitis, which can be quite severe when it occurs. It has been suggested that turning off the gland by using octreotide prior to ERCP could potentially reduce or eliminate this problem.

Caution may need to be exercised, however, when octreotide is administered as prophylaxis against ERCP pancreatitis. There are reasons to suggest that prophylactic octreotide may actually worsen acute pancreatitis. In a study by Metrakos et al. (144), prophylactic octreotide was reported to actually potentiate cerulein-induced pancreatitis in rats. This deleterious effect of octreotide was ascribed to the accumulation of proteolytic enzymes within the pancreas. They then would be released in far greater concentration than might otherwise occur. These experimental results have been borne out by a prospective randomized trial (145). Eighty-four patients were randomized to receive either 100 g of octreotide subcutaneously immediately prior to ERCP and 100 g 45 minutes after the initial dose, or placebo. Interim analysis revealed an 11% incidence of clinical pancreatitis in the control group and 35% in the treatment group, and the study was halted.

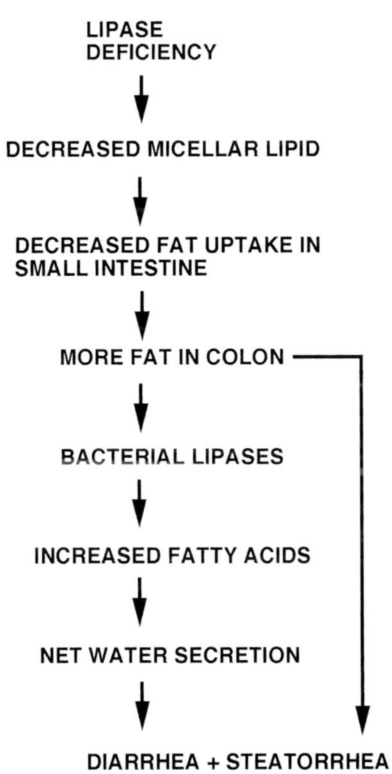


**FIG. 3.6.** Pathophysiology of the consequences of pancreatic exocrine insufficiency.

## Pancreatic Transplantation

**Problem: How to Monitor for Rejection?** One of the Achilles' heels of transplantation of the pancreas is the lack of a sensitive and specific way to monitor for acute endocrine rejection. By the time serum levels of glucose are rising, rejection is well established and the loss of graft function is likely to be permanent.

Experience has shown, however, that changes in the pancreatic exocrine secretion of the graft can be used as an indicator of rejection. To take advantage of this situation, the transplant procedure has to be performed in a manner that leads to the external drainage of exocrine secretions. There are two ways for this to be accomplished—enteric drainage of the graft with an external drainage catheter leading from the duct (146), or the more common bladder drainage technique of Sollinger (147). In the bladder drainage procedure, the donor pancreas is anastomosed to the recipient urinary bladder, and urinary amylase and pH are monitored in a routine fashion. Rejection causes a decrease in both pH (as a result of diminished bicarbonate secretion) and amylase (because of acinar cell destruction) (148), usually before there has been any change in the blood glucose level. Unfortunately, a method of monitoring rejection in an islet cell graft has yet to be found, and diagnosis of rejection remains a fundamental problem in islet transplantation.

## REFERENCES

1. Fujita T, Murakami T. Microcirculation of the monkey pancreas with special reference to the insulo-acinar portal system. A scanning electron microscope study of vascular casts. Arch Histol Jpn 1973;35:255–263.
2. Henderson JR, Daniel PM. A comparative study of the portal vessels connecting the endocrine and exocrine pancreas, with a discussion of some functional implications. Q J Exp Physiol 1979;64:267–275.
3. Fraser PA, Henderson JR. The arrangement of endocrine and exocrine pancreatic microcirculation observed in the living rabbit. Q J Exp Physiol 1980;65:151–158.
4. Lifson N, Kramlinger KG, Mayrand RR, Lender EJ. Blood flow to the rabbit pancreas with special reference to the islets of Langerhans. Gastroenterology 1980;79:466–473.
5. Bolender RP. Stereological analysis of the guinea pig pancreas. I. Analytical model and quantitative description of nonstimulated pancreatic exocrine cells. J Cell Biol 1974;61:269–287.
6. Schonfeld JV, Goebell H, Muller MK. The islet-acinar axis of the pancreas. Int J Pancreatol 1994;16:131–140.
7. Williams JA, Goldfine ID. The insulin-pancreatic axis. Diabetes 1985;34:980–986.
8. Solomon T. Physiology of the exocrine pancreas. In: Howard JM, Jordan GL, Reber H, eds. Surgical diseases of the pancreas. Baltimore: Williams & Wilkins, 1987:45–65.
9. Chung RS, Safaie-Shirazi S. The effect of secretin on pancreatic blood flow in the awake and anesthetized dog. Proc Soc Exp Biol Med 1983;173:620–625.
10. Delaney JP, Grim E. Influence of hormones and drugs on canine pancreatic blood flow. Am J Physiol 1966;211:1398–1402.
11. Said SI, Mutt V. Potent peripheral and splanchnic vasodilatation peptide from normal gut. Nature 1970;225:863–864.
12. Papp M, Feher S, Varga B, Folly G. Humoral influences on local blood flow and external secretion of the resting dog pancreas. Acta Med Acad Sci Hung 1977;34:185–188.
13. Dorigotti L, Glasser AH. Comparative effects of cerulein, pan-

creozymin and secretin on pancreatic blood flow. Experientia 1968;24:806–807.

14. Barlow TE, Greenwell JR, Harper AA, Scratcherd T. The effect of adrenaline and noradrenaline on the blood flow, electrical conductance and external secretion of the pancreas. J Physiol (Lond) 1971;217:665–678.
15. Bastie MJ, Vaysse N, Brenac B, Pasacal JP, Ribet A. Effects of catecholamines and their inhibitors on the isolated canine pancreas. II. Dopamine. Gastroenterology 1977;72:719–723.
16. Barlow TE, Greenwell JR, Harper AA, Scratcherd T. Factors influencing pancreatic flow. In: Bain WH, Harper AM, eds. Blood flow through organs and tissues. Edinburgh: E and S Livingstone, 1968.
17. Aune S, Semb LS. The effect of secretin and pancreozymin on pancreatic blood flow in the conscious and anesthetized dog. Acta Physiol 1969;76:406–414.
18. Beijer HJM, Brouwer FAS, Charbon GA. Time course and sensitivity of secretin-stimulated pancreatic secretion and blood flow in the anesthetized dog. Scand J Gastroenterol 1979;14: 295–300.
19. Legg PG. Fluorescence studies on neural structures and endocrine cells in the pancreas of the cat. Z Zellforsch Mikrosk Anat 1968;88:487–495.
20. Richins CA. The innervation of the pancreas. J Comp Neurol 1945;83:223–236.
21. Holst JJ, Fahrenkrug J, Knuhtsen S, et al. VIP and PH1 in the pig pancreas: coexistence, corelease, and cooperative effects. Am J Physiol 1987;252:G182–G189.
22. Knuhtsen S, Holst JJ, Jensen SL, Knigge SL, Nielsen OV. Gastrin releasing peptide: effect on exocrine secretion, and release from isolated perfused porcine pancreas. Am J Physiol 1985; 248:G281–G286.
23. Larsson LI. Innervation of the pancreas by substance P, enkephalin, vasoactive intestinal polypeptide and gastrin/CCK immunoreactive nerves. J Histochem Cytochem 1979;27:1283–1284.
24. Mori J, Satoh Y, Hashimoto M, Honda F. Amines and the rat exocrine pancreas: (1) effects of receptor blockers on turnover of L-dopa. Jpn J Pharmacol 1979;29:899–911.
25. Koevary SB, Azmitia EC, McEvoy RC. Rat pancreatic serotonergic nerves: morphologic, pharmacologic and physiologic studies. Brain Res 1983;265:328–332.
26. Lightwood R, Rebr HA. Micropuncture study of pancreatic secretion in the cat. Gastroenterology 1977;72:61–66.
27. Bockman DE, Boydston WR, Parsa I. Architecture of human pancreas: implications for early changes in pancreatic diseases. Gastroenterology 1983;85:55–61.
28. Ham AW. Histology. 7th ed. Philadelphia: JB Lippincott, 1974: 681–685.
29. Domschke S, Domschke W, Rosch W, Konturek SJ, Wunsch E, Demling L. Bicarbonate and cyclic AMP content of pure human pancreatic juice in response to graded doses of synthetic secretin. Gastroenterology 1976;70:533–536.
30. Scheele G, Bartlelt D, Bieger W. Characterization of human exocrine pancreatic proteins by two-dimensional isolectric focusing/sodium dodecyl sulfate gel electrophoresis. Gastroenterology 1981;80:461–473.
31. Kern HF. Fine structure of the human exocrine pancreas. In: Go VLW, Gardner JD, Brooks FP, Lebenthal E, DiMagno EP, Scheele GA, eds. The exocrine pancreas: biology, pathobiology, and diseases. New York: Raven Press, 1986:9–20.
32. Kodama T. A light and electron microscopic study on the pancreatic ductal system. Acta Pathol Jpn 1983;33:297–321.
33. Geleff S, Bock P. Pancreatic duct glands. II. Lectin binding affinities of ductular epithelium, ductular glands, and Brunner's glands. Histochemistry 1984;80:31–38.
34. Hootman SR, de Ondarza J. Mucin secretion in isolated guinea pig pancreatic ducts (Abstract). Pancreas 1992;7:742.
35. Lee SP, Choong YS, Park HZ. Isolation and partial characterization of a soluble mucin in human pancreatic juice. Biochem Cell Biol 1991;69:566–571.
36. Reber HA, Roberts C, Way LW. The pancreatic duct mucosal barrier. Am J Surg 1979;137:128–134.
37. Kanno T, Yamamoto M. Differentiation between the calcium-dependent effects of cholecystokinin-pancreozymin and the bicarbonate-dependent effects of secretin in exocrine secretion of the rat pancreas. J Physiol (Lond) 1977;264:787–799.
38. Case RM, Scratcherd T, Wynne RD. The origin and secretion of pancreatic juice bicarbonate. J Physiol (Lond) 1970;210:1–15.
39. Way LW, Diamond JM. The effect of secretin on electrical potential differences in the pancreatic duct. Biochim Biophys Acta 1970;203:298–307.
40. Ridderstrap AS, Bonting SL. Na-K-activated adenosine triphosphate and pancreatic secretion in the dog. Am J Physiol 1969;216:547–553.
41. Bundgaard M, Moller M, Poulsen JH. Localization of sodium pump sites in cat pancreas. J Physiol (Lond) 1981;313:405–414.
42. Dyck WP, Hightower NC, Janowitz HD. Effect of acetozolamide on human pancreatic secretion. Gastroenterology 1972;62: 547–552.
43. Hootman SR, de Ondarza J. Overview of pancreatic duct physiology and pathophysiology. Digestion 1993;54:323–330.
44. De Giorgio R, Sternini C, Anderson K, Brecha NC, Go VLW. Tissue distribution and innervation pattern of peptide immunoreactivities in the rat pancreas. Peptides 1992;13:91–98.
45. Holst JJ. Neural regulation of pancreatic exocrine function. In: Go VLW, Gardner JD, Brooks FP, Lebenthal E, DiMagno EP, Scheele GA, eds. The exocrine pancreas: biology, pathobiology, and diseases. New York: Raven Press, 1986:287–300.
46. Heinz E. Transport through biological membranes. Annu Rev Physiol 1967;29–21–58.
47. Scheele GA. Biosynthesis, segregation, and secretion of exportable proteins by the exocrine pancreas (Abstract). Am J Physiol 1980;238:G467.
48. Palade G. Intracellular aspects of the process of protein synthesis. Science 1975;189:347–358.
49. Bieger W, Martin-Achard A, Bassler M, Kern HF. Studies on intracellular transport of secretory proteins in the rat exocrine pancreas. IV. Stimulation by in vivo infusion of caerulein. Cell Tissue Res 1976;165:435–453.
50. Solomon TE. Regulation of exocrine pancreatic cell proliferation and enzyme synthesis. In: Johnson LR. Physiology of the gastrointestinal tract. New York: Raven Press, 1981:873–892.
51. Gardner JD, Jensen RT. Regulation of pancreatic enzyme secretion in vitro. In: Johnson LR. Physiology of the gastrointestinal tract. New York: Raven Press, 1981:831–872.
52. Heisler S, Lambert M. Dissociation of cyclic GMP synthesis from cholinergic-stimulated secretion of protein from rat exocrine pancreas. Can J Physiol Pharmacol 1978;56:395–399.
53. Debas HT, Grossman MI. Pure cholecystokinin: pancreatic protein and bicarbonate response. Digestion 1973;9:469–481.
54. Banwell JG, Northan BE, Cooke WT. Secretory response of the human pancreas to continuous intravenous infusion of pancreozymin-cholecystokinin (Cecekin). Gut 1967;8:380–387.
55. Petersen H. The effect of pure natural secretin on the bicarbonate secretion into the duodenum in man. Scand J Gastroenterol 1970;5:105–111.
56. DiMagno EP, Hendricks JC, Go VLW, Dozois RR. Relationships among canine fasting pancreatic and biliary secretions, pancreatic duct pressures, and duodenal phase III motor activity—Boldyreff revisited. Dig Dis Sci 1979;24:689–693.
57. Chen MH, Joffe SN, Magee DF, Murphy RF, Naruse S. Cyclic changes of plasma pancreatic polypeptide and pancreatic secretion in fasting dogs. J Physiol (Lond) 1983;341:453–461.
58. Lee KY, Shiratori K, Chen YF, Chang TM, Chey WY. A hormonal mechanism for the interdigestive pancreatic secretion in dogs. Am J Physiol 1986;251:G759–G764.
59. Lee KY, Park HJ, Chang TM, Chey WY. Cholinergic role on release and action of motilin. Peptides 1983;4:375–380.
60. Shiratori K, Lee KY, Change TM, Jo YH, Coy DH, Chey WY. Role of pancreatic polypeptide in the regulation of pancreatic exocrine secretion in dogs. Am J Physiol 1988;255:G837–G842.
61. DeFillipi C, Solomon TE, Valenzuela JE. Pancreatic secretory response to sham feeding in humans. Digestion 1982;23:217–223.
62. Pavlov IP. The work of the digestive glands. 2nd ed. Thompson WH, trans. Philadelphia: JB Lippincott, 1910:59–64.
63. Preshaw RM, Cooke AR, Grossman MI. Sham feeding and pancreatic secretion in the dog. Gastroenterology 1966;50: 171–178.
64. Schwartz TW, Stenquist B, Olbe L. Cephalic phase of pancreatic polypeptide secretion studied by sham feeding in man. Scand J Gastroenterol 1979;14:313–320.

65. Sarles H, Dani R, Pzezelin G, Souville C, Figarella C. Cephalic phase of pancreatic secretion in man. Gut 1968;9:214–221.
66. Cargill JM, Wormsley KG. Effect of gastric distension on human pancreatic secretion. Acta Hepato-gastroenterol 1979;26: 235–238.
67. Vagne M, Grossman MI. Gastric and pancreatic secretion in response to gastric distension in dogs. Gastroenterology 1969; 57:300–310.
68. Go VL, Hofmann AF, Summerskill WHJ. Pancreozymin bioassay in man based on pancreatic enzyme secretion: potency of specific amino acids and other digestive products. J Clin Invest 1970;49:1558–1564.
69. Malegelada JR, Go VLW, DiMagno EP, Summerskill WHJ. Interactions between luminal bile acids and digestive products on pancreatic and gallbladder function. J Clin Invest 1973;52:2160–2165.
70. Malegelada JR, DiMagno EP, Summerskill WHJ, Go VLW. Regulation of pancreatic and gallbladder functions by intraluminal fatty acids and bile acids in man. J Clin Invest 1976; 58:493–499.
71. Meyer JH, Jones RS. Canine pancreatic responses to intestinally perfused fat and products of fat digestion. Am J Physiol 1974;226:1178–1187.
72. Malegelada JR, Go VLW, Summerskil WHJ. Different gastric, pancreatic, and biliary responses to solid-liquid or homogenized meals. Dig Dis Sci 1979;24:101.
73. Fahrenkrug J, Schaffalitzky de Muckadell OB, Rune SJ. pH threshold for release of secretin in normal subjects and in patients with duodenal ulcer and patients with chronic pancreatitis. Scand J Gastroenterol 1978;13:177–186.
74. Meyer JH, Way LW, Grossman MI. Pancreatic response to acidification of various lengths of proximal intestine in the dog. Am J Physiol 1970;219:971–977.
75. Rune SJ. pH in the human duodenum. Digestion 1973;8:261–268.
76. Holtermuller KH, Malegelada JR, McCall JT, Go VLW. Pancreatic, gallbladder and gastric responses to intraduodenal calcium perfusion in man. Gastroenterology 1976;70:693–696.
77. Chey WY, Chang TM. Secretin. In: Makhlouf GM, ed. Handbook of physiology, section 6, GI system, vol II. American Physiological Society. New York: Oxford University Press, 1989:359–402.
78. Rehfeld JF. Cholecystokinin. In: Makhlouf GM, ed. Handbook of physiology, section 6, GI system, vol II. American Physiological Society. New York: Oxford University Press, 1989:337–358.
79. Reinecke M. Neurotensin. Immunohistochemical localization in central and peripheral nervous system and in endocrine cells and its functional role as a neurotransmitter and endocrine hormone (Review). Prog Histochem Cytochem 1985;16:1–172.
80. Lee KY, Lu Z, Ren XS, Chang TM, Chey WY. An important role of endogenous insulin on exocrine pancreatic secretion in rats. Am J Physiol 1990;258:G268–G274.
81. Taylor I. Pancreatic polypeptide family: pancreatic polypeptide, neuropeptide Y, and peptide Y. In: Makhlouf GM, ed. Handbook of physiology, section 6, GI system, vol II. American Physiological Society. New York: Oxford University Press, 1989: 475–543.
82. Nechles H. Effect of glucagon on external secretion of the pancreas. Am J Physiol 1957;191:595–597.
83. Boden G, Sivitz MC, Owen OE, Essa-Koumar N, Landor JH. Somatostatin suppresses secretin and pancreatic exocrine secretion. Science 1975;90:163–164.
84. Funakoshi A, Miyasaka K, Nakamura R, et al. Bioactivity of synthetic human pancreastatin on exocrine pancreas. Biochem Biophys Res Commun 1988;156:1237–1242.
85. Gullo L, Labo G. Thyrotropin-releasing hormone inhibits pancreatic enzyme secretion in humans. Gastroenterology 1981;80: 735–739.
86. Beglinger C, Koehler E, Born W, et al. Effect of calcitonin and calcitonin gene-related peptide on pancreatic function in man. Gut 1988;29:243–248.
87. Chey WY, Kim MS, Lee KY, Chang TM. Effect of rabbit antisecretin serum on post-prandial pancreatic secretion in dogs. Gastroenterology 1979;77:1268–1275.
88. Jo YH, Lee KY, Chang TM, Chey WY. The role of cholecystokinin on pancreatic bicarbonate secretion in dogs. Pancreas 1990; 6:197–201.
89. Li P, Lee KY, Chang TM, Chey WY. The hormonal mechanism of sodium oleate stimulated pancreatic secretion in rats. Am J Physiol 1990;259:G960–G965.
90. Brown JC, Harper AA, Scratcherd T. Potentiation of secretin stimulation of the pancreas. J Physiol (Lond) 1967;190:519–530.
91. You CH, Rominger JM, Chey WY. Effects of atropine on the action and release of secretin humans. Am J Physiol 1982;242: G608–G611.
92. You CH, Chey Wy. Atropine abolishes potentiation effect of secretin and cholecystokinin octapeptide on exocrine pancreatic secretion in humans. Pancreas 1988;3:99–103.
93. Byrnes DJ, Henderson L, Borody T, Rehfeld JF. Radioimmunoassay of cholecystokinin in human plasma. Clin Chim Acta 1981;111: 81–89.
94. Walsh JH, Lamers CB, Valenzuela JE. Cholecystokinin-octapeptide immunoreactivity in human plasma. Gastroenterology 1982;82:438–444.
95. Jansen JB, Lamers CB. Radioimmunoassay of cholecystokinin in human tissue and plasma. Clin Chim Acta 1983;131:305–316.
96. Singer MV, Solomon TE, Grossman MI. Effect of atropine on secretion from intact and transplanted pancreas in dog. Am J Physiol 1980;238:G18–G22.
97. Moreland HJ, Johnson LR. Effect of vagotomy on pancreatic secretion stimulated by endogenous and exogenous secretin. Gastroenterology 1971;60:425–431.
98. Konturek SJ, Becker HD, Thompson JC. Effect of vagotomy on hormones stimulating pancreatic secretion. Arch Surg 1974;108: 704–708.
99. Debas HT, Konturek SJ, Grossman MI. Effect of extragastric and truncal vagotomy on pancreatic secretion in the dog. Am J Physiol 1975;228:1172–1177.
100. Williams JA, Korc M, Dormer RL. Action of secretagogues on a new preparation of functionally intact, isolated pancreatic acini. Am J Physiol 1978;235;E517–E524.
101. Gyr K, Beglinger C, Kohler E, Trautzl U, Keller U, Bloom S. Circulating somatostatin. Physiological regulator of pancreatic function? J Clin Invest 1987;79:1595–1600.
102. Green GM, Lyman RL. Feedback regulation of pancreatic enzyme secretion as a mechanism for trypsin inhibitor-induced hypersecretion in rats. Proc Soc Exp Biol Med 1972;140: 6–12.
103. Owyang C, Louie DS, Tatum D. Feedback regulation of pancreatic enzyme secretion. Suppression of cholecystokinin by release of trypsin. J Clin Invest 1986;77:2042–2047.
104. Imamura M, Lee KY, Chang TM, Chey WY. Role of secretin in negative feedback regulation of postprandial pancreatic secretion in dogs (Abstract). Gastroenterology 1990;98(part 2): A220.
105. Li P, Lee KY, Ren XS, Chang TM, Chey WY. Effect of pancreatic proteases on plasma cholecystokinin, secretin, and pancreatic exocrine secretion in response to sodium oleate. Gastroenterology 1990;98:1642–1648.
106. Lu L, Louie D, Owyang C. A cholecystokinin releasing peptide mediates feedback regulation of pancreatic secretion. Am J Physiol 1989;19:G430–G435.
107. Miyasaka K, Guan D, Liddle RA, Green GM. Feedback regulation by trypsin: evidence for intraluminal CCK-releasing peptide. Am J Physiol 1989;257:G175–G181.
108. Ihse I, Lilja P, Lundquist I. Feedback regulation of pancreatic enzyme secretion by intestinal trypsin in man. Digestion 1977; 15:303–308.
109. Owyang C. Negative feedback control of exocrine pancreatic secretion: role of cholecystokinin and cholinergic pathway. J Nutr 1994;124:1321S–1326S.
110. Kanno T, Saito A. The potentiating influence of insulin on pancreozymin-induced hyperpolarization and amylase release in the pancreatic acinar cell. J Physiol (Lond) 1976;261: 505–521.
111. Lee YL, Lee KY, Chang TM, Chey WY. Interaction between secretin and cholecystokinin (CCK) and paracrine action of insulin on pancreatic secretion in rats (Abstract). Clin Res 1990;38:344A.
112. Reilly JJ Jr, Gerhardt AL. Modern surgical nutrition. Curr Probl Surg 1985;22:42.
113. Wang CC, Grossman MI. Physiological determination of release of secretion and pancreozymin from intestine of dogs with transplanted pancreas. Am J Physiol 1951;164:527–545.

114. Meyer JH, Grossman MI. Comparison of D- and L-phenylalanine as pancreatic stimulants. Am J Physiol 1972;222:1058–1063.
115. Ertan A, Brooks FP, Ostrow JD, et al. Effect of jejunal amino acid perfusion and exogenous cholecystokinin on the exocrine pancreatic and biliary secretions in man. Gastroenterology 1971;61:686–692.
116. Wolfe BM, Keltner RM, Kaminski DL. The effect of intraduodenal elemental diet on pancreatic secretion. Surg Gynecol Obstet 1975;140:241–245.
117. Ragins H, Levensen SM, Signer R, et al. Intrajejunal administration of an elemental diet at neutral pH avoids pancreatic stimulation. Am J Surg 1973;126:606–614.
118. Kelly GA, Nahrwold DL. Pancreatic secretion in response to an elemental diet and intravenous hyperalimentation. Surg Gynecol Obstet 1976;143:87–91.
119. McArdle AH, Echave W, Brown RA, et al. Effect of elemental diet on pancreatic secretion. Am J Surg 1974;128:690–692.
120. Cassin MM, Allardyce DB. Pancreatic secretion in response to jejunal feeding of elemental diet. Ann Surg 1974;180: 228–231.
121. Voitk A, Brown RA, Echave V, et al. Use of an elemental diet in the treatment of complicated pancreatitis. Am J Surg 1973;125: 223–227.
122. Buchler M, Friess H, Klempa I, Hermanek P, Sulkowski U, et al. Role of octreotide in the prevention of postoperative complications following pancreatic resection. Am J Surg 1992;163:125–130.
123. Klempa J, Schedes U, Usadel KH. Verutung von postoperativen pankreatitischen komplikationen nach duodenpankreatektomie durch somatostatin. Chirurg 1979;50:427–432.
124. Montorsi M, Zago M, Mosca F, Capussotti L, Zotti E, et al. Efficacy of octreotide in the prevention of pancreatic fistula after elective pancreatic resections: a prospective, controlled, randomized clinical trial. Surgery 1995;117:26–31.
125. Rosenberg L, Brown RA. Sandostatin in the management of nonendocrine gastrointestinal and pancreatic disorders: a preliminary study. Can J Surg 1991;34:223–229.
126. Rosenberg L, Dafoe DC, Schwartz R, et al. Administration of somatostatin analog (SMS 201–995) in the treatment of a fistula occurring after pancreas transplantation. Interference with cyclosporine immunosuppression. Transplantation 1987;43: 764–766.
127. Hurst RD, Modlin IM. The therapeutic role of octreotide in the management of surgical disorders. Am J Surg 1991;162:499–507.
128. Segal I, Parekh D, Lipschitz J, Gecelter G, Myburgh JA. Treatment of pancreatic ascites and external pancreatic fistulas with a long-acting somatostatin analogue (Sandostatin). Digestion 1993;54(suppl 1):53–58.
129. Steer M. Pancreatic surgery. Curr Opinions Gastroenterol 1994; 10:513–516.
130. Nealon WH, Thompson JC. Progressive loss of pancreatic function in chronic pancreatitis is delayed by main pancreatic decompression: a longitudinal prospective analysis of the modified Puestow procedure. Ann Surg 1993;217:458–468.
131. Nealon WH, Townsend CM Jr, Thompson JC. Operative drainage of the pancreatic duct delays functional impairment in patients with chronic pancreatitis: a prospective analysis. Ann Surg 1988;208:321–329.
132. Korc M, Schmiegel W. Chronic pancreatitis. Curr Opinions Gastroenterol 1994;10:502–506.
133. DiMagno EP, Layer P, Clain JE. Chronic pancreatitis. In: Go VLW, DiMagno EP, Gardner JD, Lebenthal E, Reber HA, Scheele GA, eds. The pancreas. Biology, pathobiology and disease. New York: Raven Press, 1993:665–706.
134. Toskes PP. Is there an effective nonsurgical treatment for pain in chronic pancreatitis? Gastroenterology 1991;86:28–29.
135. Slaff J, Wolfe M, Toskes PP. Elevated fasting cholecystokinin levels in pancreatic exocrine impairment: evidence to support feedback regulation. J Lab Clin Med 1995;105:282–285.
136. Slaff J, Jacobson D, Tillerman RC, et al. Protease-specific suppression of pancreatic exocrine secretion. Gastroenterology 1984;87:44–52.
137. Bozkurt T, Adler G, Koop I, et al. Plasma CCK levels in patients with chronic insufficiency. Dig Dis Sci 1988;33:276–281.
138. Korc M, Schmiegel W. Chronic pancreatitis. Curr Opinions Gastroenterol 1994;10:502–506.
139. Burroughs AK, Malagelada R. Potential indications for octreotide in gastroenterology: summary of workshop. Digestion 1993;54:59–67.
140. Matsushita K, Okabayashi Y, Hasegawa H, Koide M, Kido Y, et al. In vitro inhibitory effect of somatostatin action in exocrine pancreas of rats. Gastroenterology 1993;104:1146–1152.
141. Toskes PP, Forsmark CE, DeMeo MT, Prinz RA, Owyang C, et al. A multicenter trial of octreotide for the pain of chronic pancreatitis (Abstract). Pancreas 1993;8;774.
142. DiMagno EP, Go VLW, Summerskill WHJ. Relations between pancreatic enzyme outputs and malabsorption in severe pancreatic insufficiency. N Engl J Med 1973;288:813–815.
143. Regan PT, Malegelada JR, DiMagno EP, Glanzman SL, Go VLW. Comparative effects of antacids, cimetidine and enteric coating on the therapeutic response to oral enzymes in severe pancreatic insufficiency. N Engl J Med 1977;297:854–858.
144. Metrakos P, Rosenberg L, Duguid W, Fried GM. Prophylactic sandostatin potentiates acute pancreatitis. Surg Forum 1990;41: 160–161.
145. Sternlieb JM, Aronchik CA, Retig JN, Dabezies M, Saunders F, et al. A multicenter, randomized controlled trial to evaluate the effects of prophylactic octreotide on ERCP-induced pancreatitis. Am J Gastroenterol 1992;87:1561–1566.
146. Groth CG, Collste H, Lundgren G, et al. Successful outcome of segmental human pancreatic transplantation with enteric exocrine diversion after modifications in technique. Lancet 1982;2:522–524.
147. Sollinger HW, Cook K, Kamps D, et al. Clinical and experimental experience with pancreaticocystostomy for exocrine pancreatic drainage in pancreas transplantation. Transplant Proc 1984;16:749–751.
148. Prieto M, Sutherland DER, Fernadez-Cruz L, et al. Experimental and clinical experience with urine amylase monitoring for early diagnosis of pancreas allograft rejection in dogs. Transplantation 1987;43:71–79.

SECTION II

PREOPERATIVE APPROACHES TO PANCREATIC DISEASE

# 4

# *Conventional Radiology and Ultrasonography*

Yasutusugu Bandai and Masatoshi Makuuchi

## CONVENTIONAL RADIOLOGY

Plain film of the abdomen and chest, barium study of the upper gastrointestinal tract, and hypotonic duodenography have roles in the diagnosis of pancreatic diseases. These procedures are relatively inexpensive and readily available, but the limited accuracy of these modalities and the development of ultrasonography and computed tomographic (CT) scanning have diminished their usage.

### Plain Chest and Abdominal Film

Films of the chest and abdomen are important in the diagnosis of acute pancreatitis. Roentgenologic signs may include pleural effusions, particularly on the left side, or atelectasis of the basal lobe (1). Local intestinal distention in the region of the pancreas is famous as a "sentinel loop" (2), as is a sharp demarcation of the gas pattern in the transverse colon ("the colon cutoff sign" (3, 4)). These are not specific for acute pancreatitis and may be seen even where an irritation from an inflammatory process creates a localized ileus. An obstruction secondary to neoplasm can also create this nonspecific appearance.

Pancreatic calcification can often be demonstrated by abdominal x-ray. In chronic pancreatitis, stones in the pancreatic ductal system are demonstrated as spots of calcifications arranged transversely across the upper abdomen, reflecting advanced chronic pancreatitis. Calcification may also be rarely seen in certain tumors of the pancreas such as islet cell tumor, mucinous adenocarcinoma, cystadenomas, cystadenocarcinomas, hemangiomas, papillary cystic and solid tumors, and (after treatment) lymphomas (5).

**Upper Gastrointestinal Series.** Barium study of the esophagus, stomach, and duodenum may be helpful in the diagnosis and treatment of pancreatic diseases. Esophageal varices may be found as a sequel to obstruction of the portal vein by pancreatic carcinoma or by pancreatitis. The stomach may show an irregular contour from infiltration of tumor (6). Invasion of the second portion of the duodenum and distortion of the papilla of Vater may occur with development of the "inverted three" sign (7). The entire duodenum may appear enlarged with widening of the C loop. These findings may occur not only with malignant diseases but also with inflammatory process of the pancreas. Ductal carcinoma of the body of the pancreas may infiltrate the fourth portion of the duodenum, sometimes necessitating bypass operation when radical operation is impossible.

**Hypotonic Duodenography.** Peristalsis, including hypermotility of the duodenum, may mimic an abnormality and make diagnosis difficult. Elimination of peristalsis by pharmacologic paralysis helps to delineate the contour of the duodenum by double-contrast study with barium and air (8). Intubation of the duodenum, which facilitates the introduction of optimal amounts of barium and air, is usually done. Intubation also has the advantage of allowing opacification of the duodenum only (9). Thus hypotonic duodenography enhances the findings of an upper gastrointestinal series.

Alterations in the mucosal pattern of the duodenum may appear as "saw tooth" or "rose thorn" projections on the medial border, and in far-advanced disease, obvious filling defects may be noted. Hypotonic duodenography is seldom used since gastroduodenoscopy has become widely available, yet it occasionally remains a useful adjunct in the evaluation of partial duodenal obstruction.

## ULTRASONOGRAPHY

### The Normal Pancreas

**Sonographic Anatomy of the Pancreas.** When performing ultrasonography of the pancreas, identification of the anatomic arrangement of organs adjacent to the pancreas, especially the vascular structures, is important in obtaining definition of the pancreas itself (Fig. 4.1). The pancreas is surrounded by the inferior vena cava, aorta, superior mesenteric artery, and portal, splenic, and superior mesenteric veins. Of these, the portal vein and its tributaries provide the best landmark for localization of the pancreas, because these veins are attached to the dorsal aspect of the pancreas. The superior mesenteric artery is usually seen in cross-section posterior to the body of the pancreas and the splenic vein.

Anatomically, the pancreas has three parts: head, body, and tail. The head of the pancreas is bounded by the superior mesenteric and portal veins, with the neck of the gland overlying the superior mesenteric vein.

**Techniques for Demonstration of the Pancreas.** Ultrasonic identification of the pancreas is more difficult for the beginner than such organs as the liver, gallbladder, and kidneys. The blood vessels surrounding the pancreas are the first structures to identify. The examination is begun with the patient supine. The patient is asked to take a deep breath and to hold it, but the extent of inspiration must be adjusted as necessitated by the patient's habitus. Frequently, better images can be obtained when the breath is held at normal tidal volumes, especially in obese patients. Oblique tilting of the transducer from the transverse plane may be necessary to demonstrate the long axis of the pancreas. The gastroduodenal artery lies ventral and lateral to the pancreatic head, whereas the distal common bile duct courses through the posterior portion of the head. Except in thin patients, demonstration of the entire tail of the pancreas may be difficult because of gas in the stomach.

General factors that handicap study of the pancreas are gas in the gastrointestinal tract, alteration of anatomy after abdominal surgery, barium in the colon, and obesity. These factors may be overcome by transducer compression of the anterior abdominal

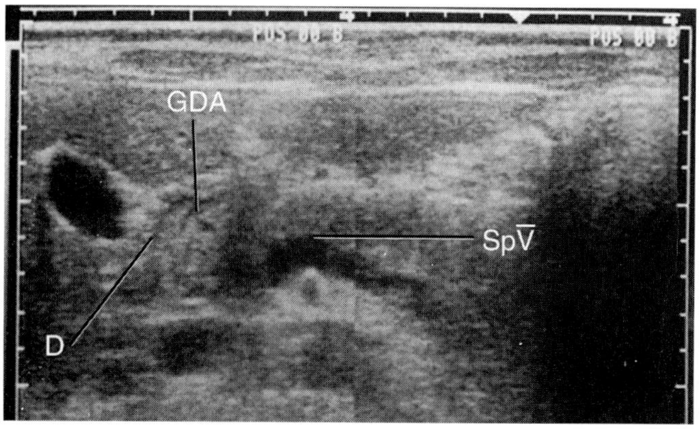


**FIG. 4.1.** Normal pancreas (transverse scan). The pancreas is surrounded by several vessels; of these, the portal and splenic veins *(SpV)* provide the best landmarks for localization. The second portion of the duodenum *(D)* and the gastroduodenal artery *(GDA)*, which mark the anterolateral margin of head of the pancreas may be depicted.

wall, changing the patient's position, and use of the spleen or the left kidney as an acoustic window. Scanning with the patient in a sitting position will shift gas in the stomach from the antrum to the fundus and thus permit better visualization of the pancreatic body and head. The distal portion of the tail of the pancreas can be detected only by longitudinal or transverse scans at the left flank through the spleen (10) (Fig. 4.2*A*). The stomach can be used as an acoustic window (11) to the body and head if the patient drinks 500 mL or more fluid and shifts to an upright position. Figure 4.2*B* demonstrates its use in the supine position to outline a tumor of the tail of the pancreas (12). Fluid in the stomach enhances echoes from posterior organs including the pancreas, although it necessitates adjustment in the gain setting and sensitivity-time control.

**Ultrasonic Patterns of the Normal Pancreas.** Sonographic diagnosis of the pancreas is based on size, intensity of echoes from the parenchyma, and shape of the main pancreatic duct. The configuration of the pancreas on sonograms differs from patient to patient. "Sausage," "dumbbell," and "tadpole" are terms used to describe the three main normal configurations of the pancreas (13). The configuration, however, may change depending on the direction of scanning, respiration, changes of position of the patient, and other factors.

***Size.*** In the supine position, the maximal thickness of the pancreas in the anterior-posterior axis is 2.5, 2.0, and 2.0 cm at the head, body, and tail, respectively (13–15). The size of the pancreas decreases in older people and may be within normal limits when a carcinoma is small. Size, therefore, has limited significance in ultrasonography.

***Intensity of echoes.*** The intensity of parenchymal echoes equals or slightly exceeds that of the liver (16). The normal pancreatic parenchyma is filled with homogeneous fine echoes. This echogenicity increases in older people; deposition of fat within the pancreas apparently being the chief cause (17).

***Main pancreatic duct.*** A normal main pancreatic duct can be demonstrated as parallel echogenic lines or one strong echoic line (18, 19). The main duct is most easily detected in the body of the pancreas, where a diameter of 2 mm is the upper limit of the normal range. Sometimes, changes in the diameter of the duct are noted during examination because of expulsion of pancreatic juice through the papilla of Vater.

### Acute Pancreatitis

The ultrasonographic examination of patients with acute pancreatitis is made more difficult by severe pain and tenderness and by accumulation of intestinal gas secondary to paralytic ileus (20). Moreover, minimal pathologic changes resulting from mild forms of acute pancreatitis may not appear on ultrasonograms. The role of ultrasound, therefore, is limited to the assessment of severity and to comparison of changes on follow-up examinations (21, 22). The examination may also reveal specific etiologic factors such as gallstones (23).

**Sonographic Findings of Acute Pancreatitis.** Sonographic findings of acute pancreatitis are divided into direct and indirect findings.

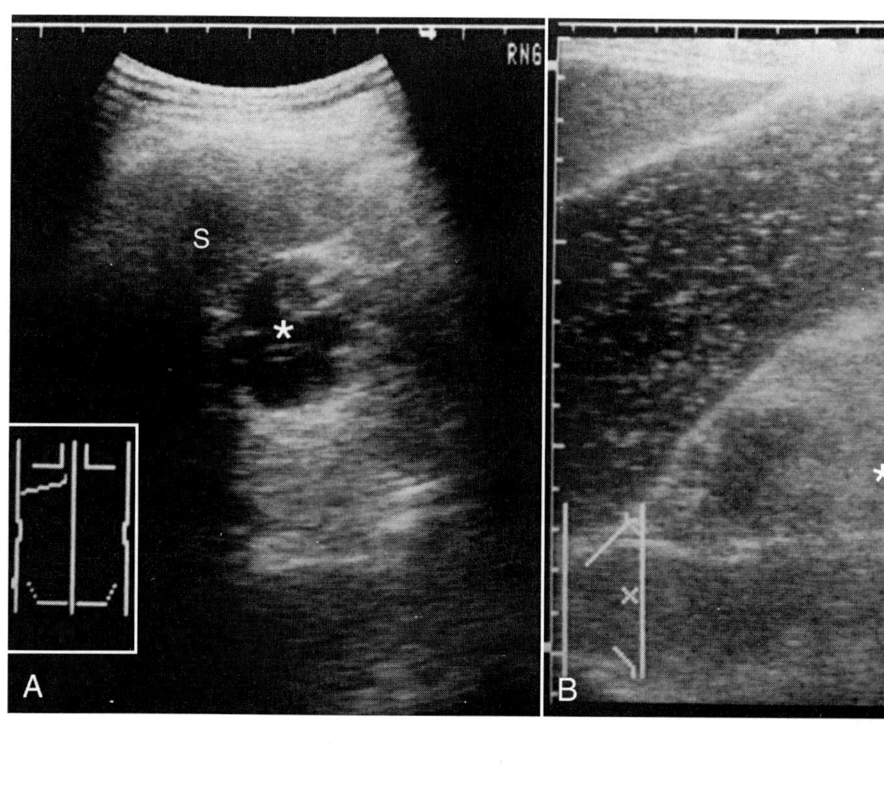


**FIG. 4.2.** Acoustic windows for the pancreas, demonstrating a cystadenoma of the tail of the pancreas. Fluid-filled stomach and the spleen are used as acoustic windows. **A.** A cystadenoma (*) of the tail of the pancreas is depicted through the spleen *(S)* on an intercostal scan. **B.** In a supine position, the cystadenoma (*) can be demonstrated through the fluid-filled stomach.

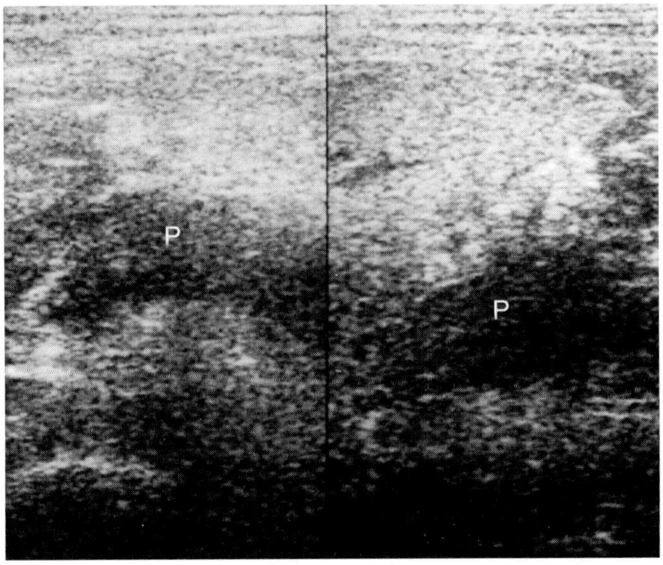


**FIG. 4.3.** Acute pancreatitis. Diffuse enlargement and diminished echogenicity indicate edematous pancreatitis *(P)*. The definition of pancreatic margin is obscure. *Left,* transverse scan; *right,* longitudinal scan.

***Direct findings.*** Although localized swelling of the pancreas may be encountered, diffuse enlargement is more characteristic and can be detected in more than 60% of patients with moderate or severe acute pancreatitis. Poor definition of the pancreatic margin may indicate extension of inflammation into adjacent structures, a finding that is noted in approximately one-third of patients. The internal echo pattern is homogeneous and less echogenic than is normal in edematous pancreatitis (24) (Fig. 4.3); a heterogeneous echo pattern is characteristic of hemorrhagic or necrotizing pancreatitis (25) (Fig. 4.4).

***Indirect findings.*** An important clue to the diagnosis of acute pancreatitis is the detection of a fluid collection around the pancreas (26, 27). A small amount of fluid may appear immediately anterior to the pancreas as a thin hypoechoic area (Fig. 4.4*A*). As the amount of fluid increases, irregularly shaped anechoic areas can be detected. As a pseudocyst evolves, this irregular fluid collection becomes encapsulated and assumes a round shape (28). Pancreatic ascites or pleural effusion is easily demonstrated on sonography, reflecting a severe form of acute pancreatitis. Biliary diseases, such as gallbladder or common bile ductal stones or cholecystitis, can be detected by ultrasound and provide significant information relative to etiology and treatment.

### Significance of Ultrasound

Ultrasound can indicate the severity of acute pancreatitis. Mild, moderate, and severe forms can be differentiated by interpretation of echoes from the parenchyma. Pancreatic abscess and thrombosis of the portal vein, which are severe complications, are often easily diagnosed by ultrasonography, although differentiating infected from noninfected peripancreatic necrosis may require percutaneous aspiration for bacterial culture. Such aspiration can be performed under ultrasonic guidance.

### Chronic Pancreatitis

The sonographic characteristics of chronic pancreatitis include dilatation of the pancreatic duct with or without calculi (29) and heterogeneous echogenicity of the parenchyma. Ultrasonographic findings of chronic pancreatitis vary, depending on the clinical stage, extent of inflammation, fibrosis, calcification, and changes in the pancreatic duct as well as in changes in adjacent organs. The exocrine function is poorly correlated with sonographic alterations (30).

**Pancreatic Calculi.** Pancreatic calculi are depicted as strong echoes, often with posterior shadowing in the main pancreatic duct or in the smaller ducts (31). Although a large stone has an acoustic shadow, smaller ones may not but occasionally combine to produce cometlike echoes (Fig. 4.5). The presence of many stones may enhance the echogenicity of the parenchyma so that it becomes difficult to distinguish the pancreas from the intestines. A calcified pseudocyst may also be confused with the intestines.

Computerized tomography is superior to ultrasonography in demonstrating pancreatic calculi, but ultrasound may have an advantage in demonstrating the relationship between stones and a dilated pancreatic duct. Protein plugs, which have been described as the precursors of stones, are also depicted as strong echoes. Echogenicity of the protein plug, however, is lower than that of calculi. Its differentiation from a tumor is mandatory.

**Dilatation of the Main Pancreatic Duct.** The wall of the dilated pancreatic duct may be smooth or irregular (32). Smooth dilatation reflects the mild changes of chronic pancreatitis; irregular dilatation reflects fibrosis of the parenchyma and is pathognomonic for severe chronic pancreatitis.

**Size, Shape, and Consistency of the Pancreas.** Enlargement of the chronically inflamed pancreas may be generalized or localized. Echogenicity is decreased by fibrosis of the parenchyma, but edema associated with acute pancreatitis, which may be superimposed on chronic pancreatitis, may also cause hypoechoic changes in the parenchyma. Ultrasonography cannot

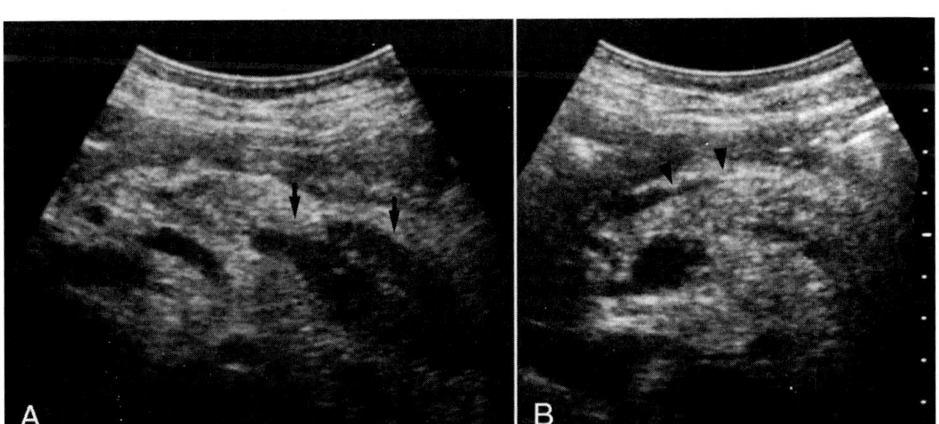


**FIG. 4.4.** Acute pancreatitis. **A.** Parenchyma of the pancreas, especially in the tail shows heterogeneity *(arrows)*. **B.** A thin collection of fluid is recognized anterior to the head of the pancreas *(arrowheads)*. The diagnosis of hemorrhagic or necrotizing pancreatitis can be made.

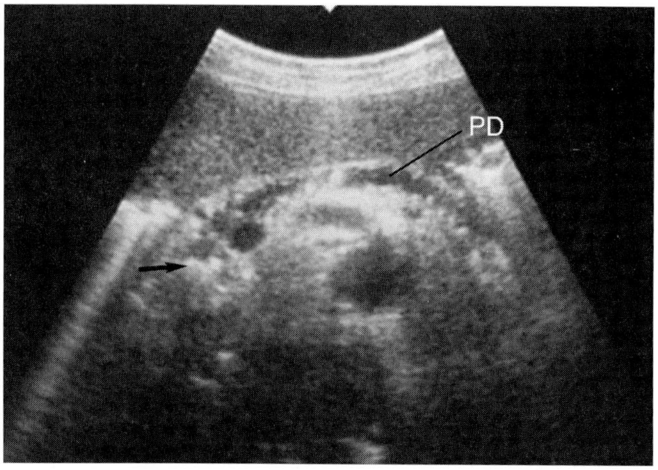


**FIG. 4.5.** Chronic pancreatitis. The main pancreatic *(PD)* duct is dilated, and pancreatic calculi are depicted as strong echoes. In the head of the pancreas, strong echoes combine cometlike echoes *(arrow)*.

differentiate between edema and fibrosis of the parenchyma; clinical findings are needed for evaluation. Edematous swelling may disappear with time.

A localized enlargement of the pancreas in chronic pancreatitis should be differentiated from carcinoma of the pancreas, which requires consideration of CT, endoscopic retrograde cholangiopancreatography (ERCP), and biopsy (33). When the main pancreatic duct penetrates deeply into the enlargement, or when upstream dilatation of the pancreatic duct is slight compared with the size of the tumor, a diagnosis of chronic pancreatitis is probable.

**Significance of Ultrasonic Findings.** Pancreatic calculi, thick-walled pseudocysts, or irregularly shaped dilatation of the main pancreatic duct are pathognomonic for chronic pancreatitis, and pseudoaneurysm of the splenic artery is highly suggestive. Coarse echoes in the parenchyma is a complementary finding, whose interpretation may require histologic definition.

### Pancreatic Neoplasm

Tumors of the pancreas can be classified into two patterns: solid and cystic tumors. Although a solid tumor may be complicated by cystic degeneration, so that the borderline between the two patterns is sometimes obscured, this classification is convenient for describing the ultrasonic patterns of pancreatic neoplasms.

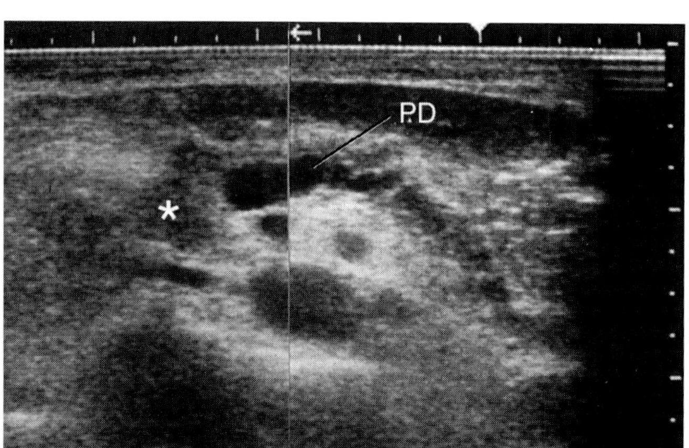


**FIG. 4.6.** Dilatation of the main pancreatic duct *(PD)* is a key to diagnosing pancreatic lesions. An irregularly shaped hypoechoic mass (*) is depicted at the point of obstruction.

**Pancreatic Screening.** A diagnosis of pancreatic tumor is made by demonstration of an area of abnormal echogenic pattern. A solid pancreatic tumor usually appears hypoechoic or reflects a mixture of hypoechoic and hyperechoic patterns. A cystic tumor is easily detected when an anechoic mass is demonstrated, but the tumor becomes echogenic, as does a hemangioma of the liver, when the tumor is composed of many tiny cysts or vascular spaces. In malignant tumors, especially in ductal carcinoma of the pancreas, the distal (upstream) segment of the main pancreatic duct may be dilated secondary to obstruction by the tumor. Dilatation may reach 8 to 10 mm in diameter, but 3 to 6 mm is more common. A highly dilated duct becomes tortuous, and a transverse scan of the dilated duct depicts it as a chain of beads. When dilatation is slight, a smooth wall is demonstrated, and two strong echoic lines, depicting its anterior and posterior walls, are noted. A dilated main pancreatic duct is usually anechoic, but cellular debris or mucus may generate echoes within it. A dilated main pancreatic duct is frequently a clue to the diagnosis of pancreatic neoplasm. Once a dilated duct is detected, the pancreatic parenchyma around the point of obstruction should be carefully defined (Fig. 4.6).

#### Solid Tumors of the Pancreas

***Ductal carcinoma.*** Ductal adenocarcinoma is the most common histologic type of pancreatic carcinoma. In more than 90% of clinically defined ductal cancers, abnormal echo pattern can be detected (34–37). Internal echoes are hypoechoic in almost all tumors smaller than 3 cm in diameter (Fig. 4.7), although precise observation may find slight heterogeneity. Tumors larger than 5 cm in diameter contain patchy hyperechoic areas, but homogeneous hyperechoic pattern is scarce (Fig. 4.8). In cancers with a rather homogeneous histologic pattern (e.g., medullary or scirrhous patterns), the echo pattern is homogeneous. The echo pattern is homogeneously hypoechoic because acoustic interfaces are scant. Necrosis or bleeding within a tumor is highly echogenic, producing heterogeneous high echoes. Cystic degeneration is another pattern of necrosis.

Localized enlargement may be the only manifestation of the tumor, but conventional ultrasonography may not demonstrate "localized enlargement" of a tumor less than 2 cm in diameter. In almost all instances, dilatation of the main pancreatic duct can be delineated. The wall of the main pancreatic duct has a smooth or beaded appearance. When a retention cyst or a pseudocyst complicates the carcinoma, it results in an associated cystic pattern. Ultrasound can also delineate vascular involvement to the portal vein (38) or the superior mesenteric artery ("cuff sign") (39).

Squamous carcinoma is another rare form of ductal carcinoma. Its margins are rather clear, and heterogeneous internal echoes are common. When cystic areas can be determined within the tumor, this lesion is a likely diagnosis.

Acinar cell carcinoma is also a rare histologic subtype among pancreatic carcinomas. The margins of the tumor are described as rather clear and smooth with heterogeneous internal echoes.

***Islet cell tumors.*** Typical findings of islet cell tumors are a round, well-circumscribed tumor with smooth margins and homogeneous internal echoes (40). With an islet cell tumor less than 2 cm in diameter, detectability depends on its location: tumors located in the body of the pancreas are most easily demonstrated (Fig. 4.9). This tumor is hypervascular, but color-flow mapping is only occasionally demonstrable. Echogenicity may be very low in some instances, so that this tumor has to be differentiated from a small cyst. Usually it does not alter the diameter of the main pancreatic duct.

Islet cell carcinomas usually show expansive growth that can be detected on ultrasonograms. The margins are smooth and

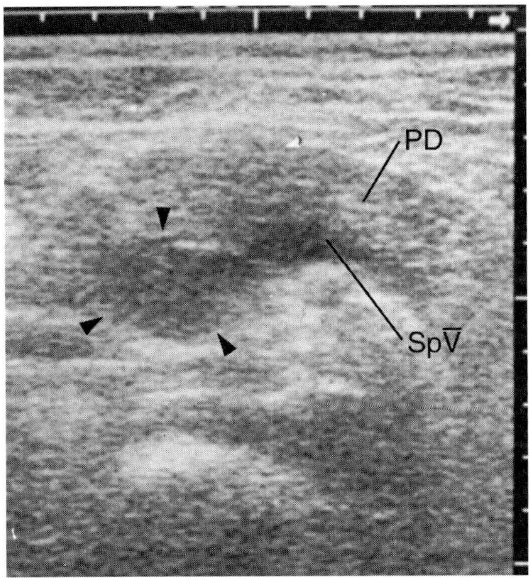


**FIG. 4.7.** Small ductal carcinoma of the pancreas. Hypoechoic mass *(arrow heads)* is depicted in the head of the pancreas. The tumor is located in the uncinate lobe and does not affect the diameter of the main pancreatic duct *(PD); SpV,* splenic vein.

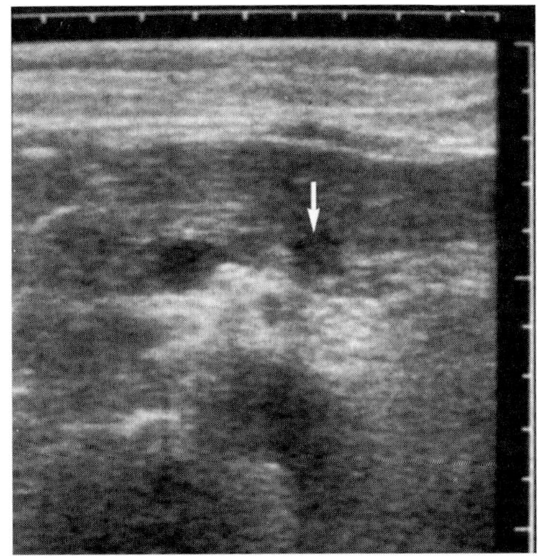

**FIG. 4.9.** Insulinoma of the pancreas. Islet cell tumors are basically hypoechoic tumors *(arrow).* Internal echoes are homogeneous, and the margin is clear.

clear, even in tumors larger than 5 cm in diameter. Bleeding or necrosis may yield echogenic spots or cystic areas within the tumor. The main pancreatic duct is often deviated by the tumor but is seldom obstructed. Dilatation of the duct is rare.

***Other rare tumors.*** Carcinoids of the pancreas show expansive growth, as do the islet cell tumors, so that this tumor also appears well circumscribed with smooth margins. When the tumor enlarges, irregular internal echoes may appear.

Papillary cystic and solid tumors of the pancreas frequently occur in females in their 2nd or 3rd decade of life. The size of the tumor at diagnosis varies from a few centimeters to 10 cm in diameter. Smooth and clear margins and a round shape are characteristic findings. Internal echoes reflect a mixture of irregularly shaped cysts and parenchymal patterns (41, 42). Calcification is common and is depicted as strong echoes. When the tumor is small, differentiation from islet cell tumor is difficult because both tumors are hypoechoic.

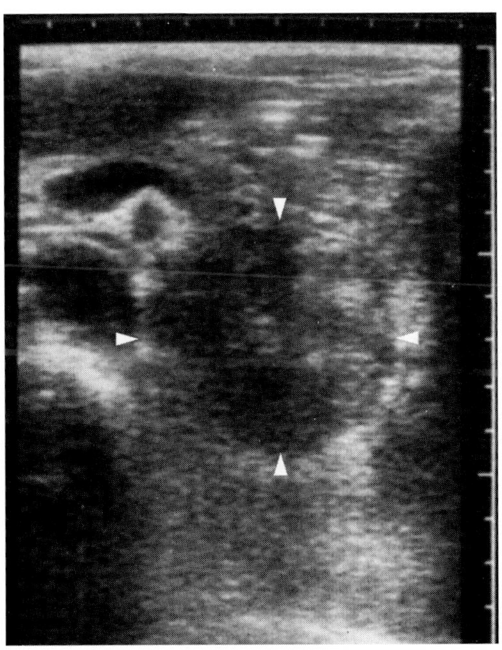

**FIG. 4.8.** Large ductal carcinoma of the tail of the pancreas. If the the tumor exceeds 5 cm *(arrowheads),* heterogeneous internal echoes become a common feature.

### Cystic Tumors of the Pancreas

***Cystadenoma and cystadenocarcinoma.*** Serous cystadenoma consists of small cysts up to 2 cm in diameter. Sonography reflects the cut surface of the tumor, which appears as a sponge, depicting a hyperechoic tumor (Fig. 4.10) (43, 44). This pattern is similar in echogenicity to that of hemangioma of the liver. Some cysts may be large enough to depict an anechoic pattern within the tumor. An atypical tumor composed of several cysts of 1 cm or more appears as a multilocular cyst (45).

Basically, mucinous cystadenomas and mucinous cystadenocarcinomas demonstrate similar sonographic patterns, as both tumors have macroscopically similar appearances. Differentiation between their benign and malignant nature is, therefore, difficult. Tumors larger than 5 cm in diameter, with well-circumscribed margins, consisting of cystic tumors of various sizes, appear sonographically as multilocular cysts (46). Hyperechoic projections into the lumen of a cyst are often noted and may indicate a malignant nature or malignant potential of the tumor. Calcification of the wall or capsule appears as a hyperechoic line (46). Changes in the main pancreatic duct are slight, seldom including ductal dilatation.

***Mucinous papillary cystic tumors with ductal ectasia.*** The mucinous papillary cystic tumors with ductal ectasia are highly productive of mucin, which causes marked dilatation of the pancreatic duct. This tumor is classified in two types: main pancreatic ductal type and branch type. Even in the branch type, the main pancreatic duct may become dilated, as mucin produced by the tumor in the ductal branches pools in the main duct. In the main ductal type, a polypoid lesion in the dilated main pancreatic duct can be detected by weak echoes on ultrasound (47). The sonographic pattern of the branch type resembles that of multilocular cysts, because transcutaneous ultrasound is unable to delineate individual dilated ducts. Histologically, the spread of atypical cells along the surface of the

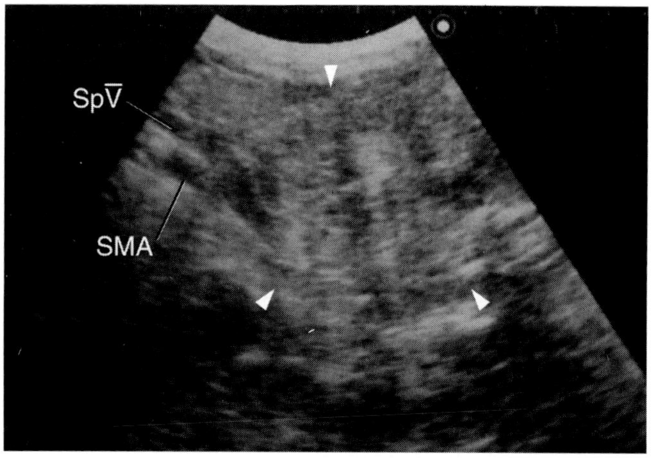


**FIG. 4.10.** Serous cystadenoma of the pancreas. Hyperechoic mass *(arrowheads)* is depicted in the tail of the pancreas on transverse scan. Because of its echogenicity, the margin is obscure. Posterior echo enhancement is also unclear, as is the number of cysts, delineated as an anechoic area. *SpV,* splenic vein; *SMA,* superior mesenteric artery.

pancreatic duct is often seen in both types, as atypical cells change to hyperplasia and then to normal epithelium. Such transitions are impossible to diagnose on sonography.

## REFERENCES

1. Fishbein R, Murphy GP, Wilder RJ. The pleuropulmonary manifestations of pancreatitis. Dis Chest 1962;41:392–397.
2. Stein GN, Kalser MH, Sapian NN, Fikelstein A. An evaluation of the roentgen changes in acute pancreatitis: correlation with clinical findings. Gastroenterology 1959;36:354–358.
3. Brascho DJ, Reynolds RN. The radiographic "colon cut-off sign" in acute pancreatitis. Radiology 1962;79:763–768.
4. Price CWR. The colon cut-off sign in acute pancreatitis. Med J Aust 1956;1:313–317.
5. Minagi H, Margolin FR. Pancreatic calcifications. Am J Gastroenterol 1972;57:139–145.
6. Sifre RA, Stenberg ES, Graybill LDS. Roentogenographic configuration of the duodenojejunal area in carcinoma of the pancreas. Geriatrics 1953;8:486–493.
7. Frostberg N. Characteristic duodenal deformity in cases of different kinds of perivaterian enlargement of the pancreas. Acta Radiol 1938;19:164–169.
8. Mallet-Guy P, Jacquemet P. Results of 500 cases of hypotonic duodenography. J Radiol Electrol 1963;44:249–255.
9. Goldstein HM, Zboralske FF. Tubeless hypotonic duodenography. JAMA 1969;210:2086–2088.
10. Goldstein HM, Katragadda CS. Prone view ultrasonography for pancreatic tail neoplasms. Am J Roentgenol 1978;131: 231–234.
11. Warren PS, Garret WJ, Kossoff G. The liquid filled stomach—an ultrasonic window to the upper abdomen J Clin Ultrasound 1978;6:315–320.
12. Wieghall SL, Wolfman NT, Watson N. The fluid-filled stomach; a new sonic window. J Clin Ultrasound 1979;7:353–356.
13. Weill F, Schraub A, Eisenscher A, Bourgoin A. Ultrasonography of the normal pancreas: success rate and criteria for normality. Radiology 1977;123:417–423.
14. de Graaff CS, Taylor KJ, Simonds BD, Rosenfield AJ. Gray-scale echography of the pancreas: re-evaluation of normal size. Radiology 1978;129:157–161.
15. Arger PH, Mulhern CB, Bonavita JA, et al. An analysis of pancreatic sonography in suspected pancreatic disease. J Clin Ultrasound 1979;7:91–97.
16. Filly RA, London SS. The normal pancreas; acoustic characteristics and frequency of imaging. J Clin Ultrasound 1979;7:121–124.
17. Marks WM, Filly RA, Callen PW. Ultrasonic evaluation of normal pancreatic echogenicity and its relationship to fat deposition. Radiology 1980;137:475–479.
18. Parulekar SG. Ultrasonic evaluation of the pancreatic duct. J Clin Ultrasound 1980;8:457–463.
19. Bryan PJ. Appearance of normal pancreatic duct: a study using real-time ultrasound. J Clin Ultrasound 1982;10:63–66.
20. Block S, Maier W, Bittner R, et al. Identification of pancreas necrosis in severe acute pancreatitis: imaging procedures versus clinical staging. Gut 1986;27:1035–1042.
21. Johnson ML, Mack LA. Ultrasonic evaluation of the pancreas. Gastrointest Radiol 1978;3:257–266.
22. McKay AJ, Imrie CW, O'Neill J, Duncan JG. Is an early ultrasound scan of value in acute pancreatitis? Br J Surg 1982;69: 369–372.
23. Neoptolemos JP, Hall AW, Finlay DF, et al. The urgent diagnosis of gallstones in acute pancreatitis: a prospective study of three methods. Br J Surg 1984;71:230–233.
24. Silverstein W, Isikoff MB, Hill MC, Barkin J. Diagnostic imaging of acute pancreatitis: prospective study using CT and sonography. AJR 1981;137:497–502.
25. Russell JG, Vallon AG, Braganza JM, Howat HT. Ultrasonic scanning in pancreatic disease. Gut 1978;19:1027–1033.
26. Hashimoto BE, Laing FC, Jeffrey RB Jr, Federle MP. Hemorrhagic pancreatic fluid collections examined by ultrasound. Radiology 1984;150:803–808.
27. Jeffrey RB JR, Laing FC, Wing VW. Extrapancreatic spread of acute pancreatitis: new observations with real-time US. Radiology 1986;159:707–711.
28. Gonzalez AC, Bradley EL, Clements JL JR. Pseudocyst formation in acute pancreatitis; ultrasonographic evaluation of 99 cases. AJR 1976;127:315–317.
29. Niederau C, Grendell JH. Diagnosis of chronic pancreatitis. Gastroenterology 1985;88:1973–1995.
30. Bolondi L, Priori P, Gullo L, et al. Relationship between morphological changes detected by ultrasonography and pancreatic exocrine function in chronic pancreatitis. Pancreas 1987;2: 222–229.
31. Weinstein BJ, Weinstein DP, Brodmerkel GJ Jr. Ultrasonography of pancreatic lithiasis. Radiology 1980;134:185–189.
32. Bastid C, Sahel J, Filho M, Sarles H. Diameter of the main pancreatic duct in chronic calcifying pancreatitis. Pancreas 1990;5:524–527.
33. Lammer J, Herlinger H, Zalaudek G, Hofler H. Pseudotumorous pancreatitis. Gastrointest Radiol 1985;10:59–67.
34. Pollock D, Taylor KJ. Ultrasound scanning in patients with clinical suspicion of pancreatic cancer: a retrospective study. Cancer 1981;47:1662–1665.
35. Wang TH, Lin JT, Chen DS, Sheu JC, Sung JL. Noninvasive diagnosis of advanced pancreatic cancer by real-time ultrasonography, carcinoembryonic antigen, and carbohydrate antigen 19-9. Pancreas 1986;1:219–223.
36. DelMaschio A, Vanzulli A, Sironi S, et al. Pancreatic cancer versus chronic pancreatitis: diagnosis with CA 19-9 assessment, US, CT, and CT-guided fine-needle biopsy. Radiology 1991;178:95–99.
37. Nakaizumi A, Tatsuta M, Uehara H, et al. A prospective trial of early detection of pancreatic cancer by ultrasonographic examination combined with measurement of serum elastase 1. Cancer 1992;69:936–940.
38. Campbell JP, Wilson SR. Pancreatic neoplasms: how useful is evaluation with US? Radiology 1988;167:341–344.
39. Kosuge T, Makuuchi M, Takayama T, et al. Thickening at the root of the superior mesenteric artery on sonography: evidence of vascular involvement in patients with cancer of the pancreas. AJR 1991;156:69–72.
40. Gunther RW, Klose KJ, Ruckert K, et al. Localization of small islet-cell tumors. Preoperative and intraoperative ultrasound, computed tomography, arteriography, digital subtraction angiography, and pancreatic venous sampling. Gastrointest Radiol 1985;10:145–152.
41. Friedman AC, Lichtenstein JE, Fishman EK, et al. Solid and papillary epithelial neoplasm of the pancreas. Radiology 1985; 154:333–337.

42. Todani T, Shimada K, Watanabe Y, et al. Frantz's tumor: a papillary and cystic tumor of the pancreas in girls. J Pediatr Surg 1988;23:116–121.
43. Itai Y, Ohhashi K, Furui S, et al. Microcystic adenoma of the pancreas: spectrum of computed tomographic findings. J Comput Assist Tomogr 1988;12:797–803.
44. Buck JL, Hayes WS. From the archives of the AFIP. Microcystic adenoma of the pancreas. Radiographics 1990;10:313–322.
45. Lewandrowski K, Warshaw A, Compton C. Macrocystic serous cystadenoma of the pancreas: a morphologic variant differing from microcystic adenoma. Hum Pathol 1992;23:871–875.
46. Bastid C, Sahel J, Sastre B, Schurger P, Sarles H. Mucinous cystadenocarcinoma of the pancreas. Ultrasonographic findings in 5 cases. Acta Radiol 1989;30:45–47.
47. Yamaguchi K, Tanaka M. Mucin-hypersecreting tumor of the pancreas with mucin extrusion through an enlarged papilla. Am J Gastroenterol 1991;86:835–839.

# 5

# Computed Tomography and Magnetic Resonance Imaging

Thomas L. Lawson, Mary C. Olson, and Harold V. Posniak

There are several methods currently available for imaging the pancreas. Sonography, a full discussion of which appears in another chapter, is inexpensive, is readily available, and in thin patients provides good images of the pancreas and biliary system. However, gas within overlying bowel loops can obscure the pancreas, and in large patients imaging is difficult and frequently limited. Endoscopic and operative ultrasound, while providing excellent images of the pancreas, provide a small field of view and are invasive. Magnetic resonance (MR) imaging provides multiplanar imaging of the upper abdomen and high soft tissue contrast. Newer pulse sequences and the use of intravenous MR contrast agents give high spatial resolution images and have improved the ability to differentiate malignant from inflammatory tissue (1–3). However, there are several disadvantages, including long imaging time, high cost, limited availability, and the high level of expertise and experience required for accurate interpretation. In some patients, it is technically difficult to obtain an examination with superior diagnostic image quality. Nevertheless, there does appear to be a developing role for MRI for problem solving in difficult cases.

Contrast-enhanced computed tomography (CT) remains the most accurate noninvasive imaging modality for pancreatic evaluation. It is readily available, diagnostic criteria are well established and accepted, and patient acceptance is high. Recent technical advancement in CT, including the development of helical (spiral) CT with slip-ring detectors and improved high heat capacity tubes, allows continuous imaging of the patient over a 30-second or longer interval (4–6). This technique has the advantage of markedly reduced total imaging time and the ability to obtain scans with high spatial resolution during peak intravascular and organ enhancement following the intravenous administration of iodinated contrast material.

With helical CT scan, there is continuous rotation of the tube and detector around the patient with continuous data acquisition as the patient is slowly advanced through the scanning gantry. With conventional axial CT, a single image is obtained during the tube and detector rotation. The table and patient are indexed to a new location and subsequent axial images are obtained. This is a much slower technique. However, it is occasionally useful in very large patients or if very narrow collimation is being utilized, as a much greater amount of x-ray can be delivered, which improves image quality.

Contrast-enhanced helical CT of the pancreas is the initial diagnostic modality of choice in patients with a high probability of pancreatic carcinoma (7). It is very accurate in the detection of pancreatic carcinoma, in part because of the relatively advanced stage of most pancreatic carcinomas at the time of initial presentation as well as the high spatial and contrast resolution of modern CT scanners and the well-established diagnostic criteria. In addition, once a mass is detected, histologic confirmation of the diagnosis may be made by CT-guided fine-needle aspiration biopsy. However, while CT is extremely accurate in the detection of pancreatic adenocarcinoma, it is much less accurate in predicting the stage and extent of disease. In a substantial number of patients, CT will under- or overestimate the extent of disease and surgical resectability (8, 9).

It may be difficult on CT to separate those patients with chronic pancreatitis from those with carcinoma. Both diseases may demonstrate focal masses, pancreatic and biliary ductal dilation, and pseudocyst. The imaging diagnosis of chronic pancreatitis usually rests with the identification of pancreatic calcifications, whereas diagnosis of pancreatic carcinoma usually rests on the identification of metastatic disease, although this may be subtle.

With current MR pulse sequences, the pancreas can be well visualized by MRI. In addition, following the administration of intravenous gadolinium contrast agents, differences in enhancement patterns between the normal pancreas, pancreatitis, and carcinoma can be identified (10). However, at the present time, CT should remain the initial imaging modality in the evaluation of pancreatic disease. Patients should be referred for MRI in the following situations: when a clinical history suggests pancreatic disease and findings at CT are equivocal, when distinguishing focal pancreatitis from pancreatic carcinoma when the CT and endoscopic retrograde cholangiopancreatography (ERCP) findings are confusing, and when impaired renal function or allergy to iodinated contrast will limit the value of CT. As MR pulse sequences continue to improve and as more experience is gained with this modality in the evaluation of pancreatic lesions and problem solving in difficult cases, a larger role for MR investigation of pancreatic disease is expected.

## TECHNIQUE

### CT Evaluation of the Pancreas

Pancreatic abnormalities may be detected during a survey examination in which the entire abdomen, as well as adjacent anatomic areas, is being imaged. Alternatively, a pancreatic lesion may be known or suspected, and a dedicated imaging sequence focused on the pancreas is performed. The technique will be different in these two situations.

The general abdominal survey examination is usually obtained following oral administration of contrast material to opacify bowel loops and eliminate any diagnostic problems that may occur when unopacified loops of bowel mimic a mass. Iodinated intravenous contrast material is also usually given if the patient's renal function is normal and there is no history of allergy. The use of intravenous contrast material markedly increases diagnostic accuracy and confidence. The intravenous contrast material should be given with a uniphasic rapid (2–4 mL/sec) injection. An appropriate time delay from contrast injection to image acquisition for a general abdominal survey examination is 50–70 seconds.

When performing a focused CT scan of the pancreas, noncontrast scans are usually first performed to localize the pancreas and to evaluate for calcifications. Once the pancreas is localized, images of the pancreas are obtained with a relatively small field of view (20–24 cm) and narrow collimation (3–5 mm) to maximize spatial resolution. Iodinated contrast material is administered intravenously at a faster rate than in a survey abdominal examination (3–5 mL/sec), and a rapid series of helical scans is obtained through the pancreas, starting approximately 30 seconds after contrast material injection (the arterial phase). The arterial phase is useful for evaluating the peripancreatic arteries as well as vascular pancreatic lesions. Immediately following the arterial phase images, a second set of images is obtained through the liver and pancreas during the portal venous phase (approximately 60–70 seconds following contrast injection). This second phase optimizes visualization of the pancreatic parenchyma as well as the liver. The normal pancreatic parenchyma enhances, while neoplasms and areas of fibrosis will enhance less and be low in attenuation.

### MRI Evaluation of the Pancreas

In the past, MRI played a limited role in detection of pancreatic abnormalities because of artifacts and poor spatial resolution. However, new techniques and the increasing experience with the use of intravenous contrast agents (gadolinium) have dramatically improved the sensitivity and usefulness of MRI (Fig. 5.1). It is beyond the scope of this chapter to discuss MR physics and the multiple pulse sequences that may be used to image the pancreas. However, the fat surrounding the pancreas provides an excellent inherent contrast to visualize the pancreas. The use of long and short pulse sequences, breath-holding sequences, gradient echo techniques, fat suppression, and intravenous gadolinium provide MR with several advantages over CT (10). Several authors have published encouraging results in the differentiation of chronic pancreatitis from carcinoma (11). However, imaging characteristics of fibrosis due to pancreatitis and fibrosis due to desmoplasia stimulated by carcinoma are similar and prevent accurate diagnosis in some cases.

The normal pancreas has a higher signal intensity than the adjacent liver, probably because of the slightly higher fluid content of the pancreas. In patients with acute pancreatitis, morphologic changes similar to those seen on CT may be demonstrated. In patients with chronic pancreatitis, signal intensity is lower because of fibrosis and calcifications. Pseudocysts will have imaging characteristics similar to those of other fluid in the upper abdomen such as bile or cerebrospinal fluid in the spinal canal. Pancreatic carcinoma has variable signal intensity, usually being low on short pulse sequences and nonhomogeneously high on long pulse sequences (12, 13). Because adenocarcinoma is relatively avascular, carcinoma will enhance less than the normal pancreas following intravenous contrast (Fig. 5.2).

## ACUTE PANCREATITIS

Although the initial diagnosis of acute pancreatitis is based upon clinical and laboratory parameters, radiology plays an important role in the subsequent evaluation of these patients. First, there are a number of radiologic findings that may help to substantiate the clinical diagnosis. Second, radiologic imaging is important for early detection of complications of acute pancreatitis (necrosis, abscess, pseudocyst) or for planning subsequent medical or surgical treatment. Third, once the primary inflammatory process has subsided, radiologic techniques may be used to identify surgically correctable anatomic abnormalities responsible for the disease.

In mild acute pancreatitis, the pancreas usually maintains a normal size and appearance. With more severe disease, there may be focal or diffuse enlargement. The contours of the gland may be well defined, or they may become indistinct because of edema and inflammation of the peripancreatic soft tissue. A halo of edema, manifested on CT by a relative increase in the attenuation of the peripancreatic fat, may surround the pancreas (Fig. 5.3). This and the presence of peripancreatic fluid are extremely important diagnostic signs. They may be the only CT abnormalities present in these patients (14). In severe pancreatitis, the gland is usually enlarged and complications may be present, including fluid collections, pseudocyst formation, or pancreatic necrosis. These are discussed later in this chapter.

Thickening of the renal fascia, edema in the peripancreatic soft tissues, and fluid collections in the lesser sac and anterior

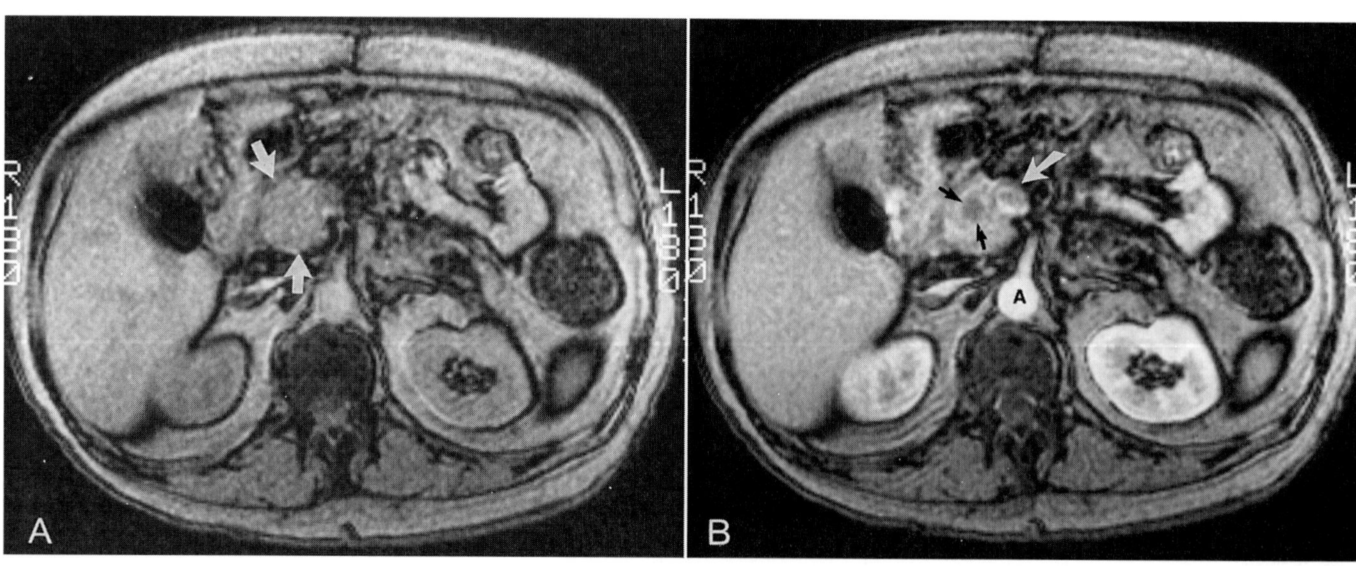


**FIG. 5.1.** Small pancreatic carcinoma. **A.** Non–contrast enhanced T1-weighted MRI of the head of the pancreas demonstrates uniform signal intensity and no pancreatic mass or enlargement *(white arrows)*. **B.** Following the administration of intravenous gadolinium, the normal pancreatic parenchyma enhances, whereas the hypovascular carcinoma *(black arrows)* remains relatively hypointense. The intravenous gadolinium increases the signal intensity in the superior mesenteric vein *(white arrow)* and aorta *(A)*.

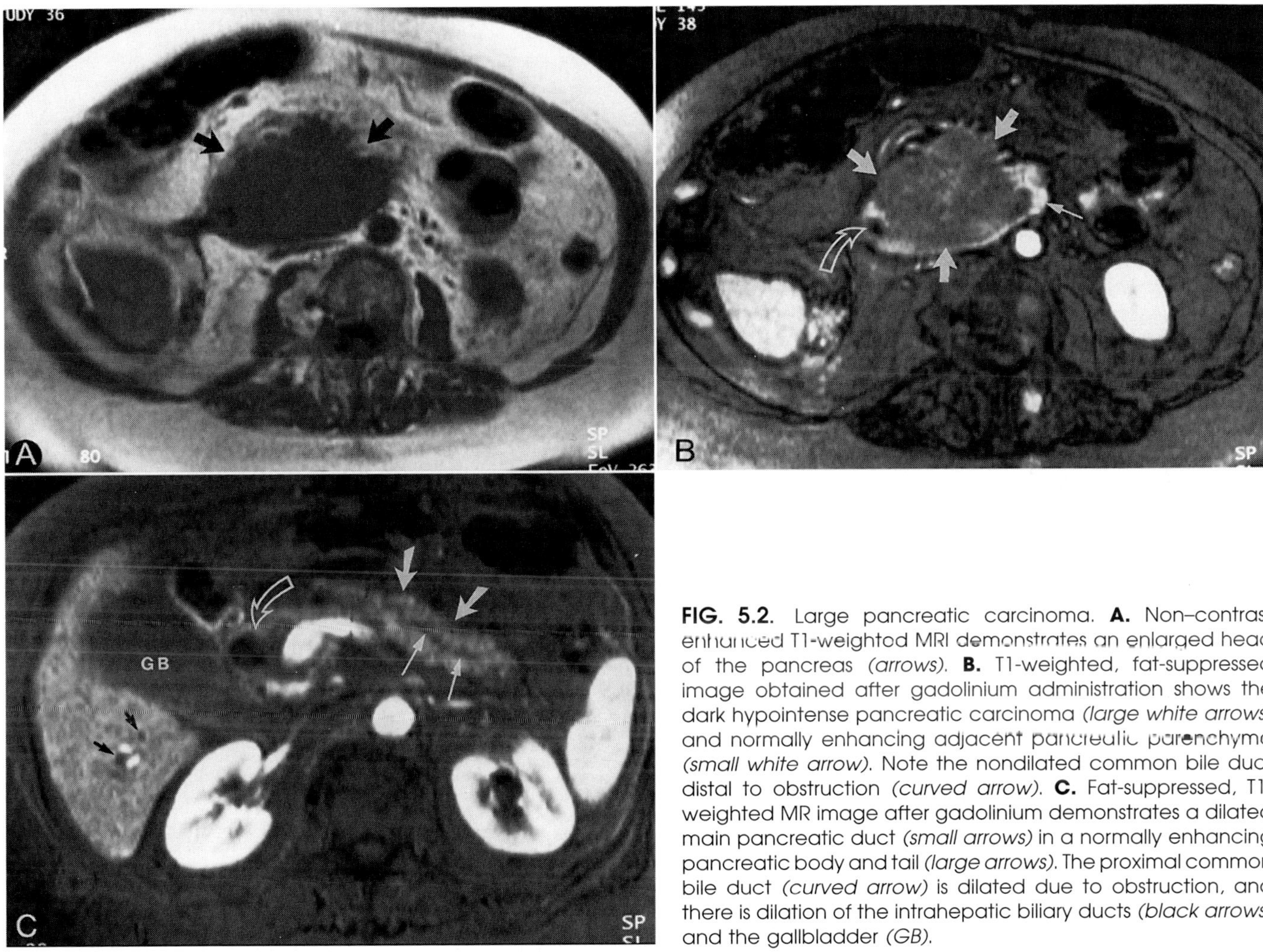


**FIG. 5.2.** Large pancreatic carcinoma. **A.** Non–contrast enhanced T1-weighted MRI demonstrates an enlarged head of the pancreas *(arrows)*. **B.** T1-weighted, fat-suppressed image obtained after gadolinium administration shows the dark hypointense pancreatic carcinoma *(large white arrows)* and normally enhancing adjacent pancreatic parenchyma *(small white arrow)*. Note the nondilated common bile duct distal to obstruction *(curved arrow)*. **C.** Fat-suppressed, T1-weighted MR image after gadolinium demonstrates a dilated main pancreatic duct *(small arrows)* in a normally enhancing pancreatic body and tail *(large arrows)*. The proximal common bile duct *(curved arrow)* is dilated due to obstruction, and there is dilation of the intrahepatic biliary ducts *(black arrows)* and the gallbladder *(GB)*.

pararenal spaces are the most commonly observed extrapancreatic findings during an early acute inflammatory episode.

## CHRONIC PANCREATITIS

Although the diagnosis of chronic pancreatitis is primarily based on clinical and laboratory findings, radiology may play several important roles in the evaluation of patients with known or suspected chronic pancreatitis. As with acute pancreatitis, it may be used to confirm the diagnosis in difficult cases. Radiologic evaluation may aid in the early diagnosis and assessment of complications resulting from the inflammatory process and may be used to identify a correctable anatomic cause of pancreatitis. Also, careful preoperative radiologic evaluation of the pancreatic and biliary ducts and vascular anatomy is essential for performing appropriate and safe surgery.

CT currently is the single best imaging modality for initial evaluation of patients with known or suspected chronic pancreatitis. The primary diagnostic features include pancreatic atrophy or enlargement, pancreatic ductal dilation, and calculi (Fig. 5.4). Thickening of peripancreatic fascia, pancreatic and extrapancreatic fluid collections, and biliary tract disease are secondary diagnostic features (15).

### Primary Diagnostic Features

Chronic pancreatitis may cause changes in the size of the pancreas, either atrophy or enlargement. The pancreas may be diffusely enlarged when recurrent acute pancreatitis is superimposed on chronic pancreatitis. However, focal enlargement, usually of the head, is common and may mimic the appearance of carcinoma (Fig. 5.5). In either case, a focal or diffuse mass without ancillary criteria to aid in specific diagnosis is nonspecific, and differentiation of inflammatory from neoplastic disease is often not possible by CT alone. In most cases, however, other findings, such as intraductal calcifications, indicate the correct diagnosis.

The pancreas is usually atrophic in patients with end-stage chronic pancreatitis. Interpretation of pancreatic size must include consideration of the age of the patient. The normal pancreas decreases in size as patients age, particularly by the seventh or eighth decade. Thus, in elderly patients, the presence of ancillary findings, such as intraductal calcifications, is helpful in diagnosis. Pancreatic atrophy also may occur as a response to ductal obstruction by neoplasm. In the latter case, an obvious pancreatic mass usually is seen, but several cases have been reported in which the mass was small and overlooked during CT evaluation. Patients with chronic pancreatitis may have a normal-size pancreas. In these cases, ancillary findings may be absent and lead to a false-negative CT diagnosis.

Evaluation of the pancreatic duct is important in examining patients with chronic pancreatitis. Current-generation helical CT scanners are able to demonstrate a portion of the normal pancreatic duct in about 80–90% of cases if optimal scan techniques and intravenous contrast are utilized. The normal pancreatic duct is seen as a thin, low-attenuation tubular structure. The measured internal diameter of the normal pancreatic duct averages up to 4 or 5 mm in the head and 2 mm in the body and tail. In addition to size, the configuration of the duct should be evaluated. The normal duct is relatively smooth in contour with parallel walls and is seen only for a short segment on one or two scan slices. When a long segment of the duct is seen, or if it is visible on many scan sections, it is likely to be dilated.

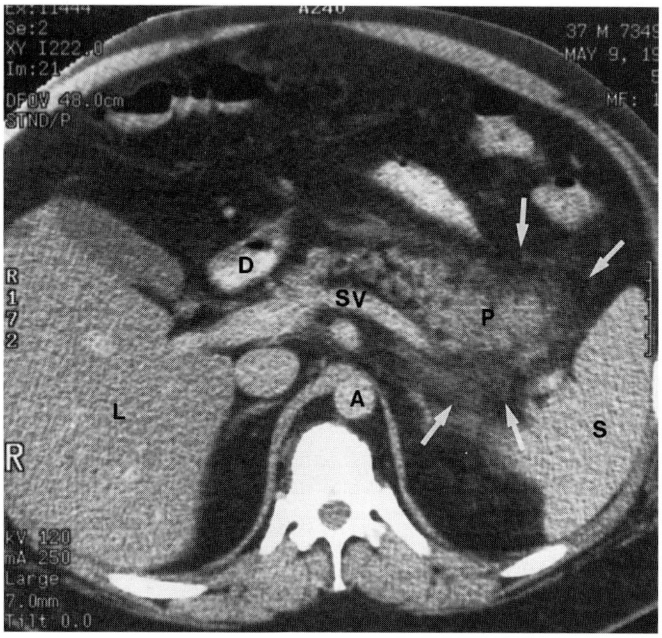


**FIG. 5.3.** Mild acute pancreatitis. Contrast-enhanced CT demonstrates a halo of edema *(arrows)* surrounding the pancreas *(P)*. The normal retroperitoneal fat is homogeneously black. The inflammatory process and edema increase the water content of the retroperitoneal fat and the attenuation, making it whiter. *A,* aorta; *L,* liver; *D,* duodenum; *S,* spleen; *SV,* splenic vein.

The normal pancreatic duct is seen most frequently by CT in cross section in the head of the gland medial to the common bile duct and in longitudinal section in the body. The duct usually is ventral to the common bile duct, cephalad to their junction, and medial to the bile duct at their periampullary confluence. One possible source of confusion is low insertion of the cystic duct into the common bile duct. The location of the pancreatic duct has been described as either central or within the dorsal one-third of the gland. However, the location is variable, and a more ventral position is not uncommon. These variations must be appreciated to avoid misinterpretation.

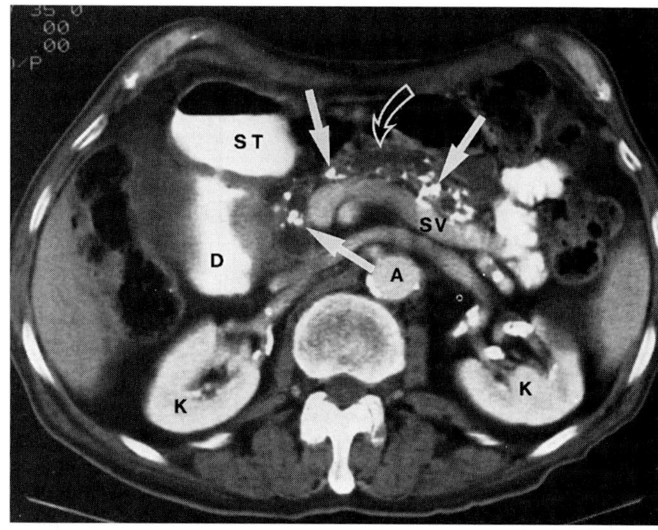


**FIG. 5.4.** Chronic calcific pancreatitis. Contrast-enhanced CT demonstrates marked pancreatic atrophy with virtually no pancreatic parenchyma identifiable. The pancreatic duct is dilated *(curved arrow)* and contains numerous calculi *(straight arrows)*. *ST,* stomach; *D,* duodenum; *A,* aorta; *K,* kidney.

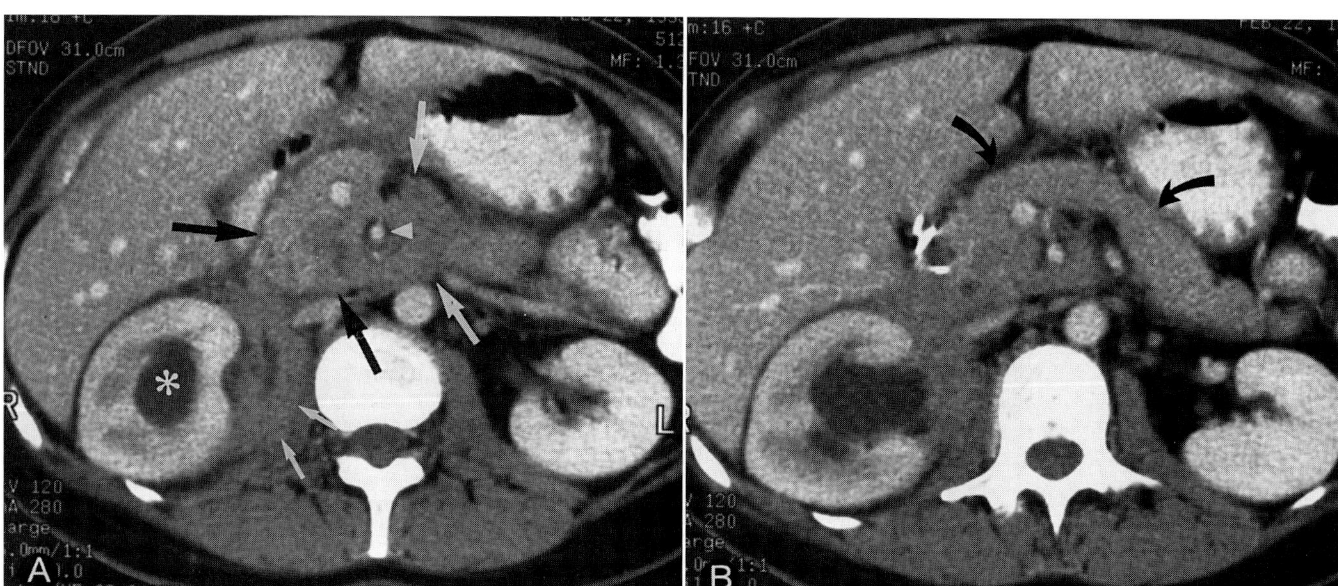


**FIG. 5.5.** Focal pancreatitis that mimics carcinoma. **A.** Contrast-enhanced CT demonstrates enlargement of the head of the pancreas *(black arrows)* with inflammatory fluid extending into the root of the mesentery *(long white arrows)* and the right perirenal space *(short white arrows)*, causing hydronephrosis *(asterisk)*. Note the halo of black low-attenuation fat that is preserved around the superior mesenteric artery *(arrowhead)*. This halo of fat is usually lost with pancreatic carcinoma. **B.** Contrast-enhanced CT 2 cm above (**A**) demonstrates normal enhancement of the body and tail of the pancreas *(curved arrows)*.

A dilated and/or irregular pancreatic duct is commonly demonstrated in cases of chronic pancreatitis. If the ductal diameter is greater than 5 mm in the head or 2 mm in the body or tail, the duct is considered dilated. The walls of the dilated duct may appear outwardly convex with small areas of focal ectasia and may be either smooth or irregular. ERCP has demonstrated that the appearance of the dilated pancreatic duct in carcinoma and chronic pancreatitis may be similar. Thus, attempts to correlate ductal diameter and wall morphology with a specific pathologic etiology have not been successful.

Pancreatic calculi are virtually pathognomonic of chronic pancreatitis (Fig. 5.6). The high sensitivity of CT to small changes in tissue attenuation values results in detection of calculi that may not be visible on the conventional roentgenogram. In some cases, the calculi may be seen to lie within the pancreatic ducts. In other cases, the calculi may form within lateral side branches, and their intraductal location may not be appreciated by CT. Calcifications within the wall of the splenic artery should not be mistaken for pancreatic calculi.

Common bile duct obstruction may be associated with pancreatic duct dilation in both carcinoma and chronic pancreatitis. As an isolated finding, biductal dilation is nonspecific, and ancillary criteria must be present for accurate differentiation of inflammatory and neoplastic disease. Carcinoma of the head of the pancreas may be diagnosed if a mass or other specific findings of tumor (metastases, regional node involvement, contiguous organ invasion, etc.) are present. Similarly, chronic pancreatitis may be diagnosed if typical intraductal calculi are seen. However, in the absence of these ancillary findings, additional diagnostic procedures such as ERCP, percutaneous transhepatic cholangiography (PTC), or percutaneous biopsy may be required to reach a specific diagnosis. In addition, chronic pancreatitis and pancreatic carcinoma may rarely coexist. In this case, preoperative radiologic diagnosis is virtually impossible.

### Secondary Diagnostic Features

The pancreas is located within the anterior pararenal space, and thickening of the fascial planes may occur as pancreatic enzymes are released during an acute episode. However, this is a nonspecific finding, and the fascia may be thickened in other upper abdominal inflammatory or neoplastic diseases. The normal renal fascia appears on CT as a thin, delicate line of slightly increased attenuation against the background of the retroperitoneal fat. Pancreatic inflammatory disease often causes thickening of the left renal fascia, but right-sided or bilateral involvement occurs in about one-third of cases. Renal fascial thickening may persist long after the acute inflammatory process has subsided.

## COMPLICATIONS OF PANCREATITIS

### Fluid Collections and Pseudocysts

The term *pseudocyst* classically has been used to refer to all intrapancreatic and peripancreatic fluid collections arising as a complication of either acute or chronic pancreatitis (16, 17). However, the terms *pancreatic fluid collection* and *extrapancreatic fluid collection* should be used to designate acute fluid collections that are only confined by, and take the shape of, the anatomic compartments in which they form (Fig. 5.7). Fluid collections that are chronic are limited by an inflammatory fibrous capsule and are round or oval. The cystlike walls are devoid of an epithelial lining and thus properly may be termed pseudocysts (Fig. 5.8).

Radiologic evaluation of patients with suspected pancreatic fluid collections is crucial for accurate diagnosis and proper management. While the clinical diagnosis of acute and chronic pancreatitis is highly accurate, the clinical diagnosis of pancreatic or peripancreatic fluid collections is notoriously inaccurate. CT can accurately localize and precisely define the full extent of pancreatic and extrapancreatic fluid collections.

Intrapancreatic fluid collections as small as 5 mm in diameter can be delineated. However, when collections smaller than 5 mm are detected, differentiation from focal pancreatic ductal ectasia or small, retention cysts may be impossible. Intrapancreatic fluid collections or pseudocysts characteristically present

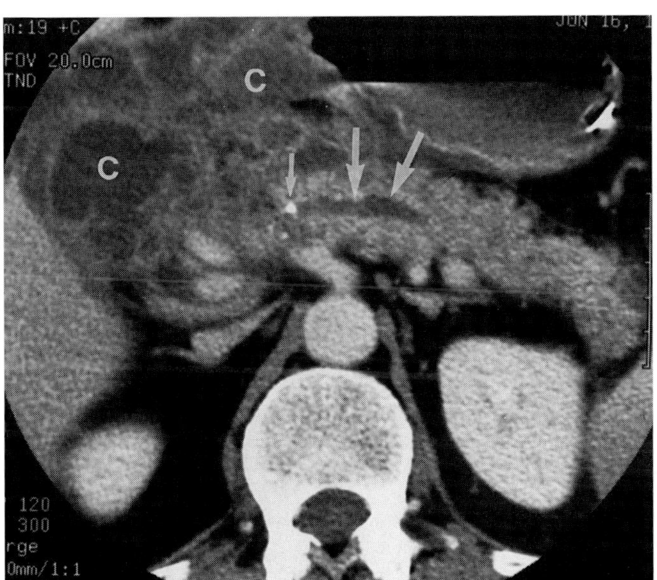


**FIG. 5.6.** Recurrent pancreatitis with pancreatic calculi. CT following intravenous contrast administration demonstrates a dilated main pancreatic duct *(long arrows)* proximal to an obstructing intraductal calculus *(short arrow)*. Multiple pseudocysts *(C)* surround the head of the pancreas.

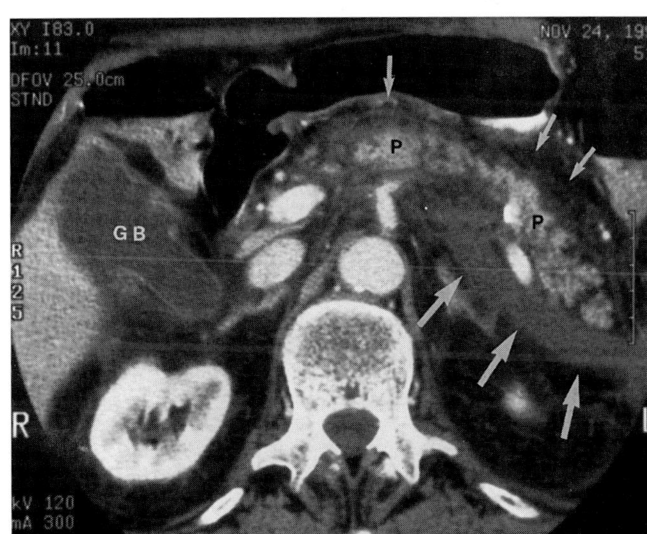


**FIG. 5.7.** Acute pancreatitis with extrapancreatic fluid collection. CT following intravenous contrast administration demonstrates enhancement of the body and tail of the pancreas *(P)*. There is fluid *(arrows)* in the anterior perirenal space surrounding the pancreas. *GB*, gallbladder.

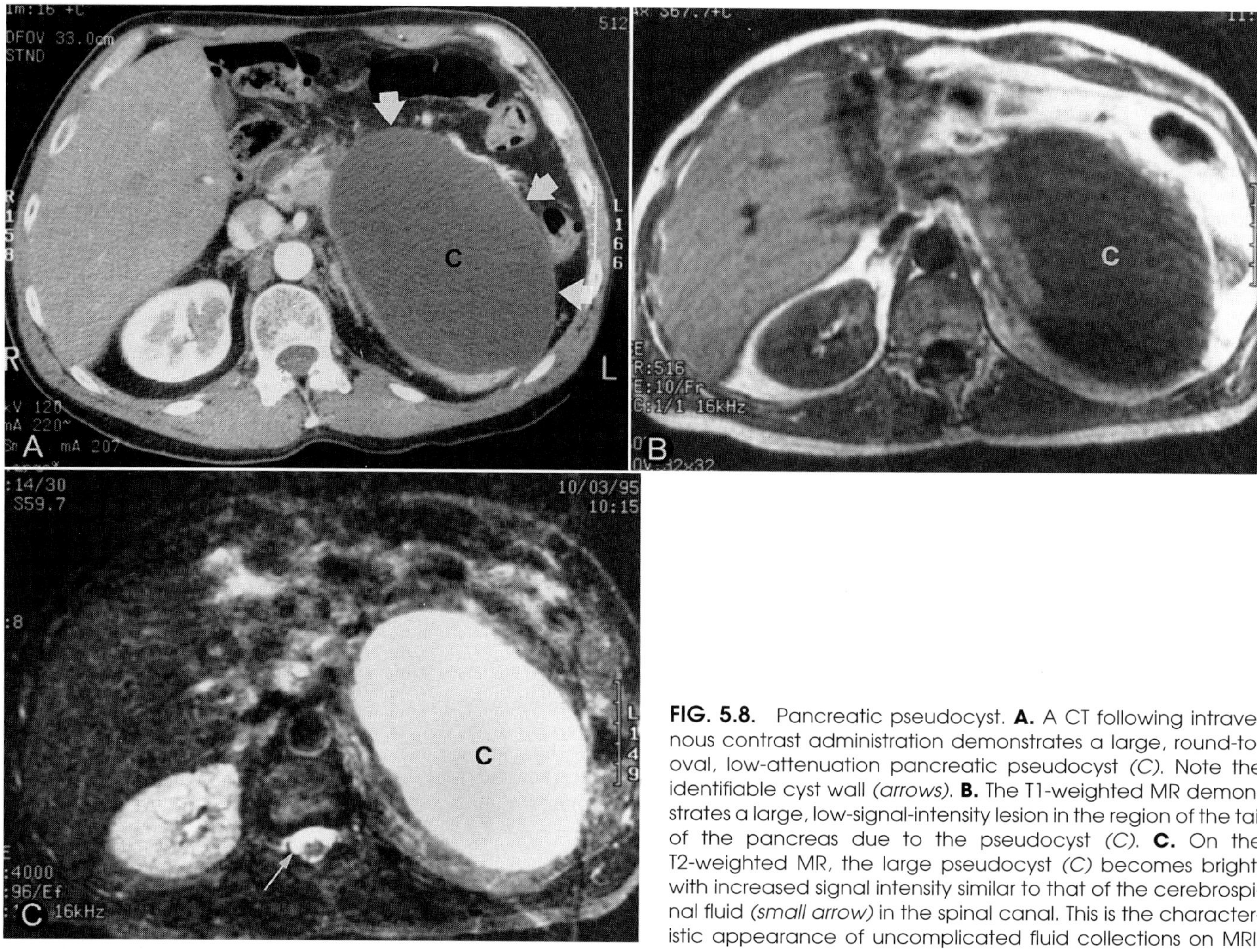


**FIG. 5.8.** Pancreatic pseudocyst. **A.** A CT following intravenous contrast administration demonstrates a large, round-to-oval, low-attenuation pancreatic pseudocyst *(C)*. Note the identifiable cyst wall *(arrows)*. **B.** The T1-weighted MR demonstrates a large, low-signal-intensity lesion in the region of the tail of the pancreas due to the pseudocyst *(C)*. **C.** On the T2-weighted MR, the large pseudocyst *(C)* becomes bright, with increased signal intensity similar to that of the cerebrospinal fluid *(small arrow)* in the spinal canal. This is the characteristic appearance of uncomplicated fluid collections on MRI.

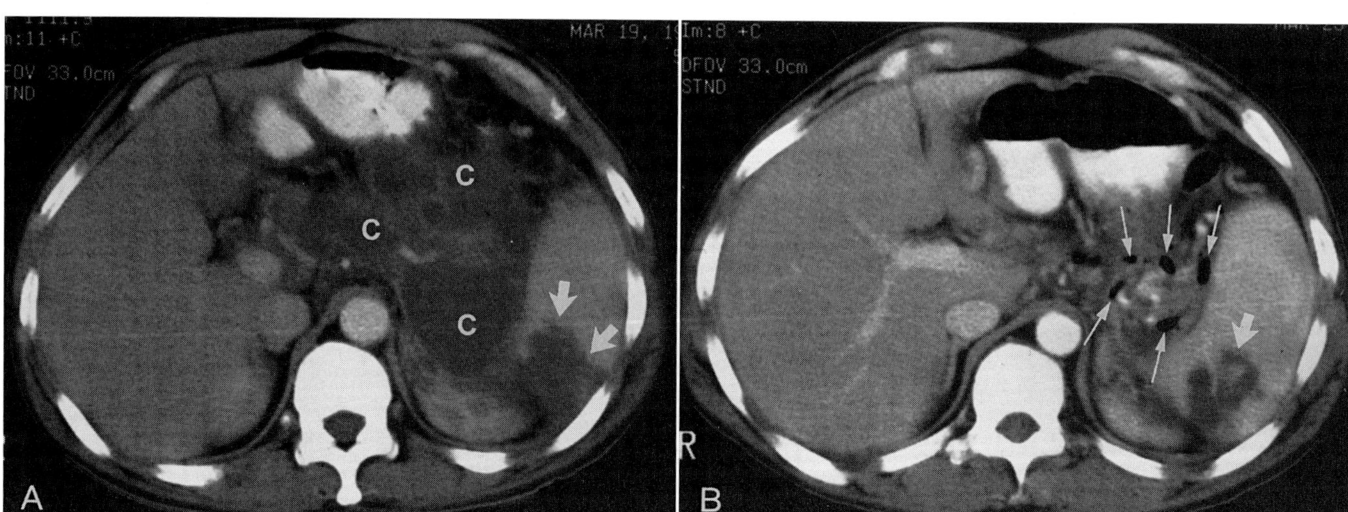


**FIG. 5.9.** Pancreatic pseudocysts with splenic penetration. **A.** Contrast-enhanced CT demonstrates multiple pancreatic pseudocysts *(C)* that distort and obscure any residual normal pancreatic tissue. The pseudocyst penetrates into the spleen *(arrows)*. **B.** CT performed 6 days after the initial examination shows partial resolution of the splenic pseudocyst *(short arrow)* and significant decrease in the size of the pseudocysts in the pancreatic bed because of spontaneous decompression into the stomach. Note gas *(long arrows)* in the pancreatic bed. This was due to the development of a fistula and not abscess formation.

as round, or oval areas of decreased attenuation relative to the pancreas, with near water attenuation on CT. The presence of blood or necrotic debris may result in a higher range of attenuation values. This is particularly evident if hemorrhage has occurred into the fluid.

Pancreatic fluid collections are dynamic, and their CT appearance depends upon their stage of development. During their early evolution, the collections have poorly defined margins and often are indistinctly separated from the pancreatic parenchyma. As they mature and develop a fibrous capsule, the walls become more distinctly marginated. The walls may be several centimeters thick, or they may be quite thin. The walls may enhance following intravenous contrast administration, particularly if the cyst becomes infected. If the cyst is confined to the pancreas and is large or septated, there is often marked pancreatic distortion. In some of these cases, it may be difficult to identify any normal pancreatic tissue.

The incursive nature of pancreatic fluid allows migration of extrapancreatic collections to virtually any location. They may penetrate into the spleen and liver (Fig. 5.9). They also may dissect superiorly and enter the mediastinum, or inferiorly and enter the lumbar, pelvic, or inguinal regions. Although sonography is quite accurate in identifying pancreatic and peripancreatic collections, unsuspected collections in these remote locations are often only recognized during CT. CT is the imaging modality of choice for precise evaluation prior to surgical drainage.

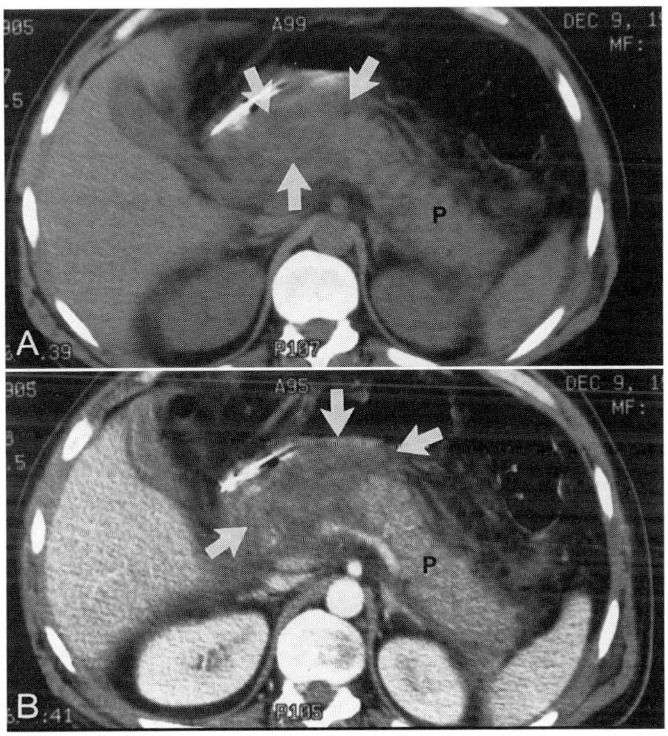


**FIG. 5.10.** Pancreatic necrosis. **A.** Noncontrast CT of the pancreas demonstrates a poorly defined area of slightly lower attenuation *(arrows)* compared with the normal pancreas *(P)*. **B.** On contrast-enhanced CT this same area of low attenuation *(arrows)* is much more clearly distinguishable from the normal pancreas *(P)*. This represents a focal area of pancreatic necrosis.

## Pancreatic Necrosis

In the most severe forms of pancreatitis, there is destruction and necrosis of pancreatic parenchyma and peripancreatic tissues. The primary CT feature of pancreatic necrosis is generalized or focal areas of low CT attenuation within the pancreas (18). Following intravenous administration of contrast, there is lack of glandular enhancement (Fig. 5.10). The pancreas is usually enlarged, and pancreatic and parapancreatic fluid collections are commonly present.

Evaluation of the extent of pancreatic necrosis by CT is important, as large areas of necrosis (>50%) are associated with higher morbidity and mortality (Fig. 5.11). Large or multiple peripancreatic fluid collections, large areas of peripancreatic inflammation, and pancreatic necrosis are associated with a poor prognosis (19–21).

Infection that develops within the gland as part of the continuum of pancreatic inflammation and necrosis may be difficult to diagnose during its acute phase. These patients are severely ill and usually have multiple complications. If CT is performed during the acute phase, the findings include diffuse pancreatic enlargement, loss of definition of the margins of the gland, obliteration of the surrounding soft tissue planes, and thickening or obscuration of the normal peripancreatic fascial

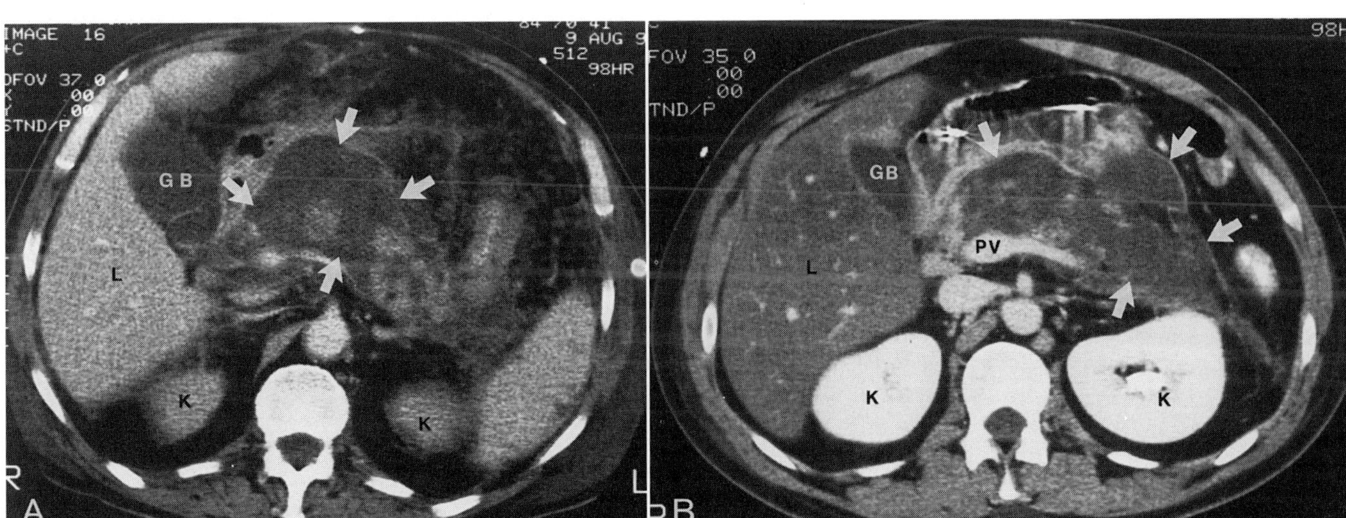


**FIG. 5.11.** Pancreatic necrosis. **A** and **B.** Contrast-enhanced CT in two different patients demonstrates pancreatic fluid collections and large areas of pancreatic necrosis *(arrows)* involving more than 50% of the gland. As predicted from the CT, both of these patients had stormy clinical courses with pseudocyst formation. *GB*, gallbladder; *PV*, portal vein confluence; *L*, liver; *K*, kidney.

layers. The attenuation values of the inflammatory pancreatic mass usually are variable and not of diagnostic help. At this early stage, detectable bubbles of gas are often absent. Thus, while CT may identify many findings suggesting infected necrosis, none are specific. A definitive diagnosis may be made only by a combination of clinical suspicion, CT findings, and percutaneous needle aspiration of the pancreatic necrosis. Increasing tissue necrosis and suppuration during the subacute and chronic phases usually are manifested by progressive clinical deterioration.

### Pancreatic Abscess

A pancreatic abscess* may arise as a complication in an existing pancreatic or extrapancreatic fluid collection (pseudocysts), or it may develop in an area of pancreatic necrosis. The initial diagnosis of a pancreatic abscess usually is based upon a combination of clinical and laboratory findings. Radiologic evaluation may aid in the detection of the abscess, define the extent of the inflammatory process, and detect complications arising from the abscess.

Diagnostic features include a fluid collection with a thick, irregular wall. The attenuation values of the fluid usually are higher than those of a pseudocyst because of the presence of necrotic debris. However, the sine qua non of the diagnosis of abscess is the presence of gas bubbles within the fluid collection. Rarely, gas may be seen within a noninfected pseudocyst that has fistulized into a contiguous loop of bowel (Fig. 5.9). With this one exception, gas-containing masses within the pancreas indicate the presence of an abscess.

### Pancreatic Ascites

Pancreatic ascites may result from either acute or chronic pancreatitis. The diagnosis of ascites may be made clinically and confirmed by sonography or CT. A specific diagnosis of pancreatic ascites may be made by paracentesis and analysis of the ascitic fluid. The fluid amylase level and albumin concentration are always high.

Patients with pancreatic ascites invariably have pancreatic ductal disruption and associated abnormalities, including segmental ductal stenosis, intraductal calculi, and periampullary ductal obstruction. The presence of stenosis or obstruction between the ampulla and the site of ductal leakage is a particularly important consideration when planning surgical or percutaneous therapy.

### Vascular Complications of Pancreatitis

Vascular complications arising from acute and chronic pancreatitis or from sequelae of pancreatic inflammation include formation of arterial pseudoaneurysms, inflammatory stenosis or obstruction (thrombosis) of peripancreatic vessels, and development of varices secondary to portal venous occlusion. Clinical manifestations of these vascular sequelae include gastrointestinal or intraabdominal hemorrhage and intestinal ischemia or infarction.

The application of helical CT in conjunction with optimal intravenous contrast administration has improved our ability to detect a thrombus within the portal venous system. In addition, collateral venous channels (varices) are easily visualized.

Abnormality of the major arteries adjacent to the pancreas can also be detected with helical CT. Pseudoaneurysms secondary to pancreatic inflammation are more accurately detected by helical CT than by conventional axial CT. This is due to the rapidity of helical scanning and the acquisition of images during peak contrast enhancement of the peripancreatic arteries.

*Editor's note: see Chapter 28 for an alternative definition of pancreatic abscess.

## ADENOCARCINOMA OF THE PANCREAS

The high degree of accuracy and reliability of CT in the detection and assessment of pancreatic carcinoma has made it the initial procedure of choice for evaluation of patients in whom there is a high clinical suspicion of pancreatic carcinoma (22). In most patients, a diagnosis of pancreatic carcinoma can be made or excluded without the use of additional imaging procedures. CT also can assess resectability and precisely guide percutaneous fine-needle aspiration biopsy to confirm the diagnosis.

The most common abnormality produced by pancreatic carcinoma is a mass (Fig. 5.12). Most neoplastic masses are focal and produce a change in the contour and/or attenuation of the gland. In about 10% of cases, pancreatic carcinoma produces diffuse enlargement of the gland, usually due to associated pancreatitis.

Pancreatic masses usually must be 1–2 cm in diameter to be detectable by CT. However, the requisite size for detection also depends upon the size of the pancreas and the location of the tumor within the gland. If carcinoma develops in a small atrophic or fatty replaced gland, it may be detected at a smaller size. Location also is important. Tumors that develop in the center of the gland must grow to larger dimensions to be detected by CT than those that arise on the periphery. Similarly, since the tail of the pancreas is usually the thinnest portion of the gland, tumors in this location may be easier to recognize than those in the body or head. The uncinate process is small and usually has a characteristic wedge-shaped tongue that extends posterior to the superior mesenteric artery and vein. Tumors that arise in this location cause rounding of the uncinate and loss of the small tongue of tissue. Tumors that arise in close proximity to the periampullary portions of the pancreatic and common bile ducts usually result in ductal obstruction and jaundice, which aids in their detection.

Tumors that arise in the head or body of the pancreas frequently produce pancreatic ductal obstruction and atrophy of

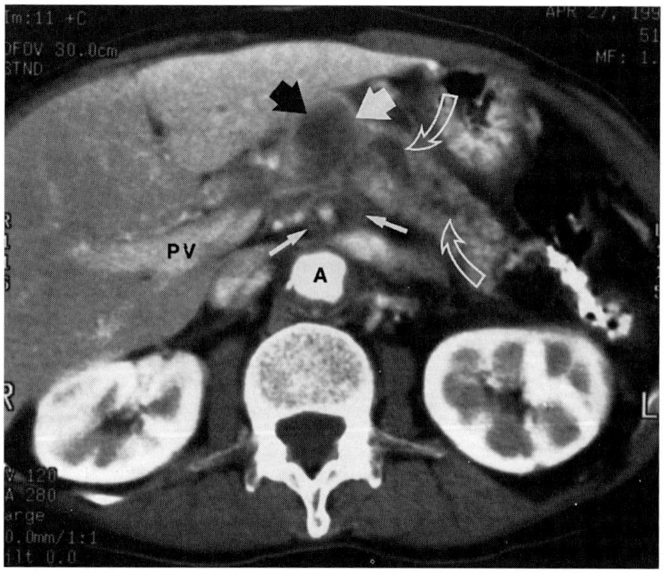


**FIG. 5.12.** Carcinoma of the pancreas. Contrast-enhanced CT demonstrates a mass in the body of the pancreas *(arrows)*. Note the poorly defined, low-attenuation center of the mass. This is the characteristic appearance of a pancreatic carcinoma on a contrast-enhanced scan. Note the dilated pancreatic duct *(curved arrows)* and the dorsal invasion of the tumor to encase the superior mesenteric artery *(small arrows)*. *A*, aorta; *PV*, portal vein.

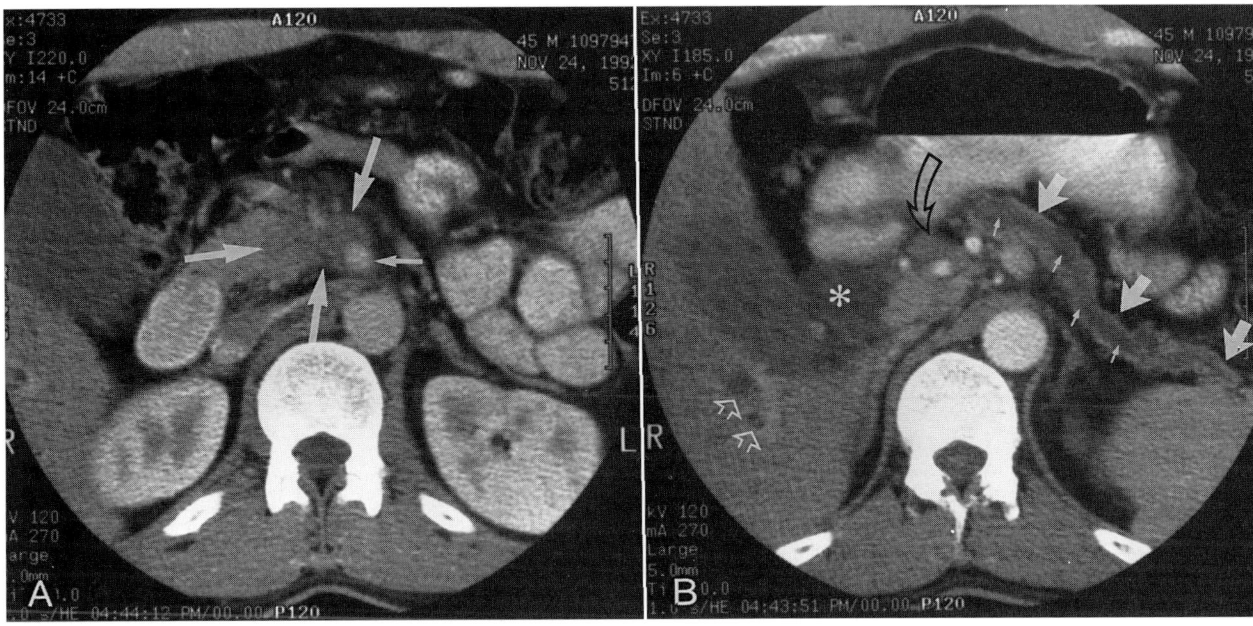


**FIG. 5.13.** Pancreatic carcinoma. **A.** Contrast-enhanced CT demonstrates a small pancreatic carcinoma *(long arrows)* that enhances slightly less than the adjacent normal pancreas. It extends into the root of the mesentery encasing the superior mesenteric artery *(short arrow)*. **B.** A contrast-enhanced CT of the pancreatic body and tail demonstrates atrophy *(large arrows)* with marked pancreatic duct dilation *(small arrows)*. An enlarged lymph node adjacent to the head of the pancreas *(curved arrow)*, a dilated common bile duct *(asterisk)*, and dilated intrahepatic bile ducts *(small open arrows)* are also seen.

the tail of the gland. In some cases, the tail simply appears small relative to the tumor mass; in other cases, the tail undergoes obstructive atrophy and the dilated pancreatic duct may be seen as an irregular tubular structure in the center of the atrophic tail (Fig. 5.13).

Pancreatic carcinoma may cause biliary obstruction by direct involvement of the intrapancreatic portion of the common bile duct, by extrinsic compression of the suprapancreatic portion due to enlarged metastatic nodes in the porta hepatis, and by intrahepatic metastases. In each case, CT may provide an accurate assessment of the presence and extent of biliary obstruction.

The attenuation values of pancreatic tumors and normal pancreatic parenchyma are similar on a non–contrast enhanced CT scan. However, after injection of intravenous iodinated contrast material, the attenuation differences between normal and neoplastic pancreatic tissue become apparent. Pancreatic ductal adenocarcinoma is an infiltrating, scirrhous hypovascular tumor. Thus, following bolus contrast injections, the neoplasm has relatively decreased attenuation compared with the normal surrounding contrast-enhanced pancreatic parenchyma (Fig. 5.14).

Some pancreatic tumors contain areas of lower attenuation that most likely represent foci of tissue necrosis. These areas may cause confusion, especially if they are associated with small calcifications, suggesting a diagnosis of chronic pancreatitis and pseudocyst formation. The areas of decreased attenuation in tumors are usually less well defined and have slightly higher CT numbers than pseudocysts. However, pancreatic carcinoma can rarely coexist with chronic pancreatitis or cause formation of a pseudocyst. Although the pathophysiology of pseudocyst formation in pancreatic carcinoma is not well understood, they probably develop as postobstructive lesions due to tumor stenosis or obstruction of the proximal pancreatic duct.

Pancreatic duct dilation can occur in both chronic pancreatitis and carcinoma, and evaluation of several findings may aid in differentiation. Carcinoma usually causes abrupt occlusion of the pancreatic duct by a mass that encases or obliterates the duct.

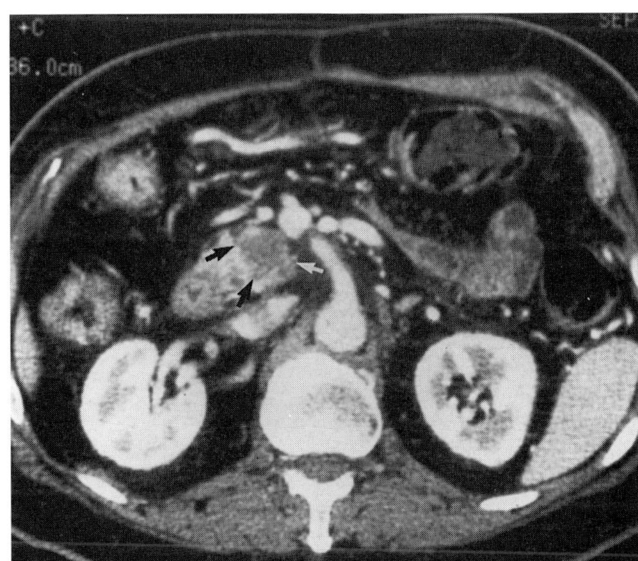

**FIG. 5.14.** Pancreatic carcinoma. Contrast-enhanced CT demonstrates a small, low-attenuation mass *(arrows)* that deforms the medial margin of the uncinate process of the pancreas. There is no CT evidence of local extension of this cancer.

The pancreatic duct is not seen within the mass. Proximal to the mass, the duct may dilate to a large caliber, and the walls are often smooth and parallel. Chronic pancreatitis may result in abrupt ductal dilation proximal to a focal inflammatory stricture and produce pancreatic duct dilation morphologically indistinguishable from carcinoma. More often, however, in chronic pancreatitis the duct is irregularly dilated with focal duct visualization. The caliber is usually less than that seen with carcinoma, and the walls tend to be beaded and nonparallel. Focal and diffuse masses may occur in chronic pancreatitis, but often the dilated duct may be seen within the mass. Intraductal debris or calculi and pseudocysts also are frequent findings in chronic pancreatitis and may aid in differential diagnosis.

In patients with suspected pancreatic carcinoma, CT also may provide information regarding the presence of metastases to the liver or lymph nodes, dilated intra- or extrahepatic biliary ducts, and gallbladder dilation (Fig. 5.15).

While the diagnosis of pancreatic carcinoma is correct in the vast majority of patients who present with a pancreatic mass and hepatic metastases, similar findings may be seen with neoplasms metastatic to both the pancreas and liver, or rarely, with pancreatic or peripancreatic lymphoma (Fig. 5.16). Multiple discrete pancreatic masses suggest metastatic disease to the pancreas, especially if they are vascular and demonstrate significant enhancement.

Pancreatic carcinoma frequently extends through the thin fascial covering of the gland and infiltrates into the peripancreatic soft tissues. The most common site of tumor extension is into the retropancreatic space. This is identified on CT by obliteration of the normal posterior fat planes. Loss of the fat planes may also be seen in patients with pancreatitis. Thus, while obliteration of the retropancreatic fat plane is a frequent finding in pancreatic carcinoma, it is nonspecific.

Pancreatic carcinoma may extend into the root of the small bowel mesentery and encase the superior mesentery artery and vein as well as the celiac axis and its branches (Fig. 5.17). Vascular encasement appears on CT as a halo of increased attenuation or thick soft tissue collar surrounding the proximal portion of the celiac or superior mesenteric vessels (Fig. 5.12). The peripheral borders of the collar usually are indistinct (23). The superior mesenteric vein also may be obstructed, and mesenteric varices may be recognized. One of the most common vascular complications of pancreatic carcinoma is splenic vein obstruction with subsequent congestive splenomegaly and formation of gastric varices.

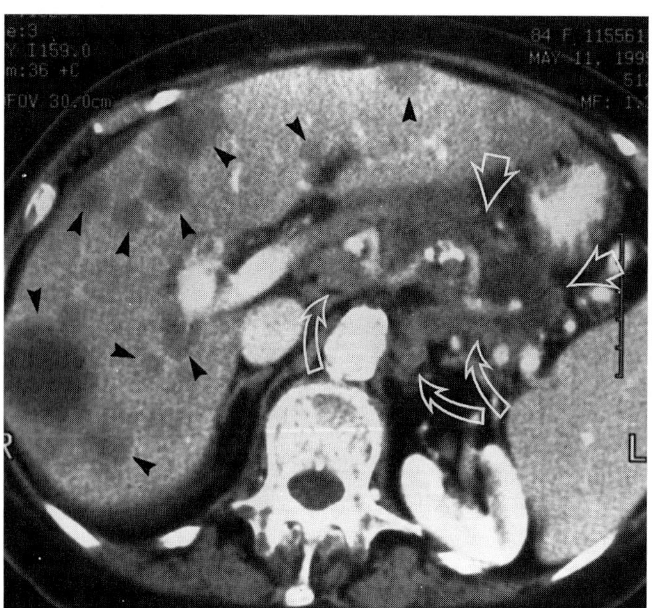

**FIG. 5.15.** Carcinoma of the pancreas with local and distant metastases. Contrast-enhanced CT demonstrates a mass in the pancreas *(arrows)*, which represents a carcinoma of the pancreas. Note the dorsal tumor invasion, *(curved arrows)* and the multiple hepatic metastases *(arrowheads)*.

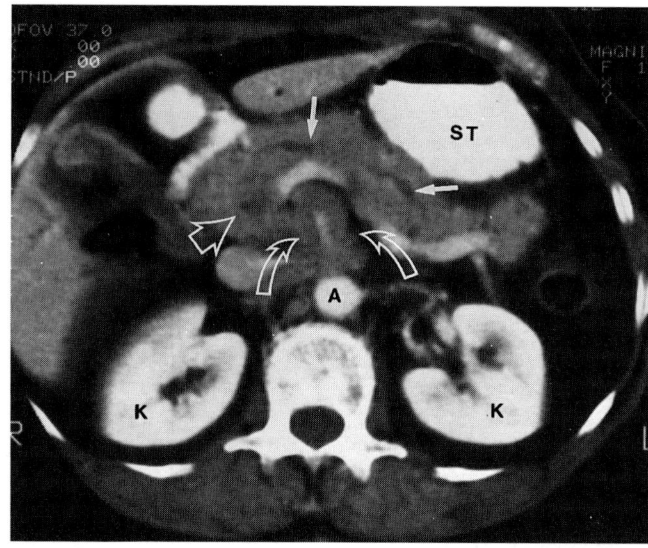


**FIG. 5.16.** Lymphoma of the pancreas that mimics a pancreatic carcinoma. Contrast-enhanced CT demonstrates a mass in the region in the head of the pancreas *(large arrow)*, dilation of the main pancreatic duct *(small arrows)*, and tumor mass surrounding the celiac artery *(curved arrows)*. Biopsy at the time of surgery revealed non-Hodgkins lymphoma. *ST*, stomach; *A*, aorta; *K*, kidney.

Pancreatic carcinoma metastasizes to regional lymph nodes early in its course. Peripancreatic, celiac, and lesser omental lymph nodes more than 5–8 mm in diameter should be considered enlarged and potential sites for metastatic tumor. However, lymph node enlargement per se is a nonspecific finding, since lymphadenopathy may be due to reactive changes or to inflammatory disease.

Malignant ascites may be associated with pancreatic carcinoma secondary to tumor obstruction of the portal vein and subsequent portal hypertension. However, it most often results from diffuse peritoneal metastases. CT accurately detects small amounts of peritoneal fluid, but actual peritoneal metastases are usually not identified unless they are quite large.

## UNCOMMON PANCREATIC NEOPLASMS

### Metastatic Disease

Metastatic disease to the pancreas may be silent or create a variety of clinical signs and symptoms that may simulate primary carcinoma of the pancreas (24). Metastatic carcinoma to the pancreas from direct extension from contiguous organs is more common than hematogenous spread of disease. Common tumors that directly invade the pancreas include carcinomas of the stomach, colon, and much less frequently, the duodenum. The most common primary carcinomas that metastasize to the pancreas by hematogenous spread, in descending order of frequency, include carcinoma of the lung, malignant melanoma, carcinoma of the kidney, and carcinoma of the breast. Lymphoma may rarely primarily involve the pancreas (25). More commonly, it involves the peripancreatic lymph nodes and does not actually invade the pancreas itself.

CT may demonstrate one or more masses in the pancreatic region, which are usually nonhomogeneous and of lower attenuation than the surrounding pancreatic tissue, and dilation of the pancreatic duct and/or biliary ductal system if the metastases are strategically located. Other evidence of metastatic disease such as

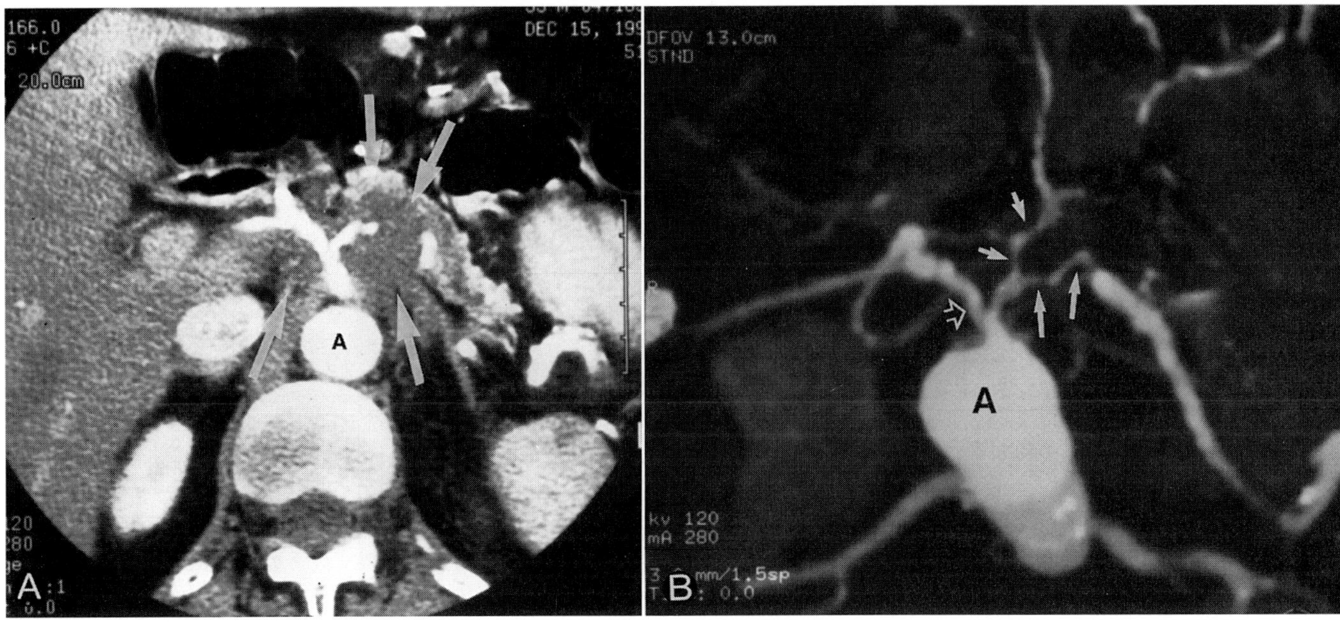


**FIG. 5.17.** Pancreatic carcinoma with vascular encasement. **A.** Contrast-enhanced CT demonstrates tumor encasement of the celiac artery and its branches *(arrows)*. **B.** CT angiogram using maximum intensity projection rendering demonstrates irregularities of the splenic artery *(long arrows)*, the left gastric artery *(short arrows)*, and the hepatic artery *(open arrow)*, caused by tumor encasement. The CT angiogram is a computer reconstruction using the original axial CT data. *A*, aorta.

hepatic metastases, peripancreatic lymphadenopathy, mesenteric tumor deposits, or ascites with peritoneal deposits may also be identified.

## Pancreatic Sarcoma

Primary sarcoma of the mesenchymal supporting structures of the pancreas is rare and may mimic the appearance of primary tumors or pseudocysts (26) (Fig. 5.18). Sarcomas may also develop in the retroperitoneum and secondarily invade the pancreas. The most commonly occurring retroperitoneal sarcomas that involve the pancreas are leiomyosarcomas and fibrosarcomas. These lesions are usually large at the time of diagnosis and easily recognizable by CT. However, they may be obscured if they are smaller than 2 cm in diameter or in patients who have small amounts of retroperitoneal fat. CT will demonstrate these tumors as having attenuation values different from the surrounding tissues, although this is usually of no help in arising at a specific histologic diagnosis. Liposarcomas may have attenuation values that are lower than those of fibrosarcomas or leiomyosarcomas.

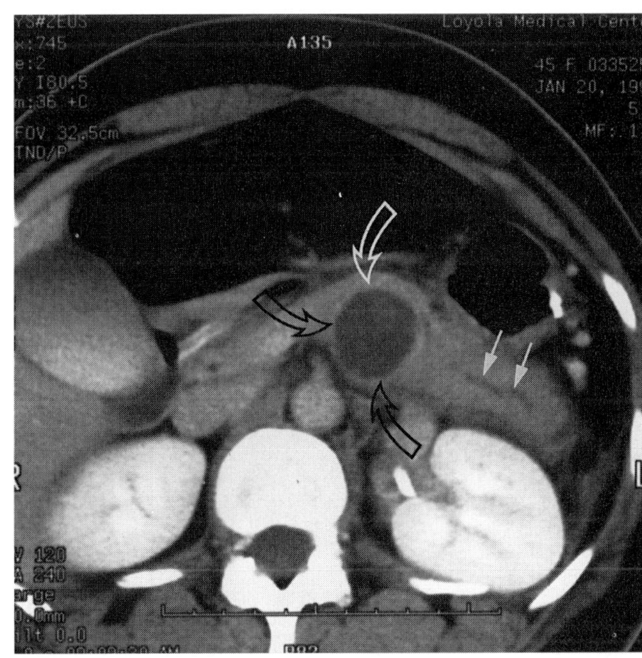


**FIG. 5.18.** Pancreatic sarcoma. Contrast-enhanced CT image demonstrates a low-attenuation mass *(curved arrows)* in the body of the pancreas, which was found at surgery to be secondary to a primary pancreatic sarcoma. Its appearance mimics that of a pseudocyst. Note the dilation of proximal pancreatic duct *(arrows)*.

## Cystic Neoplasms of the Pancreas

Cystic neoplasms are rare pancreatic tumors. There are two distinct types: mucinous cystic tumors (mucinous cystadenoma; mucinous cystadenocarcinoma), which have a high malignant potential, and microcystic adenomas (serous or glycogen-rich cystadenoma), which are generally benign (27–29).

Mucinous cystic tumors are large, predominantly cystic neoplasms that range from 2 to 24 cm in diameter. They may be found in any part of the pancreas but are most common in the body and tail. They are well encapsulated and have smooth, lobulated external surfaces. The wall is usually thick and may contain areas of peripheral dystrophic calcification (Fig. 5.19). The internal structure may be unilocular or multilocular, and the cyst lining is thrown into numerous folds with papillary excrescences (Fig. 5.20).

Microcystic adenomas represent a distinctive type of cystic pancreatic tumor that seldom demonstrates a malignant potential. While variable in size, they tend to be large, with an average diameter of 10–12 cm, and may occur in any part of the pancreas (Fig. 5.21). They are lobulated neoplasms with well-defined, thick fibrous capsules. The internal architecture consists of multiple cysts, ranging in size from several millimeters to several

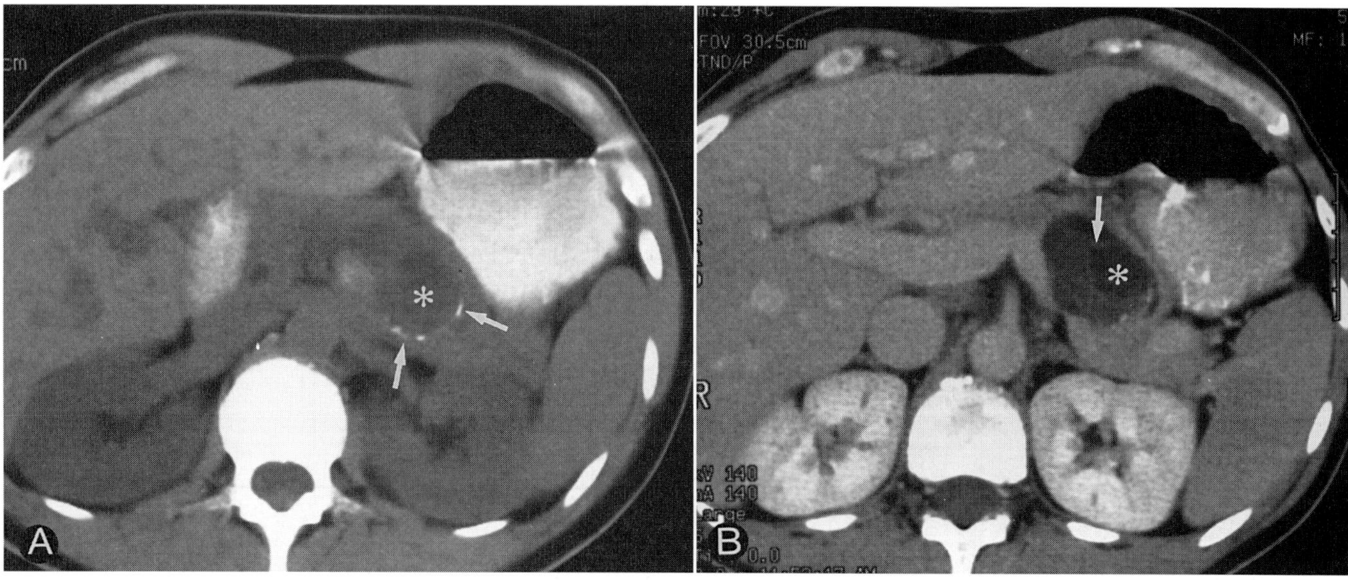


**FIG. 5.19.** Mucinous cystic neoplasm. **A.** Noncontrast CT demonstrates a low-attenuation pancreatic mass *(asterisk)* with peripheral calcification *(arrows)*. **B.** Following intravenous contrast, the mucinous cystic neoplasm *(asterisk)* is more clearly defined, and septations are now visible *(arrow)* within the cystic mass.

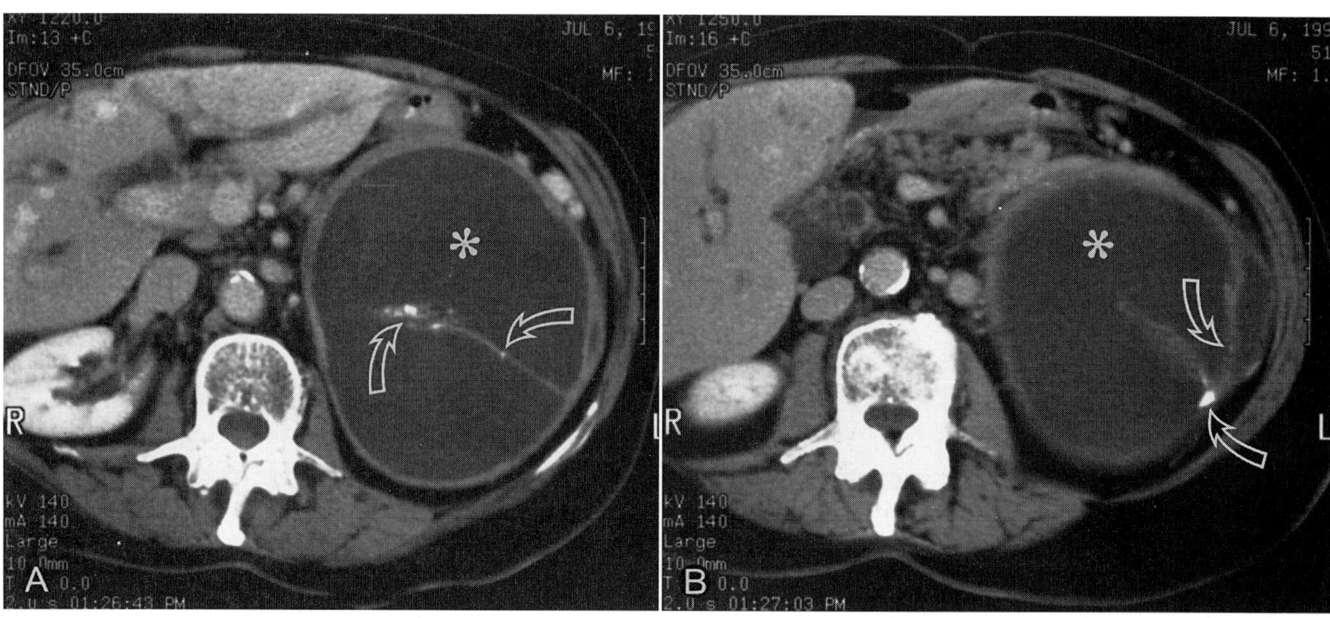


**FIG. 5.20.** Mucinous cystic neoplasm. **A** and **B.** Contrast-enhanced CTs demonstrate a large cystic mass *(asterisk)* involving the tail of the pancreas. Note the thick irregular walls of the mass and the prominent course septations containing focal calcifications *(curved arrows)*.

centimeters, which contain a clear serous fluid. A central, stellate fibrous scar is frequently seen. Calcifications occasionally form within the scar.

CT is the single best imaging procedure for initial diagnosis and differentiation of mucinous cystic tumors from microcystic adenomas. Mucinous tumors appear as large pancreatic cystic masses composed of both solid tumor tissue and varying-sized cysts containing septae and enhancing areas of tumor excrescence. Random, amorphous calcifications are often seen in the peripheral portions of the tumor, and hepatic metastases and invasion of contiguous organs may be present.

Microcystic adenomas are usually well circumscribed and show no evidence of contiguous organ invasion. Their internal architecture is characterized by numerous small cysts of varying sizes with no septation or internal tumor nodules. If the cysts are quite small, they may be difficult to resolve, and the lesion may appear to be a solid mass. If calcifications are present, they are usually arranged in a central stellate pattern.

## CT-GUIDED DIAGNOSTIC AND THERAPEUTIC PROCEDURES

### Nonoperative Pancreatic Biopsy

The primary indication for percutaneous fine-needle pancreatic biopsy is microscopic confirmation of the clinical or radiologic

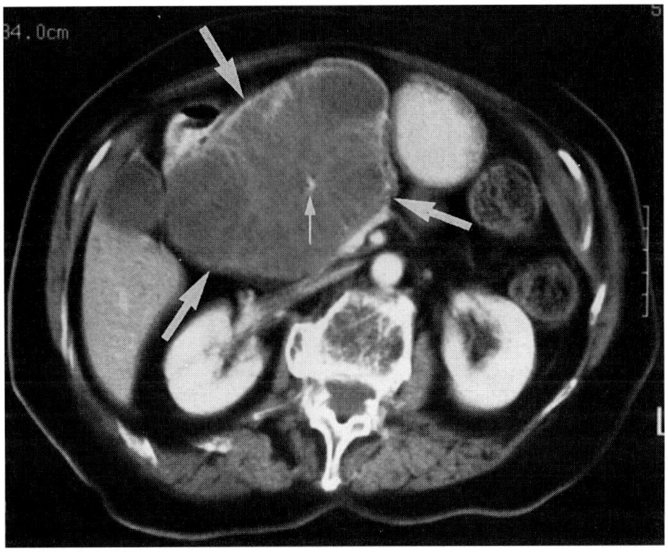

**FIG. 5.21.** Pancreatic microcystic adenoma. Contrast-enhanced CT demonstrates a large, well-defined, low-attenuation mass in the head of the pancreas *(long arrows)* with a central calcification *(short arrow)*. Note the enhancing septa radiating through the mass, creating innumerable tiny cystic spaces.

diagnosis of an unresectable pancreatic carcinoma. The question of whether to perform pancreatic biopsy prior to surgery in a patient with a potentially resectable pancreatic carcinoma is controversial (30).

Our recommendation is that percutaneous biopsy be performed to provide microscopic confirmation of the diagnosis of carcinoma only in patients judged to have unresectable tumors on the basis of either clinical evaluation or radiologic examination and who will not require surgery to relieve biliary or duodenal obstruction. Intraoperative biopsy is performed when surgery is indicated for palliation or curative reasons.

Precise localization of the tumor is crucial for obtaining a satisfactory fine-needle aspirate (31). However, localization may sometimes be difficult because of the nature of pancreatic tumors. Adenocarcinoma arises from pancreatic ductal epithelium and usually causes ductal obstruction or encasement. The point of ductal abnormality thus represents the site of the tumor. However, most tumors are enveloped by a thick rind of inflammatory tissue due to pancreatitis resulting from obstruction of the surrounding ducts. Biopsy of this peripheral area will yield only inflammatory cells. Thus, precise localization of the tumor requires either visualization of the point of pancreatic ductal abnormality or the ability to obtain a three-dimensional image of the tumor mass and subsequently guide the biopsy needle to its geometric center. The ability of CT to verify the exact location of the needle tip is reflected in the high accuracy rate (90–95%) obtained by CT-guided biopsies. The safety of percutaneous pancreatic biopsy is well established. Although there is a potential risk of needle tract seeding, it appears to be very small.

### Fluid Collection Aspiration and Catheter Drainage

CT-guided needle aspiration of pancreatic and peripancreatic fluid collections is an accurate method for diagnosis and can be followed by placement of a catheter percutaneously for therapy (32, 33). The diagnostic aspiration is performed with techniques similar to that used for solid mass aspiration biopsy. The target is localized, and a safe route to the fluid collection is selected. If at all possible, loops of bowel, lung, and pleural space are avoided. The aspirated fluid is then sent to the laboratory for analysis.

If laboratory or clinical data suggest an abscess, a catheter can be placed into the fluid collection. If a catheter is placed, it must not traverse loops of large or small bowel and should not traverse the solid upper abdominal organs or pleural space. In the latter case, traversing the pleural space may lead to empyema. Depending on the viscosity of the fluid in the collection, large catheters from 12 to 16 French may be necessary for adequate drainage. Follow-up CT examinations at regular intervals to document the resolution of the abscess are essential (34–37).

Pseudocysts may also be effectively drained percutaneously. Percutaneous drainage is most successful when the collection is unilocular, peripheral to the pancreas, and not associated with a pseudocyst-to-pancreatic-duct fistula and downstream pancreatic duct stenosis or obstruction. Even in uncomplicated cases, successful percutaneous drainage of pseudocysts takes significantly longer than other abdominal fluid collections. Percutaneous drainage may be unsuccessful or require substantially longer catheter drainage or multiple catheters if the pseudocyst is multilocular. If there is a fistula between the pancreatic duct and the pseudocyst, with associated downstream pancreatic duct stenosis or obstruction, a persistent pancreatic percutaneous fistula may occur requiring surgical intervention.

## REFERENCES

1. Mitchell DG, Winston CB, Outwater EK, Ehrilich SM. Delineation of pancreas with MR imaging: multiobserver comparison of five pulse sequences. JMRI 1995;5:193.
2. Semelka RC, Ascher SM. MR imaging of the pancreas. Radiology 1993;188:593.
3. Mitchell DG, Shapiro M, Schurich A, et al. Pancreatic disease: findings on state-of-the-art MR images. AJR 1992;159:533.
4. Fishman EK, Wyatt SH, Ney DR, Kuhlman JE, Siegelman SS. Spiral CT of the pancreas with multiplanar display. Am J Roentgenol 1992;159:1209–1215.
5. Dupuy DE, Costello P, Ecker CP. Spiral CT of the pancreas. Radiology 1992;183:815–818.
6. Wyatt SH, Fishman EK. Spiral CT of the pancreas. Semin US CT MR 1994;15:122.
7. Thoeni RF, Blankenberg F. Pancreatic imaging: computed tomography and magnetic resonance imaging. Radiol Clin North Am 1993;31:1085.
8. Nghiem HV, Freeny PC. Radiologic staging of pancreatic adenocarcinoma. Radiol Clin North Am 1994;32:71.
9. Reznek RH, Stephens DH. Review: staging of pancreatic adenocarcinoma. Clin Radiol 1993;47:373.
10. Gabata T, Matsui O, Kadoya M, Yoshikawa J, Miyayama S, et al. Small pancreatic adenocarcinomas: efficacy of MR imaging with fat suppression and gadolinium enhancement. Radiology 1994;193:683.
11. Semelka RC, Shoenut JP, Kroeker MA, Mickflikier AB. Chronic pancreatitis: MR imaging features before and after administration of gadopentetate dimeglumine. JMRI 1993;3:79.
12. Vellet AD, Romano W, Bach DB, Passi RB, Taves DH, Munk PL. Adenocarcinoma of the pancreatic ducts: comparative evaluation with CT and MR imaging at 1.5T. Radiology 1992;183:87.
13. Megibow AJ, Zhou XH, Rotterdam H, Francis IR, Zerhouni EA, et al. Pancreatic adenocarcinoma: CT versus MR imaging in the evaluation of resectability—report of the Radiology Diagnostic Oncology Group. Radiology 1995;195:327.
14. Freeny PC, Lawson TL. Acute pancreatitis. In: Radiology of the pancreas. New York: Springer-Verlag, 1982.
15. Freeny PC, Lawson TL. Chronic pancreatitis. In: Radiology of the pancreas. New York: Springer-Verlag, 1982.
16. Siegelman SS, Copeland BE, Saba GP, et al. CT of fluid collections associated with pancreatitis. AJR 1980;134:1121–1132.
17. Freeny PC, Rohrmann CA. Inflammatory disease of the pancreas. In: Freeny PC, Stevenson GW, eds. Alimentary tract radiology. 5th ed. St. Louis: CV Mosby, 1994.
18. Johnson CD, Stephens DH, Sarr MG. CT of acute pancreatitis. Correlation between lack of contrast enhancement and pancreatic necrosis. AJR 191;156:93–95.

19. Balthazar EJ, Robinson DL, Megibow AJ, et al. Acute pancreatitis: value of CT in establishing prognosis. Radiology 1990;174: 331–336.
20. Clavien PA, Hauser H, Meyer P, et al. Value of contrast enhanced computerized tomography in the early diagnosis and prognosis of acute pancreatitis. A prospective study of 202 patients. Am J Surg 1988;155:457–466.
21. Balthazar EJ. CT diagnosis and staging of acute pancreatitis. Radiol Clin North Am 1989;27:19–38.
22. Stephens DA. Pancreatic adenocarcinoma. Radiologic diagnosis and staging. In: Freeny PC, Stevenson GW, eds. Alimentary tract radiology. 5th ed. St. Louis: CV Mosby, 1994.
23. Schulte SJ, Baron RL, Greeny PC, Patten RM, Gorell HA, Maclin ML. Root of the superior mesenteric artery in pancreatitis and pancreatic carcinoma: evaluation with CT. Radiology 1991;180: 659–662.
24. Rypens F, Van Gansbeke D, Lambilliotte JP, et al. Pancreatic metastasis from renal cell carcinoma. Radiology 1992;65:547.
25. Prayer LM, Schurawitzki H, Mallek R, et al. CT in pancreatic involvement of non-Hodgkin lymphoma. Acta Radiol 1992; 33:123.
26. Laverdiere JT, vanSonnenberg E, Strum WB, et al. Pleomorphic pancreatic sarcoma mimicking pancreatic pseudocyst: CT appearance. AJR 1992;158:87.
27. Ros PR, Hamrick-Turner JR, Chiechi MV, Ros LH, Gallego P, Burton SS. Cystic masses of the pancreas. RadioGraphics 1992; 12:673.
28. Bennett GL, Chew FS. Serous cystadenoma of the pancreas. AJR 1993;161:786.
29. Healy JC, Davies SE, Reznek RH. CT of microcystic (serous) pancreatic adenoma. JCAT 1994;18:146.
30. Balen FG, Little A, Smith AC, Theis BA, Abrams KR, et al. Biopsy of inoperable pancreatic tumors does not adversely influence patient survival time. Radiology 1944;193:753.
31. Brandt KR, Charboneau JW, Stephens DH, Welch TJ, Goeliner JR. CT and US guided biopsy of the pancreas. Radiology 1993; 187:99.
32. Lee MJ, Rattner DW, Legemate DA, Saini S, Dawson SL, et al. Acute complicated pancreatitis: redefining the role of interventional radiology. Radiology 1992;183:171.
33. Balthazar EJ, Freeny PC, van Sonnenberg E. Imaging and intervention in acute pancreatitis. Radiology 1994;193:297.
34. Lambiase RE, Deyoe LA, Cronan JJ, Dorfman GS. Percutaneous drainage of 335 consecutive abscesses: results of primary drainage with 1-year follow-up. Radiology 1992;184:167.
35. Fotman N, Mathieu D, Anglade M-C, et al. Failure of percutaneous drainage of pancreatic abscesses complicating severe acute pancreatitis. Surg Gynecol Obstet 1992;174:141–147.
36. Criado E, De Stefano AA, Weiner TM, et al. Long-term results of percutaneous catheter drainage of pancreatic pseudocysts. Surg Gynecol Obstet 1992;175:293–298.
37. Feig BW, Pomerantz RA, Vogelzang R, et al. Treatment of peripancreatic fluid collections in patients with complicated acute pancreatitis. Surg Gynecol Obstet 1992;175:429–436.

# 6

# Angiography

Hans Stridbeck and Ingemar Ihse

The significance of angiography in the preoperative evaluation of pancreatic disease has diminished substantially since the introduction of cross-sectional imaging and endoscopic retrograde cholangiopancreatography (1, 2). Currently, the possible indications for preoperative angiography in pancreatic disease are to delineate vascular anatomy, to reveal a significant vascular abnormality that may require a specific preoperative or intraoperative measure, to assess vascular involvement by tumor (angiographic staging) and pancreatitis, respectively, and to aid in the localization of endocrine tumors.

## VASCULAR ANATOMY

Extensive dissection studies by Pierson, Michels, and others describe in detail the anatomy of the pancreatic vasculature (3–5). The angiographic anatomy of the pancreas has been analyzed and thoroughly described in vivo by Lunderquist, Reuter, and others (6–9).

## ARTERIES

The pancreas is supplied by the celiac and the superior mesenteric arteries and their branches (Fig. 6.1). The celiac artery arises from the front of the aorta at the level of T12-L1, forming an hepatolienogastric trunk in almost 90% of cases. In about 60% of cases, the common hepatic artery arises from the celiac artery giving off the gastroduodenal artery. The superior mesenteric artery usually has a separate origin from the aorta, slightly below the origin of the celiac artery. In some 20–25% of cases, an aberrant right hepatic artery arises from the superior mesenteric artery, and in some 10–15% of cases, the right hepatic lobe is entirely supplied from the superior mesenteric artery. The gastroduodenal artery arises from the common hepatic artery in about 75% of cases.

The main supply of the head of the pancreas is through the pancreaticoduodenal arcades originating from the gastroduodenal and superior mesenteric arteries via the superior and inferior pancreaticoduodenal arteries. The dorsal pancreatic artery that gives off branches to the whole pancreas may arise from the celiac artery or its main branches. The body and tail of the pancreas are mainly supplied by branches from the splenic artery and by the transverse pancreatic artery representing the left main branch of the dorsal pancreatic artery. Many collateral pathways exist between the arteries supplying the pancreas.

## VEINS

The anterior aspect of the head of the pancreas is mainly drained by the anterior superior pancreaticoduodenal vein into the superior mesenteric vein within a few centimeters of the confluence of the splenic and superior mesenteric veins (Fig. 6.2). The posterior aspect of the head is usually drained by the posterior superior pancreaticoduodenal vein into the portal vein, also within a few centimeters of the portal venous confluence (Fig. 6.2). The veins of the pancreatic body may drain into the superior mesenteric vein alone or its confluence with the portal vein or into the splenic vein. The veins of the tail of the pancreas usually drain into the splenic vein.

## ANGIOGRAPHIC TECHNIQUE

There are few contraindications to angiography, but caution should be exercised in patients on anticoagulant therapy or with a history of bleeding episodes. In patients with a history of suspected or proven previous adverse reaction to contrast medium, an adequate steroid prophylaxis should be administered for 48 hours prior to the examination. The patients, especially those in shock or in hepatic or renal failure, should be well hydrated, as angiography may require large doses of contrast medium. Solid foods should be discontinued 4 hours prior to the examination, to reduce the risk of aspiration if vomiting should occur.

The introduction of digital imaging and subtraction techniques in angiography has, however, further reduced the amount of contrast medium being used to obtain high-quality images of the vascular system.

Angiography is usually performed under local anesthesia. A mild sedative may be used as premedication, when needed.

## ARTERIOGRAPHY

Under local anesthesia, the femoral artery is punctured in the groin, using the Seldinger technique (10). Other routes of arterial access, such as the axillary or brachial arteries, may also be used. The axillary route may in fact facilitate the superselective catheterization of the celiac and superior mesenteric branches in many patients because of a straighter access to these vessels. Under fluoroscopic control, a 5–6.5F (1.7–2.2 mm OD) simple curved angiographic catheter is passed into the aorta over a guide wire. The celiac and superior mesenteric arteries are selectively catheterized, and angiograms are obtained for evaluation of the vascular anatomy and angiographic findings. Using superselective guide wire/catheter techniques, it is usually possible to further insert the original catheter or a coaxial catheter system into various branches of the celiac, superior mesenteric, and splenic arteries. Modern coaxial guide wire/catheter systems have to a great extent facilitated superselective catheterization of small arterial branches, and this

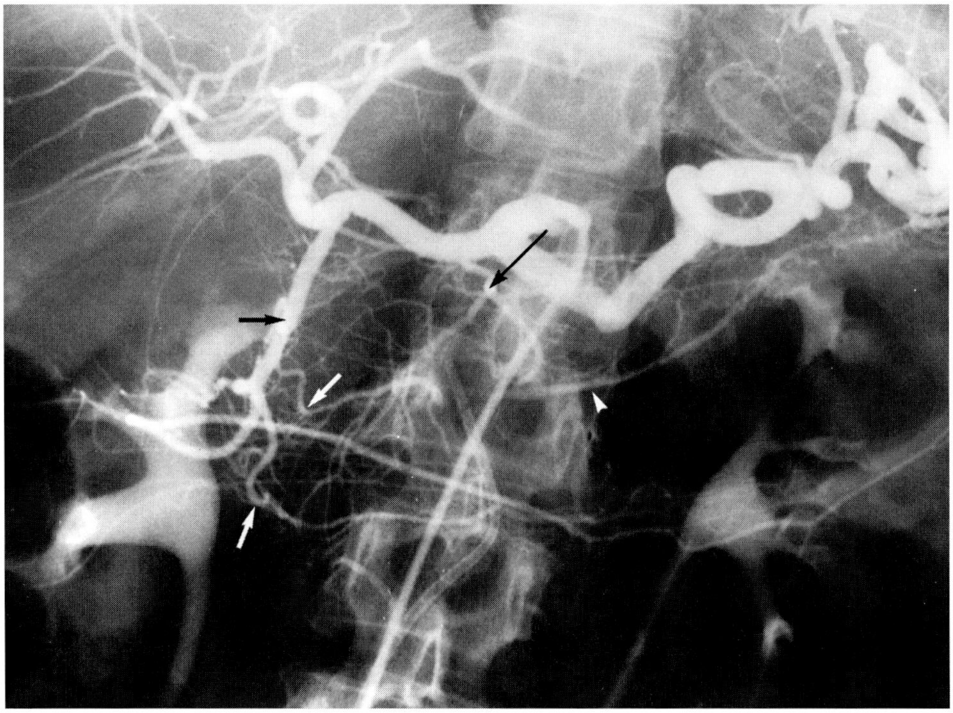

**FIG. 6.1.** Arterial blood supply of the pancreas. Selective celiac arteriogram. Gastroduodenal artery *(short black arrow)*, pancreaticoduodenal arcades *(white arrows)*, dorsal pancreatic artery *(long black arrow)*, transverse pancreatic artery *(white arrowhead)*.

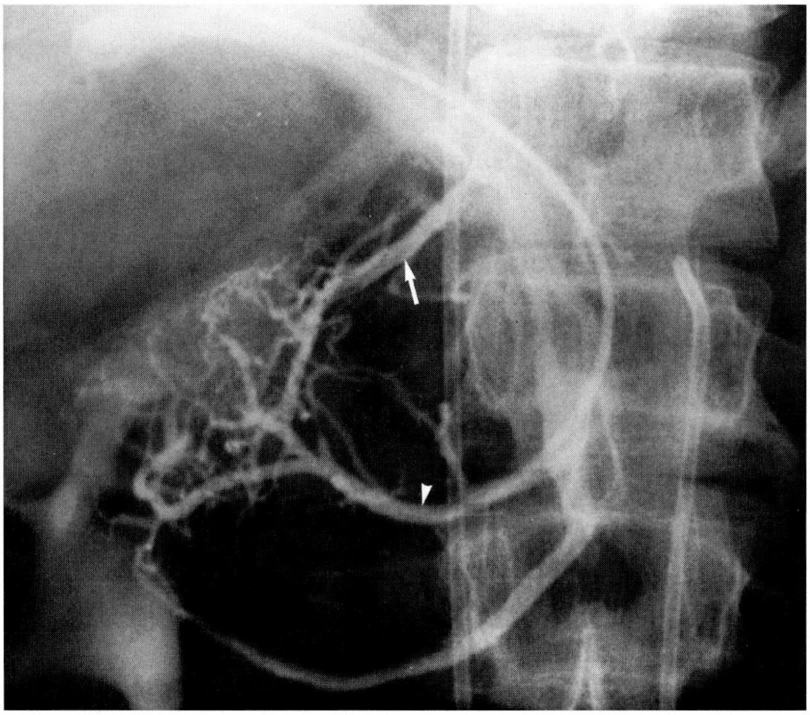

**FIG. 6.2.** The venous drainage of the head of the pancreas. The anterior *(white arrowhead)* and posterior *(white arrow)* superior pancreaticoduodenal veins.

technique is being increasingly used for embolization procedures.

For adequate opacification of the celiac and superior mesenteric territories in the adult, usually a total volume of 40–50 mL of contrast medium is injected at 8–10 mL/sec into the main stem of these arteries, using an automatic mechanical-pressure injector. To allow adequate visualization of the portal venous system, the filming sequence should continue for 16–20 seconds and sometimes longer. Exposures are usually made at a rate of 1–2/sec. The exact rate and volume of injection must, however, be individualized for each patient, depending upon the vessel size and the estimated flow in the vessel. Distension of the stomach and duodenum with gas after the administration of a smooth muscle relaxant improves the diagnostic accuracy of pancreatic angiography, since misinterpretation of folded gastric and duodenal mucosa as a pathologic process is avoided by this technique.

## PORTAL VENOGRAPHY

The portal venous system may be angiographically visualized by several techniques including indirect arterioportography and direct venography through a transhepatic, splenic, transjugular transvenous, or perioperative mesenteric puncture approach. Indirect arterioportography is usually sufficient for diagnostic purposes, but the direct transhepatic or perioperative mesenteric approach may be used also for the evaluation of the portal, mesenteric, and splenic veins by intravascular ultrasonography (11, 12).

### Indirect Portography

Indirect portography (arterioportography) is obtained following high-dose arteriograms (60–80 mL of contrast medium at 8–10 mL/sec) of the superior mesenteric and the splenic arteries, usually following an intraarterial injection of a vasodilator.

### Percutaneous Transhepatic Portography

Percutaneous transhepatic portography provides another angiographic approach (7, 13–15). Following local and sometimes intercostal anesthesia, a percutaneous approach is done in the midaxillary line through one of the lower right intercostal spaces. Under fluoroscopic control, a 25-cm sheathed needle (1.6–2.0 mm OD) is inserted in the direction of the hilum of the liver. Following withdrawal of the needle, the sheath is slowly withdrawn until blood is aspirated. When the tip is in a portal vein branch, verified by injection of contrast medium, a guide wire is introduced into the main stem of the portal vein, and the sheath subsequently further advanced over the guide wire into the splenic and superior mesenteric veins. Thereafter, angiograms are obtained of the portal venous system, using 20–40 mL of contrast medium at 6–8 mL/sec (Fig. 6.3).

At termination of the examination, during withdrawal of the angiographic catheter, the transhepatic track should be embolized to reduce the risk of bleeding complications (16).

## COMPLICATIONS

Puncture-site complications (external bleeding with hematoma, vascular thrombosis or occlusion, aneurysm formation, AV-fistula) are encountered infrequently with a good angiographic technique and with the small-size catheters recommended. Also, intimal and subintimal lesions in the aorta and the visceral arterial branches rarely occur with adequate technique.

Complications to percutaneous transhepatic portography include hemorrhage from the liver surface and within the liver, fistula formation, portal vein thrombosis, and accidental puncture of other visceral structures. A complication rate of about 9% and a mortality rate of about 0.7% have been reported, but the complication rate is lower (5–6%) in patients without cirrhosis or extrahepatic cholestasis (16).

Complications related to contrast medium (adverse reactions, local and systemic vascular changes, organ toxicity) rarely cause serious problems when a modern nonionic contrast medium is used.

## ANGIOGRAPHIC STAGING IN PANCREATIC CARCINOMA

The primary role of preoperative angiography, in those specialized centers where it is still being used, is to provide the surgeon with a map of the vascular anatomy and disclose a significant vascular abnormality; for instance, a stenosis of one of the main arteries, requiring an intraoperative move.

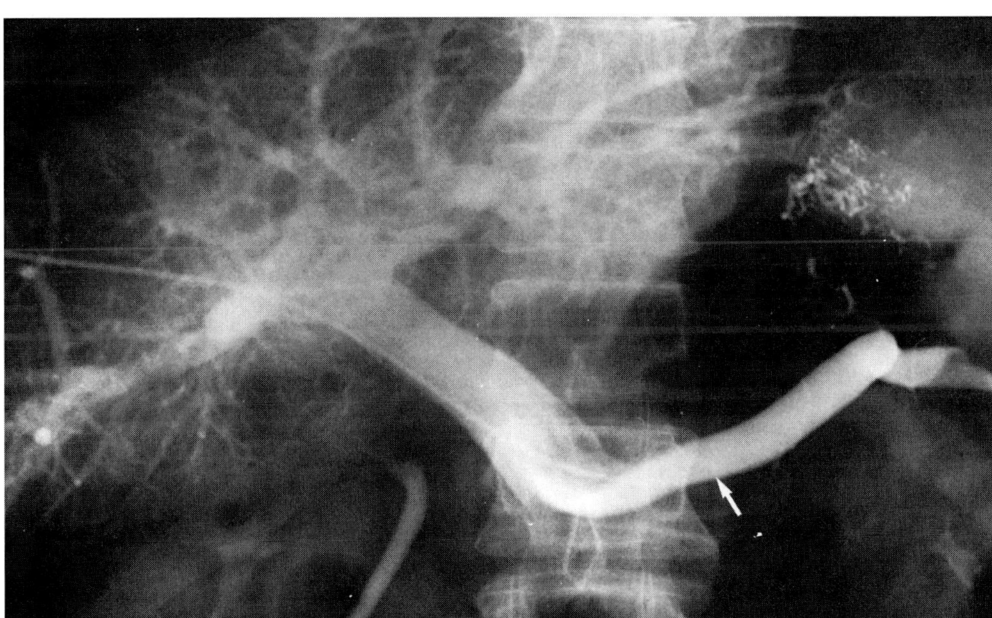

**FIG. 6.3.** Selective portal venography following a percutaneous transhepatic puncture. Catheter tip in the splenic vein *(white arrow)*.

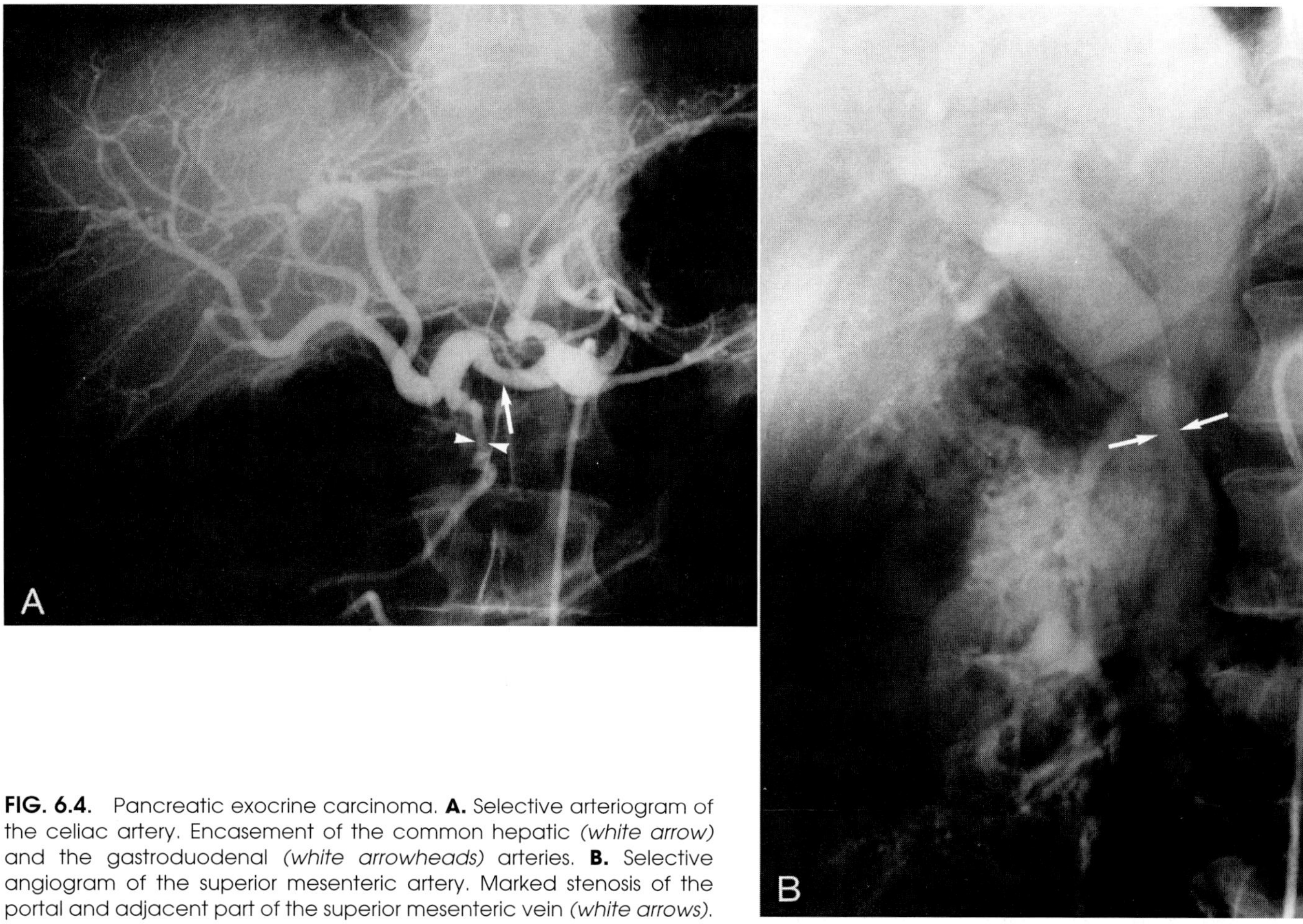


**FIG. 6.4.** Pancreatic exocrine carcinoma. **A.** Selective arteriogram of the celiac artery. Encasement of the common hepatic *(white arrow)* and the gastroduodenal *(white arrowheads)* arteries. **B.** Selective angiogram of the superior mesenteric artery. Marked stenosis of the portal and adjacent part of the superior mesenteric vein *(white arrows).*

Pancreatic exocrine carcinoma is usually hypovascular. Angiographic criteria of tumor irresectability include involvement of major extrapancreatic arteries and veins by encasement, obstruction, or occlusion (Fig. 6.4, *A* and *B*) (6, 15, 17, 18). Not rarely does a false-positive diagnosis of pancreatic carcinoma occur because of misinterpretation of the angiographic findings caused by pancreatitis or pseudocyst (18–20).

Angiography carries a diagnostic sensitivity and specificity of about 70%. Comparison of angiography and contrast-enhanced CT in patients with pancreatic carcinoma has shown that both techniques give similar information in more than 70% of the cases, but rarely do the results from angiography change the initial CT stage of a tumor (21–23).

A combination of arteriography and CT, CT arterial portography (CTAP), is commonly used for preoperative staging of pancreatic tumors. CTAP is more accurate than arteriography alone for predicting vascular involvement by tumor (23).

Preoperative assessment aims at selecting those patients with adenocarcinoma of the pancreas who are the best candidates for surgery and to identify patients with unresectable disease so that they can be spared an unnecessary operation. The demand for an accurate preoperative method of staging has been fueled by the introduction of nonoperative palliative treatment options such as endoscopic biliary stenting or laparoscopic methods for bilioenteric and gastrojejunal bypass procedures. Although Warshaw and coworkers (24) claim angiography to be complementary to CT, most recent studies, as well as their own, show a poor relationship between resectability and the angiographic features (1, 25). As these data are consistent with our own experience, we feel that angiography can no longer be advocated in the routine investigation of patients being considered for resection of pancreatic and periampullary cancer.

## ANGIOGRAPHY IN PANCREATITIS

The vascular sequelae that may follow acute and chronic pancreatitis include arterial irregularities and aneurysms as well as compression or occlusion of major veins. The vascular changes in chronic pancreatitis are in some cases indistinguishable from those seen in pancreatic carcinoma (19, 20).

## BLEEDING COMPLICATIONS IN PANCREATIC DISEASE

The most detailed information about vascular involvement in cases of arterial bleeding or thrombosis of the portal venous system is obtained by selective angiography and arterioportography, respectively. Bleeding manifests itself on angiograms as extravasation of contrast medium into a free or confined space (Fig. 6.5, *A*). It has been estimated that bleeding at a rate as low as 0.5 mL/min may be detected with selective angiography (26). When an arterial bleeding source has been identified, therapeutic transcatheter embolization can be used as a temporizing or definitive form of treatment (Fig. 6.5, *A* and *B*) (27, 28). Usually a combination of stainless steel coils and gelfoam plugs is used, but in patients with massive bleeding, balloon occlusion of the main arterial feeder may also be employed to obtain hemostasis prior to and during surgery. In cases where contrast extravasation is not appreciated, angiography may reveal an underlying vascular abnormality, such as pseudoaneurysm, aneurysm, or varices.

An immediate success rate of almost 80% has been reported with transcatheter embolotherapy in arterial complications of pancreatitis (27, 28).

When the bleeding source is a branch of a pancreaticoduodenal arcade, one has to be aware of the dual blood supply from the celiac and superior mesenteric arteries, respectively, which may require embolization from both these arteries.

## ANGIOGRAPHIC LOCALIZATION OF ENDOCRINE TUMORS OF THE PANCREAS

### Arteriography

Arteriography still has a role in the diagnosis of small endocrine pancreatic tumors. To detect a subtle tumor blush of a small tumor, a very careful angiographic technique in combination with excellent technical quality arteriograms is necessary. An islet cell tumor most often manifests itself on an angiogram as a dense, well-circumscribed, homogeneous capillary blush extending into the early venous phase (Fig. 6.6, *A* and *B*) (29–31). Selective catheterization with injection of contrast medium into the branches of the celiac and superior mesenteric arteries may localize insulinomas in 60–90%, and gastrinomas in 15–90%, of patients (32–36). When multiple tumors are present, the sensitivity for individual lesions is lower (34).

### Transhepatic Portal Venous Sampling in Endocrine Pancreatic Tumors (TPVS)

Using the technique for percutaneous transhepatic puncture of the portal venous system described above, a branch of the right portal vein is cannulated. The catheter is inserted further into the splenic vein, and samples are taken at 1.0–1.5 cm intervals in the splenic vein, in the proximal part of the portal vein, and in the superior mesenteric vein within 3–4 cm of the confluence.

TPVS yields positive results in 75–90% of patients with insulinomas and in about 40–70% of patients with gastrinomas (7, 9, 36–40). Some researchers believe that samples from the portal vein, the superior mesenteric vein, and the splenic vein are not sufficient to establish with certainty the localization of small tumors; they recommend superselective catheterization of the pancreatic veins, which may increase the sensitivity by 20–25% (13). This, however, requires great technical skill and is time consuming.

The method of transhepatic sampling is invasive and carries the risks of transhepatic puncture described above.

### Arterial Stimulation and Venous Sampling (ASVS)

Using an arterial stimulation venous sampling technique, Doppman and coworkers have presented promising results regarding the localization of insulinomas and gastrinomas by means of selective intraarterial injection of calcium and secretin, respectively, into the splenic, gastroduodenal, hepatic and superior mesenteric arteries (38, 41). Blood samples are drawn at various time intervals from the hepatic vein and a peripheral vein before and after arterial stimulation. In these studies ASVS has about the same sensitivity as portal venous sampling for the localization of insulinomas but seems superior for the localization of gastrinomas.

## CONCLUSION

Angiography can no longer be advocated in the routine preoperative investigation of patients being considered for resection of pancreatic cancer. If used at all, it should be reserved to provide a map of the vascular anatomy and to reveal significant vascular abnormalities that may influence the surgical technique. Angiography still remains as an important tool for the localization of pancreatic endocrine tumors.

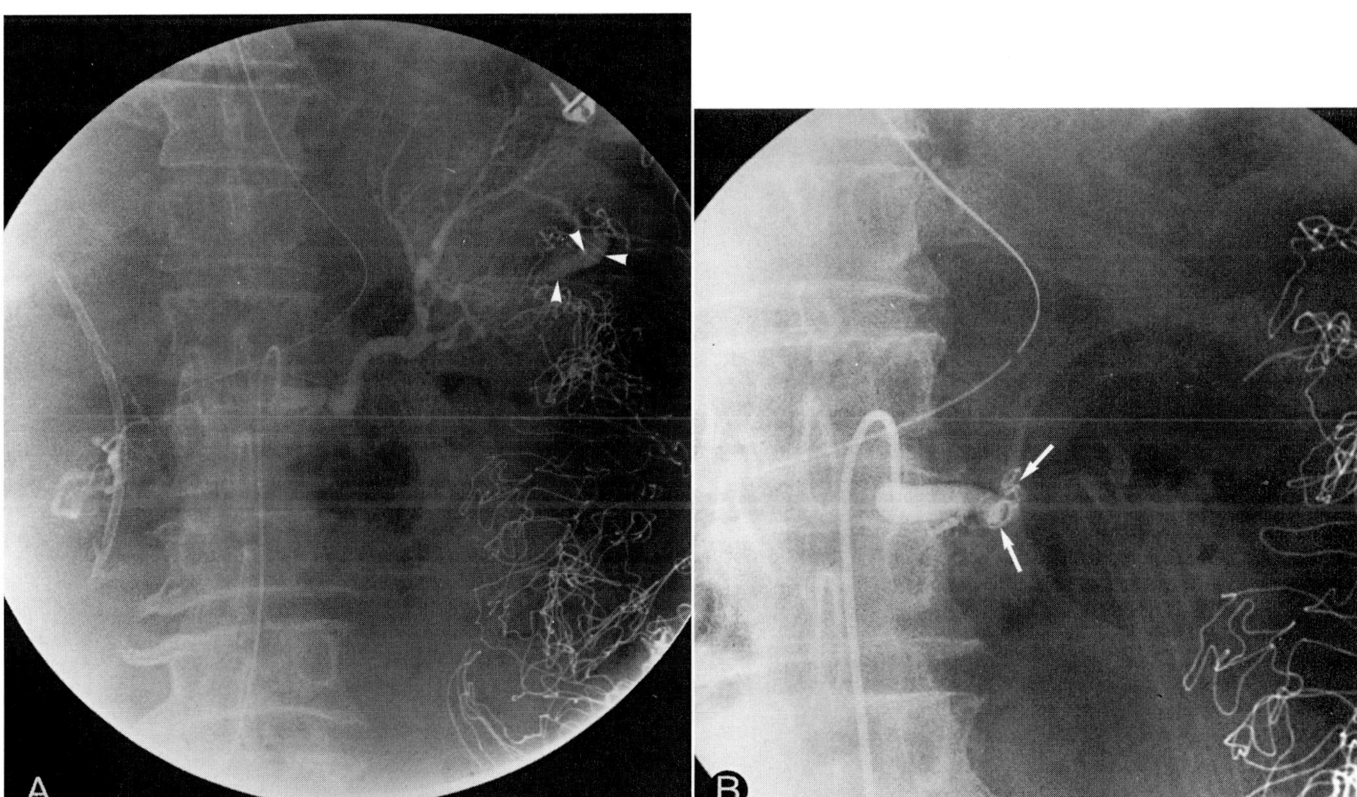

**FIG. 6.5.** Bleeding complications in acute pancreatitis. Selective arteriogram of the splenic artery. Metal strings in surgical packings. **A.** Extravasation from a branch of the splenic artery *(white arrowheads)*. **B.** The splenic artery is occluded by steel coils *(white arrows)*.

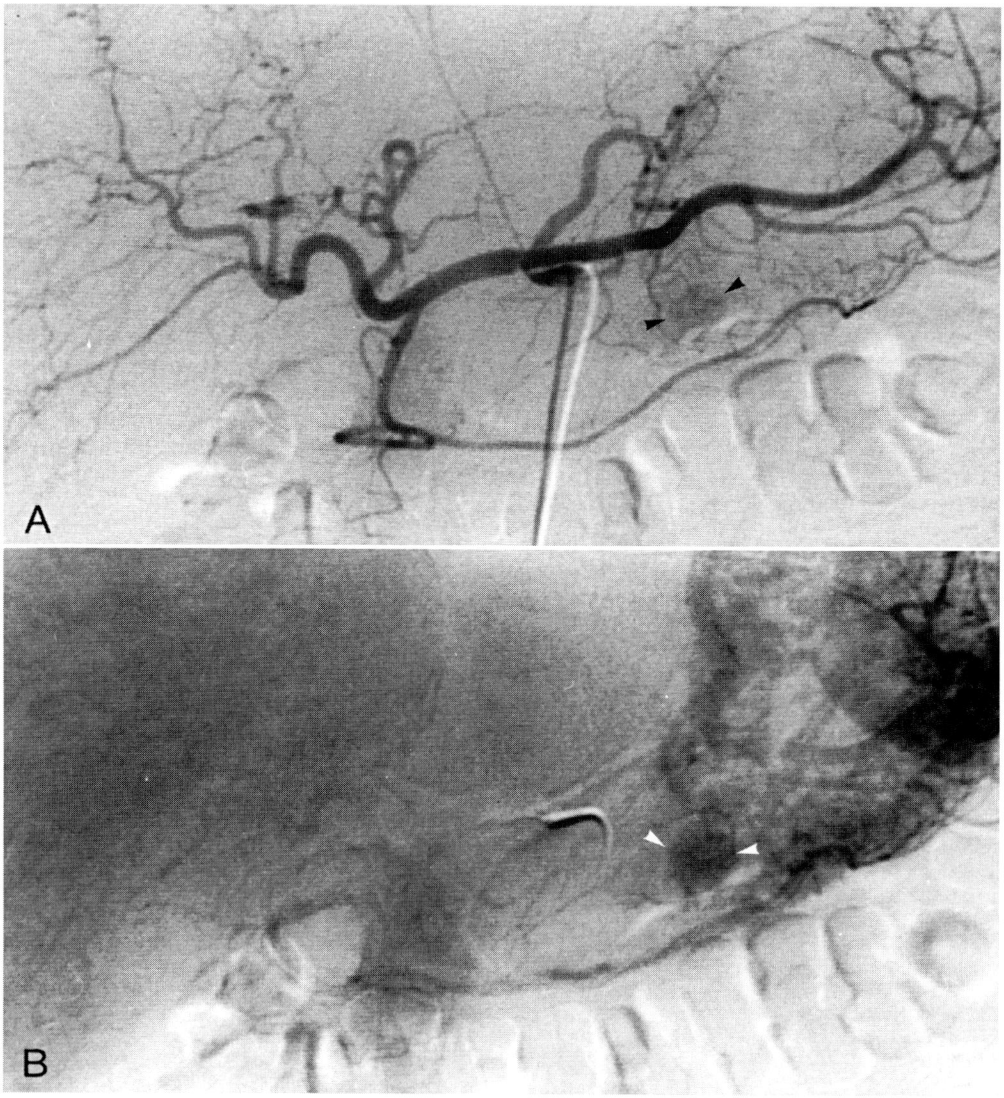


**FIG. 6.6.** Insulinoma of the body of the pancreas. Digital subtraction angiogram of the celiac artery. **A.** Early arterial phase. **B.** Late arterial phase. The tumor is seen as a well-circumscribed capillary blush *(arrowheads).*

The most detailed information about vascular involvement in cases of bleeding complications in pancreatic disease is obtained by angiography, and transcatheter embolotherapy is frequently used in such cases.

## REFERENCES

1. Murugiah M, Windsor JA, Redhead DN, et al. The role of selective visceral angiography in the management of pancreatic and periampullary cancer. World J Surg 1993;17:796–800.
2. Reznek RH, Stephens DH. Review. The staging of pancreatic adenocarcinoma. Clin Radiol 1993;47:373–381.
3. Pierson JM. The arterial blood supply of the pancreas. Surg Gynecol Obstet 1943;77:426–432.
4. Michels NA. Blood supply and anatomy of the upper abdominal organs. Philadelphia: JB Lippincott, 1955.
5. Woodburne RT, Olsen LL. The arteries of the pancreas. Anat Rec 1951;111:255–270.
6. Lunderquist A. Angiography in carcinoma of the pancreas (Thesis). Lund, Sweden. Acta Radiol 1965;(suppl 235).
7. Reichardt W. Phlebography of the pancreas. Anatomy, technique and clinical applications (Thesis). Lund, Sweden, 1979.
8. Reuter SR. Superselective pancreatic angiography. Radiology 1969;92:74–85.
9. Rösch J, Bret J. Arteriography of the pancreas. AJR 1965;94:182–193.
10. Seldinger SI. Catheter replacement of the needle in percutaneous arteriography: a new technique. Acta Radiol 1953;39:368–376.
11. Hannesson P, Stridbeck H, Lundstedt C, Andrén-Sandberg Å, Ihse I. Intravascular ultrasound of the portal vein. Normal anatomy. Acta Radiol 1995;36:388–392.
12. Hannesson PH, Stridbeck H, Lundstedt C, Dawiskiba S, Andrén-Sandberg Å, Ihse I. Intravascular ultrasound for evaluation of portal venous involvement in exocrine pancreatic cancer. Eur Radiol 1997;7:21–25.
13. Günther RW, Klose KJ, Rückert K, et al. Localization of small islet cell tumors. Preoperative and intraoperative ultrasound, computed tomography, arteriography, digital subtraction angiography and pancreatic venous sampling. Gastrointest Radiol 1985;10:145–151.
14. Hoevels J, Lunderquist A, Tylén U. Percutaneous transhepatic portography. Acta Radiol (Diagn) 1978;19:643–655.
15. Reichardt W, Ihse I. Percutaneous transhepatic portography in pancreatic carcinoma. Acta Radiol (Diagn) 1980;21:579–586.

16. Hoevels J, Lunderquist A, Owman T. Complications of percutaneous transhepatic catheterization of the portal vein and its tributaries. Acta Radiol (Diagn) 1980;21:593–601.
17. Boijsen E. Selective pancreatic angiography. Br J Radiol 1966;39: 481–487.
18. Reuter SR, Redman HC, Bookstein J. Differential problems in the angiographic diagnosis of carcinoma of the pancreas. Radiology 1970;96:93–99.
19. Boijsen E, Tylén U. Vascular changes in chronic pancreatitis. Acta Radiol (Diagn) 1972;12:34–48.
20. Reuter SR, Redman HC, Joseph RR. Angiographic findings in pancreatitis. AJR 1969;107:56–64.
21. Freeny PC, Marks WM, Ryan JA, Traverso LW. Pancreatic ductal adenocarcinoma. Diagnosis and staging with dynamic CT. Radiology 1988;166:125–133.
22. Jafri SZ, Aisen AM, Glazer GM, Weiss CA. Comparison of CT and angiography in assessing resectability of pancreatic carcinoma. AJR 1984;142:525–529.
23. Savader BL, Fishman EK, Savader SJ, Cameron JL. CT arterial portography vs pancreatic arteriography in the assessment of vascular involvement in pancreatic and periampullary tumors. J Comput Assist Tomogr 1994;18:916–920.
24. Warshaw AL, Zhuo-Yun GU, Wittenberg J, Waltman AC. Preoperative staging and assessment of resectability of pancreatic cancer. Arch Surg 1990;125:230–233.
25. Appleton GVN, Bathurst NCG, Virjee J, et al. The value of angiography in the surgical management of pancreatic disease. Ann R Coll Surg Engl 1989;71:92–96.
26. Nusbaum M, Baum S, Blakemore WS, et al. Demonstration of intraabdominal bleeding by selective arteriography. JAMA 1965; 191:389–390.
27. Mauro MA, Jaques P. Transcatheter management of pseudoaneurysms complicating pancreatitis. JVIR 1991;2:527–532.
28. Boudghéne F, L Herminé CL, Bigot J-M. Arterial complications of pancreatitis: diagnostic and therapeutic aspects in 104 cases. JVIR 1993;4:551–558.
29. Auerbach RC, Koehler PR. The many faces of islet cell tumors. AJR 1973;119:133–140.
30. Clouse ME, Costello P, Legg MA, Soeldner SJ, Cady B. Subselective angiography in localizing insulinomas of the pancreas. AJR 1977;128:741–746.
31. Fulton RE, Sheedy PF, McIlrath DC, et al. Preoperative angiographic localization of insulin-producing tumors of the pancreas. AJR 1975;123:367–377.
32. Fraker DL, Norton JA. Localization and resection of insulinomas and gastrinomas. JAMA 1988;259:3601–3605.
33. Frucht H, Doppman JL, Norton JA, et al. Gastrinomas: comparison of MR imaging with CT, angiography and US. Radiology 1989; 171:713–717.
34. Galiber AK, Reading CC, Charboneau JW, et al. Localization of pancreatic insulinoma: comparison of pre- and intraoperative US with CT and angiography. Radiology 1988;166:405–408.
35. King CM, Reznek RH, Dacie JE, Wass JA. Review. Imaging islet cell tumours. Clin Radiol 1994;49:295–303.
36. Rossi P, Allison DJ, Bezzi M, et al. Endocrine tumors of the pancreas. Radiol Clin North Am 1989;27:129–161.
37. Doherty GM; Doppman JL, Shawker TH, et al. Results of a prospective strategy to diagnose, localize and resect insulinomas. Surgery 1991;110:989–997.
38. Doppman JL, Miller DL, Chang R, et al. Gastrinomas: localization by means of selective intraarterial injection of secretin. Radiology 1990;174:25–29.
39. Pedrazzoli S, Pasquali C, Miotto D, et al. Transhepatic portal sampling for preoperative localization of insulinomas. Surg Gynecol Obstet 1987;165:101–106.
40. Vinik AI, Moattari AR, Cho K, et al. Transhepatic portal vein catheterization for localization of sporadic and MEN gastrinomas: a ten-year experience. Surgery 1990;107: 246–255.
41. Doppman JL, Miller DL, Chang R, et al. Insulinomas: localization with selective intraarterial injection of calcium. Radiology 1991; 178:237–241.

7

# Endoscopic Retrograde Cholangiopancreatography

Kogoro Kasahara and Hideo Nagai

Soon after the first report by McCune in 1968 (1), Oi published a large series of endoscopic retrograde cholangiopancreatography (ERCP) studies with a high success rate, using a lateral viewing fiberduodenoscope specifically designed for cannulating the duodenal papilla (2, 3). With its rapid widespread application throughout the world, ERCP became one of the most important diagnostic modalities for pancreatic and biliary diseases. Shortly thereafter, an endoscopic cannulation technique for ERCP brought about the development of endoscopic sphincterotomy (4, 5), bilionasal drainage (6, 7), and bilioduodenal endoprosthesis (8).

This chapter describes the overall usefulness and limitations of ECRP (not the endoscopic techniques) in managing patients with pancreatic disorders and pancreas-related diseases.

## COMPLICATIONS

Even in experienced hands, complications occur in 0.6–3.1% of examinations, with a mortality rate of 0.13–0.19% (9–11). Pancreatitis and sepsis are the two main complications. Injection of contrast may cause a transient rise in serum amylase and lipase in about 60% of patients after pancreatography, particularly in cases of acinar opacification, and may result in a pyelogram in some instances. These sequelae are asymptomatic in most instances (12–14). ERCP, however, may rarely (0–1.3%) cause acute pancreatitis, which is usually self-limited and only occasionally requires medical treatment (9–11, 15). Post-ERCP pancreatitis may be prevented to an extent by careful limitation of contrast volume and avoidance of acinar opacification (15).

Post-ERCP sepsis occurs almost exclusively in patients with poor drainage of the pancreatic and biliary systems. As the result of the bacterial contamination introduced by the procedure (16), pancreatic sepsis occurs in 0.3–1.7%, with a mortality rate of up to 0.06% in patients with recurrent pancreatitis, malignant stenosis, and pseudocysts (9–11). Resulting from dissemination of bacteria already present in the biliary tract (17, 18), septic cholangitis occurs in 0.3–0.8%, with a mortality rate of 0.05–0.1% (9–11). When ductal stricture is suspected, the volume of contrast injected should be kept to the minimum needed to confirm the presence of the stricture but not necessarily depict the lesion itself. Prophylactic antibiotics should be either used parenterally or added to the contrast material (19). However, the most effective prevention and treatment of sepsis is a prompt surgical, endoscopic, or transcutaneous decompression when ductal strictures are found.

Other complications of ERCP are either of less importance or uncommon, including instrumental injury, perforation of the biliary tree, extraluminal injection of the contrast medium, drug reaction, and aspiration pneumonia.

## THE NORMAL PANCREATOGRAM

### Common Channel

The common bile duct and the main pancreatic duct usually coalesce to form a common channel as they traverse the duodenal wall. In most cases the common channel is visualized on ERCP as a small-caliber duct, usually 1–15 mm long, with slight undulation of a villous mucosal pattern. Ampullary dilation of this portion is seen in relatively few cases, despite the prevailing terminology of "ampulla."

The sphincter of Oddi encircles the common channel as well as the terminal ends of the bile and pancreatic ducts, forming the narrow segment of each duct. These narrow segments may sometimes appear indistinguishable from "true" stenosis with neoplasm or inflammation on ERCP. Fluoroscopic observation, however, can well differentiate it from a pathologic stenosis, by demonstrating periodic contraction of each sphincter of the bile and pancreatic ducts. The exception is a noninvasive tumor, such as adenoma of the papilla, with which the sphincters may occasionally maintain phasic contractions (Fig. 7.1).

A separate opening of the bile and pancreatic ducts on the papilla is seen in 2–18% of individuals (20–22). The incidence may differ, depending on whether necropsy materials are used or the living papilla is observed endoscopically. Double papillae of Vater have been reported as a rare variant (less than 0.2%) (23).

### The Main Pancreatic Duct (Wirsung)

The three-dimensional course of the main pancreatic duct should be understood. The duct bends anteriorly approximately 2 cm before its conjunction with the accessory duct (Santorini) and changes direction to the left. An anteroposterior projection of this bending is shown on ERCP as either a smooth transition, sharp angulation, or alpha-loop formation, depending on the difference in the angle and position of the turning points.

The configuration of the main pancreatic duct has been classified on the basis of the pattern of its course through the pancreas (19, 24), but these do not appear to be of much clinical significance. An unusual course of the duct sometimes reflects compression by an extrapancreatic mass but may also only reflect a normal variation.

The length of the main pancreatic duct ranges from 95 to 240 mm, as measured on ERCP (19, 25–26) or autopsy radiograms (24). Of clinical note is the judgment of whether or not contrast medium extends to the caudal end of the pancreatic duct. The main pancreatic duct gradually tapers as it runs from the head to the tail of the pancreas. Average diameters of the main pancreatic duct in the head, body, and tail are 3.1–4.8, 2.0–3.5 and 0.9–2.4 mm, respectively, when measured by ERCP (19, 25, 27).

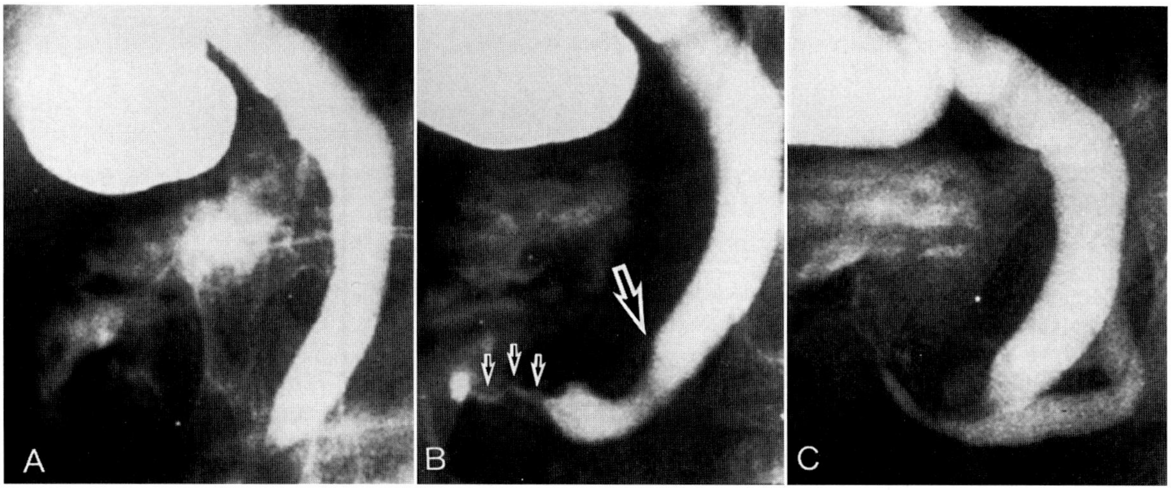


**FIG. 7.1.** Adenoma of the papilla of Vater does not diminish phasic contractions of the sphincter. The two cholangiograms during the contracting (**A**) and relaxing (**B**) phases of Oddi's sphincter around the terminal portion of the common bile duct (CBD) demonstrate that the neoplastic spread *(small arrows)* into the bile duct might not reach the uppermost edge of the sphincter *(large arrow)*. **C.** The simultaneously opacified pancreatic duct also indicates limited extension of the adenoma within the sphincter around the main pancreatic duct (MPD). These ERCP findings have enabled us to perform local resection of the papilla of Vater including the uppermost portions of Oddi's sphincter around the CBD and main pancreatic duct with clear surgical margins (33).

The main pancreatic duct usually has a slight narrowing of its caliber (fusion narrowing) near or at its junction with the accessory duct (Santorini), which sometimes looks like an abrupt, pinhole stricture on the films (28, 29). This "pseudostricture" does not cause dilation of the upstream pancreatic duct, and normal side branches arise from the side. Another rare normal variant of the main pancreatic duct is a bifid duct that bifurcates into two large paralleling ducts in the body of the pancreas (29).

### The Accessory Pancreatic Duct (Santorini)

The accessory pancreatic duct usually joins the main pancreatic duct at the uppermost part of the pancreatic genu. In most cases, it has a smaller caliber than does the main duct in the head region.

The accessory pancreatic duct usually opens on the minor papilla into the duodenum. However, the rate of its patency to the duodenal lumen has been reported as 55–60% (20, 28, 30). Ampullary or cystic dilation of the accessory duct at its duodenal end is often observed, irrespective of its patency to the duodenal lumen (31). The accessory duct, however, rarely loses a connection with the main pancreatic duct.

### Side Branches

Both the main and accessory ducts have numerous tributaries radiating chiefly at right angles from the stem duct. Some 20–30 branches are seen to join the main duct in the body of the pancreas (32). The head of the pancreas has a rather complicated ramification due to embryologic fusion of the ventral and dorsal anlagen. The lower part of the head of the pancreas, including the uncinate process, is dominated by descending branches from both the main and accessory ducts.

### Pancreatographic Changes with Aging

The pancreas, as other organs, undergoes atrophic changes with increasing age, after full development between its 20th and 40th year. Atrophy is more marked in the parenchymal tissues of the gland than in the mesenchymal ones. The ductal system tends to retain its structure despite ongoing shrinkage of the surrounding acinar tissues. These alterations may be reflected on the pancreatogram of aged people as various degrees of dilation, meandering, and irregularity of the main pancreatic duct and tributaries. Despite several reports (19, 24, 26, 27, 31), it has not been determined whether the duct elongates with aging. However, the caliber seems to change with aging as the pancreas undergoes parenchymal atrophy (31).

Epithelial changes can also affect the pancreatogram of "normal" elderly subjects. Both mucous and squamous cell metaplasia, commonly seen in small ducts, is frequently found with increasing age after 50 years of age, as shown by an autopsy study (34). The duct lined with metaplastic, often hyperplastic, epithelium usually shows segmental dilation, mostly as a small round "cyst" containing mucoid material (as in mucous cell metaplasia) or calcified stones (as in squamous cell metaplasia) (35) within its lumen (Fig. 7.2). Such small cystic or calcified lesions, 2–5 mm in diameter, as demonstrated in the peripheral ducts of asymptomatic elderly patients, almost invariably represent "senile changes" of the pancreas. These pancreatographic features should not be regarded as representing mucus-secreting cystic neoplasm or chronic calcifying pancreatitis. However, mucous metaplastic cysts occasionally require differentiation from cystic neoplasms when they are over 3 cm in diameter.

## CONGENITAL ANOMALY

ERCP can often delineate well the anomalous pancreatobiliary ductal systems. Pancreas divisum, that is, nonfusion of the dorsal and ventral pancreatic duct systems, occurs in 4–6% of the population and may be related to chronic pancreatitis if the minor papilla orifice is small compared with the large secretory volume required to drain the large dorsal pancreas (Fig. 7.3). The short ventral pancreatic duct in the congenitally short pancreas, as well as in pancreas divisum, may be mistaken for neoplastic obstruction of the main pancreatic duct at pancreatography (36). An annular pancreas may present during adult life with duodenal stenosis, peptic ulceration, or chronic pancreatitis or as an incidental finding. Its diagnosis may be established by the combined use of computed tomography (CT) and ERCP, demonstrating a duct surrounding the duodenum (37–40).

Anomalous pancreaticobiliary duct union (APBDU),

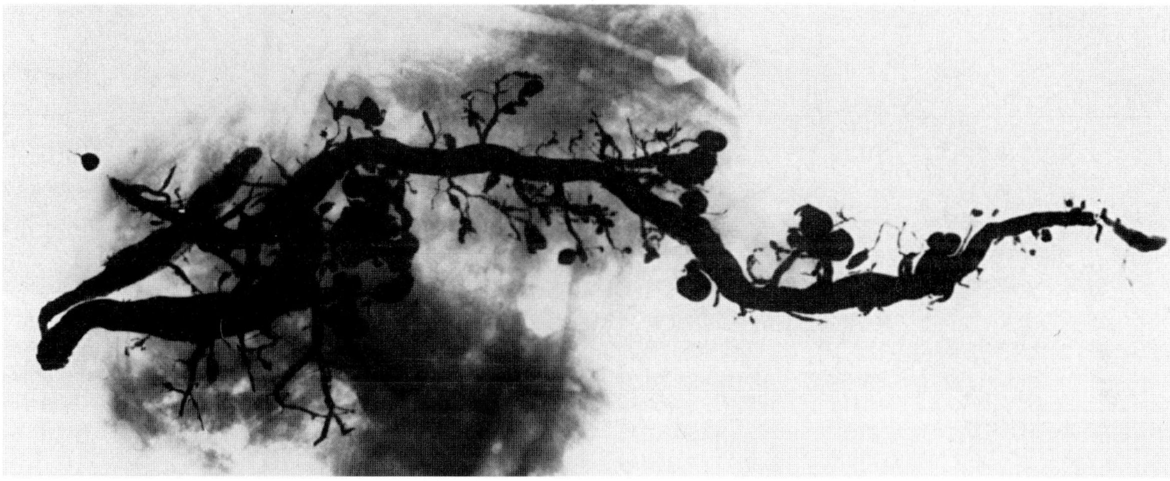

**FIG. 7.2.** Pancreatogram of autopsy material obtained from a 78-year-old man. The side branches are studded with multiple round cysts; histologic examination reveals an internal surface lined by hyperplastic epithelia with mucous cell metaplasia.

whether associated with choledochal dilation or not, results in a high rate of occurrence of cancer of the gallbladder and bile duct with increasing age (41–43). Choledochal dilation can be easily detected on ultrasound and CT, whereas APBDU itself is difficult to diagnose. Preoperative evaluation of APBDU with ERCP may be very helpful in safely achieving the standard operative procedure, that is, complete excision of the extrahepatic bile duct followed by biliary diversion (44) (Fig. 7.4).

## TRAUMA

Pancreatic trauma may lead to pancreatitis, fistulas, pseudocysts, abscesses, and retroperitoneal hemorrhage. Many of these situations resolve with conservative management, except for pancreatic ductal leakage and resultant "pseudocystic" collection. Persistent ductal leakage, which otherwise carries prolonged morbidity and high mortality, requires definitive surgical correction.

Even during laparotomy, traumatic ductal rupture may be easily overlooked because of a retroperitoneal hematoma and a seemingly intact pancreas. Therefore, for suspected pancreatic trauma, ERP should preferably be performed within 24 or 72 hours at the latest after injury, to delineate a pancreatic ductal rupture. Once a major ductal rupture is shown, immediate surgery should follow because of the possible risks of infection with contrast (45). For late posttraumatic complications, ERP is also effective to demonstrate stricture or disruption of the main pancreatic duct, with or without upstream dilation and its associated fluid collection (46, 47). On the contrary, a normal pancreatogram can prevent an unnecessary laparotomy, if a possible pancreatic injury is the only reason for exploratory laparotomy (48).

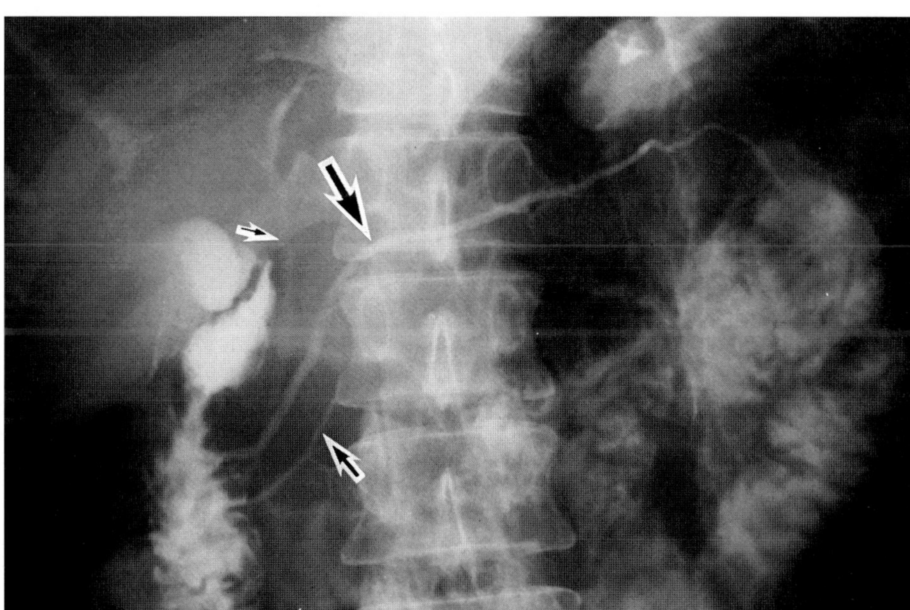

**FIG. 7.3.** Pancreas divisum. This ERCP demonstrates simultaneously the thin and short ventral pancreatic duct *(arrow)*, the thick and long dorsal pancreatic duct *(large arrow)*, and the choledochus *(small arrow)*, respectively.

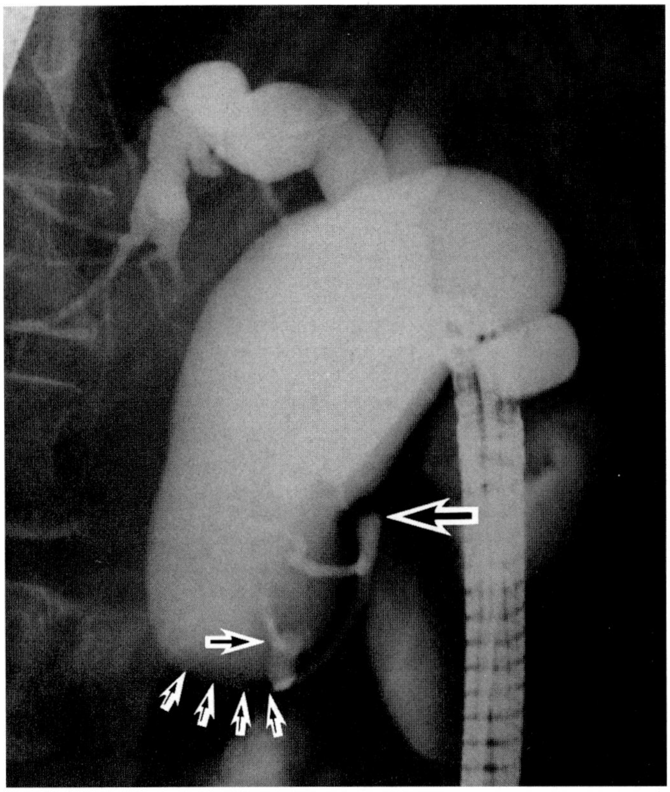

**FIG. 7.4.** Choledochal cyst. Injection of the minor papilla *(large arrow)* demonstrates that the accessory duct communicates with a thin main pancreatic duct *(small arrows)*, which appears to terminate blind distally. The choledochal cyst drains into the main pancreatic duct at a right angle *(middle arrow)*.

## ACUTE PANCREATITIS

As a rule, nonbiliary acute pancreatitis is a contraindication for ERCP. A danger of inducing necrotizing pancreatitis (about 0.1% of pancreatographies) is increased tenfold with preexisting inflammatory changes in the ductular system (49, 50). Whether or not a diagnostic ERCP should be carried out 2–4 weeks after normalization of serum amylase is under discussion (51).

While the pancreatogram is normal in most patients with acute relapsing pancreatitis, the incidence of an abnormal pancreatogram, such as minor tortuosity, saccular dilation, and obstruction of the main pancreatic duct, generalized or segmental moniliform dilation of secondary ductules, or pseudocysts (Fig. 7.5), varies from rare (52, 53) to frequent (39%) (54). This presumably reflects differences in the severity and etiologic spectrum from institution to institution. Contrary to many reports (53), Hamilton et al. (55) advocated that such an abnormal pancreatogram predicts a further recurrent attack in 50%, while no recurrent attack occurs in any patient with a normal pancreatogram, despite continued alcohol abuse.

"Idiopathic" pancreatitis, for which no causative factor can be determined despite extensive workup, is encountered in 10–30% of cases of acute pancreatitis. Within this group, ERCP can also identify potentially remediable causes in 31–46%, including biliary stones, ampullary stenosis, pancreas divisum, pancreatic ductal stricture, and pancreatic cancer (56–58).

## ACUTE BILIARY PANCREATITIS

It is widely accepted that biliary pancreatitis is initiated by a gallstone migrating along the distal common bile duct. It is also accepted that most stones spontaneously pass through the ampulla during the acute phase (59). However, it is not known with certainty whether the inflammatory process subsides or is aggravated in the presence of a persisting stone. Some advocate that for patients with suspected common bile duct (CBD) stones,

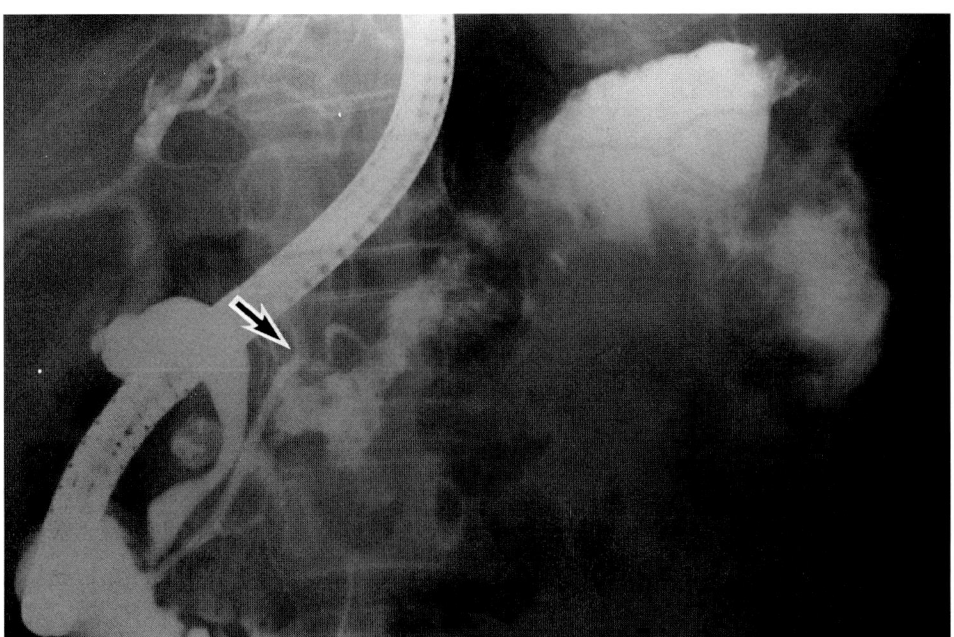

**FIG. 7.5.** Acute pancreatitis with pseudocyst formation after biliary surgery. Contrast medium leaks from the ruptured main pancreatic duct *(arrow)* and extends into the retroperitoneal space, forming a large complex pseudocyst.

selective ERC, not ERP, is indicated within 48–72 hours after admission. If biliary stones and/or papillary stenosis is confirmed as the cause of the pancreatitis, endoscopic sphincterotomy (EST) and endoscopic stone extraction should be performed in virtually all cases, in expectation of an aborted or reduced inflammatory process (60–65). The optimal timing of ERC and EST, urgent (within 72 hours after admission), or earlier, or later, is not yet clear.

Despite the fact that migrating gallstones may separately cause acute pancreatitis or acute cholangitis, the coexistence of both conditions in the same patient (14.4% of biliary pancreatitis) has received little attention. Early EST and stone extraction may significantly improve mortality (4.7%) in such patients with the coexisting problems, as compared with early surgical decompression (59, 66).

As more widely accepted, ERCP and/or EST can be employed for patients with suspected biliary stones several weeks (within 2 weeks of recovery) (51) after resolution of an attack or for those with late complications, such as pancreatic fistula or pseudocyst. ERCP can more precisely detect gallstones than other diagnostic techniques in this situation and can be immediately followed by EST and stone extraction if necessary (64, 67).

*Ascaris*-induced pancreatitis, a condition similar to biliary pancreatitis, is one of the most important causes of acute pancreatitis (23%) in endemic areas of the world (68). Urgent duodenoscopy with ERCP, followed by endoscopic or surgical worm extraction, is very effective in aborting the inflammatory process.

## CHRONIC PANCREATITIS

Pancreatographic alterations, varying from almost normal to severe, often reflect the degree of severity of the histologic and functional changes of chronic pancreatitis (69) (Fig. 7.6). However, most patients with chronic pancreatitis referred for surgical treatment have definitive abnormalities of the pancreatic ductal system, such as multiple segmental dilatations and stenoses (the chain of lakes) (Fig. 7.7), complete obstruction, cystic dilatation of side branches, stones or protein precipitations, fistulae, and pseudocysts. Preoperative ERCP is mandatory, especially for performing decompression surgery to relieve pain.

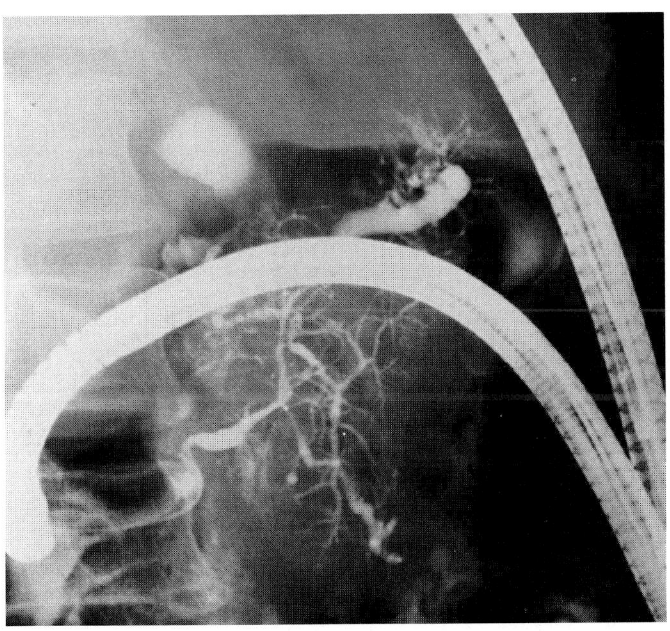

**FIG. 7.6.** Chronic pancreatitis. Pancreatography demonstrates moderate ductal and ductular changes in the pancreatic head but, proximal to this area, a remarkable dilatation of the distal main pancreatic duct.

"Groove pancreatitis" is a special form of segmental pancreatitis occurring between the pancreatic head, duodenum, and common bile duct, often causing duodenal stenosis, and presenting as a tumor of the head of the pancreas on sonography and CT scanning (70). ERCP is of great value in diagnosing this disease.

In 25% of patients with chronic pancreatitis, the common bile duct is affected, resulting in stenosis and obstruction (Fig. 7.8). Therefore, before operation for chronic pancreatitis, the bile duct should also be opacified (71).

## PANCREATIC PSEUDOCYST

CT or ultrasonography plays an important role in detecting pancreatic pseudocysts and their anatomic relations. ERCP can introduce infection in a pseudocyst, resulting in a major disaster (49, 72).

Although proposed earlier by pioneering investigators (10, 73–80), only recently has the value of a preoperative ERCP in surgical management been shown, demonstrating that ductal abnormalities are common in patients with pseudocysts, whether associated with acute or chronic pancreatitis (77, 81–84).

In the late 1980s, percutaneous and endoscopic drainage of pseudocysts were developed, providing additional therapeutic options with good results (85–97). Both techniques yielded fewer complications but more recurrences than surgical drainage, whether external or internal. As pancreatic ductal abnormalities are important factors inducing pseudocyst recurrences and persistent symptoms (78, 83), routine preoperative evaluation with ERCP was advocated to select the optimal treatment for pseudocysts. Asymptomatic isolated small pseudocysts (<5 cm in diameter) can be observed expectantly for spontaneous resolution. If ERCP shows pancreatic duct obstruction or pseudocyst communication (Fig. 7.5), surgical decompression of the main pancreatic duct and pseudocyst should be performed; otherwise, percutaneous or endoscopic decompression of pseudocysts may be indicated. For another notable ERCP finding, dilatation of the entire main pancreatic duct, so frequently seen in chronic pancreatitis, pancreaticojejunostomy has been advocated (83, 98), but its indication remains controversial unless it is associated with persistent pain due to ductal obstruction. Routine preoperative use of ERCP, along with CT scans, has almost eliminated the need for intraoperative assessment of biliary and pancreatic ductal abnormalities (99).

To minimize complications, preoperative ERCP should be followed by surgery, if necessary, within 24 hours, with parenteral antibiotics having been given before the ERCP. Contrast should be injected under low pressure and under close fluoroscopic control and terminated immediately when a cavity or ductal obstruction is identified. Fortunately, the incidence of complications with ERCP for patients with pancreatic pseudocysts, including a 4% incidence of clinical sepsis, may only be slightly higher than that for patients of all diagnoses (10, 82, 84, 100).

## CHRONIC PANCREATIC ASCITES AND PLEURAL EFFUSIONS

Pancreatic ascites and pleural effusions are uncommon complications that are postulated to result from pancreatic ductular rupture (101, 102). These complications may occur in alcoholic

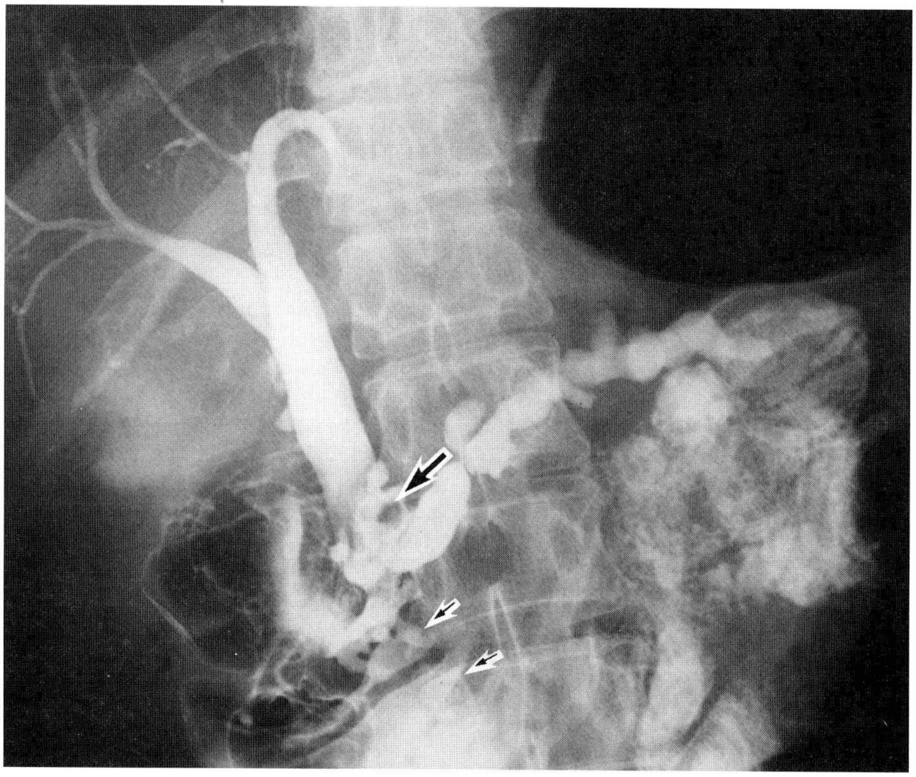

**FIG. 7.7.** Chronic pancreatitis. The pancreatogram suggests a severely atrophic pancreas due to chronic pancreatitis. *Small arrows* indicate stones in the dilated ductal branches. A *large arrow* indicates protein precipitation in the dilated main duct.

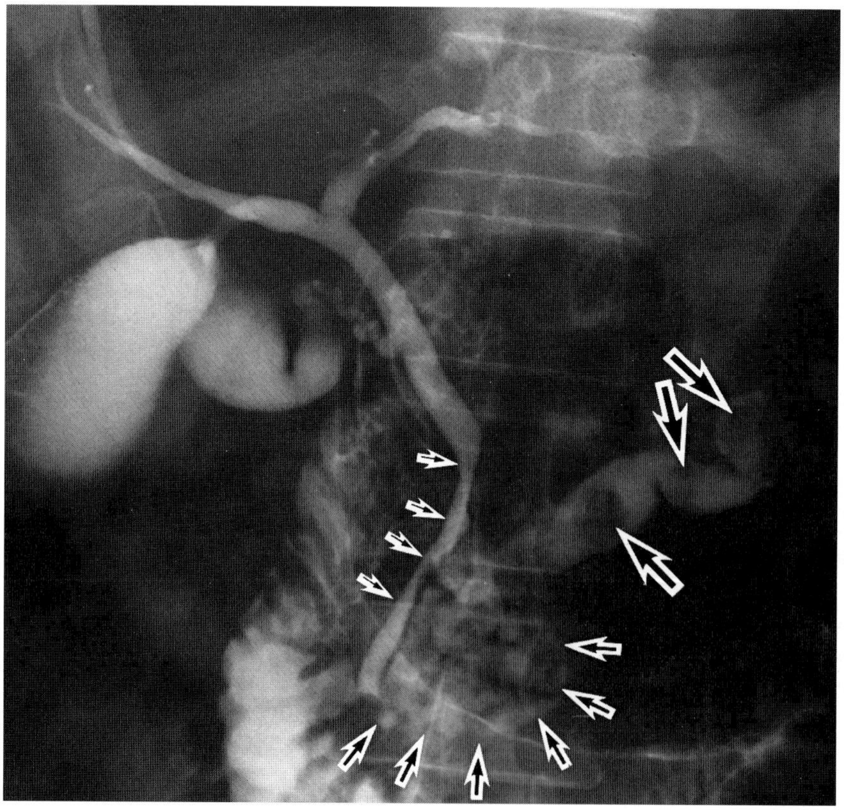

**FIG. 7.8.** Chronic pancreatitis. The cholangiogram shows a relatively smooth and long stenotic portion of the CBD *(small arrows)* with a slight upstream dilatation. The simultaneous pancreatogram demonstrates multiple dilated branches in the pancreatic head *(middle-sized arrows)* and, proximal to this, the dilated main pancreatic duct containing shadow defects *(large arrows)*, which represent immature stones.

pancreatitis, with either a recent or remote history of alcohol abuse. They may also follow pancreatic trauma in rare cases. Following a conservative regimen, such as bowel rest with total parenteral nutrition, nasogastric suction, and serial peritoneo- or thoracocenteses, most fistulas close spontaneously (101, 103). However, ERCP may provide anatomic information on the location of fistulous tracts and pancreatic duct abnormalities that is mandatory for surgical management (102, 104–106).

## OBSTRUCTIVE JAUNDICE

Management of jaundiced patients first requires confirmation that the jaundice is obstructive in type and then, determination of the site and nature of the obstruction. Ultrasound can detect the presence of biliary obstruction and of a mass lesion but fails to visualize the distal common bile duct. CT is also effective in determining bile duct obstruction and mass lesions with metastases, but is unable to define a small stone impacted in the ampulla and the precise nature of an enlarged pancreas head. For these reasons, cholangiography is indicated in every suspected case of obstructive jaundice. [*Editor's note:* Others might be more selective in this indication.]

ERCP has three distinct advantages. *(a)* the ability to visualize and biopsy ampullary lesions, *(b)* the demonstration of both biliary and pancreatic duct system, and *(c)* most importantly, better therapeutic potential such as endoscopic bilioduodenal drainage (107). However, in biliary obstruction, especially that of a neoplastic nature (108), ERCP as a diagnostic tool carries a high risk of biliary sepsis, with an incidence of 0.12–6.5% (10, 109). Therefore, bilioduodenal drainage, such as endoprostheses, is best placed during the same session as the diagnostic endoscopic study, or surgical decompression should be performed within 24 hours after ERCP to prevent biliary sepsis (100, 110, 111).

Another scheme in managing biliary obstruction is percutaneous transhepatic cholangiodrainage (PTCD) as the first step for decompression of the biliary ducts, followed after reduction of jaundice by diagnostic cholangiography.

### Cancer of the Papilla of Vater

An epithelial neoplasm of the papilla of Vater should theoretically arise from either the pancreatic duct, bile duct, common channel, duodenal mucosa, or glandular tissues surrounded by or embedded in Oddi's musculature. It is often difficult, however, to pinpoint its precise origin clinically or histopathologically. When arising from or near the orifice of the papilla, duodenoscopy can reveal a papillary, nodular, or ulcerative neoplasm, and ERCP usually shows a localized stenosis or obstruction of both the pancreatic and bile ducts at their terminal portions, accompanied by the dilated upstream ducts. If the cancer is as small as 5–10 mm in diameter, however, and is localized at the terminal portions of the pancreatic duct or choledochus, it may escape the notice of an endoscopist because of an endoscopically normal appearance of the papilla. ERCP may suggest involvement of either the pancreatic or bile duct, with an intact common channel or duodenal mucosa.

In cases of failure to visualize the orifice because of neoplastic involvement, cannulation is better attempted at the center of an ulcerative or papillary lesion, searching for a point where a catheter can be inserted without resistance.

## PANCREATIC CANCER

### Tumors of the Pancreas

The vast majority of pancreatic cancer is invasive ductal adenocarcinoma. Although its earliest nidus is believed to be in a peripheral duct or ductule, by the time of clinical detection it will have reached 2 cm or more in diameter. Even with modern diagnostic tools, it almost invariably presents with considerable anatomic alterations such as obstruction or stenosis of the main pancreatic duct with upstream dilation noted on pancreatography. ERCP can further offer useful diagnostic clues to small pancreatic cancers, defined as 2 cm or less in diameter, tumors that are found on only rare occasions (112, 113). Obstruction may be tapered or abrupt, whereas stenosis is characteristically irregular or nodular, although it may occasionally appear smooth (Fig. 7.9). In the body and tail of the pancreas, the length of stenosis depends on the size of the tumor. When the cancer is located in the periphery of the pancreatic head, especially in the uncinate process (Fig. 7.10), or when it is not large enough to produce encasement, it may cause only a very subtle or no change in the main pancreatic duct.

Although ultrasonography or CT scanning can readily show the dilated ductal system proximal to stenosis or obstruction, ERCP sometimes helps differentiate cancer from chronic pancreatitis by direct depiction of the proximal duct. Although the marked contrast between the intact distal (head) duct and the dilated proximal (tail) duct makes it easy to differentiate a neoplasm from chronic pancreatitis, the differential diagnosis often becomes difficult when stenosis begins near the papilla of Vater. The clue to differentiation may be that cancer likely causes regularly undulated dilation of the proximal (obstructed) ductal system (Fig. 7.9), whereas chronic pancreatitis presents with variegated patterns such as unevenly situated segments of dilatation and stenosis of the main duct, cystically dilated side branches, stones or protein plugs, and/or pseudocysts (113). There is a tendency toward budding of several side branches from the stenotic portion in chronic pancreatitis, while cancer seldom spawns tributaries at the very site of stenosis. Chronic pancreatitis associated with cancer, even if uncommon, provides a challenging problem in ERCP diagnosis.

More uncommon pancreatographic findings include extravasation of contrast medium into necrotic cavities of a tumor (Fig. 7.11) and focal nonvisualization of minute ductules or acini (acinar defect) without any other abnormal findings. The latter reflects a localized tumor invading and replacing the surrounding acinar tissues and small branches.

Endoscopic cholangiography also reveals irregular stenosis or occlusion of the common bile duct involved by cancer of the pancreatic head (double duct sign). Cancer of the uncinate process or the pancreatic body and tail rarely involves the bile duct until far advanced.

### Other Pancreatic Tumors

Lymphomas may involve any portion of the pancreas (Fig. 7.12). In general, islet cell tumors are expansive and slow growing, providing no or minimal pancreatographic abnormalities. ERCP is of little diagnostic value for symptomatic islet cell tumors such as insulinoma or gastrinoma, which can be diagnosed otherwise at a small size. Nonfunctioning and/or malignant large tumors may involve the pancreatic ductal system and require ERCP to diagnose.

Mucinous cystadenoma and cystadenocarcinoma of the pancreas (Fig. 7.13) also characteristically demonstrate expansive and slow growth. Owing to their asymptomatic nature, tumors often escape the notice of patients and physicians to attain a large size, usually 5–10 cm in diameter. These tumors usually demonstrate only a prominent compression of the ductal system, but, if extremely enlarged, sometimes show seemingly total obstruction of the main pancreatic duct on ERCP, despite obvious patency on mechanical examination of the resected specimen with a probe. ERCP seldom reveals communication between the pancreatic duct and the cystic lumen.

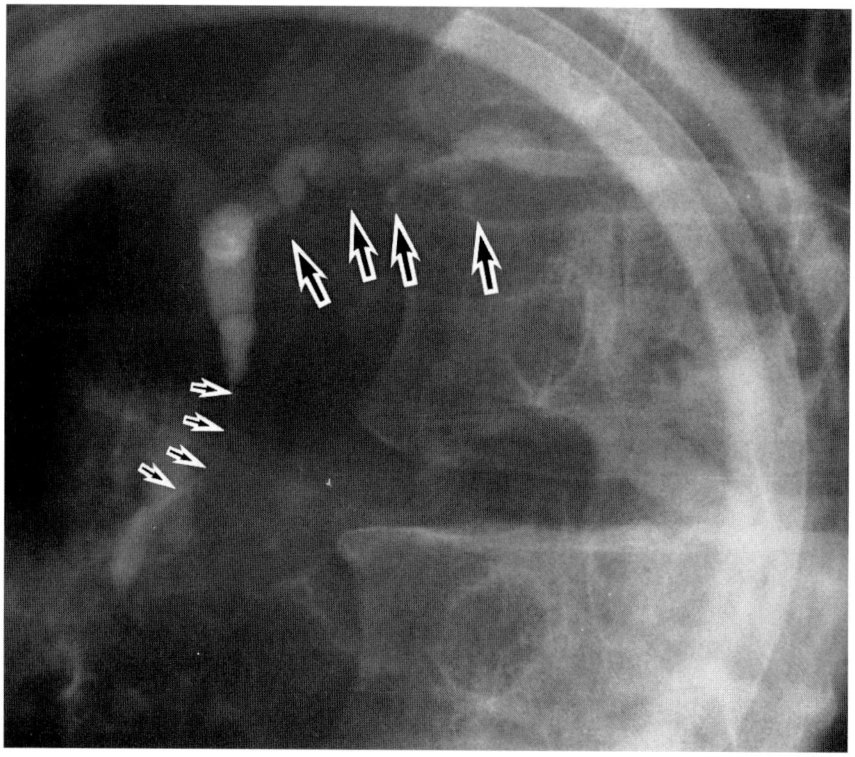

**FIG. 7.9.** Cancer of the head of the pancreas. A long, tapered, and smooth ductal stenosis *(small arrows)* in the pancreatic head with a moderate upstream dilatation of the main duct and blurred stains *(large arrows)* of branches.

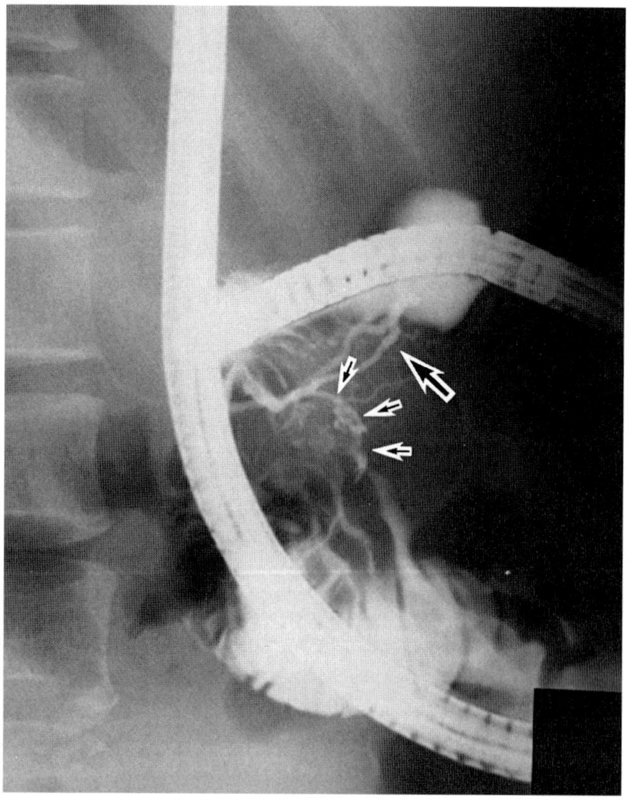

**FIG. 7.10.** Cancer of the uncinate process of the pancreas. Cancer involves the inferior cranial branch *(small arrows)* of the pancreatic duct, but does not involve the main pancreatic duct in lateral view *(large arrow)* nor, so far, the common bile duct.

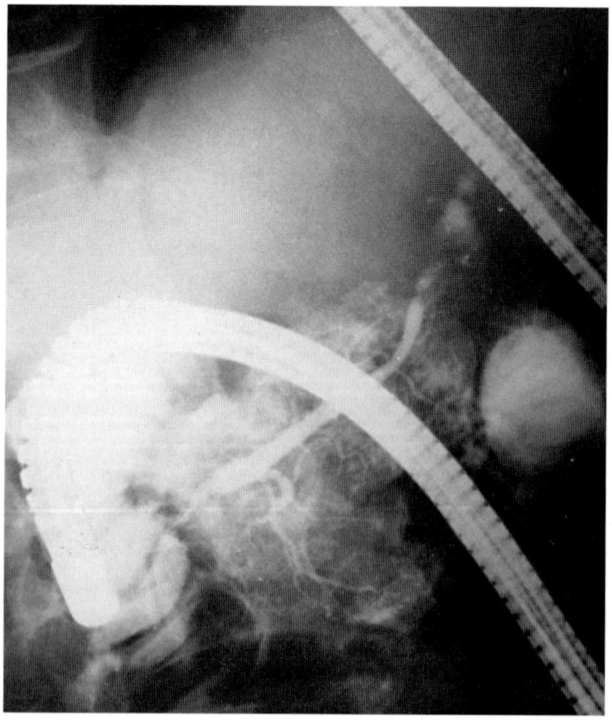

**FIG. 7.11.** Cancer of the body of the pancreas. Pancreatography shows, proximal to a cancerous stricture of the main pancreatic duct, small areas of extravasating contrast representing a necrotic cavity within the cancer. Attempts to fill the pancreatic duct led to acinarization.

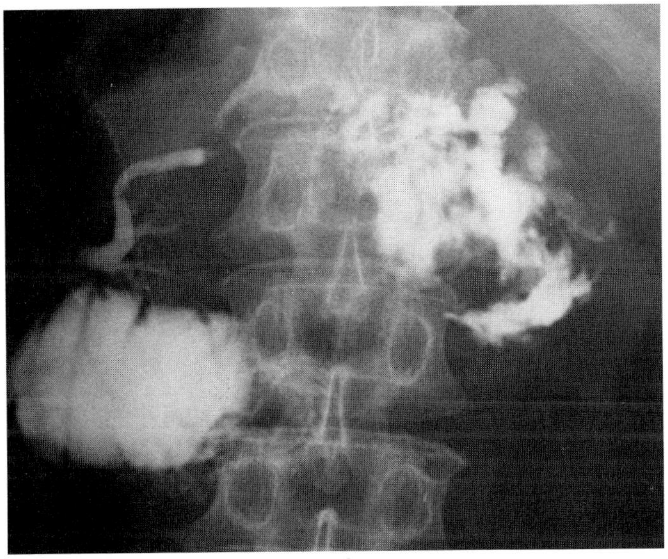

**FIG. 7.12.** Lymphoma of the body of the pancreas. Injection of the major papilla filled a large necrotic cavity of lymphoma of the body of the pancreas with contrast medium.

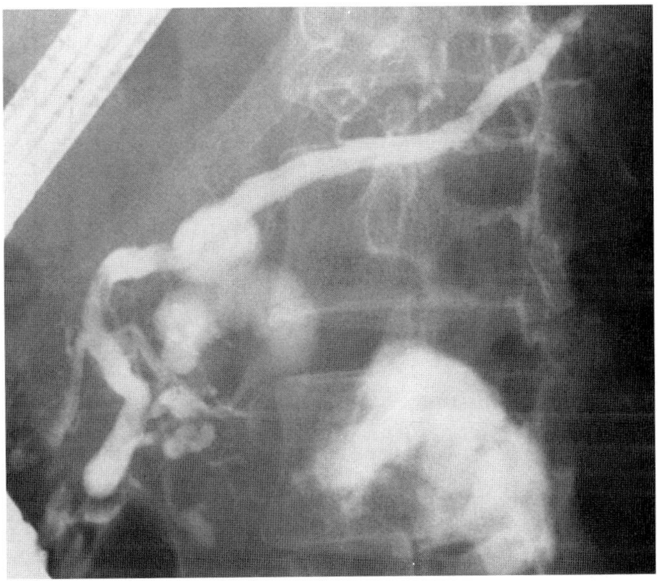

**FIG. 7.13.** Mucinous cystadenoma of the head of the pancreas. A multilocular mass involving the pancreatic head, at least some cysts of which were confirmed to communicate with the main pancreatic duct in the surgical specimen.

Serous cystadenoma of the pancreas differs macroscopically, histologically, and clinically from its mucinous counterpart. The tumor, characteristically benign, affects the neighboring duct(s) so that they are depicted at ERCP as ductal displacement. However, serous cystadenoma occasionally demonstrates an apparent stenosis of the main pancreatic duct on the pancreatogram. Histologic study of the specimen demonstrates inflammatory changes of the duct at the periphery of the tumor, whose cause still remains to be elucidated. Contrast medium does not flow into the cystic lumen.

Ductectatic mucin-producing tumor (DMPT) of the pancreas (Fig. 7.14), histopathologically intraductal papillary adenoma or adenocarcinoma, is typically characterized by no or minimal invasive and metastatic behavior and by massive thick mucus secreted from the neoplastic epithelium lining the main pancreatic duct or its side branches. Contrary to the classic mucinous cystadenoma or cystadenocarcinoma, DMPT has an obvious communication between the nontumorous, but dilated, ductal system and the ductal lumen lined with neoplastic epithelia. Thus, the orifice of the papilla of Vater often dilates to allow passage of mucoid material from the outlet into the duodenal lumen. On the other hand, too viscid mucus interferes

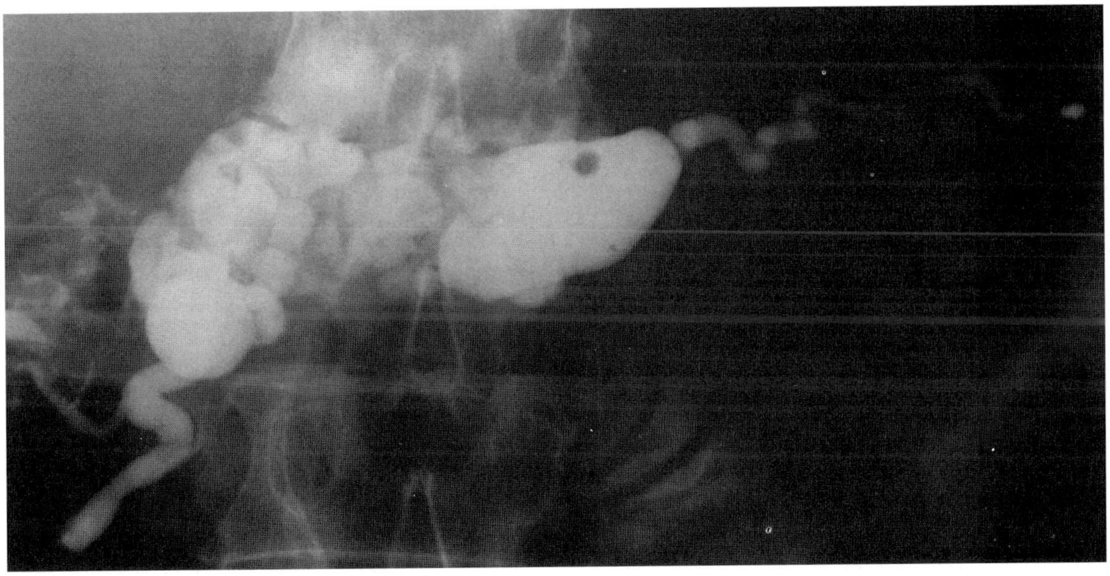

**FIG. 7.14.** Mucinous cystadenoma, ductectatic type, of the body of the pancreas. A midportion of the main pancreatic duct is segmentally involved by a multilocular lesion, the main duct, distal and proximal to this lesion, appearing intact. The patient underwent segmental pancreatectomy followed by "distal" pancreatogastrostomy.

with complete visualization of the whole pancreatic duct system at ERCP, even with use of the balloon-occlusion technique. This tumor tends to "erode" the neighboring hollow organs such as the choledochus, duodenum, or stomach to form a fistula (Fig. 7.15). This "erosion" appears to differ from invasion and rather to represent a mechanical "holding" from compression by secreted mucus.

### Extrapancreatic Diseases Affecting the Pancreatogram

The pancreatogram can be influenced by inflammatory as well as neoplastic lesions in the extrapancreatic organs; tuberculous lymphadenitis, malignant lymphoma, carcinoma of the left adrenal gland, or retroperitoneal tumor. The findings are usually deviation or compression of the pancreatic ducts by extensive or voluminous alteration of the adjacent organs.

## ENDOSCOPIC BIOPSY

Endoscopic biopsy during ERCP is essential in achieving a tissue diagnosis of tumors of the papilla of Vater (115, 116). Cytologic study of pancreatic fluid aspirated through the papilla of Vater during ERCP, even after secretin stimulation, has a rather low sensitivity of 54% in diagnosing pancreatic cancer (117). Brush cytology appears favorable in achieving adequate sampling of the tumor cells (60–85%) but is limited by the inability to reach the ductal (tail) lesions in many instances (118–120). It may be difficult to distinguish epithelial atypia due to chronic pancreatitis from well-differential neoplasms cytologically (121).

In the diagnosis of malignant biliary obstruction, brush cytology is superior to bile cytology (33%) during ERCP, providing a sensitivity of about 60%, with a range of 44–100% (119, 122–127).

Using a malleable forceps within the outer sheath and, if necessary, performing endoscopic papillotomy before biopsy, endoscopic transpapillary biopsy may provide sufficient tissue for histologic diagnosis in pancreaticobiliary strictures, with a high diagnostic accuracy of 71.4% for pancreatic cancers and 88.8% for cancer of the bile duct, respectively, without complications (128).

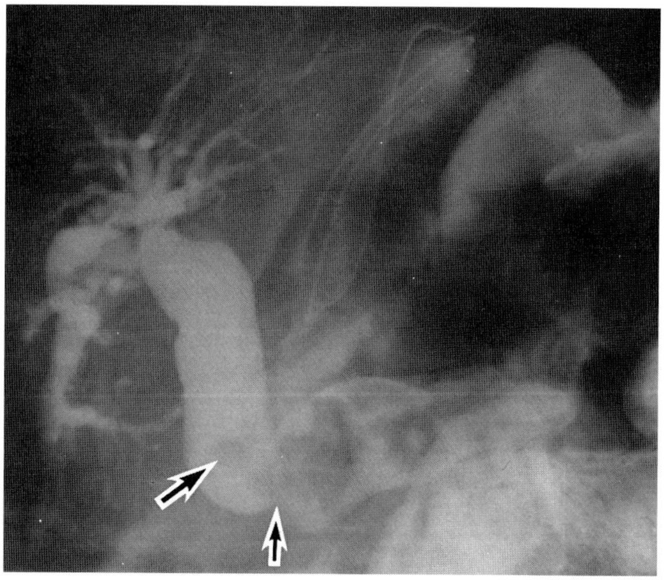

**FIG. 7.15.** Ductectatic mucin-producing cancer. A severe dilatation of the main pancreatic duct contains shadow defects representing viscid mucus. Mucus, a small round shadow defect *(large arrow)*, passes into the dilated choledochus through a fistula *(small arrow)*.

## ENDOSCOPIC SPHINCTEROTOMY

Using a diathermy papillotomy knife through a duodenoscope, a cut of 10–15 mm effectively destroys the sphincteric mechanism and allows subsequent passage of a balloon catheter or a dormia-type basket, under guidance of guide wires, if necessary, to remove retained stones. Symptomatic retained stones of the common bile duct, which are still encountered after cholecystectomy in 2% of patients despite routine intraoperative cholangiography and choledochoscopy (129), has become the prime indication for EST in not only elderly and frail patients but also young ones. EST and the subsequent retraction of retained stones provides a success rate of 85–90%, a morbidity of 6–10% (perforation, cholangitis, pancreatitis, and hemorrhage), and a mortality of less than 1% (130–136). Primary CBD stones, which arise de novo in the bile duct itself in a setting of cholestasis and bacterial colonization, also provide an indication for EST (137).

EST can also be performed for choledocholithiasis with the gallbladder in situ. However, 10–20% or more of patients will eventually require cholecystectomy for recurrent common duct stones, cholecystitis, or persistent pain after EST (138–140). Obstructive cholangitis may be an indication for emergent EST, with subsequent nasobiliary catheter insertion if necessary (66, 141).

Fibrosis, adenomyosis, or benign tumors of the papilla of Vater causing papillary stenosis are logical indications for EST. Surgery can be replaced by endoscopic treatment (71).

With correct indications, EST is almost always possible, but it should not be used for purely diagnostic ERCP, as papillary stenosis may occur due to scarring (71).

## ENDOSCOPIC BILIARY DRAINAGE

Biliary leaks usually result from surgery or penetrating trauma, less commonly from blunt trauma or native disease. These can be treated with endoscopic biliary stenting for 4–6 weeks, resulting in spontaneous closure of the fistula with a high success rate (86%) (142–144). Stent placement without sphincterotomy is widely used, although sphincterotomy can be added. Endoscopic stenting can also be applied for benign biliary strictures that result from operative or penetrating traumas, but a high recurrence rate (17%) may be seen a year after removal of the stents (145–148).

Endoscopic biliary stents or prostheses for relieving malignant obstruction, a more recent innovation, have been improved by sophisticated technical refinements. Therapeutic endoscopes with large channels permit the insertion of large stents (12 French) through obstructing neoplasms, with a high rate of relief of jaundice (78%) (107). Moreover, three developments have markedly affected the success rate of stenting: *(a)* the development of low-friction guide wires, *(b)* the precut technique of sphincterotomy, and *(c)* the use of combined endoscopic and percutaneous approaches, which improved the rate of success in placing stents up to 97% (149). Plastic stents become occluded by sludge and should be replaced on a scheduled basis (every 3–4 months). Occlusions of expandable metal stents can be managed by placement of another metal stent, placement of a plastic stent, cautery of ingrown tissue, or hydrostatic balloon dilation (150). However, it remains to be determined which of the techniques, surgical bypass, percutaneous, or endoscopic stents, is most effective in relieving malignant jaundice with the lowest morbidity and mortality.

## REFERENCES


1. McCune WS, Shorb PE, Moscovitz H. Endoscopic cannulation of the ampulla of Vater: a preliminary report. Ann Surg 1968;167: 752–756.
2. Oi I, Takemoto T, Kondo T. Fiberduodenoscope. Direct observation of the papilla of Vater. Endoscopy 1969;1:101–103.
3. Oi I. Fiberduodenoscopy and endoscopic pancreatocholangiography. Gastrointest Endosc 1970;17:59–62.
4. Kawai K, Akasaka Y, Murakami M, et al. Endoscopic sphincterotomy of the ampulla of Vater. Gastrointest Endosc 1974;20: 148–151.
5. Classen M, Demling L. Endoskopische Sphinkterotomie der Papilla Vateri und Steinextraktion aus dem Ductus choledochus. Dtsch Med Wochenschr 1974;99:496–497.
6. Nagai N, Toki N, Oi F, et al. Continuous endoscopic pancreatocholedochal catheterization. Gastrointest Endosc 1976;23: 78–80.
7. Wurbs D, Classen M. Transpapillary long standing tube for hepato-biliary drainage. Endoscopy 1977;9:192–193.
8. Soehendra N, Reynders-Frederix V. Palliative bile duct drainage—a new endoscopic method of introducing a transpapillary drain. Endoscopy 1980;12:8–11.
9. Nebel OT, Silvis SE, Rogers G, Sugawara C, Mandelstam P. Complications associated with endoscopic retrograde cholangio-pancreatography. Results of the 1974 ASGE survey. Gastrointest Endosc 1975;22:34–36.
10. Bilbao MK, Dotter CT, Lee TG, Katon RM. Complications of endoscopic retrograde cholangiopancreatography (ERCP). A study of 10,000 cases. Gastroenterology 1976;70:314–320.
11. Oi I. ERCP. In: Proceedings of practical diagnosis and treatment of gastrointestinal disease. Tokyo, 1982.
12. Blackwood W, Vennes J, Silvis S. Post-endoscopy pancreatitis and hyperamylasemia. Gastrointest Endosc 1973;20:56.
13. Skude G, Wehlin L, Maruyama T, Ariyama J. Hyperamylasemia after duodenoscopy and retrograde cholangiopancreatography. Gut 1976;17:127–132.
14. Pelot D, Berke JE, Fridhandler L. Serum isoamylase changes following endoscopy. Gastrointest Endosc 1978;24:166.
15. Koch H, Belohlavek D, Schffner O, Tympner F, Rosch W, Demling L. Prospective study for the prevention of pancreatitis following endoscopic retrograde cholangiopancreatography (ERCP). Endoscopy 1975;7:221–224.
16. Elson CO, Hattori K, Blackstone MO. Polymicrobial sepsis following endoscopic retrograde cholangiopancreatography. Gastoenterology 1975;69:509–510.
17. Parker HW, Geenan JE, Bjork JR, Stewart ET, Schaffer RD. Source of bacteraemia during ERCP (Abstract). Gastrointest Endosc 1976;22:233.
18. Keighley MRG. Micro-organisms in the bile. A preventable cause of sepsis after biliary surgery. Ann R Coll Surg Engl 1977;59: 328–334.
19. Kasugai T, Kuno N, Kobayashi S, Hattori K. Endoscopic pancreato-cholangiography. 1. The normal endoscopic pancreatocholangiogram. Gastroenterology 1972;63:217–226.
20. Hand BH. An anatomical study of the choledochoduodenal area. Br J Surg 1962;50:486–494.
21. Phillip J, Koch H, Classen M. Variations and anomalies of the papilla of Vater. The pancreas and the biliary duct system. Endoscopy 1977;6:70–77.
22. Skandalakis JE, Gray SW, Skandalakis LJ. Surgical anatomy of the pancreas. In: Howard JM, Jordan GI Jr, Reber HA, eds. Surgical diseases of the pancreas. Philadelphia: Lea & Febiger, 1987: 11–36.
23. Simon MA, Moreira VF, Menono E, et al. The double papilla of Vater. Gastrointest Endosc 1985;31:353.
24. Kreel L, Sandin B. Changes in pancreatic morphology associated with aging. Gut 1973;14:962–970.
25. Classen M, Hellwig H, Roesch W. Anatomy of the pancreatic duct. A duodenoscopic-radiological study. Endoscopy 1973;5: 14–17.
26. Cotton PB. The normal endoscopic pancreatogram. Endoscopy 1974;6:65–70.
27. Varley PF, Rohrmann CA, Silvis SE, Vennes JA. The normal pancreatogram. Radiology 1976;118:295–300.
28. Birnstingl M. A study of pancreatography. Br J Surg 1959;47: 128–139.
29. Howard JM, Short WF. An evaluation of pancreatography in suspected pancreatic disease. Surg Gynecol Obstet 1969;129: 319–324.
30. Kleitsch WP. Anatomy of the pancreas. A study with special reference to the duct system. Arch Surg 1955;71:795–802.
31. Millbourn E. Calibre and appearance of the pancreatic ducts and relevant clinical problems. A roentgenographic and anatomical study. Acta Chir Scand 1960;118:295–303.
32. Ansel HJ. The normal pancreatic duct. In: Silvis SE, Rohrmann CA Jr, Ansel HJ, eds. Text and atlas of endoscopic retrograde cholangio-pancreatography. Tokyo:Igaku-Shoin, 1995:311–335.
33. Kasahara K, Saito K, Kondo Y, et al. Case report; papillocholedochectomy in the operative management of mucosal neoplasms of the periampullary region. HPB Surg 1993;6: 211–217.
34. Suda K. Epithelial metaplasia; goblet cell metaplasia with aging. In: Naito S, ed. Pancreatic diseases. Tokyo: Dobun-Shoin, 1983:114–134.
35. Nagai H, Ohtsubo K. Pancreatic lithiasis in the aged. Its clinicopathology and pathogenesis. Gastroenterology 1984;86: 331–338.
36. Ariyama J, Shirakabe H, Sumida M, Bartram CI. Angiographic evaluation of the abnormal endoscopic pancreatogram. Gastrointest Radiol 1979;4:231–237.
37. Dharmsathaphorn K, Burrell M, Dobbins J. Diagnosis of annular pancreas with endoscopic retrograde cholangiopancreatography. Gastroenterology 1979;77:1109–1114.
38. Glazer GM, Margulis AR. Annular pancreas: etiology and diagnosis using endoscopic retrograde cholangiopancreatography. Radiology 1979;133:303–306.
39. Yogi Y, Shibue T, Hashimoto S. Annular pancreas detected in adults, diagnosed by endoscopic retrograde cholangiopancreatography: report of four cases. Gastroenterol Jpn 1987; 2292–2299.
40. Itoh Y, Hada T, Terano A, Itai Y, Harada T. Pancreatitis in the annulus of annular pancreas demonstrated by the combined use of computed tomography and endoscopic retrograde cholangio-pancreatography. Am J Gastroenterol 1989;84: 961–964.
41. Todani T, Tabuchi K, Watanabe Y, Kobayashi T. Carcinoma arising in the wall of congenital bile duct cyst. Cancer 1979;44: 1134–1141.
42. Todani T, Watanabe Y, Toki A, Urushima NN. Carcinoma related to choledochal cysts with internal drainage operations. Surg Gynecol Obstet 1987;164:61–64.
43. Morohoshi T, Kunimura T, Kanda M, et al. Multiple carcinoma associated with anomalous arrangement of the biliary and pancreatic duct system. A report of two cases with a literature survey. Acta Pathol Jpn 1990;40:755–763.
44. Chijiiwa K, Koga A. Surgical management and long-term follow-up of patients with choledochal cysts. Am J Surg 1993; 165:238–242.
45. Barkin JS, Ferstenberg RM, Panullo W, Manten HD, Davis RC. Endoscopic retrograde cholangiopancreatography in pancreatic trauma. Gastrointest Endosc 1988;34:102–105.
46. Hall RI, Lavelle MI, Venables CW. Use of ERCP to identify the site of traumatic injuries of the main pancreatic duct in children. Br J Surg 1986;73:411–412.
47. Carr ND, Cairns SJ, Lees WR, Russel RCG. Late complications of pancreatic trauma. Br J Surg 1989;76:1244–1246.
48. Stone A, Sugawa C, Lucas C, Hayward S, Nakamura R. The role of endoscopic retrograde pancreatography in blunt abdominal trauma. Am Surg 1990;56:715–720.
49. Ammann RW, Deyhle P, Butkofer E. Fatal necrotizing pancreatitis after peroral cholangiopancreatography 1973;64:320–323.
50. Ebner F, Hofler H, Kratochvil P, et al. Pankreasnekrose nach endoskopisch retrograder Pankreatikographie. Dtsch Med Wochenschr 1982;107:453–455.
51. Lee MJR, Choi TK, Lai ECS, Wong KP, Ngan H, Wong J. Endoscopic retrograde cholangiopancreatography after acute pancreatitis. Surg Gynec Obstet 1986;163:354–358.
52. Rohrmann CA Jr, Silvis SE, Vennes JA. Evaluation of the endoscopic pancreatogram. Radiology 1974;113:297–304.

53. Cotton PB, Beales JSM. Endoscopic pancreatography in management of relapsing acute pancreatitis. Br Med J 1974;1:608.
54. Zimmon DS, Falkenstein DB, Abrams RM, et al. Endoscopic retrograde cholangiopancreatography (ERCP) in the diagnosis of pancreatic inflammatory disease. Radiology 1974;113:287–292.
55. Hamilton I, Bradley P, Lintott DJ, McMahon MJ, Axon ATR. Endoscopic retrograde cholangiopancreatography in the investigation and management of patients after acute pancreatitis. Br J Surg 1982;69:504–506.
56. Katon RM, Bibao MK, Eldemiller LR, et al. Endoscopic retrograde cholangiopancreatography in the diagnosis and management of non-alcoholic pancreatitis. Surg Gynecol Obstet 1978;147:333–338.
57. Cooperman M, Ferrara JJ, Carey LC, Thomas FB, Martin EW, Fromkes JJ. Idiopathic acute pancreatitis: the value of endoscopic retrograde cholangiopancreatography. Surgery 1981;90:666–670.
58. Feller ER. Endoscopic retrograde cholangiopancreatography in the diagnosis of unexplained pancreatitis. Arch Intern Med 1984;144:1797–1799.
59. Neoptolemos JP, London N, Slater ND, Carr-Locke DL, Fossard DP, Moosa AR. A prospective study of ERCP and endoscopic sphincterotomy in the diagnosis and treatment of gallstone acute pancreatitis. A rational and safe approach to management. Arch Surg 1986;121:697–702.
60. Classen M, Osenberg FW, Wurbs D, et al. Pancreatitis—an indication for endoscopic papillotomy? Endoscopy 1978;10:223.
61. Rosseland AR, Solhaug JH. Early or delayed endoscopic papillotomy in gallstone pancreatitis. Ann Surg 1984;199:165–167.
62. Neoptolemos JP, Carr-Locke DJ, London NJ, Bailey IA, James D, Fossard DP. Controlled trial of urgent endoscopic retrograde cholangiopancreatography and endoscopic sphincterotomy versus conservative treatment for acute pancreatitis due to gallstones. Lancet 1988;29:979–983.
63. Carter DC. Pancreatitis and the biliary tree: the continuing problem. Am J Surg 1988;155:10–17.
64. Scholmerich J, Gross J, Johannessson J, et al. Detection of biliary origin of acute pancreatitis. Comparison of laboratory tests, ultrasound, computed tomography, ERCP. Dig Dis Sci 1989;34:830–833.
65. Scholmerich J, Lausen M, Lay L, et al. Value of endoscopic retrograde cholangiopancreatography in determining the cause but not course of acute pancreatitis. Endoscopy 1992;24:244–247.
66. Leese T, Neoptolemos JP, Baker AR, Carr-Locke DL. Management of acute cholangitis and the impact of endoscopic sphincterotomy. Br J Surg 1986;73:988–992.
67. Venu RP, Geenen JE, Stewart E, et al. Endoscopic retrograde cholangiopancreatography: diagnosis of cholelithiasis in patients with normal gallbladder x-ray and ultrasound studies. JAMA 1983;249:758–761.
68. Khuroo MS, Zargar SA, Yattoo GN, et al. Ascaris-induced acute pancreatitis. Br J Surg 1992;9:1335–1338.
69. Kasugai T, Kuno N, Kizu M. Manometric endoscopic retrograde cholangiopancreatography: technique, significance and evaluation. Am J Dig Dis 1974;19:485–502.
70. Stolte M, Weiss W, Volkholz H, Rosch W. A special form of segmental pancreatitis: "groove pancreatitis." Hepato-Gastroenterology 1982;29:198–208.
71. Classen M, Philip J. Endoscopic retrograde cholangiopancreatography and endoscopic therapy in pancreatic disease. Clin Gastroenterol 1984;13:819–842.
72. Galvan A, Klotz AP. Is transduodenal pancreatography ever contraindicated? Gastrointest Endosc 1973;20:28–30.
73. Siefert E, Stander H, Safrany L, et al. X-ray findings of pancreatic cysts diagnosed by ERCP. Endoscopy 1974;6:77–83.
74. Silvis SE, Vennes JA, Rohrmann CA. ERCP in the evaluation of patients with suspected pancreatic pseudocysts 1974;61:452–459.
75. Anderson BN, Hancke S, Nielsen SAD, Schmidt A. The diagnosis of pancreatic cyst by endoscopic retrograde pancreatography and ultrasonic scanning. Ann Surg 1977;185:286–289.
76. Shatney CH, Lillehei RC. Surgical treatment of pancreatic pseudocyst. Ann Surg 1979;189:386–394.
77. Sugawa C, Walt AJ. Endoscopic retrograde pancreatography in the surgery of pancreatic pseudocysts. Surgery 1979;86:639–647.
78. Aranha GV, Prinz RA, Freark RJ, et al. Evaluation of therapeutic options for pancreatic pseudocysts. Arch Surg 1982;117:717–721.
79. Beebe DS, Budrick MP, Onstad GR, et al. Management of pancreatic pseudocysts. Surg Gynecol Obstet 1984;159:562–564.
80. Wade JW. Twenty-five year experience with pancreatic pseudocysts. Are we making progress? Am J Surg 1985;149:705–708.
81. Laxson LC, Fromkes JJ, Cooperman M. Endoscopic retrograde cholangiopancreatography in the management of pancreatic pseudocysts. Am J Surg 1985;150:683–686.
82. O'Connor M, Kolars J, Ansel H, Silvis S, Vennes J. Preoperative endoscopic retrograde cholangiopancreatography in the surgical management of pancreatic pseudocysts. Am J Surg 1986;151:18–24.
83. Nealon WH, Townsend C Jr, Thompson JC. Preoperative endoscopic retrograde cholangiopancreatography in patients with pancreatic pseudocyst associated with resolving acute and chronic pancreatitis. Ann Surg 1989;209:532–540.
84. Kolars JC, Allen MO, Ansel H, Silvis SE, Vennes JA. Pancreatic pseudocysts: clinical and endoscopic experience. Am J Gastroenterol 1989;84:259–264.
85. Bernardino ME, Amerson RJ. Percutaneous gastrocystostomy: a new approach to pancreatic pseudocyst drainage. Am J Roentgenol 1984;143:1096–1097.
86. Nunez P Jr, Yrizarry JM, Russel E, et al. Transgastric drainage of pancreatic fluid collections. Am J Roentgenol 1985;145:815–818.
87. Torres WE, Evert MB, Baumgartner BR, Bernardino ME. Percutaneous aspiration and drainage of pancreatic pseudocysts. Am J Roentgenol 1986;147:1007–1009.
88. Sahel J, Batid C, Pellat B, Schurgars P, Sarles H. Endoscopic cystoduodenostomy for cysts of chronic pancreatitis: a report of 20 cases. Pancreas 1987;2:447–453.
89. Gandini G, Grosso M, Bonardi L, Cassini MC, Regge D, Righi P. Results of percutaneous treatment of sixty-three pancreatic pseudocysts. Ann Radiol (Paris) 1988;31:117–122.
90. Sacks D, Robinson MC. Transgastric percutaneous drainage of pancreatic pseudocysts. Am J Roentgenol 1988;151:303–306.
91. Spinelli P, Meroni E, Prada A. Endoscopic treatment of a pancreatic pseudocysts by naso-cystic tube. Endoscopy 1988;20:27–29.
92. Huibregste K, Schneider B, Vrij AA, Tytgat GNJ. Endoscopic pancreatic drainage in chronic pancreatitis. Gastrointest Endosc 1988;34:9–15.
93. Hyder N, Flugel H, Domschke W. Catheter drainage of pancreatic pseudocysts into the stomach. Endoscopy 1988;20:75–77.
94. Sacks BA, Greenberg JJ, Porter DH, et al. An internalized double-J catheter for percutaneous transgastric cystogastrostomy. Am J Roentgenol 1989;152:523–526.
95. van Sonnenberg E, Wittich GR, Casola G, et al. Percutaneous drainage of infected and noninfected pancreatic pseudocysts: experience with 101 cases. Radiology 1989;170:757–761.
96. Cremer M, Deviere T, Engelholm L. Endoscopic management of cysts and pseudocysts in chronic pancreatitis: long-term follow-up after 7 years of experience. Gastrointest Endosc 1989;35:1–9.
97. Grosso M, Gandini G, Cassinis MC, Regge D, Righi D, Rossi P. Percutaneous treatment (including pseudocystogastrostomy) of 74 pancreatic pseudocysts. Radiology 1989;173:493–497.
98. Ahearne PM, Baillie JM, Cotton PB, Baker ME, Meyers WC, Pappas TN. An endoscopic retrograde cholangiopancreatography (ERCP)-based algorithm for the management of pancreatic pseudocysts. Am J Surg 1992;163:111–116.
99. Adams DB, Anderson MC. Changing concepts in the surgical management of pancreatic pseudocysts. Am Surg 1992;58:173–180.
100. Brandes JW, Scheffer B, Lorenz-Meyer H, Korst HA, Littman KP. ERCP: complications and prophylaxis. A controlled study. Endoscopy 1981;13:27–30.
101. Cameron JL, Kieffer RS, Anderson WT. Internal pancreatic fistula: pancreatic ascites and pleural effusions. Ann Surg 1976;184:587.

102. Cameron JL. Chronic pancreatic ascites and pancreatic pleural effusions. Gastroenterology 1978;74:134–140.
103. Hotz J, Goebell H, Herfath C, et al. Massive pancreatic ascites. Digestion 1977;15:200.
104. Anderson WJ, Skinner DB, Zuidema GD, et al. Chronic pancreatic pleural effusion. Surg Gynecol Obstet 1973;137:827–830.
105. Horiguchi Y, Hayakawa T, Noda A, et al. Pancreatic internal fistula to the left pleural cavity. Am J Gastroenterol 1978;70: 85–88.
106. Tumen JJ, Sutton WW, Dunn GD. Bilateral pancreatic pleural effusions: a case report and literature review. Am J Gastroenterol 1983;78:284–286.
107. Summerfield JA. Biliary obstruction is best managed by endoscopists. Gut 1988;29:741–745.
108. Takada T. Cholangitis. In: Takemoto T, Kasugai T, eds. Endoscopic retrograde cholangiopancreatography. New York: Igaku-Shoin, 1978:277–293.
109. Zimmon DS, Falkenstein DB, Riccobono C, Aaron B. Complications of endoscopic retrograde cholangiopancreatography. Analysis of 300 consecutive cases. Gastroenterology 1975;69: 303–309.
110. Vennes JA, Jacobson JR, Silvis SE. Endoscopic cholangiopancreatography for biliary system diagnosis. Ann Intern Med 1974;80:61–64.
111. Davis JL, Miligan FD, Cameron JL. Septic complications following endoscopic retrograde cholangiopancreatography. Surg Gynecol Obstet 1975;140:365–367.
112. Tuchiya R, Tomioka T, Izawa K, et al. Collective review of small carcinoma of the pancreas. Ann Surg 1986;203:77–81.
113. Ariyama J, Shirakabe H, Ikenobe H, Kurosawa A, Owman T. The diagnosis of the small resectable pancreatic carcinoma. Clin Radiol 1977;28:437–444.
114. Frick MP, Feinberg SB, Goodale RL. The value of endoscopic retrograde cholangiopancreatography in patients with suspected carcinoma of the pancreas and indeterminate computed tomographic results. Surg Gynecol Obstet 1982;155: 177–182.
115. Blumgart LH, Salomon PR, Cotton PB. Endoscopy and retrograde cholangiopancreatography in the diagnosis of the patient with jaundice. Surg Gynecol Obstet 1974;138: 565–570.
116. Hall TJ, Blackstone MO, Cooper MJ, et al. Prospective evaluation of endoscopic retrograde cholangiopancreatography in the diagnosis of periampullary cancers. Ann Surg 1978;187: 313–317.
117. Goodale RL, Gaje-Peczalska K, Dressel T, Samuelson J. Cytologic studies for the diagnosis of pancreatic cancer. Cancer 1981;47: 1652–1655.
118. Osnes M, Serck-Hanssen A, Kristensen O, Swensen T, Aune S, Myren J. Endoscopic retrograde brush cytology in patients with primary and secondary malignancies of the pancreas. Gut 1979;20:279–284.
119. Venu RP, Geenen JE, Kini M, et al. Endoscopic retrograde brush cytology. A new technique. Gastroenterology 1990;99:1475–1479.
120. Sawada Y, Gonda H, Hayashida Y. Combined use of brushing cytology and endoscopic retrograde pancreatography for the early detection of pancreatic cancer. Acta Cytol 1989;33: 870–874.
121. Kocjan G, Rode J, Lees WR. Percutaneous fine needle aspiration cytology of the pancreas. Advantage and pitfalls. J Clin Pathol 1989;42:341–347.
122. Pugliese V, Barone D, Saccomanno S, Conio M, Aste H, Santi L. Tissue sampling from the common bile duct through endoscopic retrograde cholangiopancreatography, endoscopic papillo(sphinctero)tomy and drainage in juxtapapillary malignancies. Surg Endosc 1987;1:83–87.
123. Foutch PG, Kerr DM, Harlan JR, et al. Endoscopic retrograde wire-guided brush cytology for diagnosis of patients with malignant obstruction of the bile duct. Am J Gastroenterol 1990;85:791–795.
124. Rabinovitz M, Zajko AB, Hassanein T, et al. Diagnostic value of brush cytology in the diagnosis of bile duct carcinoma: a study in 65 patients with bile duct strictures. Hepatology 1990;12:747–752.
125. Foutch PG, Kerr DM, Harlen JR, Kummet TD. A prospective, controlled analysis of endoscopic cytodiagnosis for diagnosis of malignant biliary stricture. Am J Gastroenterol 1991;86: 577–580.
126. Ryan ME. Cytologic brushings of ductal lesions during ERCP. Gastrointest Endosc 1991;37:139–142.
127. Kurzawinski TR, Deery A, Dooley JS, Dick R, Hobbs KEF, Davidson BR. A prospective study of biliary cytology in 100 patients with bile duct strictures. Hepatology 1993;18:1399–1403.
128. Kubota Y, Takaoka M, Tani K, et al. Endoscopic transpapillary biopsy for diagnosis of patients with pancreaticobiliary ductal strictures. Am J Gastroenterol 1993;88:1700–1704.
129. Motson RW, Wetter LA. Operative choledochoscopy: common bile duct exploration is incomplete without it. Br J Surg 1990;77: 975–982.
130. Classen M, Safrany L. Endoscopic papillotomy and removal of gallstones. Br Med J 1975;4:371–374.
131. Rosch W. Workshop: operative endoscopy. Endoscopy 1975;7: 157–160.
132. Cotton PB, Chapman M, Whiteside CG, LeQuesne LP. Duodenoscopic papillotomy and gallstone removal. Br J Surg 1976;63: 709–714.
133. Ghazi A, McSherry CK. Endoscopic retrograde cholangio-pancreatography and sphincterotomy. Ann Surg 1984;199:21–27.
134. Miller BM, Kozarek RA, Ryan JA, Ball TJ, Traverso LO. Surgical versus endoscopic management of common bile duct stones. Ann Surg 1988;207:135–141.
135. Worthley CS, Watts JM, Toouli J. Common duct exploration or endoscopic sphincterotomy for choledocholithiasis? Aust NZ J Surg 1989;59:209–215.
136. Vitale GC. Interventional endoscopic retrograde cholangiopancreatography: state of the art (part 1). J R Coll Surg Edinb 1992;37:289–297.
137. Tanaka M, Ikeda S, Yoshimoto H, et al. Long-term fate of the gallbladder after endoscopic sphincterotomy: complete follow-up study of 122 patients. Am J Surg 1987;54:505–509.
138. Siegel JH, Safrany L, Pullano W, et al. The significance of duodenoscopic sphincterotomy on patients with gallbladder in situ: 11 year follow-up of 1272 patients (Abstract). Gastroenterology 1987;92:1385.
139. Ikeda S, Tanaka M, Matsumoto S, Yoshimoto H, Itoh H. Endoscopic sphincterotomy: long-term results in 408 patients with complete follow-up. Endoscopy 1988;20:13–17.
140. Davidson BR, Neoptolemos JP, Carr-Locke DL. Endoscopic sphincterotomy for common bile duct calculi in patients with gallbladder in situ considered unfit for surgery. Gut 1988;29: 114–120.
141. Leung JWC, Song JY, Chung SCS, et al. Urgent endoscopic drainage in acute suppurative cholangitis. Lancet 1989;1:1307–1309.
142. Mortensen J, Kruse A. Endoscopic management of postoperative bile leaks. Br J Surg 1992;79:1339–1341.
143. Foutch PG, Harlan JR, Hoefer M. Endoscopic therapy for patients with a postoperative biliary leak. Gastrointest Endosc 1993;39:416–421.
144. Sherman S, Shaked A, Cryer HM, et al. Endoscopic management of biliary fistulas complicating liver transplantation and other hepatobiliary operations. Ann Surg 1993;218:167–175.
145. Berkelhammar C, Kortan P, Haberr GB. Endoscopic biliary prostheses as treatment for benign postoperative bile duct strictures. Gastrointest Endosc 1989;35:95–101.
146. Geenen DJ, Geenen JE, Hogan WJ, et al. Endoscopic therapy for benign bile duct strictures. Gastrointest Endosc 1989;35: 367–371.
147. Deviere J, Baize M, Vandermeeren A, et al. Endoscopic stenting for biliary strictures. Acta Gastroenterol Belg 1992;55: 295–305.
148. Davids PH, Rauws EAJ, Coene PP. Endoscopic stenting for post-operative biliary strictures. Gastrointest Endosc 1992;38: 12–18.
149. Robertson DA, Ayres R, Hacking CN, et al. Experience with a combined percutaneous and endoscopic approach to stent insertion in malignant obstructive jaundice. Lancet 1987;2:1449–1452.
150. Sherman S, Hawew RH, Lehman GA. Endoscopic biliary and pancreatic drainage procedures. In: Silvis SE, Rohrmann CA, Ansel HJ, eds. Textbook and atlas of endoscopic retrograde cholangiopancreatography. Tokyo: Igaku-Shoin, 1995:413–445.

# 8

# Percutaneous Transhepatic Cholangiography and Biliary Drainage

Keiichi Kubota and Masatoshi Makuuchi

Intrahepatic cholestasis and obstruction of the common bile duct induce jaundice. When obstructive jaundice is suspected, it is necessary to visualize the whole biliary tree to clarify the site, extent, and nature of the obstruction and establish a treatment strategy. Several diagnostic imaging techniques are now available for visualization of the biliary tree, such as drip infusion cholangiography, endoscopic retrograde cholangiography (ERC), and percutaneous transhepatic cholangiography (PTC) (1–3). Of these three, PTC can reveal the biliary tree clearly and contribute to determining the nature of the obstruction with a high degree of certainty (4–7). Percutaneous transhepatic biliary drainage (PTBD) is a safe and effective means of achieving biliary decompression nonoperatively and provides a definitive palliative treatment for those patients with unresectable malignancies or for those who are too ill to undergo surgery. PTC was first performed by Huard and Do-Xuan-Hop in 1937 (8). Since then, thanks to the development of ultrasound-guided techniques and instruments such as puncture needles and drainage tubes, PTC and PTBD have become safe methods for investigating and treating biliary diseases (1, 9).

## INDICATIONS

Candidates for PTC can be divided into two groups: those requiring only PTC and those requiring biliary drainage following PTC. The first group is limited and includes patients who have elevated serum levels of biliary enzymes, such as alkaline phosphatase and γ-glutamyl transpeptidase (γ-GTP), suggesting the presence of biliary obstruction, but whose total bilirubin levels are only slightly raised (<2.0 mg/dL). In most such patients, the causes of biliary obstruction are benign; some have certain types of malignancy. The second group includes patients with significantly increased total serum bilirubin levels induced by advanced cancers of the pancreas, bile duct, gallbladder, or liver, as well as certain benign obstructions. As PTC is more invasive than ERC, ERC is the first choice for most patients. However, when ERC cannot completely visualize the bile duct or cannot be performed for technical reasons (e.g., in postoperative patients who have undergone Billroth II reconstruction), PTC is indicated. When PTC shows significant biliary obstruction and biliary drainage is considered necessary, the procedure can be converted to PTBD. In the second group, PTBD is usually carried out as a one-step procedure without performing PTC (1).

### Benign Diseases

Of the benign diseases that may cause obstructive jaundice (Table 8.1), gallstones are the most frequently encountered and are an indication for biliary drainage. However, when gallstones are present in the common bile duct, ERC, rather than PTBD, should be the treatment of choice, as the stones may be removable following endoscopic sphincterotomy (2), but when ERC is technically difficult, PTBD is an alternative. Benign strictures may result from accidental injury to the biliary tract during surgery or be a result of external trauma or pancreatitis. Surgical treatment is usually effective in most patients, but the results have been reported to be influenced by several factors, such as infection and elevated serum bilirubin levels (10). Preoperative biliary drainage temporarily relieves the obstruction and leads to subsidence of the biliary infection. PTC is also useful for visualization of a choledochal cyst, as it can clearly demonstrate the stenotic site and the size and extent of the cyst (11). Other benign causes of obstructive jaundice include Mirizzi syndrome due to an inflammatory obstruction secondary to a stone in the cystic duct, pancreatic pseudocyst, chronic pancreatitis, and sclerosing cholangitis (1–3).

### Malignant Obstructions

Several cancers, such as those of the bile duct, gallbladder, and pancreas, may cause biliary tract obstruction, which sometimes induces severe jaundice. Although recent advances in abdominal imaging techniques have led to earlier detection and diagnosis of these cancers, their first manifestation is often the appearance of jaundice, an indication that they are already at an advanced stage. Therefore, to establish a treatment strategy for a cancer, visualization of the site and extent of the lesion is mandatory. In cases of complete obstruction, ERC can only show the distal part of the bile duct, whereas PTC can yield important information about the proximal (upstream) side of the obstructed bile duct, information that may be useful in evaluating the resectability of the cancer (12).

### Cholangitis

Cholangitis is observed most frequently in patients with stones in the common bile duct. Biliary drainage generally results in prompt relief of the sepsis (13). As acute obstructive cholangitis carries a high mortality rate (14), biliary decompression should be performed promptly after diagnosis. Before the procedure, appropriate antibiotic coverage and hydration of the patient are essential. Elevation of the intraductal pressure may easily induce septic shock, and therefore, only a small volume of contrast material should be injected. Our observation is that PTBD reduces the mortality rate of severe cholangitis.

### Others

Kissin and Grundy (15) observed that PTC was more useful for identifying the site of postoperative persistent bile leakage than other diagnostic imaging techniques. Recently, PTC was also used for investigating complications following transplantation of the liver, such as stricture of the bile duct, common bile duct redundancy, bile leakage, and choledocholithiasis (16).

**TABLE 8.1. Benign Diseases Causing Obstructive Jaundice**

| |
|---|
| Bile duct stones |
| Gallbladder stones (Mirizzi syndrome)[a] |
| Bile duct injuries during previous biliary surgery |
| Chronic pancreatitis |
| Pancreatic pseudocysts |
| Choledochal cysts |
| Sclerosing cholangitis |
| Benign neoplasms |
| Papillitis |
| Juxtapapillary duodenal diverticula |
| Others |

[a] Obstruction of the common hepatic duct resulting from an inflammatory response secondary to the impaction of a gallstone in the cystic duct or in the neck of the gallbladder.

## CONTRAINDICATIONS

### Severe Bleeding Diathesis

As PTC and PTBD require hepatic puncture, patients with severe bleeding diatheses are at risk for intraabdominal bleeding from the hepatic surface or from intraductal bleeding. Moderate or marked prolongation of the prothrombin and/or partial thromboplastin time and a platelet count below 50,000/mL, therefore, are relative contraindications (2). When the procedure is clinically necessary, administration of vitamin K and fresh frozen plasma and/or platelet transfusion should precede the procedure; if the bleeding diathesis does not improve, the procedure should be abandoned.

### Ascites

When massive ascites is present, although puncture of a dilated bile duct is not difficult, manipulation of a guide wire and drainage catheter may be technically difficult, as they buckle easily in a confined space between the surface of the liver and the abdominal wall. Consequently, the risk of hemorrhage is increased, as the hepatic capsule may be lacerated. When bile leaks into the intraabdominal cavity, the presence of ascites promotes the spread of local bile peritonitis. Administration of diuretics or paracentesis should, therefore, precede PTC and PTBD to reduce the volume of ascites.

### Others

PTC and PTBD are particularly difficult and hazardous in patients in poor general condition who cannot lie still or hold their breath. Known hypersensitivity to the contrast material is also a contraindication.

## INSTRUMENTS

As PTC and PTBD are performed under ultrasonic guidance, special instruments are required. First, it is important to obtain good-quality intrahepatic ultrasonic images. In our department, a convex probe with a 3.5-MHz transducer is used routinely. This probe can yield a wide-range scan of the liver and be equipped with a needle holder, which makes it easy to puncture the bile duct, and the puncture line is demonstrated on the monitor of the ultrasound machine. We routinely use an 18- or 21-gauge puncture needle composed of an outer guide needle and a PTBD needle. The tip of the guide wire should be soft; therefore, movable-core or Radifocus (Terumo Co., Ltd., Tokyo) guide wire (0.035 inc) are best. To insert a drainage catheter smoothly into the bile duct, dilators with diameters of 6–8 Fr should be used. They can be inserted over the guide wire to dilate the anterior wall of the bile duct. We routinely leave a dilator in place for at least 2 minutes before inserting a drainage catheter. There are several types of drainage catheter, such as straight, pigtail, and balloon tipped. The latter two types best avoid having the tube slip out of the bile duct into the intraabdominal cavity.

## TECHNIQUES

### Selection of the Puncture Site

It is important to select the optimal puncture site on the abdominal wall. First, under ultrasonographic visualization, the liver should be observed in the epigastric area and from the seventh or eighth intercostal space; then it is decided where the dilated bile duct is best visualized and is closest to the body surface. When the bile duct can be visualized equally well from both sites, the epigastric site is preferable, because when a patient suddenly breathes, the target bile duct may move to greater extent relative to the intercostal space than to the epigastric area. In particular, when a catheter is inserted from the intercostal space, respiratory movements often cause the catheter to slip out of the bile duct and lie between the abdominal wall and the surface of the liver. There is less respiratory movement at the epigastrium, where the bile ducts of both the left lateral superior and inferior segments can be observed. Either duct is usually suitable for PTC, although it is generally easier to insert a drainage catheter into the bile duct of the left lateral inferior segment. Ultrasonographically, the portal venous branch is located more ventrally than the bile duct in the left lateral inferior segment and, therefore, the puncture route selected should avoid penetrating the portal venous branch (Fig. 8.1). The catheter placed in the bile duct should be long enough to prevent its slipping out of the bile duct, and as an extra precaution, the bile duct should be punctured peripherally, especially in patients with obstruction at the porta hepatis. If the left lobe is invaded by tumor or if a carcinoma of the porta hepatis has invaded far more of the left lobe than the right side, then the bile duct of the right lobe is an alternative target. In such a situation, to avoid injuring the intercostal artery and lung, the upper margin of the rib should be selected, and the puncture route should be confirmed both ultrasonographically and roentgenographically to ensure that the lung is avoided.

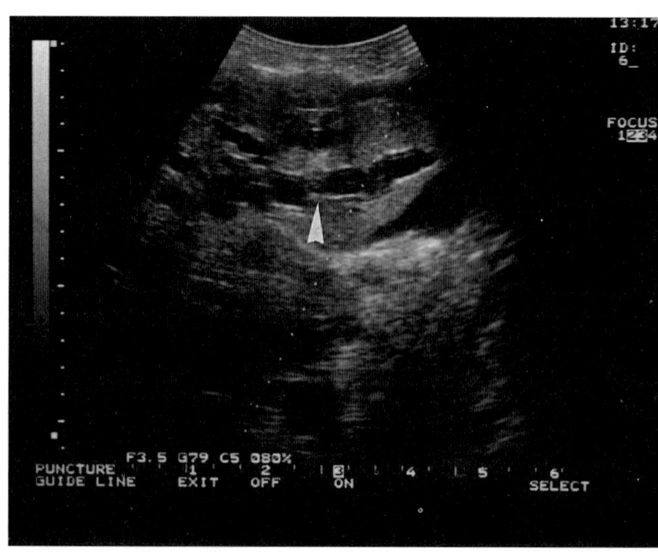


**FIG. 8.1.** Ultrasound of the liver of a patient with a cancer of the pancreatic head. A transverse view of the liver shows dilated intrahepatic bile ducts *(white arrow)*. The puncture line is demonstrated on the monitor.

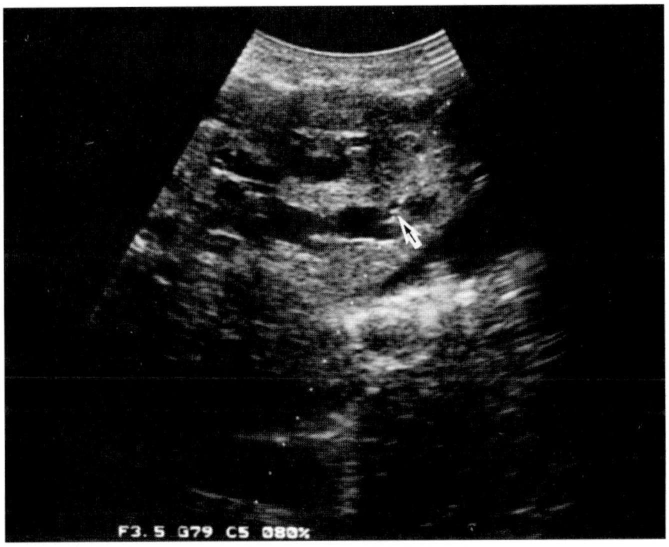


**FIG. 8.2.** Bile duct puncture. The PTBD needle is advanced to the dilated bile duct. The PTBD needle tip is shown as a glittering line *(arrow)*.

### Anesthesia

Using a fine needle, punctures are made along the guideline on the monitor, and a local anesthetic agent is injected to anesthetize the skin, subcutaneous tissue, peritoneum, and hepatic capsule. Care should be taken to avoid injecting too much anesthetic fluid or air, as they obscure ultrasonic delineation of the bile ducts.

### Puncture of the Bile Duct

While the bile duct of the lateral segment is being punctured, the patient should continue to take very shallow breaths. the bile duct of the right lobe should be punctured while the patient is exhaling slightly. After selecting the puncture site, a small skin incision is made, the outer guide needle is advanced to the peritoneum, and the PTBD needle is then advanced to the bile duct. When the tip of the needle is confirmed by ultrasound to be within the bile duct (Fig. 8.2), the stylet is removed, and bile will usually come out spontaneously. If it does not, suction should be applied by use of a syringe. If PTC is intended, contrast material can now be injected, and the biliary tree clearly visualized. Contrast material should be injected slowly after first aspirating the bile to ensure that the intraductal pressure does not suddenly increase, as this can induce bilioportal reflux, transporting infected bile into the circulation and possibly resulting in septicemia and shock (2). If biliary drainage is scheduled, one can proceed to the next step.

### Guide Wire Insertion

Under ultrasonic guidance, a guide wire can be inserted into the bile duct (Fig. 8.3). The movement of the guide wire in the bile duct can be observed easily on ultrasound, and the operator must be sure that the guide wire is not lying outside the bile duct.

### Dilator Insertion

Insertion of the dilator and all subsequent steps of the procedure should be performed under roentgenographic guidance. The dilator is fed over the guide wire into the bile duct and left there for at least 2 minutes. If an 8-Fr catheter is to be inserted, the route should be dilated gradually by use of 6- to 8-Fr dilators. If a dilator is inserted into the bile duct forcefully, bleeding from the wall of the bile duct or a vagovagal reflex may occur, resulting in a fall of blood pressure.

### Insertion of Drainage Catheter

After removing the dilator, the drainage catheter is inserted into the bile duct by feeding it over the guide wire. When the target is a long segment of dilated bile duct, a straight catheter can be used, but when the catheter can only be inserted for a short distance, a pigtail or balloon-tipped catheter should be used. After removing the guide wire, the biliary tree should be visualized by gently injecting contrast material and again evaluating whether the catheter lies in the correct position (Fig. 8.4).

### Drainage of Gallbladder

When the intrahepatic bile duct is not sufficiently dilated to permit puncture with a PTBD needle and an obstructive lesion distal to the confluence of the cystic duct is suspected, percutaneous transhepatic drainage of the gallbladder (PTGBD) should be used as an alternative method of draining the biliary tree. The technique is almost the same as that for PTBD. Gallbladders are punctured through the seventh or eighth intercostal space. For easy manipulation of the guide wire and drainage catheter that are to be inserted, the puncture route should penetrate the parenchyma of the liver to a depth of at least 2–3 cm. The fundus of the gallbladder or the borderline area between its neck and the fundus should be selected for puncture, and a drainage catheter long enough to prevent it from slipping out of the gallbladder should be inserted (Fig. 8.5, *A* to *D*).

### Biliary Stenting

When an obstructive lesion cannot be treated surgically, it is possible to place a metallic stent at the site of obstruction via a PTBD route (17, 18). Although the long-term patency of such stents is unknown, this technique is a therapeutic option for biliary obstruction.

## DRAINAGE EFFECT

The effectiveness of PTBD in reducing the serum bilirubin level and relieving symptoms of obstructive jaundice has been well documented (19–21). After adequate biliary decompression, serum bilirubin levels decrease following first-order kinetics at an average rate of 8% per day in patients without serious hepatic disease (22, 23). This rate is not influenced by the type of

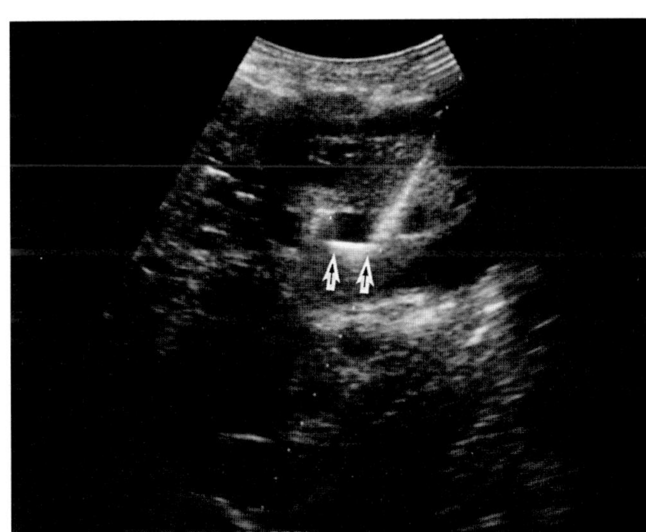


**FIG. 8.3.** Insertion of a guide wire, seen as a hyperechoic line *(arrows)* into the bile duct.

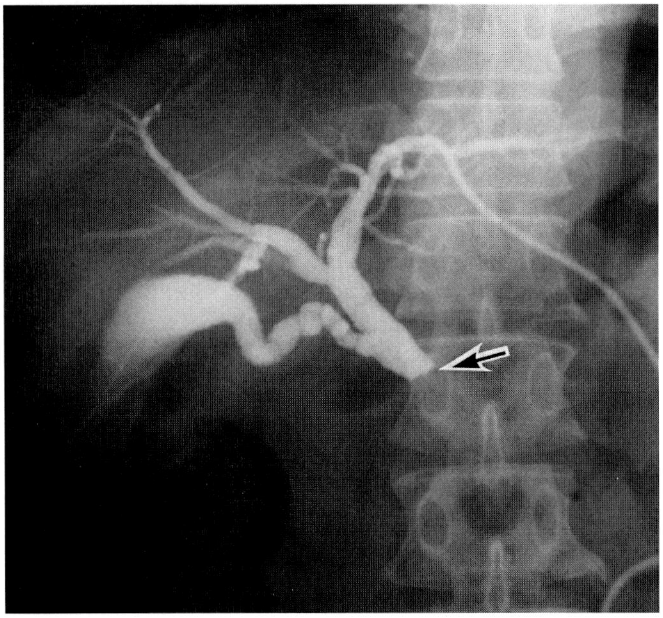

**FIG. 8.4.** Cholangiography through a drainage tube. After inserting a drainage tube, cholangiography showed an obstructive lesion clearly *(arrow)*.

obstructing disease, the duration of jaundice, or the absolute serum bilirubin level (24). We estimate "serum bilirubin decreasing rates" (b-values) using the formula shown below (25).

$$Y = ae^{bx}$$

where $Y$ = serum bilirubin level on the day before the operation, $x$ = number of days between puncture and operation, $a$ = bilirubin level on the day of puncture, $e$ = base of the natural logarithm.

The respective b-values of patients who had obstruction at the porta hepatis, between the bifurcation and cystic duct, or distal to the cystic duct, were $-0.06 \pm 0.01$ ($n = 15$), $-0.16 \pm 0.33$ ($n = 22$), and $-0.22 \pm 0.05$ ($n = 44$). There were no statistically significant differences noted among these three values. However, the b-values of patients who underwent PTBD within and over 14 days after jaundice appeared were $-0.281 \pm 0.07$ ($n = 38$) and $-0.103 \pm 0.01$ ($n = 49$), respectively, and differed significantly ($p < .05$). Thus, our results suggest that PTBD should be performed as soon as jaundice is noticed to achieve optimal drainage and reduction of jaundice and its accompanying symptoms.

## Complications

Complications of PTC and PTBD include bleeding, acute cholangitis, bile peritonitis, intraabdominal organ injuries, and/or the slipping out of the drainage catheter. Complications observed in our 134 patients who underwent biliary drainage are summarized in Table 8.2. As some complications contribute to an increased morbidity, they should be treated promptly.

### Sepsis

Sepsis is the most frequent and severe complication associated with PTC and PTBD. The presence of infected bile and biliary obstruction may induce sepsis under the conditions of elevated intraductal pressure, which sometimes follow the procedure. Sepsis is most likely to be associated with "benign" obstructions such as gallstones or benign strictures, particularly when the obstruction is incomplete; complete obstruction due to cancer is rarely associated with biliary infection. Furthermore, inadequate biliary drainage with persistent or recurrent biliary stasis, leakage of bile including procedure-related complications of occlusion or dislodgment of the drainage cather, or prolonged catheter manipulation are all factors predisposing to sepsis. Although prophylactic administration of antibiotics may reduce the incidence of sepsis, it cannot always prevent its development. Sacks-Berg et al. (26) found that although prophylactic antibiotics were given to 80 and 93% of patients undergoing cholangiographies and biliary drainage procedures, respectively, the overall incidence of sepsis was 13.5%. When sepsis is diagnosed, antibiotics should be administered, but if septic signs do not resolve, repeat biliary drainage or replacement of a drainage catheter should be performed.

### Bleeding

Intraperitoneal bleeding from the hepatic surface and intraductal bleeding from the wall of the bile duct are occasionally fatal complications and are usually associated with a severe bleeding diathesis. The former is likely to occur when the hepatic capsule is lacerated or several punctures are made and is detected by observing fluid collection by ultrasound or CT or by the development of hypotension. The latter may occur if a portal venous branch is penetrated by the catheter and result in hemobilia. Cholangiography will then usually show defects of filling in the bile ducts. Voegeli et al. (19) reported that intraductal arterial and portal venous bleeding each occurred in 1% of patients who underwent percutaneous transhepatic procedures. Subcapsular hematomas may also develop, but they cause few problems. Administration of hemostatic drugs or plasma fractions should be considered. Nevertheless, when intraperitoneal bleeding becomes severe, laparotomy may be necessary. Intraductal bleeding can usually be stopped by injecting saline into the ductal lumen, washing out the clots or debris occluding the biliary drainage catheter. When hemostasis is not achieved, abdominal angiography should be performed: transcatheter arterial embolization using a coil may stop the bleeding.

### Bile Leakage

Leakage of bile usually presents as abdominal or right shoulder pain. This complication is likely to occur when the bile duct is completely obstructed, when the extrahepatic bile duct or the peritoneal surface of the gallbladder is punctured, or when a drainage catheter tube has slipped out of the bile duct. Bile peritonitis has been reported to occur in about 1.5% of cases following PTC (5). In most instances, the signs of bile peritonitis resolve spontaneously, but when they do not, percutaneous drainage or laparotomy is required.

### Slipping out of Drainage Catheter

Drainage catheters tend to slip out when they cannot be inserted into the distal segment of the common bile duct, are placed only a short distance into the bile duct, or are inserted via the intercostal space. This complication usually occurs when the patient coughs or breathes deeply (1). When a catheter is confirmed to have slipped out of the bile duct, it should be left with its tip intraperitoneal for a few days to drain ascites, after which it should be removed.

### Others

Miscellaneous complications include pneumothorax, intraabdominal organ injuries, intrahepatic arterioportal fistula, and bile pulmonary embolism (1–3, 27). Pneumothorax may occur when the puncture is made via the intercostal space and transverses the thoracic cavity. Intraabdominal organ injuries can be avoided when the procedures are performed under ultrasonic guidance.

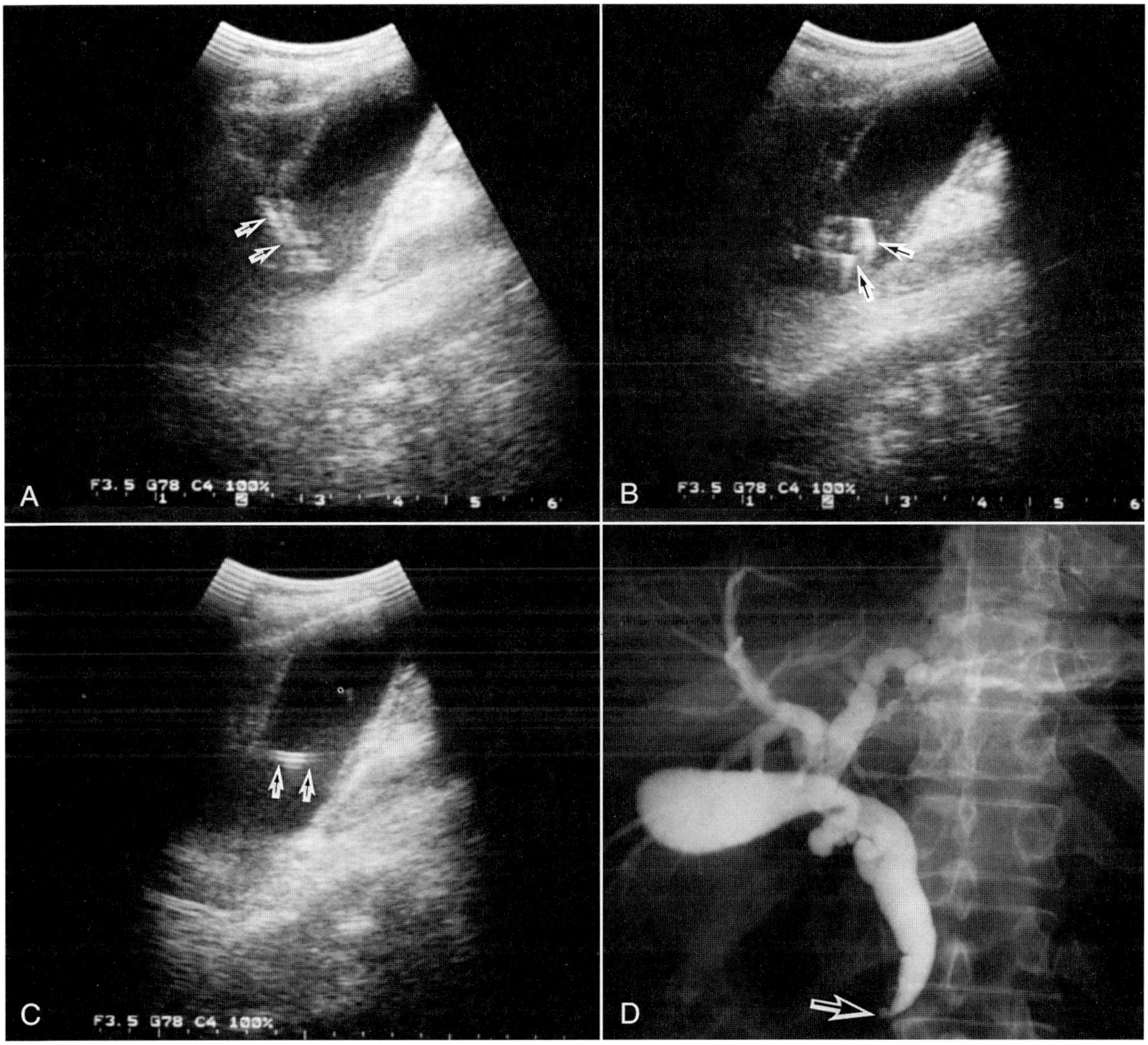


**FIG. 8.5.** **A.** Gallbladder puncture in a patient with a cancer of the papilla of Vater. The PTBD needle, the tip of which is shown clearly *(arrows)*, is advanced to the gallbladder. **B.** Insertion of a guide wire into the gallbladder *(arrows)*. **C.** Insertion of a drainage tube into the gallbladder *(arrows)*. **D.** Cholangiography through a drainage tube. After inserting a drainage tube, cholangiography showed an obstructive lesion clearly *(arrow)*.

## CONTROVERSY

Clinically, it is still controversial whether reduction of jaundice by biliary drainage should precede operative treatment. Nakayama et al. (28) found that the perioperative mortality rate in patients drained preoperatively was 8.2%, compared with 28.3% in controls who were not drained. Relief of obstruction before surgery has been reported to lead to improved hepatic function, reversal of secondary portal hypertension, improved wound healing, and a reduced incidence of postoperative acute renal tubular necrosis (10, 20–22, 29, 30). By contrast, Sirinek et al. (31) reported that preoperative biliary decompression had no therapeutic benefit compared with the outcome of patients whose jaundice was not alleviated prior to surgical intervention. Furthermore, in a randomized, controlled, prospective study, McPherson et al. (32) showed that the postoperative mortality rate was higher (32%) in patients who underwent preoperative biliary decompression than in those who underwent only an operation (19%). Similar results were reported by Dooley et al. (33) and Hatfield et al. (34). Furthermore, Pitt et al. (35) leveled the criticism that PTBD does not reduce the operative risk but does increase hospital costs and, therefore, should not be performed routinely. Thus, the clinical utility of preoperative biliary drainage has not been established. However, we believe that improved hepatic function is necessary for extended opera-

**TABLE 8.2. Complications Associated with PTBD in 134 Patients**

| Complication | Patients *(n)* |
|---|---|
| Drainage tubes slipping out | 18 |
| Hemobilia | 3 |
| Acute cholangitis | 3 |
| Hypotension | 1 |
| Biliary pleuritis | 1 |

*Editor's note:* see also section on sepsis.

tive procedures, such as hepatic trisegmentectomy and hepatectomy with pancreatoduodenectomy for cancers of the liver, bile duct, and pancreas, and therefore, PTBD, despite its attendant complications, should precede surgical treatment in these circumstances.

## SUMMARY

PTC and PTBD under ultrasound guidance have become important techniques for visualizing the biliary tree and reducing obstructive jaundice, respectively. In summary, the merits of these two procedures are *(a)* puncture of the larger blood vessels can be avoided because ultrasound can demonstrate the vessels during the procedure, *(b)* irradiation can be avoided or minimized, and *(c)* if desired, PTBD can be performed in the patient's room.

The procedures, however, also have demerits: *(a)* doctors must be trained in real-time scanning and *(b)* an appropriate real-time system and specialized instruments must be available. Taking these factors into consideration, however, we believe that both procedures have a clinical role in investigation of patients with obstructive jaundice.

## REFERENCES


1. Makuuchi M, Yamazaki S, Hasegawa H, Bandai Y, Ito T, Watanabe G. Ultrasonically guided cholangiography and bile drainage. Ultrasound Med Biol 1984;5:617–623.
2. Lintott DJ. Percutaneous transhepatic cholangiography. Clin Gastroenterol 1985;14:373–385.
3. Lunderquist A. The radiology of jaundice. Bailliere's Clinical Gastroenterology 1989;3:387–406.
4. Goldstein LI, Kadell BM, Weiner M. Thin needle cholangiography: experience with fifty patients. Ann Surg 1977;186:602–606.
5. Harbin WP, Mueller PR, Ferrucci JT Jr. Transhepatic cholangiography: complications and use patterns of the fine-needle technique. Radiology 1980;135:15–22.
6. Schiff ER. Diagnostic percutaneous transhepatic cholangiography. Semin Liver Dis 1982;2:49–56.
7. Thomas MJ, Pellegrini Ca, Way LW. Usefulness of diagnostic tests for biliary obstruction. Am J Surg 1982;144:102–108.
8. Huard P, Do-Xuan-Hop. La ponction transhepatique des canaux biliaires. Bull Soc Med Chir Indochine 1937;62:1090–1100.
9. Okuda K, Tanikawa K, Emura T, et al. Nonsurgical percutaneous transhepatic cholangiography—diagnostic significance in medical problems of the liver. Am J Dig Dis 1974;19:21–36.
10. Gundry SR, Strodel WE, Knol JA, et al. Efficacy of preoperative biliary tract decompression in patients with obstructive jaundice. Arch Surg 1984;119:703–708.
11. Savader SJ, Venbrux AC, Benenati JF, Mitchell SE, Widlus DM, et al. Choledochal cysts: role of noninvasive imaging, percutaneous transhepatic cholangiography, and percutaneous biliary drainage in diagnosis and treatment. J Vasc Intervent Radiol 1991;2: 379–385.
12. Lynn RB, Wilson JAP, Cho KJ. Cholangiocarcinoma. Role of percutaneous transhepatic cholangiography in determination of resectability. Dig Dis Sci 1988;33:587–591.
13. Huang M-H, Ker C-G. Ultrasonic guided percutaneous transhepatic bile drainage for cholangitis due to intrahepatic stones. Arch Surg 1988;123:106–109.
14. Boey JH, Way LW. Acute cholangitis. Ann Surg 1980;191:264–270.
15. Kissin CM, Grundy A. Percutaneous transhepatic cholangiography in the investigation of the persistent postoperative bile leak. Gastrointest Radiol 1987;12:215–218.
16. Zemel G, Zajko AB, Skonick ML, Bron KM, Campbell WL. The role of sonography and transhepatic cholangiography in the diagnosis of biliary complications after liver transplantation. AJR 1988;151:943–946.
17. Lameris JS, Stoker J, Nijs HGT, et al. Malignant biliary obstruction: percutaneous use of self-expandable stents. Radiology 1991;179: 703–707.
18. Gordon RL, Ring EJ, LaBerge JM, Doherty MM. Malignant biliary obstruction: treatment with expandable metallic stents—follow-up of 50 consecutive patients. Radiology 1992;182: 697–701.
19. Voegeli DR, Crummy AB, Weese JL. Percutaneous transhepatic cholangiography, drainage, and biopsy in patients with malignant biliary obstruction: an alternative to surgery. Am J Surg 1985;150:243–247.
20. Gobien RP, Stanley JH, Soucek CD, Anderson MC, Vujic I, Gobien BS. Routine preoperative biliary drainage: effect on management of obstructive jaundice. Radiology 1984;152:353–356.
21. Nagino M, Hayakawa N, Nimura Y, Dohke M, Kitagawa S. Percutaneous transhepatic biliary drainage in patients with malignant biliary obstruction of the hepatic confluence. Hepatogastroenterology 1992;39:296–300.
22. Clark RA, Mitchell SE, Colley DP, Alexander E. Percutaneous catheter biliary decompression. AJR 1981;137:503–509.
23. Pellegrini CA, Thomas MJ, Way LW. Bilirubin and alkaline phosphatase values before and after surgery for biliary obstruction. Am J Surg 1982;143:67–73.
24. Kerlan RK Jr, Ring EJ. Percutaneous transhepatic cholangiography and interventional radiology of the gallbladder and bile ducts. In: Way LW, Pellegrini CA, eds. Surgery of the gallbladder and bile ducts. Philadelphia: WB Saunders, 1987:169–186.
25. Shimizu T, Yoshida K. Evaluation of serum bilirubin decreasing rate b. Tan to Sui 1989;10:538–590 (in Japanese).
26. Sacks-Berg A, Calubiran OV, Epstein HY, Cunha BA. Sepsis associated with transhepatic cholangiography. J Hosp Infect 1992;20:43–50.
27. Kihira T, Konishi T, Shiraishi T, Yatani R, Nakano T. Fatal bile pulmonary embolism following percutaneous transhepatic cholangiodrainage: case report and literature review. Angiology 1993;44:725–730.
28. Nakayama T, Ikeda A, Okuda K. Percutaneous transhepatic drainage of the biliary tract. Gastroenterology 1978;74:554–559.
29. Denning DA, Ellison EC, Carey LC. Preoperative percutaneous transhepatic biliary decompression lowers operative morbidity in patients with obstructive jaundice. Am J Surg 1981;141:61–65.
30. Smith RC, Pooley M, George CRP, Faithful GR. Preoperative percutaneous transhepatic drainage in obstructive jaundice: a randomized, controlled trial examining renal function. Surgery 1985;97:641–647.
31. Sirinek KR, Levine BA. Percutaneous transhepatic cholangiography and biliary decompression. Arch Surg 1989;124:885–888.
32. McPherson GA, Benjamin IS, Hodgson HJ, Bowley NB, Allison DJ, Blumgart LH. Pre-operative percutaneous transhepatic biliary drainage in obstructive jaundice: the results of a controlled trial. Br J Surg 1984;71:371–375.
33. Dooley JS, Dick R, Olney J, Sherlock S. Non-surgical treatment of biliary obstruction. Lancet 1979;2:1040–1044.
34. Hatfield ARW, Tobias R, Terblanche J, et al. Preoperative external biliary drainage in obstructive jaundice. Lancet 1982;2: 896–899.
35. Pitt HA, Gomes AS, Lois JF, Mann LL, Deutsch LS, Longmire WP. Does preoperative percutaneous biliary drainage reduce operative risk or increase hospital cost? Ann Surg 1985;201:545–553.

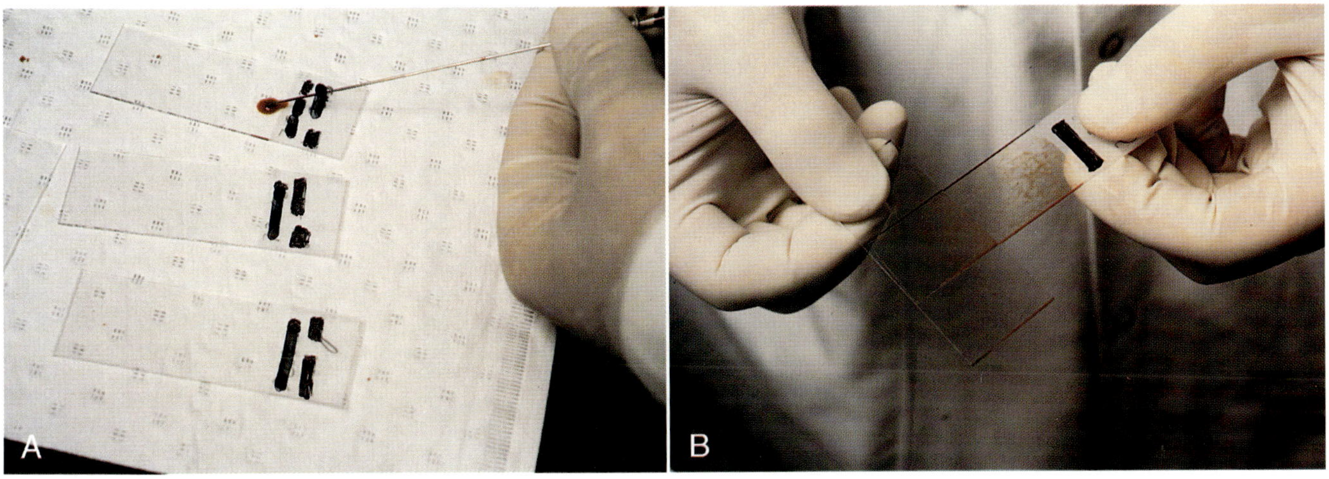

FIG. 10-2

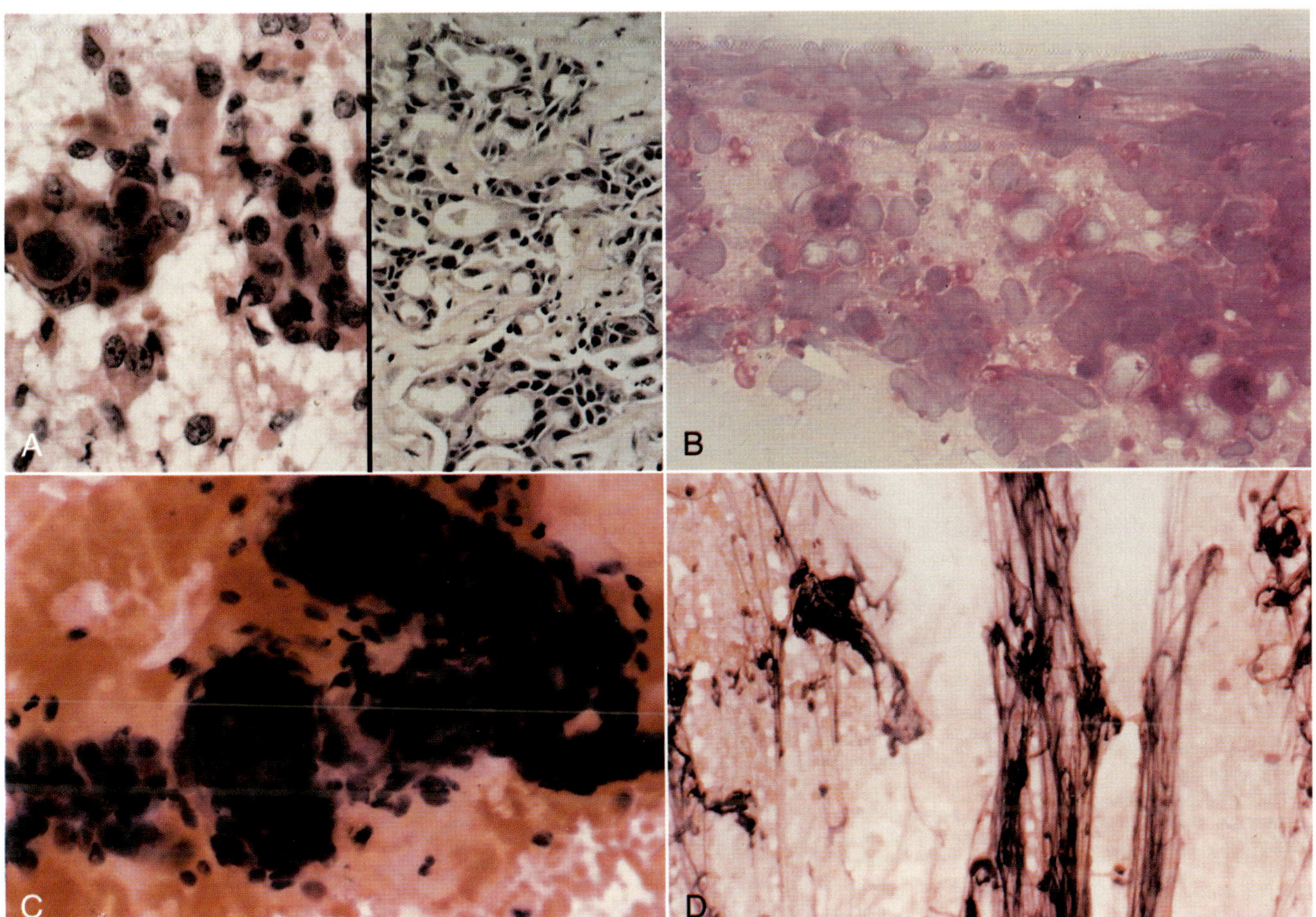

FIG. 10-3

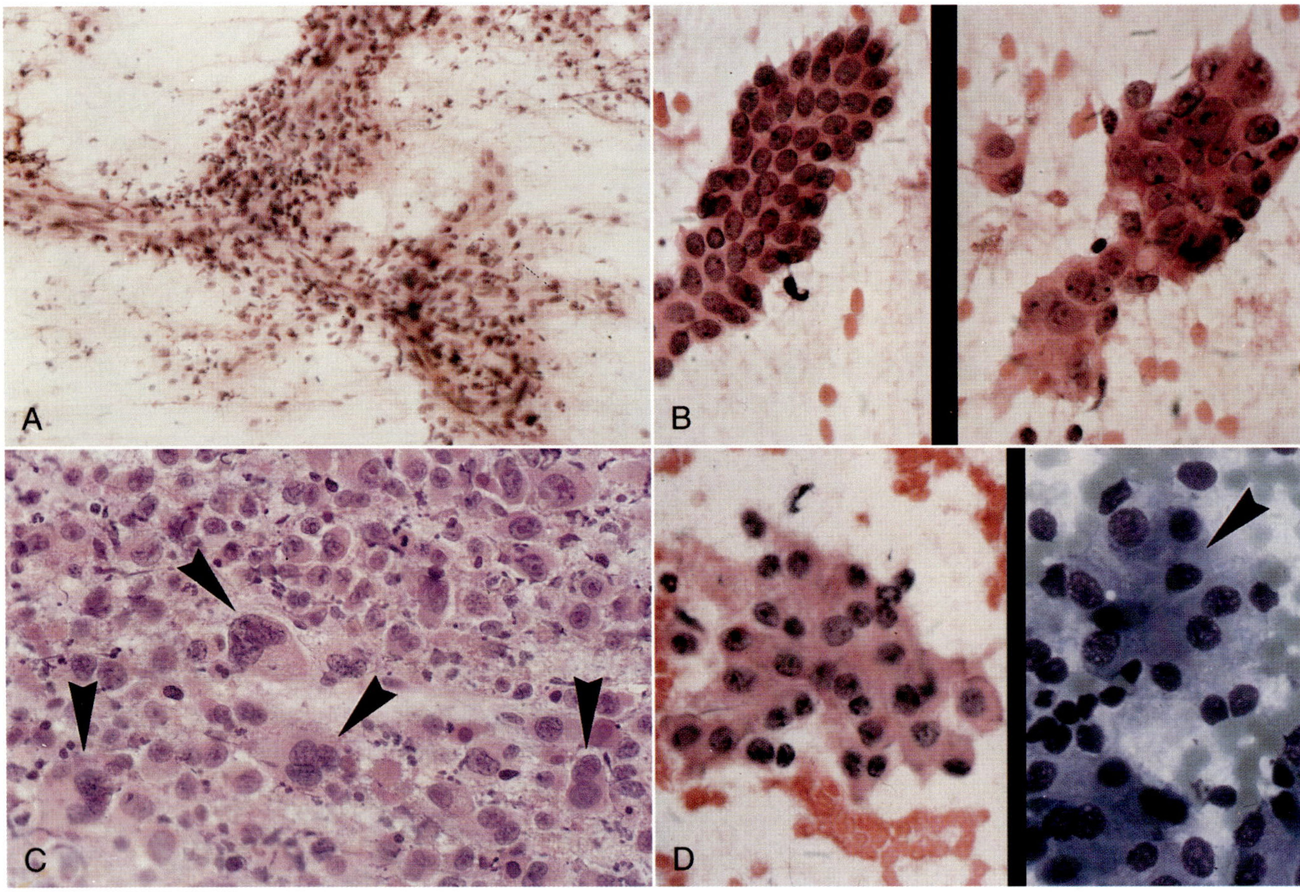

FIG. 10-4

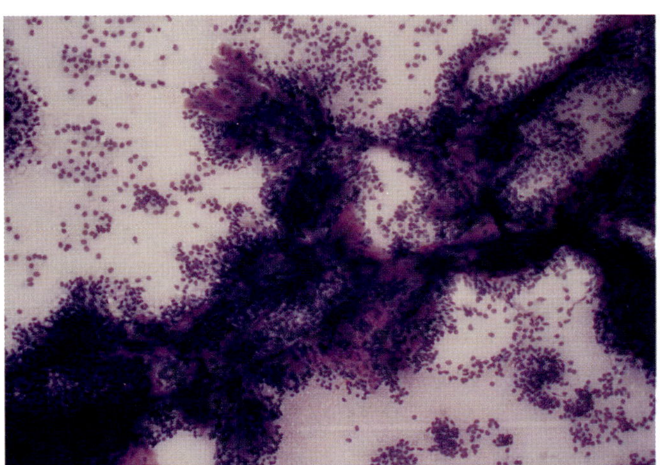
FIG. 10-5

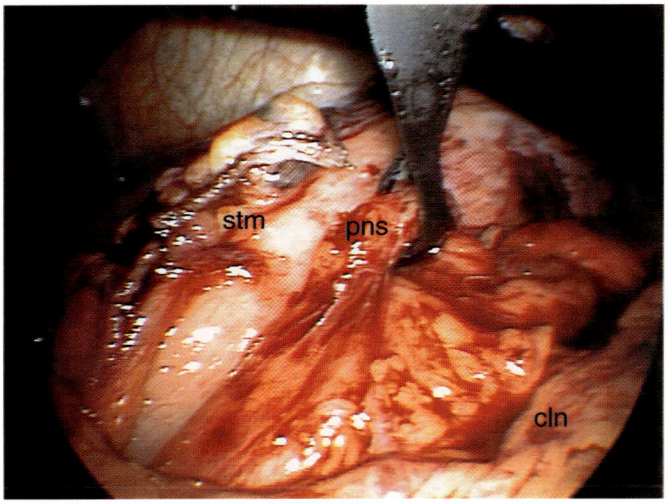

FIG. 13-1

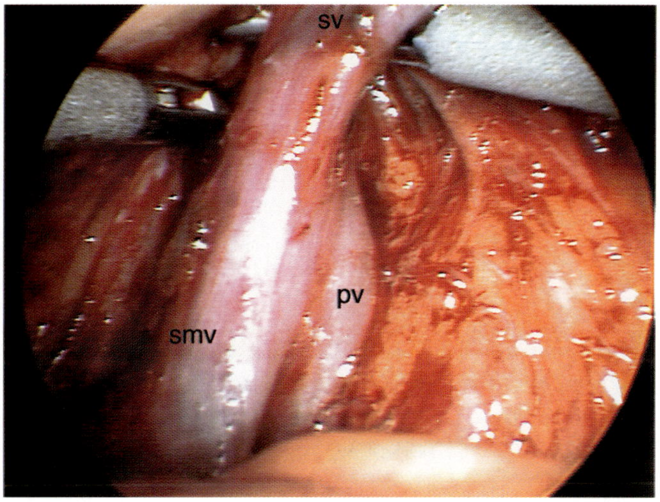

FIG. 13-2

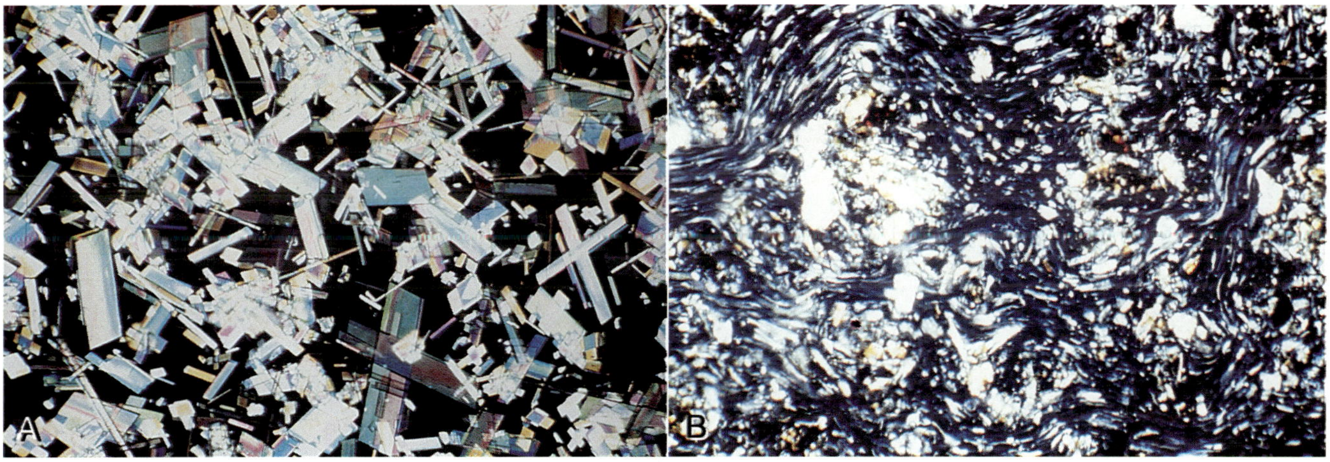

FIG. 22-1

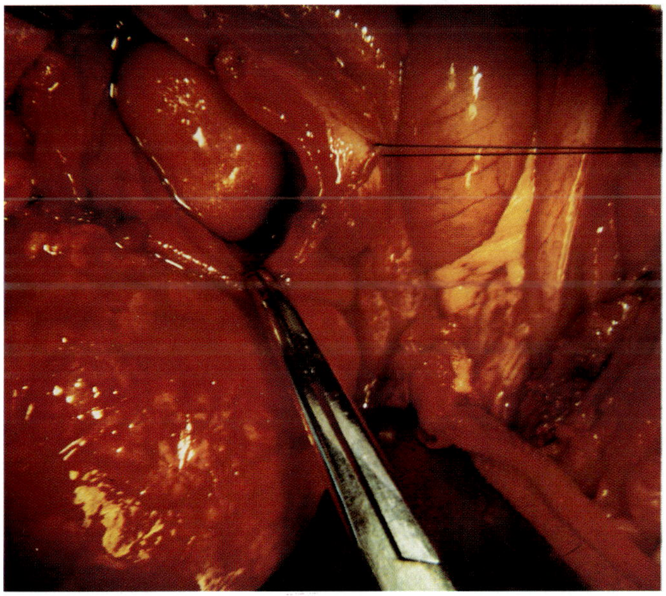
FIG. 24-8B

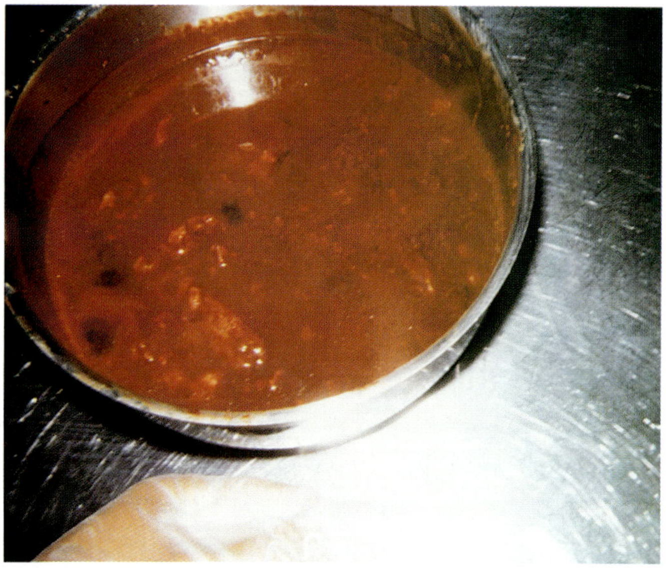

FIG. 28-3

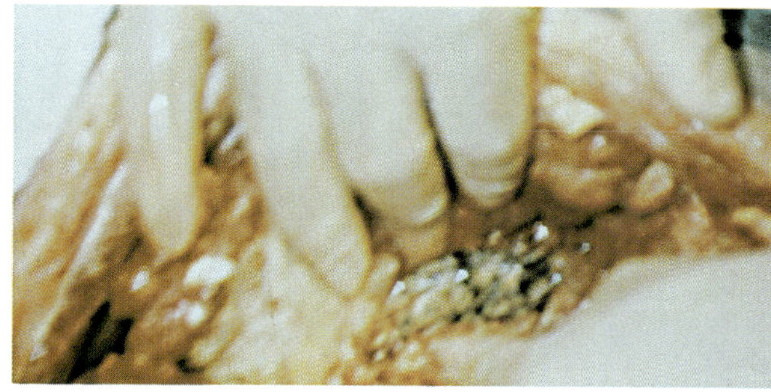

FIG. 28-4

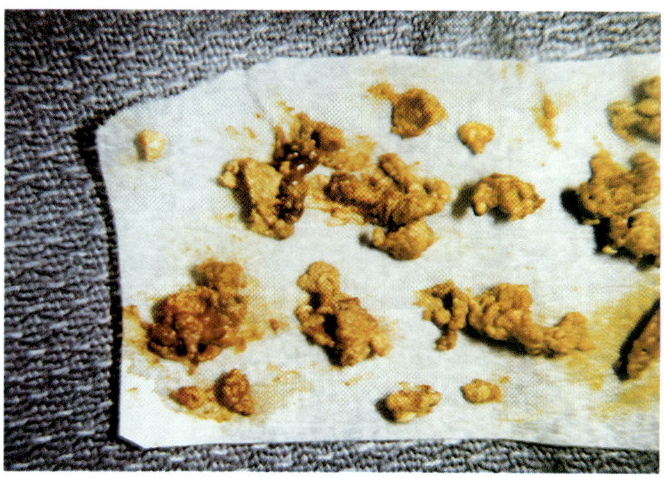

FIG. 28-5

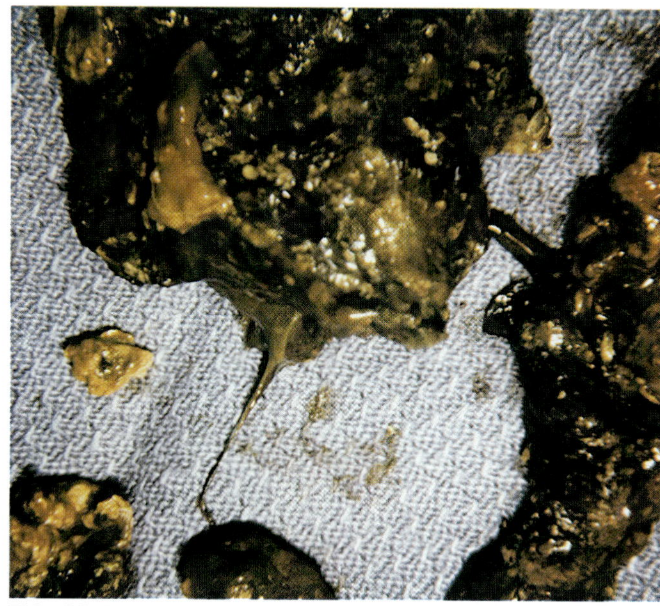

FIG. 28-6

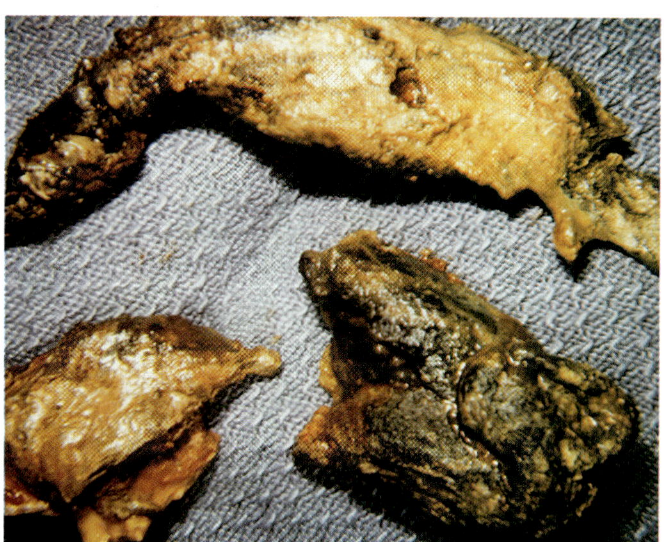

FIG. 28-7

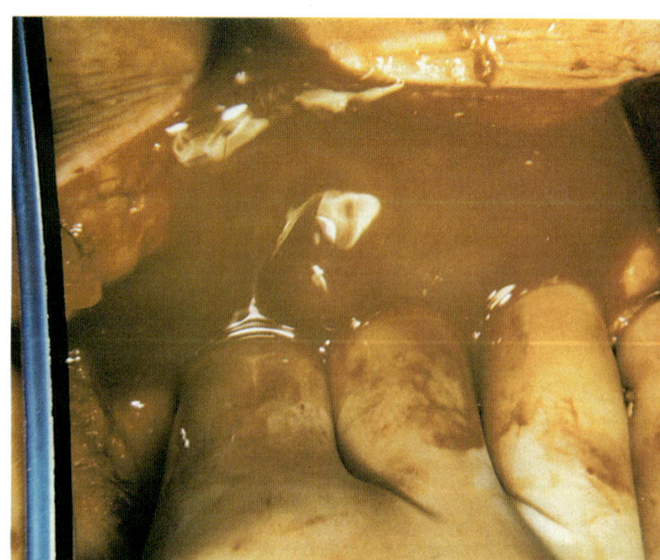

FIG. 28-8

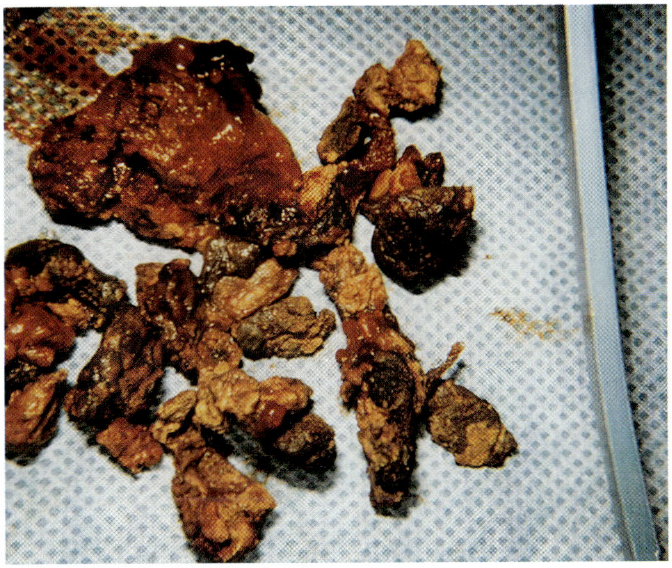

FIG. 28-9

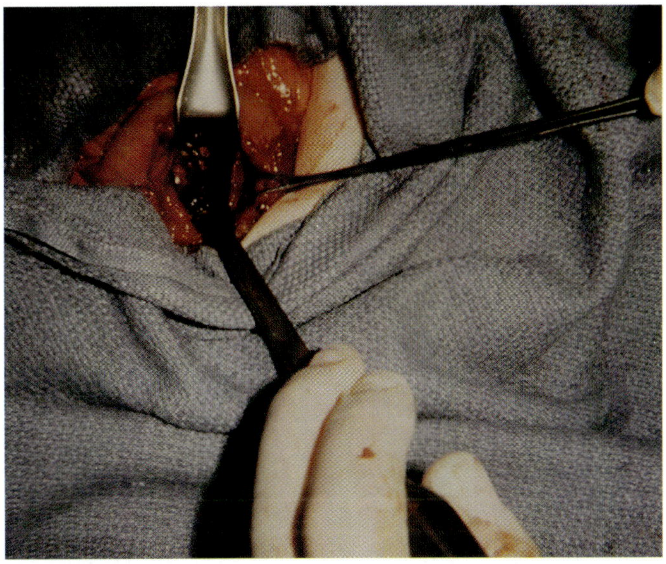

FIG. 28-10

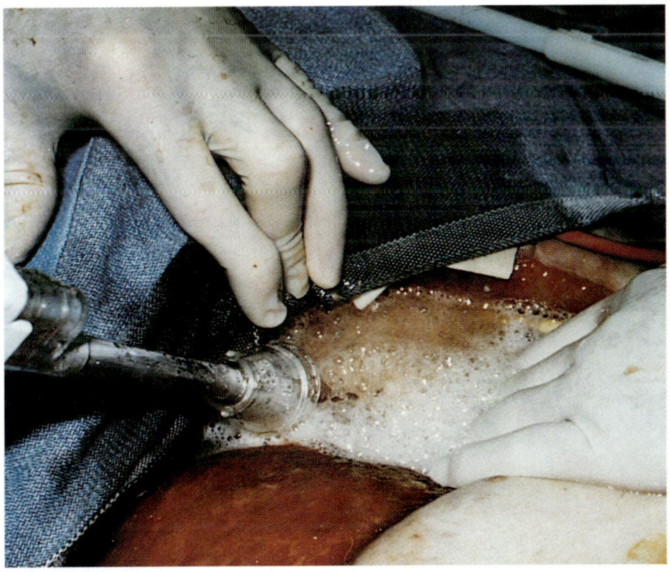

FIG. 28-11

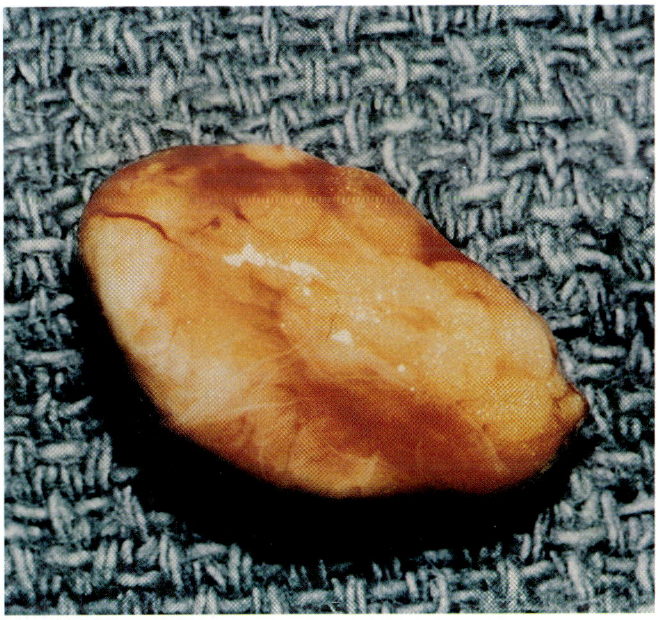

FIG. 28-16

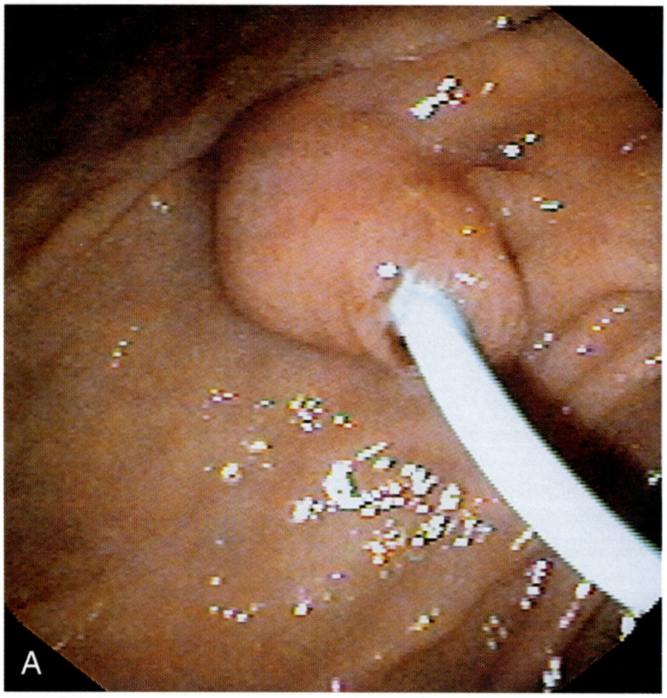


FIG. 34-4A

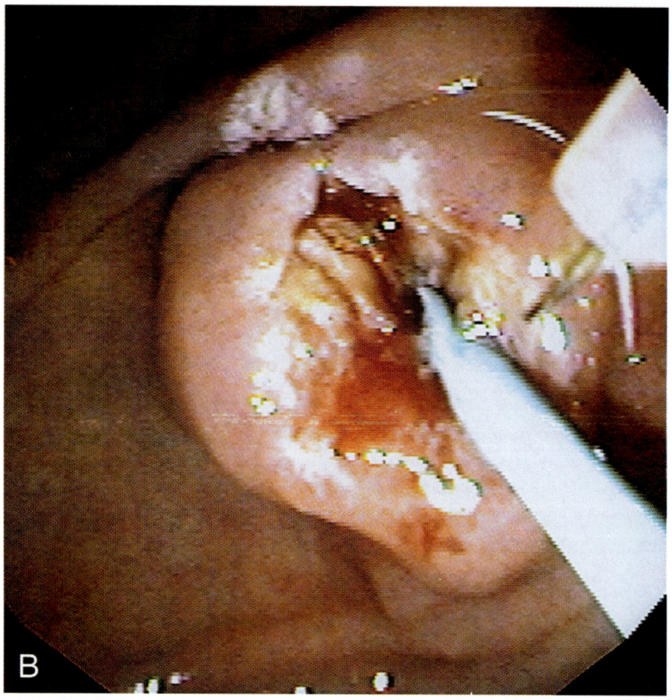


FIG. 34-4B

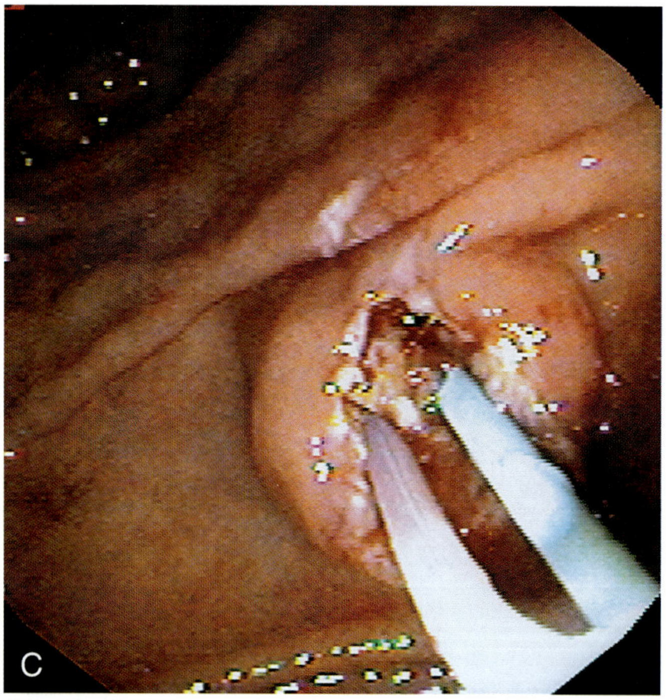


FIG. 34-4C

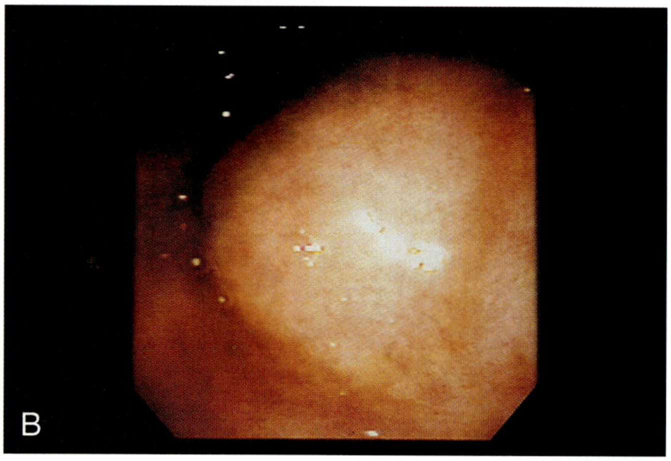


FIG. 34-6B

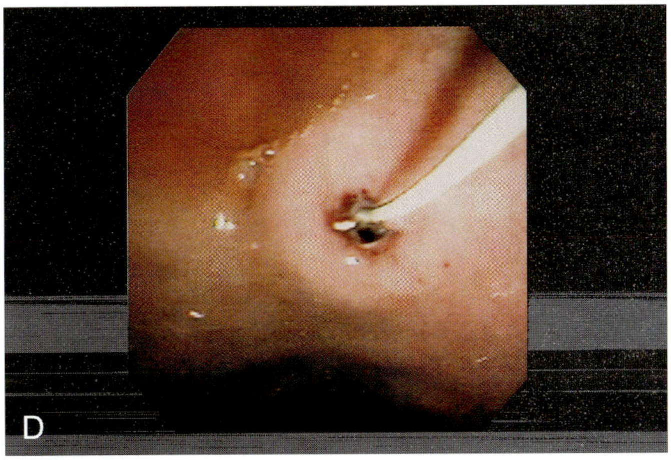


FIG. 34-6D

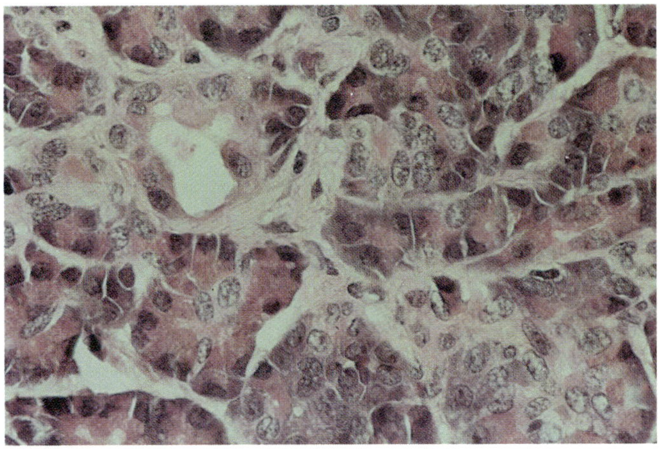

FIG. 48-3

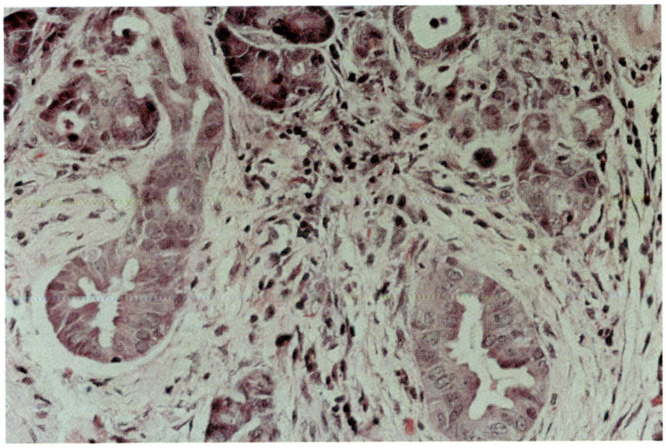

FIG. 48-4

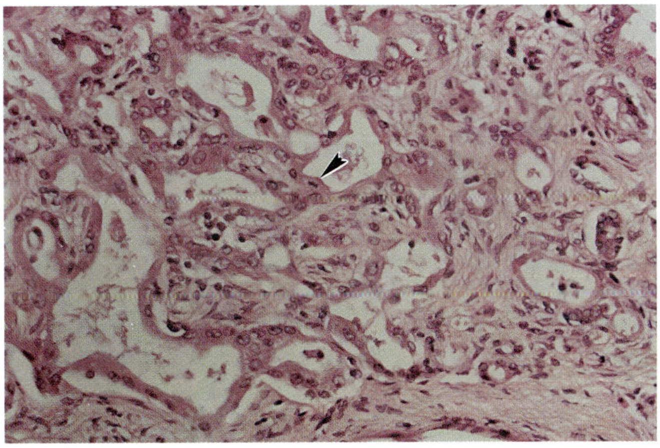

FIG. 48-5

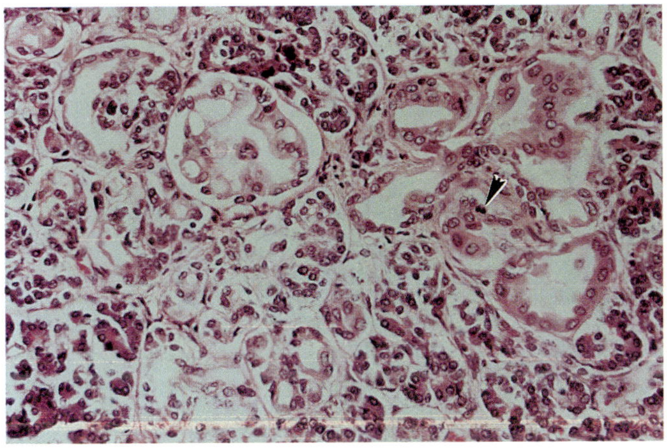

FIG. 48-7

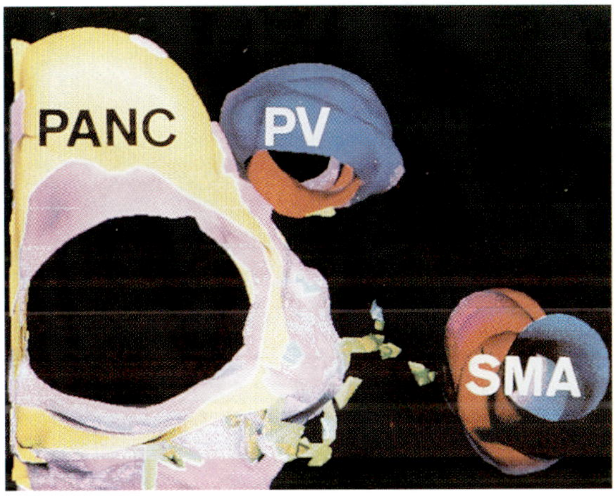


FIG. 56-18

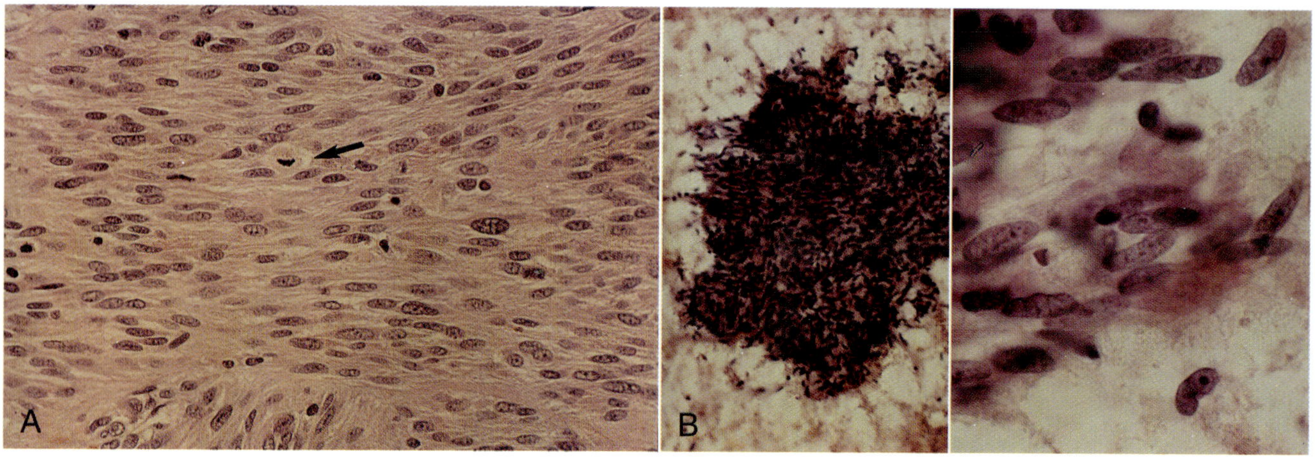


FIG. 65-1AB

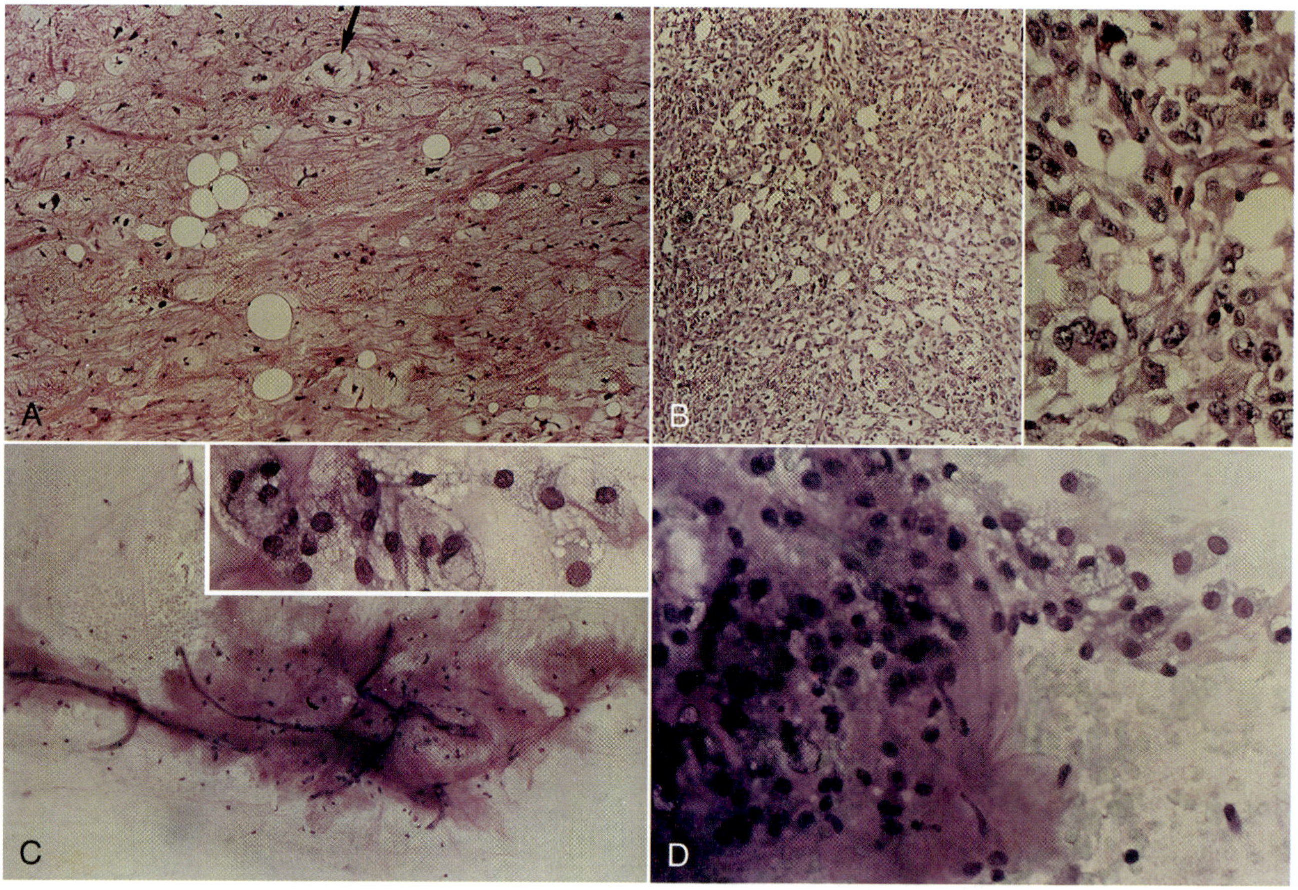


FIG. 65-2

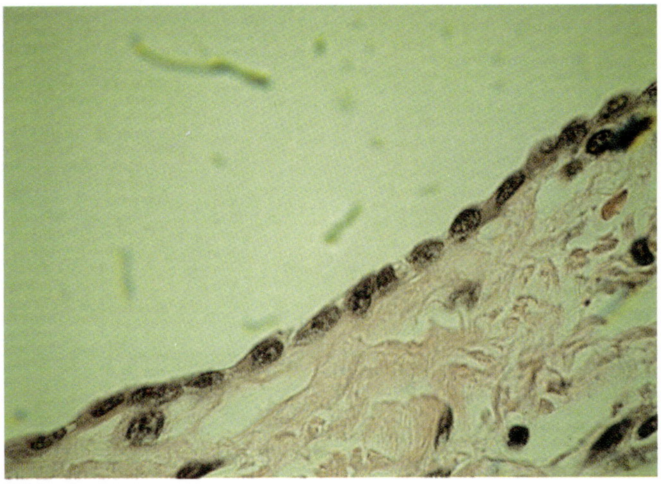

FIG. 71-1

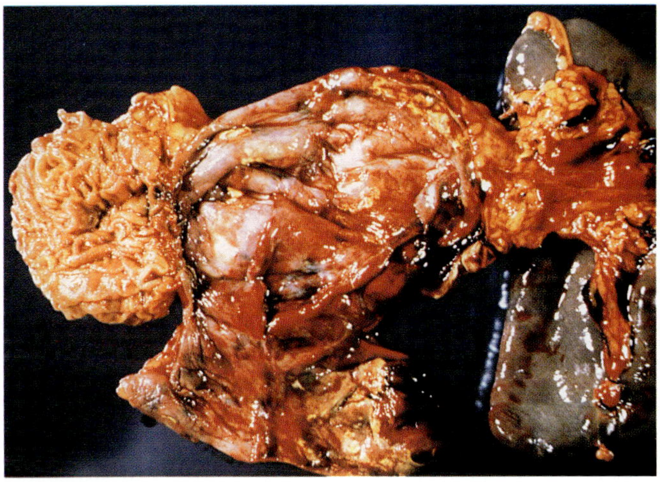

FIG. 71-4

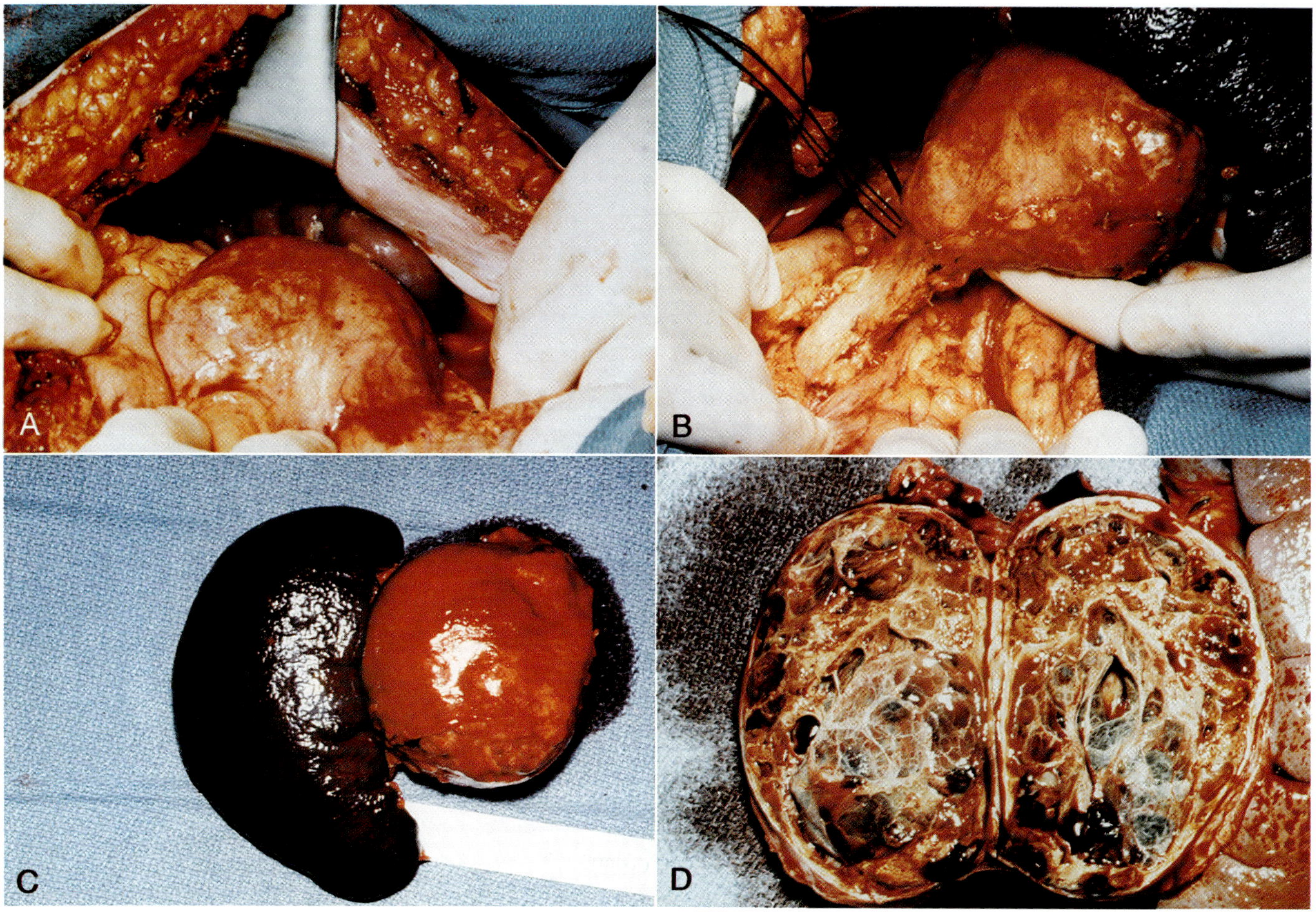

FIG. 73-3

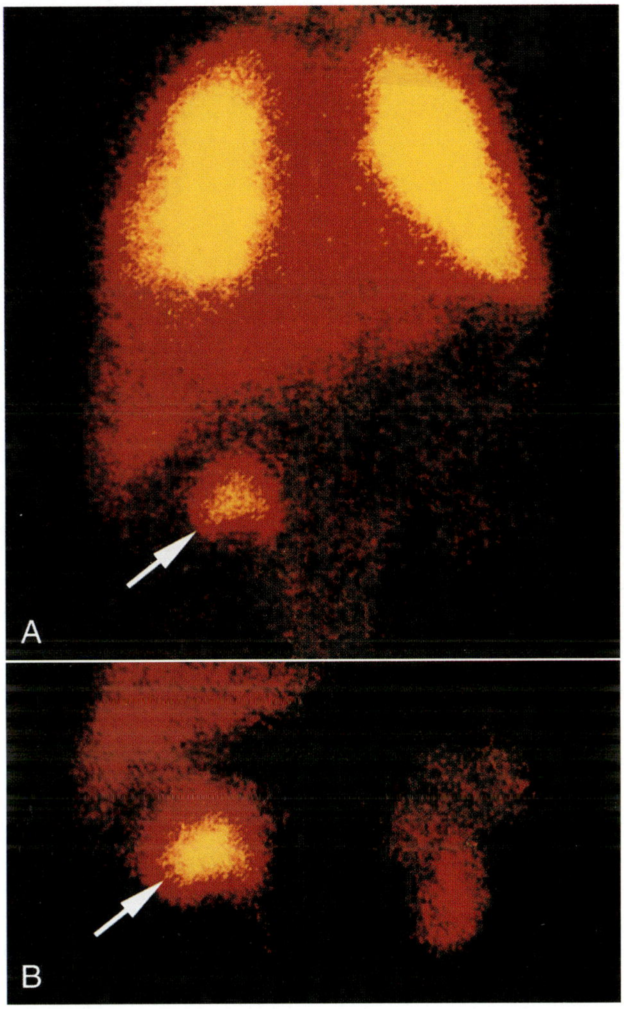


FIG. 80-7

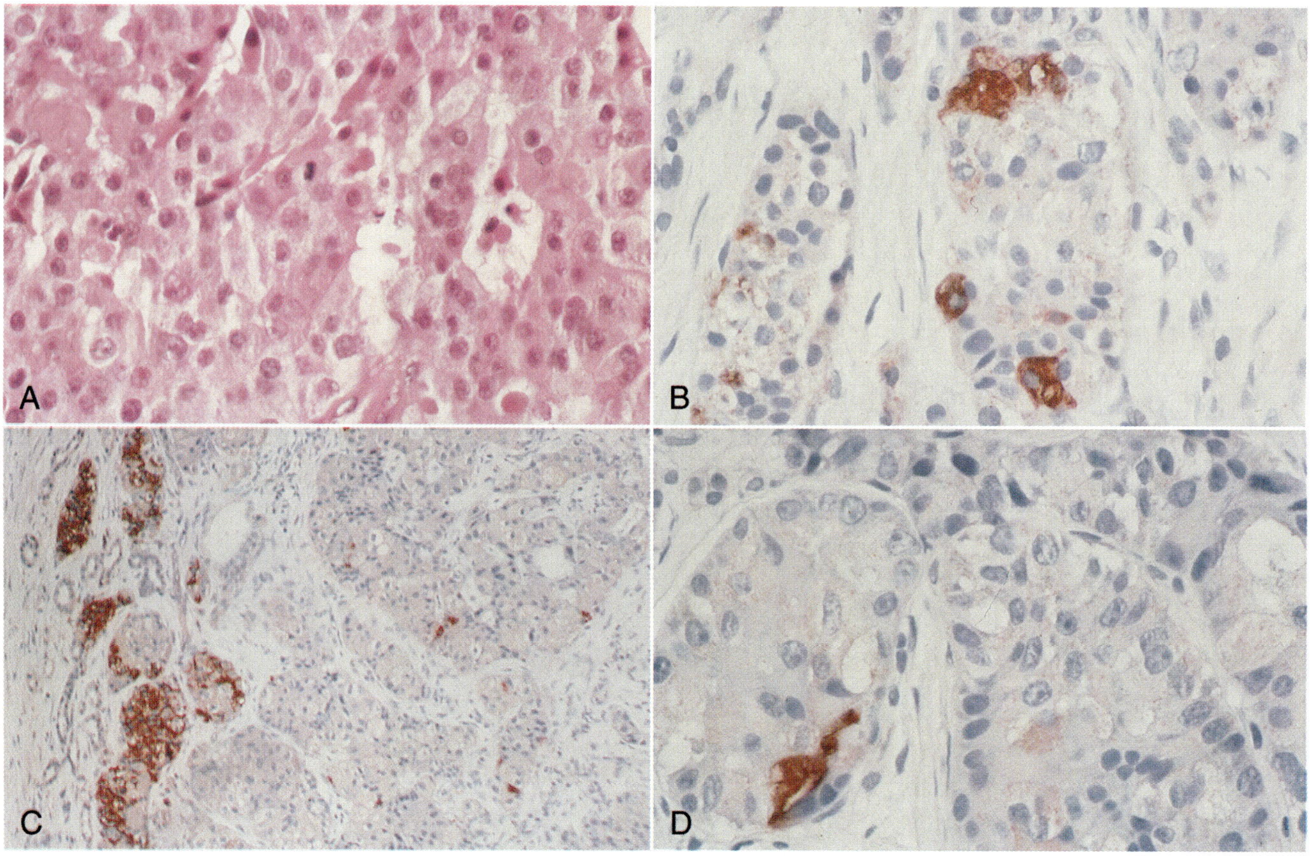


FIG. 82-7

# 9

# Endoscopic Ultrasonography

Thomas Rösch

Endoscopic ultrasonography (EUS) was introduced into the diagnostic armamentarium in gastroenterology nearly 15 years ago. Over that period, its application in the diagnosis and staging of gastrointestinal malignancies has been firmly established. A combination of endoscopy and high-frequency ultrasound, EUS has a limited penetration depth outside the gastrointestinal (GI) wall, restricting its application to organs immediately adjacent to the upper GI tract, such as the pancreas and the biliary tract. Visualization of the pancreatobiliary area is still considered one of the most difficult areas of EUS and requires considerable training and expertise. The range of normal findings, the findings and diagnostic accuracy in pancreatic disease, and the limitations of EUS are described and discussed in this chapter.

## EUS ANATOMY AND NORMAL FINDINGS OF THE PANCREAS

Echoendoscopes for the upper GI tract (including pancreatic scanning) are side-viewing endoscopes with a small ultrasonic transducer incorporated into their rigid tip. Using higher frequencies (5–20 MHz; most commonly, 7.5 MHz) than with transabdominal ultrasound (TUS), the mode of ultrasonic scanning is either radial (360° perpendicular to the shaft axis of the instrument) or linear, i.e., parallel (mostly 90–100° sector scan) to the instrument. The pancreas is visualized from the duodenum (head) and the stomach (body, tail), assuming various, imperfectly standardized positions of the ultrasonic endoscope and its tip. The normal pancreas has been described (1) as having a homogeneous echo-pattern slightly brighter than that of the adjacent liver; the ventral part of the head is considered to be more echo poor than the rest of the organ in most instances (1, 2). There are no established measures for normal pancreatic size, making it difficult to differentiate the normal pattern from early inflammation (2). As a result, there may be considerable interobserver variation in delineating and measuring the normal pancreas and in defining and interpreting the echo pattern in health and disease. The pancreatic duct can be traced in parts from different echoendoscope positions, but for visualizing the entire duct, including the side branches, EUS is inferior to endoscopic retrograde cholangiopancreatography (ERCP).

## ACUTE PANCREATITIS

The use of EUS in the diagnosis of acute pancreatitis is greatly limited, and no studies have shown its value in the diagnosis or staging of this disease; contrast-enhanced computerized tomography (CT) is generally considered the "gold standard" in differentiating between edematous and necrotic pancreatitis. EUS in general is unlikely to be as sensitive and specific as CT. However, in patients with "idiopathic" recurrent pancreatitis, EUS yields satisfactory results in the diagnosis of underlying causes (gallbladder or common bile duct minilithiasis, ampullary neoplasms, early chronic pancreatitis) in up to 50% of instances (3). Recently, EUS has been shown in several studies to be very sensitive and specific in the diagnosis of common bile duct stones (4–13)(Table 9.1); hence, its use in diagnosing gallstone pancreatitis is currently under evaluation.

## CHRONIC PANCREATITIS

EUS can delineate the features of the pancreatic parenchyma as well as the size and contour of the main duct; exclusive changes of the side branches are probably better detected by ERCP. Typical patterns of moderate-to-advanced chronic pancreatitis are ductal dilatation and irregularity, including side branches, intraductal concrements, cysts in the pancreas and the duodenal wall, parenchymal inhomogenicity including fibrotic stranding, echo-poor areas, and calcifications. These changes are seen clearly in moderate-to-advanced chronic pancreatitis, but the more subtle parenchymal abnormalities (the duct being normal) seen on EUS in early chronic pancreatitis are more difficult to distinguish from the normal parenchymal pattern (2). Several studies (Table 9.2) have therefore shown a high sensitivity and specificity of EUS in the moderate-to-advanced forms of chronic pancreatitis, whereas a very high sensitivity in early chronic pancreatitis is somewhat in contrast to a probably lower specificity. The definition of a false-positive finding of early chronic pancreatitis in EUS depends on the standard applied, which is usually ERCP. However, there have been descriptions of correct positive EUS diagnoses in patients with a normal ERCP in conjunction with a pathologic test of pancreatic function or in those with a normal ERCP accompanied by a history of alcohol abuse or recurrent attacks of pancreatitis, in whom some pancreatic damage is likely (2, 14).

EUS can be used in pancreatic pseudocysts for several purposes. EUS can help to differentiate a pseudocyst from cystic tumors (15, 16), even though larger prospective studies are still missing. Morphologic features suggesting a cystic pancreatic tumor are wall irregularities, solid regions in the cyst, and septation or lobulation, whereas a benign (pseudo)cyst should be suspected when a clear thin wall with smooth margins and no intracystic tissue is seen (15). The true predictive value of these features, however, is unknown. EUS can guide endoscopic transgastric or transduodenal endoscopic drainage of symptomatic pseudocysts; the distance between the cyst and the GI wall (in the absence of a bulging lesion) is of crucial importance. Surgeons with experience in endoscopic internal drainage have recommended that this distance should not exceed 1 cm (15). Finally, paramural vascular structures between the GI wall and the cyst—e.g., collaterals due to splenic vein thrombosis, a well-known complication of chronic pancreatitis—that would be in the potential puncture canal may preclude endoscopic drain-

**TABLE 9.1. Results of EUS in the Diagnosis of Choledocholithiasis[a]**

| First Author | *n* | Type of Study[b] | Sensitivity (%) | Specificity (%) |
|---|---|---|---|---|
| Edmundowicz (4) | 40 | Pro | 88 | 97 |
| Amouyal (5) | 62 | Pro | 97 | 100 |
| Shim (6) | 132 | Pro | 89 | 100 |
| Denis (7) | 60 | Pro | 92 | 100 |
| Palazzo (8) | 262 | Retro | 99 | 98 |
| Salmeron (9) | 211 | Retro | 96 | 96 |
| Keriven (10) | 78 | Pro | 100 | 89 |
| Canto (11,12) | 64 | Pro | 84 | 95 |
| Prat (13) | 109 | Pro | 93 | 97 |
| All cases | 1018 | | 94.5 | 97 |

[a]No cases of gallstone pancreatitis included.
[b]Pro, prospective; Retro, retrospective.

age. Cyst puncture has also been performed under EUS guidance, using linear instruments, leaving a guide wire in place for endoscopic stent insertion. Presently, the working channel of echoendoscopes is not large enough to accomodate a 7 Fr. stent, so that exchange of instruments is necessary. New prototype echoendoscopes however, will have larger instrumentation channels.

## PANCREATIC CANCER: DIAGNOSIS, DIFFERENTIATION, AND EUS-GUIDED PUNCTURE

Several endosonographic studies have described features of pancreatic cancer such as inhomogeneous and echo-poor pattern and irregular outer margins, partly with tumorous pseudopodia (17–19). However, others found that the echo features of pancreatic inflammatory masses are not significantly different (18), although some doubt this (20). The studies dealing with the differential diagnosis of cancer versus focal chronic pancreatitis show conflicting results (18, 20–23). Using various methodologic approaches, we have shown that EUS has a high sensitivity but a very low specificity (18, 23, 24) (Table 9.3). We therefore do not recommend the use of EUS for the differential diagnosis of pancreatic masses.

Most recently, EUS-guided fine-needle aspiration cytology (FNAC) was introduced, which requires the use of linear EUS instruments for proper visualization of the course of the needle. Until now, only cytologic specimens could be obtained, although some authors reported gaining "microhistology," i.e., thin cylinders of tissue for histopathologic evaluation. Instruments with larger instrumentation channels and larger needles are under development. First results using this technique are encouraging, sensitivity rates ranging from 75 to 85% for pancreatic tumors (25–28) (Table 9.4), but the clinical value and the accuracy compared with those of percutaneous ultrasound- or CT-guided puncture are not yet known. The complication rate of this new technique is very low, as can be judged from series including several hundred patients with various indications, mostly other than pancreatic masses. Tumor cell spread has been stated to occur more often in patients who have undergone percutaneous puncture (29), although confirmation of this by a prospective study is still missing. Theoretically, EUS-guided fine-needle puncture has a lower risk of spreading tumor cells because of the very short, or shallow, needle puncture, but proving this may be very difficult.

Several prospective and retrospective studies claim to demonstrate that EUS is the most sensitive method for diagnosing pancreatic mass lesions and especially small cancers. Most studies were performed with radial scanners (17–19, 21, 22, 30–38); information utilizing linear-type instruments is still limited (39). In various small-series studies, partly retrospective, EUS was shown to be superior to other imaging methods (Tables 9.5 and 9.6). In most papers, the study population consisted entirely of patients with pancreatic tumors; in some studies, there were only a few inflammatory masses; and in only very few studies, persons with a normal pancreas were included (18, 35). The high prevalence of pancreatic tumors might therefore have influenced these very good results. From the few data available, sensitivity and specificity of EUS was also high in studies including tumor patients and those with a normal pancreas and/or nonneoplastic disease (18, 23, 34, 35, 38, 39) (Table 9.7).

The other major criticism of most EUS studies in pancreatic cancer is that the endosonographic results of one experienced EUS examiner with some knowledge of the presumed diagnosis might have been compared with those of several ultrasound (US) examiners. Furthermore, in many studies, CT was done in various institutions with earlier-model technology. A recent French study claims that, when US was repeated at the time of EUS with the same information that was available to the EUS examiners, US provided the same information as EUS in 60% of cases (40).

In summary, provided the user has acquired expertise with this technique, EUS is very sensitive in diagnosing pancreatic tumors, even in less highly selected patients, but the very high sensitivity in some studies, approaching 100%, is expected to decrease slightly. The specificity of EUS depends on whether cancer is compared with focal chronic pancreatitis (low specificity) or with the normal pancreas (high specificity) (Tables 9.3 and 9.6).

**TABLE 9.2. Results of EUS in the Diagosis of Chronic Pancreatitis**

| Nattermann et al. 1993 (72) | | |
|---|---|---|
| ERCP staging of chronic pancreatitis | *n* | Rate of abnormal EUS findings (%) |
| 0 | 43 | 63 |
| I | 8 | 88 |
| II | 16 | 100 |
| III | 27 | 100 |
| **Wiersema et al. 1993 (73) n = 69** | | |
| Standard applied | Sensitivity of EUS (%) | Specificity of EUS (%) |
| ERCP alone | 100 | 79 |
| ERCP + PPJ[a] | 70 | 33 |
| ERCP + clinical criteria | 90 | 99 |

[a]PPJ, secretin-stimulated pancreatic juice collection.

## PANCREATIC CANCER: STAGING

In the locoregional staging of pancreatic cancer the tumor, node, metastasis (TNM) system and the Union Internationale Contre le Cancer (UICC) classification are used. As with other GI malignancies, detection of distant metastases is beyond the scope of EUS, but in our experience, small amounts of ascitic fluid is often seen around the duodenum or the stomach (e.g., in the lesser sac), suggesting peritoneal spread. However, the sensitivity and specificity of this sign for the diagnosis of peritoneal metastases has not been studied.

Tables 9.8 and 9.9 give an overview on staging results reported in the literature (20, 22, 35, 38, 39, 41–46). Most studies contain only small numbers of patients (no study has more than 40 cases). In the tumors that were misstaged, most errors occurred between stages T2 (overstaging) and T3 (understaging); in terms of therapeutic consequences, this differen-

**TABLE 9.3. Sensitivity (Se) and Specificity (Sp) of EUS versus Ultrasonography (US), Computed Tomography (CT), and Endoscopic Retrograde Cholangiopancreatography (ERCP) in the Differentiation between Pancreatic Cancer and Focal Chronic Pancreatitis**

| | | EUS | | US | | CT | | ERCP | |
|---|---|---|---|---|---|---|---|---|---|
| First Author | *n* | Se (%) | Sp (%) | Se (%) | Sp (%) | Se (%) | Sp (%) | Se (%) | Sp (%) |
| Forsmark (21) | 25 | 77 | 88 | 44 | 80 | 56 | 71 | 86 | 88 |
| Palazzo (22) | 49 | 96 | 73 | 65 | 60 | 69 | 53 | — | — |
| Wiersema (20) | 39 | 88 | 86 | — | — | — | — | — | — |
| Rösch (23)[a] | 38 | 64 | 50 | — | — | 45 | 50 | 71 | 50 |
| Rösch (24)[a] | 40 | | | | | | | | |
| Rösch (18)[a] | 108 | 74 | 52 | 59 | 30 | 60 | 65 | 92 | 82 |

[a]The three studies by our group use diferent methodologies; the first (18) was a prospective study with a predominance of pancreatic cancer; the second (23) performed EUS always prior to CT and ERCP, with only a third of patients having neoplasia; and the third (24) used completely blinded videotape assessment. There is partial overlap of included cases between patient groups in study 3 with those of studies 1 and 2, but none between studies 1 and 2.

**TABLE 9.4. Results of Studies Analyzing the Sensitivity and Specificity of EUS-Guided Fine-Needle Aspiration Cytology (FNAC) in the Diagnosis of Pancreatic Tumors**

| First Author | *n* | Sensitivity (%) | Specificity (%) |
|---|---|---|---|
| Giovannini (25) | 43 | 75 | 100 |
| Wiersema (26) | 11 | 82 | — |
| Bhutani (27) | 11 | 91 | — |
| Chang (28) | 10 | 90 | — |

**TABLE 9.5. Sensitivity of EUS in the Diagnosis of Pancreatic Cancer in Comparison with Transabdominal Ultrasound (US), Computed Tomography (CT), Endoscopic Retrograde Cholangiopancreatography (ERCP)**

| First author | *n* | EUS | US | CT | ERCP |
|---|---|---|---|---|---|
| Ikeda (30) | 5 | 100% | — | — | — |
| Sugiyama (31) | 5 | 100% | 100% | 20% | — |
| Fukuda (32) | 10 | 100% | — | — | — |
| Kaufman (33) | 12 | 75% | — | — | |
| Keriven-Souquet (34)[a] | 17 | 88% | — | — | — |
| Müller (35)[b] | 22 | 94% | — | 69% | — |
| Forsmark (21) | 25 | 77% | 44% | 56% | 86% |
| Hayashi (19) | 30 | 97% | 87% | — | — |
| Giovannini (39)[c] | 30 | 100% | 48% | 69% | — |
| Kallimanis (36) | 32 | 92% | 66% | 74% | 88% |
| Wiersema (37) | 39 | 88% | — | — | — |
| Palazzo (22) | 49 | 96% | 65% | 69% | — |
| Yasuda (17) | 50 | 100% | 78% | 86% | 94% |
| Rösch (18) | 76 | 99% | 67% | 77% | 90% |
| All cases | | 94% *n* = 402 | 67% *n* = 297 | 72% *n* = 289 | 91% *n* = 158 |

[a]Only patients with inconclusive US and/or CT.
[b]The sensitivity for MRI was 83%.
[c]Linear-type instrument used.

**TABLE 9.6. Sensitivity of Endoscopic Ultrasonography (EUS), Ultrasonography (US), Computed Tomography (CT), Endoscopic Retrograde Cholangiopancreatography (ERCP), and Magnetic Resonance Imaging (MRI) in Diagnosing Small Pancreatic Tumors**

| | | | Sensitivity (%) | | | | |
|---|---|---|---|---|---|---|---|
| First author | *n* | Tumor Size (cm) | EUS | US | CT | ERCP | MRI |
| Hayashi (19) | 5 | <2 | 100 | 80 | — | — | — |
| Ikeda (30) | 5 | <3 | 100 | — | — | — | — |
| Sugiyama (31) | 5 | <3 | 100 | 100 | 20 | — | — |
| Palazzo (22) | 7 | <2.5 | 100 | 14 | 14 | — | — |
| Akahoshi (38) | 10 | <3 | 90 | 80 | 50 | 67 | — |
| Yasuda (17) | 5 | <2 | 100 | 20 | 40 | 60 | — |
| | 13 | <3 | 100 | 54 | 62 | 85 | — |
| Müller (35) | 10 | <2 | 90 | — | 40 | — | 33 |
| | 15 | <3 | 93 | — | 53 | — | 67 |
| Rösch (18) | 28 | <3 | 100 | 61 | 64 | 86 | — |
| All cases | | | 99 *n* = 78 | 59 *n* = 58 | 53 *n* = 68 | 85 *n* = 40 | 67 *n* = 15 |

**TABLE 9.7. Sensitivity (Se) and Specificity (Sp) of EUS versus Ultrasound (US) and Computed Tomography (CT) in the Differentiation between Pancreatic Neoplasia and Normal Pancreas (NP) or between Pancreatic Neoplasia and Nontumorous Conditions (Normal Pancreas plus Chronic Pancreatitis (CP))**

| | | EUS | | US | | CT | | ERCP | |
|---|---|---|---|---|---|---|---|---|---|
| First author | *n* | Se | Sp | Se | Sp | Se | Sp | Se | Sp |
| Müller (35)[a] NP + CP[b] | 49 | 94% | 100% | — | — | 69% | 100% | — | — |
| Keriven-Souquet (34) NP + CP[b] | 52 | 88% | 89% | — | — | — | — | — | — |
| Rösch (23)[c] NP[b] | 57 | 95% | 95% | — | — | 90% | 63% | 90% | 84% |
| Giovannini (39)[d] NP + CP[b] | 62 | 100% | 96% | 48% | 60% | 69% | 83% | — | — |
| Rösch (18)[c] NP[b] | 128 | 99% | 100% | 67% | 40% | 77% | 53% | 90% | 73% |

[a]The respective values for MRI were 83% (Se) and 100% (Sp).
[b]Control group (nonneoplasia patients).
[c]One study (23) included only a third of neoplasia cases and EUS was performed prior to CT and ERCP; there is no overlap in cases with the previous prospective study with a predominance of tumors in the entire patient group (18).
[d]Use of linear instruments.

tiation is much more important than discrimination between stages T1 and T2. A comparison of the TN staging by EUS with results of other imaging tests is shown in Table 9.10. Only one study (38) compared EUS with CT and magnetic resonance imaging (MRI); accuracy rates were for T staging 82% (EUS), 45% (CT), and 50% (MRI) and for N staging, 64% (EUS), 50% (CT), and 56% (MRI).

Vascular invasion is probably the most important parameter for determining resectability in pancreatic cancer. Table 9.11 shows an overview on the results of EUS and other tests in predicting infiltration into the portal venous system. Table 9.12 shows the remaining studies in which vascular invasion is used as a general parameter without further differentiating between the different vessels.

There are some limitations to the above-mentioned prospective (22, 35, 38, 47) and retrospective (31, 39, 45) studies. First, in most studies there is no separate analysis of the different vessels (portal vein, splenic vein, superior mesenteric vein or arteries). Second, in most of the papers, cancers in all locations (head, body, and tail) are lumped together. From the few available data, however, it seems obvious that EUS achieves different results in diagnosing invasion of different vessels: Whereas portal vein involvement can be detected with good sensitivity and specificity, far less accurate results are achieved in diagnosing arterial encasement (47). Furthermore, the superior mesenteric vein cannot be fully traced with the radial echoendoscope, and most cases of misstaging in some studies (35, 46) were due to deficiencies in diagnosing superior mesenteric involvement. Perhaps linear-type echoendoscopes are better for visualizing the entire portal venous system, but only one initial study is available, which shows an 88% accuracy for EUS in diagnosing vascular involvement in general (39). The contribution of Doppler to the EUS staging of pancreatic cancer has not yet been evaluated. Some authors tried to determine the sensitivity and specificity of various criteria for the diagnosis of vascular involvement (48–50), but clear criteria have not yet been elucidated and agreed upon.

In contrast to the upper GI tract, in most studies EUS is either equal to CT diagnosis of vascular involvement (35, 51) or superior by only 10–15% (22, 38, 39, 47), even though the most modern CT technology such as spiral CT and CT-angioportography was not used in any of these studies.

In summary, the role of EUS in the locoregional staging and

**TABLE 9.8. Staging Results of Pancreatic Cancer in the Literature According to the Tumor, Node, Metastasis (TNM) System**

| | | Accuracy (%) of EUS in | | |
|---|---|---|---|---|
| Author | *n* | T Staging | N Staging | Ref |
| Grimm et al. 1990 | 26 | 85 | 72 | (41) |
| Tio et al. 1990 | 36 | 92 | 72 | (42) |
| Kallimanis et al. 1992 | 32 | 78 | 66 | (43) |
| Rösch et al 1992 | 35[a] | 94 | 80 | (44) |
| Palazzo et al. 1993 | 38 | — | 74 | (22) |
| Wiersema et al. 1993 | 39 | 76 | 82 | (20) |
| Yasuda et al. 1993 | 29 | — | 66 | (45) |
| Giovannini et al. 1994 | 25[b] | — | 92 | (39) |
| Müller et al. 1994 | 22[c] | 82 | 64 | (35) |
| Gress et al. 1995 | 59[d] | 87 | 80 | (74) |
| Gress et al. 1995 | 16[d] | 88 | 94 | (75) |
| Kadish et al. 1995 | 32/21[e] | 94 | 76 | (76) |
| Rösch et al. 1995 | 35/20[f] | 69 | 60 | (46) |
| All cases: T staging | 332 | 83% | | |
| N staging | 398 | | 74% | |

[a]Only pancreatic head cancer cases included.
[b]Use of linear-type instrument.
[c]22 patients with pancreatic head cancer, 65 patients with periampullary cancer.
[d]Comparative study between radial (*n* = 9) and linear instrument (*n* = 7), obviously other patients than in the other study by the same group.
[e]Only 21 cases had complete information about N staging.
[f]Only pancreatic head cancer cases included; blind reevaluation of videotapes; data on N staging only available for 20 patients.

**TABLE 9.9. Staging Accuracy of EUS in Pancreatic Cancer by Various Stages**

| Stage | *n* | EUS Correct (%) |
|---|---|---|
| T1 | 24 | 80 |
| T2 | 67 | 81 |
| T3 | 75 | 85 |
| N0 | 79 | 76 |
| N1 | 142 | 81 |

Data from (22, 35, 39, 41–44, 77).

**TABLE 9.10. Comparison of EUS, Transabdominal Ultrasound (US), and Computed Tomography (CT) in the T and N Staging of Pancreatic Carcinoma**

| Staging | n | EUS | US[a] | CT | MRI[b] |
|---|---|---|---|---|---|
| T stage | 173 | 86% | 35% | 42% | 57% |
| N stage | 223 | 71% | 42% | 53% | 59% |

Data from (22, 35, 38, 44, 45, 74, 76).
[a]Data on 60 patients (T staging) and 121 patients (N staging) were available for analysis.
[b]Data on 35 patients (T staging) and 29 patients (N staging) were available for analysis.

**TABLE 9.12. Results of Other Studies Analyzing the Accuracy of EUS in Detecting "Vascular Invasion" Without Further Specification of the Vascular System Under Consideration**

| | | Accuracy (%) | | | | |
|---|---|---|---|---|---|---|
| Author | n | EUS[a] | US | CT | ANG | Ref |
| Kobayashi et al. 1993 | 30 | 73 | — | — | — | (79) |
| Wiersema et al. 1993 | 18 | Se 100<br>Sp 80 | — | — | — | (20) |
| Yasuda et al. 1993 | 29 | 79 | 55 | 41 | 72 | (45) |
| Kadish et al. 1995 | 15 | 93 | — | — | 60 | (76) |
| Gress et al. 1995 | 16 | 100 | — | — | — | (75) |
| Gress et al. 1995 | 59 | 95 | — | 78 | — | (74) |
| All cases | 167 | 88 | | | | |

[a]Se, sensitivity; Sp, specificity.

in the assessment of resectability of pancreatic cancer has not yet been established. Since there are distinct deficiencies in the diagnosis of infiltration into the superior mesenteric vein—at least with radial instruments—and in the diagnosis of arterial involvement, the value of EUS seems limited. Initial results probably overestimated the staging value of EUS. Accuracy rates of about 80%, similar to those for upper GI EUS staging, are probably more realistic. A better definition of EUS criteria for the diagnosis of vascular involvement, the value of a combination of radial and linear scanners, and the use of Doppler EUS may be the topics of future research in this area. Nevertheless, more "objective" methods such as spiral CT or MRI could possibly provide a better three-dimensional visualization of the tumors and their relation to the surrounding vessels. Future studies will show which techniques are superior in the locoregional staging of pancreatic cancer.

## LOCALIZATION OF PANCREATIC ENDOCRINE TUMORS

Like other imaging tests, EUS can localize a tumor within the pancreas (or in other locations), but it should be performed only when the diagnosis of a tumor is firmly established or at least strongly suspected on the basis of clinical signs and symptoms and specific laboratory tests.

The typical aspect of a pancreatic endocrine tumor is a homogenous, echo-poor, and well-demarcated lesion surrounded by normal pancreatic tissue (52). An echo-free halo around the tumor or central echo-rich spots have also been described by some authors (19). Isoechoic or hyperechoic tumors have rarely been reported, as has an inhomogeneous echo-pattern with central echo-poor, echo-free, or cystic lesions, especially in large tumors. The smallest tumors localized were about 5 mm, but larger lesions have been missed on EUS.

Duodenal wall tumors and lymph node metastases are similar in appearance to submucosal tumors localized in the submucosal layer (echo-rich, homogenous, well defined) and to lymph nodes with malignant neoplasia. Every pancreatic endocrine tumor, especially gastrinomas, requires staging, looking for infiltration into adjacent organs or vessels and for lymph node metastases. Screening the duodenum for small duodenal gastrinomas *not* previously detected on careful upper GI endoscopy (which should be performed with forward- and side-viewing endoscopes) is difficult and time consuming, and EUS results have not been impressive (53). Pitfalls consist of pedunculated tumors adjacent to the pancreas (52, 54, 55) and misinterpretation of adjacent lymph nodes as endocrine tumors (52, 56).

**TABLE 9.11. Results of Endoscopic Ultrasonography (EUS) Compared with Ultrasound (US), Computed Tomography (CT), Angiography (ANG), and Magnetic Resonance Imaging (MRI) in Predicting Involvement of the Portal Venous System**

| | | Accuracy (%) of | | | | | |
|---|---|---|---|---|---|---|---|
| Author | n | EUS | US | CT | ANG | MRI | Ref |
| Sugiyama et al. 1988 | 5 | 100 | 60 | 20 | 100 | — | (31) |
| Yasuda et al. 1988 | 37 | 81 | — | — | — | — | (45) |
| Amouyal et al. 1989 | 5 | 80 | 40 | 80 | — | — | (51) |
| Snady et al. 1990 | 30 | 97 | — | 53 | 80 | — | (78) |
| Rösch et al. 1992[a] | 40 | 95 | 55 | 73 | 85 | — | (47) |
| Palazzo et al. 1993 | 38 | 87 | 47 | 75 | — | — | (22) |
| Giovannini et al. 1994[b] | 25 | 88 | 19 | 76 | — | — | (39) |
| Müller et al. 1994 | 16 | 88 | — | 88 | — | 63 | (35) |
| Rösch et al. 1995[c] | 35 | 66 | — | — | — | — | (46) |
| All cases | | 85%<br>n = 231 | 49%<br>n = 113 | 69%<br>n = 159 | 83%<br>n = 75 | 63%<br>n = 16 | |

[a]Pancreatic (n = 28) and ampullary cancer (n = 12) included.
[b]Use of linear-type echoendoscope.
[c]Only patients with pancreatic head cancer included; completely blind analysis of videotypes.

**TABLE 9.13. Literature Results in Localizing Pancreatic Endocrine Tumors by EUS**

| First Author | n[a] | Tumors[b] | Sensitivity of EUS (%) |
|---|---|---|---|
| Dancygier (57) | 3 | INS, GLU | 67 |
| Hayashi (19) | 4 | Islet cell tu | 100 |
| Lux (58) | 6 | INS, GAS | 100 |
| Lightdale (59) | 7 | INS, GAS, VIP, inactive tu | 86 |
| Rösch (60) | 9 | INS, GAS, GLU | 89 |
| Thompson (55) | 10 | INS, GAS | 70 |
| Yamada (61) | 13 | Islet cell tu | 100 |
| Schumacher (56) | 14 | INS | 57[c] |
| Ruszniewski (53) | 15 | GAS | 86 |
| Glover (62) | 16 | INS, GAS, GLU, VIP, inactive tu | 79 |
| Ruszniewski (63) | 19 | INS | 89 |
| Palazzo (64) | 23 | INS, GAS, VIP, GLU, carcinoid tu somatostatinoma | 91 |
| Zimmer (65) | 25 | INS, GAS | 88 |
| Bansal (54)[d] | 25 | INS, GAS | 80 |
| Rösch (52) | 39 | INS, GAS, GLU, Somatostatinoma | 82 |

[a]The total number of all cases cannot be given since there is partial overlap between studies, especially multicenter studies.
[b]INS, insulinoma; GAS, gastrinoma; GLU, glucagonoma; VIP, vipoma; tu, tumor.
[c]Sensitivity was better in the head (83%) than in the tail (37%).
[d]Randomized comparison between radial and linear instruments.

An overview of the results in the literature is given in Table 9.13 (19, 52–65); case reports are not included (32, 66–70). A high accuracy for EUS and superiority over other tests, at least for tumors located in the pancreas, are demonstrated (Table 9.14). The methodology of the imaging tests, especially CT, is not always clear from these studies, and it is therefore likely that more modern CT equipment with high-dose intravenous or intraarterial contrast (CT angiography) or spiral CT may prove better. However, the superiority of EUS over CT has been consistently reported, even in the most recent studies. Radial and linear echoendoscopes do not seem to differ in the ability to localize pancreatic endocrine tumors (54). EUS was also shown to be very accurate (82%) in CT- and US-negative patients, and in a subgroup of these series, EUS results were considerably superior to angiography (82 vs. 27%) (52). EUS was also superior to MRI in a report from 1994, and compared with somatostatin receptor scintigraphy, EUS was superior in insulinomas but equal in gastrinomas. One recent study, however, reported less impressive results for tumor localization, with distinct deficiencies in the pancreatic tail (56).

**TABLE 9.14. Comparison of EUS with Ultrasonography (US), Computed Tomography (CT), Magnetic resonance imaging (MRI), and Somatostatin Receptor Scintigraphy (SRS) in Localizing Pancreatic Endocrine Tumors**

| | EUS | US | CT | MRI | SRS |
|---|---|---|---|---|---|
| Sensitivity | 84% | 30% | 28% | 24% | 52% |
| No. of patients[a] | 176 | 111 | 126 | 25 | 25 |

Data from (53–56, 59–65).
[a]Not enough patients underwent angiography to be included.

## SUMMARY

EUS is the best single test available for delineating both the pancreatic duct and discrete abnormalities in the pancreatic parenchyma. This leads to an accurate diagnosis of small tumors (exocrine and endocrine) and to recognition of subtle parenchymal abnormalities, the specificity of which is not fully known. As with most sensitive imaging procedures, the clinical impact of EUS has not yet been sufficiently elucidated. EUS appears to have less impact on the differential diagnosis of pancreatic masses, and its clinical value in locoregional staging in comparison with other modern imaging methods is still uncertain. Further technical development may ultimately lead to better three-dimensional visualization of the pancreas and surrounding large vessels; the use of ultrasonic miniprobes to be introduced into the common bile and/or pancreatic duct is still experimental and provides a low penetration depth of ultrasonic scanning (71). Further progress is to be expected.

## REFERENCES

1. Rösch T, Classen M. Gastroenterologic endosonography. Stuttgart: Thieme, 1992.
2. Wiersema MJ, Wiersema LM. Endosonography of the pancreas: normal variation versus changes of early chronic pancreatitis. Gastrointest Endosc Clin North Am 1995;5:487–496.
3. Buscail L. Endoscopic ultrasonography in pancreatobiliary disease using radial instruments. Gastrointest Endosc Clin North Am 1995;5:781–788.
4. Edmundowicz SA, Neidich RL, Aliperti G, Middleton WD. A prospective comparison of endoscopic ultrasonography (EUS), ERCP and standard abdominal ultrasonography (US) for the detection of choledocholithiasis prior to laparoscopic cholecystectomy (LC) (Abstract). Gastrointest Endosc 1994;40:P63.
5. Amouyal P, Amouyal G, Levy P, Tuzet S, Palazzo L, et al. Diagnosis of choledocholithiasis by endoscopic ultrasonography. Gastroenterology 1994;106:1062–1067.
6. Shim CS, Joo JH, Park CW, Kim YS, Lee JS, et al. Effectiveness of endoscopic ultrasonography in the diagnosis of choledocholithiasis prior to laparoscopic cholecystectomy. Endoscopy 1995; 27:428–432.
7. Denis BJ, Bas V, Goudot C, Frederic M, Bigard MA, Gaucher P. Accuracy of endoscopic ultrasonography (EUS) for diagnosis of common bile duct stones (CBDS) (Abstract). Gastroenterology 1993;104:A358.
8. Palazzo L, Girollet PP, Salmeron M, Roseau G, Silvain C, et al. Is endoscopic ultrasonography (EUS) accurate for diagnosis of common bile duct stones (CBDS)—comparison with ERCP and surgical exploration (Abstract). Gastrointest Endosc 1992;38: A290.
9. Salmeron M, Simon JF, Houdart R, Lemann M, Johanet H. Endoscopic ultrasonography versus invasive methods for the diagnosis of common bile duct stones (Abstract). Gastroenterology 1994;106:A357.
10. Keriven O, Group for the Evaluation of Digestive Echoendoscopy. Prospective study of the accuracy of echoendoscopy for the diagnosis of bile duct stones (Abstract). Gastrointest Endosc 1994;40:P65.
11. Canto M, Chak A, Sivak MV, Blades E, Stellato T. Endoscopic ultrasonography (EUS) versus cholangiography for diagnosing extrahepatic biliary stones: a prospective, blinded study in pre- and post-cholecystectomy patients (Abstract). Gastrointest Endosc 1995;41:391.
12. Canto M, Chak A, Sivak MV. Clinical and sonographic predictors of choledocholithiasis in pre- and post-cholecstectomy patients (Abstract). Gastroenterology 1995;108:A7.
13. Prat F, Amouyal G, Amouyal P, Pelletier G, Fritsch J, et al. Prospective controlled study of endoscopic ultrasonography (EUS) and retrograde cholangiography (ERC) in patients with suspected common bile duct lithiasis (CBDL) (Abstract). Gastrointest Endosc 1995;41:411.
14. Dancygier H. Endoscopic ultrasonography in chronic pancreatitis. Gastrointest Endosc Clin North Am 1995;5:795–804.

15. Binmoeller KF, Soehendra N. Endoscopic ultrasonography in the diagnosis and treatment of pancreatic pseudocysts. Gastrointest Endosc Clin North Am 1995;5:805–816.
16. Napoleon B, Pujol L, Roseau G, Keriven O, Ponchon T, et al. Pancreatic cysts: potential usefulness of endoscopic ultrasonography (EUS) for their management (Abstract). Gastrointest Endosc 1993;39:A326.
17. Yasuda K, Mukai H, Fujimoto S, Nakajima M, Kawai K. The diagnosis of pancreatic cancer by endoscopic ultrasonography. Gastrointest Endosc 1988;34:1–8.
18. Rösch T, Lorenz R, Braig C, Feuerbach S, Siewert JR, et al. Endoscopic ultrasound in pancreatic tumor diagnosis. Gastrointest Endosc 1991;37:347–352.
19. Hayashi Y, Nakazawa S, Kimoto E, Naito Y, Morita K. Clinicopathological analysis of endoscopic ultrasonograms in pancreatic mass lesions. Endoscopy 1989;21:121–125.
20. Wiersema MJ, Chak A, Hawes RH, Kopecky KK. Evaluation of endosonography in distinguishing malignant from inflammatory pancreatic masses (Abstract). Gastrointest Endosc 1993;39:A336.
21. Forsmark CE, Albert CA, Lambiase L, Vogel SB, Torres GM, et al. Diagnostic tests for pancreatic cancer (Abstract). Gastrointest Endosc 1993;39:A314.
22. Palazzo L, Roseau G, Gayet B, Vilgrain V, Belghiti J, et al. Endoscopic ultrasonography in the diagnosis and staging of pancreatic adenocarcinoma. Results of a prospective study with comparison to ultrasonography and CT scan. Endoscopy 1993; 25:143–150.
23. Rösch T, Neuhaus H, Gmeinwieser J, Zapilko R, Siewert JR, Classen M. Role of endoscopic ultrasonography in the evaluation of patients with suspected pancreatic disease (Abstract). Gastroenterology 1993;104:A21.
24. Rösch T, Roder JR, Decassian T, Dittler HJ, Born P, et al. Indeterminate pancreatic tumors: still a problem even with modern diagnostic methods (Abstract). Endoscopy, in press.
25. Giovannini M, Seitz JF, Monges G, Rabbia I, Perrier H. Fine-needle aspiration biopsy guided by endoscopic ultrasonography. Results in 141 patients. Endoscopy 1995;27:171–177.
26. Wiersema MJ, Kochman ML, Cramer HM, Tao LC, Wiersema LM. Endosonography-guided real-time fine-needle aspiration biopsy. Gastrointest Endosc 1994;40:700–707.
27. Bhutani M, Hoffman B, van Velse A, Sanders-Cliette A, Hawes R. Endoscopic ultrasound (EUS) guided fine needle aspiration (FNA) of malignant pancreatic lesions: accuracy, safety and clinical utility (Abstract). Gastrointest Endosc 1995;41:298.
28. Chang K, Nguyen P, Durbin T, Katz K, Erickson R, et al. Endoscopic ultrasound (EUS) guided fine needle aspiration (FNA) in the diagnosis and staging of pancreatic carcinoma (Abstract). Gastrointest Endosc 1994;40:P62.
29. Warshaw AL. Implications of peritoneal cytology for staging of early pancreatic cancer. Am J Surg 1991;161:26–30.
30. Ikeda M, Fujino MA, Morozumi A, Sano S, Kinose T, et al. Diagnosis of small pancreatic tumor by endoscopic ultrasonography (Abstract). Gastroenterology 1989;96:225.
31. Sugiyama S, Asada M, Fujita R, Sugata F. Endoscopic ultrasonography for the diagnosis of pancreas carcinoma (Abstract). Endoscopy 1988;20:94.
32. Fukuda M, Nakano Y, Saito K, Hirata K, Terada S, Urushizaki I. Endoscopic ultrasonography in the diagnosis of pancreatic carcinoma. Scand J Gastroenterol 1984;19(suppl 94):65–76.
33. Kaufman AR, Sivak MV. Endoscopic ultrasonography in the differential diagnosis of pancreatic disease. Gastrointest Endosc 1989;35:214–219.
34. Keriven-Souquet O, Souquet JC, Ponchon T, Napoleon B, Pujol B. Endoscopic ultrasound for the diagnosis of pancreatic cancer: prospective study in 52 patients with non informative abdominal ultrasound (Abstract). Gastrointest Endosc 1995;41:425.
35. Muller MF, Meyenberger C, Bertschinger P, Schaer R, Marincek B. Pancreatic tumors: evaluation with endoscopic US, CT, and MR imaging. Radiology 1994;190:745–751.
36. Kallimanis G, Axiotis E, Papantoniou P, Kostalou E, Voudouris G, Kalantzis N. EUS, ERCP, US, CT in the diagnosis of pancreatic cancer (Abstract). Endoscopy 1992;24:656.
37. Tio TL, Sie LH, Tytgat GNJ. Endosonography and cytology in diagnosing and staging pancreatic body and tail carcinoma. Dig Dis Sci 1993;38:59–64.
38. Akahoshi K, Chijiiwa Y, Nakano I, Nawata H, Ogawa Y, et al. Role of endosonography in diagnosis and staging of pancreatic cancer. Endoscopy, in press.
39. Giovannini M, Seitz JF. Endoscopic ultrasonography with a linear type echoendoscope in the evaluation of 94 patients with pancreatobiliary disease. Endoscopy 1994;26:579–585.
40. Valette PJ, Guibal AL, Jeriven O, Souquet JC, Ternamian A, et al. "Second look" transabdominal ultrasound vs. echoendoscopy for biliopancreatic explorations: a prospective comparative study of 76 patients (Abstract). Endoscopy 1994;26:444.
41. Grimm H, Maydeo A, Soehendra N. Endoluminal ultrasound for the diagnosis and staging of pancreatic cancer. Bailliere's Clin Gastroenterol 1990;4:869–887.
42. Tio TL, Tytgat GNJ, Cikot RJLM, Houthoff HJ, Sars PRA. Ampullopancreatic carcinoma: preoperative TNM classification with endosonography. Radiology 1990;175:455–461.
43. Kallimanis G, Axiotis E, Papantoniou P, Kytridis G, Gabriel P, Kalantzis N. Endoscopic ultrasonography in preoperative TNM classification of pancreatic cancer (Abstract). Endoscopy 1992; 24:656.
44. Rösch T, Dittler HJ, Lorenz R, Braig C, Gain T, et al. Endosonographisches Staging des Pankreaskarzinoms. Dtsch Med Wochenschr 1992;117:563–569.
45. Yasuda K, Mukai H, Nakajima M, Kawai K. Staging of pancreatic carcinoma by endoscopic ultrasonography. Endoscopy 1993;25: 151–155.
46. Rösch T, Dittler HJ, Strobel K, Decassian T, Bautz W, et al. Local staging of pancreatic head cancer by endoscopic ultrasonography: a re-evaluation using blind videotape assessment (Abstract). Endoscopy 1995;27:S48.
47. Rösch T, Braig C, Gain T, Feuerbach S, Siewert JR, et al. Staging of pancreatic and ampullary carcinoma by endoscopic ultrasonography. Gastroenterology 1992;102:188–199.
48. Snady H, Bruckner H, Siegel J, Cooperman A, Neff R, Kiefer L. Endoscopic ultrasonographic criteria of vascular invasion by potentially resectable pancreatic tumors. Gastrointest Endosc 1994;40:326–333.
49. Brugge WR, Lee MJ, Warshaw AL. Endoscopic ultrasonography criteria for diagnosing vascular invasion by pancreatic masses (Abstract). Endoscopy 1994;26:825.
50. Brugge WR. Pancreatic cancer staging: endoscopic ultrasonography criteria for vascular invasion. Gastrointest Endosc Clin North Am 1995;5:741–754.
51. Amouyal P, Amouyal G, Mompoint D, Gayet B, Palazzo L, et al. Endosonography: promising method for diagnosis of extrahepatic cholestasis. Lancet 1989;II:1195–1198.
52. Rösch T, Lightdale CJ, Botet JF, Boyce GA, Sivak MV, et al. Endosonograpic localization of pancreatic endocrine tumors. N Engl J Med 1992;326:1721–1726.
53. Ruszniewski P, Amouyal P, Amouyal G, Cadiot G, Mignon M, Bernades P. Diagnostic value of endoscopic ultrasonography (EUS) for the localisation of gastrinomas (Abstract). Gastroenterology 1993;104:A331.
54. Bansal R, Nostrant TT, Elta GH, Bude R, Thompson N, Scheiman JM. Comparison of radial and sector array endoscopic endoscopic ultrasound (EUS) for localization of pancreatic endocrine tumors (PET) (Abstract). Gastrointest Endosc 1995;41:296.
55. Thompson NW, Czako PF, Fritts LL, Bude R, Bansal R, et al. Role of endoscopic ultrasonography in the localization of insulinomas and gastrinomas. Surgery 1994;116:1131–1138.
56. Schumacher B, Lübke HJ, Frieling T, Strohmeyer G, Starke AAR. Prospective detection of insulinomas by endoscopic ultrasonography. Endoscopy, in press.
57. Dancygier H, Classen M. Endosonographic diagnosis of benign pancreatic and biliary lesions. Scand J Gastroenterol 1986; 21(suppl 123):119–122.
58. Lux G, Heyder N. Endoscopic ultrasonography of the pancreas. Technical aspects. Scand J Gastroenterol 1986;21(suppl 123): 112–118.
59. Lightdale CJ, Botet JF, Woodruff JM, Brennan MF. Localization of endocrine tumors of the pancreas with endoscopic ultrasound. Cancer 1991;68:1815–1820.
60. Rösch T, Lorenz R, Braig C, Siewert JR, Classen M. Preoperative localization of endocrine tumors of the pancreas: endoscopic ultrasound is superior to transabdominal sonography and com-

puted tomography (Abstract). Gastrointest Endosc 1990;36: 199–200.

61. Yamada M, Komoto E, Naito Y, Tsukamoto Y, Mitake M. Endoscopic ultrasonography in the diagnosis of pancreatic islet cell tumors. J Ultrasound Med 1991;23:85–87.
62. Glover JR, Shover PJ, Lees WR. Endoscopic ultrasound for localisation of islet cell tumours. Gut 1992;33:108–110.
63. Ruszniewski P, Amouyal P, Amouyal G, Hautecouverture M, Grimaldi A, et al. Endoscopic ultrasonography (EUS) in the localization of insulinomas: results of a multicentre prospective study (Abstract). Gastroenterology 1993;104:A332.
64. Palazzo L, Roseau G, Salmeron M. Endoscopic ultrasonography in the preoperative localization of pancreatic endocrine tumors. Endoscopy 1992;24:350–353.
65. Zimmer T, Ziegler K, Bader M, Fett U, Hamm B, et al. Localisation of neuroendocrine tumours of the upper gastrointestinal tract. Gut 1994;35:471–475.
66. Yasuda K, Nakajima M, Mukai H, Yoshida S, Kawai K. The detection of small pancreatic cancers by endoscopic ultrasonography. In: Dancygier H, Classen M, eds. 5th International Symposium on Endoscopic Ultrasonography. Munich: Demeter Verlag (Z Gastroenterol suppl), 1989:86–91.
67. Bolondi L, Li Bassi S, Gaiani S, Campione O, Marrano D, Barbara L. Diagnosis of islet cell tumor by means of endoscopic ultrasonography. J Clin Gastroenterol 1990;12:218–221.
68. Heyder N. Localization of an insulinoma by ultrasonic endoscopy (Letter). N Engl J Med 1985;312:860–861.
69. Casanova C, Altdorfer J, Münch R, Meyenberger C, Wirth HP, et al. Endosonographie—ein Fortschritt in der Diagnostik endokriner Pankreastumoren. Schweiz Med Wochenschr 1992;81: 815–818.
70. Kobayashi M, Araki K, Ogata T. Usefulness of endoscopic ultrasonography for the localization of insulinomas (Letter). Surgery 1993;113:478.
71. Yasuda K. Development and clinical use of ultrasonic probes. Endoscopy 1994;26:816–817.
72. Nattermann C, Goldschmidt AJW, Dancygier H. Endosonography in chronic pancreatitis—a comparison between endoscopic retrograde pancreatography and endoscopic ultrasonography. Endoscopy 1993;25:565–570.
73. Wiersema MJ, Hawes RH, Lehman GA, Kochman ML, Sherman S, Kopecky KK. Prospective evaluation of endoscopic ultrasonography and endoscopic retrograde cholangiopancreatography in patients with chronic abdominal pain of suspected pancreatic origin. Endoscopy 1993;25:555–564.
74. Gress F, Savides T, Zaidi S, Sherman S, Madura J, et al. Endoscopic ultrasound (EUS) staging correlates with survival in patients with pancreatic cancer (PCa) (Abstract). Gastrointest Endosc 1995; 41:423.
75. Gress F, Ikenberry S, Zaidi S, Savides T, Sherman S, et al. A prospective randomized comparison of radial (Olympus UM-20) and linear array (Pentax FG 32UA) scanning echoendoscopes (EE) in staging pancreatic cancer (PCa) (Abstract). Gastrointest Endosc 1995;41:304.
76. Kadish SL, Kochman ML, Rosato EF, Morris JB, Smith D, Ginsberg GG. Endosonography. The modality of choice for T staging and vascular involvement in patients with pancreatic carcinoma (Abstract)? Gastroenterology 1995;108:A486.
77. Kazi S, Gunasekaran TS, Berman J, Kraut J. Gastric mucosal injury in children from inflatable balloon type G-tube (Abstract). Gastrointest Endosc 1995;41:339.
78. Snady H, Cooperman A, Siegel JH. Assessment of vascular involvement by pancreatic disease–a comparison of endoscopic ultrasonography to computerized tomography and angiography (Abstract). Gastrointest Endosc 1990;36:197.
79. Kobayashi G, Fujita N, Noda Y, Kimura K, Watanabe H, et al. The evaluation of portal venous invasion of pancreatic cancer by endoscopic ultrasonography. Jpn J Gastroenterol 1993;90:49–56.

# 10

# *Percutaneous Needle Biopsy*

Ingemar Ihse and Sigmund Dawiskiba

In spite of the introduction of a variety of diagnostic methods such as endoscopic retrograde cholangiopancreatography (ERCP), computerized tomography (CT), ultrasonography (US), and magnetic resonance imaging (MRI) during the last decades, the diagnosis of pancreatic diseases still possesses well-known difficulties. This is in part due to the uncertainty of these imaging methods in discriminating between neoplastic and inflammatory diseases. For further nonoperative characterization and classification, percutaneous biopsy was introduced in the beginning of the 1970s. This chapter discusses to what extent percutaneous guided needle biopsy for cytologic or histologic examination has reached expectations.

## INDICATIONS

The indications for percutaneous fine-needle aspiration cytology (FNAC) have varied with time, and at many centers the method has never gained full acceptance, perhaps due mainly to a lack of trained cytologists. In Scandinavia, it was practiced for many years and in many places in almost all patients with suspicion of a pancreatic lesion at imaging (1). However, there has been a swing toward a more selective policy in Scandinavia (2) as well as in other countries (3, 4). One reason for this changed attitude is the fairly high frequency of false-negative results. Another reason is that pancreaticoduodenectomy without microscopic verification of the cancer diagnosis currently is legitimate in centers with a documented low hospital mortality.

At present, thus, percutaneous cytodiagnosis is restricted to patients with suspected pancreatic cancer who are not candidates for surgery because of advanced disease, high age, and/or bad general condition. Suspected hepatic metastases as noted before initial therapy or as recurrent lesions after therapy provide a frequent indication for FNAC. Verification of the malignant diagnosis in these cases facilitates a sincere and trustful discussion with the patient on the prognosis and course of the disease, and finding, for example, an endocrine tumor or a non-Hodgkin's lymphoma may completely alter the clinical management. Another indication for FNAC refers to patients who are candidates for attempted curative surgery with planned preoperative radiation and chemotherapy (chemoradiation), as such treatment needs nonoperative histologic tumor verification. Chemoradiation is, however, currently done in only a few centers (5), and its future role is not settled.

The indications for needle core biopsy of the pancreas are about the same as those described above for cytologic investigations. Logically, core biopsy specimens should provide more accurate information about tissue characteristics. This may be of particular importance in the differential diagnosis between well-differentiated tumors and chronic pancreatitis, which sometimes is a difficult clinical decision.

## FINE-NEEDLE ASPIRATION CYTOLOGY (FNAC)

FNAC means in a strict sense a morphologic diagnosis on cellular material achieved by the needling and aspiration of a tumorous lesion by needles not thicker than 0.7 mm (≤22 gauge). The first study on percutaneous cytodiagnosis of the pancreas was published in 1972 and contained only a few patients (6). Since then, several series have been reported, and they form the basis for the following discussion.

## TECHNIQUE

Most frequently, US or CT is used for visualization of lesions of the pancreas. Under local anesthesia, a 0.7-mm (22-gauge) thin needle with stylet and clear plastic hub is advanced toward the target under fluoroscopic control. A thin, long needle produces higher capillary aspiration and decreases the risk of puncture bleeding or hematoma. It simultaneously increases the chance of obtaining more cellular material. We do not recommend the use of thicker needles because of the greater risk of unwanted blood in the aspirate, which interferes with making slides for light microscopy. Spinal needles of Westcott (22 gauge) (Becton Dickinson, Stockholm, Sweden), notched or unnotched, 12–18 cm in length, with a clear plastic hub, are best-suited for most tumors in the pancreas. Notched needles are more useful in compact, fibrotic tumor tissues. Use of the CAMECO Syringe Pistol (Fibre Medical, Vellinge, Sweden) for 10-mL disposable syringes facilitates one-hand manipulation (Fig. 10.1).

When the lesion is entered with the needle, the stylet is removed, the needle is attached to the syringe with the CAMECO handle, and the plunger of the syringe is retracted for negative pressure. The needle is moved back and forth a few times within the tumor mass. When material is observed to come up into the needle's clear plastic hub, the plunger is released, while the needle is still within the tumor. Otherwise, the aspirated material, with some air, disappears into the barrel of the syringe, and cannot be used because it quickly becomes air dried. The needle is withdrawn and detached from the syringe. The syringe is filled with air and reattached to the needle.

The bevel of the needle is directed toward the upper end of a clean glass slide, and its contents are squirted onto the slide with the needle close to the slide. The material is expelled on two to four glass slides, spread with another glass slide placed over it, and then the two slides are pulled apart (Fig. 10.2, *A* and *B*). Half of the slides are air dried, for May-Grünwald-Giemsa staining, and the others are ethanol fixed for staining with hematoxylin-erythrosin or Papanicolaou stain. For quick-staining hematoxylin, eosin-Harris staining is used. Wet fixation in 95% ethanol requires immediate fixation while the samples are still wet. This

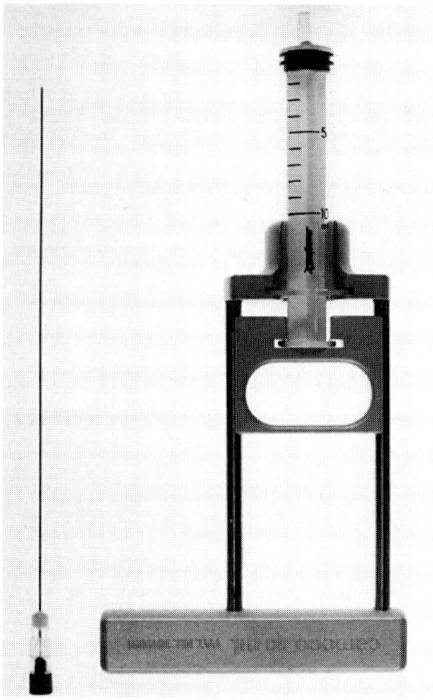

**FIG. 10.1.** The CAMECO syringe pistol for 10-mL disposable syringes. Spinal needle of Becton Dickinson, 18 cm in length and 0.7 mm outer diameter, with unnotched needle stylet.

is necessary to preserve the cellular features needed for microscopic interpretation, because even minimal air drying of the sample alters cellular features. Cells become swollen and lose details important for correct microscopic diagnosis.

Benign or normal cells with fixation artifacts can mimic malignant cells on light microscopy (Fig. 10.3*B*). During smearing of the sample on the slide, one has to apply very little pressure with the hand. Note that cells from malignant tumors are often very vulnerable to pressure. Hard smearing can completely destroy cytologic material (Fig. 10.3*D*) and make interpretation impossible. Even normal cells from lymph nodes and bone marrow are very vulnerable to pressure; cells from gastrointestinal epithelium, breast, thyroid, pancreas, and prostate are much more resistant. One has to strive to attain properly smeared, thin cell spreadings of monolayer specimens (Fig. 10.3*A*). Sometimes different errors can be seen together on the same slide; for example, the combination of hard smearing and late wet fixation in 95% ethanol. Thus, initial macroscopic examination can help one decide whether the smears are satisfactory or unsatisfactory.

If the volume of the specimen seems too great for the slide, one can tilt the slide and use absorbent tissue to remove the blood that flows to the low side. Cystic fluid is collected and enriched with centrifugation or a filter technique.

Cytologic specimens may also be used for immunocytologic staining, electron microscopy, chromosomal cytogenetic investigations, DNA measurements by means of flow cytometry or image cytometry, and microbiologic cultures. Such investigations, however, require special preparation of the smears, which is not described in detail in this chapter.

## Results

The reported sensitivity of FNAC in diagnosing pancreatic carcinoma varies between 60 and 97% (Table 10.1). Although the continuing development of available noninvasive imaging tests has improved their ability to recognize and delineate the anatomic location of pancreatic masses, there does not seem to have been any concomitant increase in the sensitivity of percutaneous cytodiagnosis. The specificity of the method is very high, reaching 100% in most series (Table 10.1). However, false-positive results do occur although rarely (13–15). We have had one false-positive finding in some 400 patients investigated (2). A risk of a false-positive diagnosis may exist in advanced chronic pancreatitis with atypical cell clusters of small ducts in the specimen, especially if the cytologist is less experienced.

A definite drawback with the method is the occurrence of false-negative results, which may be as common as one in four (11). These are due to sampling error and difficulties with the technical preparation, problems that can be counteracted in accordance with the discussion above on technique. Another cause of false-negative results is poor interpretation; the skill of the observer is of importance (1, 8, 16). Trained observers possess similar diagnostic abilities, as reflected by the small differences in interobserver kappa values in a recent study (16). Difficulties in achieving better results seem to be related more to the quality of the cytologic specimen than to the experience of the cytologist (16). Against the above backdrop, it may be concluded that percutaneous fine-needle aspiration biopsy is trustworthy in confirming the presence of a pancreatic malignancy but unreliable in excluding such a disorder. Some claim that cytologic investigation provides less accurate information about cell type and tissue characteristics than histology (17). Generally, however, a trained cytologist examining a specimen

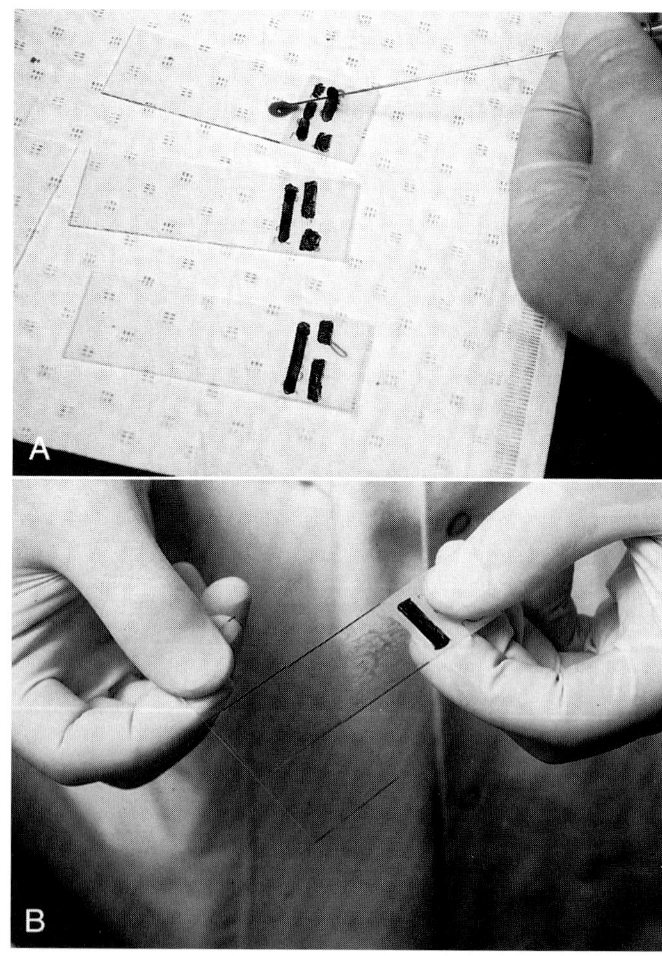

**FIG. 10.2.** The smearing technique. **A.** The needle contents are squirted onto the slide with the needle close to the slide. **B.** The second slide is placed over the first, and the two are pulled apart. See color insert.

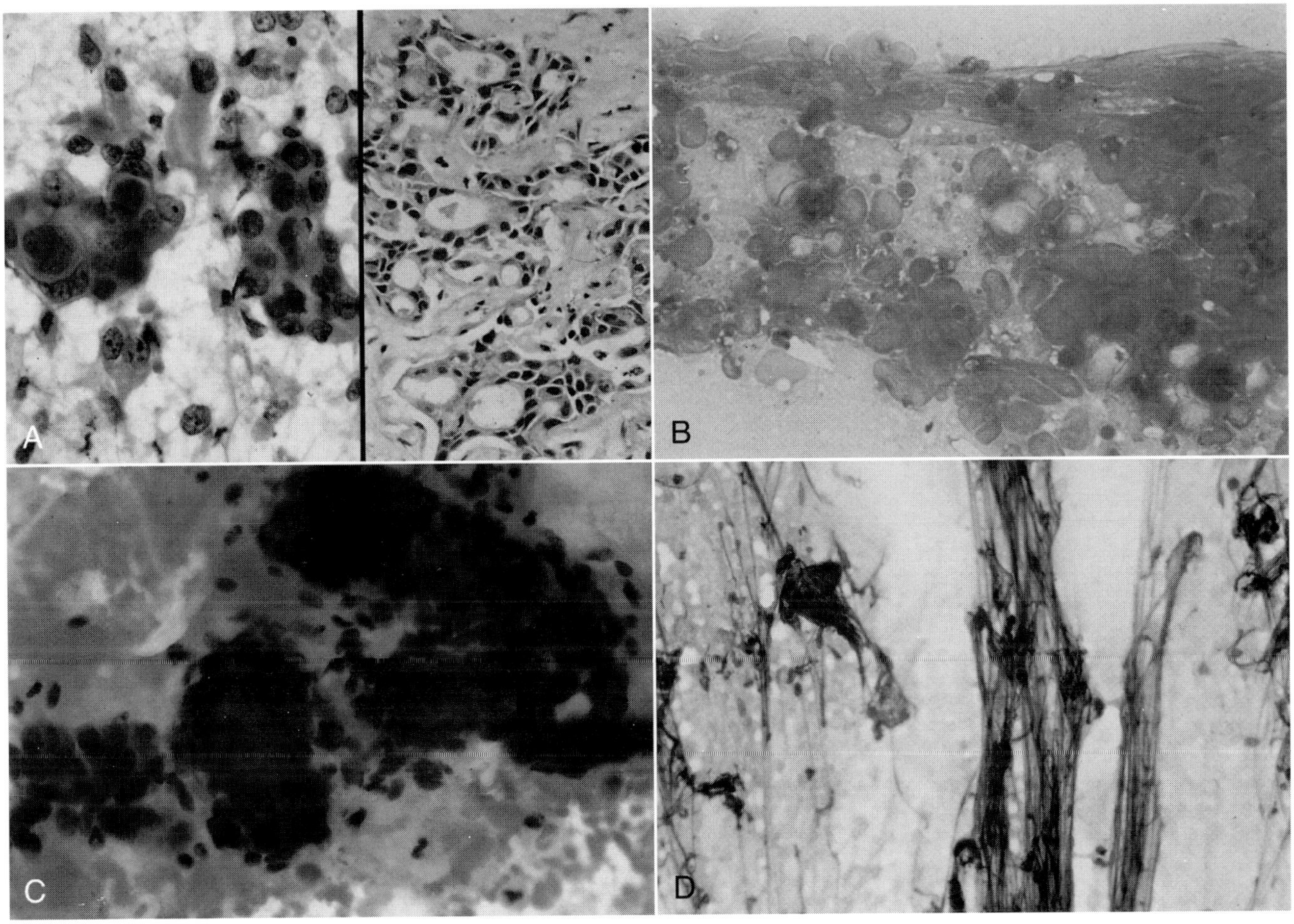


**FIG. 10.3.** **A.** Exocrine, poorly differentiated, pancreatic duct cancer cell groups of well-smeared and well-fixed (ethanol) material. Note the distinct nuclear border, nucleoli, and varying amount of cytoplasm in cancer cells with severe atypia *(left)*, and corresponding well-done needle core biopsy of the same tumor with densely packed atypical tubular malignant structures in a slight fibrotic stroma *(right)*. **B.** Ethanol fixation artifacts. Note the nonsharp cell borders and mostly indistinct nuclear morphology. The cells often become swollen, and benign or normal cells can mimic malignant cells. **C.** Thick smearing. Too much material on one glass slide leads to multilayer cell distribution, which can make the microscopic diagnosis impossible. **D.** Hard smearing. The cytologic material is completely destroyed, which makes diagnostic interpretation impossible. *A-D*, hematoxylin, erythrosin; *A (right)*, 5 μm section. *A, C, D*, ×80; *B*, ×120. See color insert.

of good quality can reliably distinguish between exocrine and endocrine tumors, and ductal carcinoma and benign pancreatic disorders (Fig. 10.4), respectively. Sometimes it may be difficult to differentiate epithelial atypia due to chronic pancreatitis and well-differentiated neoplasms, respectively (Fig. 10.4). Papillary-cystic neoplasms (see Chapter 73, Papillary Cystic and Solid Tumors) are characteristic on cytologic smears, making the diagnosis possible on cytologic aspirates only (Fig. 10.5).

## Complications

A recent review of 10,766 percutaneous fine-needle aspirations of intraabdominal masses demonstrated a mortality rate of 0.018% (18). In another review, 11,700 similar punctures were reported to have a mortality of 0.008%, with major complications registered in 0.05% (19). In a collective series of 15,777 patients, the corresponding figures were 0.006% and 0.16%, respectively (20). Of 12 mortalities reported in the literature, 3 followed pancreatic punctures (18, 21). In one study of 269

**TABLE 10.1. Literature Review of Intraoperative Fine-Needle Aspiration Cytology of the Pancreas**

| Authors | Patients *(N)* | Cancer Patients *(N)* | Sensitivity (%) | Specificity (%) |
|---|---|---|---|---|
| Elsman et al. (7) | 32 | 27 | 78 | 100 |
| Evander et al. (1) | 88 | 52 | 60 | 100 |
| Hajdu et al. (8) | 126 | 68 | 97 | 100 |
| Kocjan et al. (9) | 62 | 41 | 86 | 100 |
| Lüning et al. (10) | 141 | 45 | 71 | 84 |
| Soudah et al. (11) | 316 | 58 | 76 | — |
| Sperti et al. (12) | 83 | 67 | 91 | 100 |

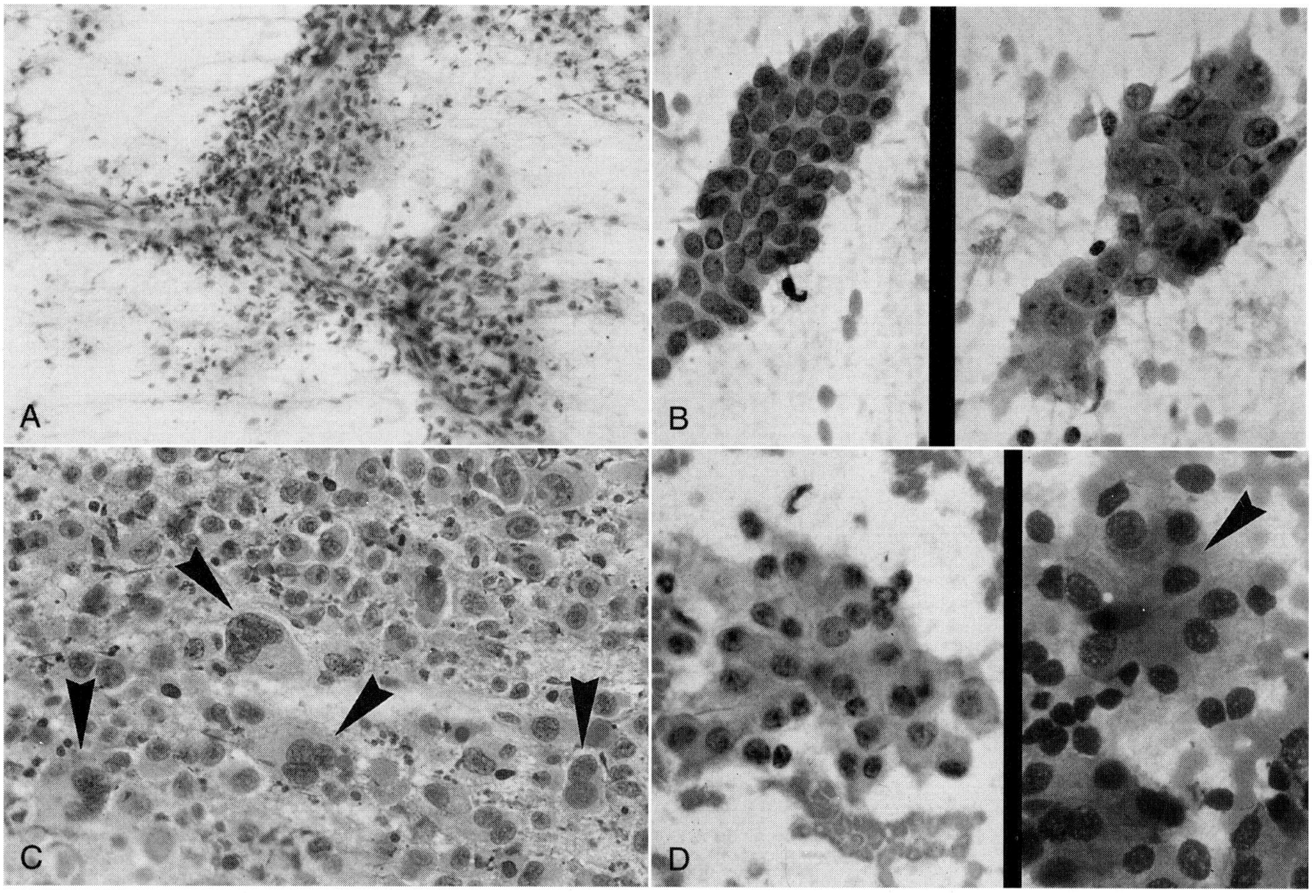


**FIG. 10.4.** Examples of fine-needle aspirates from different pancreatic lesions. **A.** Chronic pancreatitis. Aspirate of granulation tissue. Note network of capillaries surrounded by macrophages and inflammatory cells. **B.** Comparison of benign cohesive sheet of ductal pancreatic epithelium, of evenly spaced nuclei and well defined cytoplasm boundaries *(left)* with well-differentiated ductal pancreatic cancer of considerable nuclear crowding and overlapping *(right)*. **C.** Pleomorphic pancreatic carcinoma of the giant cell type. Bizarre, multinucleated giant cells *(arrow heads)* surrounded by mononuclear pleomorphic cancer cells. **D.** Islet cell tumor of the pancreas. Monolayer and sheets of polygonal cells often with eccentrically located nuclei. Note a rosette-like formation *(arrow head, right)*. *A, B, C, D,* hematoxylin, erythrosin; *D (right),* May-Grünwald-Giemsa. *A,* ×40; *B, C, D,* ×80. See color insert.

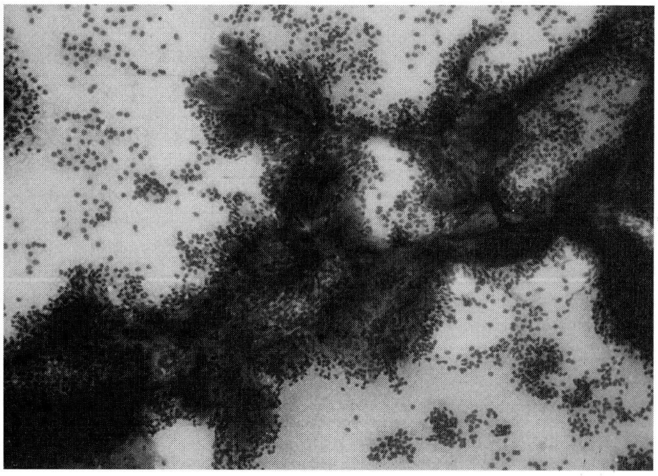

**FIG. 10.5.** Fine-needle aspirate from pancreatic papillary-cystic neoplasm. Fragment of tissue with branching capillaries and several layers of tumor cells covering clusters of amorphous mucous metachromatic material. Note solitary and clusters of oval monomorphic cells in delicate papillary formations. May-Grünwald-Giemsa, ×40. See color insert.

pancreatic punctures, major complications developed in 5 (22). Papers dealing exclusively with pancreatic examinations report without exception very low mortality and complication rates. Thus, the method is saddled with extremely few early complications. However, the risk of needle-tract seeding must not be ignored. Eight patients suffering this delayed complication have been reported (18, 23, 24).

## TISSUE CORE BIOPSY

Whereas percutaneous fine-needle aspiration for cytologic diagnosis of pancreatic diseases has been used for many years and the results from a great number of studies have been reported (see above), only a few descriptions exist of percutaneous histologic core needle biopsy for the same purposes. In the following section the current experience with this method is discussed.

### Technique

The investigation is generally done under ultrasound guidance using an 18- to 14-gauge (1.1–2.0 mm) cutting needle. Most commonly used is the Biopty-cut needle with an automatic spring-loaded sampling device (Bard Urological, Covington, GA). Release of the spring advances the central stylet, followed within a fraction of a second by the outer cutting sheath of the needle. Local anesthesia and a small skin incision are needed before puncture. The operator easily guides the needle exactly, as the device frees one hand for the ultrasound probe. The speed of the action yields clean edges on the specimen, with no crush artifacts. Depending on the macroscopic appearance of the biopsy material, one to three punctures are done. The specimens are routinely fixed in formalin and embedded individually in a paraffin block. They are generally stained with hematoxylin-erythrosin or, when required, with other histochemical and/or immunohistochemical methods.

### Results

Out of 142 pancreatic core biopsies, the sensitivity for malignancy was 91% (17). In another recent study, a correct diagnosis was obtained in 44 of the 47 patients (94%) with pancreatic cancer (25), and a Japanese series of 36 patients with pancreatic cancer and 11 with chronic pancreatitis showed conformity with the final diagnosis in 91% of the patients. In cases of pancreatic cancer with successful biopsy procedure the histologic type of carcinoma was confirmed in 91% of the tumors (26). Thus, it seems that the diagnostic accuracy of the method is high. Reported complications are discussed below.

### Complications

In the study comprising 142 patients referred to above, the only major complication was development of pancreatic ascites in one patient (17). Pain is reported as a rare side effect (25, 26), being registered in 2 of 47 investigated patients in one study (25). In the same series, hypotension due to vasovagal reaction occurred in two patients, and one had a transient rise in serum amylase. None of the patients had any signs of bleeding. Due to the differences in needle size if the puncture is done for cytologic or histologic investigation, the risk of complications can be expected to be higher with core biopsy. Still, there does not appear to be a linear increase in the number of complications with increasing needle size (25). As the Biopty-cut needle biopsy is rapid and performed during a single breath-holding, this technique is thought to further minimize the complication risk. Obviously, pancreatic core biopsy can be safely done. However, these data were collected from puncture of demarcated pancreatic masses. The low complication rate does not legitimize uncritical widening of the indications involving risk of puncture of normal pancreatic tissue, as we know from surgical practice that undue handling of a normal pancreas may lead to severe complications such as pancreatitis and fistulas.

### Comparison between Fine-Needle Aspiration Cytology and Core Biopsy

There are few comparisons reported between cytologic and histologic investigations, respectively, after percutaneous pancreatic aspiration or biopsy. In one study, 100 consecutive patients had both investigations, and the specimens were examined blindly by two trained observers (16). The predictive value of malignant diagnosis was 100% for both methods. The predictive value for benign disease was 25% for histologic specimens and 33% and 45%, respectively, for cytology. Consistent malignant diagnoses occurred more often with cytologic than with histologic specimens, and consistent diagnoses of insufficient material were more common with histologic specimens. If only one method is used, the authors recommended cytology because of its sensitivity and because it is cheaper and faster to process. It is further possible to do repeated aspirations for cytology from different areas of the lesion, which is not recommended when full-core biopsy is used.

## OTHER PERCUTANEOUS APPROACHES

Cytologic examination of peritoneal washings has been suggested as an adjunctive tool for staging pancreatic cancer (4). This recommendation was based on a study of 40 patients who had been judged as potentially resectable by CT. Malignant cells were found intraperitoneally in 30%, and their presence was more common in patients who had had percutaneous fine-needle aspiration of the pancreas. The authors concluded that FNAC promotes intraperitoneal spread of cancer cells, and there also seemed to be a correlation between the demonstration of cancer cells in the peritoneum and a worse prognosis. These data are contradicted by a recent and bigger study in radiologically resectable patients, in which positive peritoneal cytology findings were found to occur rarely (7%) and without any correlation to previous FNAC (27). When they did occur, they indicated advanced disease. The authors concluded that their findings supported continued use of FNAC when indicated (see above). Available data, however, do not suggest routine use of peritoneal washings for cytologic examination as a useful staging test in pancreatic cancer.

Another percutaneous route to study cancer cells is through bone marrow aspiration. Several groups have recently demonstrated the potential prognostic value of the presence of epithelial tumor cells in bone marrow in patients with breast, colorectal, gastric, and lung cancer (28–31). The method is based upon the development of monoclonal antibodies directed against epithelial cytokeratins (CK), making possible the immunocytochemical detection of even single disseminated tumor cells. In a recent study of 42 patients with pancreatic cancer, CK cells were found in the bone marrow of 58% of patients treated with curative intent and in 56% of those with extended disease (32). At follow-up of 24 patients after 16 months, 5 (36%) of 14 patients who had complete surgical resection but tumor cells in the bone marrow were found to have distant metastases, and 6 (43%) had local recurrence, compared with none of the corresponding patients without such cells ($p < .05$) (32). Future will tell whether the method will be of prognostic importance and useful in deciding whether systemic treatment is required in addition to the surgical removal of the tumor.

## CURRENT ROLE OF PERCUTANEOUS FINE-NEEDLE ASPIRATION CYTOLOGY AND CORE BIOPSY

Today FNAC and core biopsy are used to avoid operation and not as a method for selecting patients for operation. Their main role, thus, is to confirm the diagnosis of a pancreatic tumor in patients with signs of advanced disease or in those who are too old and/or frail for surgery. It may also have a role as a nonoperative diagnostic tool in patients planned for preoperative radiotherapy and/or chemoradiation. Irrespective, if done for cytologic or histologic purposes, the method is safe, quick, and reliable in showing the presence of malignant pancreatic disease.

Cytologic investigation of peritoneal washings does not seem to fulfill the criteria of a routine diagnostic or staging method in pancreatic disease, whereas studies of the presence of malignant cells in the bone marrow appear to be of interest in staging the disease.

## REFERENCES

1. Evander A, Ihse I, Lunderquist A, Tylén U, Åkerman M. Percutaneous cytodiagnosis of carcinoma of the pancreas and bile duct. Ann Surg 1978;188:90–92.
2. Ihse I, Andrén-Sandberg Å. Percutaneous fine needle aspiration cytology. In: Trede M, Carter D. ed. Surgery of the pancreas. Edinburgh: Churchill Livingstone, 1993:121–125.
3. Temundom T, Sarr MG, Douglas MG, Farnell MB. An argument

against routine percutaneous biopsy, ERCP, or biliary stent placement in patients with clinically resectable periampullary masses: a surgical perspective. Pancreas 1995;11:283–288.
4. Warshaw AL. Implications of peritoneal cytology for staging of early pancreatic cancer. Am J Surg 1991;161:26–30.
5. Yeung RS, Weese JL, Hoffman JP, et al. Neoadjuvant chemoradiation in pancreatic and duodenal carcinoma: a phase II study. Cancer 1993;72:2124–2133.
6. Oscarson J, Stormby N, Sundgren R. Selective angiography and fine needle aspiration cytodiagnosis of gastric and pancreatic tumors. Acta Radiol 1972;12:737–741.
7. Elsman BH, de Graaf PW, van Leeuwen MS, Obertop H. Value and risks of percutaneous cytological puncture in the preoperative assessment of pancreas tumors. Ned Tijdschr Geneeskd 1992;136: 1459–1462.
8. Hajdu EO, Kumari-Subaiya S, Phillips G. Ultrasonically guided percutaneous aspiration biopsy of the pancreas. Semin Diagn Pathol 1986;3(3):166–175.
9. Kocjan G, Rode J, Lees WR. Percutaneous fine needle aspiration cytology of the pancreas: advantages and pitfalls. J Clin Pathol 1989;42(4):341–347.
10. Lüning M, Kursawa R. Schopke W, et al. CT guided percutaneous fine needle biopsy of the pancreas. Eur J Radiol 1985;5(2): 104–108.
11. Soudah B, Fritsch RS, Witrekind C, Hilka B, Spindler B. Value of the cytologic analysis of fine needle aspiration specimens in the diagnosis of pancreatic carcinoma. Acta Cytol 1989;33:875–880.
12. Sperti C, Pasquali C, Di-Prima F, et al. Percutaneous CT-guided fine needle aspiration cytology in the differential diagnosis of pancreatic lesions. Ital J Gastroenterol 1994:26(3):126–131.
13. Holm HH, Torp-Pedersen S, Larsen T, Juul N. Percutaneous fine needle biopsy. Clin Gastroenterol 1985;14:423–449.
14. Waldner B, Dorral ED, Anghonioz P. Cytoponction pancréatique à làiguille fine. A propos de 45 observations. Gastroenterol Clin Biol 1987;11:12–16.
15. Mitchell ML, Bittner CA, Wills JS, Parker EP. Fine needle aspiration cytology of the pancreas. A retrospective study of 73 cases. Acta Cytol 1988;32:447–451.
16. Glenthöj A, Sehested M, Torp-Pedersen S. Ultrasonically guided histological and cytological fine needle biopsies of the pancreas. Reliability and reproducibility of diagnosis. Gut 1990;31:930–933.
17. Jennings PE, Coral A, Donald JJ, Rode L, Lees WR. Ultrasound-guided core biopsy. Lancet 1989;ii:1369–1371.
18. Fornari F, Civardi G, Cavanna L, et al. Complications of ultrasonically guided fine-needle abdominal biopsy. Scand J Gastroenterol 1989;24:949–955.
19. Livraghi T, Damascelli B, Lombardi C, Spagnoti J. Risk in fine-needle abdominal biopsy. J Clin Ultrasound 1983;11:77–81.
20. Smith EH. The hazards of fine-needle aspiration biopsy. Ultrasound Med Biol 1984;10:629–634.
21. Howard JM, Campbell EW. Fatal clostridial pancreatitis following ERCP and fine needle biopsy. Int J Pancreatol 1989;5:305–310.
22. Brandt KK, Charboneau JW, Stephen DH, et al. CT- and US-guided biopsy of the pancreas. Radiology 1993;187:99–104.
23. Bergenfeldt M, Genell S, Lindholm K, Ekberg D, Aspelin P. Needle-tract seeding after percutaneous fine-needle biopsy of pancreatic carcinoma. Acta Chir Scand 1988;154:77–79.
24. Ihse I, Isaksson G. Pancreatic carcinoma: diagnosis and treatment. Clin Gastroenterol 1984;13:961–984.
25. Elvin A, Andersson R, Scheibenpflug L, Lindgren PG. Biopsy of the pancreas with a biopsy gun. Radiology 1990;176:677–679.
26. Yamaguchi R, Saisho H, Ohto M, Kondo F. Diagnostic capability and clinical usefulness of percutaneous histological biopsy of the pancreas under control of ultrasound image using 21 gauge needle. Nippon Shokakibyo Gakkai Zasshi 1990:87(11):2517–2525.
27. Leach SD, Rose JA, Lowry AM, et al. Significance of peritoneal cytology in patients with potentially resectable adenocarcinoma of the pancreatic head. Surgery 1995;118:472–478.
28. Lindeman F, Schlimok G, Dischedl R, Witte J, Riehmüller G. Prognostic significance of micrometastatic tumour cells in bone marrow of colorectal cancer patients. Lancet 1992;340:685–689.
29. Pantel K, Itzbicki J, Angstwurm M, et al. Immunocytological detection of bone marrow micrometastasis in operable non-small cell lung cancer. Cancer Res 1993;52:1027–1031.
30. Gerhard M, Juhl H, Kalthogg H, Schreiber HW, Wagener Ch, Neumaier M. Specific detection of carcinoembryonic antigen-expressing tumor cells in bone marrow aspirates by polymerase chain reaction. J Clin Oncol 1994;12:725–729.
31. Mansi JL, Berger U, Easton D, et al. Micrometastases in bone marrow in patients with primary breast cancer: evaluations as an early predictor of bone metastases. Br Med J 1987;295:1093–1096.
32. Thorban St, Roder JD, Pantel K, Siewert JR. Epithelial tumour cells in bone marrow of patients with pancreatic carcinoma detected by immunocytochemical staining. Eur J Cancer 1996;32A(2): 3363–3365.

# 11

# *Pancreatic Function Tests*

Leon G. Josephs and James M. Becker

The diagnosis of pancreatic disease remains imprecise. Advances, including magnetic resonance pancreatography, continue to be made in the development of imaging techniques of both the pancreatic parenchymal and ductal anatomy, but an ideal methodology for assessing the functional status of the pancreas remains elusive. In this chapter, the laboratory methods that define disorders of pancreatic exocrine function in both acute and chronic inflammatory diseases of the pancreas as well as functional changes associated with pancreatic malignancy are discussed. Particular areas of focus include determinations of isoamylases, amylase creatinine clearance ratio, ribonuclease (RNase), trypsin, methemalbumin, C-reactive protein, pancreatic polypeptide, and amylase lipase ratio in the diagnosis of acute pancreatitis. Both standard and new techniques for the assessment of pancreatic function in patients with chronic pancreatitis are reviewed, with an emphasis on attempts to develop a noninvasive, yet sensitive and specific, test.

## TESTS OF EXOCRINE FUNCTION IN ACUTE INFLAMMATORY DISEASES OF THE PANCREAS

The diagnosis of acute pancreatitis is made primarily on the basis of clinical presentation, recognition of causative factors, and a high index of suspicion. Laboratory confirmation of pancreatitis has been imprecise, although recent advances in biochemistry have improved our ability to support the clinical diagnosis. This section focuses on biochemical techniques.

### Amylase

**Serum Amylase.** The determination of serum amylase has had extensive clinical application in the diagnosis of acute pancreatitis. Unfortunately, the test has many limitations that are often ignored.

Two isoenzymes of amylase can be differentiated by gel filtration and isoelectric focusing. Pancreatic amylase (P-type) is secreted only by the pancreas, whereas salivary amylase (S-type) can originate from various organs, including the salivary glands, liver, prostate, lungs, and fallopian tubes (1). Only about 65% of patients with an elevated serum amylase have pancreatitis. The remainder have intestinal obstruction, infarcted bowel, ectopic pregnancy, renal failure, perforated ulcer, or other illnesses (Table 11.1).

In addition to the lack of specificity of serum amylase determinations, there is also a degree of insensitivity. A normal value does not exclude the diagnosis of acute pancreatitis. In uncomplicated acute pancreatitis, the serum amylase level typically rises within 2–3 hours and returns to normal within 24–48 hours. The prevalence of a normal serum amylase level in patients with acute alcoholic pancreatitis is 32% (2).

**Urine Amylase.** To improve the sensitivity of amylase measurements, urinary amylase output is also quantified. Amylase, with a molecular weight of 50,000, is apparently filtered by the renal glomeruli. Some 25% of normal serum amylase is excreted in the urine, with P-type being cleared 50% faster than S-type isoamylase. Urinary clearance of P-type amylase is 2–3 mL/min.

Any elevation of serum amylase results in an increase in urinary amylase excretion. The level of urinary amylase may rise shortly before that of serum amylase and may remain elevated several days after the serum amylase has normalized, improving the chances of detection. When pancreatitis is suspected, a simple 2-hour urine collection of 75 mL of urine for a clearance ratio will provide a reliable index of amylase excretion (3).

**Amylase-Creatinine Clearance Ratio.** For yet unknown reasons, during episodes of acute pancreatitis, renal tubular reabsorption of amylase is decreased, resulting in increased renal clearance (4). Although currently used less frequently, the increased renal clearance can be used in diagnosing acute pancreatitis with greater specificity by measuring the ratio of amylase to creatinine clearance.

To determine this ratio (ACC), simultaneous measurements of amylase and creatinine concentrations in the serum and urine are necessary:

$$\text{ACC} = \text{urine amylase/serum amylase} \times \text{serum creatinine/urine creatinine} \times 100$$

Warshaw and Fuller demonstrated that this ratio was greater than 3–5% in acute pancreatitis and that patients with hyperamylasemia without pancreatitis had a normal clearance ratio (5). The specificity of this ratio and its clinical usefulness have been scrutinized, and the test has fallen into disfavor because of its lack of specificity in patients with hyperamylasemia secondary to renal dysfunction and because patients have had normal ratios despite an elevated serum amylase and clinical evidence of pancreatitis (6–8). Several conditions may be associated with an elevated amylase-creatinine clearance ratio despite a normal serum amylase. These include burns, diabetic ketoacidosis, duodenal perforations, Bence Jones proteinemia, and even the postoperative state in general. Pancreatitis may be most difficult to diagnose when these conditions are present.

**Isoamylase.** In patients with persistent unexplained hyperamylasemia, levels of isoamylase can be determined. The usual causes are macroamylasemia, related to the association of amylase to globulin, or elevation of S-type amylase (9). In macroamylasemia, the normal P-type amylase is bound to IgA or IgG; this molecule is not filtered by the kidney. These patients have an elevated serum amylase, low or normal urinary amylase, and a low clearance ratio. The diagnosis of macroamylasemia can now be made by direct measurement of macroamylase or S-type amylase by polyacrylamide gel filtration. Radioimmunoassays (RIA) for both P-type and S-type amylase are also available for direct measurement (10–12). *The availability of these direct tests is*

**TABLE 11.1. Incidence of Hyperamylasemia in Extrapancreatic Disease**

| Disease | Incidence (%) |
|---|---|
| Perforated peptic ulcer | 30 |
| Acute cholecystitis | 22 |
| Intestinal obstruction | 20 |
| Mesenteric thrombosis | 33 |
| Acute appendicitis | 5 |
| Following abdominal surgery | 35 |
| Neoplasms | 25 |
| Burns | 15 |
| Cirrhosis | 20 |
| Diabetic ketoacidosis | 64 |
| Renal insufficiency | 5 |
| Mumps | 85 |
| Opiates | 25 |
| Macroamylasemia | 100 |
| Acute gynecologic disease | 21 |
| Splenic rupture | 21 |
| Myocardial infarction | 21 |
| Pneumonia | 21 |

*decreasing the general use of clearance and other indirect measurements.*

**Lipase.** Serum lipase activity generally parallels that of serum amylase. Like amylase, it can be elevated in many abdominal conditions that are difficult to distinguish from acute pancreatitis. Newer assay techniques, including the measurement of pancreatic colipase, allow rapid and reliable determination of colipase and total lipase. Indirect tests of pancreatic lipase activity, utilizing the urine analysis of $^{131}$I-labeled triglyceride that is administered orally, offer a noninvasive, accurate measurement of lipase activity (13–16).

**Trypsin.** Serum trypsin, as measured by RIA, has been reported to be useful in the diagnosis of both acute and chronic pancreatitis. Trypsin levels have been shown to rise 10–40 times normal in acute pancreatitis (17). Since trypsin is confined to the pancreas, one would expect this test to have greater specificity than serum amylase or lipase. Many studies have been published on circulating immunoreactive trypsinogen levels in different conditions as measured by commercially available kits (18–21). The diagnostic accuracy of elevated serum cationic trypsinogen in pancreatic disease has been evaluated. When levels were above 80 ng/mL, there was a 95% likelihood that the patient had acute pancreatitis; however, a level below 9 ng/mL identified only 44% of patients with chronic pancreatitis (22). This test is a helpful diagnostic tool in a small minority of patients.

**C-Reactive Protein.** In several studies, the level of the acute-phase reactant, C-reactive protein (CRP), has been helpful in the assessment of the severity of acute pancreatitis. Two studies have suggested that a CRP below 120 mg/mL may predict the ability to manage necrotizing pancreatitis nonoperatively (23, 24).

**Other Tests.** Hepatic function tests with the measurement of serum bilirubin, alkaline phosphatase, and SGOT add little to the diagnosis of acute pancreatitis. McMahon and Pickford, however, have shown that significantly greater increases in the values of the liver enzymes, especially SGOT, were found in patients with gallstone pancreatitis (25).

Changes in serum calcium and glucose levels may help clarify the diagnosis of acute pancreatitis, but they are not sensitive or specific. Hyperglycemia, occurring in 30% of patients with acute pancreatitis, is likely secondary to an increased output of glucagon by the inflamed pancreas or to the release of other stress hormones. Hypocalcemia is likely multifactorial. Release of thyrocalcitonin in response to an elevated glucagon level is one potential cause.

The search has continued for specific and sensitive laboratory indicators of the severity of pancreatitis. The appearance of serum methemalbumin, suggested as an indicator of hemorrhagic or severe necrotizing pancreatitis, is both insensitive and nonspecific (26–28). In addition to measurement of CRP, early detection of necrotic pancreatic tissue in patients with acute pancreatitis may be aided by measurement of serum RNase. Finding elevated levels may assist in the decision regarding the need for debridement (29).

Serum triglycerides are elevated in 15–20% of patients with acute pancreatitis. Serum amylase activity is often inhibited in patients with both elevated serum triglycerides and pancreatitis. In fact, 85% of patients with elevated serum triglycerides will have a normal serum amylase level. Dilutional techniques must be used to get an accurate reading.

## TESTS OF EXOCRINE FUNCTION IN CHRONIC INFLAMMATORY DISEASES OF THE PANCREAS

Diagnosing chronic pancreatitis, assessing its severity and clinical relevance, and differentiating it from carcinoma of the pancreas are continuing problems. The search for simple, inexpensive, and noninvasive tests continues to be fruitless. Expensive, technically demanding, or invasive tests, such as the secretin test, remain the gold standard in the functional diagnosis of chronic pancreatitis.

### Serum Enzyme and Peptide Determinations

Elevation of serum amylase and lipase levels often does not occur in chronic inflammation of the pancreas. Estimation of the P-amylase creatinine clearance is only useful in severe pancreatic insufficiency. Studies have shown that although low levels of P-type isoamylase in the serum and urine suggest chronic pancreatitis with pancreatic insufficiency, failure to find such values does not exclude this condition. Therefore, the assay of P-amylase is of limited value in the diagnosis of chronic pancreatitis (30–33).

As with serum amylase and lipase, the measurement of trypsin has proven too insensitive to be of value in the diagnosis of chronic pancreatitis. Circulating trypsinlike activity may be reduced in pancreatic insufficiency, but like the other tests described, it occurs only in the presence of extensive pancreatic damage, when the diagnosis is usually not difficult to ascertain. The trypsin–creatinine clearance ratio has been proposed as a screening test for pancreatic cancer because this ratio is increased in most patients with this malignancy. However, Farini et al. found similar elevations in patients with calcific chronic pancreatitis (20). A new noninvasive test of exocrine function involves an $^{131}$I-labeled triglyceride analogue "MIPAG," which requires hydrolysis prior to intestinal absorption. After oral administration of MIPAG, pancreatic lipases in the small intestine digest it, releasing 15-*p*-iodophenyl pentadecanoic acid (IPPA), which is excreted and measured in the urine. In preliminary testing, this agent had a well-defined urinary excretion and effectively detected pancreatic insufficiency by simple urinalysis (34).

Serum pancreatic polypeptide (PP) is found almost exclusively in pancreatic islet tissue and exocrine parenchyma. PP is released following a meal and acts to inhibit pancreatic and biliary secretion. It was postulated that if PP correlated closely with pancreatic function, it might be useful in the detection of chronic pancreatitis. The studies of Valenzuela, however, demonstrated no correlation between PP response and pancreatic exocrine secretion and no correlation between PP and pancreatic exocrine secretion (35).

Stimulation of PP release by exogenous cholecystokinin-octapeptide (CCK-OP) appears to correlate more closely with pancreatic exocrine function than does meal-stimulated release of PP. In patients with chronic pancreatitis, increases in serum PP after CCK-OP correlated well with trypsin output into the duodenum, but the sensitivity and specificity are yet to be determined (36, 37).

## Provocative Blood Enzyme Studies

Provocative blood enzyme studies have involved pharmacologic stimulation of the flow of pancreatic juice with secretin, stimulation of pancreatic enzymes with methacholine, bethanechol, or CCK, and the blocking of pancreatic outflow with morphine. The early experience with provocative testing was extensively reviewed by Dreiling in 1954 (38), and no sound conclusions could be drawn (Table 11.2). Since then, morphine has been found to increase serum pancreatic enzymes in patients with and without pancreatic disease. Secretin-pancreomyzin stimulation has proven more successful. Burton et al. reported elevations in serum pancreatic enzymes in 53 of 57 patients with chronic pancreatitis. Mean levels were not elevated in normal subjects (39). These findings were supported by Fitzgerald, who reported a positive test in 95% of patients with chronic pancreatitis (40). Sun and Chey, on the other hand, reported that the test was clearly positive in only 29% (41, 42).

Provocative tests have been advocated in the diagnosis of chronic pancreatitis secondary to stenosis of the papilla of Vater. As described by Nardi, the test consists of measuring serum amylase and lipase before and after intramuscular (i.m.) administration of 10 mg morphine and 1 mg neostigmine (43). Induction of abdominal pain constitutes a positive test. Recent reports have failed to show any correlation between biliary manometric pressure performed at the time of endoscopic retrograde cholangiopancreatography (ERCP) or operative proof of stenosing papillitis and the morphine-neostigmine test (44).

Thus, there is no clear support in the literature for the use of provocative tests in the diagnosis of pancreatic disease. High rates of false positivity and negativity limit the clinical use of these tests. Nearly all authors conclude that duodenal drainage tests are far more accurate. The search for a noninvasive, accurate test remains elusive.

## Noninvasive Tests

Confirmation of the diagnosis of chronic pancreatitis continues to require the use of invasive and/or expensive tests. Currently available noninvasive methods lack specificity or sensitivity (45). These tests rely on decreased pancreatic enzyme secretion into the GI tract, which does not occur until more than 90% of the exocrine pancreas is not functioning. The challenge is to devise a test that detects chronic pancreatitis before frank pancreatic insufficiency occurs.

*N*-Benzoyl-L-tyrosyl-*p*-aminobenzoic acid, a synthetic peptide, has been used as a noninvasive measure of pancreatic insufficiency by indirect assessment of chymotrypsin activity. The peptide is hydrolyzed by chymotrypsin to *p*-aminobenzoic acid (PABA), which is absorbed in the gut and excreted in the urine after hepatic conjugation. Unfortunately, the test is insensitive. Separation of healthy control subjects from those with pancreatic insufficiency is possible with this test, but it is not as accurate as the secretin-CCK test (46). In addition, the test is not specific. Abnormalities of small bowel, liver, and kidney abnormalities can produce false-positive results, which can be negated by comparing excretion of the peptide with that of PABA alone, and calculating the excretion index of PABA. PABA can also be directly measured in the serum or plasma (47, 48). A similar test utilizes fluorescein dilaurate which is given orally. It is hydrolyzed by pancreatic esterases to a fluorescein dye that is absorbed by the gut, cleared by the kidneys, and measured in the urine. Unfortunately, like the PABA test, the fluorescein test is positive only in patients with severe pancreatic insufficiency and can be falsely positive in patients with hepatic, renal, or intestinal abnormalities (49).

One of the oldest and simplest tests for diagnosing pancreatic insufficiency is measurement of fecal fat and nitrogen. The use of radiolabeled fat has increased the sensitivity of fecal fat analysis. Radioactive serum tests of fat malabsorption which measure the ratio of $^{3}$H-labeled fatty acid and its $^{14}$C-triglyceride in the serum after oral administration are also available. Unfortunately, as

**TABLE 11.2. Summary of Serum Enzyme Responses to Pancreatic Secretagogues As Reported in Previous Investigations**

| | | Serum Enzyme Responses | |
|---|---|---|---|
| Observer | Drug Used As a Stimulant | Normal Patients | Patients with Pancreatic Disorders |
| Dreiling and Richman, 1954 (38) | Secretin | 0/18 | 1/15 |
| | Morphine | 2/13 | 2/10 |
| | Methacholine | 4/16 | 4/15 |
| | Bethanechol | 3/12 | 3/10 |
| | Secretin and morphine | 1/17 | 4/13 |
| | Secretin and methacholine | 0/15 | 2/11 |
| | Secretin, methacholine, morphine | 7/14 | 3/12 |
| Bogoch, 1954 (80) | Morphine | 13/41 | — |
| Mossberg, 1962 (81) | Morphine | 0/48 | 9/12 |
| Burton et al., 1960 (39) | Secretin and pancreozymin | 0/51 | 53/57 |
| Sun, 1963 (41) | Pancreozymin and secretin | — | 16/55 |
| Fitzgerald et al. 1963 (40) | Secretin and pancreozymin | — | 38/40 |
| Nardi and Acosta, 1966 (43) | Morphine and neostigmine | — | 14/15 |
| Laursen, 1966 (82) | Morphine | — | 3/3 |
| Chey et al., 1967 (42) | Pancreozymin and secretin | — | 15/81 |
| Moody, 1978 (83), 1983 (84) | Morphine and neostigmine | — | 3/11 |
| | Secretin | — | 1/29 |
| LoGiudice et al., 1979 (44) | Morphine and neostigmine | 3/6 | 6/14 |

with other tests of pancreatic function, these tests suffer from a lack of sensitivity and are nonspecific, being positive in many patients with small intestine malabsorption syndromes (50, 51).

Several tests have been devised to detect radiolabeled products of digestion in the breath. Breath hydrogen can be measured relatively easily with currently available hydrogen detectors after an oral rice-flour meal. The test will detect carbohydrate malabsorption in patients with pancreatic insufficiency, but again, only when it is severe. A breath test for fat malabsorption utilizing the detection of exhaled $^{14}CO_2$ after oral administration of $^{14}C$-triolein is available. Although Newcomer et al. reported that the test accurately separated patients with steatorrhea from normal subjects, it is only diagnostic in severe pancreatic insufficiency and is potentially invalid in patients with diabetes mellitus, obesity, or chronic pulmonary disease (52).

In the two-stage triolein breath test, the standard triolein test is conducted on patients with malabsorption before and after administration of pancreatic enzymes. The two-stage test appears to differentiate steatorrhea due to pancreatic insufficiency from other causes of steatorrhea (53). A relatively new test for noninvasive assessment of exocrine pancreatic function is the cholesteryl-[$^{14}C$] octanoate breath test which is based on the intraluminal hydrolysis of cholesteryl-[$^{14}C$]octanoate by cholesterol esterase. The lipolytic activity of cholesterol esterase is the rate-limiting step for the absorption of [$^{14}C$]octanoate, which is rapidly oxidized to $^{14}CO_2$ in the liver. As a result, the rate at which $^{14}CO_2$ appears in the breath is proportional to the rate of hydrolysis, thus providing an indirect, noninvasive assessment of pancreatic exocrine function (54). Bruno et al. confirmed the accuracy of this method by studying patients with pancreatic insufficiency as well as healthy controls, using both the cholesteryl-[$^{14}C$]octanoate breath test and plasma PABA, as a single-sample test (55). Unfortunately, the sensitivity and specificity of this test are unclear, making this a confirmatory, but perhaps not a diagnostic, test of pancreatic insufficiency.

Brugge has introduced a modification of the Schilling test as a potentially sensitive test of pancreatic function (56). Previous studies demonstrated that with the standard Schilling test, cobalamin was malabsorbed by 50% of patients with pancreatic insufficiency. This was attributed to the fact that cobalamin is bound by R protein in acidic gastric juice and is not transferred to intrinsic factor until the R protein is partially degraded by pancreatic enzymes. The standard Schilling test lacks sensitivity in pancreatic insufficiency because, at neutral pH, intrinsic factor is able to compete partially with R protein for the initial binding and retention of cobalamin. Thus, achlorhydria would result in a negative Schilling test. Because achlorhydria often coexists with chronic pancreatitis, the standard Schilling test is positive in only 50% of patients with severe pancreatic insufficiency. The dual-label Schilling test is based on the relative absorption of R protein–cobalamin and intrinsic factor–cobalamin in patients with pancreatic disease and symptoms of pancreatic insufficiency. No overlap was seen in healthy patients or in those with renal impairment, pernicious anemia, or other gastrointestinal disorders. Unfortunately, the test results are abnormal in only 50% of patients with overt pancreatic insufficiency (57).

The amino acid consumption test (AACT) is based on the premise that stimulating the pancreas increases uptake of amino acids from the circulatory pool to fuel pancreatic protein synthesis. The healthy pancreas depletes plasma amino acids to a greater extent than does an insufficient gland. Many have suggested that the AACT is an accurate diagnostic test of pancreatic exocrine function (58). More recently, however, studies comparing AACT with duodenal intubation and sampling have shown the AACT to be very nonspecific and unable to discriminate between patients with normal and impaired exocrine pancreatic secretion (59).

**TABLE 11.3. Results of Standard Secretin Test in Disorders of the Pancreas**

| | Volume | Bicarbonate | Enzyme |
|---|---|---|---|
| Acute pancreatitis | ↓ or N | ↓ or N | ↓ or N |
| Chronic pancreatitis | N or ↓ | ↓↓ | N or ↓ |
| Pancreatic CA head | ↓↓ | N | N or ↓ |
| body | ↓ | N | N |
| tail | N | N | N |

Adapted from Dreiling DA, Greenstein A. Diagnosis of pancreatic disease. In: Carey LC, ed. The pancreas. St. Louis: CV Mosby, 1973.

## Duodenal Drainage Tests

Pancreatic function in suspected chronic pancreatitis most frequently has been measured by collecting and analyzing pancreatic secretion in the duodenum in response to a standard secretory stimulus. First described in 1950 by Dreiling and Hollander, the standard secretin test remains the most reliable way to investigate pancreatic exocrine function (60).

The standard secretin test involves *(a)* gastroduodenal intubation and separate collections of gastric and duodenal secretions under constant suction; *(b)* sequential aspiration for 60–80 minutes following submaximal hormonal stimulation with secretin; and *(c)* examination of the aspirate for blood, enzymes, fluid volume, electrolytes, and cellular substances. Normal values were established on the basis of studies of 1824 patients with no evidence of pancreatic disease. Dreiling and Hollander studied over 5000 patients with pancreatic disease. As shown in Table 11.3, several diagnostic patterns emerged. Two fundamental types of secretory response were seen in patients with pancreatic disease: *(a)* a quantitative deficiency manifested by decreased volume output with maintenance of bicarbonate and enzyme secretion, which is characteristic of pancreatic ductal obstruction secondary to neoplasm, and *(b)* a qualitative deficiency with volume secretion sustained but bicarbonate response and, to a lesser extent, enzyme secretion diminished, which indicates chronic inflammatory disease. The test is 90% accurate in patients with pancreatic disease.

Attempts have been made to improve the accuracy of the secretin test by maximizing the stimulation of secretory capacity by increasing the dose of secretin or by adding CCK to stimulate both enzyme and electrolyte secretion. Neither of these additions has added substantially to the diagnostic information derived from the standard secretin test.

A further modification of the secretin test involves replacement of hormonal stimulation of pancreatic secretion with endogenous stimulation. In the Lundh test, a fasting patient is intubated with a radiopaque tube positioned fluoroscopically in the proximal jejunum (61). A test meal consisting of milk powder, vegetable oil, and dextrose is given by mouth, and the mean trypsin concentration of aspirates from the proximal jejunum is determined during the subsequent 2 hours. Lundh found that in chronic pancreatitis, the mean tryptic activity decreased to less than 6 IU/L. Gyr et al. compared the Lundh test and the secretin test in chronic pancreatic disease and found them to be comparable in accuracy (62). Unlike the secretin test, however, the Lundh test did not reliably differentiate between pancreatitis and carcinoma of the pancreas. In general, the Lundh test is simple to do, it has eliminated the need to administer hormones and is relatively accurate. Disadvantages of the test include inaccuracy secondary to dilution of the duodenal sample by small bowel, gastric, and biliary secretions, variable absorption of the test meal, and nonpancreatic conditions that lower enzyme concentration, such as sprue and various gastric operations.

Despite their expense and invasiveness, as well as the special skills necessary to perform and interpret them, the duodenal drainage tests remain the "gold standard" in the functional diagnosis of chronic pancreatic disease. These tests have been reported to be 90% sensitive and specific in diagnosing chronic pancreatitis. Nevertheless, the reliability of the tests must be approached with caution. They may be falsely negative in patients with calcific pancreatitis and falsely positive in patients with gastric or intestinal causes of malabsorption. From a surgical standpoint, the tests offer little useful information, because pain is the major indication for surgical intervention, not pancreatic insufficiency. Appropriate surgical management requires the use of function testing as a complement to imaging studies of duct morphology only when the clinical diagnosis of chronic pancreatitis is unclear.

## LABORATORY TESTS OF FUNCTIONAL CHANGES ASSOCIATED WITH PANCREATIC CANCER

Despite the availability of sophisticated diagnostic techniques, early diagnosis of pancreatic cancer is rare. In 90% of cases, by the time the patient is symptomatic, seeks medical attention, and is diagnosed, the tumor is already inoperable. New diagnostic tests continue to be developed in an attempt to establish the diagnosis and operability of pancreatic cancer more accurately and efficiently. This section focuses on serologic and pancreatic secretory tests.

### Serodiagnosis

Alterations in blood constituents have been used for many years as indicators of malignancy. A variety of enzymes, hormones, plasma proteins, protein degradation products, and immunologically related cellular substances have been used as markers in the diagnosis and management of cancer in man, including cancer of the pancreas. This has been stimulated by recent advances in radioimmunoassay and other highly sensitive immunologic techniques that allow measurement of extremely small quantities of circulating antigens. Unfortunately, for the most part, these serologic tests have provided neither the sensitivity nor the specificity needed for a definitive diagnosis of a particular tumor type. Thus, the tumor markers have been largely limited to evaluating response to therapy, determining tumor recurrence, and indicating prognosis (63).

**Serum Enzyme Tests.** Serum amylase, isoamylase, and lipase determinations are rarely useful in the diagnosis of carcinoma of the pancreas. Serum enzymes may on occasion be mildly elevated as a result of pancreatitis secondary to an obstructing tumor.

Hepatic function tests, particularly alkaline phosphatase, are useful in the differential diagnosis of jaundice. With pancreatic cancer, either bile duct obstruction or hepatic metastases may cause elevated serum alkaline phosphatase levels.

Glucose intolerance is frequently observed in carcinoma of the pancreas. Fasting serum glucose levels are significantly higher in patients with pancreatic cancer, and up to 50% of patients will have abnormal glucose tolerance tests. This may be due to the decreased and delayed insulin secretion. Decreased serum C-peptide levels suggest an abnormality of beta cell function in pancreatic cancer (64).

The Mayo Clinic, Memorial Sloan-Kettering Cancer Center, and the University of Chicago, under contract from the National Cancer Institute (NCI), collaborated to evaluate the accuracy of diagnostic procedures among patients clinically suspected of having pancreatic cancer. The three institutions enrolled 368 patients. As part of the NCI study, 48 routine and standard biochemical and immunologic tests were evaluated preoperatively (Table 11.4). This study confirmed that while patients with pancreatic disorders might have elevated serum lipase, amylase, and glucose levels, these tests did not distinguish between pancreatic inflammation and pancreatic cancer. Liver function abnormalities were also nonspecific (65).

**Peptide Hormones.** Pancreatic carcinomas may occasionally elevate peptide hormone levels. In the NCI study, systemic, venous, and portal blood was screened for peptide hormones, including gastrin, parathyroid hormone, calcitonin, glucagon, and human chorionic gonadotropin. None of these hormones was found to be significantly elevated in patients with pancreatic

**TABLE 11.4. Serologic Tests in Patients Suspected of Having Pancreatic Cancer**

| Laboratory Tests | Pancreatic Cancer *N* = 48 | Pancreatitis *N* = 9 | Other Cancers *N* = 10 | Other Benign Diseases *N* = 28 |
|---|---|---|---|---|
| Glucose mg/dL* | 122.5 ± 6.9 | 103.8 ± 8.2 | 98.9 ± 9.5 | 100.0 ± 2.9 |
| Calcium mg/dL | 9.6 ± 0.1 | 9.5 ± 0.1 | 9.2 ± 0.2 | 9.4 ± 0.1 |
| Phosphorus mg/dL | 3.5 ± 0.1 | 3.6 ± 0.2 | 3.1 ± 0.2 | 3.2 ± 0.1 |
| Total thyroxine μg/dL | 6.7 ± 0.4 | 7.8 ± 0.9 | 6.5 ± 0.5 | 6.2 ± 0.4 |
| Prothrombin time (sec) | 12.2 ± 0.3 | 11.9 ± 0.2 | 11.4 ± 0.2 | 11.4 ± 0.3 |
| Direct bilirubin mg/dL* | 2.4 ± 0.6 | 0 ± 0 | 0 ± 0 | 0.6 ± 0.5 |
| Indirect bilirubin mg/dL* | 1.9 ± 0.4 | 0.5 ± 0.1 | 0.5 ± 0.1 | 1.3 ± 0.7 |
| Alkaline phosphatase μ/L* | 565.2 ± 71.8 | 239.0 ± 76.2 | 193.6 ± 24.1 | 237.8 ± 14.1 |
| SGOT (U/L)* | 47.6 ± 6.1 | 19.1 ± 3.8 | 16.5 ± 3.2 | 20.9 ± 4.7 |
| Lipase (U/L)* | 95.8 ± 21.7 | 245.8 ± 55.2 | 61.9 ± 18.1 | 50.3 ± 12.7 |
| Amylase (U/L)* | 377.3 ± 152.4 | 609.6 ± 113.4 | 270.6 ± 49.7 | 237.8 ± 14.1 |
| Insulin (U/mL) | 16.8 ± 4.0 | 8.7 ± 2.1 | 6.8 ± 2.1 | 13.4 ± 2.3 |
| Gastrin (pg/mL) | 109.6 ± 15.3 | 150.2 ± 26.3 | 208.1 ± 55.4 | 121.2 ± 21.6 |
| Parathyroid hormone (μL eq/mL) | 25.3 ± 1.3 | 20.3 ± 4.0 | 29.7 ± 4.5 | 24.3 ± 1.4 |
| Calcitonin (pg/mL) | 78.0 ± 16.6 | 51.0 ± 11.4 | 67.0 ± 11.9 | 46.0 ± 8.3 |
| IgA (Iμ/mL) | 2.1 ± 0.2 | 2.2 ± 0.1 | 2.3 ± 0.3 | 2.4 ± 0.2 |
| IgG (Iμ/mL) | 9.5 ± 0.4 | 10.0 ± 1.2 | 9.9 ± 0.5 | 10.3 ± 0.6 |
| IgM (Iμ/mL)* | 1.2 ± 0.1 | 1.4 ± 0.3 | 0.8 ± 0.1 | 1.8 ± 0.2 |
| CEA ng/mL* | 12.4 ± 3.8 | 5.2 ± 3.8 | 18.3 ± 7.0 | 2.3 ± 0.4 |

From Go VLW, Taylor WF, DiMagno EP. Efforts at early diagnosis of pancreatic cancer: the Mayo Clinic experience. Cancer 1981; 47:1698.
*$p < .05$
Mean ± SEM

**TABLE 11.5. Serum CEA, Bilirubin, and CCK-Stimulated Pancreatic CEA, Lipase, and Bicarbonate Output (mean ± SEM)**

| Patient Group | N | Serum CEA (ng/mL) | Serum Bilirubin (mg/dL) | CEA (μg/hr) | Lipase (kU/hr) | Bicarbonate (mEq/hr) |
|---|---|---|---|---|---|---|
| Control | 19 | 2.6 ± 0.6 | <1.0 | 8.0 ± 2.1 | 139.7 ± 15.5 | 28.0 ± 3.2 |
| Pancreatic cancer | 25 | 12.5 ± 4.3 | 1.8 ± 2.8 | 9.3 ± 2.9 | 35.2 ± 8.8 | 9.3 ± 2.1 |
| Jaundiced | 12 | 12.2 ± 4.1 | 6.9 ± 1.3 | 4.2 ± 1.3 | 12.6 ± 5.7 | 5.5 ± 1.5 |
| Nonjaundiced | 13 | 12.6 ± 5.6 | 0.5 ± 0.1 | 15.1 ± 5.0 | 56.2 ± 13.8 | 12.5 ± 4.5 |
| Pancreatitis | 7 | 1.6 ± 0.3 | 0.5 ± 0.1 | 10.0 ± 2.8 | 55.6 ± 8.8 | 13.3 ± 3.8 |

From Go VLW, Taylor WF, DiMagno EP. Efforts at early diagnosis of pancreatic cancer: the Mayo Clinic experience. Cancer 1981; 47:1698.

cancer, compared with levels in patients with other cancers and benign diseases (66, 67).

**Tumor-Associated Antigens.** A concerted effort has been made to identify a pancreatic cancer-associated antigen to help in the early diagnosis of pancreatic cancer. [*Editor's note:* see also Chapter 47.] In general, the markers presently in use have shown a lack of specificity and limited sensitivity in distinguishing pancreatic cancer from benign disease or other malignancy.

Prospective studies of both carcinoembryonic antigen (CEA) and α-fetoprotein (AFP) have shown them to be of no value in the diagnosis of pancreatic cancer. Cooper et al. found that 83% of patients with pancreatic cancer had a CEA level above 2.5 ng/mL, but so did 46% of patients with benign diseases (68). This was also seen by the Mayo group (65). CEA levels may be more clinically useful in determining prognosis because extremely high levels suggest metastatic disease. AFP was elevated in only 3% of patients with pancreatic cancer and is therefore of no value (69).

A large number of additional antigens have been associated with pancreatic cancer. These include CA 19-9, CA-50, DUPAN-2, 47D10, RA96, PCAA, and SPAN. Unfortunately, an NCI consensus group concluded that their lack of tumor specificity and pancreas organ specificity made these serum markers unreliable for diagnosis. Use of multiple markers increased sensitivity in some cases but with a resultant decrease in specificity (70).

**Pancreatic Ribonuclease.** Serum RNase is one of several enzymes secreted by the pancreas. In 1976, Reddy and Holland reported that serum RNase increased in many patients with pancreatic cancer (71). Warshaw confirmed this finding, reporting significant RNase elevations in 69% of patients with pancreatic cancer, compared with elevations in only 8% of patients with other cancers, in 11% of patients with obstructive jaundice, and in no patients with chronic pancreatitis (29). These results could not be reproduced by either Mackie et al. or Fitzgerald et al. (66, 73).

**Galactosyltranferase Isoenzyme II.** Galactosyltransferase isoenzyme II (GI-II) is a tumor marker that appears to be more sensitive and specific than other serologic markers. In one study, the test was positive in 41 of 61 patients (67%) with pancreatic cancer and in only 3 of 167 with benign pancreatic disease. Unfortunately, GI-II did not distinguish between patients with pancreatic cancer and other malignancies (74).

**Micro-Leukocyte Adherence Inhibition Test.** Several immunodiagnostic tests have been used to detect the presence of specific forms of gastrointestinal cancer by measuring a specific antitumor response to tissue type-specific antigens. The Micro-LAI is one such test that can specifically detect pancreatic cancer and discriminate between cancer and pancreatitis, other forms of cancer, and the healthy state. Of the 104 subjects studied, a positive assay was found in 19 of 23 pancreatic cancer patients but in only 1 of 29 benign control patients, 2 of 26 malignant control patients, and 0 of 25 healthy patients (75).

### Pancreatic Function Tests

In pancreatic cancer, the accuracy of pancreatic function tests depends on the location of the cancer (76–78). Using a duodenal intubation and perfusion method, the Mayo group measured the rate of secretion of pancreatic CEA, bicarbonate, trypsin, and lipase into the duodenum following saline perfusion alone, with continuous intravenous infusion of secretin, or with CCK infusion. The test was performed on 57 patients with suspected pancreatic cancer. Laparotomy revealed carcinoma of the pancreas in 25 patients, pancreatitis in 7, other intraabdominal malignancies in 6, and benign nonpancreatic disorders in 19. The rate of CEA output did not differentiate cancer of pancreas patients from other patients (Table 11.5). CCK-stimulated pancreatic enzyme output was abnormal with almost 90% of cancers of the head of the pancreas and with 75% of cancers occurring in the body or tail (77). Only 23% of patients with pancreatic cancer were found to have positive cytologic studies after CCK stimulation (76).

Using a similar duodenal drainage technique, the University of Chicago group found that the secretin test accurately demonstrated abnormal pancreatic function, but did not adequately differentiate between cancer and inflammation. In their hands, however, cytologic examination of the duodenal aspirate was of much greater value. The sensitivity of duodenal cytology after secretin stimulation was 68% overall, 79% if the cancer was in the head of the pancreas; the specificity, 99%; the predictive value of a positive test, 99%; and the predictive value of a negative test, 83% (79).

Even though invasive pancreatic function testing is relatively easy to do, it requires more expertise, is cumbersome and tedious, and all too often does not distinguish between a pancreatic neoplasm and pancreatitis. Collection of duodenal contents for cytologic examination may improve the value of the test, but this material can probably be collected more accurately by direct aspiration from the pancreatic duct at the time of ERCP. With the diagnostic techniques presently available, pancreatic function tests have little to add to the diagnostic evaluation of the patient with suspected malignancy.

What is needed for the early diagnosis of pancreatic cancer is a simple, inexpensive screening test that can be applied to large populations of asymptomatic patients who may be susceptible to developing pancreatic cancer, such as smokers, chemical workers, and diabetics. Unfortunately, such a test is not available, and the high risk group not clearly defined, making screening for pancreatic cancer unwarranted.

## REFERENCES

1. Levitt MD, Ellis C, Engel RR. Isoelectric focusing of human serum and tissue isoamylases. J Lab Clin Med 1977;90:141–152.
2. Spechler SJ, Dalton JW, Robbins AH, et al. Prevalence of normal serum amylase levels in patients with acute alcoholic pancreatitis. Dig Dis Sci 1983;28:865–869.
3. Gambill EE, Mason HL. Urinary amylase excretion per hour in 100

individuals without gastrointestinal disease or renal insufficiency. J Lab Clin Med 1964;63:173–176.
4. Johnson SG, Ellis CJ, Levitt MD. Mechanisms of increased renal clearance of amylase/creatinine in acute pancreatitis. N Engl J Med 1976;295:1214–1217.
5. Warshaw AL, Fuller AF Jr. Specificity of increased renal clearance of amylase in diagnosis of acute pancreatitis. N Engl J Med 1975;292:325–328.
6. Tedesco FS, Harter HR, Alpers DH. Serum amylase determinations and amylase to creatinine clearance ratios in patients with chronic renal insufficiency. Gastroenterology 1976;71:594–598.
7. Farrar WH, Calkins G. Sensitivity of the amylase-creatinine clearance ratio in acute pancreatitis. Arch Intern Med 1978;138:958–962.
8. Lankisch PG, Koop H, Otto J, et al. Specificity of increased amylase to creatinine ratio in acute pancreatitis. Digestion 1977;16:160–164.
9. Berk JE, Kizu H, Wilding P, Searey RL. Macroamylasemia: a newly recognized cause for elevated serum amylase activity. N Engl J Med 1967;277:941–946.
10. Boehm-Truitt M, Harrison E, Wolf RO, Notkins AL. Radioimmunoassay for human salivary amylase. Anal Biochem 1978;85:476–487.
11. Takatsuka Y, Kitahara T, Matsuura K, et al. Radioimmunoassay for human pancreatic amylase: comparison of human serum amylase by measurement of enzymatic activity and by radioimmunoassay. Clin Chim Acta 1979;97:261–268.
12. Crouse SP, Hammond J, Savory J. Radioimmunoassay of human pancreatic amylase in serum and urine. Res Commun Chem Pathol Pharmacol 1980;29:513–525.
13. Song H, Tietz NW, Tan C. Usefulness of serum lipase, esterase, and amylase estimation in the diagnosis of pancreatitis—a comparison. Clin Chem 1970;16:264–268.
14. Borgstrom B, Earlanson-Albertsson C, Wieloch T. Pancreatic colipase: chemistry and physiology. J Lipid Res 1979;20:805–816.
15. Hoffmann GE, Weiss L. Specific serum pancreatic lipase determination with the use of purified colipase. Clin Chem 1980;26:1732–1733.
16. Ouagued M, Saraux B, Girard-Globa A. A rapid and reliable method for determination of colipase and total lipase in pancreatic tissue. Biochimie 1982;64:301–303.
17. Lake-Bakaar G, et al. The relative values of serum immunoreactive trypsin concentration and total amylase activity in the diagnosis of mumps, chronic renal failure, and pancreatic disease. Scand J Gastroenterol 1980;15:97–101.
18. Gullo L, Ventracci M, Bonora G, et al. Comparative study of serum trypsin levels and pancreatic exocrine function in chronic pancreatitis. Scand J Gastroenterol 1980;62:27–28.
19. Andriulli A, Masoero G, Felder G, et al. Circulating trypsin-like immunoreactivity in chronic pancreatitis. Dig Dis Sci 1981;26:532–537.
20. Farini R, Fabris C, del Favero G, et al. Role of trypsin/creatinine clearance ratio in the differential diagnosis of chronic pancreatic disease. Gastroenterology 1981;81:242–246.
21. Koop H, Lankisch PG, Stockman F, Arnold R. Trypsin radioimmunoassay in diagnosis of chronic pancreatitis. Digestion 1980;20:151–156.
22. Masoero G, Andriulli A, Bianco A, et al. Diagnostic accuracy of serum cationic trypsinogen estimation for pancreatic diseases. Dig Dis Sci 1982;27:1089–1094.
23. Wilson C, Heads A, Shenkin A, Imrie CW. C-reactive protein, antiproteases and complement factors as objective markers of severity in acute pancreatitis. Br J Surg 1989;76:177–181.
24. Rau B, Pralle U, Uhl W, Schoenberg MH, Beger HG. Management of sterile necrosis in instances of severe acute pancreatitis. J Am Coll Surg 1995;181:279–288.
25. McMahon MJ, Pickford IR. Biochemical prediction of gallstones early in an attack of acute pancreatitis. Lancet 1979;2:541–543.
26. Geokas MC, Rinderknecht H, Walberg CB, Weissman R. Methemalbumin in the diagnosis of acute hemorrhagic pancreatitis. Ann Intern Med 1974;81:483–486.
27. Goodhead B. Significance of methemalbuminemia in acute abdominal emergencies. Arch Surg 1970;101:376–378.
28. McMahon MJ, Playforth MJ, Pickford IR. A comparative study of methods for the prediction of severity of attacks of acute pancreatitis. Br J Surg 1980;67:22–25.
29. Warshaw AL, Lee KH. Serum ribonuclease elevations and pancreatic necrosis in acute pancreatitis. Surgery 1979;86:227–234.
30. Hegarty JE, O'Donnell MD, McGeeney KF, Fitzgerald O. Pancreatic and salivary amylase/creatinine clearance ratios in normal subjects and in patients with chronic pancreatitis. Gut 1978;19:350–354.
31. Aw SE, Hobbs JR, Wooten ID. Urinary isoamylases in the diagnosis of chronic pancreatitis. Gut 1967;8:402–407.
32. Berk JE, Ayulo JA, Fridhandler L. Value of pancreatic-type isoamylase assay as an index of pancreatic insufficiency. Dig Dis Sci 1979;24:6–10.
33. Johnson SG, Levitt MD. Relation between serum pancreatic isoamylase concentration and pancreatic exocrine function. Am J Dig Dis 1978;23:914–918.
34. Kropp FF, et al. Evaluation of pancreatic lipase activity by simple urine analysis after oral administration of a new iodine-131-labeled triglyceride. Eur J Nucl Med 1994;21:1227.
35. Valenzuela JE, Taylor IL, Walsh JH. Pancreatic polypeptide responses in patients with chronic pancreatitis. Dig Dis Sci 1979;24:862–864.
36. Owyang C, Scarpello JH, Vinik AI. Correlation between pancreatic enzyme secretion and plasma concentration of human pancreatic poly-peptide in health and in chronic pancreatitis. Gastroenterology 1982;83:55–62.
37. DiMagno EP, Koch MB, Go VLW. Can human pancreatic polypeptide detect pancreatic disease (Abstract). Dig Dis Sci 1983;28:932.
38. Dreiling DA, Richman A. Evaluation of provocative blood enzyme tests employed in diagnosis of pancreatic disease. Arch Intern Med 1954;94:197.
39. Burton P, et al. Serum amylase and serum lipase levels in man after administration of secretion and pancreozymin. Gut 1960;1:125.
40. Fitzgerald O, et al. A clinical study of chronic pancreatitis. Gut 1963;4:193.
41. Sun DCH. The use of pancreozymin-secretion test in the diagnosis of pancreatitis and tumors of the pancreas. Gastroenterology 1963;45:203.
42. Chey WY, Shay H, Nielsen OF. Evaluation of tests of pancreatic function in chronic pancreatic disease. JAMA 1967;201:87.
43. Nardi GL, Acosta JM. Papillitis as a cause of pancreatitis and abdominal pain: role of evocative test, operative pancreatography and histologic evaluation. Ann Surg 1966;164:611–621.
44. LoGiudice JA, Geenen JE, Hogan WJ, Dodds WJ. Efficacy of the morphine-Prostigmin test for evaluating patients with suspected papillary stenosis. Dig Dis Sci 1979;24:455–458.
45. DiMagno EP. Diagnosis of chronic pancreatitis: are noninvasive tests of exocrine pancreatic function sensitive and specific? Gastroenterology 1982;83:143–146.
46. Arvanitakis C, Greenberger NJ. Diagnosis of pancreatic disease by a synthetic peptide. A new test of exocrine pancreatic function. Lancet 1976;1:663–666.
47. Mitchell CJ, Humphrey CS, Bullen AW, et al. Improved diagnostic accuracy of a modified oral pancreatic function test. Scand J Gastroenterol 1979;14:737–741.
48. Lang C, Gyr K, Kraehenmann J, Arenz F. The oral pancreatic function test with *N*-benzoyl-L-tyrosyl-*p*-aminobenzoic acid: acute toxicity and effects of renal function on this test. J Clin Chem Clin Biochem 1980;18:551–555.
49. Lankisch PG, Schreiber A, Otto J. The pancreolauryl test (PLT)—a new tubeless pancreatic function test (Abstract). Natl Pancreatic Cancer Project Newsletter 1981;6:32.
50. Pedersen NT, Marquersen J, Skjoldborg H, Jensen E. Serum radioactivity of 14C-triolein and 3H-oleic acid ingested in a test meal—a rapid test of pancreatic exocrine insufficiency. Scand J Gastroenterol 1979;14:529–534.
51. Adlung J, Grazikowski H. Diagnosis of fat malabsorption of $^{14}$C-tripalmitate/$^{3}$H-palmitic acid. Scand J Gastroenterol 1979;14:587–592.
52. Newcomer AD, Hofmann AF, DiMagno EP, et al. Triolein breath test: a sensitive and specific test for fat malabsorption. Gastroenterology 1979;76:6–13.
53. Goff JS. Two stage triolein breath test differentiates pancreatic

insufficiency from other causes of malabsorption. Gastroenterology 1982;83:44–46.
54. Cole SG, Rossi S, Stern A, Hofmann AF. Cholesteryl octanoate breath test. Preliminary studies on a new noninvasive test of human pancreatic exocrine function. Gastroenterology 1987;93:1372–1380.
55. Bruno MJ, Hock FJ, Delzenne B, et al. Simultaneous assessments of exocrine pancreatic function by cholesteryl-($^{14}C$) octanoate breath test and measurement of plasma *p*-aminobenzoic acid. Clin Chem 1995;41:599–604.
56. Brugge WR, Goff JS, Allen NC, et al. Development of a dual label Schilling test for pancreatic exocrine function based on the differential absorption of cobalamin bound to intrinsic factor and R protein. Gastroenterology 1980;78:937–939.
57. Steer ML, Waxman I, Freedman S. Chronic pancreatitis. N Engl J Med 1995;332:1482–1490.
58. Domschke S, Heptner G, Kolb S, et al. Decrease in plasma amino acid level after secretin and pancreozymin as an indicator of exocrine pancreatic function. Gastroenterology 1986;90:1031–1038.
59. Maringhini A, Nelson DK, Jones JD, DiMagno EP. Is the plasma amino acid test an accurate test of exocrine pancreatic insufficiency? Gastroenterology 1994;106:488–493.
60. Dreiling DA, Hollander F. Studies in pancreatic function II—a statistical study of pancreatic secretion following secretion in patients with pancreatic disease. Gastroenterology 1950;15:620.
61. Lundh G. Pancreatic exocrine function in neoplastic and inflammatory disease—a simple and reliable new test. Gastroenterology 1962;42:275.
62. Gyr K, Agrawal NM, Felsenfeld O, Font RG. Comparative study of secretin and Lundh test. Am J Dig Dis 1975;20:506–512.
63. Go VL, Zamcheck N. The role of tumor markers in the management of colorectal cancer. Cancer 1982;50:2618–2623.
64. Schwartz SS, Zeidler A, Moossa AR, et al. A prospective study of glucose tolerance, insulin, C-peptide and glucagon responses in patients with pancreatic carcinoma. Am J Dig Dis 1978;23:1107–1114.
65. Go VL, Taylor WF, DiMagno EP. Efforts at early diagnosis of pancreatic cancer: the Mayo Clinic experience. Cancer 1981;47:1698–1705.
66. Mackie CR, Dhorajiwala J, Blackstone MO, et al. Value of a new diagnostic aid in relation to the disease process in pancreatic cancer. Lancet 1979;2:385–389.
67. Cooper MJ, Mackie CR, Skinner DB, Moossa AR. A reappraisal of the value of carcinoembryonic antigen in the management of patients with various neoplasms. Br J Surg 1979;66:120–123.
68. Moossa AR, Levin B. The diagnosis of ``early'' pancreatic cancer: the University of Chicago experience. Cancer 1981;47:1688–1697.
69. Banwo O, Versey J, Hobbs JR. New oncofetal antigen for human pancreas. Lancet 1974;1:643–645.
70. Metzgar RS, Asch HL. Antigens of human pancreatic adenocarcinomas: their role in the diagnosis and therapy. Pancreas 1988;3:352–371.
71. Gelder FB, Reese CJ, Moossa AR, et al. Purification, partial characterization and clinical evaluation of a pancreatic oncofetal antigen. Cancer Res 1978;38:313–324.
72. Reddi KK, Holland JF. Elevated serum ribonuclease in patients with pancreatic cancer. Proc Natl Acad Sci USA 1976;73:2308–2310.
73. Fitzgerald PJ, Fortner JG, Watson RC, et al. The value of diagnostic aids in detailing pancreas cancer. Cancer 1978;41:868–879.
74. Podolsky DK, et al. Galactosyltransferase isoenzyme II in the detection of pancreatic cancer: comparison with radiologic, endoscopic and serologic tests. N Engl J Med 1981;304:1313–1318.
75. Goldrosen MH, Russo HJ, Howell JH, et al. Evaluation of micro-leukocyte adherence inhibition as an immunodiagnostic test for pancreatic cancer. Cancer Res 1979;39:633–637.
76. DiMagno EP, Malagelada JR, Taylor WF, Go VL. A prospective comparison of current diagnostic tests for pancreatic cancer. N Engl J Med 1977;297:737–742.
77. DiMagno EP, Malagelada JR, Moertel CG, Go VL. Prospective evaluation of the pancreatic secretion of immunoreactive carcinoembryonic antigen, enzyme and bicarbonate in patients suspected of having pancreatic cancer. Gastroenterology 1977;73:457–461.
78. Dreiling DA. The early diagnosis of pancreatic cancer. Scand J Gastroenterol 1970;6:115–122.
79. Moossa AR, Levin B. Collaborative studies in the diagnosis of pancreatic cancer. Semin Oncol 1977;6:298–308.
80. Bogoch A, Roth JLA, Bockus HL. The effects of morphine on serum amylase and lipase. Gastroenterology 1954;26:697.
81. Mossberg SM, Bloom A, Berkowitz, Ross G. Serum enzyme activities following morphine. Arch Intern Med 1962;109:429.
82. Laursen T, Schmidt A. Increase in serum-GPT and serum-LDH after administration of morphine to patients suffering from bile-duct dyskinesia. Scand J Clin Lab Invest 1966;92(18 suppl):175.
83. Moody FG, Berenson MD, McCloskey D. Transampullary septectomy for post-cholecystectomy pain. Ann Surg 1977;186:415.
84. Moody FG, Becker JD, Potts JR. Transduodenal sphincteroplasty and transampullary septectomy for postcholecystectomy pain. Ann Surg 1983;197:627.

SECTION III

INTRAOPERATIVE DIAGNOSTIC PROCEDURES

# 12

# *Intraoperative Ultrasound*

Yasutsugu Bandia and Masatoshi Makuuchi

Application of ultrasound to surgery has a long history. In the 1960s, A-mode ultrasound was used to detect calculi in the kidney or common bile duct (1, 2). Late in the 1970s, with the advent of real-time ultrasonography, reappraisal of intraoperative use of ultrasound began, promoted by the development of small transducers for intraoperative usage. Studies of use at surgery for the liver (3), biliary tract (4), and pancreas (5) were reported. Intraoperative ultrasound is mandatory for hepatic resection of hepatocellular carcinoma in patients with hepatic cirrhosis (6) when precise and limited resection is necessary, because the tumor may be difficult to detect by palpation if it is located deep within the parenchyma. Stimulated by its usefulness in operations on the liver, active application of intraoperative ultrasound to the biliary tract and pancreas, as well as to the kidney, resumed.

At surgery, the transducer can be applied directly to the surface of organs, and no tissues intervene to attenuate transmission of ultrasound. High-frequency transducers are thus available, providing images with better resolution. This is the great advantage of intraoperative ultrasound. Moreover, ribs or gas in the intestine, which render portions of the body invisible with percutaneous ultrasound, are easily avoided in the intraoperative approach. The greater freedom in directing the ultrasound beam permitted by the intraoperative approach may lead to confusion in the operator's orientation. Therefore, the operator must be familiar with both the anatomy and techniques of manipulation of the transducer.

## PURPOSE AND ROLE OF INTRAOPERATIVE ULTRASOUND

Any intraoperative examination is done to obtain new information to guide the surgeon in selecting the optimal operative procedure and to minimize the need for other invasive procedures. Introduction of ultrasound during operation anticipates similar advantages. The advantage of ultrasound, compared with other imaging examinations, is its ability to delineate tubular structures, such as blood vessels or biliary and pancreatic ducts, without any contrast medium. Not only organs, but arteries, veins, and other tubular structures can be depicted simultaneously if their diameter exceeds 2 or 3 mm. Moreover, ultrasound is less invasive than roentgenographic examination.

The roles of intraoperative ultrasound can be summarized as follows:

1. Determining the location, size, and extension of a tumor
2. Assessing relationships between a tumor and adjacent organs or vessels
3. Differentiating in some instances between benign and malignant lesions
4. Detecting calculi
5. Guiding "intraoperative puncturing"
6. Guiding operation

Lateral resolution of images within 1 cm of the surface of the transducer is poor because of the thick beam width; thus direct application of the transducer to the pancreas obscures images of superficial lesions. Some "standoff" is needed to overcome this technical limitation. Although one may apply a bolus of gel to the surface of the pancreas, submerging the pancreas in 500 mL or more of warm saline is convenient and easily applicable to even wide portions of the pancreas.

## APPLICATION TO PANCREATIC SURGERY

### Chronic Pancreatitis

During operation, it may be difficult and time-consuming to localize the dilated pancreatic duct for side-to-side pancreaticojejunostomy by palpation or needle aspiration, because the pancreas may be fibrotic and inflamed and contain scattered calculi (7). This may lead to unnecessary tissue damage and additional risk of complications. Intraoperative ultrasound can not only delineate the dilated main pancreatic duct in all cases but can also identify the anatomic landmarks adjacent to the pancreas. For intraoperative localization of the main pancreatic duct for the purpose of performing a longitudinal side-to-side pancreaticojejunostomy, the pancreatic duct is first visualized in a longitudinal imaging plane to identify its most dilated segment. Thus, before any dissection, ultrasound demonstrates the most appropriate site for incision into the ductal system (8). Calculi in the pancreatic duct are seen as strong echoes with acoustic shadows. Intraoperative ultrasound has high sensitivity in detecting small calculi or areas of pancreatic calcifications, which may be demonstrated as highly reflective particles without acoustic

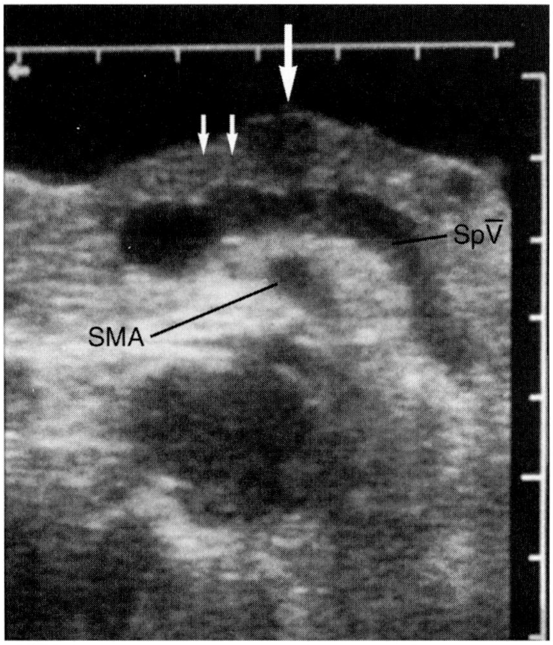


**FIG. 12.1.** A transverse image along the long axis of the pancreas demonstrates a well-defined hypoechoic mass *(arrow).* A segment of the main pancreatic duct is also depicted *(small arrows). SpV,* splenic vein; *SMA,* superior mesenteric artery.

shadows. Any residual calculi may thus be identified and removed. Intraoperative ultrasound is helpful in defining pseudocysts, especially if they are small or deeply located. In patients undergoing internal drainage of pseudocysts, the thickness of the wall of the cysts can be determined, nearby structures can be identified and protected, and potential septa within the cyst can be depicted (8, 9).

## Endocrine Tumors

Nonfunctioning endocrine tumors may become rather large before they can be diagnosed clinically and be readily localized at surgery. On the contrary, functioning endocrine tumors, especially insulinomas, often manifest symptoms even when the tumor is less than 1 cm in diameter. Sophisticated preoperative methods, such as helical CT, pharmacologic angiography, and blood sampling via percutaneous transhepatic catheterization of the portal vein, have been used to locate such tumors. However, preoperative determination of the exact position of a small tumor is frequently impossible, and its location must be reassessed at operation. Many endocrine tumors can be identified by inspection or palpation at surgery, but some are embedded within the parenchyma of the pancreas and some may be multiple. Blind distal pancreatectomy or pancreatoduodenectomy have been elected in such cases. Intraoperative ultrasound can easily demonstrate even small endocrine tumors (10–12), which decreases the necessity for large pancreatic resections of benign tumors. Enucleation, therefore, is the standard procedure for endocrine tumors of the pancreas in the era of intraoperative ultrasound. Basically, an endocrine tumor is depicted as a homogeneous, hypoechoic, round area that is easily differentiated from the pancreatic parenchyma. Even with intraoperative ultrasound, echogenicity differences between a tumor and the normal parenchyma are sometimes limited, so it should be noted that intraoperative ultrasound cannot always demonstrate a tumor (13).

Identification of the main pancreatic duct and its relationship to the tumor is a significant role of intraoperative ultrasound (Fig. 12.1). Under the guidance of intraoperative ultrasound, which can easily delineate the course of the duct, a tumor that is embedded in the head of the pancreas can be enucleated without injury to the main pancreatic duct. At surgery, even when the location of the tumor can be defined by inspection or palpation, intraoperative ultrasonography is almost mandatory for resection of a functioning endocrine tumor of the pancreas because of its high sensitivity in delineating the main pancreatic duct, thus adding a degree of safety for the patient.

## Carcinoma of the Pancreas

Intraoperative ultrasound can be used as an adjunct to identification of a malignant lesion when there is strong preoperative suspicion of cancer. A small lesion that is difficult to diagnose preoperatively may be detected by intraoperative ultrasound as a hypoechoic mass (14) (Fig. 12.2). Compared with blind biopsy,

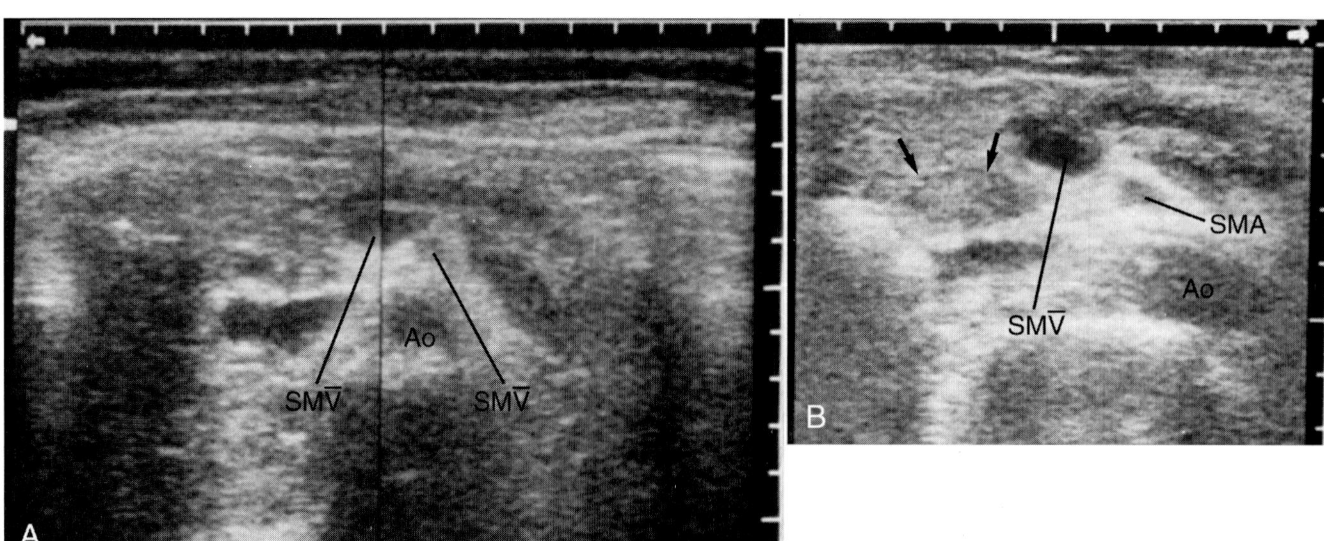


**FIG. 12.2. A.** On preoperative transverse ultrasonogram, no hypoechoic area is delineated. **B.** Intraoperative ultrasound recognizes a slightly hypoechogenic mass compared with the parenchyma of the pancreas, in the uncinate lobe *(arrows). SMA,* superior mesenteric artery; *SMV,* superior mesenteric vein; *Ao,* aorta.

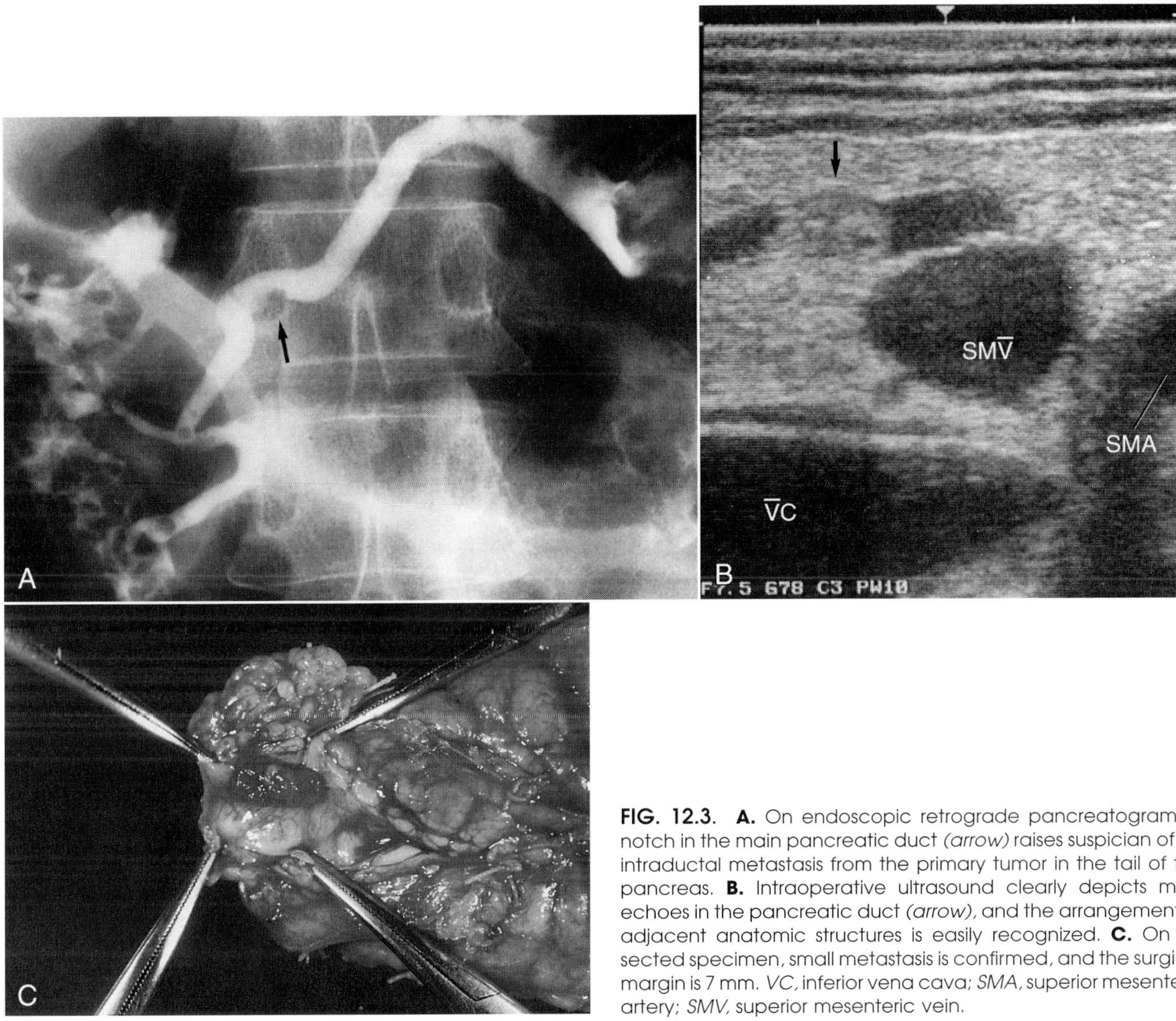


**FIG. 12.3.** **A.** On endoscopic retrograde pancreatogram, a notch in the main pancreatic duct *(arrow)* raises suspicion of an intraductal metastasis from the primary tumor in the tail of the pancreas. **B.** Intraoperative ultrasound clearly depicts mass echoes in the pancreatic duct *(arrow)*, and the arrangement of adjacent anatomic structures is easily recognized. **C.** On resected specimen, small metastasis is confirmed, and the surgical margin is 7 mm. *VC*, inferior vena cava; *SMA*, superior mesenteric artery; *SMV*, superior mesenteric vein.

ultrasound may add greater accuracy in guiding the needle for biopsy of a mass lesion.

The papillary type of ductal carcinoma and the cystadenocarcinomas may spread via the main pancreatic duct. Even though this may be recognized by endoscopic retrograde pancreatography or other imaging modalities during operation, only intraoperative ultrasound can demonstrate a papillary extension within the main duct from the surface of the pancreas and thus indicate the optimal point of resection (Fig. 12.3). Simultaneously, ultrasound alone can depict the adjacent anatomic structures. Low superficial spreading of the tumor, replacing the normal ductal mucosa, however, is difficult to delineate even by intraoperative ultrasound.

Advanced ductal carcinoma of the head of the pancreas often invades the superior mesenteric or portal veins. Intraoperative ultrasonography can not only demonstrate definite invasion of the vein by this hypoechoic tumor but can also demonstrate when the tumor only comes in contact with the wall of these veins. In the diagnosis of portal vein invasion by pancreatic carcinoma, the sensitivity of intraoperative ultrasound is superior to that of intraoperative portography or any preoperative study (15, 16). Although microscopic perineural invasion, a typical form of invasion by pancreatic carcinoma, cannot be diagnosed by ultrasound, intraoperative ultrasound can provide information early in the operation on which to base a decision whether or not to resect the portal vein. If resection of the portal vein is considered contraindicated, unnecessary dissection of tissue adjacent to the vein may be prevented.

During distal pancreatectomy for cancer, the relationship between the margins of the tumor and the superior mesenteric vein, an important anatomic landmark in this procedure, is easily demonstrated by intraoperative ultrasound prior to any dissection of those structures. Such information may provide important guidance for the surgeon's dissection (Fig. 12.4).

Finally, intraoperative ultrasonography may provide additional evidence of the presence and location of intrahepatic metastases of pancreatic cancer.

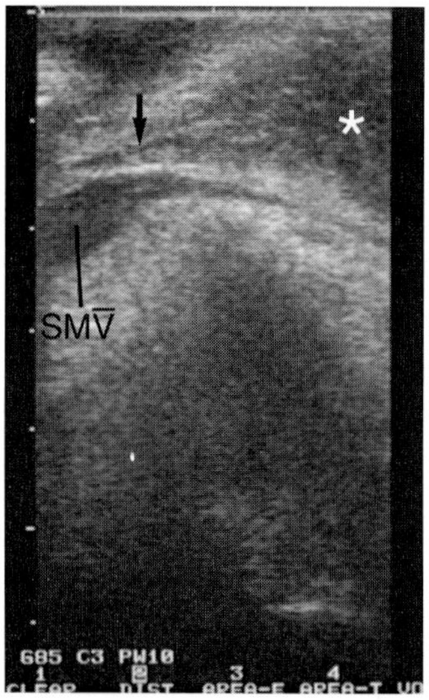


**FIG. 12.4.** Ductal carcinoma of the body of the pancreas appears as an ill-defined hypoechoic mass (*). From the course of the main pancreatic duct *(arrow)*, intraoperative ultrasound shows that 2 cm of surgical margin can be obtained when the pancreas is cut on a line in accordance with the center of the superior mesenteric vein *(SMV)*.

## REFERENCES

1. Knight PR, Newell JA. Operative use of ultrasonics in cholelithiasis. Lancet 1963;1:1023–1025.
2. Eiseman B, Greenlaw RH, Gallagher JQ. Localization of common duct stones by ultrasound. Arch Surg 1965;91:195–199.
3. Makuuchi M, Hasegawa H, Yamazaki S. Intraoperative ultrasonic examination for hepatectomy. Ultrasound Med Biol 1983;(suppl 2):493–497.
4. Lane RJ, Glazer G. Intra-operative B-mode ultrasound scanning of the extra-hepatic biliary system and pancreas. Lancet 1980; 2:334–337.
5. Sigel B, Coelho JC, Spigos DG, et al. Ultrasonic imaging during biliary and pancreatic surgery. Am J Surg 1981;141:84–89.
6. Makuuchi M, Hasegawa H, Yamazaki S. Ultrasonically guided subsegmentectomy. Surg Gynecol Obstet 1985;161:346–350.
7. Sigel B, Machi J, Kikuchi T, et al. The use of ultrasound during surgery for complications of pancreatitis. World J Surg 1987;11: 659–663.
8. Printz H, Klotter JH, Nies C, et al. Intraoperative ultrasonography in surgery for chronic pancreatitis. Int J Pancreatol 1992;12: 233–237.
9. Smith SJ, Vogelzang RL, Donovan J, et al. Intraoperative sonography of the pancreas. AJR 1985;144:557–562.
10. Sigel B, Machi J, Ramos JR, et al. The role of imaging ultrasound during pancreatic surgery. Ann Surg 1984;200:486–493.
11. Rucker KF, Klotter HJ, Kümmerle F. Intraoperative ultrasonic localization of endocrine tumors of the pancreas. Surgery 1984;96:1045–1047.
12. Norton JA, Shawker TH, Doppman JL. Localization and surgical treatment of occult insulinomas. Ann Surg 1990;212:615–620.
13. Grant CS, van Heerden J, Charboneau JW, et al. Insulinoma: the value of intraoperative ultrasonography. Arch Surg 1988;123: 843–848.
14. Rifkin MD, Weiss SM. Intraoperative sonographic identification of nonpalpable pancreatic masses. J Ultrasound Med 1984;3: 409–411.
15. Miyashita T, Suzuki T, Tani T, Uchida K, Tobe T. Ultrasonic diagnosis of portal invasion in pancreatic cancer (in Japanese). Jpn J Surg 1982;15:1338–1347.
16. Machi J, Siegel B, Zaren HA, Kjurohiji T, Yamashita Y. Operative ultrasonography during hepatobiliary and pancreatic surgery. World J Surg 1993;17:640–645.

# 13

# *Laparoscopy in the Management of Pancreatic Disease*

A. Cuschieri

Although laparoscopy was developed at the beginning of this century (1), its practice until recently has been largely restricted to gynecology, some hepatologists, and a few general surgeons with an interest in gastroenterology and hepatobiliary disease (2–6). The predominant reason for this limited use by surgeons was the lack of appreciation of the complete and detailed visual exposure of the peritoneal cavity and its contents by laparoscopy, which, with the right precautions, carries an extremely low morbidity (7–9). The turning point in the fortunes of laparoscopy was the advent of the charged couple device (CCD) endocamera and the resultant television display of the image. This immediately convinced the vast majority of surgeons of the immense practical value of this procedure. Laparoscopy is now firmly entrenched in surgical practice and will play an increasingly important role in the management of surgical disorders including oncology (10). This chapter deals with the techniques of safe laparoscopy, with special reference to pancreatic disease. Although retroperitoneal, the entire pancreas is accessible to laparoscopy. Visually guided target biopsy or fine-needle cytologic aspiration and laparoscopic contact ultrasound enhance the diagnostic and staging yield of the procedure. Certain operative procedures for benign and malignant pancreatic disease can now be performed laparoscopically. Some of these (e.g., cholecystectomy for acute pancreatitis) are established. Others, such as palliative bypass for inoperable proximal pancreatic cancer, resection of islet cell tumors, drainage of pseudocysts, and distal resections for chronic pancreatitis are under evaluation.

## General Considerations

A number of general considerations influence the practice of laparoscopy in the management of patients with surgical disorders. In the first instance, laparoscopy has to be regarded as an integral part of a surgical clinical practice, which is utilized routinely in problematic cases. In this respect, the occasional laparoscopist is both unsafe and unreliable. In the author's experience, there are a number of clinical situations the management of which will be influenced by early recourse to laparoscopy (Table 13.1). By contrast, the diagnostic yield of laparoscopy for chronic abdominal pain is much lower, although not inconsequential.

In the staging of established cancer, the problem is a logistic one, as obviously not all patients with cancer need or will benefit from a staging laparoscopy. The author's practice is outlined in Table 13.2 (11). This policy adopted over many years was subjected to a prospective audit over a 2-year period (12) in which the following outcome parameters were assessed: diagnostic yield, management benefit, and management disadvantage. In patients undergoing tumor staging, diagnostic benefit implied assessment of inoperability because of either metastatic deposits or significant local invasion. Patients were deemed to have benefited whenever the laparoscopic findings influenced the clinical decision on the management in the individual case. The results of this audit showed a diagnostic yield of 90%. Management benefit was obtained in 30% of patients, and only 4% were disadvantaged (missed hepatic secondary deposit in segment viii interpreted as no liver involvement; and involvement of the portal vein by carcinoma of the head of the pancreas, patient being deemed operable by laparoscopy). Both instances of management disadvantage occurred prior to the introduction of laparoscopic ultrasound scanning. In patients with intraabdominal malignancy, the benefit from laparoscopy often extends beyond establishing a diagnosis, as the procedure provides invaluable information on staging and often identifies inoperability, thereby avoiding needless laparotomy (13–19). In this respect, laparoscopy is the only reliable method for the detection of peritoneal deposits (13–16, 19, 20), short of exploratory laparatomy. In many of these incurable patients, palliative surgery, when indicated, can also be undertaken via the laparoscopic approach (21–24).

Experience and training in laparoscopy is essential for safety in the execution of the procedure and will avoid major iatrogenic vascular and visceral injuries. A number of situations enhance the risk of injury. These are shown in Table 13.3. They require special techniques and instrumentation.

**Techniques of Laparoscopy.** The classical technique of laparoscopy entails the initial creation of a pneumoperitoneum (usually with $CO_2$) using a Veress needle, followed by blind insertion of the trocar/cannula for the telescope. This is referred to as *closed laparoscopy*. In the unscarred abdomen, the technique is safe, provided the principles involved in its execution are strictly adhered to. Closed laparoscopy can be unsafe in the presence of adhesions, when one solution consists of the use of the *open laparoscopy* technique. In this instance, the creation of the initial pneumoperitoneum is avoided. Instead, the peritoneal cavity is entered through a small incision, and then a special olive-tipped cannula, the Hasson's cannula or one of its many disposable variants, is inserted and then connected to the $CO_2$ line. Many surgeons prefer to use open laparoscopy routinely for all their cases, which is quite acceptable and safe, although in the author's experience it does carry a number of disadvantages. It is often difficult to achieve a tight seal around the Hasson's cannula, and constant $CO_2$ leakage is inevitable. In benign cases, this carries a nuisance value only, but in malignant cases, it may predispose to tumor cell implantation. Secondly, in patients with adhesions, the initial wound may be sited inadvertently over an area of parietal adhesions. This will necessitate difficult adhesiolysis through the small access wound before the cannula can be inserted and the pneumoperitoneum established. Finally, the open laparoscopy technique can be difficult in very obese patients. The author reserves open laparoscopy for patients with abdominal distension due to intestinal obstruction.

**TABLE 13.1. Clinical Situations in Which Diagnostic Laparoscopy Offers Maximal Benefit to Patient Management**

- Suspected intraabdominal injury in a stable patient
  Both blunt and penetrating trauma
- Acute undiagnosed abdominal pain
  Patients with depressed level of consciousness
  Females of child-bearing age
  Elderly and the immunosuppressed
  Suspicion of mesenteric infarction
- Diagnosis and staging of tumors
- Ascites of unknown origin (negative cytology)

**TABLE 13.2. Indications for Diagnostic and Staging Laparoscopy in Patients with Malignant Disease**

- All patients with tumors that usually present at an advanced stage: pancreas, stomach, esophagus, liver, gallbladder
- All patients with mass lesions detected by diagnostic imaging
- Patients with ascites and a cytologically negative fluid sample
- All patients with hepatic lesions detected by the imaging tests
- All patients with unexplained weight loss
- Some patients with lymphomas

In patients with adhesions, there are a number of techniques that permit safe closed laparoscopy. With external ultrasound scanning using a 5.0-MHz linear array probe, a safe area free from adhesions can be established using the visceral slide technique (24). A visually guided technique using a beveled 5.5-mm metal cannula and a 5.0 forward-viewing telescope was first described by Semm (25). This has largely been replaced by modern disposable equivalents such as the Visiport loaded with a 10.0-mm forward-viewing optic (USSC, Norwalk, USA). Although some surgeons use the Visiport without prior pneumoperitoneum, this practice is unsafe because although the blade emerges momentarily for a distance of only 1.0 mm each time the instrument is fired, this may be sufficient to damage adherent bowel, since considerable pressure, and hence depression of the anterior abdominal wall, is needed during the penetration of the abdominal parietes by the Visiport.

Laparoscopy is of particular value in patients with ascites (26) and is indicated in patients in whom the cytologic examination of the peritoneal tap is negative or equivocal. The nature of the ascitic fluid, its cellular composition and the state of the peritoneal lining: inflammation, seedling or nodular deposits may be detected by laparoscopy. Such deposits are best biopsied by Robert's cup biopsy forceps. Special care is needed in performing diagnostic laparoscopy for ascites, as the air-filled small bowel loops float on the surface of the ascitic fluid and are therefore closely opposed to the anterior abdominal wall. This enhances the risk of bowel injury by the Veress needle during the creation of the pneumoperitoneum unless special precautions are taken. One approach is the use of open laparoscopy. The alternative is the careful insertion of the Veress needle unconnected to any tubing and with the tap opened. In this way, ascitic fluid will spurt out as soon as the tip of the Veress needle enters the peritoneal cavity. Sufficient ascitic fluid should be withdrawn to reduce the intraabdominal pressure before insufflation is started and the trocar/cannula inserted. In most instances, the primary tumor responsible for peritoneal carcinomatosis can be identified by laparoscopy. Accurate closure of the stab wounds is essential to prevent the development of a peritoneocutaneous fistula.

More recently, *gasless laparoscopy* using abdominal wall lift devices has been introduced (27). This is particularly useful in trauma cases, as it completely abolishes the risk of $CO_2$ embolism in the presence of traumatized vessels. However, with the current abdominal wall lift devices, the exposure is less adequate than that created by peritoneal insufflation. Thus gasless laparoscopy is unsuitable for elective diagnostic and staging laparoscopy.

## LAPAROSCOPIC ULTRASOUND SCANNING

Laparoscopic ultrasound scanning was first introduced by Frank et al. in 1983 (28). The technology has since been considerably improved with the advent of specifically designed laparoscopic transducer probes and real-time portable units. Modern ultrasonic transducers mainly use lead zirconate titanate (PZT), although some of the newer probes use vinylidene fluoride trifluoroethylene copolymer. In most modern scanners, mechanical or electronically controlled real-time systems are used. The speed of scanning is determined by the speed of sound, and the resolution depends on the wavelength and thus on the attenuation in the tissue. Wavelength frequency (MHz) aside, the improvement in the resolution provided by modern ultrasonic scanners is due to more sophisticated electronic signal processing by systems software of the reflected sound, providing a wider range of registration of the received signals on video storage tubes, with reduction of noise.

Contact ultrasonography employed during open and laparoscopic surgery allows the use of high-frequency probes (5.0–7.5 MHz) for maximum resolution. As the probe is in direct contact with the tissue, the sacrifice in depth of field (far field = 5.0–6.0 cm at these frequencies), which is inevitable with increased wavelength frequency, is not a problem. If the organ's depth exceeds this range (e.g., right lobe of the liver), contact scanning from the relevant two opposite surfaces ensures imaging of the entire parenchymal depth.

The value of intraoperative contact ultrasound scanning (IOCUS) in open surgery for liver tumors, biliary tract, and pancreas is beyond question (29–35). It detects deposits in the liver that are missed by preoperative imaging tests and are impalpable or invisible at operation, permits scan-guided biopsy, and assists in defining both inoperability and the extent of resection needed (29–33). In the case of pancreatic insulinomas, palpation of the pancreas together with IOCUS, permits localization of these tumors in 100% of cases (34).

The reported experience to date with laparoscopic contact ultrasonography is limited (35–37), but the results are encouraging, and the benefit should be equivalent to that accrued by IOCUS during open surgery. Laparoscopic ultrasound scanning has been used in the diagnosis of hepatic and gallbladder disease, ductal calculi, staging of cancer of the head of the pancreas and hepatic tumors, and examination of the hepatic parenchyma for secondary deposits and vascular invasion. More recently, we have extended the scope of laparoscopic ultrasound scanning to include examination of the neck and body of the pancreas (38).

Laparoscopic ultrasound examination of the liver is invaluable in the detection of focal lesions and secondary deposits and in the assessment of the resectability of primary tumors (36, 37). Contact ultrasound scanning permits the detection of deep

**TABLE 13.3. Difficult Laparoscopy**

- The very obese abdomen
- The scarred abdomen
- The distended abdomen from ascites or intestinal obstruction

lesions within the hepatic parenchyma not visualized by inspection of the surface of the liver. The technique is similar to that used in open surgery. Ultrasound scanning starts on the anterosuperior surface by identification of the vena cava at the back of the liver and subsequently the three hepatic veins that form the boundaries of the four sectors of the liver. The hepatic parenchyma of each sector is scanned from the vena cava downward to the free margin of the liver. On completion of the examination through the anterosuperior surface, the probe is placed underneath the lobes of the liver for scanning of the hepatic parenchyma from below. Examination of the entire depth of the hepatic parenchyma (especially on the right side) is ensured by this combined approach.

Cystic structures within the hepatic parenchyma are readily identified, as they contain few or no internal echoes, exhibit good transmission, and have sharply defined walls. Solid lesions (tumors) are more difficult to delineate and exhibit various sonographic patterns: hypoechoic or sonolucent, hyperechoic, or complex. The hypoechoic lesions can usually be differentiated from cysts because they have a different sound attenuation and indefinite margins. Hypoechoic lesions are usually composed of solid tumors without necrosis (39). Hyperechoic lesions exhibit intense and uniform echo reflectivity, which indicates a prominent vascular component consisting of dilated vessels (39). Hyperechoicity can also be caused by fatty change. Complex lesions have both hyper- and hypoechoic regions, which reflect viable and necrotic areas within a lesion, respectively. In some malignant tumors, alternating rings of hypo- and hyperechoic regions give rise to a "bull's eye" appearance. However, there are no reliable ultrasonographic findings that differentiate between benign and malignant tumors or between primary and metastatic hepatic disease. The most hyperechoic lesion encountered in the liver is the hemangioma. This is readily identified by its macroscopic appearance during laparoscopy and is, of course, compressible. If a solid (nonvascular) lesion is detected, an ultrasonically guided biopsy using the Bioptit or Trucut needle is performed (40).

The advent of laparoscopic contact ultrasonography has improved the diagnosis of cancer of the gallbladder, since early mucosal and intramural lesions can be identified. Better definition of the parenchymal anatomy of the gallbladder is obtained by scanning the organ from the superior surface of the liver. The gold standard preoperative investigation for the diagnosis of cancer of the gallbladder in current practice is external abdominal ultrasound scanning. A comparative study on the relative diagnostic yield of external ultrasound scanning and laparoscopy has been reported (41). In this study, 53 patients with suspected carcinoma of the gallbladder were investigated by external abdominal ultrasonography and laparoscopy. The latter correctly excluded malignancy in five patients in whom external abdominal ultrasonography was suggestive or equivocal. Cancer of the gallbladder was confirmed in the remainder ($n$ = 48 patients). Laparoscopy identified 46 of these tumors (96%), and external ultrasonography, 30 (63%). Distant metastases in the liver, parietal peritoneum, or omentum were present in 41 patients (85%) and were detected by laparoscopy in 39 (sensitivity 95%) and by ultrasonography in 21 (sensitivity 51%). The combination of external ultrasonography and laparoscopy resulted in an overall diagnostic accuracy rate of 100%. Histologic material for definitive diagnosis was provided by laparoscopy in 36 patients (75%). The procedure, by establishing the presence of advanced disease, avoided unnecessary laparotomy in 40 patients. A correct staging of resectable localized disease was made by laparoscopy in 5 out of 6 patients.

More than any other imaging modality, ultrasonography requires a skilled operator who is also an experienced interpreter. There is little doubt that with training, surgeons, by virtue of their knowledge of the structural and topographic anatomy, can become experienced, reliable ultrasound operators within a relatively short interval. The utility of laparoscopic ultrasound scanning depends as much on the acquisition of the necessary skills in manipulation of the probe and in the interpretation of the scanned images as on the quality of the equipment and probes used.

## LAPAROSCOPIC EXPOSURE OF THE PANCREAS

There are two approaches for the laparoscopic examination of the body and tail of the pancreas: the *supragastric* and the *infragastric* techniques (4, 15, 42, 43). To some extent they are complementary, in that both can be used in the same patient and the number and sites of the access ports necessary are the same. The supragastric technique provides a good exposure of the central portion of the pancreas in thin patients (Fig. 13.1). The method is difficult in obese individuals and is impossible if there are adhesions binding the pancreas to the lesser sac. In addition, the neck of the pancreas and the tail of the organ cannot be inspected adequately by this technique. By contrast, the infragastric approach is almost always technically feasible, as adhesions can be divided, and the entire region from the gastroduodenal artery on the right side to the tail of the gland and the splenic hilium on the left can be visualized (Fig. 13.2). In this technique the lesser sac is entered by ligature and division of 3–4 gastroepiploic vessels along the greater curvature of the stomach. Once inside the lesser sac, even the posterior surface of the pancreas and the confluence of the portal venous system can be visualized and inspected (Fig. 13.3). This extensive mobilization may be necessary during the search for occult islet cell tumors.

Mobilization of the head of the pancreas is carried out laparoscopically using a technique that closely approximates the Kockerisation method used in open surgery. The duodenum is grasped and pulled to the left to enable visualization of the paraduodenal gutter, the peritoneal covering of which is divided. An oblique, 30 or 45°, 10-mm telescope is essential, and the dissection is considerably expedited by the use of curved coaxial instruments (44). The pancreatic head is lifted from the retroperitoneum and the vena cava by gentle blunt dissection. Following mobilization, excellent ultrasound scanning of the proximal (head) pancreas is obtained by placement of the linear array probe behind the head of the pancreas, with the transducer facing

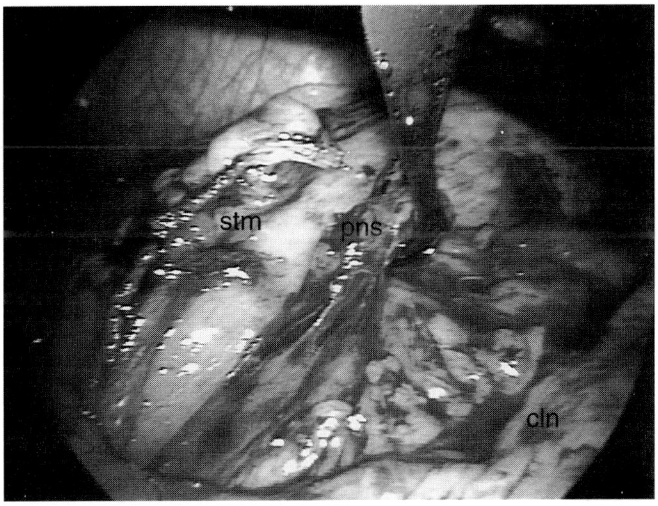


**FIG. 13.1.** Exposure of the body and tail of the pancreas by the laparoscopic infragastric approach. *Stm,* stomach; *Pns,* pancreas; *cln,* colon. See color insert.

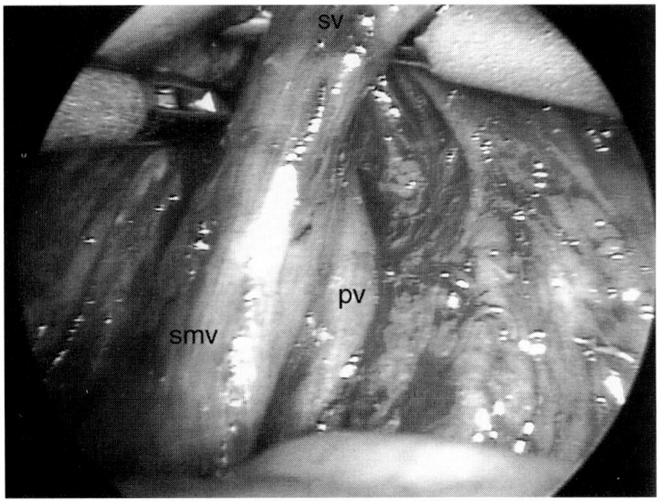


**FIG. 13.2.** Laproscopic retropancreatic exposure of the confluence of the splenic, superior mesenteric, and portal veins. *SV,* splenic vein; *SMV,* superior mesenteric vein; *PV,* portal vein. See color insert.

upward. Detailed examination of the pancreatic parenchyma, the intrapancreatic segment of the bile duct, the common channel and ampullary region, the lesion, and its encroachment on the pancreatic duct and portal vein can be determined (Fig. 13.4).

## ROLE OF LAPAROSCOPY IN ACUTE PANCREATITIS

Laparoscopic cholecystectomy is now the standard surgical treatment for gallstone-associated acute pancreatitis and, in patients with mild-to-moderate acute pancreatitis, should be performed during the same hospital admission (45). [*Editor's note:* see also Chapters 22 and 28.] This is considered preferable to interval cholecystectomy. The issue relating to the frequent presence of ductal stones remains unsettled. Currently, most surgeons resort to preoperative endoscopic retrograde cholangiopancreatography (ERCP) with endoscopic stone extraction when necessary. Others, including the author, proceed to cholecystectomy without recourse to ERCP but perform transcystic intraoperative cholangiography during the cholecystectomy. Small distal calculi, when present, can be extracted in the vast majority of cases through the cystic duct, using Dormia or Sigura baskets, with either cholangiographic control by means of an image intensifier or visually guided by means of a 3.5- to 2.8-mm flexible miniendoscope introduced into the common bile duct through the dilated cystic duct (46, 47). The merit of this approach is the avoidance of routine ERCP, which proves normal in at least 50% of cases, and a sphincterotomy, particularly in young people. After transcystic extraction of ductal calculi, it is our practice to insert a fine cystic duct drainage cannula (Fr 7–8) into the common duct, securing it to the cystic duct remnant with a catgut Roeder slipknot (48). This approach ensures immediate postoperative biliary drainage and allows a postoperative check for complete ductal clearance. There are no reported prospective clinical trials comparing these two approaches, although one such study carried out under the auspices of the European Society for Endoscopic Surgeons has completed its recruitment. At present, the management of ductal calculi in patients undergoing laparoscopic cholecystectomy depends entirely on the local expertise available.

Some of the complications of acute pancreatitis can be dealt with laparoscopically. This applies particularly to pancreatic pseudocysts. These can be drained through the transgastric approach. The infracolic technique (49) is used by the author. This approach entails proximal displacement of the transverse colon to expose the bulging inferior wall of the cyst stretching the transverse mesocolon close to the duodenojejunal junction. A small hand-sutured or stapled anastomosis is performed between the pseudocyst and the adjacent upper jejunum. Early attempts are being made on laparoscopic debridement and necrosectomy for acute necrotizing pancreatitis, but the experience is limited to one center, and no conclusions on its efficacy and benefit can be drawn. This approach to a difficult problem is attractive, since it should permit repeated interventions in these very seriously ill patients, without recourse to laparotomy (50).

## DIAGNOSIS AND STAGING OF PANCREATIC CANCER BY LAPAROSCOPY

Pancreatic cancer patients present with cholestatic jaundice, and the diagnosis is usually confirmed by external ultrasonography and computed tomography (CT) followed by ERCP. In the author's reported experience of a series of patients with pancreatic cancer in whom laparotomy was immediately preceded by laparoscopy, no instance of laparoscopically assessed inoperability was found to be incorrect at operation (15). However, some 20% of patients who were judged to be operable by laparoscopy were found to be unresectable at laparotomy because of invasion of the portal vein. This study was conducted before the advent of laparoscopic ultrasound examination, which can reliably detect vascular invasion.

A more recent seminal study by Warshaw (16) involved cytologic examination of peritoneal saline washings during laparoscopy ($n$ = 27) and laparotomy ($n$ =13) in patients with pancreatic ductal adenocarcinoma whose tumors had been judged to be potentially resectable by CT. Malignant cells were found in the peritoneal washings in 12 of 40 patients: 29% in cancers of the pancreatic head versus 40% in the body. The washings were positive for malignant cells in 33% obtained by laparoscopy and 23% at laparotomy. Malignant cells were identified in washings from 4 of 8 patients with ascites and 8 of 32 without. The cytology was positive in 6 of 8 patients who had

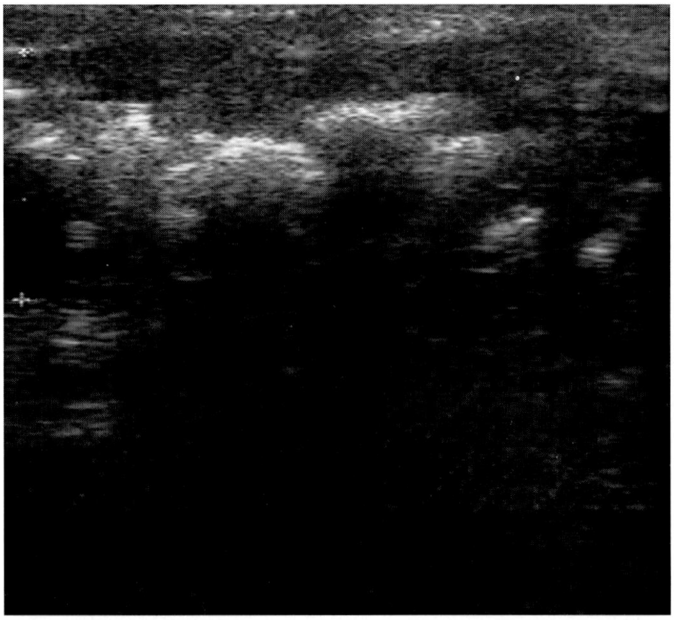

**FIG. 13.3.** Laparoscopic contact ultrasonography of the pancreas. (+), Grossly dilated duct containing calculi.

**LAPAROSCOPIC STAGING**

- **OPERABLE DISEASE:** ⇒ **LAPAROTOMY** ⇒ **PANCREATICODUODENECTOMY**
- **INOPERABLE DISEASE:**

⇓ **SUBSTANTIAL INTRAPERITONEAL ± HEPATIC DISEASE** ⇓ *ENDOSCOPIC STENTING*

⇓ **MINIMAL INTRAPERITONEAL ± MINIMAL HEPATIC DISEASE** ⇓ *LAPAROSCOPIC BILIARY BYPASS*

⇓ **GASTRIC OUTLET OBSTRUCTION** ⇓ *LAPAROSCOPIC DOUBLE BYPASS*

**FIG. 13.4.** Algorithm for the management of patients with inoperable pancreatic cancer.

a prior percutaneous needle biopsy, versus 6 of 32 in whom this procedure was not performed. Hepatic metastases were found in six patients, all with negative cytology. Only 1 of 10 cancers in the pancreatic head with positive cytology was resectable, compared with 13 of 25 with negative cytology ($p < .05$). Survival was significantly longer in patients with negative cytology. This study demonstrated that pancreatic cancer sheds malignant cells into the peritoneum early and frequently and that laparoscopic saline lavage is an effective means of cytologic study that provides an additional index of resectability and has prognostic implications. The high incidence of positive cytology in patients who had percutaneous scan-guided needle biopsy is worrisome and requires further attention.

Laparoscopic diagnosis and staging of pancreatic cancer consist of six steps:

1. Inspection of the peritoneal cavity, omentum, serosal surfaces of the small intestine, and liver with biopsy of suspect lesions
2. Inspection and palpation of the gallbladder, duodenum, and hepatoduodenal ligament
3. Biopsy/cytology of the primary lesion
4. Cholecystocholangiography
5. Mobilization of the head of the pancreas and duodenal curve
6. Ultrasonographic examination of the head of the pancreas, portal vein, and liver

The assessment of the lesion and its local infiltration to surrounding structures is carried out after the peritoneal cavity and the liver have been inspected. Suspicious or frankly metastatic lesions on the peritoneal surfaces (including the diaphragm and falciform ligament) or in the liver are biopsied and subjected to frozen section histology. If metastatic disease is confirmed in this way, detailed examination of the primary, its biopsy, and ultrasound scanning (steps 2, 3, 5, 6) are unnecessary, and the examination is limited to assessment of the duodenal encroachment by tumor. The decision should then be made to as to whether to palliate the patient by laparoscopic bilioenteric bypass or by endoscopic stenting.

The hepatoduodenal area is then inspected. Usually the dilated common bile duct is obvious, and in some cases, the upward extension of the tumor beyond the duodenal bulb can be detected. Also enlarged lymph nodes in the porta hepatis and to the right of the bile duct, low down, can be visualized. The involvement of the duodenum by the tumor is assessed by picking its anterior wall and lifting it from the mass. The degree of lift, pliability, or induration of the walls of the duodenum are determined starting at the level of the pylorus and processing along the duodenal bulb and the second part of the duodenum.

Transduodenal Trucut needle biopsy is the safest technique for biopsy of a mass lesion in the pancreatic head. Fine-needle aspiration cytology can be used instead, but the yield is lower than that obtained by the needle core biopsy technique. The advantage of fine-needle aspiration is that the small needle puncture in the anterior duodenal wall does not require suturing.

A laparoscopic cholecystocholangiogram is indicated *(a)* when the ERCP demonstrates complete or near total occlusion of the bile duct such that the proximal biliary tree is not outlined by this investigation and *(b)* before laparoscopic bilioenteric bypass, when it is essential in the selection of the appropriate bypass (cholecystojejunostomy or a choledochojejunostomy), depending on the proximity of the upper extension of the tumor to the entry of the cystic duct into the common bile duct (21). If decompression of the biliary tree is intended by an immediate laparoscopic bilioenteric bypass, then the small hole in the gallbladder can be ignored. Suture closure of the gallbladder puncture is necessary if decompression is not contemplated.

Mobilization of the duodenum and head of the pancreas is facilitated by use of the coaxial curved instruments introduced through flexible metal cannulae. The fascial plane between the posterior surface of the head of the pancreas is obliterated if there is posterior extension of the tumor, when attempts to dissect it should be resisted, as the lesion will prove to be inoperable, and persistence is likely to lead to major bleeding from damage to the vena cava, the right adrenal, or the left renal vein.

## LAPAROSCOPIC PALLIATIVE BYPASS FOR ADVANCED CANCER

There is now sufficient experience to demonstrate that palliation of obstruction of a large bile duct, as well as gastric outflow encroachment by inoperable proximal pancreatic cancer, can be obtained laparoscopically (21–23, 51). The Dundee experience indicates that these patients do well and do not require further hospital admissions other than for terminal care. The determination of efficient cystic duct drainage by operative cholecystocholangiography is essential for a functioning cholecystojeunostomy (21), and we recommend a distance of 1.5 cm or more between the entry of the cystic duct into the common bile duct and the upper limit of the common duct obstruction by the pancreatic tumor. If a laparoscopic cholecystojejunostomy (sutured or stapled) is performed in the presence of adjacent tumor, the palliation achieved will be limited and short-lived. Thus a cholecystocholangiogram is essential before a surgeon embarks on a laparoscopic cholecystojejunostomy. Patients in whom the cystic duct drainage into the common duct is compromised by the upper limit of the neoplasm, require alternative surgical drainage, choledochojejunostomy or segment III bypass, or endoscopic stenting. In patients undergoing laparoscopic biliary bypass (cholecystojejunostomy or choledochojejunostomy), gastrojejunostomy is added only if there are symptoms of gastric outlet obstruction or evidence of significant duodenal encroachment at laparoscopy. This selective policy is justified, since only 5 of 18 patients undergoing laparoscopic biliary bypass for inoperable proximal pancreatic cancer subsequently needed gastrojejunostomy for disseminated disease.

The key issue relates to the relative merits of endoscopic stenting and laparoscopic biliary bypass. In the absence of prospective randomized trials, which are needed to determine the relative merits and indications, a useful algorithm on the management of these patients is shown in Figure 13.4. This is based on two main considerations: *(a)* the extent of disease and estimated survival and *(b)* the presence or absence of gastric outlet obstruction. Thus it seems sensible and expedient to resort to endoscopic stenting in patients with advanced disease in whom the expected survival is measured in weeks and who do not have duodenal obstruction.

## LAPAROSCOPIC PANCREATIC RESECTIONS

Although technically feasible, there is no benefit to the patient in laparoscopic pancreaticoduodenectomy. Indeed, the clinical outcome may be jeopardized by the long and laborious endoscopic procedure (52). Pancreaticoduodenectomy is one instance of a major operation in which the access wound constitutes only a small proportion of the total operative trauma, and thus the benefit from reduction of the exposure wound is practically nonexistent. By contrast, distal (70–80%) pancreatectomy for chronic pancreatitis or benign cystadenomas benefits from the laparoscopic approach, provided the surgeon is experienced in both endoscopic and pancreatic surgery (53). Maximum benefit is obtained by the laparoscopic localization and enucleation of islet cell tumors of the pancreas, especially insulinomas (45).

## MORBIDITY OF LAPAROSCOPY

### Iatrogenic Injuries

Much has been written lately on the morbidity of laparoscopy and laparoscopic interventions. The injuries are sustained either *(a)* during the initial creation of the pneumoperitoneum and insertion of the first trocar cannula or *(b)* during the execution of an operative procedure. The first category of injuries, visceral or vascular (54, 55), can be substantially reduced by training and recourse to the appropriate techniques in high-risk cases (see above). Injuries during the course of an operation can result from faulty technique, e.g. misuse of thermal energy (laser or electrosurgery), by inattention trauma when the assisting instrument is out of the operative (telescope) field, and by misperception of the anatomy displayed on the television monitor. The last is probably the most important and has been largely overlooked (56). Diminished resolution, compared with direct normal vision, abnormalities in the eye fixation/refixation movements (saccades) and accommodation, and fatigue contribute to these misinterpretation errors. Research in this area together with the development of alternative image-display technology to the current television monitor will considerably enhance the safety of endoscopic surgery.

## TUMOR DISSEMINATION

Several cases have been reported of neoplastic involvement of the access cutaneous wounds, and these port site deposits usually are clinically manifest within 3–4 months after the operation (57–64). The exact incidence of these port site deposits is not known, and valid comparisons with similar incidents after open ablative procedures for intraabdominal cancer are not possible in the absence of randomized clinical trials. Reported figures vary from 1.4 to 2.0%. It is perhaps important to define a port site deposit as *a malignant localized lesion that involves the musculoaponeurotic layers of the abdominal wall with an underlying intact pneumoperitoneum, in the absence of peritoneal dissemination* (63). In this context, some reported instances of "port site deposits" simply reflect widespread tumor recurrence. Port site deposits are thought to be the result of "implantation" and subsequent growth of tumor cells rather than metastatic spread of tumor emboli to the site of fresh healing wounds, although this has not been established. Several histologic tumor types have been implicated from a variety of primary sites, and the risk is thought to be influenced by tumor grade (65). The source of these port site deposits is likely to be from exfoliated tumor cells shed from the primary tumor or secondary deposits. The exfoliation occurs naturally with certain tumors or is induced by surgical manipulation of tumors with serosal involvement during the procedure. Thus exfoliation, spontaneous or procedure-induced, would appear to be a crucial event in the process. The other theoretical source of such an inoculum may be vascular or lymphatic embolization of tumor.

Many gastrointestinal cancers shed malignant cells within the peritoneal cavity. Malignant cells are found by cytology of peritoneal saline washing fluid in 30% of patients with pancreatic ductal adenocarcinoma (66). It is more common in lesions of the body than in cancers of the pancreatic head. In pancreatic cancer, cytology is more frequently positive in patients with ascites than in those without. In patients with gastric cancer, serosal invasion is associated with positive cytology in 31% of patients, and infiltration by cancer of another organ is attended by positive cytology in 65% of patients. In addition, there is a positive correlation between the extent of the serosal area infiltrated by cancer and the tumor cell count in peritoneal washings, indicating that free cancer cells in the peritoneal cavity are mainly derived from this source. Poorly differentiated gastric adenocarcinoma is more frequently associated with positive cytology. Most free gastric cancer cells recovered from these peritoneal saline washes are viable (67). In colorectal cancer, malignant peritoneal cells were found in peritoneal washings taken prior to resection of the primary tumor in 11 of 35 patients (68) and in 13 of 287 patients with no evidence of macroscopic peritoneal dissemination (69).

Vascular permeability factor (VPF), also known as vascular endothelial growth factor, enhances vascular permeability and has endothelial cell–specific mitogenic activity. It is synthesized by many human normal and tumor cells. High levels of VPF are found in effusions with cytology-documented malignant cells. It is possible that VPF expression by tumor and mononuclear cells contributes to the plasma exudation and fluid accumulation associated with malignant and certain inflammatory effusions (70). Fibronectin is present in significantly higher concentrations in the ascitic fluid from patients with cytologically positive malignant ascites than in fluid from those with ascites but negative cytology (71). Fibronectin has been implicated in tumor cell attachment (72). Urokinase (u-PA) is a proteinase found in malignant ascites in significantly higher concentrations than in ascites due to alcoholic cirrhosis (73). Urokinase-induced proteolysis of the extracellular matrix appears to be involved in stromal invasion by tumor cells and metastasis (74).

There are several potential mechanisms by which a sustained positive-pressure $CO_2$ pneumoperitoneum may cause tumor spread within the peritoneal cavity or enhance implantation of exfoliated tumors in surgical wounds. The positive-pressure pneumoperitoneum may increase the risk of vascular or lymphatic tumor embolization. Leakage of gas around access ports causes local turbulence, which drives increasing numbers of exfoliated tumor cells into the access wounds. *For this reason, following completion of a laparoscopic procedure for malignancy, the pneumoperitoneum should be aspirated by a sucker rather than subjected to sudden deflation.* The results of animal experiments have demonstrated that during pneumoperitoneum at a pressure of 14 mm Hg, there is a significant decrease in jejunal mucosal blood flow, causing ischemia, as evidenced by a significant drop in intramural jejunal pH. In addition, portal and inferior vena cava pressures become significantly elevated, and the partial pressure of carbon dioxide in these vessels is elevated (75). After insufflation, cardiac output and blood flow in the superior mesenteric artery and portal vein decrease progressively. The net effect is a decrease in total hepatic blood flow. Mechanical compression of the splanchnic capillary beds caused by the elevated intraabdominal pressure probably accounts in part for the increase in systemic vascular resistance underlying the decreased cardiac output (76, 77). The plasma arginine vasopressin levels are elevated during positive-pressure pneumoperitoneum (78), probably consequent on a decrease in the left atrial transmural pressure gradient. The reduced superior mesenteric and jejunal mucosal blood flow (75) may be significant in the suppression of host immunity. Intestinal ischemia in dogs produces a substance that depresses platelet aggregation, which has been shown to contribute to reticuloendothelial phagocytic function (79). The effect of decreased hepatic blood flow, particularly during prolonged laparoscopic procedures, on the hepatic endothelial and Kupffer cells is not known. However, a positive correlation between phagocytic capacity and blood flow through the liver and spleen has been reported (80). The liver is the target organ in the development of hematogenous metastases from primary cancers of the GI tract. Tumor cells have been detected in hepatic sinusoids in apposition to the endothelial and parenchymal cells (81). Specific cell-surface molecules on the endothelial cells, possibly activated by local cytokine release (82), are probably involved in the adherence of these metastatic cells to the sinusoidal endothelium. Escape through the endothelial barrier appears to be necessary for the establishment of metastatic foci, since this enables the malignant cells to avoid destruction by the Kupffer and pit cells (83). The cytotoxicity of human Kupffer cells to colonic adenocarcinoma in vitro is established (84), and experimentally, suppression of the Kupffer cells increases the size and number of metastases (85). Hence, Kupffer cells may serve a useful defense role in the destruction of tumor cells that enter the portal circulation. The depression of the hepatic reticuloendothelial system by the reduced hepatic perfusion observed during laparoscopy may favor the establishment of metastatic lesions within this organ.

The raised intraabdominal pressure above capillary pressure (15 mm Hg at the venous end) and venular pressure ($<15$ mm Hg) can potentially compress these vascular beds. While compression of the venous capillary beds and lymphatics may prevent leakage of cancer cells from these vessels during pneumoperitoneum, the potential for the escape of these cells from these cut vessels after desufflation is possible and unpredictable.

The extent of surgical trauma appears to determine the degree of postoperative nonspecific immune supression (86, 87). This is important in view of the established relationship between immunocompetence and survival after cancer surgery (88). Results of experimental studies indicate a possible correlation between surgical stress and the incidence, rate, and size of subsequent metastases (89). It appears likely that the nonspecific immunosuppression following surgery may encourage both the implantation of surgically disseminated tumor cells and the growth of existing micrometastases (90). Surgery is followed by suppression of lymphocyte function (91). Documented disturbances in immune function postoperatively include decrease in lymphocyte chemotaxis, neutrophil adherence, and delayed-type hypersensitivity (92). The NK cells form an important component of the effector arm of the cellular immune response. These cells provide the first line of defense against the metastatic implantation of circulating tumor emboli (93). Surgical stress has been shown to exert a direct toxic effect on NK cell activity, localized to a specific phase of the NK cell-tumor cell lysis, i.e., postbinding programing (94).

Endoscopic surgery provides a convenient model for studying the effect of minimizing surgical trauma and thus the extent of immune suppression. In some comparative studies with open cholecystectomy, the laparoscopic operation showed a reduced acute-phase response (granulocyte count and interleukin-6 levels, glucose, C-reactive protein) at 24 hours after surgery. Likewise, phytohemagglutinin responsiveness (a sensitive indicator of T-cell function) was significantly reduced after open cholecystectomy, in contrast to laparoscopy. Further, flow cytometric analysis of blood mononuclear cells revealed a reduction of HLA-DR expression on monocytes (essential for the presentation of endocytosed antigens to T-cells (95)) after conventional, but not after laparoscopic, cholecystectomy (96). In another study, T-cell-related immune function, as measured by delayed-type hypersensitivity, was better preserved after laparoscopic than open colon resections (97). Hypochlorus acid production by neutrophils was down-regulated significantly after conventional surgery but remained similar to preoperative values after laparoscopic or laparoscopic-assisted surgery (98). Although some reports have shown abrogation of the acute-phase response after laparoscopic surgery (99), others have failed to confirm this (100, 101). While most reports suggest that laparoscopic surgery is less immunosuppressive than conventional open surgery because of the reduction of the trauma of access, most of these studies have been performed in relatively healthy patients with benign disease undergoing small ablative procedures such as cholecystectomy, and for this reason, the results have to be interpreted with caution. A practical consideration relates to the fact that major ablative surgery for cancer takes considerably longer to execute endoscopically. The total operating and anesthesia time incurred by the endoscopic approach is therefore substantially greater. This may influence the level of immune suppression in patients undergoing endoscopic ablative procedures as opposed to simple cholecystectomy for benign disease.

## REFERENCES


1. Kelling G. Zur coelioskopie. Arch Klin Chir 1923;126:226–229.
2. Henning H. Diagnostic procedures in the evaluation of hepatic disease. Laparoscopy. Lab Res Meth Biol Med 1983;7: 469–488.
3. Trujillo NP. Peritoneoscopy and guided biopsy in the diagnosis of intra-abdominal disease. Gastroenterology 1976;71:1083–1085.
4. Berci G, Shore JM, Morgenstern LM, Shapiro S. A direct approach to the differential diagnosis of jaundice. Am J Surg 1973;126:577–586.
5. Cuschieri A. Value of laparoscopy in hepatobiliary disease. Ann R Coll Surg Engl 1975;57:33–38.
6. Lightdale CJ. Clinical application of laparoscopy in patients with malignant neoplasms. Gastrointest Endosc 1982;28:99–102.
7. Villardel F, Seres I, Marti-Vincenti A. Complications of peritoneoscopy. A survey of 1455 examinations. Gastrointest Endosc 1967;14:178–180.
8. Chamberlain G, Brown JC. Gynaecological laparoscopy. The report of a working party in a confidential enquiry of gynaecological laparoscopy. London: Royal College of Obstetricians and Gynaecologists, 1978.
9. Cuschieri A. Laparoscopy in general surgery and gastroenterology. Br J Hosp Med 1980;24:252–258.
10. Greene FL. Laparoscopy in malignant disease. Surg Clin North Am 1992;72:1125–1137.
11. Cuschieri A. Diagnosis and staging of tumors by laparoscopy. Semin Laparosc Surg 1994;1:3–12.
12. Vander Velpen GC, Shimi SM, Cuschieri A. Diagnostic yield and management benefit of laparoscopy: a prospective audit. Gut 1994;1617–1621.
13. Pagliaro AL, Arinaldi F, Craxi A, et al. Percutaneous blind biopsy versus laparoscopy with guided biopsy in diagnosis of cirrhosis. Dig Dis Sci 1983;28:39–43.
14. Cuschieri A, Hall AW, Clark J. Value of laparoscopy in the diagnosis and management of pancreatic cancer. Gut 1978; 19:672–677.
15. Cuschieri A. Laparoscopy for pancreatic cancer: does it benefit the patient? Eur J Surg Oncol 1988;14:41–44.
16. Warshaw AL, Tepper JE, Shipley WU. Laparoscopy in the staging and planning of therapy for pancreatic cancer. Am J Surg 1986;151:76–79.
17. Possik RA, Franco EL, Pires DR, et al. Sensitivity, specificity and predictive value of laparoscopy for the staging of gastric cancer and for the detection of liver metastases. Cancer 1986;18:1–6.
18. Shandall A, Johnson C. Laparoscopy or scanning in oesophageal and gastric carcinoma? Br J Surg 1985;72:449–451.
19. Ishida H, Furukawa Y, Kuroda H, et al. Laparoscopic observation and biopsy of the pancreas. Endoscopy 1981;13:68–73.
20. Ishida H. Peritoneoscopy and pancreas biopsy in the diagnosis of pancreatic disease. Gastrointest Endosc 1983;29:211–216.
21. Shimi SM, Banting SB, Cuschieri A. Laparoscopy in the management of pancreatic cancer: endoscopic cholecystojejunostomy for advanced disease. Br J Surg 1992;79:317–319.
22. Hawasli A. Laparoscopic cholecysto-jejunostomy for obstructing pancreatic cancer: technique and report of two cases. J Laparoendosc Surg 1992;2:351–355.
23. Brune IB, Schonleben K. Laparoscopic side-to-side gastrojejunostomy. Chirurg 1992;63:577–580.
24. Kolecki RV, Golub RM, Sigel B, et al. Accuracy of visceral slide detection of abdominal wall adhesions by ultrasound. Surg Endosc 1994;8:871–874.
25. Semm K. Operative manual of endoscopic abdominal surgery. Chicago: Year Book Medical Publishers, 1987:141–142.
26. Berci G, Cuschieri A. Practical laparoscopy. London: Bailliere-Tindall, 1986:82–94.
27. Smith S, Eubanks S, Swanstrom L, Wolfe B. Gasless laparoscopy: the next phase of laparoscopic surgery? Contemp Surg 1994; 45:171–183.
28. Frank K, Bliesze H, Beck, et al. Laparoscopic sonography. A new dimension in the diagnostic approach to internal organs. Dtsch Med Wochenschr 1983;108:902–904.
29. Bismuth H, Castaing D, Garden OJ. The use of operative ultrasound in the surgery of primary liver cancer. World J Surg 1987:11:610–614.
30. Parker GA, Lawrence W Jr, Horsley JS, et al. Intraoperative ultrasound of the liver affects operative decision making. Ann Surg 1989;209:569–576.
31. Clarke MP, Kane RA, Steele G Jr, et al. Prospective comparison of preoperative imaging and intraoperative ultrasonography in the detection of liver tumors. Surgery 1989;106:849–855.
32. Brower ST, Dumitrescu O, Rubinoff S, et al. Operative ultrasound establishes resectability of metastases by major hepatic resection. World J Surg 1989;13:649–657.
33. Russo A, La Rosa C, Cajozzo M, et al. Screening for liver metastases of colorectal carcinoma by the routine use of intraoperative echography. Minerva Chir 1989;44:1893–1900.
34. Galiber AK, Reading CC, Charboneau JW. Localisation of pancreatic insulinoma: comparison of pre- and intraoperative US and CT and angiography. Radiology 1988:166:504–508.
35. Rothlin M, Schlumpf R, Largiader F. The technique of intraoperative ultrasonography in laparoscopic cholecystectomy. Chirurg 1991;62:899–901.
36. Fornari F, Civardi G, Cavanna L, et al. Laparoscopic ultrasonography in the study of liver disease. Preliminary results. Surg Endosc 1989;3:33–37.
37. Miles WFA, Paterson-Brown S, Garden OJ. Laparoscopic contact hepatic ultrasonography. Br J Surg 1992:79:419–420.
38. Pietrabissa A, Shimi S, Cuschieri A. Detection of occult insulinoma by laparoscopic infragastric pancreatic contact ultrasound scanning. Surg Oncol 1993;2:83–86.
39. Tanaka, S, Kitamura T, Imaoka S, et al. Hepatocellular carcinoma: sonographic and histological correlation. Am J Roentgenol 1983;140:701–707.
40. Fornari F, Rapaccini L, Cavanna L, et al. Diagnosis of hepatic lesions: ultrasonically guided fine needle biopsy or laparoscopy? Gastrointest Endosc 1988;34:231–234.
41. Kriplani AK, Jayant S, Kapur BM. Laparoscopy in primary carcinoma of the gallbladder. Gastrointest Endosc 1992;38: 326–329.
42. Meyer-Burg J, Ziegler U, Palma C. Zur supragastralen pankeaskopie. Ergebnisse aus 125 laparoskopien. Dtsch Med Wochenschr 1969;97;1969–1971.
43. Strauch M, Lux G, Ottenjann R. Infragastric pancreascopy. Endoscopy 1973;5:30–32.
44. Cuschieri A, Shimi S, Banting G, Vander Velpen G, Dunkley P. Coaxial curved instruments for minimal access surgery. Endosc Surg Allied Technol 1993;1:303–305.
45. Cuschieri A. Laparoscopic surgery of the pancreas. J R Coll Surg Edinb 1994;39:187–194.
46. Phillips EH, Rosenthal RJ, Carroll BJ, Fallas MJ. Laparoscopic trans-cystic-duct common-bile-duct exploration. Surg Endosc 1994;8:1389–1394.
47. Lezoche E, Paganini AM. Single-stage laparoscopic treatment of gallstones and common bile duct stones in 120 unselected consecutive cases. Surg Endosc 1995;9:1070–1075.
48. Shimi S, Banting S, Cuschieri A. Transcystic drainage after laparoscopic exploration of common bile duct. Min Invas Ther 1992;1:273–276.
49. Baca I, Klempa I, Gotzen V. Laparoskopische pankreatocystojejunostomie ohne entero-entero-anastomose. Chirurg 1994:65: 378–381.
50. Gagner M. Laparoscopic treatment for acute necrotizing pancreatitis. Semin Laparosc Surg, 1996;3:21–27.
51. Fingerhut A, Clideville C. Laparoscopic biliary bypass for inoperable carcinoma of the pancreas. Semin Laparosc Surg 1996;3:10–14.
52. Cuschieri A. Laparoscopic management of cancer patients. J R Coll Surg Edinb 1995;40:1–9.
53. Cuschieri A, Jakimowicz JJ, van Spreeuwel. Initial experience with laparoscopic distal 70% pancreatectomy and splenectomy for chronic pancreatitis. Ann Surg, 1996;23:280–285.
54. Crist W. Complications of laparoscopic surgery. Surg Clin North Am 1993;73:265–289.
55. Saville LE, Woods MS. Laparoscopy and major retroperitoneal vascular injuries (MRVI). Surg Endosc 1995;9:1096–1100.
56. Cuschieri A. Visual displays and visual perception in minimal access surgery. Semin Laparosc Surg 1995;2:209–214.

57. Pezet D, Fondrinier E, Rotman N, et al. Parietal seeding of carcinoma of the gallbladder after laparoscopic cholecystectomy. Br J Surg 1992;79:230.
58. Cava A, Roman J, Gonzalez Quintela A, Martin F, Aramburo P. Subcutaneous metastases following laparoscopy in gastric adenocarcinoma. Eur J Surg Oncol 1990;16:63–67.
59. Fusco MA, Paluzzi MW. Abdominal wall recurrence after laparoscopic-assisted colectomy for adenocarcinoma of the colon. Dis Colon Rectum 1993;36:858–861.
60. Ramos JM, Gupta S, Anthone GJ, et al. Laparoscopy and colon cancer. Is the port site at risk? Arch Surg 1994;129:897–899.
61. Dobronte Z, Wittmann T, Karacsony G. Rapid development of malignant metastases in the abdominal wall after laparoscopy. Endoscopy 1978;10:127–130.
62. Hsiu J, Given FT, Kemp GM. Tumor implantation after diagnostic laparoscopic biopsy of serous ovarian tumors of low malignant potential. Obstet Gynecol 1986;68:90–93.
63. Mouiel J, Gugenheim J, Toouli J, et al. Port-site recurrence of cancer associated with laparoscopic diagnosis and resection: the European experience. Semin Laparosc Surg 1995;2:167–175.
64. Bouvier S, G.R.E.G.C.O. Group. Metastases sur les trajets de trocars apres traitement coelio-chiurgical de tumor digestives. J Coelio-Chir 1994;10:13–22.
65. Addonizio JC, Kapoor SN. Perineal seeding of prostatic carcinoma after needle biopsy. Urology 1976;8:513–515.
66. Warshaw AL. Implications of peritoneal cytology for staging of early pancreatic cancer. Am J Surg 1991;161:26–29.
67. Iitsuka Y, Kaneshima S, Tanida O, Takeuchi T, Koga S. Intraperitoneal free cancer cells and their viability in gastric cancer. Cancer 1979;44:1476–1480.
68. Leather AJ, Kocjan G, Savage F, Hu W, Yiu CY, et al. Detection of free malignant cells in the peritoneal cavity before and after resection of colorectal cancer. Dis Colon Rectum 1994;37:814–819.
69. Kameyama M, Fukuda I, Imaoka S, Masutani S, Ohigashi, et al. Prevention of peritoneal dissemination after colorectal surgery—significance of MMC administration in abdominal cavity. Gan To Kagaku Ryoho 1991;18:1808–1811.
70. Yeo KT, Wang HH, Nagy JA, Sioussat TM, Ledbetter SR, et al. Vascular permeability factor (vascular endothelial growth factor) in guinea pig and human tumor and inflammatory effusions. Cancer Res 1993;53:2912–2918.
71. Siddiqui RA, Hochhar R, Singh V, Rajwanshi A, Goenka MK, Mehta SK. Evaluation of fibronectin as a marker of malignant ascites. J Gastroenterol Hepatol 1992;7:161–164.
72. Whalen GF, Ingber DE. Inhibition of tumor-cell attachment to extracellular matrix as a method of preventing tumor recurrence in a surgical wound. Ann Surg 1989;210:758.
73. Scott-Coombes DM, Whawell SA, Vipond MN, Crnojevic L, Thompson JN. Fibrinolytic activity of ascites caused by alcoholic cirrhosis and peritoneal malignancy. Gut 1993;34:1120–1122.
74. Gleeson N, Gonsalves R, Bonnar J. Uterine fibrinolytic enzymes in endometrial cancer. Eur J Gynaecol Oncol 1993;14:369–373.
75. Kotzampassi K, Kapanidis N, Kazamias P, Eleftheriadis E. Hemodynamic events in the peritoneal environment during pneumoperitoneum in dogs. Surg Endosc 1993;7:494–499.
76. Ishizaki Y, Bandai Y, Shimomura K, Abe H, Ohtomo Y, Idezuki Y. Changes in splanchnic blood flow and cardiovascular effects following peritoneal insufflation of carbon dioxide. Surg Endosc 1993;7:420–423.
77. Ishizaki Y, Bandai Y, Shimomura K, Abe H, Ohtomo Y, Idezuki Y. Safe intraabdominal pressure of carbon dioxide pneumoperitoneum during laparoscopic surgery. Surgery 1993;114:549–554.
78. Solis-Herruzo JA, Castellano G, Larrodera L, Morillas JD, Moreno Sanchez D, et al. Plasma arginine vasopressin concentration during laparoscopy. Hepatogastroenterology 1989;36:499–503.
79. Loegering D, Moon D, Kaplan J, Weber P, Blumenstock F. Reticuloendothelial-depressing substance: studies on the mechanism of action. J Leukocyte Biol 1985;38:613–624.
80. Benacerraf B, Biozzi G, Cuendet A, Halpern BN. Influence of portal blood flow and of partial hepatectomy on the granulopeptic activity of the reticuloendothelial system. J Physiol 1955;128:1–8.
81. Bresalier RS, Hujanan ES, Roll FJ, Itzkowitz SH, Martin GR, et al. An animal model for colon cancer metastases: establishment and characterization of murine cell lines with enhanced liver-metastasizing ability. Cancer Res 1987;47:1398–1406.
82. Abdela SM. Biology of disease. Role of integrins and other cell adhesion molecules in tumor progression and metastases. J Lab Invest 1993;68:4–17.
83. Bouwens L, Geerts A, Van Bossuyt H, Wisse E. Recent insights into the function of hepatic sinusoidal cells. Neth J Med 1987;31:129–148.
84. Roh MS, Wang L, Oyedeji C, LeRoux ME, Curley SA, et al. Human Kupffer cells are cytotoxic against human colon adenocarcinoma. Surgery 1990;108:400–404.
85. Phillips NC. Kupffer cells and liver metastasis. Cancer Metastasis Rev 1989;8:231–252.
86. Moss NM, Cough DB, Jordan AI, et al. Temporal correlation of impaired immune response after thermal injury with susceptibility to infection in a murine model. Surgery 1988;104:882–887.
87. Cruickshank AM, Fraser WD, Burns HJG, Van Damme J, Shenkin A. Response of serum interleukin-6 in patients undergoing elective surgery of varying severity. Clin Sci 1990;79:161–165.
88. Eilber FR, Morton DL. Impaired immunologic reactivity and recurrence following cancer surgery. Cancer 1970;25:362–367.
89. Liotta LA, Kleinerman J, Saidel GM. The significance of haematogenous tumor cell clumps on the metastatic process. Cancer Res 1976;36:889–894.
90. Colacchio TA, Yeager MP, Hildebrandt LW. Perioperative immunomodulation in cancer surgery. Am J Surg 1994;167:174–179.
91. Lundy J, Ford CM. Surgery, trauma and immune suppression. Evolving the mechanism. Ann Surg 1983;197:434–438.
92. Lennard TWJ, Shenton BK, Borzotta A. The influence of surgical operations on components of the human immune system. Br J Surg 1985;72:771–776.
93. Barlozzari T, Reynolds CW, Herberman RB. In vivo role of natural killer cells: involvement of large granular lymphocytes in the clearance of tumor cells in anti-asialo GM1-treated rats. J Immunol 1983;131:1024–1027.
94. Pollock RE, Lotzova E, Stanford SD. Surgical stress impairs natural killer cell programming of tumor for lysis in patients with sarcomas and other solid tumors. Cancer 1992;70:2192–2202.
95. Neefjes JJ, Ploegh HL. Intracellular transport of MHC class M molecules. Immunol Today 1992;13:179–184.
96. Kloosterman T, von Blomberg ME, Borgstein P, Cuesta MA, Scheper RJ, Meijer S. Unimpaired immune functions after laparoscopic cholecystectomy. Surgery 1994;115:424–428.
97. Bessler M, Whelan RL, Halverson A, Treat MR, Nowygrod R. Is immune function better preserved after laparoscopic versus open colon resection? Surg Endosc 1994;8:881–883.
98. Carey PD, Wakefield CH, Thayeb A, Monson JRT, Darzi A, Guillou PJ. Effects of minimally invasive surgery on hypochlorus acid production by neutrophils. Br J Surg 1994;81:557–560.
99. Joris J, Cigarini I, Legrand M, Jacquet N, De Groote D, et al. Metabolic and respiratory changes after cholecystectomy performed via laparotomy or laparoscopy. Br J Anaesth 1992;69:341–345.
100. McMahon AJ, O'Dwyer PJ, Cruikshank AM, McMillan DC, O'Reilly DStJ, et al. Comparison of metabolic responses to laparoscopic and minilaparotomy cholecystectomy. Br J Surg 1993;80:1255–1258.
101. Vander Velpen G, Penninckx F, Kerremans R, Van Damme J, Arnout J. Interleukin-6 and coagulation-fibrinolysis fluctuations after laparoscopic and conventional cholecystectomy. Surg Endosc 1994;8:1216–1220.

# 14

# *Biopsy of the Pancreas*

Yasuo Idezuki and Kazuyuki Shimomura

## BIOPSY OF THE PANCREAS

The pancreas is one of the organs that remains difficult to evaluate preoperatively. Even in recent years, diagnosis of pancreatic cancer depends mainly upon symptoms, clinical findings, laboratory tests, various imaging tests including ultrasonography (US) and computed tomography (CT), and the gross findings during exploratory laparotomy. The survival rate after operation for pancreatic cancer remains extremely low. These observations can be explained, in part, as follows: *(a)* the pancreas, in the retroperitoneal area, lies deeper than any other abdominal organ; *(b)* clinical symptoms tend to be apparent late in the course of pancreatic cancer, and most patients with pancreatic cancer are ineligible for radical operation at the time of diagnosis; *(c)* differentiation between cancer and inflammatory disease of the pancreas is difficult because of their similarities on clinical, laboratory, and imaging study, plus the high incidence of patients who have both malignant and inflammatory components. The prevailing opinion that pancreatic biopsy during laparotomy was dangerous and unreliable led to many diagnoses of pancreatic cancer by palpation and inspection. In the study reported in 1968 by Gillitano et al., about 40% of patients with a diagnosis of pancreatic cancer had to be excluded from the study because of a lack of histologic verification of the tumor (1). During the last two decades, the introduction of nonoperative imaging techniques (such as US, CT, endoscopic retrograde pancreatography (ERP), and magnetic resonance imaging (MRI) created new opportunities for the management of patients clinically suspected of having pancreatic disease. Among these, US is considered by many Japanese surgeons to be the most useful, not only as a diagnostic device but also as a guide to biopsy.

In 1972, Oscarson et al. reported the results of fine-needle aspiration cytology (FNAC) in pancreatic tumors (2). Since then, this technique has been widely used, as several reports showed its usefulness accompanied by relatively few complications (3–29). (See also Chapter 10).

### Percutaneous Fine-Needle Aspiration Cytology (FNAC)

Although pancreatic cancer and pancreatitis are the most prevalent diseases of the exocrine pancreas, the treatment and prognosis of these are entirely different. The two diseases are often difficult to distinguish clinically, biochemically, and morphologically, and they sometimes occur in conjunction with each other. Many patients with pancreatic cancer have inflammatory and fibrotic lesions of the pancreas, and many patients with chronic pancreatitis may have focal pancreatic cancer. Final differentiation between pancreatitis and pancreatic cancer is most often made during exploratory laparotomy, although a few surgeons still hesitate to perform direct incisional or needle biopsy of the pancreas because of the hazards of possible bleeding, fistula, or abscess formation. Others insist upon histopathologic a histologic diagnosis as the basis for radical operation in pancreatic cancer. This dilemma remains controversial.

The complication rate of intraoperative biopsy of the pancreas has been reported as 5–10%, and in recent years, percutaneous pancreatic FNAC has been introduced for preoperative cytologic diagnosis. This development has been made possible due to the rapid development of various imaging examinations, especially US (30, 31) which provides guidance of the aspiration needle. The fine needle aspiration technique, used primarily as a percutaneous method, has also been adapted for use during exploratory laparotomy. During the biopsy procedure, aspiration technique is recommended rather than nonaspiration technique because of its higher positive predictive value (33, 34). Percutaneous pancreatic biopsy can be guided by US, CT, or fluoroscopy, and occasionally by angiography, ERC, or percutaneous pancreatography. Fluoroscopy allows good visualization of the needle, but the patients usually must change position during the procedure to allow biplanar imaging, not only for the horizontal localization, but also for the depth of the tip of the needle.

If fluoroscopy is used, close monitoring of radiation levels is necessary to avoid excessive exposure of the patient and staff. CT offers an excellent image of the pancreas, as well as surrounding organs, such as small bowel, stomach, and colon, and large vessels, such as splenic and superior mesenteric artery, and the portal venous system. With a skin marker in place, a control scan enables the physician to determine the precise site of skin puncture on the patient's abdomen. However, CT-guided biopsy requires a longer time, more cooperation from the patient in breath-holding and/or positioning, and a higher dose of radiation to both physicians and patients. Helical CT scanning, introduced recently, can provide a slice of transectional image every few seconds, with somewhat fewer disadvantages than described above for standard CT.

US is a simple, inexpensive method for visualization of the pancreas and pancreatic lesions. US also has the advantages of shorter duration, less pain, and less invasion. Physicians can create a three-dimensional image of the tumor in a few minutes and, if needed, this can be done repeatedly. The insertion of the needle can be followed on the monitor throughout the procedure, when the needle holder is attached to the ultrasound probe. US has some limitations: stomach or intestine, distended with gas between the pancreas and the skin surface, will obscure images of the pancreas and needles. Between 1980 and 1985, more than 70% of studies of percutaneous FNAC were done using US. We use US in most cases, with CT or fluoroscopy being used in cases of failure of US-guided biopsy.

**Indications.** Percutaneous FNAC of the pancreas is used mainly to verify the existence of cancer cells in the lesion. The absence of cancer cells does not directly support a diagnosis of benign disease because of the high false-negative rate discussed below. Biopsies can provide the advantages of avoiding laparotomy, reducing the patients' stress, and allowing earlier initiation of chemotherapy or radiation therapy.

The accepted indication for FNAC in pancreatic lesions today is primarily to establish a definite diagnosis among aged or high-risk patients who are not suited for laparotomy. (See also Chapter 10). Biopsies (FNAC) should be avoided in patients who are to have a radical or palliative surgical procedure; we recommend that such patients undergo biopsy during laparotomy. Preoperative biopsies are not essential when pancreatic cancer is strongly suspected clinically or on the basis of image examination by an experienced physician. Percutaneous aspiration of the contents of pancreatic cystic lesions is of limited value for analysis of the fluid and has little advantage in treatment because of the high recurrence rate. The indications must also weigh the risks of hemorrhage, fistula, abscess, pancreatitis, and needle-tract dissemination of the tumor. The only relative contraindications to this procedure are bowel dilatation and abnormal coagulation parameters.

**Techniques.** US and radiologic examinations used for diagnosis of the disease are also used for localization of the puncture site on the anterior abdominal wall. Recent reports indicate that US is being used most frequently for pancreatic cancer. CT is also used, especially if US fails to demonstrate the tumor. Barium duodenography, choledochography by the presence of contrast medium after percutaneous transhepatic cholangiogram (PTC), or a catheter placed near the tumor for angiography is sometimes helpful in determining the puncture site.

Biopsies are performed on either an outpatient or inpatient basis. An inpatient procedure is recommended for the early recognition and treatment of acute complications such as bleeding or pancreatitis after the biopsy. Fasting is sometimes necessary to avoid air in the gastrointestinal tract under US scanning, and atropine (0.5 mg) and/or a minor tranquilizer are occasionally used as premedication. Both anterior and posterior approaches to the pancreas can be considered. In many cases, an anterior transabdominal approach is recommended to avoid bony interference. Biopsy of some lesions of the tail of the pancreas can be done via a posterior approach. Penetration of the liver, gastrointestinal tract, and sometimes colon may occur during the procedure. Care should be taken to avoid damage to major vessels (e.g., celiac axis, superior mesenteric artery, and portal vein).

The skin and the subcutaneous tissue down to the peritoneum are anesthetized locally with 0.5%–2% lidocaine. A small skin incision is made by a surgical blade or with an 18-gauge needle, and the subcutaneous tissue is separated for the entry of the biopsy needle. An additional 3–4 mL of local anesthetic solution should be injected in the preperitoneal layer to avoid pain at peritoneal puncture, which is usually done under US scanning after the needle tip has been inserted just superficial to the peritoneum.

A pancreatic mass that is large enough to palpate from the abdominal surface can be punctured directly. A medium-sized tumor should be punctured free hand under US guide; biopsy of a lesion smaller than 10 mm in diameter is usually performed with the needle holder attached to the commercially available US probe. The patient lies on the bed or stretcher in the supine position, with the physician on the right side of the patient.

A 17- to 23-gauge puncture needle should be used for pancreatic aspiration-biopsy. The 23-gauge needle is easily bent during the procedure, and large needles are apt to increase the risk of complications. We generally use a 22-gauge needle. Needle length varies from 7 to 20 cm and should be selected on the basis of the depth of the pancreatic lesion. A needle that is too long tends to bend and miss the tumor when pushed toward it.

When pancreatic biopsies are performed under US guidance, the needle should remain visible during the entire procedure. Pushing the needle slowly in the longitudinal direction without torsion may prevent bending of the needle tract as the needle progresses. There is no need for breath-holding, but patients should be advised to take small frequent breaths rather than a deep one that might cause the image of the needle tract to disappear on the US monitor and, perhaps, result in an unsuccessful biopsy.

When the tip of the needle reaches the tumor, the needle is attached to a 20-mL disposable plastic syringe and aspiration is performed with maximal suction with about 1 cm excursion of the needle. The aspiration gun can make this part of the procedure easy and secure.

When the tumor is hard and difficult to sample, the next aspiration trial should last approximately 30 seconds. To avoid undesirable contamination of the sample by blood, the duration of suction should not be too long. After release of the suction, the needle is withdrawn. If suction continues during or after withdrawal of the needle, the cytologic specimen will be aspirated into the syringe, making retrieval difficult. This procedure is repeated two to four times to obtain sufficient specimen. For a hard tumor, an 18- or 19-gauge needle may be helpful for taking the sample. For hemostasis, the biopsy site is pressed by an assistant's hand immediately after the needle is withdrawn.

Adding an anticoagulant to the biopsy sample is recommended, especially when it is contaminated by blood. The aspirated material is immediately ejected onto a glass slide, fixed by alcohol spray, and stained by the Papanicolaou or Giemsa method (Fig. 14.1). The results of FNAC are strongly influenced by the technique of the physician, and a skillful and experienced cytopathologist is essential.

Since 1986, a variety of automated biopsy devices using different needles has been introduced (35). The whole movement is performed instantaneously, and the biopsy itself is painless because of the speed of the movement. A recent result suggests that most 18-gauge automated biopsy devices with a biopsy excursion of at least 2.0 cm can provide a high-quality, diagnostically adequate specimen for cytologic analysis (36). Further studies are necessary to evaluate the usefulness of these devices.

During the 1970s and 1980s, the reported sensitivity of FNAC in the diagnosis of pancreatic cancer varied from 49% to 100% (36–43). These differences may be partially explained by the variations of techniques and indications in each institution as well as by the experience and diagnostic criteria of each cytopathologist. The rate of false-negative findings did not decrease in this series of reports, despite the rapid improvements in imaging during these two decades. In 1993 Paksoy et al., showed a 62% sensitivity for FNAC (44). Actually the results reported may vary depending on whether or not the authors have included "inconclusive" results as "false-negative" results.

Generally, FNAC of the pancreas seems to be an efficient alternative to intraoperative gross diagnosis or biopsy during laparotomy, which is usually associated with a certain rate of morbidity and mortality. The failure of diagnosis can be explained as sampling error, such as missing the tumor, severe fibrosis of the tumor, or aspiration of necrotic cancer tissue.

The reported specificity of FNAC of the pancreas is almost 100% in many studies. Thus, the cytologic result of FNAC can provide the basis for treatment decisions once the biopsy diagnosis of cancer is positive (45). With a positive FNA result, patients can undergo radical resection without further delay or without another diagnostic examination. Patients with unresectable disease or at high risk can avoid other invasive examinations or exploratory laparotomy and start nonoperative treatment immediately after FNAC.

According to a report by Bret et al. in 1986, the cost for the diagnostic workup of a pancreatic mass decreased at least 35%

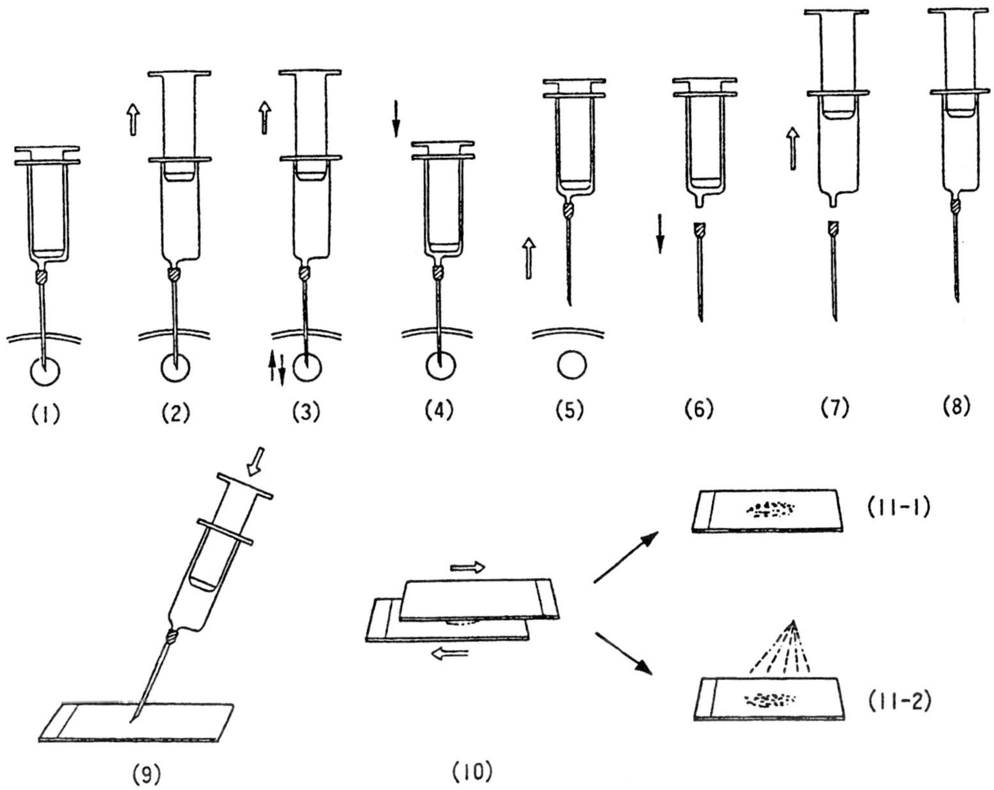


**FIG. 14.1.** Technique for FNAC of pancreas. *(1)* Tumor is punctured by the needle under US guidance or by finger fixing. *(2)* With the syringe held firmly, aspiration is performed. *(3)* For a hard tumor, a back and forth excursion of the needle during aspiration is helpful in obtaining the sample. *(4)* Suction is released before needle withdrawal. *(5)* Needle is withdrawn with syringe. *(6–8)* Needle is detached and the syringe is filled with air; then reconnected to the needle. *(9)* Cytologic sample is blown onto the glass slide. *(10, 11)* Specimens are transferred to the cytologist for Papanicolaou or Giemsa staining.

when a percutaneous biopsy was done, especially when it was performed early in the workup, as soon as a focal pancreatic lesion was detected (46). One report suggested that pancreatic biopsy does not adversely influence survival for patients with inoperable pancreatic tumors (47). Another study found needle biopsy to be less accurate than expert radiologic interpretation of CT scanning alone (48).

Although the result has not been shown to differ with the use of different needles, Wittenberg et al. stress the importance of obtaining tiny cores of tissue (49). Actually, histology and cytology are not competitive but complementary, and the association of these two techniques increased the sensitivity in a study by Chagnon et al. (50). In FNAC performed on cystic lesions of the pancreas, measurement of tumor marker values (CEA, CA19-9) in the aspirated fluid raises the sensitivity of cytodiagnosis to 95–100% (51, 52).

**Complications.** In many reports published in the 1980s, complications occurred but the rates were extremely low. In 1984, Livraghi et al. reported a mortality rate of 0.008% and a major complication rate of 0.005% following abdominal biopsies (FNAC) (53). Similar results were reported by Smith in 1984, 0.006% and 0.16%, and by Fornari, 0.018% and 0.18%, respectively (54, 55). Subsequent reports of smaller series of 100–300 cases in 1991 and 1993 showed no mortality (56, 57).

The most prevalent complication after FNAC of the pancreas is acute pancreatitis (58). Needle passage through the gastrointestinal tract, including the colon, does not seem to cause complications (56). Nevertheless, among 15 deaths after FNAC abdominal biopsies during 1980–1986, 5 followed pancreatic biopsies (59, 60). In 1990, a death was reported due to acute hemorrhagic pancreatitis after FNAC of the pancreas (61). Fornari et al. reported 8 collected cases of needle tract tumor seeding following FNAC (54).

Even with these major complications, the usefulness of FNAC in pancreatic diseases cannot be denied.

**Conclusions.** Percutaneous FNAC of the pancreas is a relatively safe and useful procedure with a low complication rate. The relatively low sensitivity and the fact that biopsy is not without risk leads to the authors'advice not to perform preoperative FNAC routinely when curative or palliative surgery is indicated (46, 62). FNAC of small and resectable pancreatic tumors is of limited value, and final diagnosis should be made by biopsy during the laparotomy.

### Intraoperative Pancreatic Biopsy

Intraoperative biopsy is the last opportunity to make a definite diagnosis before surgical treatment. The main indication for this type of biopsy is differentiating focal or tumor-forming chronic pancreatitis from pancreatic cancer or pancreatic cystic diseases. Although many specimens obtained during the laparotomy are examined as frozen sections, sometimes a limited amount of pancreatic tissue, associated with severe fibrosis, is misdiagnosed as well-differentiated adenocarcinoma. Therefore, if repeated intraoperative pancreatic biopsies are inclusive, the authors advise waiting for the permanent histologic result, because, in the authors' opinion, a histologic diagnosis of cancer is essential for radical operation of resectable diseases.

There are three usual types of intraoperative pancreatic biopsy: wedge biopsy, needle core biopsy, and intraoperative FNAC. The importance of intraoperative biopsy increases when preoperative percutaneous FNAC fails to make a definite diagnosis of cancer. Even with a negative result obtained preoperatively, intraoperative biopsy is useful for the final diagnosis of malignant disease because of the relatively low sensitivity of percutaneous FNAC.

The pancreas is situated deep within the abdominal cavity and is obscured by the stomach, duodenum, colon, and the peritoneal membrane between organs. Although US, the most powerful tool for intraoperative examination and biopsy of the pancreas, can image through the structures, the pancreas is usually best imaged after surgical exposure (63).

Surgical exposure of the pancreas for intraoperative US is usually accompanied by transection of the gastrocolic ligament and entry into the lesser omental sac. Once the surface of the pancreas is exposed, US scanning is started in the longitudinal and transverse planes along the course of the gland, moving from the head of the pancreas to the tail. Scanning of the entire pancreas may reveal unexpected findings such as a daughter lesion, enlarged lymph nodes, or vessel involvement by the pancreatic tumor, which may affect the surgical treatment. US scanning and biopsy of the pancreas should be performed immediately after laparotomy with the least manipulation of the pancreas to avoid artifacts caused by US.

Currently, in experienced hands, intraoperative US can detect a lesion smaller than 5 mm located deep in the pancreas. US is an excellent imaging tool that contributes to the detection and localization of a small tumor during operation, to the performance of a needle biopsy of the pancreas, and to the staging and characterization of the pancreatic tumor. Intraoperative FNAC has developed because of the rapid improvement in the resolution of US and because of the surgeons' concern of possible complications following core biopsy.

### Technique

***Wedge biopsy (Fig. 14.2).*** Pancreatic wedge biopsy is best indicated for tumors near the surface of the pancreas, no more than 5–6 mm below the surface. Care should be taken to avoid damaging large vessels or the main duct of the pancreas while performing US-guided biopsy.

1. A deep suture of 3-0 monofilament is placed at the point of the tumor to mark its location.
2. An encircling suture for subsequent hemostasis is placed 5 mm outside the planned line of resection.
3. Pancreatic tissue is carefully resected in a wedge shape, using a surgical blade. Electric cautery is usually not very useful for hemostasis of the pancreas. Bleeding should be controlled by finger pressure while the encircling suture is tied.
4. A few additional sutures may be required for complete hemostasis.
5. For pancreatic lesions located near the inferior edge of the pancreas, a wedge resection of the inferior border of the pancreas, including the tumor, may be preferable. The cut surface of the gland should then be oversewn with monofilament sutures.
6. The resected specimen is wrapped in gauze, moistened with saline, and transferred immediately for histologic (frozen section) examination.

Wedge biopsy is likely to be the best way to obtain a specimen of larger volume. Resection of the wrong tissue, however, may be responsible for a wrong diagnosis; a false negative report for cancer. A single normal biopsy report does not necessarily support the diagnosis of a benign disease. The wedge biopsy is performed by many surgeons with acceptably low complication rates of bleeding, acute pancreatitis, and pancreatic pseudocyst resulting from the procedure. This technique is sometimes combined with needle biopsy or lymph node biopsy to improve the sensitivity for diagnosis of malignant disease. The greatest error is made by the surgeon who accepts a pancreatic false negative report. Experienced surgeons, today may sometimes trust their interpretation of gross findings in the face of a negative frozen section report as a basis for resection (see Chapter 55).

***Core needle biopsy (Fig. 14.3).*** In the 1960s and 1970s, pancreas wedge biopsy was originally guided by palpation only (64, 65). Pancreatic cancer and chronic pancreatitis are usually difficult to distinguish when based on their gross resemblance. In the case of pancreatic cancers, the malignant lesion is often surrounded by indurated inflammatory tissue, which makes it difficult to locate the tumor, per se. Thus, wedge biopsy performed by palpation, may be imprecise, often unsuccessful, and thus less reliable. The complication rate may be significant.

In the early 1970s, surgeons started to use the Vim-Silverman needle and other varieties of needles (such as the TruCut variant, which is preferred by many surgeons), to reduce the possibility of complications (66–68). The Vim-Silverman needle can obtain a cylindrical tissue sample of 1.5 mm diameter, which can be examined histologically by frozen, as well as by paraffin section.

1. The surface of the pancreas is exposed for US scanning. The location, size, and depth of the tumor are determined.
2. A 14-gauge Vim-Silverman needle, consisting of the mandrin, external sheath, and tissue-sampling needle, is inserted into the tumor.
3. After the mandrin is pulled out, the tissue-sampling needle is inserted into the sheath.
4. The tissue-sampling needle is pressed into the tumor so that the two blades on the tip of the needle penetrate deeply enough into the tissue to obtain the specimen.
5. Holding the needle in one hand, the surgeon advances the outer sheath to cover the tip of the needle, which contains the material.
6. The sheath and needle are then withdrawn together. The material, between the two blades, is carefully extracted and sent for histopathological examination. A similar technique has been adapted for transduodenal core needle biopsy of tumors adjacent to the second portion of the duodenum.

***Fine-needle aspiration cytology.*** Intraoperative FNAC is simpler but uses the same techniques as the percutaneous method (Fig. 14.1).

1. After the location and size of the tumor are defined by intraoperative US, the lesion is punctured with an 18- to 22-gauge needle.
2. With a 20-mL syringe connected to the needle, aspiration with maximum suction is performed several times to obtain a cytologic specimen.
3. This procedure is repeated several times, shifting from the center and to the periphery of the lesion. More than three punctures are not recommended, to avoid possible complications.
4. Bleeding or leakage of pancreatic juice after the biopsy can be controlled by 4-0 nylon sutures.

Small intrapancreatic masses are best approached by aspiration cytology. If that technique is unavailable or unsuccessful, core needle biopsy may be done.

Aspiration biopsy is considered superior to core biopsy because FNAC carries a lower possibility of complications.

The ability to perform aspiration cytology should be available whenever surgery is performed for pancreatic cancer. FNAC tends to be performed during the preoperative diagnostic workup of pancreatic disease more often than during laparotomy. In addition, aspiration cytology of juice from the pancreatic duct as an extension of ERCP is currently being evaluated.

**Results.** In the 1970s, Christofersen and Poll reported the first 3 cases of intraoperative FNAC of the pancreas with 100% correct diagnosis (69). Since a 1980 study by Willems and Lowhagen, the reported accuracy of intraoperative FNAC of the pancreas, up to 1993, varied from 71 to 100%, being as high as or higher than reported accuracy of frozen-section study of tissue obtained by wedge biopsy or core needle biopsy (70–75).

The indications and circumstances of these results have significant bearing on the rates of accuracy and complications, although they are often not described in the literature. For example, a large pancreatic mass extending beyond the capsule is usually diagnosed as pancreatic cancer by gross intraoperative diagnosis and sometimes resected without biopsy. Many patients, strongly suspected by palpation of the tumor at laparotomy of having malignant disease of the pancreas associated with obstruction jaundice, have undergone primary resection. Higher

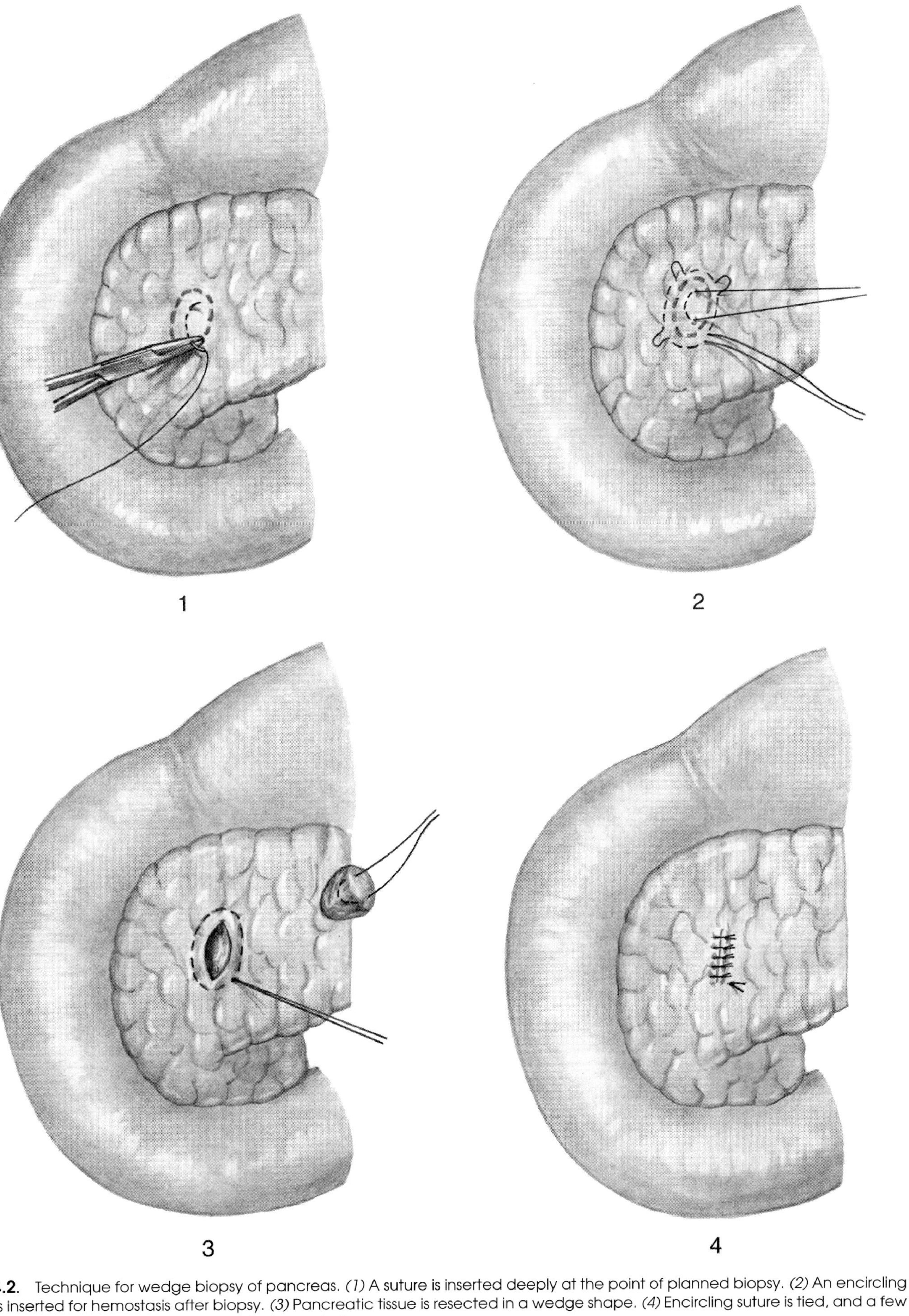


**FIG. 14.2.** Technique for wedge biopsy of pancreas. *(1)* A suture is inserted deeply at the point of planned biopsy. *(2)* An encircling suture is inserted for hemostasis after biopsy. *(3)* Pancreatic tissue is resected in a wedge shape. *(4)* Encircling suture is tied, and a few additional sutures are placed for complete hemostasis.

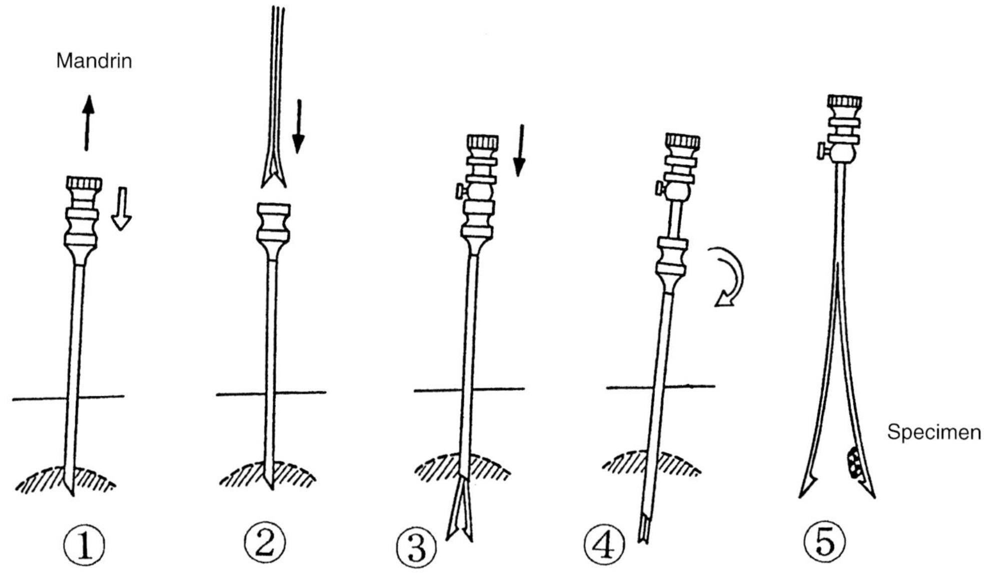


**FIG. 14.3.** Technique for core needle biopsy of the pancreas using a Vim-Silverman needle. *(1)* Puncture needle is inserted into the tumor. *(2)* After mandrin is withdrawn, the biopsy needle with cutting blades is inserted. *(3)* Biopsy needle is pushed into the tumor. *(4)* Holding the needle, the outer sheath is advanced in a twisting motion to cover the needle. *(5)* Columnar material is obtained between the blades. The Tru Cut needle provides a similar sampling.

accuracy in diagnosis is likely with lesions involving the pancreatic surface than with those in other locations. Furthermore, the skill of the cytologist performing the procedure has a significant effect on the result. Intraoperative FNAC performed by an experienced surgeon and examined by a talented pathologist is an accurate and useful technique.

With the rapid development of CT and MRI, the number of patients undergoing radical surgery with a suspected malignant tumor diagnosed merely by these imaging diagnosis is increasing, despite negative symptoms, clinical findings, and laboratory data, including the level of serum tumor markers. Intraoperative FNAC performed on these patients will be of great significance to avoid "oversurgery."

Hyoty et al. (76) showed a sensitivity of 81% in 98 patients in 1991, and Krishnaumurthy in 1993 reported a sensitivity of 90.5% and a specificity of 100% for FNAC of the pancreas by the transduodenal approach in 97 patients (72). In 1993, Earnhardt et al., on the basis of 75 cases with 90% sensitivity, 100% specificity, and 92% accuracy, concluded that intraoperative FNAC is a highly accurate diagnostic procedure and the preferred technique for obtaining an intraoperative tissue diagnosis of a pancreatic mass (73). A report in 1995 by Saez et al. showed similar excellent results in 90 cases (74).

**Complications.** Each method of tissue sampling has complications. After wedge biopsy or core needle biopsy, bleeding, fistula formation, acute pancreatitis, and pancreatic ascites have been observed. The technique of transduodenal core needle biopsy was developed to reduce the complication rate.

No major complications during intraoperative FNAC were noted in most reports during 1978–1990. However in 1984, Eggert et al. reported one case of hemorrhage after intraoperative FNAC, and a case of pancreatic fistula formation was reported in 1990 by Rosenbaum and Frost (78). Both were procedures necessary for surgical intervention.

To reduce the occurrence of the postoperative complications, external drainage at the site of biopsy is recommended, regardless of the type of biopsy.

**Conclusions.** The risk of complications from intraoperative FNAC is difficult to compare with that of percutaneous FNAC performed preoperatively, because it is primarily obscured by the risk of the exploratory laparotomy itself.

However, during intraoperative FNAC, risks of bleeding or pancreatic fistula formation can be minimized by suturing or external drainage. Percutaneous FNAC is always associated with the risk of needle-tract dissemination of the tumor. These considerations can lead one to conclude that intraoperative FNAC is a superior technique for obtaining pathologic proof of malignant disease in patients eligible for open laparotomy for radical or palliative operations. As pointed out in Chapter 55, if at laparotomy, resection of the tumor is deemed inadvisable, wedge biopsy of the primary or metastatic tumors has the advantage of providing tissue for grading, determination of policy, and studies of molecular biology.

## REFERENCES

1. Gillitano A, Fransen H, Martin RG. Carcinoma of the pancreas. Results of treatment. Cancer 1968;22:939–944.
2. Oscarson J, Stormby N, Sundgren R. Selective angiography in fine-needle aspiration cytodiagnosis of gastric and pancreatic tumors. Acta Radiol (Diagn) 1972;12:737–750.
3. Cohen MM. Early diagnosis of pancreatic cancer using ultrasound and fine-needle aspiration cytology. Am Surg 1979;45: 715–717.
4. Dekker A, Lloyd JC. Fine-needle aspiration biopsy in ampullary and pancreatic carcinoma. Arch Surg 1979;114:592–596.
5. Evander A, Ihse I, Lunderquist A, et al. Percutaneous cytodiagnosis of carcinoma of the pancreas and bile duct. Ann Surg 1978;188:90–92.
6. Ferrucci JT Jr, Wittenberg J. CT biopsy of abdominal tumors: aids for lesion localization. Radiology 1978;129:739–744.
7. Ferrucci JT Jr, Wittenberg J, Mueller J, et al. Diagnosis of abdominal malignancy by radiologic fine-needle aspiration biopsy. AJR 1980;134:323–330.
8. Freeny PC, Kidd R, Ball TJ. ERCP-guided percutaneous fine-needle pancreatic biopsy. West J Med 1980;132:283–287.
9. Goldman ML, Naib ZM, Galambos, JT, et al. Preoperative diagnosis of pancreatic carcinoma by percutaneous aspiration biopsy. Am J Dig Dis 1977;22:1076–1082.
10. Goldstein HM, Zornoza J. Percutaneous transperitoneal aspiration biopsy of pancreatic masses. Am J Dig Dis 1978;23:840–843.
11. Goldstein HM, Zornoza J, Wallace S, et al. Percutaneous fine-needle aspiration biopsy of pancreatic and other abdominal masses. Radiology 1977;123:319–322.
12. Haaga JR, Alfidi RJ. Precise biopsy localization by computed tomography. Radiology 1976;118:603–607.
13. Hancke S, Holm HH, Koch F. Ultrasonically guided percutaneous fine-needle biopsy of the pancreas. Surg Gynecol Obstet 1975; 140: 361–364.
14. Hancke S, Pederson JF. Percutaneous puncture of pancreatic cysts guided by ultrasound. Surg Gynecol Obstet 1976;142: 551–552.

15. Ho CS, McLoughlin MJ, McHattie JD, et al. Percutaneous fine needle aspiration biopsy of the pancreas following endoscopic retrograde cholangiogiopancreatography. Radiology 1977;125: 351–353.
16. Holm HH, Pedersen JF, Kristensen JK, et al. Ultrasonically guided percutaneous puncture. Radiol Clin North Am 1975;13:493–503.
17. Liberman RP, Hafez GR, Crummy AB. Histology from aspiration biopsy: Turner needle experience. Am J Roentgenol 1982;138: 561–564.
18. MacLoughlin MJ, Ho CS, Langer B, et al. Fine-needle aspiration biopsy of malignant lesions in and around the pancreas. Cancer 1978;41:2413–2419.
19. Mitty HA, Efremidis SC, Yeh HC. Impact of fine needle biopsy on management of patients with carcinoma of the pancreas. Am J Roentgenol 1981;137:1119–1121.
20. Pereiras RV, Meiers W, Kunhardt B, et al. Fluoroscopically guided thin needle aspiration biopsy of the abdomen and retroperitoneum. Am J Roentgenol 1978;131:197–202.
21. Smith EH, Bartrum RJ, Chang YC. Ultrasonically guided percutaneous aspiration biopsy of the pancreas. Radiology 1974;112: 737–738.
22. Smith EH, Bartrum RJ Jr, Chang YC, et al. Percutaneous aspiration biopsy of the pancreas under ultrasonic guidance. N Engl J Med 1975;292:825–828.
23. Tao LC, Ho CS, McLoughlin MJ, et al. Percutaneous fine-needle aspiration biopsy of the pancreas. Cytodiagnosis of pancreatic carcinoma. Acta Cytol (Baltimore) 1978;22:215–220.
24. Tylen U, Arnesjo B, Lindberg LG, et al. Percutaneous biopsy of carcinoma of the pancreas guided by angiography. Surg Gynecol Obstet 1976;142:737–739.
25. Wilson SR, Rosen IE. Abdominal biopsy with ultrasound guidance. J Can Assoc Radiol 1979;30:138–139.
26. Wittenberg J, Mueller PR, Ferrucci JT Jr, et al. Percutaneous core biopsy of abdominal tumors using 22-gauge needles: further observations. Am J Roentgenol 1982;139:75–80.
27. Yamanaka T, Kimura K. Differential diagnosis of pancreatic mass lesion with percutaneous fine-needle aspiration biopsy under ultrasonic guidance. Dig Dis Sci 1979;24:694–699.
28. Zornora J, et al. In: Zornora, ed. Percutaneous needle biopsy. Baltimore: Williams & Wilkins, 1981.
29. Zornora J, Jonsson K, Wallace S, et al. Fine needle aspiration biopsy of retroperitoneal lymph nodes and abdominal masses: an updated report. Radiology 1977;125:87–88.
30. Guidjonsson B, Livstone EM, Spiro HM. Cancer of the pancreas. Diagnostic accuracy and survival statistics. Cancer 1978;42: 2494–2506.
31. Beazley RM. Needle biopsy diagnosis of pancreatic cancer. Cancer 1981;47:1685–1687.
32. Lee YT. Tissue diagnosis for carcinoma of the pancreas and periampullary structures. Cancer 1982;49:1035–1039.
33. Hopper KD, Abendroth CS, Sturtz KW, et al. Fine-needle aspiration biopsy for cytopathologic analysis: utility of syringe handles, automated guns, and the nonsuction method. Radiology 1992; 185(3):819–824.
34. Kinney TB, Lee MJ, Filomena CA, et al. Fine-needle biopsy: prospective comparison of aspiration versus nonaspiration techniques in the abdomen. Radiology 1993;186(2):549–552.
35. Hopper KD, Abendroth CS, Sturtz KW, et al. Automated biopsy devices: a blinded evaluation. Radiology 1993;187(3):653–660.
36. Tylen U, Arnesjo B, Lindberg LG, et al. Percutaneous biopsy of carcinoma of the pancreas guided by angiography. Surg Gynecol Obstet 1976;142:737–739.
37. Evander A, Ihse I, Lunderquist A, et al. Percutaneous cytodiagnosis of carcinoma of the pancreas and the bile duct. Ann Surg 1978;188:90–92.
38. Grant EG, Richardson JD, Smirniotopoulos JG, et al. Fine-needle biopsy directed by real-time sonography: technique and accuracy. AJR 1983;141:29–32.
39. Mitchell ML, Bittner CA, Wills JS, et al. Fine needle aspiration cytology of the pancreas. A retrospective study of 73 cases. Acta Cytol 1988;32:447–451.
40. Kocjan G, Rode J, Lees WR. Percutaneous fine needle aspiration cytology of the pancreas: advantages and pitfalls. J Clin Pathol 1989;42:341–347.
41. Parsons L Jr, Palmer CH. How accurate is fine needle biopsy in malignant neoplasia of the pancreas? Arch Surg 1989;124: 681–683.
42. Soudah B, Fritsch RS, Wittekind C, et al. Value of the cytologic analysis of fine needle aspiration biopsy specimens in the diagnosis of pancreatic carcinomas. Acta Cytol 1989;33: 875–880.
43. Jeager HJ, Macfie J, Mitchell CJ, et al. Diagnosis of abdominal masses with percutaneous biopsy guided by ultrasound. BMJ 1990;301:1188–1191.
44. Paksoy N, Lilleng R, Hagmar B, et al. Diagnostic accuracy of fine needle aspiration cytology in pancreatic lesions. A review of 77 cases. Acta Cytol 1993;37(6):889–893.
45. Yamaguchi T, Saisho H, Ohto M, et al. The diagnostic process in carcinoma of the pancreas. Gan To Kagaku Ryoho 1992;19(14): 2319–2324.
46. Bret PM, Fond A, Casola G, et al. Abdominal lesions: a prospective study of clinical efficacy of percutaneous fine needle biopsy. Radiology 1986;159:345–346.
47. Balen FG, Little A, Smith AC. Biopsy of inoperable pancreatic tumors does not adversely influence patient survival time. Radiology 1994;193(3):753–755.
48. Rodriguez J, Kasberg C, Nipper M, et al. CT-guided needle biopsy of the pancreas: a retrospective analysis of diagnostic accuracy (Comment). Am J Gastroenterol 1992;87(11):1610–1613.
49. Wittenberg J, Mueller PR, Ferrucci JT Jr, et al. Percutaneous core biopsy of abdominal tumors using 22 gauge needles: further observations. AJR 1982;139:75–80.
50. Chagnon S, Cochand-Priollet B, Jacquenod P, et al. Intérêt de la cytoponction associée à la micro-biopsie dans les masses solides du pancréas. J Radiol 1987;68:733–736.
51. Pinto MM, Levine RH. Carcinoembryonic antigen assay in fine needle aspirate of pancreas: a diagnostic adjunct to cytology. Am J Gastroenterol 1992;87(4):530–533.
52. Hammel P, Levy P, Voitot H. Preoperative cyst fluid analysis is useful for the differential diagnosis of cystic lesions of the pancreas. Gastroenterology 1995;108(4):1230–1235.
53. Livraghi T, Damascelli B, Lombardi C, et al. Risk in fine needle abdominal biopsy. J Clin Ultrasound 1983;11:77–81.
54. Smith EH. The hazards of the fine-needle aspiration biopsy. Ultrasound Med Biol 1984;10:629–634.
55. Fornari F, Civardi G, Cavanna L, et al. Complications of ultrasonically guided fine-needle abdominal biopsy. Scand J Gastroenterol 1989;24:949–955.
56. Brandt KR, Charboneau JW, Stephens DH, et al. CT and US-guided biopsy of the pancreas. Radiology 1993;187(1):99–104.
57. Levin DP, Bret PM. Percutaneous fine-needle aspiration biopsy of the pancreas resulting in death. Gastrointest Radiol 1991;16(1): 67–69.
58. Evans WK, Ho CS, McLoughlin MJ, et al. Fatal necrotizing pancreatitis following fine needle aspiration biopsy of the pancreas. Radiology 1981;141:61–62.
59. Smith EH. Hazards of fine needle aspiration biopsy. Ultrasound Med Biol 1984;10(5):629–634.
60. Bergenfeldt M, Genell S, Lindholm K, et al. Needle-tract seeding after percutaneous fine-needle biopsy of pancreatic carcinoma. Acta Chir Scand 1988;154:77–79.
61. Ihse I, Isaksson G. Preoperative and operative diagnosis of pancreatic cancer. World J Surg 1984;8:846–853.
62. Nakamura R, et al. Role of fine needle aspiration cytology and endoscopic biopsy in the preoperative assessment of pancreatic and peripancreatic malignancies. Int J Pancreatol 1994;16(1): 17–21.
63. Gupta RK, Alansari AG. Aspiration cytology and immunocytochemical study of an unusual carcinoma of the pancreas with pleomorphic giant cells. Cytopathology 1994;5(5):306–309.
64. Schultz NJ, Sanders RJ. Evaluation of pancreatic biopsy. Ann Surg 1963;158:1053–1057.
65. Lightwood R, Reber HA, Way LW, et al. The risk and accuracy of pancreatic biopsy. Am J Surg 1976;132:189–194.
66. Isaacson R, Weiland LH, McIlrath DC. Biopsy of the pancreas. Arch Surg 1974;109:227–230.
67. Beazley RM. Needle biopsy diagnosis of pancreatic cancer. Cancer 1981;47:1685–1687.
68. Hermanek P. Intraoperative Diagnostik des Pankreascarcinoms. Langenbecks Arch Chir 1983;359:289–299.

69. Christofferson P, Poll P. Preoperative pancreas aspiration biopsies. Acta Pathol Microbiol Immunol Scand 1970;212:28.
70. Shorey BA. Aspiration biopsy of carcinoma of the pancreas. Gut 1975;16:645–647.
71. Soreide O, Skaarland E, Pedersen OM, et al. Fine-needle biopsy of the pancreas: results of 204 routinely performed biopsies in 190 patients. World J Surg 1985;9:960–965.
72. Krishnamurthy SC, Soni M, Jagannath KS, et al. Intraoperative fine needle aspiration cytology of pancreas: a study of 97 cases. Indian J Gastroenterol 1993;12(1):14–15.
73. Earnhardt RC, McQuone SJ, Minasi JS, et al. Intraoperative fine needle aspiration of pancreatic and extrahepatic biliary masses. Surg Gynecol Obstet 1993;177(2):147–152.
74. Saez A, Catala I, Brossa R, et al. Intraoperative fine needle aspiration cytology of pancreatic lesions. A study of 90 cases. Acta Cytol 1995;39(3):485–488.
75. Willems JS, Lowhagen T. Aspiration biopsy cytology of the pancreas. Schweiz Med Wochenschr 1980;110:845–848.
76. Hyoty MK, Mattila JJ, Salo K, et al. Intraoperative fine needle aspiration cytologic examination of pancreatic lesions. Surg Gynecol Obstet 1991;173(3):193–197.
77. Eggert A, Lattmann E, Kopf R, et al. Intraoperative Pankreaspunktionszytolozie. Zentralbl Chir 1984;109:540–544.
78. Rosenbaum DA, Frost DB. Fine needle aspiration biopsy of the pancreas complicated by pancreatic ascites. Cancer 1990; 65(11):2537–2538.

SECTION IV

SPECIAL CONSIDERATIONS

# 15

# *Obstructive Jaundice: Effects on Pancreatic Patients*

Yasuo Idezuki

Obstructive jaundice is observed in numerous pancreatic diseases, especially those involving the head of the pancreas through which the common duct passes. Obstructive jaundice in pancreatic disease is generally caused by severe stenosis or complete obstruction of the distal common bile duct, secondary to neoplasms, cystic diseases, inflammation or trauma. Impaction of a biliary stone in the distal bile duct may not only result in jaundice but it may also interfere with the outflow of the pancreatic juice into the duodenum and may cause acute pancreatitis (Chapter 22).

Obstructive jaundice may be transient or persistent, depending upon the nature of the disease. An outline of the pathologic conditions of the pancreas that may result in obstructive jaundice is shown in Table 15.1.

Jaundice in patients with pancreatic disease usually reflects not only severe pathologic changes in the pancreas but in the liver as well.

## LOCAL EFFECTS OF OBSTRUCTIVE JAUNDICE

Obstruction of the distal common bile duct caused by pancreatic diseases initially produces bile stasis and an increase in static pressure in the biliary tree. When stagnation of the bile persists and the pressure within the biliary ductal system rises above 10 cm water, secretion of bile is diminished. Biliary pressure within the common bile duct may increase as high as 30 cm water when complete obstruction persists over 2 weeks. At this pressure secretion of bile apparently ceases; at least the pressure ceases to rise (1), and dilatation of intrahepatic bile ducts is observed. Dilatation is initially observed in the extrahepatic bile duct, but as obstruction persists, intrahepatic bile ducts begin to dilate. It is often a characteristic of those pancreatic diseases that cause obstructive jaundice that flow of pancreatic juice is also obstructed. Effects of stagnation of bile may at first be local, but almost inevitably the liver, pancreas, and other adjacent organs become involved, leading to systemic effects that may disturb many vital functions.

### Derangements of Hepatic and Systemic Circulation

In patients with obstructive jaundice, hepatic blood flow initially increases. Nagorney (2) showed in the dog that biliary pressures above 25 mm Hg produced a marked increase in the hepatic arterial flow without a significant change in the portal blood flow. The mechanism for this initial hyperemia is not fully understood (3, 4). When obstruction persists for more than 3 weeks, dilatation of sinusoid (5), increase of portal pressure, and opening of intrahepatic portohepatic venous shunts are observed. As a result of these changes, effective hepatic blood flow, namely the blood perfusion through the liver, is decreased (5). In patients with obstructive jaundice, increase of cardiac output and decrease of total peripheral vascular resistance, namely, a hyperdynamic state that is also seen in patients with cirrhosis of the liver or endotoxin shock, is observed. This may be explained by the abnormalities in the sympathetic neurotransmitter, decrease of catecholamines, and increase of octopamine (false transmitter theory). These patients are characterized by an increased susceptibility to hemorrhagic shock, even with a minor hemorrhage for which normal subjects, without obstructive jaundice, could easily compensate. When the obstructive jaundice is complicated by biliary infection, endotoxin may be introduced into the bloodstream and aggravate the circulatory instability. Saito et al. have shown that when the hyperdynamic state is pronounced and the cardiac index is 3.5 L/min/m$^2$ or more, the serum bilirubin level falls slowly and tends to remain elevated even after biliary decompression. Susceptibility to multiple organ failure results (6).

In patients with obstructive jaundice, circulatory shock is often observed within 24 hours after biliary decompression by percutaneous transhepatic decompression or by other methods, without any sign of hemorrhage or infection. This postdecompression shock may be explained by *(a)* decrease of sinusoidal pressure by biliary decompression that results in increased sinusoidal perfusion (This may then trigger the extravasation of intravascular fluid and a decrease of circulatory blood volume with resulting shock); *(b)* washout of vasoactive substances by the increased blood flow through the ischemic liver; or *(c)* entrance of endotoxin and bile acids into the systemic circulation through the injured vasculature resulting from the puncture needle during PTCD (5).

Bradycardia is often observed in patients with obstructive jaundice. It results from the direct effect of bile acids on cardiac muscle and by a vagal reflex triggered by the decrease of cholinesterase seen in these patients. It is thus important in patients with obstructive jaundice to maintain fluid and acid-base balance by carefully monitoring urine volume, central venous pressure (CVP), ECG, blood gases, and cardiac index.

**TABLE 15.1. Diseases of the Pancreas and Adjacent Organs that may Cause Obstructive Jaundice**

| |
|---|
| Trauma of pancreas, common bile duct, duodenum |
| Biliary or pancreatic stone disease |
| Acute pancreatitis |
| Chronic pancreatitis |
| Inflammation |
| Ampulla of Vater |
| Diverticulitis of duodenum |
| Duodenitis |
| Cholangitis |
| Cystic disease of the pancreas |
| Genuine cysts |
| Pseudocysts |
| Tumors of pancreas, ampulla of Vater, duodenum, common bile duct |
| Benign |
| Malignant |
| Vascular diseases within the head of the pancreas |
| Aneurysm |
| Thrombophlebitis |
| Foreign bodies |
| Iatrogenic diseases |

## Endotoxemia in Obstructive Jaundice

Endotoxin, a liposaccharide derived from the coat of gram-negative enteric bacteria, is not found in the blood of normal subjects, but in obstructive jaundice, endotoxemia and bacteremia are often observed, particularly in the portal venous blood (7, 8) The absence of bile in the intestines, secondary to the obstruction of the bile duct, causes an increase in the intestinal flora (9, 10). Translocation of endotoxin may result because of an increased permeability of intestinal capillaries and the breakdown of the mucosal barrier under these conditions. The portal blood becomes contaminated with endotoxin and bacteria (12–15).

Kocsar et al. (16) and Bailey et al. (17), studying obstructive jaundice in a rat model, noted that bile acids are essential for maintaining the mucosal barrier and showed that orally administered bile acids resulted in recovery of the barrier function of the intestinal mucosa.

In obstructive jaundice, the number of Kupffer cells decreases and their phagocytic functions are impaired (18–20). The removal of bacteria and endotoxin from the blood within the liver is impaired, and the spillover or escape of endotoxin into the systemic circulation may result (21). Thus, endotoxemia in obstructive jaundice may be caused *(a)* by the lack of bile flow into the intestines and *(b)* by impairment of the functions of the Kupffer cells in the jaundiced liver.

Recently, Kunimatsu et al. (22), using a rat model, showed that a lack of bile and bile acids in the intestines resulted in morphologic changes of the intestinal mucosa: atrophic change of the intestinal villi of the proximal jejunum (10 cm distal to the pylorus ring) (Fig. 15.1). This might also be responsible for the translocation of endotoxin (Fig. 15.2). Endotoxemia may thus cause more severe systemic functional derangements: hyperdynamic circulation, septic shock, acute renal failure, or acute gastroenteropathy being triggered. Endotoxin is known to activate the complement system and cytokines (tumor necrosis factor, interleukin-1, and interleukin-6), to increase renal hypersensitivity to hypotension, and to cause fibrin deposition within the kidney.

When obstruction of the biliary ducts is complicated by biliary infection and when the intraductal pressure increases above 20 cm $H_2O$, bacteria are found to enter the regional lymphatics. When the intraductal biliary ductal pressure increases above 25 cm $H_2O$, bacteria are found in the hepatic venous blood. Infected bile contains 0.5–32 μg/mL of endotoxin, and endotoxemia may easily develop under these conditions via cholangiovenous reflux (23).

Pain and Bailey (24) measured endotoxin levels of portal blood during operation, and compared them with levels in the peripheral blood. Endotoxin levels higher than 100 pg/mL were found in 42% of portal venous blood samples, 45% of inferior mesenteric venous blood, and 35% of peripheral venous blood in the jaundiced patients. Endotoxemia and bacteremia are often observed after PTCD in which microscopic communication between the bile canaliculi and capillaries is inevitably created as the puncture needle of PTCD is passed through the hepatic parenchyma. Bacteremia and endotoxemia thus may constitute serious complications of obstructive jaundice.

## Disturbances of Intestinal Absorption and Malnutrition

In obstructive jaundice, bile flow into the duodenum is disturbed, and absorption of the nutrients from the small intestines, especially absorption of fats and fat-soluble vitamins (vitamins A, D, K, E) is impaired. Absence of bile salts in the intestines results in inability of micelle formation, which is essential for fat absorption through the intestinal mucosa. Patients with obstructive jaundice complain of diarrhea and steatorrhea. Passage of the food through the intestines is hastened, and this may contribute to the malabsorption of carbohydrates, proteins, and other nutrients, as well as fats.

Biliopancreatic secretion is considered a trophic factor for the intestinal mucosa, increasing villous density and inducing hypertrophy of the intestinal wall (25). The lack of this trophic effect of bile acids results in mucosal atrophy, the disruption of the mucosal barrier, and bacterial translocation, as discussed above (22).

Halliday et al. (26) found that body weight, midarm circumference, total body potassium, and skin test reactivity were significantly reduced in patients with obstructive jaundice who died within 1 month after operation.

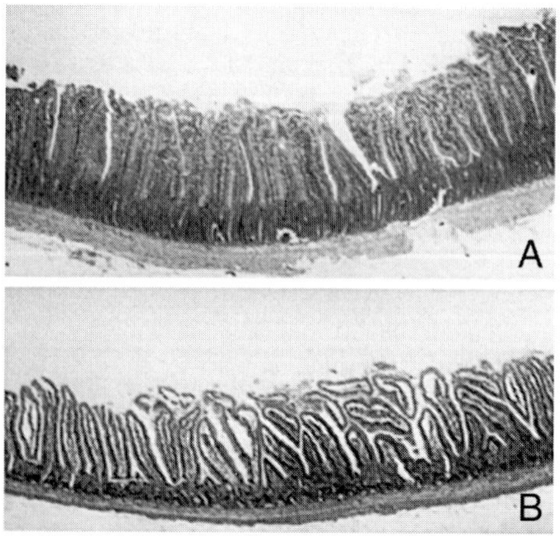


**FIG. 15.1.** Morphological changes of intestinal mucosa in obstructive jaundice. **A.** Normal rat. **B.** Duct-ligated rat. (From Aoki N, Kunimatsu N, Tamakuma S. Obstructive jaundice. Clin Gastroenterol 1992;7:119.)

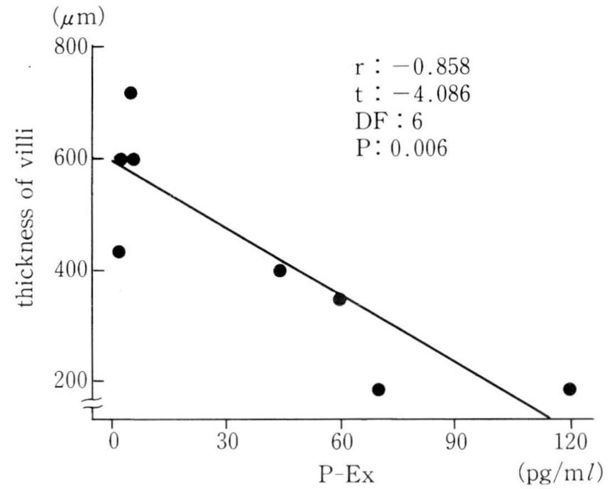


**FIG. 15.2.** Endotoxin level in portal vein and thickness of villi. (From Aoki N, Kunimatsu N, Tamakuma S. Obstructive jaundice. Clin Gastroenterol 1992;7:119.)

## Coagulation Deficiencies

Prior to the discovery of vitamin K, operative bleeding constituted a major, perhaps *the* major, complication of operating on patients with obstructive jaundice. Absorption of fat-soluble vitamin K from the intestines is impaired because of the absence in the intestine of bile and bile salts in patients with obstructive jaundice. Vitamin K is needed for production of prothrombin and factors VII, IX, and X, and deficiencies in these clotting factors are considered responsible for the bleeding tendencies and coagulopathy in jaundiced patients. Initially in obstructive jaundice, clotting is usually not markedly impaired, compared with that in jaundice caused by hepatocellular insufficiency. The prothrombin time and the thromboelastogram are usually within normal limits, but as the serum bilirubin levels rise to 20 mg/dL or more, prolongation of prothrombin time, decrease in hepaplastin and antithrombin III, and increase of fibrin degradation products are often observed. These patients may easily develop disseminated intravascular coagulopathy (DIC) and multiple organ failure (MOF). Even in patients with normal coagulation tests, clotting factors may be consumed during operation, and clotting deficiencies may develop postoperatively. Preoperative administration of vitamin K is, therefore, recommended.

It is also suggested that in obstructive jaundice, coagulopathy with impairment of fibrinolysis may be responsible for development of DIC. Many patients with obstructive jaundice show an increase of fibrinogen and factor VIII levels, decrease of antithrombin III, prolongation of euglobulin lysis time (ELT), decrease of prekallikrein level, activation of kinins, and abnormalities in complement systems (27). Patients with these abnormalities may develop coagulation deficiencies and DIC, even with minimally invasive procedures such as PTCD or biopsy or with an otherwise minor infection.

## Renal Failure

In obstructive jaundice, bilirubin in the blood is excreted to some extent by the kidney (28). Bilirubin is known to suppress mitochondrial function (oxidative phosphorylation) of the kidney and of the liver, and the renal function is impaired (29). In patients with long-standing jaundice, the glomerular filtration rate and renal plasma flow are decreased; vasoactive substances, plasma renin, and angiotensin II levels are increased. McPherson et al. (30) observed that during a prospective randomized trial of PTCD for obstructive jaundice, 40% of patients initially had impaired creatinine clearance. Adequate fluid replacement, together with infusion of mannitol, has been reported to be effective in restoring renal function (31).

The incidence of postoperative acute renal failure in jaundiced patients is higher than in patients without jaundice. Thompson et al. (32) reported that 11% of the jaundiced patients developed renal failure after biliary surgery. The incidence was higher (17.5–36%) after operations for malignancies than with benign diseases (9–12%). Mito et al. (33) reported that operative mortality rates in jaundiced patients because of acute renal failure were high, ranging from 2.4 to 6.8%. The operative mortality rates in those patients with malignancies were even higher, 11–24%. Wait and Kahng (34) reviewed 2007 cases of obstructive jaundice and reported that 4–18% of these patients developed renal failure postoperatively, with operative mortality rates among the patients with renal failure ranging from 32 to 100%. It is pointed out that the risk of postoperative acute renal failure may be predicted by the serum bilirubin levels and by the blood urea nitrogen levels (bilirubin, 10 mg/dL; BUN 80 mg/dL), but the incidence of renal failure can be significantly increased by infection. Endotoxemia has a deleterious effect on renal, cardiac, pulmonary, and other vitally important functions. Infection often associated with obstructive jaundice plays a crucial role in provoking and aggravating renal failure among jaundiced patients.

## Gastritis and Gastric Ulcers

Surgery, PTCD, biliary infection, renal failure, and other sources of stress in patients with obstructive jaundice often trigger erosive change of the gastric mucosa which results in gastric ulcers. Fukai et al. (35) reported acute ulcer in 2.3% (86 of 3697) of jaundiced patients. Higher incidences were also reported (Sato (36), 7.3%; Tamakuma (37), 16.7%). It is reported that when serum bilirubin levels rise above 10 mg/dL, the incidence of acute gastric ulcers increases (38). Others, however, found no correlation between serum bilirubin levels and the incidence of gastric ulcers. The duration of biliary obstruction may also be related with the development of upper gastrointestinal bleeding. Fukai et al. (35) reported that patients with obstructive jaundice for more than 2 months had a higher

**TABLE 15.2. Mechanisms of Endotoxemia**

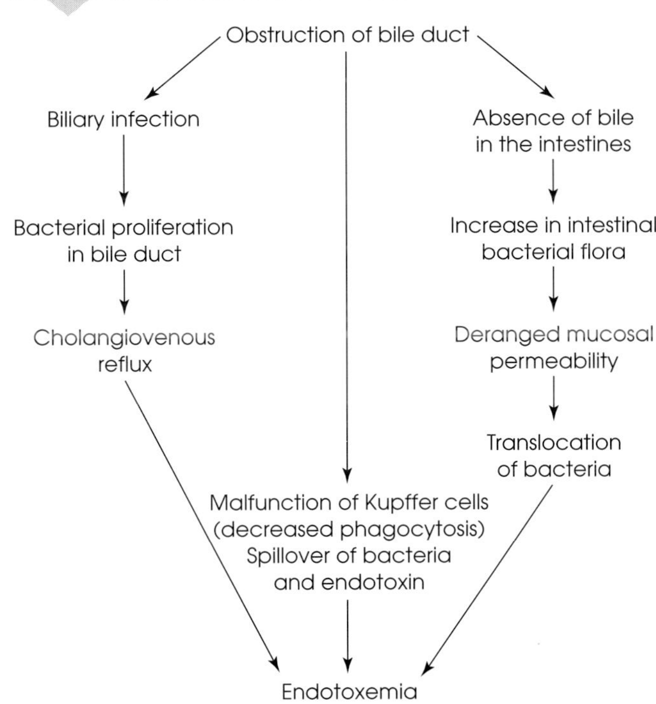

incidence (27.6%) as compared with those of less than 2 months (12.8%).

The ulcers found in obstructive jaundice are often multiple, occurring usually in the cardia or in the body of the stomach. Both an increase in the injurious factors and a diminution in defensive mechanisms are responsible for ulcer formation. Menguy (39, 40) showed in the experimental model of hemorrhagic shock, the difference of adenosine triphosphatase (ATP) synthesis between ischemic mucosa of the gastric body and antrum, but reports are conflicting.

In obstructive jaundice, prostaglandin $E_2$ ($PGE_2$) in the mucosa is decreased, and this may also be responsible for the ischemic changes of the gastric mucosa. Administration of $PGE_2$ was found to be effective in prevention of stress ulcers in the animal model. Acid content in the gastric juice may be affected by biliary diversion in the patient with obstructive jaundice. Menguy (41), Brown et al. (42), and Breen et al. (43) reported an increase of acid secretion after biliary diversion in dogs by creating a Heidenhein pouch and cholecystoileostomy. Nahrwold et al. (44) did not substantiate these findings.

Narui et al. (45) reported that capillary perfusion of gastric mucosa improved after biliary decompression. Postoperative acute hemorrhage from gastric ulcers in patients with obstructive jaundice is a serious complication and often triggers DIC and MOF, sometimes eventually leading to the death of the patient. Prophylactic use of hydrogen-ion blockers and $PGE_2$, together with careful maintenance of fluid and electrolyte balance, should be seriously considered.

## PREOPERATIVE EVALUATION OF JAUNDICED PATIENTS

The risk of surgery is no doubt greater in patients with obstructive jaundice than in patients without jaundice. Preoperative evaluation as to the operative risk is, therefore, important. Consideration of many factors, predictive of the risk of operative mortality and morbidity, has been postulated. Pitt et al. (46) stressed the following 10 risk factors for mortality after biliary surgery: *(a)* malignancy, *(b)* age over 60 years, *(c)* fever, *(d)* hematocrit less than 30%, *(e)* WBC count 10,000/mm$^3$ or more, *(f)* serum bilirubin 10 mg/dL or more, *(g)* BUN above 20 mg/dL, *(h)* serum creatinine 1.3 mg/dL or more, *(i)* serum albumin 3.0 g/dL or less, and alkaline phosphatase 100 u/L or more. When the patient had less than four of these factors, the operative mortality rate was 7%, but when more than 5 of these 10 factors existed, the operative mortality rate was 44%. It was the recommendation of the investigators that the patients with more than 5 of these factors should be considered for preoperative biliary decompression. Blamey et al. (48) reported a similar study. Dixon et al. (47) noted that the albumin level and the leucocyte count were insignificant in evaluation of operative risk but that diabetes was an important risk factor. Thompson et al. (49) reported a significant postoperative decrease of creatinine clearance among patients who had had endotoxemia preoperatively.

Evaluation of hepatic reserve in obstructive jaundice is important. Studies of ketone body ratio (50), clearance of indocyanine green, and measurement of hepatocellular volume have also been recommended for estimation of operative risk.

## REFERENCES


1. Hallenbeck GA. Biliary and pancreatic intraductal pressure. In: Code CD, ed. The handbook of physiology, section 6, the alimentary canal. Vol II: Secretion. Washington, DC: American Physiological Society, 1967:1007–1025.
2. Nagorney DM, et al. Bile duct pressure as a modulator of liver blood flow after common bile duct obstruction. Surg Forum 1982;33:206–208.
3. Alexander B, Blumgart LH, Mathie RT. The effect of propranolol on the hyperaemic response of the hepatic artery to portal venous occlusion in the dog. Br J Pharmacol 1989;96:356–362.
4. Lautt WW, et al., eds. Hepatic circulation in health and disease. New York: Raven Press, 1981:203–220.
5. Tamakuma S, et al. Pre- and postoperative management of in gastroenterological surgery (in Japanese). Tokyo: Chugai Igakusha 1991:57–58.
6. Saito H, et al. Hyperdynamic state in obstructive jaundice (in Japanese). Gekachiryo 1980;42:241–247.
7. Cahill CJ. Prevention of postoperative renal failure in patients with obstructive jaundice: the role of bile salts. Br J Surg 1983;70:590–595.
8. Diamond T, et al. Endotoxemia in obstructive jaundice: the role of gastrointestinal flow. Surg Res Commun 1989;5:11–16.
9. Bertok L. Physico-chemical defense of vertebrate organisms: the role of bile acids in defense against bacterial endotoxins. Perspect Biol Med 1977;21:70–76.
10. Deitch EA. Gut failure: its role in the multiple organ failure syndrome. In: Deitch EA, ed. Multiple organ failure. New York: Thieme Medical Publishers, 1991:40–59, 72–86.
11. Deitch EA. The role of intestinal barrier failure and bacterial translocation in the development of systemic infection and multiple organ failure. Arch Surg 1990;125:403–404.
12. Vagianos C, et al. Bacterial translocation and endotoxemia in obstructive jaundice: the protective effect of lactulose. Dis Surg 1995;12:321–326.
13. Slocum MM, Sitting KM, Specian RD, Deitch EA. Absence of intestinal bile promotes bacterial translocation. Am Surg 1992;58: 305–310.
14. Ding JW, Andersson R, Soltesz V, et al. The effect of biliary decompression on bacterial translocation in jaundiced rats. HPB Surg 1993;7:99–110.
15. Yu JL, Andersson R, Wang LQ, et al. Experimental foreign body infection in the biliary tract in rats. Scand J Gastroenterol 1995;30:478–483.
16. Kocsar LT, Bertok L, Varteresz V. Effect of bile acids on the intestinal absorption of endotoxin in rat. J Bacteriol 1969;100:220–223.
17. Bailey ME. Endotoxin, bile salts and renal function in obstructive jaundice. Br J Surg 1976;63:774–778.
18. Holman JM Jr, Rikkers LF, et al. Biliary obstruction and host defense failure. J Surg Res 1982;32:208–213.
19. Clements WD, Diamond T, McCrory DC, Rowlands BJ. Biliary drainage in obstructive jaundice: experimental and clinical aspects. Br J Surg 1993;80:834–842.
20. Ding JW, Andersson R, Soltesz V, et al. Obstructive jaundice impairs reticuloendothelial function and promotes bacterial translocation in the rat. J Surg Res 1994;57:238–245.
21. Iwasaki M, Maruyama I, Ikeziri N, et al. Endotoxin in severe liver diseases. Jpn J Gastroenterol 1980;77:386–394.
22. Kunimatsu N, et al. Bacterial translocation and intestinal mucosal atrophy in rats with bile duct ligation. Igaku No Ayumi 1990;155: 401–402.
23. Jacobsson B, et al. Cholangiovenous reflux: an experimental study. Acta Chir Scand 1962;123:316–321.
24. Pain JA, Bailey ME, et al. Measurement of operative plasma endotoxin levels in jaundiced and non-jaundiced patients. Eur Surg Res 1987;19:207–216.
25. Granger DN, Richardson PD, Kvietys PR, Mortillaro NA. Intestinal blood flow. Gastroenterology 1980;78:837–863.
26. Halliday AW, Benjamin IS, Blumgart LH. Nutritional risk factors in major hepatobiliary surgery. JPEN 1988;12:43–48.
27. Abe Y. Studies on blood coagulation, fibrinolysis and complements in patients with obstructive jaundice. J Jpn Surg Soc 1981;82:469–482.
28. Joko Y. Studies on acute renal failure in obstructive jaundice. J Jpn Surg Soc 1982;83:297–307.
29. Ozawa K, Yamada T, Tanaka J, et al. The mechanism of suppression for renal function in patients and rabbits with jaundice. Surg Gynecol Obstet 1979;149:54–60.
30. McPherson GA, Benjamin IS, Blumgart LH. Improving renal function in obstructive jaundice without preoperative drainage. Lancet 1984;1:511–512.

31. Dawson JL. The incidence of post-operative renal failure in obstructive jaundice. Br J Surg 1967;52:663–665.
32. Thompson JN, Edwards WH, Winearls CG, et al. Renal impairment following biliary tract surgery. Br J Surg 1987;74:843–847.
33. Mito M, et al. Hepatorenal syndrome in operation for hepato-pancreatic biliary diseases, portal hypertension, and diseases of spleen. Jinnai D, ed. Tokyo: Kanehara Shuppan, 1982:53.
34. Wait RB, Kahng KU. Renal failure complicating obstructive jaundice. Am J Surg 1989;157:256–263.
35. Fukai Y, Matsuyoshi R, Kasamatsu M, Yonezawa N. Obstructive jaundice and postoperative hemorrhage—with special reference to gastrointestinal hemorrhage (in Japanese). Operation 1971;25:1214–1221.
36. Sato T. Pathophysiologic and therapeutic investigation of post-operative stress ulcer in patients with obstructive jaundice (in Japanese). 1986;87:941–944.
37. Tamakuma M. Obstructive jaundice and its postoperative complication. Modern Surgery 75-D. Tokyo: Nakayama, 1975: 277–304.
38. Urakawa T, Nagahata Y, Fukuoka S, et al. Experimental study on the pathogenesis of acute ulceration in obstructive jaundice: with reference to gastric mucosal blood flow. J Jpn Surg Soc 1986;87:180–188.
39. Menguy R, Masters YF. Mechanism of stress ulcer. III: Effects of hemorrhagic shock on energy metabolism in the mucosa of the antrum, corpus, and fundus of the rabbit stomach. Gastroenterology 1974;66:1168.
40. Menguy R, Masters YF. Mechanism of stress ulcer: Influence of sodium taurocholate on gastric mucosal energy metabolism during hemorrhagic shock and on mitochondrial respiration and ATPase in gastric mucosa. Am J Dig Dis 1976;21:1001–1007.
41. Menguy R. Effect of biliary diversion from the small intestine on gastric secretory activity in dogs. Gastroenterology 1971;41:568.
42. Bowen JC, Fleming WH. Upper gastrointestinal bleeding associated with biliary diversion after hepatic injury. Ann Surg 1973;177: 420.
43. Breen JJ, Molina E, Ritchie WP. Effect of common bile duct transplantation on gastric acid secretion in the dog. Br J Surg 1968;55:282–284.
44. Nahrwold DL, Grossman MI. Effect of exclusion of bile from the intestine on gastric acid secretion. Gastroenterology 1967;52: 667–669.
45. Narui H, et al. Experimental study on acute ulceration in association with obstructive jaundice: with special reference to effect of biliary drainage on gastric mucosal blood flow and energy kinetics. J Jpn Surg Soc 1986;87:510–517.
46. Pitt HA, Cameron JL, Postier RG, Gadacz TR. Factors affecting mortality in biliary tract surgery. Am J Surg 1981;141:66–72.
47. Dixon JM, Armstrong CP, Duffy SW, Davies GC. Factors affecting morbidity and mortality after surgery for obstructive jaundice: a review of 373 patients. Gut 1983;24:845–852.
48. Blamey SL, Fearon KC, Gilmour WH, et al. Prediction of risk in biliary surgery. Br J Surg 1983;70:535–538.
49. Thompson JN, Cohen J, Moore RH, et al. Endotoxemia in obstructive jaundice. Am J Surg 1988;155:314–321.
50. Tanaka J, Ozawa K, Tobe T. Significance of blood ketone body ratio as an indicator of hepatic cellular energy status in jaundiced rabbits. Gastroenterology 1979;76:691–696.

# 16

# Chronic Obstruction of the Pancreatic Duct

C. W. Imrie

Chronic obstruction of the pancreatic duct may occur for a number of reasons, and the nature of the physical response in terms of luminal size change and total volume of pancreatic tissue change depends greatly upon the texture of the gland. Where the gland is normal in texture, considerable volume changes of the main pancreatic duct and subsidiary branches are likely to ensue with a significant change in overall pancreatic volume, whereas varying degrees of fibrosis of the gland will greatly affect the ability of the duct and surrounding tissues to respond in this manner. The texture of the pancreas will be most affected in patients with chronic pancreatitis and associated fibrosis, while the aging process itself will restrict the ability of the duct and pancreatic tissue to increase in diameter and volume, respectively, in response to chronic obstruction. In malignant disease, there may be a considerable associated fibrotic reaction within the acinar tissue of the pancreas, and this will greatly restrict the ability of the obstructed duct to change in size.

Distension and increase in pressure of the pancreatic ductal secretory system usually results in discomfort and possibly pain of considerable severity. Relief of the obstruction either by the placement of stents or by open surgical ductal decompression procedures frequently removes this discomfort and pain. Similarly, the development of a fistula from the pancreatic ductal system may also diminish the symptoms of discomfort and pain.

## Ductal Obstruction with Dilatation

The main pancreatic duct of normal size is rarely larger than 3.5–4 mm in diameter. However, in patients with focal stricture that may be due to a single area of damage to the main pancreatic duct, induced during an attack of acute pancreatitis, or less commonly, from blunt abdominal trauma, dilatation of the upstream ductal system can ensue, with a measurable increase in pancreatic ductal pressure as well as in acinar tissue pressure (1, 2). This may also occur in the patient with focal chronic pancreatitis, as shown in Figure 16.1*A*, in which gross pancreatic ductal dilatation of most of the gland took place with an associated severe painful area in the central and left upper quadrant of the abdomen. In this patient, focal chronic pancreatitis, affecting the head of the gland, had so greatly scarred the main pancreatic duct that no satisfactory pancreatogram was obtained endoscopically. However, percutaneous needle puncture of the dilated main pancreatic duct was achieved using ultrasonic guidance (Fig. 16.1*A*). Thereafter, an onlay side-to-side pancreatojejunostomy was performed, with initial symptomatic improvement. The patient returned 8 weeks later with what she described as pain in a similar location but of a different nature. Once again, a percutaneous puncture of the pancreatic duct was achieved through the onlay jejunal loop (Fig. 16.1*B*), which showed spectacular decompression of the main pancreatic duct to normal size. It was a considerable surprise to see the degree to which a markedly dilated duct had returned to normal; such a finding is not usual in the pancreatic ductal system but would not be exceptional in the biliary tree or ureteric drainage system. It certainly showed that in this particular patient it was unlikely that the later pain was derived from the pancreas. The operative decompression had been quite successful. Subsequently, it was determined that this later pain was colonic in origin and that her previous problem of chronic constipation had exacerbated. Once this problem was tackled, the pain disappeared.

## Dilated Pancreatic Duct Associated with Ampullary or Endocrine Tumors

Both ampullary and endocrine tumors grow slowly and often in the presence of normal pancreatic gland texture, so considerable dilatation of the main pancreatic duct is possible. In the case of ampullary and periampullary tumors, relief of the obstruction of the pancreatic duct depends on the age of the patient and the biologic aggression of the tumor. In older, less fit patients, laser therapy is an important advance that may be combined with endoscopic stenting. For younger patients, the most successful treatment is by pylorus-preserving pancreaticoduodenectomy.

An example of marked dilatation of the pancreatic duct is shown in a patient who had a fairly large endocrine tumor in the head of the pancreas, with considerable distal dilatation of both biliary and pancreatic ductal systems (Fig. 16.2). This gross dilatation of both systems was associated with the slow growth of a combined somatostatinoma and gastrinoma that was successfully treated by pancreaticoduodenectomy. This patient is alive and well, without major health problems more than 6 years after the resection. Ductal dilatation and raised pressures were documented many years ago by Bradley (1), and high acinar pressures by Danish physicians (2, 3).

## Chronic Obstruction of the Pancreatic Duct Associated with Fibrous Change in the Gland

Slight or moderate dilatation of the main pancreatic duct may occur in patients with chronic obstruction of the pancreatic duct associated with fibrous change in the gland, and fistula formation may result from disruption of a weak part of the obstructed ductal system, resulting in pancreatic ascites. Therapy in such patients is more difficult than in those with dilatation, because any decompression of the ductal system is unlikely to be rewarded by effective relief of symptoms. Resection may become necessary, particularly when malignancy is suspected or cannot be disproved in the case of distal chronic pancreatitis affecting the tail of the gland.

When possible, a scarred distal pancreas causing severe pain is best dealt with by resection when possible. It is best to carry this out with splenic preservation (4), the goal being to remove the gland from the splenic vessels, tying off all the many side

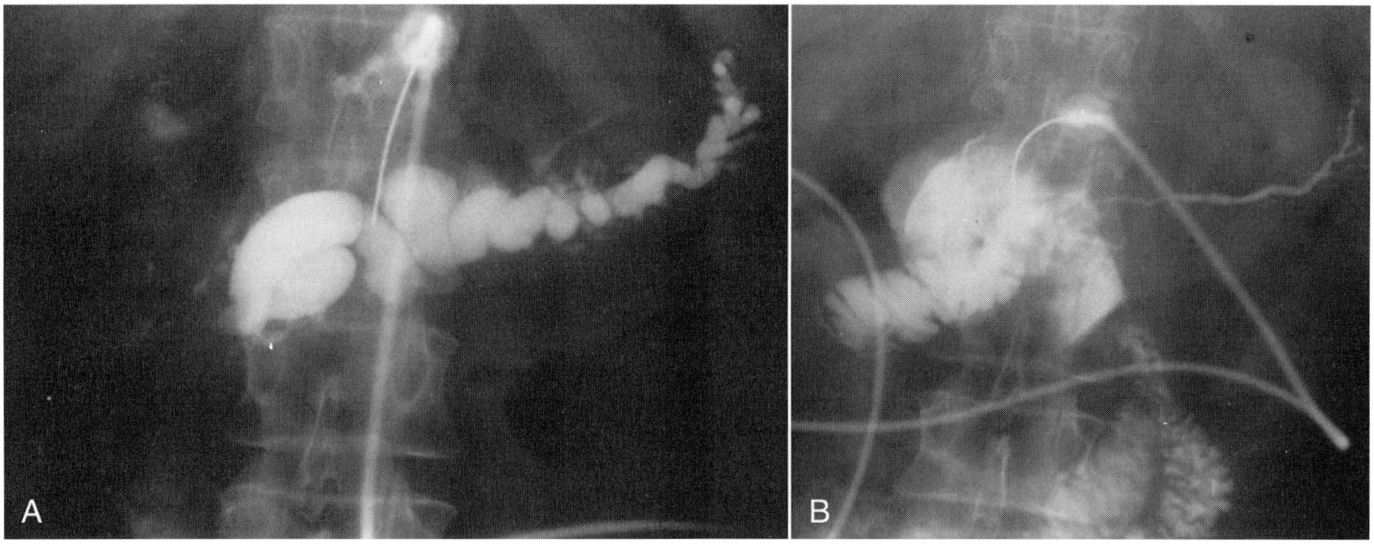


**FIG. 16.1.** **A.** A grossly distended main pancreatic ductal system associated with a focal stricture near the ampulla and demonstrated by percutaneous pancreatography. **B.** A subsequent percutaneous pancreatogram in the same patient approximately 8 weeks after onlay pancreaticojejunostomy Roux-en-Y drainage. This demonstrates the reversal to normal size of the central and distal part of the main pancreatic duct.

branches with meticulous care. Occasionally, the pancreatic scarring and fibrosis are so severe that preserving the splenic vessels is impossible; it can be hoped that the spleen will be served adequately by the vasa brevia and that it will remain viable. Should it prove necessary to resect the spleen, the reimplantation of splenic slices within the greater omentum often results in a reasonable hematologic picture with no evidence of Howell-Jolly bodies or rouleaux formations. However, such patients appear to be at risk of overwhelming postsplenectomy infection, and when splenectomy at elective surgery is considered possible, my recommendation is for triple vaccination 1 week before surgery with Pneumovax, Meningovax, and *Haemophilus influenzae* vaccines. Additionally, postoperatively, the safest routine is to give these patients 250 mg of penicillin night and morning for life.

Distal pancreatic resection is not necessarily accompanied by Roux loop drainage of the tail of the pancreas as there is no advantage over simple suture closure (4, 5). Figure 16.3 shows a typical moderately dilated distal pancreatic ductal system containing multiple stones, here associated with chronic pancreatitis. Endoscopic stone extraction was not possible, partly because of the stricture close to the ampulla. The stones were removed at open surgery when an onlay pancreaticojejunostomy was performed.

Focal main pancreatic strictures can be associated with the formation of a small cystic decompression area (or retention cyst) from the main duct as shown in Figure 16.4 in a patient with chronic pancreatitis. Considerably larger pseudocysts may also develop in the ductal tributaries in patients with chronic pancreatitis. Such pseudocysts may be managed conservatively with regular octreotide given subcutaneously to encourage spontaneous resolution or by placement of an endoscopic stent across the area of ductal disruption. Surgical therapy varies from internal drainage into the stomach, duodenum, or jejunal loop to excision of the affected area of the pancreas and is discussed in detail in other chapters.

Another type of response to increased pancreatic ductal pressure is the development of a fistula from the ductal system. Such fistulas may communicate with the main peritoneal cavity and present as pancreatic ascites, or communicate with the pleural cavity and produce an enzyme-rich pleural effusion (6, 7). Less frequently, the fistulas communicate with the bowel or with the skin.

An unusual example of a pancreatic fistula associated with cancer of the pancreas is shown in Figure 16.5; there was spontaneous drainage of pancreatic juice, which continued percutaneously after removal of a tube drain placed after a

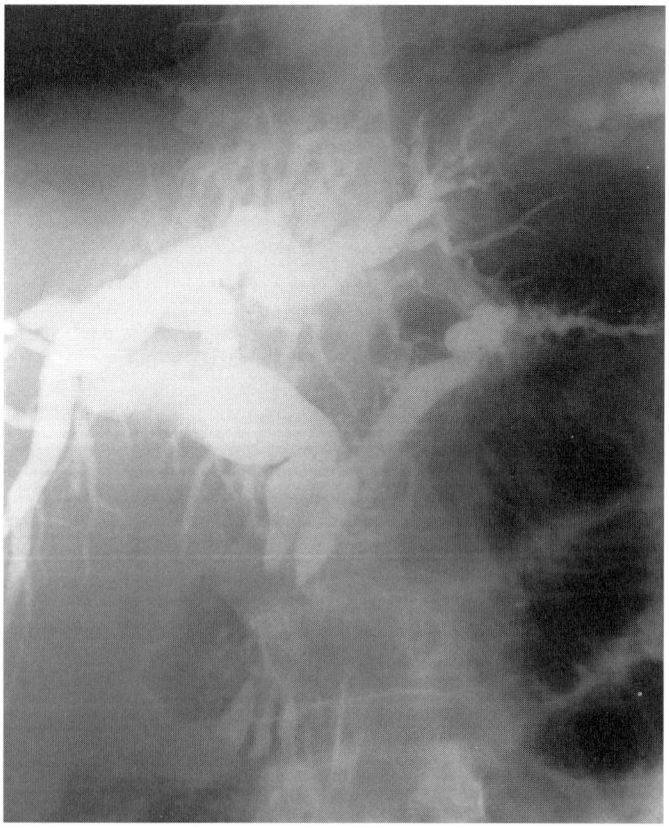

**FIG. 16.2.** An ERCP outlining both biliary and pancreatic ductal systems with gross dilatation of both associated with an unusual endocrine tumor (a combined somatostatinoma and gastrinoma).

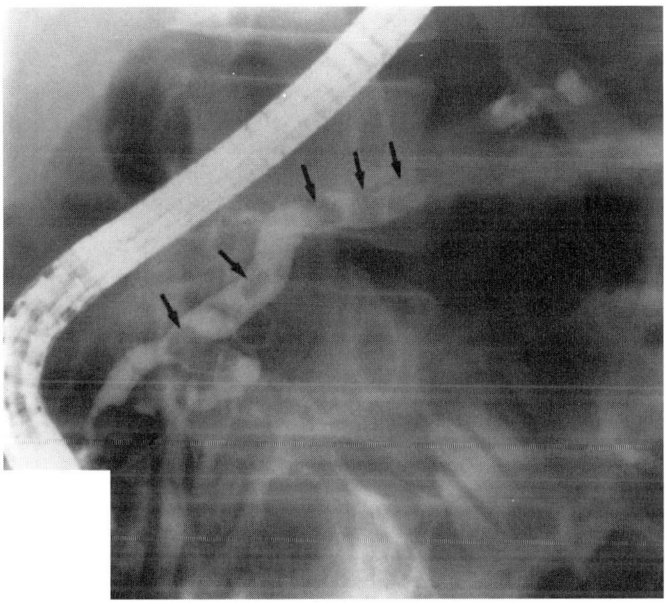

**FIG. 16.3.** A moderately distended pancreatic duct with a stricture near the ampulla and multiple stones in a patient with chronic pancreatitis.

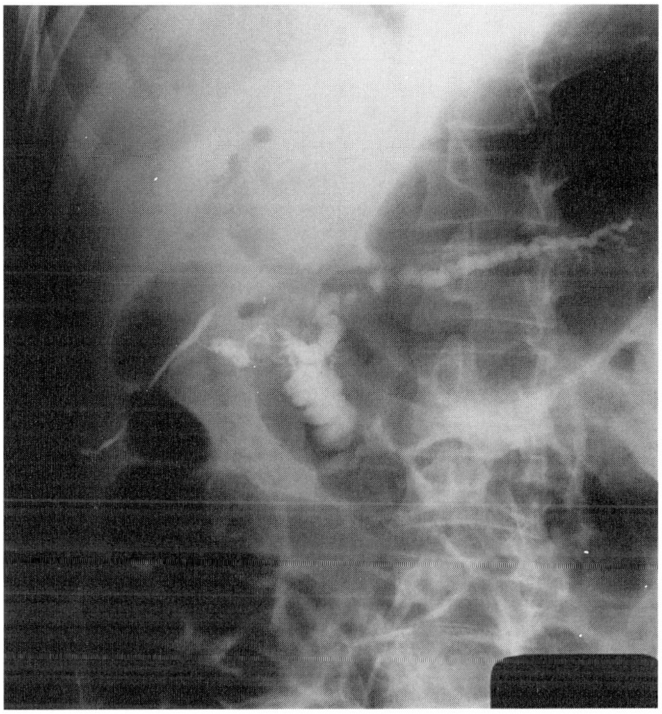

**FIG. 16.5.** A narrow pancreaticocutaneous fistula from the head of the pancreas to the skin in the right upper quadrant of the abdomen in a patient with carcinoma of the pancreas.

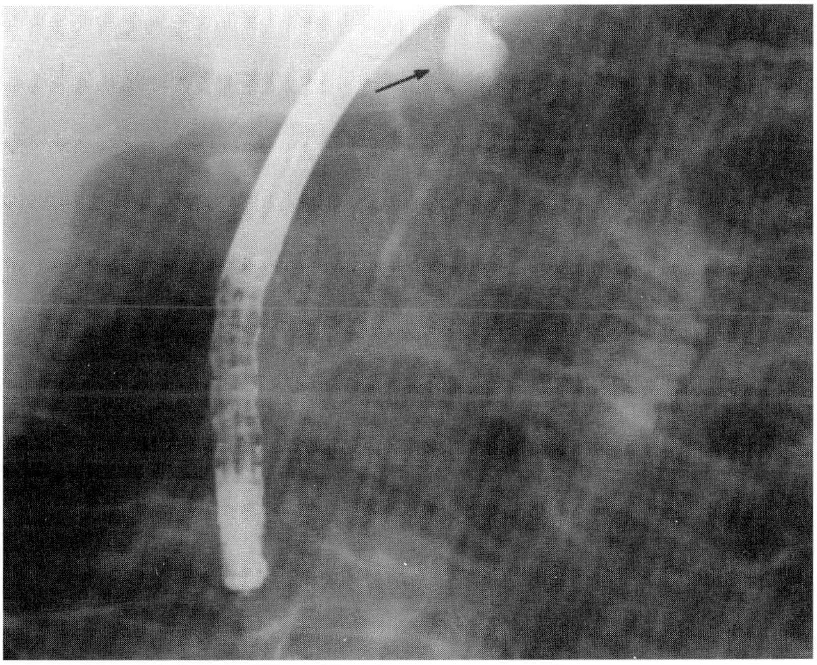

**FIG. 16.4.** A small cystic lesion leading from the main pancreatic duct in the central portion of the pancreas.

negative percutaneous biopsy. Biochemically, it was clear that this was a pancreatic fistula, but only on tertiary referral to our department was cytology performed that associated the fistula with pancreatic adenocarcinoma, by which time the disease was nonresectable, and only palliative measures were possible. This was an exceptional case, for in my experience, pancreatic ascites is almost invariably associated with disruption of the main pancreatic duct following damage from a single attack of acute pancreatitis or disruption of a weakened area of the duct associated with chronic pancreatitis.

### Chronic Ductal Obstruction without Dilatation

Over the last 18 months, we have used an alternative method to deal with pancreatic pain in patients with a nondilated ductal system. We evaluate carefully the source of pain, and after full clinical, radiologic, and psychologic assessment, perform thoracoscopic splanchnicectomy. A minimally invasive surgical approach is used through two 5-mm ports placed on each side just inferior to the lower border of the scapula, usually in the 7th and 6th interspaces. The patient is face-down, with selective intubation of the right and left bronchus so that a single lung may be nonoxygenated for part of the procedure. Collapse of the lung may be aided by injection of a small volume of carbon dioxide into the pleural space. The goal is to identify the splanchnic nerves as they cross obliquely toward the sympathetic chain and to divide the nerves by diathermy hook on each side (8, 9). We have found the procedure to involve relatively little patient trauma and to be encouragingly effective in lowering analgesic requirements and occasionally abolishing the need for analgesics. [*Editor's note:* see also Chapter 40.] We consider this an important adjunct in the management of such patients, which may represent a significant step forward in management. A randomized clinical trial is now under way to assess more fully the role of thoracoscopic splanchnic nerve division.

## REFERENCES


1. Bradley EL 3d. Pancreatic duct pressure in chronic pancreatitis. Am J Surg 1982;144:313–316.
2. Ebbehoj N, Svendsen LB, Madsen P. Pancreatic tissue pressure: techniques and pathophysiological aspects. Scand J Gastroenterol 1984;19:1066–1068.
3. Ebbehoj N, Borly L, Madsen P, Svendsen LB. Pancreatic tissue pressure and pain in chronic pancreatitis. Pancreas 1986;1: 556–558.
4. Warshaw AL. Conservation of the spleen with distal pancreatectomy. Arch Surg 1988;123:550–553.
5. Shankar S, Theis B, Russell RC. Management of the stump of the pancreas after distal pancreatic resection. Br J Surg 1990;77: 541–544.
6. Cameron JL. Chronic pancreatic ascites and pancreatic pleural effusions. Gastroenterology 1978;74:134–140.
7. Cole DJ, Bradley EL. Internal pancreatic fistulas: classification, recognition and management. In: Pederzoli P, ed. Pancreatic fistulas. Berlin: Springer-Verlag, 1993.
8. Andrén-Sandberg A. Zoucas E, Lillo-Gil R, Gyllestedt E, Ihse I. Thoracoscopic splanchnicectomy for chronic, severe pancreatic pain. Semin Laparosc Surg 1996;3:29–33.
9. Takahashi T, Kakita A, Izumika H, Iino Z, Furuta K, et al. Thoracoscopic splanchnicectomy for the relief of intractable abdominal pain. Surg Endosc 1996;10:65–68.

# 17

# Diabetes in Exocrine Pancreatic Disease: Pathophysiology and Management

Bo Ahrén

Diabetes mellitus is caused by absolute or relative deficiency of insulin. In type 1 diabetes, the B cells have been destroyed by immunologic mechanisms, whereas after total pancreatectomy, no B cells, by definition, remain. Therefore, in these two forms of diabetes, there is an absolute deficiency of insulin, and the diabetes is strictly insulin dependent. In contrast, in non-insulin-dependent (type 2) diabetes, the deficiency of insulin is relative, since peripheral insensitivity to insulin exists, and the secreted amount of insulin to retain normoglycemia, although increased, is inadequate, due to failure of the insulin-producing B cells in the pancreatic islets (1). Diseases of the exocrine pancreas might affect the endocrine function of the pancreas, ultimately leading to diabetes. This may be achieved if the disease process in the exocrine pancreas is spread into and invades the islets, ultimately destroying the endocrine cells. Alternatively, the disease process in the exocrine pancreas might produce factors that impair the function of the neighboring islet endocrine cells, causing impairment of islet function. Exocrine pancreatic diseases might also influence other regulatory pathways in the glucose metabolism, such as peripheral insulin sensitivity, ultimately leading to diabetes. This chapter presents aspects of the pathophysiology and management of diabetes when it occurs in patients with exocrine pancreatic diseases.

## DIABETES IN ACUTE PANCREATITIS

It has been demonstrated that 50% of all patients with acute pancreatitis have glucose intolerance or diabetes during their acute illness (2). The underlying reason is mainly an exaggerated stimulation of glucagon secretion rather than an inhibited insulin secretion. On the contrary, insulin secretion is often exaggerated and not inhibited during acute pancreatitis (2). The evolving hyperglucagonemia causes hyperglycemia due to stimulated glycogenolysis and release of glucose from the liver. Furthermore, very ill patients with acute pancreatitis have an impaired capacity to utilize glucose peripherally, as have severely ill patients in general, which will further exaggerate a hyperglycemia.

Due to the high risk of glucose intolerance or diabetes during acute pancreatitis, it is important to measure blood and urinary glucose levels and ketonemia in these patients and, if necessary, to initiate treatment. Usually, the diabetes is only transient, and when the patient recovers from the acute pancreatitis, the diabetes improves and in most patients disappears completely. Nevertheless, persistent diabetes is not uncommon after an episode of acute pancreatitis, and this is more prevalent if surgery has been undertaken during the acute course of the disease (3).

Another important aspect of acute pancreatitis and diabetes is that primary diabetes is associated with an increased risk of developing acute pancreatitis (4, 5), which might be due to diabetes-related vascular damage of the pancreas increasing the vulnerability of the gland. Therefore, alertness to the possibility of acute pancreatitis is warranted in diabetic patients presenting with abdominal pain. Further, preexistent diabetes significantly worsens the prognosis of acute pancreatitis (6).

## DIABETES IN CHRONIC PANCREATITIS

Diabetes is overrepresented in chronic pancreatitis, and recent publications have shown that approximately 30–70% of subjects with a well-defined chronic pancreatitis also have diabetes (7–9). The pathophysiology of diabetes in chronic pancreatitis is a progressive tissue destruction with fibrosis and sclerosis that invades the endocrine cells and causes a progressive deterioration of islet function (8, 10). The toxic action of alcohol is an additional pathogenetic factor (11). Due to the progressive nature of the disease, it could be anticipated that in the long run, all patients with chronic pancreatitis sooner or later will develop diabetes.

The importance of islet dysfunction as a key factor for the development of diabetes in chronic pancreatitis is illustrated by findings that defective insulin secretion occurs in subjects with chronic pancreatitis without diabetes (12) and that islet dysfunction progresses with time during the progressive development of the pancreatitis (13). Whether reduced peripheral insulin action contributes to diabetes in chronic pancreatitis is at present controversial, since studies both demonstrating (14, 15) and refuting (16) such a hypothesis exist.

The islet dysfunction accompanying diabetes in chronic pancreatitis is not restricted to impaired insulin secretion. Thus, glucagon and pancreatic polypeptide (PP) secretion are also impaired in severe cases (17, 18). In contrast, in mild diabetes accompanying chronic pancreatitis, glucagon secretion is exaggerated, which is probably due to low insulin secretion, since insulin inhibits glucagon secretion. Therefore, plasma glucagon levels in subjects with chronic pancreatitis and diabetes might be unaltered, lowered, or elevated. Regarding the fourth islet hormone, somatostatin, studies on its secretion in chronic pancreatitis have been difficult to interpret because circulating somatostatin is primarily extrapancreatic in origin. Elevated plasma somatostatin levels are often seen in chronic pancreatitis (18), and this is therefore probably due to increased secretion of the peptide from the gut. Nevertheless, the high somatostatin levels might be of pathophysiologic importance for the development of diabetes, since somatostatin is known to inhibit insulin secretion.

The impaired glucagon secretion accompanying diabetes in chronic pancreatitis is of clinical importance, since a main function of glucagon is to counteract the hypoglycemic action of insulin. Therefore, subjects with chronic pancreatitis and diabetes exhibit increased sensitivity to exogenous insulin and experience an increased likelihood of hypoglycemic episodes. However, counterregulation during hypoglycemia is characteristically regulated redundantly by other factors, such as catecholamines, which might explain why glucose counterregulation is only slightly impaired in subjects with chronic pancreatitis and diabetes (17). Since glucagon is also a ketogenic hormone, another consequence of the impaired glucagon secretion is a low tendency to develop diabetic ketoacidosis (19). However, ketosis might also develop in glucagon-deficient individuals during periods of declining plasma insulin levels (8). Therefore, in diabetes associated with chronic pancreatitis, ketoacidosis might also evolve, though rarely (2, 8).

An increased sensitivity to exogenous insulin with an increased tendency to develop hypoglycemia in diabetic patients with chronic pancreatitis is not only due to impaired glucagon secretion. The patients often exhibit hepatic dysfunction that impairs gluconeogenesis, to which is added a toxic alcohol-induced impairment of hepatic glucose production (8, 20). Chronic pancreatitis is also often accompanied by nutritional disturbances, caused by reduced caloric intake in combination with established malnutrition, which increases the likelihood of hypoglycemia (8).

The prevalence of secondary complications to diabetes is lower in diabetes due to chronic pancreatitis than in type 1 diabetes (8). This is probably not due to a rare occurrence of complications, per se, but rather to a shorter duration of diabetes in chronic pancreatitis. Nevertheless, secondary complications are seen in diabetes in chronic pancreatitis. In fact, retinopathy, albeit mild and not of the proliferative type, is not uncommon in diabetes in chronic pancreatitis (8, 21). This implies that regular ophthalmoscopy should be undertaken in these patients. In contrast, nephropathy and neuropathy are uncommon (8).

## DIABETES IN PANCREATIC CANCER

It has been known for several decades that subjects with pancreatic cancer have an increased prevalence of diabetes at the time of diagnosis of the cancer (22, 23). The frequency of diabetes among subjects with pancreatic cancer has varied in different studies, however, which is partially due to the retrospective nature of most studies and different diagnostic criteria. Another reason is that most patients with diabetes at the time of diagnosis of the pancreatic cancer are apparently not aware of the diagnosis of diabetes (24, 25). Thus, whereas only approximately 10–20% of patients with newly diagnosed pancreatic cancer report that they have diabetes (26), several recent studies using glucose tolerance tests for the diagnosis show that approximately 50–80% of all patients with pancreatic cancer have diabetes or impaired glucose tolerance (13, 27, 28).

The reason for the association between diabetes and pancreatic cancer has gained considerable interest during recent years. Some reports favor an assumption that diabetes precedes the cancer and may be regarded as a risk factor. Thus, a relative risk for patients with diabetes to develop pancreatic cancer has been shown to exceed four times (29, 30). This may be explained if diabetes is involved in the pathogenesis of the cancer, for example through a growth-promoting effect of insulin, during the hyperinsulinemic phase of the disease (31). Alternatively, diabetes and pancreatic cancer may share a common pathogenetic factor; alcohol has been discussed as one (30).

In contrast to this assumption, several reports have favored the concept that diabetes is a consequence of the tumor. For example, a large epidemiologic study has demonstrated that there was no clear association between the occurrence of diabetes and pancreatic cancer, except during the year preceding the onset of the malignancy (32), suggesting that diabetes evolves together with or after the development of pancreatic cancer. Several other studies have reached the same conclusion (27, 33–35). Moreover, since most patients with diabetes at the time of the diagnosis of pancreatic cancer are obviously not aware of the diabetes (25, 26), the disease is likely of recent onset. In addition, experimental studies have shown that diabetes protects from pancreatic cancer rather than being involved in its pathogenesis (25, 36). Therefore, most studies favor the view that the increased prevalence of diabetes in pancreatic cancer reflects recent-onset disease and might be a consequence of the tumor and, therefore, in some patients, an early symptom of the pancreatic cancer.

The pathogenetic mechanisms for the diabetes accompanying pancreatic cancer have been the subject of several studies. Some of these studies have demonstrated that the peripheral insulin sensitivity is reduced in these patients (27, 37, 38). Several confounding factors that accompany pancreatic cancer might cause the peripheral insulin insensitivity, such as cholestasis or weight loss, or it might be a general consequence of malignancy. No correlation has been found, however, between the reduced insulin sensitivity in pancreatic cancer and the degree of cholestasis (38), and experimentally, potentiated rather than inhibited insulin secretion has been found in cholestatic rats (39). Furthermore, although malignancy in general is associated with impaired glucose tolerance and reduced insulin sensitivity (40), the higher association between diabetes and pancreatic cancer than between diabetes and other malignancies suggests that it is the pancreatic tumor per se that initiates the reduced sensitivity to insulin rather than an association with malignancy in general.

It has therefore been hypothesized that the tumor cells in pancreatic cancer secrete a factor that inhibits the action of insulin (38). This hypothesis is also supported by studies showing that removal of the tumor improves glucose tolerance (41) and that administration of a human pancreatic cancer cell line causes hyperglycemia in immunodeficient mice (42). Recently, islet amyloid polypeptide (IAPP) was suggested to be such a factor, since the plasma level of IAPP was shown to be higher in patients with pancreatic cancer and diabetes than in patients with other malignancies or subjects with pancreatic cancer but without diabetes (43). IAPP is normally produced in pancreatic B cells together with insulin and cosecreted with insulin, and the peptide has been hypothesized to be involved in the pathogenesis of diabetes, because of both its ability to form islet amyloid and thereby possibly inhibit insulin secretion and its inhibition of the peripheral effects of insulin (44). Although this hypothesis needs to be confirmed, the idea that IAPP or some other factor is secreted from the pancreatic tumors and causes hyperglycemia or diabetes is intriguing.

Besides the existence of impaired peripheral insulin sensitivity, patients with diabetes and pancreatic cancer exhibit impaired insulin secretion (28, 45, 46). Similarly, a longitudinal experimental study of pancreatic cancer in the Syrian hamster has shown that the development of tumor is associated with a gradually developing impairment of insulin secretion (47). Impaired insulin secretion in pancreatic cancer might be induced by tumor, per se, or by a factor released from the tumor, rather than tumor tissue invading the islets, as tumor removal improves insulin secretion (41). To conclude, diabetes in pancreatic cancer seems to be caused by the tumor, perhaps by a factor released by tumor tissue, and both reduced peripheral sensitivity to insulin and impaired insulin secretion seem to contribute as pathogenetic factors.

Diabetes in subjects with pancreatic cancer shows the same clinical characteristics as type 2 diabetes in general. Thus, most patients may initially be treated with dietary regulations alone or oral hypoglycemic agents, whereas some patients require insulin (26, 27). The degree of secondary complications has not been studied in great detail, due to the short life expectancy in these patients. After total pancreatectomy for the pancreatic cancer, the diabetes by definition turns into a strict insulin-dependent type. On the contrary, following subtotal pancreatectomy, the glucose metabolism is improved (41), even though it is known that subtotal pancreatectomy per se markedly reduces the insulin secretory capacity (48).

## DIABETES AFTER SUBTOTAL AND TOTAL PANCREATECTOMY

Although the capacity to secrete insulin is inevitably reduced by subtotal pancreatectomy (48), frank diabetes rarely develops. One reason for this is that when the primary diagnosis is a pancreatic cancer, the negative influence of the tumor on glucose metabolism is ablated when the tumor is removed (41). Another reason is that islet overcapacity exists in the entire pancreas, so that the islet B cell mass has to be almost completely removed for the evolvement of diabetes (49). In fact, the rare development of diabetes after subtotal pancreatectomy has been one argument for performing subtotal rather than total pancreatectomy in pancreatic cancer (50, 51).

In contrast, after total pancreatectomy, insulin-dependent diabetes inevitably develops. In comparison with type 1 diabetes, postpancreatectomy diabetes shows certain characteristics: after pancreatectomy, the daily insulin requirement is often surprisingly low, yet the patients have a high tendency for hypoglycemic episodes and a low likelihood of developing ketosis. These characteristics have been attributed to the lack of circulating glucagon in these patients, in contrast to the often elevated plasma glucagon levels seen in type-1 diabetic patients (52). Pancreatectomized patients therefore exhibit a low gluconeogenic capacity and high circulating levels of gluconeogenic precursors (lactate, pyruvate, alanine, and glycerol) (52). Furthermore, the absence of glucagon impairs the glucose counterregulation, causing increased sensitivity to insulin, which results both in a low daily insulin requirement and in an increased likelihood of hypoglycemic episodes. Finally, the ketogenic tendency is low in the absence of glucagon, diminishing the risk of frank ketosis after pancreatectomy (19).

## MANAGEMENT OF DIABETES: GOAL OF TREATMENT AND ORGANIZATIONAL ASPECTS

The management of diabetes in exocrine pancreatic diseases or after pancreatectomy follows the same fundamental principles as the management in other diabetic patients. Thus, the tools for management are dietary adjustments, physical exercise, education of the patient, and, when required, addition of pharmacologic treatment with oral hypoglycemic agents or insulin replacement.

The goals of the treatment of diabetes in general are achievement of normal glucose and glycosylated hemoglobin levels, avoidance of hyperglycemia, glucosuria as well as hypoglycemia, prevention of complications, and the general well-being of the patient. For the diabetic patient with exocrine pancreatic diseases or after pancreatectomy, these goals should be considered in light of the special conditions of the diabetes in these diseases and the concomitant treatment of the exocrine pancreatic disease. Particularly, increased sensitivity to insulin makes hypoglycemia more hazardous than it is for other diabetic patients, and a shorter life expectancy than other diabetic patients diminishes the likelihood for development of secondary complications. Therefore, even if achievement of normoglycemia is an ultimate goal of treatment, diabetic patients with exocrine pancreatic diseases often do not require a treatment resulting in glucose levels within the normal range. For practical purposes, a realistic goal in many diabetic patients with exocrine pancreatic diseases is a fasting glucose level below 7 mmol/L (126 mg/100 mL), a postprandial glucose level below 9 mmol/L (162 mg/100 mL), and/or a glycosylated hemoglobin level below 7%.

The optimal treatment demands establishing a diabetes unit with several members: physician, diabetes nurse, nutritionist, physical therapist, social worker, psychologist etc. For patients with exocrine pancreatic diseases and for those who have been pancreatectomized, it is of great importance to have the surgeon involved in the diabetes unit, to supply knowledge of the pancreatic diseases and how they affect treatment of the diabetes. This is particularly important when surgery is planned for these subjects.

## DIETARY REGULATIONS

According to current concepts and guidelines from the American Diabetes Association (ADA), the diabetic diet should be composed of 10–20% protein, less than 30% fat, and 50–60% carbohydrates, on a caloric basis (53, 54). Other guidelines recommend a lower carbohydrate content (40–45%). If the patient is not overweight, which is seldom the case in diabetic patients with exocrine pancreatic diseases, the total caloric intake should be approximately 35 kcal/kg/day. Furthermore, the protein content should not exceed 0.8 g/kg/day, and the diet should consist of 40 g of preferably water-soluble fiber, since this type of fiber reduces the glycemia (55). Moreover, daily fat intake should be 80–100 g, the fat being (poly)unsaturated rather than saturated. Finally, the diet should contain less than 300 mg cholesterol/day and only a moderate amount of sucrose, with nonnutritive sweeteners instead. Besides the composition of the diet, it is also important to time the intake of meals. In general, a regular schedule of three meals is recommended, with 20% of calories in the morning, 20% at lunch, and 30% at dinnertime, with between-meal snacks constituting the remaining 30% (56).

Many patients with pancreatic cancer present with weight loss and are in a catabolic state; they should be treated with a high-protein and high-caloric diet initially and when diabetes is present. This is particularly important before an operation, since the metabolic response to surgery increases the utilization of fuel, which might compromise healing. In such patients, the caloric requirement should be increased by 20–35%, with a recommended daily protein intake of 1.5–2 g/kg (57). If nausea prevents the patient from eating, total parenteral nutrition (TPN) might be initiated 2–3 days before surgery. The TPN should consist of low-concentration dextrose with insulin to prevent hyperglycemia (blood glucose levels should be <14 mmol/L [252 mg/100 mL] all the time). Postoperatively, early enteral nutrition is important, and TPN should be used only during the immediate postoperative phase.

Dumping syndromes are not uncommon after pancreatic surgery. These symptoms are often difficult to manage, although they can sometimes be treated with dietary changes. The advice should include the necessity for regular and frequent intake of small meals with high protein content. The diet should be supplemented with protein, and if diarrhea is a concurrent problem, a lactose-free diet is recommended.

## PHYSICAL EXERCISE

Physical exercise is important in the treatment of diabetes because it has a beneficial effect on the general well-being, it potentially reduces long-term cardiovascular diseases, and it improves the glycemia (58, 59). The reduction of glycemia during exercise is due to increased uptake of glucose by the exercising muscle (59). Two potentially hazardous aspects of physical exercise have to be considered for patients with pancreatic diseases or after pancreatectomy. First, in insulin-treated patients, the circulating insulin concentration is usually constantly high, compared with that of nondiabetic subjects, and therefore, the increased peripheral glucose uptake in the exercising muscle increases the likelihood for hypoglycemia. Therefore, extra carbohydrate intake or a reduced insulin dose might be taken before physical exercise. Second, during phases of metabolic deterioration, for example when circulating insulin levels are low, hepatic glucose output will be increased during exercise, which will augment hyperglycemia. Therefore, the patient should not undertake physical exercise in periods of metabolic deterioration. Moreover, some patients with exocrine pancreatic diseases or after pancreatectomy are incapable of intense exercise on a regular basis. Therefore, the "dose" of exercise prescribed should be tailored for each patient, and for some patients, a simple walking program will suffice.

## ORAL HYPOGLYCEMIC AGENTS

When dietary regulations and physical exercise are not sufficient for reaching the goal of treatment, addition of pharmacologic agents is indicated. In most patients with chronic pancreatitis and pancreatic cancer, during the early stages in the development of diabetes, oral hypoglycemic agents suffice. The most commonly used oral hypoglycemic agents are the sulfonylureas, which potentiate glucose-stimulated insulin secretion from the islet B cells as well as peripheral insulin action to promote glucose uptake in muscles (60). The resulting increase in levels of plasma insulin reduces hepatic glucose delivery and exaggerates the uptake of glucose into peripheral tissues. However, during the course of both chronic pancreatitis and pancreatic cancer, treatment with sulfonylureas usually fails because of a progressive impairment in the insulin secretory capacity. Therefore, in the long run, most of these patients will require treatment with insulin.

Several different sulfonylureas are available, differing in pharmacokinetic characteristics, mode of metabolism, excretion, and adverse effects (60). Chlorpropamide and glyburide are long-acting sulfonylureas that may be taken once daily, but which carry a higher risk for hypoglycemic reactions. Glipizide, glibenclamide, and tolazamide are shorter acting, requiring intake twice daily (60). A general rule is to start sulfonylurea treatment with a low dose and then gradually increase it. Sulfonylureas are generally well accepted and with low toxicity and few adverse reactions, which occur in only approximately 3% of all patients (58). These reactions include allergic manifestations, gastrointestinal symptoms, and, in overdosage, hypoglycemia.

## INSULIN TREATMENT

Although some patients with chronic pancreatitis and pancreatic cancer with diabetes might be treated, at least temporarily, with oral hypoglycemic agents, most patients will sooner or later require exogenous insulin. The available insulin products of today are divided into short-acting insulin (Regular insulin or Semilente insulin with a peak effect 2–5 hours after administration), medium or intermediate-acting insulin (NPH insulin or Lente insulin with a peak effect at 6–12 hours), and long-acting insulin (Ultralente insulin with a peak effect at 8–20 hours) (61). For most insulin-treated diabetic patients, multiple-dose regimens are required, rather than single-dose regimens, and this is particularly true for those with chronic exocrine pancreatic diseases or after total pancreatectomy.

The optimal dose of insulin varies between patients. It varies also with time in each patient, because of temporal influences from the pancreatic disease process, concurrent nausea and catabolism, and variability in food and alcohol intake. The required amount of insulin is also altered perisurgically. Therefore, the starting dose of insulin is arbitrary, although in a newly discovered nonketotic patient or in a patient previously treated with oral hypoglycemic agent, a daily dose of medium-acting insulin in the range of 20–30 U/day is advisable as a starting dose. In contrast, higher doses (40–60 U/day) are often required for patients beginning insulin treatment postoperatively after pancreatectomy.

When starting insulin treatment, it is advisable either to give two-thirds of the required dose in the morning and one-third in the evening with dinner or to give the entire dose in the morning (58, 62). The dose should not be altered for the following 2–3 days. During these days, the glucose level in the blood should be checked three to four times daily, to provide information for continuous treatment. Following detailed instructions by the diabetic team, most patients can initiate the insulin treatment as outpatients.

The blood glucose determinations during the first few days might show that the overall glycemia is too high, suggesting that the overall daily insulin requirement has been underestimated. The insulin dose should then be increased, preferably by 5–10 U/day, and new glycemia tests performed for the following 2–3 days. However, the glycemia tests might show that the blood glucose level is too high, mainly postprandially or during the daytime, while the fasting level is adequate. If that is the case, short-acting insulin could be added, preferably with the morning dose, and if that is not sufficient, a three-dose insulin regimen with addition of a short-acting insulin, 15–20 minutes before lunch, might be initiated. If further adjustments are required, short-acting insulin 15–20 minutes before dinner may be added as well. On the other hand, if only the fasting glycemia is elevated, this could be a consequence of overcompensated glucose counterregulation to hypoglycemia at nighttime, the so-called Somogyi effect (63). Sometimes, the hypoglycemia at nighttime is accompanied by morning headache, nocturnal sweating, or nightmares. This should be handled by delaying the evening insulin dose until 11 PM, and if that is not sufficient, by reducing the evening dose and correspondingly increasing the morning dose. By careful analysis of the daily glucose profile in relation to insulin administration, it is possible to achieve an optimal insulin schedule in most patients, in terms of type, dose, and injection intervals. In the following long-term treatment, the patient should be taught to check blood glucose levels regularly at home and to report any significant fluctuations to the diabetes unit. On the basis of these home reports of the glycemia and the glycosylated hemoglobin levels, the insulin treatment should be reviewed at the regular visits at the diabetes unit.

In insulin-treated diabetic patients with exocrine pancreatic diseases, changes in the insulin requirement may be expected over time. In patients with chronic pancreatitis, this is due to the progression of the disease, which would increase the insulin requirement. Similarly, patients with pancreatic cancer might exhibit an increased insulin requirement due to continuously increased insulin resistance, although following surgery, many patients with pancreatic cancer exhibit a reduced insulin requirement (41). Also, patients with acute pancreatitis who are improving from the disease will experience a reduced insulin requirement. Therefore, regular control of blood glucose levels, both by the patient at home and by the diabetes unit, is required to achieve optimal insulin dosage in these patients.

When a patient needs both short- and medium-acting insulin, it may be tempting to use premixed insulin formulations, which exist in combinations of 70% intermediate-acting/30% short-acting or 50% intermediate-acting/50% short-acting insulin. However, these insulin combinations are optimal only for a few patients. For optimal treatment in most patients, it is preferable to tailor the mixing by the use of two different preparations. Most patients tolerate insulin treatment over a long period of time. Sometimes, however, adverse effects not related to hypoglycemia evolve after insulin treatment, the most common of which is local lipodystrophia (56, 61). This may be either of the hypertrophic or the atrophic type and is usually prevented by avoiding injecting insulin at the same place over a considerable period of time.

## MANAGEMENT OF DIABETES UNDER SPECIAL CONDITIONS

### Surgery

Surgery is associated with a variety of metabolic alterations. An important effect seen postoperatively is impairment in peripheral glucose uptake, which will cause hyperglycemia. During the postoperative phase, there is also exaggerated catabolism with lipolysis and nitrogen loss and changes in water and electrolyte balance, with sodium and water retention (64). It is advisable to prepare the insulin-treated diabetic patients with exocrine pancreatic diseases for surgery by admission to the hospital 2 days before surgery. Insulin treatment should then be changed to short-acting insulin preparations, glucose levels should be checked four times daily, potassium levels should be followed, and a close collaboration with the anesthesiologist should be initiated. If metabolic deterioration exists and persists, intravenous infusion of glucose with insulin and potassium should be undertaken to optimize the metabolism for the day of surgery. During surgery, a glucose level of 8–11 mmol/L (144–198 mg/100 mL) is advisable and is usually achieved by infusion of 5% dextrose to which is added 10–20 U insulin/L and 20–40 mmol (20–40 mEq/L) potassium/L, infused at a rate of 100–150 mL/hour. Postoperatively, the intravenous glucose/insulin/potassium administration should continue for the first 12 hours, but the patient can usually initiate the regular insulin treatment on the first postoperative day. Most important is frequent and regular monitoring of the glucose metabolic state of the patient. The insulin requirement is often higher on the first postoperative days than before surgery, because of the metabolic demand created by the surgery. However, often the insulin requirement is eventually lowered by the operation, because of relief of the disease process.

### Unstable Diabetes

Although the diabetes in most patients with exocrine pancreatic diseases or after pancreatectomy is relatively stable over a longer period of time, the disease in some patients is controlled only with great difficulty. Unstable diabetes, sometimes called "brittle diabetes," is associated with changing sensitivity to exogenous insulin over time and variable levels of blood sugar during exercise and emotional stress (65). These patients often exhibit episodes of hypoglycemia intermingled with postprandial exaggerated hyperglycemia. The cause of "brittle diabetes" is usually not clear in the individual patient; however, it is often due to a lack of endogenous insulin production causing an unopposed action of counterregulatory hormones, which creates a marked hyperglycemia following a hypoglycemic episode.

Treatment of unstable diabetes follows the same principles as treatment of diabetes in general. In difficult cases, the blood glucose changes over 24 hours should be carefully examined in relation to meals, exercise, and insulin administration. As a general rule, these patients should be encouraged to eat regularly and to undertake a moderate amount of exercise on a regular basis. In addition, careful selection of insulin types, doses, and dosing in relation to meal intake is required. For these patients, close contact between the patient, the family, and the diabetes unit is particularly important, and it is sometimes advisable to admit the patient to a metabolic ward for careful analysis of the 24-hour glucose profile.

### Acute Illnesses

During acute illnesses, the insulin requirement is increased. During a short acute illness (e.g., a few days of influenza with fever), a temporarily increased dose of insulin might be administered. As a general principle, it may be advisable to increase the morning dose of intermediate-acting insulin by 6–10 U if the afternoon urine test shows more than 0.5% sugar (56). During illnesses of longer duration, a more permanent change in the insulin dose is often necessary following a careful analysis of the glucose profile. In these cases, hospital admission of the patient is often advisable. Patients with chronic pancreatitis and pancreatic cancer sometimes exhibit nausea and anorexia, and some patients use intermittently heavy amounts of alcohol. During such periods, the insulin dose has to be reduced to avoid hypoglycemia.

### Hypoglycemia

Hypoglycemia is commonly caused by an overdose of insulin or, in some instances, of sulfonylureas, and it initiates a series of hormonal and neural compensatory mechanisms (66). The risk of hypoglycemia is increased by physical exercise, which increases the muscle uptake of glucose (58), and in hepatic dysfunction and after alcohol intake, which inhibit hepatic gluconeogenesis (8, 20). In patients with exocrine pancreatic diseases or after pancreatectomy, the likelihood for hypoglycemia is also increased, because of low circulating glucagon levels, which reduce the endogenous counterregulation (8, 17, 52). The danger of hypoglycemia resides in the fact that the brain depends solely on glucose as energy. Since the brain cannot store or synthesize glucose for a long period of time, it relies on the blood for regular delivery of glucose. Normal function in the central nervous system can be maintained for only a few minutes if glucose delivery is stopped. The most common symptoms of hypoglycemia are sweating, tachycardia, tremor, hunger, and clouded sensorium. In more severe cases, confusion, convulsions, and coma develop. The glucose level that elicits these symptoms varies from patient to patient and from time to time in each patient. In general, however, mild hypoglycemic symptoms develop at blood glucose levels below 2.5 mmol/L (45 mg/100 mL), whereas at levels below 1.8 mmol/L (32 mg/100 mL), serious symptoms usually evolve. Treatment of hypoglycemia requires increasing the blood glucose level. In mild cases, this may be achieved by the intake of an extra snack or oral glucose. In more severe cases, glucagon may be administered (0.5–1 mg intramuscularly) or glucose might be given intravenously as a bolus injection of 25 g followed by a continuous intravenous infusion.

## CONCLUDING REMARKS

Diabetes mellitus is common among patients with acute and chronic pancreatitis and pancreatic cancer, and a strict insulin-dependent diabetes evolves after total pancreatectomy. The management of the diabetes in these patients follows fundamentally the same principles as those for management of diabetes in other patients, i.e., it is based on dietary adjustments, physical exercise, education of the patient, and, when necessary, pharmacologic additions (oral hypoglycemic agents or insulin). Many specific aspects of diabetes are important considerations in patients with exocrine pancreatic diseases or after pancreatectomy. It is particularly important to consider the increased likelihood for hypoglycemic episodes and the increased sensitivity to exogenous insulin, and the lower likelihood for development of secondary complications should also be acknowledged. The management of diabetes should be the responsibility of doctors who are experienced in the management of both diabetes and the exocrine pancreatic disease and who can integrate their knowledge of the two diseases for the benefit of the patient.

## REFERENCES

1. Porte Jr D. B cells in type 2 diabetes mellitus. Diabetes 1992;40: 166–180.

2. Gorelick FS. Diabetes mellitus and the exocrine pancreas. Yale J Biol Med 1983;56:271–275.
3. Eriksson J, Doepel M, Widén E, Halme L, Ekstrand A, et al. Pancreatic surgery, not pancreatitis, is the primary cause of diabetes after acute fulminant pancreatitis. Gut 1992;33:843–847.
4. Blumenthal HT, Probstein JG, Berns AW. Interrelationship of diabetes mellitus and pancreatitis. Arch Surg 1963;87:156–162.
5. O'Sullivan JN, Norbrega FT, Morlock CG, Brown AL, Bartholomew LG. Acute and chronic pancreatitis in Rochester, Minnesota, 1940 to 1969. Gastroenterology 1972;62:373–379.
6. Renner IG, Savage WT, Pantoja JL, Renner VJ. Death due to acute pancreatitis. A retrospective analysis of 405 autopsy cases. Dig Dis Sci 1985;30:1005–1018.
7. Sarles H. Chronic pancreatitis and diabetes. Baillière's Clin Endocrinol Metab 1992;6:745–775.
8. Larsen S. Diabetes mellitus secondary to chronic pancreatitis. Dan Med Bull 1992;40:153–162.
9. Bank S. Chronic pancreatitis: clinical features and medical management. Am J Gastroenterol 1987;81:153–167.
10. Klöppel G, Bommer G, Commandeur G, Heitz P. The endocrine pancreas in chronic pancreatitis. Immunocytochemical and ultrastructural studies. Virchows Arch (A) 1978;377:157–174.
11. Noronha M, Bordalo O, Dreiling DA. Alcohol and the pancreas. II. Pancreatic morphology of advanced pancreatitis. Am J Gastroenterol 1981;76:120–124.
12. Bonora E, Rizzi G, Lesi C, Berra P, Coscelli C, Butturini U. Insulin and C-peptide plasma levels in patients with severe chronic pancreatitis and fasting normoglycemia. Dig Dis Sci 1988;6:732–736.
13. Pedersen NT, Andersen BN, Pedersen G, Worning H. Chronic pancreatitis in Copenhagen. A retrospective study of 64 consecutive patients. Scand J Gastroenterol 1982;17:925–931.
14. Cavallini G, Vaona B, Bovo P, Cigolini M, Rizo L, et al. Diabetes in chronic alcoholic pancreatitis. Role of residual beta cell function and insulin resistance. Dig Dis Sci 1993;38:497–501.
15. Yki-Järvinen H, Kiviluoto T, Taskinen MR. Insulin resistance is a prominent feature of patients with pancreatogenic diabetes. Metabolism 1986;35:718–727.
16. Nosadini R, Del Prato S, Tiengo A, Duner E, Toffolo G, et al. Insulin sensitivity, binding, and kinetics in pancreatogenic and type 1 diabetes. Diabetes 1982;31:346–355.
17. Larsen S, Hilsted J, Philipsen EK, Tronier B, Christensen NJ, et al. Glucose counterregulation in diabetes secondary to chronic pancreatitis. Metabolism 1990;39:138–143.
18. Larsen S, Hilsted J, Tronier B, Worning H. Pancreatic hormone secretion in chronic pancreatitis without residual beta-cell function. Acta Endocrinol 1988;118:357–364.
19. Barnes AJ, Bloom SR, Alberti KGMM, Smythe P, Alford FP, Chischolm DJ. Ketoacidosis in pancreatectomized man. N Engl J Med 1977;296:1250–1253.
20. Arky RA, Freinkel N. Alcohol infusion to test gluconeogenesis in starvation with special reference to obesity. N Engl J Med 1966;274:426–433.
21. Couet C, Genton P, Pointel JP, Louis J, Gross P, et al. The prevalence of retinopathy is similar in diabetes mellitus secondary to chronic pancreatitis with or without pancreatectomy and in idiopathic diabetes mellitus. Diabetes Care 1985;8:323–328.
22. Kessler II. Cancer mortality among diabetics. J Natl Cancer Inst 1970;44:673–686.
23. Karmody AJ, Kyle J. The association between carcinoma of the pancreas and diabetes mellitus. Br J Surg 1969;56:362–364.
24. Schwartz SS, Zeidler A, Moossa AR, Kuku SF, Rubenstein A. A prospective study of glucose tolerance, insulin, C-peptide, and glucagon responses in patients with pancreatic carcinoma. Dig Dis Sci 1978;23:1107–1114.
25. Permert J, Larsson J, Ihse I, Pour PM. Diagnosis of pancreatic cancer. Alteration of glucose metabolism. Int J Pancreatol 1991;9:113–117.
26. Andrén-Sandberg Å, Ahrén B, Tranberg KG, Bengmark S. Surgical treatment of pancreatic cancer. The Swedish experience. Int J Pancreatol 1991;9:145–151.
27. Permert J, Ihse I, Jorfeldt L, Arnquist H, von Schenk H, Larsson J. Pancreatic cancer is associated with impaired glucose metabolism. Eur J Surg 1993;159:101–107.
28. Fogar P, Pasquali C, Basso D, Sperti C, Panozzo MP, et al. Diabetes mellitus in pancreatic cancer follow up. Anticancer Res 1994;14: 2827–2830.
29. Ragozzino M, Melton LJ, Chu CP, Palumbo PJ. Subsequent cancer risk in the incidence cohort of Rochester, Minnesota, residents with diabetes mellitus. J Chron Dis 1982;35:13–19.
30. Balkau B, Barrett-Connor E, Eschwege E, Richard JL, Claude JR, Ducimetiere P. Diabetes and pancreatic carcinoma. Diabetes Metab 1993;19:448–462.
31. Takeda Y, Escribano MJ. Effects of insulin and somatostatin on the growth and the colony formation of two human pancreatic cancer cell lines. J Cancer Res Clin Oncol 1991;117:416–420.
32. O'Mara BA, Byers T, Schoenfeld E. Diabetes mellitus and cancer risk: a multisite case-control study. J Chron Dis 1985;38:435–441.
33. Vecchia CL, Negri E, Franceschi S, D'Avanzo B, Boyle P. Diabetes and pancreatic cancer risk. An epidemiological assessment. Int J Pancreatol 1994;16:81–82.
34. Adami HO, McLaughlin J, Ekbom A, Berne C, Silverman D, et al. Cancer risk in patients with diabetes mellitus. Cancer Causes Control 1991;2:307–314.
35. Gullo L, Pezzilli R, Morselli-Labate AM, Italian Pancreatic Cancer Study Group. Diabetes and the risk of pancreatic cancer. N Engl J Med 1994;331:81–84.
36. Pour PM. The role of Langerhans islets in exocrine pancreatic cancer. Int J Pancreatol 1995;17:217–223.
37. Cerosimo E, Pisters P, Pesola G, McDermott K, Bajorunas D, Brennan MF. Insulin secretion and action in patients with pancreatic cancer. Cancer 1991;67:468–493.
38. Permert J, Adrian TE, Jacobsson P, Jorfelt L, Fruin B, Larsson J. Is profound peripheral insulin resistance in patients with pancreatic cancer caused by a tumor-associated factor? Am J Surg 1993;165:61–67.
39. Holmberg JT, Ihse I, Lundquist I, Ahrén B. Influence of bile duct occlusion on plasma insulin responses to glucose in rats. Scand J Gastroenterol 1986;21:59–64.
40. Coupeland GP, Al-Sumidaie AM, Leinster SJ, Davis JC, Hipkin LH. Glucose metabolism in patients with gastrointestinal malignancy but without excessive weight loss. Eur J Surg Oncol 1987;13:11–16.
41. Permert J, Ihse I, Jorfeldt L, von Schenk H, Arnquist HJ, Larsson J. Improved glucose metabolism after subtotal pancreatectomy for pancreatic cancer. Br J Surg 1993;80:1047–1050.
42. DelFavero G, Basso D, Fogar P, Panozzo MP, Meggiato T, et al. Alterations of serum pancreatic hormones in pancreatic cancer patients. Int J Pancreatol 1994;16:84–86.
43. Permert J, Larsson J, Westermark GT, Herrington MK, Christmanson L, et al. Islet amyloid polypeptide in patients with pancreatic cancer and diabetes. N Engl J Med 1994;330:313–318.
44. Castillo MJ, Scheen AJ, Lefebvre PJ. Amylin/islet amyloid polypeptide: biochemistry, physiology, patho-physiology. Diabetes Metab 1995;21:3–25.
45. Fox JN, Frier BM, Armitage M, Ashby JP. Abnormal insulin secretion in carcinoma of the pancreas: response to glucagon stimulation. Diabetes Med 1985;2:113–116.
46. Basso D, Plebani M, Fogar P, Del Favero G, Briani G, et al. Beta-cell function in pancreatic adenocarcinoma. Pancreas 1994;9: 332–335.
47. Ahrén B, Andrén-Sandberg Å. Glucose tolerance and insulin secretion in experimental pancreatic cancer in the Syrian hamster. Res Exp Med 1993;193:21–26.
48. Ahrén B, Andrén-Sandberg Å. Capacity to secrete islet hormones after subtotal pancreatectomy for pancreatic cancer. Eur J Surg 1993;159:223–227.
49. Bonner-Weir S, Trent DF, Weir GC. Partial pancreatectomy in the rat and subsequent defect in glucose-induced insulin release. J Clin Invest 1983;71:1544–1553.
50. Crace PA, Pitt HA, Tompkins RK, Den Bestern L, Longmire WP. Decreased morbidity and mortality after pancreatoduodenectomy. Am J Surg 1986;151:141–149.
51. Edis AJ, Kiernam PD, Taylor AF. Attempted curative resection of ductal carcinoma of the pancreas: a review of the Mayo Clinic experience. Mayo Clin Proc 1980;55:531–534.
52. Del Prato S, Tiengo A, Baccaglini U, Tremolada C, Duner E, et al. Effect of insulin replacement on intermediary metabolism in diabetes secondary to pancreatectomy. Diabetologia 1983;25: 252–259.

53. American Diabetes Association. Nutritional principles for the management of diabetes and related complications (Technical Review). Diabetes Care 1994;17:490–518.
54. American Diabetes Association. Nutritional recommendations and principles for people with diabetes mellitus (Position Statement). Diabetes Care 1994;17:519–522.
55. Jenkins DJA. Dietary fiber, diabetes and hyperlipidemia. Lancet 1979;2:1287–1289.
56. Unger RH, Foster DW. Diabetes mellitus. In: Wilson JD, Foster DW, eds. Williams textbook of endocrinology. 8th ed. Philadelphia: WB Saunders, 1992:1255–1333.
57. McLaughlin S. Pancreatic cancer and diabetes. Diabetes Educ 1994;20:20–26.
58. Koivisto VA, Yki-Järvinen H, DeFronzo RA. Physical training and insulin sensitivity. Diabetes Metab Rev 1986;1:445–481.
59. Schneider SH, Vitug A, Ruderman NB. Atherosclerosis and physical activity. Diabetes Metab Rev 1986;1:513–553.
60. Gerich JE. Oral hypoglycemic agents. N Engl J Med 1989;321:1231–1245.
61. Marble A. Insulin in the treatment of diabetes. In: Marble A, Krall LP, Bradley RF, Christlieb AR, Soeldner JS, eds. Joslin's diabetes mellitus. 12th ed. Philadelphia: Lea & Febiger, 1985:380–405.
62. Singh I, Marshall MC. Diabetes mellitus in the elderly. Endocrinol Metab Clin North Am 1995;24:255–272.
63. Somogyi M. Exacerbation of diabetes by excess insulin action. Am J Med 1959;26:169–191.
64. Schade DS. Surgery and diabetes. Med Clin North Am 1988;72:1531–1543.
65. Tattersall R, Gregory R, Selby C, Kerr D, Heller S. Course of brittle diabetes: 12 year follow up. Br Med J 1991;302:1240–1243.
66. Cryer PE, Gerich JE. Glucose counterregulation, hypoglycaemia, and intensive insulin therapy in diabetes mellitus. N Engl J Med 1985;313:232–241.

# 18

# *Perioperative Nutritional Support in Pancreatic Disease*

Jörgen Larsson

The pancreas is essential for optimal nutritional and metabolic balance of the body and has both exocrine and endocrine functions. The exocrine function is especially important for growth and development during childhood. The endocrine function is related to many hormones essential for growth, substrate uptake, and for substrate utilization. The pancreas synthesizes and secretes enzymes and hormones important for digestion of nutrients and regulation of intraluminal transit throughout the bowel. It plays a role in modulating intestinal growth. This chapter focuses upon the background of malnutrition in pancreatic diseases, the effects of malnutrition, nutritional assessment, and perioperative nutritional support in pancreatic diseases.

The gland has a key role in nutritional metabolism and 1–2 L of pancreatic juice are produced by the cells of the exocrine pancreas each day. The juice contains bicarbonate and electrolytes and has a daily output of about 8 g of protein. Because of its role in digestion, malfunction of the exocrine pancreas may have a major impact on nutrition. Malnutrition per se also affects the gland negatively. As the enzymes released from the pancreas have considerable digestive power, their activation within the gland or within the peritoneal cavity can have severe consequences.

## GENERAL ASPECTS OF MALNUTRITION

Starvation and weight loss are seen in many diseases. A number of factors, such as changes in metabolism, anorexia, and malabsorption are associated with malnutrition (Table 18.1). Malnutrition is often regarded as a natural part of the disease process, and too little is done to recognize the problem or to restore the nutritional state in malnourished patients. Generally, one in four patients entering a medical or a surgical ward and one in two patients with malignancy develop protein-energy malnutrition (1). The problem is even greater in the group of elderly patients often seen today (2).

A correlation between malnutrition and postoperative morbidity/mortality is well documented (3–6). Fifty years ago, an American surgeon studied different factors contributing to mortality after gastric resection because of ulcers (3). A striking correlation between preoperative weight loss and postoperative mortality was seen. The main reason for mortality was infections. Protein-energy malnutrition is important clinically when it is so severe that organ function is negatively affected, which contributes to increased risk for complications and/or a prolonged rehabilitation.

Malnutrition is associated with a changed body composition, with loss of cellular protein, especially skeletal muscle protein, and accumulation of extracellular fluid in the form of edema. Organ function is affected, with both somatic and psychosomatic symptoms.

Typical somatic symptoms are impaired wound healing, immune response, and skeletal muscle function (Table 18.2). Hypoalbuminemia is associated with prolonged wound healing in man, which can be seen early in the development of protein-energy malnutrition (7). The number of T cells, the response to mitogen stimulation, and the delayed hypersensitivity reaction in skin tests are all negatively affected in a state of malnutrition (8). The phagocytic function can be impaired and the complement system affected. Muscle force is decreased during malnutrition, and a prolonged relaxation and increased endurance have been seen (9–11).

Most studies have concentrated on the metabolic effects of malnutrition, and limited attention has been given to psychologic effects and quality-of-life concerns that are of great importance for the rehabilitation of surgical patients (12) (Table 18.2). A close connection has been observed between diet and neurotransmitter function (13–14). An impaired psychologic response could hamper self-help motivation, resulting in further reduction in dietary intake. There is a clear relationship between nutritional status and quality of life (12). Weight loss and serum albumin and prealbumin levels affect the patients' outlook (12). In the Minnesota experiments on partial starvation in man conducted by Keys et al, during World War II, young adults lost approximately 24% of their body weight during a 6-month period (15). They exhibited several changes in behavior including increased fatigue, depression, and apathy. Psychologic changes induced by undernutrition seem to be just as typical as the physiologic changes. The changed biology of malnourished patients leads to a marked increase in risk for postoperative complications and to prolonged hospital stays (16).

## SPECIFIC CAUSES OF MALNUTRITION IN PANCREATIC DISEASES

Patients with pancreatic disorders frequently present with anorexia, cachexia, and abdominal pain. Malabsorption is a prominent finding in pancreatic disease. Depending on the duration of the disease, patients generally have some nutritional depletion at admission. During acute illness, nutritional needs are increased in response to metabolic stress, and fever, sepsis, organ failure, and different surgical interventions are frequent in pancreatic diseases. The nutritional problem may be further aggravated by a history of alcohol abuse.

### Cachexia

Cachexia is a syndrome that occurs during the terminal course of the disease in most cancer patients. It is characterized by weakness and weight loss, with a progressive impairment of vital functions. The typical features of these patients are pallor, severe skeletal muscle wasting, and loss of subcutaneous fat stores.

Patients with malignancies have the highest rate of malnutrition of any hospitalized population (17); more than 60% of

**TABLE 18.1. Some Factors Contributing to Malnutrition in Pancreatic Disease**

| | |
|---|---|
| • Malabsorption | • Anorexia |
| • Motility disturbance | • Decreased protein synthesis |
| • Pain | • Increased protein catabolism |
| • Drug treatment | • Increased energy expenditure |
| • Anxiety | • Insulin resistance |

patients develop weight loss during the course of their disease (18). In a study by the Eastern Cooperative Oncology Group comprising more than 3000 patients with 11 different tumor types, patients with pancreatic or gastric cancers had the highest incidence of weight loss (83–87%) (18). The severity of cachexia was not directly related to size or spread of the tumor; cachexia can be very obvious even when the tumor represents a small part of the body weight, as in pancreatic cancer.

The etiology and pathogenesis of cancer cachexia are not only related to anorexia, malabsorption, and disturbed cell metabolism but also to psychologic factors, surgery of the alimentary tract, radiotherapy, and chemotherapy.

### Anorexia

Anorexia is one of the first symptoms seen in a patient with cancer. The patient not only eats less but changes eating behavior, with a more pronounced intake of carbohydrates. Anorexia is often marked and reduces food intake profoundly. The causes of anorexia are multifactorial, and in pancreatic cancer, certain peptides such as cytokinins and islet amyloid polypeptide have been implicated (19). Among the cytokinins, tumor necrosis factor (TNF) and interleukin-1 have a pronounced anorectic effect that is dose dependent.

Other tentative mechanisms of anorexia involve intermediate metabolites such as lactate, ketones, and oligonucleotides. More recently, the existence of an amino acid imbalance with accumulation of tryptophan and serotonin in the brain has been postulated. As a consequence of malnutrition, secondary changes occur in the digestive tract that result in atrophy of the mucosa, which may be responsible for the feeling of fullness and for delayed emptying and digestion of nutrients.

Islet amyloid polypeptide (IAPP), also called amylin, is a 37-amino acid polypeptide produced by the beta cells of the endocrine pancreas. This peptide was first isolated from the amyloid associated with human insulinoma (20). Because the peptide is costored and coreleased with insulin, attention has been focused on IAPP's ability to interfere with glucose metabolism. Several studies have shown that IAPP can suppress eating when injected intrahypothalamically in the rat, intravenously in the rat, intraperitoneally in the rat and in mice, and intracerebroventricularly in mice (21–23). Thus, it has been suggested that IAPP plays a role in the regulation of appetite. Marked increases in plasma IAPP concentration have been reported in patients with diabetes associated with pancreatic cancer (24). A series of studies showed that intravenous bolus injection and short-term infusion of rat IAPP markedly suppressed food intake for up to several hours in the rat (25). This is true even for doses equivalent to those seen in patients with pancreatic cancer. Chronic increases in circulating IAPP levels can also cause marked reduction in food intake and body weight, and this fact and the reduced food intake seen after acute administration, raises the possibility that IAPP may be a satiety factor (25).

**TABLE 18.2. Somatic and Psychosomatic Changes Related to Malnutrition**

| Somatic | Psychosomatic |
|---|---|
| • Muscle weakness | • Tiredness |
| • Visceral proteins decreased | • Apathy |
| • Impaired immune response | • Depression |
| • Impaired wound healing | • Irritability |
| • Multiple organ failure | • Concentration problems |
| • Decreased adaptive ability | • Decreased self-discipline |

### Malabsorption

Malabsorption is most prominent in chronic pancreatitis secondary to irreversible fibrosis of the pancreas resulting in a reduction in exocrine pancreatic cell mass. As proteolytic, lipolytic, and amylolytic enzymes are synthesized in the gland, enzyme levels are gradually reduced. Steatorrhea secondary to incomplete digestion of ingested fat does not occur in pancreatic insufficiency until approximately 90% of pancreatic secretory function is lost (26). Malabsorption directly related to the tumor can be caused by obstruction of the biliary and pancreatic ducts. Postoperatively, absorption is a consequence of a digestive enzyme deficiency caused by pancreatectomy. Radiotherapy of the small and large intestine may cause immediate and late damage since the epithelium of the bowel is relatively radiosensitive. The radiation damage is expressed as malabsorption of glucose, fat, electrolytes, and some protein.

## CELL METABOLISM

Changes in cell metabolism are most profound in acute illnesses and in cancer. The primary purpose is to protect the entire organism and secure substrate availability. In a catabolic state, protein muscle degradation occurs to secure the energy needs of the patients. The stress response is initiated by a catecholamine release that mobilizes body fuel (27–29), principally stimulating hepatic glyconeogenesis. In the periphery, a tissue insulin resistance accompanies the glucose intolerance and hyperglycemia. In the pancreas, the catecholamines inhibit insulin production and enhance glucagon secretion. Plasma glucose levels rise, but glucose utilization is impaired. Patients with severe pancreatic disease such as acute necrotizing pancreatitis can have a 50% increase in the normal resting energy expenditure. With the severe protein catabolism, protein losses reach 150–200 g protein per day (30). The individual metabolic needs and the protein losses can be estimated by indirect calorimetry and measurement of urinary urea nitrogen.

Both acute pancreatic diseases and pancreatic cancer are associated with disturbed glucose metabolism. The extracellular concentration of glucose in normal humans is precisely controlled within a very narrow range, despite the intermittent intake of nutrients. The normal glucose homeostasis depends on sophisticated coordination of pancreatic hormone secretion, hepatic glucose production, and glucose uptake in splanchnic organs and peripheral tissues. In the fasting state and during exercise, hypoglycemia is prevented by production of glucose in the liver in response to glucagon secretion from the pancreatic $\alpha$ cells. After a meal, the influx of glucose from the bowel must be matched by an insulin-mediated uptake of glucose in peripheral tissues and splanchnic organs. Hepatic glucose production is inhibited by insulin-induced inhibition of glucagon secretion and by neutralization of the hepatic actions of glucagon. A defect in any of these processes can result in disturbed glucose homeostasis.

In pancreatic cancer, altered glucose metabolism was noted in 1833 by Wright, who described a patient who developed symptoms of diabetes mellitus 6 months before he became jaundiced and died of a pancreatic carcinoma (31). Newly diagnosed diabetes or instability in previously known and well-controlled diabetes has been reported as a characteristic of pancreatic

**TABLE 18.3. Energy Expenditure in Moderate Trauma**

| Author | No. of Patients | Energy Expenditure (kcal/24 hr) |
|---|---|---|
| Sandström et al. (39) | 300 | 1677 |
| Brandi et al. (40) | 26 | 1756 |
| Brandi et al. (41) | 22 | 1516 |
| Hansell et al. (42) | 142 | 1342 |
| Mann et al. (43) | 50 | 1768 |
| Quebberman et al. (44) | 67 | 1447 |
| Smith et al. (45) | 30 | 1923 |
| MacFie et al. (46) | 24 | 1317 |

cancer (32). Only a limited number of prospective studies using modern criteria for glucose intolerance and diabetes are available (33–35). These studies indicate that diabetes or impaired glucose tolerance occurs in most patients with pancreatic carcinoma. Two different hypotheses have been proposed to explain this association: *(a)* diabetes is a predisposing factor for pancreatic cancer, and *(b)* the high incidence of diabetes is an effect of the pancreatic tumor. Recent epidemiologic reports have concluded that even though diabetes occurs frequently in pancreatic cancer, diabetes is not a risk factor for pancreatic cancer in the sense that risk factors are generally understood to operate (35).

Permert and coworkers found diabetes or impaired glucose tolerance in 74% of the patients with pancreatic cancer, and this high frequency resulted mainly from newly diagnosed diabetes (36). The diabetic state was caused more by profound insulin resistance rather than impaired insulin secretion (37). A diagnosis of diabetes before the diagnosis of cancer in a number of patients demonstrates that the alteration in glucose metabolism can be an early sign of exocrine pancreatic cancer. Glucose tolerance and insulin sensitivity both improved in diabetic patients who underwent tumor resection by an 85% subtotal pancreatectomy, despite a marked reduction in insulin secretion postoperatively (38). These results indicate that a diabetogenic factor produced by the pancreatic adenocarcinomas may be directly or indirectly responsible for the high frequency of diabetes in these patients.

In acute pancreatic disorders such as acute pancreatitis, there is an induction of hypermetabolism, with increased calorie and nitrogen requirements at a time when gastrointestinal function is impaired and not fully able to meet these increased demands. Caloric expenditure is only minimally increased after moderate trauma (Table 18.3) (39–46). The largest increase in expenditure occurs in patients with severe multiple trauma, major thermal injury, and acute necrotizing pancreatitis. Amino acids, glucose, and fatty acids are used to cover the energy needs. Amino acids are derived from endogenous or dietary proteins or are provided exogenously by the intravenous route. Glucose is produced when carbohydrate is degraded in the gut lumen or is generated in the liver. Fatty acids are derived from hydrolysis of triglycerides.

## NUTRITION AND THE ETIOLOGY OF PANCREATIC DISEASES

The most common causes of acute pancreatitis in developed countries are gallstone disease and excessive alcohol consumption. Alcohol abuse is the most common cause of chronic pancreatitis. There is a tendency toward an increased frequency of both acute and chronic pancreatitis in the Western world.

The risk for developing chronic pancreatitis is increased by high levels of fat and proteins in the diet (47–49). There is also an association between acute pancreatitis and hyperlipidemia (50). Postoperatively, acute pancreatitis has been found in children after colon resections when fat emulsions were given intravenously (51). The role of excessive circulating lipids in the etiology of acute pancreatitis is still unknown, as is the role of fat emulsions. It has been suggested that free fatty acids are released by the activity of pancreatic lipase and the toxicity results from the pancreatic production of oxygen-derived free radicals (52, 53).

Today, adenocarcinoma of the pancreas is the fifth leading cause of death in the Western world. The main risk factor for pancreatic cancer is cigarette smoking, but dietary factors have been extensively discussed. Alcohol consumption seems not to be a real risk factor (54). The fat content of the diet, on the other hand, seems to be related to pancreatic cancer (55). Support for this association comes from both clinical and experimental studies. The relation between butter consumption and pancreatic cancer was seen in a case control study (56). Stimulatory effects of high-fat diet and cholecystokinin receptor blockade on pancreatic tumor initiation was seen in the hamster model (57). It has been claimed from a study in Japan that dietary protein can also contribute to the incidence of pancreatic cancer. Persons eating meat daily had a greater risk of developing pancreatic cancer than those who ate it less often (58); however, this has not been confirmed by other studies (59).

## NUTRITIONAL ASSESSMENT

Nutritional assessment determines the patient's current nutritional status and nutritional requirements. The nutritional status is determined primarily from the patient's history, which includes questions about disease processes, medications, dietary habits, and weight loss (60–62). To the history is added a physical examination, seeking evidence of muscle wasting, specific nutrient deficiency, and weakness. Loss of more than 15% of the patient's preillness weight is associated with an increased risk for complications.

Other tests have been used to confirm the physician's clinical evaluation of the patient (Table 18.4). Anthropometric measurements of body weight and skinfold thickness can determine fat mass. Measuring creatinine excretion in a 24-hr urine collection permits determination of the creatinine-height index, a factor that is proportional to muscle mass. Newer techniques developed to determine body composition include isotopic dilution methods, $\gamma$-neutron activation, and bioimpedance measurement. However, these methods are not generally practical for use in

**TABLE 18.4. Some Methods for Measurement of the Components of Nutritional Assessment**

| Technique | Component |
|---|---|
| Anthropometry | Body weight |
| | Skinfold thickness |
| | Arm muscle circumference |
| Proteins | Albumin |
| | Prealbumin |
| | Transferrin |
| Energy intake | Calorie and protein intake |
| Energy output | Resting energy expenditure |
| Body composition | Total body potassium |
| | Isotopic dilution $\gamma$-neutron activation |
| Skeletal muscle function | Hand grip strength |
| Respiratory function | Tidal volume—vital capacity |
| Immune function | Delayed cutaneous hypersensitivity |
| | Total lymphocyte count |
| Metabolic stress | Apache II—CRP—hormones |

clinical settings. Total peripheral lymphocyte count, delayed hypersensitivity test response to common antigens, and lymphocyte transformation have all been used as indicators of immunocompetence; however, these immunologic responses are not specific to nutrition deficiencies as they can be affected by medication, trauma, etc. Serum albumin and transferrin are the most common serum protein indicators of malnutrition. These proteins are synthesized in the liver and levels may fall during impaired hepatic synthesis. Both albumin and transferrin are negative phase reactants, with low levels resulting from trauma or infection. Increased extracellular fluid is also associated with low plasma protein levels.

A bedside nutritional assessment should include an evaluation of protein and energy balance, an assessment of body composition, an evaluation of physiologic function, and an estimate of metabolic stress. The protein and energy pattern can be assessed by comparing the frequency and size of the patient's meals with an estimate of rate change in body weight. A more detailed assessment of protein and energy balance can be performed by a dietitian. The body composition is assessed by evaluating body weight, fat stores, and protein stores. A gross loss of body weight can be observed from the patient's appearance but also by palpating skinfolds between the finger and thumb. Protein stores can be assessed by inspection and palpation of a number of muscle groups. Functional impairment related to the loss of body protein is the most important part of the assessment of nutritional status. Function should be observed during the physical examination and by watching the patient's activity.

## EFFECT OF ENTERAL AND PARENTERAL NUTRITION ON EXOCRINE SECRETION

The primary indication for use of nutritional support (enteral or parenteral) in patients with pancreatic diseases is a state of malnutrition and/or severe complications due to the disease. The secondary effect of the nutritional regimen is that nutritional treatment, especially parenteral nutrition, can diminish pancreatic secretion, which could have both positive and negative effects (see section below on intestinal permeability).

Nutrient ingestion stimulates exocrine pancreatic secretion primarily by three mechanisms: release of enteral hormones, a direct effect on the pancreas after absorption, and activation of the enteropancreatic reflexes. Parenteral nutrition has only a direct effect on the pancreas. Several studies have focused on the effect of glucose, amino acid, and fatty acid infusions. Parenteral infusion of glucose suppresses pancreatic exocrine secretion by increasing serum osmolarity (63, 64). Most studies support the conclusion that intravenous amino acid solutions do not stimulate pancreatic exocrine secretion in animals or humans (65). The role of fatty acids on secretion is of interest because of the association between certain types of hyperlipidemia and acute pancreatitis. Most studies have shown no effect of intraduodenal fat administration or parenteral infusion of fatty acids on pancreatic exocrine secretion (66, 67). When these substrates are combined for total parenteral nutrition (TPN), the data do not show any stimulation of exocrine pancreatic secretion.

Enteral nutrition stimulates less pancreatic exocrine secretion than food intake by mouth. Experimental studies in dogs with chronic pancreatic fistulas compared a full liquid diet with an elemental diet administered to the distal duodenum (68) and found that pancreatic secretion was stimulated less with the infusion than with oral administration of the same diet (60). Infusion into the proximal jejunum further reduced the stimulation of pancreatic secretion. The acidity of the diet also seems to affect pancreatic secretion—a neutral pH reduces the stimulatory effect.

## EFFECT OF DISEASE AND NUTRITIONAL SUPPORT ON INTESTINAL PERMEABILITY

In addition to absorbing nutrients by primarily transcellular mechanisms, intestinal mucosa allows flux of water and electrolytes. This transport capacity is highly regulated by the adhesive structures between the enterocytes tight junctions, desmosomes, and interconnecting gap junctions (70). The function of these regulating structures depends partly on the energy status of the cell. Permeability studies in malnourished animals have shown that the absorptive capacity decreases without any signs of barrier leakage (71). In addition to malnutrition, endotoxin or inflammatory trauma is needed to produce a permeability increase in short-term experimental studies. Bacterial translocation has been described in many animal experiments and is especially frequent after major burns, acute pancreatitis, cytotoxic treatment, and hypervolemic shock (72,73).

Evidence for bacterial translocation being a major clinical problem in humans is scarce (see also Chapter 28). Cultures from serosal and mesenteric lymph node biopsy specimens are positive in 10% of patients undergoing general abdominal surgery and in as many as 38% of patients with intestinal obstruction (74). The effect of surgery is less clear. Patients with bacterial translocation at the time of surgery are at risk of developing postoperative infectious complications (74). Both good nutritional state and intestinal integrity are considered important for optimal immunocompetence, particularly in the catabolic patient. With regard to the effect of enteral and parenteral nutrition, short-term starvation in the rat leads to loss of more than 50% of the weight of the small intestine, compared with 30% of whole-body weight. Adequate nutritional support given to the rat parenterally cannot prevent villous atrophy, and TPN results in decreased enzyme and immunoglobulin concentrations and promotes bacterial translocation if food is withheld (75). The strongest factor favoring intestinal growth is probably the existence of nutrients and fibers in the lumen. The effect of food, however, is not mainly a direct nutritive effect, but more indirect effects exerted upon different hormones, growth factors, and growth-stimulating aspects of neuromuscular activity and blood flow (76).

In humans, the exact amounts of nutrients required to avoid intestinal atrophy is unknown. In the case of intestinal injury or metabolic stress (e.g., acute pancreatitis), a combination of nutrient control and bowel rest increases the risk of complications attributable to intestinal dysfunction. Bowel rest results in an exaggerated stress-hormone response when endotoxin is administered to healthy volunteers (77). In clinical studies, enteral nutrition reduces infectious complications in trauma patients, compared with parenteral nutrition (78) (Table 18.5). Possible explanations for this include *(a)* the mucosal barrier is kept intact; *(b)* enteral nutrition is often hypocaloric, reducing the risk of hyperglycemia; or *(c)* stimulation of gut trophic hormones might affect the immune response.

## PERIOPERATIVE NUTRITIONAL SUPPORT

The goal for nutritional support in the preoperative period is to maintain or improve the nutritional state and reduce postoperative complications and/or mortality. The indications are a malnourished patient and surgery associated with a risk of postoperative complications. It is important that any delay due to preoperative nutritional support does not cause other complications. Generally it is wise to use the time available before surgery for some sort of nutritional support. Whether a surgical procedure should be postponed because of malnutrition is controversial, and a series of studies have tried to determine the efficacy of nutritional support in the preoperative period.

**TABLE 18.5. Effect of Total Parenteral Nutrition (TPN) and Total Enteral Nutrition (TEN) on Complications after Abdominal Trauma[a]**

| | TPN | TEN |
|---|---|---|
| Major infections (%) | 20 | 3 |
| Albumin (g/L) | 27 | 34 |

Data from Moore FA, Moore EE, Jones TN, McCroskey BL, Peterson VM. TEN versus TPN following major abdominal trauma reduced septic morbidity. J Trauma 1989;29:916–923.
[a] $n = 75$.

A number of prospective studies focused on gastrointestinal surgery, with the support aimed at trying to reduce postoperative complications. In 1977, Williams et al. studied esophageal or gastric cancer patients (79). One group was given 2–3 L of a standard intravenous nutrient solution for 7–10 days preoperatively. Both groups received oral multivitamin supplementation and a diet containing about 15 g of nitrogen and 3000 kcal. The two groups were matched in age, pathology, and gender. The groups had a similar mortality and a similar anastomotic leakage rate; the only statistically significant difference was an increased number of wound infections in the control group. The authors emphasized that patients with plasma albumin levels below 30–35 g/L could benefit from perioperative nutritional support.

Müller et al. studied the effect of 10 days of preoperative nutrition in patients undergoing surgery for gastrointestinal cancer (80). Both malnourished and nourished patients were included. In the latter study prophylactic antibiotics were not given. The results showed a decreased sepsis grade and decreased mortality in patients given preoperative intravenous nutrition. Mullen, in Philadelphia, studied a large group of patients in a retrospective preoperative nutritional study (81): 50 patients received at least 7 days of appropriate intravenous nutritional support, and 95 patients received no preoperative nutritional support. The two groups were considered matched in age, sex, nutritional status, and underlying disease process. The patients who received nutritional support preoperatively had fewer complications.

The Veterans Affairs Total Parenteral Nutrition Co-operative Study Group focused on perioperative TPN in 395 malnourished patients requiring laparotomy or noncardiac thoracotomy (Table 18.6) (82). They were randomly allocated to receive either TPN for 7–15 days before surgery and 3 days afterward or no perioperative TPN. The patients were followed up for 90 days after surgery. The TPN group had more infectious complications than the controls. The increased rate of infections was confined to patients categorized as either borderline or mildly malnourished according to subjective global assessment or an objective nutritional assessment. In contrast, severely malnourished patients who received TPN had fewer noninfectious complications than controls, with no concomitant increase in infectious complications. In the absence of severe malnutrition, most patients seemed best served by prompt surgery (82).

von Meyenfeldt et al. studied the effect of at least 10 days of preoperative TPN or total enteral nutrition on major postoperative complications and mortality in a homogenous patient group with signs of depletion; 50 patients served as a depleted control group, and 49 patients served as a nondepleted reference group and were operated upon without delay (83). The depleted control patients showed more septic complications than those in the nondepleted reference group. No significant difference was seen in septic complications between either of the nutritional support groups and the nondepleted control group. High-risk patients with a weight loss of more than 10% of body weight who lost more than 500 mL of blood during operation showed a significant decrease in major complications as a result of nutritional support. It was concluded that preoperative nutritional support in patients with severe depletion results in a reduction in major complications that justifies its routine use in the selected group of patients.

Thus, in the perioperative setting, nutritional support should be considered for patients with significant weight loss (10–15%) and a high risk of development of complications who are undergoing major surgery. In this group of patients, placement of jejunostomy feeding tube and initiation of enteral nutrition in the immediate postoperative period should be advocated, and TPN should be continued postoperatively only if the GI tract cannot be used for tube feeding. In well-nourished patients undergoing major abdominal surgery, a jejunostomy feeding tube can be placed if resumption of oral feeding is not anticipated for 7–10 days.

It is important to analyze the patient's nutritional state preoperatively. It is essential to use the time available before surgery for specialized nutrition to diminish further malnutrition. In a small group of severely malnourished patients (>15% weight loss), there are indications that surgery should be postponed and preoperative total nutritional support be administered for approximately 1–2 weeks.

## POSTOPERATIVE NUTRITION

The goal for nutritional support in the postoperative period is to minimize protein losses before normal bowel function has been achieved. How long a patient can tolerate postoperative starvation depends on the patient's preoperative nutritional state. A general rule is that complete nutritional support is initiated immediately postoperatively if the patient is malnourished, while a preoperatively well-nourished patient can tolerate 4–5 days of hypocaloric nutrition. Except for preexisting malnutrition, postoperative malnutrition could be an effect of the surgical procedure itself and/or a complication of the surgical procedure. Information on the effect of postoperative nutrition is limited.

In an important study evaluating 300 patients, Sandström et al. randomized patients undergoing general surgical procedures to either TPN from the first postoperative day or only prolonged glucose administration (250–300 g/day) up to 15 days after operation (39). The patients receiving TPN were individually treated according to energy and nitrogen balances. The goal was to keep the patients in a positive energy balance or close to nitrogen balance. The study evaluated the effect of the nutritional regimens on mortality rate, complications, need of addi-

**TABLE 18.6. Infectious and Noninfectious Complications in Relation to Nutritional State**

| Malnutrition | Group[a] | Infectious Complications (%) | Noninfectious Complications (%) |
|---|---|---|---|
| Borderline | TPN | 12.5 | 12.5 |
| | C | 9.1 | 23.6 |
| Mild | TPN | 14.4 * | 20.0 |
| | C | 3.7 | 19.4 |
| Severe | TPN | 15.8 * | 5.3 |
| | C | 21.4 | 42.9 |

Adapted from the Veterans Affairs Total Parenteral Nutrition Co-operative Study Group. Perioperative total parenteral nutrition in surgical patients. N Engl J Med 1991;325:525–532.
[a] TPN, total parenteral nutrition; C, control group.
* Indicates statistical significance ($p < .05$).

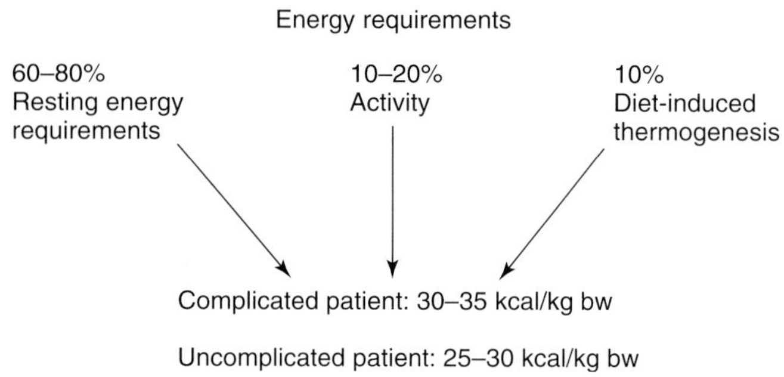


**FIG. 18.1.** Energy requirements.

tional medical support, and patient-related functional disabilities. In this study, 60% of patients started eating within 8–9 days after operation. Patients on glucose treatment for 14 days had a significantly higher mortality rate than patients on either continuous or uncomplicated TPN treatment or on short-term glucose treatment. The results demonstrated that in most surgical patients (60%), postoperative semistarvation was not a limiting factor for outcome. In the remaining 40%, inadequate nutrition was associated with both increased morbidity and mortality rates. Inadequate nutrition was defined by the authors as both too much and too little, but overfeeding seemed to be a larger problem than underfeeding. The authors concluded that TPN represents a lifesaving modality in 20% of unselected patients undergoing major surgery. However, as yet, it is not possible to identify these patients preoperatively. It seems, therefore, extremely important to try to identify those high-risk patients in need of postoperative nutritional support.

## ENERGY SUBSTRATES AND REQUIREMENTS

During the last decades the recommended energy intake for severely sick patients receiving nutritional support has decreased markedly. Previous recommendations of energy intake of up to 3000 kcal/24 hr or even more greatly exceed the energy expenditure measured by indirect calorimetry (84). The overestimation was caused by measuring resting energy expenditure close to the time of peak hypermetabolism, for example after burn injury, and then extrapolating to longer periods. Additional expenditure of energy was also added (estimated) to compensate for the effect of pyrexia, which was inappropriate.

In a number of studies, comprising more than 1000 patients, the resting energy expenditure is in the range of 1400–1800 kcal/24 hr (84). If activity is added, the energy needs could account for no more than 200 kcal/24 hr (Fig. 18.1). Both excess carbohydrate and excess lipid supplementation have been linked to complications such as hepatic steatosis and abnormal hepatic function (85). Lipid can also be deposited in the lung and impair gas exchange. Overfeeding of carbohydrates can lead to excess $CO_2$ production, which is associated with respiratory failure in patients with pulmonary problems. In animal models, overfeeding leads to increased mortality. In general, the energy requirements of patients with severe diseases are usually similar to or less than those of healthy subjects (85).

Nonprotein energy given during TPN should be a combination of glucose and fat. Glucose and fat seem to have similar nitrogen-sparing effects as long as basal glucose needs (150–200 g) are covered (86). When administering 200 kcal/24 hr, the energy proportions can be varied from 30% glucose/70% fat to 90% glucose/10% fat. However it is essential to cover basal glucose needs (150–200 g/24 hr) and essential fatty acids (100–200 g/week).

## PROTEINS AND PROTEIN REQUIREMENTS

Proteins and their amino acids have several uses in the organism. Amino acids are essential for protein synthesis in all body tissues. An adult man can synthesize about 300 g of protein per day. Amino acids are used in the synthesis of a number of nitrogen-rich molecules. An overload of amino acids undergoes degradation in the liver, with urea formation.

Increased urinary excretion of nitrogen is a typical sign after trauma or during severe disease. Such patients often have a negative nitrogen balance of 10–20 g nitrogen/24 hr during glucose infusion. Generally it is not possible to achieve a positive nitrogen balance during the acute phase of the disease. For nitrogen balance estimations, it is essential to collect urine for at least 2 days for urinary urea assay. Losses other than through the urine, namely from drainage, feces, etc., must be measured or calculated to about 2–4 g/day. It is essential to monitor the serum urea level during therapy, because an accumulation of urea in the extracellular space could influence the balance. It is also important to have the patient in energy balance so that the nitrogen balance can be calculated.

Supplementation of nitrogen (0–300 mg N/kg/day) to severely sick patients given a high energy intake has been studied. Nitrogen balance improved with increasing nitrogen intake up to 200 mg/kg/day (approximately 14 g N/day) (87). Nitrogen retention decreased markedly with a further increase in nitrogen supply and also with time after injury. It was suggested that a nitrogen supply of 200 mg/kg body weight/24 hr is optimal for severely injured patients during the first week after trauma (Table 18.7).

Amino acid therapy is one of the most important means of stimulating protein synthesis during catabolism. Another factor of great importance is physical activity, which stimulates protein synthesis; immobility is a catabolic factor.

## SPECIFIC SUBSTRATES AND BIOACTIVE SUBSTANCES IN NUTRITIONAL SUPPORT

Nutrients are deficient or missing from parenteral nutritional solution partly because of poor solubility or instability. For example, heat sterilization destroys glutamine. Glutamine is an oxidative substrate in mucosal cells and lymphocytes, and a large reduction in concentration might be critical in severe illness. Thus, it seems rational to include glutamine in amino acid solutions for critically ill patients, such as those with severe acute pancreatitis. Convincing data show that a glutamine-rich amino acid solution produces a better nitrogen economy in such patients (88). Whether glutamine supplementation improves patient outcome is unknown. The dosage of glutamine is also unclear, and up to 40 g/day of glutamine has been given to patients on intravenous nutrition, compared with an estimated normal dietary intake of only 3–5 g/day. In a study of bone marrow transplantation patients, this dosage improved nitrogen balance and significantly reduced both infection rate and hospital stay (89).

Arginine is another amino acid associated with benefit to the immune system. It has been combined with other immuno-

**TABLE 18.7. Nitrogen Needs in the Perioperative State**

| | |
|---|---|
| • Basal needs | 0.10 g N/kg body weight |
| • Malnourished—no stress | 0.15 g N/kg body weight |
| • Hypermetabolism | 0.20 g N/kg body weight |

Data from Larsson J, Lennmarken C, Mårtensson J, et al. Nitrogen requirements in severely injured patients. Br J Surg 1990;77:413–416.

modulators and has been incorporated into enteral diets with the aim of providing immunonutrition. In one of these studies, the diet significantly reduced infection and wound complications after major surgery and shortened hospital stay (90). However, it is difficult to evaluate the effect of these immunomodulators because of differences between the test and control patients.

Bioactive substances such as growth hormone have been tried in nutritional support. When recombinant human growth hormone became available, interest increased. Growth hormone in a supraphysiologic dosage results in a definite improvement in nitrogen economy in patients with critical illness (91). There is some risk of hyperglycemia and risk that insulin-dependent diabetes mellitus can be made difficult to control. Growth hormone was tried in intestinal failure, and some patients requiring long-term parenteral nutrition could be switched to an enteral diet because of improved intestinal function (92). Herndon et al. reported a significant reduction in hospital stay (from 46 to 32 days) for burned children receiving growth hormone (93). Treatment with human growth hormone is associated with increased production of insulin-like growth factor I (IGF-I), and it has been postulated that the anabolic effect of human growth hormone on protein metabolism is mainly mediated by IGF-I (94). IGF-I is structurally related to insulin and exerts similar metabolic actions. Studies in animals have shown that IGF-I, as well as affecting glucose metabolism, has protein-sparing effects and both stimulates protein synthesis and reduces its breakdown (95). IGF-I may be useful in treating catabolic patients perioperatively, especially when hyperglycemia and pronounced insulin resistance are expected (96).

Large doses of medium-chain triglycerides, which account for 50% of all fat, have been used to decrease infusional hyperlipidemia and thus reduce hepatic steatosis and avoid suppressing the reticular endothelial system (97). Triglycerides rich in N-3 fatty acids (fish oils), administered enterally or parenterally, alter membrane biology and insulin sensitivity and modify both prostaglandin and cytotoxin production (97). Certain observations suggest that administration of triglycerides rich in N-3 fatty acids can modify acute inflammatory or infectious diseases; however, clinical experience is still limited.

## NUTRITIONAL TREATMENT OF PATIENTS WITH ACUTE PANCREATITIS

Most episodes of acute pancreatitis are short, and extraordinary nutritional support is rarely indicated. Severe acute pancreatitis on the other hand produces systemic illness that could be comparable to severe sepsis or burn injury and results in severe hypermetabolism and catabolism. It is generally agreed that the systemic response is related to release of enzymes and other bioactive products from the pancreas into the surrounding tissues and the peritoneal cavity or the bloodstream. The pancreatic lesion can itself give rise to complications such as abscesses or necrosis, putting new demands on the nutritional therapy. Studies on patients with severe pancreatitis show a loss of about 25% of body weight (98). This weight loss is associated with disturbances in muscle metabolism and high peripheral insulin resistance. Energy metabolism is increased to levels near those of severe sepsis or severe burns (30–35 kcal/kg/day). Nitrogen losses could reach 15–20 g N/kg/day. The nutritional needs are usually covered by both parenteral and enteral routes. Parenteral nutrition can reduce the stimulation of pancreatic exocrine function and also provides nutritional support until enteral nutrition can be supplied or the patient can start eating.

The impact of enteral stimulation on the integrity of the gut has aroused increased interest in using enteral feeding in patients with acute pancreatitis (see "Effect of Disease and Nutritional Support on Intestinal Permeability"). The role of nutritional support in acute pancreatitis has been evaluated in a series of studies, many of them retrospective or nonrandomized. One of the few randomized prospective studies investigated the role of early TPN in acute pancreatitis (99). A group who received intravenous fluids, analgesics, and nasogastric suction was compared with a group who had conventional therapy with early TPN. No effect of nutritional supply was seen. A retrospective study evaluated the role of intravenous nutrition on the development of complications; 88% of the 44 patients underwent operative treatment and there was a 20% mortality rate (100); intravenous nutrition had no significant effect on the natural history of the attack.

In a retrospective study, Grant et al. studied the effect of TPN on pancreatic disease in 73 patients. The mean duration of treatment was 24 days. The mortality rate in subgroups with severe acute pancreatitis were the same as those in previously published series (101). A prospective nonrandomized study evaluated three TPN formulations in terms of nutrient indices, nitrogen balance, and mortality in severe acute pancreatitis (102). The patients were malnourished. After TPN, most patients had an improved nutritional status. A relationship between nitrogen balance and mortality was seen. Most patients were in positive nitrogen balance within 2 weeks of TPN. The study suggested that mortality from severe acute pancreatitis can be reduced by nutritional support. Kalfarentzos et al. performed a prospective nonrandomized study in 67 patients receiving TPN for severe acute pancreatitis. TPN seemed to be safe and effective, with a frequency of catheter-related sepsis of 8.9%. The study indicated a reduction in complications and mortality if TPN was administered within 72 hours of admission (103).

Generally the aim of nutritional support in acute severe pancreatitis is to cover the energy and nitrogen needs during the disease processes. The risk for severe malnutrition is obvious, and nutritional therapy is important to counteract complications. Initially, the nutritional supply is based on parenteral nutrition, but an early introduction of enteral nutrition could benefit gut integrity. Complications of acute pancreatitis are related to impaired integrity of the gut.

In summary, most patients with mild pancreatitis do not need nutritional support and can be handled with intravenous fluids. In severe cases, nutritional support should be introduced early, initially by parenteral nutrition including fat emulsion. A feeding jejunostomy tube should be placed at the time of operation, for enteral nutrition. The patient's energy and nitrogen needs must be covered, often both parenterally and enterally. The optimal nutritional support for patients with severe acute pancreatitis needs to be defined by further investigation. Patients with chronic pancreatitis can develop complications such as abscesses or acute pancreatitis; they should then be handled nutritionally in the perioperative period in the same way as those with acute pancreatitis.

## NUTRITIONAL MANAGEMENTS OF PATIENTS WITH PANCREATIC CANCER

Sooner or later, most patients with cancer show signs of cachexia. The cachectic state is associated with fatigue both physically and psychologically, and the quality of life declines (12). It is estimated that 25–30% of patients with cancer die more as a consequence of the cachexia than as a consequence of tumoral overgrowth of vital organ systems.

The rationale for perioperative TPN or enteral nutrition for patients with pancreatic diseases was discussed above in the section "Perioperative Nutritional Support." Many of the randomized clinical trials focusing on cancer patients have been inconclusive. Two papers pooled these trials in a meta-analysis looking at complication rates after TPN (104, 105). Only one of these studies, comprised of patients with small cell cancer of the lung receiving TPN, showed an increased but incomplete remission after the TPN treatment. In three studies, decreased survival or shortened remission was seen in subgroups after TPN treatment (106–108). Most studies showed no effect of the treatment. The statistics and methodology used in these studies were criticized, as was patient selection. Patients with gastrointestinal cancer were involved in only one or two of these studies. The nutritional supplementation varied and was sometimes inadequate. The rationale for giving TPN in these studies was poor tolerance and poor compliance when receiving chemotherapy, which means that only severely malnourished patients were included.

Some studies have compared different modalities of nutritional administration, e.g., TPN versus enteral nutrition (109). No significant differences were reported between parenteral and enteral nutrition. Comparisons of different enteral diets showed no difference between elemental diets and meal feeding in addition to standard diets (110).

In the future, new options such as anticachectic drugs, new forms of nutrient modulation, and metabolic manipulation may be considered to meet the nutritional requirements of patients.

## REFERENCES


1. Symreng T, Anderberg B, Kågedahl B, et al. Nutritional assessment and clinical course in 112 elective surgical patients. Acta Chir Scand 1983;149:657–662.
2. Larsson J, Unosson M, Ek AC, et al. Effect of dietary supplement on nutritional outcome in 501 geriatric patients—a randomized study. Clin Nutr 1990:756–772.
3. Studley HO. Percentage of weight loss. A basic indicator of surgical risk in patients with chronic peptic ulcer. JAMA 1936; 106:458–460.
4. Buzby GP, Mullen JL, Matthews DC, et al. Prognostic nutritional index in gastrointestinal surgery. Am J Surg 1980;139:160–167.
5. Mullen JL, Buzby GP, Matthew DC, et al. Reduction of operative morbidity and mortality by combined preoperative and postoperative nutritional support. Ann Surg 1980;139:160–167.
6. Warnold I, Lundholm K. Clinical significance of preoperative nutritional status in 215 non cancer patients. Ann Surg 1984;199: 299–305.
7. Haydock DA, Hill GL. Improved wound healing response in surgical patients receiving intravenous nutrition. Br J Surg 1987;74:320–323.
8. Superina R, Meakins JL. Delayed hypersensitivity, anergy and the surgical patient. J Surg Res 1984;37:151–174.
9. Lennmarken C, Sandstedt S, Larsson J. Effect of starvation in man on skeletal muscle function. Clin Nutr 1986;5:99–103.
10. Christensen T, Hougård F, Kehlet H, Influence of pre- and intraoperative factors on the occurrence of postoperative fatigue. Br J Surg 1985;72:63–65.
11. Christensen T, Kehlet H. Postoperative fatigue and changes in nutritional status. Br J Surg 1984;71:473–476.
12. Larsson J, Åkerlind J, Permert J, et al. The relation between nutritional state and quality of life in surgical patients. Eur J Surg 1994;160:329–334.
13. Wurtzman RG. Nutrients that modify brain function. Sci Am 1982;246:50–59.
14. Wurtzman RJ, Hefti F, Melamed E. Precursor control of neurotransmitter synthesis. Pharmacol Rev 1980;32:315–335.
15. Keys A, Brozek J, Gerschel A. The biology of human starvation. Minneapolis: University of Minnesota Press, 1950.
16. Jendteg S, Larsson J, Lindgren B. Clinical and economical aspects of nutritional supply. Clin Nutr 1987;6:185–190.
17. Nixon D, Mohih S, Lawson D, et al. Total parenteral nutrition as an adjunct to chemotherapy of metastatic colorectal cancer. Cancer Treat Rep 1981;65:121–128.
18. DeWys WD, Begg C, Lavin PT, et al. Prognostic effect of weight loss prior to chemotherapy in cancer patients. Am J Med 1980;69:491–497.
19. Arnelo U, Blevins JE, Larsson J, Permert J, Westermark P, et al. Effects of acute and chronic infusion of islet amyloid polypeptide on food intake in rats. Scand J Gastroenterol 1996;31:83–89.
20. Westermark P, Wernstedt C, Wilander E, Sletten K. A novel peptide in the calcitonin gene related family as an amyloid fibril protein in the endocrine pancreas. Biochim Biophys Res Commun 1996;140:827–831.
21. Balasubramaniam A, Renugopalakrishnan V, Stein M, Fischer JE, Chance WT. Syntheses, structures and anorectic effects of human and rat amylin. Peptides 1991;12:919–924.
22. Bouali SM, Wimalawansa SJ, Jolicoeur FB. In vivo central actions of rat amylin. Regul Pept 1995;56:167–174.
23. Chance WT, Balasubramaniam A, Zhang FS, Wimalawansa SJ, Fischer JE. Anorexia following the intrahypothalamic administration of amylin. Brain Res 1991;539:352–354.
24. Permert J, Larsson J, Westermark GT, Harrington MK, Christmansson L, et al. Islet amyloid polypeptide in patients with pancreatic cancer patients and diabetes. N Engl J Med 1994;330:313–318.
25. Arnelo U, Permert J, Adrian TE, et al. Chronic infusion of islet amyloid polypeptide causes anorexia in rats. Am J Physiol 1996;271:R1654–R1659.
26. DiMagno EP, Go VLW, Summerskill WHJ. Relations between pancreatic enzyme outputs and malabsorption in severe pancreatic insufficiency. N Engl J Med 1973:288:813–815.
27. Larsson J, Liljedahl S-O, Schildt B, Fürst P, Vinnars E. Metabolic studies in multiple injured patients. Clinical features, chemical analysis and nitrogen balance. Acta Chir Scand 1981:147: 317–324.
28. Kinney JM. Energy requirements in injury and sepsis. Acta Anaesth Scand 1974;55(suppl):15.
29. Shenkin A, Neuhauser M, Bergström J, et al. Biochemical changes associated with severe trauma. Am J Clin Nutr 1980;33:2119–2127.
30. Larsson J, Lennmarken C, Mårtenson J, et al. Nitrogen requirements in severely injured patients. Br J Surg 1990;77:413–416.
31. Zimmerman B. Diabetes and gross lesions of the pancreas (Editorial). J Clin Endocrinol Metab 1954;14:481–483.
32. Ihse I, Isaksson G. Pancreatic carcinoma: Diagnosis and treatment. Clin Gastroenterol 1984;13(3):961–984.
33. Schwarz SS, Zeidler A, Moossa AR, et al. A prospective study of glucose tolerance, insulin, C-peptide, and glucagon responses in patients with pancreatic carcinoma. Dig Dis 1978;23:1107–1114.
34. Cersosimo E, Pisters P, Pesola G, McDermott K, Bajorunas D, Brennan MF. Insulin secretion and action in patients with pancreatic cancer. Cancer 1991;67:468–493.
35. Boyle P, Hsieh CC, Maisonneuve P, et al. Epidemiology of pancreatic cancer. Int J Pancreatol 1989;5:327–346.
36. Permert J, Ihse I, Jorfeldt L, et al. Pancreatic cancer is associated with impaired glucose metabolism. Eur J Surg 1993;159:101–107.
37. Permert J, Adrian TE, Jacobsson P, et al. Is the profound peripheral insulin resistance in patients with pancreatic cancer caused by a tumor associated factor? Am J Surg 1993;165: 61–67.
38. Permert J, Jorfeldt L, von Schenck H, et al. Glucose metabolism improved in patients with pancreatic cancer after subtotal pancreatectomy. Br J Surg 1993;80:1047–1050.
39. Sandström R, Drott C, Hyltander A, Arfidsson B, Scherstén T, et al. The effect of postoperative intravenous feeding (TNP) on outcome following major surgery evaluated in a randomized study. Ann Surg 1993;217:185–195.
40. Brandi LS; Grana M, Massanti T, Giunta F, Natali A, Ferrannini E. Energy expenditure and gas exchange measurements in postoperative patients. Thermodilution versus indirect calorimetry. Crit Care Med 1992;20:1273–1283.
41. Brandi LS, Oleggini M, Lachi S, Frediani M, Bevilacqua S, et al. Energy metabolism of surgical patients in the early postoperative period. A reappraisal. Crit Care Med 1988;16:18–22.
42. Hansell DT, Richardson R, Davies JWL, Burns HJG. Estimation of resting energy expenditure by anthropometry. Clin Nutr 1987;6: 51–57.
43. Mann S, Westenskow D, Houstschens B. Measured and predicted caloric expenditure in the acutely ill. Crit Care Med 1985;13:173–177.
44. Quebberman E, Ausman R. Estimating energy requirements in patients receiving parenteral nutrition. Arch Surg 1982;117:1281–1284.
45. Smith RC, Burkinshaw L, Hill G. Optimal energy and nitrogen intake for gastroenterological patients requiring intravenous nutrition. Gastroenterology 1982;82:445–452.

46. MacFie J, Burkinshaw L, Oxby C, Holmfield JHM, Hill GL. The effect of gastrointestinal malignancy on resting metabolic expenditure. Br J Surg 1982;69:443–446.
47. Sarles H. An international survey on nutrition and pancreatitis. Digestion 1973;9:389–403.
48. Sarles H, Cros RC, Bidart JM. A multicenter inquiry into the aetiology of pancreatic diseases. Digestion 1979;19:110–125.
49. Durbec JP, Bidart JM, Sarles H. Interaction between alcohol and other foodstuffs: epidemiological aspects. Colloq Inserm 1980; 95:33–52.
50. Haig TH. Experimental pancreatitis intensified by a high fat diet. Surg Gynecol Obstet 1970;131:914–918.
51. Noseworthy J, Colodny AH, Eraklis AJ. Pancreatitis and intravenous fat: an association in patients with inflammatory bowel disease. J Pediatr Surg 1983;18:269–272.
52. Saharia P, Margolis S, Zuidema CD, et al. Acute pancreatitis with hyperliaemia: studies with an isolated perfused canine pancreas. Surgery 1977;82:60–67.
53. Sanfey H, Bulkley BG, Cameron JL. The role of oxygen derived free radicals in the pathogenesis of acute pancreatitis. Ann Surg 1984;200:405–413.
54. McMahan B. Risk factors for cancer of the pancreas. Cancer 1982;50:2676–2680.
55. Wynder EL. An epidemiological evaluation of the causes of cancer of the pancreas. Cancer Res 1975;35:2228–2233.
56. Gold EB, Gordis L, Drener MD, et al. Diet and other risk factors for cancer of the pancreas. Cancer 1985;55:460–467.
57. Harrington MK, Permert J, Pour PM, et al. Effect of high fat diet and cholecystokinin receptor blockade on pancreatic tumor initiation in the hamster. Carcinogenesis 1993;14:1021–1026.
58. Hirayama T. A large-scale cohort study on the relationship between diet and selected cancers of digestive organs. In: Bruce WR, et al., eds. Banbury report no. 7. Cold Spring Harbor, NY, 1981.
59. Roebuck BD, Yager JP, Longnecker DS. Dietary modulations of azaserine-induced pancreatic carcinogenesis in the rat. Cancer Res 1981;41:888–893.
60. Detsky AS, McLughlin JR, Baker P, et al. What is subjective global assessment of nutritional state. JPEN 1987;11:440.
61. Baker JP, Detsky AS, Wesson DE, et al. Nutritional assessment. A comparison of clinical judgement and objective measurements. N Engl J Med 1982;306:969.
62. Detsky AS, Smalley PS, Chang J. Is this patient malnourished? JAMA 1994;271:54.
63. Klein E, Sheinbaum S, Ben-Ari G, et al. Effects of total parenteral nutrition on exocrine pancreatic secretion. Am J Gastroenterol 1983;78:31–33.
64. Zaljchuck R, Shoemaker WC, Baker RJ. The relationship between blood glucose levels and external pancreatic secretion in man. J Trauma 1969;9:629–636.
65. Konturek SW, Tasler J, Cieszkowski M, et al. Intravenous amino acids and fat stimulate pancreatic secretion. Am J Physiol 1979;236:E678–E684.
66. Edelman K, Valenzuela JE. Effect of intravenous lipid on human pancreatic secretion. Gastroenterology 1983;85:1063–1066.
67. Grundfest S, Steiger E, Selinkoff P, Fletcher J. The effect of intravenous fat emulsions in patients with pancreatic fistula. JPEN 1980;4:27–31.
68. Stabile BE, Borzatta M, Stubbs RS. Pancreatic secretory responses to intravenous hyperalimentation and intraduodenal elemental and full liquid diets. JPEN 1984;8:377–380.
69. Kelly GA, Nahrwold DL. Pancreatic secretion in response to an elemental diet and intravenous hyperalimentation. Surg Gynecol Obstet 1976;143:87–91.
70. Mandel LJ, Bacallo R, Zampighi G. Uncoupling of the molecular "fence" and paracellular "gate" functions in epithelial tight junctions. Nature 1993;361:552–554.
71. Worthington BS, Syrotuch J. Intestinal permeability to large particles in normal and protein-deficient adult rats. J Nutr 1976;106:20–32.
72. Deitch EA, Ma WJ, Ma L, Berg R, Specian R. Protein malnutrition predisposes to inflammatory induced gut-origin septic states. Ann Surg 1990;211:560–568.
73. O'Dwyer ST, Michie HR, Ziegler TR, Revhaug A, Smith RJ, Wilmore DW. A single dose of endotoxin increases intestinal permeability in healthy humans. Arch Surg 1988;123:1459–1464.
74. Sedman PC, Macfie J, Sagar P, Mitchell CJ, May J, et al. The prevalence of gut translocation in humans. Gastroenterology 1994;107:643–649.
75. Alverdy JC, Aoys E, Moss GS. Total parenteral nutrition promotes bacterial translocation from the gut. Surgery 1988;104: 185–190.
76. Adrian TE, Bloom SR. Effect of food on the hormones of the gastrointestinal tract. In: Hunter JO, Jones V, eds. Food and the gut. Philadelphia: Baillière Tindall, 1985:13–29.
77. Fong Y, Marano MA, Barber A, et al. Total parenteral nutrition and bowel rest modify the metabolic response to endotoxin in humans. Ann Surg 1989;210:449–457.
78. Moore FA, Moore EE, Jones TN, McCroskey BL, Peterson VM. TEN versus TPN following major abdominal trauma reduced septic morbidity. J Trauma 1989;29:916–923.
79. Williams RHP, Heatley RV, Lewis MH, et al. Preoperative parenteral nutrition in patients with stomach cancer. In Baxter DH, Jackson GM, eds. Clinical parenteral nutrition. Chester, England: Geistlich Education 1977:52–59.
80. Müller JM, Brenner U, Dienst C, et al. Preoperative parenteral feeding in patients with gastrointestinal carcinoma. Lancet 1982;1:68–71.
81. Mullen JL. Consequences of malnutrition in the surgical patient. Surg Clin North Am 1981;61:465–487.
82. The Veterans Affairs Total Parenteral Nutrition Co-operative Study Group. Perioperative total parenteral nutrition in surgical patients. N Engl J Med 1991;325:525–532.
83. von Meyenfeldt MF, Jeijerink WJ, Rouflart MT, et al. Perioperative nutritional support: a randomised clinical trial. Clin Nutr 1992,11. 180–186.
84. Nordenström J, Thörne A. Benefits and complications of parenteral nutritional support. Eur J Clin Nutr 1994;48:531–537.
85. Elia M. Changing concepts of nutrient requirements in disease: implications for artificial nutritional support. Lancet 1995;345: 1279–1284.
86. Nordenström J, Askanazi J, Elwyn DH, et al. Nitrogen balance during total parenteral nutrition; glucose vs fat. Ann Surg 1983;197:27–33.
87. Larsson J, Lennmarken C, Mårtensson J, et al. Nitrogen requirements in severely injured patients. Br J Surg 1990;77:413–416.
88. Elia M. Glutamine in parenteral nutrition. Int J Food Sci Nutr 1992;43:47–59.
89. Ziegler TR, Young LS, Benfell K, et al. Clinical and metabolic efficacy of glutamine supplemented parenteral nutrition after bone marrow transplantation. Am J Clin Nutr 1991;54: 905–908.
90. Daly JM, Lickerman MD, Foldfine J, et al. Enteral nutrition with supplemental arginine, RNA and omega 3 fatty acids in patients after operation: immunologic metabolic and clinical outcomes. Surgery 1992;112:56–57.
91. Mjaaland M, Unneberg K, Larsson J, et al. Growth hormone after abdominal surgery attenuated forearm glutamine, alanine, 3-methylhistidine and total amino acid efflux in patients receiving total parenteral nutrition. Ann Surg 1993;217:413–422.
92. Byrne TA, Morrissey T, Ziegler TR, et al. Growth hormone, glutamine and fiber enhance adaptation of remnant bowel following massive intestinal resection. Surg Forum 1992;43: 151–153.
93. Herndon PN, Barrow RE, Kunkel KR, et al. Effects on recombinant human growth hormone on donor-site healing in severely burned children. Ann Surg 1990;212:424–429.
94. Daughaday WH, Rotwein P. Insulin-like growth factors I and II. Endocr Rev 1989;10:68–91.
95. Koea JB, Douglas RG, Breier BH, et al. Synergistic effects of insulin-like growth factor-1 administration on the protein-sparing effects of total parenteral nutrition in fasted lambs. Endocrinology 1992;131:643–648.
96. Leinsköld T, Permert J, Olaison G, et al. Effect of postoperative insulin-like growth factor I supplementation on protein metabolism in humans. Br J Surg 1995;82:921–925.
97. Fürst P. New parenteral substrates in clinical nutrition. Part II. New substrates in lipid nutrition. Eur J Clin Nutr 1994;48:681–691.
98. Blackburn GL, Williams LF, Bistrian BR, et al. New approaches to the management of severe acute pancreatitis. Am J Surg 1976;131:114–124.
99. Sax HC, Warner BW, Talamini MA, et al. Early total parenteral

nutrition in acute pancreatitis: lack of beneficial effects. Am J Surg 1987;153:117–124.
100. Goodgame JT, Fischer JE. Parenteral nutrition in the treatment of acute pancreatitis. Ann Surg 1977;186:651–658.
101. Grant JP, James S, Grabowski V, et al. Total parenteral nutrition in pancreatic disease. Ann Surg 1984;200:627–631.
102. Sitzman JZ, Steinborn PA, Zinner MJ, et al. TPN and alternative energy substrates in the treatment of severe acute pancreatitis. Surg Gynecol Obstet 1989;168:311–317.
103. Kalfarentzos FE, Karavias DD, Karatzas TM, et al. Total parenteral nutrition in severe acute pancreatitis. J Am Coll Nutr 1991;10: 156–162.
104. Klein S, Simes J, Blackburn GL. Total parenteral nutrition and cancer clinical trials. Cancer 1986;58:1378–1386.
105. McGeer AJ, Detsky AS, O'Rourke K. Parenteral nutritional in cancer patients undergoing chemotherapy: a meta-analysis. Nutrition 1990;6:233–240.
106. Jordan WM, Valdivieso M, Frankmann C, et al. Treatment of advanced adenocarcinoma of the lung with florafur, doxorubin, cyclophosphamide and cisplatin (FCAP) and intensive IV hyperalimentation. Cancer Treat Rep 1981;65: 197–206.
107. Nixon DW, Heymsfield SB, Lawson DG, et al. Effect of total parenteral nutrition on survival in advanced colon cancer. Cancer Detect Prev 1981;4:421–427.
108. Shamberger RC, Brennan MF, Goodgame JT, et al. A prospective, randomized study of adjuvant parenteral nutrition in the treatment of sarcomas: results of metabolic and survival studies. Surgery 1996;96:1–12.
109. Heylen AM, Lybeer MB, Penninckx FM, et al. Parenteral vs needle jejunostomy nutrition after total gastrectomy. Clin Nutr 1987;6: 131–136.
110. Douglass HO, Milliron S, Nava H, et al. Elemental diets as an adjuvant for patients with locally advanced gastrointestinal cancer receiving radiation therapy: a prospectively randomized study. JPEN 1978;2:682–686.

SECTION V

ACUTE PANCREATITIS

# 19

# The Broad Spectrum of Pancreatitis, with Etiologic Considerations: A Clinical Overview from around the World

John M. Howard

The major advance in the field of pancreatitis in the 20th century has been the understanding that pancreatitis is not a single disease. This chapter reviews the clinical basis of this concept. The author has attempted to summarize these multiple diseases to provide a framework for clinical evaluation. Certain etiologic factors may prove to be only associated but noncausal in their relationship. In areas where extensive information has accumulated, the data are presented in detail in other chapters. In more limited areas, few reports may exist, and the discussion is relatively comprehensive.

## GALLSTONE PANCREATITIS (CHAPTER 22)

The syndrome of gallstone pancreatitis rests on a solid factual basis (1). It is the most frequently recognized form of acute pancreatitis, occurring in females three times more frequently than in males. It was recognized in the early 20th century that a stone at the ampulla of Vater might sometimes be associated with acute pancreatitis (2, 3). Concepts of pathogenesis of this cause of acute pancreatitis have centered around obstruction and hypertension of the pancreatic duct as the pancreas continues to secrete. This leads to distal distension with rupture or back diffusion of pancreatitic juice into the periacinar and peripancreatic fluid spaces. Secondly, the ampullary stone might create a common channel or passageway between the common bile duct and the pancreatic duct, allowing bile to reflux into the pancreatic duct. Activation of pancreatic proenzymes, such as trypsinogen, can result in digestion of the pancreas. Thirdly, partial obstruction of the pancreatic duct might be associated with retrograde passage of bacteria or bacterial toxins into the pancreatic duct, establishing a bacterial pancreatitis.

Although it was recognized that an ampullary gallstone could cause pancreatitis, most patients who had delayed exploration of their biliary system did not have a stone in the common bile duct (4). Acosta and associates (5, 6), Kelly (7), and Stone et al. (8) provided convincing data that gallstone pancreatitis was caused by the migration of stones from the gallbladder, through the ampulla of Vater, and into the duodenum. Gallstone pancreatitis obviously results from the transitory presence of the stone near the duodenal outlet of the pancreatic duct, as Safrany and Cotton (9, 10) clearly demonstrated by emergency endoscopic visualization and removal of stones impacted in the ampulla. The migration of tiny stones or sludge, often not recognized on standard imaging techniques, can be an etiologic factor (11, 12).

## ALCOHOLIC PANCREATITIS (CHAPTER 23)

Alcohol has been recognized as a cause of pancreatitis since the reports of Friedreich (1887) (13) and Fitz (1889) (14). Pancreatitis can result from many, if not all, forms of alcoholic drinks: whiskey, beer, gin, vodka, wine, etc. The relationship may be due to the toxic effect of alcohol, per se, or to the nutritional deficits resulting from alcoholism. Since acute pancreatitis can follow a week-long drunken spree, the toxic effect is a likely factor in acute disease. On the other hand, chronic alcoholic pancreatitis, with destruction of the acini and replacement with scar tissue, is similar to tropical forms of pancreatitis.

Apparently, alcoholic pancreatitis evolves through two stages, similar to the effect of alcohol on the liver. Massive ingestion of alcohol can result in toxic (alcoholic) hepatitis with destruction of the hepatic cells, impairment of hepatic function, and the release of hepatic cellular contents into the lymphatic and venous pathways. Acute alcoholic pancreatitis with the release of pancreatic enzymes and vasoactive substances into the lymphatic and venous channels is also well recognized. In the liver, chronic alcoholism may lead to the gradual destruction of the hepatocyte and its replacement with fibrous tissue. Similarly, chronic alcoholic pancreatitis represents pancreatic cirrhosis. It appears that the direct or indirect effect of too much alcohol is the death of the pancreatic or hepatic cell. In the United States, pancreatic calcification is a frequent late complication of alcoholic pancreatic disease (15).

## PANCREATITIS ASSOCIATED WITH HYPERPARATHYROIDISM (CHAPTER 25)

Acute pancreatitis, as well as chronic pancreatitis with pancreatic calcification, has been found in association with parathyroid tumors. In 1957, Cope et al. (16) described an association between hyperparathyroidism and pancreatitis. In 1968, Carey and Fitzgerald (17) found the incidence of pancreatitis in primary hyperparathyroidism, to vary between 8 and 19%. They presented a family in whom the relationship appeared to be hereditary. The complex relationship of the parathyroid with pancreatitis is exemplified by patients hospitalized with severe acute pancreatitis who initially have a normal serum calcium level. Following recovery from acute pancreatitis, a markedly elevated serum calcium level may be found due to a parathyroid adenoma. Hyperparathyroidism caused the acute pancreatitis that, in turn, caused a transient fall in the serum calcium level to normal. In addition to hyperparathyroidism and other causes of hypercalcemia causing pancreatitis, it may also occur immediately following parathyroidectomy.

## PANCREATITIS ASSOCIATED WITH HYPERLIPIDEMIA (CHAPTER 25)

Originally described by Speck in 1865 (18), the syndromes of hyperlipidemia in association with pancreatitis have recently been better delineated. In 1960, when the author reviewed the world's literature (19), only about a dozen patients had been reported in detail. The relationship of pancreatitis and hyperlipidemia is complex concerning when the hyperlipidemia is the cause or when it is the effect of pancreatitis. The hyperlipidemia of pancreatitis may be familial, associated with alcoholism, or a result of estrogen or other hormonal therapy for prostatic malignancy.

## POSTOPERATIVE AND POSTTRANSPLANTATION PANCREATITIS (CHAPTERS 26 AND 27)

Postoperative pancreatitis develops under at least six separate conditions. It is a major problem, in part, because it is a second insult; operation having already produced a primary injury.

1. Overdistension of the pancreatic ducts by intraoperative or endoscopic retrograde pancreatography. Trapnell and Howard (20) demonstrated *at autopsy* in patients without evidence of pancreatic disease, that injection of over 2 mL of radiopaque dye caused a diffuse radiographic blush throughout the pancreas. With dilated, chronically diseased ducts, more dye is tolerated. Retrograde pancreatography of the normal pancreas is often followed immediately by hyperamylasemia; less frequently, by clinical manifestations of acute pancreatitis. Pancreatitis induced by retrograde endoscopic injection often involves bacterial contamination from the onset as endoscopic retrograde cholangiography (ERCP) is not a sterile procedure.

2. Operation on or around the pancreatic duct with resulting ductal laceration or obstruction. Obstruction may result directly from operation, or indirectly from the secondary inflammatory response. Leakage of juice or ductal hypertension may result. Secondary infection may constitute an early complication. Duodenal operations, including sphincterotomy and resection of duodenal ulcer are frequently followed by an asymptomatic rise in the serum amylase level (21). Operations near the ampulla of Vater are especially prone to produce acute pancreatitis. Pancreatitis following pancreatic biopsy may be the result of injury or transection of the pancreatic duct.

3. Aneurysmectomy, cardiac bypass, and other low-flow states. Pancreatitis may result from aortic aneurysmectomy (22), particularly if the aneurysm has ruptured. Although direct operative injury to the pancreas may be a factor, low blood flow to the pancreas may be responsible for the pancreatitis. Pancreatitis can be a complication of cardiac bypass (23). Low blood flow may also be an etiologic factor in systemic problems such as cardiac failure or septic shock or the embolization of arteriosclerotic plaques during coronary artery catheterization (24, 25).

4. Resection of parathyroid tumors. As discussed above, parathyroidectomy sometimes results in the early development of acute pancreatitis. The mechanism remains unexplained.

5. Pancreatitis following other operations distant to the pancreas, including prostatectomy, operations on the brain, thyroidectomy, biliary tract operations, and operations in the abdomen or on the abdominal wall (26). Pancreatitis may be the result of narcotic or anesthetic agents, low-flow state, or other unknown mechanisms. Levine et al. (27) and Shader and Paxton (28) reported patients with acute pancreatitis following transurethral prostatic resection. Earlier studies (29–31) demonstrated that in the postoperative state, hyperamylasemia is not synonymous with acute pancreatitis but often reflects a heterogeneity of isoenzymes of salivary as well as pancreatic origin. Increased use of isoenzyme and lipase determinations has resulted in more specific diagnosis of postoperative pancreatitis.

6. Pancreatitis following allotransplantation of organs. This is a complex problem recognized originally by Starzl following renal transplantation (32) and since noted after transplantation of liver, heart, lung, pancreas, bone marrow and other organs (Chapter 27).

## FAMILIAL PANCREATITIS (CHAPTER 41)

In 1952, Comfort and Steinberg (33) reported three generations of a family who developed acute relapsing pancreatitis that progressed to chronic calcareous disease. No predisposing metabolic syndrome was recognized. Gerber (34) described a similar family. To be classified as hereditary pancreatitis, most authors stipulate that the pancreatitis must have been recognized in three generations. The author has studied two such families. The patients presented with acute pancreatitis that recurred at frequent intervals and that finally presented in the 4th to 5th decade as chronic pancreatitis with pancreatic calcification. Retrograde pancreatography demonstrated dilatation of the pancreatic ducts in the later stages. No predisposing metabolic syndrome could be identified.

Gross, Gambill and Ulrich (35) presented an extensive study of a family over four generations. Six people definitely had pancreatitis, and four additional people probably had pancreatitis. The mode of inheritance was that of a non-sex-linked Mendelian dominant gene; the sexes being equally affected. Pancreatic calculi developed in the larger ducts. The authors described the urinary excretion of abnormally large amounts of lysine and cystine but recognized no pathogenic relationship between the aminoaciduria and the pancreatitis.

The association between hyperlipidemia and pancreatitis in the earlier literature centered around patients with familial hyperlipidemia that preceded the onset of pancreatitis. In these patients, acute pancreatitis tended to lapse into recurrent and, finally, into chronic pancreatitis with its complications.

Davies et al. (36) described four families with familial hypocalciuric hypercalcemia. Three of the four index patients presented with acute pancreatitis, which was quite severe in two. They had diminished urinary excretion of calcium and a high serum calcium level. Parathyroid hyperplasia was observed. The authors identified reports of 66 patients with this familial metabolic syndrome, only one of whom had previously been reported to have had acute pancreatitis (37). They concluded that the metabolic syndrome was compatible with an autosomal dominant inheritance. Van Haeften et al. (38) described such a family, in which a member developed severe chronic pancreatitis with pancreatolithiasis.

Jackson (39) reported six and possibly seven patients with hyperparathyroidism in two generations of one family. Associated recurrent pancreatitis was present in at least two patients. The author found an autosomal dominant type of inheritance. Two patients developed acute pancreatitis at ages 27 and 29 years, respectively; one progressing in 4 years to pancreatic calcification. Carey and Fitzgerald (40) described another such family.

Williams et al. (41), as well as Perrault (42), acknowledging various metabolic patterns associated with hereditary pancreatitis, considered the various syndromes to represent a single disease entity: hereditary pancreatitis, marked by an autosomal dominant trait. Gerard et al. (43) identified from the literature (1981) more than 40 affected families including 195 proven and another 190 suspected cases of pancreatitis. With an onset of acute pancreatitis usually in childhood, chronicity sometimes became apparent later.

### Acute Pancreatitis in Twins

Beall et al. (44) and Henderson et al. (45) separately reported the development of acute pancreatitis in identical twins. In addition, Hoste et al. (1978) (46) provided the first report of type V hyperlipoproteinemia associated with pancreatitis in monozygotic twins. The hyperlipoproteinemia was familial. Pancreatitis appeared between 20 and 30 years of age and manifested itself by relapsing episodes. Both patients developed thrombosis of the splenic vein, splenomegaly, and varices.

## PANCREATITIS OF THE TROPICS (CHAPTER 42)

Pancreatitis of the tropics, a disease of children and young adults, leading to very early onset of diabetes, pancreatic calcification, and severe chronic pancreatitis, has been reported primarily from southern India and along the equator of Africa and Southeast Asia. Its pathogenesis remains essentially unknown; but alcohol is not its cause. The disease is progressively life-threatening.

## TRAUMATIC PANCREATITIS (CHAPTER 84)

Patients who suffer direct compression of the pancreas from nonpenetrating trauma may develop extravasation of pancreatic juice and present a syndrome of acute pancreatitis with fairly widespread fat necrosis.

### "Self-Inflicted" Recurrent Pancreatitis

A 23-year-old patient with muscular dystrophy used several large books on his lap to support his rib cage so he could sit and write. An intraductal rise in pancreatic pressure, secondary to the external pressure produced by the books, was postulated as the cause of his recurrent acute pancreatitis (47).

### Electrical Burns

Sarles (48) mentions pancreatitis as having resulted from electrical burns.

### Thermal Burns

In 1956, Haigh (49) reported fatal acute pancreatitis 2–3 weeks after a severe thermal burn. Goodwin et al. (50, 51) described the autopsy finding of pancreatitis in patients who died of thermal burns. Acute pancreatitis was noted in as many as 35% of burned patients requiring therapy in an intensive care unit. Recently Ryan et al. (52) noted the high incidence (40%) of hyperamylasemia or hyperlipasemia and symptoms of pancreatitis (82% among those with elevated serum amylase levels) among 121 patients with severe burns. Three (6%) of the burned patients developed pancreatic abscesses or pseudocysts.

**TABLE 19.1. Carcinoma of the Exocrine Pancreas as a Cause of Pancreatitis**

| | Number of Patients | |
|---|---|---|
| Author (Reference) | With Exocrine CA Pancreas | With Pancreatitis (%) |
| Gambill (53) | 255 | 26 (10) |
| Köhler and Lankisch (54) | 174[a] | 24[b] (13.8) |
| Mikel and Campbell (55) | 100 | 23 (23) |
| Lin and Feller (56) | 302 | 10 (3.3) |
| Mao et al. (57) | 154 (autopsy) | 27[c] (17.5) |
| Total | 985 | 110 (11) |

[a]Includes 18 patients with carcinoma of the ampulla of Vater.
[b]Seventeen additional patients (9.8%) had hyperamylasemia without clinically evident pancreatitis.
[c]Four had acute pancreatitis and 23 had chronic pancreatitis.

**TABLE 19.2. Acute Pancreatitis**

| | Number of Patients | |
|---|---|---|
| Author (Reference) | With Acute Pancreatitis | With Exocrine CA |
| Trapnell and Duncan (58) | 590 | 7 |
| Bemman, Dunn, and Straehley (59) | 644 | 3 |
| Enquist and Gleidman (60) | 85 | 3 |
| Sharon et al. (61) | 130 | 2 |
| Weissberg et al. (62) | 139 | 1 |
| Imrie and Whyte (63) | 78 | 2 |
| Mayday and Pheils (64) | 177 | 2 |
| Total | 1843 | 20 (1%) |

## PANCREATITIS SECONDARY TO BENIGN AND MALIGNANT TUMORS

### Carcinomas of the Exocrine Pancreas

In 1971 Gambill (53) described 26 patients with pancreatitis associated with an underlying carcinoma of the pancreas. One-third had a history of acute attacks of pain suggesting acute pancreatitis. In 38%, the carcinoma had not been diagnosed antemortem. This failure to recognize that cancer of the pancreas may be a cause of pancreatitis has often led to a delay in the diagnosis of the underlying carcinoma. Table 19.1 summarizes five major series with carcinoma of the pancreas, a total of 985 patients, of whom 11% had a superimposed pancreatitis (53–57), most of which was chronic pancreatitis. It is now obvious that chronic pancreatitis may result from the gradual occlusion of the pancreatic duct by carcinoma. Acute pancreatitis as an early signal of exocrine pancreatic carcinoma has been recognized less frequently. The author has become increasingly aware of the frequency with which patients with carcinoma of the exocrine pancreas have had discreet attacks of pain, sometimes diagnosed as acute pancreatitis, within the preceding 12–24 months. In a collected series of 1843 patients, with many types of acute pancreatitis (Table 19.2), an underlying pancreatic carcinoma was found in 20 (1%) (58–64).

Greenberg and Bank (65) described four patients with pancreatic carcinoma who had severe pancreatitis with many complications requiring multiple laparotomies, in whom the diagnosis of underlying carcinoma was often delayed for several months. Köhler and Lankisch (54) retrospectively studied 174 patients with pancreatic carcinoma (including 18 with carcinoma of the ampulla of Vater), finding acute pancreatitis in 24 (14%). An additional 17 patients had hyperamylasemia without clinical manifestations of acute pancreatitis, giving a total incidence of pancreatitis of 23.6%. Patients with periampullary cancer had the highest incidence of pancreatitis. They advised that pancreatic carcinoma be considered whenever patients had relapsing and/or unexplained pancreatitis. Wilson and Imrie (66) and Tell and Brolin (67) described missing the diagnosis of carcinoma of the pancreas for prolonged periods because of superimposed acute pancreatitis. Carpentier et al. (68) pointed out the difficulty in radiographic diagnosis of pancreatic carcinoma in the setting of acute pancreatitis. Boyle and McLeod (69) noted the failure to diagnose carcinoma of the pancreas at laparotomy when the patient presented with acute pancreatitis during pregnancy. In general, pancreatitis resulting from carcinoma of the exocrine pancreas is insidious but may be episodic, severe, or catastrophic. The possibility of an underlying pancreatic malignancy should always be considered prior to making the diagnosis of idiopathic pancreatitis, especially in its chronic stage.

### Malignant and Benign Tumors of the Ampulla of Vater and Duodenum, Gardner's Syndrome

In 1987, Robertson and Imrie (70) reported that 6 (14.6%) of 41 patients with carcinoma of the ampulla had acute pancreatitis. Three additional patients, without clinical evidence of acute pancreatitis, had elevated serum amylase levels. Thus, 22% of the patients had evidence of pancreatitis or pancreatic ductal obstruction. Belghiti et al. (71) studied 28 patients with ampullary carcinoma. Four (14%) had abdominal pain and hyperamylasemia; four others had elevated serum amylase levels, giving an overall incidence of pancreatitis of 29%. Ultrasound revealed a distended pancreatic duct in 56% of those studied. Patients with congenital polyposis of the colon (Gardner's syndrome) have a high incidence of polyps of the duodenum and of carcinoma of the ampulla of Vater. Clarke et al. (72) described acute pancreatitis as a complication of ampullary carcinoma in a patient with Gardner's syndrome, as did Sener et al. (73). Several others have called attention to the relationship of ampullary cancer and acute pancreatitis (53, 54, 74).

Burt et al. (75) in 1987 described a patient with villous adenoma of the major duodenal papilla, with Gardner's syndrome, who developed necrotizing pancreatitis. Guzzardo et al. (76) described recurrent acute pancreatitis secondary to an ampullary villous adenoma, apparently in the absence of polyposis coli. They summarized eight patients, previously reported, with villous adenomas of the ampulla of Vater as the cause of acute pancreatitis. The case records of the Massachusetts General Hospital (77) describe such a patient who had experienced multiple attacks of acute pancreatitis. Meyer and Gebhardt (78) found a villous adenoma of the papilla to be the cause of acute necrotizing pancreatitis in two patients. Following conservative treatment of the pancreatitis, the adenomas were excised, and both patients remained disease free for the ensuing 6 and 18 months, respectively. Of 141 patients with familial polyposis of the colon who had undergone prophylactic colectomy, Sener et al. (73) observed that five had a history of acute pancreatitis, and one had an adenocarcinoma of the ampulla. Ohmori et al. (79) described pancreatic ductal obstruction by a benign adenoma of the ampulla of Vater. Relapsing acute pancreatitis was the presenting manifestation of an ampullary tumor with Gardner's syndrome (80). Two patients experienced iatrogenic pancreatitis related to ampullary polyps. Nugent et al. (81) reported a patient who developed acute pancreatitis within 8 hours following an endoscopic biopsy of a papillary polyp, and Mannoury et al. (82) described a fatality resulting from acute pancreatitis as a complication of laser therapy of a villous adenoma.

A 66-year-old man with acute necrotizing pancreatitis was found by ERCP to have a 10-mm polypoid tumor in the *distal common bile duct* (83). Sphincterotomy permitted endoscopic resection of the papillary adenoma. Acute relapsing and chronic pancreatitis was noted as a complication of an inflammatory polyp of the duodenum, detected 25 years after a Bilroth II resection. The polyp, which resulted from a nonabsorbable suture and chalk granuloma in the duodenal stump, occluded the duct of Santorini (84). Oh and Jemerin (85) and Griffin et al. (86) described pancreatitis secondary to adenomatous duodenal polyps.

An *intraduodenal lipoma*, adjacent to the papilla of Vater, is an unusual cause of recurrent acute pancreatitis (87). Following recovery from the pancreatitis, the lipoma was excised transduodenally without complications. Kalvaria et al. (88) described a 21-year-old woman with recurrent pancreatitis associated with a *duodenal cyst* that was obstructing the duct of Santorini.

### Pancreatitis Associated with Neuroendocrine (Islet Cell) Tumors

In 1977, Pellegrini et al. (89) reported that an islet cell carcinoma of the pancreas obstructed the main pancreatic duct and resulted in acute pancreatitis and pseudocyst. Five patients with acute pancreatitis secondary to islet cell tumors were described by Mao and Howard (90). There was a pattern of acute relapsing pancreatitis before the tumors were identified. Four of the five tumors were malignant, and it was evident in retrospect that acute pancreatitis was the first recognizable indication of the tumor. These authors summarized 21 patients in whom pancreatitis was secondary to an islet cell tumor: gastrinoma in 3, carcinoid in 6, glucagonoma in 2, insulinoma in 2, somatostatinoma in 1, nonfunctioning tumor in 5, and not determined in 2. Fifteen of the 21 tumors were malignant (71%). The pancreatitis appeared to result from obstruction of the pancreatic duct in most patients, but in at least 3, obstruction of the duct was not a related factor. Of the 21 tumors, 16 were in the body and tail, 5 in the head. In 12 of the 21 patients (57%) an attack of acute pancreatitis, usually recurrent, was the initial syndrome. Chronic pancreatitis from obstruction of the pancreatic duct by a carcinoid tumor is often diagnosed months or years before the underlying neoplasm is identified. Dixon, Chapman, and Berry (91) reported acute pancreatitis in a nonjaundiced patient with a carcinoid of the *ampulla of Vater*. Sarles et al. (92) described chronic pancreatitis in two patients secondary to tiny nonfunctioning islet cell tumors, one as small as 0.6 mm in diameter. When no other cause for pancreatitis is evident, an islet cell tumor should be considered. ERCP may help in diagnosis.

### Pancreatitis Associated with Lymphomas

Acute pancreatitis may result not only from lymphomas and leukemias but also from their treatment. Safadi et al. (93) in 1944 described subacute pancreatitis as the presenting manifestation of an immunoblastic lymphoma, and Kotwall et al. (94) noted that a man with acute pancreatitis and obstructive jaundice died of a poorly differentiated lymphocytic lymphoma. They found reports of six other patients with lymphoma-pancreatitis (95–99), five with non-Hodgkin's lymphoma; one with Hodgkin's. In each of the seven, acute pancreatitis was the presenting manifestation. A 14-year-old boy with a huge solitary Burkitt's lymphoma in the liver presented with acute pancreatitis secondary to pressure of the tumor on the ampulla of Vater (100). In another patient, 4 months after an orchidectomy for a non-Hodgkin's lymphoma, acute pancreatitis and pseudocyst developed secondary to pancreatic lymphoma (101). Halline et al. (102) described a large cell lymphoma as an ulcerating ampullary mass that resulted in pain, hyperamylasemia, and a dilated pancreatic duct. Several reports have described an association between acute pancreatitis and adult T-cell leukemia (103–107). Dazai (106) noted that at least four of the patients had hypercalcemia as the probable cause of the acute pancreatitis (104–106). Senba et al. (108) reported 632 autopsies with adult T-cell leukemia, of whom 25 (4%) showed acute pancreatitis. Adult T-cell leukemia-lymphoma is often accompanied by hypercalcemia that is difficult to treat and is the direct cause of death in 22% of such patients. L-Asparaginase and other cytotoxic drugs used in the treatment of these tumors frequently result in acute pancreatitis, so-called tumor-lytic pancreatitis (109–112).

### Pancreatitis Secondary to Metastasis to Pancreas

**Pulmonary Carcinoma.** The literature contains numerous reports of acute pancreatitis secondary to metastases of carcinoma of the lungs to the pancreas. The primary lung cancer may be squamous cell (113) or adenocarcinoma (114) but is most frequently the small cell (oat cell) type (115–123). Not infrequently, acute pancreatitis has been the initial manifestation of oat cell cancer.

### Metastases from Other Cancers

Hung and Ardalan (124) described acute pancreatitis as secondary to metastases from other tumors including gastric carcinoma, hepatocellular carcinoma, hepatoangiocarcinoma, and a diffuse large cell lymphoma. In their 1991 review, they noted that 29 patients with pancreatitis due to metastasis to the pancreas had been reported in the English language. Included were 12 from the lung, 10 lymphomas, 5 gastric carcinomas, 1 melanoma, and 1 anaplastic carcinoma of the tonsil. Often the onset of acute pancreatitis was the initial manifestation of the underlying metastasis. Scheiman, Elta, and Francis (125) described a patient with a plasmacytoma of the pancreas that caused diffuse pancreatic enlargement and obstructive jaundice. The plasmacytoma was a recurrent tumor, first treated in the maxilla. On computed tomography (CT) it had the appearance of acute pancreatitis but was actually replacement of the pancreas by tumor. In 1972, Gatchell and Minor (126) noted that a malignant melanoma of the orbit resulted in acute pancreatitis when it metastasized to the pancreas 29 years later. Zagorski and Badowski (127) described acute pancreatitis as a result of metastasis from a cutaneous melanoma.

## PANCREATITIS ASSOCIATED WITH UNUSUAL ABDOMINAL PROBLEMS

### Afferent Loop Obstruction after Gastric Resection

In 1954, Perry (128) described a patient who had previously had a subtotal gastrectomy (Bilroth II) and whose afferent (proximal) jejunal limb became obstructed in the early postoperative period. Hyperamylasemia was misinterpreted as acute pancreatitis. Autopsy revealed massive dilatation of the duodenum behind the obstruction, without pancreatitis. In 1960, Howard and Jordan (129) reported six patients who died, or almost died, from misdiagnosis of this underlying closed-loop obstruction of the duodenum. Dahlgren (130) added an additional six patients, with the syndrome sometimes occurring as late as 2 years following the Bilroth II gastrectomy. Bubrick and Hitchcock (131) described fatal acute pancreatitis, post–Bilroth II, when the second part of the duodenum became obstructed by a renal cyst.

### Volvulus and Intussusception of the Stomach

First reported in 1901 by von Wiesenger, volvulus of the stomach is a rare cause of acute pancreatitis (132, 133). The patient reported by Dine and Martin (134) was a child with malrotation of the intestine, resulting in gastric and midgut volvulus. Cuschieri and Wilson (135) and Oliver et al. (136) each reported acute pancreatitis associated with a gastric volvulus that was incarcerated in a diaphragmatic hernia. Kafka et al. (137) described acute pancreatitis secondary to an incarcerated paraesophageal hernia, but apparently volvulus of the stomach was not involved.

Herman et al. (138) described acute pancreatitis as a result of intussusception of a gastric polyp that was associated with Gardner's syndrome. He noted two other reports of gastric intussusception causing pancreatitis, (139, 140) one involved retrogastric jejunogastric intussusception following gastric surgery. Alzen et al. (141) described acute pancreatitis in association with *ileocolic* intussusception resulting from an acute gastroenteritis.

### Wandering Spleen and Pancreatitis

Parker et al. (142) described a 21-year-old female with a wandering spleen that had undergone torsion of its vascular pedicle. The tail of the pancreas had also undergone torsion and was infarcted. The diagnosis was made preoperatively by CT scan and ultrasound, with confirmation by sulfa-colloid radionuclide scan on which the spleen was barely visible. Visceral angiography demonstrated narrowing of the splenic artery with hypovascularity of both the tail of the pancreas and the spleen. Splenectomy and distal pancreatectomy were followed by an uncomplicated postoperative course. Murray, Morgan and Christie (143) described the same problem in a 3.5-year-old child.

### Gastric Duplications Causing Acute Pancreatitis

Several interesting congenital anomalies involving the stomach have presented clinically as cystic masses associated with pancreatitis. An early review of the literature was provided by Traverso et al. (143a). Black et al. (143b) described four children, aged 9–12 years, with an intestinal duplication adjacent to the pancreas. Each had abdominal pain; three had increased serum amylase levels. The cyst communicated with the pancreatic duct and was lined by gastric epithelium. Their bibliography included reports of 17 such patients with ductal communications, less than half having had an elevated serum amylase level. The authors preferred to resect the cystic structure if possible and felt that interruption of the communication of the cyst with the pancreatic duct was essential. Lavine et al. (144) described a 6-year-old girl with relapsing pancreatitis and a gastric duplication containing ectopic pancreatic tissue. Resection of the duplication was curative. Their literature review included six patients with duplications within the stomach that were connected to the pancreatic duct and were associated with relapsing pancreatitis. Two of the patients had ectopic pancreatic tissue within the cystic duplication. Hoffman et al. (145) recommended preoperative ERCP, as the diagnosis at laparotomy can be confusing unless the anatomy has been previously delineated.

### Diverticulosis of the Small Intestine

Mahida, Chapman and Jewell (146) described three patients with chronic pancreatitis resulting from small intestinal diverticulosis with bacterial overgrowth. Two of the patients developed perforation of a diverticulum. Although two of the patients also had diverticula adjacent to the ampulla of Vater, the diverticula were predominantly jejunal. No other cause for chronic pancreatitis could be identified.

### Choledochal Cyst and Pancreatitis

Choledochal cyst, a congenital dilatation of the common bile duct, is a well-recognized cause of acute pancreatitis (147–155). Unlike the choledochocele, the development of pancreatitis is related to the presence of anomalous connections between the choledochal cyst and the pancreatic duct. Since the advent of CT scanning (152), this relationship is being recognized more frequently in adults. Okada et al. (147) described pancreatitis as a complication of choledochal cyst in 48 children. Forty-six of the children underwent resection of the cyst; 41 primarily, 5 others subsequent to primary cystojejunostomy. Because of the anomalous connection of the cyst to the pancreatic duct, the related anatomy must be accurately mapped preoperatively or intraoperatively. These cysts have a malignant potential, which adds to the need for resection. Resection is usually associated with a high Roux-en-Y choledochojejunostomy.

### Pancreatitis and Other Congenital Anomalies of Pancreatic Ducts

Leese, Chiche, and Bismuth (156) described three young adults who developed pancreatitis secondary to congenital anomalies of the pancreatic duct. In one, the pancreatic duct emptied into the duodenum 3 cm distal to the common bile duct. There was a stricture of the duct of Wirsung in the isthmus of the pancreas, with cystic dilatation behind it. The spleen was congenitally absent. The liver and gallbladder were in the midline, and the inferior vena cava was to the left of the aorta. There was mirror inversion of the stomach and duodenum, and the pancreas consisted only of the head of the gland. Relief followed anastomosis of the dilated pancreatic duct to the duodenum. They also described a patient with calculi filling only the duct of Santorini (an incomplete pancreas division). A third patient had a congenital stricture of the pancreatic duct in its midsection. Cangiarella et al. (157) discussed pancreatitis associated with anomalous junctions of the pancreaticobiliary ductal systems, reporting a Whipple resection in an infant with an inflammatory mass in the head of the pancreas secondary to a 4.0-cm long common channel. Resection was based on the suspicion that the mass might represent a pancreatoblastoma. Toki et al. (158) reviewed 61 patients with anomalous junctions of the pancreatic and biliary ducts, noting pancreatitis or pancreatic pain in 14: 2 with chronic pancreatitis and 12 with acute pancreatitis. Mori et al. (159) and Fuchshuber et al. (160) made similar observations. The literature indicates that anomalous connections of the biliary and pancreatic ducts result in acute pancreatitis in 10–25% of patients and chronic pancreatitis in about 15% (158, 160). Turner described chronic pancreatitis in the distal pancreas in two patients secondary to partial obstruction of the pancreatic duct by a congenital stenosis (161).

### Annular Pancreas and Pancreatitis

Although an annular pancreas has been a cause of acute pancreatitis (162), it is more often associated with chronic pancreatitis in the adult (163–168). Mercadier et al. (169) and Itoh et al. (163) described calcification within the annulus. The limited experience hardly justifies generalization, but the cause of pancreatitis is believed to be secondary to ductal obstruction.

### Pancreas Divisum (Chapter 7)

Pancreas divisum, a frequent congenital "anomaly" of the pancreatic duct, consists of a failure of fusion of the ducts of Wirsung and Santorini. "Rediscovered" by the endoscopists, it exists in about 5% of patients (170, 171). Its importance as a cause of pancreatitis and its indications for treatment are quite controversial (172, 173–176). Principles of assessment and management have not yet evolved.

**Santorinicele.** Santorinicele, a cystic dilatation of the termination of the duct of Santorini, was described by Eisen et al. (176) as associated with pancreatitis in four patients, aged 58–80 years. In two of them, the accessory papilla was located within a duodenal diverticulum. These observations are worthy of further study.

**Ectopic Pancreatitis.** Fam et al. (177) described acute pancreatitis in ectopic pancreatic tissue in the mesentery of the small intestine of a child. In their review of the English language literature (1982), they found only seven other patients who had developed acute pancreatitis in ectopic pancreas. Two patients had been found to have mumps pancreatitis developing in both ectopic and isotopic pancreas (178). Quizilbash (180) reported acute pancreatitis in ectopic pancreatic tissue within the gallbladder. Another patient had obstruction of the common bile duct, caused by "ectopic acute pancreatitis," and in three instances, ectopic pancreatitis resulted from the proximity of adjacent inflammatory processes (179).

### Cystic Fibrosis

Cystic fibrosis can cause chronic pancreatitis and exocrine pancreatic insufficiency in both children *and adults*. Its familial transmission indicates an autosomal recessive trait. Earlier, most patients with cystic fibrosis died before the age of 10 years, but as their life expectancy has increased, it is no longer a disease of children only. Exocrine pancreatic insufficiency has been noted in 85% of patients (181) as the result primarily of a deficiency of water and electrolytic secretion, leading secondarily to a failure of enzyme "wash out." A sparse, thick, mucoid secretion results. In a review of 2000 patients with cystic fibrosis, Shwachman et al. (182) found 10 (0.5%) with recurrent pancreatitis: 9 of whom were adolescents or young adults. In two, the diagnosis of pancreatitis preceded that of cystic fibrosis, although each had bronchiectasis. Gross et al. (183) described relapsing pancreatitis as the initial manifestation of cystic fibrosis in a young adult male without pulmonary disease.

In 1961, de Sant Agnese and Lepore (184) apparently first described the relationship between cystic fibrosis and pancreatitis. Scattered reports confirmed the relationship (185, 186). Pancreatitis may occur in young children, sometimes as the first manifestation of the underlying cystic fibrosis (183, 187, 188). Although pancreatitis may be recognized initially during an acute attack, it progresses to recurrent and chronic pancreatitis. Pancreatic exocrine insufficiency may not necessarily be evident prior to the development of pancreatitis.

Schwachman et al. (182) described a patient with recurrent pancreatitis and cystic fibrosis at a stage when the pancreatic exocrine enzyme excretion was still normal, whereas del Rosario et al. (189) noted pancreatitis as a delayed manifestation, recognized in adulthood. Three children with cystic fibrosis were found to have pancreatitis before the age of 1 year (190). The diagnosis of pancreatitis was delayed in two other children in the erroneous belief that pancreatitis occurred only at an older age with cystic fibrosis. The authors concluded that pancreatitis should be considered as a possible cause of abdominal pain in children with pancreatic insufficiency and cystic fibrosis and, conversely, that the diagnosis of cystic fibrosis should be considered an unexpected cause of pancreatitis even in a young child. Moreno Gonzáles et al. (191) described what may prove to be relatively representative of the natural history of the milder form of this disease. Their patient, at age 19, was diagnosed as having cystic fibrosis, recognized primarily because of its respiratory manifestations. Six years later, she was hospitalized with acute pancreatitis. Ultrasound revealed a dilated pancreatic duct. ERCP revealed that the duct of Wirsung was dilated and obstructed with what was interpreted as deposits of thick mucus. Pancreatic exocrine insufficiency was demonstrated. She then developed multiple attacks of pain, sometimes requiring hospitalization, until a longitudinal pancreaticojejunostomy was performed. Follow-up 1 year later revealed a normal course.

### Pancreatitis Induced by Foreign Bodies

Although foreign bodies represent a rare cause of acute pancreatitis, the current widespread use of flexible duodenoscopy has increased the number of interesting observations. The distal migration of a Foley catheter-type gastrostomy tube with resultant obstruction of the pancreatic duct was first described by Bui and Dang (192). Panicek et al. (193) described a second such patient and noted reports of three patients in whom similar migration had resulted in obstructive jaundice instead of pancreatitis. A variation was described in which the gastrostomy tube had migrated distally to obstruct the duct of Santorini in a patient who had only a small rudimentary duct of Wirsung. Acute recurrent pancreatitis resulted until the gastrostomy tube was replaced with a jejunostomy feeding catheter (194).

**Metallic Foreign Bodies.** In 1983, Chamoun et al. (195)

described chronic pancreatitis in the tail of the pancreas secondary to a metallic foreign body, perhaps a chip from a tin can, in the pancreatic duct. A sharp line of demarcation existed between the normal head of the pancreas and the fibrotic tail. They postulated that the tin might have penetrated the gastric wall to enter the pancreatic duct. Danzi (196) observed a dental wire, impacted through the duodenal wall into the head of the pancreas, resulting in pancreatitis, and Dabadie et al. (197) observed (by x-ray) a paper clip in the duodenum of a patient with acute pancreatitis. Endoscopy revealed an edematous hemorrhagic duodenal papilla. The paper clip was removed endoscopically, and the patient remained well over an 18-month follow-up. Another patient with acute pancreatitis had had cholecystectomy for gallstones 5 years earlier. Retrograde cholangiography revealed a surgical hemoclip within an otherwise radiolucent stone in the common bile duct. Removal of the clip and its induced stone was apparently curative (198). Following a remote cholecystectomy, a linen suture surrounded by a concretion in the common duct caused acute pancreatitis. Endoscopic removal of the foreign body was followed by prolonged freedom from pancreatitis (199).

**Vegetable and Animal Matter.** A 44-year-old farmer who had a habit of sucking on bristles from a cornhusk broom had two attacks of acute pancreatitis. Duodenoscopy revealed a foreign body resembling a cornhusk bristle projecting from the papilla of Vater. Following its endoscopic removal, the patient remained symptom free for 3 years (196). Meltzer and Goldberg (200) described a similar finding: a 5-cm cordlike structure, apparently cellulose, protruding from the papilla of Vater into the duodenal lumen. Endoscopic removal was followed by a disease-free period of 3 years. Others (201) described pancreatitis resulting from a gastric trichobezoar. "Herbs of Provence," a mixture of herb plants, which a patient had been chewing, resulted in fatal pancreatic necrosis (202). Although the authors do not specifically state this, it appears that a side-to-side choledochoduodenostomy performed 12 years earlier permitted the herbs to pass through the choledochoduodenostomy, to fill the distal common bile duct, and to obstruct the ampulla of Vater. Bedogni et al. (203) described two similar patients with acute pancreatitis resulting from foreign bodies accumulating as part of the sump syndrome following choledochoduodenostomy. Such patients were handled by endoscopic clearance of the distal common bile duct; one of the three died. Deboever and Sels (204) removed an ingested chicken feather from the ampulla of Vater, where it was endoscopically noted to be projecting into the duodenal lumen.

**Iatrogenic Foreign Bodies.** A retained fragment of a pancreatojejunostomy splint resulted in acute pancreatitis (205), as did a metal biliary stent that had been passed transhepatically through the ampulla of Vater into the duodenum (206). Kozarek (207, 208) observed that pancreatic-duct stents, placed for treatment of various problems of sphincteric stenosis, often result in varying degrees of pancreatitis, particularly consistent with chronic pancreatitis.

### Periampullary Duodenal Diverticulum

Caos (209) described acute pancreatitis and jaundice in an 84-year-old man, secondary to a narrow-mouthed duodenal diverticulum adjacent to the papilla of Vater. The diverticulum was filled with a pastelike material. Heath et al. (210) had previously reported a very similar observation, the diverticulum being filled with a soft, tenacious material. The papilla of Vater lay within the large duodenal diverticulum. Material similar to that within the diverticulum was found within the distal common bile duct.

Because of pancreaticobiliary complications of duodenal diverticula in three patients, Crithlow et al. (211) bypassed the periampullary duodenum by creating a Roux-en-Y from the first portion of the duodenum to the jejunum, thus diverting the foodstream while allowing the bile and pancreatic juice to drain through their normal duodenojejunal pathway. Each patient experienced a transient delay in gastric emptying. Shallman and Kolts (212) performed a similar operation for persistent pancreatitis secondary to a periampullary duodenal diverticulum.

De las Heras et al. (213) studied 74 patients with duodenal diverticula, 38 of whom also had gallstones. Of these 38, 24% had acute pancreatitis. The authors concluded that duodenal diverticula are often associated with gallstones and that gallstones may cause acute pancreatitis in these patients.

## PANCREATITIS ASSOCIATED WITH UNUSUAL SALIVARY, GASTROINTESTINAL, AND PANCREATIC DISEASES

### Primary Biliary Cirrhosis and Sjögren Syndrome

In a study of 41 patients with primary biliary cirrhosis, Epstein et al. (214) detected chronic pancreatitis in over half. This was characterized by hyposecretion of the exocrine pancreas, which the authors related to Sjögren syndrome. Sjögren syndrome is a chronic inflammatory autoimmune disease, characterized in part by chronic inflammation of the salivary and lacrimal glands, leading to diminished saliva and tear formation. The pancreas, as well as the salivary and lacrimal glands, are part of this dry gland disease. In another study of 35 patients with primary biliary cirrhosis, they noted abnormal pancreatograms in almost half (215). Shibata et al. (216) described a patient with chronic sialadenitis who had a diffusely enlarged pancreas, loss of pancreatic acini, interstitial fibrosis, and diffuse narrowing of the main pancreatic duct. Fibrous replacement of the acini was striking. A retrograde sialogram and biopsy of the submandibular gland revealed pooling of the contrast medium and destruction of the acini. The common bile duct was dilated secondary to stenosis in the head of the pancreas. Decreased exocrine function of the pancreas was noted in 6 of 11 patients with primary biliary cirrhosis (217). Perisic et al. (218) described pancreatitis in association with congenital hepatic fibrosis, a recessive autosomal hepatobiliary disease. A 12-year-old girl with an enlarged liver and spleen, esophageal varices and jaundice presented with elevated serum and urinary amylase levels. Primary biliary cirrhosis and pancreatitis have also been associated with ulcerative colitis. (See "Ulcerative Colitis").

### Sclerosing Cholangitis and Chronic Pancreatitis, Lymphoplasmacytic Sclerosing Pancreatitis, and Lymphoplasmacytic Sclerosing Pancreatitis

Several reports have linked sclerosing cholangitis and chronic pancreatitis. In 1965, Smith and Loe (219) found that 8 of 25 patients (32%) with primary sclerosing cholangitis had chronic pancreatitis. In the same year, Epstein et al. (220) found that 3 (15%) of 20 patients with sclerosing cholangitis had abnormal pancreatograms. Waldram et al. (221) described severe chronic pancreatitis in siblings in association with sclerosing cholangitis and suggested that an immune mechanism might be involved. They suggested that chronic pancreatitis might also be associated with retroperitoneal fibrosis. Others described a relationship between chronic pancreatitis and sclerosing cholangitis (222–225). In 1987, Fritsch (226) reviewed and confirmed the relationship, tying the complex relationship in with Crohn's disease and ulcerative colitis. Borkje et al. (227) also discussed a relationship of chronic pancreatitis in sclerosing cholangitis and ulcerative colitis, as have others. (See section on ulcerative colitis.)

*Lymphoplasmacytic sclerosing pancreatitis* with cholangitis was described as a variant of primary sclerosing cholangitis (228). This unusual inflammation involved almost the entire pancreas. The two elderly patients presented with a masslike enlargement of the pancreas and regional lymphadenopathy. Histologically, diffuse lymphoplasmacytic infiltration with marked interstitial fibrosis and acinar atrophy of the pancreas were observed. Pancreatic veins were occluded. The bile ducts and gallbladder were inflamed. The authors called the disease lymphoplasmacytic sclerosing pancreatitis with cholangitis and noted that it could be mistaken for pancreatic carcinoma. Their 1991 literature review revealed only one other reference to this unusual inflammatory process involving the entire pancreas (229).

### Fibrosing Pancreatitis in Children

Fibrosing pancreatitis is a chronic disease of unknown etiology, presenting usually in children and characterized by severe fibrous replacement of acinar tissue. Apparently first described by Williams, Sherman and Clatworthy (230), the syndrome includes recurrent abdominal pain. Ghishan et al. (231, 232) considered 4 of 10 children with chronic relapsing pancreatitis to have fibrosing pancreatitis. They reviewed the previous literature, pointing out that the disease could lead children to painless obstructive jaundice (although only one of their patients was free of pain) (232). Obstructive jaundice developed as early as 2 years of age (234). Stephen et al. (235) described a child with fibrosing pancreatitis associated with pericholangitis and cholangitis. Histologic study of the pancreas revealed replacement of acinar tissue with dense connective tissue and nodular aggregates of lymphocytes and plasma cells. Although the child was transiently jaundiced, liver biopsy did not reveal cirrhosis or sclerosing cholangitis. In their review of the literature, they noted that 6 of 8 patients with fibrosing pancreatitis presented with nonspecific abdominal pain of 6 weeks to 3 years duration. They cautioned that this syndrome should not be confused with chronic relapsing pancreatitis nor chronic pancreatitis associated with cystic fibrosis. Others provided case reports (236, 237).

### Painless Fibrosing Pancreatitis in Adults

In 1962, Gaulston and Gallagher (238) described "chronic painless pancreatitis." Ten patients, described by Bartholomew and Comfort (239), with chronic pancreatitis had never had abdominal pain. In a series of 125 patients with chronic pancreatitis, 14% had the painless type; their mean age was 46 years (240). Others have noted the syndrome (241–244). The author has studied 5 such patients over periods up to 10 years. Two developed extensive pancreatic calcification for which no causal factor could be identified. Exocrine and endocrine insufficiency were prominent developments.

### Celiac Disease (Nontropical Sprue or Gluten-Sensitive Enteropathy) and Chronic Pancreatitis

In 1963, Fitzgerald et al. (245) described a patient with severe chronic pancreatitis in association with celiac disease. Subsequently, Regan and DiMagno (246) described a patient with celiac disease and exocrine pancreatic insufficiency. In 1993 Nanda and Anand (247) observed celiac disease associated with juvenile calcific pancreatitis. The diagnosis of celiac disease was based on biopsy of the jejunum, which showed severe villous atrophy. ERCP showed dilatation of the pancreatic ducts. The patient improved on a gluten-free diet plus pancreatic enzymes. Earlier, Pitchumoni et al. (248) had reported a similar patient with severe pancreatic insufficiency associated with untreated celiac disease. Others (249, 250) noted the relationship of exocrine pancreatic insufficiency and glutenenteropathy.

### Pancreatitis Associated with Abnormal Feeding Patterns: Ramadan Syndrome, "Starvation" and Refeeding, Acute Pancreatitis

"Ramadan syndrome" is a term introduced by Benson and Ward (251) to describe a syndrome that is familiar to clinicians in Muslim societies but not well-documented in the literature. They observed a 14-year-old Muslim boy with acute pancreatitis of 24 hours duration, with its onset 5 hours after breaking the traditional Ramadan fast. Gastric dilatation was enormous. They quote three previous reports (252–254) in which two of the four patients had anorexia nervosa. Chen et al. (255) from Suzhou, China, reviewed 596 patients with acute pancreatitis. They attributed over 40% of the pancreatitis to ingestion of a large meal of cold rice, particularly after prolonged fasting by weak individuals.

### Anorexia Nervosa, "Refeeding Pancreatitis"

Several reports have related pancreatitis to anorexia nervosa (252, 254, 256–259). Gryboski et al. (259) described three such children or adolescents who became extremely malnourished. Following sudden increased feeding by mouth or by gastric tube, mild acute pancreatitis developed in each patient. The sequence was repetitive in one patient.

### Chronic Malnutrition with Refeeding, Kwashiorkor Disease

In autopsies of 40 children dying with malnutrition during the Biafan War in Africa, Montalegre et al. (260) studied the relationship between kwashiorkor and chronic calcifying pancreatitis of the tropics. They postulated that kwashiorkor is a transitional disease between malnutrition and the classical pancreatitis of the tropics. Acinar atrophy and extensive pancreatic fibrosis probably result from a lack of dietary protein at an earlier stage. Protein plugs in the pancreatic ducts are subsequently caused by feeding a balanced diet to a previously starving child.

### Pancreatitis after Operations for Morbid Obesity

A patient who had an ileal bypass of the distal 200 cm of the small intestine for hyperlipidemia developed acute pancreatitis (261), and another patient with morbid obesity developed acute pancreatitis after a pancreaticobiliary bypass (Scopinaro operation) (262). Sorrell et al. (263) found that 3 of 24 patients undergoing intestinal bypass for treatment of morbid obesity developed acute pancreatitis 1–6 months following bypass. Two of the patients died of hemorrhagic pancreatitis, one of whom also had gallstones. Payne et al. (264) described death from acute hemorrhagic pancreatitis following intestinal bypass.

### Total Parenteral Nutrition, Intravenous Lipids

A 17-year-old boy with Crohn's disease developed acute pancreatitis while receiving total parenteral nutrition, including 500 mL/day of a 20% fat emulsion. A recurrence of pancreatitis occurred when the lipid infusion was repeated (265). Pancreatitis occurred in two other patients who were receiving 20% lipid emulsion (266). Izsak et al. (267) reported six patients on total parenteral nutrition who developed acute pancreatitis. Hypercalcemia was apparently the cause. Two of the patients developed pancreatitis while on a lipid-free regimen. Weizman and Durie (268) in their review of acute pancreatitis in childhood, noted that acute pancreatitis had resulted from hypercalcemia, secondary to total parenteral nutrition therapy. Others made similar observations (269, 270).

### Pancreatitis Associated with Chronic Inflammatory Bowel Disease: Granulomatous Enteritis (Crohn's Disease) and Ulcerative Colitis

The literature on the relationship of acute and chronic pancreatitis to Crohn's disease and ulcerative colitis is difficult to interpret because the drugs (5-aminosalicylate, sulfapyridine, combinations of the two, azathioprine, 6-mercaptopurine [6-MP], and corticosteroids) used to treat these diseases may cause pancreatitis. Acute pancreatitis may result from Crohn's disease of the duodenum or from drugs used to treat it in any segment; ulcerative colitis results in acute pancreatitis chiefly through drug induction. Either, in its natural course, may cause chronic pancreatitis. Further evaluation of such generalizations is obviously required.

### Crohn's Disease of Duodenum (Chapter 24)

Crohn's disease of the duodenum, per se, is a definite cause of pancreatitis. Of 204 patients with pancreatitis of various causes, Efron detected stenosis of the ampulla of Vater associated with Crohn's granuloma in 10 (271). In reporting two patients with Crohn's disease and pancreatitis, Eisner et al. (272) tabulated 9 reported patients with duodenal Crohn's and pancreatitis and 21 with pancreatitis in whom the Crohn's did not involve the duodenum. In one patient, the ampulla of Vater was involved, and ERCP demonstrated marked dilatation and delayed drainage of the pancreatic duct. Legge et al. reported 10 patients with regional enteritis (Crohn's disease) involving the duodenum, three of whom had acute or recurrent pancreatitis (273). In one patient, an upper gastrointestinal series showed barium outlining the biliary and pancreatic ducts. On a subsequent hospital admission, the patient died of acute hemorrhagic pancreatitis. In none of the three patients was any other etiologic factor for the pancreatitis identified. Newman et al. (274) described a 37-year-old woman with a 9-year history of Crohn's ileocolitis and a 2-year history of increasing postprandial epigastric pain and vomiting. Her serum amylase level was strikingly elevated. Studies revealed strictures of the second and fourth part of the duodenum, periampullary inflammation, a dilated pancreatic duct, and chronic pancreatitis. Roux-en-Y gastrojejunostomy resulted in improvement. A 24-year-old man developed duodenal Crohn's (275). At age 32, he developed the first of multiple episodes of pancreatitis. By age 42, he developed obstruction of the distal common duct secondary to its stricture, with a gallstone obstructing it. Pancreatitis resulted in another patient with duodenal Crohn's where a persimmon bezoar apparently obstructed the ampulla of Vater (276). Meltzer and Korelitz (277) described a 21-year-old female with duodenal Crohn's who developed pancreatitis several years after radiographic demonstration of duodenopancreatic reflux. They attributed the pathogenesis of pancreatitis with duodenal Crohn's to either obstruction or duodenal reflux into the pancreatic duct. Pancreatitis may also occur without demonstrable involvement of the duodenum or in patients not on drug treatment.

### Crohn's Disease of the Distal Intestine

Seyrig et al. (278), of Paris, reported 331 patients with Crohn's disease, of whom 5 (1.5%) developed pancreatitis; none of the 5 had evidence of duodenal Crohn's. Apparently the pancreatitis was chronic and was thought to be unrelated to drug therapy. Axon, et al. described four patients with Crohn's disease limited to the small bowel or colon who had chronic pancreatitis (222). In a review of 852 patients with Crohn's disease, Weber et al., of Germany (279), found overt pancreatitis in 12 (1.4%) during a follow-up period of 10 years. In 10 of the patients, common causes of pancreatitis were excluded. Recurrence of pancreatitis was observed in only two patients. Younger patients and those with active disease seemed at greater risk for development of pancreatitis. No autoantibodies against the exocrine pancreas were found. When prednisolone was needed for treatment of active Crohn's disease, no adverse effect on the pancreatitis was observed. Omata et al. (280) described the development of pancreatitis in a patient with granulomatous disease of the colon and anus. Treatment of the enteritis with salazosulfapyridine and prednisolone resulted in improvement of both the Crohn's and the pancreatitis. Meyers et al. (281) noted that resection of the disease of the ileum in a young woman coincided with resolution of her pancreatitis in spite of residual Crohn's of the colon.

Haber et al. (282) reported that during the 15-year period from 1969 to 1985, 400 patients with Crohn's disease or ulcerative colitis were treated with 6-MP. Of these patients, 13 developed pancreatitis; 12 with Crohn's disease and 1 with ulcerative colitis. The authors believed that the acute pancreatitis was the result of the 6-MP. Seven patients had a secondary challenge with 6-MP, and all developed recurrent pancreatitis. The authors concluded that 6-MP should not be reinstituted once it had caused pancreatitis. Azathioprine, used in therapy of Crohn's has also been reported as a likely cause of pancreatitis (283). Several other reports, however, have confirmed the observation that Crohn's disease can cause pancreatitis (284–288).

### Ulcerative Colitis

The relationship of ulcerative colitis to pancreatitis is less definite than the one between Crohn's disease and pancreatitis. Ball, Baggenstoss and Bargen studied 86 consecutive autopsies involving ulcerative colitis and noted interstitial pancreatitis of varying degrees in 46 (289). They doubted the clinical importance of the pancreatitis. Joske (290) and Davies (291) each described ulcerative colitis as a probable cause of pancreatitis in respective patients. Kondo et al. (292) described acute pancreatitis as a complication of ulcerative colitis, but the associated drug therapy was not noted. A 19-year-old man with no other recognizable predisposing factors developed chronic pancreatitis (293); 6 months later, ulcerative colitis was diagnosed. Others have reported chronic pancreatitis in association with ulcerative colitis (222, 294).

Chronic pancreatitis has been described in patients who had sclerosing cholangitis or pericholangitis with ulcerative colitis (215, 227, 278, 295, 296). Kato et al. (297) described a 65-year-old Japanese woman with primary biliary cirrhosis and chronic pancreatitis associated with ulcerative colitis. Apparently the pancreatitis was relatively asymptomatic but was associated with an abnormal pancreatogram. Veloso et al. (298) described a similar relationship. The pancreatitis discussed above tends to be painless, without calcification, with exocrine pancreatic insufficiency, and with mildly abnormal pancreatograms.

## PANCREATITIS AND VASCULITIS

Pancreatitis associated with the several forms of vasculitis is fundamentally a disease of children and young people.

### Lupus Erythematosus

Lupus erythematosus (SLE) is thought to induce pancreatitis by creating a low-flow state from vasculitis involving the pancreatic vessels. The data supporting this concept are confused by the fact that many of these patients are on corticosteroids or immunosuppression, either of which may result in pancreatitis. Thus, the basic cause of the lupus-associated pancreatitis has not been definitively established. Petri (299) reviewed the subject and observed that pancreatitis is an unusual complication of SLE, occurring in only 3% of patients with this disease at Johns Hopkins Hospital and in 4% of another group (300). Corticosteroid therapy was not the major cause of pancreatitis in these patients with SLE, since it occurred before the drug was used or after it had been discontinued. Autopsies have demonstrated arteritis, inspissated concretions within the pancreatic ducts, or vascular thrombosis. Vera Arieta (301) described two patients with generalized lupus and acute pancreatitis. In one, pancreatitis appeared to result from vasculitis in the pancreatic vessels. The other developed an infected pseudocyst. The author credits Osler with having first described (1895) the visceral manifestations of generalized lupus.

In a study of 18 patients with SLE, Odaira et al. (302) noted that 7 developed acute pancreatitis. This report reviewed 27 autopsies of patients dying of SLE, including 20 with histologic pancreatic lesions: 2 (7% of total group) with enteritis, 10 (37%) with vascular thrombosis, 6 (22%) with focal pancreatitis, 8 (29%) with periductal fibrosis, 11 (41%) with interlobular fibrosis, 6 (22%) with ductule dilatation, and 7 (26%) with pancreatic fat deposition. They found diminution of exocrine pancreatic function in several patients. The findings suggest that pancreatic damage in SLE is frequent but mild. Serrano Lopez et al. (303) described a 27-year-old woman who died of acute pancreatitis after a 12-year history of SLE. She had been off all medication for 1 year. Autopsy revealed no cause for the pancreatitis except that the pancreatic vessels were almost occluded by intimal fibrous proliferation. Their extensive review of reports of 69 patients with pancreatitis associated with SLE revealed that 30 (44%) had died. Autopsies were performed in 26, and half had evidence of vascular lesions. *Ninety percent of the patients were female, with a mean age of 28 years.* Eaker and Toskes (304) also support vasculitis as the likely cause of the pancreatitis in SLE. Their patient, a 22-year-old woman had acute pancreatitis as the initial manifestation of SLE. She had never been on steroid therapy. In their review of 67 patients with SLE who developed acute pancreatitis, 39 had been taking steroids. Others (305–308) have noted acute pancreatitis as the presenting manifestation of SLE, although most patients have had SLE for months or years prior to its development. Rupprecht et al. (309) described an 11-year-old girl who developed chronic relapsing pancreatitis 6 years prior to developing other manifestations of SLE. Similar patients have been reported, including those with autopsy findings of thrombosis (310–315). Eaker and Toskes (304) documented 10 patients who were not on drugs that might have been implicated as a cause of the pancreatitis. Kolk et al. (316) described a 16-year-old girl who died from acute hemorrhagic pancreatitis that they attributed to methotrexate therapy. Several (314, 317) have indicated that acute pancreatitis is not an indication to discontinue corticosteroid therapy.

In 1993, Borum et al. (318) described two patients with SLE who developed chronic pancreatitis with no other identifiable cause. A 24-year-old female with a history of SLE since the age of 13 had multiple calcifications of the pancreas. A Puestow operation was performed for relief of pain. The authors found no previous documentation of SLE and chronic pancreatitis in the absence of other identifiable causes for the pancreatitis. Odaira et al. (302), however, had shown functional evidence of chronic pancreatic insufficiency in two patients.

### Unusual Forms of Vasculitis Associated with Pancreatitis

Although several reports link pancreatitis to the following forms of vasculitis, the relationship is relatively tenuous.

### Wegener's Granulomatosis

Wegener's granulomatosis has been repeatedly shown histologically to include pancreatic vasculitis. Kemp et al., (319) apparently reported (1990) the first patient with acute pancreatitis associated with Wegener's granulomatosis. With a 16-year history of Wegener's granulomatosis, their patient had 6 episodes of acute pancreatitis and developed a pseudocyst. In most instances an attack of pancreatitis was associated with a reactivation of the Wegener's granulomatosis and appeared to precede and herald it.

### Henoch-Schönlein Syndrome (Nonthrombocytopenic Purpura)

Acute pancreatitis associated with nonthrombocytopenic purpura has been identified primarily in children, including one patient with hemorrhagic pancreatitis (320–325). Pancreatitis may be the initial manifestation of the purpura (324).

### Polyarteritis (Periarteritis) Nodosa and Churg-Strauss Angiitis

As early as 1926, Gruber (326) noted periarteritis in the pancreatic vessels in 26 patients with periarteritis nodosa. Several reports have since linked periarteritis or the related Churg-Strauss syndrome with pancreatitis (327–332). As a resident, the author saw a patient with periarteritis nodosa who experienced a discrete atypical attack of acute pancreatitis. She died from chronic renal failure resulting from the periarteritis.

### Kawasaki Disease

Kawasaki disease has been shown at autopsy in children to involve perivascular inflammation, medial destruction, and inflammation of the intima of medium- and large-sized arteries and veins, including those of the pancreas (333). Stoler et al. (334) apparently described the first two patients with Kawasaki disease who developed acute pancreatitis. One was a 5-year-old boy, the other a 16-year-old male who developed pancreatitis approximately 2 weeks into the Kawasaki disease. Both patients survived. Lanting et al. (335) described acute pancreatitis developing 4 days before the onset of Kawasaki syndrome in a 5-year-old boy.

### Scleroderma

In a 1979 review, Grief and Wolff (336) noted several reports associating scleroderma with pancreatic fibrosis, diabetes, or pancreatic exocrine insufficiency. The vascular lesions consisted of arteritis-associated intimal proliferation, resulting in partial obliteration of the lumen. They reported a 43-year-old man with pancreatic calcification associated with progressive scleroderma. Laparotomy and biopsy revealed fibrosis of the pancreas, stenosis of the pancreatic duct, and chronic inflammation. The patient had multiple attacks of abdominal pain associated with elevated serum amylase levels.

### Postradiation Pancreatitis

In an excellent report, "Abdominal Radiotherapy is a Cause for Chronic Pancreatitis," Levy et al. (337) described five patients with chronic pancreatitis who had undergone abdominal radiotherapy (for Hodgkin's disease in four, for seminoma in one) in doses of 3600–4050 rads, 6–20 years previously. The median time lapse between radiotherapy and recognition of pancreatitis was 7 years. Each patient was in complete remission from the malignant diseases. The symptoms of chronic pancreatitis included pancreatic pain in 5 patients, acute pancreatitis in 3, pseudocysts in 3, stenosis of the common bile duct in 2, stenosis of the duodenum in 1, splenic vein thrombosis in 1, diabetes mellitus in 4, steatorrhea in 4, and pancreatic calcification in 1. Three of the five had laparotomy for complications of chronic pancreatitis. Histologically, there was severe fibrosis and endarteritis. The authors suggested that the pathogenesis of the pancreatitis related to the changes in the vascular system. They summarized three previous reports of one patient each (338–340) in whom chronic pancreatitis had been recognized 11–24 years after radiotherapy; two of the three had marked abnormalities of the pancreatic duct on ERCP.

A 25-year follow-up of a patient who had received external irradiation with 5000 rads for treatment of seminoma (341), revealed a severely fibrotic and atrophic pancreas with scattered foci of calcification and massive dilatation of the pancreatic ducts, as well as vascular alterations. Sindelar et al. (342) reported finding similar pancreatic lesions in 5 of 22 patients following intraoperative radiotherapy. Swaroop et al. (343) reported a prospective study of radiation-induced pancreatic changes in 11 patients treated for primary gastric lymphoma. In addition to chemotherapy, they received external beam radiation therapy of 3500–5000 cGy. ERCP performed 8–50 months after completion of the radiation therapy (mean, 30.7 months) showed minimal dilatation of the main pancreatic duct in one patient but clubbing of side branches of the pancreatic duct in four. In a subsequent report (Gastroenterol 1994;107:632), they stated that none of the 11 patients developed pancreatic pain after a mean follow-up of 60 months. Experimental studies on dogs (344–348) revealed atrophy of the pancreas with severe fibrosis and variable degrees of stenosis of the pancreatic ducts.

## RENAL INSUFFICIENCY AND PANCREATITIS AND HEMOLYSIS

### Renal Insufficiency

Both acute and chronic pancreatitis may result from, or be associated with, renal failure. The relationship is complicated not only by the renal failure but by its treatment with steroids and dialysis. Before dialysis was available, Baggenstoss (349) noted at autopsy that approximately half of patients dying of renal failure had histologic evidence of pancreatitis. These patients usually had not had clinical evidence of pancreatitis. Welch (350) found that 15% of children with end-stage renal disease had evidence of pancreatitis; the incidence rose to 40% when the renal disease had been treated with steroids. Secondary hypercalcemia and hyperparathyroidism were considered to be causally involved in the pancreatitis. In chronic renal failure, Avram (351) noted histologic evidence of pancreatitis at autopsy in 21 patients; the pancreas showed chronic ductal dilatation and periductal inflammation without evidence of acute pancreatitis. Others (352–354) noted acute, as well as chronic, pancreatitis. With widespread use of chronic dialysis, patients with end-stage renal disease survived longer, thus providing an opportunity to study its continued effects on the pancreas. Vaziri et al. (355) observed pancreatitis in 28% of 78 patients treated by long-term hemodialysis; 2 had the hemorrhagic form. Eguchi et al. (356) found pancreatic fibrosis in over 90% and inflammatory infiltrate in 72% of patients treated by long-term hemodialysis. Araki et al. (357) also found that patients with end-stage renal disease often had an increased serum level of pancreatic-type amylase, which seldom rose after administration of secretin. Their autopsy findings revealed histologic changes of chronic pancreatitis in half of patients after long-term hemodialysis. Among 1001 patients with end-stage renal disease, Rutsky et al. (358) noted that 23 experienced 35 attacks of acute pancreatitis; 4 patients died with complications related to pancreatic pseudocysts and 1 died from hemorrhagic pancreatitis. The 10-year incidence of pancreatitis was 2.3%, and the overall mortality among patients developing pancreatitis was 21%. The authors concluded that clinically evident acute pancreatitis occurs more often than had been previously recognized, particularly in patients managed with peritoneal dialysis. They calculated an incidence of pancreatitis of 0.03 per patient year of peritoneal dialysis versus 0.01 per patient year of hemodialysis ($p < .001$). Others (359, 360) have reported acute pancreatitis during peritoneal dialysis. In their second report, Van Dyke et al. (361) described 54 episodes of acute pancreatitis in 34 patients with chronic renal failure, including 26 on maintenance dialysis, 6 after renal transplantation, and 2 managed conservatively; 10 (29%) died. Six children with chronic renal failure had 10 attacks of acute pancreatitis (362). Others (363, 364) made similar observations, including a large series by Padilla et al. (365) that included a patient with chronic calcific pancreatitis with end-stage renal disease secondary to systemic lupus erythematosus (SLE).

Acute pancreatitis in these patients may have had multiple causes. Evans and Slapak (366) noted a patient on home hemodialysis who developed acute pancreatitis associated with a serum calcium level of 19.6 mg/100 mL, which they attributed to hypercalcemia secondary to a failure to use a water softener properly. Others (367) made related observations.

### Hemolysis and Mismatched Blood Transfusions

Daul et al. (368) in 1994 reported acute hemolysis with life-threatening pancreatitis in 12 patients undergoing chronic hemodialysis and in 2 patients undergoing hemofiltration for chronic renal insufficiency; 6 developed necrotizing pancreatitis, of whom 3 died. The authors attributed the hemolysis to a mechanical defect in 8 patients, an osmotic mechanism in 1, and unknown causes in the others. Walker et al. (369) first described acute pancreatitis as a complication of hypotonic dialysate fluid in two patients with chronic renal failure. The patients developed acute hemolysis, complained of epigastric pain, and developed paralytic ileus. Their serum amylase levels rose extremely high, but the symptoms resolved within approximately 8 days. Pancreatitis due to mismatched blood transfusion was first described by Ackerman (370) in 1942. The patient received 200 mL of mismatched blood and died within 24 hours, with acute hemorrhagic pancreatitis. Druml et al. (371) studied 40 patients with acute hemolysis (defined as a drop in the hematocrit of more than 12% within 12 hours) and concluded that acute pancreatitis resulted in about 20–25% of patients. The pancreatitis, a diffuse edematous type, sometimes progressed to focal necrosis, but rarely (if ever) progressed to gross pancreatic hemorrhage, and rarely contributed to the patient's death. Acute renal failure and intravascular coagulation were frequent. Pancreatitis occurred during or immediately after the red cell destruction and before development of the uremic state. Although acute renal failure, per se, may cause a rise in serum amylase level, the authors observed that this rise without pancreatitis rarely exceeds 2.5 times the upper limits of normal.

## PANCREATITIS ASSOCIATED WITH MISCELLANEOUS METABOLIC AND OTHER DISEASES

### Porphyria

Saint et al. (372) and Joske (373) each reported acute pancreatitis in patients with acute porphyria. In 1995, Shiraki et al. (374) reported a patient with acute pancreatitis associated with acute intermittent porphyria. In their review they found nine cases previously reported; five had acute pancreatitis following an attack of intermittent acute porphyria and two or more had chronic pancreatitis.

### Glycogen Storage Disease Type I (von Gierke Disease)

Several patients with inherited disorders of glycogen metabolism have been reported with pancreatitis. Each patient has had the subtype of type I disease known as Von Gierke disease, which is characterized by glucose-6-phosphatase deficiency. In 1980, Michaels and Beaudet (375) described a 17-year-old female with glycogen storage disease (type 1) who died suddenly of acute hemorrhagic pancreatitis. Autopsy also demonstrated evidence of chronic pancreatitis. A similar observation in a child was described by Herman (376). Others (377) reported acute pancreatitis, including the hemorrhagic form (378). Kikuchi et al. (379) described glycogen storage disease (type 1) in an 8-year-old boy with a history of hyperlipidemia, chronic pancreatitis, and an infected pseudocyst that required resection. Too little is known to generalize beyond the predilection for the pancreatitis to be severe and to occur at an early age.

### Wilson's Disease

Wilson's disease is associated with defective excretion of copper in bile, resulting in its excessive deposition in the liver and other organs, including the pancreas. Weizman et al. (380) described acute recurrent pancreatitis in a 12-year-old boy who had an abnormally high urinary excretion of copper. Improvement was attributed to penicillamine therapy. They found two previous reports (381, 382).

### Diabetic Ketoacidosis

Diabetic ketoacidosis has been described as associated with acute pancreatitis in four patients (383). The pancreatitis was relatively mild and resolved rapidly.

### Organic Acidemias and Pancreatitis

Kahlen et al. (384) identified 9 children (8%) with pancreatitis (7 with acute type, 2 with chronic) among 108 children with branched-chain organic aminoacidemias: maple syrup urine disease or isovaleric or methylmalonic acidemia. Three children with pancreatitis died, two of acute hemorrhagic pancreatitis. Burlina et al. (385) described two children with acute pancreatitis associated with *propionic acidemia*. Pancreatitis has been noted in patients with homocystinuria (386, 387), observations that related back to the pioneer work of Gross et al. (388). Valproic acid, a major cause of drug-induced pancreatitis, is a branched-chain organic acid.

### Acute Pancreatitis in Long-Distance Runners

Ertan and Schneider (389) documented two patients who developed acute pancreatitis following runs of 5 and 17 miles, respectively. Both were females, aged 27 and 46 years, respectively. Each was a well-trained runner, who developed elevated serum amylase levels and ultrasound or CT scan evidence of pancreatitis. Follow-up ERCP was normal in each. The authors did not postulate a mechanism for this pancreatitis. From previous reports of abdominal pain while running, particularly among young women, the authors proposed that the incidence of pancreatitis among runners may be higher than has been recognized.

### Acute Pancreatitis in Sickle Cell Disease

Kumar et al. (390) in 1989 described the development of acute pancreatitis in a 51-year-old man during a sickle cell crisis, an observation made as early as 1961 (59). In 1971, Song (392) noted pancreatic fibrosis at autopsy in a patient with sickle cell disease. In a review of pancreatitis in childhood, Ziegler et al. (393) reported six children with sickle cell disease, pancreatitis, and gallstones. A 3-year-old black girl reported by Sheehan et al. (394) had acute pancreatitis during a sickle cell crisis.

### Thrombocytopenic Purpura

Olson (395) reported acute pancreatitis in a 49-year-old man with thrombocytopenic purpura. Autopsy revealed diffuse peripancreatic fat necrosis. He referenced nine other patients who had pancreatitis associated with thrombocytopenia.

### Juvenile Dermatomyositis and Ehlers-Danlos Syndrome

Petros et al. (396) described an 11-year-old girl who had recurring acute pancreatitis associated with juvenile dermatomyositis. Ehlers-Danlos syndrome is an inherited polysystemic elastic tissue disorder characterized by relaxation of joints, hyperelastic skin, and a tendency to excessive bleeding. Sarra-Carbonell and Jimenez (397) reported two siblings with this syndrome who developed acute pancreatitis.

### Polyarthritis

Ferrari et al. (398) reported a 76-year-old white male with prolonged hospitalization for a complicated hip fracture who developed pancreatitis and severe polyarthritis. Subcutaneous fat necrosis surrounded the involved joints and was limited to these areas. There were scattered nodules of acute and chronic pancreatitis with dystrophic calcification. Their bibliography included 11 references that suggest that polyarthritis may be a complication of pancreatitis rather than its cause and that widespread subcutaneous fat necrosis is not usually limited to the joint areas.

### Behcet's Disease

Behcet's disease, a syndrome of oral and genital aphthae and uveitis, was first associated with acute pancreatitis by O'Duffy and associates in 1971 (399). Huong et al. (400) described 2 such patients with acute pancreatitis and quoted Lakhanpal et al. (401) as noting 5 patients with pancreatitis among 170 autopsies in patients with Behcet's disease.

### Pancreatitis Associated with Low-Flow States, Hypothermia

Acute or chronic pancreatitis may result from reduced blood flow to the pancreas, secondary to arteriosclerosis or cardiac failure (402), vasculitis, embolization, and related systemic vascular problems. The most frequently reported cause at present is cardiac bypass operations (see Chapter 26, "Postoperative Pancreatitis").

### Hypothermia and Acute Pancreatitis

An earlier review of the literature reported numerous instances of acute pancreatitis as probably caused by hypothermia (403). The etiologic importance of hypothermia was not entirely convincing as the relationship was sometimes based on a low body temperature at the time of hospitalization. Perhaps most striking was the report by Sano and Smith (404) who treated approximately 50 patients with advanced cancer by refrigerating them for 50–230 hours at an average body temperature of 31°C (87°F). Autopsy revealed acute pancreatitis in five patients. The authors hypothesized that the pancreatitis might have resulted from low blood flow to the pancreas secondary to the hypothermia. Little has been published in the more current literature.

### Other Associations

Other possible etiologic associations include hemochromatosis (405), hereditary spherocytosis (406, 407), and gout (408).

### α-1-Antitrypsin Deficiency

α-1-Antitrypsin is a serum inhibitor of numerous proteolytic enzymes including pancreatic, leukocytic, and bacterial proteases. The deficiency is a genetic disorder, whose relationship to pancreatitis has not been clearly defined as its implication has usually been indirect. Two patients with α-1-antitrypsin deficiency developed acute pancreatitis, one a 3-year-old girl (409) and the other a 63-year-old man (410). Two others with this deficiency developed acute pancreatitis after ERCP (411). A relationship of this deficiency with chronic pancreatitis has also been observed (412–414), but again, evidence for its etiologic importance is indirect.

### Werner's Syndrome

Werner's syndrome is an inherited syndrome characterized by premature atherosclerotic changes and premature aging. Hyperlipidemia may develop. Naafs et al. (415) in 1989 described such a patient with acute pancreatitis. Hyperlipidemia might have been the precipitating factor.

### Carnitive Palmitoyl Transferase II Deficiency

Carnitive palmitoyl transferase II deficiency has recently been described as a cause of recurrent pancreatitis (416). This syndrome, often resulting in myoglobinuria and hypertriglyceridemia, is a mitochondrial disorder. The authors quote Rotig et al. (417) that pancreatitis may also occur with Pearson's pancreas-marrow syndrome, another mitochondrial disorder.

### Pancreatitis in Pregnancy and the Postpartum Period

Pregnancy may predispose to acute pancreatitis. Estrogen increases cholesterol excretion in bile, and progesterone inhibits gallbladder contraction. Thus, pregnancy may predispose to gallstone formation and hyperlipidemia. In 1951, Langmade and Edmondson (418) reported 9 patients and reviewed 53 others. Montgomery and Miller noted that pancreatitis tended to occur more frequently as pregnancy progressed, with the highest incidence in the third trimester and puerperium (419). In 1972, Corlett and Mishell (420) reported no maternal deaths among 52 patients with acute pancreatitis during pregnancy or the puerperium. They noted an incidence of pancreatitis of 1 in 1066 live births. At that time most attacks were considered idiopathic pancreatitis. Makay, O'Neill, and Imrie (421) summarized 20 patients: 18 with gallstones, 1 alcohol induced, and 1 with hyperlipoproteinemia. One of the attacks occurred 8 weeks postabortion, and 13 (65%) were postpartum.

Nine patients reported by Legro and Laifer (422) developed acute pancreatitis in the first trimester of pregnancy: 5 were due to gallstones, 1 alcohol, 4 idiopathic, and 1 low-flow state from hypotension. Apparently all mothers and infants survived, but preterm labor occurred in two. Hospitalization tended to be prolonged; one patient required 8 hospitalizations. Wilkinson (423) studied pancreatitis during pregnancy and its 8-week puerperium, reviewed 106 patients, and found the incidence of gallstone pancreatitis to be 36%.

Niess and Dreiss (424) reviewed 11 reports of hyperlipidemic pancreatitis during pregnancy. Their patient and infant survived, although the mother experienced adult respiratory distress syndrome and developed a pancreatic pseudocyst. Acute pancreatitis with pancreatic necrosis and pseudocyst formation complicating pregnancy was reported in a 20-year-old patient with a choledochal cyst (425); she was treated conservatively during a difficult pregnancy until caesarean section could be performed. Resection of the choledochal cyst was later performed. Of related interest, Flege (426) observed elevated serum amylase levels in a patient with a ruptured tubal pregnancy, and Steinmetz et al. (427) noted a possible association with in vitro fertilization. Recurrent acute pancreatitis developed in a 32-year-old woman during each of two cycles of in vitro fertilization.

In general, patients with pregnancy-associated pancreatitis are managed conservatively. Since most have gallstones, ultrasound of the gallbladder should be routine in pregnant patients. Its inclusion would add only a few minutes to their evaluation. The role of endoscopic therapy in the pregnant patient with gallstone pancreatitis is uncertain.

### Allergic Pancreatitis and Eosinophilic Pancreatitis

**Allergic Pancreatitis.** A 48-year-old welder with a history of recurrent hives had repeated attacks of abdominal pain associated with generalized urticaria (428). Laparotomy during one attack showed acute pancreatitis. Shaffer (428) cited Lindsay's description of two patients with allergic pancreatitis, one from chocolate and the second from apples. The author has had two patients with acute pancreatitis that appeared to result from an allergy to shrimp.

**Hereditary Angioedema.** Hereditary angioedema was associated with recurrent acute pancreatitis by Cutler et al. (429). The attacks of pancreatitis were mild but repetitive. Their review found only a single article, in which Brickman et al. (430) found 3 of 157 patients with hereditary angioedema to have chronic pancreatitis. Each had recurrent attacks of acute or subacute pancreatitis. The diagnosis of pancreatitis was confirmed by laparotomy in two.

**Eosinophilic Pancreatitis.** Vazquez-Rodriquez et al. (431) described a patient with eosinophilic acute pancreatitis and reviewed the literature on eosinophilic gastroenteritis prior to 1973. Of over 40 patients previously reported, only 1 had had eosinophilic infiltration of the pancreas. Their patient was a middle-aged man with acute pancreatitis with repetitive peripheral eosinophilia. The patient had a stricture of the common bile duct within the substance of the pancreas and stenosis of the gastric antrum. During an attack of acute pancreatitis, laparotomy was performed and biopsy specimens from the gastric antrum and jejunum showed striking eosinophilic infiltration. Pancreatic biopsy revealed intense eosinophilic infiltration. A 54-year-old patient with a history of alcohol abuse developed acute pancreatitis with pseudocyst formation. The attack was associated with a striking transient eosinophilia (432). This author treated a middle-aged man for a severe attack of acute pancreatitis. He previously had gastric outlet obstruction from eosinophilic gastritis and several years later developed obstruction of the common bile duct associated with eosinophilic infiltration of the terminal common bile duct. Each required operative relief. On his third admission, CT scan revealed an enlarged pancreas. The author believes that he had eosinophilic inflammatory obstruction of the pancreatic duct. He improved without operation.

Flejou et al. (433) resected the left side of the pancreas for a tumor consisting of eosinophilic pancreatitis in a 26-year-old woman. No other organ appeared be involved. The peripheral eosinophilic count was normal. A cystic mass in the tail of the pancreas was noted by Baskin et al. (434) to involve the spleen, lymph nodes, and colon. Radical resection of the mass revealed eosinophilic gastroenteritis with areas of necrosis and abscess in the pancreas. Biopsies of the stomach and duodenum revealed similar findings. Two other patients underwent Whipple resections for tumor masses resulting from eosinophilic infiltration (435, 436). Barresi et al. (437) described the autopsy finding of eosinophilic pancreatitis in a premature infant.

### Sarcoidosis and Other Granulomas

In addition to Crohn's disease, tuberculosis, and syphilis, sarcoidosis and other granulomas have occasionally been reported to result in pancreatitis (438–449). Sarcoid of the pancreas has caused obstructive jaundice (443). Becker and Lux (449) performed a Whipple resection, believing that they were doing a palliative resection for carcinoma of the pancreas. Instead, it was a granulomatous involvement of the head of the pancreas by sarcoid. Among 1000 surgical specimens of the pancreas resected for chronic pancreatitis, granulomas of varying morphologies were found by Stümer and Becker (441) in 34; 2 were sarcoidosis of the pancreas and peripancreatic lymph nodes. One patient with syphilis and common duct obstruction had undergone a Whipple resection. Granulomas containing Langerhans-type giant cells were found in the pancreas and duodenum. The diagnosis was syphilitic pancreatitis represented by a $4.5 \times 5.0$ cm mass. The authors also described pancreatitis from suture granulomas from previous operations in four patients and granulomas from prior efforts to obliterate the exocrine pancreas by endoscopic injection into the pancreatic duct of a rapidly hardening amino acid mixture (Ethibloc) in two patients (441). Numerous reports have described tuberculosis of the pancreas (see section on tuberculous pancreatitis and tuberculosis of the pancreas).

## PANCREATITIS SECONDARY TO BACTERIAL INFECTIONS

Because of the rarity of some infections (e.g., tuberculosis of the pancreas), reports are included that describe subacute or chronic pancreatitis, as well as acute pancreatitis. With two exceptions the following literature is organized by the specific bacteria involved. Veghelyi (450) summarized the early literature (1947) on secondary pancreatitis during or after typhoid fever, spirochetal jaundice, scarlet fever, diphtheria, malaria, and pneumonia.

### Acute Pancreatitis Post-ERCP

ERCP is followed by a relatively high incidence of pancreatitis, secondary to overdistension of the pancreatic ducts with a hyperosmolar fluid, but the catheter used in this procedure is contaminated and may introduce bacteria directly into the pancreatic duct. This may explain why bacterial infection of the pancreas appears to be important in patients whose post-ERCP pancreatitis is severe.

### Primary Pyogenic Cholangitis as a Cause of Acute Pancreatitis

Primary pyogenic cholangitis, which occurs predominantly in the Orient, was apparently first described in 1930 when Digby (451) reported 8 patients in Hong Kong. Its clinical features were described by Cook et al. (452) who proposed the term "recurrent pyogenic cholangitis" (453). Primary pyogenic cholangitis should not be confused with primary sclerosing cholangitis. It is associated with a high incidence of calculi in both the intrahepatic and extrahepatic bile ducts and sometimes in the gallbladder. These calculi are composed almost entirely of bile pigment. They are often quite small and ill formed, sometimes resembling "muddy flakes." Patients characteristically suffer multiple episodes of cholangitis with fever associated with jaundice. The disease results in a high incidence of acute pancreatitis (453). Although the pancreatitis is considered secondary to the biliary calculi, it is uncertain whether biliary infection, per se, plays a causal role. The cholangitis is characteristically caused by enteric gram-negative bacteria, especially *Escherichia coli.* Obstruction of the pancreatic duct by an ampullary stone and biliary-pancreatic infection require therapy.

### Staphylococci and Pancreatitis

Thal and Molestina (454) produced fulminating pancreatic necrosis by injecting staphylococcal toxin into the pancreatic duct of dogs and rabbits. This writer has also been impressed with the severe pancreatitis and widespread fat necrosis that results in the dog after injection of killed *Staphylococcus aureus* into the pancreatic duct, an approach previously taken by others (455, 456). There are few clinical data to relate these observations to man.

### Pancreatitis with Food Poisoning

*Salmonella* enteritis is a significant cause of acute pancreatitis. Renner et al. (457) reported that 29 (62%) of 47 patients with *Salmonella* enteritis developed acute pancreatitis. Of these, 7 patients had infection by *S. typhimurium* and 22 with *S. enteritidis.* Pancreatitis was usually mild to moderate. *Salmonella* pancreatitis was apparently first described by Boyd (458) (1969) and subsequently by Honegr et al. (459). Boyd reported an outbreak of *S. typhimurium* food poisoning resulting in six deaths; four had acute interstitial pancreatitis. He postulated that the pancreatitis might have resulted from endotoxic or bacterial shock rather than from an ascending pancreatic ductal infection. Of 171 patients hospitalized in Liverpool with acute gastroenteritis, Murphy et al. (460) found 64% to be due to *Salmonella* spp. None presented clinical evidence of acute pancreatitis. Andren-Sandberg and Hojer (461) described a 57-year-old man with acute pancreatic necrosis and sepsis that the authors attributed to *Salmonella* found in the blood and bile. Others have described associated pancreatitis, sometimes relatively severe (459, 462, 463). Abdullah et al. (464) reported a patient with severe *S. enteritidis* food poisoning who developed rhabdomyolysis, acute tubular necrosis, and acute pancreatitis. Pastore et al. (465) reported two patients with *Salmonella*-related pancreatitis and recommended that patients with *Salmonella* infections and upper abdominal pain be investigated for pancreatitis and *Salmonella* infection should be considered as a possible cause of hyperamylasemia and diarrhea. Three patients with *food poisoning* after eating warmed-over blue herring became violently ill; two died. Autopsy revealed severe edematous pancreatitis in both, with *hemolytic streptococcus* in pure culture from the pancreas and its exudate (466).

### Pancreatitis with Typhoid Fever *(Salmonella typhi)*

Russell et al. (467), in describing a patient with typhoid fever and acute pancreatitis, cited Osler (468) as first noting that occasionally hemorrhagic pancreatitis occurred in patients with typhoid infections. Sedallian et al. (469) subsequently reported a patient with typhoid pancreatitis in 1947, and Monad-Broca et al. (470) described a patient with laparotomy-confirmed acute typhoid pancreatitis. Writing from Russia, Borisova et al. (471) described a patient with acute abdominal pain and increased urinary amylase level but no diarrhea. Laparotomy revealed acute pancreatic necrosis from which they cultured *S. typhi.* Others have observed pancreatitis or pancreatic abscess with typhoid fever (472–479). Ginsburg and Raffenne (480) described typhoid fever complicated by acute renal failure, rhabdomyolysis, and acute pancreatitis. Elevation of serum pancreatic enzyme levels and a positive blood culture for *S. typhi* were observed in an HIV-positive patient (481).

### Pancreatitis following Typhoid and Cholera Vaccinations

Gatt (482) reported a 75-year-old female who had received vaccinations for typhoid, paratyphoid A & B, and cholera 2 years earlier. Some 48 hours after a subsequent revaccination with monovalent typhoid and cholera vaccine, she was hospitalized with severe acute pancreatitis and required 21 days of hospitalization before recovery. She had had an identical but milder episode of pain following the original vaccination.

### Leptospirosis and Pancreatitis

*Leptospira icterohaemorrhagiae,* transmitted to humans by the rat, gives rise to Weil's disease and apparently is the leptospire involved in the associated pancreatitis, first described by Stolze et al. (483) in 1959. Bell et al. (484) reported a child with leptospirosis who developed acalcalous hydrops of the gallbladder and acute edematous pancreatitis. They postulated that the pancreatitis and cholecystitis might be secondary to the "vasculitis that affects all organ symptoms." Three patients with leptospirosis and pancreatitis and two others with hyperamylasemia were reported by Edwards and Evarard (485). Edwards et al. (486) noted hyperamylasemia in up to 65% of patients with leptospirosis and jaundice. Ribiczey et al. (487) noted that although the literature would indicate that leptospirosis was an unusual cause of acute pancreatitis, they had diagnosed acute pancreatitis in four patients with malignant leptospirosis within a short time. Others have reported the association (488–491).

### *Campylobacter* Pancreatitis

Gallagher et al. (492) first attributed acute pancreatitis to *Campylobacter* when they reported a 19-year-old female with acute pancreatitis and *Campylobacter fetus* subsps. *jejuni* cultured from the stool and confirmed by antibody studies. deBois et al. (493) described a severe form of acute *Campylobacter*-associated pancreatitis. A high incidence of hyperamylasemia and hyperlipasemia in association with *Campylobacter* enteritis was noted in two studies (494–495).

### Brucellosis

Al-Awadhi et al. (496), from Kuwait, described acute pancreatitis in a 31-year-old male, with *Brucella melitensis* cultured from the blood. The patient recovered. The authors found no previous report.

### *Yersinia*-Associated Pancreatitis

At least four reports have implicated *Yersinia enterocolitica*, type 3, infection as a possible cause of pancreatitis. Pettersson and Gordin (497) reported three patients, 20–28 years of age, with acute pancreatitis associated with a rising serum agglutination titer against *Y. enterocolitica.* They found no previous report of this association. A 25-year-old female developed acute pancreatitis a few days after a family epidemic of *Yersinia* enteritis. Again, serologic tests confirmed an acute yersinosis (498). A third report, by Lindholt and Hansen (499) described a 23-year-old previously healthy female who was hospitalized with a 48-hour history of abdominal pain. Laparotomy revealed the ileum to be hyperemic. On the 5th postoperative day acute pancreatitis developed. Stool cultures were positive for *Y. enterocolitica* type 3, and the *Yersinia* agglutinin titer showed a striking and progressive rise. In reviewing the above reports, Lindholt and Hansen noted the similarity among the patients. Each was in the 3rd decade of life, had previously been healthy, and developed a relatively mild but protracted pancreatitis with no manifestation of disease in other organs. They suggested monitoring the agglutinin titer for *Y. enterocolitica* type 3 in selected patients with pancreatitis. Of 458 patients hospitalized with *Y. enterocolitica* infections in Norway, Saebo and Lassen (500) observed 8 (1.75%) with signs of acute pancreatitis and elevated serum or urine amylase levels. During follow-up of 4–14 years, four were readmitted with chronic pancreatitis and one with acute pancreatitis.

### Tuberculous Pancreatitis and Tuberculosis of the Pancreas

Numerous reports have described tuberculosis of the pancreas, sometimes presenting as acute pancreatitis. Rushing, Hanna and Selecky (501) wrote of pancreatitis as the presenting manifestation of miliary tuberculosis. Their diagnosis was based on clinical findings compatible with acute pancreatitis, associated with elevated serum amylase levels. Autopsy revealed a grossly normal pancreas with multiple intrapancreatic abscesses of acid-fast bacilli. Others (502, 503) previously described pancreatitis and hyperamylasemia in association with miliary tuberculosis. Fan et al. (504) described necrotizing tuberculosis of the pancreas as a cause of massive duodenal bleeding, and Stock et al. (505) as well as Fan described pancreatic calcification in tuberculous pancreatitis. Several authors have reported biliary obstruction from tuberculous pancreatitis (504, 506, 507). Others have described tuberculosis of the pancreas causing pancreatic abscess or acute or chronic pancreatitis (509–519). In at least one instance (506), tuberculosis of the pancreas led to pancreatoduodenectomy. Houston (520) in 1991 reviewed the literature, noting six reports of tuberculous pancreatitis and abscess in association with AIDS (521–526). At least one more has since appeared (527).

### Legionnaires' Disease and Pancreatitis

Gordon and Zmyslinski (528) (1980) first reported an association of acute pancreatitis and Legionnaires' disease. Other reports by Michel et al. (529) and Arneborn and Kallings (530) associated the diseases. Westblom and Hamory (531) described a patient with acute pancreatitis, apparently due to *Legionella pneumophila*. Jespersen and Engbaek (532) described fatal hemorrhagic pancreatitis resulting from Legionnaires' disease. From Sweden, Eitrem, Forsgren, and Nilsson (533) reported a patient with *L. longbeachae* infection who recovered from pneumonia and acute pancreatitis following erythromycin therapy. A seventh patient, a 56-year-old Jamaican who survived Legionnaire-associated acute pancreatitis, has been reported by Kesavan, Pitchumoni, and Marino (534).

### Clostridial Pancreatitis *(Clostridia perfringens)*

In 1943, Steiner and Tracy (535) described fatal pancreatic necrosis in a child with enteritis associated with *Clostridium perfringens*. Gas gangrene, per se, did not involve the pancreas. Howard and Campbell (536) described a 58-year-old female with a large necrotic pancreatic carcinoma who underwent ERCP and percutaneous biopsy of the cancer. On the 2nd day she developed a massive hemolysis, with a 50% drop in her hemoglobin level and a rise in her serum bilirubin level from 1.3 to 37.5 mg/100 mL. CT scan of the pancreas revealed pancreatic gas, and needle aspiration of the pancreas and multiple blood cultures revealed *C. perfringens*. Death resulted from sepsis on the 4th day.

Morton and Taylor (537) described fatal pancreatic necrosis following transduodenal biopsy of the pancreas with a Tru-cut needle. The biopsy was performed at laparotomy, at which time gallbladder bile was sterile. In the early postoperative period, the patient was hypotensive, complained of abdominal pain, and had a sharply rising serum amylase level. *C. perfringens* was cultured from the pancreatic slough and from blood. She died of multi-organ failure 20 days later.

## PANCREATITIS DUE TO VIRUSES

The past decade has demonstrated that viruses can cause pancreatitis. This recognition has resulted from improvements in the field of virology and to a greater extent from increased immunosuppression of organ transplant and cancer chemotherapy patients. In addition, the worldwide epidemic of AIDS has focused attention on the high incidence of pancreatitis associated with this disease and with its treatment.

Several authors have suggested that viral antibody titers should be measured in patients (especially children and the immunodepressed) whose pancreatitis might otherwise be considered idiopathic. In 1973, a controlled study of normal adults and patients with acute pancreatitis from Finland (538) measured serial antibody titers of a large number of viruses and concluded that virus-induced pancreatitis had not been definitely demonstrated. Most current reports in immunocompetent patients are in the pediatric literature. Haddock et al. (539) reviewed the incidence of acute pancreatitis over a 15-year period in three pediatric hospitals in Scotland. In the 49 children with acute pancreatitis, the most common cause was mumps (39%). Chicken pox was noted as the cause of pancreatitis in one. Capner et al. (540) could not confirm these findings in a similar study except that two of their patients with acute pancreatitis demonstrated a marked rise in the antibody titer to herpes simplex.

### Herpes Simplex (Herpesvirus Hominis)

In addition to the previous report (540), a student with severe acute pancreatitis was found to have a rising serum antibody titer to herpes simplex virus. The virus (type I) was cultured from his gastric contents (541).

### Herpesvirus Varicella-Zoster (Chickenpox and Shingles)

A 52-year-old patient who had undergone hepatic transplantation for primary biliary cirrhosis was rehospitalized 26 days later with a vesicular rash involving a single intercostal dermatome, clinically suggestive of herpes zoster infection. Autopsy revealed acute hemorrhagic pancreatitis due to herpes zoster virus (542). Wacker et al. (543) described three children with acute pancreatitis associated with generalized infection with varicella-zoster virus after autologous bone marrow transplantation. Varicella pancreatitis has also been associated with a pancreatic pseudocyst (544).

### Pancreatitis Associated with Reye Syndrome and Influenza Viruses

Balistreri (545) noted that the high incidence of Reye syndrome (acute encephalopathy and fatty degeneration of the liver) previously noted in association with viral infections has diminished from approximately 400 cases reported in the United States in 1974 to 20 cases in 1988. He attributes this fall to the recognition of the association between the Reye syndrome and the ingestion of aspirin by children who have an influenza-like illness or varicella. Influenza B was most frequently involved, influenza A and chickenpox less often. Morens et al. (546) in 1974 described two such patients who developed acute pancreatitis; one died of massive acute hemorrhagic pancreatitis. Others reported an association between Reye syndrome and acute pancreatitis (547–552). Chaves-Carballo et al. (553) in 1980 reviewed eight earlier reports on Reye pancreatitis and reported five additional patients, four of whom had died of acute pancreatitis. Of 18 previously reported patients with associated pancreatitis, 15 had died; 10 had acute hemorrhagic pancreatitis found at autopsy. In 1989, Pascual Velasco (554) described a 42-year-old patient who survived acute pancreatitis associated with an influenza A viral infection.

### Measles Virus and Pancreatitis

Miralbés et al. (555) reported (1995) a mild attack of acute pancreatitis thought to have resulted from measles. This apparently was the first report in an adult, although Sibert (556) had implicated the measles virus in acute pancreatitis in children. Sherman, Michaels, and Kenny (557) reported that a child who died of rubella encephalopathy had a mild acute hemorrhagic pancreatitis at autopsy. Bunnell et al. (558) described interstitial pancreatitis in the congenital rubella syndrome.

### Smallpox (Variola), Vaccinia, and Pancreatitis

Marczynska-Robowska reported a 5-year-old boy who died on the sixth day of smallpox. Autopsy demonstrated fat necrosis of the omentum and subcapsular hemorrhage of the pancreas (559). Progressive *vaccinia* was noted in a patient with chronic lymphatic leukemia (560); autopsy findings included areas of focal necrosis of the pancreas, an observation previously made by Hall, Cunliffe, and Dudgeon (561).

### Common Cold

Mitov and Paunov (562) described acute pancreatitis in a child as a complication of viral "common cold."

### Mumps Pancreatitis

In 1899, Harris (563) first described diabetes and pancreatitis as a sequel to mumps parotitis. By 1922, Farnam (564) identified 119 patients who met the characteristics of the mumps pancreatitis syndrome. She noted that the pancreatitis was usually mild. Haddock et al. (539) found it constituted 39% of pancreatitis among their children. Others (565–576) described acute pancreatitis as a result of the mumps virus, predominantly in children. Two patients had mumps pancreatitis precede mumps parotitis (450), and one had mumps pancreatitis in the absence of parotitis (575). Chronic pancreatitis can develop as the result of mumps pancreatitis (577–579).

### Pancreatitis Induced by Measles, Mumps, and Rubella Vaccines

Adler, Mazzota, and Barkin (580) reported an adult who survived an episode of acute pancreatitis that they attributed to the measles, mumps, and rubella vaccine. Cebriá et al. (581) reported a 17-year-old boy who received a similar triple vaccine. Two weeks later he developed fever, generalized illness, and bilateral parotid swelling, followed several days later by acute pancreatitis from which he recovered. This sequence of events led the authors to attribute the pancreatitis to the virus of the mumps vaccine.

### Enteroviruses: Coxsackie B and Echovirus Pancreatitis

In 1964, Nakao et al. (582) reported that during an epidemic of meningitis due to coxsackieviruses, 31% of the patients had an increase in serum and urinary amylase levels. Others reported the coxsackie B virus to induce acute pancreatitis (583–588). Kibrick and Benirschke (589) reported that an infant died 36 hours after birth, having developed coxsackie B4 *myocarditis* and pancreatitis in utero, and Kennedy et al. (590) described acute pancreatitis in a 3-year-old girl with coxsackie B4 virus infection and an $\alpha$-1-antitrypsin deficiency. Ozsvar et al. (591) reported that of 118 patients with acute and recurrent pancreatitis, a rise in the antibody titers of coxsackie B virus was observed in 40. Included among the 40 were 21 with chronic pancreatitis. The authors concluded that coxsackie B virus can cause acute pancreatitis and can make chronic pancreatitis worse. They recommended serial screening for coxsackie B antibodies in patients with idiopathic pancreatitis. In a study of 91 patients with acute pancreatitis, Arnesjo et al. (592) isolated an enterovirus from the feces or urine in 17, of whom 7 had a rising serum antibody titer; coxsackie B viruses and echoviruses were implicated.

### Pancreatitis Caused by *Mycoplasma pneumoniae*

Leinikki et al. (538) found a significant increase in *M. pneumoniae* antibody titers in 18 of 56 patients with acute pancreatitis. Hayflick (593) found that one-third of patients with acute pancreatitis had evidence of mycoplasma infection, and Mardh and Ursing (594) noted that 6 (9%) of 70 patients with *M. pneumoniae* infection developed pancreatitis. Others (595, 596, 596a) confirmed that *M. pneumoniae* infection can cause acute pancreatitis.

### Infectious Mononucleosis Pancreatitis

In a study of 20 patients with infectious mononucleosis, Myhre and Nesbitt (597) detected asymptomatic elevations of serum amylase and lipase levels in 2. Wislocki (598) reported the first instance of infectious mononucleosis with clinical acute pancreatitis. Others (599–602) have noted the association, but the reports to date would suggest that infectious mononucleosis plays a limited and uncertain role in the etiology of acute pancreatitis.

### Pancreatitis Associated with Infectious Hepatitis

In a survey of 1062 cases of infectious hepatitis, Lisney (603) in 1943 first described pancreatitis as a complication of hepatitis. Confirming reports were initially infrequent (577, 604), and the specific cause was not always easily identified. Of 16 patients who died of fulminating viral hepatitis, Geokas et al. (605) found autopsy evidence of acute pancreatitis in 7. Others (606) found autopsy evidence of acute pancreatitis in 13 of 35 patients who died of acute viral hepatic necrosis. Others have attributed the pancreatitis to hepatic failure rather than to the underlying viral infection (607).

Pancreatitis has been associated with hepatitis A, B, and C, respectively. Wands et al. (608) and others described pancreatitis as a complication of hepatitis A (608–611). Davis and Keeffe (612) described a young male who survived acute hepatitis of the virus A type, whose serum bilirubin peaked at 16.5 mg/100 mL. They pointed out that usually, viral hepatitis associated with acute pancreatitis has been severe. Cadranel et al. (613) described an exception.

**Hepatitis C.** Eugene et al. (614) reported a 33-year-old man, previously vaccinated against hepatitis B, who pricked himself with a patient's needle while working in a hemodialysis unit. Four weeks later he developed acute pancreatitis and acute hepatitis. A diagnosis of non-A, non-B hepatitis was documented. The authors had not found a previous report of this association in a nonfulminant hepatitis patient. Ede et al. (615) described pancreatitis in four patients with non-A, non-B hepatitis in whom the hepatitis was fulminating.

**Hepatitis B.** There is no doubt that the hepatitis B virus is a cause of acute pancreatitis. Both Shimoda et al. (616) and Cavalhari et al. (617) detected the hepatitis B antigen within the pancreatic acinar cells. With the development of hepatic transplantation, the incidence of hepatitis B–induced pancreatitis has substantially increased. (See Chapter 27, "Posttransplant Pancreatitis.")

### Cytomegalovirus (CMV) Pancreatitis

Cytomegalovirus virus causes opportunistic human infections. CMV pancreatitis has been reported chiefly in immunosuppressed patients. Among 73 patients with pancreatic transplants, Margreiter et al. (618) described 4 who developed acute pancreatitis with CMV infections. There was no fatality. Similarly, Wilcox. et al. (619) described two patients with AIDS who at autopsy had evidence of acute pancreatitis, considered to be CMV induced. Iwasaki et al. (620) described the autopsy finding of necrotizing pancreatitis and CMV infection in a patient who had been treated for a brain tumor. They quoted Takayama (621) as saying that pancreatic involvement is observed microscopically in about 10% of autopsies involving CMV infection but that the pancreatitis is usually subclinical. Other reports of the association appeared in the earlier transplant literature (622). Two reports have described CMV pancreatitis as triggering the onset of diabetes (623, 624). (See also the next section on AIDS.)

### AIDS-Associated Pancreatitis

Pancreatitis can occur in both the treated and the untreated HIV patient. It can be the result of the HIV infection in some patients, drug therapy in other patients, and opportunistic infections with other organisms (viral, yeast, bacterial, or parasitic) in others. It is difficult to identify the specific etiologic factor in the numerous reports. All clinicians who see patients with pancreatitis or with AIDS should be aware of the association. Zazzo et al. (625) reported a prospective study of 35 consecutive (32 male, 3 female) patients with AIDS-related acute pancreatitis. Although the amylase and lipase levels often remained normal, autopsy confirmed pancreatic disease in 21 (60%). They credit Bricarie et al. (626) with finding pancreatic lesions in 113 AIDS patients at autopsy; included in these lesions were opportunistic infections (CMV, *Cryptococcus, Toxoplasma gondii,* and *Candida*) as well as Kaposi's sarcoma and lymphoma. Brivet et al. (627) reported that 7 of 13 patients (54%) who were HIV positive and who came to autopsy had pancreatic involvement including CMV infiltrations and *T. gondii*. These opportunistic infections were asymptomatic. Two patients had massive tumor infiltrations of the pancreas, one by Kaposi's sarcoma and one by lymphoma. In three patients the pancreatitis was considered iatrogenic.

A review of children with AIDS over a 6-year period revealed 9 (17%) who developed pancreatitis (628). Their median age was 5.2 years with a range of 1 to 20 years. Four patients had CMV infections with the onset of pancreatitis. Four had *Cryptosporidium*, three had *Pneumocystis carinii* pneumonia, and four had *Mycobacterium avium*. The authors did not detect an increase in pancreatitis among HIV-positive patients without AIDS. Pancreatitis appeared to be an indicator of a poor prognosis, with an average survival time of 8 months after developing it. In one patient, ERP was normal but pancreatic juice was found to contain CMV. In only one patient did the pancreatitis resolve. Two developed recurrent episodes, and in several, the pancreatitis appeared to remain active until death. Five children had been receiving pentamidine at the time of onset of pancreatitis. Cappell and Marks (629) reported that 44 patients with HIV-pancreatitis constituted 4.7% of 939 patients hospitalized with HIV; 9 of the pancreatitis patients died in the hospital. Numerous other reports (630–639) describe the deadly course of HIV-induced pancreatitis.

Several authors have noted that the HIV infection has usually been recognized prior to the onset of pancreatitis (639–643). Because HIV infection is increasing, the authors suggested that clinicians include it in the differential diagnosis of acute pancreatitis. Vendrell et al. (644) reported two HIV-positive patients who developed insulin-dependent diabetes. Furthermore, a 3-year-old girl with AIDS was found to have persistent malabsorption and elevations of serum amylase and lipase levels associated with chronic pancreatitis. After a course of 6 months, autopsy revealed extensive pancreatic fibrosis without calcification (645). (See also "Drug-Induced Pancreatitis" for further information on AIDS-associated pancreatitis.)

### Adenoviral Infection with Acute Pancreatitis

Niemann et al. (646) described a 9-year-old girl with acute lymphoblastic leukemia who underwent bone marrow transplantation. Four years later, while immunosuppressed, she developed acute abdominal pain secondary to acute pancreatitis and died; autopsy revealed hemorrhagic pancreatitis and fulminating hepatic necrosis. Both the pancreas and the liver contained intranuclear inclusions consistent with adenovirus. The authors noted three other reports of adenovirus-type inclusions in the pancreas of immunosuppressed patients dying of disseminated adenovirus infection but in whom their presence in the pancreas appeared incidental.

## PANCREATITIS SECONDARY TO PARASITES

In many parts of the world parasites are being recognized as a major cause of pancreatitis.

### Roundworms *(Ascaris lumbricoides)*

In 1923, two reports of acute pancreatitis secondary to *A. lumbricoides* were published in the British Journal of Surgery. Novis described the operative finding of acute pancreatitis in a 12-year-old child (647). The surgeon incised the pancreatic duct longitudinally and extracted a full-sized, living roundworm and a second partially disintegrated one. The patient survived. In the same issue, Rigby described a patient, who at laparotomy had acute pancreatitis with widespread fat necrosis (648). Autopsy revealed an ascarid projecting into the duodenum from the pancreatic duct. By 1925, Sabrazes et al. (649) were able to collect 19 patients in whom an ascarid was found within the pancreatic duct. Following the introduction of flexible endoscopy, information about ascarid-induced acute pancreatitis increased. Two fundamental observations have emerged: first, ascarid-induced acute pancreatitis develops from transampullary invasion by the ascarid of the common bile duct. Second, but less frequently, pancreatitis results from transampullary invasion of the pancreatic duct per se. Ascarid invasion of the duct of Santorini has not been observed. In 1984 Chen et al. (650) from the People's Republic of China, described 14 patients in whom an endoscopic diagnosis was made of adult ascarids lodged in the ampulla of Vater with their caudal ends protruding from the papilla. Under endoscopic visualization in the emergency department, the worms were grasped by forceps and removed. In each patient, the colicky epigastric pain immediately abated. All patients recovered. The authors considered *Ascaris* the most common cause of pancreatitis in China. Another series of 462 patients with biliary ascariasis included 35 with acute pancreatitis, of whom 4 died (651). Others (652) clearly demonstrated the outline of an intraductal ascarid by ERCP.

Khuroo et al. (653, 654) writing from Kashmir, quoted Crompton et al. (655, 656) as stating that ascariasis is the most common helminthic disease of mankind, infecting more than one billion people worldwide, mostly in tropical and subtropical countries. In their earlier report (653) Khuroo et al. found that of 500 patients with (hepato-biliary-pancreatic) ascariasis, 171 had biliary ascarisis, 8 had gallbladder ascariasis, and 7 had pancreatic ascariasis. Many had duodenal ascariasis. Some 31 developed acute pancreatitis, including the 7 with pancreatic invasion. Of these 31, 28 had mild pancreatitis; 3 had severe disease, and 2 died. At laparotomy, one of the patients with fatal hemorrhagic pancreatitis had four worms extracted from the pancreatic duct and seven from the common bile duct. Sixteen of the patients had endoscopic removal of worms from the ampullary orifice. Dead worms were removed from the biliary tree by laparotomy or with the endoscopic basket. Reinfestation was frequent. A follow-up report (654) described *Ascaris* as the etiologic agent in 59 (23%) of 256 patients with acute pancreatitis from various causes. The mortality rate involving ascarid pancreatitis was 3%. In all studies, drug therapy was considered essential to rid the patient of further parasites. Leung, Mok, and Metreweli (657) from Hong Kong, described the removal of a 15-cm long ascarid from the pancreatic duct and stated that 5 (6%) of 84 patients with acute pancreatitis had *Ascaris* as its cause. Ramirez-Degollado et al. (658) also used endoscopic cholangiography to diagnose *Ascaris* in the common bile duct. In children, the diagnosis of *Ascaris* as the cause of pancreatitis was usually by identification of the worms in the intestinal tract, although sometimes they were caught red-handed within the pancreatic or bile ducts (659). Hsia and Chang of Taiwan (660) found the adult worms and eggs of *Ascaris* in the stool and vomitus of a child with acute pancreatitis and proceeded directly with successful anthelmintic drug therapy without endoscopy.

Of 42 patients with *Ascaris*-induced pancreatitis treated conservatively, only 2 (5%) developed necrotizing pancreatitis and required laparotomy (661). As there was no fatality, the authors recommended that laparotomy be avoided unless there is evidence of infection around the pancreas, bloody peritoneal fluid is detected on aspiration, or dead worms remain within the biliary tree. Recurrent pancreatitis can result from a calcified ascarid within the duct of Wirsung. The dead calcified worm could be seen on flat plate but required pancreatotomy (and pancreatojejunostomy), as endoscopic retrieval proved impractical. Numerous other reports reflect the rapid advances in the diagnosis and management of this disease.

### Tapeworms *(Taenia saginata)*

*T. saginata* may be a long-term inhabitant of the human small intestine, particularly of the jejunum, where it attaches itself to the wall. Acute pancreatitis is a rare complication; only three reports have been found by the author. Plane, Ronceray, and Dupin (663) first described acute pancreatitis due to this parasite when they identified segments of taenia in the duct of Wirsung. Delvaux et al. (664) reported acute pancreatitis secondary to the obstruction of the papilla of Vater by the parasite within the duodenum. The worm was extracted endoscopically. In studying an 84-year-old female with recurrent acute pancreatitis, Bouteloup (665) visualized endoscopically a taenia penetrating the ampulla from the duodenum. Unable to remove the worm, sphincterotomy was performed, permitting visualization of the worm's invasion of the duct of Wirsung. Apparently, still unable to completely remove the worm, drug therapy was followed by secondary endoscopy and pancreatography 48 hours later, revealing only debris in the duct of Wirsung. *T. saginata,* attaching itself firmly to the wall of a viscus, seems more difficult to manage endoscopically than the roundworm.

### Chinese Liver Flukes *(Clonorchis sinensis)*

*C. sinensis,* a trematode of the Orient, is transmitted by eating uncooked, freshwater fish from contaminated water. In the intestine, it swims upstream and enters the biliary tract, causing cholangitis. In 1908, Nakamura (666) found more than 30 of the parasites in a pancreatic duct. He and Kawamura (1911) (667), in their respective case reports, described extensive metaplasia of the epithelium of the pancreatic duct. In a study of 500 necropsies involving clonorchiasis, Hou (668), from Hong Kong, often found the pancreatic ducts dilated with adult worms. Histologically, the infested ducts showed adenomatous changes and squamous metaplasia but without necrosis of pancreatic tissue. In 1967, in their autopsy study of 64 patients with *Clonorchis* infestation of the liver, Chan and Teoh (669), in Hong Kong, found the parasites in the pancreatic ducts in 24 (37%). Up to 114 pancreatic worms filled the main duct and its tributaries. Dead and degenerating worms were noted. Periductal fibrosis and mild cellular infiltrates were found, but acute pancreatitis, per se, was not described.

The first description of acute pancreatitis secondary to *C. sinensis* was by McFadzean and Yeung in 1966 (670), who found *Clonorchis* in the duodenal aspirate or stool of 91 of 110 patients with acute pancreatitis of otherwise idiopathic etiology. Often asymptomatic, the most common complication of infestation is bacterial cholangitis, which may lead to acute pancreatitis. Other reports describe acute pancreatitis caused by *Clonorchis* (671, 672). Medical treatment is essential to cure the overall infestation. Shugar and Ryan (673) noted *Clonorchis*-induced pancreatitis 25 years after initial exposure.

### *Fasciola hepatica* (Another Liver Fluke)

The natural habitat of *Fasciola hepatica* is the bile of sheep and cattle. Maroy et al. (674) described a 43-year-old patient with a prolonged history of cholangitis. Laparotomy revealed acute pancreatitis with ova of *F. hepatica* in the gallbladder. Subsequently, cholangiography revealed an adult fluke in the common bile duct, which disappeared following drug therapy. Only one other report has been found (675).

### Filariasis *(Wuchereria bancrofti)*

Jesudason et al. (676) apparently presented the only report of pancreatitis of filarial origin. With a background of chronic pancreatic pain, the patient underwent laparotomy. An inflamed pancreas was found, and filariae were identified in a peripancreatic lymph node. Successful treatment was achieved using diethyl carbamazine.

### *Toxoplasma gondii*

Ahuja et al. (677) reported a 34-year-old man who was HIV-seropositive with disseminated toxoplasmosis. He died with necrotizing pancreatitis, which was not identified until autopsy. *T. gondii* cysts were found throughout the pancreas. The authors reviewed the literature prior to their report (1993) and found that pancreatic *Toxoplasma* cysts had been identified in only three previous patients, each with AIDS. The diagnosis of pancreatitis had been recognized prior to death in only one instance (678–680).

### Blood Flukes *(Schistosoma mansoni)*

As part of their overall study of schistosomiasis, three reports from Brazil related the infestation to the pancreas. Lenzi et al. (681) described the pathogenesis of experimental *S. mansoni*–induced pancreatitis in mice. The pancreatitis was subacute to chronic, marked by the development of granulomas within the pancreas. Periductal fibrosis was prominent. He reported that Lima (682) and Ladosky (683) found pancreatic involvement in *S. mansoni*–infested patients studied at autopsy, in an incidence of 11–48%.

### Leishmaniasis

*Leishmania* protozoa may not cause pancreatitis per se, but several reports have described acute pancreatitis, including fatalities, after the treatment of visceral leishmaniasis with stibogluconate or meglumine antimonate (684–687). In three instances the patients were immunodepressed following renal transplantation.

### *Echinococcus* Hydatid Disease

As early as 1955 Joske (290) described a hydatid cyst of the pancreas as a cause of pancreatitis. Pellegrini et al. (89) reported a hydatid cyst of the liver that ruptured into the bile ducts, resulting in obstructive jaundice and acute edematous pancreatitis. Another such cyst in the pancreas obstructed both the common bile duct and the pancreatic duct (688). Mestiri et al. (689), of Tunisia, described three patients who developed acute pancreatitis following rupture of hepatic cysts into the bile duct. Similar patients were described (690–693) in whom small stones (concretions) passed from the ruptured cysts into the bile ducts to contribute, in part, to the acute pancreatitis. The pancreatitis was usually an edematous type but was sometimes hemorrhagic or necrotic. Four reports described infected hydatid cysts involving the pancreatic parenchyma (694–697). Others (698, 699) observed acute pancreatitis secondary to obstruction of the pancreatic duct by the echinococcus. Mathai et al. (700) described recurrent episodes of acute abdominal pain and hyperamylasemia, with the CT finding of a cystic mass in the body and tail of the pancreas. Following drug therapy for a month, resection of the body and tail revealed multiple hydatid cysts within the dilated pancreatic duct.

### Cryptosporidiosis

Hawkins et al. (701) described acute pancreatitis as a complication of cryptosporidium enteritis in a 14-year-old farm girl. Recovery was complicated by pseudocyst formation. Kocoshis et al. (702) reported finding the parasites in the pancreatic duct of an immunodeficient infant at autopsy. The pancreatic duct showed epithelial metaplasia, but pancreatitis was not mentioned.

### *Giardia lamblia*

Kozarska et al. (703) reported a 41-year-old woman who developed acute pancreatitis that they considered to be secondary to giardiasis. Among 477 patients with acute pancreatitis observed over a 10-year period, 3 were considered to be caused by *Giardia*. Drew reported another patient whose recurrent acute pancreatitis was thought to result from *Giardia* (704).

## FUNGUS-INDUCED PANCREATITIS

Immunosuppressed transplant and cancer patients constitute populations at risk for mycotic infections. In this population, *Candida albicans* is the most frequent fungal invader, *Aspergillus* is the second.

### *Aspergillus* Pancreatitis

Guice, Lynch, and Weatherbee (705) reported a 63-year-old white man undergoing chemotherapy for diffuse histiocytic lymphoma who developed acute hemorrhagic pancreatitis. Laparotomy and autopsy revealed defuse aspergillosis. *Aspergillus* had extended through the wall of a pancreatic artery, leading to thrombosis and invasion of the adjacent pancreas. The authors indicated that this was the first report (1987) of pancreatic involvement with disseminated aspergillosis.

### Actinomycosis

Halevy et al. (706) reported a 57-year-old man with a localized inflammatory mass in the head of the pancreas from which *Actinomyces* was identified. The authors found four previous reports of actinomycosis of the pancreas.

### *Candida albicans*

Chung et al. (707) described an 88-year-old man who experienced recurrent attacks of acute pancreatitis. ERCP revealed a dilated pancreatic duct with multiple noncalcified intraluminal filling defects that proved to be *C. albicans* "fungus balls." The patient was treated with longitudinal pancreaticojejunostomy and oral fuconazole, and he remained recurrence free for 30 months. Mannell and Obers (708) described a patient with a mass in the head of the pancreas that resulted in obstruction of the common bile duct. A tentative diagnosis of pancreatic cancer was made, and a Whipple resection was performed. The mass was inflammatory, containing microabscesses of *Candida* in the pancreatic duct. Richter et al. (709) and Howard and Bieluch (710) described *C. albicans* as a primary infecting organism in patients with acute pancreatitic necrosis. Although many surgeons have noted *Candida* as a secondary pathogen following drainage of patients with pancreatic necrosis, a primary infection with this fungus is unusual.

## PANCREATITIS DUE TO SCORPION STINGS

Waterman (711) (1938) described a sting of the scorpion of Trinidad *(Tityus trinitatis)* that resulted in immediate acute pancreatitis in 12 patients. Autopsy findings were acute edematous pancreatitis in two patients and acute hemorrhagic pancreatitis in two. Pseudocysts developed in the 12 patients at varying intervals after the scorpion stings. Subsequently, Bartholomew (712) described 30 patients who were hospitalized following the sting of this scorpion; 24 developed acute pancreatitis. All made an uneventful recovery, without pseudocyst formation or hemorrhagic pancreatitis. Repetitive stinging of the same individual demonstrated no evidence of immunity. Pancreatitis occurred in seven patients who had been previously stung. Intravenous injection of the venom into the dog or into the isolated pancreas resulted in direct stimulation of pancreatic secretion (713). In the dog, the serum amylase level rose. The authors noted edema of the papilla and postulated that pancreatitis resulted from pancreatic stimulation and secretion against a partial ampullary outflow obstruction (714, 715).

Novaes et al. (716–718) demonstrated that intravenous injection of the purified venom from the scorpion *Tityus serrulatus* into mice and rats resulted in an inflamed pancreas in all animals at the end of 20 days. Others (719) showed that injection of the venom of *T. descrepans* (scorpion of Venezuela) into mice resulted in a curare-like effect and induced pancreatitis. Sofer et al. (720) observed that acute pancreatitis was found in 13 of 14 (93%) children stung by the yellow scorpion *(Leiurus quinquestriatus)*. Gueron and Yarom (721) noted elevated serum amylase levels in 14 of 16 patients complaining of abdominal pain following a sting by the yellow scorpion. Pancreatitis was confirmed at autopsy in one of their patients.

## SNAKE BITE PANCREATITIS

Kjellström (722) described a 26-year-old male who developed acute abdominal pain following a snakebite of the hand. Within

90 minutes of the onset of abdominal pain he was hospitalized. His serum amylase level was elevated. Immediate laparotomy revealed acute pancreatitis with an intense edema of the head of the pancreas. Recovery was uncomplicated. Although abdominal pain has been reported as a frequent symptom following bites by the adder *Vipera berus* in Sweden and other countries, no similar diagnosis of acute pancreatitis has been made.

## DRUG-INDUCED PANCREATITIS

Knowledge of the role of drugs in the etiology of pancreatitis has become indispensable to the clinician. The following abridged review summarizes the data predominantly from the standpoint of the indication of the drugs used.

### Antibacterial Agents

Considering the millions of patients treated, the incidence of associated pancreatitis is extremely low. (See also section on antitubercular drugs below.)

**Tetracycline.** In a 1986 review, Dobrilla et al. (723) found seven reports involving 24 patients with tetracycline-induced pancreatitis, including 14 deaths. These reports emphasized the incidence of tetracycline-induced pancreatitis during pregnancy in patients with fatty livers. Others (724–726) reported four patients in whom oral tetracycline, in the absence of hepatic dysfunction, caused pancreatitis. Among the latter, Elmore and Rogge (725) and Torosis and Vender (726) each reported a young healthy patient who developed acute pancreatitis on two separate occasions following administration of tetracycline.

**Other Antibiotics and Related Drugs.** Four reports (727–730) each described a single patient who developed acute pancreatitis after intravenous infusion of *erythromycin*. In one patient, the attack started within 40 minutes of the infusion. Acute pancreatitis as the result of an oral overdose of the drug has also been described (731).

Hanline (732) described a patient who developed pancreatitis while on *ampicillin* for treatment of a urinary tract infection. After stopping the drug, her symptoms subsided and elevated serum amylase and lipase levels returned to normal. With resumption of the drug, her serum amylase and lipase levels again rose. *Ceftriaxone* (Rocephin), a cephalosporin antibiotic, was suggested as a possible cause of acute pancreatitis in two patients (733, 734); neither involved a definite causal relationship. *Metronidazole* (Flagyl) is a synthetic antibacterial-antiprotozoal agent used in the treatment of amebiasis, trichomoniasis, and several bacterial infections. Four reports have noted metronidazole-induced acute pancreatitis (735–738). *Nitrofurantoin* (Macrodantin), used largely in the treatment of urinary tract infections, has been incriminated in two reports (739, 740).

**Sulfonamides.** In a 1986 review (741), three reports relating pancreatitis to sulfonamides involved only three patients and no deaths. Sulfapyridine, however, has been associated with numerous attacks of acute pancreatitis during the course of treatment of ulcerative colitis and Crohn's disease. Sulfasalazine (Asulfidine) and salicylazosulfapyridine consist of sulfapyridine combined with 5-aminosalicylic acid (5-ASA). The compound is split in the intestine, with most of the sulfapyridine and a smaller portion of the 5-ASA being absorbed. The literature reflects the belief that the sulfapyridine is the predominant agent causing acute pancreatitis (742–747).

Sulfamethizole-associated pancreatitis was described by Barrett and Thier (748). Sulfamethoxazole with trimethoprim (Bactrim) was reported to be etiologically associated with acute pancreatitis (749, 750). Cotrimoxazoline, a sulfonamide moiety was reported to be associated with acute pancreatitis in patients with AIDS (751, 752).

### Diuretics

Numerous reports implicate diuretics as a cause of pancreatitis. Frequently used for the treatment of hypertension, cardiac failure, and renal insufficiency, which are predisposing factors to the development of acute pancreatitis, the role of the drug is not clear-cut. Nevertheless, the clinical reports strongly suggest that these drugs predispose to pancreatitis. Cornish et al. (753) implicated chlorothiazide with pancreatitis as early as 1961. Bourke et al. (754) compared patients who were on diuretics, usually thiazide, and who developed acute pancreatitis with matched controls. The patients who were taking diuretics were 2.5 times more likely to develop pancreatitis than were the controls.

**Furosemide.**

Wilson et al. (755) (1967) first associated furosemide therapy with the development of acute pancreatitis. Thomas et al. (756) studied 12 normal subjects on a continuous intravenous secretin infusion and observed that a 20-mg bolus of furosemide increased the mean secretion of pancreatic juice from 32 to 110 mL/min. Others (757–760) reported furosemide-induced pancreatitis in 10 patients, including three fatalities.

**Thiazides and Other Diuretics.** Acute pancreatitis was attributed to hydrochlorothiazide and chlorothiazide in several reports (761–764). Chlorothalidone was associated with the development of acute hemorrhagic pancreatitis (765). Eckhauser et al. (78) in a 1987 collective review of diuretic-associated pancreatitis, reported three patients who developed severe necrotizing pancreatitis, two of whom died. They summarized 27 previously reported patients whose acute pancreatitis was attributed to the two types of diuretics: benzothiadiazine (including hydrochlorothiazide and chlorothiazide) and phthalimidine (including chlorothalidone). Seventeen patients developed pancreatitis during pregnancy. Hypertension and arteriosclerotic heart disease were present in nine patients, four of whom died from complications directly attributable to acute necrotizing pancreatitis.

*Ethacrynic acid* has been associated with development of acute pancreatitis (765, 766), as has *metalazone* (767, 768).

### Hydrogen-Ion Receptor Antagonists

**Cimetidine (Tagamet).** Several patients have developed acute pancreatitis while taking cimetidine (Tagamet) (769–772). Hainaut et al. (771) described a patient who developed acute pancreatitis while on oral cimetidine. The drug was discontinued and the pancreatitis subsided. Cimetidine was then given intravenously after which acute pancreatitis recurred. Recovery again followed cessation of cimetidine therapy.

**Ranitidine (Zantac).** An 81-year-old patient had three episodes of acute pancreatitis associated with ranitidine treatment for duodenal ulcer (773). On each occasion the pancreatitis resolved after withdrawing the drug and recurred on reexposure.

### Antiinflammatory Agents

*Sulindac* (Clinoril), a nonsteroidal antiinflammatory drug (NSAID) is used for treatment of arthritis and bursitis. Numerous reports have related its use to the onset of acute pancreatitis. Sugerman (774) reported two cases in 1989 and reviewed nine previous reports. Falling et al. (784) had previously discussed this relationship. Except for the 5-ASA preparations, it appears to be the NSAID most frequently associated with pancreatitis.

*Piroxicam* (Feldane) a NSAID used in treatment of rheumatoid and osteoarthritis was noted by Haye (785) as a possible cause of acute pancreatitis. Jick et al. (786) noted one patient. *Ketoprofen*, another NSAID and analgesic agent has been suggested as a cause of pancreatitis (787).

*Indomethacin*, a NSAID and analgesic agent used in the treatment of arthritis, was suggested to cause pancreatitis (788,

789), as were *Naprosen* (786, 790), *mefenamic acid* (791), *Ibuprofen* (792), *phenylbutazone* (793), *diclofenac salt* (786, 794), and *tiaprofenic acid* (778).

*5-Aminosalicylic acid (mesalamine, 5-ASA)* is an antiinflammatory agent often used in the treatment of ulcerative colitis and granulomatous enteritis. It is not to be confused with aspirin (acetylsalicylic acid), which also has an antiinflammatory effect but which has apparently not been associated with pancreatitis. Sachedina et al. (795) described a patient with Crohn's disease who repeatedly developed acute pancreatitis while taking 5-ASA. At that time (1989), they found no other report, although two additional cases had been reported to the drug's distributor and Poldermans and van Blankenstein (796) had reported a case associated with the dimeric form of the drug. In 1990, Fiorentini et al. (797) reported two patients with inflammatory bowel disease who had developed mild acute pancreatitis while taking 5-ASA. They reviewed four previous reports, two of patients who developed recurrent attacks of pancreatitis on rechallenge (796, 798). Others (799, 800) noted recurrence of pancreatitis with rechallenge. A subsequent review (1991) reported nine cases of acute mild-to-moderate pancreatitis associated with oral or intrarectal administration of 5-ASA or disodium azodisalicylate. In five patients, immediate relapse of pancreatitis occurred with rechallenge.

**Corticosteroids.** Corticosteroids have often been associated with the etiology of pancreatitis, but their importance has often been in doubt because of the possible etiologic role of the primary condition underlying the drug's usage. Levine and McGuire (802), in 1988, described a patient in whom an attack of pancreatitis developed following corticosteroid administration and recurred with rechallenge. The authors found over 40 reports of corticosteroid-induced pancreatitis since it had first been described in 1955 (803). No previous report had shown recurrence with rechallenge. Keefe and Munro (804) described a fatal attack of acute pancreatitis when a patient was treated with systemic corticosteroids for bullous pemphigoid. There seems little doubt that corticosteroids can cause acute pancreatitis.

## Analgesics and Narcotics

Acetaminophen (Tylenol, Paracetanol), an analgesic, when taken in overdose, resulted in acute pancreatitis in at least four patients (805–808). In three instances, the pancreatitis was the severe hemorrhagic type. In autopsies of four patients dying of fulminant hepatic failure after an overdose of acetaminophen, Gazzard et al. (809) noted fat necrosis around the pancreas or extensive hemorrhage into the gland. No report has been found of pancreatitis resulting from therapeutic dose of this drug.

**Narcotics.** Demerol and, to a greater extent, morphine and codeine cause spasm of the sphincter of Oddi and perhaps lead to pancreatitis. Mills and Goddard (810) recently described acute pancreatitis in a patient who was self-administering boluses of morphine by a PCA pump. Lankisch et al. (811) questioned whether their patient developed acute pancreatitis as a result of heroin use. They found no previous report of such a relationship.

## Psychomotor Drugs

**Valproic Acid.** Valproic acid is an anticonvulsant drug widely used in the treatment of epilepsy. In 1979, two papers reported acute pancreatitis following its administration (812, 813). A third report followed 2 years later (814). These three reports described six patients, 3–16 years old, who had been taking the drug for 3–6 months before developing acute pancreatitis. When the drug was discontinued, the five surviving patients had no further attacks; the sixth patient died of acute hemorrhagic pancreatitis. At least nine other reports followed, including the development of hemorrhagic pancreatitis in a 4-year-old child (815).

In 1991, Binek et al. (816) found 24 patients who had been reported with isolated attacks of acute pancreatitis and 6 others, including their patient, with pancreatitis and hepatic failure, all brought on by valproic acid. Most of the patients were less than 20 years of age. Pancreatitis developed during the 1st year of therapy in 72% of the patients, resulting in a mortality rate of approximately 20%. Reports of other fatalities followed (817, 818).

Asconape et al. (819) summarized 39 such patients, some collected from the literature. The mean patient age was 16.4 years. The youngest patient was 1 year old. The highest risk of pancreatitis was during the first month of treatment; 44% occurring during the first 3 months. Of the 39 patients, 33 (85%) suffered mild-to-moderate pancreatitis with prompt recovery after the valproic acid was discontinued; 6 (15%) had hemorrhagic pancreatitis, of whom 3 died; 9 were rechallenged, 6 of whom had relapses; 2 were rechallenged more than once, with relapse on each challenge. The mechanism by which valproic acid induces acute pancreatitis is unknown. Children before receiving valproic acid frequently complain of abdominal pain and gastrointestinal symptoms, so the diagnosis of pancreatitis may be delayed. Since patients on anticonvulsant therapy may be mentally retarded and may often be lethargic, monitoring for acute pancreatitis becomes important.

**Carbamazepine (Tegretol) and Phenytoin (Dilantin).** Carbamazepine, another anticonvulsant drug, is considered a specific analgesic for trigeminal neuralgia. The first report of a patient with acute pancreatitis following carbamazepine administration appeared in 1985 (820). When the authors found no other report in the literature, they called the pharmaceutical manufacturer who indicated that their files contained three unpublished patient reports of pancreatitis possibly induced by this drug. Other reports of acute (821) and chronic calcific (822) pancreatitis appeared. Others noted pancreatitis after *phenytoin* (Dilantin) therapy (823).

## Antidepressants and Antipsychotic Agents

Pancreatitis has been reported following the use of *indalpine* (824), an antidepressant, and *clozapine* (825, 826), an antipsychotic. Pancreatitis has also followed suicide attempts with overdosage. *Amineptine*, another tricyclic antidepressant induced (827) acute pancreatitis associated with mild acute drug-induced hepatitis, a known complication of amineptine therapy.

## Cardiovascular Agents

**ß-Blocking Agents.** ß-Blocking agents have been reported to cause acute pancreatitis, possibly because of hyperlipidemia (828, 829). Weaver (830) noted three hypertensive patients who developed chronic pancreatitis after being treated for long periods with *propranolol* and *reserpine* and raised the question of whether patients treated with ß-blocking drugs were likely to develop chronic pancreatitis.

**Angiotensin Converting Enzyme (ACE) Inhibitors.** Tilkemeir and Thompson (831) described a patient with *enalapril* (Vasotec)-related pancreatitis. Although they could find no previous report of such an association, they found that as of October 1987, "about 20" cases had been reported to the Food and Drug Administration. *Captopril*, another ACE inhibitor, has been associated with the development of acute pancreatitis (832, 833). Others ( 834–836) described the development of a mild acute pancreatitis associated with the administration of *lisinopril* for the treatment of hypertension. Standridge (837) described a fatality from pancreatitis in a patient who had been taking lisinopril and collected six reports of enalapril-induced pancreatitis; this 1994 report is suggested for further references.

*Procainamide*, an antiarrhythmic drug, has been associated with acute pancreatitis (838) but the data are quite limited.

**Cholesterol-Reducing Agents.** *Simvastatine*, a drug used to treat hypercholesterolemia, and *Lovastatin*, a similar cholesterol-lowering agent derived from *Aspergillus,* have been reported to cause acute pancreatitis (838–842).

### Hormones and Pancreatitis

**Octreotide.** In 1991, Gradon et al. (843) reported acute pancreatitis in a patient with AIDS who was being treated with octreotide, an analogue of somatostatin, which acts as a universal inhibitor of secretory cells. Octreotide was being given to palliate chronic diarrhea. The authors postulated that the pancreatitis resulted from the hormone's inhibition of exocrine pancreatic secretion. Others reported acute pancreatitis after octreotide treatment for acromegaly (844) and for chronic diarrhea in AIDS patients (845, 846). Sadoul et al. (847) reported acute pancreatitis following the withdrawal of octreotide.

**Growth Hormone.** Malozowski et al. (848) reported the development of acute pancreatitis following the use of growth hormone for the treatment of short stature. A 12-year-old boy with growth hormone deficiency was treated daily with growth hormone. After the sixth dose, he developed acute pancreatitis. The growth hormone was discontinued, and he improved. Approximately 1 month later, hormone therapy was resumed, but after the second injection he developed a recurrence of acute pancreatitis. The authors reported that 10 other children had developed acute pancreatitis while on growth hormone therapy for short stature.

**Adrenocorticosteroids.** The literature is replete with reports of pancreatitis secondary to adrenal steroids. These hormones are now used widely for immunosuppression in organ transplantation, where, often in association with other drugs, the incidence of acute pancreatitis is quite substantial.

**Estrogen.** Glueck et al. (849, 850) noted 31 patients on postmenopausal estrogen replacement therapy who developed high triglyceride plasma levels. Seven patients had triglyceride levels above 1500 mg/100 mL while on estrogen replacement therapy. Four were hospitalized with severe acute pancreatitis and another two had abdominal pain thought to reflect acute pancreatitis.

### Anticancer Drugs Associated with Pancreatitis

Several drugs used in the treatment of cancer have been associated with the development of acute pancreatitis. Although the pancreatitis varies in severity from patient to patient, it is a serious illness in a patient who is already sick. As reviewed by Underwood and Frye (851) the drugs include *6-mercaptopurine,* high-dose *cytosine arabinoside, corticosteroid,* and *cisplatin* (852–855). In addition, *cyclophosphamide* (Cytoxan) was associated with pancreatitis when used as part of a combination chemotherapy program (856–858). As a single agent, it has not been reported to cause pancreatitis.

**L-Asparaginase.** In their 1986 review, Dobrilla et al. (859) summarized 10 reports of 34 patients who developed acute pancreatitis while on L-asparaginase therapy; 18 of them died. Satake and Nakashima (860) noted that acute pancreatitis occurs in patients (mainly children) with acute leukemia and lymphoma during treatment with L-asparaginase, with or without prednisone therapy (861, 862). Weetman and Baehner (863) reported that among 43 children receiving this drug, 5 of the 7 patients who developed pancreatitis were females older than 9 years. Because estrogens may potentiate the activity of L-asparaginase, pubertal females may be at greater risk of pancreatitis than their male counterparts. Many other instances have been reported.

#### Other Cancer Chemotherapy Agents

***Erwinase.*** Erwinase, an enzyme reportedly less toxic than L-asparaginase, resulted in severe acute pancreatitis in an 11-year-old girl following treatment of acute lymphoblastic leukemia (864). Sotomatsu et al. (865) reported a 9-year-old girl with chronic myelogenous leukemia treated with *interferon-α* who developed acute pancreatitis. The drug was discontinued, and she recovered. No other cause for the pancreatitis could be demonstrated. Izraeli et al. (866) reported a 16-year-old girl with metastatic osteosarcoma who experienced recurrent bouts of pancreatitis beginning within 24 hours after treatment with ifosfamide administered as a single agent. Because she had responded to the drug and because pancreatitis was not known to be a complication of its use, a lower dose was used. She again developed acute pancreatitis from which she recovered.

### Immunosuppressant Drugs

Apparently all of the immunosuppressant drugs can cause pancreatitis, either directly by their toxic effects on the pancreas or indirectly by predisposing to viral or bacterial infection of the pancreas. In addition to corticosteroids, *azathioprine, mercaptopurine, cyclosporine* (867–869), *cytosine arabinoside* (868, 870), *Minnesota anti-lymphoblastic globulin* (871), and *murine monoclonal anti-CD 3 antibody (OKT3)* (871, 872) have apparently caused pancreatitis.

### Antitubercular Drugs

*Isoniazid* was implicated as a possible cause of pancreatitis in four reports (873–876). Asymptomatic hyperamylasemia was found by Mattson (874) in 20 (3.7%) of 547 patients receiving intermittent *rifampin* and daily isoniazid for treatment of tuberculosis. Nine (1.6%) of the patients developed abdominal pain with hyperamylasemia, and therapy had to be discontinued in three of them.

### Antiparasitic Drugs

*Stibogluconaten* therapy of leishmaniasis was reported to be associated with the onset of acute pancreatitis by several authors (877–879), as was *pentavalent antimony* (879).

### Antiviral (AIDS) Agents

**Pentamidine and Didanosine for Treatment of AIDS.** Murphey and Josephs (880) initially noted the relationship of pentamidine therapy, AIDS, and acute pancreatitis. Klatt (881) reported the autopsy findings of three patients with AIDS who had received pentamidine by aerosol and intravenously. Each had necrotizing pancreatitis. In one patient, the pancreas was completely black, although histologically the architecture was not completely destroyed. An infectious agent was not detected within the pancreas. Others (882, 883) reported pentamidine-associated pancreatitis of varying severity, including fatalities (884–892). Several (885, 893–895) reported acute pancreatitis in AIDS patients following treatment with pentamidine by aerosol.

2,3-Didesoxyinosine (didanosine), an antiretroviral agent, has been associated with acute pancreatitis in AIDS patients (896–899). Pancreatitis of varying severity was noted in 7 of 44 patients treated by Seidlin et al. (900). Daniels (897) pointed out that 11 of 12 patients with clinically apparent pancreatitis had received pentamidine as well as didanosine. Maxson et al. (898) noted pancreatitis in 12 of 51 patients with AIDS treated with this drug, including two fatalities. Based on the pancreatitis recognized clinically (12 patients) or detected by elevated serum amylase levels (10 patients), pancreatitis developed in 62.7%. From the frequency and severity of the pancreatitis, it would appear that all AIDS patients receiving 2,3-dideoxinosine should be monitored for development of acute pancreatitis (900).

## CHEMICALLY INDUCED PANCREATITIS

It is obvious today that specific industrial chemicals can cause pancreatitis.

### Methyl Alcohol

Methyl alcohol poisoning was first described as a cause of pancreatitis in 1944 (901). In 1952 (902), 300 people were poisoned with methyl alcohol, of whom 17 died. Acute pancreatitis was noted histologically at autopsy.

### Insecticides

Severe acute pancreatitis complicated by pseudocyst formation followed the accidental ingestion of the *anticholinesterase insecticide* (*O*-ethyl-s-phenylethylphosphenodithioate) (903). Earl et al. (904) noted hyperamylasemia and acute pancreatitis following the chronic administration of the organophosphate anticholinesterase (Diazionon) to pigs and dogs. Marsh et al. (905) described the development of acute pancreatitis following cutaneous exposure to an organophosphate insecticide. This was apparently the first such description: the previous cases resulted from oral ingestion of these agents (903, 906). Acute necrotizing pancreatitis developed following ingestion of carbamate insecticide in a suicide attempt; the patient barely survived (906a).

Lankisch et al. (906b) described acute pancreatitis following ingestion of Parathion, an anticholinesterase insecticide. This alkylphosphate is used frequently in agriculture, especially in vineyards. All nine patients hospitalized with Parathion poisoning developed a low serum cholinesterase level and required mechanical ventilation. Two of the patients developed hemorrhagic pancreatitis. One, a 42-year-old woman, had attempted suicide by ingesting 5 gm of Parathion. Hemorrhagic pancreatitis was detected by laparotomy. She died of respiratory failure on the 99th day. The second patient, also attempting suicide, took 7.5 gm of Parathion and survived following laparotomy. Weizman and Sofer (906c) reported 17 children with anticholinesterase insecticide intoxication. Five developed acute pancreatitis: caused by Parathion in two, Diazionon in one, carbamate in one, and unspecified in one. Four additional patients had serum amylase elevations but no abdominal pain. All nine patients recovered. Braganza et al. (907, 908) concluded that occupational exposure to *aromatic or chlorinated hydrocarbons* might prove relevant to the study of idiopathic pancreatitis.

## IDIOPATHIC PANCREATITIS

As the profession becomes more sophisticated in the field of pancreatitis, idiopathic pancreatitis becomes a "diagnostic crutch" on which we lean less and less frequently.

Biliary microlithiasis has been recognized as a cause of acute pancreatitis for several decades, even when stones could not be palpated at laparotomy. With increased diagnostic capability the recognition of microlithiasis-induced acute pancreatitis is increasing, thereby reducing the frequency of "idiopathic" pancreatitis (909–913). Biliary sludge (914) or limy bile (915) are being recognized as probable causes of acute pancreatitis, as is cholesterosis (909, 916). Reverting to the old technique of duodenal drainage for diagnosis, Miquel et al. (909) performed biliary drainage in 12 patients in whom ultrasonography showed no evidence of gallstones. Gallbladder bile was obtained by duodenal drainage in 8 of the 12, and cholesterol crystals were identified in 6. Cholecystectomy was performed in five, showing cholesterosis in four and microlithiasis in one. Two of the patients with negative drainage studies underwent cholecystectomy, and one was found to have cholesterol crystals and calcium bilirubinate granules along with cholesterol polyps. Overall, they found gallbladder disease in 7 of the 12 patients.

Grendell (911) pointed out that hyperlipidemia may be missed if the serum triglyceride concentration is not measured early in the patient's course. He also noted that a serum triglyceride concentration above 1000 mg/dL is unlikely to result from pancreatitis but strongly suggests a preexisting defect in lipid metabolism. Although in individual patients, it is sometimes difficult to identify a low-flow state from congestive heart failure, small arteriosclerotic emboli, vasculitis or, chronic renal failure as the cause of acute pancreatitis, this factor is becoming more widely recognized. Carcinoma of the pancreas, including islet cell carcinomas and carcinoid tumors of the pancreas are identifiable causes of pancreatitis that may be unrecognized when the physician originally sees the patient for the presenting pancreatitis. With the increasing age of our population and their increasing use of several drugs, this diagnostic consideration requires additional emphasis. Patients with cystic fibrosis of the pancreas are now living far beyond childhood with the diagnosis sometimes unrecognized until pancreatitis occurs. The future may find an increase in the number of occupational and environmental chemicals that induce pancreatitis. Viral diseases, especially AIDS, in association with pancreatitis, are being recognized with increasing frequency.

The pattern of pancreatitis for which no causative factor is recognized varies with age. Grendell (911) noted the incidence of idiopathic acute pancreatitis to be 11–45% and recommends the frequent use of upper endoscopy and ERCP to identify congenital anomalies and gallstones in children. Gross et al. (917) and others increasingly suggest that cystic fibrosis may be overlooked as a cause of pancreatitis in individuals above 21 years of age. In older patients, Venu et al. (918) described "idiopathic" recurrent pancreatitis due to neurofibromas, carcinomas, and adenomas in the ampullary area.

Browder (919) found that in 21 (23%) of 93 patients over the age of 60 years, their acute pancreatitis had no recognized cause. The "idiopathic patients" were sicker and experienced a 24% mortality rate, compared with 8% among 70 patients whose pancreatitis had a known cause. The authors cited three previous reports indicating that the cause of acute pancreatitis in the elderly is likely to be more poorly defined (21–35%) than in younger patients.

A review of 66 patients with the diagnosis of idiopathic *chronic* pancreatitis at Mayo Clinic (920) led to definition of two groups. An early onset of pancreatitis was noted in 25 patients whose median age was 19 years; 44% were males. Pain was frequently the initial manifestation. Pancreatic calcification and exocrine and endocrine insufficiency developed more slowly than in other patients. The second group of 41 patients, 56% male, had a median age at onset of 56 years. Pain was often mild and in 50% was absent. Both groups developed pancreatitis more slowly than did patients with alcoholic pancreatitis.

Although fewer and fewer illnesses are being diagnosed as "idiopathic" pancreatitis, it is evident that many of the groups discussed in this chapter are only descriptive. Nevertheless, the description of a group with features in common may permit recognition of natural histories, even in the absence of etiologic recognition. For the present, many patients included in the idiopathic group can be more clearly defined by a detailed and knowledgeable history, by reappraisal of the biliary tract, by visual inspection of the periampullary area, and by ERCP.

## REFERENCES


#### Gallstone Pancreatitis

1. Howard JM, Ehrlich EW. Gallstone pancreatitis: a clinical entity. Surgery 1962;51:177–183.
2. Opie EL. The etiology of acute hemorrhagic pancreatitis. Bull Johns Hopkins Hosp 1901;12:182–188.
3. Opie EL. The relation of choledocholithiasis in disease of the pancreas and to fat necrosis. Bull John Hopkins Hosp 1901;12: 19–20.
4. Howard JM. Pancreatitis associated with gallstones. In: Howard JM, Jordan GL Jr. Surgical diseases of the pancreas. Philadelphia: JB Lippincott, 1960:169.
5. Acosta JM, Ledesma CL. Gallstone migration as a cause of acute pancreatitis. N Engl J Med 1974;290:484–487.

6. Acosta JM, Rossi R, Galli OM, et al. Early surgery for acute gallstone pancreatitis: evaluation of a systematic approach. Surgery 1978;83:367–370.
7. Kelly TR. Gallstone pancreatitis: pathophysiology. Surgery 1976; 80:488–492.
8. Stone HH, Fabian TC, Dunlop WE. Gallstone pancreatitis: biliary tract pathology in relation to time of operation. Ann Surg 1981;194:305–312.
9. Safrany L, Cotton PB. A preliminary report: urgent duodenoscopic sphincterotomy for acute gallstone pancreatitis. Surgery 1981;89:424–428.
10. Safrany L. Controversies in acute pancreatitis. Hollender LR, ed. Heidelberg: Springer-Verlag, 1982:214–218.
11. Lee SP, Nicholls JF, Park HZ. Biliary sludge as a cause of acute pancreatitis. N Engl J Med 1992;326:589–593.
12. Levy I, Lantsberg L, Khoda J. Spontaneous disappearance of limy bile. A cause of acute pancreatitis? J Clin Gastroenterol 1994;18:220–221.

**Alcoholic Pancreatitis**

13. Friedreich N. In: von Ziemssen H. Cyclopedia of the practice of medicine (American translation). New York: William Wood, 1878:601–602.
14. Fitz RH. Acute pancreatitis: a consideration of pancreatic hemorrhage, hemorrhagic, suppurative, and gangrenous pancreatitis, and of disseminated fat necrosis. Med Rec 1889;35:197.
15. Owens JL Jr, Howard JM. Pancreatic calcification: a late sequel in the natural history of chronic alcoholism and alcoholic pancreatitis. Ann Surg 1958;147:3.

**Pancreatitis Associated with Hyperparathyroidism**

16. Cope O, Culver PJ, Mixter CG Jr, Nardi GL. Pancreatitis, a diagnostic clue to hyperparathyroidism. Ann Surg 1957;145: 857–863.
17. Carey MC, Fitzgerald O. Hyperparathyroidism associated with chronic pancreatitis in a family. Gut 1968;9:700–703.

**Pancreatitis Associated with Hyperlipidemia**

18. Speck L, Fall von Lipämie F. Arch des Verein. f. Wissenschafte. Heilkunde, 1865;I:232. (Cited in Thannhauser SJ. Lipidoses: diseases of cellular lipid metabolism. 2nd ed. New York: Oxford University Press, 1950:301.)
19. Howard JM. Pancreatitis associated with familial hyperlipidemia. In: Howard JM, Jordan GL Jr, eds. Surgical diseases of the pancreas. Philadelphia: JB Lippincott, 1960:266–267.

**Postoperative and Posttransplantation Pancreatitis**

20. Trapnell JE, Howard JM. Transduodenal pancreatography. An improved technique. Surgery 1966;60:1112–1119.
21. Mahaffey JH, Howard JM. The incidence of postoperative pancreatitis: studies of 131 surgical patients utilizing serum amylase concentration. Arch Surg 1955;70:348–352.
22. McCombs PR, Mahon DE. Acute pancreatitis following aortic aneurysm repair: report of three cases. Ann Vasc Surg 1991;5: 366–369.
23. Panebianco AC, Scott SM, Dart CH Jr, et al. Acute pancreatitis following extracorporeal circulation. Ann Thorac Surg 1970;9: 562–568.
24. Orvar K, Johlin FC. Atheromatous embolization resulting in acute pancreatitis after cardiac catheterization and angiographic studies. Arch Intern Med 1994;154:1755–1761.
25. Probstein JG, Joshi RA, Blumenthal HT. Atheromatous embolization: etiology of acute pancreatitis. Arch Surg 1957;75:566–572.
26. Howard JM, Vowles KDJ. Postoperative pancreatitis. In: Howard JM, Jordan GL Jr, eds. Surgical disease of the pancreas, Philadelphia: JB Lippincott, 1960.
27. Levine SR, Gambill EE, Greene LF. Acute pancreatitis following transurethral prostatic resection; report of 6 cases. J Urol 1962;88:657–663.
28. Shader AE, Paxton Jr. Fatal pancreatitis. Am J Surg 1966;111: 369–373.
29. Gourgoutis GD. Postoperative hyperamylasemia. Am Surg 1973; 39:111–114.
30. Harada K, Kitamura M, Ikenaga T. Isoenzyme study on postoperative transient hyperamylasemia. Am J Gastroenterol 1974; 61:121–126.
31. Morrissey R, Berk JE, Fridhandler L, Pelot D. The nature and significance of hyperamylasemia following operation. Ann Surg 1974;180:67–71.
32. Starzl TE. Experience in renal transplantation. Philadelphia: WB Saunders, 1964.

**Familial Pancreatitis**

33. Comfort MW, Steinberg AG. Pedigree of a family with heredity, chronic, relapsing pancreatitis. Gastroenterol 1952;21: 54–63.
34. Gerber BC. Hereditary pancreatitis. Arch Surg 1963;87:70–80.
35. Gross JB, Gambill EE, Ulrich JA. Hereditary pancreatitis. Am J Med 1962;33:358–364.
36. Davies M, Klimiuk PS, Adams PH, et al. Familial hypocalciuric hypercalcaemia and acute pancreatitis. Br Med J 1981;282: 1023–1025.
37. Marx SJ, Stock JL, Attie MF, et al. Familial hypocalciuric hypercalcemia: recognition among patients referred after unsuccessful parathyroid exploration. Ann Intern Med 1980;92: 351–356.
38. van Haeften TW, Hoogenberg K, van Essen LH. Acute pancreatitis in a patient with familial benign hypercalcaemia. Neth J Med 1994;45:110–113.
39. Jackson CE. Hereditary hyperparathyroidism associated with recurrent pancreatitis. Ann Intern Med 1958;49:829–836.
40. Carey MC, Fitzgerald O. Hyperparathyroidism associated with chronic pancreatitis in a family. Gut 1968;9:700–703.
41. Williams RA, Caldwell BF, Wilson SE. Idiopathic hereditary pancreatitis. Experience with surgical treatment. Arch Surg 1982; 117:408–412.
42. Perrault J. Hereditary pancreatitis (Review). Gastroenterol Clin North Am 1994;23:743–752.
43. Girard RM, Dube S, Archambault AP. Hereditary pancreatitis: report of an affected Canadian kindred and review of the disease. Can Med Assoc J 1981;125:576–580.
44. Beall JH, Bell HW, Jesseph JE, Nyhus LM. Fatal acute hemorrhagic pancreatitis occurring simultaneously in identical twins. Gastroenterology 1960;39:215.
45. Henderson J, Ingram D, House T. Acute pancreatitis in identical twins. Med J Aust 1982;1:432–434.
46. Hoste P, Lentini F, Rottiers R. Chronic relapsing pancreatitis in twin brothers with type V hyperlipoproteinemia. Acta Clin Belg 1978;33:313–322.

**Traumatic Pancreatitis**

47. Grace TW, Cammerer RC. Self inflicted recurrent pancreatitis (Letter). JAMA 1980;243:1232.
48. Sarles H. Pancreatitis. Bibl Gastroenterol Fasc, 7th ed. Basle: S Krager, 1965.
49. Haigh E. Acute pancreatitis in childhood. Arch Dis Child 1956;31:272–275.
50. Goodwin CW, Warfen GD, Wilmore DW, et al. Pancreatitis: a hidden complication in the burn patient. Presented at the 6th annual meeting of the American Burn Association, April 4–6, 1974, Cincinnati. (Quoted in ref 52.)
51. Goodwin CW, Pruitt BA Jr. Increased incidence of pancreatitis in thermally injured patients: a prospective study. Proc Am Assoc Surg Trauma 1981.
52. Ryan CM, Sheridan RL, Schoenfeld DA, et al. Postburn pancreatitis. Ann Surg 1995;222:163–170.

**Pancreatitis Secondary to Benign and Malignant Tumors: Carcinoma of the Exocrine Pancreas**

53. Gambill EE. Pancreatitis associated with pancreatic carcinoma: a study of 26 cases. Mayo Clin Proc 1971;46:174–177.
54. Köhler H, Lankisch PG. Acute pancreatitis and hyperamylasemia in pancreatic carcinoma. Pancreas 1987;2:117–119.
55. Mikel S, Campbell A. Carcinoma of the pancreas. Surgery 1950;28:963–969.
56. Lin A, Feller ER. Pancreatic carcinoma as a cause of unexplained pancreatitis: report of ten cases. Ann Intern Med 1990;113:166–167.
57. Mao C, Domenico DR, Kim K, et al. Observations on the developmental pattern and the consequences of pancreatic exocrine adenocarcinoma. Findings of 154 autopsies. Arch Surg 1995;130:125–134.

58. Trapnell JE, Duncan EH. Patterns of incidence in acute pancreatitis. Br Med J 1975;2:179–183.
59. Berman LG, Dunn E, Straehley CJ. Survey of pancreatitis, Central New York Surgical Society. Gastroenterology 1961;40:94.
60. Enquist IF, Gliedman JL. Gross autopsy findings in cases of fatal acute pancreatitis. Arch Surg 1958;77:985.
61. Sharon P, Melmed S, Neuman G. Acute pancreatitis in a community with a low alcohol intake. Int Surg 1979;64: 63–66.
62. Weissberg D, Adam YG, Volk H, State D. Acute pancreatitis: a 10-year study. Am Surg 1972;38:574–581.
63. Imrie CW, Whyte AS. A prospective study of acute pancreatitis. Br J Surg 1975;62:490–494.
64. Mayday GB, Pheils MT. Pancreatitis: a clinical review. Med J Aust 1970;1:1142–1144.
65. Greenberg RE, Bank S. Acute pancreatitis in pancreatic carcinoma (Letter). Pancreas 1987;2:495.
66. Wilson C, Imrie CW. Occult pancreatic cancer with recurrent acute pancreatitis. Postgrad Med J 1986;62:765–767.
67. Tell BL, Brolin RE. Carcinoma of the pancreas misdiagnosed as acute pancreatitis. NJ Med 1986;83:666–668.
68. Carpentier F, Coolen J, De Bie P, Nijssens M. Pancreatic carcinoma complicated by acute pancreatitis. J Belg Radiol 1990;73:512–513.
69. Boyle JM, McLeod ME. Pancreatic cancer presenting as pancreatitis of pregnancy. Case report. Am J Gastroenterol 1978; 70:371–373.

**Malignant and Benign Tumors of the Ampulla of Vater and Duodenum, Gardner's Syndrome**

70. Robertson JF, Imrie CW. Acute pancreatitis associated with carcinoma of the ampulla of Vater. Br J Surg 1987;74:395–397.
71. Belghiti J, Wind P, Bernades P, Fekete F. Acute pancreatitis associated with carcinoma of the ampulla of Vater (Letter). Br J Surg 1987;74:1067–1068.
72. Clarke DN, Smith JA, Norman JN, Brunt PW. Pancreatitis and duodenal obstruction due to periampullary carcinoma associated with familial polyposis coli. Postgrad Med J 1978;54: 418–420.
73. Sener SF, Miller HH, DeCosse JJ. The spectrum of polyposis. Surg Gynecol Obstet 1984;159:525–532.
74. Wise RH Jr, Stanley RJ. Carcinoma of the ampulla of Vater presenting as acute pancreatitis. J Comput Assist Tomogr 1984;8:158–161.
75. Burt RW, Rikkers LF, Gardner EJ, et al. Villous adenoma of the duodenal papilla presenting as necrotizing pancreatitis in a patient with Gardner's syndrome. Gastroenterol 1987;92: 532–535.
76. Guzzardo G, Kleinman MS, Krackov JH, Schwartz SI. Recurrent acute pancreatitis caused by ampullary villous adenoma (Review). J Clin Gastroenterol 1990;12:200–202.
77. Case records of the Massachusetts General Hospital. N Engl J Med 1994;330:671–676.
78. Meyer W, Gebhardt C. Villous adenoma of the papilla of Vater and acute necrotizing pancreatitis (Review, in German). Dtsch Med Wochenschr 1988;113;1557–1560.
79. Ohmori K, Kinoshita H, Shiraha Y, Satuke K. Pancreatic duct obstruction by a benign polypoid adenoma of the ampulla of Vater. Am J Surg 1976;132:662–663.
80. Berk T, Friedman LS, Goldstein SD, et al. Relapsing acute pancreatitis as the presenting manifestation of an ampullary neoplasm in a patient with familial polyposis coli. Am J Gastroenterol 1985;80:627–629.
81. Nugent KP, Spigelman AD, Williams CB, Phillips RK. Iatrogenic pancreatitis in familial adenomatous polyposis. Gut 1993;34: 1269–1270.
82. Mannoury V, Brunetaud JM, Ghisbain H, et al. Severe acute pancreatitis following laser treatment of periampullary villous adenoma (Letter). Dig Dis Sci 1993;38:382–383.
83. Mancheron H, Dupas JL, Sevestre H, et al. Acute pancreatitis caused by papillary adenoma of the distal common bile duct. Treatment by endoscopic excision. Gastroenterol Clin Biol 1988;12:259–261.
84. Sawin R, Brooks DC. Chronic pancreatitis secondary to an inflammatory polyp of the duodenum 25 years after Billroth II reconstruction. Surg 1988;104:575–576.
85. Oh C, Jemerin EE. Benign adenomatous polyp of the papilla of Vater. Surg 1965;57:495–503.
86. Griffen WO Jr, Schaefer JW, Schindler S, et al. Ampullary obstruction by benign duodenal polyps. Arch Surg 1968;97: 444–449.
87. Koninger J, Butters M, Roos U, Bittner R. Juxtapapillary intraduodenal lipoma as a rare cause of jaundice and acute pancreatitis. Z Gastroenterol 1944;3(3):1597–1599.
88. Kalvaria I, Bornman TC, Girdwood AH, Marks IN. Periampullary cyst: a surgically remediable cause of pancreatitis. Gut 1987; 28:358–362.

**Pancreatitis Associated with Neuroendocrine (Islet Cell) Tumors**

89. Pellegrini CA, Paloyan D, Acosta JM, Skinner DB. Acute pancreatitis of rare causation. Surg Gynecol Obstet 1977;144:899–902.
90. Mao CY, Howard JM. Pancreatitis associated with neuroendocrine (islet cell) tumors of the pancreas. Am J Surg 1996;171: 562–564.
91. Dixon JM, Chapman RW, Berry AR. Carcinoid tumor of the ampulla of Vater presenting as acute pancreatitis. Gut 1987; 28:1296–1297.
92. Sarles H, Cambon P, Choux R, et al. Chronic obstructive pancreatitis due to tiny (0.6 to 8 mm) benign tumors obstructing pancreatic ducts: report of three cases. Pancreas 1988;3: 232–237.

**Pancreatitis Associated with Lymphomas**

93. Safadi R, Or R, Bar Ziv J, Polliack A. Lymphoma-associated pancreatitis as a presenting manifestation of immunoblastic lymphoma. Leuk Lymph 1944;12:318–319.
94. Kotwall CA, Brow JR, Keith RG. Lymphoma pancreatitis: a real entity. Can J Surg 1989;32:375–377.
95. Anderson JH, Morran CG, Anderson JR, Carter DC. Acute pancreatitis and non-Hodgkin's lymphoma. Postgrad Med J 1987;63:137–139
96. Moossa MR, Segal I. Tumor associated acute pancreatitis (Letter). J Clin Gastroenterol 1984;6:188.
97. Cameron-Strange A. Acute pancreatitis associated with lymphosarcoma. Br J Surg 1983;70:444.
98. Freed JS, Dreiling DA, Reiner MA. Non-Hodgkin's lymphoma of the pancreas producing acute pancreatitis and pancreatic abscess. Mt Sinai J Med 1983;50:424–427.
99. Francis IR, Glazer GM. Case report. Burkitt's lymphoma of the pancreas presenting as acute pancreatitis. J Comput Assist Tomogr 1982;6:395–397.
100. Wan YL, Chen WJ, Huang SC, et al. Solitary hepatic Burkitt lymphoma presenting as acute pancreatitis. Pediatr Radiol 1988;18:160.
101. Ade C, Hatton M, Hamilton Stewart P, et al. Testicular lymphoma with pancreatitis. J R Soc Med 1991;84:309–310.
102. Halline A, Lerios M, Melissas J, et al. Primary lymphoma of the small bowel with obstructive jaundice and pancreatitis. A case report. S Afr Med J 1987;72:61–62.
103. Mansour P, Adams RD, Isaacs PE, et al. T-cell non-Hodgkin's lymphoma with uveitis, pancreatitis, digital gangrene and multiple chromosomal abnormalities (Letter). J Clin Pathol 1990;43:694–695.
104. Senba M. Adult T-cell leukemia associated with acute pancreatitis under hypercalcemic conditions (Letter; comment). Am J Med 1991;91:445–446.
105. Hosokawa T, et al. An autopsy case of adult T-cell leukemia, who died of acute hemorrhagic pancreatitis. J Kyushu Hematol Soc 1984;32:75–81.
106. Dazai Y, Katoh I, Hara Y, et al. Two cases of adult T-cell leukemia associated with acute pancreatitis due to hypercalcemia. Am J Med 1991;90:251–254.
107. Report of the Japanese Pathological Society for 1982–89. (Cited in ref 108.)
108. Senba M, Nakamura T, Kawai K, Senba MI. HTLV-1 and acute pancreatitis (Letter). Lancet 1991;337:1489.
109. Nguyen DL, Wilson DA, Engleman ED, et al. Serial sonograms to detect pancreatitis in children receiving L-asparaginase. South Med J 1987;80:1133–1136.
110. Pecquenard L, Damay M, Naveau C, et al. Delayed acute pancreatitis after treatment with L-asparaginase. A case report (Letter). Therapie 1990;45:453–454.

111. Yamada S, Ikuno Y, Okamura J, et al. A case of acute lymphoblastic leukemia with massively enlarged kidneys at diagnosis and complicated with tumor lytic syndrome, diabetes mellitus and pancreatitis with remission induction. Jpn J Clin Hematol 1988;29:249–253.
112. Batson OA, Branda RF. Acute pancreatitis complicating therapy of Hodgkin disease: a case report. Am J Hematol 1990;33:78–79.

**Pancreatitis Secondary to Metastasis to the Pancreas: Pulmonary Carcinoma**

113. McLatchie GR, Imrie CW. Acute pancreatitis associated with tumor metastases in the pancreas. Digestion 1981;21:13–17.
114. Niccolini DG, Graham JH, Banks PA. Tumor-induced acute pancreatitis. Gastroenterology 1976;71:142–145.
115. Schmitt JK. Pancreatitis and diabetes mellitus with metastatic pulmonary oat cell carcinoma (Letter). Ann Intern Med 1985; 103:638–639.
116. Hall M, Bundred NJ, Hall AW. Oat cell carcinoma of the bronchus and acute pancreatitis. Eur J Surg Oncol 1987;13:371–372.
117. Stewart KC, Dickout WJ, Urschel JD. Metastasis-induced acute pancreatitis as the initial manifestation of bronchogenic carcinoma. Chest 1993;104:98–100.
118. Noseda A, Gangji D, Cremer M. Acute pancreatitis as presenting symptom and sole manifestation of small cell lung carcinoma. Dig Dis Sci 1987;32:327–331.
119. Evans AT. Necrotising pancreatitis and diabetes associated with disseminated small cell carcinomas of lung. Scott Med J 1988;33:337.
120. Chowhan NM, Madajewicz S. Management of metastases-induced acute pancreatitis in small cell carcinoma of the lung. Cancer 1990;65:1445–1448.
121. Maclennan AC, Macleod IA. Case report: small cell carcinoma induced acute pancreatitis. Br J Radiol 1993;66:161–162.
122. Levine M, Danovitch SH. Metastatic carcinoma to the pancreas. Another cause for acute pancreatitis. Am J Gastroenterol 1973;60:290–294.
123. Hsieh TL, Chen JJ, Chien CS, et al. Small cell lung cancer with liver and bone metastasis associated with hypercalcemia and acute pancreatitis—a case report. Chang Gung Med J 1995; 18:190–193.

**Metastases from Other Cancers**

124. Hung SS, Ardalan B. Metastasis-induced acute pancreatitis. West J Med 1991;155:176–178.
125. Scheiman J, Elta G, Francis I. Biliary obstruction secondary to an extramedullary plasmacytoma of the pancreas: confusion with pancreatitis on computed tomography. Pancreas 1987;2: 237–239.
126. Gatchell FG, Minor D. Malignant melanoma of the eye, metastatic after twenty-nine years. A case report. J Okla State Med Assoc 1972;65:211–213.
127. Zagorski W, Badowski A. Acute pancreatitis and cholecystitis caused by skin melanoma metastasis. Wiad Lek 1975;28: 877–880.

**Afferent Loop Obstruction After Gastric Resection**

128. Perry T Jr. Post-gastrectomy proximal jejunal loop obstruction simulating acute pancreatitis. Ann Surg 1954;140:119–121.
129. Howard JM, Jordan GL Jr. Afferent loop obstruction after gastric resection. In: Howard JM, Jordan GL Jr, eds. Surgical diseases of the pancreas. Philadelphia: JB Lippincott, 1960.
130. Dahlgren S. The afferent loop syndrome. Stockholm: Almquist and Wiksell, 1964.
131. Bubrick MP, Hitchcock CR. Renal cyst causing afferent loop obstruction and acute pancreatitis. Am Surg 1975;41:440–443.

**Volvulus and Intussusception of the Stomach, Wandering Spleen**

132. Von Wiesenger D. Ein fall von volvulus des magens mit totalem dadurch bedingtem verschluss von cardia und pylorus in adulter futtnekrose heilung. Dtsch Med Wochenschr 1901;27:83.
133. Hailes WA. Volvulus of the stomach. Med J Aust 1923;2:544.
134. Dine MS, Martin LW. Malrotation with gastric volvulus, midgut volvulus, and pancreatitis. Am J Dis Child 1977;131:1345–1346.
135. Cuschieri RJ, Wilson WA. Incarcerated Bochdalek hernia presenting as acute pancreatitis. Br J Surg 1981;68:669.
136. Oliver MJ, Wilson AR, Kapila L. Acute pancreatitis and gastric volvulus occurring in a congenital diaphragmatic hernia. J Pediatr Surg 1990;25:1240–1241.
137. Kafka NJ, Leitman IM, Tromba J. Acute pancreatitis secondary to incarcerated paraesophageal hernia. Surgery 1994;115: 653–655.
138. Herman LL, Kurtz RC, Brennan MF, Shike M. Acute pancreatitis from intussusception of a gastric polyp in a patient with Gardner's syndrome. Dig Dis Sci 1992;37:955–960.
139. Ready AR, Downing R, Black J. Elevated serum amylase in association with jejunogastric intussusception. Br J Surg 1984; 71:844.
140. Galea MH, Mayell MJ. Gastroduodenal mucosal intussusception causing gastric outlet obstruction: a complication of gastrostomy tubes. J Pediatr Surg 1988;23:980–981.
141. Alzen G, Fass J, Riesener KP. Ileocolic invagination and pancreatitis in an adult—complications of an acute gastroenteritis. ROFO 1988;149:429–431.
142. Parker LA, Mittelstaedt CA, Mauro MA, et al. Torsion of a wandering spleen: CT appearance. J Comput Assist Tomogr 1984;8:1201–1204.
143. Murray KF, Morgan A, Christie DL. Pancreatitis caused by a wandering spleen. J Pediatr Gastroenterol Nutr 1994;18:486–489.

**Gastric Duplications Causing Acute Pancreatitis**

143a. Traverso LW, Damus PS, Longmire WL Jr. Pancreatitis of unusual origin. Surg Gynecol Obstet 1975;141:383–386.
143b. Black PR, Welch KJ, Eraklis AJ. Juxtapancreatic intestinal duplications with pancreatic ductal communication: a cause of pancreatitis and recurrent abdominal pain in childhood. J Pediatr Surg 1986;21:257–261.
144. Lavine JE, Harrison M, Heyman MB. Gastrointestinal duplications causing relapsing pancreatitis in children. Gastroenterology 1989;97:1556–1558.
145. Hoffman M, Sugarman HJ, Heuman D, et al. Gastric duplication cyst communicating with aberrant pancreatic duct: a rare cause of recurrent acute pancreatitis. Surgery 1987;101: 369–372.

**Diverticulosis of the Small Intestine**

146. Mahida YR, Chapman RW, Jewell DP. Association of small intestinal diverticulosis with chronic pancreatitis leading to severe malabsorption. Report of three cases. Postgrad Med J 1988;64:893–896.
147. Okada A, Higaki J, Nakamura T, et al. Pancreatitis associated with choledochal cyst and other anomalies in childhood. Br J Surg 1995;82:829–832.
148. Taylor RG, Auldist AW. Choledochal cyst presenting as a acute pancreatitis. Aust NZ J Surg 1985;55:611–612.
149. Rémy P, Renoirte P, De Neve De Roden A, Libon E. Pancreatitis and choledochal cyst (French). Chir Pediatr 1987;28:179–181.
150. Beattie GJ, Keay S, Muir BB, Boddy K. Acute pancreatitis with pseudocyst formation complicating pregnancy in a patient with a co-existent choledochal cyst. Br J Obstet Gynecol 1993;100:957–959.
151. Shieh CS, Eng HL, Huang SC, Chuang JH. Congenital pancreatic cyst presenting as acute pancreatitis in an adolescent. J Pediatr Gastroenterol Nutr 1994;18:490–493.
152. Swisher SG, Cates JA, Hunt KK, et al. Pancreatitis associated with adult choledochal cysts. Pancreas 1994;9:633–637.
153. Jaubert de Beaujeu M, Bonjean JA, Brusq A. Congenital cystic dilatation of the common bile duct and acute pancreatitis in children. Chir Pediatr 1979;20:325–331.
154. Yamaguchi M. Congenital choledochal cyst. Analysis of 1,433 patients in the Japanese literature. Am J Surg 1980;140:653–657.
155. Shaked G, Avinoah E, Ovnat A, et al. Anomalous biliopancreatic ductal system, recurrent pancreatitis, and choledochal cyst (Letter). Am J Gastroenterol 1989;84:685–686.

**Pancreatitis and Other Congenital Anomalies of the Pancreatic Ducts**

156. Leese T, Chiche L, Bismuth H. Pancreatitis caused by congenital anomalies of the pancreatic ducts. Surgery 1989;105:125–130.
157. Cangiarella J, Thomas PA, Genieser NB, Greco MA. Pancreatitis due to anomalous junction of the pancreaticobiliary ductal system. Pediatr Pathol 1993;13:853–861.

158. Toki F, Oi I, Takechi T. Anomaly of the pancreatic duct system: its association with pancreatitis. In: Sato T, Jamauchi H, eds. Pancreatitis: its pathophysiology and clinical aspects. Tokyo: University of Tokyo Press 1985:29–35.
159. Mori K, Nagakawa T, Ohta T, et al. Pancreatitis and anomalous union of the pancreaticobiliary ductal system in childhood. J Pediatr Surg 1993;28:67–71.
160. Fuchshuber PR, Vecchio R, Turnquest D, Moody FG. Aberrant biliopancreatic duct. A probable cause of acute pancreatitis? Arch Surg 1995;130:1139–1141.
161. Turner LJ. Chronic pancreatitis and congenital strictures of the pancreatic duct. Am J Surg 1983;145:582–584.

**Annular Pancreas and Pancreatitis**

162. Chevillotte G, Sahel J, Raillat A, Sarles H. Annular pancreas. Report of one case associated with acute pancreatitis and diagnosed by ERCP. Dig Dis Sci 1984;29:75–77.
163. Itoh Y, Hada T, Terano A, et al. Pancreatitis in the annulus of annular pancreas demonstrated by the combined use of computed tomography and endoscopic retrograde cholangiopancreatography. Am J Gastroenterol 1989;84:961–964.
164. Gilinsky NH, Lewis JW, Flueck JA, Fried AM. Annular pancreas associated with diffuse chronic pancreatitis. Am J Gastroenterol 1987;82:681–684.
165. Lloyd-Jones W, Mountain JC, Warren KW. Annular pancreas in the adult. Ann Surg 1972;176:163–170.
166. Thomford NR, Knight PR, Pace WG, Madura JA. Annular pancreas in adult: selection of operation. Ann Surg 1972;176: 159–162.
167. Drey NW. Symptomatic annular pancreas in the adult. Ann Intern Med 1957;46:750–772.
168. Etienne J, Foll Y, Volant A, Lozac'h P. Chronic segmental pancreatitis and the annular pancreas. Ann Chir 1989;43:244–247.
169. Mercadier M, Clot JP, Clot P. A case of annular pancreas associated with pancreatic calcification (French). Ann Chir 1967;21:660–665.
170. Delhaye M, Cremer M. Clinical significance of pancreas divisum. Acta Gastroenterol Belg 1992;55:306–313.
171. Stern CD. A historical perspective on the discovery of the accessory duct of the pancreas, the ampulla of Vater and pancreas divisum. Gut 1986;27:203–212.
172. Cotton PB. Pancreas divisum—curiosity or culprit? Gastroenterol 1985;89:1431–1435.
173. Carr-Locke DL. Pancreas divisum: the controversy goes on? Endoscopy 1991;23:88–90.
174. Russell RC, Wong NW, Cotton PB. Accessory sphincterotomy (endoscopic and surgical) in patients with pancreas divisum. Br J Surg 1984;71:954–957.
175. Siegel JH, Cooperman AM, Pullano W, Hammerman H. Pancreas divisum: observation, endoscopic drainage, and surgical treatment results in 65 patients. Surg Laparosc Endosc 1993;3: 281–285.
176. Eisen G, Schutz S, Metzler D, et al. Santorinicele: new evidence for obstruction in pancreas divisum. Gastrointest Endosc 1994; 40:73–76.

**Aberrant Pancreatitis**

177. Fam S, O Briain DS, Borger JA. Ectopic pancreas with acute inflammation. J Pediatr Surg 1982;17:86–87.
178. Barbosa J de C, Dockerty MB, Waugh JM. Pancreatic heterotopia: review of the literature and report of 41 authenticated surgical cases of which 25 were clinically significant. Surg Gynecol Obstet 1946;87:527–542.
179. Longmire W. Pancreas and periampullary region. In: Ackerman LV, ed. Surgical pathology. 5th ed. St. Louis: CV Mosby, 1974.
180. Qizilbash AH. Acute pancreatitis occurring in heterotopic pancreatic tissue within the gallbladder. Can J Surg 1976;19: 413–414.

**Cystic Fibrosis**

181. Stafford RJ, Grand RJ. Hereditary disease of the exocrine pancreas. Clin Gastroenterol 1982;11:141–170.
182. Shwachman H, Lebenthal E, Khaw KT. Recurrent acute pancreatitis in patients with cystic fibrosis with normal pancreatic enzymes. Pediatrics 1975;55:86–95.
183. Gross V, Schoelmerich J, Denzel K, Gerok W. Relapsing pancreatitis as initial manifestation of cystic fibrosis in a young man without pulmonary disease. Int J Pancreatol 1989;4: 221–228.
184. de Sant Angese PA, Lepore MJ. Involvement of abdominal organs in cystic fibrosis of the pancreas. Gastroenterology 1961;40:64.
185. James O, Agnew JE, Bouchier IA. Chronic pancreatitis in England: a changing picture? Br Med J 1974;2:34–38.
186. Buts JP, Scalais E, De Meyer R. Asymptomatic pancreatitis in cystic fibrosis without enzymatic achylia. Acta Paediatr Belg 1980;33:179–182.
187. Masaryk TJ, Achkar E. Pancreatitis as initial presentation of cystic fibrosis in young adults: a report of two cases. Dig Dis Sci 1983;28:874–878.
188. Caballero Plasencia AM, Casals Sanchez JL, Garcia Sanchez A, Caballero Plasencia M. Acute pancreatitis: an infrequent complication of cystic fibrosis. Rev Esp Enferm Apar Dig 1989; 75:515–518.
189. del Rosario JF, Putnam PE, Orenstein DM. Chronic pancreatitis in a patient with cystic fibrosis and clinical pancreatic insufficiency. J Pediatr 1995;126:951–952.
190. Atlas AB, Orenstein SR, Orenstein DM. Pancreatitis in young children with cystic fibrosis. J Pediatr 1992;120:756–759.
191. Moreno González E, Ibañez Aguirre J, Rico Selas P, et al. Recurrent acute pancreatitis as a complication of cystic fibrosis: report of one case treated surgically. Ann Ital Chir 1991;62: 345–347.
192. Bui HD, Dang CV. Acute pancreatitis: a complication of Foley catheter gastrostomy. J Natl Med Assoc 1986;78:779–781.
193. Panicek DM, Ewing DK, Gottlieb RH, Chew FS. Gastrostomy tube pancreatitis. Pediatr Radiol 1988;18:416–417.
194. Barthel JS, Mangum D. Recurrent acute pancreatitis in pancreas divisum secondary to minor papilla obstruction from a gastrostomy feeding tube. Gastrointest Endosc 1991;37:638–640.
195. Chamoun S, Testart J, Metayer P. Chronic segmental pancreatitis caused by a foreign body in Wirsung's duct (French). J Chir 1983;120:191–193.
196. Danzi JT. Two cases of acute pancreatitis due to a foreign body. Gastrointest Endosc 1986;32:360–361.
197. Dabadie A, Roussey M, Betremieux P, et al. Acute pancreatitis from a duodenal foreign body in a child. J Pediatr Gastroenterol Nutr 1989;8:533–535.
198. Farr CM, Larson C, Gladen HE, et al. An iatrogenic gallstone with pancreatitis (Letter). J Clin Gastroenterol 1989;11:596–597.
199. Uomo G, Manes G, Leccetti M, Rabbitti PG. Necrotizing acute pancreatitis due to a common bile duct foreign body. Am J Gastroenterol 1994;89:1109–1110.
200. Meltzer SJ, Goldberg MD. Recurrent pancreatitis caused by vegetable matter obstruction. Am J Gastroenterol 1986;81: 1091–1092.
201. Shawis RN, Doig CM. Gastric trichobezoar associated with transient pancreatitis. Arch Dis Child 1984;59:994–995.
202. David X, Bories P, Parelon G, et al. Acute pancreatitis induced by herbs of Provence (Letter). Lancet 1991;337:311.
203. Bedogni G, Meinero M, Barbieri I, et al. Foreign bodies of the biliary tract: endoscopic management, Dig Dis Sci 1986;31: 1100–1104.
204. Deboever G, Sels F. An exceptional case of foreign body induced pancreatitis (Letter). Am J Gastroenterol 1990;85: 632–633.
205. Madhaven SV, Vaughan SW. Recurrent pancreatitis: a complication secondary to a retained pancreaticojejunostomy splint. Gastrointest Endosc 1983;29:298–299.
206. van Steenbergen W, van Aken L, Ponette E. Acute pancreatitis complicating the insertion of a self-expandable biliary metal stent. Endoscopy 1992;24:440–442.
207. Kozarek RA. Pancreatic stents can induce ductal changes consistent with chronic pancreatitis. Gastrointest Endosc 1990; 36:93–95.
208. Kozarek RA. Direct cholangiopancreatoscopy and use of pancreatic duct stents and drains in the treatment of pancreatitis. In: Beger HG, Büchler M, Ditschuneit H, Malfertheiner P, eds. Chronic pancreatitis. Berlin: Springer-Verlag, 1990: 371–382.
209. Caos A. Biliary pancreatitis and jaundice associated with

obstructed peripapillary duodenal diverticulum. Am J Gastroenterol 1989;84:982–983.
210. Heath D, Leese T, Carr-Locke DL, et al. Obstructing calculous material in a periampullary duodenal diverticulum associated with primary common bile duct calculi and acute pancreatitis. Br J Surg 1987;74:648.
211. Crithlow JR, Shapiro MF, Silen M, et al. Duodenojejunostomy for the pancreaticobiliary complications of duodenal diverticulum. Ann Surg 1985;202:56–58.
212. Shallman RW, Kolts RL. Duodenojejunostomy for pancreatitis secondary to periampullary duodenal diverticula. Arch Surg 1987;122:850–851.
213. De las Heras G, González Bernal AC, García D, Dueñas C, Silván M. Asociación de divertículos duodenales y pancreatitis aguda. Rev Esp Enferm Apar Dig 1994;85:349–353.

**Primary Biliary Cirrhosis and Sjögren Syndrome: Chronic Pancreatitis**

214. Epstein O, Lake-Bakaar G, McKavanagh S, Sherlock S. Pancreatic hyposecretion in primary biliary cirrhosis: a "dry gland" disease. Gut 1979;20:A 448.
215. Epstein O, Chapman RWG, Lake-Bakaar G, et al. The pancreas in primary biliary cirrhosis and primary sclerosing cholangitis. Gastroenterology 1982;83:1177–1182.
216. Shibata T, Hayakawa T, Kondo T, et al. A case of chronic pancreatitis associated with Sjögren's syndrome. Jpn J Gastroenterol 1989;86:960–964.
217. Klass HJ, Braganza JM, Warnes TW. Pancreas in primary biliary cirrhosis. Gut 1979;20:A448.
218. Perisic VN, Mihailovic T, Filipovic D. Congenital hepatic fibrosis, bile duct abnormality, long pancreaticobiliary common channel, and pancreatitis (Letter). J Pediatr Gastroenterol Nutr 1988;7:790–791.

**Sclerosing Cholangitis and Lymphoplasmacytic Sclerosing Pancreatitis**

219. Smith MP, Loe RH. Sclerosing cholangitis. Am J Surg 1965;110:239–245.
220. Epstein O, Chapman RW, Lake-Bakaar G, et al. The pancreas in primary biliary cirrhosis and primary sclerosing cholangitis. Gastroenterology 1982;83:1177–1182.
221. Waldram R, Kopelman H, Tsantoulas D, Williams R. Chronic pancreatitis, sclerosing cholangitis and sicca complex in two siblings. Lancet 1975;1:550–552.
222. Axon AT, Ashton MG, Lintott DJ. Chronic pancreatitis and inflammatory bowel disease. Clin Radiol 1979;30:179–182.
223. Weisner RH, La Russo NF. Clinicopathologic features of primary sclerosing cholangitis. Gastroenterology 1980;79:200–206.
224. Thompson HH, Pitt HA, Tompkins RK, Longmire WP Jr. Primary sclerosing cholangitis. A heterogenous disease. Ann Surg 1982;196:128–136.
225. Sjögren I, Wengle B, Korsgren M. Primary sclerosing cholangitis associated with fibrosis of the submandibular gland and the pancreas. Acta Med Scand 1979;205:139–141.
226. Fritsch WP. Chronic pancreatitis and primary sclerosing cholangitis. Z Gastroenterol 1987;25:182–184.
227. Borkje B, Vetvik K, Odergaard S, et al. Chronic pancreatitis in patients with sclerosing cholangitis and ulcerative colitis. Scand J Gastroenterol 1985;20:539–542.
228. Kawaguchi K, Koike M, Tsuruta K, et al. Lymphoplasmacytic sclerosing pancreatitis with cholangitis: a variant of primary sclerosing cholangitis extensively involving the pancreas. Hum Pathol 1991;22:387–395.
229. Scully RE. Case records of the Mass. Gen Hosp. N Engl J Med 1982;306:349–358.

**Fibrosing Pancreatitis in Children**

230. Williams TE Jr, Sherman NJ, Clatworthy HW Jr. Chronic fibrosing pancreatitis in childhood: a cause of recurrent abdominal pain. Pediatrics 1967;40:1019–1023.
231. Ghishan FK, Green HL, Avant G, et al. Chronic relapsing pancreatitis in childhood. J Pediatr 1983;102:514–518.
232. Meneely RL, O'Neill J, Ghishan FK. Fibrosing pancreatitis—an obscure cause of painless obstructive jaundice: a case report and review of the literature. Pediatrics 1981;67:136–139.
233. Atkinson GO Jr, Wyly JB, Gay BB Jr, et al. Idiopathic fibrosing pancreatitis: a cause of obstructive jaundice in childhood. Pediatr Radiol 1988;18:28–31.
234. Elitsur Y, Siddiqui SY, Sloven D, et al. Chronic pancreatitis with diffuse fibrosis in early childhood. Pancreas 1989;4:504–510.
235. Stephen TC, Younoszai MK, Tyson RW, Groff DB. Fibrosing pancreatitis associated with pericholangitis and cholangitis in a child. J Pediatr Gastroenterol Nutr 1992;15:208–212.
236. Ingomar CJ, Terslev E. A case of chronic pancreatitis in early childhood. Dan Med Bull 1965;12:91–92.
237. Isaacs JD, Keshavarzian A, Blumgart LH, Hodgson HJ. Juvenile chronic pancreatitis—a cause of painless jaundice in a patient with multiple somatic abnormalities. J Clin Gastroenterol 1985;7:533–536.

**Painless Fibrosing Pancreatitis in Adults**

238. Gaulston SJM, Gallagher ND. Chronic painless pancreatitis. Gut 1962;3:252–254.
239. Bartholomew LG, Comfort MW. Chronic pancreatitis without pain. Gastroenterology 1956;31:724–743.
240. Buscail L, Ravaud A, Moreau J, et al. Is the incidence of painless chronic pancreatitis underestimated? Gastroenterol Clin Biol 1989;13:640–641.
241. Gross JB. Some recent developments pertaining to pancreatitis. Ann Intern Med 1958;49:796.
242. Ammann RW, Hammer B, Fumagalli I. Chronic pancreatitis in Zurich 1963–1972. Digestion 1973;9:404–415.
243. Gastard J, Joubaud F, Farbos T, et al. Etiology and course of primary chronic pancreatitis in western France. Digestion 1973;9:416–428.
244. Vantini I, Piubello W, Cavallini G, et al. Chronic pancreatitis in north-east Italy: a clinical and pathological study. Acta Hepato-Gastroenterol 1978;25:130–135.

**Celiac Disease, Chronic Pancreatitis, and Kwashiorkor Disease**

245. Fitzgerald O, Fitzgerald P, Fennelly J, et al. A clinical study of chronic pancreatitis. Gut 1963;4:193–216.
246. Regan PT, DiMagno EP. Exocrine pancreatic insufficiency in celiac sprue. A cause of treatment failure. Gastroenterology 1980;78:484–487.
247. Nanda R, Anand BS. Celiac disease and tropical calcific pancreatitis. Am J Gastroenterol 1993;88:1790–1792.
248. Pitchumoni CS, Thomas E, Balthazar E, Sherling B. Chronic calcific pancreatitis in association with celiac disease. Am J Gastroenterol 1977;68:358–361.
249. Bustos Fernanez L, De Paula A, Prizont R, et al. Exocrine pancreatic insufficiency secondary to glutenenteropathy. Am J Gastroenterol 1970;53:564–569.
250. Faulques B, Grimaud JC, Leung PP, et al. Celiac disease, autoimmune cirrhosis, chronic pancreatitis: apropos of a triple association. Gastroenterol Clin Biol 1989;13:1082–1085.

**Ramadan Syndrome**

251. Benson JR, Ward MP. Massive gastric dilatation and acute pancreatitis—a case of the Ramadan syndrome (Letter)? Postgrad Med J 1992;68:689.
252. Backett SA. Acute pancreatitis and gastric dilatation in a patient with anorexia nervosa. Postgrad Med J 1985;61:39–40.
253. Murray WJ. Massive gastric distension in acute pancreatitis—a report of two cases. Postgrad Med J 1984;60:631–633.
254. Keane FB, Fennell JS, Tomkin GH. Acute pancreatitis, acute gastric dilatation and duodenal ileus following refeeding in anorexia nervosa. Ir J Med Sci 1972:147–191.
255. Chen MZ, Yang HS, Xu QF, et al. Acute pancreatitis in Suzhou area. Predisposing causes and natural history. Chin Med J 1984;97:747–750.

**Anorexia Nervosa**

256. Schoetle UC. Pancreatitis. A complication, a concomitant, or a cause of an anorexia nervosa like syndrome. J Am Acad Child Psychiatry 1979;18:384–390.
257. Nordgren L, von Scheele C. Hepatic and pancreatic dysfunction in anorexia nervosa: a report of two cases. Biol Psychiatry 1977;12:681–686.
258. Keane FB, Fennell JS, Tomkin GH. Acute pancreatitis, acute

gastric dilation and duodenal ileus following refeeding in anorexia nervosa. Ir J Med Sci 1978;147:191–192.
259. Gryboski J, Hillemeier C, Kocoshis S, et al. Refeeding pancreatitis in malnourished children. J Pediatr 1980;97:441–443.

**Chronic Malnutrition with Refeeding: Kwashiorkor Disease**

260. Montalegre A, Sarles H, Ricosse JH, Sahel J. Pancreatic lesions due to prolonged malnutrition in IBO children: possible transition between kwashiorkor and chronic calcifying pancreatitis. Pancreas 1987;2:114–116.

**Morbid Obesity Operations**

261. Du Toit DF, Knott-Craig C, Laker L. Recurrent pancreatitis after partial ileal bypass for hyperlipidemia. A case report. S Afr Med J 1985;68:483–484.
262. Schein M. Acute pancreatitis following pancreaticobiliary bypass (Scopinaro operation) (Letter). Arch Surg 1987;122:1088.
263. Sorrell VF, Knight DH, Burcher SK. Pancreatitis following intestinal bypass for obesity. Aust NZ J Surg 1975;45:163–167.
264. Payne JH, DeWind L, Schwab CE, Kern WH. Surgical treatment of morbid obesity. Sixteen years of experience. Arch Surg 1973;106:432–437.
265. Lashner BA, Kirsner JB, Hanauer SB. Acute pancreatitis associated with high concentration lipid emulsion during total parenteral nutrition therapy for Crohn's disease. Gastroenterology 1986;90:1039–1041.
266. Noseworthy J, Colodney AH, Eraklis AJ. Pancreatitis and intravenous fat: an association in patients with inflammatory bowel disease. J Pediatr Surg 1983;18:269–272.
267. Izsak EM, Shike M, Roulet M, Jeejeebhoy KN. Pancreatitis in association with hypercalcemia in patients receiving total parenteral nutrition. Gastroenterology 1980;79:555–558.
268. Weizman Z, Durie PR. Acute pancreatitis in childhood. J Pediatr 1988;113:24–29.
269. Ülstrom RA, Brown DM. Hypercalcemia as a complication of hyperalimentation (Letter). J Pediatr 1972;81:419–420.
270. Manson RR. Acute pancreatitis secondary to iatrogenic hypercalcemia: implications of hyperalimentation. Arch Surg 1974;108:213–215.

**Pancreatitis Associated with Chronic Inflammatory Bowel Disease: Crohn's Disease of the Duodenum**

271. Efron G. The natural history of pancreatitis. Br J Surg 1966;53:702–706.
272. Eisner TD, Goldman IS, McKinley MJ. Crohn's disease and pancreatitis. Am J Gastroenterol 1993;88:583–586.
273. Legge DA, Hoffman HN 2d, Carlson HC. Pancreatitis as a complication of regional enteritis of the duodenum. Gastroenterology 1971;61:834–837.
274. Newman LH, Wellinger JR, Present DH, Aufses AH Jr. Crohn's disease of the duodenum associated with pancreatitis: a case report and review of the literature. Mt Sinai J Med 1987;54:429–432.
275. Speiss SE, Braun M, Vogelsang RL, Craig RM. Crohn's disease of the duodenum complicated by pancreatitis and common bile duct obstruction. Am J Gastroenterol 1992;87:1033–1036.
276. Eliakim R, Fich A, Libson E, et al. Crohn's disease of the duodenum presented as pancreatitis due to persimmon bezoar. J Clin Gastroenterol 1987;9:553–555.
277. Meltzer SJ, Korelitz BI. Pancreatitis and duodenopancreatic reflux in Crohn's disease. J Clin Gastroenterol 1988;10:555–558.

**Crohn's Disease of the Distal Intestine**

278. Seyrig JA, Jian R, Modigliani R, et al. Idiopathic pancreatitis associated with inflammatory bowel disease. Dig Dis Sci 1985;30:1121–1126.
279. Weber P, Seibold F, Jenss H. Acute pancreatitis in Crohn's disease. J Clin Gastroenterol 1993;17:286–291.
280. Omata F, Arakawa S, Takahashi H, Ueno F. Crohn's disease associated with pancreatitis of unknown etiology: a case report. Gastroenterol Jpn 1993;28:420–423.
281. Meyers S, Greenspan J, Greenstein AJ, et al. Pancreatitis with Crohn's ileocolitis. Report of a case and review of the literature. Dis Colon Rectum 1987;30:119–122.
282. Haber CJ, Meltzer SJ, Present DH, Korelitz BI. Nature and course of pancreatitis caused by 6-mercaptopurine in the treatment of inflammatory bowel disease. Gastroenterology 1986;91:982–986.
283. Sturdevant RA, Singleton JW, Deren JL, et al. Azathioprine-related pancreatitis in patients with Crohn's disease. Gastroenterology 1979;77:883–886.
284. Tromm A, Huppe D, Micklefield GH, et al. Acute pancreatitis complicating Crohn's disease: mere coincidence or causality? Gut 1992;33:1289–1291.
285. Matsumoto T, Matsui T, Iida M, et al. Acute pancreatitis as a complication of Crohn's disease. Am J Gastroenterol 1989;84:804–807.
286. Meyers S, Greenspan J, Greenstein AJ, et al. Pancreatitis coincident with Crohn's ileocolitis. Report of a case and review of the literature. Dis Colon Rectum 1987;30:119–122.
287. Niemala S, Lehtola J, Karttunen T, Lahde S. Pancreatitis in patients with chronic inflammatory bowel disease. Hepatogastroenterology 1989;36:175–177.
288. Dobrilla G. Regional enteritis and pancreatitis. Gastroenterology 1972;63:713–714.

**Ulcerative Colitis**

289. Ball PW, Baggenstoss AH, Bargen JA. Pancreatic lesions associated with chronic ulcerative colitis. Arch Pathol 1950;50:347–358.
290. Joske RA. Etiological factors in the pancreatitis syndrome. Br Med J 1955;2:1477–1481.
291. Davies J. The essential pathology of kwashiorkor. Lancet 1948;1:317–320.
292. Kondo K, Matsukawa M, Yamada S, et al. A case of ulcerative colitis complicated with acute pancreatitis. J Jpn Soc Intern Med (Japan) 1989;78:75–78.
293. Lysy J, Goldin E. Pancreatitis in ulcerative colitis (Review). J Clin Gastroenterol 1992;15:336–339.
294. Forbes D, Scott RB, Trevenen C, et al. Chronic pancreatitis associated wtih ulcerative colitis. Clin Invest Med 1987;10:321–324.
295. Gurian LE, Keeffe EB. Pancreatic insufficiency associated with ulcerative colitis and pericholangitis. Gastroenterology 1982;82:581–585.
296. Schrumf E, Fausa O, Forre O, et al. HLA antigens and immunoregulatory T cells in ulcerative colitis associated with hepatobiliary disease. Scand J Gastroenterol 1982;17:187–191.
297. Kato Y, Morimoto H, Unovra M. Primary biliary cirrhosis and chronic pancreatitis in a patient with ulcerative colitis. J Clin Gastroenterol 1985;7:425–427.
298. Veloso FT, Dias LM, Carvalho J, et al. Ulcerative colitis, primary biliary cirrhosis, and chronic pancreatitis: coincident or coexistent? J Clin Gastroenterol 1993;16:55–57.

**Pancreatitis and Vasculitis: Lupus Erythematosus**

299. Petri M. Pancreatitis in systemic lupus erythematosus: still in search of a mechanism. J Rheumatol 1992;19:1014–1016.
300. DiVittorio G, Wees S, Koopman WJ, Ball GV. Pancreatitis in systemic lupus erythematosus (Abstract). Arthritis Rheum 1982;24:S6.
301. Vera Arieta R. Acute pancreatitis in generalized lupus erythematosus. Rev Gastroenterol Mex 1985;50:161–167.
302. Odaira C, Koizumi M, Fujiwara A, et al. A study of pancreatic injury in patients with SLE. Jpn J Gastroenterol 1987;84:2722–2730.
303. Serrano Lopez MC, Yebra Bango M, Lopez Bonet E, et al. Acute pancreatitis and systemic lupus erythematosus: necropsy of a case and review of the pancreatic vascular lesions (Review). Am J Gastroenterol 1991;86:764–767.
304. Eaker EY, Toskes PP. Systemic lupus erythematosus presenting initially with acute pancreatitis and a review of the literature. Am J Med Sci 1989;297:38–41.
305. Falko JM, Thomas FB. Acute pancreatitis due to procainamide-induced lupus erythematosus (Letter). Ann Intern Med 1975;83:832–833.
306. Mekori YA, Yaretzky A, Schneider M, Klajman A. Pancreatitis in systemic lupus erythematosus: a case report and review of the literature. Postgrad Med J 1980;56:145–147.

307. Marino C, Lipstein-Kresch E. Pancreatitis in systemic lupus erythematosus (Letter). Arthritis Rheum 1984;27:118–119.
308. Reynolds JC, Inman RD, Kimberly RP, et al. Acute pancreatitis in systemic lupus erythematosus: report of twenty cases and a review of the literature. Medicine 1982;61:25–32.
309. Rupprecht T, Wenzel D, Michalk D. Akut rezidivierende pankreatitis als leitsymptom eines lupus erythematodes disseminatus im Kindesalter. Monatsschr Kinderheilkd 1988;136:143–145.
310. Huang JL, Huang CC, Chen CY, Hung IJ. Acute pancreatitis: an early manifestation of systemic lupus erythematosus. Pediatr Emer Care 1994;10:291–293.
311. Wolman R, de Gara C, Isenberg D. Acute pancreatitis in systemic lupus erythematosus: report of a case unrelated to drug therapy. Ann Rheum Dis 1988;47:77–79.
312. Bruijn JA, van Albada-Kuipers GA, et al. Acute pancreatitis in SLE. Scand J Rheum 1986;15:363–367.
313. Yeh TS, Wang CR, Lee YT, et al. Acute pancreatitis related to anticardiolipin antibodies in lupus patients visiting an emergency department. Am J Emer Med 1993;11:230–232.
314. Hebbar M, Gosset D, Hatron PY, Devulder B. Acute pancreatitis, systemic lupus and antiphospholipid syndrome. 2 cases (Letter). Rev Med Interne 1994;15:146–147.
315. Moalla M, Boussen K, Meddeb S. Fatal acute pancreatitis in systemic lupus erythematosus (Letter). Ann Med Interne 1991; 142:230–232.
316. Kolk A, Horneff G, Wilgenbus KK, et al. Acute lethal necrotising pancreatitis in childhood systemic lupus erythematosus—possible toxicity of immunosuppressive therapy. Clin Exp Rheum 1995;13:399–403.
317. Le Thi Huong D, Papo T, Laraki R, et al. Pancreatitis in systemic lupus erythematosus. Review of the literature apropos of 5 cases. Rev Med Interne 1994;15:89–94.
318. Borum M, Steinberg W, Steer M, et al. Chronic pancreatitis: a complication of systemic lupus erythematosus. Gastroenterology 1993;104:613–615.
319. Kemp JA, Arora S, Fawaz K. Recurrent acute pancreatitis as a manifestation of Wegener's granulomatosis. Dig Dis Sci 1990;35: 912–915.
320. Branski D, Gross V, Gross-Kieselstein E, et al. Pancreatitis as a complication of Henoch-Schonlein purpura. J Pediatr Gastroenterol Nutr 1982;1:275–276.
321. Garner JA. Acute pancreatitis as a complication of anaphylactoid (Henoch-Schönlein) purpura. Arch Dis Child 1977;52: 971–972.
322. Puppala AR, Cheng JC, Steinheber FU. Pancreatitis—a rare complication of Schönlein-Henoch purpura. Am J Gastroenterol 1978;69:101–104.
323. Toskin KD. Syndrome of hemorrhagic pancreatitis as a manifestation of Schönlein-Henoch disease. Klin Khir 1965;11:65.
324. El Alami S, Azar C, Bheane M, Derumier J. Acute pancreatitis: a rare initial clinical manifestation of Henoch-Schönlein disease (Letter). Acta Gastroenterol Belg 1994;57:264–265.
325. Diaz CF. Schönlein-Henoch purpura and pancreatitis (Letter). Dig Dis Sci 1995;40:750–751.
326. Gruber GB. Kasuistik und Kritik der periarteritis nodosa. Sentraalbl. F. Herz u Gerfasskr. 1926;18:185.
327. Brown HW, Ghosh S. Polyarteritis presenting as an acute abdomen. Int Surg 1969;5130–5135.
328. Miller HG, Daley R. Clinical aspects of polyarteritis nodosa. Q J Med 1946;15:255–283.
329. Pear BL. Radiologic recognition of extrahepatic manifestations of hepatitis B antigenemia. AJR 1981;137:135–140.
330. Guillevin L, Le Thi Huong D, Godeau P, et al. Clinical findings and prognosis of polyarteritis nodosa and Churg-Strauss angiitis. A study in 165 patients. Br J Rheum 1988;27:258–264.
331. Camilleri M, Pusey CD, Chadwick VS, Rees AJ. Gastrointestinal manifestations of systemic vasculitis. Q J Med 1983;52: 141–149.
332. Colton CL, Butler TJ. The surgical problem of polyarteritis nodosa. Br J Surg 1967;54:393–396.
333. Rowley AH, Gonzalez-Crussi F, Shulman ST. Kawasaki syndrome. Curr Probl Pediatr 1991;21:387–405.
334. Stoler J, Biller JA, Grand RJ. Pancreatitis in Kawasaki disease. Am J Dis Child 1987;141:306–308.
335. Lanting WA, Muinos WI, Kamani NR. Pancreatitis heralding Kawasaki disease. J Pediatr 1992;121:743–744.
336. Greif JM, Wolff WI. Idiopathic calcific pancreatitis, CRST syndrome and progressive systemic sclerosis. Am J Gastroenterol 1979;71:177–182.

#### Postradiation Pancreatitis

337. Levy P, Menzelxhiu A, Paillot B, et al. Abdominal radiotherapy is a cause for chronic pancreatitis. Gastroenterology 1993;105: 905–909.
338. Burbige EJ, Tarder GL, Belber JP. Malabsorption following radiation therapy. Am J Gastroenterol 1977;67:589–592.
339. Mitchell CJ, Simpson FG, Davison A, Losowsky MS. Radiation pancreatitis: a clinical entity? Digestion 1979;19:134–136.
340. Sarles H. Chronic pancreatitis and main pancreatic duct stricture following cobalt therapy. Eur J Gastroenterol Hepatol 1992;4:509–510.
341. Case records of the Mass Gen Hosp. Weekly clinical pathol exercises. N Engl J Med 1969;281:314–323.
342. Sindelar WF, Hoekstra H, Restrepo, Kinsella TJ. Pathological tissue changes following intraoperative radiotherapy. Am J Clin Oncol 1986;9:504–509.
343. Swaroop VS, Mohandas KM, Dinshaw KA, et al. A prospective study of radiation induced damage of pancreatic ducts. Indian J Gastroenterol 1992;11:124–126.
344. Ahmadu-Suka F, Gillette EL, Withrow SJ, et al. Exocrine pancreatic function following intraoperative irradiation of the canine pancreas. Cancer 1988;62:1091–1095.
345. Ahmadu-Suka F, Gillette EL, Withrow SJ, et al. Pathologic response of the pancreas and duodenum to experimental intraoperative irradiation. Int J Radiat Oncol Biol Phys 1988;14: 1197–1204.
346. Archambeau J, Griem M, Harper P. The effects of 250-kv x-rays on the dog's pancreas: morphological and functional changes. Radiat Res 1966;28:243–256.
347. Pieroni PL, Rudick J, Adler M, et al. Effect of irradiation on the canine exocrine pancreas. Ann Surg 1976;184:610–614.
348. Du Toit DF, Heydenrych JJ, Smit B, et al. The effect of ionizing radiation of the primate pancreas: an endocrine and morphologic study. J Surg Oncol 1987;34:43–52.

#### Renal Insufficiency

349. Baggenstoss AH: The pancreas in uremia: a histopathologic study. Am J Pathol 1948;24:1003.
350. Welch KJ. The pancreas. In: Ravitch MM, Welch KJ, Benson CD, et al., eds. Pediatric surgery. 3rd ed. Chicago: Year Book Medical Publishers, 1979.
351. Avram MM. High prevalence of pancreatic disease in chronic renal failure. Nephron 1977;18:68–71.
352. Robinson DO, Alp MH, Grant AK, Lawrence JR. Pancreatitis and renal disease. Scand J Gastroenterol 1977;12:17–20.
353. Berman LG, Dunn E, Straehley CJ. Survey of pancreatitis, Central New York Surgical Society. Gastroenterology 1961;40:94.
354. Lynch KM. Pancreatitis: analysis of types and causes. Ann Intern Med 1940;14:628.
355. Vaziri ND, Dure-Smith B, Miller R, Mirahmadi M. Pancreatic pathology in chronic dialysis patients—an autopsy study of 78 cases. Nephron 1987;46:347–349.
356. Eguchi M, Tamura H, Kakinuma Y, Maeda S. Pancreatic pathology in hemodialysis patients. Jpn J Clin Dial 1988;4:1859–1866.
357. Araki T, Ueda M, Ogawa K, Tsuji T. Histological pancreatitis in end-stage renal disease. Int J Pancreatol 1992;12:263–269.
358. Rutsky EA, Robards M, Van Dyke JA, Rostand SG. Acute pancreatitis in patients with end-stage renal disease without transplantation. Arch Intern Med 1986;146:1741–1745.
359. Witzel L, Bolcskei P, Porzelt R, Haasis R. Acute pancreatitis with diabetic coma during peritoneal dialysis. Med Welt 1971;20:838.
360. Olenska T, Bulhak W. Case of acute pancreatitis following peritoneal dialysis in a patient with terminal renal failure. Pol Tyg Lek 1976;31:2105–2106.
361. Van Dyke JA, Rutsky EA, Stanley RJ. Acute pancreatitis associated with end-stage renal disease. Radiol 1986;160:403–405.
362. Boudailliez B, André JL, Broyer M, et al. Acute pancreatitis in six non-transplanted uraemic children. Pediatr Nephrol 1988;2: 431–435.
363. Pitrone F, Pellegrino E, Mileto G, Consolo F. May pancreatitis represent a CAPD complication? Report of two cases with a rapid evolution to death (Letter). Int J Artif Organs 1985;8:235.

364. Singh S, Wadhwa N. Peritonitis, pancreatitis and infected pseudocyst in a continuous ambulatory peritoneal dialysis patient. Am J Kidney Dis 1987;9:84–86.
365. Padilla B, Pollak VE, Pesce A, et al. Pancreatitis in patients with end-stage renal disease. Medicine 1994;73:8–20.
366. Evans DB, Slapak M. Pancreatitis in the hard water syndrome. Br Med J 1975;3:748.
367. Hochgelerent EL, David DS. Acute pancreatitis secondary to calcium infusion in a dialysis patient. Arch Surg 1974;108: 218–219.

**Hemolysis and Mismatched Blood Transfusion**

368. Daul AE, Schafers RF, Wenzel RR, et al. Acute hemolysis with subsequent life-threatening pancreatitis in hemodialysis. A complication which is not preventable with current dialysis equipment. Dtsch Med Wochenschr 1994;119:1263–1269.
369. Walker JF, Cronin CJ, Donohoe JF, et al. Acute severe intravascular haemolysis: an unrecognized cause of pancreatitis. Br Med J 1981;282:1929.
370. Ackerman LV. Acute pancreatitis following blood transfusion. Arch Pathol 1942;34:1065.
371. Druml W, Laggner AN, Lenz K, et al. Pancreatitis in acute hemolysis. Ann Hematol 1991;63:39–41.

**Porphyria**

372. Saint EG, Curnow D, Paton R. Diagnosis of acute porphyria. Br Med J 1954;1:1182–1184.
373. Joske RA. Aetiological factors in the pancreatitis syndrome. Br Med J 1955;2:1477–1481.
374. Shiraki K, Takase K, Tameda Y, Kosaka Y. Acute pancreatitis associated with acute intermittent porphyria (Japanese). Nippon Rinsho 1995;53:1479–1483.

**Glycogen Storage Disease**

375. Michaels VV, Beaudet AL. Hemorrhagic pancreatitis in a patient with glycogen storage disease, type 1. Clin Genet 1980;17: 220–222.
376. Herman TE. Type 1A glycogenosis with acute pancreatitis. J Radiol 1995;76:51–53.
377. Yoshioka M, et al. Pancreatitis in a case of glycogen storage disease type 1. Intern Med 1982;50:765–773.
378. Ohtani T, et al. Acute hemorrhagic pancreatitis in a patient with glycogen storage disease, type 1. J Jpn Pediatr Soc 1985;89: 838–844.
379. Kikuchi M, Hasegawa K, Handa I, et al. Chronic pancreatitis in a child with glycogen storage disease (type 1). Eur J Pediatr 1991;150:852–853.
380. Weizman Z, Picard E, Barki Y, Moses S. Wilson's disease associated with pancreatitis. J Pediatr Gastroenterol Nutr 1988;7: 931–933.
381. Minns RA, Eden OB, Hendry GM. Pancreatic enlargement and Wilson's disease (Letter). Lancet 1982;2:337–338.
382. Scheinberg IH, Sternlieb I. Wilson's disease. In: Smith LH, ed. Major problems in internal medicine. Philadelphia: WB Saunders, 1984:111–113.

**Diabetic Ketoacidosis**

383. Slyper AH, Wyatt DT, Brown CW. Clinical and/or biochemical pancreatitis in diabetic ketoacidosis. J Pediatr Endocrinol 1994; 7:261–264.

**Organic Acidemias**

384. Kahlen SG, Sherwood WG, Woolf D, et al. Pancreatitis in patients with organic acidemias. J Pediatr 1944;124:239–243.
385. Burlina AB, Dionisi-Vici C, Piovan S, et al. Acute pancreatitis in propionic acidaemia. J Inherited Metab Dis 1995;18:169–172.
386. Collins JE, Brenton DP. Pancreatitis and homocystinuria. J Inherited Metab Dis 1990;13:232–233.
387. Ilan Y, Eid A, Rivkind AI, et al. Gastrointestinal involvement in homocystinuria. J Gastroenterol Hepatol 1993;8:60–62.
388. Gross JB, Gambill EE, Ulrich JA. Hereditary pancreatitis. Am J Med 1962;33:358.

**Pancreatitis in Long-Distance Runners**

389. Erlan A, Schneider FE. Acute pancreatitis in long-distance runners. Am J Gastroenterol 1995;90:70–71.

**Pancreatitis with Sickle Cell Disease**

390. Kumar A, Posner G, Marsh F, et al. Acute pancreatitis in sickle cell crisis. J Natl Med Assoc 1989;81:91–92.
391. Berman LG, Dunn E, Straehley CJ. Survey of pancreatitis, Central New York Surgical Society. Gastroenterology 1961;40:94.
392. Song J. Pathology of sickle cell disease. Springfield, IL: Charles C Thomas, 1971:355–367.
393. Ziegler DW, Long JA, Philippart AI, Klein MD. Pancreatitis in childhood. Experience with 49 patients. Arch Surg 1988;207: 257–261.
394. Sheehan AG, Machida H, Butzner JD. Acute pancreatitis in a child with sickle cell anemia. J Natl Med Assoc 1993;85:70–72.
395. Olsen H. Thrombotic thrombocytopenic purpura as a cause of pancreatitis. Report of a case and review of the literature. Am J Dig Dis 1973;18:238–246.
396. Petros P, et al. Recurrent pancreatitis in juvenile dermatomyositis. Orv Hetil 1989;130:1937–1939.

**Juvenile Dermatomyositis and Ehlers-Danlos Syndrome**

397. Sarra-Carbonell S, Jimenez SA. Ehlers-Danlos syndrome associated with acute pancreatitis. J Rheumatol 1989;16:1390–1394.

**Polyarthritis and Behcet's Syndrome**

398. Ferrari R, Wendelboe M, Ford PM, et al. Pancreatitis arthritis with periarticular fat necrosis. J Rheumatol 1993;20:1436–1437.
399. O'Duffy JD, Carney JA, Deodhar S. Behcet's disease. Report of 10 cases, 3 with new manifestation. Ann Intern Med 1971;75: 561–570.
400. LeThi HD, Wechsler B, Dell Isola B, et al. Acute pancreatitis in Behcet's disease. Dig Dis Sci 1992;37:1452–1453.
401. Lakhanpal S, Tani K, Lie JT, et al. Pathologic features of Behcet's syndrome: a review of Japanese autopsy registry data. Hum Pathol 1985;16:790–795.

**Low-Flow States**

402. Hranilovich GT, Baggenstoss AH. Lesions of the pancreas in malignant hypertension. Review of 100 cases at necropsy. Arch Pathol 1953;55:443.
403. Howard JM. Pancreatitis: multiple diseases with multiple causes. In: Howard JM, Jordan GL Jr, Reber HA, eds. Surgical diseases of the pancreas. Philadelphia: Lea & Febinger, 1987:207–208.
404. Sano ME, Smith LW. A critical histopathologic study. Fifty post-mortem patients with cancer subjected to local or generalized refrigeration. J Lab Clin Med 1940;26:443–450.
405. Joske RA. Aetiological factors in the pancreatitis syndrome. Br Med J 1955;2:1477–1481.
406. Hyman PE, Brennan MF, Head G, McCarthy DM. Hyperamylasemia, duodenal duplication, and pleural effusion in hereditary spherocytosis. Dig Dis Sci 1981;26:81–84.
407. Hendren WH, Greep JM, Patton AS. Pancreatitis in childhood: Experiences with 15 cases. Arch Dis Child 1965;40:132.
408. Tasman-Jones C. Pancreatitis-aetiological associations. NZ Med J 1971;73:283–284.
409. Kennedy JD, Talbot IC, Tanner MS. Severe pancreatitis and fatty liver progressing to cirrhosis associated with coxsackie B4 infection in a three-year-old with alpha-1-antitrypsin deficiency. Acta Pediatr Scand 1986;75:336–339.
410. Case records of the Mass Gen Hosp. N Engl J Med 1973;289: 1360.
411. Svenberg T, Haggmark T, Strandvik B, Slezak P. Haemorrhagic pancreatitis after ERCP in patients with alpha-1-antitrypsin deficiency. Lancet 1988;1:772.
412. Novis BH, Young GO, Bank S, Marks IN. Chronic pancreatitis and alpha-1-antitrypsin. Lancet 1975;2:748–749.
413. Mihas AA, Hirschowitz BI. Alpha-1-antitrypsin and chronic pancreatitis. Lancet 1976;2:1032–1033.
414. Rabassa AA, Schwartz MR, Ertan A. Alpha-1-antitrypsin deficiency and chronic pancreatitis. Dig Dis Sci 1995;40:1997–2001.

**Werner's Syndrome**

415. Naafs MA, Schouwink H, Roeleveld GG, et al. Acute pancreatitis in a case of Werner's syndrome with severe hyperlipidemia. Neth J Med 1989;34:194–199.

**Carnitive Palmitoyl Transferase Deficiency**

416. Tein I, Christodoulou J, Donner E, McInnes RR. Carnitine palmi-

toyltransferase II deficiency: a new cause of recurrent pancreatitis. J Pediatr 1994;124:938–940.
417. Rotig AA, Cormier V, Blanche S, et al. Pearson's marrow-pancreas syndrome: a multisystem mitochondrial disorder in infancy. J Clin Invest 1990;86:1601–1608.

**Pregnancy and Postpartum Period**

418. Langmade CF, Edmondson HA. Acute pancreatitis during pregnancy and the postpartum period. A report of nine cases. Surg Gynecol Obstet 1951;92:43–52.
419. Montgomery WH, Miller FC. Pancreatitis and pregnancy. Obstet Gynecol 1970;35:658–664.
420. Corlett RC Jr, Mishell DR Jr. Pancreatitis in pregnancy. Am J Obstet Gynecol 1972;113:281–290.
421. Makay AJ, O Neill J, Imrie CW. Pancreatitis, pregnancy and gallstones. Br J Obstet Gynecol 1980;87:47–50.
422. Legro RS, Laifer SA. First-trimester pancreatitis. Maternal and neonatal outcome. J Reprod Med 1995;40:689–695.
423. Wilkinson EJ. Acute pancreatitis in pregnancy, a review of 98 cases and a report of 8 new cases. Obstet Gynecol Surv 1973;28:281–303.
424. Nies BM, Dreiss RJ. Hyperlipidemic pancreatitis in pregnancy. A case report and review of the literature. Am J Perinatol 1990;7:166–169.
425. Beattie GJ, Keay S, Muir BB, Boddy K. Acute pancreatitis with pseudocyst formation complicating pregnancy in a patient with a co-existent choledochal cyst. Br J Obstet Gyncol 1993;100:957–959.
426. Flege JB. Ruptured tubal pregnancy with elevated serum amylase levels. Arch Surg 1966;92:397–398.
427. Steinmetz OK, Hashim E, Falcone T, et al. Recurrent pancreatitis associated with in vitro fertilization. Obstet Gynecol 1993;81: 890–892.
428. Shaffer J. Allergic pancreatitis. Permanente Found Med Bull 1948;6:204.
429. Cutler AF, Yousif EA, Blumenkehl ML. Hereditary angio-edema associated with pancreatitis. South Med J 1992;85:1149–1150.
430. Brickman CM, Tsokos GC, Balow JE, et al. Immunoregulatory disorders associated with hereditary angioedema. Clinical manifestations of autoimmune disease. J Allergy Clin Immunol 1986;77:749–757.
431. Vazquez-Rodriguez JJ, Soleto Saez E, Sanchez Vega J, et al. Pancreatitis and eosinophilic gastroenteritis. Int Surg 1973;58: 415–419.
432. Hashimoto F. Transient eosinophilia associated with pancreatitis and pseudocyst formation. Arch Intern Med 1980;140:1099–1100.
433. Flejou JF, Potet F, Bernades P. Eosinophilic pancreatitis: a rare manifestation of digestive allergy? Gastroenterol Clin Biol 1989; 13:731–733.
434. Bastid C, Sahel J, Choux R, et al. Eosinophilic pancreatitis: report of a case. Pancreas 1990;5:104–107.
435. Eugene C, Gury B, Bergue A, et al. Jaundice caused by eosinophilic pancreatitis as the major first symptom in a case of idiopathic hypereosinophilic syndrome. Gastroenterol Clin Biol 1984;8:966–969.
436. Ryan KG. Eosinophilic infiltration of duodenum and pancreatic head; report of a case studied arteriographically. Surgery 1975;77:321–324.
437. Barresi G, Inferrera C, DeLuca F. Eosinophilic pancreatitis in the newborn infant of a diabetic mother. Virchows Arch (A) 1978;380:341–348.
438. Chaun H, King DM, Gofton JP, et al. Sarcoidosis of the pancreas. Am J Dig Dis 1972;17:725–730.
439. Friedman HZ, Weinstein RA. Sarcoidosis of the pancreas. Arch Intern Med 1983;143;2182–2183.
440. Essop AR, Posen J, Segal I, Pantanowitz D. Isolated granulomatous pancreatitis. J Clin Gastroenterol 1984;6:61–64.
441. Stürmer J, Becker V. Granulomatous pancreatitis—granulomas in chronic pancreatitis. Virchows Arch (A) 1987;410:327–338.
442. Curran J, Curren J. Boeck's sarcoid of the pancreas. Surgery 1950;28:574–578.
443. Ryrie DR. Sarcoidosis with obstructive jaundice. Proc R Soc Med 1954;47:897.
444. Chauen H, King DM, Gofton JP, et al. Sarcoidosis of the pancreas. Am J Dig Dis 1972;17:725–730.
445. Caldwell JH, Evans WE. Granuloma (sarcoid?) of the pancreas. A case report. Am J Gastroenterol 1978;69:320–322.
446. McCormick PA, Malone D, Fitzgerald M, Fitzgerald O. Pancreatitis in sarcoidosis. Br Med J 1985;290:1472–1473.
447. Biedermann G. Differential diagnosis of a non-epithelial tumor in the region of the Bauchspeicheldruse. (Quoted in ref 441) Inaugural dissertation (med), Erlangen, 1985.
448. Stolte M. Chronic pancreatitis, morphology, pancreatogram, differential diagnosis. Erlangen: Perimed, 1984. (Cited in ref 441.)
449. Becker V, Lux G. Pathologe und Internist. Verh Dtsch Ges Inn Med 1985;91:104–114.
450. Veghelyi PV. Secondary pancreatitis. Am J Dis Child 1947;74:45.

**Primary Pyogenic Cholangitis and Pancreatitis**

451. Digby KH. Common duct stones of liver origin. Br J Surg 1930;17:578–591.
452. Cook H, et al. Recurrent pyogenic cholangitis. Br J Surg 1954;42:188.
453. Koo J, Ong GB. Pancreatitis in India and the Orient. In: Howard JM, Jordan GL, Reber HA, eds. Surgical diseases of the pancreas. Philadelphia: Lea & Febiger, 1987:250–256.

***Staphylococcus* and Pancreatitis**

454. Thal A, Molestina JE. Studies on pancreatitis; fulminating hemorrhagic pancreatic necrosis produced by means of staphylococcal toxin. Arch Pathol 1955;60:212–220.
455. Flexner S. Experimental pancreatitis. John Hopkins Hosp Rep 1900;9:743–771.
456. Hlava J. 1898. (Cited in Opie EL. Diseases of the pancreas. 2nd ed. Philadelphia: JB Lippincott, 1910:125.)

**Food Poisoning: *Salmonella* and Hemolytic *Streptococcus***

457. Renner F, Nimeth C, Demmelbauer N. High frequency of concomitant pancreatitis in salmonella enteritis. Lancet 1991; 337:1611.
458. Boyd JF. Salmonella typhimurium, colitis, and pancreatitis. Lancet 1969;2:901–902.
459. Honegr K, Dite P, Dulicek K, et al. Salmonella typhimurium in the etiology of acute pancreatitis. CS Gastroent Vyz 1981;35(8): 387–390.
460. Murphy S, Beeching NJ, Rogerson SJ, Harries AD. Pancreatitis associated with salmonella enteritis. Lancet 1991;338:571.
461. Andren-Sandberg A, Hojer H. Necrotizing acute pancreatitis induced by Salmonella infection. Int J Pancreatol 1994;15: 229–230.
462. Strand CL, Sanders SL. Salmonella typhimurium pancreatic abscess: report of a case. Am Surg 1978;44:174–176.
463. Gibb AP, Lewin CS, Garden OJ. Development of quinolone resistance and multiple antibiotic resistance in salmonella bovismorbificans in pancreatic abscess (Letter). J Antimicrob Chemother 1991;28:318–321.
464. Abdulla AJJ, Moorhead JF, Sweny P. Acute tubular necrosis due to rhabdomyolysis and pancreatitis associated with salmonella enteritidis food poisoning (Letter). Nephrol Dial Transplant 1993; 8:672–673.
465. Pastore M, Pellegrino M, Maruzzi M, et al. Pancreatitis associated with salmonella (Italian). Minerva Pediatr 1993;45:471–473.
466. Koller O. Acute interstitial pancreatitis provoked by haemolytic streptococci in infected food (fish). Acta Chir Scand 1947;95: 358–366.

**Typhoid Fever and Pancreatitis**

467. Russell IJ, Forgacs P, Geraci JE. Pancreatitis complicating typhoid fever. Report of a case. JAMA 1976;235:753–754.
468. Christian HA. Osler's principles and practice of medicine. 15th ed. New York: D. Appleton Century, 1944:145. (Quoted in 467).
469. Sedallian P, Monnet P, Brete R. A case of typhoid pancreatitis. Lyon Med 1947;177:432–434.
470. Monad-Broca P, Auzepy P, Lesourd G, et al. Pancreatitie aigue typhique verifiee operatoirement: guerison. Mem Acad Chir 1967;93:779–783.
471. Borisova MA, Krylova AM, Rybka IN, et al. Pancreatitis as a

rare complication of abdominal typhoid. Vrach Delo 1977;9: 140–142.
472. Kune GA, Coster D. Typhoid pancreatic abscess. Med J Aust 1972;1:417–418.
473. Spay G, Savoye B, Rahimi N. Typhoid and pancreatitis. Typhique pancreatitis? Apropos of a case. J Med Lyon 1971;52:1741–1742.
474. Lemanczy M, Kaminska E, Wejchert K. Adnexitis in the course of typhoid fever in a 13-year-old girl (Polish). Pediatr Pol 1974;49: 1027–1028.
475. Hermans P, Gerard M, Dewit S, van Laethem Y. Pancreatitis and typhoid fever. Am J Med 1990;89:546–547.
476. Garg P, Parashar S. Pancreatic abscess due to salmonella typhi. Postgrad Med J 1992;68:294–295.
477. Rubtzov IV. (Cited in ref 471.)
478. Hearne SE, Whigham TE, Brady CE III. Pancreatitis and typhoid fever. Am J Med 1989;86:471–473.
479. Mandell G, ed. Principles and practice of infectious disease. New York: John Wiley and Sons, 1985.
480. Ginsburg C, Raffenne L. Typhoid fever complicated by acute renal failure, by rhabdomyolysis and by acute pancreatitis (Letter). Rev Med Intern 1989;10:279–280.
481. Whigham TE, Brady CE III. Letter. Am J Med 1990;89:547.

**Pancreatitis after Typhoid and Cholera Vaccination**

482. Gatt DT. Pancreatitis following monovalent typhoid and cholera vaccinations. Br J Clin Pract 1986;40:300–301.

**Leptospirosis and Pancreatitis**

483. Stolze E, et al. Weil's disease associated with pancreatic necrosis. Trop Geogr Med 1959;2:93–95.
484. Bell MJ, Ternberg JL, Feigin RD. Surgical complications of leptospirosis in children. J Pediatr Surg 1978;13:325–330.
485. Edwards CN, Evarard CO. Hyperamylasemia in pancreatitis in leptospirosis. Am J Gastroenterol 1991;86:1665–1668.
486. Edwards CN, Nicholson GD, Hassell TA, et al. Penicillin therapy in icteric leptospirosis. Am J Trop Med Hyg 1988;39:388–390.
487. Ribiczey P, Szekeres I, Tureczi I. Acute pancreatitis as a complication of leptospirosis. Orv Hetil 1988;129:1367–1369.
488. Jasperson D, Hammar CH, Fassbinder W. Jaundice and pancreatitis in a 50 year-old patient (Leptospirosis iceterohaemorrhagica), (clinical conference) (German). Med Klin 1991;86: 518–520.
489. Jaspersen D. Pancreatitis associated with Weil's disease (Letter). Dtsch Med Wocheschr 1991;116:559.
490. Monno S, Mizushima Y. Leptospirosis with acute acalculous cholecystitis and pancreatitis. J Clin Gastroenterol 1993;16: 52–54.
491. Primachenko NB, Beliak GM, Biriukov IS. Rare complications in leptospirosis. Klin Med (Mosk) 1986;64(4):129–131.

***Campylobacter* Pancreatitis**

492. Gallagher P, Chadwick P, Jones DM, Turner L. Acute pancreatitis associated with campylobacter infection. Br J Surg 1981;68:383.
493. de Bois MHW, Schoemaker MC, van der Werf SDJ, et al. Pancreatitis associated with campylobacter jejuni infection: diagnosis by ultrasonography. Br Med J 1989;298:1004.
494. Pitkänen T, Pönkä A, Pettersson T, Kosunen TU. Campylobacter enteritis in 188 hospitalized patients. Arch Intern Med 1983;143: 215–219.
495. Felton JM, Harries AD, Beeching NJ, et al. Acute gastroenteritis: The need to remember alternative diagnoses. Postgrad Med J 1990;66:1037–1039.

**Brucellosis**

496. al-Awadhi NZ, Ashkenani F, Khalaf ES. Acute pancreatitis associated with brucellosis. Am J Gastroenterol 1989;84:1570–1574.

***Yersinia*-Associated Pancreatitis**

497. Pettersson T, Gordin R. Yersinia enterocolitica Infection as a possible cause of gallbladder and pancreatic disease. Ann Clin Res 1970;2:157–160.
498. Schultz TB. Association of pancreas affection and yersiniosis. Acta Med Scand 1979;205:255–256.
499. Lindholt J, Hansen PT. Yersiniosis as a possible cause of acute pancreatitis. Acta Chir Scand 1985;151:703.
500. Saebo A, Lassen J. Acute and chronic pancreatic disease associated with yersina enterocolitica infection. A Norwegian 10-year follow-up study of 458 hospitalized patients. J Intern Med 1992;231:537–541.

**Tuberculosis and Pancreatitis**

501. Rushing JL, Hanna CJ, Selecky PA. Pancreatitis as the presenting manifestation of military tuberculosis. West J Med 1978;129: 432–436.
502. Biehl JP. Military tuberculosis: a review of 68 adult patients admitted to a municipal general hospital. Am Rev Tuberc 1958;77:605–622.
503. Auerbach O. Acute generalized military tuberculosis. Am J Pathol 1944;20:121–136.
504. Fan ST, Yan KW, Lau WY, Wong KK. Tuberculosis of the pancreas: a rare cause of massive gastrointestinal bleeding. Br J Surg 1986;73:373.
505. Stock KP, Riemann JF, Stadler W, Rösch W. Tuberculosis of the pancreas. Endoscopy 1981;13:178–180.
506. Mann M, Stoger F. Rare case of tuberculosis of the pancreas treated by duodenopancreatectomy. Rozhl Chir 1966;45:96–99.
507. Crowson MC, Perry M, Burden E. Tuberculosis of the pancreas: a rare cause of obstructive jaundice. Br J Surg 1984;71:239.
508. Knowles KF, Saltman D, Robson HG, Lalonde R. Tuberculous pancreatitis. Tubercle 1990;71:65–68.
509. Van Valzah SL. Tuberculosis of the pancreas. Am Rev Tuberc 1924;9:409–417.
510. Little RL. Tuberculosis of the Pancreas. N Engl J Med 1949;222: 135–137.
511. Stambler JB, Klibaner MI, Bliss CM, LaMont JT. Tuberculous abscess of the pancreas. Gastroenterology 1982;83:922–925.
512. Brehant J. A case of primary tuberculosis of the pancreas. Presse Med 1950;58:1479–1481.
513. Spay G, Latif M. Tuberculosis of the pancreas. Lyon Med 1973;229:480–491.
514. de Miguel F, Beltran J, Sabas JA, et al. Tuberculous pancreatic abscess. Br J Surg 1985;72:438.
515. Pierruges R, Bories P, Marrel E, et al. Pseudo-tumeur du pancréas par tuberculose ganglionnaire bilio-pancréatique. Presse Med 1986;15:2201–2203.
516. Chandrasekhara KL, Iyer SK, Stanek AE, Herbstman H. Pancreatic tuberculosis mimicking carcinoma. Gastrointest Endosc 1985;31:386–388.
517. Danne O, Mehaut M, Gouerou H, et al. Tuberculose péri-pancréatique. Sem Hop Paris 1977;53:703–706.
518. Mourad FH, McLean A, Farthing MJ. Tuberculous pancreatitis: a diagnostic problem. Case report and review of the literature. J Clin Gastroenterol 1995;20:237–240.
519. Habscheid W. Tuberculosis of the pancreas region (Letter). Dtsch Med Wochenschr 1986;111:1988–1989.
520. Houston S. Tuberculous pancreatitis and AIDS (Letter). Tubercle 1991;72:73.
521. Pateron D, Naveau S, Brivet F, et al. Acute tuberculous pancreatitis in a patient with acquired immunodeficiency syndrome. Gastroenterol Clin Biol 1990;14:80–83.
522. Ezratty A, Gumasti V, Rose E, et al. Pancreatic tuberculosis: a frequently fatal but potentially curable disease. J Clin Gastroenterol 1990;12:74–77.
523. Cho KC, Lucak SL, Delany HM, et al. CT appearance in tuberculous pancreatic abscess. J Comput Assist Tomogr 1990; 14:152–154.
524. Berson BD, Mendelson DS, Janus CL. Tuberculous abscess of the pancreas in AIDS: CT findings. Mt Sinai J Med 1989;56:297–299.
525. Tetzeli JP, Pisegna JR, Barkin JS. Tuberculous pancreatic abscess as a manifestation of AIDS (Letter). Am J Gastroenterol 1989;84: 581–582.
526. Meinke AK. Pancreatic tuberculous abscess. Conn Med 1989; 53:139–141.
527. Mokoena T, Bairagi N. Acute tuberculous pancreatitis associated with HIV infection. Trop Doct 1994;24:172–173.

**Legionnaires' Disease and Pancreatitis**

528. Gordan V, Zmyslinski RW. Legionnaires' disease complicated by acute pancreatitis (Case Report). Milit Med 1980;145:345–347.
529. Michel O, Naeije N, Csoma M. Acute pancreatitis in legion-

naires' disease. Eur J Resp Dis 1985;66:62–64.

530. Arneborn P, Kallings I. Acute pancreatitis possibly caused by Legionella micdadei. Scand J Infect Dis 1985;17:229–231.
531. Westblom TU, Hamory BH. Acute pancreatitis caused by Legionella pneumophila. South Med J 1988;81:1200–1201.
532. Jespersen C, Engbaek K. Legionnaires' disease with pancreatic involvement. Ugeskr Laeger 1982;144:158.
533. Eitrem R, Forsgren A, Nilsson C. Pneumonia and acute pancreatitis most probably caused by Legionella longbeachae infection. Scand J Infect Dis 1987;19:381–382.
534. Kesavan CR, Pitchumoni CS, Marino WD. Acute painless pancreatitis as a rare complication in legionnaire's disease (Letter). Am J Gastroenterol 1993;88:468–469.

**Clostridial Pancreatitis**

535. Steiner MM, Tracy PC. Diabetic coma, acute pancreatitis and bacillus welchii peritonitis. Am J Dis Child 1943;65:36–45.
536. Howard JM, Campbell EW. Fatal clostridial pancreatitis following ERCP and percutaneous needle biopsy. Int J Pancreatol 1989;5:305–310.
537. Morton AL, Taylor EW. Fatal clostridial pancreatitis following transduodenal biopsy of the pancreas. J R Coll Surg Edinb 1990;35(4):254.
538. Leinikki P, Pantzar P, Tykkä H. Antibody response in patients with acute pancreatitis to mycoplasma pneumoniae. Scand J Gastroenterol 1973;8:631–635.
539. Haddock G, Coupar G, Youngson GG, et al. Acute pancreatitis in children: a 15-year review. J Pediatr Surg 1994;29:719–722.
540. Capner P, Lendrum R, Jeffries DJ, Walker G. Viral antibody studies in pancreatic disease. Gut 1975;16:866.

**Herpes Simplex**

541. Rand KH. Isolation of herpes simplex virus type 1 from gastric contents of a patient with acute pancreatitis. South Med J 1981;74:489–491.

**Herpes Varicella-Zoster**

542. Coelho JC, Wiederkehr JC, Campos AC, et al. Acute pancreatitis caused by varicella-zoster virus. J Chir (Paris) 1994;131: 96–98.
543. Wacker P, Hartmann O, Benhamou E, et al. Varicella-zoster virus infections after autologous bone marrow transplantation in children. Bone Marrow Transplant 1989;4:191–194.
544. Kirschner S, Raufman J-P. Varicella pancreatitis complicated by pancreatic pseudocyst and duodenal obstruction. Dig Dis Sci 1988;33:1192–1195.

**Pancreatitis with Reye Syndrome and Influenza Virus**

545. Balistreri WF. Reye's syndrome. In: Behrman RE, ed. Nelson textbook of pediatrics. 14th ed. Philadelphia: WB Saunders, 1992:1020–1021.
546. Morens DM, Hammar SL, Heicher DA. Idiopathic acute pancreatitis in children. Am J Dis Child 1974;128:401.
547. DeVivo DC, Keating JP. Reye's syndrome. Adv Pediatr 1976; 22:175.
548. Ellis GH, Mirkin LD, Mills MC. Pancreatitis and Reye's syndrome. Am J Dis Child 1979;133:1014.
549. Glassman M, Tahan S, Hillemeier C, et al. Pancreatitis in patients with Reye's syndrome. J Clin Gastroenterol 1981;3: 165–169.
550. Stover SL, Wanglee P, Kennedy C. Acute hemorrhagic pancreatitis and other visceral changes associated with acute encephalopathy. J Pediatr 1968;73:235–241.
551. Glick TH, Likosky WH, Levitt LP, et al. Reye's syndrome: an epidemiologic approach. Pediatrics 1970;46:371.
552. Gilboa N. Reye's syndrome and pancreatitis (Letter). Am J Dis Child 1980;134:903.
553. Chaves-Carballo E, Menezes AH, Bell WE, Hernriquez EM. Acute pancreatitis in Reye's syndrome: a fatal complication during intensive supportive care. South Med J 1980;73:152.
554. Pascual Velasco F. Influenza A virus and acute pancreatitis (Letter). Med Clin (Barc) 1989;92:516.

**Measles Pancreatitis**

555. Miralbés M, Garreta J, Manonelles A, et al. Acute pancreatitis induced by the measles virus: a case report (Letter). Pancreas 1995;11:101–102.
556. Sibert JR. Pancreatitis in children. A study in the north of England. Arch Dis Child 1975;50:443–448.
557. Sherman FE, Michaels RH, Kenny FM. Acute encephalopathy (encephalitis) complicating rubella. JAMA 1965;192:675.
558. Bunnell CE, Gilles R, Monif G. Interstitial pancreatitis in the congenital rubella syndrome. J Pediatr 1972;80:465.

**Smallpox and Pancreatitis (Variola and Vaccinia)**

559. Marczynska-Robowska M. Pancreatic necrosis in a case of Still's disease. Lancet 1957;1:815.
560. Paradinas FJ, Wiltshaw E. Necropsy findings in a case of progressive vaccinia. J Clin Pathol 1972;25:233–239.
561. Hall GFM, Cunliffe AC, Dudgeon JA. Prolonged generalized vaccinia. J Pathol Bacteriol 1953;66:25–38.

**Common Cold**

562. Mitov F, Paunov B. Acute pancreatitis in an 11-year-old boy as a complication from viral common cold. Khirurgiia (Sofiia) 1969;22:203–204.

**Mumps Pancreatitis**

563. Harris HF. A case of diabetic mellitus quickly following mumps. Boston Med Surg J 1899;140:465–469.
564. Farnam LW. Pancreatitis following mumps: report of a case with operation. Am J Med Sci 1922;163:859.
565. Trapnell JE, Duncan EHL. Patterns of incidence of acute pancreatitis. Br Med J 1975;2:179.
566. Berman LG, Dunn E, Straehley CJ. Survey of pancreatitis, Central New York Surgical Society. Gastroenterology 1961;40:94.
567. Joshi RA, Probstein JG, Blumenthal HT. A survey of experience with 300 clinical and 108 autopsy cases of acute pancreatitis. Am Surg 1957;23:34.
568. Brahdy MB, Scheffer IH. Pancreatitis complicating mumps. Am J Med Sci 1931;181:255.
569. Sharon P, Melmed S, Neuman G. Acute pancreatitis in a community with a low alcohol intake. Int Surg 1979;64: 63–66.
570. Imrie CW, Ferguson JC, Sommerville RG. Coxsackie and mumps virus infection in a prospective study of acute pancreatitis. Gut 1977;18:53.
571. Eagles AY. Analysis of a four year epidemic of the mumps. Arch Intern Med 1947;80:374.
572. Witte CL, Schanzer B. Pancreatitis due to mumps. JAMA 1968;203:1068–1069.
573. Zelman S. Blood disease values in mumps and mumps pancreatitis. JAMA 1944;207:461.
574. Tasman-Jones C. Pancreatitis-aetiological associations. NZ Med J 1971;73: 283–284.
575. Naficy K, Nategh R, Ghadimi H. Mumps pancreatitis without parotitis. Br Med J 1973;1:529.
576. Laraya-Cuasay LR, Wolfe R, Hughes WT. Acute pancreatitis and hypoglycemia. Clin Pediatr 1968;7:525–528.
577. Joske RA. Aetiological factors in the pancreatitis syndrome. Br Med J 1955;2:1477.
578. Wood CB, Bradbrook RA, Blumgart LH. Chronic pancreatitis in childhood associated with mumps virus infection. Br J Clin Pract 1974;28:67–69.
579. Graham JR. Mumps causing chronic calcific pancreatitis (Letter). Med J Aust 1980;2:454.

**Viral Vaccine–Induced Pancreatitis**

580. Adler JB, Mazzota SA, Barkin JS. Pancreatitis caused by measles, mumps, and rubella vaccine. Pancreas 1991;6:489–490.
581. Cebriá L, Roldán FP, Sánchez E, et al. Acute pancreatitis caused by parotiditis vaccine (Letter). Pancreas 1994;9:390–391.

**Coxsackie B and Echo Virus Pancreatitis**

582. Nakao T, et al. Clinical and epidemiological studies on an outbreak of aseptic meningitis caused by coxsackie B-5 and A-9 viruses in Amori in 1961. Tohoku J Exp Med 1964;83:94.
583. Ross ME, Hayashi K, Notkins AL. Virus-induced pancreatic disease: alterations and concentration of glucose and amylase in blood. J Infect Dis 1974;129:669–676.

584. Fechner RE, Smith MG, Middlekamp JN. Coxsackie B virus infection of the newborn. Am J Pathol 1963;42:493.
585. Imrie CW, Ferguson JC, Sommervile RG. Coxsackie and mumps virus infection in a prospective study of acute pancreatitis. Gut 1977;18:53–56.
586. Murphy AM, Simmul R. Coxsackie B4 virus infections in New South Wales during 1962. Med J Aust 1964;2:443.
587. Ursing B. Acute pancreatitis in coxsackie B infection. Br Med J 1973;3:524.
588. Capner P, Lendrum R, Jeffries DJ, Walker G. Viral antibody studies in pancreatic disease. Gut 1975;16:866–870.
589. Kibrick S, Benirschke K. Severe generalized disease (Encephalohepatomyocarditis) occurring in the newborn period and due to infection with coxsackie virus, group B. Pediatrics 1958; 22:857.
590. Kennedy JD, Talbot IC, Tanner MS. Severe pancreatitis and fatty liver progressing to cirrhosis associated with coxsackie B4 infection in a three-year-old with alpha-1-antitrypsin deficiency. Acta Paediatr Scand 1986;75:336–339.
591. Ozsvar Z, Deak J, Pap A. Possible role of coxsackie-B virus infection in pancreatitis. Int J Pancreatol 1992;11:105–108.
592. Arnesjo B, Eden T, Ihse I, et al. Enterovirus infections in acute pancreatitis—a possible etiological connection. Scand J Gastroenterol 1976;11:645–649.

***Mycoplasma pneumoniae***

593. Hayflick L. Biology of the mycoplasma (Opening remarks). Ann NY Acad Sci 1967;143:5–6.
594. Mardh PA, Ursing B. The occurrence of acute pancreatitis in mycoplasma pneumoniae infection. Scand J Infect Dis 1974;6: 167–171.
595. Freeman R, McMahon MJ. Acute pancreatitis and serological evidence of infection with Mycoplasma pneumoniae. Gut 1978;19:367.
596. Oderda G, Kraut JR. Rising antibody titer to mycoplasma pneumoniae in acute pancreatitis. Pediatrics 1980;66:305–306.
596a. Herbaut C, Tielemans C, Burette A, Dratwa M. Mycoplasma pneumoniae infection and acute pancreatitis. Acta Clin Belg 1983;38:186–188.

**Infectious Mononucleosis**

597. Myhre J, Nesbitt A. Pancreatitis in infectious mononucleosis. J Lab Clin Med 1949;34:1671.
598. Wislocki LC. Acute pancreatitis in infectious mononucleosis. N Engl J Med 1966;275:322–323.
599. Everett ED, Volpe JA, Bergin JJ. Pancreatitis in infectious mononucleosis. South Med J 1969;62:359–360.
600. Werbitt W, Mohsenifar Z. Mononucleosis pancreatitis. South Med J 1980;73:1094.
601. Lifschitz C, LaSala S. Pancreatitis, cholecystitis and choledocholithiasis associated with infectious mononucleosis. Clin Pediatr 1981;20:131.
602. Hedstrom SA, Belfrage I. Acute pancreatitis in two cases of infectious mononucleosis. Scand J Infect Dis 1976;8:124–126.

**Pancreatitis Associated with Infectious Hepatitis**

603. Lisney AA: Infective hepatitis in Leichestershire: a survey of 1,062 cases. Proc R Soc Med 1943;37:165.
604. Achord JL. Acute pancreatitis with infectious hepatitis. JAMA 1968;205:837–840.
605. Geokas MC, Olsen H, Swanson V, Rinderknecht H. The association of viral hepatitis and acute pancreatitis. Calif Med 1972; 117:1.
606. Ham JM, Fitzpatrick P. Acute pancreatitis in patients with acute hepatic failure. Am J Dig Dis 1973;18:1079–1083.
607. Parbhoo SP, Welch J, Sherlock S. Acute pancreatitis in patients with fulminant hepatic failure. Gut 1973;14:428.
608. Wands JR, Salyer DC, Boitnott JK, Maddrey WC. Fulminant hepatitis complicated by pancreatitis. John Hopkins Med J 1973;133:156–160.
609. Lopez Morante A, Rodriguez de Lope C, San Miguel G, Pons Romero I. Acute pancreatitis in hepatitis A infection. Postgrad Med J 1986;62:407–408.
610. Shrier LA, Karpen SJ, McEvoy C. Acute pancreatitis associated with acute hepatitis A in a young child. J Pediatr 1995;126:57–59.
611. Garty BZ, Kanner D, Danon YL. Pancreatitis associated with hepatitis A viral infection (Letter). J Pediatr 1995;127:669.
612. Davis TV, Keeffe EB. Acute pancreatitis associated with acute hepatitis A. Am J Gastroenterol 1992;87:1648–1650.
613. Cadranel JF, Guivarch P, Duvoux C, et al. Pancréatite aiguë au cours d'une hépatitie virale A bénigne. Gastroenterol Clin Biol 1987;11:344–345.
614. Eugene C, Cadranel JF, Bergue A, Anciaux ML. Acute pancreatitis associated with non-A non-B hepatitis. J Clin Gastroenterol 1990;12:195–197.
615. Ede RJ, Moore KP, Marshall WJ, Williams R. Frequency of pancreatitis in fulminant hepatic failure using isoenzyme markers. Gut 1988;29:778–781.
616. Shimoda T, Shikata T, Karasawa T, et al. Light microscopic localization of hepatitis B virus antigens in the human pancreas. Possibility of multiplication of hepatitis B virus in the human pancreas. Gastroenterology 1981;81:998–1005.
617. Cavallari A, Vivarelli M, D'Errico A, et al. Fatal necrotizing pancreatitis caused by hepatitis B virus infection in a liver transplant recipient. J Hepatol 1995;22:685–690.

**Cytomegalovirus Pancreatitis**

618. Margreiter R, Schmid T, Dunser M, et al. Cytomegalovirus (CMV)-pancreatitis: a rare complication after pancreas transplantation. Transplant Proc 1991;23:1619–1622.
619. Wilcox CM, Forsmark CE, Grendell JH, et al. Cytomegalovirus-associated acute pancreatic disease in patients with acquired immunodeficiency syndrome. Gastroenterology 1990;99: 263–267.
620. Iwasaki T, Tashiro A, Satodate R, et al. Acute pancreatitis with cytomegalovirus infection. Acta Pathol Jpn 1987;37:1661–1668.
621. Takayama S. Incidence of cytomegalic inclusion disease. Bull Tokyo Med Dental Univ 1969;16:7–15. (Quoted in ref 620.)
622. Howard JM. Pancreatitis after renal transplantation. In: Howard JM, Jordan GL Jr, Reber HA, eds. Surgical diseases of the pancreas. Philadelphia: Lea & Febinger, 1987:177–178.
623. Yoon JW, Ihm SH, Kim KW. Viruses as a triggering factor of type I diabetes and genetic markers related to the susceptibility to the virus associated diabetes (Review). Diabetes Res Clin Pract 1989;7:S47–S58.
624. Yasumoto N, Hara M, Kitamoto Y, et al. Cytomegalovirus infection associated with acute pancreatitis, rhabdomyolysis and renal failure. Intern Med 1992;31:426–430.

**HIV (AIDS) and Pancreatitis**

625. Zazzo J-F, Pichon F, Regnier B. HIV and the pancreas (Letter). Lancet 1987;2:1212–1213.
626. Bricarie et al. Pancreatic disturbances in AIDS: an anatomopathological study. III International Conference on AIDS, Washington, DC, 1987. (Quoted in ref 625.)
627. Brivet F, Coffin B, Bedossa P, et al. Pancreatic lesions in AIDS (Letter). Lancet 1987;2:570–571.
628. Miller TL, Winter HS, Luginbuhl LM, et al. Pancreatitis in pediatric human immunodeficiency virus infection. J Pediatr 1992;120: 223–227.
629. Cappell MS, Marks S. Acute pancreatitis in HIV-seropositive patients: A case control study of 44 patients. Am J Med 1995;98:243–248.
630. Iredale JP, Arthur MJP, Sterling GM. Pancreatitis in a patient with AIDS. Endoscopy 1993;25:486–487.
631. Clas D, Falutz J, Rosenberg L. Acute pancreatitis associated with HIV infection. Can Med Assoc J 1989;140:823.
632. Bengoa JM, Widgren S. Gastrointestinal manifestation of acquired immunodeficiency syndrome; case studies of 14 patients. Schweiz Med Wochenschr 1986;116:1358–1366.
633. Murthy UK, DeGregorio F, Oates RP, Blair DC. Hyperamylasemia in patients with the acquired immunodeficiency syndrome. Am J Gastroenterol 1992;87:332–336.
634. Cina SJ, Conradi SE. Acute pancreatitis in a prisoner with AIDS. Bugs or drugs? Am J Forensic Med Pathol 1994;15:28–31.
635. Grasela TH, Walawander CA, Beltangady M, et al. Analysis of potential risk factors associated with the development of pancreatitis in phase I patients with AIDS or AIDS-related complex receiving didanosine. J Infect Dis 1994;169:1250–1255.
636. Siedlin M, Lambert JS, Dolin R, Valentine FT. Pancreatitis and

pancreatic dysfunction in patients taking dideoxyinosine. AIDS 1992;6:831–835.
637. Kordossis T, Kosmopoulou O, Tzavaras A, Anevlavis E. Recurrent acute pancreatitis and pancreatic pseudocyst as the presenting manifestation of HIV infection. J Clin Gastroenterol 1995;20: 261–262.
638. Witt MD, Edwards JE Jr. Pancreatic abscess and infected pancreatic pseudocyst: diagnosis and management. In: Remington JS, Swartz MN, eds. Current clinical topics in infectious diseases. Boston: Blackwell Scientific Publications, 1992:111–137.
639. Cappell MS, Hassan T. Pancreatic disease in AIDS—a review. J Clin Gastroenterol 1993;17:254–263.
640. Seidlin M, Lambert JS, Dolin R, Valentine FT. Pancreatitis and pancreatic dysfunction in patients taking dideoxyinosine. AIDS 1992;6:831–835.
641. Lambert JS, Seidlin M, Valentine FT, et al. Didanosine: long-term follow-up of patients in a phase 1 study. Clin Infect Dis 1993;16:S40–45.
642. Moyle GJ, Nelson MR, Hawkins D, Gazzard BG. The use and toxicity of didanosine (ddI) in HIV-antibody-positive individuals intolerant to zidovudine (AZT). Q J Med 1993;86:155–163.
643. Cina SJ, Conradi SE. Acute pancreatitis in a prisoner with AIDS. Bugs or drugs? Am J Forensic Med Pathol 1994;15:28–31.
644. Vendrell J, Nubiola A, Goday A, et al. HIV and the pancreas (Letter). Lancet 1987;2:1212.
645. Torre D, Montanari M, Fiori GP, et al. HIV and the pancreas (Letter). Lancet 1987;2:1212.

**Adenoviral Pancreatitis**

646. Niemann TH, Trigg ME, Winick N, Penick GD. Disseminated adenoviral infection presenting as acute pancreatitis. Hum Pathol 1993;24:1145–1148.

**Acute Pancreatitis Secondary to Parasites Roundworms *(Ascaris lumbricoides)***

647. Novis, IMS. Partial obstruction of the pancreatitis duct by round worms. Br J Surg 1923;10:421.
648. Rigby MH. Acute hemorrhagic pancreatitis: round worm in pancreatic duct. Br J Surg 1923;10:419.
649. Sabrazes J, Parcelier A, Bonnin H. Ann Anat Pathol 1925;2:385.
650. Chen YS, Den BX, Huang BI, Xu LZ. Endoscopic diagnosis and management of ascaris-induced acute pancreatitis. Endoscopy 1986;18:127–128.
651. Shi-hui Z. The migratory ascariasis and ascaris complications-analysis. In: Ye Weifa. Progress in gastroenterology 1982:562. (Cited in ref 650.)
652. Winters C Jr, Chobanian SJ, Benjamin SB, et al. Endoscopic documentation of ascaris-induced pancreatitis. Gastrointest Endosc 1984;30:83–84.
653. Khuroo MS, Zargar SA, Mahajan R. Hepatobiliary and pancreatic ascariasis in India. Lancet 1990;335:1503–1506.
654. Khuroo MS, Zargar SA, Yattoo GN, et al. Ascaris-induced acute pancreatitis. Br J Surg 1992;79:1335–1338.
655. Crompton DW. Ascariasis and its public health significance. London: Taylor and Francis, 1985.
656. Crompton DW. Ascariasis and its prevention and control. London: Taylor and Francis, 1989.
657. Leung JW, Mok SD, Metreweli C. Ascaris-induced pancreatitis. AJR 1987;149:511–512.
658. Ramirez-Degollado J, Peniche-Bojorques J, Olvera-Perez O. Endoscopic cholangiographic diagnosis of ascaris in the common bile duct. Gastrointest Endosc 1977;24:86–87.
659. Das S. Pancreatitis in children associated with round worms. Indian Pediatr 1977;14:81–83.
660. Hsia SH, Chang MH. Ascariasis associated with acute pancreatitis in a child. Acta Pedol Sin 1995;36:128–130.
661. Chen D, Li X. Forty-two patients with acute ascaris pancreatitis in China. J Gastroenterol 1994;29:676–678.
662. Krige JE, Lewis G, Bornman PC. Recurrent pancreatitis caused by a calcified ascaris in the duct of Wirsung. Am J Gastroenterol 1987;82:256–257.

**Tape Worms: *Taenia saginata***

663. Plane P, Ronceray J, Dubin P. Acute pancreatitis from obstruction of Wirsung's canal by Taenia saginata. J Chir 1980;117: 193–194.
664. Delvaux M, Escourrou J, Frexinos J, Ribet A. A propos d'un cas de pancreatite aigue obstructive d'origine inhabituelle. Gastroenterol Clin Biol 1987;11:611–612.
665. Bouteloup C, Michel P, Desechalliers JP, et al. Recurrent acute pancreatitis caused by Taenia saginata. Gastroenterol Clin Biol 1992;16:818–820.

**Liver Fluke *(Clonorchis sinensis)***

666. Nakamura H. Kyoto Igaku Zasshi 1908;5:1. (Quoted in ref 669.)
667. Kawamura R. Arch Pathol Anat 1911;203:420. (Quoted in ref 669.)
668. Hou PC. The pathology of clonorchis sinensis infestation of the liver. J Pathol Bacteriol 1955;70:53–64.
669. Chan PH, Teoh TB. The pathology of Clonorchis sinensis infestation of the pancreas. J Pathol Bacteriol 1967;93:185–189.
670. McFadzean AJ, Yeung RT. Acute pancreatitis due to Clonorchis sinensis. Trans R Soc Trop Med Hyg 1966;60:466–470.
671. Escoffier JM, Gauthier AP, Sarles H. Acute pancreatitis: varieties, etiologies and prognosis. Rev Prat 1981;31:231–234,237–240.
672. Fontaine JP, de la Coussaye JE, Ould-Said A, et al. Acute necrotic hemorrhagic pancreatitis caused by an Asiatic distomiasis. Presse Med 1986;15:1100–1101.
673. Shugar RA, Ryan JJ. Clonorchis sinensis and pancreatitis. Twenty-five years after endemic exposure. Am J Gastroenterol 1975;64:400–403.

**Liver Fluke *(Fasciola hepatica)***

674. Maroy B, Moullot P, Daloubeix H, Mathey JC. Acute pancreatitis complicating biliary distomatosis caused by Fasciola hepatica in a patient with a choledochal diverticulum. Ann Gastroenterol Hepatol 1987;23:67–70.
675. Chitchang S, Mitarnun W, Ratananikom N. Fasciola hepatica in human pancreas. A case report. J Med Assoc Thai 1982;65:345, 348–349. (Quoted in ref 674.)

**Filiarisis *(Wuchereria bancrofti)***

676. Jesudason SR, Mathai V, Muthusami JC, Mathai E. Wuchereria bancrofti induced pancreatitis. Trop Gastroenterol 1992;13: 115–118.

***Toxoplasma gondii***

677. Ahuja SK, Ahuja SS, Thelmo W, et al. Necrotizing pancreatitis and multisystem organ failure associated with toxoplasmosis in a patient with AIDS. Clin Infect Dis 1993;16:432–434.
678. Dowell SF, Moore GW, Hutchins GM. The spectrum of pancreatic pathology in patients with AIDS. Mod Pathol 1990;3:49–53.
679. Brivet F, Coffin B, Bedossa P, et al. Pancreatic lesions in AIDS (Letter). Lancet 1987;2:570–571.
680. Zazzo JF, Pichon F, Regnier B. HIV and the pancreas (Letter). Lancet 1987;2:1212–1213.

**Blood Flukes *(Schistosoma mansoni)***

681. Lenzi HL, Lenzi JA, Rosman FC. Pancreatic Involvement in murine schistosomiasis. Braz J Med Biol Res 1989;22:1105–1109.
682. Lima JP. Study of so-called ectopic lesions in schistosomiasis mansoni. I. General incidence. Rev Inst Med Trop Sao Paulo 1966;8:167–172. (Quoted in ref 681.)
683. Ladosky W. Rev Assoc Med Bras 1958;4:141–150. (Quoted in ref 681.)

**Leishmaniasis**

684. De Lalla F, Pellizzer G, Gradoni L. Acute pancreatitis associated with administration of meglumine antimonate for the treatment of visceral leishmaniasis (Letter). Clin Infect Dis 1993;16: 730–731.
685. Donovan KL, White AD, Cooke DA, Fisher DJ. Pancreatitis and palindromic arthropathy with effusions associated with sodium stibogluconate treatment in a renal transplant recipient. J Infect 1990;21:107–110.
686. Halim MA, Alfurayh O, Kalin ME, et al. Successful treatment of visceral leishmaniasis with allopurinol plus ketoconazole in a renal transplant recipient after the occurrence of pancreatitis due to stibogluconate. Clin Infect Dis 1993;16:397–399.
687. Broeckaert van Orshoven A, Michielsen P, Vandepitte J. Fatal leishmaniasis in renal-transplant patient (Letter). Lancet 1979;2: 740–741.

### *Echinococcus*

688. Morton PCG, Terblanche JT, Bornman PC, Tyrrell JCH. Obstructive jaundice caused by an intrapancreatic hydatid cyst. Br J Surg 1981;68:474.
689. Mestiri S, Hadj Salah M, Laarif R, Kehila M. Hepatic hydatid cyst opening into the bile ducts and acute pancreatitis: etiopathogenic problems apropos of 3 cases. Med Chir Dig 1982;11:197–199.
690. Parthe S, Maier M, Kohler B, et al. Acute pancreatitis due to the rupture of an echinococcal cyst into the bile duct system. Dtsch Med Wochenschr 1994;119:624–627.
691. Fodha M, Belhadj Bettaieb N, Morjane A, et al. Acute pancreatitis and hydatid cysts of the liver opening Into the bile ducts. Apropos of a new case. Tunis Med 1989;67:201–205.
692. Seror J, Mentouri B, Daoud K, Vedrenne C. Biliary lithiasis and hydatid cysts of the liver. Experimental research and clinical studies. Ann Chir 1968;22:1269–1277.
693. Baumer R, et al. Acute pancreatitis and hydatid cysts of the liver. Med Chir Dig 1983;12:277–280.
694. Papadimitriou J. Pancreatic abscess due to infective hydatid disease. Surgery 1987;102:880–882.
695. El Mufti M. Surgical management of hydatid disease. London: Butterworths, 1989:87.
696. Albo M. Hydatid cysts of the pancreas. Surg Gynecol Obstet 1922;34:739–752.
697. Katkhouda N, Legoff D, Tricarico A, et al. Hydatid cyst of the pancreas responsible for chronic recurrent pancreatitis. Presse Med 1988;17:2021–2023.
698. Morris DL. Pre-operative albendazole therapy for hydatid cysts. Br J Surg 1987;74:805–806.
699. Cook GC. Gastroenterological problems. In: Manson-Bahr PEC, Bell DR, eds. Manson's tropical diseases. 19th ed. London: Bailliere Tindall, 1987:998–1010.
700. Mathai V, Jesudason SRB, Muthusami JC, et al. Chronic pancreatitis caused by intraductal hydatid cysts of the pancreas. Br J Surg 1994;81:1029.

### Cryptosporidiosis

701. Hawkins SP, Thomas RP, Teasdale C. Acute pancreatitis, a new finding in Cryptosporidium enteritis. Br Med J 1987;294:483–484.
702. Kocoshis SA, Cibull ML, Davies TE, et al. Intestinal and pulmonary cryptospiridiosis in an infant with severe combined immune deficiency. J Pediatr Gastroenterol Nutr 1984;3:149–157.

### *Giardia lamblia*

703. Koszarska J, Gruszczynska M, Pilarska K. Lambliasis as a cause of acute pancreatitis. Wiad Lek 1977;30:875–877.
704. Drew JH. Biliary giardiasis and pancreatitis (Letter). Med J Aust 1981;196–197.

### Fungus-Induced Pancreatitis

705. Guice KS, Lynch M, Weatherbee L. Invasive aspergillosis: an unusual cause of hemorrhagic pancreatitis. Am J Gastroenterol 1987;82:563–565.
706. Halevy A, Blenkharn JI, Christodoloupolous J, Blumgart LH. Actinomycosis of the pancreas. Br J Surg 1987;74:150.
707. Chung RT, Schapiro RH, Warshaw AL. Intraluminal pancreatic candidiasis presenting as recurrent pancreatitis. Gastroenterology 1993;104:1532–1534.
708. Mannell A, Obers V. Pancreatic candidiasis. A case report. S Afr J Surg 1990;28:26–27.
709. Richter JM, Jacoby GA, Schapiro RH, Warshaw AL. Pancreatic abscess due to Candida albicans. Ann Intern Med 1982;97:120–122.
710. Howard JM, Bieluch VM. Pancreatic abscess secondary to Candida albicans. Pancreas 1989;4:120–122.

### Scorpion Sting Pancreatitis

711. Waterman JA. Some notes on scorpion poisoning in Trinidad. Trans R Soc Trop Med Hyg 1938;31:607.
712. Bartholomew C. Acute scorpion pancreatitis in Trinidad. Br Med J 1970;1:666–668.
713. Bartholomew C, McGeeney KF, Murphy JJ, et al. Experimental studies on the aetiology of acute scorpion pancreatitis. Br J Surg 1976;63:807.
714. Bartholomew C, Murphy JJ, McGeeney KF, Fitzgerald O. Exocrine pancreatic response to the venom of the scorpion, Tityus trinitatis. Gut 1977;18:623–625.
715. Sankaran C, et al. Mechanism of the scorpion toxin-induced pancreatitis in dogs. Biochem Arch 1987;3:41–46.
716. Novaes G, Cardozo C de C, Costa NM, et al. Experimental chronic interstitial pancreatitis induced by scorpion toxin in rats. Arq Gastroenterol 1990;27:187–190.
717. Novaes G, Cabral AP, deFalco CN, de Queiroz AC. Acute pancreatitis induced by scorpion toxin, tityustoxin. Histopathological study in rats. Arq Gastroenterol 1989;26:9–12.
718. Novaes G, Cantanzaro OL, Beraldo WT, Freire-Maia L. Effect of purified scorpion toxin (tityustoxin) on the pancreatic secretion of the rat. Toxicon 1982;20:847–853.
719. D'Suze G, Sevcik C, Ramos M. Presence of curarizing polypeptides and a pancreatitis-inducing fraction without muscarinic effects in the venom of the Venezuelan scorpion Tityus discrepans (Karsch). Toxicon 1995;33:333–345.
720. Sofer S, Shalev H, Weizman Z, Shahak E. Acute pancreatitis in children following envenomation by the yellow scorpion Leiurus quinquestriatus. Toxicon 1991;29:125–128.
721. Gueron M, Yaron R. Cardiovascular manifestations of severe scorpion sting. Clinico pathologic correlations. Chest 1970;57:156–162.

### Snake Bite Pancreatitis

722. Kjellström BT. Acute pancreatitis after snake bite. Acta Chir Scand 1989;155:291–292.

### Tetracycline

723. Dobrilla G, Felder M, Chilovi F. Proven relationship between drugs and pancreatitis. Dtsch Med Wochenschr 1986;111:868–870.
724. Nicolau DP, Mengedoht DE, Kline JJ. Tetracycline-induced pancreatitis. Am J Gastroenterol 1991;86:1669–1671.
725. Elmore MF, Rogge JD. Tetracycline-induced pancreatitis. Gastroenterology 1981;81:1134–1136.
726. Torosis J, Vender R. Tetracycline-induced pancreatitis. J Clin Gastroenterol 1987;9:580–581.

### Other Antibiotics and Related Drugs

727. Gumaste VV. Erythromycin-induced pancreatitis. Am J Med 1989;86:725.
728. Teillet L, Chaussade S, Mory B, et al. Drug-induced acute pancreatitis following intravenous erythromycin antibiotherapy (Letter). Gastroenterol Clin Biol 1991;15:265–266.
729. Surinach JM, Alegre J, Fernandez de Sevilla T. Acute pancreatitis from erythromycin (Letter, in Spanish). Rev Clin Esp 1993;192:458.
730. Hawksworth CR. Acute pancreatitis associated with infusion of erythromycin lactobionate. Br Med J 1989;298:190.
731. Berger TM, Cook WJ, O Marcaigh AS, Zimmerman D. Acute pancreatitis in a 12-year-old girl after an erythromycin overdose. Pediatrics 1992;90:624–626.
732. Hanline MH, Jr. Acute pancreatitis caused by ampicillin (Letter). South Med J 1987;80:1069.
733. Zimmermann AE, Katona BG, Jodhka JS, Williams RB. Ceftriaxone-induced acute pancreatitis. Ann Pharmacother 1993;27:36–37.
734. Zinberg J, Chernaik R, Coman E, et al. Reversible symptomatic biliary obstruction associated with ceftriaxone pseudolithiasis. Am J Gastroenterol 1991;86:1251–1254.
735. Plotnick BH, Cohen I, Tsang T, Cullinane T. Metronidazole-induced pancreatitis. Ann Intern Med 1985;103:891–892.
736. Sanford KA, Mayle JE, Dean HA, Greenbaum DS. Metronidazole-induced pancreatitis. Ann Intern Med 1988;109:756–757.
737. Celifarco A, Warschauer W, Burakoff R. Metronidazole-induced pancreatitis. Am J Gastroenterol 1989;84:958–960.
738. Corey WA, Doebbeling BN, DeJong KJ, Britigan BE. Metronidazole-induced acute pancreatitis. Rev Infect Dis 1991;13:1213–1215.
739. Christophe JL. Pancreatitis induced by nitrofurantoin. Gut 1994;35:712–713.
740. Nelis GF. Nitrofurantoin-induced pancreatitis: report of a case. Gastroenterology 1983;84:1032–1034.

#### Sulfonamides

741. Dobrilla G, Felder M, Chilovi F. Proven relationship between drugs and pancreatitis. Dtsch Med Wochenschr 1986;111: 868–870.
742. Aubry P, Alandry G, Lemiere C. Acute pancreatitis in the course of treatment with salazosulfapyridine. Presse Med 1989; 18:80.
743. Block MB, Genant HK, Kirsner JB. Pancreatitis as an adverse reaction to salicylazosulfapyridine. N Engl J Med 1970;282: 380–382.
744. Garau P, Orenstein SR, Neigut DA, Kocoshis SA. Pancreatitis associated with olsalazine and sulfasalazine in children with ulcerative colitis. J Pediatr Gastroenterol Nutr 1994;18:481–485.
745. Rubin R. Sulfasalazine-induced fulminant hepatic failure and necrotizing pancreatitis. Am J Gastroenterol 1994;89:789–791.
746. Chiba M, Horie Y, Ishida H, et al. A case of salicylazosulfapyridine (Salazopyrin)-induced acute pancreatitis with positive lymphocyte stimulation test (LST). Gastroenterology Jpn 1987;22: 228–233.
747. Surypapranata H, DeVries H. Pancreatitis associated with sulphasalazine. Br Med J 1986;292:732.
748. Barrett PV, Thier SO. Meningitis and pancreatitis associated with sulfamethizole. N Engl J Med 1963;268:36–37.
749. Brazer SR, Medoff JR. Sulfonamide-induced pancreatitis. Pancreas 1988;3:583–586.
750. Antonow DR. Acute pancreatitis associated with trimethoprim-sulfamethoxazole. Ann Intern Med 1986;104:363–365.
751. Jost R, Stey C, Salomon F. Fatal drug-induced pancreatitis in HIV (Letter). Lancet 1993;341:1412.
752. Brockner J, Boisen E. Fatal multisystem toxicity after co-trimoxazole (Letter). Lancet 1978;1:831.

#### Diuretics

753. Cornish AL, McClellan JT, Johnston DH. Effects of chlorothiazide on the pancreas. N Engl J Med 1961;265:673–675.
754. Bourke JB, McIllmurray MB, Mead GM, Langman MJ. Drug-associated primary acute pancreatitis. Lancet 1978;1:706–708.
755. Wilson AE, Mehra SK, Gomersall CR, Davies DM. Acute pancreatitis associated with furosemide therapy. Lancet 1967; 1:105.
756. Thomas FB, Sinar D, Caldwell JH, et al. Stimulation of pancreatic secretion of water and electrolytes by furosemide. Gastroenterology 1977;73:221–225.
757. Jones PE, Oelbaum MH. Frusemide-induced pancreatitis. Br Med J 1975;1:133–134.
758. Call T, Malarkey WB, Thomas FB. Acute pancreatitis secondary to furosemide with associated hyperlipidemia. Am J Dig Dis 1977;22:835–838.
759. Buchanan N, Cane RD. Frusemide-induced pancreatitis (Letter). Br Med J 1977;2:1417.
760. Strung P. Furosemide-induced pancreatitis? Br Med J 1975;1:434.
761. Diamond MT. Hyperglycemic hyperosmolar coma associated with hydro-chlorothiazide and pancreatitis. NY State J Med 1972;72:1741–1742.
762. Eckhauser ML, Dokler M, Imbembo AL. Diuretic associated pancreatitis: a collective review and illustrative cases. Am J Gastroenterol 1987;82:865–870.
763. Rion RJ. Recurrent pancreatitis after treatment with hydrochlorothiazide. J Am Board Fam Pract 1994;7:74–76.
764. Johnston DH, Cornish AL. Acute pancreatitis in patients receiving chlorothiazide. JAMA 1959;170:2054–2056.
765. Jones MF, Caldwall JR. Acute hemorrhagic pancreatitis associated with administration of chlorthalidone: report of a case. N Engl J Med 1962;267:1029.
766. Cooperman LB, Rubin IL. Toxicity of ethacrynic acid and furosemide. Am Heart J 1973;85:831–834.
767. Fuchs JE Jr, Keith MR, Galands AN. Probable metolazone-induced pancreatitis. Drug Intell Clin Pharm 1989;23:711.
768. Anderson PE, Ellis GG Jr, Austin SM. Case report. Metolazone-associated hypercalcemia and acute pancreatitis. Am J Med Sci 1991;302:235–237.
769. Arnold R, Doyle PJ, Bell G. Acute pancreatitis in a patient treated with cimetidine. Lancet 1978;1:382–383.
770. Wilkinson ML, O Driscoll R, Kiernan TJ. Cimetidine and pancreatitis (Letter). Lancet 1981;1:610–611.
771. Hainaut P, et al. Cimetidine-induced pancreatitis. Rev Med Intern 1987;8:516–518.
772. Nott DM, de Sousa BA. Suspected cimetidine-induced acute pancreatitis. Br J Clin Prac 1989;43:264–265.
773. Herrmann R, Shaw RG, Fone DJ. Ranitidine-associated recurrent acute pancreatitis. Aust NZ J Med 1990;20:243–244.

#### Antiinflammatory Agents
#### Sulindac (Clinoril)

774. Sugerman HJ. Sulindac-induced acute pancreatitis mimicking gallstone pancreatitis. Am Surg 1989;55:536–538.
775. Klein SM, Kahn MA. Hepatitis, toxic epidermal necrolysis and pancreatitis in association with sulindac therapy. J Rheum 1983;10:512–513.
776. Siefkin AD. Sulindac and pancreatitis (Letter). Ann Intern Med 1980;93:932–933.
777. Memon AN. Pancreatitis and sulindac (Letter). Ann Intern Med 1982;97:139.
778. Clark BG, Vestal RE. Adverse drug reactions in the elderly: case studies. Geriatrics 1984;39:53–66.
779. Detlefs RL. Drug-induced pancreatitis presenting as subcutaneous fat necrosis (Letter). J Am Acad Dermatol 1985;13:305–307.
780. Zygmunt DJ, Williams HJ, Bienz SR. Acute pancreatitis associated with long-term sulindac therapy. West J Med 1986;144:461–462.
781. Lerche A, Vyberg M, Kirkegaard E. Acute cholangitis and pancreatitis associated with sulindac Clinoril. Histopathology 1987;11:647–653.
782. Goldstein J, Laskin DA, Ginsberg GH. Sulindac associated with pancreatitis (Letter). Ann Intern Med 1980;93:151.
783. Lilly EL. Pancreatitis after administration of sulindac. JAMA 1981;246:2680.
784. Goldstein J, Laskin DA, Ginsberg GH. Sulindac associated with pancreatitis (Letter). Ann Intern Med 1980;93:151.

#### Piroxicam (Feldane and Ketoprofen)

785. Haye OL. Drug-induced pancreatitis: a critical review. Gastroenterology 1980;8:813–820.
786. Jick H, Derby L, Garcia Rodriguez LA, Jick SS, Dean AD. Nonsteroidal anti-inflammatory drugs and certain rare, serious adverse events: a cohort study. Pharmacotherapy 1993;13: 212–217.
787. Cobb TK, Pierce JR Jr. Acute pancreatitis associated with ketoprofen. South Med J 1992;85:430–431.

#### Indomethacin and other NSAIDs

788. O'Brien WM. Adverse reactions to nonsteroidal anti-inflammatory drugs: diclofenac compared with other nonsteroidal anti-inflammatory drugs. Am J Med 1986;80:S4B:70–80.
789. Guerra M. Toxicity of indomethacin: report of a case of acute pancreatitis. JAMA 1967;200:552–553.
790. Du Ville L, Debeuckelaere S, Reynaert H, Devis G. Pancreatitis associated with naproxen (Letter). Am J Gastroenterol 1993; 88:464.
791. Van Walraven AA, Edels M, Fong S. Pancreatitis caused by mefenamic acid (Letter). Can Med Assoc J 1982;126:894.
792. Ruppert GB, Barth WF. Ibuprofen hypersensitivity in systemic lupus erythematosus. South Med J 1981;74:241–243.
793. Bathan DA, Meitus ML, Capland L. Death following phenylbutazone therapy: report of a case. Ann Intern Med 1953;39:1096–1103.
794. Khan IH, Edward N. Pancreatitis associated with diclofenac. Postgrad Med J 1993;69:486–487.

#### 5-Aminosalicylic Acid, Sulfasalazine, and Related Drugs

795. Sachedina B, Saibil F, Cohen LB, Whittey J. Acute pancreatitis due to 5-aminosalicylic. Ann Intern Med 1989;110:490–492.
796. Poldermans D, van Blankenstein M. Pancreatitis induced by disodium azodisalicylate. Am J Gastroenterol 1988;83: 578–580.
797. Fiorentini MT, Fracchia M, Galatala G, et al. Acute pancreatitis during oral 5-aminosalicylic acid therapy. Case report. Dig Dis Sci 1990;35:1180–1182.
798. Deprez P, Descamps C, Fiasse R. Pancreatitis induced by 5-aminosalicylic acid (Letter). Lancet 1989;2:445–446.
799. Erdkamp F, Houben M, Ackerman E, et al. Pancreatitis induced by mesalamine. Neth J Med 1992;41:71–73.

800. Eckardt VF, Kanzler G, Rieder H, Ewe K. Pancreatitis associated with 5-aminosalicylic acid. Dtsch Med Wochenschr 1991;116:540–542.
801. Tran K, Froguel E, Jian R, et al. Acute pancreatitis induced by Mesalazine (Letter). J Clin Gastroenterol 1991;13:715–716.

**Corticosteroids**

802. Levine RA, McGuire RF. Corticosteroid-induced pancreatitis: a case report demonstrating recurrence with rechallenge. Am J Gastroenterol 1988;83:1161–1164.
803. Zion MM, Goldberg B, Suzman MM. Corticotropin and cortisone in the treatment of scleroderma. Q J Med 1955;24:215–217.
804. Keefe M, Munro F. Acute pancreatitis: a fatal complication of treatment of bullous pemphigoid with systemic corticosteroids. Dermatologica 1989;179:73–75.

**Analgesics and Narcotics**

805. Caldarola V, Hassett JM, Hall AH, et al. Hemorrhagic pancreatitis associated with acetaminophen overdose. Am J Gastroenterol 1986;81:579–582.
806. Coward RA. Paracetamol-induced acute pancreatitis (Letter). Br Med J 1977;1:1086.
807. Gilmore IT, Tourvas E. Paracetamol-induced acute pancreatitis. Br Med J 1977;1:753–754.
808. Mofenson HC, Caraccio TR, Nawaz H, Steckler G. Acetaminophen induced pancreatitis. Clin Toxicol 1991;29:223–230.
809. Gazzard BG, Portmann B, Murray-Lyon IM, Williams R. Causes of death in fulminant hepatic failure and relationship to quantitative histological assessment of parenchymal damage. Q J Med 1975;44:615–626.
810. Mills GH, Goddard JM. A case of patient controlled analgesia exacerbating postoperative pain (Letter). Anaesthesia 1991;46:893.
811. Lankisch PG, Niederstadt H, Redlin-Kress E, et al. Acute pancreatitis: induced by heroin intoxication? Pancreas 1993;8:123–126.

**Psychomoter Drugs**

812. Batalden PB, Van Dyne BJ, Cloyd J. Pancreatitis associated with valproic acid therapy. Pediatrics 1979;64:520–522.
813. Camfield PR, Bagnell R, Camfield CS, Tibbles JA. Pancreatitis due to valproic acid (Letter). Lancet 1979;1:1198–1199.
814. Murphy MJ, Lyon IW, Taylor JW, Mitts G. Valproic acid associated pancreatitis in an adult (Letter). Lancet 1981;1:41–42.
815. Rosenberg HK, Ortega W. Hemorrhagic pancreatitis in a young child following valproic acid therapy. Clin Pediatr 1987;26:98–101.
816. Binek J, Hany A, Heer M. Valproic acid-induced pancreatitis: case report and review of the literature. J Clin Gastroenterol 1991;13:690–693.
817. Engelmann MD, Henriksen SD, Tingsgaard LK. Fatal pancreatitis associated with valproate therapy (Danish). Ugeskr Laeger 1995;157:4357–4358.
818. Evans RJ, Miranda RN, Jordan J, Krolikowski FJ. Fatal acute pancreatitis caused by valproic acid. Am J Forensic Med 1995;16:62–65.
819. Asconape JJ, Penry JK, Dreifuss FE, et al. Valproate-associated pancreatitis. Epilepsia 1993;34:177–183.

**Carbamazepine and Phenytoin**

820. Soman M, Swenson C. A possible case of carbamazepine-induced pancreatitis. Drug Intell Clin Pharm 1985;19:925–927.
821. Tsao CY, Wright FS. Acute chemical pancreatitis associated with carbamazepine intoxication. Epilepsia 1993;34:174–176.
822. Pezzilli R, Billi P, Melandri R, et al. Anticonvulsant-induced chronic pancreatitis. A case report. Ital J Gastroenterol 1992;24:245–246.
823. Yamashina T, Takeuchi H, Kawanishi J, et al. A case of drug induced pancreatitis with erythrodermia due to administration of phenytoin (Japanese). Nippon Shokakibyo Gakkai Zasshi 1991;88:1269–1274.

**Antidepressants and Antipsychotics**

824. Calmus Y, Biour M, Bodin F, et al. Hepatitis and pancreatitis due to indalpine. Gastroenterol Clin Biol 1985;9:266–268.
825. Martin A. Acute pancreatitis associated with clozapine use (Letter). Am J Psychiatry 1992;149:714.
826. Frankenburg FR, Kando J. Eosinophilia, clozapine and pancreatitis (Letter). Lancet 1992;340:251.
827. Sebastian Domingo JJ, Simon Marco MA, Uribarrena Echebarria R. Hepatic and pancreatic injury associated with amineptine therapy. J Clin Gastroenterol 1994;18:168–169.

**ß-Blocking Agents**

828. O'Donoghue DJ. Acute pancreatitis due to nadolol-induced hypertriglyceridaemia. Br J Clin Pract 1989;43:74–75.
829. Durrington PN, Cairns SA. Acute pancreatitis, a complication of beta-blockade. Br Med J 1982;284:1016.
830. Weaver GA. Do antihypertensive agents cause chronic pancreatitis? J Clin Gastroenterol 1987;9:8–11.

**Angiotensin Converting Enzyme (ACE) Inhibitors**

831. Tilkemeir P, Thompson PD. Acute pancreatitis possibly related to enalapril (Letter). N Engl J Med 1988;318:1275–1276.
832. Pedro-Botet J, Miralles R, Coll J, Rubies-Prat J. Captopril versus enalapril: cough versus pancreatitis. DICP Ann Pharmocother 1990;24:438–439.
833. Jeandidier N, Klewansky M, Pinget M. Captopril-induced acute pancreatitis. Diabetes Care 1995;18:410–411.
834. Marinella MA, Bille JE. Lisinopril therapy associated with acute pancreatitis. West J Med 1955;163:77–78.
835. Dabaghi S. ACE inhibitors and pancreatitis (Letter). Ann Intern Med 1991;115:330–331.
836. Maliekal J, Drake CF. Acute pancreatitis associated with the use of lisinopril. Ann Pharmacother 1993;27:1465–1466.
837. Standridge JB. Fulminant pancreatitis associated with lisinopril therapy. South Med J 1994;87:179–181.

**Procainamide**

838. Falko JM, Thomas FB. Acute pancreatitis due to procainamide-induced lupus erythematosus (Letter). Am Intern Med 1975;83:832–833.

**Cholesterol-Reducing Agents**

839. Lons T, Chousterman M. Simvastatine: a new drug responsible for acute pancreatitis (Letter)? Gastroenterol Clin Biol 1991;15:93–94.
840. Ramdani M, Schmitt AM, Liautard J. Simvastatin-induced acute pancreatitis: two cases (Letter). Gastroenterology Clin Biol 1991;15:986.
841. Couderc M, Blanc P, Rouillon JM, et al. A new case of simvastatin-induced acute pancreatitis (Letter). Gastroenterol Clin Biol 1991;15:986–987.
842. Pluhart W. Lovastatine as having induced acute pancreatitis. Wien Klin Wochenschr 1989;101:551–554.

**Octreotide**

843. Gradon JD, Schulman RH, Chapnick EK, Sepkowitz DV. Octreotide-induced acute pancreatitis in a patient with acquired immunodeficiency syndrome. South Med J 1991;84:1410–1411.
844. Fredenrich A, Sosset C, Bernard JL, et al. Acute pancreatitis after short-term octreotide (Letter). Lancet 1991;338:52–53.
845. Vidal J, Sacanella E, Munoz E, et al. Acute pancreatitis related to octreotide in a patient with acquired immunodeficiency syndrome (Letter). Pancreas 1994;9:395–397.
846. Romeu J, Miro JM, Sirera G, et al. Efficacy of octreotide in the management of chronic diarrhea in AIDS. AIDS 1991;5:1495–1499.
847. Sadoul JL, Benchimal D, Thyss A, Freychet P. Acute pancreatitis following octreotide withdrawal (Letter). Am J Med 1991;90:763–764.

**Growth Hormone**

848. Malozowski S, Hung W, Scott DC, Stadel BV. Acute pancreatitis associated with growth hormone therapy for short stature (Letter). N Engl J Med 1995;332:401–402.

**Estrogen**

849. Glueck CJ, Lang J, Hamer T, Tracy T. Severe hypertriglyceridemia and pancreatitis when estrogen replacement therapy is given to hypetriglyceridemic women. J Lab Clin Med 1994;123:59–64.

850. Stone NJ. Estrogen-induced pancreatitis: a caveat worth remembering. J Lab Clin Med 1994;123:18–19.

**Anticancer Drugs**

851. Underwood TW, Frye CB. Drug-induced pancreatitis (Review). Clin Pharm 1993;12:440–448.
852. Tarin F, Camps C, Berrocal A, Vicent JM. Acute pancreatitis caused by cisplatin and vindesin (Letter). Rev Esp Enferm Dig 1994;85:224–225.
853. Bunin N, Meyer WH, Christensen M, Pratt CB. Pancreatitis following cisplatin: a case report. Cancer Treat Rep 1985;69:236–237.
854. Vermorken JR, Pinedo HM. Gastrointestinal toxicity of cisdiammine dichloroplatin (II). Personal observations. Neth J Med 1982;25;270–274.
855. Chiuten D, Vogl S, Kaplan B, Camacho F. Is there cumulative or delayed toxicity from *cis*-platinum? Cancer 1983;52:211–214.
856. Balis FM, Holcenberg JS, Poplack DG. General principles of chemotherapy: oxazaphosphorines. In: Pizzo PA, Poplack DG, eds. Principles and practice of pediatric oncology. 2nd ed. Philadelphia: JB Lippincott, 1993:203–211.
857. Newman CE, Ellis DJ. Pancreatitis during combination chemotherapy. Clin Oncol 1979;5:83–84.
858. Puckett JB, Butler WM, McFarland JA. Pancreatitis and cancer chemotherapy (Letter). Ann Intern Med 1982;97:453.
859. Dobrilla G, Felder M, Chilovi F. Proven relationship between drugs and pancreatitis. Dtsch Med Wochenschr 1986;111:868–870.
860. Satake K, Nakashima Y. Drug-induced pancreatitis. In: Howard JM, Jordan GL, Jordan, Reber HA, eds. Surgical diseases of the pancreas. Philadelphia: Lea & Febiger, 1987.
861. Land VJ, Sutow WW, Fernbach DJ, et al. Toxicity of L-asparaginase in children with advance leukemia. Cancer 1972;30:339–347.
862. Oettgen HF, Stephenson PA, Schwartz MK, et al. Toxicity of E. coli L-asparaginase in man. Cancer 1970;25:253–278.
863. Weetman RM, Baehner RL. Latent onset of clinical pancreatitis in children receiving L-asparaginase therapy. Cancer 1974;34:780–785.

**Other Cancer Chemotherapy Agents**

864. Bekassy AN, Wiebe T, Hochbergs P. Erwinase-induced pancreatitis (Letter). Lancet 1992;340:1552–1553.
865. Sotomatsu M, Shimoda M, Ogawa C, Morikawa A. Acute pancreatitis associated with interferon-alpha therapy for chronic myelogenous leukemia (Letter). Am J Hematol 1995;48:211–212.
866. Izraeli S, Adamson PC, Blaney SM, Balis FM. Acute pancreatitis after ifosfamide therapy. Cancer 1994;74:1627–1628.

**Immunosuppressant Drugs**

867. Yoshimura N, Nakai I, Ohmori Y, et al. Effect of cyclosporine on the endocrine and exocrine pancreas in kidney transplant recipients. Am J Kidney Dis 1988;12:11–17.
868. Werlin SL, Casper J, Antonson D, Calabro C. Pancreatitis associated with bone marrow transplantation in children. Bone Marrow Transplant 1992;10:65–69.
869. Lorber MI, Van Buren CT, Flechner JM, et al. Hepatobiliary and pancreatic complications of cyclosporin therapy in 466 renal transplant recipients. Transplantation 1987;43:35–40.
870. Siemers RF, Friedenberg WR, Norfleet RG. High dose cytosine arabinoside associated pancreatitis. Cancer 1985;56:1940–1942.
871. Deeb GM, Bolling SF, Steimle CN, et al. A randomized prospective comparison of MALG with OKT3 for rescue therapy of acute myocardial rejection. Transplantation 1991;51:180–183.
872. Scheinin S, Radovancevic B, Frazier OH. Acute pancreatitis complicating OKT 3 administration for resistant cardiac rejection. Transplant Proc 1993;25;2368–2369.

**Antitubercular Drugs**

873. Rabassa AA, Trey G, Shukla U, et al. Isoniazid-induced acute pancreatitis. Ann Intern Med 1994;121:433–434.
874. Mattson K. Side effects of rifampicin. A clinical study. Scand J Resp Dis 1973;82(suppl):1–52.
875. Kvale PA, Parks RD. Acute abdomen. An unusual reaction to isoniazid (Letter). Chest 1975;68:271–272.
876. Chan KL, Chan HS, Lui SF, Lai KN. Recurrent acute pancreatitis induced by isoniazid. Tubercle Lung Dis 1994;75:383–385.

**Antiparasitic Drugs**

877. Donovan KL, White AD, Cooke DA, Fisher DJ. Pancreatitis and palindromic arthropathy with effusions associated with sodium stibogluconate treatment in a renal transplant recipient. J Infect 1990;21:107–110.
878. McCarthy AE, Keystone JS, Kain KC. Pancreatitis occurring during therapy with stibogluconate: two case reports. Clin Infect Dis 1993;17:952–953.
879. Gasser RA, Magill AJ, Oster CN, et al. Pancreatitis induced by pentavalent antimonial agents during treatment of leishmaniasis. Clin Infect Dis 1994;18:83–90.

**Antiviral (AIDS) Agents: Pentamidine and Didanosine**

880. Murphey SA, Josephs AS. Acute pancreatitis associated with pentamidine therapy. Arch Intern Med 1981;141:56–58.
881. Klatt EC. Pathology of pentamidine-induced pancreatitis. Arch Pathol Lab Med 1992;116:162–164.
882. Villamil A, Hammer RA, Rodriguez FH. Edematous pancreatitis associated with intravenous pentamidine. South Med J 1991;84:796–798.
883. Pais JR, Cazorla C, Novo E, Viana A. Massive hemorrhage from rupture of a pancreatic pseudocyst after pentamidine-associated pancreatitis. Eur J Med 1992;1:251–253.
884. O'Neil MG, Selub SE, Hak LJ. Pancreatitis during pentamidine therapy in patients with AIDS. Clin Pharm 1991;10:56–59.
885. Singh G, El-Gadi SM, Sparks RA. Pancreatitis associated with aerosolized pentamidine (Letter). Genitourin Med 1995;71:130–131.
886. Echinard E, Dupon M, Malou M, et al. Acute fatal pancreatitis following treatment with pentamidine (Letter). Therapie 1986;41:520.
887. Salmeron S, Petitpretz P, Katlama C, et al. Pentamidine and pancreatitis (Letter). Ann Intern Med 1986;105:140–141.
888. Zuger A, Wolf BZ, el-Sadr W, et al. Pentamidine-associated fatal acute pancreatitis (Letter). JAMA 1986;256:2383–2385.
889. Kumar S, Schnadig VJ, MacGregor MG. Fatal acute pancreatitis associated with pentamidine therapy (Letter). Am J Gastroenterol 1989;84:451–453.
890. Schwartz MS, Cappell MS. Pentamidine-associated pancreatitis. Dig Dis Sci 1989;34:1617–1620.
891. Pauwels A, Eliaszewicz M, Larrey D, et al. Pentamidine-induced acute pancreatitis in a patient with AIDS. J Gastroenterol 1990;12:457–459.
892. Sauleda J, Gea JG, Aguar MC, et al. Probable pentamidine-induced acute pancreatitis. Ann Pharmacother 1994;28:52–53.
893. Hart CC. Aerosolized pentamidine and pancreatitis (Letter). Ann Intern Med 1989;111:691.
894. Murphy RL, Noskin GA, Ehrenpreis ED. Acute pancreatitis associated with aerosolized pentamidine. Am J Med 1990;88:53N–56N.
895. Herer B, Chinet T, Labrune S, et al. Pancreatitis associated with pentamidine by aerosol (Letter). Br Med J 1989;298:605.
896. Foisy MM, Slayter KL, Hewitt RG, Morse GD. Pancreatitis during intravenous pentamidine therapy in an AIDS patient with prior exposure to didanosine. Ann Pharmocother 1994;28:1025–1028.
897. Daniels M. Pancreatitis in AIDS patients treated with didanosine (Letter). Am J Gastroenterol 1993;88:459–460.
898. Maxson CJ, Greenfield SM, Turner JL. Acute pancreatitis as a common complication of 2,3-dideoxyinosine therapy in the acquired immunodeficiency syndrome. Am J Gastroenterol 1992;87:708–713.
899. Bouvet E, Casalino E, Prevost MH, Vachon F. Fatal case of 2,3-dideoxyinosine-associated pancreatitis (Letter). Lancet 1990;336:1515.
900. Seidlin M, Lambert JS, Dolin R, Valentine FT. Pancreatitis and pancreatic dysfunction in patients taking dideoxyinosine. AIDS 1992;6:831–835.

### Chemically Induced Pancreatitis: Insecticides

901. Branch A. Pancreatic necrosis in ethyl alcohol, methyl alcohol, and arsenic poisoning. Can Med Assoc J 1944;51:428.
902. Bennett IL Jr, Nation TC, Olley JR. Pancreatitis in methyl alcohol poisoning. J Lab Clin Med 1952;40:405.
903. Dressel TD, Goodale RL, Jr, Arneson MA, Borner JW. Pancreatitis as a complication of anticholinesterase insecticide intoxication. Ann Surg 1979;189:199–204.
904. Earl F, et al.. Diazionon toxicity-comparative studies in dogs and miniature swine. Toxicol Appl Pharmacol 1971;18:285.
905. Marsh WH, Vukov GA, Conradi EC. Acute pancreatitis after cutaneous exposure to an organophosphate insecticide. Am J Gastroenterol 1988;83:1158–1160.
906. Dagli AJ, Shaikh WA. Pancreatic involvement in Malathion-anticholinesterase insecticide intoxication: a study of 75 cases. Br J Clin Prac 1983;37:270–272.
906a. Moritz F, Droy JM, Dutheil G, et al. Acute pancreatitis after carbamate insecticide intoxication. Intensive Care Med 1994; 20:49–50.
906b. Lankisch PG, Müller C-H, Niederstadt H, Brand A. Painless acute pancreatitis subsequent to antecholinesterase insecticide (Parathion) intoxication. Am J Gastroenterology 1990;85:872–875.
906c. Weizman Z, Sofer S. Acute pancreatitis in children with anticholinesterase insecticide intoxication. Pediatrics 1992;90:204–206.
907. Braganza JM, Jolley JE, Lee WR. Occupational chemicals and pancreatitis: a link? Int J Pancreatol 1986;1:9–19.
908. McNamee R. Braganza JM, Hogg, J. et al. Occupational exposure to hydrocarbons and chronic pancreatitis: a case-referent study. Occup Environ Med 1994;51:631–637.

### Idiopathic Pancreatitis

909. Miquel JF, Rollan A, Guzman S, Nervi F. Microlithiasis and cholesterolosis in idiopathic acute pancreatitis (Letter). Gastroenterology 1992;102:2188–2190.
910. Kaufman Z, Shpitz B, Denbar A. Microlithiasis of the cystic duct (Letter). Am J Gastroenterol 1986;81:303–304.
911. Grendell JH. Idiopathic acute pancreatitis. Gastroenterol Clin North Am 1990;19:843–848.
912. Houssin D, Castaing D, Lemoine J, Bismuth H. Microlithiasis of the gallbladder. Surg Gynecol Obstet 1983;157:20–24.
913. Ros E, Navarro S, Bru C, et al. Occult microlithiasis in idiopathic acute pancreatitis: prevention of relapses by cholecystectomy or ursodeoxycholic acid therapy. Gastroenterology 1991;101: 1701–1709.
914. Lee SP, Nicholls JF, Park HZ. Biliary sludge as a cause of acute pancreatitis. N Engl J Med 1992;326:589–593.
915. Levy I, Lantsberg L, Khoda J. Spontaneous disappearance of limy bile. A cause of acute pancreatitis? J Clin Gastroenterol 1994;18:220–221.
916. Parrilla P, Garcia OD, Pellicer FE, et al. Gallbladder cholesterolosis: an aetiological factor in acute pancreatitis of uncertain origin. Br J Surg 1990;77:735–736.
917. Gross V, Schoelmerich J, Denzel K, Gerok W. Relapsing pancreatitis as initial manifestation of cystic fibrosis in a young man without pulmonary disease. Int J Pancreatol 1989;4: 221–228.
918. Venu RP, Geenen JE, Hogan W, et al. Idiopathic recurrent pancreatitis. An approach to diagnosis and treatment. Dig Dis Sci 1989;34:56–60.
919. Browder W. Acute pancreatitis of unknown etiology in the elderly. Ann Surg 1993;217:469–474.
920. Layer P, Yamamoto H, Kalthoff L, et al. The different courses of early- and late-onset idiopathic and alcoholic chronic pancreatitis. Gastroenterology 1994;107:1481–1487.

# 20

# *Pathophysiologic Basis of Management*

Mark T. Toyama, Stanley W. Ashley, and Howard A. Reber

The local consequences of severe acute pancreatitis are well known and include pancreatic and peripancreatic necrosis, infection, abscess, and fluid collections. Less apparent are the distant effects of the disease, in which the function of a variety of organ systems can be impaired. Pancreatic enzymes released from the inflamed pancreas may be responsible for some of the organ dysfunction. However, recent studies suggest that the systemic alterations may also be due to release of cellular mediators, such as interleukins and tumor necrosis factor, which affect the cardiovascular, renal, pulmonary, and endocrine systems. This chapter reviews the changes that occur in various organ systems and discusses the latest concepts of their pathogenesis.

## PATHOGENESIS OF ACUTE PANCREATITIS

Pancreatitis may result from a variety of causes, but it is generally believed that these inciting factors initiate a common chain of events that lead to autodigestion of the pancreas. In all forms of acute pancreatitis, it has been proposed that pancreatic enzymes, normally inactive and confined to acinar cells or ducts, pass instead into the interstitium of the gland, where they digest the tissues (1). The mechanisms by which activation occur are poorly defined, although recent work suggests that the events may actually take place in the acinar cells themselves. In the normal pancreas, inactive enzymes are packaged in zymogen granules that fuse with the acinar cell membrane and release their contents into the ductal lumen when secretion occurs. In several animal models of acute pancreatitis, Steer (2) showed that the zymogen granules failed to fuse with the membrane and instead joined with lysosomes (colocalization). The lysosomes contain the enzyme cathepsin B, which may convert trypsinogen to trypsin within the living cell. Steer proposed that this event could initiate autodigestion and inflammation, but it has not been shown to occur in humans, and the hypothesis remains controversial.

In any case, activated enzymes and inflammatory mediators are then released into the interstitium, retroperitoneum, and peritoneal cavity. Absorption of these potential toxins is believed to account for some of the systemic effects of the disease. However, the severity of the systemic illness and the progression of changes within the gland may be related to factors other than the direct effects of pancreatic enzymes (3, 4).

## GENERAL CONSIDERATIONS

### Prediction of Severity

Most patients with acute pancreatitis have mild disease that resolves spontaneously. For these patients, medical therapy is largely supportive. Patients with more severe disease require intensive medical monitoring and care. These individuals should be identified early in the course of their disease, in an effort to institute treatment as early as possible.

Ranson et al. were the first to demonstrate that assessment of certain parameters early in the course of the disease could help predict the severity of the pancreatitis and the likelihood of death (5). The mortality rate correlated closely with the number of positive criteria found to be present during the first 48 hours of the disease. Patients with more than four positive signs were more likely to have necrotizing pancreatitis, develop major complications, and die. However, even though patients with fewer than four signs were likely to have milder disease, many still had serious complications, some of which required surgery. Because Ranson's system (as well as its numerous refinements) can be cumbersome to apply and has only been validated for the first 2 days of an attack of pancreatitis, a variety of other prognostic approaches have evolved. The APACHE II (Acute Physiologic and Chronic Health Evaluation) system also accurately predicts the severity of the disease and has the advantage of being applicable at any time during the illness (6, 7). However, it requires a computer for most effective use. Other methods, such as abdominal paracentesis (8), grading of CT scans (9, 10), and evaluation of inflammatory serum markers (11, 12) have all been used with varying degrees of success (Table 20.1).

The combination of clinical assessment and measurement of biochemical abnormalities, such as alterations in hematocrit, blood urea nitrogen (BUN), creatinine, $pO_2$, and calcium levels, gives the best initial index of the severity of pancreatitis. The magnitude of the rise in serum pancreatic enzyme levels (e.g., amylase) bears no relationship to the severity of the disease (13). Evaluation of concentrations of inflammatory markers (11, 12) such as C-reactive protein, complement factors, protease inhibitors, and leukocyte enzymes may be more helpful in predicting severity, but further evaluation is needed. Derangements in other organ systems generally indicate severe diseases and the need for aggressive management to minimize morbidity and mortality.

## LOCAL EFFECTS

### Pathology

In mild forms of acute pancreatitis, pancreatic edema is a prominent feature (14). Grossly, the pancreas appears boggy and indurated. Microscopically, the pancreatic lobules are separated by edema fluid without evidence of hemorrhage. There is a variable amount of interlobular infiltration by inflammatory cells. The acinar cells appear structurally intact, however, and blood flow appears to be maintained in the small capillaries and venules. In severe cases, the edema and accompanying inflam-

**TABLE 20.1. Predictions of Severity of Acute Pancreatitis**

| Study | Factor Studied | | Ability to Distinguish Between Severe and Mild Acute Pancreatitis: Sensitivity (%) | Specificity (%) |
|---|---|---|---|---|
| Heath (8) | IL-6 | | 100 | 71 |
| | CRP | | 90 | 79 |
| Dominguez-Munoz (60) | PMN-elastase | 0 hr | 93 | 94 |
| | | 24 hr | 93 | 99 |
| | | 48 hr | 92 | 100 |
| London (6) | Dynamic CT | | 83 | 65 |
| Dominguez-Munoz (89) | APACHE[a] score | | 70 | 79 |
| | SAPS[b] | | 67 | 79 |

[a]APACHE, Acute Physiology and Chronic Health Evaluation.
[b]SAPS, Simplified Acute Physiology Score.

mation may extend throughout the retroperitoneum and to surrounding organs. Acute fluid collections often develop. Fat necrosis from the interaction of activated pancreatic enzymes with fatty tissue is common.

If the initial inflammatory process progresses, pancreatic necrosis can occur. Grossly, the pancreas first appears hemorrhagic and then becomes necrotic. The surface of the pancreas may appear devitalized, although it may look normal if the dead tissue is located inside the gland. Necrotic areas can be found adjacent to healthy lobules, along with an intense inflammatory reaction and cellular infiltration.

The acinar cells undergo necrosis in association with thrombosis of their supplying nutrient vessels. Early in the disease, acinar cell organelles responsible for protein synthesis appear abnormal. However, zymogen granules remain intact until late. Pancreatic enzymes may be released as the terminal event of acinar cell death.

### Fluid Sequestration

Patients with acute pancreatitis may develop hypotension secondary to hypovolemia caused by fluid sequestration. In response to inflammation, 2 or more liters of fluid may be lost into the abdominal cavity and retroperitoneum (15). The most frequent site of fluid accumulation is the lesser sac; other sites include the spaces posterior to the pancreas and anterior to the kidneys. In most patients with uncomplicated edematous pancreatitis, ascitic fluid is straw colored and without necrotic debris. It becomes blood tinged or “prune juice colored” in more severe forms.

The elevated hematocrit frequently seen is indirect evidence of the relative hypovolemia that exists. Systolic blood pressure decreases early in the course of the disease and is treated by administration of intravenous fluid.

### Fat Necrosis

Fat necrosis is the result of local and/or systemic pancreatic enzyme activation (16). Locally, it is found within the intralobular septa of the pancreas, in the retroperitoneum, and in the abdominal cavity. Although the sequestered fluid contains a variety of enzymes, only lipase, in combination with colipase, causes necrosis of fat. These necrotic areas are sharply demarcated from healthy fat and appear as whitish gray, firm plaques. Analysis reveals high concentrations of lipase, calcium, and free fatty acids. Calcium binds with the free fatty acids in the process of saponification. Although this may contribute to the reduction in serum calcium seen in some patients with severe pancreatitis, there are probably multiple causes of the hypocalcemia (see below).

Fat necrosis is also occasionally found outside the abdominal cavity in the subcutaneous tissue and in the bone marrow. The subcutaneous lesions are similar morphologically and histologically to those found in the abdomen and appear during the acute disease. Peripheral fat necrosis also may occur in the joints, which provokes a synovitis. Arthrocentesis reveals a cloudy or creamy fluid with elevated concentrations of lipase. These lesions frequently disappear with resolution of the disease or following pancreatectomy.

## SYSTEMIC EFFECTS

### Cardiovascular

Oliguria, decreased cardiac output, and hypotension are common during severe acute pancreatitis. These may be the result of hypovolemia from the fluid sequestration. A systemic capillary leak may also occur secondary to the release of inflammatory mediators such as histamine or bradykinin. However, hypovolemia alone probably cannot account for all the systemic manifestations of the disease.

The usual response to fluid sequestration in mild acute pancreatitis is a compensatory increase in cardiac output. This is the result of an increase in both cardiac rate and contractility. Normally, intravenous fluid administration increases intravascular volume, and the pulse rate decreases. However, in patients with severe pancreatitis, the cardiac output often remains unchanged even if the pulse rate increases. This is due to a concomitant decrease in cardiac contractility. Even when intravascular volume is restored, there may still be an inadequate contractile response. Other abnormalities include a progressive depression of left ventricular stroke work and an increasing pulmonary capillary wedge pressure (PCWP) (17). Tissue perfusion falls (18), metabolic function is impaired, and oxygen consumption decreases (19). In spite of these abnormalities, no structural or histologic changes have been noted in the myocardium of patients who died from acute pancreatitis (14).

Transient ECG abnormalities have also been observed in patients with acute pancreatitis (20), but their cause and significance are unknown. They are more common in patients with a history of cardiac disease (21). The acidosis as well as the hypovolemia may contribute to these abnormalities of cardiac rhythm.

Humoral factors released from the pancreas may be important in the development of the cardiovascular complications. For example, bradykinin and related substances are elevated in the serum in both patients and experimental animals with acute pancreatitis. They are known to alter cardiac and vascular function in ways that could explain the changes that are seen. The pancreas is a major source of bradykinin in experimental pancreatitis, and its production is initiated by trypsin (4). The effects of pancreatic enzymes on cardiac function have not been studied.

The presence of circulating myocardial depressant factor (MDF) has been proposed in experimental animals with acute pancreatitis and with hypovolemic shock (22), two conditions associated with impairment of splanchnic blood flow. The proposed production of MDF in experimental pancreatitis is temporally related to the release of lysosomal enzymes from pancreatic acinar cells and is decreased by pancreatectomy in the experimental animals. A substance thought to be MDF has been isolated from the serum of patients with hypovolemic shock, but it has not been isolated from patients with pancreatitis. Thus, the role of MDF in mediating the impairment of cardiovascular function associated with pancreatitis has not been defined.

### Renal Alterations

Oliguria is common in patients with pancreatitis and fluid sequestrations, but the urine output usually increases when intravascular volume is repleted. In most patients with uncomplicated disease, the BUN can rise as high as 40 mg/dL, and the creatinine to about 6 mg/dL. These values return to normal with adequate fluid replacement (23). In more severe cases or when fluid replacement is inadequate, acute renal failure may ensue. When renal failure complicates acute pancreatitis, the mortality rate may be as high as 70%.

In some patients with acute pancreatitis, renal function may be impaired without any history of hypovolemia, hypotension, or sepsis. These patients often show evidence of a membranous glomerulopathy and acute tubular necrosis. Other studies have demonstrated small renal arterioles blocked by fat emboli. These observations have not been investigated experimentally. Some investigators have actually noted hypertension during the first 72 hours of acute disease (24). The cause is unknown, but in these patients, the renal and systemic resistances were both elevated, and the renal blood flow and glomerular filtration rate were decreased. The importance of these changes and the responsible mechanisms are not known.

The urine output may improve in some patients with acute pancreatitis treated with peritoneal lavage. This has suggested that a dialyzable substance may be responsible for the renal failure. However, in other studies, hemodialysis has not affected the course of either the pancreatitis or the renal failure (25). Others have suggested the use of vasodilators and natriuretic diuretics, but their efficacy is unproven. The clinical course of the renal failure associated with acute pancreatitis is similar to that associated with hemorrhagic or septic shock alone.

### Respiratory Alterations

Arterial hypoxemia is common in patients with acute pancreatitis. However, most do not require endotracheal intubation and mechanical ventilation. When respiratory support is necessary, it indicates a more severe impairment of pulmonary function, with an expected increase in associated mortality.

Measurements of arterial blood gases and serial chest x-rays should be parts of the early assessment in all patients with acute pancreatitis. Some 50–60% of patients with acute pancreatitis exhibit arterial hypoxemia, with a partial pressure of oxygen ($pO_2$) below 70 mm Hg while breathing room air (14, 26). Most improve rapidly as the disease resolves, but some patients deteriorate. Marked progression of respiratory failure within the first 48 hours is associated with an increase in mortality rate. Because hypoxemia usually precedes any observable changes in the chest x-ray, there may be a substantial time lag between the appearance of hypoxemia and x-ray evidence of pulmonary disease. Eventually, abnormalities on a chest x-ray can be seen in over half of all patients with acute pancreatitis. Pulmonary edema is evident in up to 60% of those with hypoxemia who survive the first 48 hours of pancreatitis. Reactive changes such as diaphragmatic elevation, pleural thickening, and pleural effusion are most commonly found on the left side, although they may be found on the right side or bilaterally (27). Sterile pleural effusions are common in patients with pancreatitis, and the fluid may have an elevated amylase concentration. The volume of the pleural effusion, however, usually cannot account for the ventilatory abnormalities.

Ventilation, gas exchange, and the pulmonary circulation may all be affected. Ventilation-perfusion mismatch results from the reduction in both pulmonary capillary blood flow and alveolar ventilation. This causes an increase in the amount of ventilation to nonperfused alveolar spaces and does not appear to be cardiogenic in origin. There is also an increase in the amount of pulmonary capillary blood that flows past alveoli that are not ventilated. The results of the mismatch in ventilation and perfusion are that oxygen and carbon dioxide are not exchanged, and potentially severe respiratory compromise can develop.

Many of the physiologic abnormalities observed in the respiratory failure associated with acute pancreatitis are similar to those seen in adult respiratory distress syndrome (ARDS) occurring from other causes. A transient increase in pulmonary vascular resistance has been noted on occasion (28, 29), but this does not account for the decreased capillary flow in most patients. The increase in resistance is likely due to the effect of vasoconstrictive substances released from the pancreas on the pulmonary vasculature.

Most patients with acute pancreatitis have ventilatory abnormalities. Measurement of ventilation-perfusion mismatch may reveal a right to left shunt in 10–30% of patients not requiring mechanical ventilatory support (30). The vital capacity is decreased approximately 25%, and the ratio of the forced expiratory volume per second ($FEV_1$) to forced vital capacity (FVC) is reduced by 20–35% (31, 32). The efficiency of pulmonary gas exchange, measured by the carbon monoxide diffusion capacity, is also reduced by about 25% in most patients. The oxygen-carrying capacity of hemoglobin is also impaired, but this does not appear to be related to alkalosis, decreased 2,3-diphosphoglycerate (2,3-DPG) levels, or hemoglobin concentration (33). It has been postulated that the elevated levels of free fatty acids sometimes found in acute pancreatitis may contribute to the increased affinity of oxyhemoglobin (34). Despite these ventilatory abnormalities, most patients do not require assisted ventilation, and most of these values return to normal levels after resolution of the pancreatitis.

The mechanisms of pulmonary injury in acute pancreatitis are unknown (3). Sepsis may contribute to the respiratory failure in patients with infection, but many patients who develop pulmonary dysfunction have sterile disease. High serum concentrations of pancreatic enzymes may contribute to respiratory failure. Intravenous infusion of trypsin in sheep increased pulmonary transvascular protein clearance (leakage) and pulmonary lymph flow. Pretreatment of these animals with a trypsin inhibitor (e.g., aprotinin, Trasylol) prevented the increased pulmonary vascular permeability (35). Pulmonary leukostasis with capillary sludging also results from trypsin infusion and is inhibited with aprotinin pretreatment. This suggests that proteolytic enzymes could be contributing to the pathogenesis of the pulmonary dysfunction. Cytokines released from the pancreas or liver have also been implicated (see below).

Free fatty acids in the circulation can cause respiratory failure and may be released as the result of digestion of fat by lipase. Some patients with acute pancreatitis have elevated levels of serum triglycerides, particularly patients with a history of chronic alcoholism and/or disorders of lipid metabolism. Experiments performed with isolated lungs of dogs have confirmed the injurious effects of free fatty acids (36). Histologic studies of diseased lungs in patients with acute pancreatitis demonstrated fat emboli (37). However, the mechanism by which free fatty acids actually cause pulmonary injury is now known and requires further investigation.

Phospholipase $A_2$ ($PLA_2$) has been recovered from the serum of patients with acute pancreatitis who developed respiratory failure. The magnitude of pulmonary derangement correlated with the degree of $PLA_2$ elevation. The proposed mechanism of action of $PLA_2$ is through the dissolution of pulmonary surfactant. In patients with the highest levels of $PLA_2$, neither peritoneal lavage nor pancreatectomy altered the course of the respiratory failure (38). In experimental pancreatitis, decreased surfactant activity and elevation of the metabolic products of surfactant digestion have also been observed (39).

### Endocrine Alterations

**Glucose.** Important abnormalities occur in the metabolism of glucose and calcium. Elevated blood glucose concentrations (130–200 mg/dL) are seen in 50–75% of patients with acute pancreatitis (40). However, glucosuria occurs in only about one-third of patients with hyperglycemia. Although blood glucose levels above 200 mg/dL are associated with increased mortality rates (5), this only reflects the severity of the pancreatitis. Death rarely occurs as the result of hyperglycemia or of diabetic complications alone. A number of factors contribute to the hyperglycemia (14). In general, both the serum glucagon and insulin concentrations are elevated in patients with any form of stress. However, serum insulin concentrations are not high enough to prevent hyperglycemia. In patients with acute pancreatitis, the serum glucagon concentrations are much higher, and the insulin concentrations are lower than in patients with stress from other causes. Elevated serum growth hormone and cortisol concentrations, both of which can produce hyperglycemia, are also found in patients with acute pancreatitis (41). Intravenous infusion of arginine or alanine stimulates moderate secretion of glucagon and insulin in healthy individuals. In patients with acute pancreatitis, these secretory stimuli produce an increase in serum glucagon that is up to 10 times normal and 50% higher than that seen in patients with other forms of stress. Likewise insulin concentrations after secretagogue infusion are up to 6 times those seen in the normal response to stress (42). When studied up to 4–6 weeks later, these responses return to normal. The fasting hyperglycemia, hyperglucagonemia, and the abnormal response to alanine and arginine infusion all resolve along with the pancreatitis. During the first 48–72 hours after the onset of disease, there is marked fasting hyperglycemia along with hyperglucagonemia and hypoinsulinemia. The elevated concentrations of glucagon and glucose usually return to normal within 18–21 days after resolution of pancreatitis (43).

Serum insulin concentrations do not increase to the same level as they do in normal individuals in response to arginine infusion during the first 48–72 hours. A significant decrease in both phases of arginine-stimulated insulin release is seen. The early phase of stimulated secretion returned to normal within 10 days. The second phase of insulin release after arginine infusion remained significantly impaired up to 3 weeks after the onset of pancreatitis. (Insulin is normally secreted in a biphasic pattern in response to arginine and glucose, a phenomenon thought to represent release of insulin from two compartments. The first phase is characterized by a rapid release, and the second by a more prolonged release. Primary diabetes most commonly affects the early release phase).

Hyperglycemia in patients with acute pancreatitis should not be treated unless it is severe. Administration of insulin is not very effective in lowering the serum glucose level of patients with hyperglucagonemia, so high doses of insulin may be necessary. Because the hyperglucagonemia of acute pancreatitis tends to resolve suddenly and unpredictably, administration of large amounts of insulin to these patients to correct an elevated blood glucose may produce dangerous hypoglycemia. Since the elevated blood glucose level is not a common source of either morbidity or mortality, mild hyperglycemia should be tolerated. However, patients with diabetic ketoacidosis (without acute pancreatitis) may mimic patients with acute pancreatitis and elevated blood glucose, because they both may have elevated amylase levels and complain of abdominal pain.

**Calcium.** Mild hypocalcemia is frequent in patients with pancreatitis, and while the serum calcium concentration is usually only minimally depressed, profound hypocalcemia can occur. This implies a poor prognosis. A number of factors may contribute to the hypocalcemia. Hypoalbuminemia is common in acute pancreatitis because vascular permeability is increased, and albumin is lost from the intravascular space. Since some of the serum calcium is normally bound to albumin, some of it is lost in this way. In this situation, the serum ionized calcium level is often normal, despite a low total serum calcium. Therefore, in the laboratory examination of a patient with acute pancreatitis, calcium levels should be measured in conjunction with albumin levels to determine the amount of ionized calcium accurately. If only total calcium is measured, a falsely low value for ionized calcium may be obtained. Fat necrosis, with saponification of calcium into soap, may account for the loss of as much as 1–2 g of calcium. However, this is not sufficient to account for the level of hypocalcemia sometimes seen in acute pancreatitis.

Parathyroid hormone (PTH) production, release, and peripheral activity in response to hypocalcemia are all normal in acute pancreatitis. Patients with true ionized hypocalcemia have appropriately elevated serum PTH concentrations, which decrease as serum ionized calcium returns to normal. Hypocalciuria and decreased tubular reabsorption of phosphate indicate normal action of PTH in the kidney. Infusion of PTH into patients with acute pancreatitis and hypocalcemia results in increased serum calcium and urinary cyclic adenine monophosphate (cAMP), indicating unimpaired action of the hormone. Calcitonin concentrations are elevated up to six times normal in hypocalcemic patients with pancreatitis. The increase in serum calcitonin precedes the development of hypocalcemia (45). Infusion of glucagon in normal individuals results in an increase in serum calcitonin concentration. Thus, the hyperglucagonemia present in acute pancreatitis may account for, or at least contribute to, the hypercalcitoninemia. However, infusion of glucagon in patients with acute pancreatitis does not increase serum calcitonin levels or further reduce ionized calcium concentrations (14).

Hypomagnesemia may also be present in patients with acute pancreatitis. This is important because it may be impossible to correct the hypocalcemia without also treating the hypomagnesemia. Hypomagnesemia can inhibit PTH secretion and its peripheral function.

In most patients with acute pancreatitis, hypocalcemia is transient and mild. Calcium replacement is not necessary unless the ionized calcium level is also decreased or the patient is symptomatic. Any hypokalemia should be corrected at the same time, because rapid correction of hypocalcemia in this clinical setting may precipitate cardiac arrhythmias.

### Coagulation Abnormalities

Clinically important coagulopathy is uncommon in acute pancreatitis, and there are no consistent alterations in coagulation parameters. However, thromboses of capillaries and small vessels of the pancreas, lung, and kidney as well as disseminated intravascular coagulopathy (DIC) can occur in these patients, and the effect of acute pancreatitis on the coagulation process has been studied. The association of a hypercoagulable state with elevated levels of fibrinogen and factor VIII in patients with acute pancreatitis was first noted more than 20 years ago (46). Subsequent studies confirmed these findings (47, 48). Abnormalities included a rise in serum fibrinogen with peak values occurring around 1 week after disease onset, as well as elevations in platelet count and fibrinogen-related antigen. However, alterations of prothrombin time, partial thromboplastin time, thrombin time, and levels of factors II, V, and VII to X showed no consistent pattern. Other studies noted the occurrence of DIC with a consumptive coagulopathy and excess fibrinolysis (49, 50).

The mechanisms by which acute pancreatitis alters coagulation parameters are unknown. Ranson et al. (48) theorized that trypsin was responsible and experimental studies have shown that trypsin activates fibrinogen (51). Other potential mechanisms include increased reactivity of the reticuloendothelial system, protease-antiprotease imbalance, and loss of fibrinogen from the circulation secondary to vascular injury.

Some studies have attempted to correlate the changes in coagulation parameters with the severity of the acute pancreatitis

(48, 52). They showed that alterations in coagulation status, including fibrinogen, fibrinogen-related antigen, platelet count, and prothrombin time were the greatest in patients with the most severe forms of acute pancreatitis.

Success in the treatment of coagulation abnormalities in acute pancreatitis has been limited. Heparin administration to treat the DIC has not been beneficial. Aprotinin (Trasylol), a protease inhibitor, has also not been of any value (53).

## NEW DIRECTIONS IN THE PATHOGENESIS OF ACUTE PANCREATITIS

### Role of Cytokines and Inflammatory Mediators

Although the release of activated pancreatic enzymes into the circulation undoubtedly accounts for some of the manifestations of acute pancreatitis, this cannot explain all the systemic effects of severe disease. Recent studies suggest that the production and release of a variety of inflammatory mediators by the inflamed pancreas contributes as well.

For example, acute pancreatitis is associated with the rapid release of interleukin-1 (IL-1), IL-6, and tumor necrosis factor alpha (TNF-$\alpha$) into the serum, and the serum levels of these cytokines correlate well with the degree of pancreatic inflammation. One study found that serum from patients admitted with a diagnosis of acute pancreatitis had elevations of IL-6 that correlated with the severity of the disease (12). IL-6 levels correlated with those of two other markers, C-reactive protein and $PLA_2$ activity, suggesting a causal role for IL-6 in the acute-phase response (54). IL-1, IL-6, and TNF-$\alpha$ are all elevated in the serum of animals with acute pancreatitis. One study demonstrated that pretreatment with anti-TNF antibodies attenuated the expected rise of serum TNF, glucose, and amylase (55).

Platelet activating factor (PAF), another inflammatory mediator, also seems to play an important role in the pathogenesis of acute disease. PAF is a low-molecular-weight phospholipid that stimulates platelet, macrophage, and neutrophil aggregation and promotes hypotension and capillary leakage (56, 57). Treatment with PAF-antibodies appears to ameliorate the severity of acute pancreatitis (58).

The mechanisms of cytokine production are only beginning to be defined. In the pancreas, cytokines appear to be released primarily from tissue macrophages, although recruitment of leukocytes and other inflammatory cells may contribute to the process as well. The release of histamine and other secretory proteins into the interstitial space from the inflamed pancreas may cause the initial macrophage and endothelial cell activation, with release of such cytokines as IL-8 and PAF and neutrophil recruitment. Cytokines derived from the pancreas may travel to the liver via the portal venous circulation. There, they could cause hepatic injury and additional release of cytokines derived from the hepatic Kupffer cells. These could enter the systemic circulation via the hepatic venous drainage and be responsible for the widespread effects on the other organ systems.

One of the primary effects of the cytokines is to activate neutrophils, which then mediate the destructive events associated with inflammation. IL-8, a product of tissue macrophages, also contributes to initial neutrophil activation, and its release correlates with circulating levels of neutrophil elastase. The ability of neutrophils to produce tissue damage comes, at least in part, from their tendency to form free radicals and to release proteolytic enzymes. One of the most abundant is PMN-elastase, which can degrade components of the extracellular matrix, cleanse various plasma proteins, and even attach intact cells (59). PMN-elastase has also been studied as a potential prognostic marker in acute pancreatitis. Three clinical (60–62) and one experimental study (63) suggest that it may predict the severity of the clinical course of the disease.

The complement system can be activated by trypsin and other proteolytic enzymes. Activation of complement results in the formation of factors C3a and C5a. These can contribute to increases in vascular permeability, induce smooth muscle contraction, release histamine from mast cells and basophils, and impair cardiac function. Despite these known effects, there is no consensus on the role of complement activation in acute pancreatitis (64, 65). C3a also has been proposed as a useful marker for assessing the severity of acute pancreatitis, but further studies are needed.

### Nitric Oxide

Nitric oxide (NO) is a potent vasodilator that has been shown to have a wide variety of biologic effects, some of which may relate to the pathogenesis of acute pancreatitis. For example, NO is known to increase pancreatic secretion as well as improve pancreatic perfusion (66). NO decreases microvascular permeability and white blood cell emigration (67, 68). It may also influence free radical formation and cytokine release (69, 70).

Although some studies have concluded that NO may be harmful in the course of acute pancreatitis (71, 72), they focused on the very early stages of the disease process. Other workers found that NO administration in established acute pancreatitis can benefit both the pancreatitis and the associated pulmonary injury (73, 74). These beneficial effects may be due to NO's inhibitory effects on neutrophil emigration. Its vasodilatory effects may also contribute by improving pancreatic perfusion.

### Bacterial Translocation

Secondary infection of necrotic pancreatic and peripancreatic tissue is a common source of morbidity in acute pancreatitis. The origin of the bacteria is generally thought to be the gastrointestinal tract, although hematogenous seeding from infected intravenous lines or other sources could occur.

Bacterial overgrowth of indigenous enteric organisms may be common in association with the ileus associated with acute pancreatitis. One study demonstrated that enteric bacteria within the gut and in adjacent mesenteric lymph nodes increased as interstitial transit decreased during experimental pancreatitis in rats (75).

Other studies investigated the origin of the bacteria that caused pancreatic infection. Either plasmid or radiolabeled *Escherichia coli* were placed into the intestinal tracts of the animals to be studied. After pancreatitis was induced, cultures of the mesenteric lymph nodes and pancreas of the animals were positive for the labeled bacteria, suggesting that the gut was the source (76, 77).

Antibiotic prophylaxis has been proposed for all patients with severe acute pancreatitis to prevent subsequent infection. One study found that early pancreatic infection in severe experimental pancreatitis was reduced with a full-gut decontamination regimen or with an antibiotic that was concentrated in pancreatic tissue (imipenem) (78) (See also Chapters 21 and 28). Clinically, this form of therapy appears to decrease the frequency of pancreatic infection, as well.

### Ischemia-Reperfusion and the Role of the Microcirculation

In acute pancreatitis, pancreatic blood flow is reduced, and the interstitial pH of the pancreatic tissue is also low, which suggests ischemia (79). Pancreatic microcirculatory changes such as vasoconstriction, capillary stasis, decreased oxygen saturation, and progressive ischemia seem to occur early in the course of experimental acute pancreatitis (80, 81). If aerobic metabolism is impaired, high-energy phosphates would be reduced to adenosine, inosine, and hypoxanthine via anaerobic metabolic pathways.

In a canine model of pancreatitis, a 45% drop in ATP levels was seen after a severe reduction in blood flow. With total ischemia and also with the pancreatitis produced by intraductal injection of oleic acid into dogs, a drop in high-energy phosphates measured by nuclear magnetic resonance was seen within 1 hour (82). The hypoxanthine produced in this setting is metabolized on reperfusion and reoxygenation to produce superoxide. This reaction is catalyzed by xanthine oxidase, produced from xanthine dehydrogenase under hypoxic conditions.

There also is evidence that ischemia-reperfusion (IR) may produce acute pancreatitis in animal models that incorporate complete pancreatic ischemia for varying lengths of time, followed by reperfusion (83–85). However, the magnitude or duration of ischemia necessary to initiate IR injury is unknown.

Experimental acute pancreatitis can be modified by the early use of free radical scavengers or antioxidants (84, 86). For example, superoxide dismutase decreased the arterial vasoconstriction and leukocyte adherence associated with experimental acute pancreatitis (84). This was associated with a reduction in disease severity, suggesting that initially, pancreatitis depends on reactive oxygen metabolites (ROMs) for its progression. Sources of ROMs include xanthine oxygenase, neutrophil myeloperoxidase, prostaglandin synthetase, flavoproteins, and hemoglobin (87). Of these, the first two are probably the most important in pathologic states.

Superoxide produced by IR is a potent oxidant that exists with its conjugate acid, the hydroperoxyl radical ($HOO^-$). Together, they generate additional secondary ROMs (88). Under normal physiologic circumstances, the ROMs are relatively noncytotoxic because of endogenous enzymatic antioxidants such as superoxide dismutase and catalase, which degrade them rapidly. Other endogenous substances also have antioxidant properties (ascorbate, urate, bilirubin, albumin, and sulfhydryl groups on proteins). However, during IR, the normal tissue protective mechanisms are overwhelmed, and cells are injured by the cytotoxic oxidation reactions. In addition, ROMs react with cell lipids to generate potent chemotoxins (87). This results in further cytokine release, complement activation, endothelial expression of intercellular adhesion molecules, and neutrophil activation and emigration. The myeloperoxidase released by activated neutrophils combines with hydrogen peroxide to produce more free radicals and cellular damage.

There are two reasons why free radical injury may be worse in the pancreas than in other tissues. First, the pancreatic interstitial pH is low, especially in the stimulated gland (89). At low pH, more of the superoxide radical exists as its conjugate acid, the hydroperoxyl radical. This is a more potent oxidant, which can initiate lipid peroxidation (90). Second, ROMs derived from neutrophil myeloperoxidase inactivate interstitial proteinase inhibitors. Acinar cell damage causes extravasation of intracellular proteases into the interstitium where these protease inhibitors normally protect tissues from autodigestion. Indeed, the concentration of interstitial proteases can reach very high levels following ductal and acinar damage.

## SUMMARY

Acute pancreatitis is a complex disease whose pathogenesis is incompletely understood. Research has suggested the possibility that enzyme activation may occur intracellularly to initiate the disease and that interleukins and other inflammatory mediators may be important in its propagation.

Once the disease is established, its prognosis depends, in part, on the degree of involvement of other organs and organ systems. These include the cardiovascular, renal, pulmonary, and endocrine organs, and the coagulation mechanism. Treatment should be based on these pathophysiologic alterations.

## REFERENCES


1. Wedgewood K, Reber HA. Acute pancreatitis: the concepts of pathogenesis. In: Howard J, Jordan G, Reber HA, eds. Surgical diseases of the pancreas. Philadelphia: Lea & Febiger, 1986.
2. Steer ML. How and where does acute pancreatitis begin? Arch Surg 1992;123(11):1350–1353.
3. Malik AB. Pulmonary edema after pancreatitis: role of humoral factors. Circ Shock 1983;10:71.
4. Popieruitis AS, Thompson AG. The site of bradykinin release in acute experimental pancreatitis. Arch Surg 1969;98:73.
5. Ranson JH, Rifkind KM, Roses DF, Fink DS, Eng K, Spencer FC. Prognostic signs and the role of operative management in acute pancreatitis. Surg Gynecol Obstet 1974;139:69–81.
6. Tran DD, Cuesta MA. Evaluation of severity in patients with acute pancreatitis. Am J Gastroenterol 1992;87(5):604–608.
7. Wilson C, Heath DI, Imrie CW. Prediction of outcome in acute pancreatitis: a comparative study of APACHE II, clinical assessment and multiple factor scoring systems. Br J Surg 1990;77(11): 1260–1264.
8. Ranson JHC, Spencer F. The role of peritoneal lavage in severe acute pancreatitis. Ann Surg 1978;187:565.
9. Freeny PC. Angio-CT: diagnosis and detection of complications of acute pancreatitis. Hepatogastroenterology 1991;38(2): 109–115.
10. London NJM, Leese T, Lavelle JM, et al. Rapid-bolus contrast-enhanced dynamic computed tomography in acute pancreatitis: a prospective study. Br J Surg 1991;78:1452–1456.
11. Dominguez-Munoz JE, Carballo F, Garcia MJ, et al. Monitoring of serum proteinase-antiproteinase balance and systemic inflammatory response in prognostic evaluation of acute pancreatitis; results of a prospective multicenter trial. Dig Dis Sci 1993;38(3): 507–513.
12. Heath DI, Cruickshank A, Gudgeon M, Jehanli A, Shenkin A, Imrie CW. Role of interleukin-6 in mediating the acute phase protein response and potential as an early means of severity assessment in acute pancreatitis. Gut 1993;34(1):41–45.
13. Pezzilli R, Billi P, Miglioli M, Gullo L. Serum amylase and lipase concentrations and lipase/amylase ration in assessment of etiology and severity of acute pancreatitis. Dig Dis Sci 1993;38(7): 1265–1269.
14. Austin J, Reber HA. The pathologic features of acute pancreatitis. In: Howard J, Jordan G, Reber HA, eds. Surgical diseases of the pancreas. Philadelphia: Lea & Febiger, 1986.
15. Carey LC. Extra-abdominal manifestations of acute pancreatitis. Surgery 1979;86:337.
16. Lee PC, Howard JM. Fat necrosis. Surg Gynecol Obstet 1979; 148:785.
17. Bradley EL, Hall JR, Lutz J, Hamner L, Lattouf O. Hemodynamic consequences of severe pancreatitis. Ann Surg 1983;198: 130–133.
18. DiCarlo V, Nespoli A, Chiesa R, et al. Hemodynamic and metabolic impairment in acute pancreatitis. World J Surg 1981; 5:329–339.
19. Bevilacqua G, et al. Hemodynamics and metabolic impairment in acute pancreatitis. In: Hollender LF, ed. Controversies in acute pancreatitis. Berlin: Springer-Verlag, 1982.
20. Buch J, Buch A, Schmidt A. Transient ECG changes during attacks of pancreatitis. Acta Cardiol 1980;35:381.
21. Mautner RK, Siegel LA, Giles TD, Kayser J. Electrocardiographic changes in acute pancreatitis. South Med J 1982;75:317.
22. Lefer AM. Vascular mediators in ischemia and shock. In: Cowley RA, Trump BF, eds. Pathophysiology of shock; anoxia, and ischemia. Baltimore: Williams & Wilkins, 1982.
23. Goldstein DA, Llach F, Massry SG. Acute renal failure in patients with acute pancreatitis. Arch Intern Med 1976;136:1363.
24. Sankaran S, Lucas CE, Walt AJ. Transient hypertension with acute pancreatitis. Surg Gynecol Obstet 1974;138:225.
25. Balsov JT, Jorgensen HE, Neilsen R. Acute renal failure complicating acute pancreatitis. Acta Chir Scand 1962;124:348.

26. Nath BJ, Warshaw AL. Pulmonary insufficiency. In: Bradley EL, ed. Complications of pancreatitis. Philadelphia: WB Saunders, 1982.
27. Kaye MD. Pleuropulmonary complications of pancreatitis. Thorax 1968;23:297.
28. Halmagyi DF, Karis JH, Stenning FG, Varga D. Pulmonary hypertension in acute hemorrhagic pancreatitis. Surgery 1974;76: 637–642.
29. Miyashiro A, Grosberg SJ, Wapnick S. Reversible pulmonary hypertension and cardiac failure with recurrent pancreatitis. Chest 1977;71:669–671.
30. DeTroyer A, Naerje R, Yernault JC, Englert M. Impairment of pulmonary function in acute pancreatitis. Chest 1979;73:360.
31. Berry AR, Taylor TV, Davies GC. Pulmonary function and fibrinogen metabolism in acute pancreatitis. Br J Surg 1981;68:870.
32. Murphy D, Pack AI, Imrie CW. The mechanisms of arterial hypoxia occurring in acute pancreatitis. Q J Med 1980;194:151.
33. Greenburg AG, Terlizzi L, Peskin GW. Oxyhemoglobin affinity in acute pancreatitis. J Surg Res 1977;22:561.
34. Cameron JL, Capuzzi DM, Zuidema GD, Margolis S. Acute pancreatitis with hyperlipidemia: evidence for a persistent defect in lipid metabolism. Ann Surg 1973;177:483.
35. Tahamont MV, Barie PS, Blumenstock FA, et al. Increased lung vascular permeability after pancreatitis and trypsin infusion. Am J Pathol 1982;109:15–26.
36. Kimura T, Toung JK, Margolis S, Permutt S, Cameron JL. Respiratory failure in acute pancreatitis. Ann Surg 1979;189:509–514.
37. Lankisch PG, Rahlf G, Koop H. Pulmonary complications in fatal acute hemorrhagic pancreatitis. Dig Dis Sci 1983;28:111.
38. Schroder T, Lempinen M, Kivilaakso E, Nikki P. Serum phospholipase A2 and pulmonary changes in acute fulminant pancreatitis. Resuscitation 1982;10:79.
39. Maciver AG, Metcalfe IL, Possmayer F, et al. Alteration of surfactant chemistry in experimental hemorrhagic pancreatitis. J Surg Res 1977;23:311–314.
40. Wellman KF, Volk VW. Pancreatitis, pancreatic lithiasis, and diabetes mellitus. In: Wellman FK, Volk BW, eds. The diabetic pancreas. New York: Plenum Press, 1977.
41. Drew SI, Joff B, Vinik A, et al. First 24 hours of acute pancreatitis. Changes in biochemical and endocrine homeostasis in patients with pancreatitis compared with those in control subjects undergoing stress for reasons other than pancreatitis. Am J Med 1978;64:795–803.
42. Donowitz M, Hendler R, Spiro HM, et al. Glucagon secretion in acute and chronic pancreatitis. Ann Intern Med 1975;83:778–781.
43. Solomon SS, Duckworth WC, Jallepalli P, et al. The glucose intolerance of acute pancreatitis: hormonal response to arginine. Diabetes 1980;29:22–26.
44. Imrie CW, Beastall GH, Allam BF, O'Neil J, Benjamin IS, McKay AJ. Parathyroid hormone and calcium homeostasis in acute pancreatitis. Br J Surg 1978;655:717–720.
45. Canale DD, Donabedian RK. Hypercalcitoninemia in acute pancreatitis. J Clin Endocrinol Metab 1975;49:738.
46. Sinowara GY, Stutman LH, Walters JI, et al. Hypercoagulability in acute pancreatitis. Am J Surg 1963;105:714–719.
47. Florkiewicz H, Korolko A, Bielak J. Disturbances of blood coagulation in acute pancreatitis. Pol Med J 1969;8:1292–1295.
48. Ranson JHC, Lackner H, Berman IR. The relationship of coagulation factors to clinical complications of acute pancreatitis. Surgery 1977;81:502–511.
49. Lasson A, Ohlsson K. Disseminated intravascular coagulation and antiprotease activity in acute human pancreatitis. Scand J Gastroenterol 1986;21(suppl 126):35–39.
50. Lasson A, Ohlsson K. Systemic involvement in pancreatic damage: coagulation and fibrinolysis. Int J Pancreatol 1988;(suppl 3):S79–S86.
51. Kwaan HC, Anderson M, Gramatica L. A study of pancreatic enzymes as a factor in the pathogenesis of disseminated intravascular coagulation during acute pancreatitis. Surgery 1971;69:663–672.
52. Berry AR, Taylor TV, Davies GC. Diagnostic tests and prognostic indicators in acute pancreatitis. J R Coll Surg Edinb 1982;27: 345–352.
53. Izquierdo R, Squillaci G, Hoppensteadt D, et al. Effects of protease inhibitors on coagulation abnormalities in acute canine pancreatitis. Am Surg 1984;50:317–323.
54. Viedema JA, Perez-Mateo M, Dominguez JE, Carballo F. Role of interleukin-6 in acute pancreatitis: comparison with C-reactive protein and phospholipase A. Gut 1992;33:1264–1267.
55. Grewal HP, Mohey EDA, Gaber L, Kotb M, Gaber A. Amelioration of the physiologic and biochemical changes of acute pancreatitis using an anti-TNF-alpha polyclonal antibody. Am J Surg 1994;167:214–219.
56. Hahahan DJ. Platelet activating factor: a biologically active phosphoglyceride. Annu Rev Biochem 1986;35:493–509.
57. Camussi G, Tetta C, Bussolino F, Caligaris-Cappio F, Masera C, Segoloni G. Mediators of immune complex induced aggregation of polymorphonuclear neutrophils: II platelet-activation factor as the effector substance of immune-induced aggregation. Int Arch Allergy Appl Immunol 1981;64:25–41.
58. Konturek SJ, Dembinski A, Konturek PJ, et al. Role of platelet activating factor in the pathogenesis of acute pancreatitis in rats. Gut 1992;33:1268–1274.
59. Smedley LA, Tennessen MG, Sandhouse RA, et al. Neutrophil mediated injury of endothelial cells: enhancement by endotoxin and essential role of neutrophil elastase. J Clin Invest 1986;77: 1233–1243.
60. Gross V. Scholemrich J, Leser HG, et al. Granulocyte elastase in assessment of severity of acute pancreatitis. Dig Dis Sci 1990;36: 97–105.
61. Uhl W, Buchler M, Malfertheiner P, Martini M, Beger JG. PMN-elastase in comparison with CRP, antiproteases and LDH as indicators of necrosis in human acute pancreatitis. Pancreas 1991;6:253–259.
62. Dominguez-Munoz JE, Carballo JEF, Garcia MJ, et al. Clinical usefulness of polymorphonuclear elastase in predicting the severity of acute pancreatitis: results of a multicenter study. Br J Surg 1991;78:1230–1234.
63. Axelsson L, Bergenfeldt M, Bjork P, Olsson R, Ohlsson K. Release of immunoreactive canine leukocyte elastase normally and in endotoxin and pancreatic shock. Scand J Clin Lab Invest 1990;50:35–42.
64. Foulis AK, Murray WR, Galloway D, et al. Endotoxemia and complement activation in acute pancreatitis in man. Gut 1982;23:656–661.
65. Whicher JT, Barnes MP, Brown A, et al. Complement activation and complement control proteins in acute pancreatitis. Gut 1982;23:944–950.
66. Patel AG, Toyama MT, Nguyen TN, et al. Role of nitric oxide in the relationship of pancreatic blood flow and exocrine secretion in cats. Gastroenterology 1995;108:1215–1220.
67. Kubes P, Granger DN. Nitric oxide modulates microvascular permeability. Am J Physiol 1992;262(31):H611–H615.
68. Kubes P, Suzuki M, Granger DN. Nitric oxide: an endogenous modulator of leukocyte adhesion. Proc Natl Acad Sci 1991;88: 4651–4655.
69. Clancy RM, Leszcynska-Piziak J, Abromson SB. Nitric oxide, and endothelial cell relaxation factor, inhibits neutrophil superoxide anion production via a direct action on the NADPH oxidase. J Clin Invest 1992;90:1116–1121.
70. Stark ME, Szurszewski JH. Role of nitric oxide in gastrointestinal and hepatic function and disease. Gastroenterology 1992;103:1928–1949.
71. Dabrowski A, Gabryelewicz A. Nitric oxide contributes to multi-organ oxidative stress in acute experimental pancreatitis. Scand J Gastroenterol 1994;29:943–948.
72. Closa D, Hotter G, Prats N, et al. Prostanoid generation in early stages of acute pancreatitis: a role for nitric oxide. Inflammation 1994;18(5):469–480.
73. O'Donovan DA, Kelly CJ, Abdih H, et al. Role of nitric oxide in lung injury associated with experimental acute pancreatitis. Br J Surg 1995;82:1122–1126.
74. Toyama MT, Kusske AM, Reber PU, et al. Administration of a nitric oxide donor decreases the severity of acute pancreatitis. Pancreas 1995;11(4):451.
75. Moody FG, Haley-Russell D, Muncy DM. Intestinal transit and bacterial translocation in obstructive pancreatitis. Dig Dis Sci 1995;40(8):1798–1804.
76. Kazsantsev GB, Hecht DW, Rao R, et al. Plasmid labeling confirms bacterial translocation in pancreatitis. Am J Surg 1994;167(1): 201–206.

77. Gianotti L, Munda R, Alexander JW, Tchervenkov JI, Babcock GF. Bacterial translocation: a potential source for infection in acute pancreatitis. Pancreas 1993;8(5):551–558.
78. Foitzik T, Castillo CF-D, Ferraro MJ, Mithofer K, Rattner DW, Warshaw AL. Pathogenesis and prevention of early pancreatic infection in experimental necrotizing pancreatitis. Ann Surg 1995;222(2):179–185.
79. Toyama MT, Kusske AM, Patel AG, Reber PU, Reber HA, Ashley SW. Inhibition of nitric oxide synthesis increases the severity of acute pancreatitis. Surg Forum 1995;46:142–144.
80. Klar E, Messmer K, Warshaw AL, Herfarth C. Pancreatic ischemia in experimental acute pancreatitis; mechanism, significance, and therapy. Br J Surg 1990;77(11):1205–1210.
81. Knoefel WT, Kollias N, Warshaw AL, Waldner H, Nishioka NS, Rattner DW. Pancreatic microcirculatory changes in experimental pancreatitis of graded severity in the rat. Surgery 1994;116(5):904–913.
82. Nordback IH, Clemens JA, Chacko VP, Olson JL, Cameron JL. Changes in high-energy phosphate metabolism and cell morphology in four models of acute experimental pancreatitis. Ann Surg 1991;213(4):341–349.
83. Prinz RA. Mechanisms of acute pancreatitis; vascular etiology. Int J Pancreatol 1991;9:31–38.
84. Kusterer K, Poschmann T, Friedmann A, Enghofer M, Zendler S, Usadel KH. Arterial constriction, ischemia-reperfusion, and leukocyte adherence in acute pancreatitis. Am J Physiol 1993;265: G165–G171.
85. Tamura K, Manabe T, Kyogoku T, Andoh K, Ohshio G, Tobe T. Effect of postischemic reperfusion on the pancreas. Hepatogastroenterology 1993;40:452–456.
86. Sanfey H, Bulkley GB, Cameron JL. The role of oxygen-derived free radicals in the pathogenesis of acute pancreatitis. Ann Surg 1984;200(4):405–413.
87. Granger D, Grisham M, Kvietys P. Mechanisms of microvascular injury. In: Physiology of the gastrointestinal tract. Johnson LR, ed. New York: Raven Press, 1994:1693–1722.
88. Granger DN, Hollwarth ME, Parks DA. Ischemia-reperfusion injury: role of oxygen-derived free radicals. Acta Physiol Scand 1986; 548(47):47–63.
89. Ashley SW, Schwartz M, Alvarez C, Nguyen TN, Vdovenko A, Reber HA. Pancreatic interstitial pH regulation: effects of secretory stimulation. Surgery 1994;115:503–509.
90. Aikens J, Dix T. Peroxyl radical initiated lipid peroxidation; the role of fatty acid hydroperoxidases. J Biol Chem 1991;266:15091–15098.

# 21

# *Assessment, Diagnosis, and Initial Treatment*

John Webber and David Fromm

## CLINICAL DIAGNOSIS

The diagnosis of acute pancreatitis is not always straightforward, because of its variable presentation and severity. Although much has been written about making the diagnosis of acute pancreatitis on the basis of objective criteria that include an array of laboratory and radiographic tests, it often hinges on the patient's clinical presentation. However, overreliance on clinical presentation is also fraught with problems, because pancreatitis mimics other intraabdominal diseases, and the latter also mimic acute pancreatitis (1, 2).

The history often suggests the diagnosis. Usually, patients present with the complaint of mild-to-severe epigastric pain that frequently radiates to the midback and flanks (3). On occasion, the pain can even present in the left lower abdominal quadrant. Classically, the pain begins after a heavy meal or during an alcoholic binge. In most patients, the pain radiates to the back and may be relieved by assuming the fetal position or sitting forward (4). Pain, the major symptom of acute pancreatitis, is encountered in practically all cases (5). Various investigators have reported that pain is present in 96–100% of patients (4, 5). The pain may be present for several days with a gradual increase in severity, or the onset may be relatively sudden and excruciating. The pain of acute pancreatitis is usually constant, dull, or boring and is worse in the supine position (6). The pain is often accompanied by sweating, tachycardia, nausea, vomiting, anorexia, and mild-to-severe prostration (3, 7). Nausea and/or vomiting occur in more than half of patients and is present early in the disease. A history of previous episodes of acute pancreatitis or excessive alcohol intake can be helpful.

The diagnosis of acute pancreatitis should be considered in any patient who presents with acute onset or increasing abdominal pain. It is also helpful to be aware of the multiple etiologies of the disease, of which alcohol and gallstone disease are the most common. Less obvious causes include drugs, trauma, collagen vascular disease, hyperlipidemia, idiopathic, duodenal diverticulum, and postoperative states (4). It cannot be overemphasized that acute pancreatitis can masquerade as biliary tract disease, alcoholic gastritis, penetrating peptic ulcer, or almost any other abdominal condition (8). Failure to recognize other treatable life-threatening abdominal emergencies such as ruptured aortic aneurysm, acute afferent loop obstruction, acute mesenteric vascular occlusion, and intestinal necrosis obviously has profound consequences for the patient (9).

Physical examination usually reveals an acutely ill patient with tachycardia, low-grade fever (the initial presence of fever is quite variable), and variable degrees of dehydration or vascular instability. Abdominal tenderness, which is mild to severe, is usually confined to the upper portion of the abdomen. Abdominal distention is common; it is usually moderate and often associated with epigastric fullness (7). The quality and frequency of bowel sounds add nothing to the diagnosis. Jaundice may be seen in 15–25% of cases (10) and is due to obstruction either from accompanying biliary tract disease or from edema of surrounding structures. Necrosis in the retroperitoneum can result in hemorrhage, with dissection of blood along different tissue planes. This can result in ecchymosis of the flanks (Grey-Turner's sign) or in the periumbilical area (Cullen's sign), but these signs occur infrequently. Peritoneal irritation, elevation of the diaphragm, basilar atelectasis, and pleural effusion (4) are other findings that are not specific.

The initial approach is to consider the possibility of acute pancreatitis, which then sets in motion a variable algorithm to establish the diagnosis. It is not necessary for every patient to undergo a large number of costly studies to confirm the diagnosis. However, if the diagnosis is made primarily on clinical grounds, one must be prepared to change it or seek confirmation if the patient does not respond to treatment. Overreliance on imaging studies may miss the diagnosis, especially in mild cases of pancreatitis (which some refer to as acute interstitial pancreatitis). Our practice is not to apply the same diagnostic algorithm to every patient, as this is costly, is unnecessary, and may even be too time consuming, thus delaying effective treatment. However, it is important to know what means are available to confirm one's clinical impression and to identify complications of the disease. In essence, the diagnosis of acute pancreatitis is often based on a constellation of "soft" findings, which when considered in the appropriate clinical context, leads to the correct diagnosis. Equally important, but not the subject of this chapter, is establishing the etiology of the disease, to perhaps avoid future morbidity from recurrence.

## LABORATORY DIAGNOSIS

Acute pancreatitis is often suspected on the basis of clinical presentation. The clinical impression can be confirmed unequivocally only by invasive measures, such as laparotomy and pancreatic biopsy, which usually are unnecessary and even hazardous. Laboratory determinations and radiographic findings are used to support the clinical diagnosis in most patients with acute abdominal pain. Currently, there are a host of serum markers and tests in use clinically or under evaluation in an attempt to find the elusive gold standard for diagnosing acute pancreatitis (Table 21.1). Curiously, substantial improvements in available diagnostic procedures have not been paralleled by a decrease in the rate of undiagnosed fatal acute pancreatitis. A contemporary autopsy review found that for patients with a past history of acute pancreatitis, 30% of the recurrent episodes of acute pancreatitis were diagnosed first at autopsy (11). This observation does not differ greatly from that in an earlier review.

**TABLE 21.1. Diagnostic Procedures Used for Acute Pancreatitis**

| |
|---|
| Laboratory diagnosis |
| Nonspecific laboratory determinations |
| Serum amylase |
| Isoamylase |
| Lipase |
| Combined use of serum amylase and lipase |
| Urine amylase |
| Amylase/creatinine clearance ratio |
| Trypsin |
| Elastase |
| Pancreas-specific protein |
| Imaging studies |
| Plain radiographs |
| Upper gastrointestinal radiographs |
| Ultrasound |
| Computed tomographic scans |
| Peritoneal lavage |
| Laparotomy |

### Nonspecific Laboratory Determinations

Most patients with acute pancreatitis have leukocytosis, usually in the range of 10–25 × $10^9$/L, but higher values may occur. The hematocrit may be increased early in the course of the disease, because of hemoconcentration. Hyperglycemia along with prerenal azotemia, altered hepatic functions, hypoalbuminemia, and hypoxia tends to correlate with the severity of illness (12).

### Serum Amylase

Measurement of amylase has been the cornerstone of diagnosis since 1929 (13), even though this enzyme is not specific for the pancreas. Serum amylase in normal individuals consists of 40% pancreatic (P-isoamylase) and 60% salivary (S-isoamylase) isoamylases (14). Although the secretions of several organs (fallopian tubes, lungs, prostate, breast, sweat and tear glands, genital epithelium, and some malignant tumors) contain S-isoamylase, they do not contribute substantially to the normal serum amylase concentration (14–16). The half-life of amylase in the baboon is approximately 130 minutes, with 24% of it being excreted intact in the urine and the rest cleared by an extrarenal mechanism, possibly through the reticuloendothelial system (17). Smokers have twice the basal serum amylase level of nonsmokers, which suggests that a different normal range for the serum amylase level should be used for smokers and nonsmokers (18).

Typically, in acute pancreatitis, amylase and lipase levels become elevated within the first 24–48 hours of the onset of symptoms and return to normal in 5–8 days. Amylase is the first enzyme to return toward normal (19–22). There is a loss of diagnostic sensitivity of amylase 24 hours after the onset of acute pancreatitis (19–21, 23). Serum amylase in one study had a sensitivity of only 67% on the 4th day after admission for acute pancreatitis (24). However, if a symptomatic patient has persistent hyperamylasemia (defined as a failure of serum amylase to return to normal within 7–10 days), the presence of a pancreatic pseudocyst, fistula, or ongoing pancreatic inflammation is suggested (25, 26).

Even though serum amylase is the most widely used test to diagnose acute pancreatitis (23), normal levels can occur in the presence of acute pancreatitis. Normoamylasemia has been reported in 19–32% of patients with acute pancreatitis confirmed by computed tomographic (CT) scans (27, 28). Normoamylasemia can occur as a result of increased urinary clearance, delayed admission, extensive destruction of the pancreas, or an association with hyperlipemia, in which case there may be circulating inhibitors of amylase (29–31). Thus, hyperamylasemia is not a sine qua non for diagnosing acute pancreatitis (27).

Older studies report that the sensitivity of the serum amylase test lies between 95 and 100%. However, most of these studies used serum amylase as the diagnostic standard, which accounts for this falsely high sensitivity (32, 33). Contemporary studies suggest that the sensitivity of the serum amylase test varies between 55 and 80% (27, 28, 34, 35).

The greatest limitation of the serum amylase test is its lack of specificity, which is even lower than its sensitivity. Only 68% of patients with hyperamylasemia and abdominal pain were eventually found to have acute pancreatitis in one study (36). This was confirmed by other investigators who found that serum amylase had a diagnostic specificity approaching 70% (37). This is due in part to the many causes of hyperamylasemia, which include renal insufficiency, salivary gland disease, perforation of the gastrointestinal tract, intestinal obstruction, ruptured ectopic pregnancy, ruptured aortic aneurysm, mesenteric thrombosis, and macroamylasemia (38) (Table 21.2). Furthermore, elevations of S-isoamylase occur in conditions in which there is no evidence of salivary gland disease, such as after coronary bypass surgery (39, 40), during lactic acidosis (41), and with eating disorders (e.g., anorexia nervosa, bulimia) (42). Certain causes of hyperamylasemia result from reduced metabolic clearance of amylase, such as chronic renal failure and macroamylasemia. The frequency and degree of elevation of amylase in chronic renal failure is controversial. However, the serum amylase level is seldom more than twice the upper limit of normal in patients with renal insufficiency (38).

Reliance on serum amylase is further compounded in alcoholics. Between 9 and 39% of alcoholics admitted for acute intoxication or for detoxification have elevated amylase levels, usually nonpancreatic in origin (43, 44). This elevation of S-isoamylase may reflect a mild injury to the salivary glands and other tissues from alcohol. The fairly frequent occurrence of nonpancreatic hyperamylasemia in alcoholic patients emphasizes the lack of specificity of the test, even when there is an etiologic predilection for acute pancreatitis. Thus, hyperamylasemia in intoxicated alcoholics does not always signify the presence of pancreatitis.

Some individuals have persistent elevations of both P- and/or S-isoamylases, lasting for weeks to months and even years, without obvious clinical cause (45, 46). Hyperamylasemia is common in HIV-infected patients, but the amylase is often of salivary origin, making routine, extensive evaluation of hyperamylasemia unproductive in this patient population (47).

Several studies have tried to reexamine lower limits of normal for serum amylase to see if this would improve diagnostic accuracy. As might be expected, if the lower limit of normal is increased, so is the specificity, but at the expense of sensitivity (20). Our view of serum amylase testing is that it must be interpreted in the context of the history and/or physical examination. At the very least, an abnormal value raises an array of differential diagnoses. On the other hand, a normal value, like being afebrile, does not indicate the patient is not sick, especially with pancreatitis. Whether serial serum amylase determinations are more valuable for diagnosis (48) is debatable, but an abnormal value in the appropriate setting can be helpful.

### Amylase in Differentiating between Gallstone and Alcoholic Pancreatitis

Although the magnitude of serum amylase elevation does not correlate with either the severity or the prognosis of the pancreatitis (49), it may provide a clue about the cause of the pancreatitis. It is generally agreed that most patients with biliary pancreatitis have substantially higher initial serum amylase levels than do those with pancreatitis from other causes (20). Some 89% of patients with biliary pancreatitis in one report had an initial serum amylase level above 1000 u/L, whereas only 6% of patients with alcoholic pancreatitis had a level in this range (50). However, few would place undue reliance on the degree of amylase elevation being pathognomonic of gallstone pancreatitis; there are a number of previously discussed confounding variables. Thus, additional laboratory criteria have been sought.

Two studies indicate that a series of seven clinical and biochemical factors showed significant differences between gallstone and alcoholic pancreatitis (51, 52). The findings that argued for a gallstone were an alkaline phosphatase level above 300 u/L, patient age above 50 years, alanine aminotransferase above 100 u/L, female gender, amylase level above 4000 u/L, bilirubin above 25 mol/L, and an aspartate aminotransferase level above 100 u/L (53). A scoring system was devised, and patients with zero to one positive factor had alcoholic pancreatitis 95–96% of the time. In contrast, if three or more factors were present, there was a greater than 86% association with gallstones. This scoring system could not discriminate the cause of an episode of acute pancreatitis if only two factors were present.

A meta-analysis involving four factors (serum bilirubin, alkaline phosphatase, alanine aminotransferase (ALT), and aspartate aminotransferase (AST)) found that bilirubin and alkaline phosphatase were not useful in diagnosing gallstone pancreatitis (54). However, serum ALT was highly specific. A 3-fold elevation or more of ALT in the presence of acute pancreatitis had a positive predictive value of 95% in diagnosing acute gallstone pancreatitis. This finding corroborates an earlier report (55). In another study, a more than 3-fold elevation of ALT was present in over one-third of patients with an initial diagnosis of idiopathic pancreatitis who were subsequently found to have gallstones as the cause of their disease (56).

**TABLE 21.2. Differential Diagnosis of Hyperamylasemia**

| Disease | Predominant Type of Serum Amylase[a] |
|---|---|
| Pancreatic diseases | |
| Pancreatitis—acute or chronic | P |
| Pseudocyst | P |
| Pancreatic ascites | P |
| Pancreatic trauma | |
| Blunt trauma | P |
| Abdominal or retroperitoneal surgery | P |
| Endoscopic retrograde cholangio-pancreatography | P |
| Choledocholithiasis | P |
| Pancreatic cancer | P |
| Early cystic fibrosis | P |
| Salivary diseases | |
| Parotitis | S |
| Trauma/surgery | S |
| Radiation | S |
| Impacted calculi | S |
| Gastrointestinal diseases | |
| Perforated bowel | P |
| Mesenteric infarction | P |
| Intestinal obstruction | P |
| Appendicitis | P |
| Peritonitis | P |
| Liver diseases | |
| Hepatitis | S and P |
| Cirrhosis | S and P |
| Alcoholism | S or P |
| Ectopic amylase production by malignancies | S |
| Acidosis | |
| Ketoacidosis | S or P |
| Nonketotic | S |
| Renal failure | S and P |
| Macroamylasemia | M |
| Female genital tract | |
| Ruptured ectopic pregnancy | S |
| Fallopian or ovarian cysts | S |
| Salpingitis | S |
| Postoperative | |
| Extracorporeal circulation | S or P |
| Nonabdominal surgery | S or P |
| Miscellaneous | |
| Pneumonia | S |
| Cerebral trauma | |
| Burns | |
| Ruptured abdominal aortic aneurysm | P |
| Drugs | S or P |
| Anorexia nervosa and/or bulimia | S |

[a]S, salivary; P, pancreatic; M, macro.

## Isoamylase

Older assays for P-isoamylase showed that its measurement provides little improvement in sensitivity and specificity for the diagnosis of acute pancreatitis (33, 57), but this is controversial (58, 59). Newer P-isoamylase assays show a sensitivity between 89 and 100% and a specificity between 88 and 91% in diagnosing acute pancreatitis (60, 61). The current consensus is that the isoamylase assay confers a small increase in sensitivity but an even greater boost in specificity (23). Another advantage of P-isoamylase determination is that it remains elevated longer than total amylase (20).

Serum P-amylase does seem useful in verifying the cause of an elevated serum amylase level. Nearly one-third of patients admitted with hyperamylasemia and the diagnosis of acute pancreatitis did not have the disease, and the initial measurement of P-amylase could have saved time and money in determining this (36, 62). While P-isoamylase measurement may have its greatest utility in situations in which the diagnosis of acute pancreatitis is in question (62, 63), it is not completely specific for diseases of the pancreas. Elevated levels can occur in mesenteric infarction, intestinal obstruction, perforated peptic ulcer (64), and ovarian neoplasms (65). It remains to be seen if fractionation of P-isoamylase will improve its diagnostic value (66).

## Lipase

Lipase was originally believed to originate exclusively from the pancreas, but it can also emanate from other tissues such as the liver and stomach (37). Earlier methods for determining serum lipase required 24 hours to complete and were technically difficult (67). This resulted in conflicting reports concerning its clinical utility (68). With newer assays, lipase has a greater sensitivity and specificity in the diagnosis of acute pancreatitis than does serum amylase (19, 21, 34, 69, 70). The sensitivity of the lipase assay ranges from 86.5 to 100% (20). Several studies show that serum lipase remains elevated longer than does amylase, making the lipase assay more sensitive after the first hospital day (19, 21, 69) and a better test in patients with a late clinical presentation. In contrast, others find that the serum lipase assay is slightly less sensitive than amylase (12, 33).

Lipase levels can be elevated in a number of diseases that may be confused clinically with acute pancreatitis, such as acute cholecystitis, perforated peptic ulcer, and intestinal infarction (71). Lipase levels can also be elevated in other disease states, such as mumps, malignant neoplasms of the pancreas, acute renal failure, types I and IV hyperlipoproteinemias, bone fractures, and fat embolism (48). In the presence of abdominal pain unrelated to the pancreas, 11–17% of patients have elevate serum lipase levels (57, 72). However, if the serum lipase level is more than three times normal, its sensitivity is reported to be 100% and its specificity 99% for the detection of pancreatitis (72).

Serum lipase determination may have greater value in the diagnosis of acute alcoholic pancreatitis (32, 73), a situation in which the sensitivity of serum amylase is low (28, 73). The sensitivity and specificity of serum lipase assay in acute alcoholic pancreatitis have been reported to be 100 and 99%, respectively. In a study comparing enzyme levels in 202 asymptomatic chronic alcoholics with those in 29 patients with acute pancreatitis proven by radiologic imaging, a considerable overlap between serum amylase levels was noted for both groups, but there was no overlap of lipase levels (34). Measurement of serum lipase correctly diagnosed acute pancreatitis in 68% of normoamylasemic patients whose pancreatitis was demonstrated by CT scan (27).

Thus, lipase determination appears to have three advantages over serum amylase. It has an increased sensitivity in the diagnosis of acute alcoholic pancreatitis. Second, it is more accurate for detecting pancreatitis in patients with a late clinical presentation. Finally, it is useful in detecting pancreatitis when the serum amylase level is normal (32).

### Combined Use of Serum Amylase and Lipase

While it has been suggested that the serum lipase assay should replace serum amylase determination (19, 21, 34), most clinicians order both tests. Amylase may be a better test for gallstone pancreatitis (73), and lipase may be better for other causes of pancreatitis (34, 73). Since both tests have limitations, simultaneous use has been advocated to optimize sensitivity and specificity (48, 74). However, not all investigators have been able to confirm an improvement in diagnostic accuracy using both enzyme tests (75). Still others suggest algorithms using amylase, lipase, isoamylase, and serum creatinine determinations to discriminate among the various causes of elevated amylase levels (76). As mentioned above, there are conditions other than acute pancreatitis that can cause simultaneous elevations of amylase and lipase (77).

There is controversy also about using serum lipase levels to distinguish between alcoholic and nonalcoholic causes of pancreatitis. Some report that a lipase/amylase ratio greater than two suggests acute alcoholic pancreatitis and a ratio of less than two indicates gallstone pancreatitis (78). While this has been confirmed by others (79), there is not general agreement that a lipase/amylase ratio of two is a precise cutoff point. Other studies conclude that the serum lipase/amylase ratio is neither useful nor sufficiently sensitive or specific in differentiating between alcoholic and nonalcoholic acute pancreatitis (80–82). A recent review of this issue concluded that a ratio of less than two suggests that alcohol is not the cause of the pancreatitis, that a ratio of more than three is very suggestive of alcohol, but that a ratio between two and three is indeterminate (83).

### Urine Amylase and Amylase/Creatinine Clearance Ratio

Although earlier studies considered an isolated urine amylase test more sensitive than a serum amylase determination as an indicator of acute pancreatitis (84), urine amylase measurements suffer from the same disadvantages as serum amylase. In one study, hyperamylasuria in 16% of patients was attributed to nonpancreatic disorders associated with an elevated serum amylase (85). Thus, hyperamylasuria, like hyperamylasemia, is not absolutely diagnostic of acute pancreatitis. In addition, a normal urine amylase level does not exclude the diagnosis of pancreatitis (86). The clearance of amylase is influenced by the hydrational status of the patient. This reduces the diagnostic accuracy of urine amylase unless it is measured against creatinine clearance (87).

The amylase to creatinine clearance ratio was found to be elevated in earlier studies (88), suggesting that it might be useful in differentiating the hyperamylasemia of pancreatitis from nonpancreatic disease (89). However, enthusiasm for this test has diminished, since the amylase to creatinine clearance ratio may be elevated in a number of conditions other than acute pancreatitis (90, 91). In fact, a rise in the amylase/creatinine clearance ratio can be a nonspecific response to acute illness and is found with perforated peptic ulcer and biliary colic (92). In addition, a normal amylase to creatinine clearance ratio has been reported in patients with documented acute pancreatitis (93). Two recent reviews agree that these measurements do not seem to add any important diagnostic information or practical clinical advantage over serum amylase, isoamylase, and lipase determinations (12, 94). In difficult patients, it may be helpful, since the amylase to creatinine clearance ratio remains elevated for several days after serum amylase levels have returned to normal (86).

### Trypsin

Trypsin is the major enzyme responsible for the activation of other pancreatic proenzymes, including its own proenzyme trypsinogen. However, since active trypsin is rapidly inactivated by $\alpha_1$-antiproteases in the blood, it is necessary to measure the quantity of immunoreactive trypsin (IRT), which is not affected by proteolytic digestion (20). Until recently, the pancreas was considered the only source of trypsin, but it has been identified in the basal cells of the crypts in the small intestinal mucosa (Paneth cells) (37). Thus, trypsin does not fulfill the ideal criterion of organ specificity. In fact, IRT levels can be elevated with malignant neoplasms of the pancreas, diabetes mellitus, cirrhosis of the liver, and chronic pancreatitis (48). False positives have also been reported with choledocholithiasis and chronic renal failure (37). Studies comparing the sensitivities and specificities of amylase, P-isoamylase, lipase, trypsin, and elastase-1 have found that trypsin was the least specific (33, 60). However, trypsin appears to have a very high sensitivity in detecting acute pancreatitis. The sensitivity of trypsin was 100% and 97%, respectively, in two studies (33, 60). Furthermore, trypsin and elastase-1 levels remain elevated longer than other enzymes, making these markers better late in the course of disease (22, 60). Elastase-1 appears to be the more sensitive of the two (60). However, IRT measurement is probably no better as a single diagnostic test in acute pancreatitis than amylase or lipase. IRT is more difficult to perform and requires 24 hours to complete (20). This and the limited number of studies that have evaluated it make the routine use of trypsin measurements unclear at present (37).

There has been recent interest in trypsin activity. Trypsin in the serum is complexed by its two main inhibitors, $\alpha_1$-protease inhibitor and $\alpha_2$-macroglobulin. In contrast, IRT reflects mainly circulating trypsinogen and $\alpha_1$-protease inhibitor–trypsin complexes and not the $\alpha_2$-macroglobulin–trypsin complex. The latter is the only form that retains its enzyme activity toward small peptides. Using an assay for $\alpha_2$-macroglobulin-bound trypsin activity, plasma trypsin activity was elevated in active alcoholics with acute pancreatitis, even when amylase levels were normal (95). Trypsin activity may become an increasingly important test, especially in view of the observation that the incidence of normoamylasemia in acute alcoholic pancreatitis can be as high as 32% (28).

### Elastase

Serum elastase-1 has been implicated in the development of vascular complications of acute pancreatitis, since it has specific elastolytic properties (96). Over a decade ago, a new radioimmunoassay for elastase was developed that required only 4 hours to complete (97). Although extremely high levels of serum elastase-1 occur in acute pancreatitis, most studies do not show any important advantages of this enzyme over amylase, lipase, and IRT in the diagnosis of acute pancreatitis (22, 32, 37). Furthermore, high levels of elastase-1 have been described in up to two-thirds of patients with pancreatic cancer and less frequently in chronic pancreatitis (32, 37). Serum elastase levels may be meaningful in those patients who present late and in whom the diagnosis of pancreatitis is in doubt. One study showed that both trypsin and elastase levels remain elevated in 90% of patients 10 days after the onset of symptoms, while other enzyme levels returned to normal (22). Elevated elastase-1 levels were found in another report of patients studied 7 days after the onset of symptoms (60). As with trypsin, technical difficulties and limited studies leave the value of elastase measurements open to question (37).

### Pancreas-Specific Protein

Pancreas-specific protein (PASP) exists in the exocrine gland cytosol as a procarboxypeptidase B (98–100). PASP is believed to be a good marker in the diagnosis of acute pancreatitis, with high sensitivity, specificity, and accuracy (101, 102). Patients with hyperamylasemia due to S-isoenzyme have normal PASP levels. Although the pattern of rise and fall of PASP mirrors that of amylase and lipase in the serum of patients with acute pancreatitis, there appears to be no advantage of PASP over isoamylase and lipase (32, 100).

## IMAGING STUDIES

The role of imaging in patients with acute pancreatitis is usually not to make the diagnosis, since this can be done on the basis of clinical and laboratory data, but rather to help identify complications (103). Yet, there are instances in which the clinical presentation is unclear and imaging techniques can aid in the diagnosis.

### Plain Radiographs

Abdominal radiographs can suggest pancreatitis but are not diagnostic. Such radiographs are usually done to exclude other conditions such as a perforated viscus or small bowel obstruction, which may mimic acute pancreatitis. Abnormalities associated with acute pancreatitis include ileus, sentinel loop (localized segments of gas-filled dilated small bowel), colon cutoff sign (distention of the right and transverse colon with abrupt cutoff at the splenic flexure), distortion of the gastric air bubble, increased gastrocolic separation, and loss of the psoas muscle outline. However, none of these findings are specific for acute pancreatitis.

Chest radiographic findings suggesting acute pancreatitis include left pleural effusion, basal atelectasis, and left diaphragmatic elevation, which are reflections of a subdiaphragmatic and retroperitoneal inflammatory process (86).

### Upper Gastrointestinal Radiographs

Upper gastrointestinal contrast studies may reveal widening of the duodenal C loop with anterior displacement of the stomach by an inflamed and edematous pancreas. However, these findings are not specific for acute pancreatitis (86).

### Ultrasound

[*Editor's note:* see also Chapter 4.]

Pancreatic enlargement greater than 3 cm in width is the most sensitive and reproducible criterion for diagnosing acute pancreatitis by ultrasound (US). Other criteria include reduction in glandular echogenicity and dilatation of the pancreatic duct beyond 2-mm diameter (20). Unfortunately, the presence of overlying intestinal gas limits the usefulness of US, obscuring the gland and making it impossible to visualize in 30–40% of patients (103). Even in normal persons, where ileus and distended loops of bowel are not present, the head of the pancreas is seen in only 80–90% of examinations, the body in 70%, and the tail even less often (104, 105). When examination of the gland is possible, the sensitivity of US in diagnosing pancreatitis varies between 62 and 95% (106, 107), whereas the specificity is higher, reaching 97–98% (104, 107). By comparison, US accurately diagnosed only 75–92% of fluid collections detected by CT scanning (103, 108). US is very operator dependent, making it difficult to compare different series. US lacks accuracy for determining pancreatic necrosis, assessing the other retroperitoneal structures, identifying pancreatic abscesses (109), and distinguishing between an abscess and a phlegmon (20).

Despite its drawbacks, US remains the best noninvasive means of ascertaining a gallstone etiology for acute pancreatitis (110, 111). The main role of US in pancreatitis is to determine the presence or absence of gallstones as well as dilation of the biliary tree. US performed within 1 week of admission for acute pancreatitis was found to be 96% accurate in predicting the presence of gallstones, but the gall bladder could only be visualized in 69% of patients (110). Others have shown that the initial US study has a sensitivity of 67% in the urgent diagnosis of gallstones in acute pancreatitis and a specificity of 100% (112). However, the sensitivity improved to 78% when the US study was repeated after clinical improvement. False-negative rates of about 30% are generally attributed to overlying intestinal gas and soft stones that do not cause acoustic shadowing (113). Furthermore, US may also miss microlithiasis (56) and cholesterol crystals, which may be important etiologic factors in acute pancreatitis.

### Computed Tomographic Scans

CT scanning is probably the best available method to image the pancreas during acute pancreatitis, with visualization rates varying from 64 to 100% (103, 111, 114). Most agree that CT scans are superior to ultrasonography for detecting acute pancreatitis (20, 28, 103, 114, 115), because overlying bowel gas from paralytic ileus can obscure the pancreas with US (103). CT scans performed within 72 hours of admission are abnormal in 91% of patients with acute pancreatitis (111). The most common abnormalities include loss of peripancreatic tissue planes, decreased enhancement, and a diffuse increase in pancreatic size. Another study reported similar findings, with CT scanning having a sensitivity of 92% and a specificity of 100% (116). Serial CT scans done 1 week after admission are still abnormal in 84% of patients with acute pancreatitis and thus may be of value in establishing the diagnosis late, when conventional laboratory studies may be normal. Even at 6 weeks, abnormal CT scans occur in 51% of patients (111). Others note abnormal CT scans in 81% of patients at the time of discharge, even though the patients were asymptomatic (117). Furthermore, serum amylase and lipase levels do not necessarily correlate with CT scan findings at discharge (117). It has been asserted that the cause of acute pancreatitis can be inferred 27% of the time from admission CT scans (111).

The sensitivity of CT in detecting gallstones in patients with biliary pancreatitis is relatively low, with reports ranging from 34% (111) to 53% (115). The specificity of CT for identifying gallstones has been reported to be 100% (111, 115). US has the highest sensitivity for detecting gallstones early in acute pancreatitis (110, 112) and, unlike CT, the sensitivity of US for finding gallstones increases 6 weeks after the onset of the disease (118).

While there is little disagreement about the value of CT scanning in diagnosing acute pancreatitis, the study is not necessary in most patients. It can be very helpful when there is uncertainty about the diagnosis (116) and for searching for complications of acute pancreatitis (see "Treatment").

Certainly, a normal CT scan in a patient thought to have severe pancreatitis should raise concern that the diagnosis is incorrect.

One report found that early CT scanning detected 18 of 25 false-positive acute pancreatitis diagnoses (116). In these cases, the CT scan provided other diagnoses, such as pseudocyst, cholecystitis, intraabdominal abscess, and carcinoma of the colon. It is economically impractical to recommend CT scanning as a routine modality in acute pancreatitis. Some suggest reserving it for patients who demonstrate persistent toxicity over 2–7 days (109, 119).

### Magnetic Resonance Imaging

Magnetic resonance imaging (MRI) currently provides no advantage over CT scanning and is inferior to CT scanning for assessing acute pancreatitis (115). The emerging improvements in MRI technology, however, remain to be evaluated.

## PERITONEAL LAVAGE

Peritoneal lavage may on occasion help establish the diagnosis of acute pancreatitis, especially if it contains amylase substantially in excess of the serum value and does not contain bacteria or fluid that looks like intestinal contents or bilirubin in excess of serum levels.

## LAPAROTOMY

In occasional patients, the diagnosis is not clear and the diagnostic studies are equivocal. Since the mimicking diseases can be potentially fatal, an operation may be necessary to establish the correct diagnosis.

## TREATMENT

There are no major recent breakthroughs in the treatment of acute pancreatitis. However, outcomes are thought to be better because of earlier recognition and better intensive management of complications. While many believe that newer diagnostic modalities and more aggressive use of parenteral nutrition are beneficial, substantive data are lacking.

Acute pancreatitis is a variable disease. The patient may be minimally ill on presentation or be in or progress to a critical state with an acute abdomen and signs of shock and respiratory and renal failure. Some patients are well within a few days, and others die within the first week or develop a protracted, complicated course with a variable outcome. Acute fulminant pancreatitis represents 5–15% of all cases of pancreatitis and is associated with a high mortality rate, ranging from 13 to 64% (120). The overall mortality of clinically diagnosed pancreatitis remains about 10%. Obese patients seem to be at greater risk for peripancreatic fat necrosis, abscess, and death (121).

The function of every major organ system is affected in severe acute pancreatitis. Since there is no specific modality presently available to reverse acute pancreatic inflammation, treatment is aimed at organ support. While prophylactic treatment of specific complications has been suggested, the data supporting this approach are highly controversial.

The use of the available prognostic schemes (e.g., Ranson, Imrie or Glasgow, APACHE II, computed tomography) is not to define treatment, but rather to compare the severity of disease and the treatment outcomes between different series. Aside from maintaining plasma volume and general metabolic support as is required for any seriously ill patient, an important aspect of management is the early diagnosis of potentially treatable organ failure or complications related to the pancreas per se.

Guidelines for treatment tend to be variable. While all agree that the mainstay of therapy is general physiologic support, treatment measures beyond that remain controversial. Certainly, the necessity for operation in uncomplicated forms of the disease is rare. There are three sequential phases in the treatment of acute pancreatitis: *(a)* providing physiologic support; *(b)* diagnosing and treating complications; and *(c)* establishing the cause.

### Intravenous Fluids

Up to one-third of the plasma volume may be sequestered into the third space (122). Other sources of plasma volume loss include vomiting and ascites. It is generally held that the initial adverse effects of acute pancreatitis on cardiovascular function are hypovolemia and reduced cardiac filling (123). Early, aggressive fluid administration usually averts or reverses shock. Experimental data indicate that the initial decrease in pancreatic blood flow associated with acute pancreatitis can be moderated by vigorous fluid administration. However, pancreatic oxygen consumption is less responsive to maintenance of intravascular volume (124). Experimental studies suggest that isovolemic hemodilution and use of ultra-high-molecular-weight dextrans may improve the microcirculatory disturbances occurring in acute pancreatitis (125–127), but the benefits of such treatment in man require further study (128).

### Hemodynamic Function

There are surprisingly few published studies of uniform groups of patients. In one study, 16 patients with necrotizing pancreatitis had a hyperdynamic picture with a significantly higher cardiac index (mean, 4.5 vs. 3.1 L/min-m$^2$) and significantly lower peripheral vascular resistance (mean, 884 vs. 1338 dyn-s/cm$^2$) than 6 patients with interstitial pancreatitis (129). While such a picture is typical of sepsis in certain clinical settings, the hemodynamic picture does not distinguish between septic and nonseptic necrosis. Another study found a high cardiac index and decreased systemic vascular resistance in patients with severe pancreatitis uncomplicated by infected retroperitoneal necrosis or abscess (130).

Because a few patients die in shock despite aggressive fluid therapy, some have suggested that there is a myocardial depressant factor. However, more creditable data supports a significant decrease in vascular tone as the major cardiovascular abnormality in severe pancreatitis (131).

In theory, it is advisable to avoid inappropriate vasoconstriction, since ischemia of the pancreas may aggravate the disease. Thus, support of the cardiovascular system is primarily directed at organ perfusion.

### Renal Function

The best known renal abnormality is increased amylase clearance, but this is of little consequence in terms of treatment. More important are the decreases in glomerular filtration rate and renal blood and plasma flow as well as the increase in vascular resistance (132). Serum phospholipase $A_2$ catalytic activity may play a role in addition to hypovolemia in the renal dysfunction associated with acute pancreatitis (133).

Renal dialysis is occasionally necessary and may be successful (134). However, most surviving patients who develop impaired renal function tend to have high-output renal failure, with blood urea nitrogen levels stabilizing in a range as high as 50–70 mg/dL. Renal function then progressively returns to normal.

### Pulmonary Function

Patients with associated pulmonary complications have significantly higher phospholipase A and pancreatic immunoreactive phospholipase $A_2$ catalytic activity in their sera, which affects surfactant (135). Other contributing factors may be the presence of pancreatic proteases, free fatty acids, activated complement, kinin components, and activated neutrophils (136). Diaphragmatic elevation related to inflammatory retroperitoneal processes, abdominal distention related to ileus, atelectasis, pleural effusion, intravascular coagulation, and microemboli in the pulmonary vascular bed may also play a role. A restrictive lung disturbance has been observed in many patients, but given the variability of preexisting factors, dynamic ventilatory tests can be quite variable (137).

Respiratory problems were once considered relatively rare, with mild hypoxia occurring in only 5% of patients, and even fewer developing progressive respiratory failure (138). It is now recognized that respiratory failure is quite common. Respiratory insufficiency occurs in two phases (139). The early phase (first 48 hours of illness) can be insidious in onset and frequently occurs not only with severe disease (42% with $PaO_2 < 66$ mm Hg) but also with mild disease (24% with $PaO_2 < 66$ mm Hg). The second phase involves clinically and radiographically apparent respiratory complications. Neither age nor mortality are related to early respiratory failure. The later occurrence of respiratory failure reflects severe or continuing disease, which is usually preceded by early arterial hypoxemia and is related to age. It is not clear how often an arterial blood gas should be obtained, even though measurements have been proposed at no less than 12-hour intervals during the first 2–3 days of acute illness. Our usual practice is to obtain a baseline value at admission, which, if normal, is not repeated unless there is *any* worsening of vital signs or clinical condition.

### Nutrition

Patients with severe pancreatitis are metabolically similar to septic patients (140). They have an impaired ability to oxidize infused glucose and an elevated rate of net protein catabolism. Hypoproteinemia frequently occurs and is a result of albumin sequestration in the retroperitoneal space and in the abdominal and thoracic cavities. Patients with severe acute pancreatitis are less sensitive to the protein-sparing effects of glucose. Despite this, the elevated rate of net protein catabolism can be substantially ameliorated by 2 hours of glucose infusion. These patients are also able to adapt to an increase in glucose availability by increasing the percentage of glucose uptake oxidized during parenteral nutrition (140). Initially, glucose intolerance is common, 25% in one series (141), but this can usually be controlled by decreasing the glucose infusion and/or by adding insulin.

Parenteral nutrition does not appear to have any effect on the incidence of complications related to acute pancreatitis per se (141). Furthermore, a prospective randomized study showed no benefit of parenteral nutrition in terms of the number of days to oral intake, total length of hospital stay, and the number of complications from pancreatitis (142). Thus, it has been recommended that parenteral nutrition should be limited to those patients who experience prolonged periods without oral intake or for the treatment of specific complications related to the pancreatitis. However, this study consisted mainly of patients with mild pancreatitis, and at least one nonrandomized study suggests that parenteral nutrition may be beneficial in patients with more severe pancreatitis (143). Use of intravenous lipid does not exacerbate pancreatitis and does not cause hypertriglyceridemia (143). Catheter-related sepsis (11–17%) appears to be more common within 7 days of initiation of treatment (141, 142).

While some maintain that it is dangerous to perform a feeding jejunostomy in the presence of pancreatitis because they are prone to breakdown, this has not been our experience using an elemental diet low in fat (144).

Oral diet is generally resumed when clinical and laboratory evidence indicates resolution of the pancreatitis. Some patients will develop recurrence of their pain and abnormal laboratory values (e.g., elevation of amylase, lipase levels) upon resumption of feeding. Most of these patients will be able to eat after the acute exacerbation subsides. Those that are unable to resume diet may have an underlying anatomic cause for recurrence that is demonstrable by endoscopic retrograde cholangiopancreatography (ERCP).

### Vitamins

Ascorbic acid, an antioxidant in plasma, is active against oxidants released by activated leukocytes and macrophages. These phagocytes have been implicated in the progression of edematous pancreatitis to more severe forms of the disease. Ascorbic acid levels are significantly lower in patients with acute pancreatitis than in patients with acute abdominal crises resulting from other diseases (145). While a principle of general metabolic care is to give vitamins to critically ill patients, it is not known whether ascorbic acid supplementation affects the course of acute pancreatitis in man.

### Pain Relief

It is traditional to administer meperidine rather than morphine because of the lesser effect of the drug on sphincter of Oddi spasm. Epidural anesthesia is also effective, but one must be mindful of associated altered circulatory dynamics.

### Resting the Pancreas

A time-honored concept in treating acute pancreatitis is to put the pancreas at rest, even though the validity of this assumption has not been established. Methods to inhibit pancreatic secretion may not be based on pathophysiologic principles. However, in some models of experimental pancreatitis, stimulation of the pancreas prevents extrusion of zymogen granules (which contain pancreatic enzymes) from acinar cells, suggesting that secretory blockade may be an important characteristic of the disease (146, 147). However, this does not explain why premature feeding can cause recurrence of signs and symptoms, unless, possibly, acinar function recovers as the clinical improvement occurs.

**Nasogastric Suction.** It was assumed for many years that aspiration of gastric contents helps to "decompress" ileus and put the pancreas at rest. Three prospective randomized studies of mild-to-moderate pancreatitis concluded that there was no clear advantage in the use of nasogastric suction (148–150). Thus, a nasogastric tube is used mostly to relieve gastric distention or vomiting in patients with acute pancreatitis.

**$H_2$-Receptor Antagonism.** The concept behind the use of a $H_2$-receptor antagonist, (similar to the concept relating to a nasogastric tube) is that by reducing the acid load in the duodenum there would be a decrease in hormonal stimulation of the pancreas. However, three prospective randomized studies involving mild-to-moderate cases of acute pancreatitis found no effect of cimetidine on the course of disease (151–153). Nevertheless, $H_2$-receptor antagonism does have a role in the prophylaxis of stress gastritis in patients with severe forms of acute pancreatitis.

**Anticholinergics.** Administration of anticholinergics used to be popular because it was thought that inhibition of pancreatic secretion and relaxation of the sphincter of Oddi would be beneficial. In a prospective randomized study using atropine, no significant difference in clinical course was noted (154). Even though this study did not classify patients by severity of disease, the results are still accepted by most.

**Glucagon.** Glucagon normally inhibits gastric acid and pancreatic exocrine secretion and relaxes the sphincter of Oddi. It was hoped that glucagon administration might ameliorate pancreatitis by physiologically resting the pancreas. However, in a double-blind randomized study of severely and moderately ill patients with acute pancreatitis, there was no major difference in the frequency of expected complications in patients treated with glucagon or anticholinergics (155). Glucagon had no significant influence on mortality rate or course of disease in three other prospective randomized trials (156–158).

**Somatostatin.** Somatostatin reduces pancreatic secretion by 70% in healthy patients. Thus, there was hope that somatostatin administration might decrease the work of the pancreas by decreasing secretion. However, the secretory state of the pancreas during acute pancreatitis in man is unknown. While pancreatic secretion is impaired after patients recover from necrotizing pancreatitis (159), there is little information about other forms of acute pancreatitis. Somatostatin may in theory make pancreatitis worse, because this hormone is known to reduce pancreatic blood flow by vasoconstriction. In general, vasoconstrictors exacerbate the histologic severity of pancreatitis in animal models (159).

A critical review of somatostatin therapy has concluded that a sufficiently large trial has not yet been published to support firm conclusions for or against the use of this agent in acute pancreatitis (159–160). However, a meta-analysis of controlled trials reports a survival advantage (161). The use of somatostatin or its long-acting synthetic analogue octreotide in preventing acute pancreatitis following ERCP is controversial (159). A prospective study using octreotide in severe acute pancreatitis found a reduction in sepsis from 74 to 26% and a reduction in adult respiratory distress syndrome from 63 to 37% in treated patients (162). However, the number of patients in the study was small, and another study has suggested that the disease is exacerbated.

**Calcitonin.** Calcitonin, which depresses both gastric acid secretion and stimulated pancreatic enzyme secretion, had no influence on mortality in a double-blind treatment trial for acute pancreatitis (163).

### Antiproteases

Experimental studies have shown that intracellular activation of proteases may represent an important pathophysiologic sequence in initiating acute pancreatitis. Furthermore, proteolytic enzymes are released into the blood and retroperitoneum. However, attempts at protease inhibition in humans have not significantly influenced the course of disease in most patients.

**Fresh Frozen Plasma (FFP).** FFP has been suggested as a means of replenishing levels of naturally occurring antiproteases. In a prospective randomized study, two units of FFP daily for 3 days did not have any noticeable effect on the course of pancreatitis, compared with controls receiving human albumin (164). The dose was based on a retrospective study suggesting benefit. While FFP did result in some improvement in antiprotease and related profiles, it is possible that greater volumes of FFP or specific concentrates might be more beneficial. However, a very large number of patients would seem to be required to show even a 10% difference in outcome.

**Aprotinin (Trasylol).** Aprotinin, an antiprotease drug used in early clinical trials, has had disappointing results (157, 165). A randomized controlled trial of aprotinin, 200,000 units intravenously every 6 hours for 5 days, in the treatment of gallstone or idiopathic pancreatitis concluded that the enzyme inhibitor reduced mortality from 25 to 7.5% (166). While the dose was considered sufficient in contrast to previous reports, the data suggest that the treated and controlled groups may not have been as comparable as the authors suggest. Another prospective randomized trial, using somewhat higher doses for 5 days, found that aprotinin had no effect on mortality (157).

**Gabexate Mesilate.** At least two prospective randomized trials involving a lower-molecular-weight antiprotease, gabexate mesilate, which may better enter acinar cells, showed no significant effect on complications or mortality (167, 168). In contrast, a meta-analysis of gabexate mesilate concluded that this drug did not affect mortality from acute pancreatitis but appeared to reduce the incidence of complications requiring surgery (169). This discrepancy remains unexplained.

### Prophylactic Antibiotic(s)

A devastating complication of acute pancreatitis is the development of a secondary infection in necrotic glandular and/or peripancreatic tissue. Prophylactic antibiotics have been administered in hopes of minimizing the incidence of this problem. About two-thirds of the bacteria in pancreatic necrosis and pancreatic abscesses are gram-negative enteric organisms, 20% are gram positive, and 15% are anaerobes (170). Bacterial contamination of the retroperitoneum is most often believed to come primarily from the intestine by one or more potential routes (e.g., blood, lymphatics, ascites). The routine use of a prophylactic antibiotic regimen remains controversial, and even though recent studies suggest there may be some benefit, more data are essential.

Randomized clinical studies, published in the 1970s, used either cephazolin (171) or ampicillin (172–174) and found no significant difference in the incidence of intraabdominal infection. These studies have been criticized not only for having too few patients but also for including patients who were at low risk for infection. They have also been criticized for using antibiotics that penetrate poorly into the pancreas (170, 175). It is not clear if the latter point is valid, because it is often peripancreatic tissue rather than the pancreas that becomes infected. There is information about penetration of antibiotics into the human pancreas. Concentrations of antibiotics in the human pancreas obtained at surgery (170) show that the administration of aminoglycosides (tobramycin and netilmicin) results in tissue concentrations below the minimal inhibitory concentrations for most bacteria found in pancreatic infection. In contrast, broad-spectrum penicillins (mezlocillin, piperacillin) and third-generation cephalosporins (cefotaxime, ceftizoxime) achieve high enough tissue concentrations to inhibit some, but not all, bacteria present in pancreatic infection. On the other hand, quinolones (ofloxacin, ciprofloxacin) and imipenem achieve high tissue levels effective against most aerobic bacteria present in pancreatic infection. Metronidazole tissue levels were found to be effective against anaerobic bacteria. The drugs were administered in doses according to the manufacturer's recommendation for intravenous therapeutic application in Germany. On the basis of these data, it has been recommended that the first-choice drugs are those with sufficient tissue bacterial inhibitory concentrations. Metronidazole should also be used in combination with the chosen antibiotics for its activity against anaerobes.

There is very little information about the pharmacokinetics of antibiotics in acute pancreatitis. A study of pharmacokinetic parameters using gentamicin in patients with acute pancreatitis indicates that such patients require approximately a 25% greater dose than controls to achieve therapeutic serum concentrations (176). This is primarily due to fluid sequestration, which results in greater total body clearance rather than faster rates of elimination.

A recent randomized multicenter prospective trial using imipenem, 0.5 g intravenously every 8 hours for 14 days, found a lower incidence of pancreatic sepsis (12.2 vs. 30.3%) in treated patients (177). The mean Ranson score was 3.7, and all patients had evidence of necrotizing pancreatitis as defined by CT scan. However, the incidence of multiorgan system failure, necessity for operation, or mortality appeared to be unaffected by antibiotic treatment. This discrepancy remains unexplained.

A prospective randomized study of selective decontamination of the gut in severe pancreatitis found a reduction in mortality after 2 weeks from 35 to 22% (178). The regimen consisted of colistin sulfate, amphotericin, and norfloxacin in a paste smeared on the gums every 6 hours and at the tracheostomy site, if present. The drugs were given orally every 6 hours and daily in a rectal enema. Cefotaxime sodium was given intravenously every 8 hours until gram-negative bacteria were eliminated from the rectum and oral cavity. The drugs were continued until the patient recovered. Secondary pancreatic infection occurred in 18% of patients who received selective decontamination and in 38% of controls. Only gram-positive bacteria were noted in patients with infected necrosis who were treated with the antibiotic regimen. The authors of this study advocate selective decontamination for patients with Imrie (Glasgow) scores of 3 or more, regardless of the CT findings at admission. The results of this study require confirmation, especially in view of the controversy concerning whether selective decontamination prevents other complications in critically ill patients.

### Peritoneal Dialysis

Peritoneal fluid obtained from patients with acute pancreatitis contains many substances, including amylase, lipase, phospholipase-A, protease-antiprotease complexes, trypsinogen, proteolytic proenzymes, prostaglandin-like activity, and kinin-forming enzymes, some of which are believed to be absorbed into the circulation (as opposed to released into pancreatic venous drainage) (179, 180). Not surprisingly, peritoneal fluid obtained during acute pancreatitis in humans is toxic to mitochondrial respiration (181). Experimental studies show that intravenous infusion of ascitic fluid causes a fall in mean arterial blood pressure and peripheral vascular resistance, however, pulmonary artery pressure increases (182). To minimize the peritoneal absorption of biologically active agents that affect the cardiovascular-pulmonary system, some consider peritoneal lavage as a means of preventing local and systemic effects of this transudate.

Unquestionably, some patients sustain immediate benefits from peritoneal lavage, which causes an improvement in vital signs within 24 hours (171). Some authors even claim that lavage decreases early mortality (183). However, a prospective randomized study found no significant effect of 4 days of lavage on mortality, on the incidence of major complications, or on the length of hospital stay in patients with 2 or fewer or 3 or more of Ranson's criteria (184). Furthermore, another controlled clinical trial found no significant beneficial effect of dialysis (175). In spite of these data, some continue to use peritoneal lavage for the first 48 hours in patients with fulminant disease when hypotension and hyperdynamic cardiorespiratory collapse fail to respond to aggressive therapy (185). One study suggests that a long cycle of peritoneal lavage, 14 days, may reduce the frequency and mortality of pancreatic sepsis (180). However, the latter study involved a small number of patients and required 9 years to complete. Given this time span, it is not clear if the beneficial effects of prolonged lavage were influenced by improvements in overall patient management that had occurred over the 9-year interval.

Peritoneal dialysis can be associated with complications that include injury to distended bowel during catheter insertion, hypothermia caused by the perfusate, puncture site bleeding, secondary infection, hypoalbuminemia, respiratory depression, and severe swelling in the lower abdomen and scrotum (171, 175, 186).

### Prophylactic Drainage

At one time it was popular to decompress the biliary tree, place a gastrostomy and feeding jejunostomy, and drain the peripancreatic region as a prophylactic procedure to minimize complications (187, 188). This is no longer advocated, as these procedures provide little, if any, prophylactic benefit.

### Plain Abdominal Radiographs Once the Diagnosis of Acute Pancreatitis Is Made

Flat and upright abdominal radiographs are of little value in following the course of acute pancreatitis. Although on occasion evidence suggesting abscess or retroperitoneal necrosis (e.g., soap bubbles) is demonstrated, our experience is that these are usually late findings in patients with septic courses or progressively enlarging masses.

### CT Scanning Once the Diagnosis of Acute Pancreatitis Is Made

CT scans are most valuable in assessing the local complications of acute pancreatitis (189). An ordinary CT scan with contrast will miss the diagnosis of retroperitoneal necrosis in 77% of patients in our experience (144). There has been enthusiasm for a rapid bolus infusion of intravenous contrast (dynamic pancreatography), which identifies areas of reduced pancreatic perfusion that are thought to represent sites at risk for necrosis, if not already necrotic (190, 191). The importance of determining the extent of hypoperfusion is that it helps to identify those patients who are at risk for bacterial infection of the retroperitoneum. However, the identification of areas of hypoperfusion or lack of perfusion does not indicate that pancreatic resection is necessary.

Experimental studies suggest that dynamic pancreatography may convert borderline ischemic areas to irreversible necrosis (192), but this observation, made in rats, does not occur in the opossum (193). It is likely that this discrepancy is related to the differing experimental models of pancreatitis. Progression of disease following dynamic pancreatography has not been confirmed in humans.

There appears to be a growing consensus that neither routine nor emergent dynamic CT scanning is justified in every patient with acute pancreatitis. However, there are strong advocates for dynamic CT scanning in patients who are classified as severe by one scoring system or another, since this is the group at risk for infection.

In most situations of acute pancreatitis diagnosed by clinical and laboratory criteria, we find CT scanning to be of greatest value later in the course of disease. This is especially true of patients who do not progressively improve.

### Diagnostic ERCP Once the Diagnosis of Acute Pancreatitis Is Made

ERCP is not necessary in all cases. Certainly for *recurrent episodes* of acute pancreatitis, especially in the absence of a history of alcohol intake and demonstrable gallstones, ERCP is worthwhile. This may reveal ductal abnormalities, duodenal diverticula, unsuspected gallstones, cholesterol crystals (on aspirated duodenal specimen), periampullary CA, and congenital as well as other abnormalities. In the past there was enthusiasm for pancreas divisum as a cause of acute pancreatitis, but this is now doubtful (194). Patients with carcinoma of the ampulla (195) or pancreas can initially present with mild or severe pancreatitis only to recover and present months later with more traditional manifestations of malignancy (196). In these asymptomatic patients, CT scans can be misleading because the residual inflammation, which may take months to resolve, can obscure the underlying carcinoma.

There are generally no accepted indications for ERCP early in the course of acute pancreatitis, even though some advocate this study early for gallstone pancreatitis. It is generally accepted that in most such patients, the onset of pancreatitis is related to passage of a stone through the ampulla into the duodenal lumen. This being the case, ERCP can be negative, since a single offending stone may have already passed. However, when there is concern about cholangitis accompanying acute pancreatitis, ERCP can be of value. The procedure as well as endoscopic papillotomy can be done without complications in patients suspected of having pancreatitis from gallstones (159) [*Editor's note:* serious complications have occasionally been noted in other series]. Nevertheless, we are reluctant to do ERCP early in the course of acute pancreatitis for fear of intensifying the disease.

## PREDICTION OF SEVERITY OF ILLNESS

A shortcoming of scoring systems to predict the severity of acute pancreatitis is the time it usually takes (e.g., 48 hours in the Ranson and Imrie scoring system) (165, 197) to obtain all the data. Clinical assessment, by then, is believed by some to be probably just as good (49). Overreliance on scores to predict a severe episode can result in mismanagement of the relatively small number of patients who were initially judged to have mild pancreatitis and who subsequently develop severe disease. Unfortunately, approximately 5% of these patients will eventually die. This underscores the fact that while the course of acute pancreatitis is predictable in many instances, there are those patients who will rapidly and unexpectedly deteriorate. This is in stark contrast to other patients who will improve contrary to their initial assessment.

**Ranson, Glasgow, APACHE.** Scoring systems (e.g., Ranson, Glasgow, APACHE) based primarily on multiple laboratory criteria to detect complicated episodes of acute pancreatitis are more useful in comparing treatment regimens than in the actual management of the individual patient. Patients with a mild episode according to various criteria can still die (198). However, scoring systems can be of value in determining the necessity for admission to a critical care unit and can be used to predict mortality. For example, patients with Ranson scores (Table 21.3) of 3–4 have a mortality approaching 20%, which roughly doubles with 5 to 6 positive signs. The mortality becomes 100% when 7 to 8 signs are present (197), but this is not universally true.

The Ranson scoring system is the most popular one in the United States today (Table 21.3). The Glasgow scoring system includes similar parameters (Table 21.4) (53). If three or more factors are positive in either the Ranson or Glasgow systems, it predicts severe disease. The APACHE II severity-of-disease classification system involves 12 variables, which include temperature, cardiovascular and respiratory parameters, serum electrolytes, creatinine, blood count, and Glasgow Coma score (199). The scoring system is complicated by the fact that it also involves the determination of assigned values for certain ranges of physiologic variables.

A study comparing scoring systems found no significant differences in the Ranson, Glasgow, or APACHE II classifications (200). The Ranson and Glasgow scoring systems provide a one-time prediction within the first 48 hours of admission, whereas the APACHE II grading system can be gathered within a few hours. Daily monitoring of the APACHE II score showed that patients dying within 4 days of admission had scores that continued to rise, whereas survivors had scores that decreased during the first 7 days of illness (201). Although the admission APACHE II score appeared to be less accurate than either the Ranson or Glasgow score, APACHE II scores recorded during the first 3 days of admission (when peak values were set at more than 9 and 12) appeared to be similar in predictive value to the Ranson and Glasgow scores. The APACHE II system may be more accurate in patients with gallstone pancreatitis, whereas the Ranson system may be more accurate in patients with alcoholic pancreatitis (201). More data are required to resolve this issue.

**TABLE 21.3. Ranson's Criteria**

| |
|---|
| At admission or diagnosis |
| Age > 55 years |
| WBC > 16,000 mm$^3$ |
| Blood glucose > 200 mg/dL (no i.v. glucose or diabetes) |
| Serum lactic dehydrogenase > 350 IU/L |
| Serum glutamic oxaloacetic transaminase > 250 Sigma-Frankel units % |
| During initial 48 hours |
| Hematocrit fall > 10 percentage points |
| Blood urea nitrogen rise > 5 mg/dL |
| Serum calcium level < 8 mg/dL |
| Arterial $pO_2$ < 60 mm Hg |
| Base deficit > 4 mEq/L |
| Estimated fluid sequestration > 6 L |

Modified from Ranson JHC. Acute pancreatitis. In: Cameron JL, ed. Current surgical therapy. St. Louis: Mosby-Year Book, 1995:409.

**TABLE 21.4. Glasgow Scoring System**

| |
|---|
| Within 48 hours |
| Albumin < 3.2 g/dL |
| WBC > 15,000 mm$^3$ |
| Lactic dehydrogenase > 600 u/L |
| Aspartate transaminase/alanine transaminase > 200 units/L |
| Glucose > 10 mmol/L |
| Calcium < 2 mmol/L |
| Urea > 16 mmol/L |
| $p_aO_2$ < 60 mm Hg |

**Clinical Scoring System.** Many clinicians do not use scoring systems, relying instead on clinical signs. Clinical assessment based on the presence or absence of shock, adequacy of peripheral perfusion, urinary output, respiratory distress, fever, body wall ecchymosis, abdominal distention, tenderness, and ileus have been found to be more accurate than the Ranson and Glasgow scoring systems in predicting severity of illness at admission. However, overreliance on clinical assessment has failed to identify two-thirds of patients who ultimately had a complicated course or fatal outcome (201). A composite clinical staging system that does not rely on laboratory tests has been shown to compare reasonably well with the Ranson criteria (202). The composite clinical staging system is primarily based on the presence of ileus and peritonitis as well as the Charlson Weighted Index of Comorbidity (Table 21.5). This new system requires additional verification, and a significant variable involves the definition of ileus.

**C-Reactive Protein.** Another means of determining severity of disease is C-reactive protein (CRP) measurement. Raised serum levels of C-reactive protein are a measure of the acute-phase response (203). CRP has been evaluated as a prognostic index and prognosticator of the course of disease in acute pancreatitis. C-reactive protein can differentiate between mild and severe cases of acute pancreatitis (204, 205) and is at least as accurate as either the Ranson or Glasgow scoring systems in predicting the severity of acute pancreatitis (206). The sensitivity and specificity of CRP in predicting severe disease are high, 83–84% and 74–85%, respectively (206, 207). CRP has been reported to have an overall accuracy of 93% in detecting pancreatic necrosis. When using a serum CRP concentration of 100 mg/L or more, one study distinguished between patients with a better or worse prognosis with 100% sensitivity and 86% specificity (208). CRP may be the single best serum parameter for distinguishing between mild and severe episodes of acute pancreatitis (203, 205, 206, 208). A major drawback of CRP is that it shares a similar delay to the other methods used for severity assessment in acute pancreatitis (209). That is, peak CRP levels are not attained until 48–72 hours after disease onset. To circumvent this delay in severity assessment, recent interest has focused on the cytokines, particularly interleukin-6 (IL-6).

**Interleukin-6.** Since cytokines are inducers of all major acute-phase proteins in the liver, including C-reactive protein, measurement of IL-6 was proposed as an early means of severity assessment in acute pancreatitis. In fact, IL-6, like CRP, was found to correlate well with the severity of acute pancreatitis, the advantage being that peak serum IL-6 levels preceded peak CRP levels by 12–24 hours (209–211). IL-6 levels showed only slight initial elevations in patients with mild disease and decreased within 4 days (210). On the other hand, patients with lethal disease had marked initial IL-6 elevations, which subsequently decreased but were still elevated on the 7th day of hospitalization. Thus, the apparent advantage of measuring IL-6 is that it may provide an even earlier clue to detecting and measuring the acute-phase response (203). Unfortunately, assay of IL-6 can be time consuming (209).

**Interleukin-8.** Interleukin-8 (IL-8) is a neutrophil-activating peptide (212). Since polymorphonuclear cells (PMNs) play a major role in the pathogenesis of pancreatitis, there should be a correlation between IL-8 levels and plasma concentrations of PMN-elastase and the clinical course of acute pancreatitis. Patients with complicated pancreatitis are reported to have significantly higher values of IL-8 and PMN-elastase than patients with mild pancreatitis (213). Furthermore, a decrease in IL-8 levels correlates with clinical improvement.

**Elastase.** PMN elastase has 43% homology in its primary structure with elastase-1 (214). Acute pancreatitis is heralded by the infiltration of PMNs into the interstitial pancreatic space, which could be the fundamental stage in the development of the disease (215). There is a correlation between the severity of disease and leukocyte infiltration (216). PMNs can produce

**TABLE 21.5. Composite Clinical Staging System**

Overall scheme

| | | Comorbidity Score ≥ 3 | Stage |
|---|---|---|---|
| Ileus | No | No | I |
| | Yes | Yes | II |
| Peritonitis | No | No | II |
| | Yes | Yes | III |

Comorbidity score (the score for each condition is summed and the total score = comorbidity score)

| Score | Condition |
|---|---|
| 1 | Myocardial infarct |
| | Congestive heart failure |
| | Peripheral vascular disease |
| | Cerebrovascular disease |
| | Dementia |
| | Chronic pulmonary disease |
| | Connective tissue disease |
| | Ulcer disease |
| | Mild liver disease |
| | Diabetes |
| 2 | Hemiplegia |
| | Moderate or severe renal disease (creatinine > 3 mg/dL; dialysis; transplant; uremia) |
| | Diabetes with end-organ damage |
| | Any tumor |
| | Leukemia |
| 3 | Moderate or severe liver disease |
| 6 | Metastatic solid tumor |
| | AIDS |

Mortality

| Stage | Mortality % |
|---|---|
| I | 7 |
| II | 23 |
| III | 67 |

Modified from Rabeneck L, Feinstein AR, Horwitz RI, Wells CK. A new clinical prognostic staging system for acute pancreatitis. Am J Med 1993;95:61–70.

excessive tissue damage by release of lysosomal proteases such as elastase and oxygen free radicals (217). Elastase, in addition to causing local tissue damage, is also capable of activating complement, kinins, and fibrinolytic systems, which are believed to be important in the evolution of multisystem failure. Among inflammatory cells, neutrophils are the largest producer of oxygen free radicals (218), which also are suspected of playing a role in the pathogenesis of acute pancreatitis. Both pancreatic- and PMN-elastase cause increased production of superoxide by stimulated neutrophils. Thus, PMN-elastase levels would be expected to correlate with the severity of pancreatitis (218, 219).

PMN-elastase levels have been used to differentiate between edematous and necrotizing pancreatitis (220). PMN-elastase has a reported sensitivity and specificity of higher than 90% in predicting the severity of acute pancreatitis, compared with the Ranson and Glasgow criteria, which have a sensitivity and specificity in the range of 70 to 80% (221). PMN-elastase also has a positive predictive value of severity approaching 97% on the first morning of hospitalization. Thus, the probability that a patient with acute pancreatitis will have a severe episode is great if the PMN-elastase levels are elevated (300 g/L). Furthermore, the value of the test in ruling out severity was 98% from the onset (negative predictive value of severity). Severe acute pancreatitis reportedly occurs only exceptionally in patients with normal or only slightly elevated levels of PMN-elastase (221). However, a series containing a larger number of patients with severe pancreatitis found that the predictive value for severity of PMN-elastase was 82% (222), which approaches the predictions derived from more commonly used scoring systems.

PMN-elastase and CRP are comparable as indicators of necrosis in acute pancreatitis (223). However, two advantages of PMN-elastase over CRP appear to be its earlier increase in the blood (median peak value reached on day 1 after the onset of pancreatitis, compared with days 3 and 4 for CRP) and the greater dynamism of its serum course (PMN-elastase levels decreased rapidly in patients with edematous pancreatitis, compared with CRP values, which remained elevated). Another study showed that the PMN-elastase level on the 1st day and the CRP value on the 2nd day were the most useful variables in predicting the severity of acute pancreatitis (224). However, more data are required to determine the superiority of PMN-elastase to the more easily obtained scoring systems.

**Phospholipase $A_2$.** Phospholipase $A_2$ ($PLA_2$) is a lipolytic enzyme that hydrolyzes phospholipids. It is produced by the pancreatic acinar cells as an inactive precursor, prophospholipase $A_2$ (pro-$PLA_2$), which is activated by trypsin. In addition to the pancreas, the enzyme is also found in synovial fluid, placenta, platelets, and almost every tissue studied (225). Large amounts of lysophosphatidylcholine are found in necrotic pancreatic tissue taken from patients who die of acute pancreatitis (226). Extremely high serum levels of $PLA_2$ (more than 500 times) have been found in patients with acute pancreatitis (32). Subsequently, it was postulated that $PLA_2$ might play an important role in the pathology of acute pancreatitis.

Elevated serum $PLA_2$ levels correlate well with the severity of acute pancreatitis, and estimation of $PLA_2$ may provide a more rapid prediction of severity of disease (227). However, serum $PLA_2$ levels in acute pancreatitis are of two types: synovial and pancreatic (225). Pancreatic $PLA_2$ circulates mostly as the inactive enzyme in patients with acute pancreatitis; the synovial $PLA_2$ is responsible for the increased enzyme activity. It is the level of synovial $PLA_2$, not pancreatic $PLA_2$, that appears to correlate best with the severity of acute pancreatitis. Serum $PLA_2$ levels are significantly higher in patients with hemorrhagic pancreatitis than in those with spontaneously resolving disease (228). Thus, serum $PLA_2$ might help to identify those patients with necrosis in contrast to those with milder forms of the disease. However, the assay for $PLA_2$ is time consuming and not specific. Elevated levels of $PLA_2$ can occur in other conditions, such as septic shock, rheumatoid arthritis, pancreatic cancer, chronic renal failure, and multiple injuries (225, 229, 230).

Pro-$PLA_2$ the inactive form of $PLA_2$, is the major form of circulating enzyme in healthy subjects. The proportion of pro-$PLA_2$ is decreased in acute pancreatitis, the active phase of chronic relapsing pancreatitis, and the early stage of pancreatic cancer, conditions associated with markedly elevated levels of serum total $PLA_2$ (229). This suggests that the ratio of pro-$PLA_2$ to total $PLA_2$ in patients with acute pancreatitis also may reflect the severity of the disease.

**Ribonuclease.** It has been reported that an acid ribonuclease of low molecular weight is an indicator of pancreatic necrosis (231). While this has been confirmed by additional reports, others find considerable overlap between patients with and without necrosis, which lessens the discriminatory value of this test (32). Another problem with acid ribonuclease is that it is not entirely of pancreatic origin. Ribonuclease levels tend to remain elevated, even after pancreatectomy, indicating that extrapancreatic sources must exist (232).

**Methemalbuminemia.** Methemalbuminemia was once considered useful in the diagnosis of acute hemorrhagic pancreatitis (233). However, this breakdown product of hemoglobin may also be associated with other conditions in which there is extravasated blood in the peritoneal cavity, such as mesenteric infarction or hemolysis (234, 235). Methemalbumin is formed when pancreatic enzymes split hemoglobin from extravasated blood into heme and globin. When heme is oxidized to hematin and absorbed into the circulation, it combines with albumin to form methemalbumin (86). Elevated methemalbumin in the serum during acute pancreatitis is associated with the subsequent development of complications and mortality (236), but a clinically severe course can also occur in the absence of methemalbuminemia. One study showed that only 29% of patients with severe acute pancreatitis had methemalbumin in the serum (237). Both false-positive and false-negative methemalbumin results can occur (234, 238, 239).

**$\alpha_2$-Macroglobulin.** $\alpha_2$-Macroglobulin is the key antiprotease that prevents free proteolytic enzymes, such as trypsin and elastase, from circulating in plasma. Levels of $\alpha_2$-macroglobulin decrease during acute pancreatitis, and there is a relationship between the magnitude of decrease and the severity of pancreatitis (240). $\alpha_2$-2 Macroglobulin levels are lower in patients with severe attacks of pancreatitis than in those with mild attacks and lower yet in patients who have fatal attacks (241). This may be due to the formation of rapidly cleared $\alpha_2$-macroglobulin complexes and active proteases. Other enzyme inhibitors, such as $\alpha_1$-protease inhibitor and antichymotrypsin, have also been evaluated, but the results are less encouraging (32).

**Diagnostic Peritoneal Lavage.** Diagnostic peritoneal lavage is a rapid but invasive means of predicting severity. Criteria that predict a severe episode of pancreatitis include aspiration of more than 10 mL of free peritoneal fluid or free fluid of a dark to "mid-straw" color (237). Lavage correctly predicted severe disease at 8 hours in 72% of patients, which compares with 82% for Ranson and 71% for Glasgow scores at 48 hours. Lavage correctly predicted mild cases at 8 hours in 95% of patients, compared with 79% for Ranson and 83% for Glasgow scores.

**CT Scan.** Clinical scoring systems based primarily on multiple laboratory data appear to be better predictors of mortality than CT scores (178). Contrast-enhanced CT scanning does not necessarily improve on the prognostic value of a plain scan and is similar in its predictive value to the Glasgow scoring system (189). This is somewhat controversial, as other authors believe that CT scanning findings are more accurate than clinical criteria in predicting outcome (114). Nevertheless, it is generally agreed that clinical scoring systems are composed of more inherent criteria, such as physiologic response parameters, which are probably more important than the anatomic features seen on CT scans.

The pancreatic size index (maximum anteroposterior measurement of head times maximum anteroposterior measurement of the body) in patients with severe episodes is significantly greater than in those with mild attacks (111). The mean index of severe cases at admission was 12.6 $cm^2$ (range, 3.4–47.6 $cm^2$) which is slightly more than twice the mean of mild episodes (range, 1.0–30 $cm^2$). Significant differences in the index were also apparent at 1 and 6 weeks. Although even more elaborate CT classification schemes have been used to assess severity (242), they are not required for all patients with acute pancreatitis. This is primarily because scoring systems based on CT scans have been shown to have similar predictive value to clinical scoring systems that depend primarily on laboratory data (189).

**CT Scan, C-Reactive Protein, and Scoring Systems.** In a prospective comparison of contrast-enhanced CT scans, Ranson score, and CRP levels for predicting the development of sepsis in acute pancreatitis, CT scanning was the best predictor of septic outcome (243). This finding was primarily due to the presumed ability of CT scans to determine the presence and extent of necrosis. Nevertheless, the same study showed that Ranson scores and CRP levels still correlated significantly with pancreatic sepsis (243). Similarly, it has been suggested that a Glasgow score in the first 24 hours predicting a severe attack combined with blood CRP levels above 120 mg/L within the first 72 hours or a failure of clinical resolution within 7 days has a high positive predictive value for CT scan–diagnosed necrosis (244). The combined criteria (Glasgow score plus CRP) were better than either alone.

It is generally held that dynamic pancreatography is the best method for discriminating between edematous and necrotizing pancreatitis. However, if one must rely on a serum indicator of pancreatic necrosis, CRP is probably the best in this regard and may well serve as an alternative to contrast-enhanced CT scanning.

**CT Scan and Ranson Score.** Another proposed scoring system is based on a modified Ranson score combined with CT scan findings (116). In the modified Ranson scores, 1 indicates zero to one positive signs, 2 indicates two to four signs, and 3 indicates five or more signs (245). Patients are then classified into three groups based on CT scan findings: group I, no phlegmonous extrapancreatic spread (none died); group II, phlegmonous extrapancreatic spread in one or two areas (4% died); and group III, phlegmonous extrapancreatic spread in three or more areas (42% died). Patients in group III with a modified Ranson score of 3 or 2 had mortality rates of 58 and 32%, respectively. Except for two cases, all patients who developed pancreatic abscess were found in group III. This study suggests that an early CT scan may be of value in patients with a modified Ranson score of 2 or 3 (116).

Another study also showed that early CT can identify patients who are at increased risk of infection related to pancreatitis (246). CT scan findings were graded into A, normal; B, pancreatic enlargement alone; C, inflammation confined to the pancreas and peripancreatic fat; D, one peripancreatic fluid collection; and E, two or more fluid collections. The severity of pancreatitis was also graded by Ranson's prognostic signs as mild (0–2 signs), moderate (3–5 signs), and severe (≥6 signs) (245). CT scan findings correlated reasonably well with the prognostic signs. The incidence of abscesses in mild disease was 13%; in moderate, 32%; and in severe, 80%. Patients with three or more prognostic signs and CT grade C, D, or E had a 57% rate of abscess. Patients with grade A or B disease tended to have self-limited disease.

While the combination of CT grades and various scoring systems can be a good predictor of infection (114, 116, 246), there are no data indicating that the knowledge derived from

**TABLE 21.6. Time and Mode of Death in Acute Pancreatitis**

| | % | % Pulmonary Congestion and/or Edema | % Infection |
|---|---|---|---|
| Dead < 24 hr | 20.5 | 95.2 | 26.5 |
| 1–7 days | 39.5 | 93.8 | 28.1 |
| > 7 days | 40.0 | 61.6 | 79.6 |

Modified from Renner IG, Savage WT III, Pantoja JL, Renner VJ. Death due to acute pancreatitis. Dig Dis Sci 1985;30:1005–1108.

accurate prediction of complications alters morbidity or mortality. Despite the paucity of such data, the use of scoring systems by whatever means should at the very least heighten sensitivity toward more aggressive diagnostic and/or therapeutic procedures (i.e., operation) in patients who do not progressively improve after 48–72 hours of resuscitation.

## COMPLICATIONS

Many of the errors in management are from a failure to recognize complications, especially after the 1st week of hospitalization. The overall mortality from acute pancreatitis ranges from 6 to 23%, and in the more severe forms, mortality ranges from 20 to 50% (247). In an autopsy series of 405 patients who died from acute pancreatitis, 21% of those autopsied died within 24 hours of admission, and 60% died within 7 days (Table 21.6). Most (94%) patients who died within 7 days of admission had pulmonary edema and congestion. Pulmonary complications were the most significant factor in patients who died early. In contrast, those who survived longer than 7 days had a reduced incidence of pulmonary edema, 62%. Infection (pneumonia, abscess, peritonitis, septicemia) was the major contributing factor to death in those who lived longer than 7 days.

A multicenter study found that 32% of patients died within the first 7 days and that approximately 5% of these died within 24 hours (198); 12 and 19% died during the 2nd and 3rd weeks, respectively, and the remainder, 37%, died during or after the 4th week. One-third of deaths that occurred during the 1st week were from fulminant multisystem organ failure, manifested as the adult respiratory distress syndrome and acute renal failure (198). After the 1st week, the most common cause of death was infection. Although only 5% of patients with pancreatitis develop infected pancreatic and/or peripancreatic necrosis, the latter accounts for more than 70–80% of all deaths from this disease in some series (190, 198).

The discussion of complications below is neither inclusive nor presented in order of frequency.

**Hyperglycemia.** Hyperglycemia occurs presumably as a result of the altered hormonal milieu, which includes increased release of pancreatic glucagon, glucocorticoids, and catecholamines as well as altered insulin resistance during acute pancreatitis. Significant hyperglycemia is treated with insulin. About 7% of nondiabetic patients will have a blood sugar level in excess of 300 mg/dL. In general, hyperglycemia is transient, occurring predominantly within the first few days of disease.

**Hypocalcemia.** It is generally agreed that a fall in serum calcium to less than 7 mg/dL is an ominous sign. Hypocalcemia in most cases is related to the loss of calcium bound to serum albumin, which leaks into the retroperitoneum or peritoneal cavity. However, ionized calcium may also be diminished by its deposition as complexes of fatty acids and calcium in areas of fat necrosis. Hypocalcemia may also be secondary to altered parathormone secretion, altered receptors, or hypomagnesemia. The value of supplemental intravenous calcium is debatable, except in rare cases of neuromuscular irritability (248). The low serum calcium levels that are frequently seen initially tend to self-correct within a few days of resuscitation.

**Hypomagnesemia.** A decrease in serum magnesium may occur as a result of vomiting and urinary losses and from magnesium deposition in areas of fat necrosis.

**Hyperlipemia.** Increased levels of serum triglyceride, cholesterol, and phospholipids may precede or occur during an acute episode of pancreatitis. This is either a result of alcohol or hyperlipoproteinemia. The association of alcohol with pancreatitis is well established, and the most common cause of hyperlipemia in an alcoholic is mild hepatic cell damage (249). As many as 22–38% of patients with acute pancreatitis have elevated serum triglyceride levels during the acute episode (250). Most of these patients have either type I or type V primary hyperlipidemia. After recovery from acute pancreatitis, serum triglycerides may remain elevated in as many as 23% of patients (250). Those patients with persistently elevated serum triglyceride levels after recovery usually exhibit type IV hyperlipidemia (250). Hyperlipemia occurring during pancreatitis does not appear to affect the outcome of the acute episode (29).

**Pseudohyponatremia.** Dilutional hyponatremia can occur in the presence of hyperlipemia (251). The importance of recognizing this condition is to avoid resuscitating a patient for a falsely low sodium, which could result in an hyperosmolar syndrome causing cerebral dysfunction.

**Ketoacidosis.** While the most common cause of acidosis during acute pancreatitis is hypovolemia, ketoacidosis that is unrelated to starvation, alcohol, or diabetes mellitus can occur (252). This ketoacidosis appears to be associated with very high serum lipase levels.

**Coagulopathy.** Disseminated intravascular coagulation may occur, and its initiating factors may be the release of proteolytic enzymes (253, 254) as well as sepsis and/or tissue necrosis and liver disease. Marked changes in coagulation can occur in pancreatitis, and there is a strong correlation with overall morbidity (255).

**Hepatic Disease.** While it is generally believed that hepatic disease is infrequent in patients with alcoholic pancreatitis, 28% of patients dying from severe alcoholic disease of the liver have histologic evidence of pancreatitis (256). However, it is unusual for both conditions to be of clinical importance simultaneously.

**Jaundice.** Mild, transient jaundice occurs in 15–30% of patients with acute pancreatitis (257, 258). The presence of jaundice does not necessarily mean the patient has choledocholithiasis or cholangitis. In an autopsy series of acute pancreatitis, obstruction of the common bile duct was found in 41% of patients (259). Gallstones were the cause of obstruction in 61% of patients, and edema near the common bile duct from an inflamed pancreas was the cause in another 32%. Hepatitis and cirrhosis generally account for 89% of jaundiced patients without common bile duct obstruction. Jaundice caused by pancreatic inflammation tends to appear several days after the onset of disease, whereas in patients with cirrhosis, the jaundice often precedes the onset of the pancreatitis. On the other hand, the time to detectable jaundice from choledocholithiasis is variable.

**Pleural Effusion.** Most pleural effusions related to acute pancreatitis occur within 48 hours of admission and are associated with an increased rate of complications from the disease (259, 260). Most effusions resolve without further problem.

**Pericardial Effusion.** Clinically relevant pericardial effusions with a high amylase content are rare (261). Presumably these can result from lymphatic extravasation or small fistulas, but generally they are associated with a communicating pseudocyst (262).

**Neuropsychiatric Disturbance.** Neuropsychiatric disturbances are unusual but can include paralysis, seizures, coma, confusion, and psychoses. How much of this is secondary to toxic psychosis related to drug intake (alcohol or prescribed medications), sepsis, hypoxia, fat emboli, or focal pathology in the cerebral cortex (263) is difficult to determine (258). Cerebral demyelination is seen histologically and may contribute to the constellation of manifestations (264).

**Gastrointestinal Hemorrhage.** When upper gastrointestinal hemorrhage occurs during an episode of acute pancreatitis, it is usually due to stress gastritis. Although this is numerically true, it is dangerous to make this assumption, since there may be other coexistent disease processes, such as peptic ulcer disease. Endoscopy is generally required to confirm the cause. With massive gastrointestinal hemorrhage, arteriography may be useful to establish the source of bleeding.

When either upper or lower gastrointestinal hemorrhage occurs in a patient who presents with recurrent episodes of acute pancreatitis, a splenic or gastroduodenal artery pseudoaneurysm, either alone or in association with a pseudocyst, may be the cause (265). Gastrointestinal hemorrhage from pseudoaneurysms may initially manifest as a self-limited episode of brisk bleeding. It is more common in patients who have recurring episodes of pancreatitis rather than in those who have clinically overt retroperitoneal necrosis (266, 267). Operative mortality rates for this condition vary with the bleeding site. Distal pancreatectomy has a lower mortality rate than resection of the pancreatic head. Because of the high operative risk, arteriographic localization and catheter embolization are often preferable for this problem (261).

Another cause of lower gastrointestinal hemorrhage is ischemic colitis associated with retroperitoneal necrosis. However, erosion by a drainage catheter or operative injury are more frequent causes of gastrointestinal perforation.

**Gastrointestinal and Hepatic Ischemia and Infarction.** Infarction of the stomach or small or large intestine is uncommon, but when retroperitoneal necrosis is present, it can cause thrombosis of the celiac axis or superior mesenteric artery and their branches may develop (144, 268, 269). Superior mesenteric artery occlusion without infarction may manifest itself as prolonged ileus if vascular collateralization occurs. Intestinal infarction most often involves the transverse colon, because extension of retroperitoneal necrosis can digest and thrombose its mesenteric blood supply. This is not necessarily a fatal condition provided it is recognized early and treated appropriately by resection, which should include a proximal colostomy as well as meticulous debridement of the retroperitoneum (144). A fixed colonic stricture can be diagnosed months after the patient recovers. It is presumably due to ischemia and most commonly involves the area around the splenic flexure (270).

**Intestinal Obstruction.** Obstruction generally involves the duodenum or stomach as a result of pancreatic and peripancreatic inflammation. A rare patient may develop adhesions of the mid small intestine to the posterior parietal peritoneum overlying an area of retroperitoneal necrosis.

**Retroperitoneal Hemorrhage.** Massive retroperitoneal hemorrhage occurring during an acute episode of pancreatitis is rare, developing in less than 3% of patients. In one series, all of the patients with massive retroperitoneal hemorrhage had at least one operation (Puestow, pseudocyst, debridement and drainage of necrotic tissue) (271). Depending on the cause of the hemorrhage, transcatheter embolization can be effective in its control.

**Hemorrhagic Pancreatitis.** The older literature frequently referred to hemorrhagic pancreatitis, which included those patients with blood in the peritoneal cavity and/or in the retroperitoneum. The term hemorrhagic pancreatitis is little used today and has been encompassed by the term necrotizing or severe pancreatitis.

**Pancreatic Phlegmon.** The term pancreatic phlegmon was initially defined as indurated pancreatic and peripancreatic tissue associated with necrosis. However, this term has been used imprecisely (275). Phlegmon should not be used by clinicians because of its lack of definition.

**Pancreatic Fistula.** Most patients who develop a fistula do so following surgical debridement of the retroperitoneum, and most of these are low-output types that will usually close spontaneously (258, 273). However, spontaneous internal fistulas can occur and be pancreaticopleural, pancreaticopericardial, or pancreaticogastric or result in pancreatic ascites.

**Splenic Rupture.** Spontaneous rupture of the spleen is an unusual complication (258). It is unclear whether this is associated with acute splenic vein thrombosis.

**Retinopathy.** Retinopathy occurring during acute pancreatitis is very rare and is suggested by complaints of visual impairment (274). This is usually Purtscher's retinopathy (cotton wool spots, or edema, and hemorrhages) confined to the optic disk and macula. Sudden blindness may occur and is presumably due to aggregated granulocyte microemboli (275).

**Subcutaneous Fat Necrosis.** Erythema nodosum–like lesions of fat necrosis occurring in the course of acute pancreatitis are rare (276). These lesions develop most often in the lower extremities but can be diffuse. Healing tends to occur with scarring and hyperpigmentation. The skin lesions may also occur with polyserositis (arthritis, pleural effusion). The etiology is unclear and is not merely related to elevated serum enzyme levels. Curiously, subcutaneous fat necrosis does not recur with subsequent episodes of pancreatitis.

**Skeletal Lesions.** Medullary bone can be affected by metastatic fat necrosis (277) and present as intramedullary calcification, osteolytic lesions, and periosteal reactions (280). Fragmentation of cartilage following end-artery thrombosis may manifest itself later as aseptic necrosis.

**Acute Cholecystitis and Cholangitis.** Even though they are not direct complications of acute pancreatitis, acute cholecystitis and/or cholangitis can accompany gallstone pancreatitis (278, 279). The symptoms and physical findings of these conditions can mimic those associated with acute pancreatitis and its complications. Ultrasonographic detection of pericholecystic fluid and a thickened gallbladder wall should be interpreted with caution, as these findings may be due to the inflammatory reaction relating to the pancreatitis rather than the acute cholecystitis.

**The Unresuscitable Patient.** An area of controversy is what to do with the patient who does not respond to initial, aggressive resuscitative measures. Some believe this is a fatal situation no matter what is done, while others believe that it may be an indication for emergent operation. Support for the latter is based on anecdotes, but one may find infected retroperitoneal necrosis or even more rarely, an overtly necrotic pancreas. The incidence of potentially treatable complications that can be corrected by surgery in patients who do not respond to resuscitation is not well known.

**Abscess.** The currently accepted definition of pancreatic abscess is a walled-off collection of pus. Its diagnosis usually is made late, during the 3rd to 5th weeks after onset of the pancreatitis, when the acute pancreatitis has clinically subsided (280). An abscess resulting from infected peritoneal fluid may be difficult to distinguish from an infected pseudocyst, which is usually diagnosed a bit later, during the 3rd to 6th weeks. If there is doubt about the diagnosis clinically, it can be established by radiographically controlled aspiration. There appears to be an increasing tendency to treat these at least initially with percutaneous drainage.

**Retroperitoneal Necrosis.** Unfortunately, there continues to be confusion about the definition and use of the term retroperitoneal necrosis, making comparison of series difficult. Necrotizing pancreatitis is defined as active inflammation associated with either devitalized pancreatic or peripancreatic tissue or both (281). Yet, these two conditions can exist grossly independent of one another. Furthermore, varying criteria are used to diagnose devitalization of the pancreas. These include dynamic pancreatography, in which areas of poor perfusion may be reversible; gross findings, in which necrotic retroperitoneal fat may be mistaken for necrotic pancreas (282); and/or histologic findings, in which the extent or severity of the microscopic findings may or may not be defined. An example of the importance of these distinctions is that pancreatic necrosis defined by dynamic pancreatography often does not require debridement or resection of the pancreas. The lack of a precise definition of what is actually necrotic in several studies and the lack of contemporary autopsy series add to the difficulty in knowing if early operation is indicated at all for the patient in difficulty during the initial stages of the disease.

It is not clear if infected retroperitoneal fat necrosis was missed in studies showing a high mortality associated with operation done early in patients with acute pancreatitis who were not responding to nonoperative treatment. Merely examining the retroperitoneum by superficial inspection and palpation can be deceptive for determining the presence of necrosis (144). The retroperitoneum around the pancreas must be opened widely to make the diagnosis. At least one series of infected retroperitoneal necrosis suggests that early surgery (within the 1st week) in patients who do not respond to treatment or who reach a clinical plateau in their course is associated with both survival and decreased morbidity (144).

It is not entirely clear whether all or most patients with multisystem organ failure have retroperitoneal necrosis. However, every patient with retroperitoneal necrosis does not require operative debridement. There is no argument about the necessity for operative intervention for infected retroperitoneal necrosis, but there is considerable controversy about the indications for operation in patients with sterile retroperitoneal necrosis.

Early severe, fatal infection is suggested by a semicomatose or obtunded state at the time of admission (247). While infection can occur during the 1st week with less impressive signs in as many as 20–22% of patients (144, 282), the incidence increases over the next several weeks. Retroperitoneal infection can be difficult to diagnose, since the symptoms and signs of acute pancreatitis are so similar. This had led to enthusiasm for fine-needle aspiration (FNA) of the retroperitoneum. When suspicious retroperitoneal (peripancreatic) areas are targeted under CT guidance, however, undue reliance should not be placed on the results of FNA, as aspiration can lead to false-positive and false-negative conclusions. FNA should be used as an adjunct when it is necessary to support the clinical assessment of the patient's status.

Most use dynamic pancreatography to help decide if FNA of the retroperitoneum should be done. In one study of patients with evidence of pancreatic necrosis on dynamic pancreatography, 74% of patients who had clinical suspicion of sepsis had infected necrosis diagnosed by FNA (283). However, another study, which appears to have used similar criteria, found a 30% incidence of sepsis (177). It is generally accepted, however, that there is a 40–60% risk of infection in patients with necrotizing pancreatitis (170).

There is considerable controversy about the indications for operation in patients with sterile retroperitoneal necrosis. The mortality was 38% in one series of sterile necrosis (284). Surgical debridement did not appear to benefit patients with unfavorable prognostic signs, but the operation was performed many days after the onset of such signs. Unfavorable prognostic signs rarely develop suddenly in our experience. They usually are added insults during a progressively downhill course. Thus, our practice is to try to intervene before shock occurs. However, the importance of systemic signs (e.g., pulmonary insufficiency and renal failure) as indications for operation is not borne out by all studies (129).

In one of the largest series (172 patients) with sterile necrosis determined by FNA or at operation, 107 patients underwent operation with the indications of persisting or advanced organ complications, abdominal complications, or both, despite aggressive intensive care measures over a 3- to 5-day period (288). Operation consisted of "necrosectomy," but neither the extent of necrosis nor which tissues were involved with necrosis were stated. Patients who underwent operation were sicker than, and had roughly twice the mortality rate (13.1%) of, the nonoperative group (6.2%). It is not clear whether the higher mortality rate occurring after surgery would have been lower without operation, because the operated patients were clearly sicker than those who did not undergo surgery. Continuous postoperative closed lavage of the peritoneal cavity was also used. Thus, it is not clear if the higher incidence of postoperative sepsis (42% vs. 8% without operation) was due to operation per se and/or the postoperative lavage. An important conclusion of this retrospective study was that operation should not be based on CT morphology but rather on persisting or increasing organ complications occurring in spite of aggressive care. Herein lies another problem—definition of "aggressive care," which may be a more important variable than generally appreciated.

ERCP with papillotomy has been advocated in patients who require surgery for necrosis, because biliary exploration at the time of operation is hazardous and difficult (286). There are few data to support this contention.

Our approach to patients with acute pancreatitis who do not show some signs of improvement by 48–72 hours of aggressive resuscitation or whose clinical course reaches a plateau with no improvement or regression is to seriously consider operation. We have not relied on either dynamic pancreatography or FNA, primarily because of the dilemma of what to do if the FNA shows no evidence of bacteria in a patient who is not doing well. This approach appears to decrease morbidity, which is considerable following delayed operations for infected retroperitoneal necrosis (144). The high mortality rate reported by several series dealing with retroperitoneal necrosis, in our opinion, may be due to lack of thorough exploration of the retroperitoneum and meticulous debridement of the obviously necrotic tissue (144). This aggressive operative approach early in the course of a patient who does not respond to treatment remains controversial. Well-designed prospective randomized studies are needed, since other investigators believe that a nonoperative approach is best when infection can not be documented.

## SPECIAL SITUATIONS

**Pregnancy.** Fortunately, acute pancreatitis occurring during pregnancy is relatively rare (1 in 1000–3333 deliveries) and is mild in most cases (287). However, severe episodes do occur and are associated with high mortality. Fetal loss is as high as 14%. Indications for operation and endoscopic intervention to the biliary tract are not altered, providing measures to protect the fetus are undertaken.

**Systemic Lupus Erythematosus.** While corticosteroids have been implicated as a rare cause of pancreatitis, patients with SLE can develop pancreatitis related to associated vasculitis. Corticosteroids need not be discontinued and should be started if necessary in most patients with SLE (288).

**AIDS.** The prevalence of pancreatitis in hospitalized patients with AIDS varies widely, ranging from 4% to 31%. Causes of pancreatitis specifically related to AIDS include medications (e.g., pentamidine, trimethoprim-sulfamethoxazole, 2′,3′-dideoxyinosine), associated infections (e.g., cytomegalovirus, *Toxoplasma gondii, Candida, Cryptococcus neoformans,* and other opportunistic infections) as well as infections that can cause a pancreatic abscess (e.g., *Mycobacterium tuberculosis, Mycobacterium avium-intracellulare, Aspergillus*) (289). These are best diagnosed by aspiration under radiographic guidance but may require external drainage. One should be suspicious of a developing abscess if small multicystic areas occur with pancreatitis. Some of these are infected lymph nodes undergoing degenerative changes.

**Prior Billroth II Gastrectomy.** A condition associated with acute pancreatitis that requires emergent operation is *acute* obstruction of an afferent limb (290). This is a closed loop obstruction that can either mimic or cause acute pancreatitis (290, 291). It is essential to demonstrate patency of the afferent limb by whatever means are appropriate in a patient who has acute pancreatitis and a prior Billroth II gastrectomy.

**Postoperative Pancreatitis.** Patients with no prior evidence of pancreatitis appear to develop a more fulminant form of the disease if it occurs postoperatively (292). As many as one-half of these patients require operation for complications related to the pancreatitis (293). Postoperative pancreatitis can occur after any operation, even those far removed from the pancreas (e.g., head and neck procedures such as parathyroidectomy). In the abdominal cavity, it can follow operations on biliary or gastrointestinal tracts (292), but more often an operation related to the pancreas is involved.

## REFERENCES


1. Cogbill CL, Song KT. Acute pancreatitis. Arch Surg 1970;100: 673–680.
2. Diaco JF, Miller LD, Copeland EM. The role of early diagnostic laparotomy in acute pancreatitis. Surg Gynecol Obstet 1969; 129:263–269.
3. Black WS, Sutterfield TC, Martin JD Jr. Acute pancreatitis. Am Surg 1967;33:94–99.
4. Olsen H. Pancreatitis: a prospective clinical evaluation of 100 cases and review of the literature. Am J Dig Dis 1974;19:1077–1090.
5. Tuzhilin SA. The clinical features of pancreatic inflammation. Am J Gastroenterol 1974;61:97–112.
6. Fromm D. Pancreas. In: Gastrointestinal surgery. New York: Churchill Livingstone, 1985:872.
7. Geokas MC, Van Lancker JL, Kadell BM, et al. Acute pancreatitis: UCLA conference. Ann Intern Med 1972;76:105–117.
8. Warshaw AL. Acute pancreatitis. Viewpoints Dig Dis 1977;9:5.
9. Zimberg YH. Pancreatitis: principles of management. Surg Clin North Am 1968;48:889–905.
10. Weinstein BR, Korn RJ, Zimmerman HJ. Obstructive jaundice as a complication of pancreatitis. Ann Intern Med 1963;58:245.
11. Lankisch PG, Schirren CA, Kunze E. Undetected fatal acute pancreatitis: why is the disease so frequently overlooked? Am J Gastroenterol 1991;86:322–326.
12. Marshall JB. Acute pancreatitis: a review with an emphasis on new developments. Arch Intern Med 1993;153:1185–1198.
13. Elman R, Arneson, N, Graham EA. Value of blood amylase estimations in the diagnosis of pancreatic disease: a clinical study. Arch Surg 1929;19:943–967.
14. Warshaw AL, Lee K-H. Characteristic alterations of serum isoenzymes of amylase in diseases of liver, pancreas, salivary gland, lung, and genitalia. J Surg Res 1977;22:362–369.
15. Skude G. On human amylase isoenzymes. Scand J Gastroenterol 1977;44:1–37.
16. Pieper-Bigelow C, Strocchi A, Levitt MD. Where does serum amylase come from and where does it go? Gastroenterol Clin North Am 1990;19:793–810.
17. Duane WC, Frerichs R, Levitt MD. Distribution, turnover, and mechanism of renal excretion of amylase in the baboon. J Clin Invest 1971;50:156–165.
18. Dubick MA, Conteas CN, Billy HT, et al. Raised serum concentrations of pancreatic enzymes in cigarette smokers. Gut 1987;28:330–335.
19. Kolars JC, Ellis CJ, Levitt MD. Comparison of serum amylase, pancreatic isoamylase and lipase in patients with hyperamylasemia. Dig Dis Sci 1984;29:289–293.
20. Agarwal N, Pitchumoni CS, Sivaprasad AV. Evaluating tests for acute pancreatitis. Am J Gastroenterol 1990;85:356–366.
21. Eckfeldt JH, Kolars JC, Elson MK, et al. Serum tests for pancreatitis in patients with abdominal pain. Arch Pathol Lab Med 1985; 109:316–319.
22. Flamion B, Delhaye M, Horanyi Z, et al. Comparison of elastase-1 with amylase, lipase, and trypsin-like immunoreactivity in the diagnosis of acute pancreatitis. Am J Gastroenterol 1987;82: 532–535.
23. Moossa AR. Diagnostic tests and procedures in acute pancreatitis. N Engl J Med 1984;311:639–643.
24. Ventrucci M, Pezzilli R, Naldoni P, et al. Serum pancreatic enzyme behavior during the course of acute pancreatitis. Pancreas 1987;2:506–509.
25. Veith FJ, Filler RM, Berard CW. Significance of prolonged elevation of the serum amylase. Ann Surg 1963;158:20–26.
26. Bockus HL, Kalser MH, Roth JLA, et al. Clinical features of acute inflammation of the pancreas. Arch Intern Med 1955;96:308.
27. Clavien P-A, Robert J, Meyer P, et al. Acute pancreatitis and normoamylasemia: not an uncommon combination. Ann Surg 1989;210:614–620.
28. Spechler SJ, Dalton JW, Robbins AH, et al. Prevalence of normal serum amylase levels in patients with acute alcoholic pancreatitis. Dig Dis Sci 1983;28:865–869.
29. Cameron JL, Capuzzi MD, Zuidema GD, et al. Acute pancreatitis with hyperlipemia: the incidence of lipid abnormalities in acute pancreatitis. Ann Surg 1973;177:483–489.
30. Warshaw AL, Bellini CA, Lesser PB. Inhibition of serum amylase and urine amylase activity in pancreatitis with hyperlipemia. Ann Surg 1975;182:72–75.
31. Zieve L. Clinical value of determinations of various pancreatic enzymes in serum. Gastroenterology 1964;46:62–67.
32. Gumaste VV. Diagnostic tests for acute pancreatitis. Gastroenterologist 1994;2:119–130.
33. Steinberg WM, Goldstein SS, Davis ND, et al. Diagnostic assays in acute pancreatitis: a study of sensitivity and specificity. Ann Intern Med 1985;102:576–580.
34. Gumaste VV, Dave P, Sereny G. Serum lipase: a better test to diagnose acute alcoholic pancreatitis. Am J Med 1992;92: 239–242.
35. Orebaugh SL. Normal amylase levels in the presentation of acute pancreatitis. Am J Emerg Med 1994;12:21–24.
36. Weaver DW, Bouwman DL, Walt AJ, et al. A correlation between clinical pancreatitis and isoenzyme patterns of amylase. Surgery 1982;92:576–580.
37. Clavien P-A, Burgan S, Moossa AR. Serum enzymes and other laboratory tests in acute pancreatitis. Br J Surg 1989;76:1234–1243.
38. Salt WB II, Schenker S. Amylase—its clinical significance: a review of the literature. Medicine 1976;55:269–289.
39. Rattner DW, Gu Z-Y, Vlahakes GJ, et al. Hyperamylasemia after cardiac surgery: incidence, significance, and management. Ann Surg 1989;209:279–283.
40. Kazmierczak SC, Van Lente F. Incidence and source of hyperamylasemia after cardiac surgery. Clin Chem 1988;34:916–919.
41. Eckfeldt JH, Leatherman JW, Levitt MD. High prevalence of hyperamylasemia in patients with acidemia. Ann Intern Med 1986;104:362–363.
42. Humphries LL, Adams LJ, Eckfeldt JH, et al. Hyperamylasemia in patients with eating disorders. Ann Intern Med 1987;106: 50–52.
43. Dutta SK, Douglass W, Smalls UA, et al. Prevalence and nature of hyperamylasemia in acute alcoholism. Dig Dis Sci 1981;26: 136–141.
44. Berk JE, Fridhandler L, Webb SF. Does hyperamylasemia in the drunken alcoholic signify pancreatitis? Am J Gastroenterol 1979;71:557–562.
45. Warshaw AL, Hawboldt MM. Puzzling persistent hyperamylasemia, probably neither pancreatic nor pathologic. Am J Surg 1988;155:453–456.
46. Ventrucci M, Pezzilli R, Festi D. Clinical significance of chronic hyperamylasemia. Dig Dis Sci 1991;36:1517–1522.
47. Murthy UK, DeGregorio F, Oates RP, et al. Hyperamylasemia in patients with the acquired immunodeficiency syndrome. Am J Gastroenterol 1992;87:332–336.
48. Lott JA, Speicher CE, Nemesanszky E. Is serum amylase an obsolete test in the diagnosis of acute pancreatitis? Arch Pathol Lab Med 1985;109:314–315.

49. Williamson RCN. Early assessment of severity in acute pancreatitis. Gut 1984;25:1331–1339.
50. Hiatt JR, Calabria RP, Passaro E, et al. The amylase profile: a discriminant in biliary and pancreatic disease. Am J Surg 1987;154:490–492.
51. Carter DC. Pancreatitis and the biliary tree: the continuing problem. Am J Surg 1988;155:10–17.
52. Blamey SL, Osborne DH, Gilmour WH, et al. The early identification of patients with gallstone associated pancreatitis using clinical and biochemical factors only. Ann Surg 1983;198: 574–578.
53. Osborne DH, Imrie CW, Carter DC. Biliary surgery in the same admission for gallstone-associated acute pancreatitis. Br J Surg 1981;68:758–761.
54. Tenner S, Dubner H, Steinberg W. Predicting gallstone pancreatitis with laboratory parameters: a meta-analysis. Am J Gastroenterol 1994;89:1863–1866.
55. Van Gossum A, Seferain V, Rodzynek JJ, et al. Early detection of biliary pancreatitis. Dig Dis Sci 1984;29:97–101.
56. Ros E, Navarro S, Bru C, et al. Occult microlithiasis in idiopathic acute pancreatitis: prevention of relapses by cholecystectomy or ursodeoxycholic acid therapy. Gastroenterology 1991;101: 1701–1709.
57. Lin X-Z, Wang S-S, Tsai Y-T, et al. Serum amylase, isoamylase, and lipase in the acute abdomen: their diagnostic value for acute pancreatitis. J Clin Gastroenterol 1989;11:47–52.
58. Ventrucci M, Pezzilli R, Gullo L, et al. Role of serum pancreatic enzyme assays in diagnosis of pancreatic disease. Dig Dis Sci 1989;34:39–45.
59. Apple F, Benson P, Preese L, et al. Lipase and pancreatic amylase activities in tissues and in patients with hyperamylasemia. Am J Clin Pathol 1991;96:610–614.
60. Ventrucci M, Pezzilli R, Gullo L. Comparison of a new immunoassay for determining serum pancreatic isoamylase with two standard techniques. Am J Gastroenterol 1990;85:1381–1385.
61. Van Lente F, Kazmierczak SC. Immunologically-derived pancreatic amylase, pancreatic lipase, and total amylase compared as predictors of pancreatic inflammation. Clin Chem 1989;35: 1542.
62. Pace BW, Bank S, Wise L, et al. Amylase isoenzymes in the acute abdomen: an adjunct in those patients with elevated total amylase. Am J Gastroenterol 1985;80:898–901.
63. Jensen DM, Royse VL, Bonello JN, et al. Use of amylase isoenzymes in laboratory evaluation of hyperamylasemia. Dig Dis Sci 1987;32:561–568.
64. Banks PA, Warshaw AL, Wolfe GZ, et al. Identification of amylase isoenzymes in intestinal contents. Dig Dis Sci 1984;29:297–299.
65. Corlette MB, Dratch M, Sorger K. Amylase elevation attributable to an ovarian neoplasm. Gastroenterology 1978;74:907–909.
66. Massey JH. Efficiency in the diagnosis of acute pancreatitis is increased by improved electrophoresis of amylase isoenzyme P3 on cellulose acetate. Clin Chem 1985;31:70–75.
67. Lifton LJ, Slickers KA, Pragay DA, et al. Pancreatitis and lipase: a reevaluation with a five-minute turbidimetric lipase determination. JAMA 1974;229:47–50.
68. Tietz NW, Huang WY, Rauh DF, et al. Laboratory tests in the differential diagnosis of hyperamylasemia. Clin Chem 1986;32: 301–307.
69. Gwozdz GP, Steinberg WM, Werner M, et al. Comparative evaluation of the diagnosis of acute pancreatitis based on serum and urine enzyme assays. Clin Chim Acta 1990;187: 243–254.
70. Lott JA, Patel ST, Sawhney AK, et al. Assays of serum lipase: analytical and clinical considerations. Clin Chem 1986;32:1290–1302.
71. Patt HH, Kramer SP, Woel G, et al. Serum lipase determinations in acute pancreatitis. Arch Surg 1966;92:718–723.
72. Gumaste VV, Roditis N, Mehta D, et al. Serum lipase levels in nonpancreatic abdominal pain versus acute pancreatitis. Am J Gastroenterol 1993;88:2051–2055.
73. Winslet M, Hall C, London NJM, et al. Relation of diagnostic serum amylase levels to etiology and severity of acute pancreatitis. Gut 1992;33:982–986.
74. Kazmierczak SC, Van Lente F, Hodges ED. Diagnostic and prognostic utility of phospholipase A activity in patients with acute pancreatitis: comparison with amylase and lipase. Clin Chem 1991;37:356–360.
75. Werner M, Steinberg WM, Pauley C. Strategic use of individual and combined enzyme indicators for acute pancreatitis analyzed by receiver-operator characteristics. Clin Chem 1989;35: 967–971.
76. Panteghini M, Pagani F. Clinical evaluation of an algorithm for the interpretation of hyperamylasemia. Arch Pathol Lab Med 1991;115:355–358.
77. Lott JA. The value of clinical laboratory studies in acute pancreatitis. Arch Pathol Lab Med 1991;115:325–326.
78. Gumaste VV, Dave PB, Weissman D, et al. Lipase/amylase ratio: a new index that distinguishes acute episodes of alcoholic from nonalcoholic acute pancreatitis. Gastroenterology 1991;101: 1361–1366.
79. Tenner SM, Steinberg W. The admission serum lipase:amylase ratio differentiates alcoholic from nonalcoholic acute pancreatitis. Am J Gastroenterol 1992;87:1755–1758.
80. Sadowski DC, Todd JK, Sutherland LR. Biochemical models as early predictors of the etiology of acute pancreatitis. Dig Dis Sci 1993;38:637–643.
81. Pezzilli R, Billi P, Miglioli M, et al. Serum amylase and lipase concentrations and lipase/amylase ratio in assessment of etiology and severity of acute pancreatitis. Dig Dis Sci 1993;38: 1265–1269.
82. King LG, Seelig CB, Ranney JE. The lipase to amylase ratio in acute pancreatitis. Am J Gastroenterol 1995;90:67–69.
83. Gumaste VV. Lipase/amylase ratio: a review. Pancreas 1995;10: 210–212.
84. Seward CW. Diagnosing pancreatitis the first day: a comparison of urinary amylase and serum enzymes in pancreatic dysfunction. South Med J 1970;63:285–289.
85. Waller SL, Ralston AJ. The hourly rate of urinary amylase excretion, serum amylase and serum lipase: part II: patients with gastrointestinal and pancreatic disorders. Gut 1971;12: 884–890.
86. Crist DW, Cameron JL. The current management of acute pancreatitis. Adv Surg 1987;20:69–124.
87. Calleja GA, Barkin JS. Acute pancreatitis. Med Clin North Am 1993;77:1037–1056.
88. Levitt MD, Rapoport M, Cooperband SR. The renal clearance of amylase in renal insufficiency, acute pancreatitis, and macroamylasemia. Ann Intern Med 1969;71:919–925.
89. Warshaw AL, Fuller AF. Specificity of increased renal clearance of amylase in the diagnosis of acute pancreatitis. N Engl J Med 1975;292:325–328.
90. Levitt MD, Gross JB Jr. Postoperative elevation of amylase/creatinine clearance ratio in patients without pancreatitis. Gastroenterology 1979;77:497–499.
91. Levine RI, Glauser FL, Berk JE. Enhancement of the amylase-creatinine clearance ratio in disorders other than acute pancreatitis. N Engl J Med 1975;292:329–332.
92. McMahon MJ, Playforth MJ, Rashid SA, et al. The amylase to creatinine clearance ratio: a non-specific response to acute illness? Br J Surg 1982;69:29–32.
93. Berry AR, Taylor TV, Davies GC. Diagnostic tests and prognostic indicators in acute pancreatitis. J R Coll Surg Edinb 1982;27: 345–352.
94. Steinberg W, Tenner S. Acute pancreatitis. N Engl J Med 1994;330:1198–1210.
95. Le Moine O, Devaster J-M, Deviere J, et al. Trypsin activity: a new marker of acute alcoholic pancreatitis. Dig Dis Sci 1994;39:2634–2638.
96. Geokas MC. The role of elastase in acute pancreatitis. Arch Pathol 1968;86:135–141.
97. Satake K, Chung Y-S, Umeyama K. Serum elastase-1 levels in pancreatic disease. Am J Surg 1982;144:239–242.
98. Pousette A, Fernstad R, Skoldefors H, et al. Novel assay for pancreatic cellular damage: 1. Characterization of protein profiles in human pancreatic cytosol and purification and characterization of a pancreatic specific protein. Pancreas 1988;3:421–426.
99. Yamamoto KK, Pousette A, Chow P, et al. Isolation of a cDNA encoding a human serum marker of acute pancreatitis. Identification of pancreas-specific protein as pancreatic procarboxypeptidase B. J Biol Chem 1992;267:2575–2581.

100. Printz H, Siegmund H, Wojte C, et al. "Human pancreas-specific protein" (procarboxypeptidase B): a valuable marker in pancreatitis? Pancreas 1995;10:222–230.
101. Chen C-C, Wang S-S, Chao Y, et al. Serum pancreas-specific protein in acute pancreatitis: its clinical utility in comparison with serum amylase. Scand J Gastroenterol 1994;29:87–90.
102. Fernstad R, Pousette A, Carlstorm K, et al. A novel assay for pancreatic cellular damage: serum concentrations of pancreas specific protein (PASP) in acute pancreatitis and other abdominal diseases. Pancreas 1990;5:42–49.
103. Silverstein W, Isikoff MB, Hill MC, et al. Diagnostic imaging of acute pancreatitis: prospective study using CT and sonography. AJR 1981;137:497–502.
104. Arger PH, Mulhern CB, Bonavita JA, et al. An analysis of pancreatic sonography in suspected pancreatic disease. J Clin Ultrasound 1979;7:91–97.
105. Levitt RG, Geisse GG, Sagel SS, et al. Complementary use of ultrasound and computed tomography in studies of the pancreas and kidney. Radiology 1978;126:149–152.
106. Fleischer AC, Parker P, Kirschner SG, et al. Sonographic findings of pancreatitis in children. Radiology 1983;146:151–155.
107. Williford ME, Foster WL, Halvorsen RA. Pancreatic pseudocyst: comparative evaluation by sonography and computed tomography. Am J Radiol 1983;140:53–57.
108. Gonzalez AC, Bradley EL, Clements JL Jr. Pseudocyst formation in acute pancreatitis: ultrasonographic evaluation of 99 cases. AJR 1976;127:315–317.
109. Warshaw AL, Gongliang J. Improved survival in 45 patients with pancreatic abscess. Ann Surg 1985;202:408–417.
110. McKay AJ, Imrie CW, O'Neill J, et al. Is an early ultrasound scan of value in acute pancreatitis? Br J Surg 1982;69:369–372.
111. London NJM, Neoptolemos JP, Lavelle J, et al. Serial computed tomography scanning in acute pancreatitis: a prospective study. Gut 1989;30:397–403.
112. Neoptolemos JP, Hall AW, Finlay DF, et al. The urgent diagnosis of gallstones in acute pancreatitis: a prospective study of three methods. Br J Surg 1984;71:230–233.
113. Wang S-S, Lin X-Z, Tsai Y-T, et al. Clinical significance of ultrasonography, computed tomography, and biochemical tests in the rapid diagnosis of gallstone-related pancreatitis: a prospective study. Pancreas 1988;3:153–158.
114. Nordestgaard AG, Wilson SE, Williams RA. Early computed tomography as a predictor of outcome in acute pancreatitis. Am J Surg 1986;152:127–132.
115. Thoeni RF, Gorczyca DP. Non-invasive pancreatic imaging in inflammatory diseases. Semin Gastrointest Dis 1991;2:152–164.
116. Clavien P-A, Hauser H, Meyer P, et al. Value of contrast-enhanced computerized tomography in the early diagnosis and prognosis of acute pancreatitis: a prospective study of 202 patients. Am J Surg 1988;155:457–466.
117. Lankisch PG, Haseloff M, Becher R. No parallel between the biochemical course of acute pancreatitis and morphologic findings. Pancreas 1994;9:240–243.
118. Goodman AJ, Neoptolemos JP, Carr-Locke DL, et al. Detection of gallstones after acute pancreatitis. Gut 1985;26:125–132.
119. Steer ML. The value of CT in acute pancreatitis. Gastroenterology 1986;90:1303–1304.
120. Eriksson J, Doepel M, Widen E, et al. Pancreatic surgery, not pancreatitis, is the primary cause of diabetes after acute fulminant pancreatitis. Gut 1992;33:843–847.
121. Funnell IC, Bornman PC, Weakley SP, Terblanche J, Marks IN. Obesity: an important prognostic factor in acute pancreatitis. Br J Surg 1993;80:484–486.
122. Poston GJ, Williamson RCN. Surgical management of acute pancreatitis. Br J Surg 1990;77:5–12.
123. Horton JW, Burnweit A. Hemodynamic function in acute pancreatitis. Surgery 1988;103:538–546.
124. Knol JA, Inman MG, Strodel WE, Eckhauser FE. Pancreatic response to crystalloid resuscitation in experimental pancreatitis. J Surg Res 1987;43:387–392.
125. Klar E, Mall G, Messmer K, et al. Improvement in impaired pancreatic microcirculation by isovolemic hemodilution protects pancreatic morphology in acute biliary pancreatitis. Surg Gynecol Obstet 1993;174:144–150.
126. Schmidt J, Fernandez-del Castillo C, Rattner DW, et al. Hyperoncotic ultrahigh molecular weight dextran solutions reduce trypsinogen activation, prevent acinar necrosis, and lower mortality in rodent pancreatitis. Am J Surg 1993;165:40–45.
127. Klar E, Herfarth C, Messmer K. Therapeutic effect of isovolemic hemodilution with dextran 60 on the impairment of pancreatic microcirculation in acute biliary pancreatitis. Ann Surg 1990;211:346–353.
128. Klar E, Foitzik T, Buhr H, et al. Isovolemic hemodilution with dextran 60 as treatment of pancreatic ischemia in acute pancreatitis. Ann Surg 1993;217:369–374.
129. Beger HG, Bittner R, Buchler M, Hess W, Schmitz J. Hemodynamic data pattern in patients with acute pancreatitis. Gastroenterology 1986;90:74–79.
130. Bradley EL III, Hall HR, Lutz J, Hamner L, Lattouf O. Hemodynamic consequences of severe pancreatitis. Ann Surg 1983;198:130–133.
131. Cobo JC, Abraham E, Bland RD, Schoemaker WC. Sequential hemodynamic and oxygen transport abnormalities in patients with acute pancreatitis. Surgery 1984;95:324–330.
132. Werner MH, Hayes DF, Lucas C, Rosenberg IK. Renal vasoconstriction in association with acute pancreatitis. Am J Surg 1974;127:185–190.
133. Grömroos JM, Hietaranta AJ, Nevalainen TJ. Renal tubular cell injury and serum phospholipase $A_2$ activity in acute pancreatitis. Br J Surg 1992;79:800–801.
134. Gordon D, Calne RY. Renal failure in acute pancreatitis. Br Med J 1972;3:801–802.
135. Buchler M, Malfertheiner P, Schadlich H, et al. Role of phospholipase $A_2$ in human acute pancreatitis. Gastroenterology 1989;97:1521–1526.
136. Guice K, Oldham KT, Johson KJ, et al. Pancreatitis-induced acute lung injury: an ARDS model. Ann Surg 1988;208:71–77.
137. Berry AR, Taylor TV, Davies GC. Pulmonary function and fibrinogen metabolism in acute pancreatitis. Br J Surg 1981;68:870–873.
138. Balart LS, Ferrante WA. Pathophysiology of acute and chronic pancreatitis. Arch Intern Med 1982;142:113–117.
139. Ranson JHC, Turner JW, Roses DF, et al. Respiratory complications in acute pancreatitis. Ann Surg 1974;179:557–565.
140. Shaw JHF, Wolfe RR. Glucose, fatty acid, and urea kinetics in patients with severe pancreatitis. Ann Surg 1986;204:665–672.
141. Goodgame JT, Fischer JE. Parenteral nutrition in the treatment of acute pancreatitis: effect on complications and mortality. Ann Surg 1977;186:651–658.
142. Sax HC, Warner BW, Talamini MA, et al. Early total parenteral nutrition in acute pancreatitis: lack of beneficial effects. Am J Surg 1987;153:117–124.
143. Sitzmann JV, Steinborn PA, Zinner MJ, Cameron JL. Total parenteral nutrition and alternate energy substrates in treatment of severe acute pancreatitis. Surg Gynecol Obstet 1989;168:311–317.
144. Madry S, Fromm D. Infected retroperitoneal fat necrosis associated with acute pancreatitis. J Am Coll Surg 1994;178:277–282.
145. Scott P, Bruce C, Schofield D, et al. Vitamin C status in patients with acute pancreatitis. Br J Surg 1993;80:750–754.
146. Steer ML, Meldolesi J. The cell biology of experimental pancreatitis. N Engl J Med 1987;316:144–150.
147. Niederau C, Neiderau M, Luthen R, et al. Pancreatic exocrine secretion in acute experimental pancreatitis. Gastroenterology 1990;99:1120–1127.
148. Levant JA, Secrist DM, Resin H, et al. Nasogastric suction in the treatment of alcoholic pancreatitis. JAMA 1974;229:51–52.
149. Naeije R, Salingret E, Clumeck N, DeTroyer A, Devis G. Is nasogastric suction necessary in acute pancreatitis? Br Med J 1978;2:659–660.
150. Sarr MG, Sanfey H, Cameron JL. Prospective randomized trial of nasogastric suction in patients with acute pancreatitis. Surgery 1986;100:500–504.
151. Broe PJ, Zinner MJ, Cameron J. a clinical trial of cimetidine in acute pancreatitis. Surg Gynecol Obstet 1982;154:13–16.
152. Meshkinpour H, Molinari MD, Gardner L, Berk JE, Hoehler FK. Cimetidine in the treatment of acute alcoholic pancreatitis: a randomized, double-blind study. Gastroenterology 1979;77:687–690.
153. Goff JS, Feinberg LE, Brugge WR. A randomized trial comparing

cimetidine to nasogastric suction in acute pancreatitis. Dig Dis Sci 1982;27:1085–1088.
154. Cameron JL, Mehigan D, Zuidema G. Evaluation of atropine in acute pancreatitis. Surg Gynecol Obstet 1979;148:206–208.
155. Gilsanz V, Oteyza CP, Rebollar JL. Glucagon vs anticholinergics in the treatment of pancreatitis. Arch Intern Med 1978;138: 535–538.
156. Durr HK, Maroske D, Zelder O, Bode JCH. glucagon therapy in acute pancreatitis: report of a double-blind trial. Gut 1978;19: 175–179.
157. M.R.C. Multicentre trial of glucagon and aprotinin. Death from acute pancreatitis. Lancet 1977;2:632–635.
158. Olazabal A, Fuller R. Failure of glucagon in the treatment of alcoholic pancreatitis. Gastroenterology 1978;74:489–491.
159. McKay CJ, Imrie CW, Baxter JN. Somatostatin and somatostatin analogues—are they indicated in the management of acute pancreatitis? Gut 1993;34:1622–1626.
160. Raptis SA, Ladas SD. Therapy of acute pancreatitis with somatostatin. Scand J Gastroenterol (Suppl) 1994;207:34–38.
161. Carballo F, Dominguez E, Fernandez-Calvet L, et al. Is somatostatin useful in the treatment of acute pancreatitis? A meta-analysis. Digestion 1991;49:12–13.
162. Paran H, Neufeld D, Mayo A, et al. Preliminary report of a prospective randomized study of octreotide in the treatment of severe acute pancreatitis. Surg Gynecol Obstet 1995;181: 121–124.
163. Goebell H, Ammann R, Herfarth CH, et al. A double-blind trial of synthetic salmon calcitonin in the treatment of acute pancreatitis. Scand J Gastroenterol 1979;14:881–889.
164. Leese T, Holliday M, Heath D, Hall AW, Bell PRF. Multicentre clinical trial of low volume fresh frozen plasma therapy in acute pancreatitis. Br J Surg 1987;74:907–911.
165. Imrie CW, Benjamin IS, Ferguson JC, et al. A single-centre double-blind trial of Trasylol therapy in primary acute pancreatitis. Br J Surg 1978;65:337–341.
166. Trapnell JE, Rigby CC, Talbot CG, Duncan EHL. A controlled trial of Trasylol in the treatment of acute pancreatitis. Br J Surg 1974;61:177–182.
167. Buchler M, Malfertheiner, Uhl W, et al. Gabexate mesilate in human acute pancreatitis. Gastroenterology 1993;104:1165–1170.
168. Valderama R, Perez-Mateo M, Narrro S, et al. Multicenter double-blind trial of gabexate mesylate (FOY) in unselected patients with acute pancreatitis. Digestion 1992;51:65–70.
169. Messori A, Rampazzo R, Scroccaro G, et al. Effectiveness of gabexate mesilate in acute pancreatitis: a meta-analysis. Dig Dis Sci 1995;40:734–738.
170. Buchler M, Malfertheiner P, Freis H, et al. Human pancreatic tissue concentration of bactericidal antibiotics. Gastroenterology 1992;103:1902–1908.
171. Stone HH, Fabian TC. Peritoneal dialysis in the treatment of acute alcoholic pancreatitis. Surg Gynecol Obstet 1980;150: 878–882.
172. Craig RM, Dordal E, Myles L. The use of ampicillin in acute pancreatitis. Ann Intern Med 1975;83:831–832.
173. Howes R, Zuidema GD, Cameron JL. Evaluation of prophylactic antibiotics in acute pancreatitis. J Surg Res 1975;18:197–200.
174. Finch WT, Sawyers JL, Schenker S. A prospective study to determine the efficacy of antibiotics in acute pancreatitis. Ann Surg 1976;183:667–671.
175. Mayer D, McMahon MJ, Cornfield AP, et al. Controlled clinical trial of peritoneal lavage for the treatment of severe acute pancreatitis. N Engl J Med 1985;312:399–404.
176. Carr MR, Dick SP, Brodley J IV, Bertino JS. Gentamicin dosing requirements in patients with acute pancreatitis. Surgery 1988; 103:533–537.
177. Pederzoli P, Bassi C, Vesentini S, Campedelli A. A randomized multicenter clinical trial of antibiotic prophylaxis of septic complications in acute necrotizing pancreatitis with imipenem. Surg Gynecol Obstet 1993;176:480–483.
178. Luiten EJT, Hop WCJ, Lange JF, Bruining HA. Controlled clinical trial of selective decontamination for the treatment of severe acute pancreatitis. Ann Surg 1995;222:57–65.
179. Dubick MA, Mayer D, Majumdar APN, et al. Biochemical studies in peritoneal fluid from patients with acute pancreatitis. Dig Dis Sci 1987;32:305–312.
180. Ranson JHC, Berman RS. Long peritoneal lavage decreases pancreatitis sepsis in acute pancreatitis. Ann Surg 1990;311: 708–716.
181. Coticchia JM, Lessler MA, Carey LC, et al. Peritoneal fluid in human acute pancreatitis blocks hepatic mitochondrial respiration. Surgery 1986;100:850–855.
182. Innes J, Fraser I, Carey LC. The vasoactive properties of ascitic fluid in acute pancreatitis in a porcine model. Arch Surg 1986;121:665–668.
183. Ranson JHC, Spencer FC. The role of peritoneal lavage in severe acute pancreatitis. Ann Surg 1978;187:565–573.
184. Ihse I, Evander A, Holmberg JT, Gustafson I. Influence of peritoneal lavage on objective prognostic signs in acute pancreatitis. Ann Surg 1986;204:122–127.
185. Fernandez-del Castillo C, Rattner DW, Warshaw AL. Acute pancreatitis. Lancet 1993;342:475–479.
186. Ranson JHC, Rikfind KM, Turner JW. Prognostic signs and nonoperative peritoneal lavage in acute pancreatitis. Surg Gynecol Obstet 1976;143:209–219.
187. Lawson DW, Daggett WM, Civetta JM, Corry RJ, Bartlett MK. Surgical treatment of acute necrotizing pancreatitis. Ann Surg 1970;172:605–615.
188. Warshaw AL, Imbembo AL, Civetta JM, Dagget WM. Surgical intervention in acute necrotizing pancreatitis. Am J Surg 1974; 127:484–490.
189. London NJM, Neoptolemos JP, Lavelle J, Bailey I, James D. Contrast-enhanced computed tomography scanning and prediction of severity of acute pancreatitis: a prospective study. Br J Surg 1989;76:268–272.
190. Bradley EL, Murphy F, Ferguson C. Prediction of pancreatic necrosis by dynamic pancreatography. Ann Surg 1989;504: 495–504.
191. London NJM, Leese T, Lavelle JM, et al. Rapid-bolus contrast-enhanced dynamic computed tomography in acute pancreatitis: a prospective study. Br J Surg 1991;78:1452–1456.
192. Foitzik T, Bassi DG, Schmidt J, et al. Intravenous contrast medium accentuates the severity of acute necrotizing pancreatitis in the rat. Gastroenterology 1994;106:207–214.
193. Keiser AM, Grady T, Gerdes D, Saluja M, Steer ML. Intravenous contrast medium does not increase the severity of acute necrotizing pancreatitis in the opossum. Dig Dis Sci 1995;40: 1547–1553.
194. Delhaye M, Engelholm L, Cremer M. Pancreas divisum: congenital anatomic variant an anomaly? Contribution of endoscopic retrograde dorsal pancreatography. Gastroenterology 1985;89: 951–958.
195. Roberston JFR, Imrie CW. Acute pancreatitis associated with carcinoma of the ampulla of Vater. Br J Surg 1987;74:395–397.
196. Lin A, Feller ER. Pancreatic carcinoma as a cause of unexplained pancreatitis: report of ten cases. Ann Intern Med 1990;113:166–167.
197. Ranson JHC. Acute pancreatitis. In: Cameron JL, ed. Current surgical therapy. St. Louis: Mosby-Year Book, 1995:409.
198. Mann DV, Hershman MJ, Hittinger R, Glazer G. Multicentre audit of death from acute pancreatitis. Br J Surg 1994;81: 890–893.
199. Knaus WA, Draper EA, Wagner DP, Zimmerman JE. APACHE II: a severity of disease classification system. Crit Care Med 1985;13: 818–829.
200. Demmy T, Burch JM, Feliciano DV, Mattox KL, Jordan GL Jr. Comparison of multiple-parameter prognostic systems in acute pancreatitis. Am J Surg 1988;156:492–495.
201. Wilson C, Heath DI, Imrie CW. Prediction of outcome in acute pancreatitis: a comparative study of APACHE II, clinical assessment and multiple factor scoring systems. Br J Surg 1990;77:1260–1264.
202. Rabeneck L, Feinstein AR, Horwitz RI, Wells CK. A new clinical prognostic staging system for acute pancreatitis. Am J Med 1993;95:61–70.
203. Mazlam MZ, Hodgson HJF. Why measure C reactive protein? Gut 1994;35:5–7.
204. Mayer AD, McMahon MJ, Bowen M, et al. C reactive protein: an aid to assessment and monitoring of acute pancreatitis. J Clin Pathol 1984;37:207–211.
205. Puolakkainen P, Valtonen V, Paananen A, et al. C-reactive

protein (CRP) and serum phospholipase A2 in the assessment of the severity of acute pancreatitis. Gut 1987;28:764–771.
206. Wilson C, Heads A, Shenkin A, et al. C-reactive protein, antiproteases and complement factors as objective markers of severity in acute pancreatitis. Br J Surg 1989;76:177–181.
207. Paajanen H, Laato M, Jaakkola M, et al. Serum tumour necrosis factor compared with C-reactive protein in the early assessment of severity of acute pancreatitis. Br J Surg 1995;82:271–273.
208. Buchler M. Objectification of the severity of acute pancreatitis. Hepatogastroenterology 1991;38:101–108.
209. Heath DI, Cruickshank A, Gudgeon M, et al. Role of interleukin-6 in mediating the acute phase protein response and potential as an early means of severity assessment in acute pancreatitis. Gut 1993;34:41–45.
210. Leser H-G, Gross V, Scheibenbogen C, et al. Elevation of serum interleukin-6 concentration precedes acute-phase response and reflects severity in acute pancreatitis. Gastroenterology 1991;101:782–785.
211. Viedma JA, Perez-Mateo M, Dominguez JE, et al. Role of interleukin-6 in acute pancreatitis. Comparison with C-reactive protein and phospholipase A. Gut 1992;33:1264–1267.
212. Baggiolini M, Walz A, Kunkel SL. Neutrophil-activating peptide-1/interleukin 8, a novel cytokine that activates neutrophils. J Clin Invest 1989;84:1045–1049.
213. Gross V, Andreesen R, Leser H-G, et al. Interleukin-8 and neutrophil activation in acute pancreatitis. Eur J Clin Invest 1992;22:200–203.
214. Sinha S, Watorek W, Karr S, et al. Primary structure of human neutrophil elastase. Proc Natl Acad Sci USA 1987;84:2228–2232.
215. Sanfey H, Bulkley GB, Cameron JL. The role of oxygen-derived free radicals in the pathogenesis of acute pancreatitis. Ann Surg 1984;200:405–413.
216. Scholmerich J, Schumichen C, Lausen M, et al. Scintigraphic assessment of leukocyte infiltration in acute pancreatitis using technetium-99m-hexamethyl propylene amine oxine as leukocyte label. Dig Dis Sci 1991;36:65–70.
217. Henson PM, Johnston RB Jr. Tissue injury in inflammation: oxidants, proteinases, and cationic proteins. J Clin Invest 1987;79:669–674.
218. Tsuji N, Watanabe N, Okamoto T, et al. Specific interaction of pancreatic elastase and leucocytes to produce oxygen radicals and its implication in pancreatitis. Gut 1994;35:1659–1664.
219. Kusner DJ, King CH. Protease-modulation of neutrophil superoxide response. J Immunol 1989;143:1696–1702.
220. Uhl W, Buchler M, Malfertheiner P, et al. PMN-elastase: a new serum marker for the staging of acute pancreatitis. Digestion 1989;43:176–177.
221. Dominguez-Munoz JE, Carballo F, Garcia MJ, et al. Clinical usefulness of polymorphonuclear elastase in predicting the severity of acute pancreatitis: results of a multicentre study. Br J Surg 1991;78:1230–1234.
222. Gross V, Scholmerich J, Leser H-G, et al. Granulocyte elastase in assessment of severity of acute pancreatitis: comparison with acute-phase proteins C-reactive protein, $\alpha_1$-antitrypsin, and protease inhibitor $\alpha_2$-macroglobulin. Dig Dis Sci 1990;35:97–105.
223. Uhl W, Buchler M, Malfertheiner P, et al. PMN-elastase in comparison with CRP, antiproteases, and LDH as indicators of necrosis in human acute pancreatitis. Pancreas 1991;6:253–259.
224. Viedma JA, Perez-Mateo M, Agullo J, et al. Inflammatory response in the early prediction of severity in human acute pancreatitis. Gut 1994;35:822–827.
225. Nevalainen TJ, Gronroos JM, Kortesuo PT. Pancreatic and synovial type phospholipases A2 in serum samples from patients with severe acute pancreatitis. Gut 1993;34:1133–1136.
226. Schmidt H, Creutzfeldt W. The possible role of phospholipase A in the pathogenesis of acute pancreatitis. Scand J Gastroenterol 1969;4:39–48.
227. Bird NC, Goodman AJ, Johnson AG. Serum phospholipase A2 activity in acute pancreatitis: an early guide to severity. Br J Surg 1989;76:731–732.
228. Schroder T, Kivilaakso E, Kinnunen PKJ, et al. Serum phospholipase A2 in human acute pancreatitis. Scand J Gastroenterol 1980;15:633–636.
229. Funakoshi A, Yamada Y, Migita Y, et al. Simultaneous determinations of pancreatic phospholipase A2 and prophospholipase A2 in various pancreatic diseases. Dig Dis Sci 1993;38:502–506.
230. Uhl W, Buchler M, Nevalainen TJ, et al. Serum phospholipase A2 in patients with multiple injuries. J Trauma 1990;30:1285–1290.
231. Warshaw AL, Lee K-H. Serum ribonuclease elevations and pancreatic necrosis in acute pancreatitis. Surgery 1979;86:227–234.
232. Abramson SB, Rinderknecht H, Renner IG. Ribonuclease C and pancreatic secretory proteins in the peripheral circulation before and after pancreatectomy for pancreatic cancer. Dig Dis Sci 1982;27:889–896.
233. Northam BE, Rowe DS, Winstone NE. Methaemalbumin in the differential diagnosis of acute haemorrhagic and oedematous pancreatitis. Lancet 1963;1:348–352.
234. Battersby C, Green MK. The surgical significance of methaemalbuminaemia. Gut 1971;12:995–1000.
235. Schow PD, Englert E. Methemalbumin and pancreatitis: a warning. Ann Intern Med 1975;82:281–282.
236. Lankisch PG, Schirren CA, Otto J. Methemalbumin in acute pancreatitis: an evaluation of its prognostic value and comparison with multiple prognostic parameters. Am J Gastroenterol 1989;84:1391–1395.
237. McMahon MJ, Playforth MJ, Pickford IR. A comparative study of methods for the prediction of severity of attacks of acute pancreatitis. Br J Surg 1980;67:22–25.
238. Anderson MC, Toronto IR, Needleman SB, et al. Assessment of methemalbumin as a diagnostic test for acute pancreatitis. Arch Surg 1969;98:776–780.
239. Goodhead B. Significance of methemalbuminemia in acute abdominal emergencies. Arch Surg 1970;101:376–378.
240. Lasson A, Ohlsson K. Protease inhibitors in acute human pancreatitis: correlation between biochemical changes and clinical course. Scand J Gastroenterol 1984;19:779–786.
241. McMahon MJ, Bowen M, Mayer AD, et al. Relation of $\alpha_2$-macroglobulin and other antiproteases to the clinical features of acute pancreatitis. Am J Surg 1984;147:164–170.
242. Balthazar EJ, Ranson JHC, Naidich DP, Megibow AJ, Caccavale R, Cooper MM. Acute pancreatitis: prognostic value of CT. Radiology 1985;156:767–772.
243. Vesentini S, Bassi C, Talamini G, et al. Prospective comparison of C-reactive protein level, Ranson score and contrast-enhanced computed tomography in the prediction of septic complications of acute pancreatitis. Br J Surg 1993;80:755–757.
244. Lucarotti ME, Virjee J, Alderson D. Patient selection and timing of dynamic computed tomography in acute pancreatitis. Br J Surg 1993;80:1393–1395.
245. Ranson J HC, Pasternak BS. Statistical methods for quantifying the severity of clinical acute pancreatitis. J Surg Res 1977;22:79–91.
246. Ranson J HC, Balthazar E, Caccavale R, et al. Computed tomography and the prediction of pancreatic abscess in acute pancreatitis. Ann Surg 1985;201:656–665.
247. Renner IG, Savage WT III, Pantoja JL, Renner VJ. Death due to acute pancreatitis. Dig Dis Sci 1985;30:1005–1108.
248. Nardi G. Pancreatitis. N Engl J Med 1963;268:1065–1072.
249. Zieve L. Invited commentary. World J Surg 1980;4:313–314.
250. Guzman S, Nervi F, Llanos O, Leion P, Valdevieso V. Impaired lipid clearance in patients with previous acute pancreatitis. Gut 1985;26:888–891.
251. Howard JM, Reed J. Pseudohyponatremia in acute hyperlipemic pancreatitis: a potential pitfall in therapy. Arch Surg 1985;120:1053–1055.
252. Kabadi UM. Pancreatic ketoacidosis: ketonemia associated with acute pancreatitis. Postgrad Med J 1995;71:32–35.
253. Satake K, Uchima K, Umeyama K, Appert HR, Howard JM. The effects upon blood coagulation in dogs of experimentally induced pancreatitis and the infusion of pancreatic juice. Surg Gynecol Obstet 1981;153:341–345.
254. Kwan HC, Anderson MC, Gramatica L. A study of pancreatic enzymes as a factor in the pathogenesis of disseminated intravascular coagulation during acute pancreatitis. Surgery 1971;69:663–672.
255. Ranson JHC, Lackner H, Berman IR, Schinella R. The relationship of coagulation factors to clinical complications of acute pancreatitis. Surgery 1977;81:502–511.
256. Renner IG, Savage WT III, Stace NH, et al. Pancreatitis associated

with alcoholic liver disease: a review of 1022 autopsy cases. Dig Dis Sci 1984;29:593–599.
257. Friden JH. The significance of jaundice in acute pancreatitis. Arch Surg 1965;90:422–426.
258. Lukash WM. Complications of acute pancreatitis. Arch Surg 1967;94:848–852.
259. Gumaste V, Singh V, Dave P. Significance of pleural effusion in patients with acute pancreatitis. Am J Gastroenterol 1992;87: 871–874.
260. Lankisch PG, Droge M, Becher R. Pleural effusions: a new negative prognostic parameter for acute pancreatitis. Am J Gastroenterol 1994;89:1849–1851.
261. Withrington R, Collins P. Cardiac tamponade in acute pancreatitis. Thorax 1980;35:959–960.
262. Louie S, McGahan JP, Frey C, Cross CE. Pancreatic pleuropericardial effusions: fistulous tracts demonstrated by computed tomography. Arch Intern Med 1985;145:1231–1234.
263. Carey LC. Extra-abdominal manifestations of acute pancreatitis. Surgery 1979;86:337–342.
264. Vogel FS. Cerebral demyelination and focal visceral lesions in cases of acute hemorrhagic pancreatitis with consideration of possible role of circulating enzymes in causation of lesions. Arch Pathol Lab Med 1951;52:355–362.
265. Poole GV Jr, Wallenhaupt SL. Massive rectal bleeding from colonic fistula in pancreatitis. Arch Surg 1984;119:732–735.
266. Haller JD, Pena C, Dragan EL. Massive upper-gastrointestinal hemorrhage due to pancreatitis. Arch Surg 1966;93:567–572.
267. Steckman ML, Dooley MC, Jaques PF, Powell DW. Major gastrointestinal hemorrhage from peripancreatic blood vessel in pancreatitis: treatment by embolotherapy. Dig Dis Sci 1984; 29:486–497.
268. Bloodworth LL, Stevens PE, Bury RF, Arm JP, Rainford DJ. Emphysematous gastritis after acute pancreatitis. Gut 1987;28: 900–902.
269. Collins JJ, Peterson LM, Wilson RE. Small intestinal infarction as a complication of pancreatitis. Ann Surg 1968;167:433–436.
270. Grodsinsky C, Ponk JL. The spectrum of colonic involvement in pancreatitis. Dis Colon Rectum 1978;21:66–70.
271. Waltman AC, Leurs PR, Athanasoulis CA, Warshaw A. Massive arterial hemorrhage in patients with pancreatitis. Arch Surg 1986;121:439–443.
272. Sostre CF, Flournoy JG, Bova JG, et al. Pancreatic phlegmon: clinical features and course. Dig Dis Sci 1985;30:918–927.
273. Fielding GA, McLatchie GR, Wilson C, Imrie CW, Carter DC. Acute pancreatitis and pancreatic fistula formation. Br J Surg 1989;76:1126–1128.
274. Wells AD, McDonnell PJ, Burnand KG. Purtscher's retinopathy in acute pancreatitis. Br J Surg 1990;77:820.
275. Jacob HS, Goldstein IM, Shapiro I, et al. Sudden blindness in acute pancreatitis: possible role of complement-induced retinal leukoembolization. Arch Intern Med 1981;141:134–136.
276. Higgins E, Ive FA. Subcutaneous fat necrosis in pancreatic disease. Br J Surg 1990;77:532–533.
277. Sperling MA. Bone lesions in pancreatitis. Australas Ann Med 1968;17:340–344.
278. Choi TK, Ng WS, Wong J. Surgery during acute pancreatitis. Am J Surg 1987;153:369–373.
279. Semel L, Schrieber D, Fromm D. Gallstone pancreatitis: support for a flexible approach. Arch Surg 1983;118:901–903.
280. Frey CF, Bradley EL III, Beger HG. Progress in acute pancreatitis. Surg Gynecol Obstet 1988;167:282–286.
281. Nordback I, Pessi T, Auvinen O, Autio V. Determination of necrosis in necrotizing pancreatitis. Br J Surg 1985;72:225–227.
282. Gerzof SG, Banks PA, Robbins AH, et al. Early diagnosis of pancreatic infection by computed tomography-guided aspiration. Gastroenterology 1987;93:1315–1320.
283. Bradley EL III, Allen K. A prospective longitudinal study of observation versus surgical intervention in the management of necrotizing pancreatitis. Am J Surg 1991;161:19–24.
284. Karimgani I, Porter KA, Langevin RE, Banks PA. Prognostic factors in sterile pancreatic necrosis. Gastroenterology 1992;103:1636–1640.
285. Rau B, Pralle U, Uhl W, et al. Management of sterile necrosis in instances of severe acute pancreatitis. J Am Coll Surg 1995;181: 279–288.
286. Neoptolemos JP. Endoscopic sphincterotomy in acute gallstone pancreatitis. Br J Surg 1993;80:547–549.
287. Ramin KD, Ramin SM, Richey SD, Cunninham EG. Acute pancreatitis in pregnancy. Am J Obstet Gynecol 1995;173: 187–191.
288. Reynolds JC, Inman RD, Kimberly RP, et al. Acute pancreatitis in systemic lupus erythematosus: report of twenty cases and a review of the literature. Medicine 1982;61:25–32.
289. Cappell MS, Hassan T. Pancreatic disease in patients with the acquired immuno-deficiency syndrome. Pract Gastroenterol 1993;17:18–24.
290. Fromm, D. Complications of gastric surgery. New York: John Wiley & Sons, 1977.
291. Perry T Jr. Post-gastrectomy proximal jejunal loop obstruction simulating acute pancreatitis. Ann Surg 1954;140:119–121.
292. Peterson LM, Collins JJ Jr, Wilson RE. Acute pancreatitis occurring after operation. Surg Gynecol Obstet 1968;127:23–28.
293. Bragg LE, Thompson JS, Burnett DA, Hodgson PE, Rikkers LF. Increased incidence of pancreas-related complications in patients with postoperative pancreatitis. Am J Surg 1985;150: 694–696.

# 22

# *Gallstone-Associated Acute Pancreatitis*

Paul G. Wilson and John P. Neoptolemos

Gallstones are the single most common identifiable cause of acute pancreatitis worldwide, with an overall relative incidence of about 50%. The diagnosis of gallstone-associated acute pancreatitis is made when acute pancreatitis occurs in the presence of gallstones and no other etiologic factor can be identified.

Opie, in 1901, first recognized the association between acute pancreatitis and gallstones (1) when he described a patient who had died of acute pancreatitis and was found to have a gallstone impacted at the ampulla of Vater at postmortem examination. Opie assumed that there was bile reflux into the pancreas (2) which had led to the overwhelming inflammatory reaction observed at necropsy. Despite this initial description, it became apparent over the years that the features described by Opie of an impacted stone at the ampulla of Vater were actually unusual findings in those dying of acute pancreatitis (3–5). During this time, other causes of pancreatitis became recognized (6, 7), and the concept that acute gallstone pancreatitis was a distinct clinical entity developed.

Ideas on the pathogenesis of gallstone pancreatitis evolved further when, in 1974, Acosta and Ledesma proposed that it was the passage of a gallstone through the ampulla of Vater that led to an attack of acute pancreatitis rather than the impaction of a stone (8), a concept that was supported by subsequent studies (9, 10). These observations have stimulated therapeutic trials of both surgery and endoscopic sphincterotomy to remove gallstones from the biliary tree in patients with acute pancreatitis, and because of these trials, treatment of acute gallstone pancreatitis has become much more clearly defined.

## EPIDEMIOLOGY

The true incidence of acute pancreatitis due to gallstones may be difficult to ascertain accurately, as the diagnosis of acute pancreatitis is not always clear-cut, and the methods for detecting gallstones are not always efficient. Nevertheless, it is clear that the incidence of gallstone-associated acute pancreatitis varies with the ethnic, cultural, and geographic background of the patients. Reports from Western countries show a wide variation in the incidence of acute pancreatitis, ranging from 50 to 465 per million population (Table 22.1), and the incidence is probably increasing (11–14). The reasons for this increase are unclear, but it may be due to rising alcohol consumption (14) and a rising prevalence of gallstones (15–17) as well as improved diagnostic techniques. The relative incidence (percentage) of patients with gallstone-induced disease is of the order of 50%, although this varies considerably depending on the type of study and the population investigated (Table 22.2). A study from Italy suggested that the risk from gallstone-associated pancreatitis is directly proportional to the estimated daily alcohol consumption once the consumption exceeds 40 g/day (18). This suggests that moderate alcohol consumption may increase the sensitivity to an attack of acute pancreatitis specifically triggered by gallstones.

There are three main types of gallstones, the most common being cholesterol gallstones, which form in the gallbladder and are most commonly found in the West. Cholesterol stones can be subdivided into pure cholesterol stones, which are usually solitary, and mixed stones, which contain a mixture of cholesterol, calcium, and nonpolymerized bile pigment. Black-pigment stones are formed in the gallbladder and are more common with hemolytic disorders, cirrhosis, chronic bile duct obstruction, and malaria. The black-pigment stones are made of tightly packed polymerized bilirubinate crystals. The third type is the brown-pigment stone, which tends to form in the main bile ducts. These stones form secondary to infection and stasis or in the presence of retained foreign bodies such as suture material and biliary stents. They are composed of loosely packed calcium bilirubinate crystals and biliary sludge; primary brown-pigment stones are particularly prevalent in the Far East.

Cholesterol gallstones occur more commonly in women, but the incidence increases in both men and women with advancing age (19). In addition, obesity, certain drugs (e.g., clofibrate), and gastrointestinal diseases such as Crohn's disease are associated with a higher incidence of gallstones than is found in the general population. Any condition predisposing to black-pigment gallstones, such as hemolysis, also puts individuals at greater risk of acute pancreatitis, and this has been observed in children and teenagers (20). Although gallstones are much commoner in females, the relative proportion of men with symptomatic gallstones who suffer an attack of acute pancreatitis is higher (21). Taylor et al. found that of 664 patients with gallstones, 490 (74%) were women, of whom 27 (5.5%) suffered an attack of acute pancreatitis, compared with 25 (14.4%) of 174 men. Following treatment of gallbladder stones by extracorporeal shock-wave lithotripsy (ESWL), the incidence of an attack of acute pancreatitis, which is probably due to the smaller stone fragments passing more easily down the biliary tree, is about 1.4% (22). This represents the true potential risk for developing acute pancreatitis from gallstones and should equal the proportion of patients with a common channel if Opie's concepts are correct.

Increasing age is a factor in the incidence of acute pancreatitis. In the older patient, the common bile duct is of a greater diameter (23, 24) and is more likely therefore to allow the passage of gallstones and a subsequent attack of acute pancreatitis. Patients with an attack of gallstone pancreatitis have a relatively larger main bile duct (MBD) and main pancreatic duct (MPD) than those who have other causes for their pancreatitis (25). Of 94 patients with an attack of gallstone-associated acute pancreatitis, the mean diameter of the MBD was 9.2 mm, compared with a mean of 5.0 mm in 26 patients who had other causes of their acute pancreatitis. As patients get older, the proportion of men with gallstones increases, so that the ratio in some populations is close to 1 : 1 in those over the age of 60 (26, 27). This may explain

**TABLE 22.1. Incidence of Acute Pancreatitis (cases per $10^6$ population) Reported by Different Authors**

| Author | Number of Cases | Country/Area | Period | Incidence per $10^6$ Population |
|---|---|---|---|---|
| O'Sullivan et al. | 116 | USA/Rochester | 1940–1969 | 110 |
| Trapnell and Duncan | 590 | England/Bristol | 1961–1967 | 54 |
| Corfield et al. | 737 | England/Bristol | 1968–1979 | 73 |
| Bourke et al. | 214 | England/Nottingham | 1969–1974 | 47 |
| McMahon | 35 | England/Leeds | 1976 | 110 |
| Neoptolemos[a] | 600 | England/Birmingham | 1987–1992 | 350 |
| Thomson | 632 | Scotland/North-East | 1972–1979 | 94 |
| Thomson et al. | 378 | Scotland/North-East | 1983–1985 | 242 |
| CPSG[b] | 343 | Denmark/Copenhagen | 1978–1979 | 281 |
| Gatell et al. | NA | Spain/Barcelona | 1975–1977 | 50 |
| Grilo et al. | NA | Spain/Cordoba | 1983–1986 | 385 |
| Carballo[b] | NA | Spain/Guadalajara | 1989 | 465 |

[a]Unpublished data.
[b]Prospective studies.

**TABLE 22.2. Relative Incidence of Gallstone-Associated Acute Pancreatitis**

| Author/Country | Year | Number of Patients: Acute Pancreatitis | Number of Patients: Gallstones (%) |
|---|---|---|---|
| USA | | | |
| Enquist and Gleidman | 1958 | 85[a] | 31 (36) |
| Berman et al. | 1961 | 644 | 357[b] (55) |
| Howard & Ehrlich | 1962 | 454 | 251 (55) |
| Weissberg et al. | 1972 | 139 | 47 (34) |
| Kelly | 1974 | 100 | 52 (52) |
| Kelly | 1976 | 125 | 56 (45) |
| Kelly | 1980 | 275 | 172 (63) |
| Acosta et al. | 1980 | 78 | 59 (76) |
| Great Britain | | | |
| Efron | 1966 | 204 | 40 (20) |
| Gillespie | 1973 | 93 | 32 (34) |
| Trapnell and Duncan | 1975 | 590 | 316 (54) |
| Bourke | 1975 | 202 | 94 (47) |
| Imrie and Whyte | 1975 | 78 | 40 (51) |
| Imrie et al. | 1978 | 161 | 84 (52) |
| Winslet et al. | 1992 | 417 | 258 (62) |
| Sweden | | | |
| Edlund et al. | 1968 | 460 | 342[c] (74) |
| Storck et al. | 1976 | 116[a] | 50 (43) |
| Svensson et al. | 1979 | | |
| | 1956–1960 | 454[d] | 309 (68) |
| | 1968–1969 | 105[d] | 21 (20) |
| | 1974–1975 | 204[d] | 54 (26) |
| South Africa | | | |
| Kessler and Mieny | 1975 | 71 | 17 (24) |
| Australia | | | |
| Battersby and Chapuis | 1977 | 100 | 43 (43) |
| Reid and Kune | 1980 | 113 | 30 (27) |
| Israel | | | |
| Sharon et al. | 1979 | 130 | 90 (69) |
| Switzerland | | | |
| Tondelli et al. | 1982 | 523 | 114 (22) |
| Italy | | | |
| Pezzilli et al. | 1993 | 66 | 42 (63) |
| Pederzoli et al. | 1995 | 182 | 102 (56) |
| Germany | | | |
| Lankisch et al. | 1995 | 1613 | 635 (39) |
| Total | | 7782 | 3738 (48) |

[a]All cases autopsied.
[b]Includes 14 patients with acute noncalculous cholecystitis.
[c]Includes 32 patients with a prior cholecystectomy.
[d]Limited to patients with their first recognizable attack of acute pancreatitis.

**TABLE 22.3. Causes of Biliary Acute Pancreatitis**

| | |
|---|---|
| Gallstones | Choledochocele |
| Cholesterolosis | Choledochal cyst |
| Sludge (?) | Periampullary diverticulum |
| Complications of ERCP and ES[a] | Intraluminal diverticulum |
| ESWL[b] for gallstones | AUPBD[c] |
| Biliary tract surgery | Parasitic infestation |
| Ampullary tumors | Sclerosing cholangitis |
| Cholangiocarcinoma | Sphincter of Oddi dysfunction |
| Microlithiasis/biliary crystals | Pancreas divisum (?) |

[a]ERCP, endoscopic retrograde cholangiopancreatography; ES, endoscopic sphincterotomy.
[b]ESWL, extracorporeal shock-wave lithotripsy.
[c]AUPBD, anomalous union of the pancreatic and biliary ducts.

why the sex difference in the incidence of gallstone-associated acute pancreatitis disappears in older age groups (28).

## PATHOGENESIS

Although gallstone-associated acute pancreatitis is a distinct disease necessitating a specific management regimen, many of the clinical and biochemical features of gallstone-induced disease can be mimicked by other, less common, biliary tract diseases. These include parasitic infections, anatomic abnormalities, tumors, and instrumentation of the biliary tract (Table 22.3).

### Gallstones, Microlithiasis, and Cholesterolosis

Acute pancreatitis affects between 3 and 8% of all patients with symptomatic gallstones (29, 30), although this may increase to as high as 20–30% in those with microlithiasis (defined as stones less than 3 mm in diameter) (31, 32). In addition to gallstones and microlithiasis, cholesterolosis may also be a risk factor for the development of acute pancreatitis. In 1990 it was reported that 434 (11%) gallbladders removed from patients by cholecystectomy had cholesterolosis, and acute pancreatitis was clearly documented in 125 (29%) cases (33). Acute pancreatitis had been diagnosed in 26% of patients with cholesterolosis and gallstones, compared with 49% of 55 patients with cholesterolosis and no gallstones. The precise cause of acute pancreatitis in these patients is unclear. The authors (33) suggested that the responsible mechanism involved the shedding of small cholesterol polyps from the gallbladder followed by shedding into the biliary tree, but it is probably more likely that the concomitant presence of microlithiasis is responsible.

### Biliary Sludge and Crystals

Biliary sludge consists of bile supersaturated with cholesterol, cholesterol monohydrate crystals, mucin, glycoprotein, calcium bilirubinate crystals, cell debris, and proteinaceous material (34) and is a risk factor for the development of gallstones (35). Ultrasound (US) can detect sludge in the gallbladder and is associated with any condition that reduces contractility of the gallbladder.

The presence of cholesterol crystals on microscopy of bile indicates that the bile is capable of forming gallstones within the biliary tree (Fig. 22.1). The discovery of cholesterol crystals in the gallbladder, bile duct, or duodenal bile permits the diagnosis of "gallstone"-associated acute pancreatitis in those patients who were previously labeled "idiopathic" because of normal radiology and the absence of any other known causative factor (36). A cholecystectomy specimen from these patients frequently demonstrates microlithiasis in association with chronic inflammation.

From the data presently available, however, it is unclear if biliary sludge without cholesterol crystals or calcium bilirubinate granules on biliary microscopy is a risk factor for the development of acute pancreatitis or not. In a study in 1991 by Ros et al. (37), 50 patients of a total of 51 patients who were labeled as having "idiopathic" acute pancreatitis had microscopic bile abnormalities and/or gallstones on follow-up by US. In 1992, a further study (38) of 31 patients with acute pancreatitis found that 23 patients had sludge on US and/or abnormal bile microscopy, although 2 of these patients were excluded from the analysis on the grounds of MBD obstruction. Of the 21 remaining patients, 11 were found to have sludge on US, and of these, 10 had calcium bilirubinate crystals on bile microscopy. The authors unfortunately did not quantify the calcium bilirubinate crystals, which is important, as healthy individuals can also have bilirubinate crystals in their bile (39). The 10 patients who did not have sludge on US had bile crystals on microscopy. Moreover, 3 of 14 patients with alcohol-induced acute pancreatitis had sludge detected on US but not abnormalities of bile on microscopy. Thus, one interpretation of the findings is that sludge formation is secondary to the attack of acute pancreatitis rather than a cause and may have been present because of the coexistent ileus and reduced gallbladder contractility. Until more data are available, patients with sludge alone on US should not be

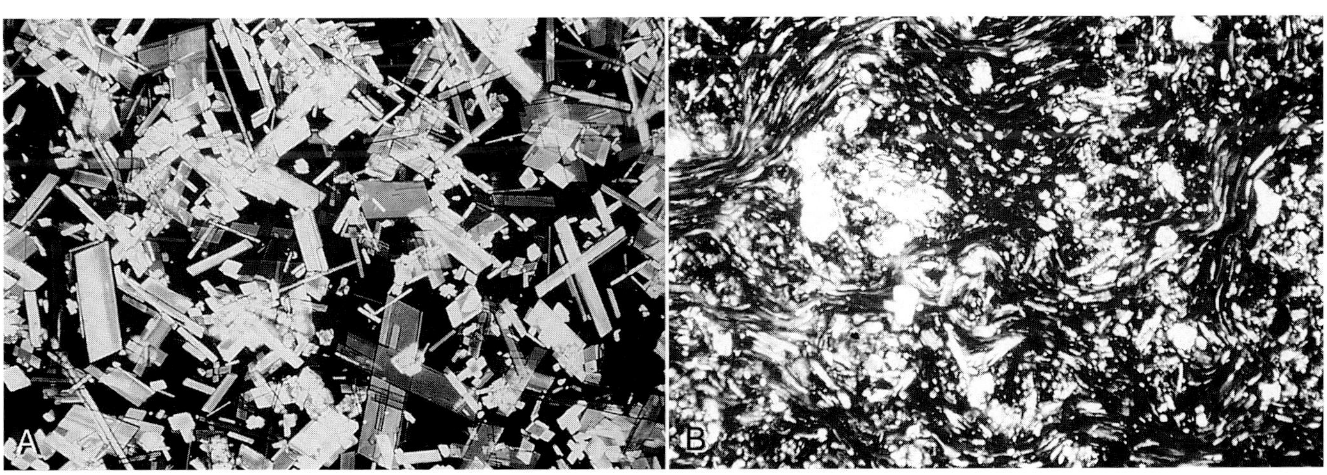


**FIG. 22.1.** **A.** Cholesterol crystals seen under polarizing microscopy following duodenal bile collection. **B.** Calcium bilirubinate granules seen amid biliary sludge. See color insert.

regarded as having gallstone-associated or biliary acute pancreatitis. Instead, they warrant the detailed investigations of any patient in whom the cause of acute pancreatitis has not been resolved by initial assessment.

## Migration of Stones

In 1974, Acosta and Ledesma showed a relationship between the migration of gallstones down the biliary tree and attacks of acute pancreatitis (8). They studied 36 patients with gallstone-associated acute pancreatitis and compared them with 36 patients with preceding attacks of acute pancreatitis, but in the control group only 3 (8%) patients were found to have gallstones in their feces. These findings have since been confirmed by other studies (9, 10). How the passage of a gallstone precipitates an attack of pancreatitis continues to be the subject of some debate. Presently, the weight of evidence is in favor of Opie's early theory of the common channel with bile reflux (Table 22.4).

## The Common Channel

The theory of the common channel has been criticized by some as too simplistic, particularly as ampullary obstruction is found in less than 5% of patients with acute pancreatitis (40), and furthermore, the union of the MPD and MBD is too short in most patients to allow the common channel situation to arise (41). There are, however, certain anatomic features that are more frequently associated with the development of gallstone-induced acute pancreatitis. Armstrong and Taylor (42) studied 614 consecutive patients undergoing cholecystectomy and operative cholangiography for biliary stones (Fig. 22.2). Some 53 of the patients had had a previous attack of gallstone-associated acute pancreatitis; the other 561 patients without acute pancreatitis were termed controls. Pancreatic duct reflux was noted on the cholangiograms of 115 patients (18.7%). Of the 53 patients with a previous history of acute pancreatitis, 33 (62.3%) had pancreatic duct reflux on their operative cholangiograms, compared with 82 (14.6%) of the 561 controls ($p < .0001$). In addition, in the acute pancreatitis group, the mean (±SD) diameter of the pancreatic duct was greater (4.9 ± 1.0 mm vs. 2.6 ± 1.3 mm; $p < .001$), the mean (±SD) angle of reflux was greater (40 ± 12° vs. 21 ± 15°; $p < .02$), and the common channel was longer (median length [range], 8 [4–16] mm vs. 4 [2–44] mm). Not all patients with gallstones develop acute pancreatitis as a consequence, but it is apparent that there are important anatomic variations that permit development of gallstone-associated acute pancreatitis.

**TABLE 22.4. Factors Linking Gallstone-Associated Acute Pancreatitis to the Presence of Biliary-Pancreatic Reflux**

- Necessary factors
  - Passage of gallstones
  - Presence of gallstones
  - Ampullary obstruction
- Predisposing factors
  - Multiple gallstones
  - Smaller gallstones
  - Cholesterolosis
  - Biliary sludge
  - Microlithiasis
  - Larger-diameter cystic duct
  - Larger-diameter main pancreatic duct
  - Greater pancreaticobiliary angle
  - Anatomic pancreaticobiliary channel
  - Functional pancreaticobiliary channel
- Associated factors
  - Dilated main bile duct
  - Dilated main pancreatic duct
  - Increased incidence of radiographic biliary-pancreatic reflux
  - Increased incidence of infected bile
  - Early pancreatic duct changes
  - Early ampullary changes
  - Periductular acinar necrosis
  - Pancreatic necrosis >36 hours after onset of attack
  - Higher incidence of bile duct stones in severe attacks
  - Higher incidence of acute cholangitis in severe pancreatitis
  - Decreased patency of the duct of Santorini
  - Serum amylase remains elevated longer with severe attacks
  - Sphincter of Oddi dysfunction
  - Experimental pancreatic duct obstruction increases severity
  - Bile-induced experimental acute edematous pancreatitis
  - Gallbladder bile bacteria colonize the pancreas in experimental pancreatitis

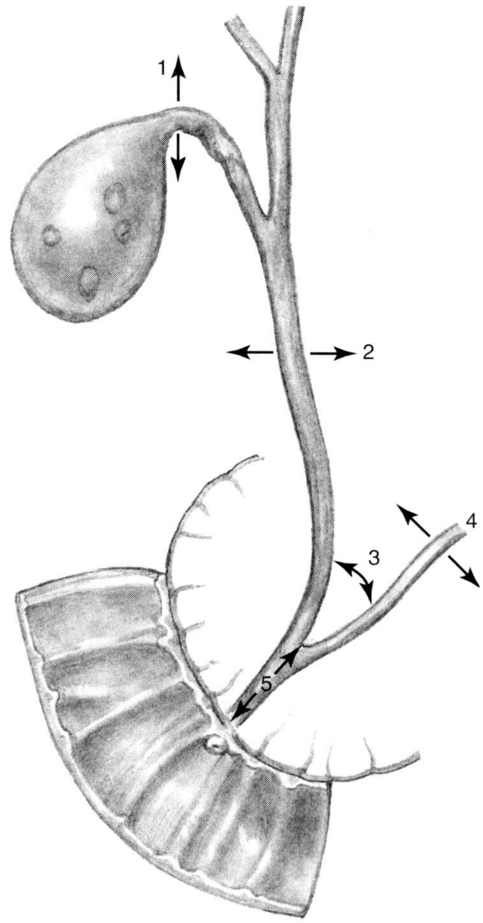


**FIG. 22.2.** Measurements of the biliary tract taken from the intraoperative cholangiogram. *1,* Diameter of the cystic duct; *2,* diameter of the common bile duct; *3,* angle of reflux; *4,* diameter of the pancreatic duct; *5,* length of the common channel.

Despite criticism of the common channel theory, two studies have demonstrated that a functional common channel can arise in patients who have suffered an attack of gallstone-associated acute pancreatitis, (43–44). The larger of the two studies (43) investigated 21 patients who had undergone open cholecystectomy and common bile duct exploration. All patients had a T tube in situ following their surgery, and they were divided into three groups: *(a)* those with gallbladder stones alone; *(b)* those with gallbladder stones and MBD stones; *(c)* those with gallbladder stones and a recent attack of gallstone-associated pancreatitis. Patients were given a standard meal, and the bile from the T tube was collected and analyzed for the presence of pancreatic enzymes. In those with a recent attack of gallstone-induced acute pancreatitis, the resting and stimulated amylase activity was up to 100 times greater than in the other two groups of patients. Moreover, none of the three groups of patients had any detectable duodenal enzymes in the T-tube fluid, which significantly undermines the duodenal reflux theory as a cause of acute pancreatitis (45).

In the normal situation, the pressure in the MBD is exceeded by that of the MPD (46), suggesting that if there were a common channel that pancreatic juice would flow into the biliary tree. However, pressures within the biliary tree are known to be higher when the MBD is obstructed, as in obstructive acute cholangitis (47). Thus under certain pathologic conditions, bile from the biliary tree may be forced into the MPD. Furthermore, contraction of the gallbladder against an obstructed papilla would raise the pressures in the MBD above that in the MPD, if only for a short time. To lend further weight to this argument, patients who have had gallstone-associated acute pancreatitis have biliopancreatic reflux more commonly demonstrated by operative cholangiography (29).

Does bile in the MPD lead to acute pancreatitis? Evidence is a little conflicting, and the bulk of information is from animal models. Infusion of large volumes of taurocholic acid into the pancreatic duct leads to a fatal form of hemorrhagic pancreatitis (48). It is unlikely, however, that this experimental model mirrors the situation in the human disease; in the model, there is retrograde injection of volumes that exceed those that might occur with bile reflux, and ductal pressures greatly exceed those that could normally be generated (49). Perfusion of the pancreatic duct with bile under physiologic pressure does not lead to damage of the pancreatic duct or to acute pancreatitis in the dog (50). In the rat, however, the presence of bile in the MPD under physiologic pressure and without causing physical disruption of pancreatic acini leads to edematous pancreatitis with recruitment of neutrophils into the pancreatic parenchyma (51). Indeed, low concentrations of certain bile salts can increase the autocatalytic activity of trypsinogen to over 50 times the normal rate (52). Thus, the reflux of bile into the MPD could activate trypsinogen locally and saturate the capacity of the pancreatic trypsin inhibitors. Although trypsin has never been shown to be directly cytotoxic to pancreatic acinar cells in vivo, it may cause its destructive effects by activating prophospholipase $A_2$ (52), which is capable of generating various lipid inflammatory mediators.

Some workers have suggested that bacteria within bile are required to induce severe acute pancreatitis and that under physiologic pressure, bile alone will not precipitate a severe attack (53). In male Sprague-Dawley rats, infusion of sterile bile into the pancreatic duct caused a mild pancreatitis similar to that observed by Arendt and Broschewitz (51). Infusion of bile infected with *Escherichia coli*, however, produced acute hemorrhagic pancreatitis with large quantities of peritoneal fluid and fat necrosis in 19 of 30 animals. The presence of gallstones in the biliary tree is associated with a high incidence of bile-induced bacteremia (54) in patients, and bacteria may be an essential factor in the progression of disease from mild to severe. Bacteria-specific enzymes (amidases) present in infected bile can damage cell-membrane phospholipids (55), with the resultant formation of lysolecithin. Lysolecithin is cytotoxic to pancreatic acinar cells and can induce fat necrosis when injected into the peritoneal cavity (56).

### Pancreatic Ductal Obstruction

In certain animal models, pancreatic ductal obstruction without bile reflux can lead to acute pancreatitis (57–59). Steer's group (57), using the American opossum, which has a long common channel, carried out a comparative evaluation of the severity of pancreatitis occurring after ligation of the MPD alone, the MPD and MBD separately (preventing the reflux of bile into the pancreatic duct), and the common biliopancreatic duct. They found similarly severe acute hemorrhagic pancreatitis in all three groups of animals and concluded that the MPD obstruction was the critical event. However, these observations conflict with earlier studies (60–62) in the same animal model that demonstrated that combined MPD and MBD obstruction, irrespective of the presence of a common channel, led to the most severe attack of pancreatitis. Moody's group noted that up to a third of all the animals had salmonella prior to induction of pancreatitis (62) and that infectious complications occurred in up to 61% of all their animals (61). In contrast, Steer's group did not observe any bacterial infections in their animals (57), and it may be that infection exacerbates pancreatitis in animals with obstructive jaundice.

Repeated short-term obstruction of the pancreatic duct in rats leads to a more severe form of pancreatitis than if the duct is obstructed in a single episode (63). In this study, the pancreaticobiliary duct was ligated with a metal clip. In the first group, the clip was released after 2 hours for a period of 1 hour, then reapplied for a further 2 hours. In the second group of animals, the clip was left on continuously for 4 hours. The animals with the single episode of obstruction had a less severe form of pancreatitis. Steer's group also showed that the more prolonged the pancreatic duct obstruction, the more severe the attack of hemorrhagic pancreatitis (64). They used a balloon catheter introduced into the pancreatic duct of the animal and inflated it to induce pancreatitis. The attacks of pancreatitis could be arrested and their severity reduced by deflation of the balloon.

Despite these observations in animal models, obstruction of the pancreatic duct alone in humans rarely leads to acute pancreatitis. Tumors in the head of the pancreas that obstruct the pancreatic duct tend to cause distal atrophy of the pancreas rather than acute pancreatitis, although a tumor of the ampulla of Vater may present as acute pancreatitis in about 6% of cases (65). In humans, an ampullary tumor can potentially give rise to a common channel, which suggests that there are factors more important than pancreatic ductal obstruction that lead to acute pancreatitis in humans. A tumor rarely obstructs the pancreatic duct precipitously, unlike a stone, and the rate at which the duct is obstructed may also be of importance.

The early use of endoscopic retrograde cholangiopancreatography (ERCP) during an attack of acute pancreatitis allows accurate measurement of the MBD and MPD (25). In 94 patients with gallstone-associated acute pancreatitis, the mean (SD) diameter of the MBD was 9.2 (4.5) mm, and the mean (SD) MPD diameter was 3.63 (1.21) mm. In 26 patients with non-gallstone-induced acute pancreatitis, these measurements were 5.0 (1.9) mm and 3.10 (1.57) mm, respectively. Moreover, patients with "persisting" bile duct stones had a larger-diameter MBD (12.5 [49] mm) and MPD (4.02 [1.43]) than those with gallbladder stones only (7.1 [2.7] mm and 3.45 [1.06] mm, respectively). Similar findings were reported in a study by Oria et al. (66) using US examination of the MPD and MBD in gallstone-associated acute pancreatitis. When confounding factors such as age, the presence of gallbladder stones, and the presence of bile duct stone are taken into account, the diameters of the MPD and MBD are still greater in those with gallstone-associated acute pancreatitis.

Histologic examination of the liver in 26 patients with gallstone-associated acute pancreatitis showed evidence of acute cholangitis in 65% and some degree of hepatocyte necrosis in 96% of cases (67). Electron microscopy revealed a disorganized liver plate, inspissated bile in dilated canaliculi, and shedding of cellular cytoplasm into the space of Disse. These pathologic findings probably account for the transient increases in serum transaminase levels that occur within 48 hours of an attack of acute biliary pancreatitis and subside once the temporary obstruction of the ampulla is relieved as a small calculus is passed (68). The serum bilirubin, in contrast, reflects the degree of "persisting" bile duct obstruction due to the continued presence of bile duct stones (68).

The serum amylase level falls rapidly in most patients with acute pancreatitis and returns to normal within about 5 days. The exception is the patient with severe gallstone-induced acute pancreatitis, in whom the amylase level remains elevated after an initial decline (40). This probably represents continuing obstruction of the MPD by persisting gallstones. It has been suggested that if the duct of Santorini is patent and communicates with the duct of Wirsung, then an alternative route of pancreatic decompression is available so that the attack of gallstone-associated acute pancreatitis is less severe (69).

From these data, the most reasonable conclusion is that there is a degree of obstruction of both the main bile and pancreatic ducts, and despite the experimental evidence that acute pancreatitis can be induced in animals by MPD obstruction alone, human gallstone-associated acute pancreatitis appears to require partial obstruction of both systems.

### Cellular Events

It has been reported that the lysosomal enzyme cathepsin B can activate trypsinogen in animals (70), and more recently, human cathepsin B has been reported to be able to activate human trypsinogen in acidic conditions (71). Lysosomal enzymes are synthesized along with digestive enzymes in the rough endoplasmic reticulum, and both proteins are transported together to the Golgi area of the acinar cell; from there, protein trafficking segregates lysosomal from digestive enzymes (72). It has been suggested that errors in protein trafficking may occur early on in acute pancreatitis (73), resulting in colocalization of cathepsin B with trypsinogen, thus leading to intracellular activation of digestive enzymes (59). However, other evidence suggests that colocalization is purely an epiphenomenon occurring as a result of the pancreatitis (74). In addition, the potent cathepsin B inhibitor E-64 has no protective effect against diet-induced or secretagogue-induced pancreatitis (75), which implies that cathepsin B is of little importance in these models of acute pancreatitis.

Once the digestive zymogens have been packaged into condensing vacuoles, they mature into zymogen granules during migration toward the luminal surface. The limiting membrane of the zymogen granule fuses with the cell membrane, thus discharging its contents into the ductal space (exocytosis) (76). The zymogen granule membrane is rapidly recycled from the cell surface via vesicles to the Golgi apparatus (endocytosis) (77). Lerch et al. (78) showed that in the opossum, luminal endocytosis continues in the presence of pancreatic ductal obstruction. If trypsinogen has been activated by refluxing bile, as in gallstone-associated acute pancreatitis, continued endocytosis would result in reinternalization of activated digestive enzymes from the lumen and might initiate the process of autodigestion.

### Two-Phase Hypothesis of Gallstone-Induced Acute Pancreatitis

The passage of gallstones is a universal event in patients developing gallstone-associated acute pancreatitis, though this does not explain why the severity of an attack varies between patients. A two-phase hypothesis has been proposed to explain the different aspects of gallstone-associated acute pancreatitis (79), which can explain why some patients may develop a severe attack. In the first phase, passage of a gallstone precipitates an attack of acute pancreatitis in the minority of individuals with the necessary pancreaticobiliary anatomy that predisposes them to biliary-pancreatic reflux. Once the stone has migrated through the ampulla of Vater, there is free drainage of pancreatic juice from the MPD, allowing the release of activated enzymes and limiting the damage to the gland. This is the most common situation, leading to an attack of mild acute pancreatitis (Fig. 22.3).

A further episode of obstruction that leads to retention of pancreatic enzymes that have already been activated will result in more extensive pancreatitis and may account for damage to the larger peripheral ducts as well as the main pancreatic duct. The obstruction may occur for a number of reasons: *(a)* edema of the pancreatic head or ampulla of Vater following the passage of a gallstone; *(b)* repeated passage of small stones through the ampulla, giving rise to transient obstruction on each occasion; *(c)* a large stone in the distal MBD compressing the MPD as these ducts run parallel to each other—this may even occur repeatedly with impact and disimpaction of the stone without its passage through the ampulla; or *(d)* impaction of a large stone in the ampulla of Vater itself, although the frequency of this event is only 5%. These are the situations that would more typically progress to a severe attack, with more episodes of obstruction giving rise to the worst attacks. The time between the two phases may be minutes, hours, or days. The inference from this hypothesis is that for some patients, there is a window of opportunity to alter the natural history of the disease by preventing or relieving the MPD obstruction.

## DIAGNOSIS

Three elements are essential for the diagnosis of acute pancreatitis secondary to gallstones to be made: *(a)* a diagnosis of acute pancreatitis is required, *(b)* gallstones must be detected, and *(c)* other etiologic factors must be excluded.

### Diagnosis of Acute Pancreatitis

The diagnosis of acute pancreatitis presently depends upon the presence of a compatible clinical picture with an amylase (or lipase) level 3–4 times the upper limit of normal (ULN). Commonly, a serum amylase level above 1000 IU/L (given an ULN of 300 IU/L) is taken as the diagnostic cutoff point if the sample is taken within 48 hours of the onset of the attack (40). The pain of pancreatitis is initially located in the epigastric region and is of sudden onset. The pain may spread to the whole abdomen and have associated signs of peritonism. Nausea and vomiting are frequent features, with an associated anorexia. In addition, there is usually a tachycardia and mild pyrexia. In severe cases, there may be oliguria, respiratory distress, mental obtundation, and cardiovascular collapse. The level of serum amylase reflects the degree of pancreatic inflammation, the presence of any outflow obstruction of the pancreatic duct, and to a variable degree its clearance from the systemic circulation. A serum amylase level above 1000 IU/L (given an ULN of 300 IU/L) carries a diagnostic sensitivity in excess of 98%, provided it is measured within 24 hours of the onset of symptoms (40). The serum amylase level then falls steadily and is usually in the normal range by 5–7 days. The serum amylase level tends to remain elevated longer in severe cases of acute pancreatitis associated with gallstones (but not alcohol), although occasionally in cases with extensive pancreatic necrosis, the serum amylase values may be unusually low (40).

The specificity of the diagnostic amylase level is also in excess of 98%, although this varies to some extent with the referral pattern of the receiving hospital. Common conditions that may be difficult to distinguish from acute pancreatitis include upper gastrointestinal perforation in which leaking pancreatic and salivary amylases are absorbed directly from the peritoneal cavity; mesenteric infarction, which also allows amylase to leak into the peritoneal cavity, and various causes of retroperitoneal hemorrhage. An erect chest X-ray is thus mandatory to exclude

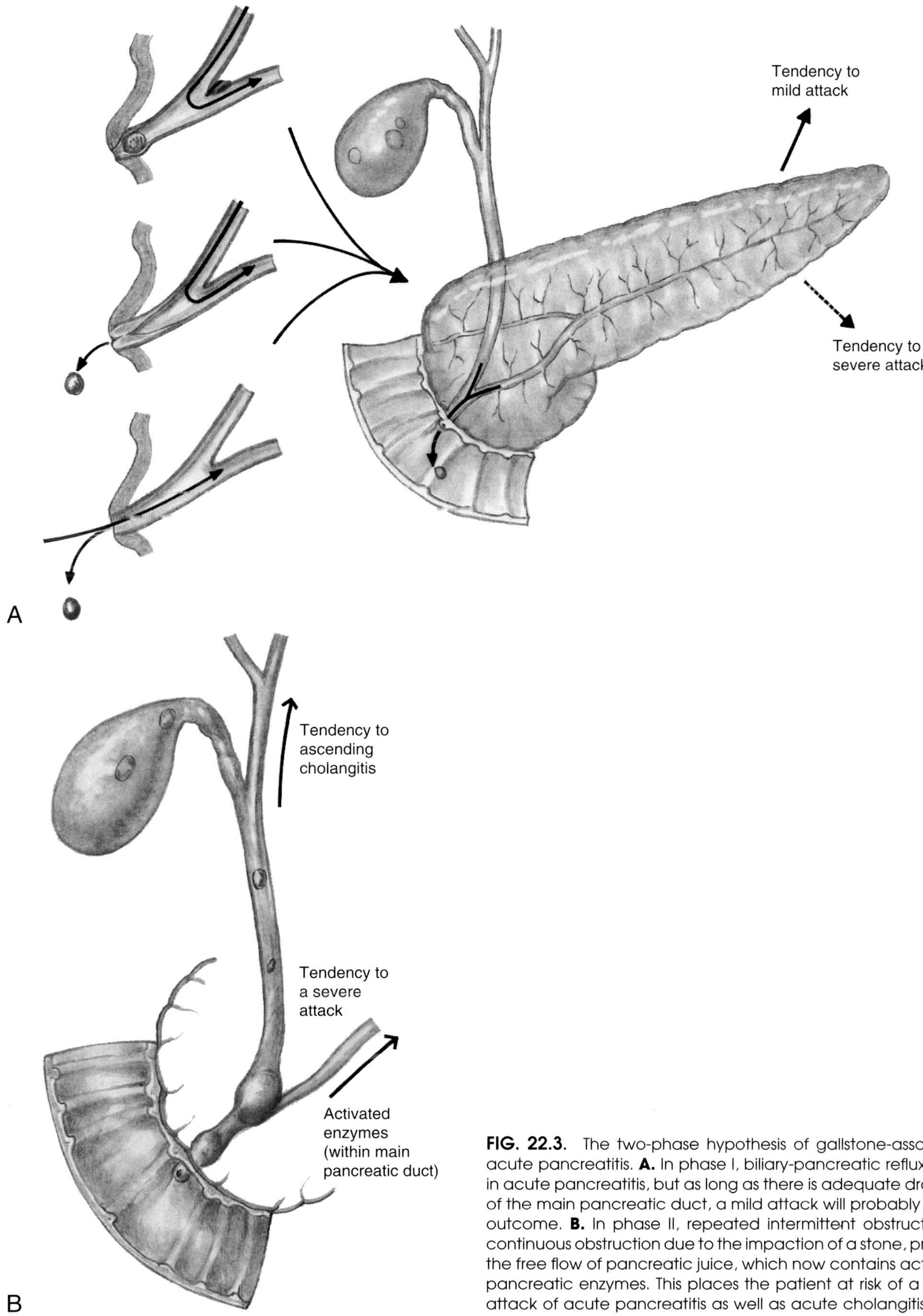


**FIG. 22.3.** The two-phase hypothesis of gallstone-associated acute pancreatitis. **A.** In phase I, biliary-pancreatic reflux results in acute pancreatitis, but as long as there is adequate drainage of the main pancreatic duct, a mild attack will probably be the outcome. **B.** In phase II, repeated intermittent obstruction, or continuous obstruction due to the impaction of a stone, prevents the free flow of pancreatic juice, which now contains activated pancreatic enzymes. This places the patient at risk of a severe attack of acute pancreatitis as well as acute cholangitis.

perforation of a viscus by detection of free gas, and any doubt about the diagnosis must be resolved by an emergency contrast-enhanced computed tomography (CE-CT) scan. This has a sensitivity of at least 90% and a specificity of nearly 100% in detecting acute pancreatitis (80).

The serum lipase level tends to remain elevated slightly longer than the amylase level but is more of an issue in alcoholic rather than in gallstone-associated acute pancreatitis (81). A urinary amylase level above 3000 IU/L is sometimes of use in diagnosing acute pancreatitis if the serum amylase level is above the normal range but less than 1000 IU/L (82), although in routine diagnosis, this is inferior to measurement of the serum amylase or lipase level (83). Although other biochemical markers of acute pancreatitis are available, in general, the routine use of serum amylase plus CE-CT scanning in more difficult cases is the most practical approach to confirming the diagnosis.

### Detection of Gallstones

Ultrasound (US) has a detection rate for gallstones in excess of 95% in patients with uncomplicated disease, but in acute pancreatitis, this rate falls to 70–80% (84–85). The main reason for this is that gas-filled loops of bowel obscure the view for the ultrasonographer, and in addition, there is a tendency for smaller stones to cause attacks of acute pancreatitis (8, 86, 87). In 1983, Houssin et al. pointed out the difficulty of demonstrating microlithiasis by US or cholecystography (31). Up to 30% of gallstones causing pancreatitis fall into this category and may go undetected by US (84). The sensitivity of detection may be increased by another 10–20% by measuring the serum levels of the liver transaminases within 48 hours of an attack. If either the aspartate aminotransferase (AST) or the alanine aminotransferase (ALT) level exceeds 60 IU/L, it is highly likely that the cause of the acute pancreatitis is gallstones (84, 85), and the degree of certainty is directly proportional to the level of the transaminases (88).

Although it has been suggested that radionuclide scanning of the biliary tract is reliable in the differentiation of gallstone-induced acute pancreatitis from other causes (89), no subsequent trials have come close to the 100% accuracy of this initial study (90–92). Nonfilling of the gallbladder does occur more commonly in gallstone-associated acute pancreatitis (45–63%) than in other causes of acute pancreatitis (25–31%), but it is not of sufficient diagnostic accuracy to warrant its use over other methods (84, 92).

If other etiologic factors can be identified, then a potentially time-consuming search for gallstones can probably be avoided. There has been interest in the use of simple biochemical tests for the detection of alcoholic pancreatitis. In 1991, it was reported that the serum lipase/amylase ratio might be of use in detecting alcohol as a cause for acute pancreatitis (93), but subsequent studies showed this ratio to be of no diagnostic value (94–96). However, a more useful-looking biochemical discriminate is in the form of serum carbohydrate–deficient transferrin (CDT). Jaakkola et al. (96) prospectively investigated 86 consecutive patients admitted with the diagnosis of acute pancreatitis to a single unit. They found that the level of CDT positively correlated with the weekly alcohol intake and was more specific in this respect than either the mean erythrocyte volume or the serum $\gamma$-glutamyl transferase level. A CDT level above 17 U/L was found only in patients with alcohol-induced acute pancreatitis, and the sensitivity of CDT to detect a weekly ethanol intake above 560 g was 75%. If further studies confirm these findings, estimating the serum CDT will be an important biochemical test in patients presenting with acute pancreatitis.

ERCP is the most accurate way to diagnose gallstones in acute pancreatitis, with a sensitivity for both MBD stones and gallbladder stones in excess of 95%, but it is invasive (25). ERCP is associated with a small but significant morbidity and mortality (97) and should not be undertaken in the acute phase of an attack unless some form of therapeutic intervention is being considered.

### Detection of Gallstones in the Convalescent Phase

If there is no other biochemical cause of pancreatitis, such as hyperlipidemia or hypercalcemia, and alcohol and drugs have been excluded as a factor, a patient should only be referred to as having "idiopathic" acute pancreatitis if an ERCP has excluded cholelithiasis (98). The advantage of ERCP in this setting is that as well as improving the detection rate for stones, other more unusual biliary causes can be identified (Table 22.3). However, ERCP will still miss a small number of patients with microlithiasis (84, 98) and those who have passed all their gallstones into the duodenum during the attack of acute pancreatitis. These patients are likely to develop more stones, and when the clinical suspicion is high, US should be performed every 4–6 months (36, 98).

The diagnosis of biliary microlithiasis can also be made by sampling gallbladder bile and finding cholesterol crystals on polarizing light microscopy. The presence of significant amounts of calcium bilirubinate granules indicates the presence of pigment stones (36). Practically, the easiest way to obtain gallbladder bile is to aspirate bile from the second part of the duodenum with a forward-viewing endoscope following stimulation of the gallbladder with an intravenous injection of cholecystokinin-pancreozymin (CCK-PZ). Alternatively, bile can be aspirated directly from the MBD at ERCP (37). Dynamic radionuclide scanning of the biliary tree may have a role in the detection of cholesterolosis (99) when no other cause of an attack of acute pancreatitis is found. This method identifies cholesterolosis by demonstrating disordered gallbladder contraction and is surprisingly sensitive, but only in highly selected cases (99).

Despite the array of diagnostic procedures presently available to the clinician for the detection of gallstones, there will still be a small number of patients in whom gallstones, microlithiasis, or cholesterolosis will only be discovered in a cholecystectomy specimen. For this reason, any patient who has recurrent attacks of pancreatitis in the absence of any identifiable etiologic factor should be considered for cholecystectomy.

## SEVERITY ASSESSMENT

Predicting the severity of an attack of acute pancreatitis is important for a number of reasons: *(a)* it allows identification of those patients who will benefit from close monitoring; *(b)* it permits institution of specific treatment; *(c)* clinical trials can be

**TABLE 22.5. Original Ranson Scoring System for the Prediction of Severity in Acute Pancreatitis**

Admission or diagnosis
1. Age >55 years
2. White blood cell count >16 × $10^9$/L
3. Blood glucose >200 mg/100 mL
4. Serum lactate dehydrogenase >350 IU/L
5. Serum glutamic oxaloacetic transaminase >250 Sigma Frankel Units%

During initial 48 hours
6. Hematocrit fall >10%
7. Blood urea nitrogen rise >5 mg/100 mL
8. Serum calcium <8 mg/100 mL
9. $PaO_2$ <60 mm Hg (8 kPa)
10. Base deficit >4 mmol/L
11. Estimated fluid sequestration >6 L

0–2 factors = mild attack
3–11 factors = severe attack

**TABLE 22.6. Modified Ranson Scoring System for the Prediction of Severity in Patients with Acute Pancreatitis Due to Gallstones[a]**

Admission or diagnosis
1. Age >70 years[b]
2. White blood cell count >18 × $10^9$/L[b]
3. Blood glucose >220 mg/mL[b]
4. Serum lactate dehydrogenase >400 IU/L[b]
5. Serum glutamic oxaloacetic transaminase >250 Sigma Frankel Units%

During initial 48 hours
6. Hematocrit fall >10%
7. Blood urea nitrogen rise >2 mg/100 mL[b]
8. Serum calcium <8 mg/100 mL
9. Base deficit >5 mmol/L[b]
10. Estimated fluid sequestration >4 L[b]

[a]Key: 0–2 factors, mild; 3–11 factors, severe.
[b]These values are different from those in the general scoring system (Table 22.4). *Note:* the $PaO_2$ has been excluded from this system.

interpreted much more clearly, and new therapies evaluated more objectively.

## Ranson Scores

The original Ranson scoring system (Table 22.5) was based on a study of 200 patients with acute pancreatitis, of whom only 14 had gallstones (100). Because patients with gallstone pancreatitis were underrepresented in the group, there was some dissatisfaction with this system for such patients (101). A further review by Ranson himself confirmed the general value of the system in that the mortality in 347 patients with fewer than three prognostic signs was 0.9%, compared with 28% in 103 patients with three or more prognostic signs. There were, however, only 74 patients with gallstones of the total 450 patients with acute pancreatitis from all causes. Some 53 of the 74 patients with gallstone-induced acute pancreatitis had fewer than three prognostic signs, of whom 1 (1.9%) died, and of 21 patients with three or more prognostic signs there were 4 (19%) deaths. Based on this review, a new scoring system was devised specifically for patients with gallstone-induced acute pancreatitis (Table 22.6). Only three factors have the same cutoff point for the two systems, and the $PaO_2$ factor has been removed from the gallstone group. Moreover, the number of patients with gallstone-induced acute pancreatitis ($n$ = 74) and the number of events (deaths = 5) was far too small to permit accurate development of a prognostic system for this group of patients. Despite the serious shortcomings of the modified Ranson scoring system, it is often used indiscriminately and without adequate scientific justification in studies of patients with acute pancreatitis that include a large, if not exclusive, proportion with gallstone-induced acute pancreatitis.

## The Glasgow or Imrie System

The original Imrie system (Table 22.7) was based on the work performed by Ranson and was introduced to stratify patients into a major clinical trial in Glasgow (Scotland) examining the effects of aprotinin (103). This study was of extreme importance; it demonstrated not only that aprotinin (which was being prescribed widely at the time) was of no benefit in acute pancreatitis but also the necessity for prognostic scoring for data analysis and comparisons of randomized groups of patients. The new system was far simpler than the Ranson system and thus was seen as a very attractive alternative. Prospective analysis of the Glasgow system in 47 patients with gallstone pancreatitis showed that to improve predictability, age could be eliminated as a factor and the serum transaminase cutoff level should be increased from 100 IU/L to 200 IU/L. In preparation for a trial of endoscopic sphincterotomy (ES) in gallstone-associated acute pancreatitis, the Leicester group (England) found that serum transaminase level was not predictive of severity but that age was predictive in a large number of patients. Based on these observations, the Glasgow (Imrie) score was modified and introduced in 1983 (Table 22.8). The accuracy of the Glasgow system in predicting severity of acute pancreatitis has been repeatedly confirmed, and although entirely empirical, it appears as accurate in gallstone-associated acute pancreatitis as in alcohol-induced acute pancreatitis (104–107).

## Acute Physiology and Sepsis Scores (APACHE II, SAPS, and MRCSS)

In 1989, Larvin and McMahon (107) compared the Acute Physiology and Chronic Health Enquiry (APACHE II) score, the Simplified Physiology Score (SAPS), and the Medical Research Council Sepsis Score (MRCSS) with clinical assessment by a single experienced clinician, the Ranson score, and the Imrie system in predicting the outcome in patients with 290 attacks of acute pancreatitis, of which 124 were due to gallstones. An APACHE II score above 9 was shown to be accurate not only at 48 hours but also on admission and at 24 hours, thus demonstrating clear advantages over the Ranson and Imrie systems, which can only be applied 48 hours after admission. Clinical assessment by an experienced clinician had a sensitivity of 66% and an overall accuracy of 89%. This contrasts quite markedly with clinicians in general, whose severity prediction is often incorrect (105). A direct comparison between the gallstone-induced and alcohol-induced episodes of acute pancreatitis showed that the predictive power of the APACHE II system was equally good. Although this approach allows prediction of severity outcome at admission, it is more complicated than the Glasgow score and is thus less useful in routine clinical practice.

## Contrast-Enhanced Computed Tomography (CE-CT)

CE-CT of the pancreas is of great importance in detecting acute pancreatitis, determining the degree of necrosis, and identifying local complications (108). As discussed above, nonimaging methods are good at predicting overall outcome in pancreatitis, but CE-CT on admission may also predict the clinical course (109).

A direct comparison between the modified Glasgow system and CE-CT within 72 hours of the onset of an attack was undertaken on 126 patients with acute pancreatitis; results were reported in 1989 (110). In 78 patients, the cause was gallstones, and 34 patients had a severe attack. The modified Glasgow score predicted a severe attack with a sensitivity of 85% and a

**TABLE 22.7. Glasgow (Imrie) System for Severity Prediction in Acute Pancreatitis**

| Prognostic Factors[a] | Value at Which Factor is Present |
|---|---|
| Age | >55 years |
| Serum transaminases | >100 IU/L |
| White cell count | >15 × $10^9$/L |
| Blood glucose | >100 mmol/L (in the absence of diabetes mellitus) |
| Serum urea | >16 mmol/L (not responding to intravenous fluids) |
| $PaO_2$ | <7.5 kPa (60 mm Hg) |
| Serum calcium | <2.0 mmol/L |
| Serum albumin | <32 g/L |
| Serum lactate dehydrogenase | >600 IU/L |

[a]Three or more of the factors present within the first 48 hours predicts a severe attack.

**TABLE 22.8. Modified Glasgow (Imrie) System**

| Prognostic Factors[a] | Value at Which Factor is Present |
|---|---|
| Age | >55 years |
| White cell count | >15 × $10^9$/L |
| Blood glucose | >10 mmol/L (in the absence of diabetes mellitus) |
| Serum urea | >16 mmol/L (not responding to intravenous fluids) |
| $PaO_2$ | <8 kPa[b] |
| Serum calcium | <2 mmol/L |
| Serum albumin | <32 g/L |
| Serum lactate dehydrogenase | >600 IU/L |

[a]The presence of three or more factors within the first 48 hours predicts a severe attack. Note the absence of serum transaminase levels from the modified system.
[b]Value different from that in the original system.

specificity of 79%, versus 71% and 77%, respectively, for CE-CT. Thus CE-CT within 72 hours is not quite as accurate as the modified Glasgow system in predicting severity, and although useful in acute pancreatitis, CE-CT does not replace well-validated scoring systems. The major role of CE-CT lies in confirmation of the diagnosis when there is doubt and in the detection of local complications (109). Using both methods together, results routinely in increased specificity (97%) but a loss in sensitivity (56%). Using either CE-CT and/or the modified Glasgow score improves sensitivity to 100%, but specificity drops to 58% (110). This is mainly because the degree of local pancreatic inflammation does not correlate perfectly with the systemic complications of acute pancreatitis.

### Other Markers of Severity

A number of biochemical markers can be related to overall outcome and the development of multiple-system organ failure. These include C-reactive protein, circulating pancreatic enzymes such as phospholipase $A_2$, elastase, and lipase, and a variety of cytokines, including interleukin (IL)-2, IL-6, IL-8 and tumor necrosis factor (TNF). None of these markers is of any specific use in gallstone pancreatitis, and their role in everyday clinical practice is still being defined.

## COMPLICATIONS AND NATURAL HISTORY

### Morbidity and Mortality

All but one of the principal complications developing in patients with gallstone-associated acute pancreatitis are the same as, and occur at a similar frequency to, those with any other cause of acute pancreatitis (Table 22.9); the one exception is acute cholangitis (40). As in acute pancreatitis from other causes, a mild attack of acute pancreatitis due to gallstones resolves quickly. The median (range) hospital stay in one randomized study for patients acting as controls was 11 (4–27) days for those with mild acute pancreatitis and 17 (4–74) days for those with a severe attack (111).

The overall mortality rate for acute pancreatitis due to gallstones varies from 0 (112) to 25% (113) (Table 22.10). These variations are due to population differences, the proportion of true cases of acute pancreatitis (i.e., diagnosed not just on the basis of hyperamylasemia), the proportion of severe cases, the standard of supportive care, and the extent of specific therapeutic intervention. The best estimate of mortality from the disease is the outcome of the control arms of prospective therapeutic intervention trials: in seven controlled trials, there were 31 (6.1%) deaths among 507 patients (Table 22.11), but mortality is nearly always lower in patients entered into clinical trials than in those excluded.

### Coexisting Acute Cholangitis

The incidence of acute cholangitis with gallstone-associated acute pancreatitis is about 10% (40, 114, 115). Up to 12% of patients with acute cholangitis also have acute pancreatitis (116, 117), and as many as 63% of patients with coexisting acute cholangitis and acute pancreatitis have a severe attack of acute pancreatitis, with a mortality at least twice that of pancreatitis

**TABLE 22.9. Incidence of Complications in Acute Pancreatitis Comparing Gallstone-Induced Disease with All Other Causes**

| Complication | Gallstones (*n* = 258) | Alcohol (*n* = 104) | Miscellaneous (*n* = 55) | Total (*n* = 417) |
|---|---|---|---|---|
| Systemic[a] | | | | |
| Respiratory failure | 18 | 15 | 6 | 39 |
| Pleural effusion | 7 | 6 | 1 | 14 |
| Cardiac failure | 5 | 0 | 2 | 7 |
| Renal failure | 3 | 1 | 2 | 6 |
| Disseminated intravascular coagulation | 1 | 0 | 0 | 1 |
| Cerebrovascular accident | 1 | 0 | 1 | 2 |
| Pulmonary embolus | 1 | 1 | 0 | 2 |
| Multiorgan failure | 7 | 3 | 3 | 13 |
| Abdominal[b] | | | | |
| Pancreatic necrosis | 11 | 4 | 5 | 20 |
| Pseudocyst | 22 | 9 | 2 | 33 |
| Pancreatic abscess | 3 | 4 | 2 | 9 |
| Duodenal obstruction | 1 | 0 | 0 | 1 |
| Gross ascites | 3 | 2 | 4 | 9 |
| Portal vein thrombosis | 1 | 2 | 0 | 3 |
| Acute cholangitis | 25 | 0 | 1 | 26 |
| Deaths | 21 (8.1%) | 5 (4.1%) | 8 (14.5%) | 34 (8.1%) |

[a]Complications despite clinical measures.
[b]Clinically significant complications (i.e., not purely based on imaging).

**TABLE 22.10. Mortality Rate of Gallstone-Associated Acute Pancreatitis**

| Series | Period | Number of Patients | Mortality |
|---|---|---|---|
| Trapnell and Duncan | 1950–1969 | 316 | 63 (20%) |
| Weissberg et al. | 1955–1964 | 47 | 12 (26%) |
| Edlund, Norback, and Risholm | 1956–1960 | 310 | 28 (9%) |
| Kelly | 1958–1973 | 52 | 0 |
| Kelly | 1960–1979 | 172 | 4 (2%) |
| Paloyan, Simonowitz, and Skinner | 1962–1974 | 64 | 0 |
| Acosta et al. | 1964–1975 | 132 | 15 (11%) |
| Berlinski, Dorazio, and Winkley | 1967–1977 | 100 | 0 |
| Tondelli et al. | 1969–1978 | 114 | 7 (6%) |
| Imrie and White | 1971–1972 | 40 | 5 (13%) |
| Elfstrom | 1972–1976 | 89 | 2 (2%) |
| Semel, Schreiber, and Fromm | 1974–1979 | 63 | 2 (3%) |
| Farinon et al. | 1977–1984 | 108 | 7 (7%) |
| Stone, Fabian, and Dunlop | 1978–1981 | 65 | 3 (5%) |
| Winslet et al. | 1980–1990 | 258 | 21 (8%) |
| Oría et al. | 1986–1990 | 51 | 3 (6%) |

alone (116–120). This might be related to a greater incidence of cholangiovenous reflux in acute cholangitis, which results in septicemia, leading to an increased risk of infection in necrotic pancreatic tissue as well as the general effects of septicemic shock.

### Recurrent Attacks

The patient who survives an attack of gallstone-associated acute pancreatitis has a 30–50% risk of a recurrent attack (Table 22.12). This risk was first described by Opie in 1903 (121), but the routine use of prophylactic cholecystectomy immediately following an attack is still not universal.

The notion that recurrent acute pancreatitis due to gallstones can progress to chronic pancreatitis is not accepted generally. A study by Reid and Kune (122) on the natural history of acute pancreatitis in Australia, however, found that with delayed operation, a mild form of chronic pancreatitis ensued. They described the development of chronic pancreatitis in nine patients with gallstone pancreatitis in whom surgery was delayed, although only two of the nine had chronic pain, and the others had a benign form of chronic pancreatitis. Most other studies suggest that if there is progression to chronic pancreatitis, it is in the patients with alcohol-induced acute pancreatitis. Howard and Erhlich detected pancreatic calcification in only 4 of 251 patients with gallstone-induced acute pancreatitis, but 3 of these patients had an excessive alcohol intake, and only 1 of those 3 had steatorrhea and diabetes (123). Unless an attack of acute pancreatitis due to gallstones results in extensive pancreatic necrosis (from which there can be no parenchymal regeneration), full functional recovery is typical, and the progression to a chronic cycle of pain and pancreatic insufficiency that may occur following repeated attacks secondary to alcohol does not occur.

## TREATMENT

Treatment of acute pancreatitis of any cause requires aggressive therapy in terms of fluid management, parenteral analgesia, and organ-system support if necessary. There is increasing evidence that prophylactic antibiotic therapy benefits those with predicted severe attacks, resulting in reduced septic complications and mortality (124, 125). No other form of medical treatment has been shown to be of benefit in randomized trials, including the use of somatostatin, fresh frozen plasma, glucagon, anticholinergics, and $H_2$-receptor blockade. There is some evidence that early treatment with a platelet-activating-factor antagonist can reduce the development of multiple-organ failure and even reduce mortality (126). This is a field of intensive clinical investigation at present.

### Urgent versus Delayed Surgery

In the 1980s there were two randomized trials of urgent versus delayed surgery for gallstone-induced acute pancreatitis, with a view to decompressing the biliary tree. In the first study, reported in 1981 (90), Stone et al. randomized 65 patients to undergo either transduodenal sphincteroplasty and biliary decompression within 73 hours or delayed surgery, which was performed once the patient was well. Some 36 patients were randomized to urgent surgery, and 4 (11%) of them had complications, with 1

**TABLE 22.11. Mortality From Gallstone-Associated Acute Pancreatitis Based on the Conservative Arms of Randomized Clinical Trials**

| Type of Study | Authors | Year | No. of Patients | Deaths (%) |
|---|---|---|---|---|
| Medical therapy | MRC Trial | 1977 | 72 | 5 (7%) |
| Surgery | Stone et al. | 1981 | 31 | 1 (3%) |
| | Kelly and Wagner | 1988 | 82 | 2 (2.4%) |
| Endoscopic therapy | Neoptolemos et al. | 1988 | 53 | 3 (5.7%) |
| | Fan et al. | 1993 | 63 | 5 (7.9%) |
| | Fölsch et al. | 1995 | 112 | 6 (5.4%) |
| | Nowak et al. | 1995 | 94 | 9 (10.4%) |
| Total | | | 507 | 31 (6.1%) |

**TABLE 22.12. Recurrence Rate of Gallstone-Associated Acute Pancreatitis in Patients without Operation**

| Author | Year | Number of Patients with First Attack | Number of Patients with One or More Recurrent Attacks (%) |
|---|---|---|---|
| Howard and Ehrlich | 1962 | 251 | 90 (36%) |
| Paloyan et al. | 1975 | 64 | 31 (48%) |
| Trapnell and Duncan | 1975 | 232 | 88 (38%) |
| Elfstrom | 1978 | 63 | 16 (25%) |
| Sharon et al. | 1979 | 90 | 30 (33%) |
| Ranson | 1979 | 21 | 7 (33%) |
| Berlinski et al. | 1979 | 39 | 8 (20%) |
| Kelly | 1980 | 14 | 5 (36%) |
| Osborne et al. | 1981 | 100 | 26 (26%) |
| Welch and White | 1982 | 25 | 6 (24%) |
| Mayer et al. | 1984 | 37 | 4 (11%) |
| Burch et al. | 1990 | 102 | 23 (23%) |
| Total | | 1038 | 334 (32%) |

(3%) death. In the conservatively managed group, there were 3 (10%) patients with complications and 2 (7%) deaths. These differences were not significant, but no predictive score of severity was used.

The second study, published in 1988, was reported by Kelly and Wagner (127). They randomized 165 patients to *(a)* surgery within 48 hours of presentation or *(b)* surgery delayed beyond this time. Ranson's criteria for severity prediction were used, but patients were defined as severe if they had 4 or more factors present and mild if fewer than 4 (as opposed to the usual predictive scores of 3 or more for severe and less than 3 for mild). Some 83 patients were randomized to have urgent surgery; 25 (30%) had complications, and 13 (15%) died. In the delayed group, 5 (5%) had complications and 2 (2.4%) died. These differences were statistically significant. When analyzed separately, the patients with predicted mild attacks showed no significant difference in outcome, but among those with a predicted severe attack, there were 11 (48%) deaths in the urgent surgery group and only 2 (11%) deaths in the delayed surgery group. Of particular concern, the incidence of bile duct stones in relation to severity was not given in this study, and there were no data presented concerning the success or failure of adequate decompression and clearance of the biliary tract in either group. Another major criticism is that patients in the active arm were operated on before a full Ranson score could be ascertained at 48 hours, which means that those undergoing urgent surgery were significantly underscored for severity. Moreover, as Ranson himself subsequently noted, using the original Ranson score with this group of patients was inappropriate.

An important difference between these two studies is the type of surgical technique employed. In the first study, the biliary tree was decompressed by transduodenal sphincteroplasty; in the latter, supraduodenal exploration and biliary decompression using a T tube was performed. The apparent improved survival in the earlier study may be due to the differences in surgical method. Transduodenal sphincteroplasty decompresses both the MPD and MBD, whereas supraduodenal exploration with insertion of a T tube without clearance of the MBD is not going to ensure a freely draining MBD and MPD.

Thus there is increased morbidity and mortality in patients with severe acute pancreatitis who are operated on soon after the onset of the acute attack without sufficient attention to full stone clearance of the biliary tract and adequate decompression.

### Emergency Endoscopic Sphincterotomy

ERCP and endoscopic sphincterotomy (ES) was first reported for MBD stone extraction in the face of acute pancreatitis by Classen et al. in 1978 (128) but at the time was dismissed by many. In 1981, Safrany and Cotton (129) also reported a dramatic improvement in some patients with acute pancreatitis due to gallstones who underwent emergency sphincterotomy to disimpact and remove stones from the MBD. Not surprisingly, and in the absence of controlled trials, there was still enormous resistance to interfering with the biliary system in acute pancreatitis, and ERCP with ES was still considered contraindicated in this condition (130). However, the way had been paved for randomized controlled trials to study the efficacy of ERCP and ES in acute pancreatitis due to gallstones.

### Randomized Trials of Emergency ERCP and ES

Four studies were reported from 1988 to 1995, all of which differed in study design and thus, conclusions. The first study was reported in 1988 by Neoptolemos et al. from Leicester (111). This study used US and biochemical parameters to screen 223 consecutive patients for gallstones and then prospectively scored them for severity with the modified Glasgow score. Subjects were then designated mild or severe and randomized to undergo urgent ERCP-ES within 72 hours or conservative treatment, in which they were prohibited from ERCP for at least 5 days. Some 146 patients were diagnosed as having gallstones, of whom 15 could not be randomized because of incomplete data or the unavailability of ERCP within the 72 hours specified; 10 other patients were subsequently excluded because of an alternative diagnosis. This left 121 patients who were eligible for analysis, 59 in the urgent ERCP ± ES arm (34 mild and 25 severe) and 62 randomized to the conservative arm (34 mild and 28 severe).

Overall, patients significantly benefited from urgent ERCP ± ES, with a morbidity of 12% and mortality of 2%, compared with the conventionally treated group with a complication rate of 34% and a mortality of 8% ($p = .03$). In the patients with a predicted mild attack, the outcomes were identical, with a morbidity of 12% and a mortality of 0%. The predicted severe group of patients undergoing urgent ERCP ± ES had a morbidity of 24% and a mortality of 1.7%, compared with 61 and 18%, respectively, in the conservatively managed group ($p < .001$). Some 63 patients in the urgent group had ES following ERCP for confirmed MBD stones.

The study was criticized because it was suggested that the observed benefits in the interventional group were due to the relief of concomitant acute cholangitis rather than an impact on the acute pancreatitis. There were six patients with cholangitis in the urgent ERCP group and five in the conservatively managed group, and if these patients are excluded from analysis, there is

**TABLE 22.13. Results of the Leicester and Hong Kong Studies of ERCP and ES in Acute Pancreatitis, Comparing Only Those with Proven Gallstones, Comparing Mild with Severe Cases**

| | Numbers of Patients | | | | | | | |
|---|---|---|---|---|---|---|---|---|
| | | Complications | | | | Complications | | |
| City Treatment | Mild | Local | Systemic | Deaths | Severe | Local | Systemic | Deaths |
| Hong Kong | | | | | | | | |
| ERCP/ES | 34 | 4 (12%) | 2 (6%) | 0 | 30 | 3 (10%)[b] | 3 (10%)[f] | 1 (3%)[j] |
| Conventional | 35 | 1 (3%) | 5 (14%)(4)[a] | 0 | 28 | 8 (29%)[c] | 16 (57%)[g] (8)[a] | 5 (18%)[k] |
| Leicester | | | | | | | | |
| ERCP/ES | 28 | 3 (11%) | 1 (4%) | 0 | 22 | 3 (14%)[d] | 1 (5%)[h] | 0[l] |
| Conventional | 29 | 4 (14%) | 0 | 0 | 24 | 6 (25%)[e] | 9 (38%)[i] | 3 (13%)[m] |

[a]() Numbers of patients with biliary sepsis.
*Note:* Statistical differences for the mild groups of patients were not significant.
(b + d) vs. (c + e): $p < .05$; (f + h) vs. (g + i): $p < .01$; (j + l) vs. (k + m): $p < .05$.

still an overall benefit for the urgent ERCP group, which is even more pronounced in the predicted severe cases (complication rate, 15 vs. 60%; $p = .003$). Active intervention also significantly reduced the length of hospital stay: the severe group that had urgent ERCP had a mean hospital stay of 9.5 days, compared with 17 days for the conservatively managed group.

The second trial, from Katowice in Poland (131, 132), involved 250 patients who all underwent upper gastrointestinal endoscopy within 24 hours of admission to hospital with an acute attack of gallstone-induced acute pancreatitis. All 62 patients with the endoscopic appearances of an impacted stone at the ampulla of Vater had an ES performed. The remaining 188 patients with a normal ampullary appearance were randomized to ES or conventional treatment, although there was no predicted scoring of severity prior to randomization. The 156 patients in whom ES was performed had significantly lower morbidity and mortality than the 94 patients in the control group (morbidity, 14 vs. 34%; mortality, 1 vs. 11%). The patients were mainly tertiary referrals and the mean time of delay was 3.5 days between the onset of symptoms and the ES. This suggests that even if ES is delayed in these patients, there is still some therapeutic benefit.

In the third trial, from Hong Kong (114), reported in 1993, 195 patients with acute pancreatitis probably due to gallstones were randomized to undergo ERCP with or without ES within 24 hours of presentation. Control patients were permitted to have ERCP and ES at any time if they deteriorated. Overall, the authors found less biliary sepsis in the urgent ERCP/ES group than in the conservatively managed group (0 vs. 12%), but no significant differences were reported in mortality or other complications. The patients were scored for predicted severity by two methods, though not prior to randomization. As well as the Ranson score, they also applied the Hong Kong score, which is based on two parameters only: a blood glucose level above 11 mmol/L and a serum urea level above 7.4 mmol/L (20.7 mg/100 mL) (133). The Hong Kong system was devised from retrospectively collected data, but when investigated by the Glasgow group, it was found to be inadequate, with a sensitivity of 33% and a specificity of 88% (134). Moreover, the Hong Kong group also found little correlation between their system and either the Ranson score or the Glasgow score (135). Finally, since the Ranson score can only be fully ascertained at 48 hours and therapeutic intervention was undertaken within 24 hours, this method of severity assessment was seriously flawed.

The problem in interpreting this study is further compounded by the fact that only 127 of the 195 patients enrolled actually had gallstones as the cause of their pancreatitis, the others have a variety of diagnoses including alcoholism, hyperlipidemia, ascariasis, gallbladder carcinoma, and hepatoma. If these nongallstone patients are excluded, the results are reasonably similar to those of the Leicester study (Table 22.13), with clinical benefits being obvious in terms of the local and systemic complications of acute pancreatitis and not just from relieving biliary sepsis.

The fourth study, a multicenter investigation from Germany, enrolled 206 patients over a 5-year period (115). Patients were randomized to ERCP and ES within 72 hours of admission or to conventional treatment (Table 22.14). Patients with jaundice were excluded from the trial, as they all underwent urgent ES. This is of great importance, because patients with a serum bilirubin above 40 μmol/L (2.3 mg/100 mL) are those most likely to have persisting MBD stones (25, 68) and thus to derive greatest benefit from ES. Severity was undefined for some patients from both groups, indicating that patients were not prospectively stratified prior to randomization. The recruitment rate from the 22 hospitals was poor, especially considering that the other studies were all from single centers. Further, 11 patients in each group developed acute cholangitis, which adequate ES and biliary drainage should have prevented, suggesting that the ES was of poor quality in at least some of the centers involved in the study. Moreover, there were 11 (52%) deaths in a group that included only 21 severe cases treated by ES, which is in strong contradistinction to every other study of ES in acute pancreatitis (Table 22.15). Thus, whether biliary decompression is attempted surgically (127) or endoscopically

**TABLE 22.14. Details of the 238 Patients Entered into the German Multicenter Randomized Trial of Urgent ERCP/ES versus Conservative Treatment in Acute Gallstone Pancreatitis**

| Clinical Details[a] | ERCP <72 Hours | Conservative |
|---|---|---|
| Patients | | |
| Entered | 126 | 112 |
| Excluded | 19 | 13 |
| Randomized | 107 | 99 |
| Predicted severity | | |
| Severe | 21 | 20 |
| Undefined | 17 | 14 |
| Mild | 69 | 65 |
| Respiratory failure | 12 | 5 |
| Renal failure | 7 | 4 |
| Acute cholangitis | 11 | 11[b] |
| Sepsis | 10 | 13 |
| Deaths | | |
| "Related" | 7 | 4 |
| "Unrelated" | 4 | 2 |
| Total | 11 | 6 |

[a]No details of any local pancreatic complications are available.
[b]8 patients underwent delayed ERCP/ES.

**TABLE 22.15. Results of Endoscopic Sphincterotomy for Gallstone-Associated Acute Pancreatitis in Worldwide Series from 1978 to 1993**

| Series | Year | Number | Complications | Deaths |
|---|---|---|---|---|
| Classen et al. | 1978 | 17 | 0 | 0 |
| Van der Spuy | 1981 | 10 | 1 | 0 |
| Kautz et al. | 1982 | 21 | 1 | 1 |
| Riemann and Lux | 1984 | 15 | 0 | 0 |
| Rosseland and Solhaug | 1984 | 29 | 2 | 1 |
| Van Husen | 1986 | 44 | 2 | 1 |
| Leung et al. | 1987 | 15 | 0 | 1 |
| Escourrou et al.[a] | 1987 | 92 | 2 | 2 |
| Neoptolemos et al. | 1988 | 37 | 3 | 0 |
| Farkas et al.[a] | 1988 | 284 | 15 | 5 |
| Lygren et al. | 1990 | 21 | 0 | 1 |
| Dufek et al. | 1990 | 76 | 1 | 0 |
| Shemesh et al. | 1990 | 18 | 1 | 0 |
| Saowaros | 1990 | 16 | 3 | 0 |
| Nowak et al.[b] | 1990 | 156 | 22 | 2 |
| Karjalainen et al. | 1992 | 21 | 9 | 0 |
| Safrany and Fritscher-Ravens | 1992 | 201 | 12 | 7 |
| Deus et al.[c] | 1993 | 87 | NA | 7 |
| Manes et al. | 1993 | 76 | 11 | 1 |
| Fan et al. | 1993 | 37 | 7 | 1 |
| Total | | 1273 | 92 (7.7%) | 30 (2.4%) |

[a]Multicenter studies.
[b]Plus personal communication.
[c]Personal communication.

(115), it appears that the results are poor if the techniques used to clear the biliary tree and ensure adequate pancreatic juice outflow are not efficient.

Finally, a significant feature of the Leicester study was that all patients received prophylactic antibiotics, cefuroxime and metronidazole, for 5 days (111); administration of prophylactic cefuroxime reduced the incidence of complications and death in patients with severe acute pancreatitis in a randomized study of patients with alcohol-induced acute pancreatitis (125).

## PREVENTION OF FURTHER ATTACKS

### Open Cholecystectomy

The natural history of gallstone acute pancreatitis is that patients have a 30–50% chance of having a further attack if there is no therapeutic intervention (10, 136, 137) (Table 22.12). Most recurrences of acute pancreatitis occur within the first month of the index attack (137), and for this reason, patients should have a cholecystectomy on the same admission once the attack has resolved (101, 127). There are now many studies confirming that open cholecystectomy reduces the incidence of recurrent attacks of acute gallstone pancreatitis (30, 112, 123, 138) (Table 22.16). MBD stones found at the time of surgery need to be extracted to minimize the risk of a further attack of pancreatitis.

### Laparoscopic Cholecystectomy

Laparoscopic cholecystectomy is a viable, and in most cases a preferable, alternative to open cholecystectomy following an attack of acute pancreatitis due to gallstones (139), with an incidence of complications that compares favorably with that of open cholecystectomy (140) (Table 22.17). A prospective study of 24 patients with acute pancreatitis with three or more Ranson's

**TABLE 22.16. Recurrence of Acute Pancreatitis Following Open Cholecystectomy**

| Series | Year | Number | Recurrent Attacks | Follow-up Median (Range) in Years |
|---|---|---|---|---|
| Raker and Bartlett | 1953 | 43 | 2.9% | (1–6) |
| Berman et al. | 1961 | 12 | 10% | 2 |
| Howard and Ehrlich | 1962 | 160 | 4% | (1–7) |
| Albo et al. | 1963 | 15 | 0 | (0–7) |
| Glenn and Frey | 1964 | 119 | 16% | (1–30) |
| Dixon and Hillam | 1970 | 62 | 8% | (1–10) |
| Kelly | 1974 | 52 | 4% | (1–7) |
| Paloyan | 1975 | 100 | 0 | (1–12) |
| Berlinski et al. | 1979 | 100 | 0 | (1–10) |
| Sharon et al. | 1979 | 48 | 10%[a] | (3–13) |
| Moreau et al. | 1988 | 58 | 0 | 15 |

[a]Of the 5 patients with recurrent pancreatitis, 3 had residual duct stones.

**TABLE 22.17. Experience with Laparoscopic Cholecystectomy for Gallstone-Induced Acute Pancreatitis**

| Authors | No. of Patients | Complications[a] | Conversion Rate |
|---|---|---|---|
| Rhodes et al. | 16 | 0 | 0 |
| Graham et al. | 29 | 7 (24%) | 0 |
| Soper et al. | 49 | 5 (10%) | 0 |
| Canal and Broadie | 29 | 1 (3%) | 0 |
| Tate et al.[b] | 24 | 1 (4%) | 3 (13%) |
| Tang et al. | 142 | 1 (0.7%)[c] | 16 (11%) |
| Taylor et al. | 29 | NA | 7 (24%) |
| Total | 318 | 15/289 (5%) | 26 (8%) |

[a]There were no deaths reported in any of the series.
[b]Prospective study.
[c]Intraoperative complication; the postoperative complications were not reported.

criteria, was reported by Tate et al. (141). ERCP was successful in 23 patients, and when choledocholithiasis was identified ($n = 7$), the MBD was cleared. Laparoscopic cholecystectomy was performed 3–24 days after admission by an experienced laparoscopist, and mean technical difficulty was assessed using a visual analogue scale. The technical difficulty was significantly greater in patients recovering from acute pancreatitis than in control patients undergoing elective surgery for symptomatic gallstones unrelated to pancreatitis (difficulty scores, 5.4 vs, 3.6, respectively; $p < .002$). The one major complication was a subhepatic hematoma, which was managed conservatively.

The timing of laparoscopic cholecystectomy following an attack of acute pancreatitis due to gallstones is as important as in open cholecystectomy. In a study by Tang et al. of 142 patients undergoing laparoscopic cholecystectomy for gallstone-associated acute pancreatitis, morbidity increased if the procedure was carried out within a week of an attack of *severe* pancreatitis (142). All patients, including 20 patients with three or more Ranson's criteria, were operated on at least 48 hours after clinical and biochemical resolution of the pancreatitis. The 11 severe patients operated on more than 1 week after admission had a significantly shorter mean hospital stay following laparoscopic cholecystectomy than did the 9 severe patients operated on earlier (2.3 vs. 5.4 days, respectively). Moreover, in 6 of the 9 patients operated on within a week, procedures had to be converted to an open procedure, compared with only 2 of the 11 patients in the delayed group. In the 122 patients with predicted mild disease, there was no difference in the mean hospital stay between the early and late groups (2.4 vs. 3.9 days, respectively), and there was no significant difference in the conversion rate. Thus, the mild group of patients who were operated on early had a significantly shorter overall mean hospital stay (7.8 vs. 14 days, respectively).

When cholecystectomy is performed laparoscopically, the MBD still needs to be imaged to ensure that there are no more stones, which will increase the risk of a recurrent pancreatitis. Stones discovered at the time of surgery can be removed intraoperatively or by performing postoperative ES.

Some authors recommend that the efficiency of MBD stone management can be increased by selecting those with a high probability of MBD stones for preoperative ERCP. This can be done on the basis of a combination of clinical, biochemical, and US findings (143, 144). Patients with a high probability of MBD stones at the time of surgery include those with acute cholangitis, obstructive jaundice, persistent hyperamylasemia, or MBD stones seen on US. Selecting patients by use of these criteria may reduce the unnecessary preoperative ERCP rate to less than 10% (144).

### ERCP and ES with Gallbladder Left in Situ

Some patients will be at a very high surgical risk following an attack of acute gallstone pancreatitis, and in these patients, ES is an important alternative to surgery in the prevention of further attacks (145). There is now an increasing experience with this method of preventing recurrent acute pancreatitis (Table 22.18). Most patients with a recurrent attack after ES will have stenosed the papilla, but they will benefit from a further ES. Despite this, approximately 10% of patients with bile duct stones treated by ES without cholecystectomy will develop gallbladder-related complications that will sometimes require surgery or may result in death (146). For these reasons, patients should have a cholecystectomy performed in preference to ES, if they are fit for surgery.

The success of ES in preventing recurrent acute pancreatitis effectively destroys McCutheon's theory of retrograde reflux of enterokinase from the duodenum into the pancreatic duct (45) and reaffirms Opie's theories (1, 2).

**TABLE 22.18. Endoscopic Sphincterotomy for Gallstone-Induced Acute Pancreatitis in Patients with Gallbladder in Situ**

| Authors | Year | Number | Recurrent Attacks | Gallbladder Complications | Unrelated Deaths | Follow-up Mean (Range) |
|---|---|---|---|---|---|---|
| Davidson et al. | 1988 | 19 | 0 | 0 | 0 | 39 months (1–8 years) |
| Shemesh et al. | 1990 | 9 | 0 | 0 | 0 | 22 months |
| Hill et al. | 1991 | 14 | 0 | NA | NA | 38 months (1–8 years) |
| Deus et al.[a] | 1993 | 34 | 1 | 0 | 4 | (1–10 years) |
| Nowak et al. | 1994 | 33 | 0 | NA | NA | (1–10 years) |
| Welbourn et al. | 1995 | 48 | 0 | 2 | 16 | 27 months (1–10 years) |

[a]Personal communication.

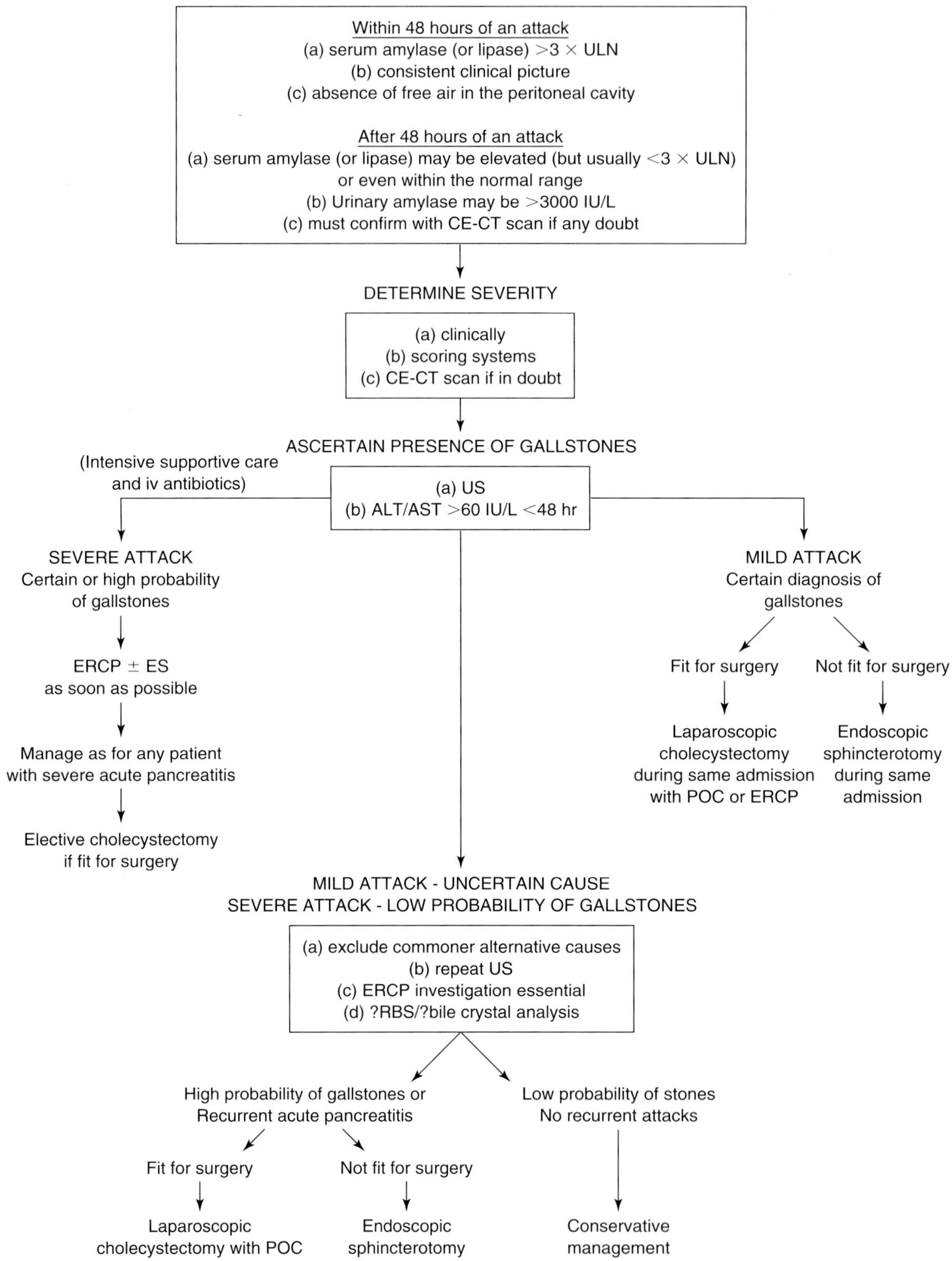


ULN = upper limit of normal
CE-CT = Contrast-enhanced computerized tomography
US = ultrasound
POC = preoperative cholangiogram
RBS = radionuclide biliary scanning

**FIG. 22.4.** Management strategy for patients with gallstone-associated acute pancreatitis.

## CONCLUSIONS

Successful management of patients with acute pancreatitis depends on establishing a confident diagnosis, determining severity, instituting relevant supportive measures, and ascertaining the presence or absence of gallstones. The latter is particularly important in patients with a severe attack (Fig. 22.4), since intensive supportive measures, systemic antibiotics, and urgent clearance of the bile duct are mandatory. The preferred approach to ductal clearance is endoscopic, as outcome by this means is relatively independent of the general fitness of the patient—in contrast to open surgery (147). Nevertheless, if ERCP/ES has failed or is not readily available, the use of emergency surgery in a surgically fit patient (particularly with evidence of obstructive jaundice) may be warranted. However, endoscopic treatment requires equally the skills of an experienced surgeon and peri-operative imaging of the biliary tree. All stones must be cleared from the biliary tree and effective drainage established. Such a policy is only effective in reducing morbidity and mortality if the patients are subsequently managed appropriately, as for any patient with severe acute pancreatitis, because of the high probability of organ failure and local pancreatic complications, especially infected pancreatic necrosis.

Patients with mild acute pancreatitis may be managed less aggressively, but if gallstones have been established as the cause of the acute attack, effective treatment should be undertaken to prevent further attacks before the patient is discharged from hospital. Laparoscopic cholecystectomy with biliary imaging is preferred, but the alternative is endoscopic sphincterotomy if the patient is a high surgical risk case. Patients with an attack of acute pancreatitis of uncertain cause require continued follow-up and further investigation.

Despite the wealth of investigations and technology available for the management of patients with gallstone-associated acute pancreatitis, clinical judgment and technical expertise remain of paramount importance. [*Editor's note:* The authors have presented a very scholarly review of acute gallstone pancreatitis, including the current frontier of its treatment. In the previous edition of this book, one of the editors presented a review of the more traditional approach of deferring operative intervention until the inflammatory response had begun to subside ("Gallstone Pancreatitis," Chapter 20 in *Surgical Diseases of the Pancreas,* Philadelphia: Lea & Febiger, 1987). Technology has progressed in the past decade, and the purpose of this comment is to maintain, under review, the timing of operation, and perhaps, the route of operative intervention, as experience continues to accumulate. J. M. Howard, M.D.]

## REFERENCES


1. Opie EL. The relation of cholelithiasis to disease of the pancreas and to fat necrosis. Am J Med Sci 1901;121:27–43.
2. Opie EL. The etiology of acute haemorrhagic pancreatitis. Bull Johns Hopkins Hosp 1901;121:182–188.
3. Bell ET. Pancreatitis: a study of 179 fatal cases. Surgery 1958;43: 527–537.
4. Shader AE, Paxton JR. Fatal pancreatitis. Am J Surg1966;111: 369–373.
5. Storck G, Pettersson G, Edlund Y. A study of autopsies upon 116 patients with acute pancreatitis. Surg Gynecol Obstet 1976;143: 241–245.
6. Kaden VG, Howard JM. Clinical studies of the natural history of acute pancreatitis. Arch Surg 1956;73:269–271.
7. Howard JM, Ehrlich EW. The etiology of pancreatitis. Ann Surg 1960;152:135–146.
8. Acosta JL, Ledesma CL. Gallstone migration as a cause for acute pancreatitis. N Engl J Med 1974;190:484–487.
9. Kelly TR. Gallstone pancreatitis: pathophysiology. Surgery 1976; 80:488–492.
10. Kelly TR. Gallstone pancreatitis: the timing of surgery. Surgery 1980;88:345–349.
11. Bourke JB. Variation in annual incidence of primary acute pancreatitis in Nottingham (1969–1974). Lancet 1975;2:967–969.
12. Thomson SR, Hendry WS, McFarlane GA, Davidson AI. Epidemiology and outcome of acute pancreatitis. Br J Surg 1987;74: 398–401.
13. Wilson C, Imrie CW. Changing patterns of incidence and mortality from acute pancreatitis in Scotland. Br J Surg 1990;79: 731–734.
14. Jaakkola M, Nordback I. Pancreatitis in Finland between 1970 and 1989. Gut 1993;34:1255–1260.
15. Acalovschi M, Dumitrascu D, Calser I, Ban A. Comparative prevalence of gallstone disease at 100-year interval in a large Romanian town, a necropsy study. Dig Dis Sci 1987;32:354–357.
16. Teilum D. The prevalence of gallstones in autopsies from a Danish urban area. Frederiksberg 1914–1955. Acta Chir Scand 1989;155:103–106.
17. Bates T, Harrison M, Lowe D, Lawson C, Padley N. Longitudinal incidence of gallstone prevelance at necropsy. Gut 1992;33: 103–107.
18. Cavallini G, Riela A, Brocco G, Bertelli G, Falconi M, et al. Epidemiology of acute pancreatitis. In: Beger HG, Buchler M, eds. Acute pancreatitis. Berlin: Springer-Verlag, 1987.
19. Lowenfels AB, Velema JP. Estimating gallstone incidence from prevalence data. Scand J Gastroenterol 1993;27:984–986.
20. Eichelberger MR, Hoelzer DJ, Koop CE. Acute pancreatitis: the difficulties of diagnosis and therapy. J Pediatr Surg 1982;17: 244–254.
21. Taylor TV, Rimmer S, Holt S, Jeacock J, Lucas S. Sex differences in gallstone pancreatitis. Ann Surg 1991;214:667–670.
22. Norwold DL. Gallstone lithotripsy. Am J Surg 1993;165:431–434.
23. Faris I, Thompson JPS, Grundy DJ, LeQuense LP. Operative cholangiography: a reappraisal based on a review of 400 cholangiograms. Br J Surg 1975;62:966–972.
24. Neoptolemos JP, Carr-Locke DL, Kelly K. Factors affecting the diameters of the common bile duct and pancreatic duct using endoscopic retrograde cholangiopancreatography. Hepatogastroenterology 1991;38:243–247.
25. Neoptolemos JP, Carr-Locke DL, London N, Bailey I, Fossard DP. ERCP findings and the role of endoscopic sphincterotomy in acute gallstone pancreatitis. Br J Surg 1988;75:954–960.
26. Jensen KH, Jorgensen T. Incidence of gallstones in a Danish population. Gastroenterology 1991;100:790–794.
27. Maram ES, Linos DA, Thistle JL, Linos A, O'Fallon WM, Kurland LT. The incidence of cholelithiasis and cholecystitis in Rochester, Minn, 1950 through 1969. Arch Intern Med 1990;150:1833–1836.
28. Imrie CW, Whyte AS. A prospective study of acute pancreatitis. Br J Surg 1975;62:490–494.
29. Armstrong CP, Taylor TV, Jeacock J, Lucas S. The biliary tract in patients with acute gallstone pancreatitis. Br J Surg 1985;72: 551–555.
30. Moreau JA, Zinsmeister AR, Melton LJ, Dimagno EP. Gallstone pancreatitis and the effect of cholecystectomy: a population-based cohort study. Mayo Clin Proc 1988;63:466–473.
31. Houssin D, Castain GD, Lemoine J, Bismuth H. Microlithiasis of the gallbladder. Surg Gynecol Obstet 1983;157:20–40.
32. Farinon AM, Ricci GL, Sianesi M, Percudani M, Zannella E. Physiopathological role of microlithiasis in gallstone pancreatitis. Surg Gynecol Obstet 1987;164:252–256.
33. Parrilla PP, Garcia OD, Pellicer FE, et al. Gallbladder cholesterolosis: an aetiological factor in acute pancreatitis of uncertain origin. Br J Surg 1990;77:735–736.
34. Lee SP, Nicholls JF. Nature and composition of biliary sludge. Gastroenterology 1986;90:677–686.
35. Paumgartner G, Sauerbruch T. Gallstones: pathogenesis. Lancet 1991;338:1117–1121.
36. Neoptolemos JP, Davidson BR, Winder AF, Vallance D. Role of duodenal bile crystal analysis in the investigation of idiopathic pancreatitis. Br J Surg 1988;75:954–960.
37. Ros E, Navarro S, Bru C, Garcia-Puges A, Valderama R. Occult microlithiasis in "idiopathic" acute pancreatitis: prevention of relapse by cholecystectomy or ursodeoxycholic acid therapy. Gastroenterology 1991;101:1701–1709.
38. Lee SP, Nicholls JF, Park HZ. Biliary sludge as a cause of acute pancreatitis. N Engl J Med 1992;326:589–593.
39. Juniper K, Burson EN. Biliary tract studies II: the significance of biliary crystals. Gastroenterology 1957;32:175–209.

40. Winslet MC, Hall C, Lodon NJM, Neoptolemos JP. Relation of diagnostic serum amylase levels to aetiology and severity of acute pancreatitis. Gut 1992;33:982–986.
41. Elliot DW, Williams RD, Zollinger RM. Alterations in the pancreatic resistance to bile in the pathogenesis of acute pancreatitis. Ann Surg 1957;146:669–682.
42. Armstrong CP, Taylor TV. Pancreatic-duct reflux and acute gallstone pancreatitis. Ann Surg 1986;204:59–64.
43. Hernandez CA, Lerch MM. Sphincter stenosis and gallstone migration through the biliary tract. Lancet 1993;341:1371–1373.
44. Lerch MM, Weidenbach H, Hernandez CA, Preclik G, Adler G. Pancreatic outflow obstruction as the critical event for human gallstone induced pancreatitis. Gut 1994;35:1501–1503.
45. McCutheon AD. Aetiological factors in pancreatitis. Lancet 1962:710–712.
46. Robinson TM, Dunpy JE. Continuous perfusion of bile protease through the pancreas. JAMA 1963;183:530–583.
47. Csendes A, Sepulveda A, Burdiles P, Bradheetto I, Basitiias J, et al. Common bile duct pressure in patients with common bile duct stones with or without suppurative cholangitis. Arch Surg 1988;123:697–699.
48. Aho HJ, Nevalainen TJ. Experimental pancreatitis in the rat. Ultrastructure of sodium taurocholate induced pancreatic lesions. Scand J Gastroenterol 1980;15:417–424.
49. Armstrong CP, Taylor TV, Torrance HB. Pressure, volume and the pancreas. Gut 1985;26:615–624.
50. White TT, Magee DF. Perfusion of the dog pancreas with bile without producing pancreatitis. Ann Surg 1960;131:245–250.
51. Arendt T, Broschewitz U. Bile induced acute oedematous pancreatitis in rats: non-parallel changes in pancreatic morphology and amylase release in vitro. Gut 1994;35:1127–1131.
52. Sarkany RPE, Moreland BH. Enhancement of the autocatalytic activation of trypsinogen to trypsin by bile and bile acids. Biochim Biophys Acta 1985;839:262–267.
53. Armstrong CP, Taylor TV. Bile, bacteria and pancreatitis. Surg Res Commun 1988;2:323–331.
54. Suzuki Y, Kobayashi A, Ohto M. Bacteriological study of transhepatically aspirated bile. Relation to cholangiographic findings in 296 patients. Dig Dis Sci 1984;29:109–115.
55. Keynes WM. A non-pancreatic source of proteolytic-enzyme amidase and bacteriology in experimental pancreatitis. Ann Surg 1980;191:187–199.
56. Schmidt H, Creutzfeldt W. The possible role of phospholipase A in the pathogenesis of acute pancreatitis. Scand J Gastroenterol 1969;4:39–48.
57. Lerch MM, Saluja AK, Runzi M, Dawra R, Saluja M, Steer ML. Pancreatic duct obstruction triggers acute necrotising pancreatitis in the opossum. Gastroenterology 1993;104:853–861.
58. Ohshio G, Saluja A, Steer ML. Effects of short-term pancreatic duct obstruction in rats. Gastroenterology 1991;100:196–202.
59. Saluja A, Saluja M, Villa A, Leli U, Rutledge A, et al. Pancreatic duct obstruction in rabbits causes digestive zymogen and lysosomal enzyme colocalization. J Clin Invest 1989;84:1260–1266.
60. Senniger N, Moody FG, Coelho JCU, Van Buren DH. The role of biliary obstruction in the pathogenesis of acute pancreatitis in the opossum. Surgery 1986;99:688–693.
61. Runkel NS, Rodrigues LF, LaRocco MT, Moody FG. Mechanisms of pancreatic infection in acute pancreatitis in opossums. Curr Surg 1990;47:460–462.
62. Runkel NS, Rodrigues LF, Moody FG, LaRocco MT, Blasdel T. Salmonella infection of the biliary and intestinal tract of wild opossums. Lab Anim Sci 1991;41:54–56.
63. Hirano T, Manabe T. A possible mechanism for gallstone pancreatitis: repeated short-term pancreaticobiliary duct obstruction with exocrine stimulation in rats. Proc Soc Exp Biol Med 1993;202:246–252.
64. Runzi M, Saluja A, Lerch MM, Dawra R, Nishino H, Steer ML. Early ductal decompression prevents the progression of biliary pancreatitis: an experimental study in the opossum. Gastroenterology 1993;105:157–164.
65. Leese T, Neoptolemos JP, West KP, Talbot IC, Carr-Locke DL. Tumours and pseudotumours or the region of the ampulla of Vater: an endoscopic, clinical and pathological study. Gut 1986;27:1186–1192.
66. Oria A, Frider B, Alvarez J, Chiappetta L, Souto N, Fontana JJ. Biliary and pancreatic obstruction during gallstone migration. Int J Pancreatol 1988;3:157–164.
67. Isogai M, Yamaguchi A, Hori A, Nakano S. Hepatic histopathologic changes in biliary pancreatitis. 10th World Conference of Gastroenterology, 1994.
68. Neoptolemos JP, London NN, Bailey I, Shaw D, Carr-Locke DL, et al. The role of clinical and biochemical criteria and endoscopic retrograde cholangiopancreatography in the urgent diagnosis of common bile duct stones in acute pancreatitis. Surgery 1956;100:732–742.
69. Nowak A, Nowakowska-Dulaw E, Rybicka J. Patency of the Santorini duct and acute biliary pancreatitis. A prospective ERCP study. Endoscopy 1990;22:124–126.
70. Greenbaum LA, Hirshkowitz A. Endogenous cathepsin activates trypsinogen in extracts of dog pancreas. Proc Soc Exp Biol Med 1961;107:74–76.
71. Figarella C, Miszczuk-Jamisica B, Barrett AJ. Possible lysosomal activation of pancreatic digestive zymogens. I: Activation of both human trypsinogens by cathepsin B and spontaneous acid activation of human trypsinogen. Biol Chem Hoppe Seyler 1988;369(suppl):293–298.
72. Kornfield S. Trafficking of lysosomal enzymes in normal and disease states. J Clin Invest 1986;77:1–6.
73. Saluja M, Saluja A, Lerch MM, Steer ML. A plasma protease which is expressed during supramaximal stimulation causes in vitro subcellular distribution of lysosomal enzymes in rat exocrine pancreas. J Clin Invest 1991;87:1280–1285.
74. Lerch MM, Adler G. Therapeutic strategies in experimental acute pancreatitis. In: Pederzoli P, Covallin G, Bassi C, eds. Facing the pancreatic dilemma. Berlin: Springer-Verlag, 1994: 487–497.
75. Saluja A, Steer D, Lerch MM, Dawra R, Saluja M, Steer ML. Failure of the cathepsin B inhibitor, E-64, to protect against cerulein and CDE-diet induced pancreatitis. Pancreas 1991;6:718.
76. Palade G. Intracellular aspects of the process of protein secretion. Science 1975;189:347–358.
77. Herzog V, Farquhar MG. Luminal membrane retrieved after exocytosis reaches most Golgi cisternae in secretory cells. Proc Natl Acad Sci USA 1977;74:5073–5077.
78. Lerch MM, Saluja AK, Runzi M, Dawra R, Steer ML. Luminal endocytosis and intracellular targeting by acinar cells during early biliary pancreatitis in the opossum. J Clin Invest 1995;95: 2222–2231.
79. Neoptolemos JP. The theory of ''persisting'' common bile duct stones in severe gallstone pancreatitis. Ann R Coll Surg Engl 1989;71:326–331.
80. London NJM, Neoptolemos JP, Lavelle J, Bailey I, James D. Serial computed tomography scanning in acute pancreatitis: a prospective study. Gut 1989;30:397–403.
81. Clavien PA, Burgan S, Moossa AR. Serum enzymes and other laboratory tests in acute pancreatitis. Br J Surg 1989;76:1234–1243.
82. Moller-Petersen J, Lamsten J, Laerke M. Serum and urinary pancreatic enzymes in differential diagnosis of acute pancreatitis. In: Malfertheimer P, Ditshumeit H, eds. Diagnostic procedures in pancreatic disease. Berlin: Springer-Verlag, 1986: 95–106.
83. Gwozdz GA, Steinberg WM, Werner M, Henry JM, Pauley C. Comparative evaluation of the diagnosis of acute pancreatitis based on serum and urine enzyme assays. Clin Chim Acta 1990;187:243–254.
84. Neoptolemos JP, Hall A, Finlay DF, Berry JM, Carr-Locke DL, Fossard DP. The urgent diagnosis of gallstones in acute pancreatitis: a prospective study of the methods. Br J Surg 1984;71: 230–247.
85. Wang SS, Lin XZ, Tsai YT, Lee S, Pan HB, et al. Clinical significance of ultrasonography, computed tomography, and biochemical tests in the rapid diagnosis of gallstone-related pancreatitis: a prospective study. Pancreas 1988;3:153–158.
86. McMahon MJ, Playforth MJ, Booth EW. Identification of risk factors for acute pancreatitis from routine radiological investigation of the biliary tract. Br J Surg 1981;68:465–467.
87. Kelly TR. Gallstone pancreatitis. Local predisposing factors. Ann Surg 1984;200:479–485.

88. Kazmierczak SC, Catrou PG, Van Lente F. Enzymatic markers of gallstone-induced pancreatitis identified by ROC curve analysis, discriminant analysis, logistic regression, likelihood ratios and information theory. Clin Chem 1995;41:523–531.
89. Glazer G, Murphy F, Clayden GS, et al. Radionuclide biliary scanning in acute pancreatitis. Br J Surg 1981;68:766.
90. Stone HH, Fabian TC, Dunlop WE. Gallstone pancreatitis: biliary tract pathology in relation to time of operation. Ann Surg 1981;194:305–310.
91. Zemanm RK, Burrell MI, Cahow CE, Caride U, et al. Diagnostic utility of cholescintigraphy and ultrasonography in acute cholecystitis. Am J Surg 1981;141:446–451.
92. Neoptolemos JP, Fossard DP, Berry JM. A prospective study of radionuclide biliary scanning in acute pancreatitis. Ann R Coll Surg Engl 1983;65:180–183.
93. Gumaste VV, Dave PB, Weissman D, Messer J. Lipase/amylase ratio. A new index that distinguishes acute episodes of alcoholic from nonalcoholic acute pancreatitis. Gastroenterology 1991; 101:1361–1366.
94. Pezzilli R, Billi P, Migliola M, Gullo L. Serum amylase and lipase concentrations and lipase/amylase ratio in assessment of etiology and severity of acute pancreatitis. Dig Dis Sci 1993;38: 1265–1269.
95. Sadowski DC, Todd JK, Sutherland LR. Biochemical models as early predictors of the etiology of acute pancreatitis. Dig Dis Sci 1993;38:637–643.
96. Jaakkola M, Sillanaukee P, Lof K, Koivula T, Norback I. Blood tests for detection of alcoholic cause of acute pancreatitis. Lancet 1994;343:1328–1329.
97. Ostroff JW, Shapiro HA. Complications of endoscopic sphincterotomy. In: Jacobsen I, ed. ERCP: diagnostic and therapeutic applications. New York: Elsevier, 1989:61–73.
98. Goodman AJ, Neoptolemos JP, Carr-Locke DL, Finlay DBL, Fossard DP. Detection of gallstones after acute pancreatitis. Gut 1985;26:125–132.
99. Kmiot WA, Perry EP, Donovan IA, et al. Cholesterolosis in patients with chronic acalculous biliary pain. Br J Surg 1994;81: 112–115.
100. Ranson JHC, Rifkind KM, Roses DF, Fink SD, Eng K, Spencer FC. Prognostic signs and the role of operative management in acute pancreatitis. Surg Gynecol Obstet 1974;139:69–81.
101. Ranson JHC. The timing of biliary surgery in acute pancreatitis. Ann Surg 1979;189:654–662.
102. Ranson JHC. Etiological and prognostic factors in human acute pancreatitis: a review. Am J Gastroenterol 1982;77:633–638.
103. Imrie CW, Benjamin IS, Ferguson JC, McKay AJ, Mackenzie I, et al. A single-centre double-blind trial of Trasylol therapy in primary acute pancreatitis. Br J Surg 1978;65:337–341.
104. Blamey SL, Imrie CW, O'Neill J, Gilmour WH, Carter DC. Prognostic factors in acute pancreatitis. Gut 1974;25:1340–1360.
105. Corfield AP, Cooper MJ, Williamson RCN, Mayer AD, McMahon MJ, et al. Prediction of severity in acute pancreatitis: a prospective comparison of three prognostic indices. Lancet 1985: 403–407.
106. Leese T, Shaw D. Comparison of three Glasgow multifactor prognostic scoring systems in acute pancreatitis. Br J Surg 1988;75:460–462.
107. Larvin M, McMahon MJ. APACHE II score for assessment and monitoring of acute pancreatitis. Lancet 1989;ii:201–204.
108. Block S, Maier W, Bittner R, Buchler M, Malfertheiner P, Beger H. Identification of pancreatic necrosis in severe acute pancreatitis: imaging procedures versus clinical staging. Gut 1986;27: 1035–1042.
109. Balthazar EJ, Robinson DL, Megibow ASJ, Ranson JHC. Acute pancreatitis: value of CT in establishing prognosis. Radiology 1990;174:331–336.
110. London NJM, Neoptolemos JP, Lavelle J, Bailey I, James D. Contrast-enhanced abdominal computed tomography scanning and prediction of severity of acute pancreatitis: a prospective study. Br J Surg 1989;76:268–272.
111. Neoptolemos JP, London NJ, James D, Carr-Locke DL, Bailey IA, Fossard DP. Controlled trial of urgent endoscopic retrograde cholangiopancreatography and endoscopic sphincterotomy versus conservative treatment for acute pancreatitis due to gallstones. Lancet 1988;ii:979–983.
112. Berlinski LS, Dorazio RA, Winkley JH. Gallstone pancreatitis. Mount Sinai J Med 1979;46:364–366.
113. Weissberg D, Adam YG, Volk H, State D. Acute pancreatitis: a ten year study. Am Surg 1972;38:574–581.
114. Fan ST, Lai CS, Mok FPT, Lo CM, Rheng SS, Wong J. Early treatment of acute biliary pancreatitis by endoscopic papillotomy. N Engl J Med 1993;328:228–232.
115. Folsch UR, Nitsche R, Ludtke R, Hilgers RA, Creutzfeldt W. Early ERCP and papillotomy compared with conservative treatment for acute biliary pancreatitis. The German Study Group of Acute Biliary Pancreatitis. N Engl J Med 1997;336:237–242.
116. Andrew DJ, Johnson SE. Acute suppurative cholangitis, a medical and surgical emergency. Am J Gastroenterol 1979;54:141–154.
117. Neoptolemos JP, Carr-Locke DL, Leese T, James D. Acute cholangitis in association with acute pancreatitis: incidence, clinical features and outcome in relation to ERCP and endoscopic sphincterotomy. Br J Surg 1987;74:1103–1106.
118. McMahon MJ, Mayer AD, Shearer MG, Corfield AP, Cooper MJ, et al. Cholangitis and acute pancreatitis (Abstract). Gut 1985; 26:A648.
119. Neoptolemos JP, Carr-Locke DL. ERCP in acute cholangitis and pancreatitis. In: Jacobson IM, ed. ERCP: diagnostic and therapeutic applications. New York: Elsevier, 1989.
120. Nowak A, Dzlurkowska-Marek E, Nowakowska-Dulawa E, Marek A, Kaczor R. Does acute biliary pancreatitis (ABP) worsen the results of urgent endoscopic treatment of acute obstructive cholangitis (AOC) (Abstract)? 10th World Congress of Gastroenterology 68EC, 1994.
121. Opie EL. Diseases of the pancreas. Its cause and nature. Philadelphia: JB Lippincott, 1903.
122. Reid BG, Kune GA. Natural history of acute pancreatitis. A long term study. Med J Aust 1980;2:555–558.
123. Howard JM, Ehrlich EW. Gallstone pancreatitis: a clinical entity. Surgery 1962;51:177–184.
124. Luiten EJT, Hop WCJ, Lange JF, Bruining HA. Controlled clinical trial of selective decontamination for the treatment of severe acute pancreatitis. Ann Surg 1995;22:57–65.
125. Sainio V, Kemppainen E, Puolakkainen P, Taavitsainen M, Kivisaari L, et al. Early antibiotic treatment in acute necrotising pancreatitis. Lancet 1995;346:663–667.
126. Kingsnorth AN, Galloway SW, Formela LJ. Randomized, double-blind phase II trial of Lexipafant, a platelet-activating factor antagonist, in human acute pancreatitis. Br J Surg 1995;82:1414–1420.
127. Kelly TR, Wagner DS. Gallstone pancreatitis: a prospective randomised trial of timing of surgery. Surgery 1988;104:600–605.
128. Classen M, Ossenberg W, Wurbs D, Dammermann R, Hagenmuller F. Pancreatitis—an indication for endoscopic papillotomy (Abstract)? Endoscopy 1978;10:223.
129. Safrany L, Cotton PB. A preliminary report: urgent duodenoscopic sphincterotomy for acute gallstone pancreatitis. Surgery 1981;89:424–428.
130. Bouchier IAD. Biochemical tests for acute pancreatitis. Br Med J 1985;291:1669–1670.
131. Nowak A, Nowakowska-Duzawa E, Rybicka J. Urgent endoscopic sphincterotomy vs conservative treatment in acute biliary pancreatitis—a prospective, controlled trial (Abstract). Hepatogastroenterology 1990;37(suppl II):A5.
132. Nowak A, Nowakowska-Dulaw E, Marek TA, Rybicka J. Final results of the prospective, randomized, controlled study on endoscopic sphincterotomy versus conventional treatment in acute biliary pancreatitis (Abstract). Gastroenterology 1995; 108:A380.
133. Fan ST, Choi TK, Lai ECS, Wong J. Prediction of severity of acute pancreatitis: an alternative approach. Gut 1989;30:1591–1595.
134. Heath DI, Imrie CW. The Hong Kong criteria and severity prediction in acute pancreatitis. Int J Pancreatol 1994;15: 179–185.
135. Fan ST, Lai CS, Mok FPT, Lo CM, Zheng SS, Wong J. Prediction of the severity of acute pancreatitis. Am J Surg 1993;166:262–268.
136. Osborne DH, Imrie CW, Carter DC. Biliary surgery in the same admission for gallstone-associated acute pancreatitis. Br J Surg 1981;68:758–761.
137. Windsor JA. Gallstone pancreatitis: a proposed management strategy. Aust NZ J Surg 1990;60:589–594.

138. Kelly TR. Gallstone pancreatitis. Arch Surg 1974;109:294–297.
139. Canal DF, Broadie TA. Results of laparoscopic cholecystectomy for the treatment of gallstone pancreatitis. Am Surg 1994;60: 495–499.
140. Graham LD, Burrus RG, Burns RP, Chandler KE, Barker DE. Laparoscopic cholecystectomy in biliary pancreatitis. Am Surg 1994;6:40–43.
141. Tate JJT, Lau WY, Li AKC. Laparoscopic cholecystectomy for biliary pancreatitis. Br J Surg 1994;81:720–722.
142. Tang E, Stain SC, Tange G, Froes E, Berne TV. Timing of laparoscopic surgery in gallstone pancreatitis. Arch Surg 1995; 130:496–500.
143. de Virgilio C, Verbin C, Chang L, Linder S, Stabile BE, Klein S. Gallstone pancreatitis: the role of preoperative endoscopic retrograde cholangiopancreatography. Arch Surg 1994;129: 909–913.
144. Rijna H, Borgstein PJ, Meuwissen SGM, de Brauw LM, Wildenborg NP, Cuesta MA. Selective preoperative endoscopic retrograde cholangiopancreatography in laparoscopic biliary surgery. Br J Surg 1994;129:909–913.
145. Welbourn CRB, Beckley DE, Eyre-Brook IA. Endoscopic sphincterotomy without cholecystectomy for gallstone pancreatitis. Gut 1995;37:119–120.
146. Winslet MC, Neoptolemos JP. The place of endoscopy in the management of gallstones. Clin Gastroenterol 1991;5:99–129.
147. Neoptolemos JP, Shaw D, Carr-Locke DL. A multivariate analysis of preoperative risk factors in patients with common bile duct stones—implications for treatment. Ann Surg 1989;209:157–161.
148. O'Sullivan JN, Nobrega FT, Morlock CG, Brown ALJ, Bartholomew LG. Acute and chronic pancreatitis in Rochester, Minnesota, 1940–1969. Gastroenterology 1972;62:373–379.
149. Trapnell JE, Duncan EH. Patterns of incidence of acute pancreatitis. Br Med J 1975;2(5964):179–183.
150. Corfield AP, Cooper MJ, Williamson RCN. Acute pancreatitis: a lethal disease of increasing incidence. Gut 1985;26:724–729.
151. Bourke JB, Giggs JA, Ebdon DS. Variations in the incidence and spatial distribution of patients with primary acute pancreatitis in Nottingham 1969–1976. Gut 1979;20:366–371.
152. McMahon MJ. Incidence and mortality of acute pancreatitis. Br Med J 1977;2:1350.
153. Thomson HJ. Acute pancreatitis in North and North-East Scotland. J R Coll Surg Edinb 1987;30:104–111.
154. Copenhagen Pancreatitis Study Group. An interim report from a prospective epidemiological multicentre study. Scand J Gastroenterol 1981;16:305–312.
155. Gatell JM, Galindo F, Camps J, Milla J. Pancreatitis aguda en el area de Barcelona. Consideaciones epidepiologicas. Gastroenterol Hepatol 1979;2:136–140.
156. Grilo A, Criado J, Martin M. Caracteristicas epidemiologicas de las pancreatitis agudas en la comarca de Moriles-Cabra. Gastroenterol Hepatol 1989;12:123–128.
157. Carballo F. Estudio multicentrico ACAD sobre evaluation pronostica precoz en pancreatitis aguda: casuistica y aspectos epidemiologicos. Rev Asoc Castellana Apar Digest 1990;6: 96–100.
158. Enquist IF, Gliedman ML. Gross autopsy findings in cases of fatal acute pancreatitis. Arch Surg 1958;77:985–991.
159. Berman LG, Dunn E, Straehley CJ. Survey of pancreatitis. Central N.Y. Surgical Society. Gastroenterology 1961;40:94–108.
160. Acosta JM, Pellegrini CA, Skinner DB. Etiology and pathogenesis of acute biliary pancreatitis. Surgery 1980;88:118–125.
161. Efron G. The natural history of pancreatitis. Br J Surg 1966;53: 702–706.
162. Gillespie WJ. Observations of acute pancreatitis. A retrospective clinical study. Br J Surg 1973;60:63–65.
163. Edlund Y, Noback B, Risholm L. Acute pancreatitis, etiology and prevention of recurrence. Follow up study of 188 patients. Rev Surg 1968;25:153–157.
164. Svensson JO, Norback B, Bokey EL, Edlund Y. Changing patterns in aetiology of pancreatitis in an urban Swedish area. Br J Surg 1979;66:159–161.
165. Kessler E, Mieny CJ. Biliary pancreatitis. S Afr Med J 1975;49:2046–2048.
166. Battersby C, Chapuis P. Acute pancreatitis: the Queensland scene. Aust NZ J Surg 1977;47:204–209.
167. Sharon T, Melmed S, Neuman G. Acute pancreatitis in a community with a low alcohol intake. Int Surg 1979;64:63–66.
168. Tondleli P, Stutz K, Harder F, Schuppisser JP, Allgower M. Acute gallstone pancreatitis: best timing for surgery. Br J Surg 1982;69: 709–710.
169. Pederzoli P, Bassi C, Falconi M, De Santis L, Uomo G, et al. Gabexate mesilate in the treatment of acute pancreatitis. Ann Ital Chir 1995;66:191–195.
170. Lankisch PG, Droge M, Gottesleben F. Drug induced acute pancreatitis: incidence and severity. Gut 1995;37:565–567.
171. Wilson D, Imrie CW, Carter DC. Fatal acute pancreatitis. Gut 1988;29:782–788.
172. Acosta JM, Rossi R, Galli OMR, Pelegrini CA, Skinner DB. Early surgery for acute gallstone pancreatitis: evaluation of a systematic approach. Surgery 1978;83:367–370.
173. McMahon MJ, Shefta JR. Physical characteristics of gallstones and the calibre of the cystic duct in patients with acute pancreatitis. Br J Surg 1980;67:6–9.
174. Uomo G, Rabitti PG, Laccetti M, Visconti M. Pancreatico-choledochal junction and pancreatic duct system morphology in acute biliary pancreatitis. A prospective study with early ERCP. Int J Pancreatol 1993;13:187–191.
175. Neoptolemos JP, London NJM, Carr-Locke DL. Assessment of main pancreatic duct integrity by endoscopic retrograde pancreatography in patients with acute pancreatitis. Br J Surg 1993;80:94–99.
176. Schmitz-Moorman P, Schwerk W, Sinn P. Histological alteration of the preampullary common bile and pancreatic duct in acute biliary and nonbiliary pancreatitis. Digestion 1986;34:93–100.
177. Foulis AK. Histological evidence of initiating factors in acute necrotising pancreatitis in man. J Clin Pathol 1980;33:1125–1131.
178. Guelrud M, Mendoza S, Vincent S, Gomez M, Villalta B. Pressures in the sphincter of Oddi in patients with gallstones, common duct stones and recurrent pancreatitis. J Clin Gastroenterol 1983;5:37–41.
179. Widdison AL, Karanjia ND, Reber HA. Routes of spread of pathogens into the pancreas in a feline model of acute pancreatitis. Gut 1994;35:1306–1310.
180. Paloyan D, Simonowitz D, Skinner DB. The timing of biliary tract operations in patients with pancreatitis associated with gallstones. Surg Gynecol Obstet 1975;141:737–739.
181. Elfstrom J. The timing of cholecystectomy in patients with gallstone pancreatitis. Acta Chir Scand 1978;144:487–490.
182. Semel L, Schrieber D, Fromm D. Gallstone pancreatitis. Support for a flexible approach. Arch Surg 1983;118:901–903.
183. Oria A, Alvarez J, Chiappetta L, Spina JC, Hernadez N, et al. Choledocholithiasis in acute gallstone pancreatitis. Incidence and clinical significance. Arch Surg 1991;126:566–568.
184. Anonymous. Death from acute pancreatitis. M. R. C. multicentre trial of alucagon and aprotinin. Lancet 1977;2:632–635.
185. Welch JP, White CE. Acute pancreatitis of biliary origin: is urgent operation necessary? Am J Surg 1982;143:120.
186. Mayer AD, McMahon MJ, Benson EA, Axon ATR. Operations upon the biliary tract in patients with acute pancreatitis: aims indications and timing. Ann R Coll Surg Engl 1984;66:179–183.
187. Burch JM, Felaciano DV, Mattox KL, Jordan GL. Gallstone pancreatitis. Arch Surg 1990;125:853–860.
188. Van der Spuy S. Endoscopic sphincterotomy in the management of gallstone pancreatitis. Endoscopy 1981;13:25–26.
189. Kautz G, Kohaus H, Keferstein RD, Bunte H. Zur pathogenese und endoskopischen therapic der okuten pankreatitis. Klinikarzt 1982;11:1202–1212.
190. Riemann JF, Lux G. Therapeutische strategie bei der akuten pankreatitis. Fortschr Med 1984;102:179–182.
191. Rosseland AR, Solhaug JH. Early or delayed endoscopic papillotomy (EPT) in gallstone pancreatitis. Ann Surg 1984;199: 165–167.
192. Van Husen N. Endoscopic sphincterotomy of Vater's ampulla in acute biliary pancreatitis. Schweiz Rundsch Med Prax 1986;75: 249–251.
193. Leung JWC, Chung SCS, Mok SD, Li AKC. Role of early ERCP and sphincterotomy in acute biliary pancreatitis (Abstract). Gut 1987;28:A1384–1385.
194. Escourrou J, Ligoury C, Boyer J, Sahel J. Emergency endoscopic

sphincterotomy in acute biliary pancreatitis: results of a multicenter study (Abstract). Gastrointest Endosc 1987;33:187–188.

195. Farkas IE, Tulassay Z, Papp J. Endoscopic sphincterotomy in acute biliary pancreatitis: results of an international study (Abstract). Digestion 1988;40:80.
196. Lygrn I, Jacobsen CD, Rosseland AR, Tronnes S. Endoscopic retrograde cholangiopancreatography in patients with suspected acute gallstone pancreatitis. Tidsskr Nor Laegeforen 1990;110:1216–1218.
197. Dufek V, Spicek J, Kodadova J. Endoscopic treatment of acute biliary pancreatitis (Abstract). Hepatogastroenterology 1990; 37(suppl II):A5.
198. Shemesh E, Czerniak A, Schneabaum S, Nass S. Early endoscopic sphincterotomy in the management of acute gallstone pancreatitis in elderly patients. J Am Geriatr Soc 1990;38:893–896.
199. Saowaros V. Endoscopic sphincterotomy in the treatment of acute gallstone pancreatitis. J Med Assoc Thai 1990:629–633.
200. Karjalainen J, Airo I, Nordback I. Routine early endoscopic cholangiography, sphincterotomy and removal of common duct stones in acute gallstone pancreatitis. Eur J Surg 1992;158: 549–553.
201. Safrany L, Fritscher-Ravens A. Endoscopische papillotomie in der behandlung der akuten biliaren panckreatitis. In: Kozuschek W, Paquet KJ, eds. Pankreas: dignostik, therapie. Munich: Karger, 1992:119–125.
202. Manes G, Nomo G, Rabitti PG, Carraturd I, Pacelli I, et al. Role of ERCP and endoscopic sphincterotomy (ES) in the management of acute biliary pancreatitis (ABP). Ital J Gastroenterol 1993;25:287–288.
203. Raker JW, Bartlett MK. Acute pancreatitis: the fate of the patient surviving one or more acute attacks. N Engl J Med 1953;249:751.
204. Albo R, Silen W, Goldmann L. A critical clinical analysis of acute pancreatitis. Arch Surg 1963;86:1032.
205. Glenn F, Frey C. Re-evaluation of the treatment of pancreatitis associated with biliary tract disease. Ann Surg 1964;160:723–726.
206. Dixon JA, Hillam JD. Surgical treatment of biliary tract disease associated with acute pancreatitis. Am J Surg 1970;120:371–375.
207. Rhodes M, Armstrong CP, Longstaff A, Cawthorn S. Laparoscopic cholecystectomy with endoscopic retrograde cholangiopancreatography for acute gallstone pancreatitis. Br J Surg 1993;80:247.
208. Soper NJ, Brunt LM, Callery MP, Edmundowicz SA, Aliperti G. Role of laparoscopic cholecystectomy in the management of acute gallstone pancreatitis. Am J Surg 1994;167:42–51.
209. Taylor EW, Dunham RH, Bloch JH. Laparscopic management of gallstone pancreatitis. J Laparoendosc Surg 1994;4:121–125.
210. Davidson BR, Neoptolemos JP, Carr-Locke DL. Endoscopic sphincterotomy for common bile duct calculi in patients with gallbladder in situ considered unfit for surgery. Gut 1988;29: 114–120.
211. Hill J, Martin DF, Tweedle DE. Risks of leaving the gallbladder in situ after endoscopic sphincterotomy for bile duct stones. Br J Surg 1991;78:554–557.
212. Nowak A, Blaszczynska M, Nowakowska-Dulaw AE, Marek TA. Endoscopic sphincterotomy applied for acute biliary pancreatitis prevents further attacks of this disease. A prospective follow-up study. 10th World Congress of Gastroenterology, 1994.

# 23

# *Acute Alcoholic Pancreatitis*

K. Z'graggen, W. Uhl, and M. W. Büchler

The most frequently reported causes of acute pancreatitis are gallstones and alcohol, in 60–80% of all patients (Table 23.1). The incidence of the two causes varies with geographic and cultural factors. However, whether acute pancreatitis due to alcohol occurs in an otherwise healthy pancreas has been discussed for more than 30 years (1–3). This controversy was initiated by Sarles et al. (1). Today we know that in most patients, alcohol causes chronic pancreatitis, and most episodes of acute alcoholic pancreatitis are bouts of the underlying chronic pancreatitis (4). However, it is also becoming increasingly clear that alcohol can cause a true acute pancreatitis in a small percentage of patients (5). Autopsy studies have shown that acute pancreatitis caused by alcohol may occur without histologic changes that typically are observed in chronic pancreatitis (6, 7). This chapter discusses the relevant acute effects of alcohol on the pancreas and the incidence, treatment, prognosis and follow-up of acute alcoholic pancreatitis.

### Definition

Acute alcoholic pancreatitis is defined as *an episode of acute upper abdominal pain in combination with elevated pancreatic serum enzymes (a threefold increase above the upper normal limit) caused by alcohol. A biliary cause has to be excluded by ultrasonography and/or endoscopic retrograde cholangiopancreatography (ERCP). However, in a few patients suffering from acute pancreatitis, both causal factors can be present.*

Considering this definition, one has to keep in mind that isolated binge drinking of alcohol with consecutive high blood ethanol levels is rarely associated with pancreatic injury or acute alcoholic pancreatitis (8–11). Acute pancreatitis is rather precipitated by an alcoholic binge after a long history of chronic alcohol abuse. A careful evaluation of the patient's history usually reveals a daily consumption of more than 40 g of alcohol (12). In clinical practice, the diagnosis of acute pancreatitis is complicated by the fact that in 10% of alcohol intoxications, the salivary amylase level in serum is elevated (13, 14). On the other hand, a long history of alcohol abuse does not necessarily mean that a patient has an underlying chronic pancreatitis. There is an individually variable organ sensibility to alcohol toxicity. Among alcoholics, 80% do not develop a clinically apparent disease. The incidence of cirrhosis is 15%, pancreatitis is encountered in 5%, and a combination of the two occurs in only 1% (15).

## INCIDENCE

The real incidence of acute alcoholic pancreatitis is difficult to determine. Bradley tried to calculate the attack rate in alcoholic patients and reported an incidence of 7.6 per 1000 alcoholics per year (16). However, this figure is thought to underestimate the problem, (17) and the exact incidence is not available. Furthermore, the known incidence rates always include acute alcoholic pancreatitis with and without underlying chronic pancreatitis.

The percentage of acute alcoholic pancreatitis varies in reported series of acute pancreatitis from 4.4% to more than 60% (18–24) and is difficult to analyze. Many factors influence these figures, such as cultural drinking habits, geographic area, the population analyzed, nutritional factors, and the incidence of gallstone disease. Patient populations of metropolitan areas with high rates of malnourished alcoholics obviously demonstrate higher rates of acute alcoholic pancreatitis (25) than mixed general patient populations of rural areas. However, most studies investigating acute pancreatitis in comparable populations over periods of many years indicate a relative and absolute increase of the alcoholic type of acute pancreatitis (19, 26) and also indicate that acute alcoholic pancreatitis is largely a disease of males below the age of 60 years (27). An interesting recent Swedish publication reported that the incidence of acute alcoholic pancreatitis paralleled the amount of consumed distilled spirits but not that of wine or beer. Therefore, the authors suggested that spirit consumption is a risk factor for both acute alcoholic pancreatitis and other alcohol-associated diseases in Sweden (28).

Even more difficult than determining the incidence of acute attacks of chronic pancreatitis is evaluating the percentage of acute alcoholic pancreatitis attacks in patients with an otherwise healthy pancreas. Considering the data from autopsy studies and the incidence of alcoholic pancreatitis in series of acute pancreatitis, this figure has been found to be below 15% (3).

## ACUTE EFFECTS OF ALCOHOL ON THE NORMAL PANCREAS

To investigate the direct effects of ethanol on pancreatic function in vivo, ethanol has to be administered by the intravenous route, because intragastric administration probably involves additional physiologic reflex responses. In vivo experiments showed that ethanol given intravenously did not influence pancreatic secretion in nonalcoholic humans or animals (5). The "physiologic" effect of alcohol in healthy nonalcoholics is inhibition of pancreatic secretion. This effect was observed when gastric acid production was diverted from the duodenum and was thought to be predominantly mediated by cholinergic nerves (29, 30). In contrast, ethanol administered to chronically alcoholic animals stimulates pancreatic secretion (31), an effect possibly induced by a change of muscarinic receptors at the acinar level (32).

The issue is far more complicated when the effects of gastric administration of alcohol are investigated. In contrast to the intravenous route, this results in weak stimulation of the exocrine function (33), an effect that is almost reversed when alcohol is ingested in combination with a meal (34). Although the results of different investigations are contradictory, alcohol probably induces a slight exocrine hypersecretion in patients with a pancreas

**TABLE 23.1. Etiologies in Acute Pancreatitis Excluding Patients with Pancreatic Abscess (29 patients) and Pancreatic Pseudocysts (63 patients)**

| Etiology | Acute Edematous Pancreatitis (*n* = 925) | Acute Necrotizing Pancreatitis (*n* = 226) |
|---|---|---|
| Alcoholic | 52% | 50% |
| Biliary | 32% | 28% |
| Other | 16% | 22% |

Data from the University of Ulm, 1130 patients from 5/82 to 5/92, Departments of Gastroenterology and General Surgery.

preconditioned by ethanol. Additionally, in vitro studies on isolated pancreatic acini also indicate a general stimulatory effect of alcohol on the pancreas (5, 35).

## HYPOTHESIS ON THE PATHOPHYSIOLOGY OF ACUTE ALCOHOLIC PANCREATITIS

Different pathogenetic hypotheses have been proposed with respect to the development of acute alcoholic pancreatitis: *(a)* ductal factors, *(b)* cellular factors, and *(c)* vascular factors (Table 23.2).

### Ductal Factors

Theories that suggested *duodenopancreatic reflux* as a possible pathogenetic mechanism for acute alcoholic pancreatitis were based on the Pfeffer loop preparations and hypothesized that alcohol reduced the tone of the sphincter of Oddi, allowing reflux of activated enzymes into the pancreatic duct (36–38). These models do not represent physiologic conditions, and the concentration of alcohol in the duodenal loop required to induce acute alcoholic pancreatitis far exceeded the 1–3% concentration in the duodenum observed in man after ethanol consumption. Alcohol and bile in common were also accused of being an important factor in the induction of acute alcoholic pancreatitis, but experiments in the rat did not support this hypothesis (39). In addition, the duodenal pressure does not increase enough to allow duodenopancreatic reflux, and pancreatic duct pressures are usually higher than those in the biliary tract system. Furthermore, intraduodenal pressure showed only a slight and transient increase after gastric ethanol administration in a cat model (40). A strong clinical argument also discounts reflux as a possible important pathophysiologic factor in acute alcoholic pancreatitis. After sphincterotomy, pancreatitis does not occur more frequently, although reflux of the duodenal contents is greatly facilitated.

*Ductal hypertension* is thought to be a major mechanism responsible for the induction of biliary pancreatitis (41). In acute alcoholic pancreatitis, different factors may alter the flow and lead to pancreatic duct hypertension. The acute effect of ethanol leads to an increase of the muscular tone of the sphincter of Oddi in humans as well as in animals (40, 42, 43). In addition, the observed pancreatic *hypersecretion* in response to alcohol in preconditioned animals supports the importance of a hypertensive factor (31). However, ductal hypertension is probably not the only pathogenetic mechanism, as a pressure of up to 80 mm Hg is needed for the disruption of ductal integrity (44). In a rat model, the importance of the sphincter mechanism was not supported, rather a state of *exocrine hyperstimulation* was thought to increase the susceptibility to alcohol-related injury in the pancreas (45). Grönroos et al. published a new theory of the pathogenesis of alcoholic pancreatitis, the *cholinergic hypothesis,* which was supported by a series of investigations (46–49). The theory was based on the idea that chronic alcohol intake resulted in dysregulation of pancreatic secretion. Tiscornia et al. had previously shown that chronic alcohol intake diminished responsiveness to cholinergic stimulation, an effect that was thought to involve muscarinic receptors (50, 51). Grönroos demonstrated that the number of pancreatic muscarinic receptors decreased by 60% after chronic intake of alcohol (47). On the other hand, the concentration of pancreatic acetylcholine after chronic alcohol intake increased significantly, a finding in keeping with decreased acetylcholine esterase activity (50–53). This led to the hypothesis that chronic ethanol consumption resulted in an increased acetylcholine concentration relative to the muscarinic receptor density, mimicking the induction mechanism of acute hyperstimulation pancreatitis. This mechanism, known to induce acute pancreatitis in animals and man (48), is similar to the mechanism triggering human acute pancreatitis by scorpion venom or insecticides (49).

Harvey et al. (40) introduced an attractive hypothesis that combines different experimental aspects of acute alcoholic pancreatitis. In a series of experiments, they demonstrated that intragastric alcohol resulted in increased ductal pressure, probably mediated by increased tone in the sphincter of Oddi. The combination of elevated ductal pressure with ethanol concentrations similar to those found after intragastric alcohol administration led to an increase in *duct permeability.* Finally, perfusion of the ducts of these animals by activated pancreatic enzymes initiated an acute edematous pancreatitis.

Sarles and coworkers isolated a pancreatic protein, subsequently termed "pancreatic stone protein" (54–56). The *ductal plug hypothesis* states that in patients and animals with chronic ethanol consumption, the basal secretion of pancreatic enzymes increases, whereas water and bicarbonate content decreases (57). In combination with an expected decrease in pancreatic stone protein concentration, plugs result, leading to obstruction and consequent inflammation of the small ducts. The composition of pancreatic juice is also altered by an increase in mucus content as well as by viscosity and trypsin activity changes (58, 59). Although the principal components of these precipitates have been shown to be "pancreatic stone proteins" (60, 61), whether these proteins are key elements in the induction of alcoholic pancreatitis is not resolved (5).

### Cellular Factors

Ethanol or one of its metabolites may cause toxic injury of pancreatic acinar cells. With respect to *ethanol toxicity,* many alterations of pancreatic cell functions have been described. These include changes in the cytoplasmic deposition of fat, and in rats fed a protein-deficient diet, the cellular accumulation of cholesteryl ester was more pronounced (62). A decrease in the trypsin-inhibiting capacity together with a specific increase of proteolytic as well as lysosomal enzymes has been demonstrated

**TABLE 23.2. Possible Pathophysiologic Factors and Hypotheses Involved in Acute Alcoholic Pancreatitis**

| | |
|---|---|
| Ductal factors | Duodenopancreatic reflux |
| | Ductal hypertension |
| | Secretory changes |
| | Cholinergic hypothesis |
| | Increased ductal permeability |
| | Ductal plug hypothesis |
| Cellular factors | Ethanol toxicity |
| | Acetaldehyde toxicity |
| | Inappropriate enzyme activation |
| | Toxic oxygen metabolites |
| Vascular factors | Pancreatic blood flow reduction |
| | Increased microvascular permeability |

(63, 64). The latter findings led to the hypothesis that proteolytic and lysosomal enzymes were mixed intracellularly, leading to *inappropriate enzyme activation* that resulted in autodigestion of the gland (65, 66). Nordback et al. investigated the *effect of acetaldehyde,* the major metabolite of ethanol, and suggested that acetaldehyde has a toxic effect on the pancreatic parenchyma in the presence of xanthine oxidase (67). Furthermore, *toxic oxygen metabolites* are thought to play an important intermediary role in the induction of acute alcoholic pancreatitis. These findings have been confirmed in studies recently published (68–70).

### Vascular Factors

The importance of circulatory changes, either in the pancreas itself or hemodynamic changes as a result of acute pancreatitis, have been discussed as initiating factors of the disease. Many complications and lethal outcomes may result from the amplifying effects of microcirculatory disturbances with decreased capillary perfusion in the pancreas (71–73). On the other hand, patients developing necrotizing pancreatitis demonstrate a hyperdynamic vascular pattern during the initial phase of the disease in contrast to patients with acute edematous pancreatitis (74). These changes do not depend upon the cause of acute pancreatitis. However, the question of whether vascular changes in the pancreas are of pathogenetic importance or the result of the progressing inflammation, especially in acute alcoholic pancreatitis, is more difficult to address.

An alcohol-induced reduction of pancreatic blood flow has been suggested to play a role in pancreatic lesions associated with alcohol abuse (75–77). Alcohol-mediated reduction of capillary flow associated with a decreased oxygen saturation of hemoglobin has been shown in animal experiments (78). In addition, microvascular permeability probably increases as a result of local regulatory mechanisms by vasoactive agents during the inflammation (79). These microvascular changes can be reduced by stimulation of dopaminergic and ß-adrenergic receptors (80, 81). As a consequence, administration of dopamine reduces the inflammation in the cat model of alcoholic pancreatitis (82).

Considering the aforementioned data that help explain important events in the pathogenesis of acute alcoholic pancreatitis, probably many different factors rather than isolated mechanisms are responsible for the initiation and progression of the disease. However, their relative pathophysiologic importance needs further experimental and clinical investigation.

## CLINICAL PRESENTATION AND DIAGNOSIS

The diagnosis of acute alcoholic pancreatitis still relies on the clinical presentation and laboratory parameters, as does the diagnosis of the other etiologic forms of acute pancreatitis (83–85). However, some specific clinical features have to be mentioned. A detailed history usually reveals that the patient has been abusing alcohol for several years, and a history of repeated pain episodes also points to alcohol as the cause of the presented complaints. Few patients present with acute alcoholic pancreatitis after their first acute abuse of alcohol. Upper gastrointestinal bleeding is usually caused by an accompanying alcoholic gastritis. If pronounced pain leading to alcohol withdrawal has been present for a few days, patients may demonstrate increased irritability or even clear signs of delirium tremens. Radiologic evaluation by either plain abdominal x-ray or computed tomography (CT) scan may show calcifications of the pancreas, a rare but pathognomonic sign of an underlying chronic pancreatitis. The characteristic ERCP findings of chronic pancreatitis are usually not known when the patient is hospitalized with a first attack of acute alcoholic pancreatitis.

### Pancreatic Enzymes and Specific Laboratory Tests

The laboratory diagnosis of acute alcoholic pancreatitis is still based on the measurement of specific pancreatic enzymes. The most widely used tests are pancreatic amylase and lipase, but normal serum amylase levels are more frequently encountered in alcoholic than in nonalcoholic pancreatitis (86). In contrast to published reports (87–89), serum lipase levels did not differ among etiologic groups in a recently published prospective study (Fig. 23.1) (12). Tests with higher diagnostic sensitivity for acute pancreatitis, such as measurement of carboxylic ester hydrolase, have been described but did not allow an etiologic differentiation (90).

Assessment of the severity of acute pancreatitis, whether of alcoholic or of other origin, is facilitated by serum parameters

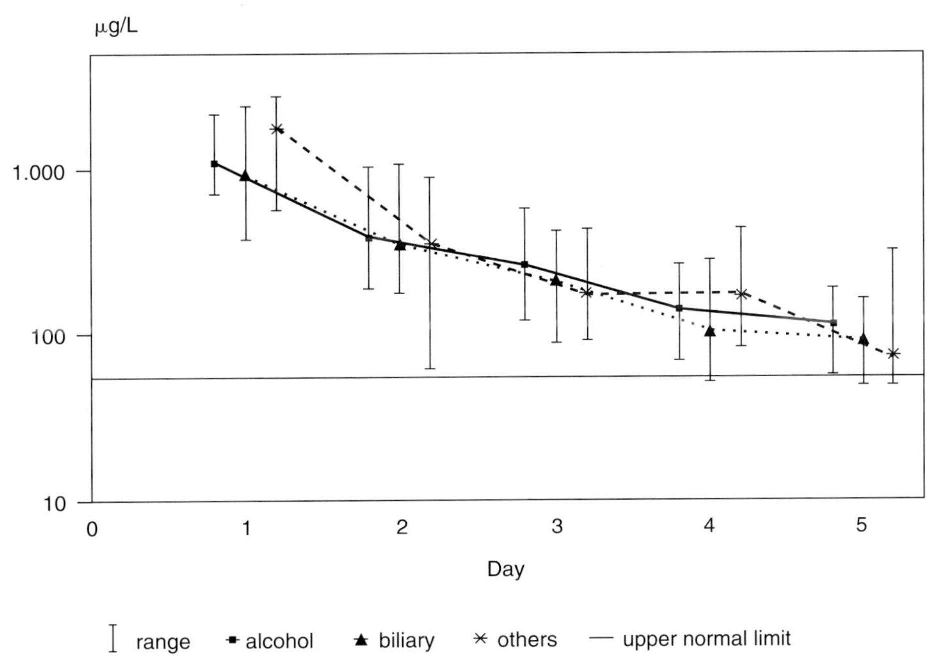


**FIG. 23.1.** Serum lipase in relation to the main causes of acute pancreatitis (normal <56 mg/L).

such as C-reactive protein (CRP), antiproteases, complement factors, and phospholipase $A_2$ (91, 92). Determination of CRP was shown to be the most valuable single serum parameter in this respect, but in our experience, none of the examined parameters could differentiate between acute alcoholic pancreatitis and nonalcoholic pancreatitis (Fig. 23.2).

Whether alcoholic pancreatitis can be distinguished from that caused by gallstones or that of other etiologies has been discussed for a long time (93). Indeed, gallstone pancreatitis is sometimes characterized by an elevation of hepatic enzymes. An increase of serum aspartate aminotransaminase (ASAT) above 80 U/L is a particularly strong indicator for a biliary cause (94). The question of whether acute alcoholic pancreatitis can be characterized by standardized laboratory parameters is still open. Renewed interest in this topic was stimulated by various recent publications.

Gumaste et al. (95) showed that the lipase:amylase ratio distinguished acute episodes of alcoholic pancreatitis from nonalcoholic pancreatitis. The sensitivity, specificity, and positive predictive value of a lipase:amylase ratio above 2 in detecting acute alcoholic pancreatitis were 91, 78, and 85%, respectively. The authors stressed the importance of an early assessment (i.e., within a day or two after the onset of symptoms). The value of this ratio for the diagnosis of acute alcoholic pancreatitis was supported by a retrospective study by Tenner and Steinberg (96), but others could not confirm its usefulness (94, 97). Jaakola et al. showed that the level of carbohydrate-deficient transferrin (CDT) correlated with ethanol consumption and that elevated levels detected an alcoholic cause of disease with a specificity of 100% and a sensitivity of 75%, with a cutoff level of 17 U/L.

Finally, trypsin activity was proposed as a new marker of acute alcoholic pancreatitis (98). The rationale of this test is that chronic alcohol consumption increases trypsinogen synthesis and that acute alcoholic pancreatitis results in a higher basal trypsinogen output in pancreatic juice (99–101). A concurrent decreased activity of $\alpha_2$-macroglobulin (102), the main inhibitor of trypsin, leads to high circulating trypsin activity levels.

## PROGNOSIS

Several studies examining the influence of the cause in acute pancreatitis suggest that the course of the disease in acute alcoholic pancreatitis differs with respect to severity, complications, and mortality rates from pancreatitis of other origins (75–77, 88). This is attributed to different pathophysiologic mechanisms in pancreatitis from different causes (103). These studies support the view that alcoholic pancreatitis, in contrast to biliary pancreatitis, more often is mild and self-limiting. This difference was only in part explained by demographic factors, as acute alcoholic pancreatitis is usually seen in relatively young males (less than 50 years), compared with acute biliary pancreatitis, which is observed in elderly women, with higher comorbidity. However, this hypothesis relies mainly on the results of retrospective studies. Our prospective analysis in patients with acute pancreatitis did not detect differences in the severity and course among etiologic subgroups (12). All patients included in the study had a first attack of acute pancreatitis and were admitted to the hospital within 72 hours after the onset of clinical symptoms. A contrast-enhanced CT scan was performed in all patients within 24 hours after admission.

Comparison of the three etiologic groups—alcoholic pancreatitis, biliary pancreatitis, and pancreatitis of other origins—demonstrated no differences with regard to the severity of the disease when assessed by two scoring systems, Ranson and Bank (104, 105). Analysis by age and sex confirmed the expected differences: male predominance and a mean age of 43 years in alcoholic pancreatitis, compared with female sex and a mean age of 59 years in biliary pancreatitis. The analyzed serum parameters (lipase, CRP, antiproteases, ASAT) showed no differences in the various etiologic groups with the exception of ASAT, which showed a significant increase in the biliary acute pancreatitis group during the first 2 days. Serum lipase levels as a diagnostic marker and CRP values as an indicator for necrotizing pancreatitis are demonstrated in Figures 23.1 and 23.2. Morphologic evaluation of the different groups (edematous pancreatitis,

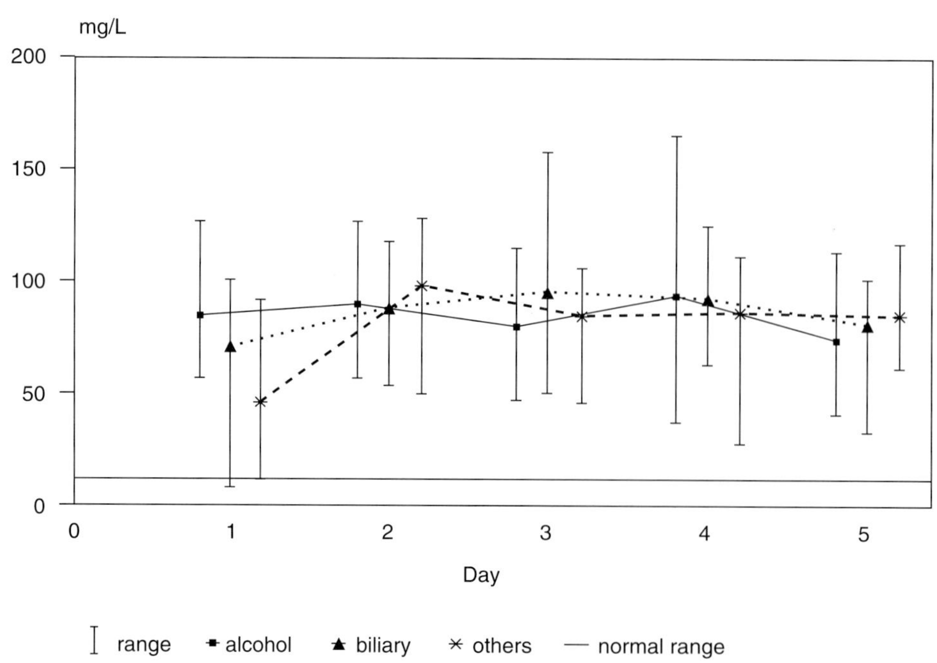


**FIG. 23.2.** Serum CRP in relation to the main causes of acute pancreatitis (normal range <12 mg/L).

**TABLE 23.3. Morphologic Findings, Frequency of Infected Necroses, and Mortality Rates in the Three Etiologic Subgroups**

| | Acute Alcoholic Pancreatitis *n* = 94 (50%) | Acute Biliary Pancreatitis *n* = 60 (31%) | Other Acute Pancreatitis *n* = 36 (19%) |
|---|---|---|---|
| Acute edematous pancreatitis | 58/94 (62%) | 36/60 (60%) | 22/36 (61%) |
| Acute necrotizing pancreatitis | 36/94 (38%) | 24/60 (40%) | 14/36 (39%) |
| Infected pancreatic necroses | 11/36 (31%) | 9/24 (38%) | 6/14 (43%) |
| Mortality | 5.3% | 10% | 5.5% |

necrotizing pancreatitis), as shown in Table 23.3, revealed comparable percentages of pancreatic necroses in the three etiologic groups and no significant differences in the relative numbers of infected pancreatic necroses.

Finally, no significant differences in organ complications (Table 23.4)or morbidity and mortality rates (Table 23.3) have been found. Although a tendency to a decreased mortality rate in the alcoholic pancreatitis group was observed, the number of patients was too small to reach significance. In addition, the patients in the biliary pancreatitis group were older, and the difference in mortality may be attributed to an increase in comorbidity. We therefore concluded that the cause had no influence on the course and severity of acute pancreatitis.

The course of acute pancreatitis depends mainly on the extent of pancreatic and peripancreatic necroses and their infection with bacteria, irrespective of the underlying cause (106–108). The necroses usually develop within 4 days after the clinical onset of acute pancreatitis and are best detected by a contrast-enhanced CT scan (109, 110).

## TREATMENT

Most patients with acute pancreatitis can be managed conservatively and according to standard treatment protocols (111). Management follows the same principles as that in other types of acute pancreatitis (see Chapters 21, 22, and 28). Strict observation of the patient in an intensive care unit during the first few days of the disease, with regular measurements of the markers of necrosis, is usually indicated. In severe necrotizing pancreatitis, repetitive fine-needle aspirations, guided by CT scan or ultrasonography, prove the bacterial infection (112). The bacterial infection determines the course and outcome of acute pancreatitis and is usually the indication for operative treatment (111, 113, 114). Different operative procedures have been shown to reduce the mortality to 10–15% (107, 115–117); our preference, with equally good results, is necrosectomy with postoperative closed local lavage of the retroperitoneum (118).

## FOLLOW-UP

Data on the evolution of the pancreas after acute pancreatitis are scarce. A full regeneration of the pancreas after a necrotizing course is particularly difficult to imagine. In patients with acute alcoholic pancreatitis, the accuracy of the functional results is reduced because the pancreatic function may have been impaired before the attack by chronic alcohol abuse (119). The reported results of exocrine and endocrine pancreatic dysfunctions are conflicting (120–122), mostly because the investigated populations with acute pancreatitis included different percentages of alcoholic patients. Assessment of the exocrine pancreas, for example, showed dysfunction in 30–86% in follow-up after severe pancreatitis (120–122); impaired endocrine function was reported in up to 90%. Our own results after acute necrotizing pancreatitis revealed endocrine and exocrine dysfunction in 57%; normal morphologic findings assessed by CT scan and ERCP were found in only 24% (119). A second study, including patients with acute edematous and necrotizing pancreatitis, examined the functional and morphologic results in relation to the etiology (123). Patients after acute edematous pancreatitis demonstrated the expected full functional and morphologic recovery after a follow-up of more than 12 months, irrespective of the underlying cause. But during the initial 12 months, 57% of patients with edematous pancreatitis and 14% of patients with mild biliary pancreatitis had impaired exocrine function as assessed by three different tests. The endocrine function investigated by an oral glucose tolerance test was normal in both groups.

The results of the follow-up studies of patients after necrotizing pancreatitis are summarized in Table 23.5. About two-thirds of patients showed endocrine and exocrine dysfunction as well as morphologic changes. The difference in exocrine function between patients with alcoholic and biliary etiologies was significant. These results are in accordance with reports of Dormeyer et al. and Seligson et al. (120, 122) but contradict a report of Angelini et al. (124). The latter analysis indicated that the

**TABLE 23.4. Complications in 190 Patients Suffering from Acute Pancreatitis in Relation to the Main Etiologies of the Disease**

| Complications | Acute Alcoholic Pancreatitis *n* = 94 (50%) | Acute Biliary Pancreatitis *n* = 60 (31%) | Other Acute Pancreatitis *n* = 36 (19%) |
|---|---|---|---|
| Pulmonary insufficiency[a] | 29/94 (31%) | 23/60 (38%) | 15/36 (42%) |
| Renal insufficiency[b] | 17/94 (18%) | 10/60 (17%) | 8/36 (22%) |
| Cardiocirculatory insufficiency[c] | 6/94 (6%) | 3/60 (5%) | 4/36 (11%) |
| Sepsis[d] | 12/94 (13%) | 3/60 (5%) | 2/36 (6%) |
| Jaundice[e] | 21/94 (22%) | 22/60 (37%) | 7/36 (19%) |
| Ileus[f] | 62/94 (66%) | 41/60 (68%) | 26/36 (72%) |

[a]Need for oxygen supply and/or artificial ventilation.
[b]Serum creatinine >2-fold upper normal limit and/or need for hemodialysis/hemofiltration.
[c]Shock and/or necessity for administration of catecholamines.
[d]Infected pancreatic necrosis diagnosed by fine-needle aspiration and culture or intraoperatively.
[e]Serum total bilirubin >2-fold normal upper limit.
[f]Absence of bowel sounds and distended small bowel loops with air/fluid levels in a plain abdominal x-ray.

**TABLE 23.5. Acute Necrotizing Pancreatitis: Follow-up Results in Relation to the Etiology, Expressed as Percentages of Pathologic Results**

| | Acute Alcoholic Pancreatitis % of Pathological Results | | | Acute Biliary Pancreatitis % of Pathological Results | | |
|---|---|---|---|---|---|---|
| Follow-up | Exocrine | Endocrine | Morphology | Exocrine | Endocrine | Morphology |
| 2–12 months | 95 | 60 | 95 | 72 | 44 | 81 |
| 13–40 months | 68 | 44 | 89 | 30 | 22 | 47 |

From Büchler M, Hauke A, Malfertheiner P. Follow up after acute pancreatitis: morphology and function. In: Beger HG, Büchler M, eds. Acute pancreatitis. Berlin: Springer-Verlag, 1987:367–374.

initially impaired exocrine function was almost completely recovered in long-term follow-up, although endocrine dysfunction and residual morphologic changes were comparable to those in our study.

In contrast to the widespread opinion that a morphologically and functionally complete recovery is more the rule than the exception after acute pancreatitis, one can conclude that the degree and duration of functional and morphologic damage depends on the severity of acute pancreatitis. The changes after necrotizing pancreatitis are mostly irreversible, with the exception of recovery of the exocrine function. Furthermore, differences between alcoholic and biliary pancreatitis can be demonstrated. Alcoholic, rather than biliary, pancreatitis leads to functional and morphologic alterations. These differences are probably due to preexisting changes of an underlying chronic pancreatitis.

## REFERENCES


1. Sarles H, Sarles JC, Camatte R, Muratore R, Gaini M, et al. Observations on 205 confirmed cases of acute pancreatitis, recurring pancreatitis, and chronic pancreatitis. Gut 1965;6:545–559.
2. Skinazi F, Lévy P, Bernardes P. Les pancréatitis aigues alcooliques révèlent-elles toujours une pancréatite chronique? Gastroenterol Clin Biol 1995;19:266–269.
3. Blackstone MO. Can alcohol cause true acute pancreatitis? Gastroenterology 1990;99:1544–1546.
4. Malagelada JR. The pathophysiology of alcoholic pancreatitis. Pancreas 1986;1:270–278.
5. Singh M, Simsek H. Ethanol and the pancreas. Gastroenterology 1990;98:1052–1062.
6. Seligson U, Cho J-W, Ihre T, Lundh G. Clinical course and autopsy findings in acute and chronic pancreatitis. Acta Chir Scand 1982;148:269–274.
7. Renner JG, Savage WT, Pantoja JL, Renner VJ. Death due to acute pancreatitis. A retrospective analysis of 405 autopsy cases. Dig Dis Sci 1985;30:1005–1018.
8. Hammond KB, Rumack BH, Rodgerson DO. Blood ethanol. A report of unusually high levels in a living patient. JAMA 1973;226:63–64.
9. Löwenfels AB, March B, Lee TCM, Rohmann M. Effect of intravenous alcohol on the pancreas. Arch Surg 1968;96:440–441.
10. Löhr J-M, Rabenstein T, Strauss R, Hahn EG, Schneider MU. Does acute ingestion of large amounts of alcohol cause pancreatic injury? Int J Pancreatol 1995;17:155–166.
11. Niederau C, Niederau M, Strohmeyer G, Bertling L, Sonnenberg A. Does acute alcohol consumption of large alcohol amounts lead to pancreatic injury? A prospective study of serum pancreatic enzymes in 300 drunken drivers. Digestion 1990;45:115–120.
12. Uhl W, Isenmann R, Curti G, Vogel R, Beger HG, Büchler MW. Influence of the etiology on the course and outcome of acute pancreatitis. Pancreas, in press.
13. Dutta SK, Douglass W, Smalls UA, Nipper HC, Levitt MD. Prevalence and the nature of hyperamylasemia in acute alcoholism. Dig Dis Sci 1981;26:136–141.
14. Berk JE, Fridhandler L, Webb SF. Does hyperamylasemia in the drunken alcoholic signify pancreatitis. Am J Gastroenterol 1979;71:557.
15. Dreiling DA, Koller M. The natural history of alcoholic pancreatitis: update 1985. Mt Sinai J Med 1985;52:340–342.
16. Bradley EL III. Complications of pancreatitis: medical and surgical management. Philadelphia: WB Saunders, 1982.
17. Reber HA. Alcoholic pancreatitis. In: Howard JM, Jordan GL, Reber HA, eds. Surgical diseases of the pancreas. Philadelphia: Lea & Febiger, 1987:284–296.
18. Edelmann G, Boutellier P. Le traitement des pancréatites aigues par l'ablation chirurgicales précoce des portions nécrosés. Chirurgie 1974;100:155–160.
19. Trapnell JE, Duncan EHL. Patterns of incidence in acute pancreatitis. Br Med J 1975;2:179–183.
20. Svensson JO, Nordback, Key EL, Edlund Y. Changing pattern in aetiology in an urban Swedish area. Br J Surg 1979;66:159–161.
21. Imrie CW, Whyte AS. A prospective study of acute pancreatitis. Br J Surg 1975;62:490–494.
22. Gillespie WJ. Observations on acute pancreatitis. A retrospective clinical study. Br J Surg 1973;60:63–65.
23. Bragg LE, Thompson JS, Burnett DA. Increased incidence of pancreas related complications in patients with postoperative pancreatitis. Am J Surg 1985;150:694–697.
24. Bourke JB. Variation in annual incidence of primary acute pancreatitis in Nottingham 1969–1974. Lancet 1975;2:967–969.
25. Satiani B, Stone HH. Predictability of present outcome and future recurrence in acute pancreatitis. Arch Surg 1979;114:711–715.
26. Corfield AP, Cooper MJ, Williamson RCN. Acute pancreatitis: a lethal disease of increasing incidence. Gut 1985;26:724–729.
27. Thompson SR, Hendry WS, McFarlane GA, Davidson AI. Epidemiology and outcome of acute pancreatitis. Br J Surg 1987;74:398–401.
28. Schmidt DN. Apparent risk factors for chronic and acute pancreatitis in Stockholm County. Spirits but not wine and beer. Int J Pancreatol 1991;8:45–50.
29. Kolbel CBM, Singer MV, Mohle T, Heinzel C, Eysselein V, Goebell H. Action of intravenous ethanol and atropine on the secretion of gastric acid, pancreatic enzymes and bile acids and the motility of the upper gastrointestinal tract in nonalcoholic humans. Pancreas 1986;1:211–218.
30. Bayer M, Rudick J, Lieber SC. Inhibitory effect of ethanol on canine exocrine pancreatic secretion. Gastroenterology 1972;63:619–626.
31. Robles-Diaz G, Devaux MA, Sarles H. Effect of acute and chronic oral administration of ethanol on canine exocrine pancreatic secretion. Digestion 1985;32:77–85.
32. Schmidt DN. Does ethanol exert its effect on the canine pancreas by mediation of cholinergic nerves. Scand J Gastroenterol 1986;21:69–74.
33. Demol P, Singer MV, Hotz J, Hofmann U, Hanssen LE, et al. Action of intragastric ethanol on pancreatic secretion in relation to the interdigestive gastrointestinal motility in humans. Arch Int Physiol Biochem 1986;94:251–259.
34. Jian R, Cortot A, Ducrot F, Jobin G, Chayvialle JA, Modigliani R. Effect of ethanol ingestion on postprandial gastric emptying and secretion, biliopancreatic secretions, and duodenal absorption in man. Dig Dis Sci 1986;31:604–614.
35. Steer ML, Glazer G, Manabe T. Direct effects of ethanol on exocrine secretion from the in vitro rabbit pancreas. Dig Dis Sci 1979;24:769–774.

36. Johnson RH, Doppman J. Duodenal reflux and the etiology of pancreatitis. Surgery 1967;62:462–467.
37. Rosato EF, Oram-Smitz JC, Reber HA, Czernobilsky B, Rosato FE. Papillary integrity as a factor in pancreatic reflux. Am J Surg 1971;121:13–15.
38. Pfeffer RB, Stasior O, Hinton JW. The clinical picture of the sequential developement of acute hemorrhagic pancreatitis in the dog. Surg Forum 1957;8:248–251.
39. Jalovaara P, Rämo OJ, Apaja-Sarkkinen M. Alcoholic bile does not intensify acute pancreatitis in rats. Res Exp Med 1988;188: 235–238.
40. Harvey MH, Cates MC, Reber HA. Possible mechanisms of acute pancreatitis induced by ethanol. Am J Surg 1988;155:49–56.
41. Lerch MM, Saluja AK, Rünzi M, Dawra R, Saluja M, Steer ML. Pancreatic duct obstruction triggers acute necrotizing pancreatitis in the opossum. Gastroenterology 1993;104:853–861.
42. Sarles JC, Midejean R. Electromyographic study of the action of alcohol upon the Oddi's sphincter. Digestion 1973;9:83–85.
43. Capitaine Y, de Barros Mott C, Gullo L, Sarles H. Action de l'ethanol sur la sécretion pancréatique chez l'homme. Biol Gastroenterol 1971;3:193–198.
44. Aho HJ, Suonpaa K, Nevalainen TJ. Experimental pancreatitis in the rat: ductal factors in the sodium taurocholate induced acute pancreatitis. Exp Pathol 1984;25:73–79.
45. Foitzik T, Lewandrowski KB, Fernandez-del Castillo C, Rattner DW, Klar E, Warshaw AL. Exocrine hyperstimulation but not pancreatic duct obstruction increases the susceptibility to alcohol-related pancreatic injury. Arch Surg 1994;129:1081–1085.
46. Grönroos JM. Pathogenesis of acute alcoholic pancreatitis. Lancet 1990;335:1046.
47. Grönroos JM, Kaila T, Aho HJ, et al. Decrease in the number of muscarinic receptors in rat pancreas after chronic alcohol intake. Pharmacol Toxicol 1989;64:356–359.
48. Grönroos JM, Aho HJ, Nevalainen TJ. Cholinergic hypothesis of alcoholic pancreatitis. Dig Dis 1992;10:38–45.
49. Grönroos JM, Kaila T, Hietaranta AJ. Alcohol, pancreatic muscarinic receptors and acute pancreatitis. Exp Toxic Pathol 1993;45:503–505.
50. Tiscornia OM, Dreiling DA. Physiopathogenic hypothesis of alcoholic pancreatitis: supranormal ecbolic stimulation of the "pancreon" units secondary to the loss of the negative component of pancreas innervation. Pancreas 1987;2: 604–612.
51. Perec CJ, Celener D, Tiscornia OM. Effects of chronic ethanol administration on the autonomic innervation of salivary glands, pancreas and heart. Am J Gastroenterol 1979;72:46–59.
52. Baratti C, Rubio M, Perec CJ, et al. Effect of chronic alcohol feeding on adrenergic and cholinergic neurotransmission mechanisms. Gastroenterology 1980;73:21–27.
53. Celener P, de la Porte P, Tiscornia OM, et al. Histochemical study of cholinergic activities in exocrine pancreas of dogs: modifications related to chronic alcoholism. Biomedicine 1977;27: 161–165.
54. Multigner L, deCaro A, Lombardo D, Campese D, Sarles H. Pancreatic stone protein, a phosphoprotein which inhibits calcium carbonate precipitation from human pancreatic juice. Biochem Biophys Res Commun 1983;110:69–74.
55. Guy O, Robles-Diaz G, Adrich Z, Sahel J, Sarles H. Protein content of precipitates present in pancreatic juice of alcoholic subjects and patients with chronic calcifying pancreatitis. Gastroenterology 1983;84:102–107.
56. de Caro A, Lohse J, Sarles H. Characterisation of a protein isolated from pancreatic calculi of men suffering from chronic calcifying pancreatitis. Biochem Biophys Res Commun 1979;87: 1176–1182.
57. Renner IG, Rinderknecht H, Douglas AP. Profiles of pure pancreatic secretions in patients with acute pancreatitis: the possible role of proteolytic enzymes in pathogenesis. Gastroenterology 1978;75:1090–1098.
58. Wakabayashi A, Takeda Y. The behavior of mucopolysaccharide in the pancreatic juice of in chronic pancreatitis. Dig Dis Sci 1976;21:607–612.
59. Tympner F, Rosch W. Viscosity and trypsin activity of pure pancreatic juice in chronic pancreatitis. Acta Hepatogastroenterol 1978;25:73–76.
60. Sarles H, deCaro A, Multigner L, Dagorn J-C. Pancreatic stone protein. Dig Dis Sci 1985;30:905.
61. Schmiegel W, Heringlake S, Kalthoff H, Baisch H, Thiele HG, Greten H. Pancreatic stone protein in chronic pancreatitis. Comparative biochemical and quantitative analyses in sera and in pancreatic secretions (Abstract). Gastroenterology 1989; 96:A451.
62. Wilson JS, Korsten MA, Leo MA, Lieber CS. Combined effect of protein deficiency and chronic ethanol consumption on rat pancreas. Dig Dis Sci 1988;33:1250–1259.
63. Rinderknecht H, Renner IG, Koyama HH. Lysosomal enzymes in pure pancreatic juice from normal healthy volunteers and chronic alcoholics. Dig Dis Sci 1979;24:180–186.
64. Singh M. Alcoholic pancreatitis in rats fed ethanol in a nutritionally adequate liquid diet. Int J Pancreatol 1987;2:311–324.
65. Steer ML, Meldolesi J. The cell biology of experimental pancreatitis. N Engl J Med 1987;316:144–150.
66. Grönroos JM, Meklin LS, Yoshida Y, et al. Changes in zymogen granule membrane and pancreatic juice after supramaximal stimulation with caerulein in the rat. Int J Pancreatol 1988;3: 389–400.
67. Nordback IH, MacGowan S, Potter JJ, Cameron JL. The role of acetaldehyde in the pathogenesis of acute alcoholic pancreatitis. Ann Surg 1991;214:671–678.
68. Schoenberg MH, Büchler MW, Beger HG. Oxygen radicals in experimental acute pancreatitis. Hepatogastroenterology 1994;41:313–319.
69. Schoenberg MH, Büchler MW, Younes M, et al. Effect of antioxidant treatment in rats with acute hemorrhagic pancreatitis. Dig Dis Sci 1994;39:1034–1040.
70. Nordback IH, Olson JL, Chacko VP, Cameron JL. Detailed characterization of experimental acute alcoholic pancreatitis. Surgery 1995;117:41–49.
71. Warshaw AL. Damage prevention versus damage control in acute pancreatitis. Gastroenterology 1993;104:1216–1219.
72. Klar E, Messmer K, Warshaw AL, Herfarth C. Pancreatic ischaemia in experimental acute pancreatitis: mechanism, significance and therapy. Br J Surg 1990;77:1205–1210.
73. Klar E, Endrich B, Messmer K. Microcirculation of the pancreas. A quantitative study of physiology and changes in pancreatitis. Int J Microcirc 1990;9:85–101.
74. Beger HG, Bittner R, Büchler M, Hess W, Schmitz JE. Hemodynamic data pattern in patients with acute pancreatitis. Gastroenterology 1986;90:74–79.
75. Dib JA, Cooper-Vastola SA, Meirelles RF. Acute effects of ethanol and ethanol plus furosemide on pancreatic capillary blood flow in rats. Am J Surg 1993;166:18–23.
76. Horowitz LD, Myers JH. Ethanol-induced alterations in pancreatic blood flow in conscious dogs. Circulation 1982;50: 250–256.
77. Widdison AL, Alvarez C, Schwarz M, Reber HA. The influence of ethanol on pancreatic blood flow in cats with chronic pancreatitis. Surgery 1992;112:201–210.
78. Foitzik T, Fernandez-del Castillo C, Rattner DW, Klar E, Warshaw AL. Alcohol selectively impairs oxygenation of the pancreas. Arch Surg 1995;130:357–361.
79. Glazer G, Bennett A, Dudley HAF. Elevation of prostaglandin like activity in the blood and peritoneal exudate of dogs with acute pancreatitis. Br J Surg 1974;61:922–925.
80. Karanjia ND, Luttrin FJ, Chang YB, Duong T, Reber HA. The effect of alcohol, prostaglandin E2 and dopamine on pancreatic duct and or vascular permeability in cats. Pancreas 1989;4:A622.
81. Karanjia ND, Widdison AL, Lutrin FJ, Chang YB, Reber HA. The anti inflammatory effect of dopamine in alcoholic haemorrhagic pancreatitis in cats. Gastroenterology 1991;101:1635–1641.
82. Karanjia ND, Widdison AL, Lutrin FJ, Reber HA. Dopamine in models of alcoholic acute pancreatitis. Gut 1994;35:547–551.
83. Büchler M. Objectification of the severity of acute pancreatitis. Hepatogastroenterology 1991;38:101–108.
84. Malfertheiner P, Dominguez-Munoz JE. Diagnosis and staging of acute pancreatitis. Dig Surg 1994;11:198–208.
85. Malfertheiner P, Büchler M. Clinical symptoms and signs and diagnostic requirements in acute pancreatitis. In: Beger HG, Büchler M, eds. Acute pancreatitis. Berlin: Springer, 1987: 103–109.

86. Spechler SJ. Prevalence of normal serum amylase levels in patients with acute alcoholic pancreatitis. Dig Dis Sci 1983;28: 865–869.
87. Ranson JHC, Rifkind KM, Roses DF, Fink SD, Eng KE, Spencer FC. Prognostic signs and the role of operative management in acute pancreatitis. Surg Gynecol Obstet 1974;139:69–81.
88. McMahon MJ, Mayer AD. Comparison of the clinical features of acute pancreatitis due to gallstones and alcohol. In: Gyr K, Singer MV, Sarles H, eds. Pancreatitis—concept and classification. Amsterdam: Elsevier, 1984:379–388.
89. Imrie CW. Observations on acute pancreatitis. Br J Surg 1974; 61:539–544.
90. Blind JP, Büchler M, Bläckberg L, Andersson Y, Uhl W, et al. Carboxylic ester hydrolase. A sensitive serum marker and indicator of severity of acute pancreatitis. Int J Pancreatol 1991;8:65–73.
91. Büchler M, Malfertheiner P, Schädlich H, Nevalainen TJ, Friess H, Beger HG. Role of phospholipase $A_2$ in human acute pancreatitis. Gastroenterology 1989;97:1521–1526.
92. Büchler M, Malfertheiner P, Schoetensack C, Uhl W, Beger HG. Sensitivity of antiproteases, complement factors and C-reactive protein in detecting pancreatic necrosis. Results of a prospective clinical study. Int J Pancreatol 1986;1:227–235.
93. Davidson BR, Neoptolemos JP, Leese T, Carr-Locke DL. Biochemical prediction of gallstones in acute pancreatitis: a prospective study of three systems. Br J Surg 1988;75:213–215.
94. Sadowski DC, Todd JK, Sutherland LR. Biochemical models as early predictors of the etiology of acute pancreatitis. Dig Dis Sci 1993;38:637–643.
95. Gumaste VV, Dave PB, Weissman D, Messer J. Lipase/amylase ratio. A new index that distinguishes acute episodes of alcoholic from nonalcoholic acute pancreatitis. Gastroenterology 1991; 101:1361–1366.
96. Tenner SM, Steinberg W. The admission serum lipase:amylase ratio differentiates alcoholic from nonalcoholic acute pancreatitis. Am J Gastroenterol 1992;87:1755–1758.
97. Jaakkola M, Sillanaukee P, Löf K, Koivula T, Nordback I. Blood tests for detection of alcoholic cause of acute pancreatitis. Lancet 1994;343:1328–1329.
98. LeMoine O, Devaster J-M, Devière J, Thiry P, Cremer M, Ooms H-A. Trypsin activity. A new marker of acute alcoholic pancreatitis. Dig Dis Sci 1994;39:2634–2638.
99. Brugge WR, Burke CA, Brand DL, Chey WY. Increased interdigestive pancreatic trypsin secretion in alcoholic pancreatic disease. Dig Dis Sci 1985;30:431–439.
100. Rinderknecht H, Stace NH, Renner IG. Effects of chronic alcohol abuse on exocrine pancreatic secretion in man. Dig Dis Sci 1985;30:65–71.
101. Sahel J, Sarles H. Modifications of pure human pancreatic juice by chronic alcohol consumption. Dig Dis Sci 1979;24:897–905.
102. McMahon MJ, Bowen M, Mayer AD, Cooper EH. Relation of alpha-2 macroglobulin and other antiproteases to the clinical features of acute pancreatitis. Am J Surg 1984;147: 164–170.
103. Steer ML, Saluja AK. Etiology and pathogenesis of acute pancreatitis. In: Beger HG, Büchler M, Malfertheiner P, eds. Standards in pancreatic surgery. Berlin: Springer Verlag, 1993: 13–24.
104. Bank S, Wise L, Gerstein M. Risk factors in acute pancreatitis. Am J Surg 1983;78:737–740.
105. Ranson JHC. Timing of biliary surgery in acute pancreatitis. Ann Surg 1979;189:645–652.
106. Isenmann R, Büchler M, Uhl W, Malfertheiner P, Martini M, Beger HG. Pancreatic necrosis: an early finding in severe acute pancreatitis. Pancreas 1993;8:358–361.
107. Bradley EL III, Allen K. A prospective longitudinal study of observation versus surgical intervention in the management of necrotizing pancreatitis. Am J Surg 1991;161:19–25.
108. Beger HG. Surgical management of necrotizing pancreatitis. Surg Clin North Am 1989;69:529–549.
109. Balthazar EJ. CT diagnosis and staging of acute pancreatitis. Radiol Clin North Am 1989;27:19–37.
110. Block S, Maier W, Bittner R, Büchler M, Malfertheiner P, Beger HG. Identification of pancreatic necrosis in severe acute pancreatitis: imaging procedures versus clinical staging. Gut 1986;27: 1035–1042.
111. Büchler MW, Uhl W, Malfertheiner P. Therapie der akuten Pankreatitis. Dtsch Med Wochenschr 1994;119:1739–1744.
112. Gerzof FG, Banks PA, Robbins HA, Johnson WC, Spechler SJ, et al. Early diagnosis of pancreatic infection by CT guided aspiration. Gastroenterology 1987;93:1315–1320.
113. Beger HG, Bittner R, Block S, Büchler M. Bacterial contamination of pancreatic necroses. Gastroenterology 1986;91:433–438.
114. Uhl W, Schrag HJ, Wheatley AM, Büchler MW. The role of infection in acute pancreatitis. Dig Surg 1994;11:214–219.
115. Bradley EL III. Management of infected pancreatic necroses by open drainage. Ann Surg 1987;206:542–550.
116. Sarr MG. Planned reoperative necrosectomy/debridement for necrotizing acute pancreatitis with delayed primary closure. Dig Surg 1994;11:252–256.
117. Beger HG, Krautzberger W, Bittner R, Block S, Büchler M. Results of surgical treatment of necrotizing pancreatitis. World J Surg 1984;9:972–979.
118. Beger HG, Büchler M, Bittner R, Block S, Nevalainen T, Roscher R. Necrosectomy and postoperative local lavage in necrotizing pancreatitis. Br J Surg 1988;75:207–221.
119. Büchler M, Malfertheiner P, Block S, Maier W, Beger HG. Morphologische und funktionelle Veränderungen des Pankreas nach akuter nekrotisierender Pankreatitis. Z Gastroenterol 1985; 23:79–83.
120. Seligson U, Ihre T, Lundh G. Prognosis in acute haemorrhagic necrotizing pancreatitis. Acta Chir Scand 1982;148:423–429.
121. Mitchell CJ, Playforth M, Kelleher J, McMahon JJ. Functional recovery of the exocrine pancreas after acute pancreatitis. Scand J Gastroenterol 1983;18:5–8.
122. Dormeyer HH, Neher M, Schönborn H, Röhrich H, Prellwitz W, et al. Langzeitergebnisse nach operativer Therapie der akuten hämorrhagischen-nekrotisierenden Pankreatitis. Dtsch Med Wochenschr 1979;104:1670–1673.
123. Büchler M, Hauke A, Malfertheiner P. Follow up after acute pancreatitis: morphology and function. In: Beger HG, Büchler M, eds. Acute pancreatitis. Berlin: Springer-Verlag, 1987: 367–374.
124. Angelini G, Pederzoli P, Caliari S, Fratton S, Brocco G, et al. Long term outcome of acute necrohaemorrhagic pancreatitis. Digestion 1984;30:131–137.

# 24

# Duodenal Anomalies and Other Conditions Associated with Pancreatitis

Scott Engum and Jay Grosfeld

A number of duodenal anomalies and other duodenal conditions are occasionally associated with pancreatitis. This chapter focuses on the occurrence of pancreatitis in patients with duplication, ulcer, atresia, stenosis, polypoid lesions, diverticula, choledochocele, intussusception, inflammatory bowel disease, lymphoma, and traumatic hematoma affecting the duodenum.

## DUODENAL DUPLICATION

Duplications of the gastrointestinal (GI) tract may be found anywhere from the mouth to the anus but most commonly occur in the terminal ileum, esophagus, and colon (1). Duodenal duplication cyst was first described by Sanger in 1880 (2). These cysts represent 4–12% of all intestinal duplications (3–7). Duplications may be either spherical or tubular, be paramesenteric, share a common muscular wall (8), and in 20% of the cases communicate with the normal intestinal tract (9, 10).

Several theories have been proposed for the formation of a duplication at various sites, including the aberrant luminal recanalization theory espoused by Bremer (11) and the diverticular theory of Lewis and Thyng. (12) Bentley postulated the split notochord theory to explain the formation of neurenteric duplications and associated vertebral anomalies (13). Finally, Mellish and Koop (14) suggested that environmental factors such as trauma or hypoxia in early fetal development may be responsible when multiple duplications are found in association with anomalies such as malrotation or intestinal atresia.

Duodenal duplication cysts are found primarily in the first and the second portions of the duodenum and frequently lie behind the duodenum. A rare case of intrapancreatic duodenal duplication causing pancreatitis has been reported by Okuyama et al. (5). As with other duplication cysts of the intestinal tract, the external appearance of the mass is that of bowel, the wall contains both smooth muscle layers, and the mucosa is similar to the normal duodenum, with occasional ectopic gastric mucosa present. Most duodenal duplications associated with pancreatitis have had some communication with the pancreatic ductal system (4, 5, 7, 15–17). Presumably, pancreatitis in these patients is due to intermittent filling of the duplication cyst with biliary or secretory mucus, and this causes subsequent obstruction of the pancreatic duct at the ampulla of Vater. This hypothesis is supported by Lavine et al. (7) who observed elevated aspartate and alanine aminotransferase and alkaline phosphatase levels in the cyst fluid, which may indicate conjoint obstruction to biliary outflow. Traverso et al. (16) suggested that viscous mucoid secretions from the aberrant mucosa may obstruct the pancreatic duct and could induce pancreatitis.

With rare exception, at birth the duodenal duplication cysts have caused obstructive symptoms, initially thought to be related to pyloric stenosis unless the palpable mass is excessively large (3, 18). Vomiting, relapsing pancreatitis, bowel obstruction, or pain during the first 2–4 years of life are possible early presenting symptoms (4, 5, 18). Occasionally a patient may present with hemorrhage and associated hematemesis. Instances of relapsing pancreatitis as a result of duodenal duplication are relatively rare (5, 7, 15–17). Occasionally, patients remain asymptomatic until well into adult life.

On physical examination, a mass is usually palpable. A plain roentgenogram of the abdomen may show a soft tissue mass in the right upper quadrant. An upper GI contrast study may reveal duodenal obstruction (Fig. 24.1) and may show duodenal communication in 10–20% of cases (19). In addition, a barium enema may show displacement of the hepatic flexure of the colon (14). Computed tomography (CT) and ultrasound (Fig. 24.2), although demonstrating a cyst (duplication), often fail to determine the exact site of origin (7, 15–17, 20). Endoscopic retrograde cholangiopancreatography (ERCP) may provide accurate information about the exact location and size of the cyst and whether it communicates to the pancreatic and biliary ductal system. The relationship between the cyst and the biliary and pancreatic ducts is best determined by ERCP. Although there are rare reports of malignant change in adults (21, 22), duplication cysts in children are benign.

Surgical management of duplications depends on their type (spherical or tubular) and location. The surgical procedure should not be more radical than necessary to eliminate the patient's complaints and prevent recurrence. Operative treatment is tailored to the anatomic relationship that the cyst bears to the biliary and pancreatic ducts, the duodenal blood supply, and the potential presence of gastric mucosa. Although Gardner and Hart (2) initially performed a classic cystoduodenostomy for duodenal duplication, segmental resection of the bowel containing the duplication cyst has become the preferred technique, since gastric mucosa can be present in the wall. However, complete surgical resection for a duodenal duplication cyst may require pancreaticoduodenectomy because of its proximity to the biliary and pancreatic ductal system. Aspiration alone, external drainage, and marsupialization procedures are unsatisfactory methods of treatment. When complete surgical excision is not possible, a cyst mucosectomy (to remove ectopic gastric mucosa) and marsupialization by internal drainage either into the duodenum (by creating a window between the cyst and the adjacent duodenal lumen) or a Roux-en-Y loop of jejunum is recommended. Because of the location of the duplication cyst next to the ampulla of Vater, Lang et al. (23) described the use of an electrocoagulation papillotome and endoscopic drainage, thus alleviating the need for open surgery. In rare cases of intrapancreatic duodenal duplication, excision with ligation of the communicating duct is indicated. Operative cholangiography and pancreatography may be needed to determine the relationship of these ductal systems and to avoid inadvertent injury to these structures.

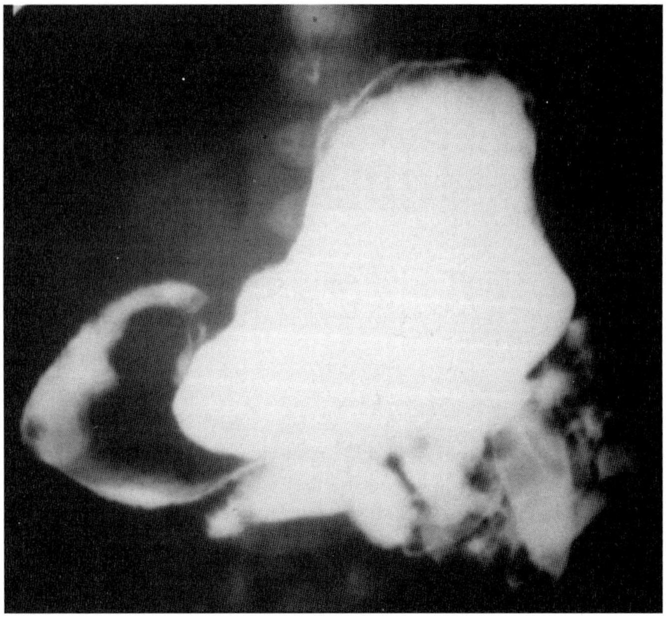

**FIG. 24.1.** Upper gastrointestinal contrast study showing lateral displacement of the second and third portion of the duodenum by a duodenal duplication cyst.

## DUODENAL ULCER

Pancreatitis secondary to a duodenal ulcer remains quite infrequent (2–15%) (24, 25). The ulcer is usually located on the posterior portion of the duodenal wall and penetrates into the head of the pancreas proximal to the ampulla of Vater (Fig. 24.3). It is presumed that the edema surrounding the ulcer bed may contribute to obstruction of the main pancreatic duct, resulting in pancreatitis. Occasionally, penetration of the ulcer into the pancreas is associated with fat necrosis and formation of a pancreatic abscess. Pancreatitis secondary to a duodenal ulcer usually responds favorably after treatment of the underlying disease (either medical or surgical management). Duodenitis may be associated with hyperamylasemia but is not considered an etiologic factor in pancreatitis. Clink et al. (26) have proposed two hypotheses to explain the occurrence of hyperamylasemia in association with duodenitis. The first theory suggests that hyperamylasemia is caused by abnormal absorption of isoamylases through areas of mucosal disruption. Upper GI bleeding is an incidental marker of the disruption. In the second theory, hyperamylasemia is caused by a central autonomic stimulation of multiple amylase-producing organs during associated upper GI bleeding. Neither hypothesis has been substantiated.

## DUODENAL OBSTRUCTION

Obstruction may increase intraduodenal pressure and result in reflux of duodenal contents into the pancreatic duct, which initiates an episode of pancreatitis (27). There are a number of causes of duodenal obstruction, including a web, atresia or stenosis, malrotation and associated midgut volvulus, and superior mesenteric artery syndrome.

Duodenal atresia, stenosis, and web (Fig. 24.4) are frequent causes of intestinal obstruction in the newborn. The first description of duodenal atresia is credited to Calder in 1733 (28). However, the first survivor was not recorded until 1916, by Ernst in Denmark (29). The etiology of duodenal atresia, web, and stenosis is probably related to a failure of recanalization of the duodenal lumen from its solid cord stage, as proposed by Tandler in 1902 (30). Failure of canalization occurs most often near the ampulla of Vater. Duodenal stenosis and atresia are frequently associated with an annular pancreas (25–30% of patients); however, some cases are not detected until laparotomy for other conditions in adult life (31). Whether annular pancreas is the cause of obstruction or is just an associated finding is not entirely clear.

Stenosis and atresia of the duodenum are usually limited to the first and second parts of the duodenum. Their most common site is at the ampulla. Frequently, the distal end of the common duct is incorporated in the intraluminal membrane. These obstructive conditions require surgical correction. A duodenal web or diaphragm may be easily excised through a longitudinal incision across the area of obstruction. Care must be taken not to injure the ampulla of Vater, which may open into the medial aspect of the membrane. In the past, the standard bypass procedure for duodenal atresia or stenosis was a retrocolic side-to-side duodenojejunostomy (32, 33); however, a more physiologic bypass procedure, side-to-side duodenoduodenostomy or diamond-shaped duodenoduodenostomy (34), is now favored because of lower complication rates, improved survival (35–39), and a shorter postoperative recovery (40). In patients with annular pancreas, one must always resist the temptation to divide the pancreatic ring, because there is often an intrinsic duodenal obstruction, pancreatic tissue may be intramural, and pancreatitis and/or a pancreatic fistula may result. A second distal duodenal web is present in 2–3% of patients. This can be recognized by passing a soft red rubber catheter into the distal duodenum and proximal jejunum.

Anomalies of bowel rotation and fixation with a high-riding cecum in the right upper quadrant associated with Ladd's bands passing across the duodenum and fixing the cecum to the right lateral abdominal wall can result in extrinsic duodenal obstruction (Fig. 24.5). Because of the narrow mesenteric vascular pedicle that exists in this situation, there is a risk of midgut volvulus. Pancreatitis has been reported in association with gastric volvulus (41, 42), as well as malrotation (43, 44). Acute hemorrhagic pancreatitis (45, 46) has been reproduced in experimental animals by creating a closed duodenal loop (47, 48), which produces reflux of duodenal contents into the pancreatic ducts (45). This reflux activates phospholipase A (49). Its reaction products, lysolecithin and lysocephalin, then may cause pancreatic necrosis (42, 50, 51). The association of malrotation and pancreatitis is very rare, but, if unrecognized, it

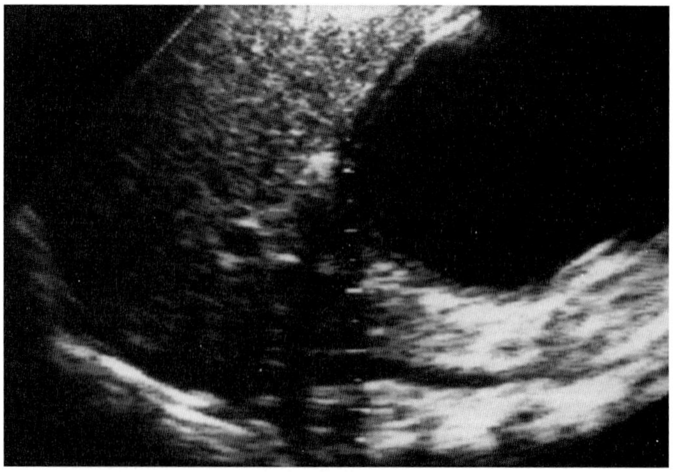

**FIG. 24.2.** Ultrasonogram of an abdominal mass showing lateral displacement of duodenal lumen and near obstruction by a duodenal duplication cyst.

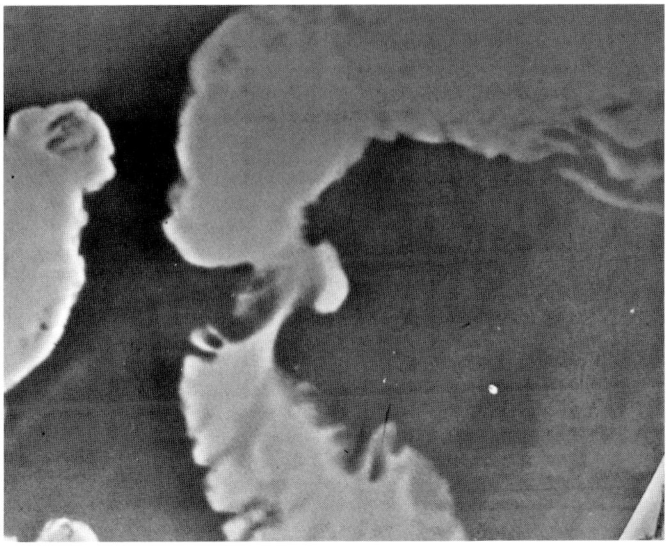

**FIG. 24.3.** Contrast radiograph shows a large collection of barium in a postbulbar duodenal ulcer crater in the second portion of the duodenum.

can lead to substantial morbidity and possible mortality. This condition, associated with a closed duodenal loop, can be treated by a counterclockwise reduction of the midgut volvulus and a classic Ladd's procedure and appendectomy.

Wilkie first described an autopsy finding of acute hemorrhagic pancreatitis secondary to chronic obstruction of the duodenum, caused by the overlying superior mesenteric artery (52). Dreiling et al. (43) reported six additional patients with chronic duodenal obstruction who developed acute and chronic pancreatitis because of superior mesenteric artery compression, afferent loop obstruction after a Billroth II partial gastrectomy, inflammatory stricture, and carcinoma of the distal duodenum.

## DUODENAL POLYPS/ADENOMA

Polypoid lesions involving the ampulla of Vater are rare, found in 0.04–0.12% of postmortem examinations (53). These lesions may result in obstruction of the bile duct, bleeding, and instances of acute and recurrent pancreatitis (54–58). The association between these benign tumors and acute pancreatitis is not well established, but transient obstruction of the pancreatic duct may be responsible (53, 55, 57, 59, 60).

Acute pancreatitis is well described in patients with ampullary neoplasms (61) but has been reported less frequently among patients with familial adenomatoid polyposis coli (FAP) who, in addition to their colonic polyps, develop adenomatous polyps in the duodenum (62, 63). Most patients with FAP and ampullary neoplasms associated with Gardner's syndrome have presented with jaundice caused by obstruction of the common bile duct, abdominal pain, or both (64–66). Ten to 15% of patients with FAP will develop polyps in the duodenum, which are usually small (<5 mm), are commonly found in the second portion of the duodenum (67, 68), and may involve the duodenal papilla (69). Children with Peutz-Jeghers syndrome also are at risk for developing duodenal hamartomatous polyps; however, these are usually associated with bleeding rather than pancreatitis (Fig. 24.6).

Neurofibromatosis, or von Recklinghausen's disease, is another hereditary disorder characterized by skin pigmentation, skeletal deformities, and/or multiple neurofibromas involving the skin, nervous system, or GI tract. GI involvement in neurofibromatosis is relatively common, with estimates ranging from 11 to 25% of patients (70, 71). Ampullary neurofibromas can not only cause mechanical obstruction of the distal pancreatic duct but also alter the neuromuscular function of the sphincter of Oddi, which may result in pancreatitis (72). Therapy for enteric neurofibromas is controversial. Most authors advocate surgical resection, especially for bulky tumors that present with hemorrhage, obstruction, or intussusception. One often sees multiple neurofibromata studding the intestine. Most of these lesions are left in place, and only symptomatic neurofibromas are resected. Endoscopic surveillance every 6 months is suggested because of the high risk of recurrence. In addition, the surgeon must also screen (endoscopically or contrast radiography) the upper and lower intestinal tracts for further polypoid disease.

Invasive or in situ carcinoma has been reported in approximately 30% of villous tumors involving the periampullary region (59, 60) (Fig. 24.7, *A* and *B*). Patients with FAP and Gardner syndrome have an increased risk of developing periampullary carcinoma. Recent studies have also demonstrated a high frequency (>50%) of multiple polyps of the stomach and duodenum, including adenomas of the ampulla, in patients with FAP (67, 72). Open biopsy of the polyp is indicated unless an unequivocal nonmalignant histologic diagnosis is obtained with endoscopic biopsy. Galandiuk et al. (73) proposed a treatment strategy involving a Whipple procedure if biopsy demonstrates malignant tissue and if the lesion is resectable. If the lesion is unresectable, a biliary enteric bypass and gastroenterostomy is suggested. If the lesion is benign, one should proceed with endoscopic or open surgical removal.

Inflammatory polyps occur in the upper GI tract, especially near suture lines after gastric and duodenal surgery. Histologic examination has shown a giant cell granulomatous reaction with associated talc and suture material (74). Acute pancreatitis occurs in the early postoperative period as a complication of gastric surgery in 0.5–2% of cases (75–77). Unlike pancreatitis in the early postoperative period, pancreatitis secondary to an inflammatory polyp tends to occur late and may be years remote from the initial surgery. Sawin described an inflammatory polyp that developed at the suture line of the duodenal stump closure adjacent to the pancreatic duct orifice, causing pancreatitis 24 years after a Billroth II procedure. They performed a submucosal resection of the polyp along with a sphincteroplasty, and the patient had an uneventful postoperative course (74).

The approach to duodenal polyps involves an initial upper GI contrast study, endoscopy with biopsy or cholecystectomy, and cholangiography to evaluate the anatomy of the distal common bile duct. This is followed by duodenotomy and direct examina-

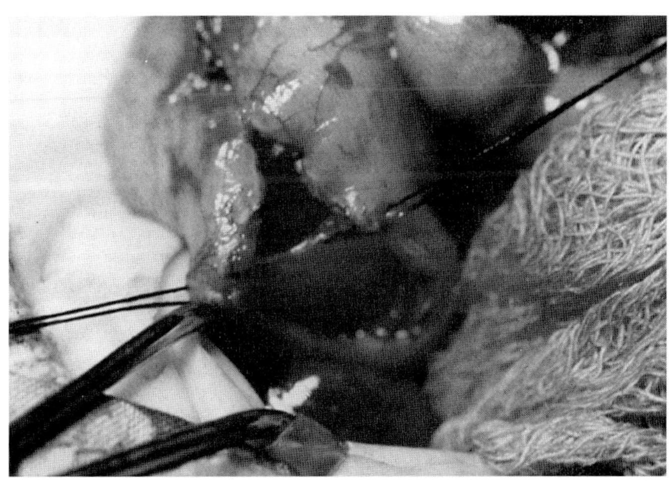

**FIG. 24.4.** Intraoperative photograph illustrating a duodenal web causing obstruction.

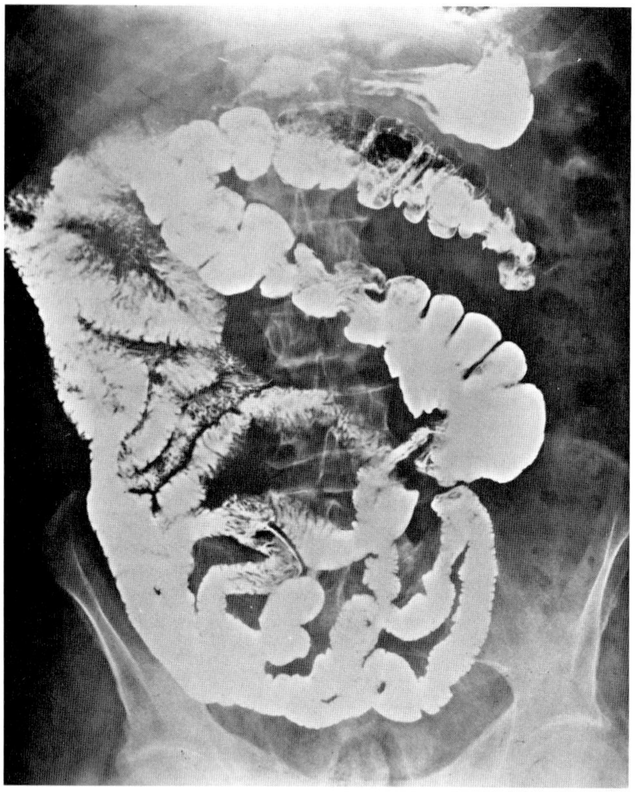

**FIG. 24.5.** Contrast radiograph showing the small intestine in the *right half* of the abdomen, the colon on the *left*, and the cecum in the *left lower quadrant*, consistent with malrotation.

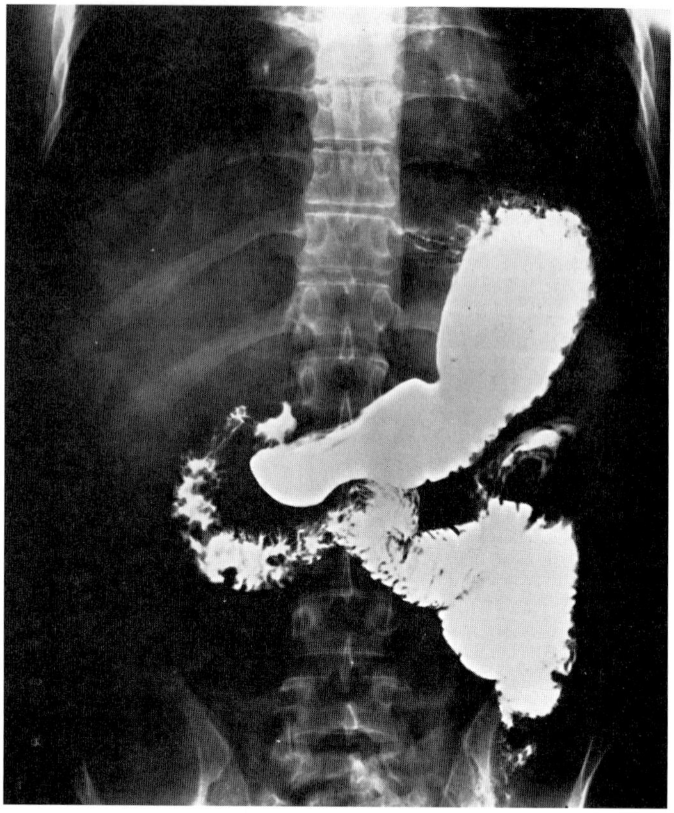

**FIG. 24.6.** Contrast radiograph showing multiple duodenal polypoid hamartomas in a patient with Peutz-Jeghers syndrome.

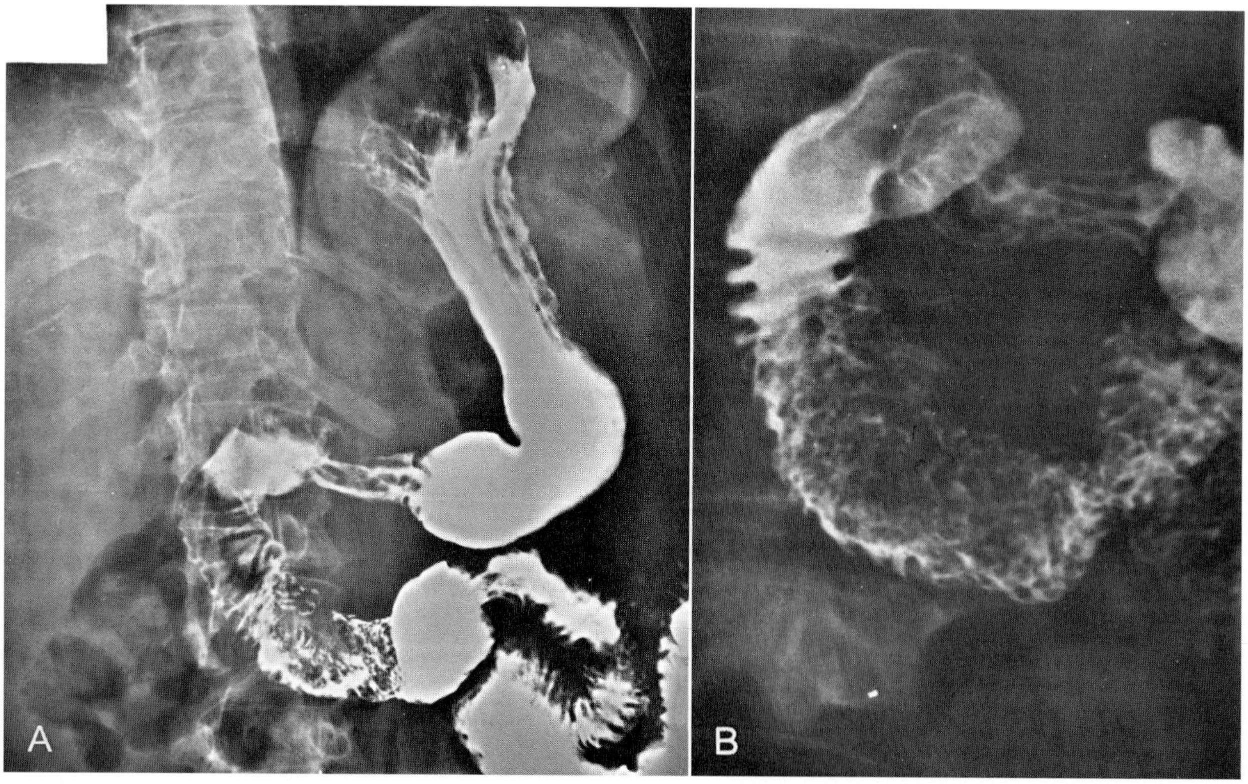


**FIG. 24.7. A.** Contrast radiograph showing a large intraluminal defect due to an adenocarcinoma of the duodenum in the second and third part of the duodenum. **B.** The mass has an irregular surface and appears to have originated from the medial aspect of the duodenum.

tion of the ampulla. If a periampullary polypoid lesion is identified, it should be excised for frozen section analysis. A probe can be placed into the papilla prior to excision, to prevent injury to the duct. If the lesion is benign, then local excision combined with a sphincteroplasty should cure the symptoms. Pancreatography may be done at this time to guarantee adequate drainage. If malignancy is present, then one must proceed with a pancreaticoduodenectomy. With the availability of modern endoscopic equipment and experienced endoscopists, a benign polypoid lesion away from the ductal system can be treated with endoscopic resection. Certainly, ERCP may be necessary prior to endoscopic resection, to define the anatomy and minimize the risk of injury to either the pancreatic or biliary duct system.

## INTRALUMINAL DUODENAL DIVERTICULUM

Intraluminal diverticula of the duodenum are rare congenital lesions that were initially described by Boyd (78) in 1845 and later given the term intraduodenal diverticulum by Kinzer in 1949 (79). There have been more than 50 cases reported (Fig. 24.8, *A* and *B*) in the world literature, with 40% having coexistent anatomic abnormalities such as a choledochocele or annular pancreas (80).

The theories of embryonic development have not been clearly established. In the 7-week-old embryo, the duodenum becomes occluded and then recanalizes. Incomplete recanalization causes either duodenal atresia, stenosis, a diaphragm (81), or duodenal duplication (82). It is postulated that a duodenal diverticulum may arise by ballooning of a diaphragm or may represent a remnant of dual recanalization (83). However, there is debate as to whether these lesions could result from gradual peristaltic pulsion acting on a duodenal diaphragm (82). The reason for this second hypothesis is the lack of occurrence in children; however, in 20% of patients, symptoms date back to childhood (84, 85). These lesions typically arise at or near the ampulla of Vater and extend intraluminally and distally in the duodenum. The diverticula are mucosal in nature and are not covered by smooth muscle. They may attach to the entire circumference of the duodenal wall or to only a part of it. The common bile duct and pancreatic duct usually empty into the diverticulum, and then a second orifice in the diverticulum allows drainage from the lumen of the diverticulum into the intestinal tract (86).

Patients with this lesion may remain asymptomatic for many years. Eventually, patients develop problems, most commonly in the 3rd to 5th decades. These include intermittent partial duodenal obstruction, most likely secondary to food trapping within the diverticular lumen; GI bleeding, either alone or in association with peptic ulcer disease; abdominal pain; or rarely (20%) (87) acute pancreatitis (88, 89). The cause of acute pancreatitis is not clear, but, it is likely the result of occlusion of the pancreatic duct from impaction of food within the diverticulum, reflux of duodenal contents into the pancreatic duct secondary to a deformed ampulla, or collapse of the diverticulum onto the papilla (90, 91). The diverticulum, because of the lack of smooth muscle, can passively distend as much as three to four times its original size, creating a duodenal obstruction. When the duodenum is empty, the diverticulum has a tendency to collapse, which explains the asymptomatic periods described by affected patients. Association with other congenital lesions including Down's syndrome, intestinal malrotation, internal hernias, and vascular abnormalities has been reported (92–95).

Although this lesion is very rare, it is a curable cause of pancreatitis and, if recognized, can be safely and effectively treated without damage to the pancreatic or biliary ductal system. Diagnosis may be suspected at endoscopy when a blind sac is noted. Endoscopy alone may not always distinguish between extra- and intraluminal diverticula, and barium contrast studies may be needed in addition to ERCP. Without excising the lesion or performing full-thickness biopsies, it is not possible to make an unequivocal diagnosis of intraluminal duodenal diverticulum, but the presence of a diverticular orifice, absence of peristalsis of the sac, and the collection of food and barium within the sac noted at endoscopy strongly suggest this diagnosis (96). With the increasing use of ERCP for the investigation of pancreatic pathology, this abnormality may be encountered more frequently than in the past.

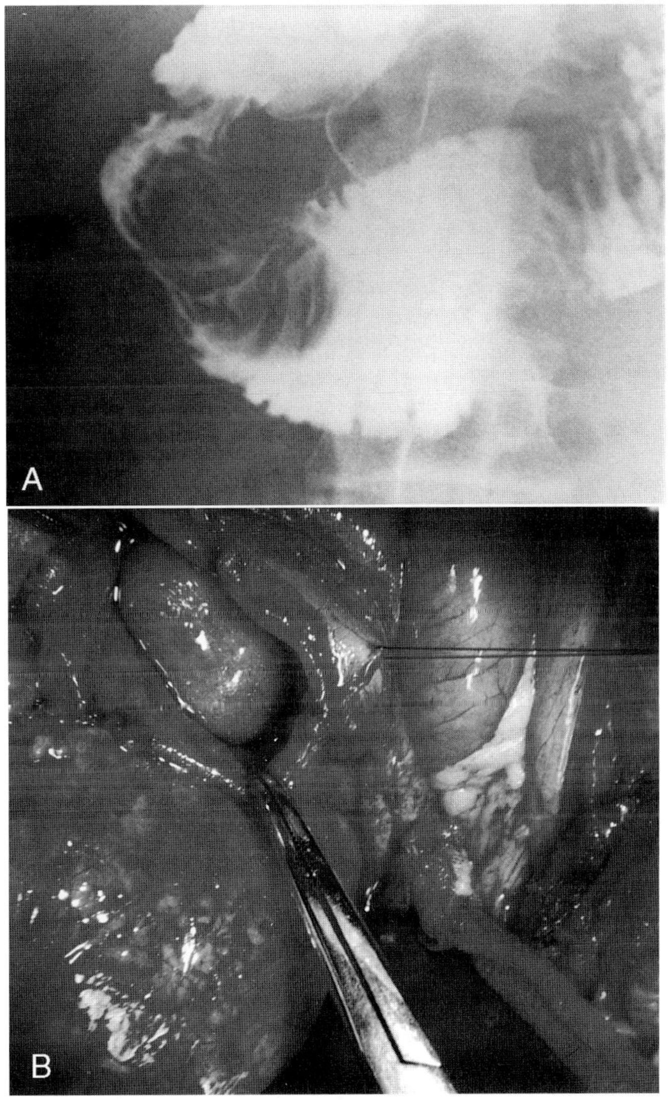

**FIG. 24.8.** **A.** Contrast radiograph of the upper gastrointestinal tract illustrating a large periampullary mass. The mass changed in size, and serial radiographs showed a small amount of barium entering a diverticulum through an inferior orifice. **B.** Operative photograph illustrating a polyplike diverticulum filling the duodenal lumen. (Reprinted by permission of the publisher from Howard JM, et al. Intraluminal duodenal diverticulum: an unusual cause of acute pancreatitis. Am J Surg 1986;151:506. Copyright 1986 by Excerpta Medica Inc.) See color insert.

Several therapeutic measures have been proposed. In some elderly or poor-risk patients with symptoms, removal of the impacted, undigested food by endoscopy, along with strict instructions regarding mastication, may suffice (40% success rate) (93). However, most symptomatic patients will require a definitive endoscopic or surgical procedure (96). The apex of the

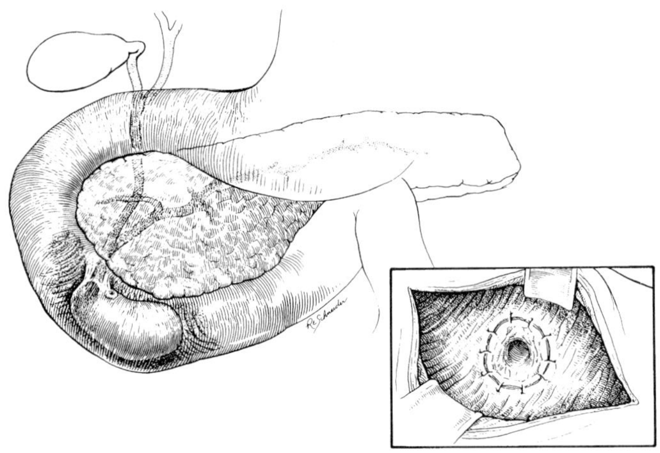

**FIG. 24.9.** Graphic illustration of a situation reported by Howard et al. (86) in which the common biliary-pancreatic channel emptied into the diverticulum. The orifice between the diverticulum and the duodenum is shown distal to the orifice of the common channel. The *inset* illustrates the opened duodenum along with the button (central common channel emptying into the duodenum) after subtotal resection of the diverticulum. (Reprinted by permission of the publisher from Howard JM, et al. Intraluminal duodenal diverticulum: an unusual cause of acute pancreatitis. Am J Surg 1986;151:506. Copyright 1986 by Excerpta Medica Inc.)

diverticulum can be opened endoscopically with an incision using a sphincterotomy knife (97) or a diathermic polypectomy snare (98, 99), followed by extension of this incision as described for the treatment of duplication cysts (100, 101). Surgical excision has been advocated by most authors (80, 85) and is required in most instances. (102) However, extreme caution must be taken to minimize injury to other local structures. The procedure of choice is a duodenotomy with excision of the diverticulum (103, 104). The duodenum is exposed, and a Kocher maneuver is performed to obtain optimal duodenal mobilization. The lesion is palpated initially. Following anterior duodenotomy, the papilla of Vater is identified, and the diverticulum is carefully excised near its base and removed. Identification of the location of the pancreatic and biliary ducts in relation to the diverticulum is essential to prevent injury.

Howard et al. (86) described partial excision with the base being saucerized in two patients with a common channel drainage system. Both patients remained well 6 years postoperatively (Fig. 24.9). In general, surgical excision of intraluminal duodenal diverticula results in complete relief of symptoms (102). Other authors have advocated a pyloric sparing Roux-en-Y duodenojejunostomy with a cholecystectomy, with or without a tube gastrostomy, for pancreaticobiliary complications of duodenal diverticulum. They suggest that diversion of food from the diverticulum will lessen complications. Transient intestinal dysmotility and poor gastric emptying resulting from disconnection of the proximal small intestinal pacemaker may occur postoperatively (105, 106).

## PERI- (JUXTA) AMPULLARY BILE-FILLED DUODENAL DUPLICATION CYST

Periampullary bile-filled duodenal duplication cyst is similar to intraluminal duodenal diverticulum, except that there is no orifice connecting the cyst and the duodenum; this cyst communicates with the common bile duct. Previous reports indicate that the mucosa of this cyst may be lined by duodenal, biliary, or other varied cell types. Treatment of these lesions involves partial excision and sphincteroplasty.

## EXTRALUMINAL PERIAMPULLARY DUODENAL DIVERTICULA

Periampullary duodenal diverticula are acquired anomalies that occur more frequently in elderly persons and have a prevalence range of 0.015–23% (107, 108). Although the diverticulum itself is rarely symptomatic (109), abnormalities of the pancreatic and biliary systems are frequently encountered (107) as a result of a mechanical obstruction (110) and/or dysfunction of Oddi's muscle (107). These events may cause stasis in the ductal system, resulting in inflammation or infection and reflux of bacteria from the diverticulum into the ductal system. Approximately two-thirds of these acquired lesions are periampullary (111). Most are on the concave pancreatic surface of the duodenum and project posteriorly (111, 112). Rosenthal first described this condition in 1893 (113). Extraluminal duodenal diverticula are associated with pancreatitis just like the intraluminal type, because of intermittent obstruction of the pancreatic duct (Fig. 24.10). Excision of the diverticulum and a sphincteroplasty are frequently efficacious and associated with long-term success.

## CHOLEDOCHOCELE

Choledochal cyst was first described by Vater in the 1700s; however, the entity was not well classified until Alonzo-Lej's report in 1959 (114). There are five anatomic variants (types I–V). The first three types were described by Alonzo-Lej, and the remaining two by various Japanese workers. The most common variant is a fusiform dilation of the common bile duct (type II). A type III choledochal cyst is usually intraduodenal but can

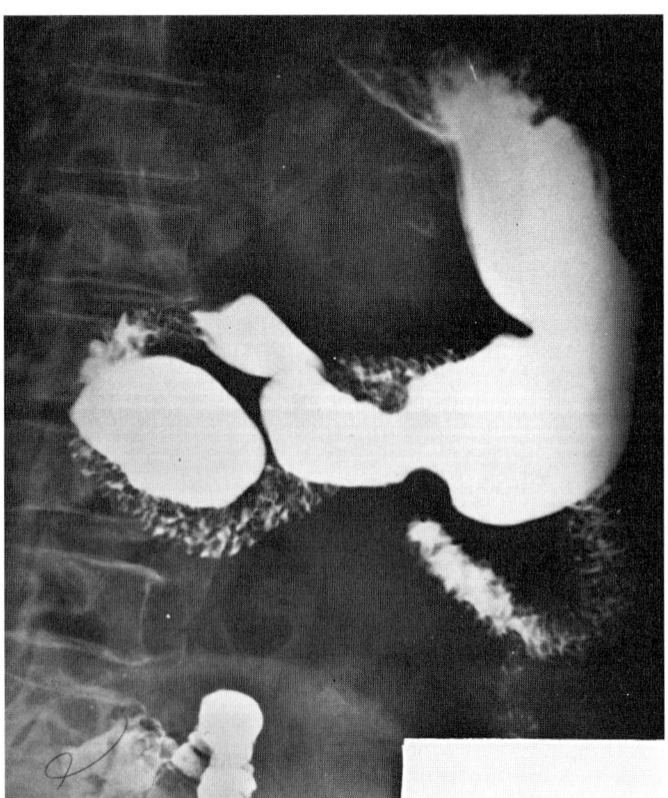

**FIG. 24.10.** Upper gastrointestinal contrast study showing a large duodenal diverticulum.

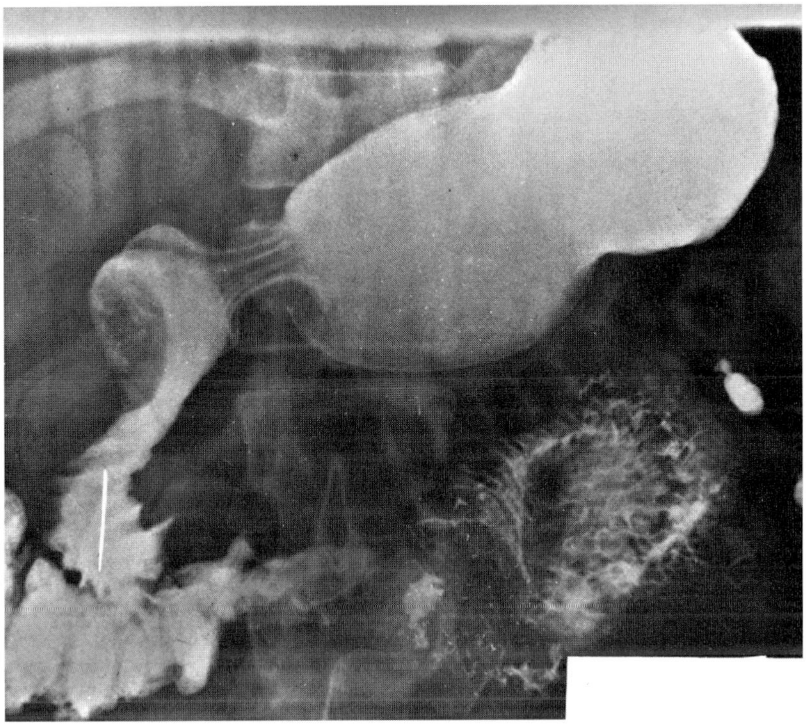

**FIG. 24.11.** Upper gastrointestinal contrast study showing a large intraluminal hematoma in the duodenal cap extending into the second part of the duodenum.

occasionally be seen in an intrapancreatic position. Some believe this represents a form of duodenal duplication rather than a true bile duct anomaly. In most cases, the common bile duct and the main pancreatic duct enter into the choledochocele separately through stenotic orifices. The choledochocele then empties into the duodenum through a single narrow orifice. The choledochocele is usually lined by duodenal mucosa; however, in some instances, the lining resembles that of the bile duct. This condition may result from either primary ectasia or possible longstanding obstruction at the point of entry into the duodenum. This region of stenosis or narrowing predisposes to stasis of biliary and pancreatic secretions, along with increased intraductal pressures, resulting in associated pancreatitis.

Stephens and Pauline first described the association of a choledochocele and pancreatitis (115). Patients with a choledochocele are best managed after the anatomy has been defined by cholangiography. Most procedures require surgical intervention with a lateral duodenotomy followed by "unroofing" of the choledochocele, which allows free drainage of the biliary and pancreatic ducts. In instances when there is an associated stenosis of the biliary and/or pancreatic duct, a sphincteroplasty may be required in addition to the "unroofing."

## DUODENAL HEMATOMA

Fiberoptic upper gastrointestinal (UGI) endoscopy is commonly performed in all age groups that present with GI bleeding, recurrent abdominal pain, and foreign body ingestion. The complication rate associated with this procedure is less than 2% (116); however, perforation, bleeding, and hematoma may occur (116, 117).

Karjoo (118) reported an adolescent with chronic diarrhea, anorexia, and abdominal pain who developed acute pancreatitis (amylase, 1165 units; lipase, 8650 units) following UGI endoscopy with biopsies of the duodenum. The pancreatitis was related to a large postprocedure duodenal hematoma. All bleeding parameters were normal on evaluation. A postprocedure UGI series showed complete postbulbar obstruction, with a cupping defect consistent with a duodenal mass, which was confirmed by ultrasonography. Treatment with nasogastric decompression and total parenteral nutrition (TPN) allowed the hematoma to resolve in 3 weeks. Pancreatitis was probably due to compression of the pancreatic duct by the duodenal hematoma (Fig. 24.11). Zinelis (119) described an adult who developed obstructive jaundice and pancreatitis associated with a duodenal hematoma following a similar endoscopic procedure, which resolved after 23 days of nasogastric decompression and TPN.

Obstructing intramural hematomas of the duodenum have also been reported after blunt trauma (120, 121), child abuse (122), blood dyscrasia (123), and small bowel biopsy (124). In blunt trauma, the duodenum (which has a rich submucosal vascular plexus, a short mesentery, and limited mobility) (122) is compressed against the vertebral column (125) (Fig. 24.12).

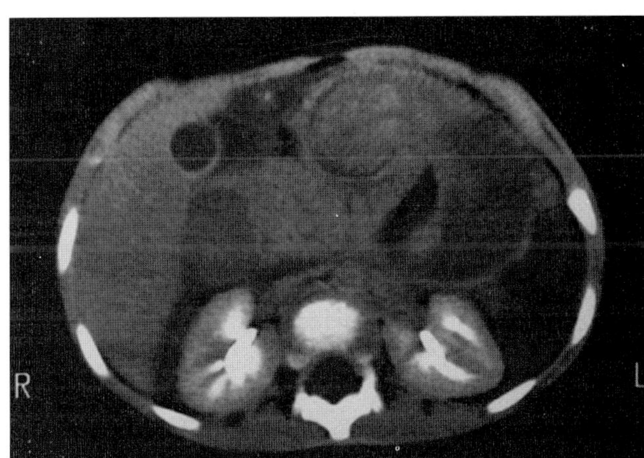


**FIG. 24.12.** Computerized tomography of a patient with elevated serum amylase and lipase levels due to a large duodenal hematoma of unknown etiology involving the second through fourth portions of the duodenum. Trauma was suspected as the etiology.

The preferred management of pancreatitis associated with a duodenal hematoma is observation and supportive therapy with nasogastric decompression, no oral intake, and intravenous hyperalimentation. Most cases treated in this manner will resolve within 2–3 weeks. In the event of persistent obstruction or an uncertain diagnosis, exploratory laparotomy may be necessary to evaluate and evacuate the hematoma.

## INTUSSUSCEPTION

Intussusception occurs much less frequently in the duodenum than in other regions of the bowel because of its fixed position in the retroperitoneum and because tumors that act as lead points are relatively rare in this location (126). Most often the cause is a benign tumor such as a lipoma, because they are more mobile and originate from either the first part of the duodenum or at the junction of the third and fourth portions of the duodenum, where it becomes intraperitoneal (127). Duodenal intussusception rarely involves the pediatric age group. McGrath et al. (128) described a 12-year-old boy who presented with signs and symptoms of acute pancreatitis resulting from a mass effect upon the ampulla of Vater by a duodenal lipoma. This resulted in a duodenojejunal intussusception that required resection followed by full recovery.

Villous adenomas represent a very small proportion of duodenal tumors, occurring primarily in the periampullary region, and show a marked propensity for malignant change. Obstruction, intussusception, and pancreatitis are infrequent clinical presentations. The characteristic appearance of a villous adenoma on barium contrast studies is an intraluminal filling defect with a "soap-bubble" appearance produced by barium trapped in the fronds of the tumor. However, this classical appearance is present in only 30% of some series (129). The diagnostic sensitivity can be increased with the use of hypotonic duodenography (130). Ultrasound, endoscopy, and CT scanning may be useful for diagnosis. In the absence of malignant change, local excision, whether open or endoscopic, is usually curative. Regular endoscopic surveillance is needed postoperatively, given the propensity of these tumors for recurrence (131).

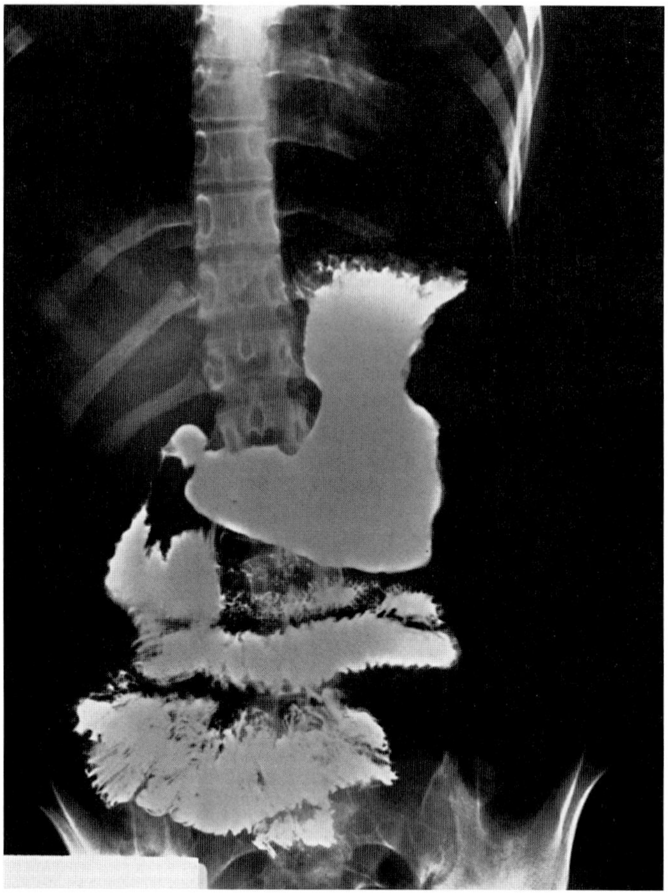

**FIG. 24.13.** Upper gastrointestinal contrast series showing the second portion of the duodenum with diffuse narrowing, irregularity, and nodular folds causing compression and stenosis in a patient with Crohn's disease.

## CROHN'S DISEASE

Once thought to be rare, duodenal involvement in Crohn's disease is being reported with increasing frequency (1.5–4%) (132–134) (Fig. 24.13). Numerous cases have been described since Gottlieb and Alpert (135) first reported duodenal involvement in regional enteritis in 1937. Most patients will have the diagnosis established in other areas of the GI tract months to years before the duodenal involvement becomes apparent (136). Although Crohn's disease is associated with numerous extraintestinal manifestations, including arthritic, dermatologic, ocular, and hepatobiliary changes, pancreatitis has rarely been reported (137–139). The first patient with Crohn's disease associated with pancreatitis was described in 1956 by Chapin et al. (140). Crohn's disease associated with pancreatitis is often attributed to the adverse effects of the drugs used in its treatment, which include prednisone and 6-mercaptopurine. However, in a small subset of patients, the timing of the administration of medication or the lack of use of the drug is inconsistent with the occurrence of pancreatitis, and duodenal involvement with Crohn's disease is the only documented cause for its development. Crohn's disease complicated by pancreatitis can be divided into that with duodenal involvement and that without. Most episodes of pancreatitis have an inciting factor (cholelithiasis, drug exposure, sclerosing cholangitis); however, some have no other obvious cause of pancreatitis other than duodenal Crohn's disease. This is the population of patients covered in this text.

Three mechanisms have been suggested for pancreatitis associated with Crohn's disease. Reflux of duodenal contents through an incompetent ampulla is supported by the occasional passage of barium into the pancreatic and biliary ducts during upper GI contrast studies (133, 141, 142). Others have described a duodenal pancreatic duct fistula with distal Crohn's disease (143); however, no episodes of pancreatitis occurred in this patient. Direct ampullary involvement with stenosis and intermittent obstruction of the duct from inflammation, resulting in sudden increase in pressure within the pancreatic duct, has also been implicated (144). Pancreatic duct outflow obstruction due to a foreign body such as bile sludge, protein plug, or stone disease has also been proposed (145).

A pathophysiologic mechanism associating inflammatory bowel disease and pancreatitis is unknown. Some authors postulate that undetected gallstones or sludge may be the cause of the pancreatitis (146, 147) and that the incidence of this relationship may be underestimated (148). Following resection of the terminal ileum, lithogenic bile and gallstone formation are noted in more than 30% of patients with Crohn's disease. Treatment with oral bile acids might be considered in selected patients in an effort to prevent recurrent pancreatitis (139). However, the unusual chronic interstitial pancreatitis seen in these patients differs substantially from the clinicopathologic entity seen with recurrent gallstone- (or sludge-) induced pancreatitis and suggests another etiology (149).

An immunologic basis for this form of pancreatitis has been suggested (150); however, one would expect diffuse involvement, chronicity, and possibly chronic pancreatic insufficiency, none of which are usually present (138). Whether the pancreas is involved by granulomatous inflammation in Crohn's disease is not known. Granulomatous lesions of the pancreas have been described in patients with sarcoidosis (151, 152) and tuberculosis; however, these patients did not develop pancreatitis.

Acute pancreatitis in Crohn's disease occurs more commonly than in a control population (138). The clinical course of pancreatitis is usually benign and self-limited. Steroid therapy is beneficial for patients with active Crohn's disease and pancreatitis; however, other possible causative factors leading to pancreatitis (drugs, alcohol, biliary tract disease) must be excluded prior to initiation of therapy. The prognosis for Crohn's disease of the duodenum (153) may be worse than Crohn's disease in general, because of its association with extensive and severe lesions elsewhere in the GI tract. The addition of a histamine-blocking antiulcer medication may minimize steroid-induced peptic ulceration. Unfortunately, not all patients respond to conservative therapy. If obstruction supervenes, a bypass procedure (gastrojejunostomy) will usually give favorable long-term results (154), obviating the need for pancreaticoduodenectomy (which is usually unwarranted for this condition). If a stricture is present secondary to inflammation, the traditional approach has been surgical; however, interventional radiologists and endoscopists have become increasingly skilled with the use of balloon catheters and stent insertion in both locations, with some success. These methods deserve consideration as an alternative treatment option in selected Crohn's disease patients with duct stenosis.

## LYMPHOMA

Primary GI lymphoma accounts for approximately 1–4% of all GI malignancies (155). However, lymphoma accounts for a higher percentage of primary small bowel malignancies (156, 157). Primary lymphoma of the duodenum with pancreatic or bile ductal obstruction is very uncommon (156, 158), and pancreatic duct obstruction resulting in pancreatitis even more rare (158, 159). Generalized B-cell lymphoma with secondary involvement of the GI tract is more common and can cause biliary tract obstruction as a result of malignant lymph node involvement, extension into the head of the pancreas, and/or infiltration of the ampulla of Vater.

Once the diagnosis of lymphoma and associated pancreatitis is confirmed, treatment with multimodal chemotherapy is initiated in an effort to relieve the obstruction of the pancreatic duct and effect subsequent improvement in pancreatitis.

## REFERENCES


1. Gross RE, Holcomb G, Farber S. Duplication of the alimentary tract. Pediatrics 1952;9:449.
2. Gardner CE, Hart D. Enterogenous cysts of the duodenum. JAMA 1935;104:1809.
3. Soper RT, Selke AC. Duplication cyst of the duodenum: case report and discussion. Surgery 1970;68:562–566.
4. Romero-Torres R. Duplication of the duodenum. Int Surg 1972; 57:337–338.
5. Okuyama H, Matsuo Y, Fukui Y, Imura K, Kamata S, Okada A. Intrapancreatic duodenal duplication associated with pancreatic pseudocysts. J Pediatr Surg 1992;27:1573–1574.
6. Acherman MB. Duodenal duplication cysts: diagnosis and operative management. Surgery 1974;76:330–333.
7. Lavine JE, Harrison M, Heyman MB. Gastrointestinal duplications causing relapsing pancreatitis in children. Gastroenterology 1989;97:1556–1558.
8. Smith JR. Accessory enteric formations: a classification and nomenclature. Arch Dis Child 1960;35:87–89.
9. Bower RJ, Sieber WK, Kiesewetter WB. Alimentary tract duplications in children. Ann Surg 1978;188:669–674.
10. Grosfeld JL, O'Neill JA Jr, Clatworthy HW Jr. Enteric duplications in infancy and childhood: an 18 year review. Ann Surg 1970; 172:83–90.
11. Bremer JL. Diverticula and duplications of the intestinal tract. Arch Pathol 1944;38:132–140.
12. Lewis FT, Thyng FW. Regular occurrence of intestinal diverticula in embryos of pig, rabbit, and man. Am J Anat 1908;7:505–519.
13. Bentley JFR, Smith JR. Developmental posterior enteric remnants and spinal malformations. Arch Dis Child 1960;35:76–86.
14. Mellish P, Koop CE. Clinical manifestations of duplication of the bowel. Pediatrics 1961;27:397.
15. Traif IA, Khan MH. Endoscopic drainage of a duodenal duplication cyst. Gastrointest Endosc 1992;38:64–65.
16. Traverso LW, Damus PS, Longmire WP. Pancreatitis of unusual origin. Surg Gynecol Obstet 1975;141:383–386.
17. Black PR, Welch KJ, Eraklis AJ. Juxtapancreatic intestinal duplication with pancreatic ductal communication: a cause of pancreatitis and recurrent abdominal pain in childhood. J Pediatr Surg 1986;21:257–261.
18. Tihansky DP, Sukarochana K, Hanrahan JB. Pyloroduodenal duplication cyst. Am J Gastroenterol 1986;81:189–191.
19. Caffey J. Pediatric x-ray diagnosis. Vol I. Chicago: Year Book, 1972.
20. McAlister WH, Siegel MJ. Pediatric radiology case of the day. Am J Radiol 1989;152:1328–1332.
21. Orr MM, Edwards AJ. Neoplastic change in duplications of the alimentary tract. Br J Surg 1975;62:269–274.
22. Adair HM, Trowell JE. Squamous cell carcinoma arising in a duplication of the small bowel. J Pathol 1981;133:25–31.
23. Lang T, Gerquist W, Rich K, et al. Treatment of recurrent pancreatitis by endoscopic drainage of a duodenal duplication. J Pediatr Gastroenterol Nutr 1994;18:494–496.
24. Berman LG, Dunn E, Straehley CJ. Survey of pancreatitis: Central New York Surgical Society. Gastroenterology 1961;40:94.
25. Sharon P, Melmed S, Neuman G. Acute pancreatitis in a community with a low alcohol intake. Int Surg 1979;64:63–66.
26. Clink DW, Bouwman DL, Weaver DW. Foregut mucosal defects: an etiology of hyperamylasemia. J Surg Res 1983;34:576–580.
27. Johnson RH, Doppman J. Duodenal reflux and the etiology of pancreatitis. Surgery 1967;62:462–467.
28. Calder J. Two examples of children born with preternatural conformation of the guts. Med Essays (Edinb) 1733;1:203.
29. Ernst NP. A case of congenital atresia of the duodenum treated successfully by operation. Br Med J 1916;1:1644.
30. Tandler J. Entwicklungsgeschichte des menschlichen Duodenum. Morphol Jahrb 1902;29:187.
31. Kiernan PD, Remine SG, Kiernan PC, Remine WH. Annular pancreas: Mayo Clinic experience from 1957 to 1976 with review of the literature. Arch Surg 1980;115:46.
32. Kraeger RR, Gromoljez P, Lewis JE. Congenital duodenal atresia. Am J Surg 1973;126:762–764.
33. Harberg FJ, Poxany WJ, Hahn H. Congenital duodenal obstruction. Am J Surg 1979;138:825–828.
34. Kimura K, Tsugawa C, Ogawa K, et al. Diamond-shaped anastomosis for congenital duodenal obstruction. Arch Surg 1977;112:1262–1263.
35. Weitzman JJ, Brennan LP. An improved technique for the correction of congenital duodenal obstruction in the neonate. J Pediatr Surg 1974;9:385–386.
36. Girvan DP, Stephens DA. Congenital intrinsic duodenal obstruction: a twenty-year review of its surgical management and consequences. J Pediatr Surg 1974;9:833–839.
37. Wayne ER, Burrington JD. Management of 97 children with duodenal obstruction. Arch Surg 1973;107:857–861.
38. Stauffer UG, Irving I. Duodenal atresia and stenosis: long-term results. Prog Pediatr Surg 1977:49–58.
39. Wesley JR, Mahour GH. Congenital intrinsic duodenal obstruction: a twenty-five year review. Surgery 1977;82:716–720.
40. Weber TR, Lewis JE, Mooney D, Connors R. Duodenal atresia: a comparison of techniques of repair. J Pediatr Surg 1986;21:1133–1136.
41. Wiesenger Von D. Ein Fall von Volvulus des Magens mit totalem dadurch bedingtem Verschluss von Cardia and Pylorus und aduter Fettnekrose Heilung. Dtsch Med Wochenschr 1901; 27:83.
42. Hailes WA. Volvulus of the stomach. Med J Aust 1923;2:544–545.

43. Dreiling DA, Kirschner PA, Nemser H. Chronic duodenal obstruction: a mechanovascular etiology of pancreatitis. Am J Dig Dis 1960;5:991–1005.
44. Dine MS, Martin LW. Malrotation with gastric volvulus, midgut volvulus, and pancreatitis. Am J Dis Child 1977;131:1345–1346.
45. McCutcheon AD. A fresh approach to the pathogenesis of pancreatitis. Gut 1968;9:286–310.
46. Banks PA. Acute pancreatitis. Gastroenterology 1971;61:382–397.
47. Pfeffer RB, Stasior O, Hinton JW. The clinical picture of the sequential development of acute hemorrhagic pancreatitis in the dog. Surg Forum 1957;8:248–251.
48. Ferrie MM, O'Hare R, Joffe SN. Acute and chronic pancreatitis in the rat caused by a closed duodenal loop. Digestion 1978;18:280–285.
49. Schmidt H, Creutzfeldt W. The possible role of phospholipase A in the pathogenesis of acute pancreatitis. Scand J Gastroenterol 1969;4:39–48.
50. Johnson RH, Doppman J. Duodenal reflux and the etiology of pancreatitis. Surgery 1967;62:462–467.
51. White T, McAlexander RA, Magee DF. The effect of gastric distention and duodenal aspirates in man. Gastroenterology 1963;44:48–51.
52. Wilkie DPD. Chronic duodenal ileus. Br Med J 1921;2:793.
53. Sobel S, Cooperman A. Villous adenoma of the ampulla of Vater. An unusual cause of biliary colic and obstructive jaundice. Gastroenterology 1978;75:107–109.
54. Griffin W, Schaefer J, Schindler S, Hyde G, Bryant L. Ampullary obstruction by benign duodenal polyps. Arch Surg 1968;97:444–449.
55. Ohmori K, Kinoshita H, Shiraha Y, Satake K. Pancreatic duct obstruction by a benign polypoid andenoma of the ampulla of Vater. Am J Surg 1976;132:662–663.
56. White SH, Nazarian NA, Smith AM, et al. Periampullary adenoma causing pancreatitis. Br Med J 1981;283:527.
57. Reynolds R, Lloyd D, Sweeney J, Stamm B, Slinger R. Villous adenoma of the duodenum presenting as acute pancreatitis. J Clin Gastroenterol 1982;4:533–536.
58. Ryan D, Schapiro R, Warshaw A. Villous tumors of the duodenum. Ann Surg 1986;203:301–306.
59. Kutin ND, Ranson B, Gouge TH, Localio SA. Villous tumors of the duodenum. Ann Surg 1975;181:164–168.
60. Perzin KH, Bridge MF. Adenomas of the small intestine: a clinicopathologic review of 51 cases and a study of their relationship to carcinoma. Cancer 1981;48:799–808.
61. Langer B, Lipson R, McHattie JD, et al. Periampullary tumors: advances in diagnosis and surgical treatment. Can J Surg 1979;22:34–37.
62. Clarke DN, Norman JN, Smith JAR, et al. Pancreatitis and duodenal obstruction due to periampullary carcinoma associated with familial polyposis coli. Postgrad Med 1978;54:418–420.
63. Sener SF, Miller HH, DeCosse JJ. The spectrum of polyposis. Surg Gynecol Obstet 1984;159:525–532.
64. Jones TR, Nance FC. Periampullary malignancy in Gardner's syndrome. Ann Surg 1977;185:565–573.
65. Lees CD, Hermann RE. Familial polyposis coli associated with bile duct cancer. Am J Surg 1981;141:378–380.
66. Harned RK, Williams SM. Familial polyposis coli and periampullary malignancy. Dis Colon Rectum 1982;25:227–229.
67. Yao T, Iada M, Ohsato K, Watanabe H, Omae T. Duodenal lesions in familial polyposis of the colon. Gastroenterology 1977;73:1086–1092.
68. Bulow S, Lauritsen KB, Johansen A, Svendsen LB, Sondergaard JO. Gastroduodenal polyps in familial polyposis coli. Dis Colon Rectum 1985;28:90–93.
69. Iada M, Yao T, Itoh H, Ohsato K, Watanabe H. Endoscopic features of adenoma of the duodenal papilla in familial polyposis of the colon. Gastrointest Endosc 1981;27:6–8.
70. Das Gupta TK. Multiple neurofibromatosis (von Recklinghausen's disease). Proc Inst Med Chicago 1969;27:254–255.
71. Davis GB, Berk RN. Intestinal neurofibromatosis in von Recklinghausen's disease. Am J Gastroenterol 1973;60:410–414.
72. Burt RW, Berenson MM, Lee RG, et al. Upper gastrointestinal polyps in Gardner's syndrome. Gastroenterology 1984;86:295–301.
73. Galandiuk S, Hermann RE, Jagelmen DG, Fazio V, Sivak M. Villous tumors of the duodenum. Ann Surg 1988;207:234–239.
74. Sawin R, Brooks DC. Chronic pancreatitis secondary to an inflammatory polyp of the duodenum 25 years after Billroth II reconstruction. Surgery 1988;104:575–576.
75. Warren KW. Acute pancreatitis and pancreatic injuries following subtotal gastrectomy. Surgery 1951;29:643–651.
76. Miller SF, Whitaker JR, Snyder RD. Incidence of elevated serum amylase levels and pancreatitis after upper abdominal surgery. Am J Surg 1973;125:535–537.
77. White TT, Morgan A, Hopton D. Postoperative pancreatitis. Am J Surg 1970;120:132–136.
78. Boyd R. Description of malformation of the duodenum. Lancet 1845;1:648.
79. Kinzer RE. Intraluminal diverticulum and other lesions producing intermittent duodenal obstruction or stasis. AJR 1949;61:212–218.
80. Adams DB. Management of the intraluminal duodenal diverticulum: endoscopy or duodenotomy. Am J Surg 1986;151:524–526.
81. Krieg EG. Duodenal diverticulum. Ann Surg 1937;106:33–41.
82. Wiot JF, Spiro E. Intraluminal diverticulum: a form of duplication. Radiology 1963;80:46–49.
83. Heilbrun N, Boyden EA. Intraluminal duodenal diverticula. Radiology 1964;82:887–894.
84. Nance FC. Intraluminal duodenal diverticula. Surg Gynecol Obstet 1967;124:613–618.
85. Navab F, Coleman, Caldwell F. Resection of intraluminal duodenal diverticulum. Am J Gastroenterol 1988;83:761–764.
86. Howard JM, Wynn OB, Lenhart FM, Chandnani PC. Intraluminal duodenal diverticulum: an unusual case of acute pancreatitis. Am J Surg 1986;151:505–508.
87. Zatzkin HR, Macy JJ, Kveton FW. Intraluminal duodenal diverticulum and report of a case. AJR 1959;82:1036–1037.
88. Griffin M, Carey WD, Hermann R, Buonocore E. Recurrent acute pancreatitis and intussusception complicating an intraluminal duodenal diverticulum. Gastroenterology 1981;81:345–348.
89. Hirch F, Halet W, Piront A. Diverticule interne du duodenum forme de duplication. Arch Mal Appar Dig 1964;53:839–844.
90. Nance FC, Cocchiara J, Kinder JL. Acute pancreatitis associated with an intraluminal duodenal diverticulum. Gastroenterology 1967;52:544–547.
91. Hartley RH, Barlow AP, Kilby JO. Intraluminal duodenal diverticulum: an unusual cause of acute pancreatitis. Br J Surg 1993;80:488.
92. Fleming CR, Newcomer AD, Stephens DH, Carlson HC. Intraluminal duodenal diverticulum: report of two cases and review of the literature. Mayo Clin Proc 1975;50:244–248.
93. Economides NG, McBurney RP, Hamilton FH. Intraluminal duodenal diverticulum in the adult. Ann Surg 1977;185:147–152.
94. Rowe MI, Buckner D, Clatworthy HW Jr. Windsock web of the duodenum. Am J Surg 1968;116:444–449.
95. Economides NG, Fortner TM, Dunavant WD. Duodenal diaphragm associated with superior mesenteric artery syndrome. Am J Surg 1981;141:274–276.
96. Karoll MP, Ghahremani GG, Port RB, Rosenberg JL. Diagnosis and management of intraluminal duodenal diverticulum. Dig Dis Sci 1983;28:84–85.
97. Finnie IA, Ghosh P, Garvey C, Poston GJ, Rhodes JM. Intraluminal duodenal diverticulum causing recurrent pancreatitis: treatment by endoscopic incision. Gut 1994;35:557–559.
98. Hajiro K, Yamamoto H, Matsui H, Yamamoto T. Endoscopic diagnosis and excision of intraluminal duodenal diverticulum. Gastrointest Endosc 1979;25:151–154.
99. Hiraoka T, Nakamura M, Ohno K. Endoscopic excision of intraluminal duodenal diverticulum. Dig Dis Sci 1985;30:274–280.
100. Johanson JF, Geenen JE, Hogan WJ, Huibregtse K. Endoscopic therapy of a duodenal duplication cyst. Gastrointest Endosc 1992;38:60–64.
101. Traif IA, Khan MH. Endoscopic therapy of a duodenal duplication cyst. Gastrointest Endosc 1992;38:64–65.
102. Willemer S, Dombrowski H, Adler G, Bussmann JF, Arnold R. Recurrent acute pancreatitis and intraluminal duodenal diverticulum. Pancreas 1992;7:257–261.

103. Cooperman AM, Adachi M, Rankin GB, Sivak M. Congenital duodenal diaphragm in adults. Ann Surg 1975;182:739–742.
104. Richardson WR, Martin LW. Pitfalls in the surgical management of the incomplete duodenal diaphragm. J Pediatr Surg 1969;4: 303–312.
105. Critchlow JF, Shapiro ME, Silen W. Duodenojejunostomy for the pancreaticobiliary complications of duodenal diverticulum. Ann Surg 1985;202:56–58.
106. Shallman RW, Kolts RL. Duodenojejunostomy for pancreatitis secondary to periampullary duodenal diverticula. Arch Surg 1987;122:850–851.
107. Lotveit T, Osnes M. Duodenal diverticula. Scand J Gastroenterol 1980;19:579–581.
108. Osnes M, Myren J, Lotveit T, et al. Juxtapapillary duodenal diverticula and abnormalities by endoscopic retrograde cholangiopancreatography (ERCP). Scand J Gastroenterol 1977; 12:347–351.
109. Brian JE, Stair JM. Noncolonic diverticular disease. Surg Gynecol Obstet 1985;161:189–195.
110. Manny J, Muga M, Eyal Z. The continuing enigma of duodenal diverticulum. Am J Surg 1981;142:595–600.
111. Jones TW, Merendino KA. The perplexing duodenal diverticulum. Surgery 1960;48:1068.
112. Landor JH, Fulkerson CC. Duodenal diverticula. Arch Surg 1966;93:182.
113. Odgers PNB. Duodenal diverticulosis. Br J Surg 1930;17:592.
114. Alonso-Lej F, Rever WR Jr, Pessagno DJ. Congenital choledochal cyst, with a report of 2, and an analysis of 94 cases. Int Abstr Surg 1959;108:1–30.
115. Stephens FO, Pauline GJ. Choledochocele: an unusual type of choledochal cyst which presented as acute pancreatitis. Aust NZ J Surg 1966;36:124.
116. Ament ME, Vargas J. Fiberoptic upper intestinal endoscopy. Pediatr Gastrointest Dis 1991;2:1247–1255.
117. Silvis SE, Nebel O, Rogers G, Sugawa C, Mandelstam P. Endoscopic complications: results of the 1974 American Society for Gastrointestinal Endoscopy survey. JAMA 1976;235: 928–930.
118. Karjoo M, Luisire A, Silberstein M, Kane RE. Duodenal hematoma and acute pancreatitis after upper gastrointestinal endoscopy. Gastrointest Endosc 1994;40:493–495.
119. Zinelis SA, Hershenson LM, Ennis MF, Boller M, Ismail-Beigi F. Intramural duodenal hematoma following upper gastrointestinal endoscopic biopsy. Dig Dis Sci 1989;34:289–291.
120. Babbi HD, Hussain MI, Gavino P, et al. Intramural duodenal hematoma in children. Am J Dis Child 1968;6:37–42.
121. Margolis I, Carnazzo A, Finn M. Intramural hematoma of the duodenum. Am J Surg 1983;132:779–783.
122. Jones WR, Hardin WJ, Davis JT, Hardy JD. Intramural hematoma of the duodenum: a review of the literature and case report. Ann Surg 1971;173:534–544.
123. Devroede GJ, Tirol FT, LoRusso VA, et al. Intramural hematoma of the duodenum and jejunum. Am J Surg 1966;112:9747–9752.
124. Tobin JO, Schlang HA, James DR. Intramural hematoma of the duodenum associated with peroral small-bowel biopsy. JAMA 1966;198:787–789.
125. Ghishan FJ, Werner M, Vieira P, Kuttesch J, DeHaro R. Intramural duodenal hematoma: an unusual complication of endoscopic small bowel biopsy. Am J Gastroenterol 1987;82:368–370.
126. Van Beers B, Trigaux J, Pringot J. Duodenojejunal intussusception secondary to duodenal tumors. Gastrointest Radiol 1988;13: 24–26.
127. Vinnicombe S, Grundy A. Case report: obstructive jaundice secondary to an intussuscepting duodenal villous adenoma. Clin Radiol 1992;46:63–65.
128. McGrath FP, Moote DJ, Langer JC, Orr W, Somers S. Duodenojejunal intussusception secondary to a duodenal lipoma presenting in a young boy. Pediatr Radiol 1991;21:590–591.
129. Schulten MF, Oyasu R, Beal J. Villous adenoma of the duodenum. Am J Surg 1976;132:90–96.
130. Geier GE, Gashti EN, Houin HP, Johnloz D, Madura JA. Villous adenoma of the duodenum. Am Surg 1984;50:617–621.
131. Miller JH, Gisvold JJ, Weiland LH, McIlrath DC. Upper gastrointestinal tract: villous tumors. Am J Roentgenol 1980;134: 933–936.
132. Nugent FW, Richmond M, Park Sk. Crohn's disease of the duodenum. Gut 1977;18:115–120.
133. Legge DA, Hoffman HN, Carlson HC. Pancreatitis as a complication of regional enteritis of the duodenum. Gastroenterology 1971;61:834–837.
134. Rutgeerts P, Onette E, Vantrappen G, et al. Crohn's disease of the stomach and duodenum: a clinical study with emphasis on the value of endoscopy and endoscopic biopsies. Endoscopy 1980;12:288–294.
135. Gottlieb C, Alpert S. Regional jejunitis. Am J Roentgenol Radium Ther Nucl Med 1937;38:881–883.
136. Thompson WM, Cockrill H Jr, Rice RP. Regional enteritis of the duodenum. Am J Roentgenol Radium Ther Nucl Med 1975;123: 252–262.
137. Tromm A, Huppe D, Micklefield GH, Schwegler U, May B. Acute pancreatitis complicating Crohn's disease: mere coincidence or causality? Gut 1992;33:1289–1291.
138. Weber P, Seibold F, Jenss H. Acute pancreatitis in Crohn's disease. J Clin Gastroenterol 1993;17:286–291.
139. Eisner TD, Goldman IS, McKinley MJ. Crohn's disease and pancreatitis. Am J Gastroenterol 1993;88:583–586.
140. Chapin LE, Scudamore HH, Baggenstoss AH, Bargen JA. Regional enteritis associated visceral changes. Gastroenterology 1956;30:404–415.
141. Barthelemy CR. Crohn's disease of the duodenum with spontaneous reflux into the pancreatic duct. Gastrointest Radiol 1983;8:319–320.
142. McCutcheon AD. A fresh approach to the pathogenesis of pancreatitis. Gut 1968;9:296–310.
143. Simmonds S, Pitman R, Machan L, et al. Duodenopancreatic fistula accompanying Crohn's disease of the distal duodenum. Am J Gastroenterol 1989;84:800–803.
144. Altman HS, Phillipps G, Bank S, Klotz H. Pancreatitis associated with duodenal Crohn's disease. Am J Gastroenterol 1983;78: 174–177.
145. Eliakim R, Fich A, Libson E, Katz E, Rachmilewitz D. Crohn's disease of the duodenum presented as pancreatitis due to persimmon bezoar. J Clin Gastroenterol 1987;9:553–555.
146. Matsumato T, Matsui T, Iida M, et al. Acute pancreatitis as a complication of Crohn's disease. Am J Gastroenterol 1989;84: 804–807.
147. Axon ATR, Ashton MG, Lindott DJ. Chronic pancreatitis and inflammatory bowel disease. Clin Radiol 1979;30:179–182.
148. Lee SP, Nicholls JF, Park HZ. Biliary sludge as a cause of acute pancreatitis. N Engl J Med 1992;326:589–593.
149. Ball WP, Baggenstoss AH, Bargen JA. Pancreatic lesions associated with chronic ulcerative colitis. Arch Pathol 1950;50: 345–348.
150. Stocker W, Otte M, Ulrich S, et al. Autoimmunity to pancreatic juice in Crohn's disease. Scand J Gastroenterol 1987;22:41–52.
151. Caldwell JH, Evans EE. Granuloma (sarcoid?) of the pancreas. Am J Gastroenterol 1978;69:320–322.
152. Curran JF Jr, Curran JF Sr. Boeck's sarcoid of the pancreas. Surgery 1950;28:574–578.
153. Frandsen PJ, Jarnum S, Malmstrom J. Crohn's disease of the duodenum. Scand J Gastroenterol 1980;15:683–688.
154. Crohn's disease of the duodenum (Editorial). Br Med J 1977;2:282.
155. Loehr WJ, Mujahed F, Fahn D, Gray GF, Thorbjarnarson B. Primary lymphoma of the gastrointestinal tract: a review of 100 cases. Ann Surg 1969;170:232–238.
156. Burgerman A, Baggenstoss AH, Cain JC. Primary malignant neoplasms of the duodenum excluding the papilla of Vater: clinicopathologic study of 31 cases. Gastroenterology 1956;30: 421–431.
157. Reyes EL, Tally RW. Primary malignant tumors of the small intestine. Am J Gastroenterol 1970;54:30–43.
158. Lewin KJ, Ranchod M, Dorfman RF. Lymphomas of the gastrointestinal tract: a study of 117 cases presenting with gastrointestinal disease. Cancer 1978;42:693–707.
159. Freed JS, Dreiling DA, Reiner MA. Non-Hodgkin's lymphoma of the pancreas producing acute pancreatitis and pancreatic abscess. Mt Sinai J Med (NY) 1983;50:424–427.

# 25

# Pancreatitis Associated with Hyperlipidemia or Hyperparathyroidism

Qiang Liu and Richard A Prinz

## PART A: HYPERLIPIDEMIA

Since Speck's first publication in 1865 (1), the association of pancreatitis and hyperlipidemia (HL) has become well established. The incidence of HL in patients with pancreatitis ranges from 4 to 53% (2–7). The broad range depends on how HL is defined. Lactescent serum is found in only 4–21% of patients with acute pancreatitis (2, 4). On the other hand, an elevated serum cholesterol level can be found in more than 50% of patients with acute pancreatitis (7). The principal question is whether the lipid abnormalities that are seen in acute pancreatitis are a primary cause or secondary effect of the disease. Since a wide variety of changes in circulating lipids are found in patients with pancreatitis, it is likely that both are true. Clinically, HL does not seem to cause acute pancreatitis unless plasma triglyceride levels are markedly elevated to values over 1000 mg/dL. Elevated cholesterol levels have not been found to cause acute pancreatitis.

Both clinical observations and experimental studies implicate HL as an etiologic factor for pancreatitis. Clinical data show that three of the five familial hyperlipidemias (types I, IV, and V) are associated with the development of pancreatitis (Table 25A.1). Recurrent attacks of pancreatitis occur in patients with marked hypertriglyceridemia, and these can be prevented if triglyceride (TG) levels are controlled (8–10). In animals, a high-fat diet can provoke an attack of pancreatitis (11, 12). Experimental evidence suggests that hypertriglyceridemia can initiate pancreatic injury through the release of free fatty acids (FFAs) (12). High serum levels of chylomicrons (CMs) and chylomicron remnants may also damage the pancreas by the release of cholesterol crystals (13).

Most patients with pancreatitis do not have a primary lipid disorder. Nevertheless, transient HL often occurs during an attack of pancreatitis and tends to clear as the pancreatitis resolves. Elevated serum lipid levels occur in most animals with acute pancreatitis (14–16). Therefore, pancreatitis seems to be the cause of HL in most patients rather than the reverse. The mechanism for this secondary HL is unclear. Caren and Carbo postulated that the inflammatory process of pancreatitis causes an acute glucagon deficiency by direct injury to the alpha cells. A lack of glucagon can cause defects in lipid metabolism that result in HL (17). This theory is not supported by experimental and clinical data that show that glucagon levels are increased in acute pancreatitis (18). Inactivation or inhibition of lipoprotein lipase (LPL) during the acute phase of disease has also been suggested as a mechanism for secondary HL in pancreatitis. Once again, experimental studies have shown conflicting results. Some investigators have found marked inhibition of LPL (15, 16, 19), while others have found normal levels of this enzyme during pancreatitis (20).

### Etiology

Serum lipids such as cholesterol and TGs are insoluble in water, and they are transported in the blood in combination with soluble lipoproteins. Lipoproteins are composed of both lipids and proteins. The lipids in lipoproteins include cholesterol, TGs, and phospholipids. The protein components of the lipoproteins are called apoproteins. The apoproteins are designated by both capital letters (A, B, and so forth) and Roman numerals (I, II and so forth). In addition to their structural role, apoproteins have other important functions. Some, such as apoproteins E and B-100, can function as ligands or binding proteins that permit the lipoproteins to bind to specific cell-surface receptors. Others can activate (e.g., apoproteins A-I and C-II) as well as inhibit (e.g., apoprotein C-III) a number of enzymes that are critical to normal lipid metabolism. Lipoproteins vary in the amount and kind of lipids and proteins that they transport (21). For example, chylomicrons contain mostly TGs (85–90%) and little cholesterol (5%); so, a marked increase in the chylomicron fraction in the blood is usually associated with hypertriglyceridemia and normal or only mildly elevated cholesterol levels. Very low density lipoproteins (VLDLs) are rich in TGs (60–70%) and also contain considerable cholesterol (20%). Therefore, an increase in the VLDL fraction in the blood is associated with both hypertriglyceridemia and hypercholesterolemia. Both low-density lipoproteins (LDL) and high-density lipoproteins (HDL) contain little TG (<8%), and marked elevation in levels of either of these circulating lipoproteins is only associated with hypercholesterolemia. Chylomicron remnants and VLDL remnants contain equal amounts of cholesterol and TGs (both 30%) and are associated with both hypertriglyceridemia and hypercholesterolemia when increased in blood.

There are two predominant pathways in lipoprotein metabolism (21). The exogenous pathway involves the absorption of dietary cholesterol and TG-derived FFAs from the intestinal tract and their transport to the liver and peripheral tissue. Chylomicrons are produced in the gut and serve as the lipid transport system through the intestinal lymphatics and mesenteric venous systems. In the capillaries of adipose tissue and muscle, the TGs in chylomicrons are hydrolyzed by endothelial LPL to produce monoglycerides, diglycerides, and FFAs. This decreases the size of chylomicrons, which are then called chylomicron remnants. The monoglycerides, diglycerides, and FFAs are taken up by the surrounding tissues, and the remnants are taken up by the liver.

The endogenous pathway begins with the synthesis and secretion of VLDLs by the liver. The TGs in these VLDLs are also hydrolyzed to produce glycerides, FFAs, and VLDL remnants (IDLs). The IDLs can be taken up by the liver or can be converted to LDLs. The LDLs deliver cholesterol to tissues for metabolic and structural needs. HDLs are also synthesized in the

**TABLE 25A.1. Phenotype Classification of Primary and Secondary Hyperlipidemia (HL)**

| Phenotype | Lipoprotein Abnormality | Lipid Abnormality[a] TG | CHOL | Genetic Disorder or Primary HL | Related Conditions of Secondary HL |
|---|---|---|---|---|---|
| I | CM | ↑ | → | LPL deficiency, apoprotein C-II deficiency | Systemic lupus erythematosus |
| $II_a$ | LDL | → | ↑ | Familial hypercholesterolemia (heterozygote, homozygote), polygenic hypercholestrolemia, familial defective apoprotein B, familial combined hyperlipidemia | Obesity, hypothyroidism, nephrotic syndrome, hepatoma |
| $II_b$ | LDL VLDL | ↑ | ↑ | Familial combined hyperlipidemia Polygenic hypercholesterolemia or familial hypercholesterolemia plus familial hypertriglyceridemia | Cushing's syndrome, dysglobulinemia, acute intermittent porphyria, anorexia nervosa, Werner's syndrome |
| III | β-VLDL, IDL | ↑ | ↑ | Familial dysbetalipoproteinemia | Dysglobulinemia |
| IV | VLDL | ↑ | → | Familial combined hyperlipidemia, familial hypertriglyceridemia | Obesity, diabetes mellitus, estrogen therapy, acromegaly, Cushing's syndrome, uremia, nephrotic syndrome, acute viral hepatitis, dysglobulinemia, alcoholic hyperlipidemia, third-trimester pregnancy |
| V | CM VLDL | ↑ | ↑ | Familial combined hyperlipidemia plus LPL deficiency LPL deficiency, apoprotein C-II deficiency | Poorly controlled diabetes mellitus, estrogen therapy, alcoholic hyperlipidemia |

[a]TGH, triglyceride; CHOL, cholesterol; LPL, lipoprotein lipase; ↑, elevated; →, no effect.
Adapted from Oberman A, Kreisberg RA, Henkin Y, eds. Principles and management of lipid disorders: a primary care approach. Baltimore: Williams & Wilkins, 1992:137–185.

liver and are products of LPL hydrolysis of chylomicrons and VLDLs. High blood levels of HDL-cholesterol are associated with a lower risk of developing coronary artery disease. HDLs participate in reverse cholesterol transport from peripheral tissues to the liver. Since this facilitates cholesterol excretion from the body, it protects against HL and its complications.

Lipid disorders were initially classified according to five lipoprotein phenotypes (I–V) by Lees and Fredrickson. This subsequently was modified to include six different phenotypes by dividing type II into type $II_a$ and type $II_b$. Secondary HL can be classified into the same phenotypes as primary HL. Phenotypic categories of primary and secondary HL are summarized in Table 25A.1 (21).

Pancreatitis has been found in patients with primary and secondary types I, IV, and V HL. In type I HL, excessive TGs are found in the form of chylomicrons. The presence of excess chylomicrons gives a diffuse cloudy appearance to the serum of these patients. If the serum has this lactescent appearance and is refrigerated (4°C) overnight (18–24 hours), chylomicrons will rise to the surface, forming a creamy layer and leaving a clear layer below. The chemical basis for type IV HL is an increase in endogenous TG that is reflected by an increase in VLDLs. When the serum of patients with type IV HL is refrigerated overnight, VLDLs usually cause the fluid to become turbid, but no creamy layer is found on top. In type V HL, both serum chylomicrons and endogenous TGs are increased. The endogenous TGs are transported in the serum as VLDLs. When the serum of patients with type V HL is refrigerated overnight, a creamy layer of chylomicrons appears on top, but the fluid below appears turbid from the VLDLs (22). The incidence of pancreatitis in patients with HL is reported as 41% in type V, 37.5% in type I, and 16% in type IV (22). Type V is the most frequent lipoprotein pattern found during an acute attack of pancreatitis, and type I is the second most common pattern. After an acute attack has resolved, most patients do not have fasting chylomicronemia, and the most common pattern is changed to type IV (13, 23).

Genetic disorders of lipid metabolism can cause primary HL and acute pancreatitis (21). Hyperchylomicronemia and hypertriglyceridemia from lipoprotein lipase (LPL) deficiency or from apoprotein C-II deficiency (type I) are uncommon genetic disorders that are seen in infants and children. LPL deficiency results in hypertriglyceridemia from delayed chylomicron metabolism. A deficiency of apoprotein C-II, which activates LPL, can also produce this lipid disorder. Familial hypertriglyceridemia (type IV) is a common autosomal dominant lipid abnormality that occurs in 1–2% of the population and accounts for about 15–25% of patients who have increased VLDL levels and hypertriglyceridemia. Typically, hypertriglyceridemia develops in early adulthood and is often associated with obesity, glucose intolerance, hyperinsulinemia, hyperuricemia, and hypertension. Chylomicronemia with elevated VLDLs (type V) is a primary genetic disorder of TG metabolism. Patients with this disorder usually have a secondary cause of hypertriglyceridemia. In primary HL, patients with the same phenotype do not necessarily have the same genetic abnormality or biochemical defect, for example, type V hyperlipoproteinemia can result from LPL deficiency, apoprotein C-II deficiency, or familial combined hyperlipidemia. Likewise, patients with the same genetic disorder may have different phenotypes, for example, LPL deficiency can cause both type I and type V hyperlipoproteinemia (Table 25A.1).

When coupled with a preexisting genetic disorder of lipid metabolism, a secondary cause of HL can cause marked hypertriglyceridemia. Common causes of secondary HL include pregnancy, diabetes mellitus, obesity, alcohol ingestion, the nephrotic syndrome, chronic renal failure, hypothyroidism, and hepatic disease. Drugs known to induce secondary HL include estrogens, progestins, androgens, glucocorticoids, retinoids, ß-blockers, thiazide and loop diuretics, and cyclosporine. Almost all of these causes of HL have been associated with pancreatitis (Table 25A.2).

Lipid abnormalities are common in diabetes mellitus,

particularly in non-insulin-dependent diabetes mellitus. Diabetics frequently have increased blood insulin levels because of peripheral insulin resistance. This hyperinsulinemia stimulates increased hepatic synthesis of VLDL and leads to hypertriglyceridemia. Obesity induces HL by increasing hepatic production of VLDL and decreasing production of HDL-cholesterol. Consumption of a high-fat diet may also lead to the accumulation of both chylomicrons and VLDL.

Alcohol ingestion, which is of course a frequent cause of pancreatitis, can cause hypertriglyceridemia both by increasing synthesis of VLDLs and by decreasing their removal from the circulation by LPL (21). The reported incidence of lipid abnormalities in alcoholic patients with pancreatitis ranges from 35% to 41% (5, 24). The pathogenesis of alcoholic pancreatitis is not completely clear. In addition to a direct toxic effect of alcohol on the acinar cells and the induction of duodenitis, which may cause partial obstruction of the pancreatic duct, hypertriglyceridemia itself has been suggested as a possible mechanism for pancreatitis after alcohol ingestion (24).

Most patients with the nephrotic syndrome also have increased blood cholesterol and TG levels. Hypercholesterolemia in the nephrotic syndrome is a result of increased apolipoprotein-B, which causes an increased LDL concentration. The hypertriglyceridemia is the result of acquired insulin resistance, which increases the rates of VLDL secretion. Hypertriglyceridemia in chronic renal failure is due to a combination of increased VLDL secretion and reduced rates of VLDL removal. Hypothyroidism can decrease LPL activity and produce acquired defects in the removal of VLDL and chylomicrons. With acute hepatocellular disease, hypertriglyceridemia and decreased HDL-cholesterol levels may result from decreased hepatic triglyceride lipase activity.

Serum TG levels increase during normal pregnancy because of an estrogen-induced increase in TG and VLDL synthesis, an increase in insulin secretion, and/or a decrease in the level of apoprotein-CII, which is a cofactor for the hydrolysis of lipoprotein TGs by LPL (25). Serum TG elevations are most marked in the third trimester. Estrogen therapy causes modest to marked elevations of serum TG levels by increasing hepatic synthesis of VLDL and inhibiting VLDL removal from the circulation by LPL (21). ß-Blockers often increase TGs and reduce HDL-cholesterol levels by decreasing LPL activity. Hypertriglyceridemia induced by vitamin A (26, 27) is due to an increase in hepatic synthesis and secretion of TGs and a decrease in tissue uptake of TGs. Elevated TG levels have been found in 17% of patients taking vitamin A for 20 weeks or more (27).

Clinically acute pancreatitis does not seem to occur unless the serum TG level is markedly elevated (1000–2000 mg/dL) (5, 9, 21). Although primary and secondary lipid disorders alone can induce HL and pancreatitis, the interaction of a familial lipid disorder with one of the above-mentioned secondary factors is more likely to cause an attack of acute pancreatitis because of the marked hypertriglyceridemia induced by this combination (9, 21, 23, 28).

**TABLE 25A.2. Common Causes of Secondary Hyperlipidemia (HL)**

| Primary Disorders | Drugs |
|---|---|
| Diabetes mellitus | Estrogens |
| Obesity | Progestins |
| Alcohol ingestion | Androgens |
| Nephrotic syndrome | Glucocorticoids |
| Chronic renal failure | Vitamin A and vitamin A derivatives |
| Hypothyroidism | β-Blockers |
| Liver disease | Thiazide and loop diuretics |
| Pregnancy | Cyclosporine |

**TABLE 25A.3. Clinical and Laboratory Features of Marked Hypertriglyceridemia**

| Clinical Features | Laboratory Features |
|---|---|
| Pancreatitis | Hyperlipoproteinemia (types I, IV or V) |
| Eruptive xanthoma | ↑ Triglyceride and/or ↑ cholesterol |
| Lipemia retinalis | Spurious blood tests (pseudohypo-amylasemia, pseudohyponatremia) |
| Hepatosplenomegaly | |
| Glucose intolerance | |
| Hyperuricemia | |

## Pathogenesis of Pancreatitis in HL Patients

Periacinar release and activation of pancreatic proteases have been traditionally considered early and essential steps in the pathogenesis of acute pancreatitis. Phospholipase $A_2$ activation and pancreatic lipase activation are regarded as important events in this inflammatory process since they cause the release of cytotoxic lysolecithins and FFAs (29–31). Lysolecithins and FFAs stimulate thrombogenesis and are lytic to cell membranes, causing the local liberation of pancreatic enzymes that initiate a self-propagating chemical pancreatitis (8).

The role of HL in the pathogenesis of acute pancreatitis is still not completely understood. In 1969, Havel (32) proposed that increased hydrolysis of TGs in and around the gland by pancreatic lipase could initiate acute pancreatitis. The local accumulation of high levels of FFAs has a number of potentially noxious effects. Excess FFAs can damage cell membranes and proteins and have toxic effects on capillary endothelium and alveolar capillary membranes. They can decrease pancreatic blood flow and induce small-vessel thrombosis. In acute pancreatitis, FFAs can produce acinar cell injury directly (33) or as a secondary phenomenon. They can initiate or aggravate the adult respiratory distress syndrome (34). In patients with acute necrotizing pancreatitis, the degree and duration of the elevation of serum FFAs seems to correlate with the severity of pancreatic parenchymal damage and extrapancreatic fat necrosis (35). Elevated chylomicrons and chylomicron remnants in type I and V HL patients may release cholesterol crystals during lipolysis. These cholesterol crystals, which are involved in the pathogenesis of atherosclerosis, can cause mechanical damage to the capillaries in the pancreas, and this can imitate or aggravate acute pancreatitis (13).

## Clinical Features and Diagnosis

There are no distinguishing features of acute pancreatitis associated with HL. The clinical presentation consists of abdominal pain, nausea, vomiting, fever, and leukocytosis just as is seen in pancreatitis from other causes (12). The abdominal pain may or may not be very severe during a spontaneous attack of acute pancreatitis (21). Other clinical features of marked hypertriglyceridemia (>1000–2000 mg/dL) that may suggest that a patient with abdominal pain has pancreatitis include eruptive xanthoma, lipemia retinalis, hepatosplenomegaly, and increased levels of serum glucose and serum uric acid (Table 25A.3). The frequency of pancreatitis in this type of patient is reduced substantially when TG levels are lowered. Rarely, a patient who has attacks of acute pancreatitis provoked by hypertriglyceridemia will not have markedly elevated TG levels because the associated nausea, vomiting, and abdominal pain prevent food intake and allow the TGs to decrease. Thus, the disease itself may obscure the relationship between HL and pancreatitis. However, fasting must last more than 24 hours to affect TGs, and most patients with pancreatitis present well before this because of abdominal pain.

Serum and urinary amylase levels are often normal in pancreatitis associated with HL. As many as 50% of patients with abdominal pain and hypertriglyceridemia who are believed clinically to have acute pancreatitis may not have elevated serum or urinary levels of amylase or lipase (3, 9). These patients will have lactescent serum because of marked hypertriglyceridemia, with serum TG levels above 300–400 mg/dL (4). Lipemic serum may either interfere with the laboratory procedure for amylase determination or may contain an amylase inhibitor (18, 36–38). Studies have shown a relative increase in amylase activity after serial dilution of hyperlipemic serum in patients with acute pancreatitis (36, 38). In acute pancreatitis, the renal clearance of amylase rises. The amylase clearance is not affected by HL, so the amylase/creatinine clearance ratio may be helpful in diagnosing acute pancreatitis in patients with HL (39). HL may also cause a pseudohyponatremia because of the space-occupying effect of lipid in the blood (37).

Patients with HL who present with symptoms and signs of acute pancreatitis but have a normal serum amylase level should usually be assumed to have this disease until proven otherwise. The tentative diagnosis can be confirmed by using the amylase/creatinine clearance ratio and/or serial dilution of hyperlipemic serum. Patients with marked hypertriglyceridemia may also present with the complications of acute pancreatitis such as pancreatic pseudocyst and pancreatic infection or with chronic pancreatitis and pancreatic insufficiency (9). Pancreatic exocrine insufficiency has been found in patients with types I, IV, and V familial hyperlipoproteinemias after repeated attacks of pancreatitis (40, 41).

### Treatment

The general principles of therapy for the acute pancreatitis are applicable in patients with HL. Once the acute attack has resolved, decreasing the serum TG levels is crucial to preventing recurrent attacks. Hypolipidemic therapy begins with an appropriate diet. In both types I and V hyperlipoproteinemia, a low-fat diet is essential to limit chylomicron formation from long-chain fatty acids in food. A low-fat diet of less than 10 g/day should be instituted in type I familial HL. In type V HL, a low-fat diet of less than 50 g/day is administered (10, 12). Limiting carbohydrate intake is also important to reduce endogenous hypertriglyceridemia, which originates from carbohydrate sources. During a severe acute attack, parenteral nutrition may be beneficial by preventing FFA release from adipose tissue or other sources (35).

Lipid-lowering drugs, such as fibrates (gemfibrozil, clofibrate, and fenofibrate), nicotinic acid, and omega-3 fatty acids can be effective in patients with hypertriglyceridemia who do not have familial LPL deficiency and may be instituted after the attack has resolved (42). Fibrates are the primary drugs used for hypertriglyceridemia. Fibrates reduce TGs by inhibiting VLDL production as well as by enhancing VLDL clearance. They also reduce LDL-cholesterol and increase HDL-cholesterol. Nicotinic acid has a favorable effect on lipoprotein metabolism, causing LDL-cholesterol and VLDL-cholesterol levels to decrease and HDL-cholesterol levels to increase. Nicotinic acid affects lipoprotein metabolism by inhibiting lipolysis in adipocytes, inhibiting the hepatic synthesis of TGs, and reducing the rate of HDL-cholesterol catabolism. The combination of fibrates and nicotinic acid may be synergistic in the treatment of hypertriglyceridemia. Fish oils that are rich in polyunsaturated fatty acids, including omega-3 polyunsaturated fatty acid, eicosapentanoic acid, and docosahexanoic acid, have been used to treat hypertriglyceridemia. The triglyceride-lowering effect of fish oils is due to inhibition of VLDL-triglyceride synthesis. Since fish oils can increase chylomicron formation, they should be used with caution. Fish oils are usually reserved for patients who are refractory to fibrates and nicotinic acid or who are intolerant to side effects of these drugs (21). Caution is required when using fish oil or nicotinic acid in diabetic patients because they may worsen glucose control.

In patients who fail to have their abdominal pain relieved with lipid-lowering drugs, feedback inhibition of pancreatic exocrine secretion can be used. Pancreatic proteases in the duodenum inhibit pancreatic enzyme secretion. Enzyme replacement therapy when effective should reduce acinar cell stimulation, decrease intraductal pressure, and alleviate associated nausea and abdominal pain (9, 43).

In patients with refractory HL, and especially in those with hyperlipidemic gestational pancreatitis, which carries a high risk of death for both mother and fetus, plasma exchange and lipoprotein apheresis have been used to reduce circulating lipid levels rapidly and halt the progression of associated pancreatitis (44–47). Plasma exchange can lower lipid and pancreatic enzyme levels and improve the signs and symptoms of acute pancreatitis. Plasma exchange also removes proteins other than lipoproteins and can increase the potential risk of bleeding and infection. Lipoprotein apheresis (pheresis), which has the same effect of decreasing serum lipids, removes only large-molecular-weight complexes from plasma such as lipoproteins and retains immunoglobulins, albumin, and clotting factors (46, 47). A combination of plasma exchange and apheresis techniques has been highly effective in some patients.

Diseases known to cause secondary HL should be treated and controlled. Alcohol should be avoided. Drugs known to increase serum TG levels such as estrogens, vitamin A, ß-blockers, thiazide, and loop diuretics should be discontinued whenever possible. Hypolipidemic therapy may be needed long term. Patients should be advised to exercise, reduce body weight, quit cigarette smoking, and limit intake of caffeine (9, 12). Regular exercise can reduce serum TG concentrations by increasing LPL activity.

## REFERENCES: PART A. HYPERLIPIDEMIA

1. Speck L. Fall von Lipämie. Arch Verein Wissenschaftl Heilkunde 1865;1:232. Quoted in: Thannhauser SJ, ed. Lipidoses, diseases of the intracellular lipid metabolism. 3rd ed. New York: Grune & Stratton, 1958:307.
2. Coffey RJ. Unusual features of pancreatic disease. Ann Surg 1952;135:715–720.
3. Greenberger NJ, Hatch FT, Drummey GD, Isselbacher KJ. Pancreatitis and hyperlipemia: a study of serum lipid alterations in 25 patients with acute pancreatitis. Medicine 1966;45:161–174.
4. Cameron JL, Capuzzi DM, Zuidema GD, Margolis S. Acute pancreatitis with hyperlipemia: the incidence of lipid abnormalities in acute pancreatitis. Ann Surg 1973;177:483–489.
5. Buch A, Buch J, Carlsen A, Schmidt A. Hyperlipidemia and pancreatitis. World J Surg 1980;4:307–314.
6. Dominguez-Munoz JE, Malfertheiner P, Ditschuneit HH, et al. Hyperlipidemia in acute pancreatitis. Relationship with etiology, onset, and severity of the disease. Int J Pancreatol 1991;10: 261–267.
7. Wang C, Adlersberg D, Feldman EB. Serum lipids in acute pancreatitis. Gastroenterology 1959;36:832–840.
8. Malloy MJ, Kane JP. Medical management of hyperlipidemic states. Adv Intern Med 1994;39:603–631.
9. Toskes PP. Hyperlipidemic pancreatitis. Gastroenterol Clin North Am 1990;19:783–791.
10. Farmer RG, Winkelman EI, Brown HB, Lewis LA. Hyperlipoproteinemia and pancreatitis. Am J Med 1973;54:161–165.
11. Brian Haig TH. Experimental pancreatitis intensified by a high fat diet. Surg Gynecol Obstet 1970;131:914–918.
12. Sanfey H, Cameron JL. Pancreatitis associated with hyperlipemia. In: Howard JM, Jordan GL Jr, Reber HA, eds. Surgical diseases of the pancreas. Philadelphia: Lea & Febiger, 1987: 297–309.
13. Ditschuneit H: Hyperlipoproteinemia in the pathogenesis of acute pancreatitis. In: Beger HG, Buchler M, eds. Acute pancreatitis. Research and clinical management. Berlin: Springer-Verlag, 1987:32–40.

14. Wang C, Strauss L, Adlersberg D. Experimental pancreatitis and plasma lipids. Gastroenterology 1958;35:465–472.
15. Stackhouse KL, Glass DD, Zimmermann B. Relationships of lipoprotein lipase and hyperlipaemia in pancreatitis. Surg Forum 1966;17:343–344.
16. Kessler JI, Finkel M, Ho P, Janowitz HD. Lipoprotein lipase inhibition in rabbits with experimental pancreatitis. Proc Soc Exp Biol Med 1962;110:24–26.
17. Caren R, Carbo L. Pancreatic alpha-cell function in relation to cholesterol metabolism. J Clin Endocr Metab 1956;16:507–516.
18. Cameron JL, Crisler C, Margolis S, DeMeester TR, Zuidema GD. Acute pancreatitis with hyperlipemia. Surgery 1971;70:53–61.
19. Kessler JI, Kniffen JC, Janowitz HD. Lipoprotein lipase inhibition in the hyperlipemia of acute alcoholic pancreatitis. N Engl J Med 1963;269:943–948.
20. Bagdade JD. Diabetic lipemia complicating acute pancreatitis. Lancet 1969;2:1041–1043.
21. Oberman A, Kreisberg RA, Henkin Y, ed. Principles and management of lipid disorders: a primary care approach. Baltimore: Williams & Wilkins, 1992:87–105, 137–185, 246–267.
22. Fredrickson DS, Levy RI. Familial hyperlipoproteinemia. In: Stangury JB, Wyngaarden JB, Fredrickson DS 3rd, eds. The metabolic basis of inherited disease. New York: McGraw-Hill, 1972:545–614.
23. Cameron JL, Capuzzi DM, Zuidema GD, Margolis S. Acute pancreatitis with hyperlipemia. Evidence for a persistent defect in lipid metabolism. Am J Med 1974;56:482–487.
24. Cameron JL. Lipid abnormalities and acute pancreatitis. Hosp Pract 1977;12:95–101.
25. De Chalain TM, Michell WL, Beger GMR. Hyperlipemia, pregnancy and pancreatitis. Surg Gynecol Obstet 1988;167:469–473.
26. Flynn WJ, Freeman PC, Wickbolat LG. Pancreatitis associated with isotretinoin-induced hypertriglyceridemia. Ann Intern Med 1987;107:63.
27. Bershad S, Rubinstein A, Paterniti JR Jr, et al. Changes in plasma lipid and lipoproteins during isotretinoin therapy for acne. N Engl J Med 1985;313:981–985.
28. Brunzell JD, Schrott HG. The interaction of familial and secondary causes of hypertriglyceridemia: role in pancreatitis. Trans Assoc Am Physicians 1973;86:245–254.
29. Nevalainen TJ. The role of phospholipase A in acute pancreatitis. Scand J Gastroenterol 1980;15:641–650.
30. Lee PC, Howard JM. Fat necrosis. Surg Gynecol Obstet 1979;148: 785–789.
31. Nagai H, Henrich H, Wunsch PH, Fischbach W, Mossner J. Role of pancreatic enzymes and their substrates in autodigestion of the pancreas. In vitro studies with isolated rat pancreatic acini. Gastroenterology 1989;96:838–847.
32. Havel RJ. Pathogenesis, differentiation, and management of hypertriglyceridemia. Adv Intern Med 1969;15:117–154.
33. Saharia P, Margolis S, Zuidema GD, Cameron JL. Acute pancreatitis with hyperlipemia: studies with an isolated perfused canine pancreas. Surgery 1977;82:60–67.
34. Kimura T, Toung JK, Margolis S, Permutt S, Cameron JL. Respiratory failure in acute pancreatitis. A possible role for triglycerides. Ann Surg 1979;189:509–514.
35. Domschke S, Malfertheiner P, Uhl W, Buchler M, Domschke W. Free fatty acids in serum of patients with acute necrotizing or, edematous pancreatitis. Int J Pancreatol 1993;13:105–110.
36. Fallat RW, Vester JW, Glueck CJ. Suppression of amylase activity by hypertriglyceridemia. JAMA 1973;225:1331–1334.
37. Dunne MJ, Shenkin A, Imrie CW. Misleading hyponatraemia in acute pancreatitis with hyperlipaemia. Lancet 1979;1:221.
38. Warshaw AL, Bellini CA, Lesser PB. Inhibition of serum and urine amylase activity in pancreatitis with hyperlipemia. Ann Surg 1975;182:72–75.
39. Lesser PB, Warshaw AL. Diagnosis of pancreatitis masked by hyperlipemia. Ann Intern Med 1975;82:795–798.
40. Herfort K, Sobra J, Fric P, Heyrovsky A. Familial hyperlipoproteinemia and exocrine pancreas. Scand J Gastroenterol 1971;6; 139–143.
41. Krauss RM, Levy AG. Subclinical chronic pancreatitis in type I hyperlipoproteinemia. Am J Med 1977;62:144–149.
42. Durrington PN. Hyperlipidaemia: diagnosis and management. London: Wright, 1989:135–156.
43. Owyang C, Louie DS, Tatum D. Feedback regulation of pancreatic enzyme secretion. Suppression of cholestokinin release by trypsin. J Clin Invest 1986;77:2042–2047.
44. Gerard A, Schooneman F, Guine JM, et al. Treatment by plasma exchange of a patient with hyperlipidemia and diabetic ketoacidosis with lesional pulmonary, edema and acute pancreatitis. Vox Sang 1982;43:147–150.
45. Achard JM, Westeel PF, Moriniere P, Lalau JD, de Cagny B, Fournier A. Pancreatitis related to severe acute hypertriglyceridemia during pregnancy: treatment with lipoprotein apheresis. Intensive Care Med 1991;17:236–237.
46. Roberts IM. Hyperlipidemic gestational pancreatitis. Gastroenterology 1993;104:1560–1562.
47. Swoboda K, Derfler K, Koppensteiner R, et al. Extracorporeal lipid elimination for treatment of gestational hyperlipidemic pancreatitis. Gastroenterology 1993;104:1527–1531.

## PART B: HYPERPARATHYROIDISM

A cause and effect relationship between hyperparathyroidism (HPT) and pancreatitis was first suggested by Cope et al. in 1957 (1). Numerous subsequent reports and reviews have supported this association. The incidence of pancreatitis in patients with HPT has ranged from 0% to 34% (2–13). With higher levels of hypercalcemia, the association is more prominent. Hyperparathyroid crisis, which occurs when the serum calcium is 15 mg/dL or greater has a 26–34% incidence of pancreatitis (2, 7). The frequency of coexistent pancreatitis was higher in early series of patients with HPT, but it has decreased substantially in more recent reports (Table 25B.1). This decrease has been attributed to the introduction of multichannel biochemical screening analysis, which has increased the overall recognition of HPT and has done so at a much earlier stage of the disease.

The association between HPT and pancreatitis may reflect a subtle selection bias that occurred before the advent of routine serum chemistry survey analysis (10, 12). Patients with pancreatitis had their serum calcium measured because of the clinical possibility of hypocalcemia, and this may have increased the relative frequency of diagnosing HPT in patients with pancreatitis (10, 14). With routine screening of serum calcium, HPT is being diagnosed at a much earlier stage. The hypercalcemia that is seen in present-day patients with HPT may not be severe enough to cause pancreatitis. Since HPT is recognized and treated sooner, the additive effects that may be necessary to cause pancreatitis never occur (15, 16). The coexistence of HPT and pancreatitis has also been identified by determining the occur-

**TABLE 25B.1. Incidence of Pancreatitis in Patients with Hyperparathyroidism**

| Year | Author | Pancreatitis (*n*)/HPT (*n*) | Incidence (%) |
|---|---|---|---|
| 1961 | Fink et al. | 19/56[a] | 34 |
| 1962 | Mixter et al. | 11/155 | 7 |
| 1962 | Kyle et al. | 5/40 | 12 |
| 1966 | Anglem. | 8/69 | 11.5 |
| 1966 | Ludwig et al. | 7/37 | 19 |
| 1967 | Herskovic et al. | 15/450 | 3.3 |
| 1968 | Kelly et al. | 23/87[a] | 26 |
| 1970 | Schmidt et al. | 24/370 | 6.5 |
| 1975 | Paloyan et al. | 6/150 | 4 |
| 1976 | Rosin. | 9/1000 | 0.9 |
| 1980 | Bess et al. | 17/1153 | 1.5 |
| 1980 | Kelly. | 7/242 | 3 |
| 1982 | Paloyan et al. | 0/26 | 0 |
| 1988 | Sitges-Serra et al. | 7/86 | 8 |

[a]Cases of hyperparathyroid crisis.

rence of HPT in patients with pancreatitis. The incidence of HPT in patients with pancreatitis has ranged from 0.2% to 0.4% in two studies (14, 17).

### Etiology and Pathogenesis

Since the first description of pancreatitis as a complication of HPT, investigators have debated whether this is a causal relationship or merely a chance coincidence. From their original experience, Cope et al. postulated that HPT might be a cause of pancreatitis and that pancreatitis might be a diagnostic clue for HPT (1). This hypothesis was soon supported by subsequent reports that as many as 7–12% of patients with HPT had associated pancreatitis (3). However, since serum calcium has been routinely measured as a part of the survey of blood chemistry, the frequency of coexistent pancreatitis appears to be much lower. In most recent series of surgically proven HPT, the frequency of coexistent pancreatitis has decreased to 1.5% or less (9, 10, 12). Because of this marked decrease, the causal relationship between HPT and pancreatitis has again been questioned. Some investigators have suggested that the association of those two disorders can be explained by the chance occurrence of two common abnormalities (10, 12).

A causal relationship is still suggested by the fact that parathyroidectomy seems to prevent recurrence of pancreatitis in patients presenting in this manner (12, 14). Three possible mechanisms have been postulated for a causal relationship between the two.

First, hypercalcemia increases the likelihood of precipitation of calcium phosphate in alkaline environs (3) such as are found in the cells and ducts of the pancreas. Longstanding hypercalcemia may also lead to inspissation and precipitation of protein plugs within the pancreatic duct (18). The resulting calculi can lead to pancreatic ductal obstruction and secretory stasis. If ductal pressure is increased, pancreatitis can result.

Second, hypercalcemia can stimulate the secretion of pancreatic enzymes (19, 20) and can increase the conversion of trypsinogen to trypsin (21). Acute hypercalcemia increases the permeability of the pancreatic duct to large dextran molecules that approximate the size of pancreatic enzymes (22). The combination of increased enzyme secretion, increased trypsin activity, and increased ductal permeability can result in an increased presence of activated pancreatic enzymes in the parenchyma and interstitium of the gland. These enzymes can then initiate an attack of pancreatitis.

The third mechanism is a direct toxic effect of parathyroid hormone on the pancreas. Excess parathyroid hormone in animals can produce thromboarteritis, necrosis, and calcification in the pancreas (23, 24). Although HPT is now rarely associated with pancreatitis, the inflammatory process in the pancreas is likely to be severe when this combination does occur.

Clinically, the attacks of pancreatitis usually precede the diagnosis of HPT (12, 14). This has prompted some investigators to postulate that HPT is secondary to the pancreatitis. Plough and Kyle (25) suggested that HPT was the end result of poor calcium absorption secondary to pancreatic exocrine insufficiency. Dent (26) noted that calcium deficiency due to steatorrhea in patients with chronic pancreatitis may result in HPT. Elevated serum glucagon levels that occur in pancreatitis may be another pertinent factor (27). Increased levels of circulating glucagon can cause hypocalcemia, which then induces a secondary stimulation of the parathyroid glands.

Both the hypercalcemia and the increase in circulating parathyroid hormone in HPT can result in pancreatitis. Supporting hypercalcemia as a cause of pancreatitis are reports of pancreatic inflammation in patients with a variety of conditions associated with elevated serum calcium levels (Table 25B.2)(16, 28–48). These include familial hypocalciuric hypercalcemia, vitamin D intoxication, excess intravenous calcium infusion in hyperalimentation solutions, increased calcium gluconate in dialysis solutions, the milk-alkali syndrome, and some malignant diseases such as multiple myeloma, adult T-cell leukemia, metastatic breast carcinoma, metastatic pancreatic islet cell carcinoma, and leiomyosarcoma. Pancreatitis has been reported after cardiopulmonary bypass. Administration of more than 800 mg of calcium chloride per square meter of body-surface area induces pancreatic cellular injury and has been implicated as a risk factor in the development of pancreatitis after cardiac surgery (41). On the other hand, acute relapsing pancreatitis has been reported in patients with HPT who have elevated parathyroid hormone levels but are normocalcemic (49). Recurrent pancreatitis has been cured by the removal of a parathyroid adenoma, even though elevation of serum calcium was never noted (50). Acute pancreatitis has also occurred in patients with secondary HPT (15, 51) who have high levels of parathyroid hormone but no apparent hypercalcemia. This same situation has been reported in a pregnant patient with HPT who developed acute pancreatitis (52). Therefore, elevated circulating parathyroid hormone may cause pancreatitis with or without hypercalcemia.

### Clinical Features and Diagnosis

Sitges-Serra et al. reviewed 107 patients with pancreatitis associated with HPT, collected from series reported between 1947 to 1985 (13). The clinical characteristics of these patients are shown in Table 25B.3. Patients presented with all of the typical manifestations of both acute and chronic pancreatitis. The symptoms of acute HPT were also typical and involved the renal, skeletal, neuromuscular, and/or gastrointestinal systems. Almost a quarter of the patients in this review had hypercalcemic or hyperparathyroid crisis, the severest form of the disease. The most common initial symptoms of hyperparathyroid crisis are muscular weakness, nausea, vomiting, weight loss, confusion, abdominal pain, and constipation (7). As the acute phase progresses, oliguria leads to renal failure, coma, and finally, death, unless effective treatment is instituted. The laboratory findings of acute pancreatitis associated with HPT are those of each disease. Serum amylase and lipase levels are elevated, indicating pancreatitis. HPT is diagnosed by elevated serum calcium, decreased serum phosphorus, and elevated serum levels of intact parathyroid hormone. Since hypocalcemia often occurs with a severe attack of pancreatitis, a normal serum calcium level may be a clue for HPT in patients extremely ill from pancreatitis.

The same criteria are used to diagnose pancreatic inflamma-

**TABLE 25B.2. Causes of Hypercalcemia Associated with Pancreatitis**

Familial hypocalciuric hypercalcemia (28–30)
Malignancy
- Multiple myeloma (31-33)
- Adult T-cell leukemia (34)
- Metastatic breast carcinoma (35)
- Metastatic islet cell carcinoma of the pancreas (36)
- Leiomyosarcoma (humoral hypercalcemia of malignancy) (37)

Calcium infusion
Calcium gluconate during dialysis (38)
"Hard water syndrome"—improper hemodialysis (42)
Total parenteral nutrition infusion (39-40)
Calcium chloride during cardiopulmonary bypass (41)
Vitamin D poisoning (43, 44)
Thyrotoxicosis (45)
Sarcoidosis (46)
Renal transplant (47)
Metolazone-induced hypercalcemia (48)
Milk-alkali syndrome (16)

**TABLE 25B.3. Clinical Characteristics of 107 Patients with Pancreatitis Associated with Primary Hyperparathyroidism (HPT)**

| Pancreatitis | % | PTH | % |
|---|---|---|---|
| **Symptoms** | | **Symptoms** | |
| Abdominal pain | 67.3 | Nephrolithiasis | 40 |
| Nausea and vomiting | 100 | Bone disease | 26.5 |
| | | Hypercalcemic crisis | 23.5 |
| Steatorrhea | 14 | Metastatic calcification | 14.7 |
| Weight loss | 8 | | |
| **Type of pancreatitis** | | **Parathyroid pathology** | |
| Acute | 35.4 | Adenoma | 67.3 |
| Acute relapsing | 12.1 | Hyperplasia | 10.3 |
| Chronic | 37.4 | Carcinoma | 9.3 |
| Unknown | 15 | Unknown | 13 |

Modified from Sitges-Serra A, Alonso M, de Lecea C, Gores PF, Sutherland DER. Pancreatitis and hyperparathyroidism. Br J Surg 1988;75:158–160.

tory disease in patients who have HPT. These include *(a)* acute or chronic abdominal pain accompanied by elevation of serum or urinary amylase levels; *(b)* a known complication of pancreatitis, such as pseudocyst formation; *(c)* radiographically proven pancreatic calcifications; and *(d)* presence of chronic pancreatic exocrine insufficiency. The diagnosis of HPT is established in the usual manner by biochemical documentation of the disease and exclusion of other causes of hypercalcemia. An elevated level of serum calcium is usually the first finding suggesting HPT. However, in some HPT patients with severe pancreatitis, serum calcium levels may be normal or below normal. Pancreatitis can cause a drop in serum calcium within 24–48 hours of the onset of the attack, which may hide chronically elevated levels (15). Therefore, follow-up serum calcium determinations are necessary after the acute attack of pancreatitis has resolved. In the absence of hypercalcemia, a low serum phosphate level may provide a clue for the diagnosis of HPT. Measurement of intact parathyroid hormone levels can establish the diagnosis in these patients.

### Treatment

The general principles of therapy for acute pancreatitis should be followed in patients with HPT. These include giving sufficient analgesics for pain, replacing fluid and electrolyte losses, and refraining from oral feeding until the inflammation improves. Patients should be monitored for local and systemic complications. Hypercalcemia can develop into a life-threatening crisis, especially when complicated by a dehydrating condition like pancreatitis. In patients with severe hypercalcemia (calcium ≥ 13 mg/dL), urgent treatment is needed to lower the serum calcium level. The principal approaches for this include decreasing the gastrointestinal (GI) absorption of calcium, increasing its renal excretion, and increasing the ratio of bone accretion to resorption (53) (Fig. 25B.1). Measures to decrease GI absorption include decreasing dietary intake of calcium and administration of corticosteroids. Treatment with intravenous saline infusion, natriuretic agents such as furosemide and ethacrynic acid, chelating or binding agents such as sodium citrate and ethylenediaminetetraacetate (EDTA), and dialysis can increase the loss or excretion of calcium from the body. Hypercalcemia is associated with an increased resorption of skeletal calcium. Therefore, increasing the ratio of bone accretion to resorption by the use of corticosteroids, calcitonin, mithramycin, and bisphosphonates can also decrease serum calcium levels.

Hypercalcemia is often associated with a reduced glomerular filtration rate and depletion of sodium and water due to abnormal tubular function. Rehydration with intravenous saline infusion can increase renal excretion of calcium by restoring the glomerular filtration rate and inducing a diuresis. Therefore, intravenous hydration is the first step in treating patients with severe hypercalcemia (54). The intravenous fluid of choice is normal saline. Up to 1 L/hr can be given. In older patients, invasive monitoring including a central venous pressure (CVP) catheter and/or a pulmonary artery (Swan-Ganz) catheter may be needed to assess cardiac function and the amount of intravascular fluid. Intravenous diuretics should only be administered when the patient is well hydrated. Emergency dialysis is an effective and safe alternative to remove calcium from the body immediately in patients with compromised renal function.

Rehydration with saline infusion will usually improve the patient's general state and reduce serum calcium levels. However, in severe hypercalcemia, saline infusion, even combined with diuretics, may not be enough to normalize serum calcium. Other calcium-lowering agents such as corticosteroids, calcitonin, mithramycin, and bisphosphonates may be needed. Patients with hypercalcemia caused by vitamin D intoxication, sarcoidosis, and some malignancies such as myeloma and lymphoma respond best to steroids, while patients with HPT are usually resistant to this therapy. Calcitonin is a relatively safe calcium-lowering agent, but its effects are often short-lived. Mithramycin is extremely effective when given as an intravenous infusion. It is a cytotoxic drug with hepatic and bone marrow toxicity, and it can cause severe side effects such as hemorrhage. Bisphosphonates are the newest calcium lowering agents. These pyrophosphate analogues bind to hydroxyapatite in bone and act as potent inhibitors of osteoclastic bone resorption (55, 56). Treatment with the bisphosphonate aminohydroxypropylidene pamidronate (APD) has been effective in lowering elevated calcium

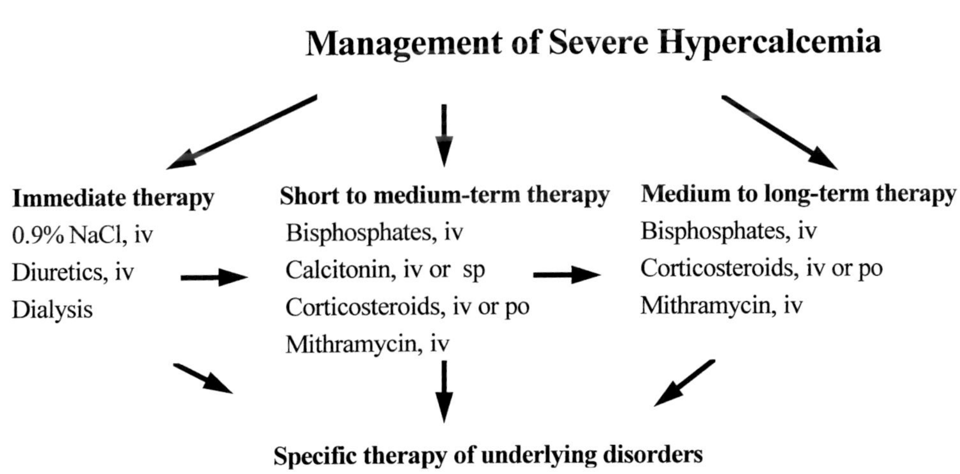


**FIG. 25B.1.** Algorithm for management of severe hypercalcemia.

levels in patients with malignancy and in primary HPT (56, 57). A recent study of nine patients with primary HPT who had moderate or severe hypercalcemia found that 1 week after a single infusion of 15–60 mg APD, serum calcium levels had decreased to normal or near normal without side effects. Repeated infusions of APD for 6- to 9-month periods were also effective and well tolerated in patients with primary HPT (56). Since APD has been very efficacious for both short- and long-term therapy of hypercalcemia without any appreciable side effects, it should be the first-line treatment for hyperparathyroid crisis that has failed to respond to basic therapy with saline infusion and diuretics. It can also be used preoperatively to lower serum calcium levels before surgery for HPT and for the long-term treatment of hypercalcemia in patients in whom parathyroid surgery is contraindicated. Therapy directed at HPT or other conditions that cause hypercalcemia is also an important measure to lower hypercalcemia. An emergency neck exploration may be needed to correct hyperparathyroid crisis and avoid deterioration of pancreatitis if laboratory and/or clinical response to medical treatment of hypercalcemia is inadequate (58). In most patients, successful parathyroidectomy will prevent recurrent attacks of pancreatitis (12, 14).

A high incidence of postoperative pancreatitis (9.3%) has been reported in a series of 86 patients undergoing parathyroidectomy for primary HPT (59). Pancreatitis following parathyroid surgery may result from hypercalcemia caused by manipulation of the parathyroid gland or by a decrease in calcitonin secretion by the thyroid C-cells (59). Postoperative monitoring and control of hypercalcemia by adequate hydration are also important until the serum calcium level has normalized.

Pancreatic pseudocysts may develop in patients with pancreatitis associated with HPT. Pseudocysts in this setting have resolved spontaneously after the removal of a parathyroid adenoma (60). Therefore, surgical treatment of HPT and normalization of serum calcium should precede any elective operation on the pancreas in patients with pancreatitis associated with HPT. If the pseudocyst is associated with a complication such as infection, hemorrhage, or gastric outlet obstruction, it may require therapy before the HPT can be treated. In this setting, care must be taken to monitor serum calcium and avoid dehydration, which may precipitate a hypercalcemic crisis.

HPT and hypercalcemia have also been associated with chronic pancreatitis. Correction of hypercalcemia with parathyroidectomy can reverse the effects of pancreatitis only if there is no permanent damage to the pancreas. Chronic pancreatitis is a progressive inflammatory disease that destroys both exocrine and endocrine tissue. Pain is the predominant symptom of chronic pancreatitis. In patients with HPT complicated by irreversible chronic pancreatitis, correction of hypercalcemia and HPT may not rectify the pancreatic abnormality. Nevertheless, it seems reasonable to recommend parathyroidectomy as the first step in treating patients with HPT and chronic pancreatitis, for two reasons: *(a)* to evaluate the potential beneficial effect of correcting the patient's hypercalcemia and HPT on ameliorating their pain of chronic pancreatitis and *(b)* to avoid the problems of controlling hypercalcemia during the perioperative period that is inherent in patients with HPT undergoing major operative intervention. Pancreatic ductal drainage or resection may be required to control the abdominal pain of chronic pancreatitis after parathyroidectomy, but this can be done more safely in a normocalcemic patient (60, 61).

## REFERENCES: PART B. HYPERPARATHYROIDISM


1. Cope O, Culver PJ, Mixter CG, Nardi GL. Pancreatitis, a diagnostic clue to hyperparathyroidism. Ann Surg 1957;145:857–863.
2. Fink WJ, Finfrock JD. Fatal hyperparathyroid crisis associated with pancreatitis. Am Surg 1961;27:424–430.
3. Mixter CG, Keynes WM, Cope O. Further experience with pancreatitis as a diagnostic clue to hyperparathyroidism. N Engl J Med 1962;266:265–272.
4. Anglem TJ. Acute hyperparathyroidism: a surgical emergency. Surg Clin North Am 1966;46:727–746.
5. Ludwig GD, Chaykin LB. Pancreatitis associated with primary hyperparathyroidism. Med Clin North Am 1966;50:1403–1418.
6. Herskovic T, Keating FR, Gross JB. Coexistent pancreatitis and hyperparathyroidism: observation on 15 cases (Abstract). Gastroenterology 1967;52:1093.
7. Kelly TR, Falor WH. Hyperparathyroid crisis associated with pancreatitis. Ann Surg 1968;168:917–920.
8. Schmidt H, Creutzfeldt W. Calciphylactic pancreatitis and pancreatitis in hyperparathyroidism. Clin Orthop 1970;69:135–145.
9. Rosin RD. Pancreatitis and hyperparathyroidism. Postgrad Med J 1976;52:95–101.
10. Bess MA, Edis AJ, van Heerden JA. Hyperparathyroidism and pancreatitis: chance or a causal association? JAMA 1980;243: 246–247.
11. Kelly TR. Primary hyperparathyroidism. A personal experience with 242 cases. Am J Surg 1980;140:632–635.
12. Paloyan D, Simonowitz D, Paloyan E, Snyder TJ. Pancreatitis associated with primary hyperparathyroidism. Am Surg 1982;48: 366–368.
13. Sitges-Serra A, Alonso M, de Lecea C, Gores PF, Sutherland DER. Pancreatitis and hyperparathyroidism. Br J Surg 1988;75:158–160.
14. Prinz RA, Aranha GV. The association of primary hyperparathyroidism and pancreatitis. Am Surg 1985;51:325–329.
15. Elliott DW. Pancreatitis associated with hyperparathyroidism. In: Howard JM, Jordan GL Jr, Reber HA, eds. Surgical diseases of the pancreas. Philadelphia: Lea & Febiger, 1987;310–315.
16. Brandwein SL, Sigman KM. Case report: milk-alkali syndrome and pancreatitis. Am J Med Sci 1994;308:173–176.
17. Shearer MG, Imrie CW. Parathyroid hormone levels, hyperparathyroidism and acute pancreatitis. Br J Surg 1986;73:282–284.
18. Cho JW, Seligson U, Somell A. Pancreatic function in patients with hyperparathyroidism. A study with the Lundh test. Acta Chir Scand 1985;151:323–325.
19. Goebell H, Steffen C, Baltzer G, Bode C. Stimulation of pancreatic secretion of enzymes by acute hypercalcemia in man. Eur J Clin Invest 1973;3:98–104.
20. Malagelada JR, Holtermuller KH, Sizemore GW, Go VLW. The influence of hypercalcemia on basal and cholecystokinin-stimulated pancreatic, gallbladder, and gastric functions in man. Gastroenterology 1976;71:405–408.
21. Haverback BJ, Dyce B, Bundy H, Edmondson HA. Trypsin, trypsinogen and trypsin inhibitor in human pancreatic juice: mechanism for pancreatitis associated with hyperparathyroidism. Am J Med 1960;29:424–433.
22. Gates MC, Singh SM, Peick AL, Harvey MH, Reber HA. Acute hypercalcemia, pancreatic duct permeability, and pancreatitis in cats. Surgery 1988;104:137–141.
23. Hueper W. Metastatic calcification in organs of the dog after injections of parathyroid extract. Arch Pathol Lab Med 1927;3: 14–25.
24. McJunkin FA, Tweedy WR, Breuhaus HC. The parathyroid hormone: its regulatory action on parathyroid glands and toxic effect on tissues of rat. Arch Pathol 1932;14:649–659.
25. Plough IC, Kyle LH. Pancreatic insufficiency and hyperparathyroidism. Ann Intern Med 1957;47:590–598.
26. Dent CE. Some problems of hyperparathyroidism. Br Med J 1962;2:1419–1425.
27. Paloyan E, Paloyan D, Harper PV. The role of glucagon hypersecretion in the relationship of pancreatitis and hyperparathyroidism. Surgery 1967;62:167–173.
28. Davies M, Klimiuk PS, Adams PH, Lumb GA, Large DM, Anderson DC. Familial hypocalciuric hypercalcemia and acute pancreatitis. Br Med J (Clin Res) 1981;282:1023–1025.
29. Stuckey BG, Gutteridge DH, Kent GN, Reed WD. Familial hypocalciuric hypercalcemia and pancreatitis: no casual link proven. Aust NZ J Med 1990;20:718–719.
30. Marx SJ, Attie MF, Levine MA, Spiegel AM, Downs RW Jr, Lasker RD. The hypocalciuric or benign variant of familial hypercalcemia: clinical and biochemical features in fifteen kindreds. Medicine 1981;60:397–412.

31. Aldis AS. Clinical experiences of the lesser known manifestations of hyperparathyroidism. Proc R Soc Med 1961;54:489–492.
32. Meltzer LE, Palmon FP Jr, Paik YK, Custer RP. Acute pancreatitis secondary to hypercalcemia of multiple myeloma. Ann Intern Med 1962;57:1008–1012.
33. Lee KH, Lee JS, Kim SH. Acute pancreatitis in a case of multiple myeloma with hypercalcemia. Korean J Intern Med 1989;4: 178–180.
34. Dazai Y, Katoh I, Hara Y, Yoshida R, Kurihara K. Two cases of adult T-cell leukemia associated with acute pancreatitis due to hypercalcemia. Am J Med 1991;90:251–254.
35. Gafter U, Mandel EM, Har-Zahav L, Weiss S. Acute pancreatitis secondary to hypercalcemia. Occurrence in a patient with breast carcinoma. JAMA 1976;235:2004–2005.
36. Goldberg LD, Herschmann EM. Hypercalcemia and pancreatitis. JAMA 1976;236:1352.
37. Nagata N, Takeda J, Kugai N, et al. A case of leiomyosarcoma associated with humoral hypercalcemia of malignancy: demonstration of biological and immunological activities of parathyroid hormone-related protein in the tumor extract. Jpn J Cancer Res 1989;80:643–648.
38. Hochgelerent EL, David DS. Acute pancreatitis secondary to calcium infusion in a dialysis patient. Arch Surg 1974;108:218–219.
39. Manson RR. Acute pancreatitis secondary to iatrogenic hypercalcemia. Implications of hyperalimentation. Arch Surg 1974;108: 213–215.
40. Izsak EM, Shike M, Roulet M, Jeejeebhoy KN. Pancreatitis in association with hypercalcemia in patients receiving total parenteral nutrition. Gastroenterology 1980;79:555–558.
41. Fernandez-del Castillo C, Harringer W, Warshaw AL, et al. Risk factors for pancreatic cellular injury after cardiopulmonary bypass. N Engl J Med 1991;325:382–387.
42. Evans DB, Slapak M. Pancreatitis in the hard water syndrome. Br Med J 1975;3:748.
43. Leeson PM, Fourman P. Acute pancreatitis from vitamin-D poisoning in a patient with parathyroid deficiency. Lancet 1966;1:1185–1186.
44. Waele BD, Smitz J, Willems G. Recurrent pancreatitis secondary to hypercalcemia following vitamin D poisoning. Pancreas 1989;4: 378–380.
45. May P, Levy RP. Thyrotoxicosis associated with renal tubular acidosis and acute pancreatitis: a case report. Ann Intern Med 1976;84:569–570.
46. McCormick PA, Malone D, Fitzgerald MX, Fitzgerald O. Pancreatitis in sarcoidosis. Br Med J (Clin Res) 1985;290:1472–1473.
47. Frick TW, Fryd DS, Sutherland DE, Goodale RL, Simmons RL, Najarian JS. Hypercalcemia associated with pancreatitis and hyperamylasemia in renal transplant recipients. Data from the Minnesota randomized trial of cyclosporine versus antilymphoblast azathioprine. Am J Surg 1987;154:487–489.
48. Anderson PE, Ellis GG Jr, Austin SM. Case report: metolazone-associated hypercalcemia and acute pancreatitis. Am J Med Sci 1991;302:235–237.
49. Danzi JT, Farmer RG, Esselstyn CB Jr. Recurrent pancreatitis associated with normocalcemia, parathyroid hyperplasia, and increased serum parathormone. Case report. Cleve Clin Q 1974;41:39–43.
50. Ballon S, Cohen H, Strasberg Z. Recurrent pancreatitis due to a parathyroid adenoma in a normocalcemic patient. Can Med Assoc J 1972;106:51–54.
51. 51 Penn I, Durst AL, Machado M, et al. Acute pancreatitis and hyperamylasemia in renal homograft recipients. Arch Surg 1972; 105:167–172.
52. Inabnet WB, Baldwin D, Daniel RO, Staren ED. Hyperparathyroidism and pancreatitis during pregnancy. Surgery 1996;119: 710–713.
53. Goldsmith RS. Treatment of hypercalcemia. Med Clin North Am 1972;56:951–960.
54. Hosking DJ, Cowley A, Bucknall CA. Rehydration in the treatment of severe hypercalcemia. Q J Med 1981;200:473–481.
55. Altmann P, Cunningham J. The management of severe hypercalcaemia. Postgrad Med J 1987;63:77–79.
56. Jansson S, Tisell LE, Lindstedt G, Lundberg PA. Disodium pamidronate in the preoperative treatment of hypercalcemia in patients with primary hyperparathyroidism. Surgery 1991;110:480–486.
57. Morton AR, Cantrill JA, Craig AE, Howell A, Davies M, Anderson DC. Single dose versus daily intravenous aminohydroxpropylidene biphosphate (APD) for the hypercalcemia of malignancy. Br Med J (Clin Res) 1988;296:811–814.
58. Daum F, Rosen JF, Boley SJ. Parathyroid adenoma, parathyroid crisis, and acute pancreatitis in an adolescent. J Pediatr 1973; 83:275–277.
59. Reeve TS, Delbridge LW. Pancreatitis following parathyroid surgery. Ann Surg 1982;195:158–162.
60. Kazantsev GB, Nash DW, Prinz RA. Pancreatic pseudocyst resolution after parathyroidectomy for hyperparathyroidism. Arch Surg 1994;129:655–658.
61. Karanjia ND, Reber HA. The cause and management of the pain of chronic pancreatitis. Gastroenterol Clin North Am 1990; 19:895–904.

# 26

# *Postoperative Pancreatitis*

Yoshifumi Kawarada

Acute pancreatitis has various causes, and one of them is a direct or indirect effect of surgical operations (Table 26.1). This chapter discusses the form of acute pancreatitis that develops postoperatively or is in some way related to surgery, usually termed postoperative pancreatitis. Many factors may contribute to postoperative pancreatitis, and it certainly is not a rare disease. Nevertheless, early diagnosis is difficult, and for that reason, comparisons with the earlier literature show that the mortality remains high. This chapter discusses the recent literature regarding the frequency of postoperative pancreatitis in relation to the surgical procedures and techniques used.

## INCIDENCE

Some 290 patients with acute pancreatitis were seen in the First Department of Surgery, Mie University Hospital, and affiliated hospitals during the 10-year period from January 1983 to August 1993 (1), and in 63 of these cases, the pancreatitis was severe. Etiologically, the 63 severe illnesses could be classified into 22 cases caused by gallstones, 12 due to alcohol, 6 cases of postoperative pancreatitis, 3 caused by trauma, and 6 due to other specific causes; 14 cases were idiopathic. There were 23 deaths (36.5%) among the severe cases, with the mortality rates according to cause being for idiopathic pancreatitis 57.1%, postoperative pancreatitis 50%, alcoholic pancreatitis 41.2%, traumatic pancreatitis 33.1%, and gallstone pancreatitis 13.6%.

Imrie and Dickson reviewed the literature and reported 291 cases of postoperative pancreatitis (8%) in a total of 3874 cases of acute pancreatitis (2). Bragg et al. (3) reported that the cause of acute pancreatitis in 100 cases was alcohol in 40%, biliary in 20%, and postoperative in 15%, with an overall mortality rate of 8%. Thus, the incidence of postoperative pancreatitis was high in both series. In our series, postoperative acute pancreatitis constituted the etiological form in 9.5% of all cases of acute pancreatitis.

In contrast, 40 cases of acute pancreatitis in elderly patients (over 70 years old) (4), were biliary in 35% (14 cases), idiopathic in 30% (12 cases), postoperative in 12.5% (5 cases), embolic in 7.5% (3 cases), alcoholic in 5% (2 cases), and secondary to endoscopic retrograde cholangiopancreatography (ERCP) in 1%, with an overall mortality rate of 20%.

Thompson et al. (5) reported 52 cases of severe postoperative pancreatitis (from 1979 to 1987), 30 in men and 22 in women, developing after a biliary tract procedure in 10 cases, colectomy in 9, intestinal resection in 9, gastrectomy in 8, vascular surgery in 5, appendectomy in 4, pancreatic surgery in 3, and other operations in 4. Thirty of the procedures involved surgery in the vicinity of the pancreas. Pancreas-related operations were performed in 16 (31%) of these 52 patients and non-pancreas-related operations in 36 (69%); 9 patients died: 4 (25%) of the 16 patients who had undergone pancreas-related operations and 5 (14%) of the 36 who had undergone non-pancreas-related operations. The mortality rate was significantly higher in patients with postoperative pancreatitis than in those with pancreatitis whose cause was biliary, alcoholic, etc. (3).

## BILIARY TRACT SURGERY

In 1928, Schmieden and Sehening (6) documented the development of pancreatitis following biliary tract operations, and in 1957, Thompson et al. (7) determined that the occurrence of pancreatitis following biliary tract operations was primarily related to common duct exploration. In 1968, Bardenheier et al. (8) reported an incidence of postoperative pancreatitis of 1.8% following cholecystectomy and 12.2% following common duct exploration.

In 1987, Vernava et al. (9) scrutinized the results of biliary tract operations performed on 1256 patieints for the presence of postoperative hyperamylesemia and pancreatitis persisting in 113 (9%) after 48 hours. They reported an incidence following cholecystectomy of only 0.6%, versus 8.4% after common duct exploration. They stated that the incidence of postoperative pancreatitis following cholecystectomy in patients with no history of pancreatic dysfunction was 0.3% and that the incidence following common duct exploration with no pancreatic dysfunction was 5%. One of the 970 patients who underwent cholecystectomy and had pancreatitis at the time of operation died of postoperative pancreatitis (9). Seven of the 286 patients who underwent common duct exploration died of pancreatitis: 4 patients had had preoperative pancreatitis and 3 had not. Among the patients with preoperative pancreatic dysfunction, cholecystectomy alone was associated with a 2.7% incidence of postoperative pancreatitis and common duct exploration with a 17% incidence. The relationship of the timing of operational therapy to the persistence of postoperative pancreatitis was evaluated. No significant differences were found in patients with pancreatitis when those who were operated on within 48 hours of hospitalization were compared with those operated on later than 48 hours.

## GASTRECTOMY

Over 25 years ago, when I was a surgical resident in the United States, postoperative pancreatitis was a common complication after gastrectomy, and I had the opportunity to observe several cases. At that time I felt that one of the factors causing postoperative pancreatitis was leakage from the anastomosis of a partial gastrectomy, directly affecting the pancreas. Postoperative pancreatitis occurred after Billroth I and Billroth II gastrectomies. Another potential factor was leakage from the duodenal stump of Billroth II gastrectomies (2, 10, 11).

We have had no instance of duodenal stump leakage recog-

**TABLE 26.1. Etiology and Mechanisms of Postoperative Pancreatitis**

I. Surgical trauma to the pancreas
  A. Direct trauma to the pancreas
    1. Biliary surgery
      a. Common duct exploration
      b. Cholecystectomy
    2. Surgery for papilla of Vater
      a. Sphincteroplasty
      b. EST (endoscopic sphincterotomy)
      c. Passing dilator or stone
    3. Pancreatic surgery
      a. Pancreatic resection
      b. Pancreatic biopsy
    4. Gastric surgery
      Difficult case, rare
    5. Other operations
      Splenectomy, hepatectomy, colectomy, transplantation etc.
  B. Indirect trauma to the pancreas
    1. Extended Kocher's maneuver
    2. Afferent loop syndrome with Billroth II operation
    3. Dissection of lymph nodes around the celiac artery and its branches
    4. Cardiac surgery and cardiopulmonary bypass
II. Indirect causes of postoperative pancreatitis
  1. Circulatory shock (bleeding, circulatory disorders, acidosis, etc.)
  2. Ischemia (cardiopulmonary bypass)
  3. Metabolic effects (uremia, diabetes mellitus)
  4. Septic shock
  5. Steroid therapy
  6. Hyperparathyroidism
  7. Pregnancy and obstetric-gynecologic surgery

nized in the 448 partial gastrectomies performed in our department of surgery at Mie University during the last 10 years, but there have been two cases (0.4%) of anastomotic leakage. There have been no instances of postoperative pancreatitis after gastrectomy, nor were we able to find any cases of postoperative pancreatitis of any degree of severity after gastrectomy in the Japanese literature during the last 10 years.

In contrast, there have been many recent reports in the Russian literature of postoperative pancreatitis after gastrectomy. In 373 surgical cases, Kulazhenkov et al. (12) reported that postoperative acute pancreatitis developed following gastrectomy for gastric carcinoma in 51.5%, gastrectomy for gastric ulcer in 26.8%, and biliary tract operations in 17.2%, with a morbidity of 25.2% and mortality of 30.4%. Veronskii and Viskunov (13) reported that acute postoperative pancreatitis developed in 60 (3.7%) of 1602 patients (3.9% mortality) who underwent gastric surgery; 20 patients died of acute postoperative pancreatitis (mortality 1.2%).

## DIRECT OPERATIVE INJURY TO PANCREAS

Reilly et al. (14) reported the results of using the transabdominal medial visceral rotation (MVR) approach to expose the paramesenteric and pararenal aorta in operations on aneurysms of the abdominal aorta. The postoperative complications in 108 cases of MVR included 5 cases of acute pancreatitis, and this technique of exposure may have been one of the factors causing postoperative acute pancreatitis. Aneurysmectomy, however, is recognized to result in pancreatitis also when performed by other exposures.

Pancreatic resection involves true direct trauma to the pancreas. While many complications after pancreatoduodenectomy have been reported, no reports of postoperative acute pancreatitis could be found in the literature, nor were there any in our own series of 115 pancreatoduodenectomies. According to the data of the Japanese Pancreas Society (15), the incidence of postoperative pancreatitis among 3743 cases of pancreatectomy for pancreatic carcinoma during the last 10 years was only 2.8%. The syndrome of acute pancreatitis associated with an elevated serum amylase level is a recognized complication heralding leakage of the pancreatojejunostomy following pancreatoduodenal resection (15a).

### Pancreatic Biopsy

Percutaneous biopsy of pancreatic lesions has become a routine procedure to establish or exclude the presence of carcinoma. (See also Chapters 10 and 14.) In 1982, Smith (16) presented data based on 15,000 biopsies of the pancreas collected from a multiinstitutional survey and reported finding one death from postoperative pancreatitis.

Mueller et al. (17) reported performing a retrospective review of 184 pancreatic biopsies in 178 patients to assess the prevalence of severe postbiopsy pancreatitis. Severe pancreatitis developed after five (3%) of these biopsies, usually within 24–48 hours. Three of the five patients who developed pancreatitis had a true-negative biopsy result (normal pancreas) corroborated either at surgery (two cases) or during clinical follow-up (one case). They concluded that although the risk of pancreatitis as a complication of percutaneous needle biopsy is exceedingly small, it may occur, and at a higher rate than previously reported.

Levin et al. (18) reported three cases of postbiopsy pancreatitis that resulted in death. In one of these cases, hemorrhagic pancreatitis developed after percutaneous fine-needle aspiration biopsy, while the other two cases had been reported in the literature. They concluded that complications were apt to occur when biopsy was performed on small pancreatic neoplasms under 3 cm in diameter, that patients with small or questionable lesions have a higher risk of complications, and that caution must be exercised in such cases.

## ENDOSCOPY

Pancreatitis may develop as a complication of routine gastroduodenoscopy without cannulation of the papilla of Vater. Various etiologic factors are involved in pancreatitis induced by ERCP and endoscopic sphincterotomy (EST). ERCP has recently become the most common diagnostic procedure for evaluation of hepatobiliary-pancreatic diseases.

### Endoscopic Sphincterotomy (EST)

Varezka et al. (19) reported that choledocholithiasis was the indication for EST in 270 (74.4%) of a total of 363 patients who underwent successful EST, and that EST was performed in four patients with acute pancreatitis. Complications were observed in 17 (4.7%) of the 363 patients, with a mortality rate of 1.1%. The most common complications were bleeding and perforation. They encountered two cases of acute pancreatitis and two cases of acute cholangitis with impacted stone in the hepatocholedochus. Sarr et al. (20) reviewed 254 patients who underwent endoscopic sphincterotomy. Six of them (2.4%) had clinically significant pancreatitis, one of whom (0.4%) died after multiple pancreatic debridements. Five patients (2.0%) had duodenal (peri-Vaterian) perforation as a complication.

### ERCP

Doherty et. al. (21) reported a case of life-threatening acute pancreatitis with *Pseudomonas aeruginosa* sepsis immediately following ERCP. Culture of the patient's blood, the inner

**TABLE 26.2. Pancreatitis after ERCP**

| Author | Reference No. (Date of Publication) | No. of ERCP Cases | No. of Pts. with Acute Pancreatitis (%) | No. of Surgical Cases | No. of Deaths |
|---|---|---|---|---|---|
| Nebel et al. | 24 (1975) | 3,884 | 51 (1.3) | 0 | 2 |
| Skude et al. | 25 (1976) | 216 | 2 (0.9) | 0 | 0 |
| Montori et al. | 26 (1979) | 8,636 | 10 (0.1) | 1 | 2 |
| Branders et al. | 27 (1981) | 118 | 3 (2.5) | — | 0 |
| Hamilton et al. | 28 (1983) | 1,118 | 15 (1.3) | 1 | 0 |
| Roszler and Campbell | 29 (1985) | 140 | 18 (12.9) | 0 | 0 |
| Reiertsen et al. | 30 (1987) | 1,950 | 8 (0.4) | 4 | 0 |
| Japanese series (Kasugai et al.) | 31 (1995) | 133,828 | 112 (0.08) | 5 | 4 |
| Japanese series (Kaneko et al.) | 32 (1995) | 209,147 | 193 (0.09) | — | 9 |

channel of the duodenoscope, and the irrigating water bottles were all positive for *Pseudomonas.* Barkin et al. (22) concluded that the risk of post-ERP acute pancreatitis was significantly lower when a nonionic contrast agent (Omnipaque) was used than when ionic agents were used.

Imrie reviewed over 15,992 cases of ERCP in the literature and found that pancreatitis had occurred after the procedure in 236 cases, an incidence of post-ERCP pancreatitis of 1.5% (2). In the prospective British study (1981–1984) (23) 34 cases (2.2%) of acute pancreatitis were observed among 1546 cases of diagnostic ERCP without any deaths, while among 721 cases of ERCP with sphincterotomy, there were 21 cases (2.9%) of acute pancreatitis with two deaths. Many authors have reported on complications after ERCP (Table 26.2) (24–32).

In a Japanese series of 133,828 cases of ERCP from 1983 to 1987, accidents occurred in 143 cases (0.107%), with 14 deaths (0.0105%) (33). In a more recent Japanese series of 209,147 cases from 1988 to 1992, accidents occurred in 245 cases (0.117%), with 14 deaths (0.0067%) (32). The most common complication in the 245 cases was acute pancreatitis (Table 26.3).

(See also Chapter 34.)

## SURGERY OF THE COLON

Elevation of serum amylase levels and pancreatitis may develop following a variety of operations, especially after upper abdominal surgery. The incidence and magnitude of these problems after colonic surgery, however, are still unknown. Sakanoue et al. (33) checked serum amylase levels after colonic surgery and reported that 27 of 70 patients exhibited hyperamylasemia on the 14th postoperative day after total colectomy and that their serum amylase levels had returned to normal by the 30th postoperative day. Postoperative elevation of serum amylase levels was observed in 3 of 37 patients after ileoanal anastomosis and in 8 of 70 patients after stomal closure. Postoperative hyperamylasemia itself, however, does not necessarily require treatment.

## HEPATIC SURGERY

Tsuzuki et al. (34) reported hyperamylasemia in 57 (42%) of 136 patients following resection of hepatocellular carcinoma and in 13 (32%) of 41 patients with metastatic liver carcinoma. They classified the hyperamylasemia into three patterns: type I (salivary type), type II (pancreatic type), and type III (mixed type). It is important to determine whether the amylase is type II or III. If type II and/or III hyperamylasemia is present after hepatectomy, then postoperative pancreatitis should be considered. Although the pathogenesis of the hyperamylasemia remains unclear, surgeons should be alert to the possible occurrence of this complication (34, 35).

Soravia et al. (36) reported on 10 women with adult polycystic liver disease who were examined and surgically treated by partial hepatic resection with cystic fenestration. Postoperative morbidity consisted of one case of pneumonia and one case of acute pancreatitis with deep vein thrombosis of the leg.

In a somewhat related field, postoperative pancreatitis has been reported after distal splenorenal shunt (37). Fegiz et al. (38) reported 286 cases of shunt surgery for portal hypertension, with complications occurring in 149 cases (52%); only one case of postoperative acute pancreatitis was observed.

## SPLENECTOMY

Splenectomy is a common operative procedure and is performed alone or in combination with resection of other organs such as the stomach, colon, and distal pancreas. Occasionally during splenectomy, the tail of the pancreas is damaged. After splenectomy, the following may be seen: pancreatic fistula, abscess, bleeding, high serum amylase levels, and other complications (39). No cases of postoperative acute pancreatitis following splenectomy could be found in the recent literature.

## OBSTETRIC AND GYNECOLOGIC SURGERY

Pregnancy is considered a predisposing condition for development of acute pancreatitis (40, 41). While manipulation of female internal genitalia is said to be followed sometimes by hyperamylasemia, Fröhlich et al. (42) evaluated the incidence of postoperative hyperamylasemia in 131 patients who underwent obstetric or gynecologic procedures and concluded that manipulation, per se, of the female internal genitalia, pregnant or not, does not induce hyperamylasemia. Thus, hyperamylasemia in postoperative obstetric and gynecologic patients should alert the clinician to the possibility of postoperative pancreatitis. In 1993, Steinmetz et al. (44) reported a case of recurrent pancreatitis associated with in vitro fertilization (IVF), which he described as apparently a unique report.

**TABLE 26.3. Complications of ERCP in 209,147 Examinations 1988–1992**

| | No. of Accidents after ERCP (%) | Deaths (%) |
|---|---|---|
| Complications | 245 (0.1171) | 14 (0.0067) |
| Acute pancreatitis | 193 (0.0922) | 9 |
| Perforation | 16 (0.0029) | 2 |
| Acute cholangitis | 13 (0.0062) | 2 |
| Shock | 4 (0.0019) | 1 |
| Others | 19 | 0 |

## CARDIOVASCULAR SURGERY

### Cardiac Surgery

The incidence of pancreatitis following cardiac surgery differs from the incidence following alcohol ingestion and cholelithiasis. Feiner (44) reported an incidence of 16% in 182 cardiac surgical patients, and Warshaw and O'Hara (45) reported an incidence of 11% in 101 patients in whom an autopsy was performed following cardiac surgery. The incidence of postoperative pancreatitis after cardiac surgery is probably higher than the 0.13% reported by Hanks et al. (46). Haas et al. (47) reported finding evidence of acute pancreatitis after cardiac surgery in 12 (0.2%) of 5400 patients: mild pancreatitis in 3, necrotizing pancreatitis in 9. The diagnosis in these nine patients had been missed because of an apparent lack of pain, tenderness, or hyperamylasemia. Eight cases were diagnosed at laparotomy and one at autopsy. Only two of these nine patients survived. The authors reported discovering acute necrotizing pancreatitis in 25% of 138 autopsies after cardiac surgery.

Krasna et al. (48) reported finding 31 gastrointestinal complications in 25 (2.0%) of 1279 patients after cardiac surgery; the mortality rate was 44%. Acute acalculous cholecystitis was the most fatal complication (86%), and acute pancreatitis was the most common complication (8 patients). Rose et al. (49) reported encountering 14 patients with severe pancreatitis since 1977; 6 developed acute fulminant pancreatitis following cardiac surgery. Possible factors in its etiology included prolonged cardiac bypass and low cardiac output syndrome. Pancreatic ischemia is a possible mechanism.

### Vascular Surgery and Angiography

Warshaw and O'Hara (45) reported a 2% incidence of acute pancreatitis after aortic resection. Gruber et al. (50) and Bagley et al. (51) reported similar cases. Bergqvist et al. (52) reported severe acute pancreatitis in 3 (0.9%) of 332 patients after renovascular surgery. Orvar et al. (53) reported a rare cases of acute pancreatitis after cardiac catheterization, apparently the result of atheromatous emboli.

## ORTHOPAEDIC SURGERY

Leichtner et al. (54) reported four cases of pancreatitis following scoliosis surgery. They pointed to a significantly high mean intraoperative blood loss in the group who developed pancreatitis.

## UROLOGIC SURGERY

In 1951, Renner (55) reported the first case of fatal acute pancreatitis, proved by necropsy, after transurethral resection of the prostate (TURP). He attributed the pathologic changes of acute pancreatitis to the proteolytic enzymatic activity of trypsin and noted that the tissues of the prostate gland have considerable proteolytic enzymatic activity and that a pronounced increase in proteolytic enzyme activity occurs during TURP.

In 1993, Lee et al. (56) reported three cases of acute pancreatitis occurring after TURP and indicated that acute pancreatitis should be considered in the differential diagnosis in the presence of abdominal pain with vomiting azotemia or oliguria after TURP. Hyperamylasemia and hyperamylasuria in postoperative urologic patients should alert the clinician to the possibility of postoperative pancreatitis.

## HYPERPARATHYROIDISM

Bess et al. (57) reported an incidence of acute pancreatitis in hyperparathyroidism of 1.5%. Vanlanschot and Bruining (58) analyzed a series of 686 patients with primary hyperparathyroidism and found concomitant pancreatitis in 1.5% of them (10 cases). Three of the cases of pancreatitis developed immediately after neck exploration, which is more than one would expect after an unrelated operation. Bess et al. (57) analyzed a much larger number of patients and found a poor correlation between hypercalcemia and pancreatitis and that most patients who suffer acute pancreatitis complicating hyperparathyroidism have either biliary disease or alcohol abuse as the more likely cause of their pancreatitis.

Watson et al. (59) reviewed 100 patients with biochemically proved primary hyperparathyroidism and found that according to the results of this prospective study, parathyroidectomy, with or without concomitant thyroid surgery, is unlikely to be complicated by postoperative pancreatitis. They reported four cases of hyperamylasemia in these 100 patients after parathyroidectomy. The elevated amylase was the S type. These findings suggest altered renal handling of amylase in the immediate postoperative period. The same finding has been observed in nonabdominal surgery.

Willems et al. (60) reported a 16% incidence of hyperamylasemia during the first 5 postoperative days after parathyroidectomy for primary hyperparathyroidism (196 patients), 3% after thyroidectomy (100 patients), and 2% after other extraabdominal operations (100 patients). They observed acute pancreatitis in 3% of patients after parathyroidectomy (6 of 196), compared with 37% of patients after pancreatic surgery (19 of 51) but never after thyroidectomy or other extraabdominal operations.

Whenever serum amylase levels are high after an operation, the type of serum amylase should be identified for diagnostic and treatment purposes.

### Posttransplantation Pancreatitis

There have been many reports of acute postoperative pancreatitis occurring after transplantation of heart, kidney, pancreas, and other organs as discussed in Chapter 27 of this book.

### Treatment and Prognosis

Early diagnosis and treatment should be performed. Causes of postoperative pancreatitis should be excluded. Nothing by mouth (NPO), nasogastric tube induction (NG), suction, intravenous nutrition, central venous catheterization, $H_2$ antagonists, and proton-pump inhibitors are usual treatments, and some people use protease inhibitors to inhibit pancreatic secretion. General care, intensive care, percutaneous biliary drainage, peritoneal lavage, and plasma exchange should be considered if necessary. When infected necrotic pancreatitis develops after postoperative pancreatitis, surgical intervention should be considered. Usually 10–14 days after the development of acute pancreatitis, pancreatectomy or necrosectomy with closed or open drain is carried out. However the mortality rate of pancreatectomy or necrosectomy for postoperative pancreatitis is about 20–50%. Therefore prevention is better than surgery, and one should know the mechanism of postoperative pancreatitis and its outcome as discussed above.

## CONCLUSION

The incidence of postoperative acute pancreatitis has decreased in the last decade, but the difficulty of diagnosis and the high mortality rate have changed very little. Whenever surgical operations are performed beyond the vicinity of the pancreas, surgeons must consider the possibility of postoperative acute pancreatitis, especially when ischemia of the pancreas, hypotension, sepsis, etc., occur during or after surgery. Clinical manifestations such as pain, tenderness, and fever are extremely difficult to assess in the postoperative period, because many factors affect these surgical patients after major surgery.

If there is any possibility that a surgical operation might be followed by acute pancreatitis, serum amylase levels should be checked postoperatively, and if they are high, the amylase should be identified as "salivary type" or "pancreatic type."

## REFERENCES


1. Naganuma T, Kawarada Y. Scoring the grading of severe acute pancreatitis and selection of early treatment (in Japanese). Geka Chiryo (Surgical Therapy) 1994;71:639–645.
2. Imrie CW, Dickson AP. Postoperative pancreatitis. In: Howard JM, ed. Surgical diseases of the pancreas. 2nd ed. Philadelphia: Lea & Febiger, 1987:332–341.
3. Bragg LE, Thompson JS, Burnett DA, Hodgson PE, Rikkers LF. Increased incidence of pancreas-related complications in patients with postoperative pancreatitis. Am J Surg 1985;150:694–697.
4. Park J, Fromkes J, Cooperman M. Acute pancreatitis in elderly patients. Pathogenesis and outcome. Am J Surg 1986;152: 638–642.
5. Thompson JS, Bragg LE, Hodgson PE, Rikkers LF. Postoperative pancreatitis. Surg Gynecol Obstet 1988;167:377–380.
6. Schmieden V, Sehening W. Surgery of the pancreas with special condition of acute pancreatic necrosis. Surg Gynecol Obstet 1928;46:735–751.
7. Thompson JA, Howard JM, Voweles KDJ. Acute pancreatitis following cholecystectomy. Surg Gynecol Obstet 1957;105: 706–710.
8. Bardenheier JA III, Kaminski DW, Willman VL. Pancreatitis after biliary tract surgery. Am J Surg 1968;116:773–776.
9. Vernava A, Andrus C, Herrmann VM, Kaminski DL. Pancreatitis after biliary tract surgery. Arch Surg 1987;122:575–580.
10. Warren KW. Pancreatic consideration in gastric surgery. JAMA 1954;154:803.
11. Jakab F, Regöly-Mérey J, Zavodszky Z, Rath Z. Postoperative pancreatitis after biliary and gastric operations. Acta Chir Hung 1988;29:241–249.
12. Kulazhenkov SA, Anisimov MA, Fedorov VN, Kuznetsov EV. Ostryi posleoperatsionnyi pankreatit. (Acute postoperative pancreatitis) Khirurgiia 1994;Jan(1):6–10.
13. Veronskii GI, Viskunov VG. Ostryi pankreatit posle operatsii na zheludke. (Acute pancreatitis after operations on the stomach) Khirurgiia-Mosk 1993;Jul(7):17–21.
14. Reilly LM, Ramos TK, Murray SP, Cheng SW, Stoney RJ. Optimal exposure of the proximal abdominal aorta: a critical appraisal of transabdominal medial visceral rotation. J Vasc Surg 1994;19: 375–389.
15. Pancreatic Cancer Registration Committee of the Japan Pancreas Society. Report of nationwide registration of pancreatic cancer patients in 1981–1990 (in Japanese). Japan Pancreas Society, 1991:49–92.

15a. Trede M, Schwall G. The complications of pancreatectomy. Ann Surg 1988;207:39–47.

16. Smith EH. Hazards of fine-needle aspiration biopsy. Ultrasound Med Biol 1984;10:629–634.
17. Mueller PR, Miketic LM, Simeone JF, Silverman SG, Saini S, et al. Severe acute pancreatitis after percutaneous biopsy of the pancreas. Am J Roentgenol 1988;151:493–494.
18. Levin DP, Bret PM. Percutaneous fine-needle aspiration biopsy of the pancreas resulting in death. Gastrointest Radiol 1991;16: 67–69.
19. Vavrecka A, Lesny P, Batovsky M. Endoscopic treatment of choledocholithiasis. Czech Med 1987;10:226–235.
20. Sarr MG, Fishman EK, Milligan FD, Siegelman SS, Cameron JL. Pancreatitis or duodenal perforation after peri-Vaterian therapeutic endoscopic procedures: diagnosis, differentiation, and management. Surg 1986;100:461–466.
21. Doherty DE, Falko JM, Lefkovitz N, Rogers J, Fromkes J. *Pseudomonas aeruginosa* sepsis following retrograde cholangiopancreatography (ERCP). Dig Dis Sci 1982;27:169–170.
22. Barkin JS, Casal GL, Reiner DK, Goldberg RI, Phillips RS, Kaplan S. A comparative study of contrast agents for endoscopic retrograde pancreatography. Am J Gastroenterol 1991;86:1437–1441.
23. Frost RA. Prospective multicentre study of British sphincterotomy: initial results and complications. Gut 1984;25:A549.
24. Nebel OT, Silvius SE, Rogers G, Sugawa C, Mandelstam P. Complication associated with endoscopic retrograde cholangiopancreatography: results of the 1974 ASGE survey. Gastrointest Endosc 1975;22:34–36.
25. Skude G, Wehlin L, Maruyama T, Ariyama J. Hyperamylasaemia after duodenoscopy and retrograde cholangiopancreatography. Gut 1976;17:127–132.
26. Montori A, Viceconte G, Viceconte GW, Bogliolo G. ERCP and EPT: Italian experience. Endoscopy 1979;11:142–145.
27. Brandes JW, Scheffer B, Lorenz-Meyer H, Korst HA, Littmann KP. ERCP: complications and prophylaxis; a controlled study. Endoscopy 1981;13:27–30.
28. Hamilton I, Lintott DJ, Rothwell J, Axon AT. Acute pancreatitis following endoscopic retrograde cholangiopancreatography. Clin Radiol 1983;34:543–546.
29. Roszler MH, Campbell WL. Post-ERCP pancreatitis: association with urographic visualization during ERCP. Radiology 1985;157: 595–598.
30. Reiertsen O, Skjoto J, Jacobsen CD, Rosseland AR. Complications of fiberoptic gastrointestinal endoscopy—five years' experience in a central hospital. Endoscopy 1987;19:1–6.
31. Kasugai T, Namiki M, Honda T, Kawai K, Takemoto T. Report on a nationwide questionnaire survey on complications of gastrointestinal endoscopy in Japan during the 5-year period from 1983 to 1987 (in Japanese). Gastroenterol Endosc 1989;31: 2214–2229.
32. Kaneko E, Harada H, Kasugai T, Sakita T. Report on a nationwide questionnaire survey on complications of gastrointestinal endoscopy in Japan during the 5-year period from 1988 to 1992 (in Japanese). Gastroenterol Endosc 1995;37:642–652.
33. Sakanoue Y, Kusunoki M, Shoji Y, Yanagi H, Yamamura T, Utsunomiya J. Transitory elevation of serum amylase levels after restorative proctocolectomy. Int J Colorectal Dis 1992;7:210–213.
34. Tsuzuki T, Shimizu S, Takahashi S, Iio H. Hyperamylasemia after hepatic resection. Am J Gastroenterol 1993;88:734–736.
35. Bernald HB, Criscione JR, Moyer CA. The pathological significance of the serum amylase concentration. Arch Surg 1959;59: 311–318.
36. Soravia C, Mentha G, Giostra E, Morel P, Rohner A. Surgery for adult polycystic liver disease. Surgery 1995;117:272–275.
37. McDermott WV, Kane RA, Vollman RW, O'Hara ET. Pseudocyst of the pancreas complicating distal splenorenal shunt: a report of three cases with successful percutaneous drainage. Ann Surg 1981;193:176–179.
38. Fegiz G, Bracci F, Trenti A, Grassini G, Collizza S, De Fazio S. Operative morbidity after shunt surgery for portal hypertension. Int Surg 1985;70:301–303.
39. White TT, Morgan A, Hopton D. Postoperative pancreatitis. A study of seventy cases. Am J Surg 1970;120:132–137.
40. Salt WB II, Schenker S. Amylase—its clinical significance. Medicine 1976;55:269–289.
41. Wyatt AP. Diagnosis and management of acute pancreatitis. Ann R Coll Surg Engl 1974;54:229–235.
42. Fröhlich EP, Herz C, van der Merwe FJ, Schein M, Smyth AE. Serum amylase levels after obstetric and gynecologic operations. Surg Gynecol Obstet 1990;170:292–294.
43. Feiner H. Pancreatitis after cardiac surgery; a morphologic study. Am J Surg 1976;131:684–688.
44. Steinmetz KO, Hashim E, Falcome T, et al. Recurrent pancreatitis associated with in vitro fertilization. Obstet Gynecol 1993;81(5): 890–892.
45. Warshaw AL, O'Hara PJ. Susceptibility of the pancreas to ischemic injury in shock. Ann Surg 1978;188:197–201.
46. Hanks JB, Curtis SE, Hanks BB, et al. Gastrointestinal complications after cardiopulmonary bypass. Surgery 1982;92:394–400.
47. Haas GS, Warshaw AL, Daggett WM, Aretz HT. Acute pancreatitis after cardiopulmonary bypass. Am J Surg 1985;149:508–515.
48. Krasna MJ, Flancbaum L, Trooskin SZ, Fitzpatrick JC, Scholz PM, et al. Gastrointestinal complications after cardiac surgery. Surgery 1988;104:773–780.
49. Rose DM, Ranson JH, Cunningham JN Jr, Spencer FC. Patterns of severe pancreatic injury following cardiopulmonary bypass. Ann Surg 1984;199:168–172.
50. Gruber HP, Fasol R, Schlosser V. Necrotising pancreatitis due to a ruptured abdominal aortic aneurysm. Eur Vasc Surg 1994;8:521–523.
51. Bagley JS, Tyler MP, Cooper GG. Hyperamylasaemia in ruptured aortic aneurysm: incidence and prognostic implications. Br J Surg 1994;81:31–32.

52. Bergqvist D, Weibull H, Bergentz SE. Acute necrotizing pancreatitis complicating surgery for renovascular hypertension. Acta Chir Scand 1989;155:489–492.
53. Orvar K, Johlin FC. Atheromatous embolization resulting in acute pancreatitis after cardiac catheterization and angiographic studies. Arch Intern Med 1994;154:1755–1761.
54. Leichtner AM, Banta JV, Etienne M, et al. Pancreatitis following scoliosis surgery in children and young adults. J Pediatr Orthop 1991;11:594–598.
55. Renner WF. Postoperative acute pancreatitis and lower nephron syndrome. JAMA 1951;147:1654–1660.
56. Lee MH, Chen KK, Lin AT, et al. Acute pancreatitis following transurethral resection of prostate. Eur Urol 1993;23:419–422.
57. Bess MA, Edis AJ, van Heerden JA. Hyperparathyroidism and pancreatitis: chance or a causal association? JAMA 1980;243: 246–247.
58. van Lanschot JJ, Bruining HA. Primary hyperparathyroidism and pancreatitis. Neth J Surg 1984;36:38–41.
59. Watson RGK, van Heerden JA, Grant CS, Klee GG. Postoperative hyperamylasemia, pancreatitis, and primary hyperparathyroidism. Surgery 1984;56:1151–1157.
60. Reference deleted.

# 27

# *Posttransplant Pancreatitis*

Keiichi Kubota and Finn P. Reinholt

Posttransplant pancreatitis, considered one of the diseases typical of the posttransplant condition, may result from various causes. Acute pancreatitis is defined as an acute condition of the pancreas, typically presenting with abdominal pain and usually associated with increased activity of pancreatic enzymes in the blood or urine, owing to inflammatory destruction of the pancreatic parenchyma. Clinically, posttransplant pancreatitis is an infrequent but severe complication (1, 2). This chapter describes the clinical features of posttransplant pancreatitis, focusing particularly on the etiology.

Posttransplant pancreatitis was first recognized as a complication of renal transplantation by Starzl (3). Since then, this type of pancreatitis has been frequently reported in the literature, and it is now well established that pancreatitis may develop after the transplantation of kidney, pancreas, liver, heart, lung, or bone marrow (1–10).

## Clinical Features

The characteristic clinical features of posttransplant pancreatitis are the same as those of acute pancreatitis in nontransplant patients. Most patients suffer from at least one of several symptoms, including epigastric pain, nausea with vomiting, high fever, and back pain, and their serum or urinary pancreatic enzyme activities are elevated (1–21). However, during steroid treatment, these symptoms may not be obvious. This type of pancreatitis can occur at any time after surgery; in particular, when the pancreatitis is associated with operative procedures, it may develop at an early phase, as in kidney, heart, and heart-lung transplantation (1, 11, 13, 16, 21). The interval between renal transplantation and the onset of pancreatitis ranges from 1 day to 570 days, with an average of 216 days (8). Johnson and Nabseth (22) found the prognosis was worse among patients who developed pancreatitis 3 months or more after renal transplantation than in those who developed it earlier.

## Incidence and Mortality

The incidence and mortality rates of posttransplant pancreatitis differ according to the organs transplanted (Table 27.1). Inflammatory changes in the pancreas are common in uremia; necropsy findings in patients with chronic renal failure show inflammatory pancreatic lesions in up to 52% of patients who had not received immunosuppressive therapy or shown any clinical evidence of pancreatic disease (19, 24, 25). Fernandez-Cruz et al. (1) reported incidence and mortality rates of 2.3% and 61.3%, respectively, in 3253 renal transplant patients. Lober et al. (23) reported clinically evident pancreatic disease in only 6 of 466 patients (1.3%) who had received renal allografts under cyclosporine/prednisone immunosuppression; of these 6 patients, 2 had clinically apparent pancreatitis, and 1 died of pancreatic abscess. Overall, the incidence of pancreatitis following renal transplantation has been reported to vary between 0.4 and 7% and to be associated with a mortality rate between 20 and 70% (1, 2, 4, 7–9, 24, 25).

Pancreatitis has also been reported as a complication in other types of transplantation. Acute pancreatitis sometimes complicates heart and heart-lung transplantation, particularly when cardiopulmonary bypass is used (26, 27). Colon et al. (13) reported incidence and mortality rates of 18.6 and 40%, respectively, in 86 heart transplant patients. Others have reported an incidence of 10% for heart transplantation (11) and 2.3–4% for heart-lung transplantation (16, 21). Acute pancreatitis has not been recognized as a frequent problem in liver transplantation in the few reports published so far (12, 28, 29), but recently, Camargo et al. (20) reported incidence and mortality rates of 5.9 and 33.3%, respectively. In bone marrow transplantation, pancreatitis is also associated with some morbidity and mortality. Werlin et al. (17) reported incidence and mortality rates of 3.5 and 42.9%. Finally, in combined renal-pancreas transplantation, one report described posttransplant pancreatitis in 2 of 60 patients (3.3%) (2). Thus, although this condition is rare, it is severe and potentially fatal.

## Etiology

Several etiological factors have been proposed for posttransplant "native" pancreatitis (Table 27.2). (The term *native pancreatitis* denotes pancreatitis in the patient's original pancreas, in contradistinction to pancreatitis developing in a transplanted pancreas.) However, clinically, it is usually difficult to determine a specific cause in a particular case. Specific causes related to the posttransplant state are described below.

**Drugs.** Many drugs have been reported to cause hyperamylasemia, abdominal pain, or both, but it is not clear whether or not this condition is really a form of acute pancreatitis. Included in this category are immunosuppressive drugs, thiazide diuretics, furosemide, estrogen, L-asparaginase, 6-mercaptopurine, methyldopa, and procainamide. The intensive immunosuppressive regimen administered after a transplant operation may explain posttransplant pancreatitis (30, 31). Azathioprine, corticosteroids, and FK506 have been reported to cause pancreatitis that usually improves after discontinuation of the drugs (14, 32–34). Nogueira and Freedman (35) and Kawanishi et al. (36) reported that patients with Crohn's disease who received only azathioprine sometimes developed pancreatitis. Nevertheless, a clear-cut relationship between the drug in question and a specific episode of pancreatitis is difficult to establish.

Although cyclosporine has a toxic effect on the pancreas in both humans and rats (32, 33, 37, 38), frank acute pancreatitis attributable to cyclosporine treatment has not been reported. However, Lober et al. (23) have reported that asymptomatic hyperamylasemia is frequently observed in renal transplant recipients under cyclosporine immunosuppression. Cyclosporine is metabolized in the liver and recirculated via the enterohe-

**TABLE 27.1. Incidence and Mortality Rate of Posttransplant Pancreatitis**

| Transplanted Organ | Incidence (%) | Mortality Rate (%) |
|---|---|---|
| Kidney (1, 2, 4, 7–9, 24, 25) | 0.4–7 | 20–70 |
| Liver (12, 20, 28, 29) | 5.9 | 33.3 |
| Heart and heart-lung (11, 13, 16, 21) | 2.3–18.6 | 40 |
| Bone marrow (17) | 3.5 | 42.9 |
| Kidney-pancreas (2) | 3.3 | |

patic route. The pancreas ranks second to the liver as a cyclosporine store (39). Thus cyclosporine is considered to be related to pancreatitis and to asymptomatic hyperamylasemia. The recently developed immunosuppressive drug, FK506, also has a toxic effect on the pancreas and is suspected of being associated with pancreatitis (34, 40). However, details of the responsible mechanism are not known.

In addition to immunosuppressive drugs, diuretics such as thiazides and furosemide have been reported to cause pancreatitis (1, 41). Thiazides may act directly on the pancreas or indirectly by altering calcium metabolism (41). The structural similarity of furosemide and chlorothiazide supports an association with pancreatitis. Recently, Halim et al. (42) reported that a renal transplant recipient developed pancreatitis during treatment with stibogluconate for visceral leishmaniasis. However, how these drugs induce acute pancreatitis is unknown.

**Infection.** Viral infection is one of the severe complications that may follow a transplant operation, and there is a well-known relationship between pancreatitis and cytomegalovirus and herpesvirus infections, respectively (5, 15, 43, 44). Such viruses may directly colonize the pancreas (5). Increased serum titers of anticytomegalovirus antibodies as well as cytomegalic nuclear inclusions in the pancreatic cells of renal transplant recipients have been reported (15, 19, 43, 44). Peterson et al. (43) reported that 59 of 141 renal transplant recipients showed symptomatic cytomegalovirus infection, and 4 of the 59 developed pancreatitis. Pancreatitis caused by cytomegalovirus is severe and may be hemorrhagic or necrotic, thus associated with high morbidity and mortality rates (16). Damage to the ductal epithelium or vasculitis caused by the virus may induce parenchymal inflammation. Adenovirus, mumps virus, Coxsackie B virus, and *Mycoplasma pneumoniae* have also been reported to cause pancreatitis (18, 45, 46). Considerable evidence suggests that both naturally acquired and experimentally induced Coxsackie B virus infections may damage the pancreas (47, 48). Furthermore, Alexander et al. (12) reported that pancreatitis in at least some patients after hepatic transplantation for viral disease of the liver may result from hepatitis B virus infection of the pancreas; Camargo et al. (20) supported the observation that hepatitis B virus may play a role in the pathogenesis of acute pancreatitis in some patients. Hepatitis B viral antigens have been detected in pancreatic acinar cells in some patients with chronic hepatitis B (49). It is conceivable that immunosuppressive therapy could facilitate not only viral replication in hepatic tissue, but also dissemination and replication in extrahepatic sites (50).

**TABLE 27.2. Specific Causes Related to Posttransplant Pancreatitis**

| |
|---|
| Drugs (e.g., azathioprine, corticosteroid, thiazide) |
| Infection (e.g., cytomegalovirus, herpesvirus, mumps virus, *Mycoplasma pneumoniae*) |
| Surgical procedures |
| Acute rejection |
| Hyperparathyroidism (in renal transplantation) |

**Surgical Procedures.** A relationship between pancreatitis and certain surgical procedures has been reported. Fernandez-Cruz et al. (1) reported that 2 of 132 orthotopic renal transplant patients had developed pancreatitis, and they suggested that injury to the pancreas might occur during removal of the left kidney when revascularization of the graft is obtained by use of the splenic vessels of the recipient. In heart and heart-lung transplantation, cardiopulmonary bypass is suspected to cause pancreatitis (13, 16). Feiner (51) noted that 15% of patients who died after cardiopulmonary bypass had evidence of pancreatitis at autopsy, and this was believed to be related to ischemia and hypothermia during bypass. Several etiologic factors have been proposed for pancreatitis in the early postoperative period after cardiac surgery: low perfusion states, splanchnic vasoconstriction secondary to use of pressor agents, hypothermia, and thromboembolic phenomena (13, 16, 51). Low perfusion states secondary to low cardiac output before transplantation may predispose the pancreas to injury caused by further episodes of ischemia or other insults during the perioperative period, but they do not explain events occurring later.

**Immunologic Response.** Posttransplant pancreatitis occasionally occurs during acute rejection episodes after renal transplantation. Corticosteroid administration for treatment of acute rejection is a possible cause. On the other hand, the host may form an antibody that recognizes pancreatic cell surfaces, destroying the pancreas and inducing "rejection pancreatitis." This notion is supported by observations of vasculitis in pancreatic biopsy specimens taken from patients after renal transplantation (4–6, 9, 24, 25, 52). Prior to transplant, Jaray et al. (10) cultured a mixture of lymphocytes from the recipient and the donor. Of the patients who developed posttransplant pancreatitis, none had demonstrated reactivity of his or her lymphocytes when cultured with either donor lymphocytes or with positive control lymphocytes. None of the other patients showed this phenomenon, and none of them developed acute pancreatitis. This suggests that the recipient's immune responsiveness (or lack or responsiveness) may be involved in the etiology of acute pancreatitis after renal transplantation.

In bone marrow transplantation, graft-versus-host disease is a possible cause. Foulis et al. (53) described autopsy findings in four patients with presumed pancreatic graft-versus-host disease. Although Werlin et al. (17) also reported pancreatitis associated with bone marrow transplantation in children, they could not determine whether it occurred secondary to transplantation, graft-versus-host disease, or other factors.

**Hyperparathyroidism.** Secondary hyperparathyroidism frequently occurs after renal transplantation and usually resolves spontaneously, although some patients develop tertiary hyperparathyroidism. Fernandez-Cruz et al. (1) noted that although it is questionable whether pancreatitis in renal transplant patients is caused by elevated serum calcium levels, acute pancreatitis is certainly associated with high serum calcium levels. Haverbood et al. (54) demonstrated that activation of pancreatic trypsin is controlled by calcium ions and that an increase in trypsin activity may account for the association of pancreatitis with hyperparathyroidism.

**Other Factors.** Total body irradiation is often used in bone marrow transplantation, but it has not been reported to cause pancreatitis. Werlin et al. (17) reported that in their series of bone marrow transplants, four patients developed pancreatitis in the peritransplant period. However, other patients developed pancreatitis as long as 2 years after receiving total body irradiation, making it unlikely that the procedure can be implicated in the etiology of pancreatitis.

**TABLE 27.3. Diagnosis of Posttransplant Pancreatitis**

| |
|---|
| Blood analysis (e.g., white blood cell count, amylase, lipase, trypsin, elastase, phospholipase) |
| Urine analysis (e.g., amylase) |
| Diagnostic imaging modalities (e.g., ultrasound, computed tomography) |
| Laparotomy, if warranted |

## Diagnosis

In principle, the diagnostic process for posttransplant pancreatitis is the same as that for "conventional" acute pancreatitis (Table 27.3).

**Blood and Urine Analysis.** Blood analysis shows an elevation not only of the white blood cell count but also of plasma levels of pancreatic enzymes such as amylase, lipase, trypsin, elastase, and phospholipase. Decreased calcium levels and elevated C-reactive protein values in the serum are also usually observed. Increased pancreatic enzyme activities are also observed in the urine. During severe pancreatitis, disseminated intravascular coagulation may occur. Therefore, serum levels of fibrinogen, fibrinogen degradation products, antithrombin III, and platelets should be checked frequently.

**Diagnostic Imaging Modalities.** Several diagnostic imaging modalities such as ultrasound and computed tomography are available for diagnosing acute pancreatitis (55). Pancreatic swelling and peripancreatic fluid accumulation visualized by these methods suggest the presence of pancreatitis. During obstructive pancreatitis, a dilated pancreatic duct may be observed.

**Laparotomy.** When a diagnosis of posttransplant pancreatitis cannot be established on the basis of blood analysis and diagnostic imaging, laparotomy is recommended (13, 16). Watson et al. (16) reported that after heart and heart-lung transplantation, 20 patients underwent laparotomy; 2 of whom were found to have acute pancreatitis. Timely emergency laparotomy may permit a definite diagnosis, and if it produces negative findings, it is preferable to running the risk of allowing generalized peritonitis to develop in an immunosuppressed patient (11).

## Treatment

When posttransplant pancreatitis is suspected, the patient should refrain from oral intake. External drainage of the gastric juice via a nasogastric tube reduces the stimulation of exocrine pancreatic secretion. Antibiotics should be administered for suspected abdominal infection. The patient usually reports abdominal pain, which should be treated with narcotics intramuscularly (or, if needed, intravenously). Fluid replacement is necessary; and the amount given should be guided by the vital signs and urinary output. The dosage of immunosuppressive drugs should be carefully adjusted to minimize the risk of infectious complications and allograft rejection. When required, a Swan-Ganz catheter should be inserted for monitoring the cardiovascular status. Severe pancreatitis necessitates careful observation and treatment of respiratory and cardiovascular function and correction of metabolic acidosis. Pancreatic necrosis causes severe inflammation and is occasionally complicated by infection with abscess formation, which may require surgical intervention for drainage and debridement of the necrotic tissue. A low-fat diet should be started after the serum amylase and lipase levels have normalized and pain has resolved (Table 27.4).

**TABLE 27.4. Treatment of Posttransplant Pancreatitis**

| |
|---|
| No oral intake |
| External drainage of gastric juice |
| Anodyne (e.g., pentadin) |
| Antibiotics (if needed) |
| Fluid replacement |
| Adjustment of immunosuppressive drugs |
| Hemodynamic monitoring |
| Drainage operations (if needed) |

# PANCREATITIS IN A PANCREATIC GRAFT

Most pancreatic grafts are placed in the right lower abdominal cavity and are anastomosed to either the small bowel or the urinary bladder. Pancreatitis in a pancreatic graft (graft pancreatitis) is a severe complication that is sometimes difficult to diagnose correctly (56).

## Clinical Features

In principle, the clinical features of graft pancreatitis are the same as those of acute pancreatitis, including one or more of the following: hyperamylasemia, increased white blood cell count, tenderness over the graft, fever, lower abdominal pain, and abdominal distension. However, these signs are not always observed, and therefore, the diagnosis of graft pancreatitis can be difficult. Acute rejection is the most difficult condition to distinguish from graft pancreatitis. Acute rejection is usually, at least initially, not accompanied by hyperamylasemia or tenderness over the graft; observations that may provide some guidance in differentiating between the two conditions (2).

## Diagnosis

Graft pancreatitis can be diagnosed by employing the measures listed in Table 27.5.

**Analysis of Blood Samples.** Increased amylase and lipase activities with normal or reduced fasting blood glucose levels are observed in association with graft pancreatitis (56). Stratta et al. (57) reported that only 17.7% of the rejection episodes are associated with hyperamylasemia.

**Cytology of Pancreatic Juice.** Cytologic analysis of pancreatic juice from pancreatic grafts has been reported to show specific signs of immunoactivation and graft pancreatitis (58–60). The characteristic cytologic signs of graft pancreatitis include increased numbers of polymorphonuclear leukocytes, degenerating cells (probably of both epithelial and inflammatory cell origin), monocytes, epithelial cells, and some macrophages, with or without necrotic tissue fragments, following a period of low cellularity (58–60). Clinically, cytologic signs of graft pancreatitis seem to be associated with a poor prognosis (59, 60).

**Amylase Activity in Pancreatic Juice or Urine.** Although decreased amylase activity in pancreatic juice has been reported to be a reliable marker of pancreatic graft rejection (58, 62, 63), no specific pattern of change in the amylase activity of the juice has been observed during graft pancreatitis (61).

**Diagnostic Imaging Modalities.** In addition to the findings described previously, graft pancreatitis is occasionally accompanied by thrombosis, which can be diagnosed by angiography or scintigraphy (64, 65).

**Graft Biopsy.** Under ultrasonic guidance, the pancreatic graft can be punctured by a core biopsy needle. Histologically,

**TABLE 27.5. Diagnosis of Pancreatitis in a Pancreatic Graft**

| |
|---|
| Blood analysis (e.g., amylase, blood sugar) |
| Pancreatic juice cytology |
| Amylase activity in the pancreatic juice or urine |
| Diagnostic imaging modalities (e.g., ultrasound, computed tomography) |
| Graft biopsy |

characteristic features of graft pancreatitis include focal inflammation with a cellular infiltrate dominated by polymorphonuclear leukocytes, often related to ducts and accompanied by necrosis, and an absence of vasculitis.

### Etiology

Table 27.6 summarizes etiologic factors for graft pancreatitis. However, in any particular case, it is difficult to determine the specific cause.

**Preservation Damage.** Busing et al. (66) reported that ischemia/reperfusion injury to the graft during preservation and surgery induces a form of acute graft pancreatitis. Clinically, patients report no tenderness over the grafts; thus, this type of pancreatitis seems to differ from graft pancreatitis that appears late in the course.

**Drugs.** As described above, drugs may also induce graft pancreatitis.

**Rejection.** Graft pancreatitis is occasionally accompanied by graft rejection (57). The causal relationship between the two conditions is not clear. Acute rejection causes inflammation in the pancreas, and therefore, graft pancreatitis may occur simultaneously.

**Infection.** Viral infection, particularly involving cytomegalovirus or herpes simplex, also causes graft pancreatitis. Backman et al. (67) reported a series of 124 pancreatic transplantations: 8 patients suffered from graft pancreatitis associated with ongoing cytomegaloviral infection; 5 patients developed intrapancreatic abscesses, and 4 grafts were lost. In addition, when the pancreatic juice has been diverted into the urinary bladder, urinary infection may cause graft pancreatitis (57).

**Other Causes.** Linder et al. (68) reported late graft pancreatitis occurring more than 1 year after segmental pancreatic transplantation. Mental stress, which is suspected of inducing hormonal stimulation of the graft, and mechanical pressure may trigger such episodes (68). Alcohol and food intake have also been reported to induce graft pancreatitis (68).

### Treatment

When graft pancreatitis is suspected, the graft should be protected from all types of stress; the patient should refrain from oral food intake and should be given antibiotics. Mittal et al. (56) reported that most cases of mild pancreatitis resolve without the wound being reopened and that only a small percentage require pancreatectomy. Moderate pancreatitis requires more aggressive treatment, including wound reexploration and debridement, which results in a 60% rate of graft salvage. In cases of severe pancreatitis, reexploration of the graft and debridement are also performed with relatively good results. Thus, resolution of pancreatitis without pancreatectomy can be achieved for 60% of grafts. When cytomegaloviral infection is thought to have induced the graft pancreatitis, antiviral drugs such as ganciclovir or acyclovir or immunoglobulin should be administered (67). When these measures are not effective, some grafts develop vascular thrombosis and cease to function. In this instance, the graft should be removed.

**TABLE 27.6. Etiologic Factors in Pancreatitis in a Pancreatic Graft**

| |
|---|
| Preservation damage |
| Drugs (azathioprine, corticosteroid, thiazides) |
| Acute rejection |
| Infection (cytomegalovirus, fungi, bacteria) |
| Mental stress |
| Mechanical pressure |
| Reflux (in bladder drainage technique) |
| Alcoholism |

## SUMMARY

Under the special conditions of the immunosuppressive state in transplant recipients, acute pancreatitis is a rare but severe condition with a high mortality rate. When pancreatitis is suspected clinically, the cause should be sought and, if possible, eliminated. In most cases, this will ameliorate the pancreatitis. If the treatment is unsuccessful or instituted too late, the patient will become severely ill, and the graft may have to be removed. Therefore, surgeons should aim for early diagnosis of posttransplant pancreatitis and institute early treatment.

## REFERENCES


1. Fernandez-Cruz L, Targarona EM, Cugat E, Alcaraz A, Oppenheimer F. Acute pancreatitis after renal transplantation. Br J Surg 1989;76:1132–1135.
2. Fernandez-Cruz L, Sabater L, Gilabert R, Ricart MJ, Saenz A, Astudillo E. Native and graft pancreatitis following combined pancreas-renal transplantation. Br J Surg 1993;80:1429–1432.
3. Starzl TE. Experience in renal transplantation. Philadelphia: WB Saunders, 1964.
4. Johnson WC, Nabseth DC. Pancreatitis in renal transplantation. Ann Surg 1970;171:309–314.
5. Renning JA, Warden GD, Stevens LE, et al. Pancreatitis after renal transplantation. Am J Surg 1972;123:293–296.
6. Woods JE, Anderson CF, Frohnert PP, Petrie CR. Pancreatitis in renal allografted patients. Mayo Clin Proc 1972;47:193–195.
7. Corrodi P, Knoblauch M, Binswanger J, et al. Pancreatitis after renal transplantation. Gut 1975;16:285–289.
8. Fernandez JA, Rosenberg JC. Post transplantation pancreatitis. Surg Gynecol Obstet 1976;143:795–798.
9. Taft PM, Jones AC, Geoffrey RN, Collins M, Halasz NA. Acute pancreatitis following renal allotransplantation. Dig Dis 1978;23:541–544.
10. Jaray J, Perner F, Alfoldy F, Onody K. Mixed lymphocyte cultures (MLC) and acute pancreatitis after renal transplantation. Int Urol Nephrol 1981;13:391–394.
11. Adiseshiah M, Wells FC, Cory-Pearce R, et al. Acute pancreatitis after cardiac transplantation. World J Surg 1983;7:519–521.
12. Alexander JA, Demetris AJ, Gavaler JS, Makowka L, Starzl TE, Van Thiel DH. Pancreatitis following liver transplantation. Transplantation 1988;45:1062–1065.
13. Colon R, Franzier OH, Kahan BD, et al. Complications in cardiac transplant patients requiring general surgery. Surgery 1988;103:32–38.
14. Przepiorka D, Shapiro S, Schwinghammer TL, et al. Cyclosporine and methylprednisolone after allogenic marrow transplantation: association between low cyclosporine concentration and risk of acute-versus-host disease. Bone Marrow Transplant 1991;7:461–465.
15. Schiller GJ, Niemer SD, Gajewski JL, Golde DW. Abdominal presentation of varicella-zoster infection in recipients of allogenic bone marrow transplantation. Bone Marrow Transplant 1991;7:489–491.
16. Watson CJE, Jamieson NV, Johnston PS, et al. Early abdominal complications following heart and heart-lung transplantation. Br J Surg 1991;78:699–704.
17. Werlin SL, Casper J, Antonson D, Calabro C. Pancreatitis associated with bone marrow transplantation in children. Bone Marrow Transplant 1992;10:65–69.
18. Niemann TH, Trigg ME, Winick N, Penick GD. Disseminated adenoviral infection presenting as acute pancreatitis. Hum Pathol 1993;24:1145–1148.
19. Washington K, Gossage DL, Gottfried MR. Pathology of the pancreas in severe combined immunodeficiency and DiGeorge syndrome: acute graft-versus-host disease and unusual viral infections. Hum Pathol 1994;25:908–914.
20. Camargo CA Jr, Greig PD, Levy GA, Clavien P-A. Acute pancreatitis following liver transplantation. J Am Coll Surg 1995;181:249–256.
21. Whitehead BF, Rees PG, Sorenson K, et al. Results of heart-lung transplantation in children with cystic fibrosis. Eur J Cardiothorac Surg 1995;9:1–6.

22. Johnson WC, Nabseth DC. Pancreatitis in renal transplantation. Ann Surg 1970;171:309–317.
23. Lober MI, Van Buren CT, Kahan BD, et al. Hepatobiliary and pancreatic complications of cyclosporin therapy in 466 renal transplant recipients. Transplantation 1987;43:35–40.
24. Penn I, Durst AL, Machado M, et al. Acute pancreatitis and hyperamylasemia in renal homograft recipients. Arch Surg 1972; 105:167–172.
25. Robinson DO, Alp MH, Grant AK, Lawrence JR. Pancreatitis and renal disease. Scand J Gastroenterol 1977;12:17–20.
26. Huddy S, Joyce W, Pepper J. Gastrointestinal complications in 4473 patients who underwent cardiopulmonary bypass surgery. Br J Srug 1991;78:293–296.
27. Del Castilloi F, Harringer W, Warshaw A, et al. Risk factors for pancreatic cellular injury after cardiopulmonary bypass. N Engl J Med 1991;325:382–387.
28. Lebeau G, Yanaga K, Marsh JW, et al. Analysis of surgical complications after 397 hepatic transplantations. Surg Gynecol Obstet 1990;170:317–322.
29. Krokos N, Karavias D, Tzakis A, et al. Acute pancreatitis after liver transplantation: incidence and contributing factors. Transplant Int 1995;8:1–7.
30. Sturdevant RAL, Singleton JW, Deren JJ. et al. Azathioprine-related pancreatitis in patients with Crohn's disease. Gastroenterology 1979;77:883–886.
31. Mallory A, Kern F. Drug induced pancreatitis: a critical review. Gastroenterology 1980;78:813–820.
32. Gunnarsson R, Klintmalm R, Lundgren C, Wilczeck H, Ostman J, Groth CG. Deterioration in glucose metabolism in pancreatic transplant recipients given cyclosporin. Lancet 1983;2:571–572.
33. Fernandez-Cruz L, Targarona EM, Robera MT, Casas A, Hotter G. The effect of immunosuppressive drugs on rat exocrine pancreas secretion. Eur Surg Res 1986;18(suppl):53–54.
34. Ito E, Kimura T, Furukawa M, et al. Protective effects of gabexate mesilate on acute pancreatitis induced by tacrolimus (FK-506) in rats in which the pancreas was stimulated by caerulein. J Gastroenterol 1994;29:305–313.
35. Nogueira JR, Freedman MA. Acute pancreatitis as a complication of Imuran therapy in regional enteritis. Gastroenterology 1972;62:1040–1041.
36. Kawanishi H, Rudolph E, Bull FE. Azathioprine-induced acute pancreatitis. N Engl J Med 1973;289:357.
37. Hahn HJ, Laube F, Lucke S, Klotking I, Kohnert KD, Warzock K. Toxic effects of cyclosporin on the endocrine pancreas of Wistar rats. Transplantation 1986;41:44–47.
38. Ribera MT, Targarona EM, Casas A, et al. The influence of cyclosporin and cyclosporin plus corticoids on the exocrine pancreas function in the rat. Digestion 1986;32:49.
39. Rogers AJ, Kahan BD. Mechanism of action and clinical applications of cyclosporine in organ transplantation. Clin Immunol Allergy 1984;4:217–258.
40. Ricordi C, Zeng Y, Alejandro R, et al. In vivo effect of FK506 on human pancreatic islets. Transplantation 1991;52:519–522.
41. Steer ML. Etiology and pathophysiology of acute pancreatitis. In: Go VLW, ed. The exocrine pancreas. New York: Raven, 1986:465.
42. Halim MA, Alfurayh O, Kalin ME, et al. Successful treatment of visceral leishmaniasis with allopurinol plus ketoconazole in a renal transplant recipient after the occurrence of pancreatitis due to stibogluconate. Clin Infect Dis 1993;16:397–399.
43. Peterson PK, Balfour HH Jr, Marker SC. Cytomegalovirus disease in renal allograft recipients: a prospective study of the clinical features, risk factors and impact on renal transplantation. Medicine (Baltimore) 1980;59:283–300.
44. Parham DM. Post-transplantation pancreatitis associated with cytomegalovirus. Hum Pathol 1981;12:63–65.
45. Imrie CW, Ferguson JC, Sommerville RG. Coxsackie and mumps virus infection in a prospective study of acute pancreatitis. Gut 1977;18:53–56.
46. Freeman R, McMahon MJ. Acute pancreatitis and serological evidence of infection with Mycoplasma pneumoniae. Gut 1978;19:367–370.
47. Ursing B. Acute pancreatitis in Coxsackie B infection. Br Med J 1973;3:524–525.
48. Arnesjo B, Eden T, Ihse I, et al. Enterovirus infections in acute pancreatitis—a possible aetiological connection. Scand J Gastroenterol 1976;II:645–649.
49. Shimoda T, Shikata T, Karasawa T, Tsukagoshi S, Yoshimura M, Sakurai I. Light microscopic localization of hepatitis B virus antigens in the human pancreas. Gastroenterology 1981;81:998–1005.
50. Lake JR, Wright TL. Liver transplantation for patients with hepatitis B: what we learned from our results. Hepatology 1991;13:796–799.
51. Feiner H. Pancreatitis after cardiac surgery. Am J Surg 1976;131: 684–688.
52. Salem PR, Williams G, Blumgart LH. Acute pancreatitis following renal transplantation. Dig Surg 1985;2:126–130.
53. Foulis AK, Farquharson MA, Sale GE. The pancreas in acute graft versus host disease in man. Histopathology 1989;14:121–128.
54. Haverbood BI, et al. Trypsin, trypsinogen and trypsin inhibitor in human pancreatic juice; mechanism for pancreatitis associated with hyperparathyroidism. Am J Med 1960;29:424.
55. Day DL, Carpenter BLM. Abdominal complications in pediatric bone marrow transplant recipients. Radiographics 1993;13:1101–1112.
56. Mittal VK, Toledo-Pereyra LH, Prough D, Frantzis P. Effect of graft pancreatitis on the outcome of whole pancreatic transplants. Transplant Proc 1989;21:2856–2857.
57. Stratta RJ, Sollinger HW, Groshek M, et al. Differential diagnosis of hyperamylasemia in pancreas allograft recipients. Transplant Proc 1990;22:675–677.
58. Reinholt FP, Tyden G, Bohman S-O, Brattstrom C, Groth CG. Pancreatic juice cytology in the diagnosis of pancreatic graft rejection. Clin Transplant 1988;2:127–133.
59. Kubota K, Reinholt FP, Tyden G, Bohman S-O, Groth CG. Cytologic patterns in juice from human pancreatic transplants: correlation with histologic findings in the graft. Surgery 1991;109:507–514.
60. Kubota K, Noie T, Itoh T, Idezuki Y. Pancreatic juice cytology can diagnose both rejection and pancreatitis. Transplant Proc 1992; 24:924.
61. Kubota K, Reinholt FP, Tyden G, Groth CG. Pancreatic juice cytology in monitoring pancreatic grafts in the early postoperative period. Transplant Int 1992;5:133–138.
62. Corry RJ. University of Iowa experience in pancreatic transplantation. Transplant Proc 1987;19(suppl 4):37–39.
63. Radio SJ, Stratta RJ, Taylor RJ, Linder J. The utility of urine cytology in the diagnosis of allograft rejection after combined pancreas-kidney transplantation. Transplantation 1993;55:509–516.
64. Patel B, Markivee CR, Mahanta B, Vas W, George E, Garvin P. Pancreatic transplantation: scintigraphy, US, and CT. Radiology 1988;167:685–687.
65. van der Hem LG, van der Linden, Ticheler CHJM, Hoitsma AJ, Corstens FHM. Early detection of post-transplant pancreatic graft dysfunction with technetium-99m-HMPAO scintigraphy. J Nucl Med 1994;35:1488–1490.
66. Busing M, Hopt UT, Quacken M, Becker HD, Morgenroth K. Morphological studies of graft pancreatitis following pancreas transplantation. Br J Surg 1993;80:1170–1173.
67. Backman L, Brattstrom C, Reinholt FP, Andersson J, Tyden G. Development of intrapancreatic abscess—a consequence of CMV pancreatitis? Transplant Int 1991;4:116–121.
68. Linder R, Tyden G, Tibell A, Groth CG. Late graft pancreatitis. Transplantation 1990;50:257–261.

# 28

# *Acute Necrotizing Pancreatitis*

John M. Howard

## Historical Notes

In 1835, J. J. Bigsby, M.D., S.L.S., "Senior Physician to the Newark Dispensary" in a cumulative review on diseases of the pancreas (1) quoted Portal in what may have been an early description of peripancreatic necrosis: "Steatoma . . . in examining the body of a man 40 years old, M. Portal . . . discovered the pancreas . . . had a coating of a consistency of suet, about half an inch thick." Bigsby continues, "in large purulent deposits, the matter is commonly inodorous and creamy. Portal has collected two pounds of it from one sac . . . Bartholin found it very fetid, but the abscess opened into the intestines. Gendrin once saw a vast sac full of grayish very fetid pus, formed in the situation of the pancreas, and in communication with the jejunum, which was perforated at its origin to the extent of an inch." A half century later (1886), Nicholas Senn, a Swiss emigre, later to be professor of surgery at Rush Medical College, proposed that "timely removal of the necrosed (pancreas) . . . would add to the chances of recovery" (2, 3).

Reginald Fitz (4) studied hemorrhagic pancreatitis from patients who died suddenly. He compiled a series from the literature of 17 cases of pancreatic hemorrhage and inflammation that he deemed hemorrhagic pancreatitis and emphasized that sudden death from hemorrhagic pancreatitis was characteristic of the patients; collapse was noted in 13 of the 17 patients, usually between the second and fourth day of the disease. Eleven of the patients died between the second and fourth day of illness. To quote him, "The hemorrhagic infiltration may be found beyond the pancreas, both in the parapancreatic tissue, mesentery, meso-colon, and in the omentum. It may extend downward behind the descending colon, nearly to Poupart's ligament, and may be found at the outer border of the left kidney." These were autopsy findings made early in the course of the disease.

A century later, surgeons performing delayed necrosectomy for massive pancreatitis and peripancreatic necrosis sometimes thought that they had performed a "gloved hand total or near total pancreatectomy" (5, 6) until the author demonstrated that follow-up endoscopic retrograde cholangiography (ERCP) often revealed a normal pancreatogram (7), the necrosis being predominantly massive retroperitoneal necrosis of adipose tissue.

## Definition of Terms

The term acute necrotizing pancreatitis, as currently used (and as used throughout this chapter), includes, but may not be limited to, those conditions earlier described as acute hemorrhagic pancreatitis. Today, early death is largely prevented, and the findings are those described at operations at a later stage of the disease. The gross findings may have changed from those typically noted at laparotomy 50 years ago, when "fat necrosis" was described as superficial white plaques of necrosis on peritoneal surfaces on and around the pancreas. Such observations obviously are still made and the term "fat necrosis" still applies to these lesions, but "necrotizing pancreatitis," currently delineates a more massive necrosis of tissue, predominantly adipose tissue, associated with life-threatening pancreatitis.

Necrosis means gangrene, irreversible death of tissue, whether digested or not. At present, there may be confusion in the use of this term, when hypoperfusion of areas of the pancreas, noted on enhanced computed tomography (CT) perfusion scans, is often interpreted as "necrosis"—gangrene and death of the pancreas. This interpretation may prove valid but a cautionary note is suggested. The author uses the term chiefly to describe the necrosis (gangrene) of peripancreatic tissues, primarily adipose tissue, which is associated with severe acute pancreatitis. The term also describes the pancreas with parenchymal spots of necrosis (gangrene) scattered on its surface and superficially involving its parenchyma but only occasionally involving gangrene of the overall pancreas or of major segments of the gland. In this latter observation, there is presently a lack of clarity.

The term "necrotizing pancreatitis" does not include acute pancreatitis in which necrosis is marked macroscopically only by spots of white fat necrosis on peritoneal surfaces.

Phlegmon is an ill-defined term, used predominantly by radiologists in the interpretation of CT scans. It implies a CT picture of a diffuse inflammatory process, edema without fluid collections. Most surgeons prefer to avoid the term as lacking specificity.

Acute postoperative pancreatitis has been largely excluded from discussion about initial management because the multiple problems associated specifically with the "prepancreatitis" causative operation, sometimes involving errors of technique or diagnosis, make it difficult to define principles of management in this important but diverse group of patients.

The terms *debridement* and *necrosectomy* have been used almost interchangeably and refer to the removal of dead tissue only, not tissue of questionable viability. The term "pancreatic necrosectomy" refers chiefly to the removal of dead tissue that is around or near the pancreas rather than to the removal of dead pancreas, per se. A few authors use the term debridement when referring to sharp resection of pancreatic tissue of questionable viability, and a few others use the term debridement when referring to formal pancreatic resection. In general, however, the term debridement, like necrosectomy, is used to denote the removal of the dead, sequestrating tissue.

## Considerations in Initial Management

It is generally agreed that *no* significant pancreatic or retroperitoneal necrosis occurs in approximately 80–85% of patients with acute pancreatitis and that, in general, these patients should be treated by supportive therapy alone. The exception may be the management of the patient with a stone in the common bile duct, in which many recommend urgent imaging of the biliary system followed by laparoscopic cholecystectomy and appropriate exploration of the common bile duct. Others recommend emergency endoscopic sphincterotomy and retrieval of stones in the common bile duct (see Chapter 22). A third, traditional option, practiced by the author, is ultrasound and CT imaging of the biliary tract followed by open biliary tract operation a few days after the acute inflammation has subsided. The experience in patients with acute gallstone pancreatitis presenting with severe peripancreatic necrosis has not been adequately evaluated to permit confident recommendations (8). To reiterate, there is agreement that most *patients with severe acute pancreatitis and peripancreatic necrosis* should be initially managed by supportive therapy. The mortality rate for the patient without necrosis approaches zero.

Inadequate consideration may have been given to the possibility of prevention of necrosis following the onset of an attack of acute pancreatitis. The time of onset of necrosis after onset of acute pancreatitis has not been clearly established. Isenmann et al. (9), using contrast-enhanced CT scan and elevated serum C-reactive protein levels as the primary indices for diagnosis of pancreatic necrosis, noted that necrosis occurred within 4 days of onset of acute pancreatitis, sometimes within the first few hours. Also unknown is whether the necrosis is completed within a period of hours after it begins or whether it continues over days or weeks. Finally, the relative role of toxic necrotizing products of pancreatic origin versus that of secondary ischemia as the cause of necrosis in selected instances continues to be debated.

It would appear that maintenance or early restoration of capillary perfusion in and around the pancreas might minimize or prevent the progression of inflammation to necrosis and gangrene. The possible effect of low-dose dopamine or sympathetic nerve (celiac ganglia) blockade on enhancement of pancreatic capillary flow and prevention of necrosis has apparently not been documented.

In a few patients, such as those with pancreatitis secondary to ERCP, bacterial contamination may be present at the onset of pancreatitis, and immediate administration of antibiotics might ameliorate or prevent necrosis of tissue. Emergency endoscopic sphincterotomy and extraction of ampullary gallstones have been suggested as possible means of interrupting the progression from inflammation to necrosis. Endoscopic decompressive stenting of the pancreatic duct might find a place in therapy (8, 10), paralleling the role of cholecystostomy in the interruption of the progression of acute cholecystitis to gangrene of the gallbladder. Regional intraarterial administration of the protease inhibitor *nafamostat mesilate* and the antibiotic *imipenem* has been evaluated, but not specifically in its role in interrupting the progression from inflammation to necrosis (11). Although there have been attempts to interrupt the progression of necrosis by the administration of antiproteases, others have indicated that fat necrosis results from the action of lipase and colipase (12, 13). The background studies have been based largely on the enzymatic effects on dead tissues with limited evidence that they are destructive to living cells. At a practical level, few patients have been recognized as presenting without evidence of necrosis in whom necrosis subsequently evolves under clinical observation. In the author's experience, with an occasional exception, patients with necrosis essentially all had necrosis at, or soon after, the time of hospital admission.

In most instances, the pancreatic/peripancreatic necrosis is initially sterile; the incidence of secondary infection rises during the second and third weeks after onset (14). In one study (15), approximately 40% became contaminated within the first week. Madry and Fromm (16) observed infection in all their patients, most of whom were operated upon late in the course of retroperitoneal necrosis. Although not of proven value, most surgeons have used intravenous antibiotic therapy following the onset of acute pancreatitis during the initial phase of therapy (17).

Four observations appear to the author to emerge as facts: *(a)* necrotic tissue predisposes to infection; *(b)* sterile necrotic pancreatic or peripancreatic tissue is usually toxic, although to varying degrees and not always clinically obvious; *(c)* the presence or absence of necrosis is not always detectable prior to operation; and *(d)* necrosis of the pancreas, per se, is not always clearly detectable, even at laparotomy (18).

Various scoring systems, used to "semiquantitate" degrees of severity, often fail to parallel bedside and radiologic observations. The study by Balthazar et al. (19), based on CT findings, has proved of greatest help in assessing the patient with necrotizing pancreatitis. Necrosis is proof of severity. Secondary factors of prognostic importance appear to include the biologic age of the patient, the overall extent of tissue necrosis as revealed by CT (Figs. 28.1, 28.2, *A* and *B*), and whether or not the necrotic tissue is infected. Factors of probable importance include the presence of necrosis of the pancreas per se, the degree of obesity of the patient, and a history of cigarette smoking. Possibly of great importance is whether or not the patient has undergone initial laparotomy prior to transfer for definitive therapy.

The most widely accepted modality for preoperative detection of necrosis of the pancreas has been contrast-enhanced CT. While valuable for detecting necrosis in the pancreas, it has not proved uniformly reliable in delineating necrosis outside the pancreas. Necrotic tissue outside the pancreas is usually associated with large fluid collections, which may mask large volumes of necrotic adipose tissue in the retroperitoneum. Although contrast-enhanced CT was introduced by Mödder et al. (20) and Isikoff et al. (21) in 1981, the first systemic study of the detection of necrosis by contrast-enhanced CT was published by Kivisaari et al. (22), who found that in nine patients with fulminant acute pancreatitis, the pancreas failed to enhance following a rapid intravenous bolus injection of contrast followed by rapid CT exposures. Laparotomy was interpreted as showing evidence of pancreatic necrosis in each instance. Other studies followed. Studies at Ulm (23) noted the effectiveness of the method in demonstrating tissue perfusion of the pancreas and related the

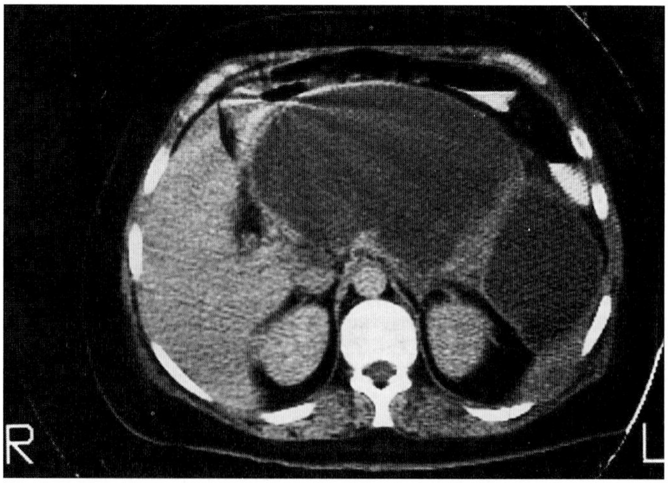


**FIG. 28.1.** CT scan reveals a massive fluid collection masking a large mass of peripancreatic necrotic tissue. The scan was taken 32 days after onset of acute gallstone pancreatitis. (Reproduced from Howard JM. Delayed debridement and external drainage of massive pancreatic or peripancreatic necrosis. Surg Gynecol Obstet 1989;168:25–29, by permission of Franklin H. Martin Foundation.)

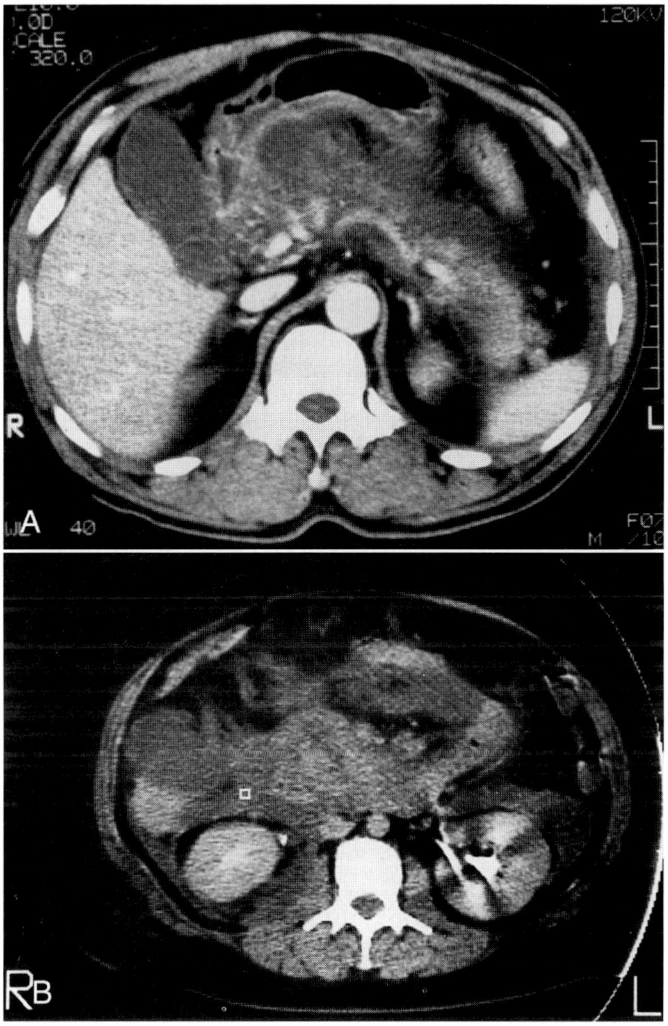

**FIG. 28.2. A.** Contrast-enhanced CT shows massive acute pancreatitis with hypoperfusion of most of the pancras. Dr. Takeda and colleagues have shown that selective arteriography of the pancreatic vessels in patients with massive necrosis, as indicated on contrast-enhanced CT, reveals patency of the major pancreatic arteries and often a mottled parenchymal blush from the contrast perfusion. This suggests that the pancreas might remain viable in spite of hypoperfusion. (Photo courtesy of Dr. Kazunori Takeda and Professor Matsuno of Tohoku University, from Takeda K, Matsuno S, Sunamura M, Kakergawa Y. Continuous regional arterial infusion of protease inhibitor and antibiotics in acute necrotizing pancreatitis. Am J Surg 1996;171:394–398.) **B.** CT shows massive peripancreatic and retroperitoneal necrosis.

anatomic areas of hypoperfusion of the pancreas to the anatomic extent of necrosis. Thus, the extent of "necrosis" was staged, varying from 0 to 100% of the pancreas.

Although the method clearly demonstrates areas of diminished perfusion by the failure to enhance, the findings may have been erroneously interpreted in some patients as reflecting gangrene or death of major segments of the pancreas. This has led to a high incidence of false-positive results when the latter interpretation has been made. By the same technique, pancreatic adenocarcinoma may show relative hypoperfusion yet not be necrotic. Nevertheless, the study is useful as an adjunct to the demonstration of severity. It has not, in the author's opinion, provided a basis for surgical intervention. Indeed, gangrene of 50–100% of the pancreas is a rarity.

Bradley et al. (24) concluded that dynamic pancreatography offers prognostic information and provides a safe and reliable technique for predicting the presence or absence of pancreatic parenchymal necrosis. In discussing the above presentation, Trede (25) noted that malperfusion of the pancreas had been documented in several patients who were subsequently well on their way to recovery. Few, if any investigators, including Bradley (24), would subject a patient to operation on the basis of dynamic pancreatography alone.

Several investigators (26, 27) have observed that an elevated serum C-reactive protein level indicates pancreatic necrosis and is useful in monitoring such patients.

## Pathology of Acute Necrotizing Pancreatitis

The following observations are intended as a progress report of the field. It is written from the viewpoint of surgical management and is not intended to detail the complete field of scientific investigation.

**Necrosis of the Pancreas.** The distinction between "pancreatic necrosis" and a viable pancreas is usually indeterminate, even at the time of early laparotomy. In a 1985 clinical pathologic study of 46 patients who underwent pancreatic resection for acute necrotizing pancreatitis, Nordback et al. (18) noted "the macroscopic appearance correlated poorly with its histology." Each pancreas when inspected at operation was considered totally or subtotally necrotic. In the resected pancreas, however, parenchymal necrosis varied from 0% to 100% of the gland. The authors concluded "in contrast to our previous tactics we think that resection should be limited to extreme cases in order to avoid resection of glands with limited necrosis and thus mainly reversible parenchymal damage." In 5 of their 46 patients (11%), there was no histologic evidence of parenchymal necrosis, and few showed as much necrosis as was anticipated. In a subsequent report, Nordbeck and Lauslaht (28) described another (overlapping) series of patients who were deemed at laparotomy to have extensive pancreatic necrosis and who underwent pancreatic resection. Postoperative study of 8 of the resected pancreases showed no parenchymal necrosis; three of the 8 patients died postoperatively. Fagniez, Rotman, and Kracht (29), in operations on 39 patients, noted that parenchymal necrosis was localized in the periphery of the gland in most patients, leaving a central healthy portion. Only one patient had necrosis of the entire head of the gland. Based on the appearance of "pancreatic necrosis" at laparotomy, Leger et al. (1977) (30) resected the pancreas in seven patients and demonstrated that "acute necrosis" begins at the periphery of the pancreas and may be extremely superficial. Thus, even biopsy of the pancreas at the time of operation may lead to erroneous interpretation of the severity of necrosis.

Complete liquefaction necrosis of the pancreas or any significant portion of it has seldom, if ever, been observed by the author at the primary operation. In one patient, the pancreas at the time of primary debridement, 2 to 3 weeks after onset, appeared absolutely black throughout its visible surface. The author misinterpreted this as gangrene, but on superficial debridement, the pancreas bled and its debridement was aborted. With open packing and repetitive explorations the surface of the pancreas turned pink, and it became obvious that it was anatomically intact.

Necrosis of the pancreas is often overestimated by the surgeon; the necrosis can be superficial or spotty and may only occasionally lead to gangrene of major segments of the organ itself.

**Peripancreatic Necrosis.** The findings at delayed operation vary significantly from patient to patient. The necrotic peripancreatic tissue, as observed at delayed operation, approximately 3 to 4 weeks after onset, appears to reflect three different processes, or patterns, any one of which may predominate in an individual patient:

1. Digestion of adipose tissue, presumably secondary to the escape of enzymes or other toxins of pancreatic origin; this is the most frequent pattern observed
2. Persistent hematomas, nonorganized and not liquefied
3. Ischemic, undigested blocks of adipose tissue

The three patterns may have different, although interwoven, natural histories. The secondary development of infection further alters the appearance of the dead tissue; adding a fourth dimension to the evolution of the "local lesion." The volume of necrotic tissue may range from a few grams to several kilograms.

In almost all patients, there is a peripancreatic collection of fluid. In the author's experience this has varied from 300 to 6000 mL (5). The fluid may sometimes appear flocculent, containing suspended bits of dead tissue. Sometimes the fluid has a dilute bloody appearance. In association with a gram-negative bacterial infection, it may be obviously purulent or have a thin, blackish appearance. At times, the fluid may appear obviously purulent, yet may or may not be infected (Fig. 28.3).

In most patients, the necrotic tissue appears "puttylike," also described as "wet peat moss" or "canned dog food" in appearance (Figs. 28.4 and 28.5). It apparently is digested adipose tissue. This "puttylike" necrotic material tends to radiate like the spokes of a wheel from its hub at the pancreas. These "spokes" or "veins" of necrotic tissue may extend like the fingers of the hand in many directions: behind the duodenum toward the right kidney, upward behind the gallbladder, behind the stomach and up to the diaphragm, behind the splenic flexure of the colon, around the spleen and up to the diaphragm, behind the transverse colon and down toward the left kidney, into the mesenteries of the transverse colon and small intestine, retroperitoneally down to the pelvis or behind the right colon and over the right kidney. Seldom does the necrosis extend anterior to the stomach or anterior to the liver, and it seldom extends intraperitoneally to a comparable extent. Gangrene of the omentum, if it exists except for superficial spots of "fat necrosis," is unusual.

At the time of delayed operation, 2 weeks or more after onset, demarcation between dead and viable tissue is relatively clear-cut. The "puttylike" necrotic material is minimally cohesive. The dead, digested tissue, when picked up with forceps, comes out in small "broken" pieces, sometimes only a cubic centimeter or less in size. By such mechanisms of debridement, one may find it difficult or impossible to cleanse all the "nooks and crannies" of the necrotic tissue, as the dead tissue is insufficiently cohesive. When pulled at its apparent point of origin near the pancreas, the necrotic tissue does not come out completely like a shrimp from its shell.

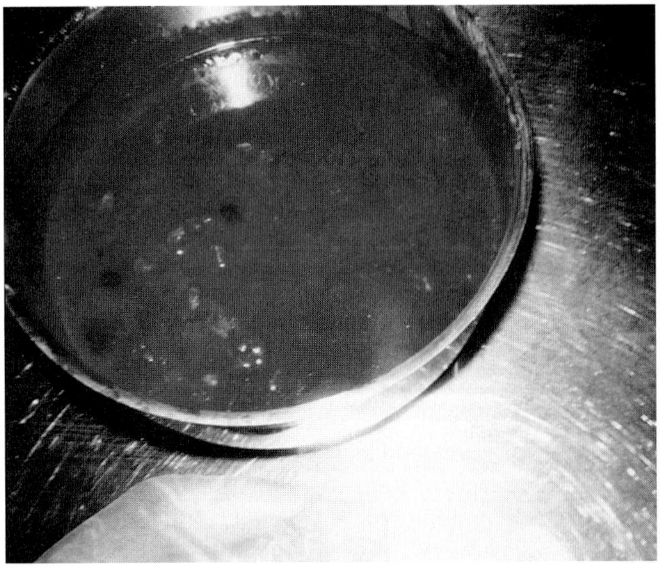

**FIG. 28.3.** Liquefied sterile peripancreatic necrotic tissue drained at the initial debridement. See color insert.

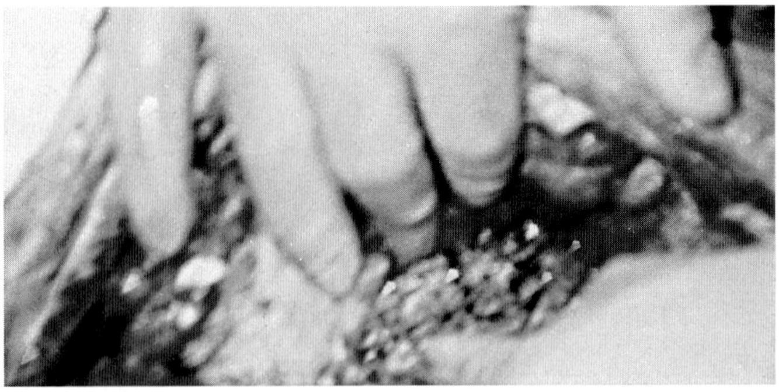

**FIG. 28.4.** Operative photograph of necrotic, digested tissue beneath gastrocolic omentum. Variations of this type of necrotic tissue have been described as "canned dog meat" or "wet peat moss" in appearance. See color insert.

In a minority of patients, the dead tissue appears to be the residue of large hematomas. Several weeks after onset of the disease, an occasional sequestrum will be found that is formed, soft, and black, suggesting a nonliquified, nonorganized hematoma (Fig. 28.6).

In some patients, the dead tissue, particularly in the paraspinal areas, is ischemic, with the appearance of suet and can be removed in blocks (Fig. 28.7), undigested and without blood supply. Whatever the gross appearance of the dead tissue, the pathologist can only describe the specimen as "necrotic tissue."

Occasionally, the necrotic tissue is rather well loculated in a single cavity, like dead tissue in an evolving pseudocyst, so that the edges of the cavity are rather well demarcated and nonradiating. Under these circumstances, debridement may appear essentially complete at the initial exploration.

Glazer and Dudley (31) delineated three separate forms of pancreatic infections: *(a)* secondary infection of peripancreatic necrotic tissue, *(b)* infection of a pseudocyst, and *(c)* pancreatic abscess. Infection of a well-formed pseudocyst is rare. It permits easy external drainage and results today in a low mortality rate. Pancreatic abscess is a walled-off purulent collection, often a complication of postoperative pancreatitis, with a higher incidence of staphylococcal infections. Pancreatic abscess is relatively rare and, within the context of this definition, has historically resulted in a lower mortality rate than infected peripancreatic necrotic tissue. It may, however, result in a higher incidence of pancreatic fistula (32).

### Pathology of the Colon

As with the pancreas, the associated inflammation of the transverse colon has often been erroneously interpreted as gangrene when the inflammation was mainly a pericolitis with superficial necrosis but with a viable viscus. As with the pancreas, however, areas of gangrene of the colon may occasionally result. In addition to the acute inflammation and necrosis of the transverse colon, subsequent iatrogenic damage to the colon may result from erosion by firm drains.

### Microbiology of Infected Pancreatic Necrosis

Now that we can effectively treat the hemodynamic instability resulting from severe necrotizing pancreatitis, infection has become the major threat. Infection is seldom a primary factor; instead, it results from secondary invasion of the preexisting necrotic tissue. Farthmann et al. (33) noted that 30–88% of patients with sterile necrosis subsequently developed secondary infection. They concluded that the incidence of secondary infection of peripancreatic necrotic tissue increases with time, particularly among those patients lacking evidence of significant improvement. In this author's experience, 23 (32%) of 71 patients undergoing initial necrosectomy had positive peripancreatic cultures: 21 with gram-negative bacilli and 2 with *Streptococcus faecalis* (34).

In a prospective study of 114 patients, diagnosed on the basis of contrast-enhanced CT studies as having acute pancreatic necrosis, Beger et al. (15) found at the initial laparotomy that 45 (31%) were infected. Some 39 (87%) of the infected (necrotic tissue) cultures revealed a single strain of organism; only six patients harbored a mixed flora. Most cultures revealed gram-negative bacilli (Table 28.1). The high incidence of infection by gram-negative bacilli is a common finding. Pederzoli et al. (35), in a study of 93 patients, found comparable results except that they found *Staphylococcus aureus* in 14%. Warshaw and Jin (32), in writing of pancreatic abscesses, but related partially to infected peripancreatic necrosis, found *S. aureus* in 35% of 45 infections.

In the aforementioned study by Beger et al. (15), the effect of infection on patient outcome was striking. Of the 45 patients with infection, 17 died (38%) and 8 (18%) developed gastrointestinal bleeding. Among the 69 patients whose original cultures were negative, 6 patients (8.7%) died; 4 (6%) experienced gastrointestinal bleeding.

Although infection is often not present at an initial necrosectomy, bacterial contamination universally results from necrosectomy and open drainage and often follows necrosectomy and closed (lavage) drainage. Bassi et al. (36) demonstrated that pancreatic juice has an inherent antibacterial influence.

**Studies of Translocation of Intestinal Flora to Infect Peripancreatic Necrotic Tissue.** What is the source of the secondary infection of the sterile peripancreatic necrotic tissue? In 1993, Gianotti et al. (37) studied the effect of experimental acute pancreatitis on the translocation of bacteria from the intestinal tract of the rat. Compared with appropriate controls, animals with induced acute pancreatitis developed increased numbers of *Escherichia coli* and, to a lesser extent, enterococci and *Klebsiella* spp. in intraperitoneal organs, including the pancreas. An early *E. coli* bacteremia was observed. The authors concluded that their data were consistent with the hypothesis that acute pancreatitis increased the permeability of the animal's intestine to bacteria and facilitated translocation of bacteria from the gastrointestinal tract. They suggested that the blood, peritoneal fluid, and mesenteric lymphatics might be the principal routes for bacterial spread from the intestinal lumen.

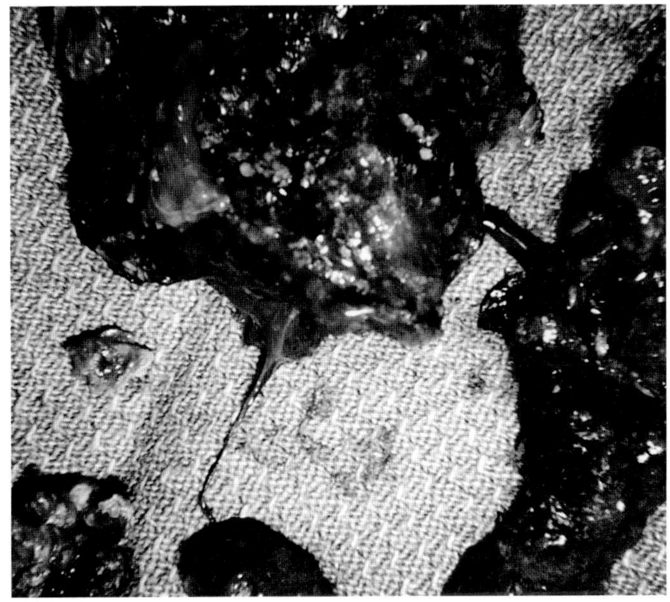

**FIG. 28.6.** Necrotic peripancreatic necrotic tissue removed 19 days after onset of pancreatitis. Appearance suggests old hematoma. See color insert.

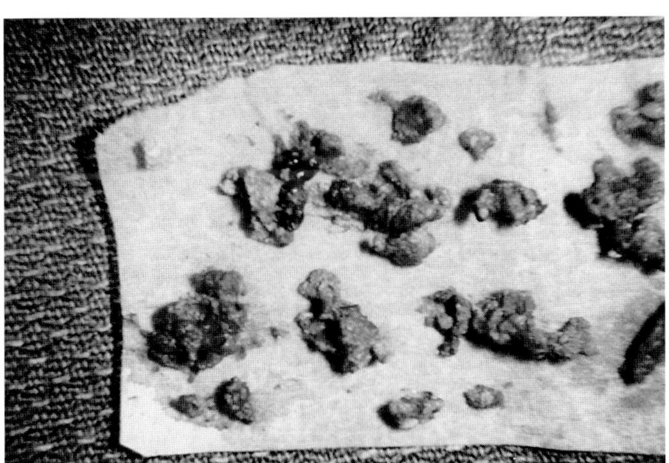

**FIG. 28.5.** Digested peripancreatic necrotic tissue removed at initial debridement. See color insert.

In 1995, Luiten et al. (38) reported a randomized, controlled, multicenter study of 102 patients with objective evidence of severe acute pancreatitis, to evaluate whether selective decontamination of the intestinal lumen might result in a reduced mortality rate. The patients were randomly divided into a control group of 52 patients who received standard treatment and 50 patients who received selective intestinal decontamination with norfloxacin, colistin, and amphotericin. The treatment group received the antibiotics repetitively, orally and by enema. In addition, they received applications of a paste containing the antibiotics in a 2% concentration, along the gums every 6 hours. The duration of antibiotic therapy apparently depended upon the patient's progress. In addition, the "decontamination" group received short-term systemic prophylaxis with cefotaxime sodium until gram-negative bacteria were eliminated from the oral cavity and rectum. There were 18 deaths in the control group (35%) and 11 deaths (22%) in the selective decontamination group. The difference in mortality was related predominantly to a reduction in the late mortality (after 2 weeks) because of a significant reduction in gram-negative pancreatic infections. Secondary pancreatic infections occurred in 20 patients (38%) in the control group and in 9 patients (18%) in the decontamination group. Gram-negative pancreatic infection occurred in 17 patients (33%) in the control group and only 4 patients (8%) in the decontamination group. The differences were statistically highly significant. The authors concluded that reduction of the intestinal flora reduced the incidence of pancreatic infections and significantly reduced the mortality and morbidity resulting from acute necrotizing pancreatitis. If confirmed, these observations may provide an additional avenue of support for these critically ill patients.

### Failure of Earlier Operative Approaches

Three operative approaches have been evaluated and abandoned. Formal planned *pancreatectomy*, a direct approach to the problem, was evaluated by numerous investigators (18, 30,

39–42). Two conclusions were reached: *(a)* the resulting mortality was unacceptably high, 42–60% in a cumulative review (43), and *(b)* neither preoperative studies (at the times of study) nor macroscopic examination of the pancreas at laparotomy could determine the severity of the pancreatic necrosis. Study of the resected pancreas sometimes revealed essentially no histologic evidence of necrosis; in others the necrosis was extremely superficial. The observers could not reliably determine the extent of necrosis and thus the possible need for resection in many patients until *after* the pancreas had been removed.

A second therapeutic approach that was evaluated is percutaneous peritoneal lavage (44). The method proved ineffective, in part because severe necrotizing pancreatitis is associated predominantly with retroperitoneal necrosis. In addition, intraabdominal tissues that undergo necrosis and infection may rapidly become sealed off from the free peritoneal cavity.

A third operative approach that was evaluated is drainage of infected, toxic fluid and peripancreatic necrosis via the insertion of drainage catheters (45). The method does not permit adequate drainage of multiloculated collections nor the masses of necrotic tissue that are too large to be removed by such means; conversion to operative debridement was required in approximately 85% of patients (45).

**TABLE 28.1. Organisms Infecting Necrotizing Pancreatitis in 45 Patients at the Initial Necrosectomy**

| Organism | |
|---|---|
| Gram-negative aerobic | |
| *Escherichia coli* | 24 |
| *Enterobacter aerogenes* | 16 |
| *Pseudomonas aeruginosa* | 5 |
| *Proteus* spp. | 5 |
| *Klebsiella pneumoniae* | 3 |
| *Citrobacter freundii* | 1 |
| Gram negative anaerobic | |
| *Bacteroides* spp. | 5 |
| Gram positive aerobic | |
| *Streptococcus faecalis* | 6 |
| *Staphylococcus aureus* | 4 |
| *Streptococcus viridans* | 1 |
| *Staphylococcus epidermis* | 1 |
| Other organisms | |
| *Mycobacterium tuberculosis* | 1 |
| *Candida* spp. | 3 |

Adapted from Beger HG, Bittner R, Block S, Büchler M. Bacterial contamination of pancreatic necrosis. A prospective clinical study. Gastroenterology 1986;91:433–438.

## NECROSECTOMY

Necrosectomy—or debridement—refers to the removal of dead tissue (and its surrounding fluid) in the peripancreatic area. The tissue surrounding the pancreas makes up most of the mass of dead tissue, and it is largely this tissue that is debrided. The pancreas, per se, is infrequently debrided. Indeed, Smadja and Bismuth (39), in their report of a 42% mortality rate following their early efforts at "debridement" of the pancreas (involving pancreatic resection), noted that in each instance the tissues removed were sterile at the time of initial early debridement, although 14 of the 38 patients subsequently developed secondary infection of residual necrotic tissue. Referring to the fact that they had sometimes resected viable pancreas and had experienced a high mortality rate, the authors concluded "therefore, it is reasonable to suggest that pancreatic debridement probably has limited indications." This author agrees with that conclusion.

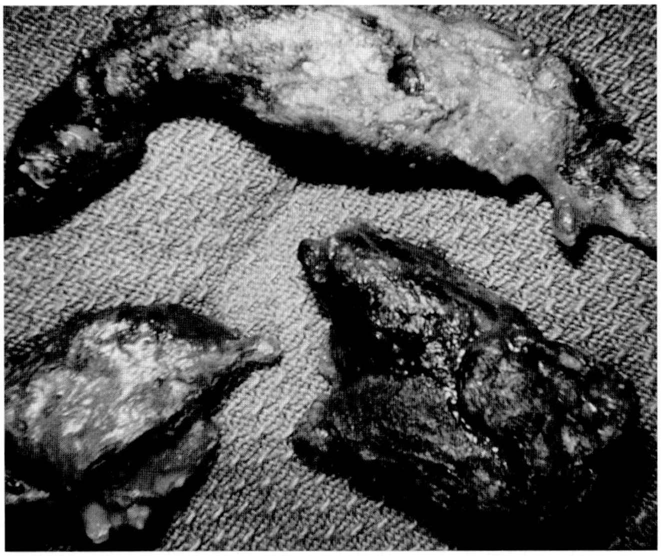

**FIG. 28.7.** Necrotic, nondigested paravertebral adipose tissue, "the suet syndrome." Appearance suggests ischemic necrosis. See color insert.

Debridement of the pancreas, per se, by sharp dissection or resection has limited indications.

### Basis and Timing of Necrosectomy

The foundation on which necrosectomy and drainage rests is that the removal of infected or noninfected dead tissue with drainage of its surrounding toxic fluid is characteristically followed by clinical improvement, including improvement in the depressed functions of the kidneys, liver, lungs, and intestinal tract as well as improvement in sensorium and sense of well-being. The converse, on which necrosectomy also rests, is that failure to achieve timely and adequate removal of the dead tissue, including drainage, often leads to the death of the patient.

Although numerous points of management require continued refinement, it is well established that severe necrotizing pancreatitis requires operative removal of toxic dead tissue and drainage of the related toxic fluids. Whatever technique is adopted, necrosectomy and drainage are the fundamental principles of treatment, particularly when the necrotic tissue is infected. Characteristically, but not inevitably, noninfected peripancreatic necrotic tissue results in varying degrees of toxicity, and when there are large quantities of necrotic tissue, it must be removed. This generalization may not be true if necrosis of the pancreas, per se, is defined on the basis of hypoperfusion noted by CT imaging; a basis which is not yet fully accepted. The current frontiers are the continuing efforts to define the optimal *timing* for operation and the best *methods* of achieving debridement and drainage. Assuming necrosis to be a continuing process, the local infusion of antiproteases into the necrotic cavities following initial debridement has been suggested (35). Further confirmation is awaited.

After treating the patient for hemodynamic instability, providing nutritional and other appropriate supportive care, and identifying peripancreatic necrotic tissue bathed in fluid, by clinical evaluation and CT scan, what and when are the indications for operative intervention? The answers are not yet completely clear because the natural history, or histories, of the process are not clearly defined. Certainly, continuing sepsis is a clear-cut indication for operation. After excluding certain iatrogenic sources of infection such as an infected central venous catheter and *Clostridia difficile* enteritis, the usual conclusion is that the necrotic tissue has become secondarily infected. Beger

(46) recommends percutaneous aspiration of the fluid bathing the necrotic tissue for Gram staining and bacterial culture. Serial aspiration for bacteriologic study has been suggested, beginning in an early phase of the disease. This author seldom uses this method because the toxic patient with infected or noninfected necrotic tissue requires operative debridement and because percutaneous aspiration, no matter how carefully done, involves the risk of introducing contamination to necrotic tissue. Gas bubbles in the peripancreatic fluid, seen best on CT scans, are a clear indication of infection. A low-grade fever, a white blood cell count as high as 30,000–50,000, and tachycardia are compatible with the toxemia sometimes associated with sterile peripancreatic necrosis, which in itself often becomes an indication for debridement (5, 34). Paralytic ileus, rising serum creatinine and bilirubin levels, deterioration of pulmonary function, and recurrence of hemodynamic instability may precede the recognition of septicemia by positive blood cultures or positive peripancreatic fluid cultures. *Sepsis secondary to infection of peripancreatic necrotic tissue is the universally accepted indication for operative debridement.* Percutaneous drainage is inadequate. This method clearly cannot evacuate large masses of dead tissue.

*A second indication for operation is continuing toxicity in the absence of infection.* As indicated above, dead tissue may be quite toxic, even in the retroperitoneum, and in the absence of infection, removal of the dead tissue may result in significant clinical improvement. In the author's experience, this is the most frequent indication for operation.

The third indication, overlapping with the second, is *the ill-defined "failure to thrive"* or "failure to improve" syndrome, which often merges with, and may sometimes be synonymous with, continuing "toxemia of dead tissue." This syndrome consists essentially of failure to improve during continued supportive care. It is marked by the maintenance of paralytic ileus, inability to eat, and thus continued parenteral feeding; low-grade fever; often a moderate leukocytosis; and persistence of the peripancreatic mass as observed clinically and by serial CT scans. The syndrome may result, in part, from mechanical pressure of the inflammatory mass on the stomach, duodenum, diaphragm, and visceral circulation, as well as from an unrecognized component of toxemia. Beger (46) observed that the continued presence of a tender upper abdominal mass, requiring analgesics; a persistent paralytic ileus; and fever, unremitting after 8–10 days of intensive care provide a strong basis for surgical intervention. This author (JMH) usually persists with nonoperative care for a longer period; only 3 of 71 patients were explored within the first 2 weeks of illness. Optimal timing, however, remains uncertain.

A fourth (unusual) indication is the clinical picture of an *acute abdominal catastrophe*, witnessed by the author in three patients. In two patients, a large peripancreatic fluid collection had ruptured into the generalized peritoneal cavity; the third had an intraabdominal hemorrhage from a delayed erosion of a splenic artery. A fifth indication, not easily defined, may be the occurrence of otherwise unexplained *gastrointestinal hemorrhage*.

Even though the above indications are generally accepted, the optimal timing of operation is not always obvious. As indicated above, the author has pursued a conservative course, usually waiting beyond 2 weeks and often significantly longer in the absence of infection or emergency before recommending operation.

Most investigators have found that in many patients, complete necrosectomy cannot be achieved at a single operation without the operation becoming life threatening. Thus, continued or repetitive debridement is frequently necessary. Since the surgeon is seldom certain that debridement has been complete, postoperative drainage is necessary and has become a standard facet of operative management.

Studies to date have led to the conclusion that initial nonoperative supportive care of the patient with life-threatening acute pancreatitis results in the lowest mortality rates. This approach, however, requires that operative debridement and drainage be available when necrosis results in continuing disability and a threat to the patient's life. Optimal care provides that the patient be in a tertiary care hospital under the care of the surgeon who is responsible for making and implementing the decisions for operation. This then is the current overall plan of management.

## OPERATION

Since the nature and extent of necrosis cannot always be predicted prior to operation, the technique of necrosectomy and drainage can not be defined prior to operation. Thus, a single protocol can hardly be used for operative management of such patients. The operative philosophy must be to achieve debridement and drainage in the simplest and safest manner compatible with removal of all of the dead tissue and drainage of infection, exudate, and secretion.

The application of the above principles has led to diverse techniques:

1. Necrosectomy and open packing of the wound with the intent of planned reoperations for secondary debridement and drainage
2. Operative necrosectomy followed by insertion of irrigating catheters for continued rinsing and drainage of the necrotic areas
3. Combinations and modifications of the above two methods

Although no single approach consistently provides effective treatment of the patient with severe necrosis, operative debridement with open packing followed by planned, repeated reexploration is the technique most frequently used by the author. Since the surgeon cannot consistently plan the overall operation prior to laparotomy and since open packing remains a likely possibility, *vertical incisions are avoided.*

Operation is performed through a bilateral subcostal incision. Although the greatest mass of necrotic tissue is likely to be in the epigastric and left upper quadrant areas, inspection of the entire area of the pancreas and its adjacent structures is desirable. If areas of necrosis in the lower retroperitoneum or pelvis are demonstrated by CT, their debridement is performed through separate retroperitoneal approaches. *Exploration of the free peritoneal cavity is usually avoided,* a practice with which Poston and Williamson (47) disagree.

At the time of delayed necrosectomy, 2–3 weeks after onset, the stomach, transverse colon, and gastrocolic omentum are usually attached by adhesions to the anterior parietal peritoneum. These are gently separated, but only enough to identify the stomach and transverse colon. The landmarks may be so obscured that the colon and stomach are not easily identified, so care must be taken to avoid perforating either viscus. When identified, the gastrocolic omentum is divided over a short distance to permit entrance into the obliterated lesser peritoneal space. Catgut suture ligatures are used to control small vessels. Fluid collections, whose exact location is not initially obvious, are identified by aspiration with a needle and syringe. The aspirate is used for Gram staining and bacterial culture. As the needle is withdrawn, fluid often exudes from the puncture site. Suction to this site permits its exact identification so that a hemostat can be inserted to widen the tract. This can be further enlarged with the exploring finger. Great volumes of fluid, usually containing bits of necrotic tissue (Fig. 28.8) pour forth. *Great care is required* to avoid tearing a viscus or a major vein. Introduction of the suction catheter into the fluid-filled cavity, irrigation with saline, and gentle blunt dissection permit a gradual increase in exposure of the necrotic debris. Dissection must be gentle and preferably performed by the surgeon only, not

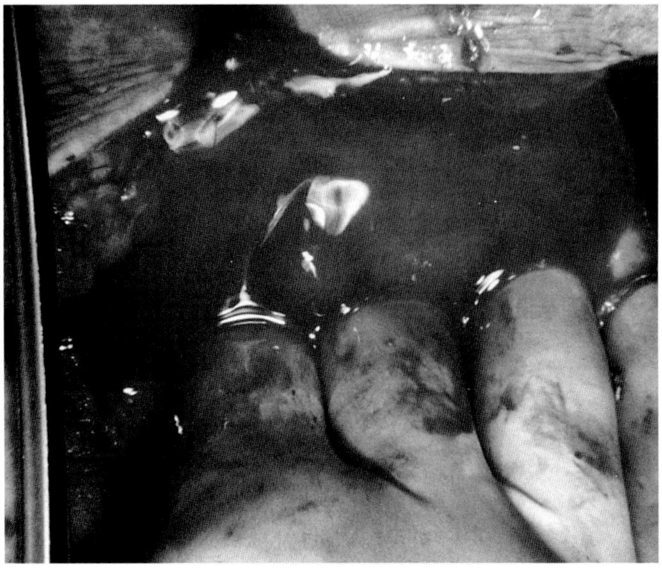

**FIG. 28.8.** Large volumes of purulent fluid often pour forth as the finger enters the peripancreatic collection. Such fluid, although purulent, may be either sterile or infected. See color insert.

by an assistant. Exploration is initially directed between the stomach and the transverse colon. Masses of semidigested necrotic tissue can be picked out of the fluid cavities (Fig. 28.9). Often the pancreas can be clearly identified but, to reiterate, in his earlier experience, this author thought at times that he had achieved a total "gloved-hand" pancreatectomy (5, 6) although subsequent observations by ERCP sometimes revealed an anatomically intact pancreas (7). As the dissection progresses, the transverse colon, still adherent to the anterior parietal peritoneum, is packed inferiorly in an effort to minimize or prevent intraperitoneal contamination. Again, unless specifically indicated, the free peritoneal cavity is *not* explored. The direction of the subsequent dissection is determined by the location of the remaining fluid and necrotic debris. This may be retrogastric, behind the splenic flexure of the colon and around the spleen and, if so, these areas are gently explored with the fingers, "peanuts" on curved clamps, blunt forceps, bulb-syringe irrigation and suction, and subsequently by power spray. Very dilute hydrogen peroxide solution may be used for its mechanical debriding effect. At times, the hidden channels of dead tissue may seem completely debrided, only to have bits of necrotic tissue subsequently removed by further finger probing or exploration with long forceps or irrigation. The ends of these "spokes" of necrotic tissue are often not visualized. In early stages of the disease, the pancreas can be clearly visualized and mobilized along its inferior aspect, where retropancreatic dead tissue may be identified and removed. Similarly, conservative, retrocolic exploration toward the left kidney can be achieved. One of the most difficult areas to debride is the transverse mesocolon. The arteries and veins within the transverse mesocolon may be surrounded by dead, semidigested tissue. In such instances, the branches of the blood vessels prevent a "sweeping" clearance of dead tissue and instead require picking necrotic tissue from between and behind the vascular branches. Hemorrhage from the middle colic vein occurred once in the author's experience and required a hazardous but successful lateral repair.

This approach does not provide good exposure of the mesentery of the small intestine, so debridement has been approached with the finger, from the retroperitoneum into the small bowel mesentery, without direct visualization. Drainage, perhaps more than debridement, has resulted. Although necrosis of adipose tissue of the small bowel mesentery occurs, it is seldom as severe as that found within the transverse mesocolon. If necrosis cephalad to the lesser curvature of the stomach is observed, it can be debrided via a direct approach anteriorly, as well as retrogastrically. One advantage in delaying debridement is that dead tissue will have become clearly demarcated. At this time, little of the necrotic tissue is firmly adherent to adjacent viable tissue. Sharp dissection can be avoided, so bleeding can be minimized. Under these circumstances, the author has not recognized a gangrenous pancreas at operation. Large hematomas (Fig. 28.6) have presented as masses, not as slender sheets of clots following along tissue planes.

Necrotic adipose tissue, particularly in the paravertebral areas, may not always be digested, lending itself to the removal of "blocks of suet" (Fig. 28.7). Such tissue appears ischemic and undigested, which allows more complete necrosectomy than is possible in other areas of necrosis. Since the paravertebral spaces close early in the open-packing sequence, it is helpful to debride the paravertebral spaces as completely as possible at the initial operation.

## Open Packing

When all of the dead tissue identifiable through this conservative exposure has been removed by digital exploration (Fig. 28.10) and manual and power spray irrigation (Fig. 28.11) and no further areas of necrosis are found, such an abdomen (described above) will be packed open. In such instances, the greater omentum at its origin at the transverse colon is superficially sutured to the anterior parietal peritoneum along the inferior lip of the incision. This is done with a continuous 3.0 chromic catgut suture. To prevent evisceration of small bowel, this suture is carried to the patient's far left side. Sometimes the sealing-off of the free peritoneal cavity at the left extent of the wound is incomplete. Consideration is then given to using small interrupted chromic sutures to tack the anterior parietal peritoneum to the serosa of the transverse colon, per se. Obviously this is hazardous; no fistula has resulted to date in the author's experience, but alternative maneuvers such as the use of packs are sought, and packing this small area to retain the small bowel is

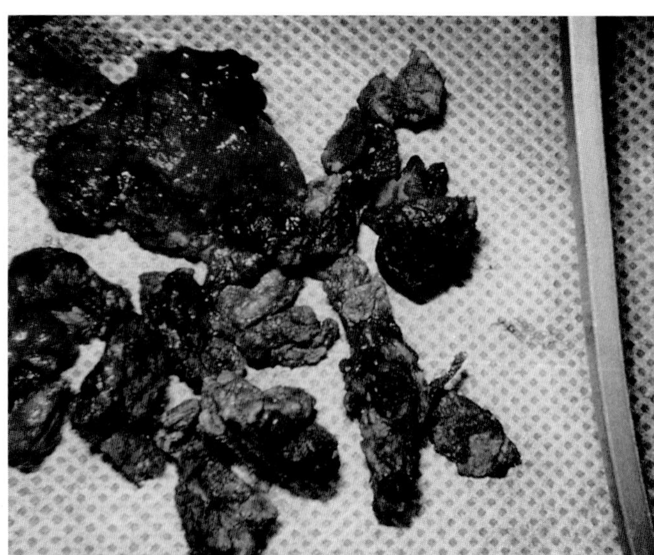

**FIG. 28.9.** Necrotic, semidigested necrotic adipose tissue may be picked out of the necrotic cavities. Such tissue led the author initially to erroneously believe that he had performed a "gloved hand total pancreatectomy." See color insert.

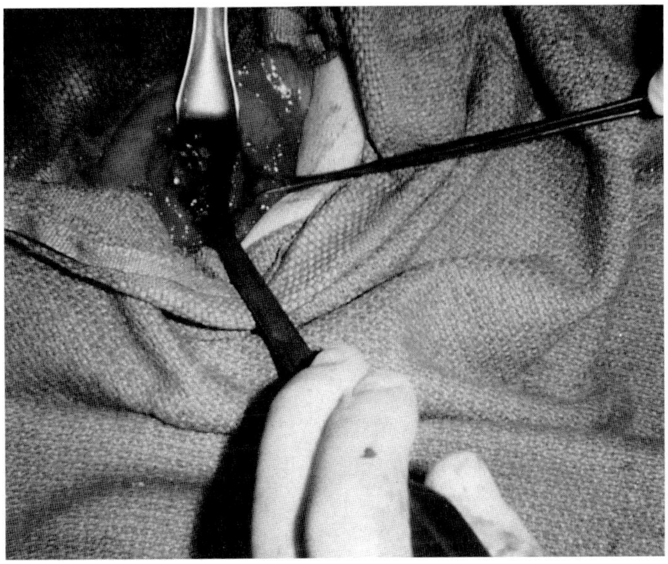

**FIG. 28.10.** Operative photograph of necrotic cavity during initial debridement. The stomach is retracted upward. The pancreas has been only partially visualized. See color insert.

probably safer. Thus the plan has been to exclude the general peritoneal cavity from the upper peritoneal and retroperitoneal spaces.

The wound is now temporarily covered with a sterile adhesive drape. The lower abdomen is reprepared, and the surgical team changes to sterile gowns, gloves, and equipment. A short transverse, left-sided abdominal incision is made for placement of a jejunal feeding tube. A small Foley catheter with a 5-mL bag is characteristically used. The tip of the catheter is amputated to minimize subsequent obstruction secondary to encrustation of feedings. The catheter is inserted through a "stab wound" in the abdominal wall and through a "Witzel tunnel" into the jejunum, the latter being tacked to the anterior parietal peritoneum. This wound is then closed and sealed with an overlying sterile plastic dressing.

Returning then to the open upper abdominal incision, the wound is packed open over Penrose drains and small, relatively soft, red rubber irrigation catheters. Over these drains, 4-inch Kerlex gauze rolls are used to pack the wound. These packs are used to fill each crevice in the depth of the wound, continuing until the wound is filled to or above the level of the skin. Each pack and drain is sutured to the edge of the wound. Large occlusive dressings are placed over the wound and are held firmly in place by two wide Velcro abdominal binders (Fig. 28.12). It is important to place the Velcro binders while the patient is still asleep; otherwise, as the patient retches during awakening, evisceration of the small bowel may result. During retching, the binder, supported by the hands of the surgical team, has prevented small bowel evisceration except in one or two instances, when 6–8 inches of small bowel were found above the left transverse colon at the time of secondary explorations.

The operative packs tend to adhere to the tissues and must be removed at an early time. In removal, they provide an element of superficial debridement that has not led to significant bleeding. Others have recommended covering the surface of the organs with nonadherent dressings. Unless small bowel is exposed in the open wound, the author prefers adherent dressings with the intent that they be changed within 48 hours. Thus, the planned approach is to take the patient back to the operating room at 48-hour intervals, including weekends and holidays, where, under general anesthesia, a formal reexploration of the wound is achieved. All dressings are removed, and the entire sequence of exploration, debridement, and repacking is repeated (Figs. 28.13 and 28.14). The initial packs, even in the presence of wound catheters, prevent adequate drainage over a longer period, even with low-volume saline irrigation of the wound. Thus the packs should be removed at short, planned intervals without waiting for clinical manifestations of infection; once packed open, bacterial contamination of the wound inevitably results. Four or five reexplorations are not infrequent; two patients underwent a total of 16 and 24 debridements, respectively, in the operating room. The serial explorations are continued so long as necrotic tissue or infection persists.

As sequential explorations proceed, the depth of the wound tends to close. The wall of the stomach becomes adherent posteriorly, closing the retrogastric space. The transverse mesocolon adheres to retroperitoneal tissues. As a result, the space between the colon and stomach narrows (Fig. 28.13). Exploration of the retroperitoneum becomes progressively limited to the extent that soft drains and packs cannot fill the retroperitoneal space. This usually coincides, however, with the clearing of infection and devitalized tissue. There may come a time when debridement can be done at the bedside without anesthesia and often without analgesia. In such instances, as noted below, it is sometimes practical to close the abdominal wall secondarily over Penrose and soft irrigating drains. The author usually prefers to let the wounds completely close by contracture and reepithelialization, resulting, however, in a large incisional hernia.

### Secondary Pelvic and Other Approaches

When a CT scan demonstrates a pelvic collection of fluid and necrotic tissue, particularly when the patient is septic, debridement and drainage of this area become essential. Rather than explore the peritoneal cavity, single or bilateral incisions are made along the crest of the ilium, and a retroperitoneal dissection over the iliac vessels is performed. The area is debrided, irrigated, and packed open or left open around drains, to be reexplored as

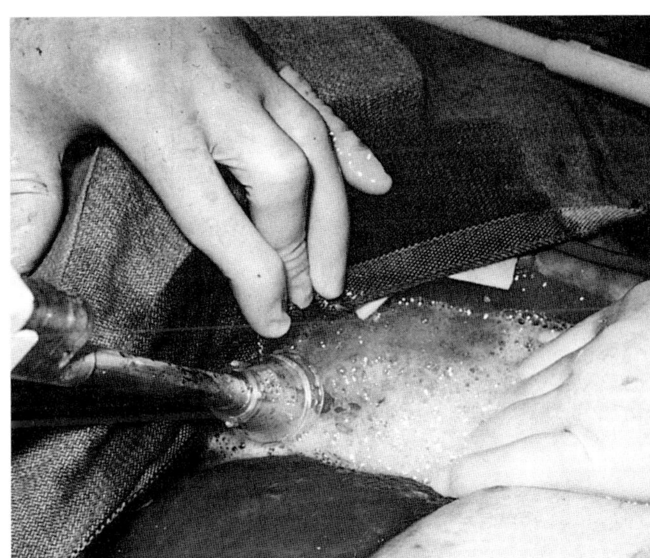

**FIG. 28.11.** The power spray provides a useful adjunct to debridement, but most of the dead tissue has to be "picked out." The spray is used primarily for a final cleansing of the wound at the end of the debridement. Very dilute hydrogen peroxide adds a further element of mechanical debridement. Manual debridement of necrotic tissue, however, is the keystone of the earlier operations. See color insert.

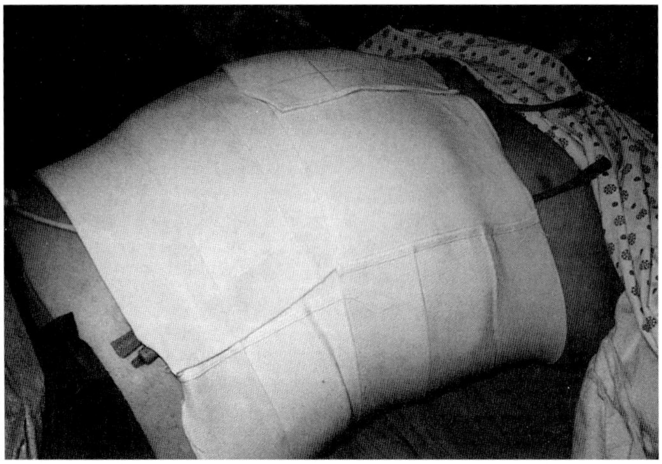

**FIG. 28.12.** Wide Velcro binders are applied while the patient is still anesthetized. These binders support the underlying bulky packing and overlying wound dressings.

above. With a single exception, the course of the pelvic collection has been shorter than that of the upper collections.

The clinical course of the patient and follow-up CT scans have occasionally indicated persistent perirenal, retrocolic, or subdiaphragmatic collections that have required retroperitoneal drainage through a flank incision, occasionally including resection of a lower rib. Such wounds have been handled by open packing, sometimes with a Penrose drain extending beyond the pack. A subdiaphragmatic collection with empyema occurred on two occasions: a left empyema developed over a subdiaphragmatic abscess, requiring resection of the 7th or 8th rib for a two-step drainage of the empyema and the underlying subhepatic collection.

**Closed Lavage Method.** Earlier, following exploration and debridement as described above, the author frequently inserted several large multichannel irrigating catheters, the wound being closed primarily. This method has been widely used under the stimulating influence of the Ulm school led by Professor Beger (14). In this method, 2–4 large, multiport, silicon rubber catheters are brought out from the necrotic catheters through stab wounds (Fig. 28.15). The catheters permit continuous irrigation and drainage, a continuous "rinsing of the necrotic tissues." Begun as a continuous infusion of a saline-based solution at a rate of 24 L during the first 24 hours, the rate is subsequently slowed to 2–4 L per 24 hours. Irrigation is maintained as long as necrotic tissue is noted in the effluent solution. Significant debridement is achieved by this method, although 40% of patients require reoperation (14).

Following exploration and debridement as indicated above, sometimes one finds unilocular or multilocular fluid collections with well-defined walls, often infected, but with a limited amount of dead tissue, most of which can be clearly identified and mechanically debrided. Under such circumstances, after meticulous debridement, the multilumen lavage catheters may be used preferentially and the wound closed. Continuous irrigation and drainage is then used to rinse the wound, permitting the drainage of small pieces of residual necrotic tissue. Although the incidence of reoperation is significant, it does not approach that of the open packing method. The author has used this method frequently, but because of the incomplete debridement of the "hub and spoke" pattern of necrosis that is often found, the frequent need for reoperation, and the relatively high incidence of subsequent fistulas of the colon in the author's hands, he has used it less frequently in recent years.

Because many patients are obese and the necrotic tissue is often infected, the skin and subcutaneous tissues are often left open. A feeding jejunostomy has also been used frequently with both closed lavage and the "open-packing" form of management.

### Debridement and Primary or Delayed Closure around Penrose Drains

Occasionally the surgeon encounters single, small, well-circumscribed areas of necrotic tissue, bathed in fluid, which can be completely debrided. Consideration may be given to the insertion of Penrose drains, with the wound closed primarily. These are the unusual exceptions in which a small cystlike cavity appears more stable, although it contains necrotic tissue. In other patients, after open packing, when all necrotic tissue and infection have been cleared, the wound may be closed around drains or irrigation tubes (48).

### Internal Drainage

Necrotizing pancreatitis may or may not prove to be an ongoing process in terms of progressive necrosis. Internal drainage (i.e., the drainage of the acute necrotic cavity into a viscus) is dangerous, and the author recognizes no indications for its use at this early stage of severe necrosis. Cystogastrostomy has occasionally been used electively, even though bits of necrotic tissue were unexpectedly found posteriorly in a chronic pseudocyst—but not under the circumstance of active necrotizing pancreatitis.

### Primary Retroperitoneal Approach

Recognizing that the disease process is predominantly located in the retroperitoneum, many have considered a primary retrocolic, retroperitoneal approach through the flank, usually from the left side. Evaluated by Fagniez, Rotman, and Kracht (29), the incidence of resulting colonic fistula was 20%, and the overall mortality rate was 33%. Exposure is difficult and often limited, so the method is seldom used as the primary approach and is reserved more for secondary approach to the pelvic or other residual areas of retroperitoneal infection.

### Avoidance of Necrosectomy

Necrosectomy is not an inevitable step in management (3, 6, 34, 49). In 5 of 76 (7%) patients with severe necrotizing pancreatitis treated by the author, continued observation, without necrosectomy, permitted the evolution of chronic pseudocysts that were

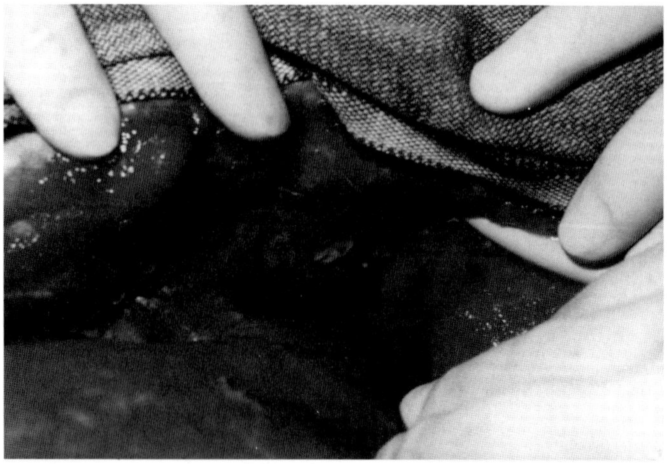

**FIG. 28.13.** Appearance of residual superficial necrotic tissue lining the necrotic cavity of the lesser sac at the time of repetitive debridement and change of packs.

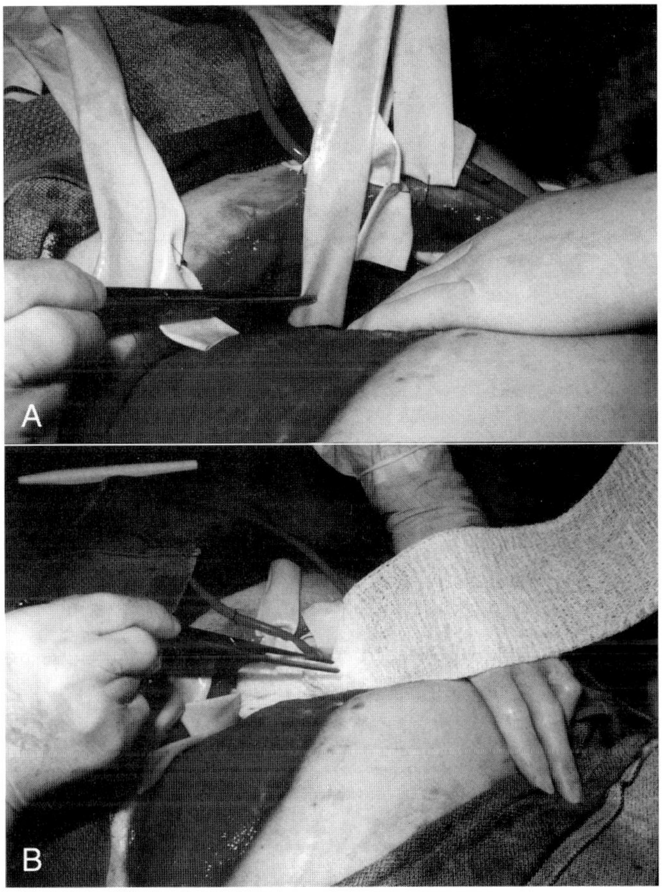

**FIG. 28.14. A** and **B.** Repacking of the open wound over Penrose drains and small irrigation catheters after secondary debridement. Penrose drains and Kerlex gauze are placed in every nook and recess of the necrotic spaces. The Kerlex gauze keeps the Penrose drains in place and packs the wound open. Note that the transverse colon is firmly adherent to the inferior lip of the bilateral subcostal incision. The colon loses its typical appearance in the open wound as its surface granulates. The wound will be completely filled with the Kerlex rolls.

ultimately treated electively by internal drainage. This further illustrates the fact that a single management protocol for these patients is impractical.

## POSTOPERATIVE COMPLICATIONS

In our present stage of knowledge, the morbidity of necrotizing pancreatitis is high, with a high incidence of pulmonary, cardiovascular, renal, metabolic, nutritional, and cerebral complications as well as complications related to the pancreas and the wound. The following discussion centers primarily around the abdominal pancreatic and wound complications.

In a 1991 collective review of 556 patients, D'Egidio and Schein (51) related the incidence of complications to the type of operative debridement and drainage performed. Their tabulation (Table 28.2) is useful. Under "reoperation as needed" and under "open packing," the reviewers included a category of patients who had undergone primary pancreatic resection, although most had been managed by delayed necrosectomy.

In the discussion of complications below, times as listed are approximate, because variations in the preoperative duration of illness and in the incidence of operations performed prior to transfer for definitive care may influence the timing of events "after operation."

### Early Complications (First 2 Weeks after Debridement)

Complications presenting prior to debridement—paralytic ileus, delayed gastric emptying, respiratory depression, and impaired renal and hepatic function—are likely to be exacerbated immediately after anesthesia and operation, but renal, hepatic, and sometimes pulmonary function may soon improve, particularly if sepsis was the indication for exploration.

Gastric emptying has been a continuing problem, possibly more often following open packing of the wound. This has led to the routine insertion of the jejunostomy feeding tube, which has proved a life-saving adjuvant to management. Paralytic ileus is seldom a serious enough problem to prevent jejunostomy feeding, and in fact, the diagnosis of paralytic ileus has been confused with that of inadequate gastric emptying. Erythromycin therapy, evaluated in the treatment of delayed gastric emptying after the Whipple resection, (50) has not, to the author's knowledge, been evaluated under these conditions. Persistent pulmonary insufficiency is often a persistent life-threatening problem, even after initial debridement. Almost two-thirds (62%) of the author's patients required endotracheal ventilatory support beyond 48 hours of the operation (34). Prolonged ventilatory support has been most frequently required for long-term cigarette smokers.

Two of the author's patients had delayed bleeding from the debrided wound within the first week and required transfusion and early, although not emergency, reexploration. A bleeding point was not identified, but bleeding was not a continuing problem. In the collected review of 556 patients with necrotizing pancreatitis treated by necrosectomy, D'Egidio and Schein (51) noted 7% incidence of subsequent hemorrhage. In their experi-

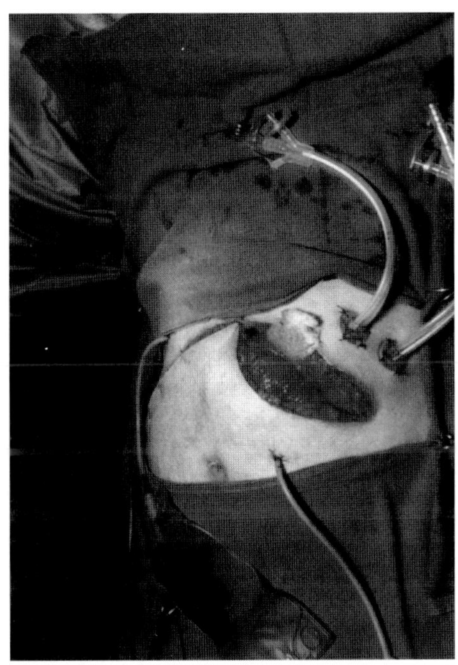

**FIG. 28.15.** Closed lavage-drainage in a patient with necrotizing gallstone pancreatitis. Operation included cholecystectomy, choledochostomy, necrosectomy, and jejunostomy. Superficially, the bilateral subcostal wound incision is left partially open. Note the jejunostomy and T tubes as well as the multichannel irrigation/drainage tubes.

**TABLE 28.2. Complications of Necrotizing Pancreatitis: Collective Review of 556 Patients**

| | Necrosectomy or Pancreatic Resection and Drainage; Reoperation as Needed | Necrosectomy and Lavage | Necrosectomy or Pancreatic Resection with Open Packing | Total |
|---|---|---|---|---|
| Number of patients | 256 | 166 | 134 | 555 |
| Small bowel complications | 5 | 4 | 14 | 4% |
| Colonic complications | 8 | 2 | 13 | 4% |
| Hemorrhage | 14 | 8 | 16 | 7% |
| Pancreatic fistula | 16 | 17 | 17 | 9% |

Adapted from 51. D'Egidio A, Schein M. Surgical strategies in the treatment of pancreatic necrosis and infection. Br J Surg 1991;78:133–137.

ence with 191 patients, Pederzoli et al. (35) noted postdebridement hemorrhage in 18 (9.4%), of whom 7 (39%) died.

A third patient of the author's who had undergone endoscopic sphincterotomy and stone retrieval and subsequent open cholecystectomy for stones was subsequently rehospitalized, vomiting blood and passing bloody stools. Acute necrotizing pancreatitis had evolved. After stabilization and negative studies for any source of bleeding, necrosectomy and drainage for massive peripancreatic necrosis were performed. Vomiting of blood recurred, and upper endoscopy was again negative. Arteriography revealed a fistula between the left hepatic artery and the left hepatic duct. Embolization of the artery resulted in gangrene of the left lobe and subsequent left hepatic lobectomy. The patient's course had been complicated by a duodenal perforation at the time of the initial necrosectomy. Whether this was due to the severe pancreatic necrosis or to a leak resulting from the endoscopic sphincterotomy could not be determined with certainty. It was treated by suture, end-to-side (bypassing) gastrojejunostomy, and insertion of a jejunostomy tube for feeding. A persistent common duct stone, missed at the time of cholecystectomy and common duct exploration for acute gallstone pancreatitis prior to transfer to our hospital, was not identified and contributed to continuing pancreatitis, with pancreatic necrosis (gangrene) and death 5 months after the initial operation.

Persisting infection has been the most frequent complication related to necrosectomy. It has been a more serious problem following debridement and closed drainage. Following debridement and open packing, infection occurs almost routinely, but repetitive debridements permit better control. In addition to excluding line sepsis, urinary and pulmonary infections, and clostridial enteritis, repeated CT scanning has been used to identify persistent or secondary collections and to "map out" a reoperative approach. An "early" pancreatic fistula was noted in a single patient who presented 3 weeks after the onset of acute gallstone pancreatitis with an abscess in the epigastrium. Since CT was not available, the epigastric abscess was treated by limited incision and drainage. A pancreatic fistula resulted and persisted for 12 months before spontaneous closure. A pancreatic fistula evolved after a longer interval in a second patient. The author has considered the diagnosis of pancreatic fistula in seven other patients on the basis of transient amylase-rich fluid drainage from the wound. No fistulograms were performed in these patients, and the possibility exists that amylase-rich lymph from necrosed or severed peripancreatic lymphatics might have been falsely interpreted as pancreatic fistulas (34).

**TABLE 28.3. Fistulas among 61 Patients with Acute Necrotizing Pancreatitis Requiring Operative Necrosectomy**

| | Number of Patients | Percentage of Total Patients | Recognized at First Operation | Number & Percentage Closed Spontaneously | Mortality Rate (Number & %)[a] |
|---|---|---|---|---|---|
| Total number of patients | 61 | 100% | — | — | 26% |
| Number with fistulas | 25 | 41% | | | 6 (24%) |
| Number without fistulas | 36 | | | | 10 (28%) |
| Number of fistulas | 33[b] | | | | |
| Pancreatic fistulas | 14 | 23% | 0 | 9[c] (64%) | 4 (29%) |
| Gastrointestinal fistulas | 19 | 31% | | | |
| Colonic | 8[d] | 13% | 1 | 2 (25%) | 3 (38%) |
| Duodenal | 5 | 8% | 3 | 4 (80%) | |
| Jejunal | 4[e] | 7% | 0 | 3[f] | 1 (25%) |
| Gastric | 2[g] | 3% | 0 | 2 (100%) | |

Modified from Tsiotos GG, Smith D, Sarr MG. Incidence and management of pancreatic and enteric fistulas after surgical management of severe necrotizing pancreatitis. Arch Surg 1995;130:48–52.
[a] Percentage of patients with fistulas.
[b] Some patients developed multiple fistulas.
[c] Time to spontaneous closure; mean, 129 days (range, 46–274 days).
[d] Time of development after initial operation: mean, 32 days (range, 4–60 days).
[e] Time of development after initial operation: mean, 26 days (range, 14–42 days).
[f] Time to spontaneous closure: 31, 125, 335 days.
[g] Recognized 30 and 33 days after initial operation.

**TABLE 28.4. Incidence of Pancreatic Fistulas in Acute Necrotizing Pancreatitis (Selected References)**

| | Total Number of Patients | Percentage with Fistulas |
|---|---|---|
| D'Egidio and Stein (51) 1991 (collected series) | 556 | 16.5% |
| Pederzoli et al. (35) 1990 | 191 | 8.4% |
| Tsiotos et al. (48) 1995 | 61 | 23% |
| Howard (34) 1996 | 71 | 3%[a] (13%) |

[a]7 other patients had transient drainage of amylase-rich wound fluid; a total incidence of 13%.

Among teams who performed pancreatic resections for acute pancreatitis, several identified a high incidence of necrosis of the colon and resected it, often as part of the original operation. The resulting incidence of sepsis, colonic fistula, and fatality was high (51–53).

### Intermediate Complications (2–4 Weeks after Operation)

With the exception of the patient described with a duodenal perforation of uncertain etiology, the author has recognized no patient with duodenal perforation from necrotizing pancreatitis. Although the author has recognized only two definite and seven suspected pancreatic fistulas, others have reported a higher (but delayed) incidence (Tables 28.3 and 28.4). Most pancreatic fistulas close spontaneously. Each of the author's did so, although, as indicated, one closed only after 12 months; a fistulogram had shown communication of the fistula to the duct of the pancreatic tail with obstruction of the duct toward the head. The patient declined a recommendation for late-stage operative repair; the fistula ultimately closed spontaneously by fibrosis of the wound with presumed acinar atrophy of the tail (a "Banting and Best preparation"). Fielding et al. (54) reported spontaneous closure of 11 (73%) pancreatic fistulas among 15 surviving patients. Octreotide does not fundamentally appear to alter the course of the complications fundamentally (48, 54).

Among the patients operated on for peripancreatic necrosis, the author has never recognized gangrene of the omentum. This would seldom have been overlooked as a primary phenomena because the omentum would have been partially inspected at the time of insertion of the feeding jejunostomy tube.

### Late Complications (One Month or Later after Initial Operation)

Hypercalcemia, apparently the result of prolonged immobilization while the patient was unconscious, was noted by the author in a single patient.

In the author's experience, only two patients have required late-stage hemodialysis; the dialysis was needed to correct a severe acid-base imbalance and remove water rather than for acute oliguric renal failure.

Gastric fistulas were not recognized by the author, although they were noted in two patients (3%) by Tsiotos, Smith, and Sarr (Table 28.3). Ranson (55) observed that necrosis of the duodenum may occur on its medial wall near the ampulla and may best be managed by drainage. Consideration should also be given to diversion of the foodstream and insertion of a feeding jejunostomy tube. The author has not observed necrosis of the common bile duct, for which Bradley (56) recommended insertion of a T tube into the common bile duct.

A single patient of the author's developed an external fistula of the first part of the jejunum where the jejunum lay exposed for a prolonged period in the base of an open wound. This was never adequately controlled for closure of the perforation, plus closure of the abdominal wall resulted each time in infection. The author has accepted as a working principle that repair of a visceral wound will not heal unless it is covered by peritoneum.

Although others have recorded primary necrosis of the colon (16, 29, 48, 52–54) at the time of initial exploration, the author has recognized it only once at the time of exploration, when it required resection and proximal colostomy. Instead, the colonic fistulas in six patients appeared to have been iatrogenic; they developed weeks after the onset of pancreatitis and manifested themselves as fecal drainage along irrigating catheters (Table 28.5). These fistulas were either proximal or distal (but close) to the splenic flexure of the colon and did not result in peritonitis (nor abscess, except in one patient) but led to fecal fistulas along the drains. A seventh patient had a cystogastrostomy 4 months after the initial attack of pancreatitis. Postoperative diarrhea led to barium studies, which demonstrated a fistula between the stomach, the "cyst," and the colon, resulting in a gastrocystocolonic fistula. One of the patients with a fistula at the splenic flexure subsequently developed stenosis of the descending colon, requiring resection. In a 1982 review, Bradley (56) found reports of only 34 patients with delayed colonic obstruction, primarily in the transverse colon.

One patient developed delayed ileal stenosis that required intestinal bypass. The stenosis, over a distance of 5–6 inches, was of uncertain etiology. Neither history nor gross examination of the intestine suggested granulomatous enteritis. Although thrombosis of branches of the superior mesenteric artery was not recognized, enteric fibrosis secondary to chronic ischemia was considered a possible cause.

Thrombosis of the superior mesenteric or portal vein was not proved in any of the author's patients, but splenic vein thrombosis was diagnosed in 6 (17%) of 36 patients (5). Portal vein occlusion was strongly suspected in the patient with the jejunal fistula, mentioned above, who developed small serosal varices of the exposed jejunum that led to their troublesome bleeding.

Occlusion of the feeding jejunostomy tube by encrustation is a troublesome, repetitive nuisance, not adequately prevented by prophylactic irrigation. When occlusion cannot be relieved by irrigation, inserting an arteriographic catheter is useful for unplugging the lumen. The catheter is maintained at the bedside for repetitive use.

Persistent dead tissue in the retroperitoneum, apparently present for over a year (34), was recognized in three patients, having been indolent in two. The necrotic tissue was recognized incidentally at the time of repair of a colostomy in one patient (Fig. 28.16), and in another, at exploration for what was erroneously considered to be acute appendicitis. In the first patient, the necrotic mass was well encapsulated; in the second, it appeared entirely dormant. Neither had a demonstrable blood supply. A third patient, who had had acute gallstone pancreatitis 11 months earlier, was initially seen by the author following erosion of the splenic artery with life-threatening hemorrhage associated with massive retroperitoneal necrosis, apparently residual from her original acute pancreatitis. She had been

**TABLE 28.5. Colonic Fistulas (Selected References)**

| | Total # Patients | Percentage with Fistula |
|---|---|---|
| Fagniez et al. (29) | 39 | 20% |
| Howard (34) | 71 | 10% |
| Tsiotos et al. (48) | 61 | 13%[a] |

[a]In addition to 3 patients who were found to have early necrosis of the right colon after anterior approach.

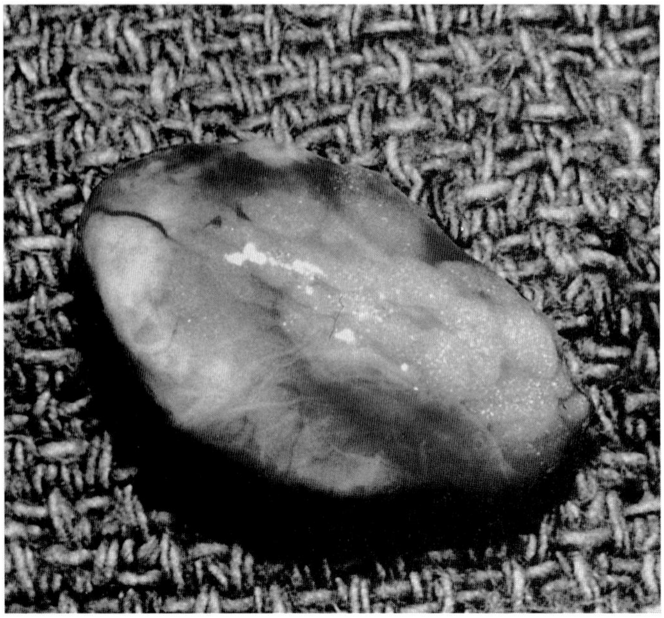

**FIG. 28.16.** Necrotic undigested retroperitoneal adipose tissue, discovered approximately 1 year after acute necrotizing pancreatitis. Apparently inert, the mass was found at the time of closure of a colostomy performed because of a colonic fistula. The solid mass, approximately 5 × 3 cm, could be enucleated. No blood supply was detected. (Reproduced from Howard JM. Studies of acute pancreatitis with retroperitoneal necrosis; "the suet syndrome." Improvements in patient survival. J Hepatobiliary Pancreat Surg 1996;3:195–202. Courtesy of Springer-Verlag Publishers.) See color insert.

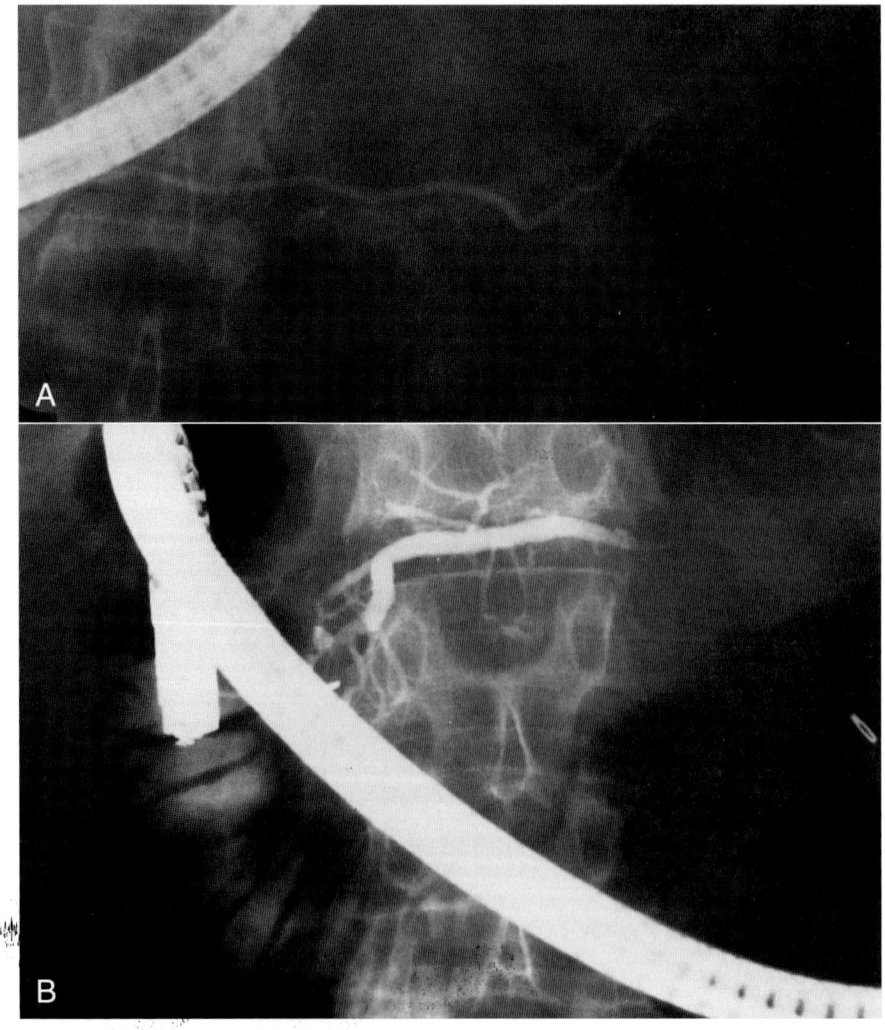


**FIG. 28.17.** Endoscopic retrograde pancreatograms in two patients approximately 1 year after recovery from acute necrotizing pancreatitis with massive peripancreatic liquefaction necrosis. At that time (the early 1980s), the author had erroneously thought that necrosectomy, performed 1 month after onset, had resulted in "gloved-hand total pancreatectomies." **A.** Normal contour of the pancreatic duct, as most frequently noted. **B.** The duct appears mildly dilated, perhaps fibrotic, and possibly obstructed in its caudal tip. Obstruction of the duct was an infrequent finding. (Reproduced from Howard JM, Wagner SM. Pancreatography after recovery from massive pancreatic necrosis. Ann Surg 1989;209:31–35, with permission of JB Lippincott.)

**TABLE 28.6. Time and Cause of Death from Acute Pancreatitis: A Multicenter Audit 1988–1992 (631 Patients, 57 Deaths)**

| | Time of Death (Weeks) after Onset of Attack | | | | |
|---|---|---|---|---|---|
| Cause of Death | 1 | 2 | 3 | >4 | Total |
| Multiple organ failure | 15 | 0 | 0 | 0 | 15 (26%)[a] |
| Infection | 0 | 3 | 7 | 16 | 26 (46%) |
| Other complications | 1 | 2 | 1 | 1 | 5 (9%) |
| Comorbid factors | 2 | 2 | 3 | 4 | 11 (19%) |
| Total | 18 (32%) | 7 (12%) | 11 (19%) | 21 (37%) | 57 (100%) |

Modified from Mann DV, Hershman MJ, Hittinger R, Glazer G. Multicenter audit of death from acute pancreatitis. Br J Surg 1994;81:890–893.
[a]Percentage of deaths.

asymptomatic during the intervening 11 months, but the "clinically indolent" necrotic mass must have been associated with low-grade necrotizing activity.

Follow-up ERCP following recovery from massive necrotizing pancreatitis revealed stenosis or obstruction of the pancreatic duct in several patients, while normal-appearing ducts were observed in most (Fig. 28.17, *A* and *B*) (7).

When treated by open packing, incisional hernia is inevitable unless secondary closure of the wound was elected. The hernias are sometimes large enough to create a significant nuisance. Repair has usually been required.

One of the author's patients developed chylous ascites 3 years after life-threatening peripancreatic necrosis that had resulted from ERCP (57). Over a period of months, the ascites spontaneously cleared. Diabetes and steatorrhea have occasionally been noted, but the relationship to the acute pancreatitis has not always been obvious.

One patient had carcinoma of the ampulla of Vater 5 years after severe pancreatitis with necrosis. This was considered probably unrelated to the acute pancreatitis, either as a cause or as a result of the pancreatitis.

No patient has been recognized by the author to have severe recurrent acute pancreatitis following recovery from necrosectomy.

## MORTALITY

Postoperative mortality rates are improving. The highest mortality rates, in the range of 50%, were associated with radical debridement, especially resectional debridement, at the first operation. Although attractive in concept, many patients were too ill to survive an "all out" operative approach. Furthermore, radical debridement requires exploratory laparotomy with varying degrees of resultant peritonitis. Those series with higher incidences of colon resection at the primary operation have been among those with the higher fatality rates. Whether this is the result of more severe disease or whether it reflects a lower clinical threshold for the diagnosis of necrosis deserves continued consideration. Experience clearly demonstrates that necrosis of the colon and pancreas is usually superficial, with the organ remaining viable.

Most deaths are related to continuing infection associated with the continued presence of dead tissue following initial debridement. Infection was reported to be responsible for over 70% of deaths in two series (58, 59).

In a broadly based audit of 631 patients with acute pancreatitis, not necessarily necrotizing in type, Mann et al. observed 57 deaths, of which at least 46% were the result of infection (60) (Table 28.6). In their collective review in 1991, D'Egidio and Schein (51) observed a mortality rate of 25% in patients with peripancreatic necrosis but more than 50% in patients with pancreatic necrosis. The spectrum of overlap between the two groups, however, is quite large.

Postoperatively, recent mortality rates have been about 20–25% (Table 28.7), but they are improving and should continue to improve as experience increases. The author's experience is that conservatism in the timing and in the aggressiveness of debridement, in gentleness and perseverance in debridement, and in the

**TABLE 28.7. Hospital Fatality Rates: Patients Requiring Necrosectomy (Selected References)**

| Author | No. Patients | Operative Treatment | Mortality Rate |
|---|---|---|---|
| D'Egidio and Schein (51) 1991 (collective review) | 216 | Debridement and closed lavage | 22.7% |
| | 118 | Resection or debridement; open packing | 24.5% |
| Bradley (61) 1994 (collected series) | 176 | Debridement and closed lavage | 25.6% |
| Bradley and Whitaker (62) 1992 (collected series) | 233 | Open packing | 16.7% |
| Pederzoli et al. (35) 1990 | 191 | Debridement and closed lavage with antiprotease | 10.5% |
| Madry and Fromm (16) 1994 | 40 | Debridement and closed drainage | 2.5% |
| Tsiotos et al. (48) 1995 | 61 | Debridement with open or closed drainage | 26% |
| Howard (34) 1996 | 71 | Debridement with open or closed drainage | 2.6% |
| Beger et al. (14) 1996 | 212 | Debridement and closed (lavage) drainage | <20%[a] |

[a]Exact mortality rate not stated.

maintenance of responsibility at all levels of care by a single surgeon can lead to the survival of most of these patients. The resulting mortality rate has been 3% among 71 patients treated by necrosectomy.

We are dealing with some of the sickest patients treated by the surgeon. Their care requires the resources of a major institution. Ideally, the first and each succeeding operation should be performed by the same surgeon. Primary laparotomy, followed by transfer to a tertiary care hospital, surely results in a higher mortality rate than might be achieved if transfer had occurred prior to the first operation. The responsible surgeon needs to be totally committed to the welfare of these critically ill patients. If not literally attending at bedside or sleeping in the intensive care unit on critical nights, there are times when the surgeon must be in direct communication with the bedside nurse throughout the critical periods, sometimes in contradistinction to communicating through the house staff. The author has not hesitated to cancel other operations and, indeed, to cancel overseas professional commitments to remain at the bedside. These are times, possibly more frequent than with any other illnesses, when care cannot be delegated.

Our morbidity remains too high, and as in most dynamic frontiers of surgery, the number of observations and tests required for optimal care remains high. The principles of care of these critically ill patients have been, or, are being, better defined. It is on the application of these principles that the lives of our patients currently depend.

## REFERENCES

1. Bigsby JJ. Observations, pathological and therapeutic, on diseases of the pancreas. Edinb Med Surg J 1835;44:85–102.
2. Senn N. The surgery of the pancreas as based upon experiments and clinical researches. Philadelphia: WJ Dornan, 1886:79.
3. Cited by Ashley SW. Sterile pancreatic necrosis: is operation necessary? J Am Coll Surg 1995;181:363–364.
4. Fitz RH. Acute pancreatitis: a consideration of pancreatic hemorrhage, hemorrhagic, suppurative and gangrenous pancreatitis, and of disseminated fat necrosis. Boston Med Surg J 1889;120: 181–188.
5. Howard JM. Delayed debridement and external drainage of massive pancreatic or peripancreatic necrosis. Surg Gynecol Obstet 1989;168:25–29.
6. Howard JM. Discussion of Warshaw AL, Jin G. Improved survival in 45 patients with pancreatic abscess. Ann Surg 1985;202:408–417.
7. Howard JM, Wagner SM. Pancreatography after recovery from massive pancreatic necrosis. Ann Surg 1989;209:31–35.
8. Neoptolemos JP, Stonelake P, Radley S. Endoscopic sphincterotomy for acute pancreatitis. Hepatogastroenterology 1993;40: 550–555.
9. Isenmann R, Büchler M, Uhl W, et al. Pancreatic necrosis: an early finding in severe acute pancreatitis. Pancreas 1993;8:358–361.
10. Kozarek RA, Ball TJ, Patterson DJ, et al. Endoscopic transpapillary therapy for disrupted pancreatic duct and peripancreatic fluid collections. Gastroenterology 1991;100:1362–1370.
11. Takeda K, Yamauchi J-I, Sunamura M, et al. Strategy for treatment of acute necrotizing pancreatitis: importance of continuous regional perfusion of protease inhibitor and antibiotics in the early phase. J Hepatobiliary Pancreatic Surg 1996;3:220–226.
12. Lee PC, Nakashima Y, Appert HE, Howard JM. Lipase and colipase in canine pancreatic juice as etiologic factors in fat necrosis. Surg Gynecol Obstet 1979;148:39–44.
13. Lee PC, Howard JM. Fat necrosis. Surg Gynecol Obstet 1979;148: 785–789.
14. Beger HG, Rau B, Mayer J. Necrotizing pancreatitis: indications for surgery and surgical techniques. J Hepatobiliary Pancreat Surg 1996;3:247–252.
15. Beger HG, Bittner R, Block S, Büchler M. Bacterial contamination of pancreatic necrosis. A prospective clinical study. Gastroenterology 1986;91:433–438.
16. Madry S, Fromm D. Infected retroperitoneal fat necrosis associated with acute pancreatitis. J Am Coll Surg 1994;178:277–282.
17. Pederzoli P, Bassi C, Vesentini S, Campedelli A. A randomized multicenter clinical trial of antibiotic prophylaxis of septic complications in acute necrotizing pancreatitis with imipenem. Surg Gynecol Obstet 1993;176:480–483.
18. Nordback I, Pessi T, Auuvinen O, Autic V. Determination of necrosis in necrotizing pancreatitis. Br J Surg 1985;72:225–227.
19. Balthazar EJ, Robinson DL, Megibow AJ, Ranson JHC. Acute pancreatitis: value of CT in establishing prognosis. Radiology 1990;174:331–337.
20. Mödder U, Friedmann G, Rosenberger J. The value of angio-CT for staging observation and treatment of acute pancreatitis. Fortschr Geb Rontgenstr Erganzungsband 1981;134:22–27.
21. Isikoff HB, Hill MC, Silverstein W, Barkin J. AJR 1981;136:679–684.
22. Kivisaari L, Somer K, Standertskijold-Nordenstam CG, et al. Early detection of acute fulminant pancreatitis by contrast-enhanced computed tomography. Scand J Gastroenterol 1983;18:39–41.
23. Maier W. Early objective diagnosis and staging of acute pancreatitis by contrast-enhanced computed tomography. In: Beger HG, Büchler M, eds. Acute pancreatitis. Berlin: Springer-Verlag 1987:132–140.
24. Bradley EL III, Murphy F, Ferguson C. Prediction of pancreatic necrosis by dynamic pancreatography. Ann Surg 1989;210: 495–504.
25. Trede M. Discussion of Bradley EL III, Murphy F, Ferguson C. Prediction of pancreatic necrosis by dynamic pancreatography. Ann Surg 1989;210:495–504.
26. Wilson C, Heads A, Shenkin A, Imrie C. C-reactive protein, antiproteases and complement factors as objective markers of severity in acute pancreatitis. Br J Surg 1989;76:177–181.
27. Uhl W, Büchler M, Malfertheiner P, et al. PNM-elastase in comparison with CRP, antiproteases and LDH as indicators in human acute pancreatitis. Pancreas 1991;6:253–259.
28. Nordback I, Lauslaht K. Clinical pathology of acute necrotizing pancreatitis. J Clin Pathol 1986;39:68–74.
29. Fagniez P-L, Rotman N, Kracht M. Direct retroperitoneal approach to necrosis in severe acute pancreatitis. Br J Surg 1989;76:264–267.
30. Leger L, Chicke B, Louvel A. Necrosis in acute pancreatitis; surgical and anatomicopathological comparisons. Seven cases. Nouv Presse Med 1977;6:337–340.
31. Glazer G, Dudley HAF. Pancreatic abscess. Letter to the editor. Br J Surg 1984;71:401.
32. Warshaw AL, Jin G. Improved survival in 45 patients with pancreatic abscess. Ann Surg 1985;202:408–417.
33. Farthmann EH, Lausen M, Schüoffel U. Indications for surgical treatment of acute pancreatitis. Hepatogastroenterology 1993; 40:556–562.
34. Howard JM. Studies of acute pancreatitis with retroperitoneal necrosis; ''the suet syndrome.'' Improvements in patient survival. J Hepatobiliary Pancreat Surg 1996;3:195–202.
35. Pederzoli P, Bassi C, Vesentini S, et al. Retroperitoneal and peritoneal drainage and lavage in the treatment of severe necrotizing pancreatitis. Surg Gynecol Obstet 1990;170:197–203.
36. Bassi C, Fontana R, Vesentini S, et al. Antibacterial and mezlocillin-enhancing activity of pure human pancreatic fluid. Int J Pancreatol 1991;10:293–297.
37. Gianotti L, Munda R, Alexander JW, et al. Bacterial translocation: a potential source for infection in acute pancreatitis. Pancreas 1993;8:551–558.
38. Luiten EJT, Hop WCJ, Lange JF, Bruining HA. Controlled clinical trial of selected decontamination for the treatment of severe acute pancreatitis. Ann Surg 1995;222:57–65.
39. Smadja C, Bismuth H. Pancreatic debridement in acute necrotizing pancreatitis: an obsolete procedure? Br J Surg 1980;73; 408–410.
40. Hollender LF, Meyer C, Marrie A, Papastratis G. Indications and long-term results after surgical treatment of hemorrhagic necrotic acute pancreatitis. Acta Chir Belg 1981;80:387–395.
41. Kestens PJ, Otte JB, Haot J, Reynaert M. Acute necrotizing hemorrhagic pancreatitis. Surgical treatment. Acta Chir Belg 1981;80:373–385.
42. Kivilaakso E, Fraki O, Nikki P, Lempinen M. Resection of the pancreas for acute fulminant pancreatitis. Surg Gynecol Obstet 1981;152:493–498.
43. Hollender LF, Meyer C, Keller D. Planned operations for necrotizing pancreatitis: the continental experience. In: Howard JM, Jerdeau

GL Jr, Reber HA, eds. Surgical diseases of the pancreas. Philadelphia: Lea & Febiger, 1987:450–460.
44. Reynaert M, Otte JB, Kestens PJ, Tremouroux J. Treatment of 30 cases of acute necrotizing hemorrhagic pancreatitis by peritoneal dialysis. Acta Chir Belg 1981;80:363–371.
45. Rotman N, Mathieu D, Anglade M-C, Fagniez PL. Failure of percutaneous drainage of pancreatic abscess complicating severe acute pancreatitis. Surg Gynecol Obstet 1992;174:141–144.
46. Beger HG. Surgical management of necrotizing pancreatitis. Surg Clin North Am 1989;69:529–549.
47. Poston GJ, Williamson RCN. Surgical management of acute pancreatitis. Br J Surg 1990;77:5–12.
48. Tsiotos GG, Smith D, Sarr MG. Incidence and management of pancreatic and enteric fistulas after surgical management of severe necrotizing pancreatitis. Arch Surg 1995;130:48–52.
49. Rau B, Pralle U, Uhl W, Schoenberg MH, Beger HG. Management of sterile necrosis in instances of severe acute pancreatitis. J Am Coll Surg 1995;181:279–288.
50. Yeo CJ, Barry MK, Sauter PK, et al. Erythromycin accelerates gastric emptying after pancreaticoduodenectomy. Ann Surg 1993;218:229–237.
51. D'Egidio A, Schein M. Surgical strategies in the treatment of pancreatic necrosis and infection. Br J Surg 1991;78:133–137.
52. Bouillot JL, Alexandre JH, Vuong NP. Colonic involvement in acute necrotizing pancreatitis. World J Surg 1989;13:83–87.
53. Aldridge MC, Francis ND, Glazer G, Dudley HAF. Colonic complications of severe acute pancreatitis. Br J Surg 1989;76:362–367.
54. Fielding GA, McLatchie GR, Wilson C, Imrie CW, Carter DC. Acute pancreatitis and pancreatic fistula formation. Br J Surg 1989;76:1126–1128.
55. Ranson JHC. Necrosis and abscess. In: Bradley EL III, ed. Complications of pancreatitis. Medical and surgical management. Philadelphia: WB Saunders, 1982:72–95.
56. Bradley EL III. Enteropathies. In: Bradley EL III, ed. Complications of pancreatitis. Medical and surgical management. Philadelphia: WB Saunders, 1982:265–292.
57. Zhang Z-Y, Howard JM. Chylous ascites: a late complication of massive peripancreatic necrosis. Int J Pancreatol, in press.
58. Ranson JHC, Balthazar E, Caccavale R, Cooper M. Computed tomography and the prediction of pancreatic abscess in acute pancreatitis. Ann Surg 1985;201:656–665.
59. Allardyce DB. Incidence of necrotizing pancreatitis and factors related to mortality. Am J Surg 1987;154:295–299.
60. Mann DV, Hershman MJ, Hittinger R, Glazer G. Multicenter audit of death from acute pancreatitis. Br J Surg 1994;81:890–893.
61. Bradley EL III. Necrosectomy in acute pancreatitis. J Hepatobiliary Pancreat Surg 1994;2:152–154.
62. Bradley EL, Whitaker WG Jr. Necrotizing pancreatitis. Significance, detection and treatment. Jpn J Gastroent Surg 1992;25:2280–2290.

29

# Treatment of Rare Complications of Acute Pancreatitis

I. B. Rasmussen and D. C. Carter

The common complications of acute pancreatitis such as necrosis, multiple organ failure, pseudocyst, and abscess formation are dealt with elsewhere (Chapters 20, 28, 43); this chapter is devoted to the rarer local complications of bleeding, pancreatic fistula, biliary obstruction, and intestinal involvement.

## HEMORRHAGE

Acute pancreatitis is complicated by life-threatening hemorrhage into the gastrointestinal tract, retroperitoneum, or peritoneal cavity in some 1–3% of patients (1, 2). Major bleeding has traditionally carried a mortality rate of 50–80% (3–6), but improvements in overall patient care, diagnosis, and management have almost certainly reduced the number of patients who succumb from hemorrhage. Review of 279 patients with acute pancreatitis managed in our own unit over the 4-year period 1989–1993 showed that major bleeding was only encountered in four patients; all four had undergone early necrosectomy, and bleeding was a major factor in the three who died (7). Major bleeding that complicates acute necrotizing pancreatitis has a particularly bad reputation and, in a recent review of 44 such cases, revealed a mortality rate of 61% (6).

### Stress Erosions and Peptic Ulceration

Routine early endoscopy will reveal gastric ulcerative lesions in almost all patients admitted to an intensive care unit, regardless of the cause of illness (8). Hemorrhage from superficial mucosal erosions was once common in severe acute pancreatitis, particularly in patients with sepsis, but the need to intervene because of significant bleeding appears to have been reduced by prophylactic measures designed to raise gastric pH or protect the gastric mucosa in critically ill patients (9, 10). Antacids given by nasogastric tube to maintain a pH above 4 are undoubtedly effective, but the approach is time consuming, and there is a danger of aspiration when large volumes of antacids are instilled. A further anxiety is that antacids and antisecretory agents such as $H_2$-receptor antagonists remove the natural bacteriocidal activity of gastric acid, and the consequent increase in gastric colonization has been linked to a high incidence of nosocomial pneumonia caused by the same microorganisms (10–12). Sucralfate is a direct mucosal protectant that appears to release cytoprotective agents such as prostaglandin $E_2$ ($PGE_2$) and inhibit bacterial colonization. Controlled studies in intensive care patients have shown that sucralfate (1 g every 6 hours by nasogastric tube) is as efficacious as $H_2$-receptor antagonist (ranitidine) plus antacid in preventing stress ulcer bleeding, reduces cost, and is associated with a lower (20.8 vs. 27.5%) incidence of pneumonia, although this last difference was not statistically significant (8).

The onset of major upper gastrointestinal hemorrhage is an indication for urgent endoscopy. Bleeding from peptic ulcers can now be arrested in most cases by endoscopic methods such as local injection of adrenaline or sclerosants (13), whereas bleeding from mucosal lesions can rarely be controlled in this way. Surgery may have to be considered if bleeding continues despite optimal medical therapy, although radical measures such as gastrectomy have a high mortality in these critically ill patients.

### Splenic Vein Thrombosis and Variceal Hemorrhage

The widespread use of dynamic computed tomography (CT) scanning has shown that splenic vein thrombosis is a much more common complication of acute and chronic pancreatitis than had been appreciated. The radiologic signs include failure of the splenic vein to outline with contrast, enlargement of the spleen, and the development of collaterals in the region of the short gastric vessels. While the exact incidence of splenic vein thrombosis is still uncertain, one autopsy study found that it occurred in 13% of 405 patients dying with acute pancreatitis, the complication affecting patients with pancreatitis due to all causes (14). Left-sided segmental portal hypertension (Fig. 29.1) leads to the development of gastric, esophageal, and even colonic (15) varices, and the gastroesophageal varices may be apparent on upper gastrointestinal endoscopy. Although variceal hemorrhage is reported in 30–70% of patients with longstanding splenic vein thrombosis (16–18), many of the reported patients have had chronic pancreatitis, and variceal hemorrhage is unusual during an episode of acute pancreatitis.

At laparotomy, splenic vein thrombosis is suggested by dilation of the gastroepiploic vein (and short gastric veins) in the absence of cirrhosis of the liver. If bleeding occurs, it almost always emanates from gastric varices, and splenectomy rather than portosystemic shunting is indicated. In patients making an otherwise good recovery from severe acute pancreatitis, the development of significant gastric varices and splenomegaly is an indication for prophylactic splenectomy to remove the risk of variceal bleeding.

### Vessel Necrosis

Vessel necrosis, a potentially lethal complication, develops when pancreatic and peripancreatic vessels come in contact with activated proteolytic enzymes in the presence of infection. The histologic changes in the affected vessels include splitting of the internal elastic lamina and arteritis (19), and inflammatory thrombosis of the nutritive vasa vasorum in the arterial wall hastens the development of full-thickness necrosis. Thrombosis, vessel rupture, or pseudoaneurysm formation may result. The splenic artery is the commonest source of bleeding in all forms of pancreatitis and in one review was the site of bleeding in 36% of patients in whom the bleeding vessel was defined (6); on the other hand, the mortality rate of splenic arterial bleeding (21.5%) was low relative to the overall mortality rate of bleeding (40%).

Pseudoaneurysms most commonly affect the splenic artery, but the gastroduodenal, pancreaticoduodenal, gastric, and he-

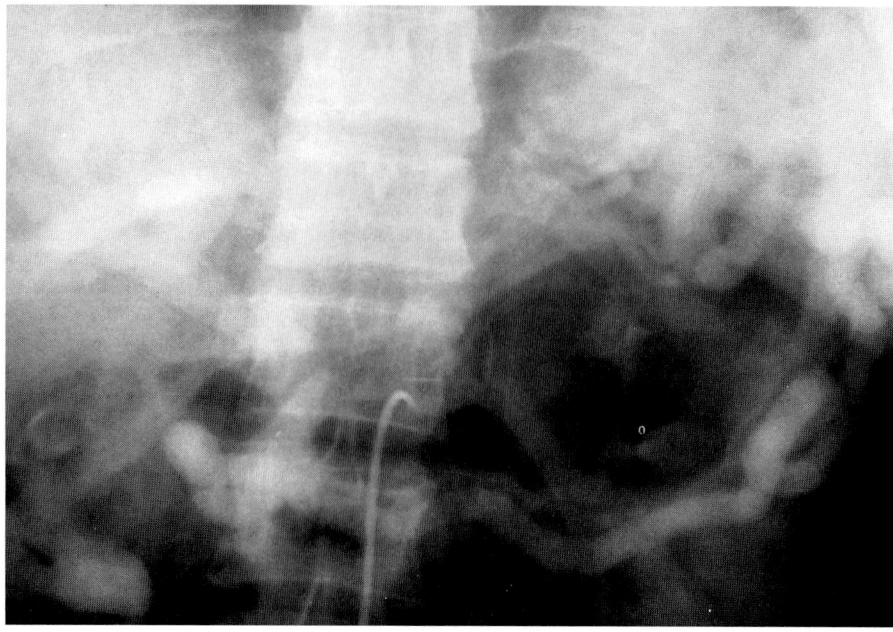

**FIG. 29.1.** Venous phase of a selective celiac angiogram in a patient with chronic pancreatitis. The venous phase reveals absence of filling of the splenic vein with the presence of large collaterals filling gastric varices. The portal vein eventually fills by a collateral route.

patic arteries may be involved in descending order of frequency (5, 20, 21). The incidence of pseudoaneurysm formation is uncertain, as many of them are small and escape detection unless a selective arteriogram is performed (5, 22). They can also be detected on CT when intravenous contrast is used, and lesions thought at first to be pseudocysts on scanning are revealed as pseudoaneurysms if intravascular contrast leaks into their lumen (Fig. 29.2)

Fatal hemorrhage may follow rupture into the gastrointestinal tract (4), pseudocyst, pancreatic duct, peritoneal cavity, or retroperitoneum. The final catastrophic bleeding is typically predated by self-limiting episodes of "herald bleeding" (23, 24). Bleeding into a preexisting pseudocyst converts it into a pseudoaneurysm, with the sudden development of a painful pulsatile abdominal mass, often in association with a bruit (25). In one

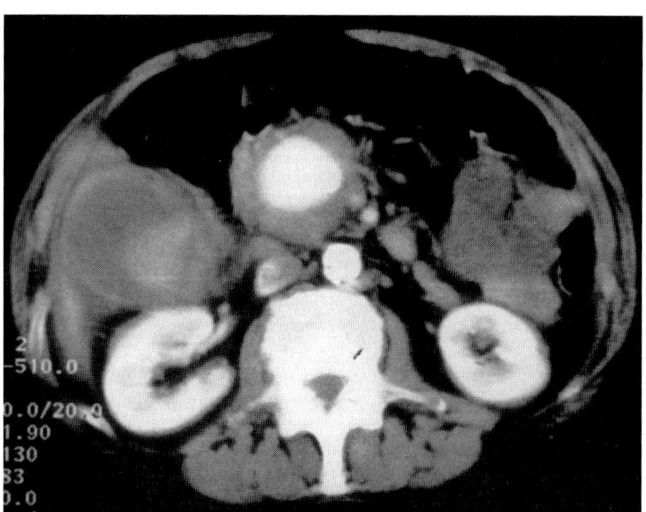

**FIG. 29.2.** Dynamic rapid-bolus contrast-enhanced CT scan in a patient with a pseudoaneurysm of the pancreas. The patient presented with alcoholic pancreatitis and was thought to have a pseudocyst before the enhanced scan was undertaken.

review of 11 series involving 596 patients with pseudocysts, such hemorrhage occurred in 39 cases (6.5%) (26). Blood loss can be prodigious, with transfusion requirements of two to three times the patient's blood volume in some cases. Bleeding due to infected necrosis or abscess has a worse prognosis than bleeding from a pseudocyst or pseudoaneurysm, and bleeding into the colon in acute pancreatitis is particularly dangerous, having a mortality rate of 86% in one review (6).

In the rare complication "hemosuccus pancreaticus" (27), the vessel or pseudoaneurysm ruptures into the pancreatic ductal system, and blood is then lost into the gastrointestinal tract via the papilla of Vater. Bleeding into the pancreatic ductal system was responsible for 11% of cases of pancreatitis-associated bleeding in the review of Flati et al. (6) and had a mortality rate of 27%.

Conservative treatment of major bleeding has a mortality rate of approximately 90% (5, 6), whereas surgery has been associated with rates of 25–53% (3, 6, 20, 21). Angiographic embolization offers an alternative means of arresting hemorrhage (22, 24, 28), and our initial approach in patients with massive hemorrhage is to perform diagnostic angiography if time permits (Fig. 29.3) and embolize the offending artery with autologous clot, sponge pledgets, or coils. In the presence of infected pancreatic and peripancreatic necrosis, embolization is followed by a high incidence of recurrent hemorrhage due to continued vascular erosion (29), and timely surgical intervention is still usually indicated. Intravascular balloon occlusion or vasopressin infusion has also been used as an aid to hemostasis pending surgical intervention (22), but we have no experience of this approach.

If surgery has to be undertaken without prior angiographic or CT localization of the source of bleeding, Bradley and Allen (30) recommend the following plan of action. If blood is seen within the gastric lumen, a longitudinal prepyloric gastrotomy is performed to search for duodenal, gastric, or variceal hemorrhage. If this fails to detect a bleeding source, "hemosuccus pancreaticus" is excluded by inspecting the papilla of Vater. If hemorrhage is coming from a pseudocyst or a pseudoaneurysm that has eroded into the gastrointestinal tract, the vessel responsible can often be identified from the location of the inflammatory mass. Pulsation in the wall of a presumed pseudocyst points to the true nature of the pathology, and needle aspiration is always advisable before a pseudocyst is incised. Masses within the head of the pancreas usually involve the gastroduodenal or pancreaticoduodenal arteries, while those in the body and tail of pancreas involve the splenic artery. The vessel responsible is controlled initially by compression, followed by ligation at its origin if local conditions permit. In some cases where the splenic artery has eroded into a pseudocyst, control can be obtained by underrunning the artery on either side of the point of rupture. Distal vascular lesions can be managed definitively by distal pancreatectomy and splenectomy, but proximal pancreatic resection is a formidable undertaking in such sick patients and is best avoided if at all possible.

## PANCREATIC FISTULA

A fistula is usually defined as an abnormal communication between two surfaces lined by epithelium. In the case of pancreatic disease, the definition is extended to include communication between the pancreatic duct and peritoneal cavity (pancreatic ascites) or pleural cavities (pancreaticopleural fistula), as well as communications between the duct and hollow viscera or skin. External pancreatic fistulas are usually the result of surgical or radiologic intervention to deal with necrotizing pancreatitis, abscess, or pseudocysts, whereas internal fistulas typically arise spontaneously. Pancreatic ascites and pancreaticopleural fistulas are known as internal pancreatic fistulas and result from disruption of the pancreatic duct or leakage from a pseudocyst. Over the past 30 years, such internal pancreatic fistulas have been diagnosed increasingly as a result of increased awareness and the availability of endoscopic retrograde pancreatography (ERP) (32, 33). Sankaran and Walt (33) found a 14.5% incidence of pancreatic ascites in 131 patients with pseudocysts treated over a 17-year period, while Iacono et al. (34) reported a 1.3% incidence of massive pancreaticopleural effusion in 670 patients with inflammatory pancreatic disease. Although the exact incidence of internal pancreatic fistulas is unknown, the frequency of recognition is directly related to the degree of clinical suspicion and diagnostic awareness. While this chapter is concerned with complications of acute pancreatitis, much of the literature dealing with pancreatic fistulas is based on patients with chronic inflammation. Internal pancreatic fistulas are relatively rare during the initial stages of acute pancreatitis and are more commonly caused by an acute exacerbation of underlying chronic pancreatitis.

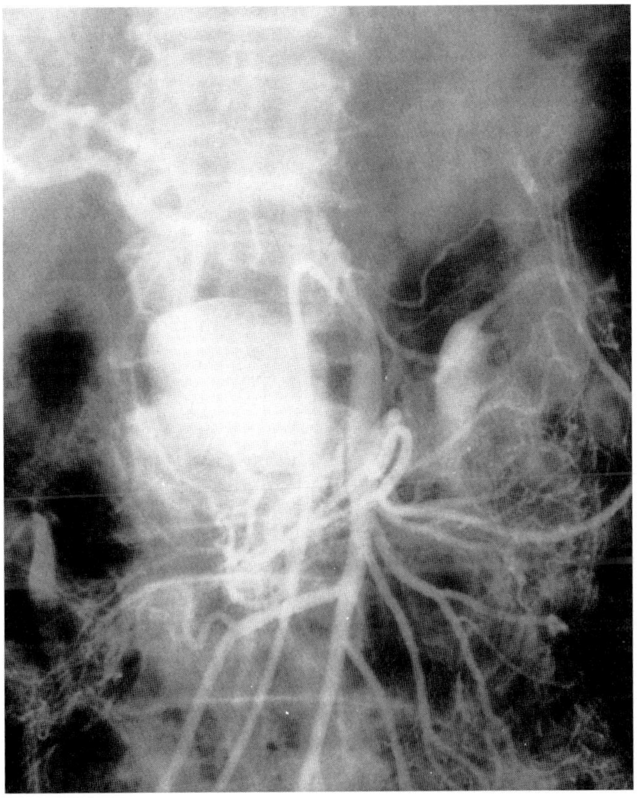

**FIG. 29.3.** Selective superior mesenteric angiogram in a patient with a pseudoaneurysm of the head of the pancreas. The pseudoaneurysm derives its blood supply from the pancreaticojejunal arcade.

Anterior disruption of a pseudocyst or the pancreatic duct is thought to result in pancreatic ascites (35), whereas posterior leaks may track through the esophageal or aortic hiatus to create a pseudocyst in the mediastinum (36). Massive pleural effusion results when such mediastinal pseudocysts rupture into one or both pleural cavities. Alternatively, leaking pancreatic juice may track through the retroperitoneum to gain direct access to one or both pleural cavities. On rare occasions, a pancreaticopleural fistula develops into a pancreaticobronchial fistula, and pancreaticocholedochal fistulas have also been described (37). As the pancreas normally produces over a liter of fluid a day, ascites and effusions are typically massive, and the absence of an appropriate inflammatory response in a patient who is often malnourished means that spontaneous closure is unlikely.

Internal pancreatic fistulas have not been reported in patients with acute gallstone pancreatitis, and most patients have underlying alcohol-associated pancreatitis. Trauma is implicated in approximately 10% of adults with internal fistulas and is responsible for virtually all cases involving children (38). In a review of 185 cases, Broe and Cameron (38) identified the typical patient as a male alcoholic, aged 20–50 years, who presents with tense ascites, mild abdominal discomfort, and malnutrition, often without a clear history of pancreatitis. It is possible that the increasing use of interventional radiology to deal with pancreatic pseudocysts has increased the incidence of pancreatic ascites, and we have encountered two patients recently in whom pancreatic ascites followed attempts at pseudocyst aspiration.

As many patients are alcoholics, pancreatic ascites is often misdiagnosed initially as a consequence of alcoholic disease of the liver. Once the true diagnosis is suspected, internal pancreatic fistulas can be distinguished readily from other forms of ascites and pleural effusions by aspiration. The straw-colored or serosanguinous fluid obtained has a grossly elevated amylase concentration, and its protein concentration usually exceeds 25 g/L (33, 39).

Chest radiography will define the presence and size of pleural effusions (Fig. 29.4), while a CT scan provides useful information regarding the pancreas, liver, and biliary system and demonstrates free peritoneal and pleural fluid. If a pancreatic fistula has an external component, fistulography can be used to delineate the track and display the pancreatic duct system. However, ERP is usually required for optimal definition of the fistula and its relationship to the pancreatic duct (Fig. 29.5). Rapid leakage of contrast sometimes prevents full visualization. Multiple sites of contrast extravasation is an occasional finding that predicts that conservative management is unlikely to succeed (40).

Management is initially conservative and consists of "resting" the pancreas by avoiding oral intake and establishing total parenteral nutrition. Nasogastric suction is probably unnecessary unless the patient has persistent vomiting and gastric outlet or duodenal obstruction. Pharmacologic inhibition of pancreatic secretion by long-acting somatostatin analogues such as octreotide will allow spontaneous closure in some cases. However, the fistula cannot be expected to close if there is "downstream" obstruction of the pancreatic duct, underlining the importance

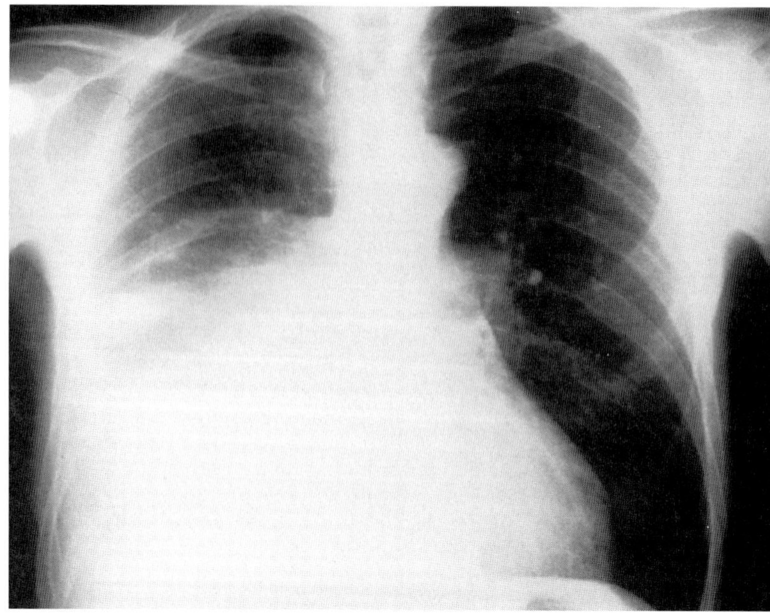

**FIG. 29.4.** Chest x-ray in the same patient as in Figure 29.5. The chest x-ray taken on admission reveals a large right-sided pleural effusion that proved to have a high amylase content on aspiration.

of defining pancreatic ductal anatomy by ERP. Other factors that predict failure of conservative treatment are severe underlying pancreatic disease, low serum sodium and albumin levels, and a high ratio of ascitic fluid protein to serum protein (40) (Table 29.1). The relatively high ascitic fluid protein concentrations may reverse Starling's forces, establishing a vicious cycle that progressively depletes the intravascular compartment. The rapid rise in serum albumin that follows fistula closure probably reflects lymphatic reabsorption of protein from the peritoneal cavity once the vicious cycle has been broken.

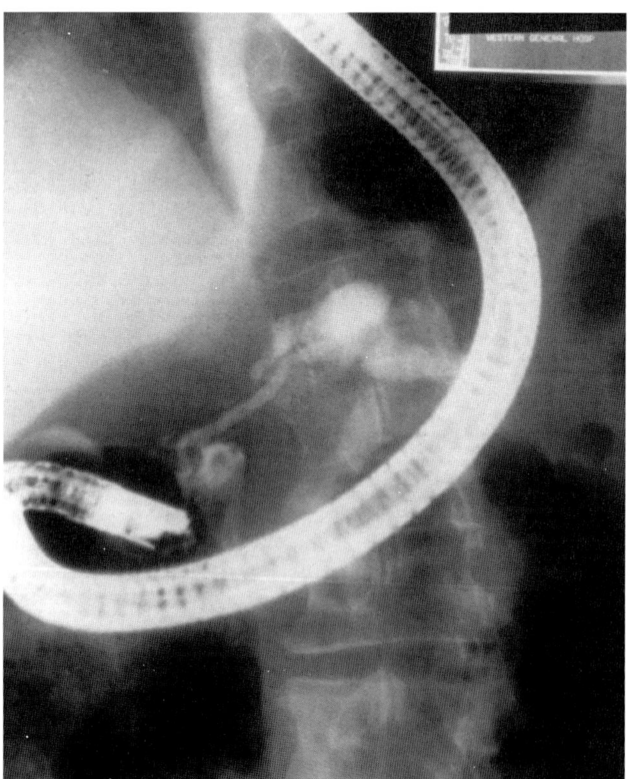

**FIG. 29.5.** Endoscopic retrograde cholangiopancreatogram in a patient with chronic alcohol-associated pancreatitis who presented with a right-sided pleural effusion. The pancreatogram shows leakage of contrast from the duct in the body of the gland.

Paracentesis or even, on occasions, chest tube placement will deal temporarily with peritoneal or pleural fluid accumulation, but it is doubtful whether this helps to promote closure of the fistula, and it may favor the entry of infection while serving as a drain on the body's stores of protein. Some 40–65% of patients experience spontaneous remission with conservative management (41–45), the prospects for closure being increased if octreotide is used. However, it is probably unwise to persist with medical management for more than 2–3 weeks, particularly when there is distal obstruction in the pancreatic duct. Sudden unexplained death has been reported after prolonged supportive care (38), and the mortality rate in some early series approached 20% (33, 46). Low-dose irradiation of the pancreas was once used to diminish pancreatic secretion in patients at prohibitive operative risk (32, 47), but this approach is now obsolete. Similarly, the need to consider peritoneovenous shunting (48) has been obviated by the availability of potent inhibitors of pancreatic secretion (40, 49, 50), improved definition of the anatomy of the fistula, and the selective use of pancreatic surgery.

Persistence of pancreatic ascites or pleural effusion after 2–3 weeks of conservative treatment is, in our view, an indication for surgery, and as discussed, ERP is an invaluable aid to surgical planning. Operative mortality in the 130 surgical patients collected by Broe and Cameron (38) was 14%, but a recent review of 50 collected cases suggests that surgical closure now has an overall success rate of 83%, with a mortality rate of 8% (51). Leakage from the body and tail of the pancreas is best managed by resecting the distal pancreas. Leakage from the head of the pancreas is better treated by drainage into a Roux loop of jejunum than by proximal pancreatic resection. The jejunal loop is applied directly to the site of ductal rupture; the pancreatic duct upstream from the point of rupture is frequently distended, and the opening in the duct should be extended to create a wide pancreaticojejunostomy. If pancreatic fluid is leaking from a pseudocyst, Roux-en-Y cystojejunostomy may be preferred to direct drainage of the pancreatic ductal system. In the case of pancreaticopleural fistula, there is no need to dissect out the fistulous track; disconnection of the fistula by surgery directed at the pancreas will prevent continuing passage of pancreatic fluid into the pleural cavities (Fig. 29.6).

Endoscopic placement of stents across the site of ductal disruption has recently been reported in patients who fail to respond to conservative management. The fistula resolved in all five patients treated by Saeed et al. (37), and none recurred within a follow-up of 14–30 months. Four of these patients had alcoholic pancreatitis, and in three cases, there was evidence of chronic inflammation. The stents were removed after approximately 6 weeks and were thought to have promoted fistula closure by providing a path of least resistance that allowed the fistulous track to collapse. The role of endoscopic stenting in fistulas associated with acute pancreatitis remains uncertain, but stenting may allow surgery to be avoided or deferred in high-risk patients, particularly when ERP has shown a narrowing in the pancreatic duct.

When an external pancreatic fistula is the consequence of radiologic or surgical intervention, much depends on the state of the remaining pancreas and its ductal system. In contrast to fistulas of the small bowel, the fluid emanating from a "pure" pancreatic fistula does not contain activated proteolytic enzymes and does not excoriate the skin. Most such fistulas are low output (i.e., less than 200 mL/day) and, in the absence of downstream pancreatic ductal obstruction, will close on conservative management. Fistulography may demonstrate the extent of the fistula and the state of the pancreatic ductal system without recourse to ERP. In our experience of 23 patients with pancreatic fistulas as a consequence of acute pancreatitis, 19 had an external fistula after necrosectomy or drainage of an abscess or pseudocyst; of the 15 patients who survived, all 11 with low-output fistulas had spontaneous closure of the fistula (52).

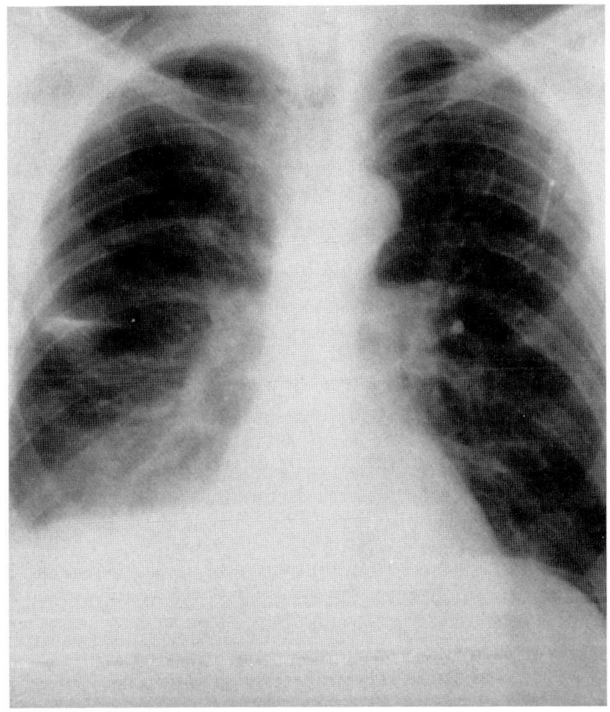

**FIG. 29.6.** Chest x-ray showing a resolving pleural effusion following surgical drainage of the pancreatic duct system in the patient shown in Figures 29.4 and 29.5.

## BILIARY OBSTRUCTION

Approximately 20% of patients with acute pancreatitis become jaundiced at some stage (53). While obstructing gallstones are often responsible (Chapter 22), the cause of cholestasis is uncertain in as many as 50% of cases. This so-called acute pancreatic cholangiopathy is usually mild and transient and has been attributed to periductular edema and cholangitis (53). In the absence of a demonstrable cause, spontaneous resolution is usual, and surgical intervention is unnecessary. Ductal compression by pancreatic abscess (54) or pseudocyst (55, 56) has been described, but as Warshaw and Rattner (57) point out, obstructive jaundice in patients with pseudocysts is usually caused by fibrosis in association with chronic inflammation and is not simply a matter of ductal compression by the pseudocyst.

**TABLE 29.1. Relationship Between Clinical and Biochemical Factors and Response to Conservative Treatment in 23 Patients with Internal Pancreatic Fistulas (Parekh and Segal, 1992)**

| | Healed | Failed to Heal |
|---|---|---|
| *n* | 15 | 8 |
| Mean age (±SEM) | 45.2 ± 3.8 | 47.4 ± 27 |
| Length of history (months) | 2.0 | 2.5 |
| Serum sodium mmol/L | 133.7 ± 1.1 | 125.5 ± 1.8[a] |
| Serum albumin g/L | 31.1 ± 1.7 | 22.0 ± 1.5[a] |
| Total serum protein g/L | 76.6 ± 2.6 | 64.9 ± 3.6[a] |
| Ascitic fluid protein g/L | 39.6 ± 3.1 | 41.1 ± 1.9[a] |
| Fluid protein: serum protein | 0.54 ± 0.03 | 0.86 ± 0.3[a] |

Adapted from Parekh D, Segal I. Pancreatic ascites and effusion. Risk factors for failure of conservative therapy and the role of octreotide. Arch Surg 1992;127:707–712.

[a]$p \leq 0.5$.

## INTESTINAL COMPLICATIONS

### Ileus

A degree of local ileus is common in acute pancreatitis and accounts for the classical but unreliable diagnostic signs of a gas-filled "sentinel" loop of jejunum in the left upper abdomen and the "colon cutoff" sign, in which a distended hepatic and splenic flexure are separated by a gasless transverse colon (58). Focal ileus frequently affects the duodenum, given its intimate anatomic relationship with the inflamed pancreas, and inflammation tracking within the transverse mesocolon is usually held responsible for colonic ileus.

### Small Bowel Obstruction

Frank duodenal obstruction is rare, affecting 1% of patients in one series of 878 patients, and usually resolves with conservative management (59). Duodenal edema or intramural hematoma is usually responsible, and surgical intervention to deal with duodenal fibrosis is only indicated if obstruction fails to resolve after some 4 weeks. Mechanical obstruction of the jejunum and ileum is also extremely uncommon unless peritonitis develops with adhesion formation (60).

### Intestinal Necrosis

Intestinal necrosis is another rare complication of acute pancreatitis, although its true incidence is almost certainly underestimated. Aldridge et al. (68) found 36 cases of colonic necrosis and/or perforation in a 22-year review of the world literature but were able to add 10 further cases of their own. Focal intestinal necrosis probably develops when parts of the gut lie in contact with a pancreatic abscess or localized area of infected pancreatic necrosis (60, 61). The intestinal wall may be eroded by activated enzymes (62, 63), and vasculitis and arterial and venous thrombosis have been implicated (64–68). Inflammatory pancreatic exudate diffusing between the leaves of the mesentery may explain involvement of the transverse colon and small bowel, and the strategic location of the pancreas in the base of the mesocolon and root of the mesentery may favor the onset of segmental vascular occlusion (30). On histopathologic examination, more patients show pericolitis with mesenteric fat necrosis and serosal and subserosal inflammation than show ischemic necrosis of the intestinal wall (65). When ischemic necrosis develops, it may progress to perforation or to the formation of an internal fistula (although this may pass unnoticed clinically), and it can give rise to major hemorrhage.

Necrosis of segments of bowel remote from the pancreas has also been reported, and hypercoagulability and disseminated intravascular coagulation could favor the development of mesenteric arterial or venous thrombosis (67, 69).

The diagnosis of intestinal necrosis requires a high index of suspicion. An abdominal mass, sepsis, and gastrointestinal bleeding are present in approximately 50% of reported cases (60). Supportive radiologic findings include the presence of edematous mucosal folds ("thumbprinting") on contrast radiology, gas within the bowel wall or peritoneal cavity, and the appearances of toxic megacolon (70). Untreated intestinal necrosis is invariably fatal, so surgical intervention is mandatory whenever it is suspected. The involved bowel is resected with creation of a proximal stoma. Despite increasing awareness, improved diagnosis, and improved perioperative and surgical care, intestinal necrosis still has a mortality rate that exceeds 50% (60, 61, 65, 68).

### Colonic Stenosis

Mechanical obstruction of the colon from inflammatory stenosis is also rare. The stenosis may present as obstruction of the large bowel during the attack of acute pancreatitis or some months later as a "pseudocarcinoma" with rectal bleeding and an "apple-core" lesion on barium enema (68). Histologically, such stenoses show an inflammatory infiltrate with muscle destruction and fibrosis. The splenic flexure is the site of stenosis in 84% of cases (71), which may reflect its proximity to the tail of the pancreas or the fact that it is the watershed between the middle and left colic arteries. Surgical intervention is rarely required, and in many cases, the obstruction resolves spontaneously (60, 72). Proximal colostomy without resection is indicated if surgery is unavoidable in the acute phase of the illness, and resection is only indicated if a stricture persists once the acute inflammatory episode has settled. In practice, it may be extremely difficult to differentiate between pericolitis and ischemic necrosis in patients coming to surgery with necrotizing pancreatitis, and resection is indicated when in doubt. In patients treated conservatively, barium enema can be used to monitor the stenosed colon, and carcinoma can be excluded by using colonoscopy to demonstrate that the mucosa is normal. Considerable skill and judgment are required in the management of these patients.

## REFERENCES


1. Marks IN, Bank S, Louw JH, et al. Peptic ulceration and gastrointestinal bleeding in pancreatitis. Gut 1967;8:253–259.
2. Trapnell JT. Management of the complications of acute pancreatitis. J R Coll Surg Engl 1971;49:361–372.
3. Stroud WH, Cullom JW, Anderson MC. Hemorrhagic complication of severe pancreatitis. Surgery 1981;90:658–665.
4. Frey CF, Stanley JC, Eckhauser F. Hemorrhage. In: Bradley EL III, ed. Complications of pancreatitis. Philadelphia: WB Saunders, 1982: 96–119.
5. Stabile BE, Wilson SE, Debas HT. Reduced mortality from bleeding pseudocysts and pseudoaneurysms caused by pancreatitis. Arch Surg 1983;118:45–51.
6. Flati G, Negro P, Porowska B, Flati D, Carboni M. Hemorrhagic complications of pancreatitis. In: Beger HG, Buchler M, Malfertheiner P, eds. Standards in pancreatic surgery. Heidelberg: Springer-Verlag, 1993:314–324.
7. DeBeaux AC, Palmer KL, Carter DC. Factors influencing morbidity and mortality in acute pancreatitis; an analysis of 279 cases. Gut 1995;37:121–126.
8. Maier RV, Mitchell D, Gentilello L. Optimal therapy for stress gastritis. Ann Surg 1994;220:353–363.
9. Borrero S, Bank S, Margolis I, et al. Antacid versus sucralfate in preventing gastrointestinal bleeding; a randomized trial in 100 critically ill patients. Am J Surg 1984;148:809–812.
10. Tryba M. Sucralfate versus antacids or $H_2$-antagonists for stress ulcer prophylaxis: a meta-analysis on efficacy and pneumonia rate. Crit Care Med 1991;19:942–949.
11. Hillman KM, Riordan T, O'Farrell SM, et al. Colonization of the gastric contents in critically ill patients. Crit Care Med 1982;10: 444–447.
12. Driks MR, Craven DE, Celli BR. Nosocomial pneumonia in intubated patients given sucralfate as compared with antacids or histamine type 2 blockers. N Engl J Med 1987;317:1376–1382.
13. Palmer KR, Choudari CP. Endoscopic intervention in bleeding peptic ulcer. Gut 1995;37:161–164.
14. Renner IG, Savage WT III, Pantoja JL, Renner VJ. Death due to acute pancreatitis. A retrospective analysis of 405 autopsy cases. Dig Dis Sci 1985;30:1005–1017.
15. Burbidge ER, Tarder G, Carson S, Eugene J, Frey CF. Colonic varices: a complication of pancreatitis with splenic vein thrombosis. Am J Dig Dis 1978;23:752–755.
16. Longstreth GF, Newcomer AD, Green PA. Extrahepatic portal hypertension caused by chronic pancreatitis. Ann Intern Med 1971;75:903–908.
17. Salam AA, Warren WD, Tyras DH. Splenic vein thrombosis: a diagnosable and curable form of portal hypertention. Surgery 1973;74:961–972.
18. Little AG, Moossa AR. Gastrointestinal hemorrhage from leftsided portal hypertension: an unappreciated complication of pancreatitis. Am J Surg 1981;141:153–158.
19. Rich AR, Duff GL. Experimental and pathologic studies on pathogenesis of acute hemorrhagic pancreatitis. Johns Hopkins Med J 1936;58:212–228.
20. Stanley JC, Frey CF, Miller TA, Lindenauer SM, Child CG. Major arterial hemorrhage: a complication of pancreatic pseudocysts and chronic pancreatitis. Arch Surg 1976;111:435–440.
21. Eckhauser FE, Stanley JC, Zelenock GB, Borlaza GS, Ferier DT, Lindenauer SM. Gastroduodenal and pancreaticoduodenal artery aneurysms: a complication of pancreatitis causing spontaneous gastrointestinal hemorrhage. Surgery 1980;88:335–344.
22. Vugic I. Vascular complications of pancreatitis. Radiol Clin North Am 1989:27:81–91.
23. Gadacz TR, Trunkey D, Kieffer RF. Visceral vessel erosion associated with pancreatitis. Arch Surg 1978;63:698–704.
24. Steckman ML, Dooley MC, Jaques PF, Powell DW. Major gastrointestinal hemorrhage from peripancreatic blood vessels in pancreatitis: treatment by embolotherapy. Dig Dis Sci 1984;29: 486–497.
25. Bradley EL III. Later complications of acute pancreatitis. In: Glazer G, Ranson JHC, eds. Acute pancreatitis: experimental and clinical aspects of pathogenesis and management. Philadelphia: WB Saunders, 1988:390–431.
26. Maule WF, Reber HA. Diagnosis and management of pancreatic pseudocysts, pancreatic ascites, and pancreatic fistula. In: Go VLW, DiMagno EP, Gardner JD, et al., eds. The exocrine pancreas: biology, pathobiology, and diseases. New York: Raven Press, 1986:601–610.
27. Sandblom P. Gastroduodenal hemorrhage through the pancreatic duct. Ann Surg 1970;171:61–66.
28. Mandel SR, Jacques PJ, Mauro MA, Sonofsky S. Nonoperative management of peripancreatic arterial aneurysms: a 10 year experience. Ann Surg 1987;205:126–128.
29. Waltman AC, Luers PR, Athanasoulis CA, Warshaw AL. Massive arterial hemorrhage in patients with pancreatitis: complementary roles of surgery and transcatheter occlusive techniques. Arch Surg 1986;121:439–443.
30. Bradley EL, Allen KA. Complications of acute pancreatitis and

their management. In: Trede M, Carter DC, eds. Surgery of the pancreas. Edinburgh: Churchill Livingstone, 1993:245–259.
31. Sankaran S, Sugawa C, Walt AJ. Value of endoscopic retrograde pancreatography in pancreatic ascites. Surg Gynecol Obstet 1979;148:185–192.
32. Greenwald RA, Deluca RF, Raskin JB. Pancreatic-pleural fistula. Demonstration by endoscopic retrograde cholangiopancreatography (ERCP) and successful treatment with radiation therapy. Dig Dis Sci 1979;24:240–244.
33. Sankaran S, Walt AJ. Pancreatic ascites; recognition and management. Arch Surg 1976;111:430–434.
34. Iacono C, Procacci C, Frigo F, et al. Thoracic complications of pancreatitis. Pancreas 1989;4:228–236.
35. Smith RB III, Warren WD, Rivard AA, Amerson RJ. Pancreatic ascites: diagnosis and management with particular reference to surgical technique. Ann Surg 1973;177:538–546.
36. Jaffe BM, Ferguso TB, Holtz S, Shields JB. Mediastinal pancreatic pseudocysts. Am J Surg 1972;124:600–606.
37. Saeed ZA, Ramirez FC, Hepps KS. Endoscopic stent placement for internal and external pancreatic fistulas. Gastroenterology 1993; 105:1213–1217.
38. Broe PJ, Cameron JL. Pancreatic ascites and pancreatic pleural effusion. In: Bradley EL III, ed. Complications of pancreatitis. Philadelphia: WB Saunders, 1982:245–264.
39. Cameron JL, Anderson RP, Zuidema GD. Pancreatic ascites. Surg Gynecol Obstet 1967;125:328–332.
40. Parekh D, Segal I. Pancreatic ascites and effusion. Risk factors for failure of conservative therapy and the role of octreotide. Arch Surg 1992;127:707–712.
41. Cameron JL. Chronic pancreatic ascites and pancreatic pleural effusion. Gastroenterology 1978;74:134–140.
42. Weaver DW, Walt AJ, Sugawa C, Bouwman DL. A continuing appraisal of pancreatic ascites. Surg Gynecol Obstet 1982;154: 845–848.
43. Moossa AR. Surgical treatment of chronic pancreatitis: an overview. Br J Surg 1987;74:661–667.
44. Dewan N, Kinney W, O'Donohue WJ. Chronic massive pancreatic effusion. Chest 1984;85:497–501.
45. Pottmeyer EW III, Frey CF, Matsuno S. Pancreaticopleural fistulas. Arch Surg 1987;122:648–654.
46. Donowitz M, Kerstein MD, Spiro HM. Pancreatic ascites. Medicine 1974;53:183–195.
47. Morton RE, Deluca R, Reisman TN. Pancreatic ascites: successful treatment with pancreatic radiation. Am J Dig Dis 1976;21: 333–336.
48. De Waele B, van der Spek P, Devis G. Peritoneovenous shunt for pancreatic ascites. Dig Dis Sci 1987;32:550–553.
49. Ellison EC, Garner WL, Mekhjian HS. Successful treatment of pancreatic ascites with somatostatin analog. Gastroenterology 1988;90:1405.
50. Øktedalen O, Nygaard K, Osnes M. Somatostatin in the treatment of pancreas ascites. Gastroenterology 1990;99:1520–1521.
51. Lippsett PA, Cameron JL. Internal pancreatic fistula. Am J Surg 1992;163:216–220.
52. Fielding GA, McLatchie GR, Wilson C, Imrie CW, Carter DC. Acute pancreatitis and pancreatic fistula formation. Br J Surg 1989;76: 1126–1128.
53. Bradley EL III, Salam AA. Hyperbilirubinemia in inflammatory pancreatic disease: natural history and management. Ann Surg 1978;188:626–629.
54. Holden JL, Berne TV, Rosoff L. Pancreatic abscess following acute pancreatitis. Arch Surg 1976;111:858–867.
55. Bradley EL III, Clements LJ, Gonzales AC. The natural history of pancreatic pseudocysts: a unified concept of management. Am J Surg 1979;137:135–141.
56. Skellinger ME, Patterson D, Foley MT, Jordan PH. Cholestasis due to compression of the common bile duct by pancreatic pseudocysts. Am J Surg 1983;145:343–348.
57. Warshaw AL, Rattner DW. Facts and fallacies of common bile duct obstruction by pancreatic pseudocysts. Ann Surg 1980;192: 33–37.
58. Price CW. The 'colon cut-off' sign in acute pancreatitis. Med J Aust 1956;1:313–314.
59. Bradley EL III, Clements LJ. Idiopathic duodenal obstruction: an unappreciated complication of pancreatitis. Ann Surg 1981;193: 638–648.
60. Bradley EL III. Enteropathies. In: Bradley EL III, ed. Complications of pancreatitis. Philadelphia: WB Saunders, 1982:265–292.
61. Schein M, Saadia R, Decker G. Colonic necrosis in acute pancreatitis: a complication of massive retroperitoneal suppuration. Dis Colon Rectum 1985;28:948–950.
62. Schroeder T, Kivilakso E, Kianunen DKJ, Lempinen M. Serum phospholipase A2 in human acute pancreatitis. Scand J Gastroenterol 1980;15:633–635.
63. Dubnick MA, Geokas MC, Mar G, McMahon MJ, Mayer AD, Majmudar APN. Digestive enzymes and protease inhibitors in ascites fluid from patients with acute pancreatitis. Gastroenterology 1985;88:1370.
64. Kukora JS. Extensive colonic necrosis complicating acute pancreatitis. Surgery 1985;97:290–293.
65. Bouillot JL, Alexander JH, Vuong NP. Colonic involvement in acute necrotizing pancreatitis: results of surgical treatment. World J Surg 1989;13:84–87.
66. Nordback I, Sisto T. Peripancreatic vascular occlusions as a complication of pancreatitis. Int Surg 1989;74:36–39.
67. Jensen K, Bradley EL III. Mesenteric venous infarction in acute pancreatitis. Int J Pancreatol 1989;5:213–219.
68. Aldridge MC, Francis ND, Glazer G, Dudley HAF. Colonic complications of severe acute pancreatitis. Br J Surg 1989;76: 362–367.
69. Carey LC. Extra-abdominal manifestations of acute pancreatitis. Surgery 1979;86:337–342.
70. Miller WT, Scott J, Rosato EF, Rosato FE, Crow H. Ischemic colitis with gangrene. Radiology 1970;94:291–297.
71. Carboni M, Negro P, Tuscano D, de Bernardinis G, Flati D, Flati G. Secondary colonic lesions in acute pancreatitis. In: Hollender LF, ed. Controversies in acute pancreatitis. Berlin: Springer-Verlag, 1982:302–315.
72. Hudson DA, De Beer JV. Acute large bowel obstruction complicating acute pancreatitis. South Med J 1988;81:804–805.

# 30

# Chronic Pancreatitis: Multiple Diseases with Multiple Etiologies

John M. Howard

*Acute* pancreatitis is now internationally recognized as consisting of multiple diseases stemming from multiple causes. This was not true in our earlier careers. This brief chapter extends the concept of multiple causes, already widely recognized, to the *chronic* disease state. Instead of writing of the treatment of "chronic pancreatitis," the time has come to write on the treatment, for example, of chronic alcoholic pancreatitis, chronic hereditary pancreatitis, or chronic obstructive pancreatitis.

The distinguished gastroenterologists, Sarles, Bernard, and Gullo (1) have classified chronic pancreatitis into two forms: *(a)* obstructive pancreatitis, which results from obstruction of the pancreatic duct, and *(b)* chronic calcifying pancreatitis, which results mainly from metabolic diseases such as alcoholism. Chronic pancreatitis seems to be etiologically much more complex. Clinical reports from around the world are gradually providing the basis for expanding these concepts. Chapter 19 documents that chronic pancreatitis may result from the following factors.

## Obstruction of the Pancreatic Duct

Numerous factors may cause obstruction of the pancreatic duct. Included are carcinoma of the head of the pancreas, carcinoma of the ampulla of Vater, islet cell tumors, carcinoid tumors of the pancreas or ampulla, benign periampullary tumors such as polyps adenomata, cysts, either benign or malignant duodenal tumors, duodenal cysts, pancreatic cysts including congenital cysts, foreign bodies (including the therapeutic use of intraductal polymer), intentional or accidental ligation of the pancreatic duct, obstruction of the duct secondary to duodenal ulcer or to operative procedures near the ampulla of Vater. Obstruction of the duct may also result from the use of pancreatic stents or from inflammatory stenosis at the ampulla of Vater or at the minor ampulla (pancreas divisum) and may result from stricture secondary to acute pancreatitis itself. It may also result from several of the anomalies or infections discussed below.

Chronic pancreatitis secondary to obstructive pancreatitis is usually remedial by operation, and the prognosis (with the exception of pancreatitis secondary to adenocarcinoma of the exocrine pancreas) tends to be better than that of most other forms of the disease. Although acute pancreatitis, not chronic pancreatitis, is the characteristic complication of an ampullary gallstone, the long-term presence of such a stone occasionally leads to chronic inflammation of the pancreas; an observation most frequently described in China. Obstruction of the pancreatic duct leads to stasis of pancreatic juice, dilatation of the pancreatic duct and its tributaries, secondary atrophy of the acini, and their replacement with scar tissue. Pancreatic calcification is unusual. Cellular infiltration may, or may not, be a resulting feature. Resultant diabetes is infrequent and mild.

## Alcoholic Pancreatitis

In North America, Europe, and Australia, alcoholic pancreatitis is a major form of chronic pancreatitis, resulting apparently from the toxic effects of alcohol. This disease goes through phases of recurrent acute pancreatitis, leading to atrophy of the acini and replacement by fibrous tissue, often associated with changes in the caliber of the pancreatic ducts, pseudocyst formation, and development of calcium carbonate stones within the pancreatic ductal system. Exocrine pancreatic insufficiency develops as the acini atrophy and are replaced by scar tissue. Diabetes often develops without histologic evidence of destruction of the islets of Langerhans. Obstruction of the pancreatic ducts is secondary to the underlying disease and, when it occurs, is usually incomplete. Today, operation seldom affects the course of the disease, being reserved for the treatment of pain.

## Tropical Pancreatitis

Tropical pancreatitis, developing in areas north and south along the equator, occurs in cultures in which alcohol is characteristically seldom used. It develops at a young age and results in atrophy of the acini, extensive fibrosis, dilatation of the pancreatic ducts, pancreatic ductal calculi, and severe diabetes. It apparently predisposes to exocrine pancreatic cancer. Operation does not alter the course of the disease and, again, is reserved largely for the treatment of pain. In many ways the disease parallels the course of alcoholic pancreatitis, except that it has an earlier onset, progresses more rapidly, and results in death at an earlier age.

## Metabolic Pancreatitis

Metabolic pancreatitis, including hyperparathyroidism, may lead to similar although less marked changes, including fibrosis with or without pancreatic calculi. Hyperlipidemia may result in chronic pancreatitis as may hemochromatosis, porphyria, Wilson's disease, glycogen storage disease type 1, and organic acidemias.

### Hereditary Pancreatitis

The general classification of hereditary pancreatitis apparently includes numerous genetic defects, resulting in multiple syndromes. Chronic pancreatitis in this setting may take several forms, often going through phases of acute recurrent pancreatitis leading to atrophy of the acini, fibrous replacement, changes in the caliber of the pancreatic duct, and formation of pancreatic calculi. In addition, patients may be seen at a young age with a strikingly diffusely dilated pancreatic duct without obstruction, and sometimes they have acute attacks of pancreatitis. Familial groups of such patients have been observed in the presence or absence of any recognizable hereditary factor. As mentioned above, several of the metabolic diseases are hereditary. $\alpha$-1-antitrypsin deficiency is a genetic disorder that leads to chronic pancreatitis as may hereditary angioedema.

### Vasculitis Including Chronic End-Stage Renal Failure

Both acute and chronic pancreatitis are occurring more frequently in patients with far-advanced chronic renal failure as hemodialysis, peritoneal dialysis, and renal transplantation prolong the lives of these patients. In addition, several other forms of vasculitis may result in chronic pancreatitis among young people. This group includes lupus erythematosus, Wegener's granulomatosis, and polyarteritis.

### Congenital Defects

Cystic fibrosis of the pancreas appears to be in part a deficiency in pancreatic development, on which chronic pancreatitis becomes superimposed, accentuating the pancreatic deficiency and presenting the clinical syndrome of an inflammatory disease. Anomalies of the pancreatic and biliary ducts may result in obstructive forms of chronic pancreatitis. An annular pancreas may sometimes result in chronic pancreatitis, recognized in middle-aged adults. Choledochal cysts, with their anomalous connections with the pancreatic ducts, may lead to both chronic and acute pancreatitis.

### Granulomatous Disease of the Pancreas or Adjacent Organs

Crohn's disease, particularly when it occurs in the duodenum, has repeatedly been shown to cause chronic pancreatitis. Tuberculosis of the pancreas, particularly in the head of the gland, has been described in numerous reports, including treatment by Whipple resection in several instances. Syphilitic granuloma has been reported as resulting in a pancreatic mass, treated by pancreaticoduodenectomy. Sarcoidosis has resulted in pancreaticoduodenectomy in several instances.

### Other Diseases

Other diseases of the gastrointestinal and biliary tracts, in addition to Crohn's granulomatous enteritis, have been associated with chronic pancreatitis. Ulcerative colitis has occasionally been noted, as has celiac disease (nontropical sprue), primary biliary cirrhosis, and sclerosing cholangitis.

### Other Ill-Defined but Related Syndromes

Other ill-defined but related syndromes include eosinophilic pancreatitis, which has presented as a mass leading to pancreaticoduodenectomy in a least two patients and a radical distal pancreatectomy in one. Fibrosing pancreatitis in children and "painless pancreatitis" in adults appear to be separate syndromes without etiologic recognition that result in chronic pancreatitis.

### Postradiation Pancreatitis

Radiation therapy has been used on a widening scale, including particularly treatment of lymphomas in and around the pancreas. Good response to therapy has resulted in longevity of more patients, permitting recognition of the long-term effects of radiation. Chronic pancreatitis has been a sequel.

### Other Infections and Infestations

Mumps, coxsackievirus, and AIDS represent viral infections that have occasionally resulted in chronic pancreatitis. *Candida*-induced chronic pancreatitis has lead to Whipple resection. The parasitic hydatid disease has been reported as a cause of chronic pancreatitis.

### Drug-Induced Chronic Pancreatitis

Although drugs, with the exception of ethyl alcohol, have infrequently been recognized as a cause of chronic pancreatitis, carbamazepine and the ß-blocking drugs have possibly been incriminated.

### Idiopathic

In a significant group of patients, chronic pancreatitis remains idiopathic. Recognition of the many causes of pancreatitis or, in some instances, only the syndromes associated with pancreatitis may, as with acute pancreatitis, decrease the need for this incomplete diagnosis.

As clinicians increasingly focus on the specific forms of chronic pancreatitis and delineate their separate natural histories, physicians may be progressively better able to diagnose the numerous specific subgroups, and surgeons may be better able to define not the treatment of a conglomerate group with chronic pancreatitis, but the principles of treatment of the various diseases involved.

## REFERENCES

1. Sarles H, Bernard JP, Gullo L. Pathogenesis of chronic pancreatitis. Gut 1990;31:629–632.

# 31

# *Etiology, Pathophysiology, and Pathology*

Günter Klöppel

## DEFINITION AND EPIDEMIOLOGY

Chronic pancreatitis is the result of fibroinflammatory changes in the pancreas from various causes. In Western countries, the incidence of chronic pancreatitis ranges between 3 and 4 per 100,000 persons (1, 2), with an increasing tendency (2). Some 70–80% of the patients presenting with chronic pancreatitis are young to middle-aged men (range, 25–50 years) who are heavy drinkers (1, 3–5). Some 20% of patients have idiopathic chronic pancreatitis, which occurs in either a young (first 2 decades of life) or an old age group and affects both genders equally (6, 7). Hereditary pancreatitis, which may occur in childhood, accounts for about 1–2% of all cases. It is an autosomal dominant trait with limited penetrance (80%) and no sex predilection (8). Uncommon causes of chronic pancreatitis are autoimmune diseases and trauma. Gallstone-related chronic pancreatitis seems to be the exception. Tropical chronic pancreatitis is frequently seen in parts of India and Africa (1, 9). It is predominantly a disease of youth, occasionally starting in the 1st decade of life, and is more common in males than in females (10).

## ETIOLOGY

A classification of chronic pancreatitis based on the most important etiologic factors is presented in Table 31.1. In all westernized countries, alcohol is the most common cause of chronic pancreatitis (1, 2). However, the number of affected individuals is far lower than that of individuals with alcoholic disease of the liver. The reason why less than 10% of alcoholics develop chronic pancreatitis is unclear (11). Presumably there is an additional (genetic?) factor in the development of alcoholic chronic pancreatitis that makes certain patients more susceptible to the disease than others. Whether the alcoholic who remains free of chronic pancreatitis may develop some particular kind of diffuse fibrosis of the pancreas (12) distinct from what can be seen in elderly patients without any known risk factors for chronic pancreatitis has yet to be established.

The group of nonalcoholic types of chronic pancreatitis is heterogeneous. The various types of chronic pancreatitis in this group are characterized by either a particular genetic background (e.g., hereditary pancreatitis), a distinct natural history (e.g., idiopathic chronic pancreatitis), or special metabolic (e.g., hypercalcemic or hyperlipidemic chronic pancreatitis) or environmental factors (e.g., tropical chronic pancreatitis). In hereditary chronic pancreatitis, the gene has recently been located on chromosome 7q23. In hypercalcemia and hyperlipidemia, the metabolic disturbances seem to play a role. In tropical pancreatitis, which occurs almost exclusively among impoverished populations, malnutrition has been discussed as an initiating factor (1). The role of cassava in the etiology of tropical pancreatitis has never been established.

## PATHOPHYSIOLOGY

Several theories have been put forth to explain the pathogenesis of alcoholic chronic pancreatitis. The most popular hypothesis is that of Sarles, who suggested that chronic ethanol consumption increases the protein concentration in the pancreatic juice, with subsequent precipitation of plug-forming secretions in the ducts, which later calcify (13). More recently, Sarles' group (14–16) identified a protein in pancreatic juice that prevented $CaCO_3$ precipitation and was therefore called lithostatin (formerly, pancreatic stone protein). It is thought that abnormal secretion of lithostatin due to either an acquired or an inherited defect in its biosynthesis contributes to the calcification of protein plugs in the pancreatic ducts. The formation of stones leads in turn to ductal obstruction and ulceration of ductal epithelium, two mechanisms that cause acinar atrophy and fibrosis upstream of the obstruction, as well as periductular inflammation.

Although this hypothesis is attractive, it has been criticized for several reasons. First, the findings concerning altered biosynthesis and function of lithostatin in chronic pancreatitis have not been universally confirmed (17–19). Second, the hypothesis only recognizes chronic pancreatitis as an alcohol-induced disease and neglects the fact that *acute* pancreatitis may also be caused by alcohol (20–23). Third, alcoholic acute and chronic pancreatitis have many features in common, such as clinical symptoms and the presence of pseudocysts. Fourth, in alcoholic acute pancreatitis, no preexistent changes due to chronic pancreatitis have been found, whereas the pancreas of patients with chronic pancreatitis may show signs of acute pancreatitis, such as autodigestive tissue necrosis (24, 25). Fifth, in its early stages, chronic pancreatitis lacks calcifications (26).

For these reasons, the plug hypothesis has been challenged by the necrosis-fibrosis sequence concept (27, 28), which postulates that alcoholic chronic pancreatitis is the result of relapsing severe acute pancreatitis (26, 29). The resorption of large areas of fat necrosis and hemorrhagic necrosis, which are the main events in severe acute (necrotizing) pancreatitis (30), induce fibrosis, possibly through the action of growth factors such as TGF$\alpha$ and TGFß (31, 32). The fibrosis develops primarily in the perilobular space, where fat necrosis and most of the hemorrhagic necrosis occur (30). Perilobular fibrosis in turn affects the structure of the interlobular ducts, gradually creating ductal dilations and strictures. In these altered ducts, the flow of secretions is most likely impaired, a situation that may trigger the spontaneous precipitation of proteins, with subsequent calcification. In addition, the impaired and eventually interrupted flow of pancreatic secretions leads to fibrotic replacement of the acinar cells upstream from the occluded duct and finally results in intralobular fibrosis.

Although the necrosis-fibrosis sequence nicely explains the perilobular fibrosis pattern, the patchy distribution of fibrosis,

**TABLE 31.1. Etiologic Classification of Chronic Pancreatitis and Pancreatic Fibrosis with or without Pancreatic Insufficiency but without Chronic Pancreatitis**

| |
|---|
| Chronic pancreatitis[a] |
| Alcoholic |
| Nonalcoholic |
| Hereditary |
| Metabolic (hypercalcemia, hyperlipidemia) |
| Autoimmune |
| Idiopathic |
| Tropical |
| Other forms |
| Chronic pancreatitis associated with anatomic abnormalities[a] |
| Obstructive chronic pancreatitis[b] |
| Periampullary duodenal wall cysts |
| Pancreas divisum |
| Posttraumatic pancreatic scars |
| Pancreatic fibrosis not associated with chronic pancreatitis[a] |
| Pancreatic fibrosis in the elderly |
| Cystic fibrosis[c] |
| Insulin-dependent diabetes mellitus |
| Hemochromatosis |

[a]Clinically defined by the occurrence of symptoms such as pain, pancreatic exocrine deficiency and diabetes.
[b]Usually only associated with pancreatic insufficiency.
[c]Associated with pancreatic insufficiency.
(*Editor's note:* see also Chapter 30.)

and the late occurrence of calcifications in the pancreas of patients with alcoholic chronic pancreatitis, certain questions remain. First, it is difficult to reconcile the fact that the necrosis-fibrosis sequence also holds true for the primary painless chronic pancreatitis that may be observed in 5–10% of alcoholics (33–35). Second, biliary acute pancreatitis, which may occasionally be as severe as alcoholic pancreatitis, virtually never progresses to chronic pancreatitis.

A third hypothesis, called the "toxic-metabolic hypothesis" was put forth by Bordalo et al. (36, 37). This hypothesis postulates that chronic consumption of alcohol induces progressive acinar lipid deposition with acinar atrophy and intrapancreatic fibrosis by exerting direct toxic and metabolic effects on the acinar cells. Because the described pancreatic changes, particularly the fatty degeneration of acinar cells, have not been confirmed by others, the significance of this concept for the pathogenesis of alcoholic chronic pancreatitis seems to be minor.

The fourth hypothesis, the "oxidative stress hypothesis" (38), postulates that oxidative stress in pancreatic acinar cells induced by excess free radicals causes a blockade of the intracellular pathway, fusion of lysosomal and zymogenic compartments, and membrane lipid oxidation. These events then lead to an inflammatory response. The hypothesis focuses on possible functional disturbances underlying acinar failure but fails to explain the particular fibroinflammatory process that characterizes chronic pancreatitis.

The pathogenesis of the various types of chronic pancreatitis that are grouped under the term nonalcoholic chronic pancreatitis is not known. In particular, we do not know the pathophysiology of hereditary, idiopathic, or tropical pancreatitis. In chronic pancreatitis associated with an autoimmune background, the pancreatic changes seem to be caused by an inflammatory destructive process involving the ducts.

### Pathology of Alcoholic Chronic Pancreatitis

**Macroscopy.** In the early stages of alcoholic chronic pancreatitis, the gland shows unevenly distributed fibrosis. The involved parts of the gland appear indurated and may be enlarged, showing coarse lobulation and/or nodular scarring on the cut surface. Only the ducts that are affected by fibrosis show irregularities (with occasional calculus formation). In 30–50% of patients there may be pseudocysts, which are usually extrapancreatic (24, 26), or foci of recent necrosis in the vicinity of scars (28). Pseudocysts occur more commonly in the pancreatic body and tail than in the region of the head (39).

In advanced chronic pancreatitis, the pancreas has a firm consistency and usually shows an irregular contour, with loss of normal lobulation (25, 30). Although fibrosis affects the entire gland, parenchymal scarring is still uneven and patchy, and occasionally the lobular pattern of the organ is preserved in some areas. The severity of the duct changes correlates closely with the extent of fibrosis. The main duct may therefore be only focally obstructed and/or dilated or diffusely involved, with irregular dilatation and distortion. Usually (80%) it contains calculi. The calculi, which consist of calcium carbonate, vary in size from less than 1 mm to more than 1 cm in diameter. They may be impacted in the ducts and therefore difficult to remove. In some cases, they may disappear during the course of the disease (40). Fibrosis in the pancreatic head may cause a tapering stenosis of the common bile duct. Thick-walled pseudocysts, usually attached to the pancreas, are present in one-quarter to one-half of cases (24). They vary in size (3–10 cm in diameter) and are filled with necrotic material and/or turbid fluid rich in enzymes. The pseudocysts may be connected with the ductal system. Occasionally they may erode the major portal veins, causing thrombosis, bleeding, and, rarely, disseminated fat necrosis with subcutaneous nodular panniculitis, polyarthritis, and necrotic lesions of the bone marrow.

**Microscopy.** Histologic examination of the early stages of the disease reveals interlobular (perilobular) cell-rich fibrosis (26, 41). The involved intralobular ducts are distorted and may contain eosinophilic secretions, so-called protein plugs. In addition, the epithelium may display metaplastic or hyperplastic changes. Moderate numbers of lymphocytes, plasma cells, and macrophages are present, either in local accumulations or scattered diffusely throughout the fibrous tissue. In the perilobular tissue, there may be foci of resolving fat necrosis with large numbers of vacuolated macrophages (foam cells) in the immediate vicinity and cell-rich fibrosis in the surrounding area (Fig. 31.1). The necrotic foci are often in the vicinity of large pseudocysts, which lie outside the pancreatic parenchyma.

In advanced chronic pancreatitis, fibrosis affects most of the parenchyma but to varying degrees (26, 41, 42). In some areas there is only perilobular fibrosis, while others show diffuse intralobular fibrosis with sparse lymphocytic infiltrates. Perilobular fibrosis causes duct distortions and dilatation, with occasional formation of a retention cyst. The lumens of these intralobular ducts are often filled with protein plugs and calculi (Fig. 31.2*A*). The ductal epithelium is either atrophic or completely replaced by polymorphocellular inflammatory tissue. In areas with intralobular fibrosis, the elements that remain are islets, thick-walled blood vessels, prominent nerves, and remnants of acinar cells, which may be atrophic, undergo apoptosis, or form so-called tubular complexes (43) (Fig. 31.2*B*). The nerves have been found to be damaged by the inflammatory process (44). The islets may form large ("adenomatoid") aggregates, which are sometimes in close contact with ductules that show islet cell neoformation (45). The number of beta cells in these islets was found to be slightly reduced (45).

**Immunopathology.** The ductal epithelium commonly expresses human leukocyte antigen (HLA-DR) MHC II, epithelial growth factor receptor (EGFR), transforming growth factor

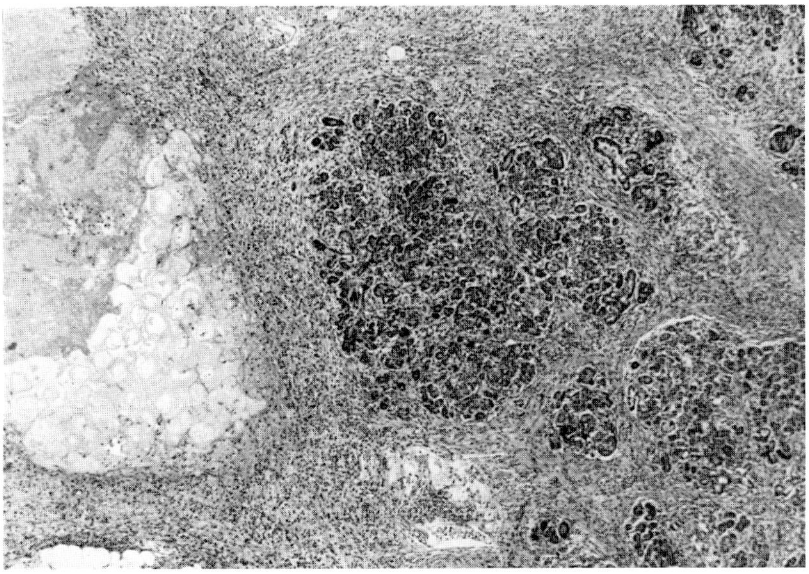

**FIG. 31.1.** Alcoholic chronic pancreatitis, early stage. Cell-rich perilobular fibrosis with fat necrosis in resorption. H & E, ×60.

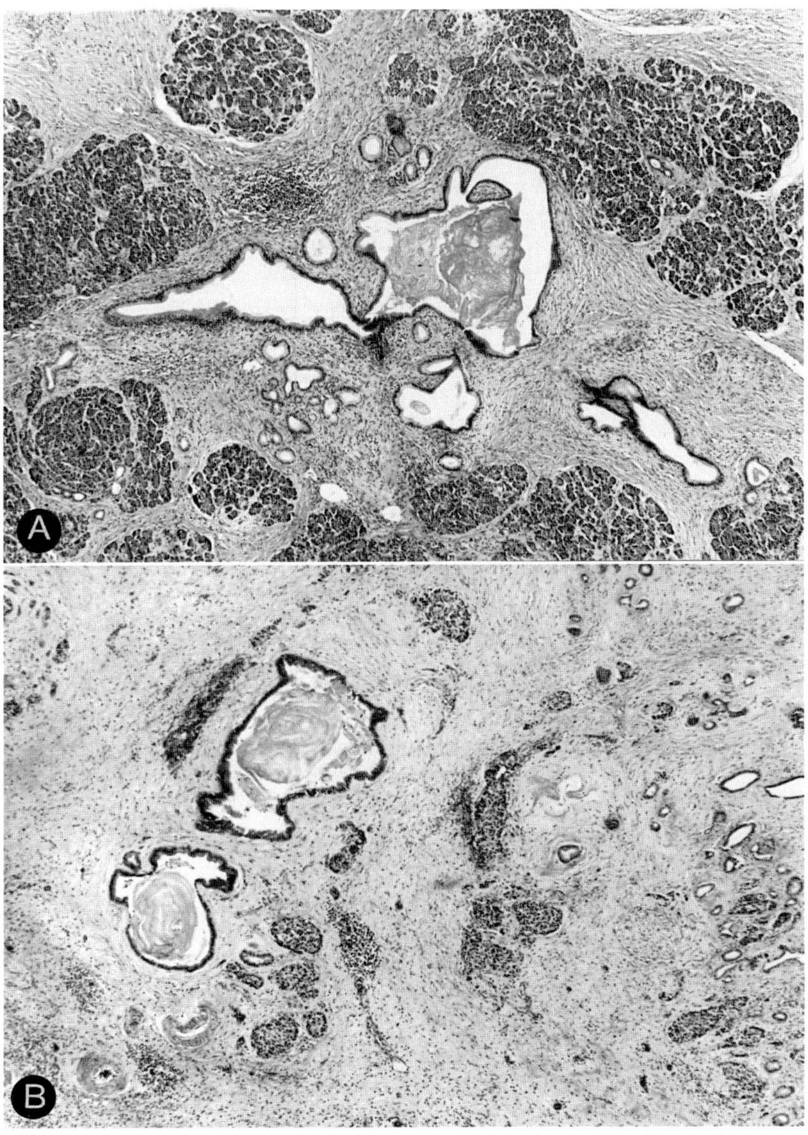


**FIG. 31.2.** Alcoholic chronic pancreatitis, advanced stage. **A.** Extensive perilobular fibrosis and distorted interlobular duct containing a protein plug. **B.** Diffuse fibrosis, distorted ducts with calculi, groups of small ducts and aggregates of islets. H & E, ×60.

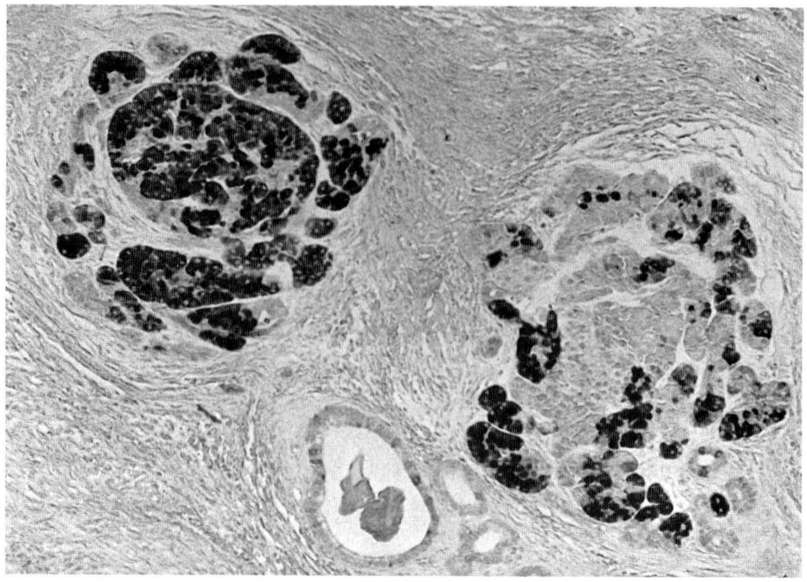

**FIG. 31.3.** Alcoholic chronic pancreatitis. Remnants of acinar lobuli embedded in fibrous tissue. The acinar cells stain strongly for α-amylase, ×120.

alpha (TGFα), c-erb B-2, TGFß, and fibroblast growth factor (FGF) (31, 32, 46–49). The lymphocytic infiltrate consists largely of T lymphocytes (46, 47). The remaining acinar cells stain brightly for pancreatic enzymes (Fig. 31.3) and PSP (50, 51). The nerves that appear enlarged express CGRP and substance P (52). Both the endothelial cells and endocrine beta and alpha cells show strong endothelin-1 expression in chronic pancreatitis (53).

**Complications.** Persistent stenosis of the bile duct develops in approximately 10% of cases (54), duodenal stenosis in about 3% (42). These complications are due to either intensive scarring or the development of a pseudocyst in the head of the pancreas.

Pseudocysts are found in 30–50% of patients with chronic pancreatitis (24, 26). They usually have a thick wall that consists of granulation and fibrous tissue and lacks an epithelial lining (24). Identical features are observed in pseudocysts associated with acute pancreatitis. Pseudocysts are usually connected with the ductal system and are therefore rich in pancreatic enzymes. They may expand and exert pressure on the surrounding organs. Further complications are fistulas into the pleura, leakage of pancreatic juice into the peritoneal cavity (pancreatic ascites), or hemorrhages from eroded vessels into the cysts and the pancreatic ductal system. Pancreatic stents inserted into the duct for the treatment of chronic pancreatitis can cause changes in the ductal system that may aggravate the chronic pancreatitis they are treating (55, 56).

With increasing fibrosis of the pancreas, the patients develop exocrine and endocrine insufficiency (26). Exocrine insufficiency results in maldigestion, which usually becomes obvious after 80–90% of the parenchyma has been replaced by fibrosis. The incidence of diabetes increases with the duration and severity of chronic pancreatitis (26).

Whether chronic pancreatitis involves an increased risk for the development of pancreatic carcinoma has been a controversial issue for years. It now appears that patients with chronic pancreatitis, particularly if they have the hereditary form (57), have a higher risk of developing pancreatic carcinoma than the normal population (58, 59).

### Pathology of Nonalcoholic Chronic Pancreatitis

**Hereditary Chronic Pancreatitis.** Since cases of hereditary chronic pancreatitis with morphologic data are limited, little is known about its pathologic features. It seems, however, that advanced disease is characterized by massive dilatation of the major and minor ducts, with occasional calculi. In addition, there may be pseudocysts (60). Histologically, there is extensive perilobular fibrosis, with some intralobular fibrosis and loss of the glandular parenchyma. It has been suggested that the dilatation of the ducts is inherited in the form of a structural or anatomic defect of the sphincter of Oddi (61).

**Autoimmune Chronic Pancreatitis.** Chronic pancreatitis associated with autoimmune diseases such as autoimmune sialadenitis, primary sclerosing cholangitis, or idiopathic inflammatory bowel disease has been described in a few patients (62–70). Recently, this type of chronic pancreatitis was also observed in patients with idiopathic chronic pancreatitis (71). The pancreatic changes are characterized by an intense mononuclear inflammation around interlobular ducts, leading to periductal fibrosis and occasionally ductal destruction (Fig. 31.4). In some cases, the inflammation also involves the intrapancreatic segment of the bile duct. The ductal lesions may resemble those seen in the liver in primary sclerosing cholangitis or the salivary glands in autoimmune sialadenitis (Sjögren's syndrome). We termed this type of pancreatic inflammation *chronic duct-destructive pancreatitis* (71). Clinically and macroscopically this disease may be mistaken for carcinoma. To date not much is known about its course and outcome.

**Idiopathic Chronic Pancreatitis.** Idiopathic chronic pancreatitis is a form of chronic pancreatitis that so far is only defined clinically (72). It can be divided into an early-onset type, which occurs within the first 2 decades of life, and a late-onset form. The disease affects both genders equally. It leads less frequently to calcifications (7). The morphologic substrate of idiopathic chronic pancreatitis has not yet been systematically studied. It appears, however, that a number of cases show pancreatic changes similar to those described in association with autoimmune diseases (see above).

**Tropical Pancreatitis.** The morphology of tropical pancreatitis at an early stage is not known. At an advanced stage, it appears to be macroscopically and microscopically indistinguishable from alcoholic chronic pancreatitis (73).

**Secondary Chronic Pancreatitis.** Obstructive chronic pancreatitis is due to focal obstruction of the main pancreatic duct leading to ductal dilatation proximal (upstream) to the stenosis and to fibrous atrophy of the acinar cells. The most common cause of ductal obstruction is a tumor in the head of the pancreas. Morphologically, the main difference between alcoholic chronic pancreatitis and obstructive chronic pancreatitis is a more generalized involvement of the gland in the obstructive type. Moreover, there usually is no formation of calculi in the dilated ductal system.

**Chronic Pancreatitis due to Duodenal Wall Cysts.** Chronic pancreatitis due to cysts of the duodenal wall or pancreas divisum shows a special pattern of changes. Cysts of the duodenal wall are rare lesions occurring either singly or multiply in the submucosal or intramuscular layers of the duodenum in close proximity to the ampulla of Vater and the intrapancreatic portion of the common bile duct. Chronic inflammation of the cysts may lead to stenosis of the common bile duct because of chronic inflammatory changes in the surrounding pancreatic tissue (74–76).

**Pancreas Divisum Pancreatitis.** Pancreas divisum connotes the situation in which the duct of Wirsung and the duct of Santorini remain separated, and the duct of Santorini drains the body and tail of the pancreas. This congenital defect is found in about 6% of an unselected population, but chronic pancreatitis develops in only a small percentage of them (77, 78). It is therefore not clear whether the pancreas divisum constellation predisposes to chronic pancreatitis. However, in individuals with a pancreas divisum who develop chronic pancreatitis, the disease involves exclusively the portion of the gland that is derived embryologically from the dorsal anlage. This suggests that relative obstruction at the accessory (minor) papilla causes acute and later chronic inflammation and fibrosis in the part of the pancreas drained by the dorsal duct.

**Pancreatic Fibrosis without the Clinical Symptoms of Chronic Pancreatitis.** Pancreatic lobular fibrosis, often combined with some degree of lipomatosis, is a frequent finding in elderly persons (79). Its intensity increases with age. Typically, fibrosis is restricted to a few lobules, whose draining ducts show obstructive changes, such as ductal papillary hyperplasia with prestenotic duct dilatation (80). This association suggests that lobular fibrosis in elderly persons results from obstruction of small peripheral ducts by hyperplastic changes in the ductal epithelium. The occurrence of small calculi in single secondary ducts of pancreases from elderly persons also seems to be related to the obstructive duct changes (81). The latter observations are of particular interest for the pathogenesis of calculus formation (pancreatic lithiasis) in the pancreas.

**Pancreatic Fibrosis Related to Hemochromatosis or Diabetes.** In primary hemochromatosis, the pancreas may be harder than normal and brown. Histologically, large quantities of iron are deposited in the acinar and ductal cells, as well as in islet beta cells and interstitial cells. This is accompanied by diffuse

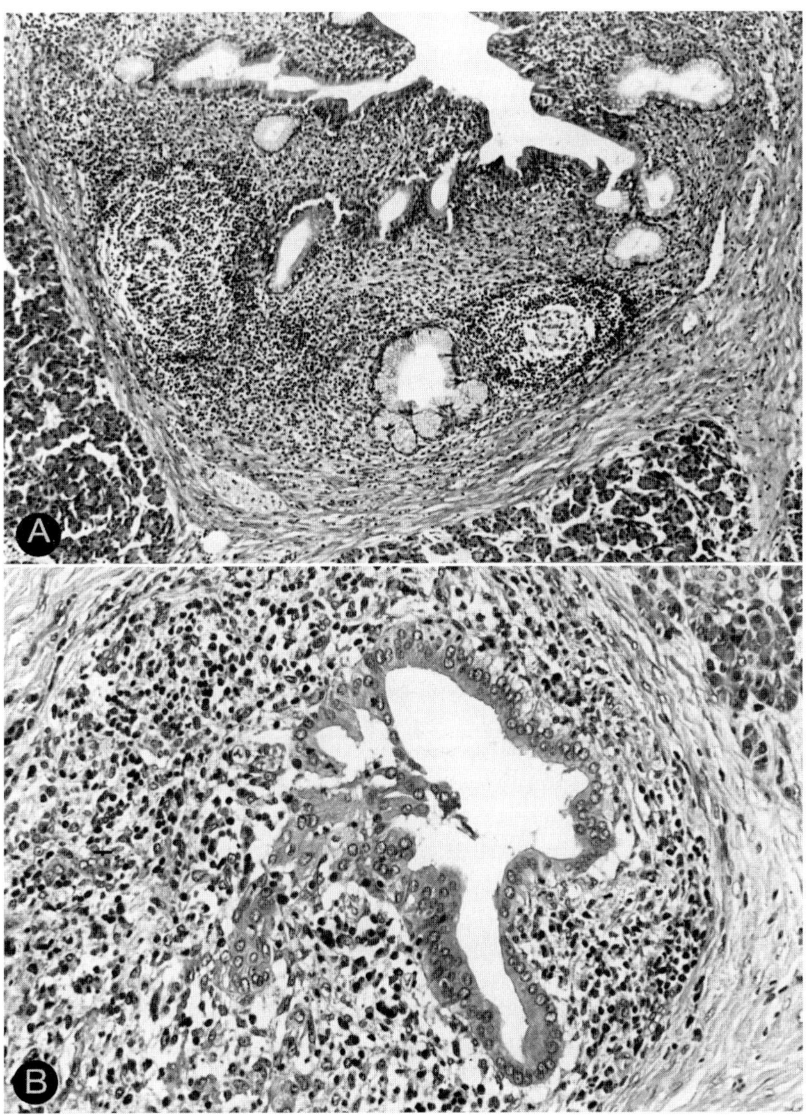


**FIG. 31.4.** Chronic duct-destructive pancreatitis. **A.** Interlobular duct encased by lymphocytic infiltrate showing lymph follicles, H & E, ×60. **B.** Inflammatory destruction of the duct epithelium. H & E, ×120.

fine intralobular (periacinar) fibrosis (82). Although fibrosis may be extensive, exocrine pancreatic insufficiency is not observed.

In longstanding insulin-dependent diabetes mellitus (IDDM), the pancreas is usually much smaller than in normal subjects. This is due to atrophy of the acinar cells, which is attributed to the missing trophic effects of insulin from beta cells. Acinar atrophy in IDDM is commonly associated with diffuse intralobular fibrosis and a sparse lymphocytic infiltrate. These changes may lead to reduced secretion of pancreatic enzymes but do not cause overt pancreatic insufficiency.

**Eosinophilic Pancreatitis.** Eosinophilic infiltration of the pancreas has been reported in a few patients with eosinophilic gastroenteritis (76, 83), idiopathic hypereosinophilic syndrome (84), and Baroquer-Simon's progressive lipodystrophy (85). The described changes consist of a focal infiltration of the pancreas by eosinophils and plasma cells, with destruction and fibrosis of the involved parenchyma.

**Graft-versus-Host Disease.** In graft-versus-host disease, marked ductal changes with lymphocytic infiltration, ductal ulceration, and intraluminal hemorrhage have been observed (86, 87).

**Pancreatitis in Miscellaneous Conditions and in Children.** Sarcoidosis may (rarely) involve the pancreas and lead to fibrosis in the vicinity of epithelioid granulomas (88). Malacoplakia has been described in association with chronic pancreatitis (89). In the acquired immunodeficiency syndrome (AIDS), the pancreas may be affected by opportunistic infections, such as cytomegalovirus (CMV) (90, 91). Radiation injury to the pancreas has been very rarely reported (92, 93). Most affected patients had undergone abdominal radiotherapy for Hodgkin's or non-Hodgkin's lymphoma and had a long delay between radiotherapy and the occurrence of chronic pancreatitis. Morphologically, the pancreas showed severe fibrosis with massive ductal dilatation and vascular changes but rarely calcifications. Chronic pancreatitis in childhood is rare (94). Most often it is of the hereditary or idiopathic form, the pathogenesis of which is obscure (see Etiology and Hereditary Pancreatitis). Other causes of chronic pancreatitis in childhood are malnutrition (see Tropical Pancreatitis), viral infections, or trauma. Severe abdominal trauma may involve the pancreas, leading to hematoma and/or disruption of the pancreatic ducts or parenchyma. Complications of such trauma are pseudocysts, fistulas, and ductal strictures leading to pancreatitis (95).

## REFERENCES


1. Mössner J. Epidemiology of chronic pancreatitis. In: Beger HG, Büchler M, Malfertheiner P, eds. Standards in pancreatic surgery. Berlin: Springer-Verlag, 1993:263–271.
2. Worning H. Incidence and prevalence of chronic pancreatitis. In: Beger HG, Büchler M, Ditschuneit H, Malfertheiner P, eds. Chronic pancreatitis. Berlin: Springer-Verlag, 1990:8–14.
3. Ammann RW, Akovbiantz A, Largiader F, Schueler G. Course and outcome of chronic pancreatitis. Longitudinal study of a mixed medical-surgical series of 245 patients. Gastroenterology 1984; 86:820–828.
4. Durbec JP, Sarles H. Multicenter survey on the etiology of pancreatic diseases. Relationship between the relative risk of developing chronic pancreatitis and alcohol, protein, and lipid consumption. Digestion 1978;18:337–350.
5. Worning H. Chronic pancreatitis: pathogenesis, natural history and conservative treatment. Clin Gastroenterol 1984;13:871–894.
6. Layer P, Singer MV. Non-alcohol-related etiologies in chronic pancreatitis. In: Beger HG, Büchler M, Ditschuneit H, Malfertheiner P, eds. Chronic pancreatitis. Berlin: Springer-Verlag, 1990:35–40.
7. Layer P, Yamamoto H, Kalthoff L, Clain JE, Bakken LJ, DiMagno EP. The different courses of early- and late-onset idiopathic and alcoholic chronic pancreatitis. Gastroenterology 1994;107:1481–1487.
8. Whitcomb DC, Preston RA, Aston CE, et al. A gene for hereditary pancreatitis maps to chromosome 7q35. Gastroenterology 1996; 110:1975–1980.
9. Pitchumoni CS, Glasser M, Saran RM, Panchacharam P, Thelmo W. Pancreatic fibrosis in chronic alcoholics and non-alcoholics without clinical pancreatitis. Am J Gastroenterol 1984;79:382–388.
10. Balaji LN, Tandon RK, Tandon BN, Banks PA. Prevalence and clinical features of chronic pancreatitis in southern India. Int J Pancreatol 1994;15:29–34.
11. Dreiling DA, Koller M. The natural history of alcoholic pancreatitis: update 1985. Mt Sinai J Med 1985;52:340–342.
12. Suda K, Takase M, Takei K, Nakamura T, Akai J, Nakamura T. Histopathologic study of coexistent pathologic states in pancreatic fibrosis in patients with chronic alcohol abuse: two distinct pathologic fibrosis entities with different mechanisms. Pancreas 1996;12:369–372.
13. Sarles H, Payan H, Tasso F, Sahel J. Chronic pancreatitis, relapsing pancreatitis, calcification of the pancreas. In: Bockus HL, ed. Gastroenterology. Philadelphia: WB Saunders, 1976:1040–1051.
14. Multigner I, Sarles H, Lombardo D, de Caro A. Pancreatic stone protein II: implication in stone formation during the course of chronic calcifying pancreatitis. Gastroenterology 1985;89: 387–391.
15. Sarles H, Bernard JP, Gullo L. Pathogenesis of chronic pancreatitis. Gut 1990;31:629–632.
16. Sarles H, Muratore R, Sarles JC, et al. Aetiology and pathology of chronic pancreatitis. In: Sarles H, ed. Pancreatitis (Bibliotheca Gastroenterologica no. 7). Basel: Karger, 1965:75–120.
17. Schmiegel W, Burchert M, Kalthoff H, et al. Immunochemical characterization and quantitative distribution of pancreatic stone protein in sera and pancreatic secretions in pancreatic disorders. Gastroenterology 1990;99:1421–1430.
18. Schmiegel W. PSP, PTP, or REG protein? The role of pancreatic stone protein. In: Beger HG, Büchler M, Malfertheiner P, eds. Standards in pancreatic surgery. Berlin: Springer-Verlag, 1993: 281–289.
19. Hayakawa T, Naruse S, Kitagawa M, et al. Pancreatic stone protein and lactoferrin in human pancreatic juice in chronic pancreatitis. Pancreas 1995;10:137–142.
20. Seligson U, Cho JW, Ihre I, Lundh G. Clinical course and autopsy findings in acute and chronic pancreatitis. Acta Chir Scand 1982;148:269–274.
21. Renner IG, Savage WT, Pantoja JL, Renner VJ. Death due to acute pancreatitis. A retrospective analysis of 405 autopsy cases. Dig Dis Sci 1985;30:1005–1018.
22. Klöppel G, Dreyer T, Willemer S, Kern HF, Adler G. Human acute pancreatitis: its pathogenesis in the light of immunocytochemical and ultrastructural findings in acinar cells. Virchows Arch (A) Pathol Anat 1986;409:791–803.
23. Marks IN, Bornman PC. Acute alcoholic pancreatitis: a South African view point. In: Bradley EL, III, ed. Acute pancreatitis. New York: Raven Press, 1994:271–277.
24. Klöppel G, Maillet B. Pseudocysts in chronic pancreatitis: a morphological analysis of 57 resection specimens and 9 autopsy pancreata. Pancreas 1991;6:266–274.
25. Uys CJ, Bank S, Marks IN. The pathology of chronic pancreatitis in Cape Town. Digestion 1973;9:454–468.
26. Ammann RW, Heitz PU, Klöppel G. Course of alcoholic chronic pancreatitis: a prospective clinicomorphological long-term study. Gastroenterology 1996;111:224–231.
27. Comfort MW, Gambill EE, Baggenstoss AH. Chronic relapsing pancreatitis. A study of 29 cases without associated disease of the biliary or gastrointestinal tract. Gastroenterology 1946;6:239–285, 376–408.
28. Klöppel G, Maillet B. Pathology of acute and chronic pancreatitis. Pancreas 1993;8:659–670.
29. Ammann RW, Muellhaupt B. Progression of alcoholic acute to chronic pancreatitis. Gut 1994;35:552–556.
30. Klöppel G, Maillet B. The morphological basis for the evolution of acute pancreatitis into chronic pancreatitis. Virchows Arch (A) Pathol Anat 1992;420:1–4.
31. van Laethem JL, Devière J, Resibois A, et al. Localizing of transforming growth factor b1 and its latent binding protein in human chronic pancreatitis. Gastroenterology 1995;108:1873–1881.
32. Korc M, Friess H, Yamanaka Y, Kobrin MS, Buchler M, Beger HG.

Chronic pancreatitis is associated with increased concentrations of epidermal growth factor receptor, transforming growth factor α, and phospholipase C gamma. Gut 1994;35:1468–1473.
33. Tabata T, Fujimoro T, Maeda S, Yamamoto M, Saitoh Y. The role of *ras* mutation in pancreatic cancer, precancerous lesions, and chronic pancreatitis. Int J Pancreatol 1993;14:237–244.
34. DiMagno EP, Layer P, Clain JE. Chronic pancreatitis. In: Go VLW, DiMagno EP, Gardner JD, Lebenthal E, Reber HA, Scheele GA, eds. The pancreas: biology, pathobiology, and disease. New York: Raven Press, 1993:665–706.
35. Bank S. Chronic pancreatitis: clinical features and medical management. Am J Gastroenterol 1986;81:153–167.
36. Bordalo O, Bapista A, Dreiling D, Noronha M. Early pathomorphological pancreatic changes in chronic alcoholism. In: Gyr KE, Singer MV, Sarles H, eds. Pancreatitis—concepts and classification. Amsterdam: Elsevier (Exerpta Medica, International Congress series no. 642), 1984.
37. Noronha M, Bordalo O, Dreiling DA. Alcohol and the pancreas. II. Pancreatic morphology of advanced alcoholic pancreatitis. Am J Gastroenterol 1981;76:120–124.
38. Braganza JM. Pancreatic disease: a casualty of hepatic "detoxification"? Lancet 1983;ii:1000–1003.
39. Bradley EL, III. Pseudocysts in chronic pancreatitis: development and clinical implications. In: Beger HG, Büchler M, Ditschuneit H, Malfertheiner P, eds. Chronic pancreatitis. Berlin: Springer-Verlag, 1990:260–268.
40. Ammann RW, Muench R, Otto R, Buehler H, Freiburghaus AU, Siegenthaler W. Evolution and regression of pancreatic calcification in chronic pancreatitis. A prospective long-term study of 107 patients. Gastroenterology 1988;95:1018–1028.
41. Howard JM, Nedwich A. Correlation of the histologic observations and operative findings in patients with chronic pancreatitis. Surg Gynecol Obstet 1971;132:387–395.
42. Gullo L, Costa PL, Labò G. Chronic pancreatitis in Italy. Aetiological, clinical and histological observations based on 253 cases. Rend Gastroenterol 1977;9:97–104.
43. Bockman DE, Boydston WR, Anderson MC. Origin of tubular complexes in human chronic pancreatitis. Am J Surg 1982;144: 243–249.
44. Bockman DE, Büchler M, Malfertheiner P, Beger HG. Analysis of nerves in chronic pancreatitis. Gastroenterology 1988;94:1459–1469.
45. Klöppel G, Bommer G, Commandeur G, Heitz PU. The endocrine pancreas in chronic pancreatitis. Immunocytochemical and ultrastructural studies. Virchows Arch (A) Pathol Anat 1978;377: 157–174.
46. Bedossa P, Bacci J, Lemaigre G, Martin E. Lymphocyte subsets and HLA-DR expression in normal pancreas and chronic pancreatitis. Pancreas 1990;5:415–420.
47. Jalleh RP, Gilbertson JA, Williamson RC, Slater SD, Foster CS. Expression of major histocompatibility antigens in human chronic pancreatitis. Gut 1993;34:1452–1457.
48. Friess H, Yamanaka Y, Büchler M, et al. A subgroup of patients with chronic pancreatitis overexpress the c-erb B-2 protooncogene. Ann Surg 1994;220:183–192.
49. Friess H, Yamanaka Y, Büchler M, et al. Increased expression of acidic and basic fibroblast growth factors in chronic pancreatitis. Am J Pathol 1994;144:117–128.
50. Klöppel G, Dreyer T, Willemer S, Kern HF, Adler G. Human acute pancreatitis: its pathogenesis in the light of immunocytochemical and ultrastructural findings in acinar cells. Virchows Arch (A) Pathol Anat 1986;409:791–803.
51. Lechene de la Porte P, de Caro A, Lafont H, Sarles H. Immunocytochemical localization of pancreatic stone protein in the human digestive tract. Pancreas 1986;1:301–308.
52. Büchler M, Weihe D, Friess H, et al. Changes in peptidergic innervation in chronic pancreatitis. Pancreas 1992;7:183–192.
53. Kakugawa Y, Giaid A, Yanagisawa M, et al. Expression of endothelin-1 in pancreatic tissue of patients with chronic pancreatitis. J Pathol 1996;178:78–83.
54. Yadegar J, Williams RA, Passaro E Jr, Wilson SE. Common duct stricture from chronic pancreatitis. Arch Surg 1980;115:582–586.
55. Kozarek RA. Pancreatic stents can induce ductal changes consistent with chronic pancreatitis. Gastrointest Endosc 1990; 36:93–95.
56. Sherman S, Alvarez C, Robert M, Ashley SW, Reber HA, Lehman GA. Polyethylene pancreatic duct stent-induced changes in the normal dog pancreas. Gastrointest Endosc 1993;39:658–664.
57. Pour PM. Is there a link between chronic pancreatitis and pancreatic cancer? In: Beger HG, Büchler M, Ditschuneit H, Malfertheiner P, eds. Chronic pancreatitis. Berlin: Springer-Verlag, 1990–106–112.
58. Lowenfels AB, Maisonneuve P, Cavallini G, et al. Pancreatitis and the risk of pancreatic cancer. N Engl J Med 1993;328:1433–1437.
59. Sgambati SA, Lawton GP, Modlin IM. Chronic pancreatitis: a precursor to pancreatic carcinoma? Dig Surg 1994;11: 275–285.
60. Konzen KM, Perrault J, Moir C, Zinsmeister AR. Long-term follow-up of young patients with chronic hereditary or idiopathic pancreatitis. Mayo Clin Proc 1993;68:449–453.
61. Malik SA, van Kley H, Knight WA Jr. Inherited defect in hereditary pancreatitis. Am J Dig Dis 1977;22:999–1004.
62. Ball WP, Baggenstoss AH, Bargen JA. Pancreatic lesions associated with chronic ulcerative colitis. Arch Pathol 1950;50:347–358.
63. Waldram R, Kopelman H, Tsantoulas D, Williams R. Chronic pancreatitis, sclerosing cholangitis, and sicca complex in two siblings. Lancet 1975;550–552.
64. Lászik GZ, Pap A, Farkas G. A case of primary sclerosing cholangitis mimicking chronic pancreatitis. Int J Pancreatol 1988;3:503–508.
65. Kawagushi K, Koike M, Tsuruta K, Okamoto A, Tabata I, Fukita N. Lymphoplasmacytic sclerosing pancreatitis with cholangitis: a variant of primary sclerosing cholangitis extensively involving pancreas. Hum Pathol 1991;22:387–395.
66. Sjögren I, Wengle B, Korsgren M. Primary sclerosing cholangitis associated with fibrosis of the submandibular glands and the pancreas. Acta Med Scand 1979;205:139–141.
67. Marrano D, Gullo L, Casadei T, Santini D, Leone O, Campione O. An unusual case of chronic pancreatitis of possible immune origin. Letter to the editor. Pancreas 1996;12:202–213.
68. Sood S, Fossard DP, Shorrock K. Chronic sclerosing pancreatitis in Sjögren's syndrome: a case report. Pancreas 1995;10:419–421.
69. Lysy J, Goldin E. Pancreatitis in ulcerative colitis. J Clin Gastroenterol 1992;15:336–339.
70. Seyrig JA, Jian R, Modigliani R, et al. Idiopathic pancreatitis as associated with inflammatory bowel disease. Dig Dis Sci 1985;30: 1121–1126.
71. Ectors N, Maillet B, Aerts R, et al. Non-alcoholic duct-destructive chronic pancreatitis. Gut 1997, in press.
72. Ammann RW, Buehler H, Muench R, Freiburghaus AU, Siegenthaler W. Differences in the natural history of idiopathic (nonalcoholic) and alcoholic chronic pancreatitis. A comparative long-term study of 287 patients. Pancreas 1987;2:368–377.
73. Viswanathan M. Pancreatic diabetes in India: an overview. In: Podolsky S, Viswanathan M, eds. Secondary diabetes: the spectrum of the diabetic syndromes. New York: Raven Press, 1980:105–116.
74. Stolte M, Weiss W, Volkholz H, Rösch W. A special form of segmental pancreatitis: "groove pancreatitis." Hepatogastroenterology 1982;29:198–208.
75. Stolte M, Zink W, Schaffner O. Duodenalwandzysten und Erkrankungen der Bauchspeicheldrüsen. Leber Magen Darm 1983;13:140–149.
76. Flejou JF, Potet F, Molas G, Bernades P, Amouyal P, Fekete F. Cystic dystrophy of the gastric and duodenal wall developing in heterotopic pancreas: an unrecognized entity. Gut 1993;34: 343–347.
77. Cotton PB. Pancreas divisum. Pancreas 1988;3:245–247.
78. Warshaw AL, Simeone JF, Schapiro RH, Flavin-Warshaw B. Evaluation and treatment of the dominant dorsal duct syndrome. Am J Surg 1990;159:59–66.
79. Olsen TS. The incidence and clinical relevance of chronic inflammation in the pancreas in autopsy material. Acta Pathol Microbiol Scand Sect A 1978;86:361–365.
80. Schmitz-Moormann P, Hein J. Changes of the pancreatic duct system associated with ageing. Virchows Arch (A) Pathol Anat 1976;371:145–152.
81. Nagai H, Ohtsubo K. Pancreatic lithiasis in the aged. Its clinicopathology and pathogenesis. Gastroenterology 1984;86: 331–338.

82. Suda K. Hemosiderin deposition in the pancreas. Arch Pathol Lab Med 1985;109:996–999.
83. Bastid C, Sahel J, Choux R, Payan MJ, Sarles H. Eosinophilic pancreatitis: report of a case. Pancreas 1990;5:104–107.
84. Eugene C, Gury B, Bergue A, Quevauvilliers J. Ictère révélant une atteinte pancréatique au cours d'un syndrome hyperéosinophilique idiopathique. Gastroenterol Clin Biol 1984;8: 966–969.
85. Smith PM, Morgan ME, Clark GC, Lennard-Jones JE, Gunnlaugsson O, Jonasson TA. Lipodystrophy, pancreatitis and eosinophilia. Gut 1975;16:230–234.
86. Foulis AK, Marquharson MA, Sale GE. The pancreas in acute graft *versus* host disease in man. Histopathology 1989;14:121–128.
87. Washington K, Gossage DL, Gottfried MR. Pathology of the pancreas in severe combined immunodeficiency and DiGeorge syndrome: acute graft-versus-host disease and unusual viral infections. Hum Pathol 1994;25:908–914.
88. Friedman HZ, Weinstein RA. Sarcoidosis of the pancreas. Arch Intern Med 1983;143:2182–2183.
89. Zuk RJ, Neal JW, Baithun SI. Malakoplakia of the pancreas. Virchows Arch (A) Pathol Anat 1990;417:181–184.
90. Hui AN, Koss MN, Meyer PR. Necropsy findings in the acquired immunodeficiency syndrome: a comparison of premortem diagnoses with postmortem findings. Hum Pathol 1984;15:670–676.
91. Kahn E, Anderson VM, Greco MA, Magid M. Pancreatic disorders in pediatric acquired immune deficiency syndrome. Hum Pathol 1995;26:765–770.
92. Lévy P, Menzelxhiu A, Paillot B, Bretagne JF, Fléjou JF, Bernades P. Abdominal radiotherapy is a cause for chronic pancreatitis. Gastroenterology 1993;105:905–909.
93. Schoonbroodt D, Zipf A, Herrmann G, Jung M. Histological findings in chronic pancreatitis after abdominal radiotherapy. Letter to the editor. Pancreas 1996;12:313–320.
94. Lewin-Smith MR, Dipalma JS, Hoy GR, Colon AR, Garvin DF. Chronic fibrosing pancreatitis in childhood: report of a case and literature review. Pediatr Pathol Lab Med 1996;16:681–690.
95. Carr ND, Cairns SJ, Lees WR, Russell RCG. Late complications of pancreatic trauma. Br J Surg 1989;76:1244–1246.

# 32

# Diagnosis of Chronic Pancreatitis

Peter Layer, Michael Rünzi, and Vay Liang W. Go

Despite remarkable technical advances in diagnostic procedures within the last decade, the diagnosis of chronic pancreatitis often remains difficult for two main reasons. First, it requires evidence of irreversible structural damage or functional impairment, yet it may take years or even decades before morphologic changes can be recognized or manifestation of exocrine or endocrine insufficiency can be detected. In contrast to most other organs, histologic evidence is usually unavailable to confirm or exclude the clinical suspicion. Second, chronic pancreatitis is characterized by a variable and often unpredictable clinical course, with dominant symptoms changing over time. Thus, most patients have intermittent or continuous pain or often recurrent attacks of acute pancreatitis for several years. For many, the severity and frequency of pain decrease over time, but it persists in a substantial proportion. In the course of this disease, exocrine and/or endocrine insufficiency may develop, but again for some patients, pancreatic function remains adequate for 20 or 30 years. On the other hand, a minority of patients have no, or only mild, pain and may present with symptoms of functional impairment as a primary symptom, a constellation frequently encountered in patients with late-onset idiopathic chronic pancreatitis, but also present in a small proportion of patients with alcoholic pancreatitis (1–3).

Generally, the diagnosis of chronic pancreatitis is easy when patients present in end-stage disease with characteristic morphologic changes or severe functional impairment, but it may be difficult or even impossible in patients presenting in early stages of the disease without such changes. A practical and rational diagnostic approach needs to be based on the primary presenting symptom. In a patient with pain and no evidence of steatorrhea, a sequence of imaging procedures is usually the most rational way to establish the diagnosis and exclude possible conditions such as pancreatic malignancy. On the other hand, in a patient with symptoms of steatorrhea, pancreatic function should be assessed and pancreatic insufficiency verified or excluded early in the diagnostic workup (Fig. 32.1).

The evaluation of a patient with suspected chronic pancreatitis should address several points (Table 32.1). The diagnosis of chronic pancreatitis must be established, and other differential diagnoses should be excluded, especially carcinoma of the pancreas. The latter is of particular importance, because carcinoma can mimic many clinical features of chronic pancreatitis, and its prevalence is increased in patients with longstanding chronic pancreatitis (4). Further, the cause of the disease (alcohol consumption, hyperparathyroidism, detection of hereditary forms of pancreatitis) should be determined so that it can be treated appropriately. Local complications of pancreatitis, such as pancreatic ductal strictures or pseudocysts, should be diagnosed early because they are potential causes of intractable pain and further complications, such as intestinal obstruction, sepsis, and hemorrhage, which may prompt additional surgery or other interventions. Finally, the severity of pancreatic functional impairment should be determined, and the efficacy of enzyme supplementation and treatment of diabetes should be assessed.

## CLINICAL FEATURES

In most patients, the earliest and dominant clinical symptom is abdominal pain, which may be severe, moderate, or mild. The pain is usually intermittent and may be elicited or aggravated by meals or consumption of alcohol. Many patients develop attacks of clinical pancreatitis. In patients with early-onset idiopathic pancreatitis, pain invariably is the leading symptom (2). It is often accompanied by weight loss, which in the early stages is more likely to be due to decreased food intake from postprandial pain rather than malabsorption. On the other hand, patients may present with signs of abnormal pancreatic exocrine and/or endocrine function, such as steatorrhea, diarrhea, diabetes mellitus and weight loss. In 5–10% of patients, these will be the primary symptoms of the disease, while in others, a history of longstanding, mild or nonspecific, abdominal pain may precede these symptoms.

Acute attacks of pancreatitis may or may not be accompanied by increased serum concentrations of pancreatic enzymes (amylase, lipase), and normal values do not exclude chronic pancreatitis. Overall, serum enzyme determinations are of limited value in the diagnosis of chronic pancreatitis, and pancreas-specific enzyme assays (pancreatic isoamylase, immunoreactive trypsin, and immunoreactive lipase) have also produced disappointing results (1, 5–7).

## IMAGING PROCEDURES

### Abdominal X-Ray

In addition to an x-ray of the chest, patients suspected of having chronic pancreatitis will usually have an abdominal roentgenogram. Plain films will detect pancreatic calcifications that are diagnostic of chronic pancreatitis in 30–70% of patients (1, 8–9). The median time from the onset of symptoms to the development of diagnostic features of chronic alcoholic pancreatitis is between 8 and 9 years (2). Calcifications are frequent in patients with chronic pancreatitis due to hyperparathyroidism. In contrast, calcifications develop rarely or very late in patients with idiopathic chronic pancreatitis. In the juvenile form, the median time from the onset of the initial symptoms of pancreatitis to the development of calcifications is about 25 years (2). Thus, the presence or absence of calcification may add a further clue regarding the etiology of pancreatitis.

### Ultrasound

Abdominal ultrasound may be useful in some patients with suspected pancreatic disease. Apart from calcifications, the echo pattern of the chronically inflamed pancreas may differ in texture and echogenicity from that of the normal pancreas. Moreover, ductal dilatation and calcification may be demonstrated. However, normal findings do not exclude chronic pancreatitis. The sensitivity and specificity of ultrasonography may reach 90% in the presence of advanced disease but is low (<50%) in early stages. Ultrasound can detect fluid collections, inflammatory masses, and other complications (10–12), but its primary role is the detection of gallstones, which may be a cause of acute pancreatitis.

### Computed Tomography (CT)

Primary findings in chronic pancreatitis are changes in pancreatic size and shape (focal or diffuse enlargement or atrophy), detection of calculi (with greater sensitivity than with conventional x-ray), and irregularities of the pancreatic ducts. The sensitivity of CT (like that of ultrasound) depends on the stage of the disease, varying between 70 and 90%, but it is higher than that of ultrasound. CT also has a high specificity of more than 95% (1).

### Endoscopic Retrograde Cholangiopancreatography (ERCP)

Whereas ultrasound and computed tomography are well suited for detecting mainly parenchymal, peripancreatic, and main duct changes, ERCP visualizes the entire ductal system. Chronic pancreatitis is considered a disease involving primarily the small ducts, which explains why ERCP may be more efficacious in detecting changes earlier than other imaging procedures. According to the classical criteria of Kasugai (13), the earliest changes in chronic pancreatitis occur in the ductal branches, which appear irregular, with dilated and narrowed segments. As the disease progresses, dilatation increases, leading to irregularities of the main pancreatic duct. In advanced pancreatitis, changes also involve the main pancreatic duct and include such major abnormalities as dilatation, strictures, and calculi. Sensitivity has been reported to be between 70 and 90%, and specificity from 90 to 100%. The major differential diagnoses are pancreatic carcinoma with proximal ductal dilatation, or pancreatic carcinoma that has developed in preexisting chronic pancreatitis (1, 14).

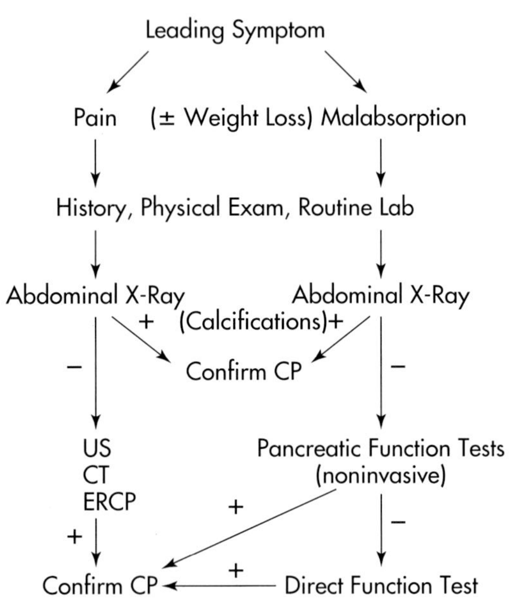


**FIG. 32.1.** Algorithm for diagnosis of chronic pancreatitis.

### Endoscopic Ultrasound (EUS)

The value of EUS, which allows high-resolution imaging of gastrointestinal organs and their immediate surroundings, has been proven for the diagnosis of pancreatic exocrine and endocrine tumors. However, in patients with chronic pancreatitis, the role of EUS has not yet been fully established, although sensitivity and specificity have been reported to reach 80 and 100%, respectively. EUS holds promise for the possible future detection of early chronic pancreatitis not presently diagnosable by conventional techniques (15–17). At present, its use is investigational, however.

### Other Methods

*Magnetic resonance imaging (MRI)* of the pancreas requires specialized sequences that diminish upper abdominal artifacts. Despite considerable technical progress, including the introduction of contrast media such as gadopentetate-dimeglumine (Gd-DTPH), the role of MRI in the diagnosis of chronic pancreatitis still needs to be further clarified.

*Echo-duplex-sonography* of the superior mesenteric artery has been suggested as helpful in chronic pancreatitis, but its value has not been proven (18).

## PANCREATIC FUNCTION TESTS

Function tests of the pancreas are described in detail in Chapter 11; their role in the diagnostic workup of patients with suspected chronic pancreatitis is briefly summarized below.

### Direct Function Test

The most precise method of determining pancreatic exocrine function is direct measurement of pancreatic enzyme output in response to a defined hormonal stimulus (usually a CCK analogue, such as cerulein, either alone or in combination with secretin). Without doubt this test has the highest sensitivity and specificity (both >90%), but because of its invasiveness and cost, it has been restricted to specialized institutions (1, 19). The same holds true for the Lundh test, which uses an endogenous rather

**TABLE 32.1. Diagnosis of Chronic Pancreatitis: Major Aims**

| Aim | Consequence |
|---|---|
| 1. Establish diagnosis | Exclude differential diagnoses, especially *cancer!* |
| 2. Determine etiology (alcohol, hypercalcemia, hereditary) | Remove or treat etiologic factors, assess course and prognosis, family workup |
| 3. Diagnose/exclude local complications (strictures, pseudocysts: potential causes of pain or further complications) | Determine indication for surgical or interventional treatment |
| 4. Stage severity of functional impairment and assess potential effect of treatment | Determine mode of conservative therapy |

than exogenous stimulus of pancreatic enzyme secretion and has a somewhat lower accuracy. Suspected chronic pancreatitis is the main indication for these tests, with ambiguous results in noninvasive tests and/or imaging procedures (Fig. 32.1).

### Fecal Tests

Examination of feces may serve two main purposes in the diagnostic workup of chronic pancreatitis: *(a)* measurement of increased fecal output of undigested substrates, resulting in steatorrhea and increased stool weight, and *(b)* measurement of decreased stool concentrations of pancreatic enzymes, such as chymotrypsin or, more recently, pancreas elastase-1.

**Stool Weight, Stool Lipids.** The combined measurement of daily cumulative stool weights collected on 3 consecutive days (while the patient takes a normal balanced diet) and of fecal weights and lipid concentrations allows determination of quantitative fecal lipid excretion. Whereas excretion of up to 7 g of lipid per day is normal, consistently greater quantities indicate steatorrhea and point to chronic pancreatitis as one of the major differential diagnoses. Additionally, the ratio between stool lipid and stool weight can be calculated. A fecal fat concentration below 10% suggests a nonpancreatic condition, and a ratio above 10% suggests a pancreatic origin of steatorrhea (20). Alternatively, qualitative fecal fat determination (concentration: grams of fat per gram of stool weight) has been reported to have nearly the same sensitivity as quantitative measurements (21). By contrast, determination of fecal nitrogen has a lower accuracy (1).

**Fecal Chymotrypsin.** Another simple diagnostic method is a colorimetric measurement of fecal chymotrypsin concentration. This enzyme is stable in stool for days, even at room temperature. The diagnostic accuracy in advanced pancreatitis is 70–90%, but not surprisingly, accuracy is low (<50%) in mild/early chronic pancreatitis. Moreover, the tests may produce false-positive results with other diseases associated with malabsorption (22–24).

**Pancreas Elastase-1.** Recently, fecal determination of human pancreas-specific elastase-1 has been proposed as another parameter to diagnose chronic pancreatitis. The advantages of this enzyme are its stability in feces, its specificity for humans (i.e., it can be used even in the presence of enzyme supplementation using porcine pancreatic extracts), and a higher diagnostic accuracy than other methods (25–30). However, the test is expensive and time consuming, and its superiority to other conventional tests has been questioned in recent studies (31–32). Overall, while determination of fecal pancreatic elastase has several theoretical advantages, its practical value needs to be further established.

### Noninvasive Pancreatic Function Tests

**Oral Function Tests.** Oral pancreatic function tests are widely used to assess pancreatic exocrine function indirectly. They are based on the recovery of substrate metabolites in urine or serum that are generated by, and correlated with, pancreatic enzyme actions in the intestinal lumen and with subsequent absorption. Two tests (namely, the NBT-PABA test and the pancreolauryl test) have been established and are described in detail in Chapter 11. Overall, both tests are reliable for detecting advanced exocrine pancreatic insufficiency but are of little predictive value in mild-to-moderate disease and in most patients with early-stage pancreatitis (33–34). Substantial impairment of intraluminal digestion occurs only after destruction of at least 90–95% of pancreatic parenchymal tissue (35), which explains the inability of these tests to detect early pancreatic insufficiency.

**Breath Test.** The exhaled concentration of labeled $CO_2$ correlates with digestion of a correspondingly labeled substrate in the intestinal lumen. Based on this principle, several breath tests have been developed for the detection of lipid malabsorption and maldigestion. For example, the triolein breath test, the cholesteryl octanoate breath test, and the mixed triglyceride breath test use either $^{14}C$ or $^{13}C$ as the isotope, respectively. Overall, most of these tests show results comparable with those of simple, noninvasive investigations, as described above, in severe disease and have similar difficulties in detecting earlier stages of exocrine insufficiency. So far, none of these tests has demonstrated any advantages over simpler tests, and they are expensive and time consuming.

A simpler test is the measurement of unlabeled hydrogen in expired breath in response to a rice starch test meal. This meal is virtually completely absorbed by normal subjects but produces increased breath hydrogen levels in the presence of starch maldigestion, with a sensitivity of about 70% (36). Other investigators have reported less favorable results (37), possibly because amylase activity has considerable stability in the intestinal lumen (38–39), and measurable starch malabsorption occurs only after disappearance of nearly all pancreatic amylase within the small intestine (40).

In summary, breath tests have not achieved a major role in the standard diagnostic workup of chronic pancreatitis.

**Other Tests.** The plasma amino acid consumption test has been suggested as a reliable noninvasive method to demonstrate exocrine pancreatic insufficiency (41–42). However, more recent studies have not confirmed its promising initial results (43–44).

### Endocrine Function Tests

Although diabetes mellitus is one of the key symptoms of end-stage chronic pancreatitis, and although abnormalities of endocrine pancreatic function are detected frequently in these patients, determination of these parameters is of little value in its diagnosis. In particular, blood glucose concentrations and glucose tolerance testing, as well as insulin and C-peptide plasma concentrations, may corroborate the diagnosis but, as sole findings, usually are not able to establish it (Table 32.2). Plasma pancreatic polypeptide (PP) is decreased in end-stage chronic pancreatitis (45) but has no advantage over simpler function tests in detecting early stages of chronic pancreatitis (19).

## PRACTICAL DIAGNOSTIC APPROACH IN PATIENTS WITH SUSPECTED CHRONIC PANCREATITIS

As mentioned above, history, clinical presentation, and major symptoms in patients with chronic pancreatitis can be very variable. Most patients will have pain as a leading symptom; a minority will present initially with symptoms of malabsorption and/or diabetes mellitus. Both presentations are frequently combined with a recent history of weight loss.

The basic diagnostic strategy includes a careful history and physical examination combined with basic imaging tests, such as abdominal x-rays and CT. In the absence of diagnostic calcifications, additional invasive imaging procedures should be performed, such as ERCP, if the clinical picture suggests abdominal pain of chronic pancreatitis.

If, on the other hand, the clinical constellation suggests malabsorption, a test revealing abnormal pancreatic function may establish the diagnosis of exocrine pancreatic insufficiency at an early stage. However, because of the pathophysiology of chronic pancreatitis, neither normal imaging tests nor normal tests of function can exclude the diagnosis (Fig. 32.1). In many cases, a variable combination of symptoms and findings has to be used to establish the diagnosis (Table 32.2).

**TABLE 32.2. Criteria for Chronic Pancreatitis**

| | Score if Present |
|---|---|
| Pancreatic calcification (x-ray, CT, ERCP) | 4 |
| Histology (chronic inflammation, fibrosis, calcification) | 4 |
| ERCP (typical duct changes, calculi) | 3 |
| Exocrine function (CCK test, fecal test) | 2 |
| Clinical symptoms/history (chronic upper abdominal pain, acute attacks of pancreatitis) | 2 |
| Endocrine function (diabetes mellitus) | 1 |
| Score ≥ 4: Chronic pancreatitis | |

From Layer P, Yamamoto H, Kalthoff L, et al. The different courses of early- and late-onset idiopathic and alcoholic chronic pancreatitis. Gastroenterology 1994;107:1481–1487, with permission.

## Acknowledgment

The authors express their gratitude to Ms. Anita M. Stein for her skillful editorial assistance and coordination of chapter submission.

## REFERENCES

1. Di Magno EP, Layer P, Clain JE. Chronic pancreatitis. In: Go VLW, et al., eds. The pancreas: biology, pathobiology, and diseases. 2nd ed. New York: Raven Press, 1993:665–706.
2. Layer P, Yamamoto H, Kalthoff L, Clain JE, Bakken LJ, DiMagno EP. The different courses of early- and late-onset idiopathic and alcoholic chronic pancreatitis. Gastroenterology 1994;107:1481–1487.
3. Ammann RW, Akovbiantz A, Largiader F, Schueler G. Course and outcome of chronic pancreatitis. Gastroenterology 1984;86: 820–828.
4. Lowenfels AB, Maisonneuve P, Cavallini G, Ammann RW, Lankisch PG, et al. and the International Pancreatitis Study Group. Pancreatitis and the risk of pancreatic cancer. N Engl J Med 1993;328:1433–1437.
5. Koop H. Serum levels of pancreatic enzymes and their clinical significance. In: Creutzfeld W, ed. Clinics in gastroenterology. London: WB Saunders, 1984:739–761.
6. Jacobsen DG, Curington C, Connery K, Toskes PP. Trypsin-like immunoreactivity as a test for pancreatic insufficiency. N Engl J Med 1984;31:1307–1308.
7. Ammann RW, Buehler H, Pei P. Comparative diagnostic accuracy for four tubeless pancreatic function tests in chronic pancreatitis. Scand J Gastroenterol 1982;17:997–1002.
8. Braganza JM, Hunt LP, Warwick F. Relationship between pancreatic exocrine function and ductal morphology in chronic pancreatitis. Gastroenterology 1982;82:1341–1347.
9. Valentini M, Cavallini G, Vantini I, et al. A comparative evaluation of endoscopic retrograde cholangiopancreatography and the secretin-cholecystokinin test in the diagnosis of chronic pancreatitis: a multicentre study in 124 patients. Endoscopy 1981;13: 64–67.
10. Swobodnik W, Meyer W, Brecht-Kraus D, et al. Ultrasound computed tomography and endoscopic retrograde cholangiopancreatography in the morphologic diagnosis of pancreatic disease. Klin Wochenschr 1983;61:291–296.
11. Gmelin E, Weiss HD, Fuchs HD, Reiser M. Vergleich der diagnostischen Treffsicherheit von Ultraschall, Computertomographie und ERCP bei der chronischen Pankreatitis und beim Pankreaskarzinom. Fortschr Rontgenstr 1981;134:136–141.
12. Hessel SJ, Siegelmann SS, McNeil BJ, et al. A prospective evaluation of computed tomography and ultrasound of the pancreas. Radiology 1982;143:129–133.
13. Kasugai T, Nobuyoshi K, Kizu M, Kobayaski S, Kattori K. Endoscopic pancreatocholangiography. Gastroenterology 1972;63: 227–234.
14. Buscail L, Escourrou J, Moreau J, Delvaux M, Louvel D, et al. Endoscopic ultrasonography in chronic pancreatitis: a comparative prospective study with conventional ultrasonography, computed tomography, and ERCP. Pancreas 1995;10:251–257.
15. Nattermann C, Goldschmidt AJW, Dancygier H. Endosonography in chronic pancreatitis. A comparison between endoscopic retrograde pancreatography and endoscopic ultrasonography. Endoscopy 1993;25:565–570.
16. Rösch T, Classen M. Endoscopic ultrasonography: an added advantage in pancreatic diagnosis? Schweiz Med Woschenschr 1993;123:1059–1068.
17. Giovannini M, Seitz JF. Endoscopic ultrasonography with a linear-type echoendoscope in the evaluation of 94 patients with pancreatobiliary disease. Endoscopy 1994;26:579–585.
18. Brambati M, Solmi L, Di-Stefano M, Gullo L, Gandolfi L. Echo-duplex evaluation of the superior mesenteric artery in chronic pancreatitis. Eur J Gastroenterol Hepatol 1994;6:617–620.
19. Malfertheiner P, Dominguez-Munoz JE, Büchler M. Diagnosis and staging of chronic pancreatitis. In: Beger HG, Büchler M, Malfertheiner P, eds. Standards in pancreatic surgery. Berlin: Springer-Verlag, 1993:297–313.
20. Bo-Linn GW, Fordtran JS. Fecal fat concentration in patients with steatorrhea. Gastroenterology 1984;87:319–322.
21. Newcomer AD, Hofmann AF, DiMagno EP, Thomas PJ, Carlson GL. Triolein breath test: a sensitive and specific test for fat malabsorption. Gastroenterology 1979;76:6–13.
22. Ammann RW, Akovbiantz A, Haecki W, Largiader F, Schmid M. Diagnostic value of the fecal chymotrypsin test in pancreatic insufficiency, particularly chronic pancreatitis: correlation with the pancreozymin-secretion test, fecal fat excretion and final clinical diagnosis. Digestion 1981;21:281–289.
23. Tympner F, Reiner TH, Domschke W. Pankreas-Funktionsanalyse. Chymotrypsin-Bestimmung im Stuhl und Sekretin-Pankreozymin Test. Eine vergleichende Untersuchung. Fortschr Med 1977;95: 1709–1750.
24. Lankisch PG, Schreiber A, Otto J. Pancreolauryl test. Evaluation of a tubeless pancreatic function test in comparison with other indirect and direct tests for exocrine pancreatic function. Dig Dis Sci 1983;28:490–493.
25. Stein J, Jung M, Zeuzem S, Lembcke B, Caspary W. Fecal elastase-1. A new tubeless test in the diagnosis of pancreatic insufficiency (Abstract). Gastroenterology 1994;106:A325.
26. Löser C, Molgaarda A, Folsch UR. Fecal elastase 1—an easy, inexpensive and highly sensitive and specific, tubeless routine test in pancreatic insufficiency (Abstract). Gut 1995;37:A140.
27. Katschinski M, Schirra J, Bross A, Arnold R, Göke B. Fecal concentration of pancreatic elastase-1 accurately indicates exocrine pancreatic insufficiency (Abstract). Gastroenterology 1994;106:A300.
28. Sziegoleit A, Krause E, Klör H, Kranacher L, Linder D. Elastase 1 and chymotrypsin B in pancreatic juice and feces. Clin Biochem 1989;22:85–89.
29. Scheefers-Borchel U, Scheefers H, Arnold R, Fischer P, Sziegoleit A. Pankreatische Elastase 1: Parameter für die chronische und akute Pankreatitis. Lab Med 1992;16:427–432.
30. Stein J, Jung M, Bienek U, Scheefers H, Lembcke B, Caspary WF. Fäkale Pankreas-Elastase 1 (E1). Ein neuer zuverlässiger Parameter zur Diagnose der exokrinen Pankreasinsuffizienz. Gastroenterology 1993;31:543.
31. Amann ST, Bishop M, Toskes PP. Fecal pancreatic elastase 1: is it the test we have been looking for? (Abstract). Gastroenterology 1995;108:A341.
32. Lankisch PG, Löhr M, König H, Schmidt I, Knollmann R, Liebe S. Fecal elastase-1: not helpful in diagnosing slight to moderate exocrine pancreatic insufficiency (Abstract). Pancreas 1995; 11(4):436.
33. Toskes PP. Bentiromide as a test of exocrine pancreatic function in adult patients with pancreatic exocrine insufficiency. Determination of appropriate dose and urinary collection interval. Gastroenterology 1983;85:565–569.
34. Malfertheiner P, Peter M, Junge U, Ditschuneit H. Indirect pancreatic function test pancreolauryl—its value in diagnosis of chronic pancreatitis. Klin Wochenschr 1983;61:193–198.
35. DiMagno EG, Go VLW, Summerskill WHJ. Relation between pancreatic enzyme outputs and malabsorption in severe pancreatic insufficiency. N Engl J Med 1973;288:813–815.

36. Kerlin P, Wong L, Harris B, Capra S. Rice flour, breath hydrogen and malabsorption. Gastroenterology 1984;87:578.
37. Hiele M, Ghoos Y, Rutgeerts P, Vantrappen G. Starch digestion in normal subjects and patients with pancreatic disease, using a $^{13}CO_2$ breath test. Gastroenterology 1989;96:503.
38. Layer P, Go VLW, DiMagno EP. Fate of pancreatic enzymes during aboral small intestinal transit in humans. Am J Physiol 1986;251: G475–G480.
39. Layer P, Jansen JBMJ, Cherian L, Lamers CBHW, Goebell H. Feedback regulation of human pancreatic secretion: effects of protease inhibition on duodenal delivery and small intestinal transit of pancreatic enzymes. Gastroenterology 1990;98:1311–1319.
40. Layer P, Zinsmeister AR, DiMagno EP. Effects of decreasing intraluminal amylase activity on starch digestion and postprandial gastrointestinal function in humans. Gastroenterology 1986; 91:41–48.
41. Domschke S, Heptner G, Kolb S, et al. Decrease in plasma amino acids level after secretin and pancreozymin as an indicator of exocrine pancreatic function. Gastroenterology 1986;90:1031–1038.
42. Gullo L, Pezzilli R, Ventrucci M, Barbara L. Caerulein induced plasma amino acid decrease: a simple, sensitive, and specific test of pancreatic function. Gut 1990;31:926–929.
43. Maringhini A, Nelson DK, Jones JD, DiMagno EP. Is the plasma amino acid consumption test an accurate test of exocrine pancreatic insufficiency? Gastroenterology 1994;106:488–493.
44. Lembcke B, Konle O, Duan LP, Caspary WF. Lack of accuracy of plasma α-amino nitrogen profiles as an indicator of exocrine pancreatic function both after continuous and bolus stimulation of the pancreas with secretin and cholecystokinin-pancreozymin. Z Gastroenterol 1994;32:679–683.
45. Adrian TE, Besterman HS, Mallinson CM, Caralotis C, Bloom SR. Impaired pancreatic polypeptide release in chronic pancreatitis with steatorrhea. Gut 1979;20:98–101.

# 33

# *Medical Management of Chronic Pancreatitis*

Jeffrey L. Barnett and Chung Owyang

Chronic pancreatitis is characterized by glandular damage resulting in pain and variable degrees of clinically important exocrine and endocrine dysfunction. The medical treatment of chronic pancreatitis consists primarily of pain control, correction of maldigestion, and management of glucose intolerance.

## PAIN MANAGEMENT

### The Natural Course of Pain

The great majority of patients with chronic pancreatitis complain of pain (1, 2). Patients with early-onset (age < 35 years) idiopathic chronic pancreatitis tend to present with pain as an initial symptom, and the pain tends to be of greater severity than that of those with late-onset (age > 35 years) idiopathic or alcoholic chronic pancreatitis (3). Long-term follow-up studies show that the number of pain-free patients with chronic pancreatitis increases over time, suggesting that pain may "burn out" after years of disease (1, 4). However, a recent study showed that although the total percentage of patients with pain attacks decreased, most alcoholics and nonalcoholics continued to complain of pain even after more than 10 years of follow-up (4). Pain improvement appears to correlate with worsening exocrine pancreatic insufficiency, especially in alcoholics (1, 4).

### Avoidance of Alcohol and Other Precipitants

Rarely, hyperparathyroidism, elevated triglycerides, and implicated drugs may cause or contribute to pancreatitis. It makes sense to eliminate these precipitants as possible causes of ongoing inflammation and pain. The same is true of alcohol, the most common cause of chronic pancreatitis. Alcohol may theoretically produce persistent pain by stimulating pancreatic secretion of an already compromised organ. Although some report that the pain of chronic alcoholic pancreatitis is reduced when patients stop drinking (1, 5, 6), others cannot confirm this (2, 7). Clearly, some continue to complain of pain even after years of abstinence. Perhaps alcohol acting as a secretagogue is more likely to induce pain in those with only moderately impaired pancreatic function, and those with end-stage disease are less likely to be affected (8). In any case, abstinence from alcohol should be strongly encouraged as a first step in the management of chronic pain.

To avoid "overstimulating" the diseased pancreas, a diet consisting of small meals containing modest amounts of fat and protein is usually advised. Acid-suppressing agents are sometimes prescribed to reduce the acid load delivered to the duodenum, which may theoretically reduce pancreatic stimulation by decreasing the release of secretin and cholecystokinin (CCK). Although these measures make some physiologic sense, their practical value in preventing pancreatic pain is unproven.

### Analgesics

Nonspecific pain control by use of analgesics remains the most common method of pain management, despite the use of more specific physiologic therapies such as pancreatic enzymes and octreotide. Initial agents should be restricted to salicylates, acetaminophen, or nonsteroidal antiinflammatory drugs. Those with moderate or severe pain who have failed these drugs may require narcotic analgesics. The need for pain relief in the compliant patient should outweigh the physician's natural reluctance to prescribe potentially addicting medications. Usually, analgesics should be given in anticipation of mealtime to prevent postprandial exacerbation of pain. Narcotic prescriptions should be carefully monitored so that the lowest effective dose can be determined and the chance of abuse minimized. The use of low-dose antidepressant medication may serve an adjunctive role to modulate pain and reduce overall analgesic use.

### Pancreatic Enzyme Therapy

Normal pancreatic enzyme secretion is subject to physiologic feedback regulation. The hormone CCK stimulates pancreatic enzyme secretion. Proteases, such as trypsin and chymotrypsin, secreted by the pancreas into the duodenal lumen eventually inhibit CCK, which, in turn, shuts off further enzyme secretion. Investigators have shown that exogenous administration of trypsin or chymotrypsin inhibits pancreatic enzyme secretion (9–13). Theoretically, patients with chronic pancreatitis produce decreased amounts of pancreatic proteases, which may cause elevated levels of CCK. Chronically elevated CCK levels may hyperstimulate the pancreas, producing ongoing or recurrent attacks of pain. Several, but not all, studies support this concept by documenting elevated CCK levels in patients with chronic pancreatitis (14–18). The practical application of this concept is that administration of oral pancreatic enzymes to these patients should reduce CCK levels, reduce chronic pancreatic hyperstimulation and intraductal pressures, and, ultimately, relieve pain (Figs. 33.1 and 33.2).

Clinical studies suggest this to be true. A 1-week, double-blinded, placebo-controlled study of 19 patients found a 30% reduction in pain during the enzyme-treated week (19). These findings were confirmed in a 1-month crossover design study in 20 patients (10). The best responses were seen in women, those with idiopathic rather than alcoholic pancreatitis, and those with only mild-to-moderate pancreatic insufficiency. Trials using enteric-coated tablets have shown mixed results. A 1-month, blinded trial allowing self-administration of pancreatic enzymes showed significant benefit, but another 1-month, double-blinded, crossover study revealed a trend toward, but no

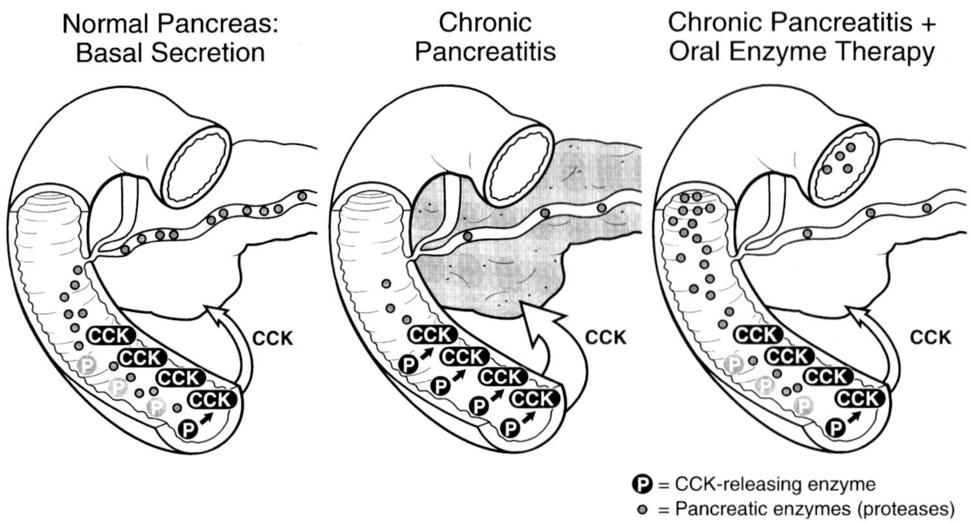


**FIG. 33.1.** Overview of the mechanism by which oral pancreatic enzyme therapy may reduce the pain of chronic pancreatitis.

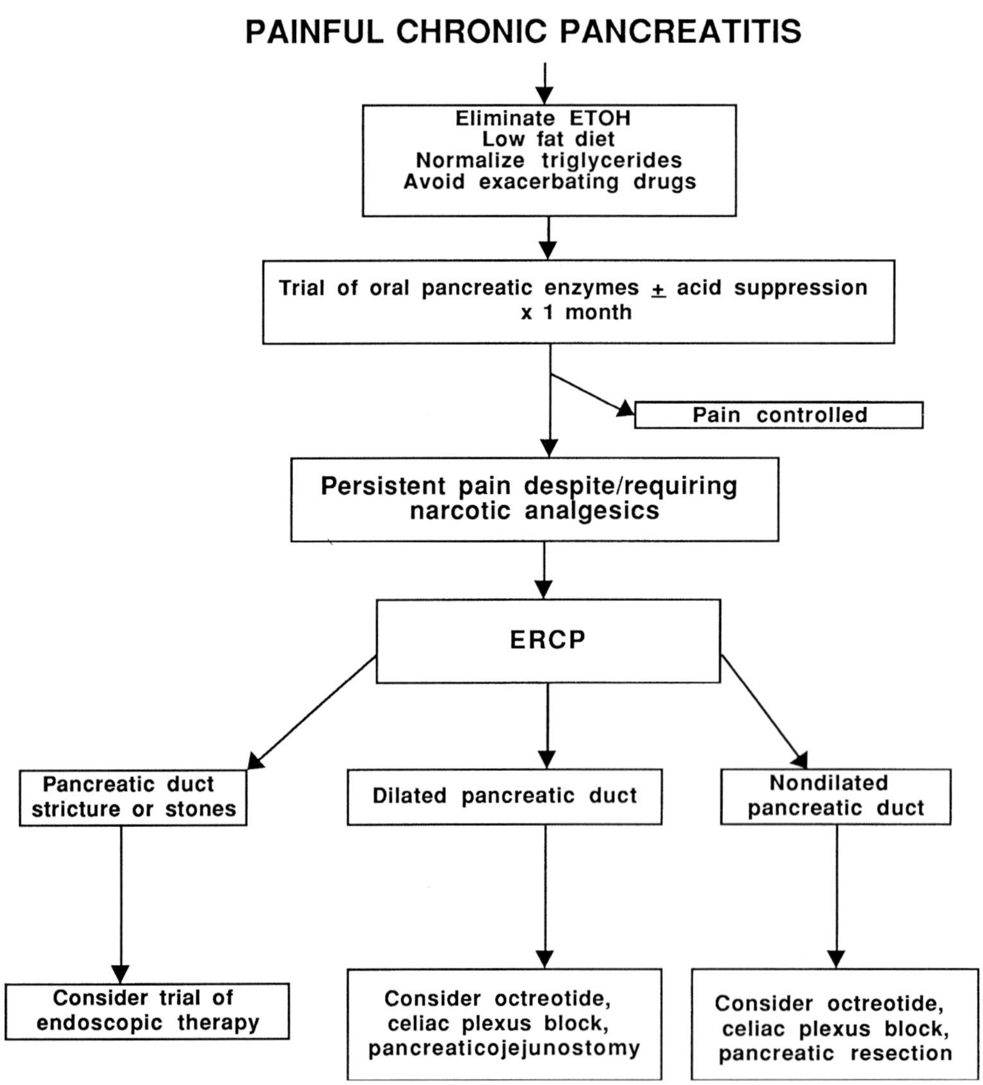


**FIG. 33.2.** Management algorithm for the patient with painful chronic pancreatitis.

significant benefit for, pain relief (20, 21). A multicenter 2-week controlled study in more than 40 patients using an enteric-coated supplement also showed no benefit (22). Feedback inhibition of pancreatic enzyme secretion depends upon delivery of high concentrations of protease to the duodenal lumen. Enteric-coated preparations preferentially release most of their enzymes distal to the duodenum and may therefore be less effective at suppressing CCK levels and producing pain relief (23). Finally, a recent 4-month, double-blinded, crossover study used an enteric-coated preparation with microspheres that release their contents at a lower pH (>5) than most commonly used microspheres (pH > 6). Despite a high delivery rate of trypsin into the duodenum, this study showed no benefit in pain scores in patients receiving pancreatic enzymes, compared with placebo (24). However, this study contained a small number of females and evaluated patients with recurrent rather than chronic pain. Long-term trials comparing non-enteric- and enteric-coated preparations in patients stratified for the etiology, severity, and pattern of disease should help clarify these issues. Until then, it seems reasonable to initiate a trial of high-dose, non-enteric-coated oral pancreatic enzymes taken with meals for several weeks in any patient with painful chronic pancreatitis. The best results may be seen in pancreatitis of nonalcoholic etiology, with symptoms of constant, rather than recurrent, pain and only mild-to-moderate pancreatic insufficiency.

### Somatostatin and Octreotide

Somatostatin is a naturally occurring hormone that has been shown to inhibit pancreatic secretion (25). Theoretically, it may also have cytoprotective action and beneficial effects on the reticuloendothelial system in the setting of pancreatic inflammation (26–28). For these reasons, somatostatin has been used for the treatment of acute pancreatitis, pancreatic fistulas, and pseudocysts. In addition, clinical studies have shown that somatostatin has antinociceptive activity in human and animal models of pain. Epidural somatostatin infusion relieves intraoperative and postoperative pain in patients who have undergone abdominal surgery (29). Intraventricular somatostatin relieves intractable pain from disseminated malignancy (30–32). In cats, perfusion of the dorsal surface of the spinal cord with somatostatin reduces neural responses to noxious heat stimulation of the extremities (33). These antinociceptive properties of somatostatin suggest that this peptide may be helpful for pain control in chronic pancreatitis.

Octreotide is a synthetic long-acting analogue of somatostatin that has been shown to inhibit CCK release and both basal and meal-stimulated pancreatic secretion (34–36). Limited data suggest that octreotide, like somatostatin, may be beneficial for a variety of pancreatic diseases, although octreotide appears to increase contractility of the sphincter of Oddi, as opposed to somatostatin, which relaxes it (37–39). Octreotide's long duration of action allows subcutaneous dosing and makes it a more practical alternative for the treatment of chronic pancreatitis than the short-acting native somatostatin. The drug is usually well tolerated, although long-term therapy predisposes to cholesterol gallstones. Unfortunately, controlled trials using octreotide for chronic pancreatitis pain are limited. Short 3-day studies using 100 and 250 μg t.i.d. showed no benefit (40, 41). Recently, a multicenter randomized 4-week study of 91 patients with advanced chronic pancreatitis and severe pain was performed (42). Octreotide at doses ranging from 40 to 200 μg t.i.d. was compared with placebo. Although results in this pilot study did not reach statistical significance, 200 μg t.i.d. of octreotide produced the greatest pain relief (65%, vs. 35% of patients with placebo), especially in patients with constant, as opposed to intermittent, pain. Additional studies are necessary to sort out the potentially confounding effect of octreotide on sphincter of Oddi function and to clarify its role in the management of chronic pancreatitis pain.

### Nerve Block Techniques

Electroacupuncture and transcutaneous electric nerve stimulation (TENS) have been effective techniques for a variety of conditions of chronic pain. A prospective, randomized, crossover-design study explored these two techniques individually in 23 patients with painful chronic pancreatitis. Unfortunately, neither electroacupuncture nor TENS was effective in reducing pain scores or the need for analgesics (43).

Celiac plexus blocks using radiologic guidance sometimes produce relief of chronic refractory visceral pain. These blocks have produced initial and sometimes extended pain relief in most patients with pancreatic cancer. For unclear reasons, the benefit is usually limited in those with chronic pancreatitis (44, 45). The benefit is least in those with previous pancreatic surgery (45). Pain reduction, when it does occur, lasts for a few months at best. The risk of procedure-induced transient hypotension, nerve root pain, and focal neuropathic damage combined with the need for repeated blocks, even if successful, make this an unattractive technique for most patients (45). A recent open trial of celiac plexus block using botulinum toxin A instead of alcohol was unsuccessful (46). Nerve ablation procedures are discussed in more detail in Chapter 40.

## TREATMENT OF MALDIGESTION

Diarrhea, steatorrhea, and azotorrhea occur when the exocrine secretion of pancreatic enzymes is insufficient to maintain normal digestion. Typically, this occurs late in the course of chronic pancreatitis, because malabsorption does not occur until enzyme secretion is reduced to less than 10% of normal (Fig. 33.3) (47, 48).

Though maldigestion affects all nutrients, the most clinically important problem is with fat maldigestion. Maldigestion of fat is caused by insufficient secretion of lipase resulting in the incomplete digestion of triglycerides. Deficient delivery of bicarbonate may also contribute to steatorrhea, because gastric acid may be inadequately neutralized and cause inactivation of digestive enzymes when the pH falls below 4.0. Low duodenal

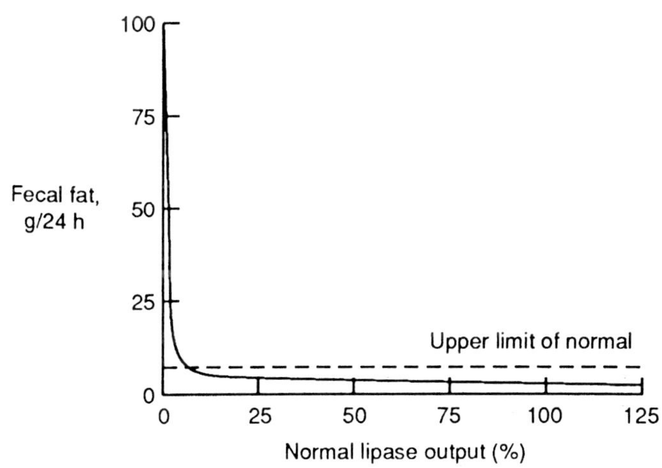


**FIG. 33.3.** Relationship between steatorrhea and lipase output. Steatorrhea does not occur until lipase output is reduced below 10% of normal. (Adapted from DiMagno EP, Go VLW, Summerskill WHJ. Relations between pancreatic enzyme outputs and malabsorption in severe pancreatic insufficiency. N Engl J Med 1973;288:813.)

**TABLE 33.1. Commercial Pancreatic Enzyme Preparations**

| Preparation | Type[a] | Content (Units) | | |
|---|---|---|---|---|
| | | Lipase | Amylase | Protease |
| Cotazyme | C | 8,000 | 30,000 | 30,000 |
| Cotazyme-S | ECMS | 5,000 | 20,000 | 20,000 |
| Creon 10 | ECMS | 10,000 | 33,200 | 37,500 |
| Creon 25 | ECMS | 25,000 | 74,700 | 62,500 |
| Ilozyme | UCT | 11,000 | 30,000 | 30,000 |
| Ku-zyme HP | ECMS | 8,000 | 30,000 | 30,000 |
| Pancrease | ECMS | 4,000 | 20,000 | 25,000 |
| Pancrease MT-4 | ECMT | 4,000 | 12,000 | 12,000 |
| Pancrease MT-10 | ECMT | 10,000 | 30,000 | 30,000 |
| Pancrease MT-16 | ECMT | 16,000 | 48,000 | 48,000 |
| Protilase | ECMS | 4,000 | 20,000 | 25,000 |
| Viokase | UCT | 8,000 | 30,000 | 30,000 |
| Viokase | P | 16,800 | 70,000 | 70,000 |
| Zymase | ECMS | 12,000 | 24,000 | 24,000 |

Adapted from Berardi RR, Dunn-Kucharski VA. Pancreatitis and cholelithiasis. In: DiPiro JT, Talbert RL, Hayes PE, et al., eds. Pharmacotherapy: a pathophysiologic approach. Norwalk, CT: Appleton & Lange, 1993:614.

[a]C, capsule; ECMS, enteric-coated microspheres encased in a cellulose capsule; ECMT, enteric-coated microtablets encased in a cellulose capsule; UCT, uncoated tablet; P, powder.

pH in patients with chronic pancreatitis will also cause precipitation of bile acids, further contributing to impaired fat absorption (49, 50).

At first glance, treating malabsorption secondary to pancreatic insufficiency appears to be relatively easy. It would seem that the simple oral replacement of pancreatic enzymes would be efficacious. However, complete correction of steatorrhea is rarely achieved. This is related to insufficient amounts of enzyme in oral supplements and acid pepsin inactivation of pancreatic enzymes.

Postprandially, the maximal pancreatic lipase output is 140,000 IU/hr for 4 hours (47), and clinical studies have shown that maldigestion does not occur if more than 5% of the normal maximal enzyme output is delivered to the duodenum. Therefore, to prevent steatorrhea, 28,000 IU of lipase should be delivered during the postprandial period. The lipase content of pancreatic enzyme preparations is highly variable, ranging from 0 to 8000 IU per tablet (51, 52). If one should choose to use a preparation such as Viokase, which contains 3000 IU of lipase per tablet, then one should expect that at least 8 tablets would be needed per meal to abolish maldigestion and malabsorption. Therefore, when prescribing pancreatic enzyme replacement, it is important to choose enzyme preparations that have higher lipase activity and to ensure that sufficient amounts are being used (Table 33.1).

Another important factor to consider is that pancreatic enzymes are highly sensitive to acid and pepsin inactivation. It has been demonstrated that following oral ingestion of pancreatic enzyme preparations such as Viokase, only 8% of ingested lipase and 22% of ingested trypsin are recovered in the duodenum. This amounts to less than 1% and 1.4% of meal-stimulated lipase and trypsin output, respectively. However, even these small increases in pancreatic enzymes in the duodenum are sufficient to reduce stool fat by 60% and stool nitrogen by 75% (53). Therefore, to eliminate steatorrhea in pancreatic insufficiency, a large number of enzyme tablets is needed. Hyperglycosuria (54) and renal stones have been reported with high doses of pancreatic supplements secondary to their high purine content. Furthermore, large amounts of enzyme supplement may lead to increased bloating and cramping because of the high lactose content of many commercial pancreatic enzyme preparations.

To improve therapeutic efficacy, efforts have been made to prevent acid peptic inactivation of ingested pancreatic enzymes. These include the use of antacids or $H_2$-receptor antagonists to raise the gastric and duodenal pH and the use of pancreatic enzymes in enteric-pH-coated forms. The use of antacids has produced mixed results. Although the use of sodium bicarbonate or aluminum hydroxide have resulted in the improvement of steatorrhea in some studies (55), in most cases there has been little success with oral antacids. Antacids increase gastric volume, and dilution of enzyme concentrations below critical levels may explain the relative ineffectiveness of antacids (58). There are also reports that the use of calcium carbonate or magnesium-aluminum hydroxide may actually lead to the worsening of steatorrhea because of the formation of poorly soluble calcium or magnesium soaps and the precipitation of glycine-conjugated bile salts (56, 57).

$H_2$-receptor antagonists decrease acid production, pepsin activity, and gastric secretory volume simultaneously and should optimize pancreatic enzyme concentration (58, 59). Duodenal lipase and trypsin activities have been shown to increase with concomitant enzyme replacement and $H_2$-receptor antagonist treatment. However acid suppression with the use of $H_2$ blockers such as cimetidine should be considered only in patients who do not respond to standard oral pancreatic supplements, because of the cost of lifelong use and potential unknown long-term side effects. Proton pump inhibitors such as omeprazole further reduce fecal fat excretion in patients with cystic fibrosis receiving enzyme replacement for pancreatic insufficiency (60). Therefore, for patients in whom the $H_2$-receptor antagonist fails to improve steatorrhea, use of a proton pump inhibitor should be considered.

Enteric coating has been used to overcome some of the problems associated with conventional tablets, powders, and capsules. Microspheres coated with a pH-sensitive covering have been developed to protect the enzyme contents from gastric acid. This theoretically may help to reduce the number of capsules needed daily and can eliminate the need for adjunctive antacid or acid suppression with $H_2$-receptor antagonists or proton pump inhibitors. Enteric-coated enzyme preparations that are stable at an acidic pH (<4) and dissolve at a pH above 5 are most effective in patients who maintain acidic gastric pH levels postprandially. This method delivers pancreatic enzymes to the duodenum intact, whereas standard supplements are irreversibly inactivated. However, enteric coating is effective only if pancreatic enzymes are delivered into the duodenum simultaneously with ingested food from the stomach and when adequate intraduodenal dissolution occurs. Because emptying of large microspheres from the stomach may differ from that of typical antral contents and the duodenal and gastric pH levels are low (<4) for prolonged periods in many patients with pancreatic insufficiency (61, 62), enteric coating may not be an effective improvement over oral pancreatic supplements alone. In fact, several studies have shown that the mean reduction of steatorrhea with the use of enteric-coated preparations such as Pancrease is not better than that with Viokase given with meals (58, 63). In these patients, the gastric pH may increase above 5 in the early postprandial period and then decrease below 4. Under these circumstances an enteric-coated preparation initially will liberate its enzymes, but the enzyme activities will be inactivated when the intragastric pH falls below 4. On the other hand, in patients who secrete more acid, the gastric and duodenal pH levels will remain low (<4) throughout the postprandial period, the enteric coat will remain intact as it traverses to the duodenum, and the pancreatic enzymes will be liberated only as the microspheres reach the jejenum, where the intraluminal pH is above 5. This may explain the effectiveness of enteric-coated preparations in abolishing steatorrhea in some patients who are secreting more acid and are able to maintain an acidified duodenum during the immediate postprandial period.

The size of the microspheres significantly influences the timing of enzyme delivery to the duodenum and hence the efficacy of the enteric-coated enzyme preparations. Microspheres with a diameter of approximately 1.4 mm appear to mix with chyme most thoroughly and are emptied from the stomach at the same rate as food. Microspheres with larger diameters tend to remain in the stomach after food has emptied into the small intestine and are therefore less efficacious in correcting steatorrhea in patients with pancreatic insufficiency (64). Some of the enteric-coated enzyme preparations contain microspheres that are too large and thus empty too slowly to be effective in the digestion of food. This may explain why some enteric-coated preparations are not effective in correcting pancreatic steatorrhea. An ideal enzyme supplement should contain a high concentration of lipase, to maximize fat digestion, and a high concentration of protease, to evoke the negative feedback mechanism for pain control. If one uses an enteric-coated preparation to avoid destruction by gastric acid, the microspheres should have a diameter of approximately 1.4 mm to allow efficient delivery of enzyme to the small bowel.

In treating patients with pancreatic steatorrhea, we recommend the following approach. A sufficient number of enzyme tablets must be given, based on the assumption that a minimum of 28,000 IU of lipase is needed during the postprandial period. For example, to abolish azotorrhea and substantially reduce steatorrhea, a patient will need 8 tablets per meal if the preparation contains 3000 IU of lipase per tablet. Most patients on this regimen will be relatively asymptomatic and achieve satisfactory nutritional status. In some patients who produce large amounts of gastric acid, the use of enteric-coated preparations may be necessary. Most of these preparations contain higher amounts of lipase and trypsin (Table 33.1), and the enzymes are coated with a pH-sensitive covering; as a result, fewer capsules are needed (–23/meal) to provide sufficient enzyme activity in the duodenum. Alternatively, the addition of an $H_2$-receptor antagonist or a proton pump inhibitor may be used for those patients who fail to respond to standard enzyme replacement. If these measures are ineffective, other contributing causes such as celiac sprue, bacterial overgrowth, or terminal ileal disease should be excluded.

## MANAGEMENT OF DIABETES

The incidence of overt diabetes in chronic pancreatitis is approximately 40% (65, 66). After the initial symptoms of pancreatitis occur, alcoholics tend to develop diabetes more rapidly than nonalcoholics, and patients with chronic calcific pancreatitis have a particularly high incidence of diabetes (70%) (67). In certain tropical regions, pancreatic diabetes related to protein malnutrition and consumption of toxic factors is particularly common (68). Although it has generally been appreciated that the vascular complications are less severe in pancreatic diabetes than in primary diabetes, this may not be the case when large numbers of patients are studied and the duration of diabetes is taken into account (69, 70). For example, the incidence and characteristics of retinopathy appear to be similar in those with pancreatic and primary diabetes (70, 71).

The therapy of pancreatic diabetes differs little from the standard management of diabetes. Blood glucose levels should be monitored and controlled, and dietary intake regulated in hope of preventing both short-term metabolic, and long-term vascular, complications of the disease. Patients with chronic pancreatitis and diabetes may be particularly sensitive to insulin and prone to episodes of hypoglycemia. Continued alcohol ingestion, maldigestion, erratic oral intake because of postprandial pain, and abnormal release of regulatory hormones such as glucagon may also contribute to hypoglycemic episodes. For these reasons, it may be prudent to control blood glucose values less intensively in pancreatic than in primary diabetes. Diabetes secondary to pancreatectomy is more likely to cause ketosis and less likely to result in hypoglycemia. Insulin requirements are likely to be greater, and thus these patients can usually be treated similarly to those with primary diabetes mellitus (72).

## REFERENCES

1. Ammann RW, Akovbiantz A, Largiader F, Schueler G. Course and outcome of chronic pancreatitis. Longitudinal study of a mixed medical-surgical series of 245 patients. Gastroenterology 1984; 86:820–828.
2. Lankisch PG, Lohr-Happe A, Otto J, Creutzfeldt W. Natural course in chronic pancreatitis. Digestion 1993;54:148–155.
3. Layer P, Yamamoto H, Kalthoff L, Clain JE, Bakken LJ, DiMagno EP. The different courses of early- and late-onset idiopathic and alcoholic chronic pancreatitis. Gastroenterology 1994;107:1481–1487.
4. Lankisch PG, Seidensticker F, Lohr-Happe A, Otto J, Creutzfeldt W. The course of pain is the same in alcohol- and nonalcohol-induced chronic pancreatitis. Pancreas 1995;10(4):338–341.
5. Trapnell JE. Chronic relapsing pancreatitis: a review of 64 cases. Br J Surg 1979;66:471–475.
6. Hayakawa T, Kondo T, Shibata T, Sugimuto Y, Kitagawa M. Chronic alcoholism and evolution of pain and prognosis in chronic pancreatitis. Dig Dis Sci 1989;34:33–38.
7. Bornman PC, Marks IN, Girdwood AH, et al. Is pancreatic duct obstruction or stricture a major cause of pain in calcific pancreatitis. Br J Surg 1980;67:425–428.
8. de las Heras G, de la Pena J, Arias MJL, Gonzalez-Bernal AC, Martin-Ramos L, Pons-Romero F. Drinking habits and pain in chronic pancreatitis. J Clin Gastroenterol 1995;20(1):33–36.
9. Ihse I, Lilja P, Lundquist I. Feedback regulation of pancreatic enzyme secretion by intestinal trypsin in man. Digestion 1977;15: 303–308.
10. Slaff J, Jacobson D, Tillman CR, Curington C, Toskes P. Protease-specific suppression of pancreatic exocrine secretion. Gastroenterology 1984;87:44–52.
11. Owyang C, Louie D, Tatum D. Feedback regulation of pancreatic enzyme secretion. J Clin Invest 1986;77:2042–2047.
12. Calam J, Bojarski JC, Springer CJ. Raw soya-bean flour increases cholecystokinin release in man. Br J Nutr 1987;58:175–179.
13. Liener JE, Goodale RL, Deshmukh A, et al. Effect of a trypsin inhibitor from soy-beans (Bowman-Birk) on the secretory activity of the human pancreas. Gastroenterology 1988;94:419–427.

14. Schafmayer A, Becker HD, Werner M, Folsch UR, Creutzfeldt W. Plasma cholecystokinin levels in patients with chronic pancreatitis. Digestion 1985;32:136–139.
15. Slaff JI, Wolfe MM, Toskes PP. Elevated fasting cholecystokinin levels in pancreatic exocrine impairment; evidence to support feedback regulation. J Lab Clin Med 1985;105:282–285.
16. Gomez Cerezo J, Codoceo R, Fernandez Calle P, Molina F, Tenias JM, Vasquez JJ. Basal and postprandial cholecystokinin values in chronic pancreatitis with and without abdominal pain. Digestion 1991;48:134–140.
17. Funakoshi A, Nakano I, Shinozake H, Ibayashi H, Tateishi K, Hamaoka T. Low plasma cholecystokinin response after ingestion of a test meal in patients with chronic pancreatitis. Am J Gastroenterol 1985;80:937–940.
18. Jansen JBMJ, Jebbink MCW, Mulders HJA, Lamers CBHW. Effect of pancreatic enzyme supplementation on postprandial plasma cholecystokinin secretion in patients with pancreatic insufficiency. Regul Pept 1989;25:333–342.
19. Isaksson G, Ihse I. Pain reduction by an oral pancreatic enzyme preparation in chronic pancreatitis. Dig Dis Sci 1983;28(2):97–102.
20. Ramo OJ, Puolakkainen PA, Seppala K, Schroder TM. Self-administration of enzyme substitution in the treatment of exocrine pancreatic insufficiency. Scand J Gastroenterol 1989;24:688–692.
21. Halgreen H, Pedersen NT, Worning H. Symptomatic effect of pancreatic enzyme therapy in patients with chronic pancreatitis. Scand J Gastroenterol 1986;21:104–108.
22. Mossner J, Secknus R, Meyer J, Niederau C, Adler G. Treatment of pain with pancreatic extracts in chronic pancreatitis: results of a prospective placebo-controlled multicenter trial. Digestion 1992; 53:54–66.
23. Campbell D, Jadunandan I, Curington C, Liddle R, Solomon T, Toskes P. Alcoholic and idiopathic patients with painful chronic pancreatitis do not experience suppression of CCK levels or pain relief following treatment with enteric-coated pancreatin (Abstract). Gastroenterology 1992;102:259.
24. Malesci A, Gaia E, Fioretta A, et al. No effect of long-term treatment with pancreatic extract on recurrent abdominal pain in patients with chronic pancreatitis. Scand J Gastroenterol 1995;30:392–398.
25. Gullo L, Priory P, Scarpignato C, Baldon F, Mattioli G, Barbara L. Effect of somatostatin 14 on pure human pancreatic secretion. Dig Dis Sci 1987;32:1065–1070.
26. Szabo S, Usadel KH. Cytoprotection-organoprotection by somatostatin; gastric and hepatic lesions. Experientia 1982;38: 254–256.
27. Usadel KH, Kessler H, Rohr G, Kusterer K, Palitzsch K, Schwedes U. Cytoprotective properties of somatostatins. Klin Wochenschr 1986;64(suppl 7):59–63.
28. Baxter JN, Jenkins SA, Day DW, Shields R. Effects of a somatostatin analogue on hepatic and splenic reticuloendothelial function in the rat. Br J Surg 1985;72:1005–1008.
29. Chrubasik J, Meynadier J, Scherpereel P, Wunsch E. The effect of epidural somatostatin on postoperative pain. Anesth Analg 1985;64:1085–1088.
30. Madrazo I, Franco-Bourland RE, Leon-Maza VM, Mena I. Intraventricular somatostatin-14, arginine vasopressin, and oxytocin: analgesic effect in a patient with intractable cancer pain. Appl Neurophysiol 1987;50:427–431.
31. Penn RD, Paice JA, Kroin JS. Intrathecal octreotide for cancer pain (Letter). Lancet 1990;335:738.
32. Mollenholt P, Post C, Paulsson I, Rawal N. Intrathecal and epidural somatostatin in rats: can antinociception, motor effects, and neurotoxicity be separated? Pain 1990;43:363–370.
33. Sandkuhler J, Fu QG, Helmchen C. Spinal somatostatin superfusion in vivo affects activity of cat nociceptive dorsal horn neurons: comparison with spinal morphine. Neuroscience 1990; 34:565–576.
34. Creutzfeldt W, Lembke B, Folsch UR, Schleser S, Koop I. Effect of somatostatin analogue (SMS 201-995, Sandostatin) on pancreatic secretion in humans. Am J Med 1987;82(suppl 5B):49–54.
35. Lembke B, Creutzfeldt W, Schleser S, Ebert R, Shaw C, Koop I. Effect of the somatostatin analogue Sandostatin (SMS 201-995) on gastrointestinal, pancreatic, and biliary function and hormone release in normal men. Digestion 1987;36:108–124.
36. Williams ST, Woltering EA, O'Dorisio TM, Fletcher WS. Effect of octreotide acetate on pancreatic exocrine function. Am J Surg 1989;157:459–462.
37. McKay CJ, Imrie CW, Baxter JN. Somatostatin and somatostatin analogues—are they indicated in the management of acute pancreatitis? Gut 1993;34:1622–1626.
38. Binmoeller KF, Dumas R, Harris AG, Delmont JP. Effect of somatostatin analogue octreotide on human sphincter of Oddi. Dig Dis Sci 1992;37:773–777.
39. Jenkins SA, Berein A. Review article: the relative effectiveness of somatostatin and octreotide therapy in pancreatic disease. Aliment Pharmacol Ther 1995;9:349–361.
40. Malfertheiner P, Mayer D, Buchler M, Dominguez-Munoz JE, Scheifer B, Ditschuneit H. Treatment of pain in chronic pancreatitis by inhibition of pancreatic secretion with octreotide. Gut 1995; 36:450–454.
41. Malfertheiner P, Mayer D, Scheifer B, Buchler M, Ditschuneit H. Does inhibition of pancreatic secretion alleviate chronic pain in chronic pancreatitis? Gastroenterology 1992;102:A277.
42. Toskes PP, Forsmark CE, DeMeo MT, et al. A multicenter controlled trial of octreotide for the pain of chronic pancreatitis (Abstract). Pancreas 1993;8(6):774.
43. Ballegaard S, Christophersen SJ, Dawids SG, Hesse J, Olsen NV. Acupuncture and transcutaneous electric nerve stimulation in the treatment of pain associated with chronic pancreatitis. Scand J Gastroenterol 1985;20:1249–1254.
44. Bengtsson M, Lofstrom JB. Nerve block in pancreatic pain. Acta Chir Scand 1990;156:285–291.
45. Leung JWC, Bowen-Wright M, Aveling W, Shorvon PJ, Cotton PB. Celiac plexus block for pain in pancreatic cancer and chronic pancreatitis. Br J Surg 1983;70;730–732.
46. Sherman S, Kopecky KK, Brashear A, Lehman GA. Percutaneous celiac plexus block with botulinum toxin A did not help the pain of chronic pancreatitis. J Clin Gastroenterol 1995;20(4): 343–344.
47. Di Magno EP, Go VLW, Summerskill WHJ. Relations between pancreatic enzyme outputs and malabsorption in severe pancreatic insufficiency. N Engl J Med 1973;288:813–815.
48. Di Magno EP, Malagelada JR, Go VLW. Relationship between alcoholism and pancreatic insufficiency. Ann NY Acad Sci 1975;252:200–207.
49. Regan PT, Malagelada JR, Di Magno EP, Go VLW. Reduced intraluminal bile acid concentrations and fat maldigestion in pancreatic insufficiency: correction by treatment. Gastroenterology 1979;77:285–289.
50. Andersen JR, Bendtsen F, Oversen L, Pedersen NT, Rune SJ, Tage-Jensen V. Pancreatic insufficiency. Duodenal pH and jejunal pH, bile acid activity, and micellar lipid solubilization. Int J Pancreatol 1990;6:263–270.
51. Graham DY. Enzyme replacement therapy of exocrine pancreatic insufficiency in man: relation between in vitro enzyme activities and in vivo potency in commercial pancreatic extracts. N Engl J Med 1977;296:1314–1317.
52. Whitehead AM. Study to compare the enzyme activity acid resistance and dissolution characteristics of currently available pancreatic enzyme preparations. Pharm Weekbl (Sci) 1988;10: (1)12–16.
53. Di Magno EP, Malagelada JR, Go VLW, Moertel CG. Fate of orally ingested enzymes in pancreatic insufficiency. Comparison of two dosage schedules. N Engl J Med 1977;296:1318–1322.
54. Stapleton FB, Kenedy J, Nousia-Arvanitakis S, et al. Hyperuricosuria due to high dose pancreatic extract therapy in cystic fibrosis. N Engl J Med 1976;295:246–248.
55. Graham DY. Pancreatic enzyme replacement. The effect of antacid or cimetidine. Dig Dis Sci 1982;27:485–490.
56. Hofmann AF, Small DM. Detergent properties of bile salts: correlation with physiological function. Annu Rev Med 1967;18: 333–376.
57. Graham DY, Sackman JW. Mechanism of increase in steatorrhea with calcium and magnesium in exocrine pancreatic insufficiency: an animal model. Gastroenterology 1982;83:638–644.
58. Regan PT, Malagelada JR, Di Magno EP, et al. Comparative effects of antacids, cimetidine, and enteric coating on the therapeutic response to oral enzymes in severe pancreatic insufficiency. N Engl J Med 1977;297:854–858.
59. Regan PT, Malageleda JR, Di Magno EP, et al. Rationale or the use

of cimetidine in pancreatic insufficiency. Mayo Clin Proc 1978; 53(2):79–83.
60. Heijerman HG, Lamers CB, Bakker W. Omeprazole enhances the efficacy of pancreatin (Pancrease) in cystic fibrosis. Ann Intern Med 1991;114:200–201.
61. Benn A, Cooke WT. Intraluminal pH of duodenum and jejunum in fasting subjects with normal and abnormal gastric and pancreatic function. Scand J Gastroenterol 1971;6:313–317.
62. Dutta SK, Russell RM, Iber FL. Influence of exocrine pancreatic insufficiency on the intraluminal pH of proximal small intestine. Dig Dis Sci 1979;24:529–534.
63. Dutta SK, Rubin J, Harvey J. Comparative evaluation of the therapeutic efficacy of a pH-sensitive enteric coated pancreatic enzyme preparation with conventional pancreatic enzyme therapy in treatment of exocrine pancreatic insufficiency. Gastroenterology 1983;84:476–482.
64. Meyer JM, Elashoff J, Porter-Fing V, et al. Human postprandial gastric emptying of 1–3 mm spheres. Gastroenterology 1988;94: 1315–1325.
65. Marks IN, Bank S. The etiology, clinical features and diagnosis of pancreatitis in S. W. Cape. S Afr Med J 1963;37:1039–1053.
66. Kalthoff L, Layer P, Clain JE, DiMagno EP. The course of alcoholic and nonalcoholic chronic pancreatitis. Dig Dis Sci 1984;29:953.
67. Marks IN, Bank S, Vinik AI. Clinical and hormonal aspects of pancreatic diabetes. Am J Gastroenterol 1975;64:13–22.
68. Hartford JD, Skyler JS, Barkin JS. Diabetes and the gastrointestinal system. In: Rifkin H, Porte D, eds. Diabetes mellitus: theory and practice. 4th ed. New York: Elsevier, 1990:824–837.
69. DiMagno EP, Clain JE. Chronic pancreatitis. In: Go VLW, Brooks FP, DiMagno EP, Gardner JD, Lebenthal E, Scheele GA, eds. The exocrine pancreas: biology, pathobiology, and diseases. New York: Raven, 1986:541–575.
70. Gullo L, Parenti M, Monti L, Pezzilli R, Barbara L. Diabetic retinopathy in chronic pancreatitis. Gastroenterology 1990;98: 1577–1581.
71. Couet C, Genton P, Pointel JP, Louis J, et al. The prevalence of retinopathy is similar in diabetes mellitus secondary to chronic pancreatitis with or without pancreatectomy and in idiopathic diabetes mellitus. Diabetes Care 1985;8:323–328.
72. Catanese VM, Kahn CR. Secondary forms of diabetes mellitus. In: Becker KL, ed. Principles and practice of endocrinology and metabolism. Philadelphia: JB Lippincott, 1995:1220–1227.

# 34

# *Endoscopic Treatment of Chronic Pancreatitis*

Stuart Sherman and Glen A. Lehman

## ENDOSCOPIC THERAPY OF CHRONIC PANCREATITIS

Chronic pancreatitis is an inflammatory process manifested by destruction of pancreatic parenchyma and ductal structures with formation of fibrosis. These changes may be associated with varying degrees of dilatation and stricture of the ductal system, as well as intraductal protein plugs and calculi (1). Pain is the predominant symptom of chronic pancreatitis, and its origin appears to be multifactorial. The pain may arise from pancreatic, neural, and extrapancreatic causes (2). Pancreatic interductal pressure is commonly increased in patients with chronic pancreatitis regardless of the cause and whether or not the main pancreatic duct is dilated (3). Increasing evidence suggests that ductal and parenchymal hypertension and possibly pancreatic ischemia are important factors in the pathogenesis of pancreatic pain (4, 5). The multiple causes of pain helps explain the mixed results achieved by current methods of therapy.

Most therapeutic efforts in the treatment of chronic pancreatitis are directed toward control of symptoms. Medical therapy consisting of dietary alterations, analgesics, nerve blocks, oral enzyme supplements, and octreotide are variably effective in relieving pain (2). Surgical therapy has been the main therapeutic option for patients who fail to improve with standard medical therapy. A surgical drainage procedure is usually performed in the setting of a dilated main pancreatic duct, whereas pancreatic resection and/or denervation are reserved for those patients with ducts of normal or small diameter. Early postoperative pain relief is seen in 80–90% of patients. However, pain recurs in 20–50% during long-term follow-up (6, 7). Surgical drainage procedures are associated with a morbidity of 20–40% and mortality averaging 4% (4).

Endoscopic therapy has revolutionized the approach to a variety of biliary tract disorders. Only recently have similar techniques been applied to disorders of the pancreas. Not until the relative safety of ERCP and endoscopic sphincterotomy in acute gallstone pancreatitis was recognized were the indications for endoscopic therapy in pancreatic disorders expanded (8–10). Endoscopic therapy is now being applied in the setting of chronic pancreatitis for patients presenting with pain and/or clinical episodes of acute pancreatitis (11, 12). Certain pathologic alterations of the pancreatic duct, the bile duct, and/or the sphincter lend themselves to endoscopic therapy. Outflow obstruction may be caused by ductal strictures (biliary or pancreatic), pancreatic stones, pseudocysts, and minor or major papilla stenosis. Although the endoscopic approach has not been directly compared with surgery, endoscopic drainage is appealing because it may offer an alternative to surgical drainage procedures with generally less morbidity and mortality. Furthermore, endoscopic procedures do not preclude subsequent surgery should it be necessary. Moreover, the outcome from reducing the intraductal pressure by endoscopic methods may be a predictor for the success of surgical drainage (13).

Outcome data following endoscopic therapy in chronic pancreatitis are rapidly accumulating. However, data are often difficult to interpret because of the heterogeneous populations with one or more pathologic processes being treated (e.g., pancreatic duct stones, strictures, pseudocysts) and because of the multiple therapies performed in a given patient (e.g., dilation of strictures, extraction of biliary stone, biliary and/or pancreatic sphincterotomy). Controlled studies are awaited.

Table 34.1 lists the currently available endoscopic techniques for the treatment of acute and chronic pancreatitis and their complications. This table intentionally includes other conditions, as differentiating acute recurrent pancreatitis from exacerbations of chronic pancreatitis may be clinically difficult. This chapter reviews current state-of-the-art endoscopy in the treatment of chronic pancreatitis.

## PANCREATIC DUCTAL STRICTURES

Benign strictures of the pancreatic duct are generally due to inflammation or necrosis around the main pancreatic duct. Given the putative role of ductal hypertension in the genesis of symptoms (at least in a subpopulation of patients), the use of stents in the pancreatic duct for treatment of dominant pancreatic ductal strictures is being evaluated (14–21). In experimental models, pancreatic ductal stents significantly reduce elevated ductal pressures, though not as effectively as surgical measures (22). The best candidates for stenting are patients with stricture in the pancreatic head with upstream dilatation (type IV pancreatitis (14).

**Pancreatic Stent Placement Techniques.** Most pancreatic stents are just standard polyethylene biliary stents with extra side holes at approximately 1-cm intervals to permit better drainage of juice from side branches (Fig. 34.1). The technique for placing such stents in the pancreatic duct is similar to that used for inserting a biliary stent. In most patients, a pancreatic sphincterotomy (with or without a biliary sphincterotomy) via the major or minor papilla is performed to facilitate placement of accessories and stents. A guide wire must be maneuvered upstream to the point of narrowing. Hydrophilic flexible-tipped and torqueable wires are especially helpful for bypassing strictures. High-grade strictures will require dilation prior to insertion of the endoprosthesis. This may be performed with graduated dilating catheters or hydrostatic balloon dilating catheters (Fig. 34.2).

In general, the diameter of the stent should not exceed the size of the more normal adjacent downstream duct. Therefore, 5- to 7-French stents are commonly used in small ducts, whereas 10- to 11.5-French stents can be used in patients with advanced chronic pancreatitis and grossly dilated ducts. Most diagnostic

**TABLE 34.1. Endoscopic Interventions for Benign Pancreatic Diseases**

| Clinical Condition | Endoscopic Therapy |
|---|---|
| Acute pancreatitis | Endoscopic sphincterotomy (bile duct and/or pancreatic duct, gallstone removal, sphincter dilation, stent, parasite (*Ascaris*) removal |
| Chronic pancreatitis | Endoscopic sphincterotomy (bile duct and/or pancreatic duct, stone extraction ± extracorporeal shock wave lithotripsy (ESWL), bile duct and/or pancreatic duct stents, stricture dilation, endoscopic ultrasound-guided celiac plexus block |
| Pancreatic pseudocysts, pancreatic duct disruption/ascites | Cystogastrostomy, cystoduodenostomy, transpapillary stenting |
| Pancreas divisum | Minor papilla endoscopic sphincterotomy, stent, and/or dilation |

trial or short-term therapy stents are left in place for 2–4 weeks. In contrast, long-term therapy stents have been left in place for 3–116 months (14, 20). Although most pancreatic stents have luminal occlusion in the first few weeks (23), clinical improvement may persist much longer than this (perhaps by pancreatic juice siphoning along the stent).

**Efficacy of Stenting of the Pancreatic Duct.** The results of pancreatic stent placement (usually with ancillary procedures) are detailed in Table 34.2 (14–21). Successful stent placement was achieved in 82–100% of patients. Sixty-six percent of patients with successful stent placement were reported to benefit from therapy during a mean follow-up to 8–39 months.

Cremer et al. (14) reported their experience with pancreatic duct stenting in 76 patients with primarily alcohol-related severe chronic pancreatitis complicated by a distal pancreatic duct stricture and upstream dilatation. A 10-French stent was successfully placed in 75 patients (98.7%) via the major ($n$ = 54) or minor papilla ($n$ = 21). All patients had undergone biliary and pancreatic sphincterotomy, stricture dilation, and extracorporeal shock-wave lithotripsy (in most patients) to fragment stones in the pancreatic duct. A dramatic decrease or complete relief of pain was initially observed in 94% of patients and was associated with a decrease in the diameter of the main pancreatic duct. Stents were *clinically* judged to give therapeutic benefit for a mean time of 12 months (range, 2–38 months). Disappearance of the stricture was observed in only 7 of 64 nonoperated patients after 13 months (range, 2–30 months). Eleven patients underwent pancreatojejunostomy after confirmation of reduction of pain following decompression of the main pancreatic duct. The remainder required repeated change of the stents. Some 55% of nonoperated patients remained largely symptom free after stenting at a mean follow-up of 3 years. Early complications were related to pancreatic and/or biliary sphincterotomy (cholangitis in 3 patients and hemobilia in 10). Intraductal infection caused by clogging of the stent developed in 8 patients, and 3 had their stents migrate inwardly. Stent therapy was believed by the authors to be an acceptable medium-term treatment of pain associated with stricture of the main pancreatic duct. Unfortunately, because the stricture persists in most patients, multiple stent changes are required. As a result, the expandable stents (18-French diameter, 23 mm long) have been tried in 29 patients. Unfortunately, mucosal hyperplasia (i.e., tissue ingrowth) resulted in stent occlusion in most (24). Since these stents are not removable by endoscopic techniques, their use should be limited, perhaps, only to patients with high surgical risk. Evaluation of covered and removable metal stents is in progress.

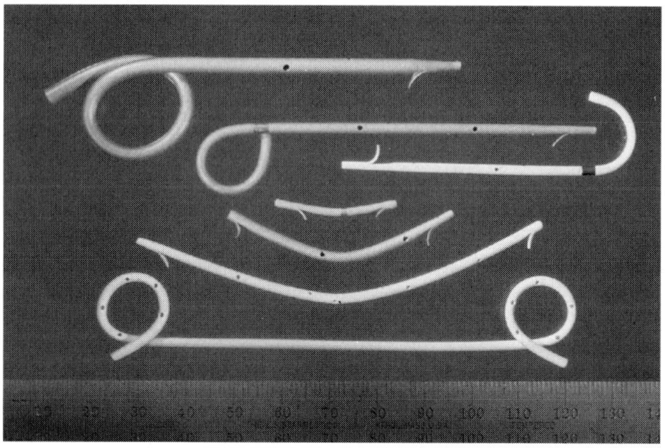

**FIG. 34.1.** A variety of commercially available pancreatic duct stents (straight and full-pigtail). Stents longer than 2 cm usually have multiple side holes to drain the main pancreatic duct side branches.

Ponchon et al. (21) successfully placed 10-French multiside-hole stents after biliary and pancreatic sphincterotomy and balloon dilation of strictures in 28 of 33 patients (85%) with a distal pancreatic duct stricture and upstream dilation. This was a highly selected subgroup; patients with multiple strictures, pancreatic calculi, pancreas divisum, common bile duct narrowing with cholestasis, any duodenal impingement, or a pseudocyst larger than 1 cm were excluded. The stents were exchanged at 2-month intervals, for a total stenting duration of 6 months. The report was based on 23 patients observed for at least 1 year after removal of the stent. During the stenting period, 21 patients (91%) had resolution or reduction in pain, usually within days of insertion of the stent, and 17 discontinued analgesic medications. Initial relief of symptoms correlated with a decreased diameter (≥2 mm; $p < .01$) of the main pancreatic duct. Twelve patients (52%) had a persistent beneficial outcome for at least 1 year after stent removal. Disappearance of the stenosis on pancreatography at stent removal ($p < .05$) and 1 year later ($p < .005$) and reduction in the diameter of the pancreatic duct (≥2 mm) were significantly associated with relief of pain. Complications of therapy were mild pancreatitis (resolved within 48 hours) in nine and a communicating pseudocyst in one.

Smits et al. (20) evaluated the long-term efficacy of pancreatic stenting (5- or 7-French in 9, and 10-French in 40) in a heterogeneous group of 51 patients with pancreatic ductal strictures (44 dominant, 7 multiple) located in the head ($n$ = 38), body ($n$ = 14), or tail ($n$ = 6) and upstream dilation. Associated pancreatic pathology treated at the time of stenting included pancreatic calculi ($n$ = 17), pseudocysts ($n$ = 10), common bile duct strictures with cholestasis ($n$ = 12) and pancreas divisum ($n$ = 3), and dilation of strictures ($n$ = 9). Patients were followed for a median of 34 months. Responders underwent stent exchanges (approximately every 3 months) until ductographic stricture patency was improved. Clinical benefit was noted in 40 of 49 patients (82%) during the stenting period. In 16 of these 40

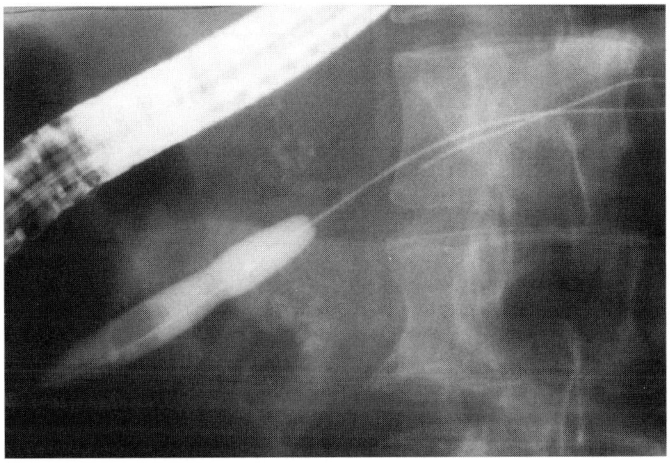

**FIG. 34.2.** A 55-year-old male with alcohol-induced chronic pancreatitis. A stricture of the main duct in the head is associated with adjacent calcifications. A guide wire has been advanced to the tail, and a 6-mm diameter hydrostatic balloon has been inflated to 12 atm, with nearly full waistline ablation.

patients, the stents were still in situ at the time of the report and offered continued clinical improvement over periods ranging from 6 to 116 months. In 22 of the 40 patients, the stents were electively removed. All 22 experienced persistent clinical improvement during periods ranging between 6 to 41 months (median, 28.5 months) after stent removal. There were no specific demographic, ductographic, or interventional factors that predicted the clinical outcome.

The appropriate duration of the pancreatic stent placement is currently unknown. A variety of options are available: *(a)* the stent can be left in place until symptoms or complications occur or *(b)* the stent can be left in place for a predetermined interval (e.g., 3 months). If the patient fails to improve, the stent should be removed, as ductal hypertension is unlikely to be the cause for pain. If the patient has benefited from stenting, then one can remove the stent and follow the patient clinically, continue stenting for a longer time, or perform a surgical drainage procedure. The latter option assumes that the results of endoscopic stenting will predict the surgical outcome. Two preliminary small reports (25, 26) support this concept, but longer-term results are awaited.

Several institutions have recently reported that symptomatic improvement may persist after removal of the pancreatic stent despite persistence of the stricture (14, 19–21). Summarizing the results of two studies ($n$ = 54) that evaluated the efficacy of pancreatic ductal stenting for dominant strictures, 65% of patients had persistent improvement of symptoms after removal of the stent, although the stricture resolved in only 33% (Table 34.3). While these data suggest that stricture resolution is not a prerequisite for symptomatic improvement, several other factors may account for this outcome. First, other therapies performed at the time of stenting (e.g., pancreatic stone removal, pancreatic sphincterotomy) may contribute to patient benefit. Second, many of the unresolved strictures had improved luminal patency (but without return of lumen diameter to normal). Third, the pain of chronic pancreatitis tends to decrease with time and may resolve when marked deterioration of pancreatic function occurs (27).

**Complications Associated with Pancreatic Stents.** True complication rates are difficult to decipher because of *(a)* the simultaneous performance of other procedures (e.g., pancreatic sphincterotomy, stricture dilation), *(b)* the heterogeneous patient populations treated (i.e., patients with acute or chronic pancreatitis), and *(c)* the lack of a uniform definition of a complication and a grading system of their severity (28). Complications related directly to stent therapy are listed in Table 34.4 (29, 38). The incidence of occlusion of pancreatic stents appears to be similar to that for biliary stents (26). We found that 50% of pancreatic stents (primarily 5- to 7-French) were occluded within 8 weeks of placement when carefully evaluated by water flow methods. More than 80% of these early occlusions were not associated with adverse clinical events. In such circumstances, the stent is perhaps serving as a dilator or a wick. Similarly, stents reported to be clinically patent for as long as 38 months (14) are clearly occluded by water flow testing.

Stent migration may be upstream (into the duct) or downstream (into the duodenum). Migration in either direction may be heralded by return of pain or pancreatitis. Johanson et al. (31) reported inward migration in 5.2% of patients and duodenal migration in 7.5%. Proximal stent migration into the duct is especially problematic and may require surgical, percutaneous, or tedious endoscopic removal. Modifications in the design of pancreatic stents may reduce the frequency of such occurrences. Dean et al. (32) reported no inward migration in 112 patients stented with a 4-barbed (2 internal and 2 external) straight polyethylene design.

Although, therapeutic benefit has been reported for pancre-

**TABLE 34.2. Main Pancreatic Duct Stenting for Dominant Strictures**

| Author/Year | Number Patients Attempted | Technical Success[a] | Mean Follow-up (Months) | No. Patients Symptomatically Improved | Major Complications | Deaths |
|---|---|---|---|---|---|---|
| Binmoeller/1995 | 93 | 84 | 39 | 61 | 6 | 0 |
| Cremer/1991 | 76 | 75 | 37 | 41 | 12 | 1 |
| Grimm/1989 | 63 | 55 | 19 | 31[b] | 20[b] | 1 |
| Kozarek/1994 | ND[c] | 17 | 8 | 13 | 3 | 0 |
| McCarthy/1988 | 5 | 5 | 14 | 4 | 2[b] | 0 |
| Ponchon/1995 | 28 | 23 | 26 | 12 | 10 | 0 |
| Smits/1995 | 51 | 49 | 34 | 40 | 8 | 0 |
| Total | 328[d] | 308 | 34[b] | 202[e] (66%) | 61[b] (19%) | 2 (1%) |

[a]Technical success refers to the number of patients successfully stented.
[b]Estimate.
[c]ND, no data avaiable.
[d]Kozarek study tallied as 17.
[e]Percentage improved refers to the percentage of patients who benefited (during the follow-up period) of those successfully stented.

**TABLE 34.3. Clinical Outcome and Main Pancreatic Duct Stricture Resolution after Endoscopic Stent Removal**

| Author/Year | Persistent Symptom Improvement after Endoscopic Stent Removal | Median Follow-up after Stent Removal (Months) | Stricture Resolution by Ductographic Appearance |
|---|---|---|---|
| Ponchon/1995 | 12/21 (57%) | 14 | 8/21 (38%) |
| Smits/1995 | 23/33 (70%) | 29 | 10/33 (20%) |
| Total | 35/54 (65%) | 23 | 18/54 (33%) |

atic stenting, morphologic changes of the pancreatic duct, directly related to this therapy, occur in most patients (Fig. 34.3). Summarizing the results of seven published series (33–39), new ductal changes were seen in 54% (range, 33–83%) of 297 patients. Limited observations to date indicate a tendency of these ductal changes to improve with time following stent change and/or removal (33, 34, 36–39). What the long-term consequences of these stent-induced ductal changes are in most patients remains uncertain; however, permanent strictures have been seen in a small number of patients. Moreover, the long-term parenchymal effects have not been studied in humans.

In a pilot study, six mongrel dogs underwent stenting of the pancreatic duct for 2–4 months (30). Radiographic, gross, and histologic abnormalities developed in all dogs. The radiographic findings (stenosis in the stented region with upstream dilation) were associated with gross evidence of fibrosis, which increased in proportion to the length of the stenting period. Histologic changes of obstructive pancreatitis were present in most experimental dogs. Although follow-up after stent removal was short, the atrophy and fibrosis seen were not likely to be reversible.

In a recently reported study (40), parenchymal changes (hypoechoic area around the stent, heterogeneity, and cystic changes) were seen on endoscopic ultrasound in 17 of 25 patients undergoing short-term pancreatic duct stenting. Four patients who had parenchymal changes at stent removal had a follow-up study at a mean time of 16 months. Two patients had (new) changes suggesting chronic pancreatitis (heterogeneous echotexture, echogenic foci in the parenchyma, and a thickened hyperechoic irregular pancreatic duct) in the stented region. While such damage in a normal pancreas may have important long-term consequences, the outcome in patients with advanced chronic pancreatitis may be inconsequential.

Further studies addressing issues of the diameter and composition of the stent as well as the duration of therapy as they relate to safety and efficacy are needed. Because of these potentially serious stent-induced ductal changes, the endoscopist is strongly encouraged not to place long-term plastic stents into patients with a normal downstream duct. Long-term trials comparing endoscopic, surgical, and medical management of stricture patients would be of great interest.

**TABLE 34.4. Complications Directly Related to Pancreatic Duct Stents or Guide Wires Used to Place Stents**

| | |
|---|---|
| • Stent occlusion or foreign body–induced pain and/or pancreatitis | • Migration into or out of duct |
| • Duodenal erosions | • Pancreatic infection |
| • Ductal perforation | • Ductal and parenchymal changes |
| • Stone formation | • Pseudocysts |

## PANCREATIC DUCTAL STONES

Alcohol-induced, tropical, and idiopathic pancreatitis are the main categories of chronic calcifying pancreatitis. Alcohol appears to be directly toxic to the pancreas and produces a dysregulation of secretion of pancreatic enzymes (including zymogens), citrate (a potent calcium chelator), lithostathine (pancreatic stone protein), and calcium. These changes favor the formation of a nidus (a protein plug) followed by precipitation of calcium carbonate to form a stone (41, 42).

There is debate about whether pancreatic calculi aggravate the clinical course of chronic pancreatitis (manifested as increased abdominal pain or recurrent attacks of acute pancreatitis) or are just the inevitable sequelae of ongoing destruction of the gland. The rationale for intervention is based on the premise that pancreatic stones increase the intraductal and parenchymal pressure with resultant pain and ischemia proximal (upstream) to the obstructed focus. Reports indicating that endoscopic removal, with or without extracorporeal shock-wave lithotripsy (ESWL), or surgical removal of pancreatic calculi results in improvement of symptoms support this notion (13). Moreover, stone impaction may cause further trauma to the pancreatic duct, with epithelial destruction and stricture formation (41, 43). Thus, identification of main pancreatic ductal stones in a symptomatic patient warrants consideration of removal.

**Endoscopic Techniques.** A sphincterotomy of the major pancreatic papilla (in patients with normal anatomy, i.e., no pancreas divisum) is usually required to facilitate access to the duct prior to attempts at stone removal. There are two methods to cut the major pancreatic sphincter (44, 45). A standard pull-type sphincterotome is inserted into the pancreatic duct and

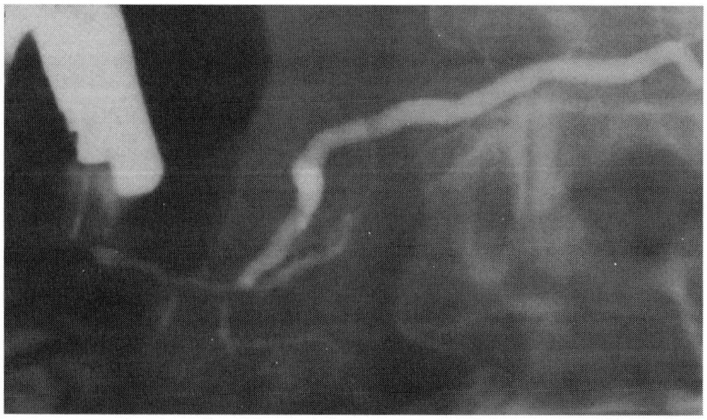

**FIG. 34.3.** This 40-year-old female with pancreas divisum had a normal dorsal pancreatogram 2 weeks previously. After minor papilla endoscopic sphincterotomy and brief-interval stenting (2 cm, 5 French), narrowing and irregularity of the main duct in the stented zone is seen.

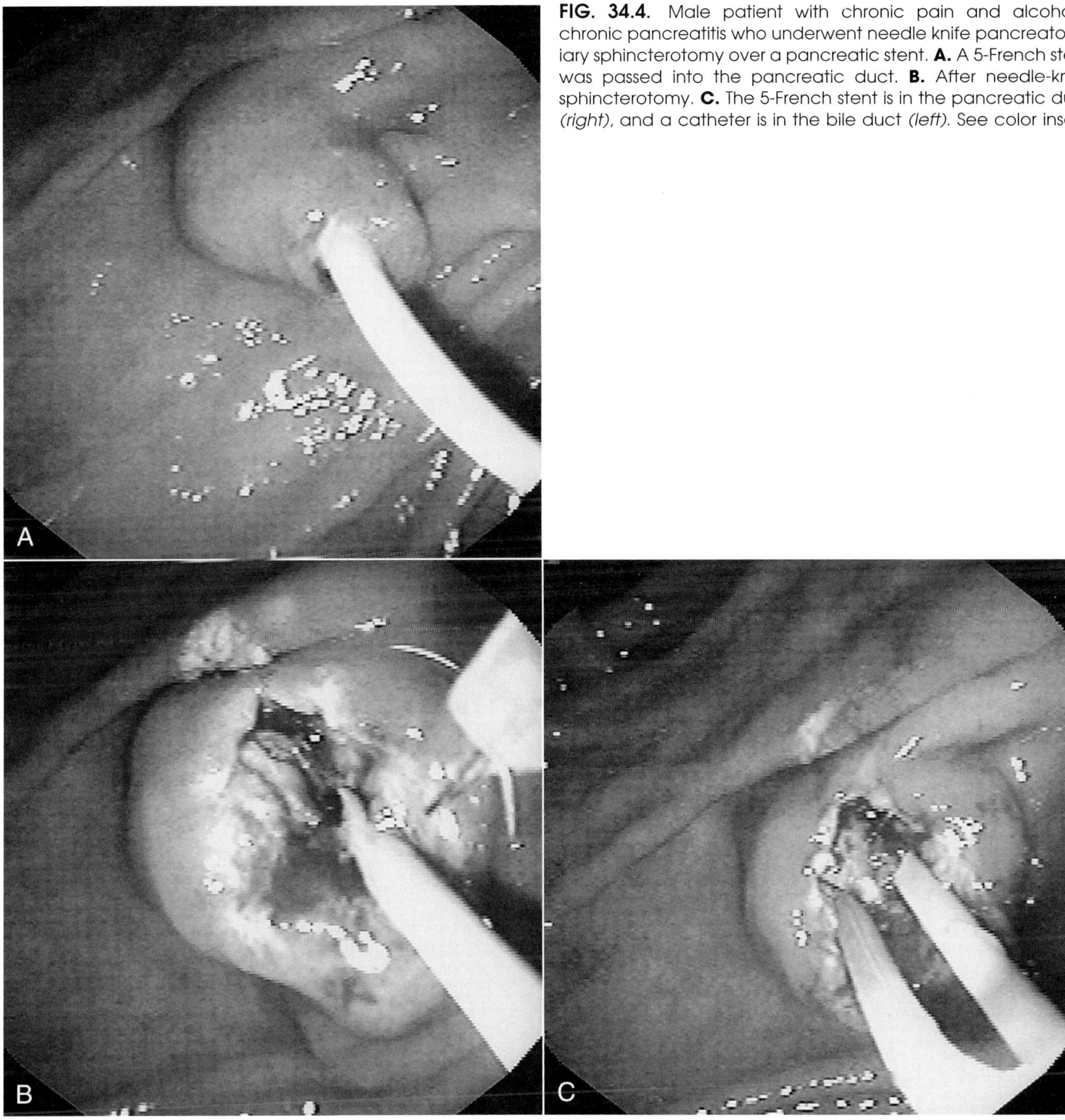


**FIG. 34.4.** Male patient with chronic pain and alcoholic chronic pancreatitis who underwent needle knife pancreatobiliary sphincterotomy over a pancreatic stent. **A.** A 5-French stent was passed into the pancreatic duct. **B.** After needle-knife sphincterotomy. **C.** The 5-French stent is in the pancreatic duct *(right)*, and a catheter is in the bile duct *(left)*. See color insert.

oriented along the axis of the pancreatic duct (usually in the 1–2 o'clock position). Although the landmarks to determine the length of incision are imprecise, authorities recommend cutting 5–10 mm (44) (Fig. 34.4). The cutting wire should not extend more than 6–7 mm up the duct when applying electrocautery, to prevent deep ductal injury. Alternatively, a needle knife can be used to perform the sphincterotomy over a previously placed pancreatic stent (44, 45). Some authorities favor performing a biliary sphincterotomy if needed for stone removal prior to the pancreatic sphincterotomy, because of the concern for cholangitis if this is not done (46). Such complications were not found by others (19, 20, 44). However, performing a biliary sphincterotomy first can expose the pancreaticobiliary septum and allow the length of the cut to be gauged more accurately. In patients with pancreas divisum, a minor papilla sphincterotomy is needed for stone removal. The technique is similar to sphincterotomy of the major papilla, except that the direction of the incision is usually in the 10–12 o'clock position and the length of the sphincterotomy is limited to 4–8 mm. The ability to remove a stone by endoscopic methods alone depends on the size and number of stones, the location of the duct, the presence of a downstream stricture, and the degree of impaction (47).

Downstream strictures usually require dilation either with catheters or hydrostatic balloons. Standard stone retrieval balloons and baskets are the most common accessories used to remove stones. Passage of these instruments around a tortuous duct can be difficult, but over-the-wire accessories are usually helpful. Stone removal is then performed in a fashion similar to extraction of biliary stones (Fig. 34.5).

**Endoscopic Results.** Sherman et al. attempted to identify those patients with stones predominately in the main pancreatic duct which were most amenable to endoscopic removal and to determine the effects of such removal on the patients' clinical course (47). Some 32 patients with ductographic evidence of chronic pancreatitis and stones in the pancreatic duct underwent attempted endoscopic removal by various techniques, including bile duct and/or pancreatic duct sphincterotomy, stricture dilation, pancreatic stenting, stone basketing, balloon extraction, and/or flushing. Of these patients, 72% had complete or partial stone removal, and 68% improved after endoscopic therapy. Symptomatic improvement was most evident (83%) in those with chronic relapsing pancreatitis versus those (46%) presenting with chronic continuous pain alone. Factors favoring complete stone removal included *(a)* 3 or fewer stones, *(b)* stones confined to the head or body of the pancreas, *(c)* absence of a downstream stricture, *(d)* stone diameter of 10 mm or less, and *(e)* absence of impacted stones. After successful stone removal, 25% of patients had regression of the ductographic changes of

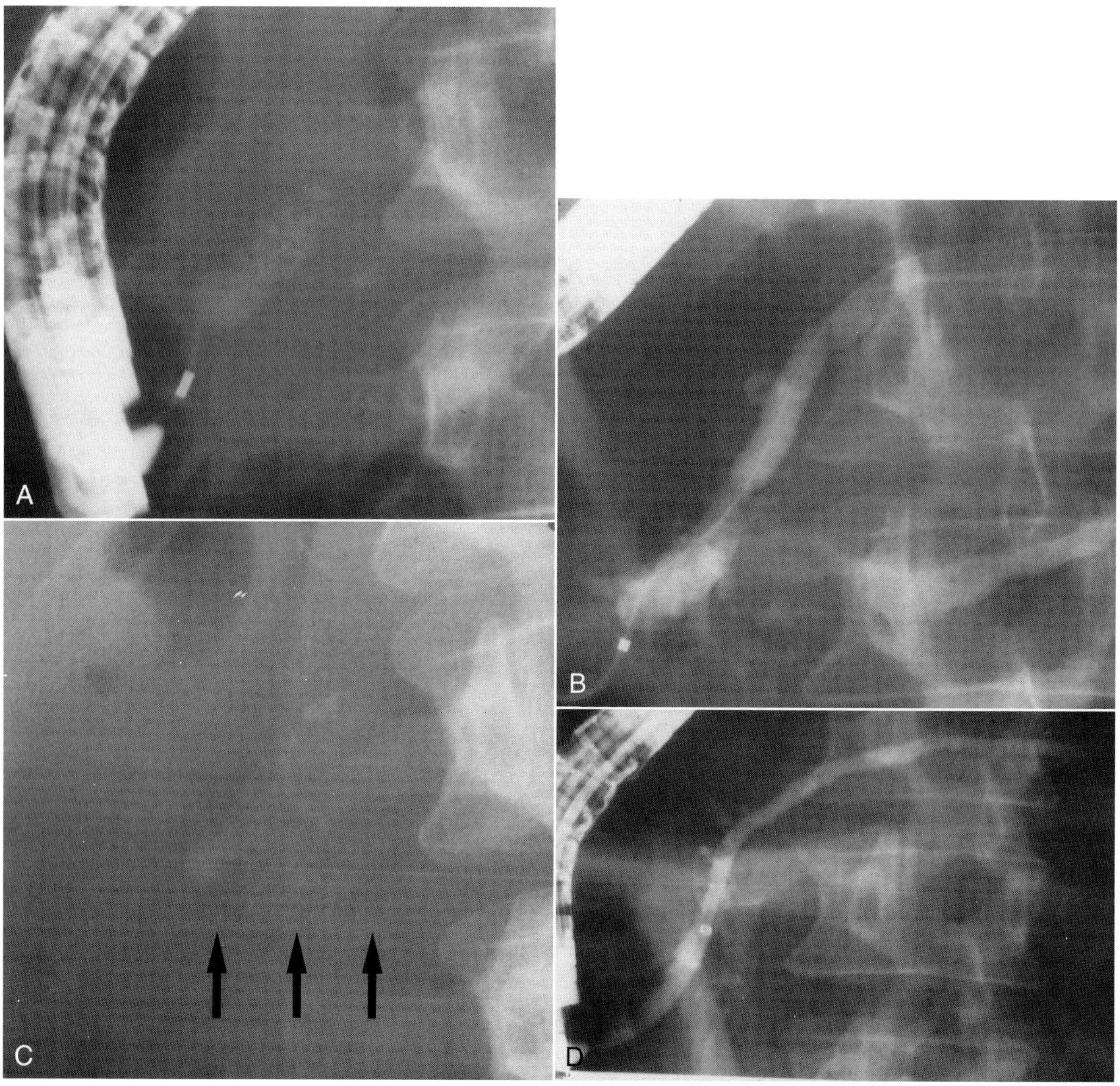


**FIG. 34.5. A.** A 47-year-old woman with chronic pancreatitis and chronic abdominal pain has a calcified stone in the terminal main pancreatic duct (no contrast has been injected). **B.** Pancreatogram. Note the limited visibility of the stone after contrast injection. The stone could not be removed via endoscopic basketing. **C.** Stone fragments seen after ESWL. **D.** Nearly normal pancreatogram after stone fragment removal.

**TABLE 34.5. Endoscopic therapy of Pancreatic Ductal Stones (Using ERCP Techniques Alone)**

| Author, Year | N | Complete Stone Clearance (%) | Major Complications[a] (%) | Mean Follow-up (Months) | Symptomatic Improvement (%) |
|---|---|---|---|---|---|
| Cremer, 1993 | 40 | 45 | 10 | 36 | 63 |
| Fuji, 1989 | 11 | 55 | 0 | ND[b] | 90 |
| Kozarek, 1992 | 8 | 88 | 13 | 17 | 88 |
| Schneider, 1985 | 3 | 100 | 0 | ND | ND |
| Sherman, 1991 | 32 | 59 | 8 | 26 | 68 |
| Smits, 1995 | 53[c] | 74 | 9 | 33 | 81 |
| Total | 147 | 63 | 9 | 31[d] | 74 |

[a] No series reported any mortalities.
[b] ND, no data.
[c] 8 also had ESWL.
[d] Estimate.

chronic pancreatitis, and 42% had a decrease in the diameter of the main pancreatic duct. The only complication from therapy was mild pancreatitis in 8%.

Smits et al. recently reported (48) their results in 53 patients with pancreatic ductal stones treated primarily by endoscopic methods alone (8 had ESWL). Removal of stones was successful in 42 patients (79%), complete in 39 and partial in 3, with initial relief of symptoms in 38 (90%). Similar to the results reported by Sherman et al. (47), in this series, 3 of 11 patients (27%) with failure of removal of the stone had improvement in symptoms, suggesting that some of the clinical response may be related to other therapies performed at the time of attempted stone removal (e.g., pancreatic sphincterotomy). During a median follow-up period of 33 months, 13 patients had recurrent symptoms caused by recurrence of the stone. The stones were successfully removed in 10 (77%). No factor evaluated (cause of pancreatitis, presentation with pain or pancreatitis, presence of single or multiple stones, location of stones, presence or absence of a stricture) was shown to predict successful stone treatment (defined as complete or partial removal of stones resulting in relief of symptoms).

Cremer et al. (24) reported 40 patients with pancreatic ductal stones who were treated by endoscopic methods alone. Complete clearance of stones was achieved in only 18 (45%). However, immediate resolution of pain occurred in 77%. During a 3-year follow-up, 63% remained symptom free. Clinical steatorrhea improved in 11 of 15 patients (73%).

Table 34.5 summarizes six selected series (24, 47–51) reporting the results of removal of pancreatic stones by endoscopic methods alone. Complete clearance of stones was achieved in 93 of 147 patients (63%). The major complication rate was 9% (primarily pancreatitis), and the mortality rate was 0%. Cremer et al. (24) reported bleeding in 3% and retroperitoneal perforation in 1.4%. Sepsis was an infrequent complication. During a 2.5-year (approximate) follow-up period, 74% of patients had improvement in their symptoms.

**Lithotripsy.** As noted, endoscopic methods alone will likely fail in the presence of large or impacted stones and stones proximal to a stricture. Extracorporeal shock-wave lithotripsy (ESWL) can be used to fragment stones and facilitate their removal (Fig. 34.6). Thus, this procedure complements endoscopic techniques and improves the success of nonsurgical ductal decompression.

In 1987, Sauerbruch et al. (52) were the first to report the successful use of ESWL in the treatment of pancreatic stones. Since then, more than 300 patients have been reported in the literature (53–59). Patients with obstructing prepapillary concrement and upstream ductal dilation appear to be the best candidates for ESWL. In the largest reported series, 123 patients with main pancreatic ductal stones and proximal dilatation were treated with an electromagnetic lithotriptor, usually before pancreatic sphincterotomy (46). Stones were successfully fragmented in 99%, resulting in a decrease in dilatation of the duct in 90%. The main pancreatic duct was completely cleared of all stones in 59%. Some 85% of patients noted improvement in pain during a mean follow-up of 14 months. However, 41% of patients had a clinical relapse because of migration of a stone into the main pancreatic duct, progressive stricture, or occlusion of the stent. This same center compared their results of pancreatic stone removal prior to the availability of ESWL and after the introduction of adjunctive ESWL therapy (24). Stones were successfully cleared in 18 of 40 patients (45%) by endoscopic methods alone, compared with 22 of 28 (78.6%) with ESWL. Table 34.6 summarizes the results of seven series reporting the efficacy and safety of adjunctive ESWL. Complications in these series were primarily related to the endoscopic procedure, although a large renal subcapsular hematoma was observed in one patient.

Although ultrasound-focused ESWL has been reported to achieve stone fragmentation, such focusing is clearly more difficult. In the series reported by Schneider et al. (57), stone localization was achieved in 17 of 119 sessions (14%) when only ultrasonography was used to monitor the position of the stone.

The Brussels group (60) studied 70 patients with pancreatic calculi who underwent attempts at endoscopic removal; adjunctive ESWL was used in 41 (59%). This was a fairly homogeneous group of patients; those with strictures, previous pancreatic surgery, and failed pancreatic sphincterotomy were excluded. The authors evaluated the immediate technical and clinical results and reviewed the long-term outcome in patients followed for more than 2 years. Complete ($n = 35$) or partial ($n = 20$) stone removal was achieved in 79% and was more frequently observed when ESWL was performed ($p < .005$) and in the absence of nonpapillary ductal substenosis or complete obstruction of the main duct ($p < .05$). Complete stone clearance was most frequently observed with single stones or stones confined to the head ($p < .05$). In the multivariate analysis, ESWL was the only independent factor influencing the technical results of endoscopic management. In this series, the number of ERCPs performed per patient was reduced from 3.4 to 2.7 after the introduction of ESWL ($p < .01$). Of the 56 patients with pain on admission, 53 (95%) were pain free ($n = 41$) or had a reduction in pain ($n = 12$). A significant association was found between immediate disappearance of pain and complete or partial clearance of the main pancreatic duct in both the univariate and multivariate analyses. During the first 2 years of follow-up after therapy, 25 of 46 (54%) patients were totally free of pain, and the

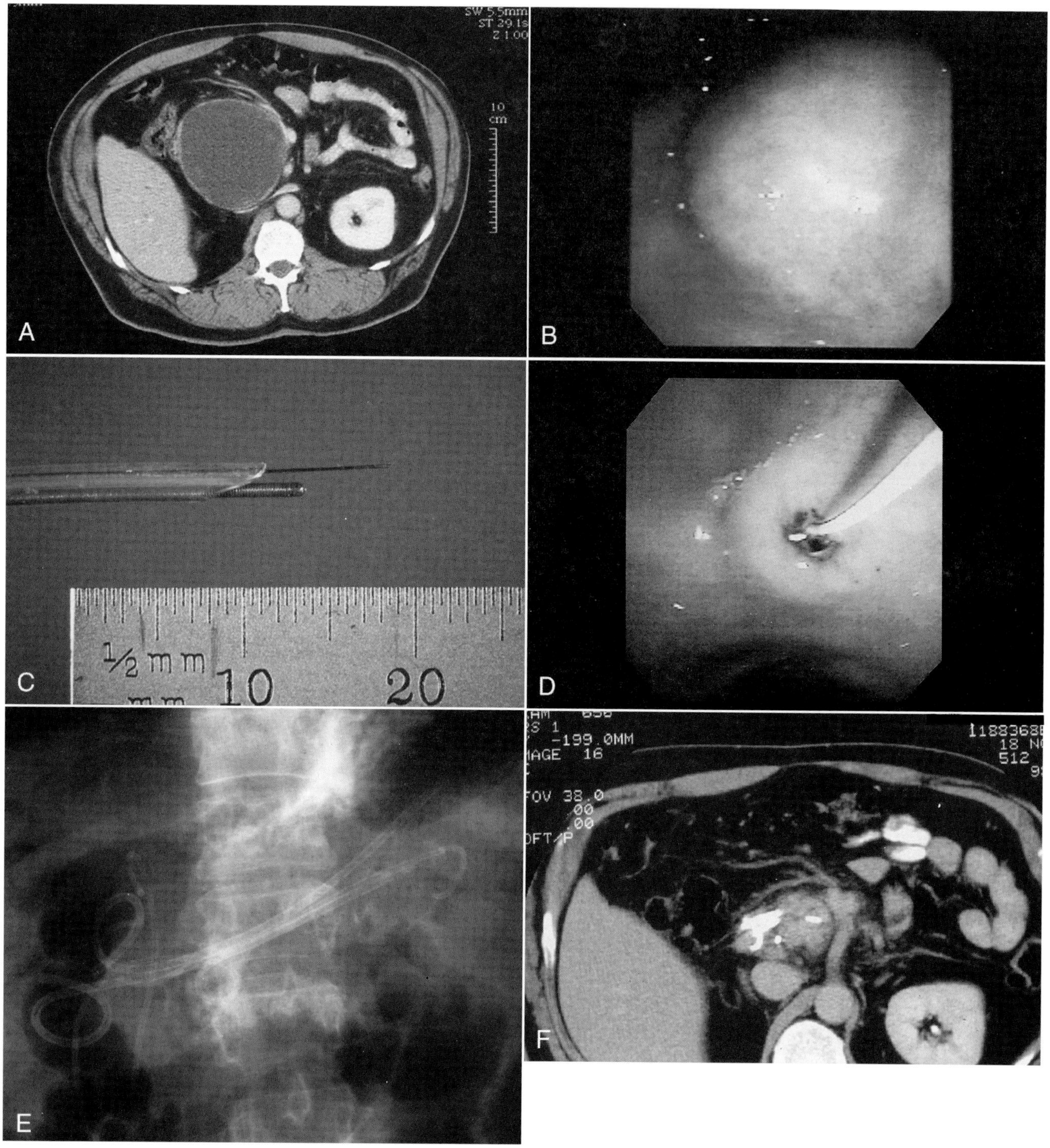


**FIG. 34.6.** **A.** A 53-year-old man with pancreatitis complicated by pseudocyst. **B.** Bulge from pseudocyst as seen from duodenum. **C.** Pseudocystotome (variant of needle knife). **D.** Guide wire passing transmurally into pseudocyst after puncture and tract dilation with 10-mm balloon. **E.** Multiple stents in place. **F.** CT scan showing residual stents in situ and cyst resolution. See color insert.

frequency of pain attacks in the remaining 21 was halved. This frequency of recurrent symptoms (46%) is comparable to that of surgical series (61). Long-term pain relief was associated with *(a)* earlier treatment after disease onset ($p < .005$), *(b)* a low frequency of pain attacks before therapy ($p < .05$), and *(c)* absence of nonpapillary substenosis in the main duct ($p < .05$).

Intraductal laser lithotripsy has received very limited use. Fluoroscopically guided catheters have limited efficacy (59). Pancreatoscopy (via a "mother-baby" scope system) can be used to visualize both laser fiber contact with the stone and fragmentation directly, although intraductal manipulation remains very limited (51, 62).

Stone dissolution via ductal irrigation (contact dissolution) or an oral agent is an attractive endoscopic adjunct for stone removal. Sahel and Sarles found that intraduodenal infusion of citrate in dogs significantly increased the citrate concentration in pancreatic juice (63). This led to a nonrandomized study of oral citrate in 18 patients with chronic pancreatitis, 17 of whom had pancreatic stones. During therapy for a mean duration of 9.5 months, 7 patients responded, with a mean stone size reduction of 21% and an improvement in symptoms (41). Berger et al. (64) performed nasopancreatic drainage in six patients with stones in the main pancreatic duct. The pancreatic duct was perfused with a mixture of isotonic citrate and saline at 3 mL/min for 4 days. A stone-free state was achieved in all cases. Pancreatic pain disappeared during the perfusion, and four patients remained free of pain during the follow-up period (1–12 months). The remaining two patients had repeat therapy, which resulted in pain resolution. Pancreatic exocrine function was improved in three of five evaluated patients.

Trimethadione, an epileptic agent and a weak organic acid, induces a concentration-dependent increase in calcium solubility in vitro (41). Noda et al. (65) showed promising results for trimethadione in a canine model of pancreatic stones. Unfortunately, the doses used in the dogs, if extrapolated to humans, could potentially be toxic. At the present time, no rapidly effective solvent for human use is available to treat pancreatic stones. Further trials in humans are needed to establish a role for medical therapy (either alone or as an aid to endoscopic measures) in treating patients with symptomatic pancreatic calculi.

These data suggest that removal of pancreatic calculi may result in symptomatic benefit. Longer follow-up will be necessary to determine the recurrence rate of stones and whether endoscopic success results in longstanding clinical improvement or permanent regression of the morphologic changes. Overall, endoscopists are encouraged to remove pancreatic calculi in symptomatic patients when they are located in the main duct (in the head, body or both) and are thus readily accessible. The currently available data suggest that the clinical outcome after successful endoscopic removal is similar to surgical outcome, with lower morbidity and mortality (66). Moreover, recurrence of symptoms because of migration of stone fragments can be treated again by endoscopy, with or without ESWL. On the other hand, rates of reoperation for recurrent pain after surgery are as high as 20%, with a striking increase in morbidity and mortality after repeated surgery (60). Controlled trials comparing endoscopic, surgical, and medical therapies are awaited.

## PANCREATIC PSEUDOCYSTS

Pancreatic pseudocysts may complicate the course of chronic pancreatitis in 20–40% of cases (67, 68). Traditionally, surgery has been the treatment of choice for such patients whose fluid collection did not resolve with observation and medical management. The introduction of ultrasound- and computed tomography (CT)-guided needle and catheter drainage techniques provided a nonoperative alternative for managing patients with pseudocysts. More recently, an endoscopic approach has been applied to this indication. Endoscopic therapy aims to create a communication between the pseudocyst cavity and the bowel lumen. This can be done by a transpapillary and/or a transmural approach. The route taken depends on the location of the pseudocyst and whether it communicates with the main pancreatic duct or compresses the gastrointestinal lumen.

Appropriate management of peripancreatic fluid collections must include consideration of multiple factors: *(a)* general clinical toxicity, *(b)* medical risk factors including obesity and diabetes, *(c)* the likelihood of infection, *(d)* the degree of associated necrosis, *(e)* size, *(f)* location, *(g)* chronicity of the collection, *(h)* underlying ductal anatomy, *(i)* cause of pancreatitis, and *(j)* associated portal hypertension (hepatic disease or portal venopathy). Optimal candidates for endoscopic transmural (transgastric or transduodenal) drainage of cysts are patients who have cysts with mature walls that are ≤1 cm from the gut lumen and have an obvious compression on the gut lumen. If location of the cyst is uncertain, localization by endoscopic ultrasound or transmural needle puncture of the cyst with injection of contrast may be helpful. The techniques recommended for drainage is outlined in Table 34.7. Follow-up CT or ultrasound monitoring is recommended at approximately monthly intervals until total resolution of the cyst indicates the time for removal of the stent. Repeat ERCP with replacement or reposition of the stent is needed in 25% of cases.

More than 400 cases of endoscopically managed pseudocysts have been reported (Table 34.8) (69–73). The results indicate that endoscopic therapy is associated with a high technical success rate (80–95%), acceptably low complication rates (equal to or less than surgical rates), and a pseudocyst recurrence rate of 10–20% (73). In the largest series reported (74, 75), 100 of 108 patients (93%) had their pseudocysts successfully drained. Pseudocysts recurred in 13 (13%). The presence of chronic pancreatitis, obstructed pancreatic duct, ductal stricture, necrosis noted on CT scan, and a pseudocyst smaller than 10 cm were not predictors of recurrent pseudocyst disease. Endoscopic therapy is also effective in the management of partial (76) and complete pancreatic ductal disruptions (77), pancreatocutaneous fistulas, pancreatic ascites, and pancreaticopleural effusions (78).

**TABLE 34.6. Endoscopic Therapy of Pancreatic Ductal Stones Using Adjunctive Extracorporeal Shock Wave Lithotripsy**

| Author/Year | Number of Patients Treated | Mean No. ESWL Sessions | Percentage of Patients with Complete Stone Clearance % | Major Complications[a] (%) | Mean Follow-up (Months) | % Patients with Symptom Improvement |
|---|---|---|---|---|---|---|
| Delhaye, 1992 | 123 | 1.8 | 59 | 36 | 14 | 63 |
| Neuhaus, 1989 | 12 | 1.6 | 67 | 0 | 8 | 91 |
| Sauerbruch, 1992 | 24 | 1.5 | 42 | 9 | 24 | 83 |
| Schneider, 1994 | 50 | 2.4 | 60 | 0 | 20 | 90 |
| Sherman, 1995 | 26 | 1.2 | 61 | 12 | 26 | 81 |
| Soehendra, 1989 | 8 | ND[b] | 100 | 0 | 6 | 75 |
| van der Hul, 1994 | 17 | 1.9 | 41 | 6 | 30 | 65 |
| Total | 260 | 1.8 | 59 | 19 | 18[c] | 72 |

[a] No series reported any mortalities.
[b] ND, no data.
[c] Estimate.

**TABLE 34.7. Drainage Technique for Pseudocysts That Compress the Gastric or Duodenal Wall**

1. Identify site of bulge against the stomach or duodenal wall with certainty
2. Align endoscope to permit perpendicular puncture of the bulge
3. If uncertain, puncture with needle catheter and aspirate juice first; use pseudocystotome (modified needle knife)
4. Perpendicularly puncture needle knife with single 1-second coagulation current and puncture full 6–10 mm into the wall
5. Advance polyethylene tubing into pseudocyst
6. Advance 0.035-inch diameter guide wire into cyst and advance 1–2 complete circles to outline cyst diameter and to ensure site location
7. Withdraw polyethylene catheter and advance 10-mm hydrostatic balloon and inflate to maximum diameter
8. While maintaining guide wire within pseudocyst withdraw balloon
9. Advance (preferably) 10-French, double-pigtail stent halfway into pseudocyst and drop other pigtail into gut lumen; place second stent alongside first after advancing 0.035-inch diameter guide wire through cystoenterostomy

## BILIARY OBSTRUCTION IN CHRONIC PANCREATITIS

Intrapancreatic strictures of the common bile duct have been reported to occur in 2.7–45.6% of patients with chronic pancreatitis (Fig. 34.7). Such strictures result from a fibrotic inflammatory restriction or compression by a pseudocyst (79, 80). In one ERCP series, a stricture of the common bile duct was seen in 30% of patients and was associated with persistent cholestasis, jaundice, or cholangitis in 9% (80). Since longstanding biliary obstruction can lead to secondary biliary cirrhosis and/or recurrent cholangitis, biliary decompression has been recommended. Surgical therapy has been the traditional approach. However, based on the excellent outcome (with low morbidity) from endoscopic biliary stenting in postoperative strictures, evaluation of similar techniques for bile duct strictures complicating chronic pancreatitis was undertaken.

Deviere et al. (80) evaluated the use of biliary stenting (one or two Biotrol 10-French C-shaped stents) in 25 patients with chronic pancreatitis with bile duct obstruction and substantial cholestasis (alkaline phosphatase levels more than twice the upper limits of normal). Nineteen patients had jaundice, and seven presented with cholangitis. Cholestasis, hyperbilirubinemia, and cholangitis resolved in all patients following stent placement. Results of late follow-up (mean, 14 months; range, 4–72 months) of 22 patients were much less satisfactory. One patient died from acute cholecystitis and postsurgical complications; a second died 10 months after stenting, of sepsis that was believed to be due to stent blockage or dislodgment. Stent migration occurred in 10 patients, and stent occlusion in 8, resulting in cholestasis with or without jaundice ($n$ = 12), cholangitis ($n$ = 4), or no symptoms ($n$ = 2). These patients were treated with stent replacement, surgery, or both ($n$ = 7). Ten patients continued to have a stent in place (mean follow-up, 8 months) and remained asymptomatic. Only three patients required no further stents because of resolution of their biliary stricture. The salient point of this study is that biliary drainage is effective for resolving cholangitis or jaundice in patients with chronic pancreatitis and a biliary stricture. However, the long-term efficacy of this treatment is much less satisfactory, because stricture resolution rarely occurs.

Barthet et al. (81) also found that biliary stenting is not a definitive therapy for the chronic pancreatitis patient with distal common bile duct stricture. In their series of 19 patients (mean duration of stenting, 20 months), only 2 had complete clinical (resolution of symptoms), biologic (normalization of cholestasis liver tests), and radiologic (resolution of biliary stricture and upstream dilatation) recovery; thus 6 of 10 (60%) were possible clinical successes, 8 of 19 (42%) possible biologic successes, and 3 of 19 (16%) possible radiologic successes.

Because of the disappointing results with plastic stents and concern about the high morbidity associated with surgically performed biliary drainage procedures in alcoholic (frequently debilitated) patients, uncoated expandable metal stents were tried (82). Twenty patients were treated with a 34-mm long metal stent that becomes 10 mm in diameter when fully expanded. The short length was chosen so that surgical bypass (e.g., choledochoduodenostomy) would still be possible if necessary. Cholestasis ($n$ = 20), jaundice ($n$ = 7), and cholangitis ($n$ = 3) resolved in all patients; 18 patients had no further biliary problems during a follow-up period of 33 months (range, 24–42 months). Two patients (10%) developed epithelial hyperplasia within the stent, resulting in recurrent cholestasis in one and jaundice in the other. These patients were treated endoscopically with standard plastic

**TABLE 34.8. Results of Endoscopic Therapy of Pseudocysts**

| | | Method of Pseudocyst Decompression | | | | |
|---|---|---|---|---|---|---|
| Author/Year | Technical Success | Transpapillary (*n*) | Cystogastrostomy (*n*) | Cystoduodenoscopy (*n*) | Complications (*n*) | Deaths (*n*) |
| Binmoeller, 1995 | 47/53[a] | 31 | 6 | 10 | 6 | 0 |
| Catalano, 1995 | 17/21 | 17 | 0 | 9 | 1 | 0 |
| Cremer, 1989 | 32/33 | 0 | 11 | 21 | 3 | 0 |
| Grimm, 1989 | 14/16 | 5 | 1 | 8 | 5 | 1 |
| Howell, 1995 | 100/108 | 37 | 38 | 25 | 25 | 0 |
| Kozarek, 1991 | 12/14 | 12 | 0 | 0 | 5 | 0 |
| Sahel, 1991, 1995 | 58/67[a] | 26 | 1 | 31 | 9 | 1 |
| Smits, 1995 | 31/37[a] | 16 | 8 | 7 | 6 | 0 |
| Total | 311/249 (89%) | 144 | 65 | 102 | 66 (17%) | 2 (1%) |

[a]Combination therapy in several.

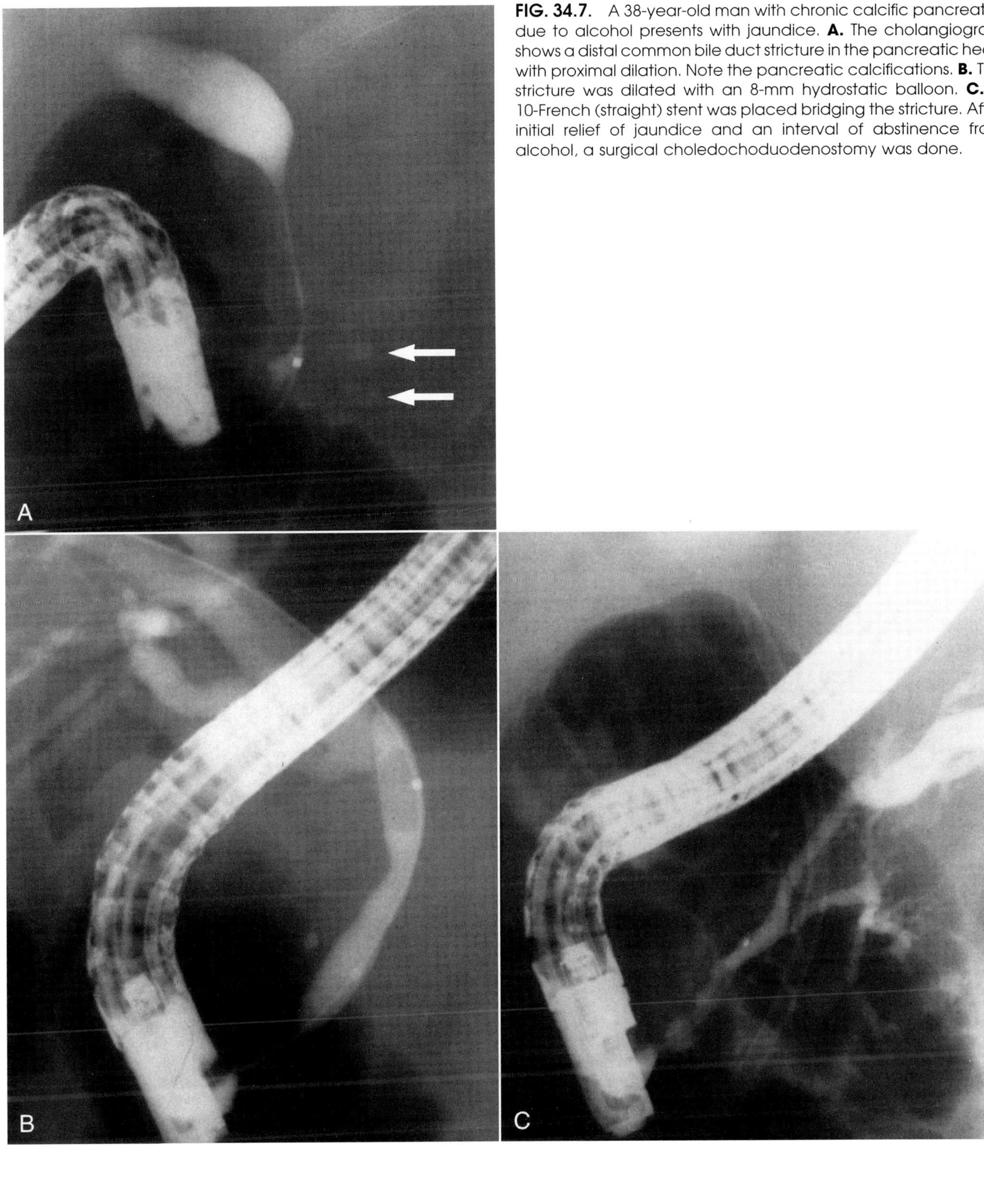


**FIG. 34.7.** A 38-year-old man with chronic calcific pancreatitis due to alcohol presents with jaundice. **A.** The cholangiogram shows a distal common bile duct stricture in the pancreatic head with proximal dilation. Note the pancreatic calcifications. **B.** The stricture was dilated with an 8-mm hydrostatic balloon. **C.** A 10-French (straight) stent was placed bridging the stricture. After initial relief of jaundice and an interval of abstinence from alcohol, a surgical choledochoduodenostomy was done.

stents, and one of them ultimately required surgical drainage. The authors concluded that this therapy could be an effective alternative to surgical biliary diversion, but longer follow-up and controlled trials will be necessary to confirm these results.

The Amsterdam group recently reported their results of placing 10-French biliary stents in 52 chronic pancreatitis patients with cholestasis (13). Jaundice and cholestasis disappeared within 2 weeks after stent insertion in all patients. During a median follow-up of 32 months (range, 3 months to 10 years), 17 patients (33%) had the stent removed without return of cholestasis. Complete resolution of the stricture was seen in 10 of the 17 patients. This suggested that complete resolution of the stricture was not necessary for long-term relief of symptoms and cholestasis.

The above studies indicate that plastic biliary stents are a useful alternative to surgery for short-term treatment of chronic pancreatitis–induced common bile duct strictures complicated by cholestasis, jaundice, and cholangitis. This therapy should also be considered for high-risk surgical patients. However, since the long-term efficacy of this treatment is much less satisfactory, operative intervention appears to be a better long-term solution for this problem in average-risk patients. More data on the long-term outcome, preferably in controlled trials, are necessary before the expandable stents can be advocated for this indication. Trials of membrane-coated metal stents and removable coil spring stents are awaited.

## SPHINCTER OF ODDI DYSFUNCTION

Although sphincter of Oddi dysfunction is a known cause of acute recurrent pancreatitis, its role in the pathogenesis of chronic pancreatitis is much less certain. A direct effect of alcohol on the sphincter of Oddi has been postulated (83). The authors suggested that alcohol increased motor activity of the sphincter of Oddi and raised the intraductular pancreatic pressure with subsequent disruption of small pancreatic ductules and backflow of pancreatic juice into the parenchyma with injury. Other studies show that intravenous or intragastric administration of alcohol in humans results in decreased sphincter of Oddi basal pressures at manometry. In a recently reported preliminary study, Morita et al. (84) showed that chronic alcohol administration in the Japanese monkey resulted in an increase in sphincter of Oddi mean basal pressure from 9 to 20 mm Hg ($p < .01$), while phasic amplitude decreased by 75%, and pancreatic ductal secretory rate nearly doubled. Two of three more recent studies using modern manometric techniques have shown a high frequency of basal sphincter pressure abnormalities, especially the pancreatic sphincter, in patients with established chronic pancreatitis (85, 86). Review of pancreatic basal sphincter pressure in 106 patients with ductographic abnormalities showed an elevated basal pressure (≥40 mm Hg) in 61%. Thus, it remains unknown whether the sphincter, at times, becomes dysfunctional as part of the overall general scarring process or has a role in the pathogenesis of chronic pancreatitis.

The surgical literature, although limited, suggests that sphincter ablation therapy (both the biliary and pancreatic sphincter) alone for patients with chronic pancreatitis and manometrically documented or suspected sphincter of Oddi dysfunction benefits 30–60% of patients (87, 88). Bagley et al. reported a surgical series (89) of 67 patients with mild-to-moderate chronic pancreatitis who underwent empiric biliary and pancreatic sphincterotomy ($n = 33$) or sphincteroplasty ($n = 34$). During a 5-year follow-up period, 44% of patients had relief of pain. The outcome for patients with idiopathic chronic pancreatitis was similar to that of patients with alcohol-induced chronic pancreatitis. However, 92% (11 of 12) of patients who stopped alcohol consumption were clinically improved, compared with 12.5% (2 of 16) of those who continued to drink.

Since endoscopic pancreatic sphincterotomy has been performed infrequently in most institutions, its role in the management of stenosis of the pancreatic sphincter has not been defined. Kozarek et al. reported resolution of pain and clinical episodes of pancreatitis and suspected or manometrically documented pancreatic sphincter of Oddi dysfunction. The utility of endoscopic sphincter ablation as the only therapy in patients with chronic pancreatitis awaits further study, preferably in controlled randomized trials.

## PANCREAS DIVISUM

Pancreas divisum is the most common congenital variant of pancreatic ductal anatomy, occurring in 7% of autopsy series (90). Usually, in the setting of chronic pancreatitis, minor papilla sphincterotomy is performed to provide access to the duct to effect stone retrieval or facilitate endoprosthesis placement (19). It has been postulated that in a subpopulation of pancreas divisum patients, the orifice of the minor papilla is critically small, so that excessively high intrapancreatic dorsal duct pressures occur during active secretion (91). This may result in pancreatic pain or pancreatitis. While most authorities agree that pancreas divisum is a definite cause of acute recurrent pancreatitis, its role in the pathogenesis of chronic pancreatitis is much more controversial. Several lines of evidence favor the association of pancreas divisum and pancreatitis including *(a)* the presence of pancreatographic and histologic changes of chronic pancreatitis isolated to the dorsal pancreas, *(b)* an increased incidence of pancreas divisum in patients with idiopathic pancreatitis, and *(c)* symptomatic benefit following endoscopic or surgical drainage of the dorsal duct.

Although ablation of the sphincter of the minor papilla by endoscopic or surgical techniques is effective for patients with pancreas divisum and acute recurrent pancreatitis, the outcome for patients with chronic pancreatitis has been much less satisfactory (17, 42, 92–97) (Table 34.9). Of 54 patients undergoing dorsal duct decompressive therapy by minor papilla sphincterotomy and/or dorsal duct stenting, only 44% of chronic pancreatitis patients improved during a mean follow-up period of 22 months. These data suggest that methods of selecting patients with pancreas divisum and chronic pancreatitis who are likely to benefit from endoscopic therapy need further investigation.

**TABLE 34.9. Selected Series Reporting the Results of Minor Papilla Therapy for Pancreas Divisum**[a]

| | | | Acute Recurrent Pancreatitis | | Pain Alone | | Chronic Pancreatitis | |
|---|---|---|---|---|---|---|---|---|
| Author | Year | Mean Follow-up (mos) | *n* | % Improved | *n* | % Improved | *n* | % Improved |
| Coleman | 1994 | 23 | 9 | 78 | 5 | 0 | 20 | 60 |
| Kozarek | 1995 | 20 | 15 | 73 | 5 | 20 | 19 | 32 |
| Lans | 1992 | 30 | 10 | 90 | 0 | — | 0 | — |
| Lehman | 1993 | 22 | 17 | 76 | 23 | 26 | 11 | 27 |
| Liguory | 1986 | 24 | 8 | 63 | 0 | — | 0 | — |
| McCarthy | 1988 | 21 | 19 | 89 | 0 | — | 0 | — |
| Sherman | 1994 | 28 | 0 | — | 16 | 44 | 0 | — |
| Soehendra | 1986 | 3 | 2 | 100 | 0 | — | 4 | 75 |
| Total | | | 80 | 80 | 49 | 29 | 54 | 44 |

[a]Endoscopic methods included minor papilla sphincterotomy and/or dorsal duct stenting

## CONCLUSION

Endoscopic therapy of chronic pancreatitis is gaining wider application. Selection of appropriate candidates for the various methods of treatment appears important for optimal results. Endoscopic management should be considered as one segment of our management options along with medical, percutaneous, and surgical treatments. Firm guidelines for application of such therapy are difficult because there are no controlled studies, follow-up in most series is brief, and there are no studies comparing endoscopic and surgical therapy. The future role of pancreatic endoscopic therapy will depend on evolving technology and the long-term results of further comparative controlled trials that address clinical outcomes. Cost efficacy studies are awaited. Endoscopists should exercise caution in the application of newer pancreatic techniques, as complications appear to be higher than those for comparable biliary procedures.

## REFERENCES

1. Sarles H, Bernard JP, Johnson C. Pathogenesis and epidemiology of chronic pancreatitis. Annu Rev Med 1989;40:453–468.
2. Steer ML, Waxman I, Freedman S. Chronic pancreatitis. N Engl J Med 1995;332:1482–1490.
3. Widdison AL, Alvarez C, Karanjia ND, Reber HA. Experimental evidence of beneficial effects of ductal decompression in chronic pancreatitis. Endoscopy 1991;23:151–154.
4. Karanjia ND, Reber HA. The cause and management of the pain of chronic pancreatitis. Gastrointest Clin North Am 1990;19: 895–904.
5. Lo SK, Lewis MPN, Reber PU, et al. In-vivo endoscopic transsphincteric measurement of pancreatic blood flow (PBF) in humans. Gastrointest Endosc 1996;43:409A.
6. Bradley EL. Long-term results of pancreatojejunostomy in patients with chronic pancreatitis. Am J Surg 1987;153:207–213.
7. Malfertheiner P, Buchler M. Indications for endoscopic or surgical therapy in chronic pancreatitis. Endoscopy 1991;23:185–190.
8. Bedford RA, Howerton DH, Geenen JE. The current role of ERCP in the treatment of benign pancreatic disease. Endoscopy 1994;26:113–119.
9. Kozarek RA, Traverso LW. Endotherapy of chronic pancreatitis. Int J Pancreatol 1996;19:93–102.
10. Kaikaus RM, Geenen JE. Current role of ERCP in the management of benign pancreatic disease. Endoscopy 1996;28:131–137.
11. Sherman S, Lehman GA. Endoscopic therapy of pancreatic disease. Gastroenterologist 1993;1:5–17.
12. Kozarek RA. Chronic pancreatitis in 1994: is there a role for endoscopic treatment? Endoscopy 1994;26:625–628.
13. Huibregtse K, Smits ME. Endoscopic management of diseases of the pancreas. Am J Gastroenterol 1994;89(suppl):S66–S77.
14. Cremer M, Deviere J, Delhaye M, Baize M, Vandermeeren A. Stenting in severe chronic pancreatitis; results of medium-term follow-up in 76 patients. Endoscopy 1991;23:171–176.
15. Grimm H, Meyer WH, Nam VC, Soehendra N. New modalities for treating chronic pancreatitis. Endoscopy 1989;21:70–74.
16. Kozarek RA, Patterson DJ, Ball TJ, Traverso LW. Endoscopic placement of pancreatic stents and drains in the management of pancreatitis. Ann Surg 1989;209:261–266.
17. McCarthy J, Geenen JE, Hogan WJ. Preliminary experience with stent placement in benign pancreatic diseases. Gastrointest Endosc 1988;34:16–18.
18. Geenen JE, Rolny P. Endoscopic therapy of acute and chronic pancreatitis. Gastrointest Endosc 1991;37:377–382.
19. Binmoeller KF, Jue P, Seifert H, Nam WC, Soehendra N. Endoscopic pancreatic stent drainage in chronic pancreatitis and a dominant stricture: long-term results. Endoscopy 1995;27: 638–644.
20. Smits ME, Badiga SM, Rauws EAJ, Tytgat GNJ, Huibregtse K. Long-term results of pancreatic stents in chronic pancreatitis. Gastrointest Endosc 1995;42:461–467.
21. Ponchon T, Bory R, Hedelius F, et al. Endoscopic stenting for pain relief in chronic pancreatitis: results of a standardized protocol. Gastrointest Endosc 1995;42:452–456.
22. Reber PU, Patel AG, Kusske AM, Toyama MT, Ashley SW, Reber HA. Stenting does not decompress the pancreatic duct as effectively as surgery in experimental chronic pancreatitis. Gastroenterology 1995;128:386A.
23. Ikenberry SO, Sherman S, Hawes RH, Smith M, Lehman GA. The occlusion rate of pancreatic stents. Gastrointest Endosc 1994;40: 611–613.
24. Cremer M, Deviere J, Delhaye M, Vandermeeren A, Baize M. Endoscopic management of chronic pancreatitis. Acta Gastroenterol Belg 1993;56:192–200.
25. McHenry L, Gore DC, DeMaria EJ, Zfass AM. Endoscopic treatment of dilated-duct chronic pancreatitis with pancreatic stents: preliminary results of a sham-controlled, blinded, crossover trial to predict surgical outcome. Am J Gastroenterol 1993;88:1536A.
26. DuVall GA, Schneider DM, Kortan P, Haber GB. Is the outcome of endoscopic therapy of chronic pancreatitis predictive of surgical success. Gastrointest Endosc 1996;43:405A.
27. Ammann RW, Akovbiantz A, Larglader F, Schueler G. Course and outcome of chronic pancreatitis: longitudinal study of a mixed medical-surgical series of 245 patients. Gastroenterology 1984; 86:820–828.
28. Cotton PB, Lehman G, Vennes J, et al. Endoscopic sphincterotomy complications and their management: an attempt at consensus. Gastrointest Endosc 1991;37:383–393.
29. Siegel J, Veerappan A. Endoscopic management of pancreatic disorders; potential risks of pancreatic prosthesis. Endoscopy 1991;23:177–180.
30. Sherman S, Alvarez C, Robert M, Ashley SW, Reber HA, Lehman GA. Polyethylene pancreatic stent-induced changes in the normal dog pancreas. Gastrointest Endosc 1993;39:658–664.
31. Johanson JF, Schmalz MJ, Geenen JE. Incidence and risk factors for biliary and pancreatic stent migration. Gastrointest Endosc 1992;38:341–346.
32. Dean RS, Geenen JE, Hogan WJ, Johnson GK, Schmalz MJ, Catalano MF. Pancreatic stent modification to prevent stent migration in patients with benign pancreatic disease. Gastrointest Endosc 1994;40:19A.
33. Kozarek RA. Pancreatic stents can induct ductal changes consistent with chronic pancreatitis. Gastrointest Endosc 1990; 36:93–95.
34. Derfus GA, Geenen JE, Hogan WJ. Effect of endoscopic pancreatic duct stent placement on pancreatic ductal morphology. Gastrointest Endosc 1990;36:206A.
35. Rossos PG, Kortan P, Haber GB. Complications associated with pancreatic duct stenting. Gastrointest Endosc 1992:38:252A.
36. Burdick JS, Geenen JE, Venu RP, et al. Ductal morphological changes due to pancreatic stent therapy—a randomized controlled study. Am J Gastroenterol 1992:87:155A.
37. Lehman GA, Sherman S, Nisi R, Hawes RH. Pancreas divisum: results of minor papilla sphincterotomy. Gastrointest Endosc 1993;39:1–8.
38. Smith MT, Sherman S, Ikenberry SO, Hawes RH, Lehman GA. Alterations in pancreatic ductal morphology following polyethylene pancreatic duct stenting. Gastrointest Endosc 1996;44: 268–275.
39. Eisen G, Coleman S, Troughton A, Cotton PB. Morphological changes in the pancreatic duct after stent placement for benign pancreatic disease. Gastrointest Endosc 1994;40:107A.
40. Sherman S, Hawes RH, Savides TJ, et al. Stent-induced pancreatic ductal and parenchymal changes: correlation of endoscopic ultrasound with ERCP. Gastrointest Endosc 1997;45,in press.
41. Alhalel R, Haber GB. Endoscopic therapy of pancreatic stones. Gastrointest Endosc Clin North Am 1995;5:195–215.
42. Sarles A, Bernard JP. Lithostathine and pancreatic lithogenesis. Viewpoints Dig Dis 1991;23:7–12.
43. Suda K, Mogaki M, Oyama T, Matsumoto Y. Histopathologic and immunohistochemical studies on alcoholic pancreatitis and chronic obstructive pancreatitis: special emphasis on ductal obstruction and genesis of pancreatitis. Am J Gastroenterol 1990;85:271–276.
44. Kozarek R, Ball TJ, Patterson DJ, Brandabur JJ, Traverso LW, Raltz S. Endoscopic pancreatic duct sphincterotomy: indications, technique, and analysis of results. Gastrointest Endosc 1994:40: 592–598.
45. Esber E, Sherman S, Earle D, Pezzi J, Gottlieb K, Lehman G.

Complications of major papilla pancreatic sphincterotomy: a review of 106 patients. Gastrointest Endosc 1995;41:422A.
46. Delhaye M, Vandermeeren A, Baize M, Cremer M. Extracorporeal shock-wave lithotripsy of pancreatic calculi. Gastroenterology 1992;102:610–620.
47. Sherman S, Lehman GA, Hawes RH, et al. Pancreatic duct stones: frequency of successful endoscopic removal and improvement in symptoms. Gastrointest Endosc 1991;37:511–517.
48. Smits ME, Rauws EA, Tytgat GNJ, Huibregtse K. Endoscopic treatment of pancreatic stones in patients with chronic pancreatitis. Gastrointest Endosc 1996;43:556–560.
49. Schneider MU, Lux G. Floating pancreatic duct concrements in chronic pancreatitis. Endoscopy 1985;17:8–10.
50. Fuji T, Amano H, Ohmura R, Akiyama T, Aibe T, Takemoto T. Endoscopic pancreatic sphincterotomy—technique and evaluation. Endoscopy 1989;21:27–30.
51. Kozarek RA, Ball TJ, Patterson DJ. Endoscopic approach to pancreatic duct calculi and obstructive pancreatitis. Am J Gastroenterol 1992;87:600–603.
52. Sauerbruch T, Holl J, Sackman M, Werner R, Wotzka R, Paumgartner G. Disintegration of a pancreatic duct stone with extracorporeal shockwaves in a patient with chronic pancreatitis. Endoscopy 1987;19:207–208.
53. Soehendra N, Grimm H, Meyer HW, et al. Extrakorporale stobwellen lithotripsie bei chronischer pankreatitis. Dtsch Med Wochenschr 1989;114:1402–1406.
54. Neuhaus H. Fragmentation of pancreatic stones by extracorporeal shock wave lithotripsy. Endoscopy 1989;23:161–165.
55. den Toom R, Nijs HG, van Blankenstein M, Schroder FH, Jeekel J, Terpstra OT. Extracorporeal shock wave lithotripsy of pancreatic duct stones. Am J Gastroenterol 1991;86:1033–1036.
56. Sauerbruch T, Holl J, Sackmann M, Paumgartner G. Extracorporeal lithotripsy of pancreatic stones in patients with chronic pancreatitis and pain: a prospective follow-up study. Gut 1992; 33:969–972.
57. Schneider HT, May A, Benninger J, et al. Piezoelectric shock wave lithotripsy of pancreatic duct stones. Am J Gastroenterol 1994; 89:2042–2048.
58. van der Hul R, Plaiser P, Jeekel J, Terpstra O, den Toom R, Bruining H. Extracorporeal shock-wave lithotripsy of pancreatic duct stones: immediate and long-term results. Endoscopy 1994;26: 573–578.
59. Sherman S, Rahaman S, Gottlieb K, et al. Lithotripsy in the management of pancreatic duct (PD) stones. Gastrointest Endosc 1995;41:429A.
60. Dumonceau J-E, Deviere J, LeMoine O, et al. Endoscopic pancreatic drainage in chronic pancreatitis associated with ductal stones: long-term results. Gastrointest Endosc 1996;43: 547–555.
61. Alvarez C, Widdison AL, Reber HA. New perspectives in the surgical management of chronic pancreatitis. Pancreas 1991; 6(suppl 1):576–581.
62. Neuhaus H, Hoffman W, Classen M. Laser lithotripsy of pancreatic and biliary stones via 3.4 mm and 3.7 mm miniscopes: first clinical results. Endoscopy 1992;24:208–214.
63. Sahel J, Sarles H. Citrate therapy in chronic calcifying pancreatitis: preliminary results. In: Mitchell CJ, Keeleheer J, eds. Pancreatic disease in clinical practice. London: Pitman, 1981:346–353.
64. Berger Z, Topa L, Takacs T, Pap A. Nasopancreatic drainage for chronic calcifying pancreatitis (CCP). Digestion 1992;52:70A.
65. Noda A, Shibata T, Ogawa Y, et al. Dissolution of pancreatic stones by oral trimethadione in a dog experimental model. Gastroenterology 1987;93:1002–1008.
66. Lehman GA, Sherman S. Pancreatic stones: to treat or not to treat? Gastrointest Endosc 1996;43:625–626.
67. Grace PA, Williamson RCN. Modern management of pancreatic pseudocysts. Br J Surg 1993;80:573–581.
68. Gumaste VV, Pitchumoni CS. Pancreatic pseudocysts. Gastroenterologist 1996;4:33–43.
69. Smits ME, Rauws EAJ, Tytgat GNJ, Huibregtse K. The efficacy of endoscopic treatment of pancreatic pseudocysts. Gastrointest Endosc 1995;42:202–207.
70. Barthet M, Sahel J, Bodiou-Bertel C, Bernard JP. Endoscopic transpapillary drainage of pancreatic pseudocysts. Gastrointest Endosc 1995;42:208–213.
71. Catalano MF, Geenen JE, Schmalz MJ, Johnson GK, Dean RS, Hogan WJ. Treatment of pancreatic pseudocysts with ductal communication by transpapillary pancreatic duct endoprosthesis. Gastrointest Endosc 1995;42:214–218.
72. Binmoeller KF, Seifert H, Walter A, Soehendra N. Transpapillary and transmural drainage of pancreatic pseudocysts. Gastrointest Endosc 1995;42:219–224.
73. Lehman GA. Endoscopic management of pancreatic pseudocysts continues to evolve. Gastrointest Endosc 1995;42: 273–275.
74. Howell DA, Lehman GA, Baron TH, et al. Endoscopic treatment of pancreatic pseudocysts: a retrospective multicenter analysis. Gastrointest Endosc 1995;41:424A.
75. Howell DA, Lehman GA, Baron TH, et al. Recurrent pseudocyst formation in patients managed with endoscopic drainage: pre-drainage features and management. Gastrointest Endosc 1996;43:407A.
76. Kozarek RA, Ball TJ, Patterson DJ, Freeny PC, Ryan JA, Traverso LW. Endoscopic transpapillary therapy for disrupted pancreatic duct and parapancreatic fluid collection. Gastroenterology 1991;100: 1362–1370.
77. Deviere J, Buseo H, Baize M, et al. Complete disruption of the main pancreatic duct: endoscopic management. Gastrointest Endosc 1995;42:445–451.
78. Kozarek RA, Jiranek G, Traverso LW. Endoscopic treatment of pancreatic ascites. Am J Surg 1994;168:223–228.
79. Frey CF, Suzuki M, Isaji S. Treatment of chronic pancreatitis complicated by obstruction of the common bile duct or duodenum. World J Surg 1990;14:59–69.
80. Deviere J, Devaere S, Baize M, Cremer M. Endoscopic biliary drainage in chronic pancreatitis. Gastrointest Endosc 1990;36: 96–100.
81. Barthet M, Bernard JP, Duval JL, Affriat C, Sahel J. Biliary stenting in benign biliary stenosis complicating chronic calcifying pancreatitis. Endoscopy 1994;26:569–572.
82. Deviere J, Cremer M, Love J, Sugai B, Vandermeeren A. Management of common bile duct strictures caused by chronic pancreatitis with metal mesh self expandable stents. Gut 1994; 35:122–126.
83. Guelrud M. How good is sphincter of Oddi manometry for chronic pancreatitis. Endoscopy 1994;26:265–267.
84. Morita M, Okazaki K, Yamasaki K, et al. Effects of long term administration of ethanol on the papillary sphincter and exocrine pancreas in the monkey. Gastroenterology 1194;106:309A.
85. Vestergaard H, Krause A, Rokkjaer M, Frombert O, Thommesen P, Funch-Jensen P. Endoscopic manometry of the sphincter of Oddi and the pancreatic and biliary ducts in patients with chronic pancreatitis. Scand J Gastroenterol 1994;29:188–192.
86. Ugljesic M, Bulajic M, Milosavljevic T, Stimec B. Endoscopic manometry of the sphincter of Oddi and pancreatic duct in patients with chronic pancreatitis. Int J Pancreatol 1996;19: 191–195.
87. Sherman S, Hawes RH, Madura JA, Lehman GA. Comparison of intraoperative and endoscopic manometry of the sphincter of Oddi. Surg Gynecol Obstet 1992;175:410–418.
88. Williamson RCN. Pancreatic sphincteroplasty: indications and outcome. Ann R Coll Surg 1988;70:205–211.
89. Bagley FH, Braasch JW, Taylor RH, Warren KW. Sphincterotomy or sphincteroplasty in the treatment of pathologically mild chronic pancreatitis. Am J Surg 1981;141:418–422.
90. Lehman GA, Sherman S. Pancreas divisum: diagnosis, clinical significance, and management alternatives. Gastrointest Endosc Clin North Am 1995;5:145–170.
91. Cotton PB. Congenital anomaly of pancreas divisum as cause of obstructive pain and pancreatitis. Gut 1980;21:105–114.
92. Soehendra N, Kempeneers I, Nam VCH, Grimm H. Endoscopic dilation and papillotomy of the accessory papilla and internal drainage in pancreas divisum. Endoscopy 1986;18: 129–132.
93. Liguory C, Lefebvre JF, Canard JM, Bonnel D, Fritsch J, Etienne JP. Le pancreas divisum: etude clinique et therapeutique chez l'homme: a propos de 87 cas. Gastroenterol Clin Biol 1986;10: 820–825.
94. Lans JI, Geenen JE, Johanson JF, Hogan WJ. Endoscopic therapy in patients with pancreas divisum and acute pancreatitis: a

prospective, randomized, controlled clinical trial. Gastrointest Endosc 1992;38:430–434.

95. Coleman SD, Eisen GM, Troughton AB, Cotton PB. Endoscopic treatment in pancreas divisum. Am J Gastroenterol 1994;89:1152–1155.
96. Sherman S, Hawes R, Nisi R, Bucksot L, Earle D, Lehman G. Randomized controlled trial of minor papilla sphincterotomy (MiES) in pancreas divisum (Pdiv) patients with pain only. Gastrointest Endosc 1994;40:125A.
97. Kozarek RA, Ball TJ, Patterson DJ, Brandabur JJ, Raltz SL. Endoscopic approach to pancreas divisum. Dig Dis Sci 1995;40:1974–1981.

# 35

# Surgical Drainage Procedures

Richard A. Prinz

Chronic pancreatitis is an inflammatory disease in which there is irreversible and usually progressive damage to the morphology and function of the gland. The gross and histologic findings that characterize this disease include fibrosis, acinar replacement, and inflammatory cell infiltrates (1). Structural abnormalities such as obstructing calculi and areas of stricture and dilatation are frequently seen in the main pancreatic duct. Ductal disruption with leakage of exocrine fluid can lead to the formation of pseudocysts, pancreatic ascites, or fistula. These morphologic changes eventually cause acinar and islet cell damage and dysfunction.

As the disease progresses, it manifests clinically with abdominal pain, steatorrhea, and/or diabetes mellitus. These are not typically surgical problems, and chronic pancreatitis should be managed medically until a surgically correctable disorder develops. An operation is clearly indicated when an anatomic problem such as a pseudocyst, pancreatic abscess, ascites, fistula, obstruction of the common bile duct or duodenum, or variceal hemorrhage secondary to splenic vein thromboses develops in a patient with chronic pancreatitis (Table 35.1). However, the main indication for operation in patients with chronic pancreatitis has been severe and intractable abdominal pain.

The goal of surgery for chronic pancreatitis is to relieve incapacitating abdominal pain while preserving as much endocrine and exocrine function as possible. A wide variety of procedures has been tried to achieve this end, but only direct operations on the pancreas have proven beneficial. These pancreatic procedures fall into two categories: drainage of a dilated duct system or resection of all or part of the gland. Since chronic pancreatitis consists of a wide spectrum of clinical, anatomic, and functional findings, no one operative approach is suitable for all patients with this disease. The challenge for the surgeon treating chronic pancreatitis is to select the procedure that best suits the anatomic and functional situation found in each individual patient. Since draining a dilated pancreatic duct is a less formidable procedure than pancreatic resection and since it preserves as much exocrine and exocrine function as possible, pancreatic ductal drainage is usually favored whenever possible.

Initially, surgeons thought that the sphincter of Oddi was the site of obstruction that led to dilatation of the pancreatic duct and to chronic pain. Sphincterotomy was popularized by Doubilet and Mulholland as a method for treating chronic pancreatitis (2). It was soon realized that this procedure provided inadequate drainage of the pancreatic duct. Link is credited with first performing retrograde drainage of the pancreatic duct when he created a pancreaticocutaneous fistula with the tail of the gland in a patient with pancreatitis (3). A more direct approach to duct decompression was introduced by Cattell in 1947 when he anastomosed the jejunum to the pancreatic duct to palliate the pain of duct-obstructing cancer in the head of the gland (4). Retrograde or caudal drainage of the pancreatic duct into a defunctionalized limb of jejunum, after resecting the spleen and a small portion of the tail of the pancreas, was reported almost simultaneously by DuVal and Zollinger et al. in 1954 (5, 6). Puestow et al. pointed out that multiple strictures and dilations often formed a "chain of lakes" throughout the ductal system and could prevent adequate ductal decompression with a caudal pancreaticojejunostomy (7). They recommended that wider drainage could be achieved by opening the pancreatic duct longitudinally from the transected tail to a point just to the right of the superior mesenteric vessels. The tail and body of the gland where the duct was opened was stuffed into, and anastomosed to, the end of the Roux-Y loop of jejunum. In 1960, Partington and Rochelle described lateral, or side-to-side, pancreaticojejunostomy, which allowed the pancreatic duct to be unroofed all the way from its origin in the tail of the pancreas to its entry into the duodenum (8). This method did not require resection of the spleen or any of the pancreatic tail. Thus, side-to-side pancreaticojejunostomy achieved more effective drainage of the pancreatic duct but did not unnecessarily sacrifice any pancreatic tissue. The importance of complete and thorough drainage has been reemphasized by Frey and Smith, who recommend resecting the anterior portion of the head of the gland where the duct courses posteriorly (9). Thick overlying tissue in this area can limit the effectiveness of ductal decompression into the jejunal loop.

## PREOPERATIVE ASSESSMENT

Appropriate patient selection is a crucial first step for a successful outcome with lateral pancreaticojejunostomy. Preoperative assessment should rule out other causes of pain, confirm the diagnosis of chronic pancreatitis, evaluate the patient's physiologic and psychosocial fitness for surgery, and assess the anatomic status of the pancreas and its ductal system, as well as the status of the duodenum and common bile duct.

The diagnosis of chronic pancreatitis should be confirmed by identification of characteristic clinical features. The nature of the patient's pain and the disability that it causes should be established with a careful history. The pain of chronic pancreatitis is usually located in the epigastrium and upper abdomen and commonly bores through or is referred to the back. It can be constant or episodic. Attacks are brought on by alcohol or food ingestion. The intensity and duration of the pain should be characterized in as much detail as possible not only to decide on the need for therapeutic intervention but also to document outcome benefit (10). The frequency of the pain and the medication required to control it should be recorded in detail. Objective measures such as analogue scales should be used to document the disabling nature of the pain and to serve as a standard for postoperative comparison. Excessive intake of alcohol will be identified as the cause of chronic pancreatitis in

**TABLE 35.1. Indications for Operation in Chronic Pancreatitis**

| |
|---|
| Incapacitating pain refractory to medical management |
| Common bile duct obstruction |
| Duodenal obstruction |
| Pseudocyst |
| Pancreatic fistula, abscess, or ascites |
| Upper gastrointestinal hemorrhage from splenic vein thrombosis |
| Inability to rule out cancer |

most patients. Physical examination may not be very revealing in uncomplicated chronic pancreatitis, but an abdominal mass, tenderness, and jaundice should be sought as well as signs of malnutrition and hepatic disease.

Extrapancreatic causes of abdominal pain, such as biliary tract or peptic ulcer disease, should be identified and treated whenever possible. Pancreatic cancer must be considered, especially in patients with masslike enlargement of the pancreatic head or substantial weight loss. Tumor markers including CA 19-9 and CEA can be assayed when malignancy is suspected. Unfortunately these markers are not specific for cancer and are also elevated in chronic pancreatitis.

Preoperative evaluation must include an assessment of the patient's metabolic and nutritional status. The endocrine function of the pancreas should be checked by measuring a fasting blood sugar level. An oral or intravenous glucose tolerance test can be obtained if there is further need to clarify the patient's ability to secrete insulin. The presence of diabetes mellitus and its method of treatment should be recorded. Pancreatic exocrine function should be assessed by determining the presence or absence of steatorrhea. The need for pancreatic enzyme replacement therapy should be documented. Malnutrition and weight loss are common in chronic pancreatitis, because of alcohol abuse, malabsorption, and pain induced by eating. Hypoalbuminemia is present in about one-third of patients who undergo pancreatic ductal drainage (11). Short-term preoperative parenteral hyperalimentation may be needed for patients with pronounced nutritional deficits. The patient's general cardiorespiratory status must be able to tolerate a major upper abdominal operation.

Determining an individual patient's suitability for pancreaticojejunostomy must also include an evaluation of his or her psychosocial status. The extent to which the patient's quality of life has been impaired should be assessed as objectively as possible. An analogue scale should be used preoperatively and postoperatively to determine the efficacy of therapeutic interventions (12). Patients who are employed, have stopped drinking, and are surrounded by a supportive family structure fare the best. Less favorable outcomes can be anticipated in patients who cannot be rehabilitated from their alcohol or drug addiction. Potential consequences of postoperative diabetes or exocrine insufficiency in these latter patients may also jeopardize their long-term outcome. Pancreaticojejunostomy preserves endocrine and exocrine function better than resective procedures, but the progressive nature of chronic pancreatitis will continue to take an adverse toll on these metabolic functions. Finally, patients must have a realistic expectation of the outcome that can be expected with pancreatic ductal drainage.

Pancreatic ductal drainage can only be expected to relieve pain if the pancreatic duct is dilated. The question then becomes at what size should the pancreatic duct be considered dilated. The minimum caliber of the main duct that various authors have suggested to be suitable for drainage has ranged from 5 to 10 mm (13). I consider doing pancreaticojejunostomy in patients whose duct diameter exceeds 5 mm. If the duct is only 3–4 mm in its greatest diameter, I regard it as normal size, and I would not recommend a pancreatic duct drainage procedure.

Since our operative approach hinges on the presence of a dilated duct, it is important to have accurate knowledge of its anatomy before taking the patient to the operating room. Radiologic imaging provides this information in most patients. Plain abdominal x-rays show pancreatic calcifications in about half of patients with chronic pancreatitis but rarely reveal any additional findings. Dynamic or spiral computed tomography (CT) that takes 3-mm cuts through the pancreas after bolus intravenous contrast has been infused should be obtained in all patients. CT provides sufficient anatomic information for surgical decision making in most patients. It is the most accurate means of detecting pancreatic calcifications, and it is a reliable method of demonstrating dilatation of the pancreatic duct. CT can also alert the surgeon to associated abnormalities such as a pseudocyst, mass lesions, obstruction of the intrapancreatic common bile duct and/or the duodenum, and splenic vein thrombosis with splenomegaly and left-sided portal hypertension. Endoscopic retrograde cholangiopancreatography (ERCP) was once considered an essential study for demonstrating the anatomy of the pancreatic duct. However, improvements in CT scanning have made it possible to avoid performing this invasive procedure in many patients with chronic pancreatitis. ERCP may fail to visualize the pancreatic duct in patients who have a tight stricture or impacted stone near the ampulla of Vater. CT can usually demonstrate a dilated duct distal (upstream) to these seemingly complete obstructions. In our practice, ERCP is no longer routinely performed before pancreaticojejunostomy. It is reserved for patients with suspected chronic pancreatitis who do not have a dilated duct demonstrated by CT or who have associated abnormalities that require further evaluation. Endoscopic ultrasound (EUS) may have some use in demonstrating the anatomy of the pancreatic duct in a less invasive manner than ERCP. It is not yet widely available, and its role in the evaluation of patients with chronic pancreatitis remains to be clarified.

## OPERATIVE PROCEDURE

The technical aspects of performing lateral pancreaticojejunostomy are an important factor in achieving complete ductal decompression and have a substantial bearing on long-term results. Prophylactic intravenous antibiotics that cover a broad spectrum of gram-negative organisms are usually given. A bowel preparation is advisable, particularly in reoperative cases, because the transverse colon and its vascular supply may be drawn in and become adherent to the inflammatory process in the retroperitoneum. One or two units of autologous blood should be obtained to avoid the need for a homologous transfusion. Perioperative use of octreotide is probably unnecessary since pancreatic exocrine secretion is already diminished in these patients and the fibrotic gland allows a relatively safe and secure anastomosis. X-ray capability should be available in case intraoperative cholangiography or pancreatography is needed. Usually the preoperative imaging evaluation makes these studies unnecessary, but it is prudent to be prepared for unexpected intraoperative findings.

## OPERATIVE TECHNIQUE

When performing pancreaticojejunostomy, I prefer to enter the peritoneal cavity through a bilateral subcostal incision. In patients with a narrow costal margin or a previous midline incision, a vertical midline incision extending from the xiphoid to just below the umbilicus may be a better alternative. A thorough exploration is performed to confirm the diagnosis of chronic pancreatitis and to rule out any unexpected findings such as malignancy. Biopsy specimens should be taken from any suspicious nodules or lymph nodes and evaluated by frozen section. The hepatic flexure and transverse colon are mobilized inferiorly. This allows an extended Kocher maneuver to be performed so that the entire head of the gland can be visualized and bimanually palpated. The lesser sac is entered by separating the greater omentum from the transverse colon and dividing the gastrocolic vessels as needed. The entire anterior surface of the pancreas is exposed by transecting the fibrous adhesions between the pancreas and the posterior wall of the stomach. This can be technically demanding if there has been a great deal of inflammatory scarring or if a prior pseudocyst has been treated by a cystogastrostomy. A branch of the superior mesenteric vein or middle colic vein may extend superiorly along the anterior surface of the pancreas. It should be ligated and divided before it is avulsed by traction and causes troublesome bleeding. This extensive exposure of the pancreas is necessary for adequate visual and manual evaluation.

The next step is to locate the pancreatic duct (Fig. 35.1). It can usually be palpated on the anterior surface of the pancreas as a fluctuant depression in the parenchyma. Its presence is confirmed by aspiration of water-clear pancreatic juice with a 20-gauge needle attached to a 10-mL syringe. If the duct is not located with these maneuvers, intraoperative ultrasound can be used (14). Before it was available, a vertical incision would be made perpendicular to the expected course of the duct in an area away from major vessels. The incision is carried down until the intersected duct is identified. Once the duct is found, the overlying pancreas is incised to splay it open and prepare it for the pancreaticojejunostomy (Fig. 35.2). This can be done with cautery to control minor bleeding. Suture ligatures are used for vessels not controlled by cautery. A right-angle dissecting forceps or metal probe is used to identify the course of the duct as it is unroofed. In the body and tail, the duct has a relatively anterior position. While in the head, it dives more posteriorly, so the

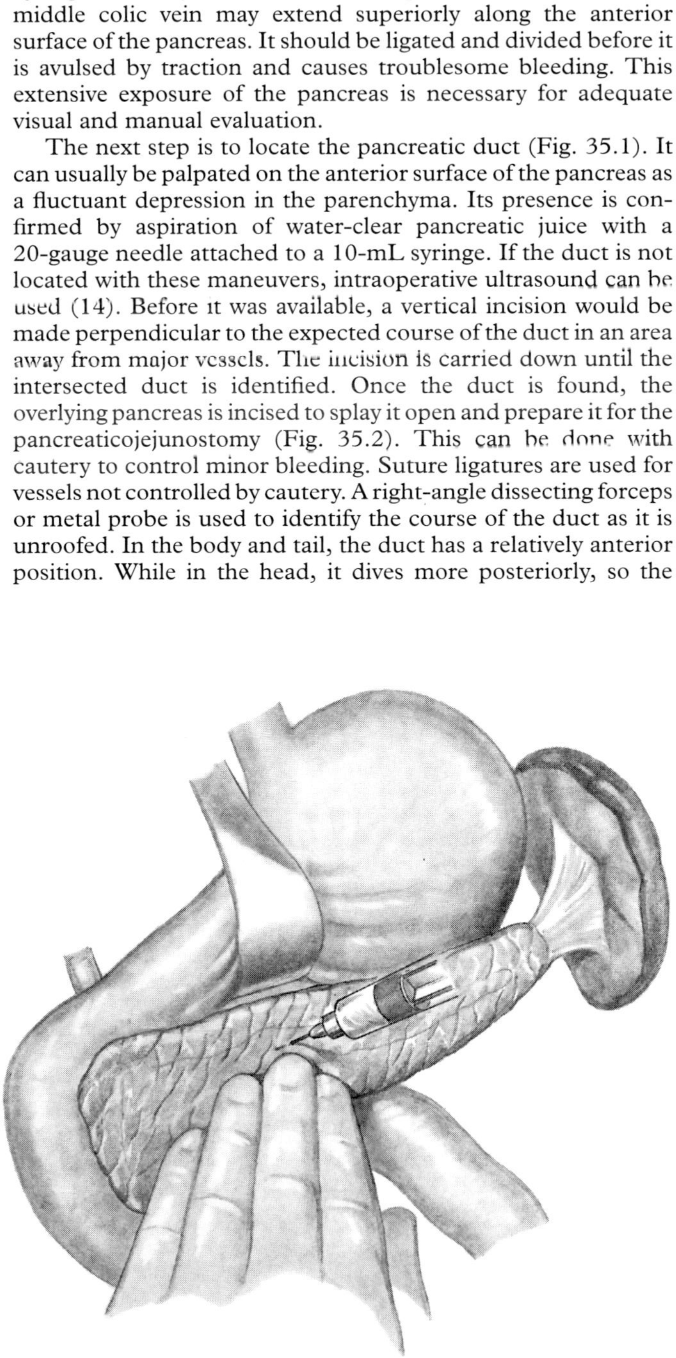

**FIG. 35.1.** The pancreatic duct can usually be palpated on the anterior surface of the pancreas as a fluctuant area. This is confirmed by needle aspiration of water-clear pancreatic exocrine fluid.

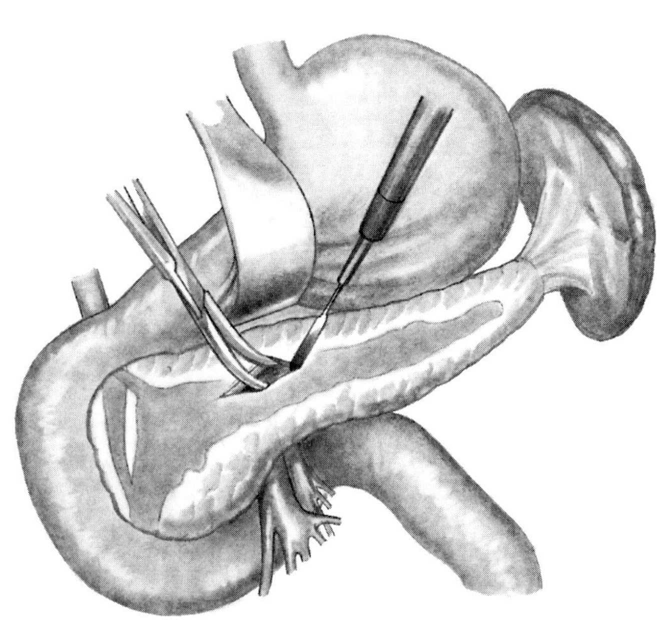

**FIG. 35.2.** Once the pancreatic duct has been located, it is entered by cutting through the pancreatic parenchyma with either a scalpel or cautery. Cautery can be used to incise the overlying parenchyma and open the entire duct system.

overlying parenchyma may be quite substantial. Both the duct of Wirsung and the duct of Santorini should be opened from the tail to as close as possible to their entry into the duodenum. All accessible stones that are found in these two ducts should be removed, especially those in the head of the gland, since they may cause persistent or recurrent obstruction. Stones impacted where these ducts enter the duodenum should be removed unless substantial bleeding is encountered. Such bleeding can usually be controlled by prolonged direct pressure.

Recent reports have focused attention on the importance of the pancreatic head and uncinate process as a source of pain in chronic pancreatitis. This area of the gland can be the most critical yet most difficult site to decompress the pancreatic duct. Anterior pancreaticoduodenal or gastroepiploic vessels that run vertically over the pancreatic head toward the superior mesenteric vein must be ligated and divided as the ductotomy is extended to the duodenum, if this has not already been done. Since the head of the gland is often enlarged and bulky in chronic pancreatitis, anterior ductotomy may not provide adequate drainage as the main pancreatic duct dives posteriorly to the right of the superior mesenteric vein. Local resection of overlying tissue as described by Frey and Smith may be necessary in this situation (9). The need for this can be assessed by bimanual examination of the Kocherized head and uncinate process. If the surrounding parenchyma extends more than 1 cm from the duct, there is a potential for undrained areas. The tissue can be cored out or locally resected to ensure complete drainage of the head. Failure to achieve adequate drainage in the juxtaduodenal head of the gland is the most common cause for failure of ductal drainage in our experience (15).

A frozen section is routinely taken from tissue removed during ductotomy and/or locally resected from the pancreatic head. A biopsy is done on any area that is suspicious for malignancy and a frozen section is evaluated. The surgeon's dilemma is that a prominent area of fibrosis and scarring may mimic a tumor, while the diffuse changes of chronic pancreatitis may obscure a cancer. In spite of routine biopsy to confirm the diagnosis of chronic pancreatitis and rule out malignancy, 4 of the first 200 patients who had pancreatic ductal drainage at our center died within a year from unsuspected pancreatic cancer (16).

After the pancreatic duct has been unroofed and decompressed, the jejunal limb is prepared for Roux-en-Y drainage. The jejunum is divided approximately 20–30 cm distal to the ligament of Treitz, where its mesentery is mobile enough to allow it to reach the pancreas. This can be done with a gastrointestinal stapler or with standard methods of suture closure, depending on the surgeon's preference. We reinforce the staple line on the distal limb with a few interrupted nonabsorbable Lembert sutures. The Roux limb is brought through the transverse mesocolon after making a window in an avascular space that provides the most direct access to the pancreas. The closed end of the jejunal limb is positioned in the splenic hilum (Fig. 35.3). The anastomosis is begun here because it is the most difficult area for exposure. At approximately 5 cm from the oversewn end of the jejunum, a single row of interrupted nonabsorbable sutures are placed to anastomose the antimesenteric surface of the jejunum to the tough fibrous capsule of the pancreas inferior to the open duct. A single-layer continuous anastomosis with nonabsorbable monofilament suture can also be used. No attempt is made to bring the mucosa of the jejunum down to the mucosa of the duct, since there is no evidence that long-term patency of this anastomosis depends on mucosal apposition. In fact, bringing the jejunal mucosa down to the narrowed or obliterated mucosa of the pancreatic duct in areas of stricture or stenosis may actually compromise the anastomotic orifice. The anastomosis is completed with interrupted sutures passed through the full thickness of the jejunal wall and the fibrotic tissue and capsule of the superior edge of the incised pancreatic duct. Sutures that are placed too deep in the gland may occlude side branches and limit pancreatic decompression.

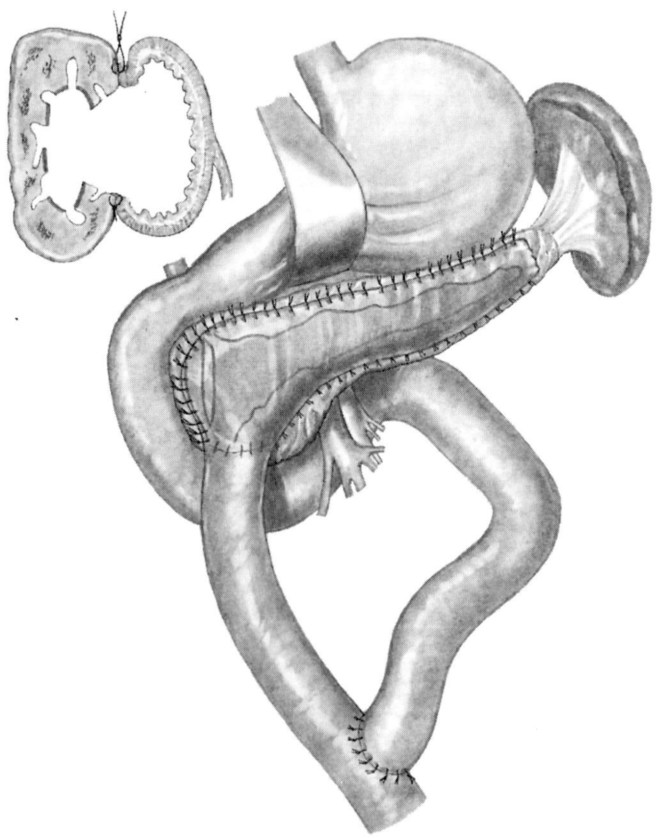

**FIG. 35.3.** The lateral pancreaticojejunostomy is performed by anastomosing the jejunum to the anterior capsule of the pancreas. Nonabsorbable suture material is used to make this anastomosis. It can be done in a continuous or interrupted manner. The jejunojejunostomy is made approximately 40 cm distal to the pancreaticojejunostomy.

Intestinal continuity is reestablished with an end-to-side jejunojejunostomy placed approximately 40 cm distal to the pancreaticojejunostomy. The opening in the transverse mesocolon is closed around the Roux limb to prevent internal small bowel herniation. Likewise, the small bowel mesenteric defect adjacent to the enteroenterostomy is closed. A cholecystectomy is usually performed along with pancreaticojejunostomy even if calculous disease is not present. This eliminates the gallbladder as a source of persistent or recurrent pain should this develop after operation. A jejunostomy tube is placed selectively for enteral feeding in patients who are malnourished or who may have gastroparesis because of an associated gastric outlet obstruction. Closed suction drains are placed if there is concern about leakage of bile or pancreatic secretions. The likelihood of this is small, and drains are rarely needed.

Postoperative management is similar to that for any abdominal operation involving an anastomosis of the small intestine. Nasogastric suction is continued until gastrointestinal function returns. Oral intake is then resumed, and the diet is advanced as tolerated. If drains are placed, they are removed when their daily output remains below 100 mL after feeding has been resumed.

## OUTCOME

Lateral pancreaticojejunostomy is a reasonably safe procedure that has an operative mortality rate of 0–4% and an associated complication rate of 10–25%. In a series of 200 patients that I reported with symptomatic chronic pancreatitis, operative mortality was 3.5%, and the complication rate was 20% (17). Long-term follow-up has been reported on the first 100 patients in this series (18). After a mean follow-up of 7.9 years (range, 1–25 years), pain was improved in 82% of patients. Frey and Amikura followed 47 patients an average of 37 months after local resection of the head of the pancreas combined with longitudinal pancreaticojejunostomy (11); 16 patients (34%) had no pain and required no narcotics, 8 (17%) had minimal pain and took no narcotics, and 11 (23%) had minimal pain and required minimal narcotics. Overall 74% of the patients had excellent pain relief, 13% had some improvement, and 13% were unimproved.

Wilson et al. compared 20 patients with chronic pancreatitis treated by pancreaticojejunostomy with 43 patients who were treated by various medical and other surgical therapies because their pancreatic duct was 7 mm or less in diameter (19). After a mean follow-up of 5 years, pain was improved in 76% of the patients who had pancreatic ductal drainage, compared with only 48% in the group with small duct disease. Most reported series indicate that 65–85% of patients have amelioration of their pain after pancreatic ductal decompression. These findings have been replicated at centers in the United States (20, 21), Europe (22), and Japan (23).

Even though endocrine and exocrine insufficiency are recognized sequelae of untreated chronic pancreatitis, diabetes and steatorrhea are not inevitable consequences of pancreatic drainage. Nealon et al. prospectively studied 68 patients with chronic pancreatitis and used a five-point system consisting of tests of morphology (ERCP), endocrine function (oral glucose tolerance test and fat-stimulated release of pancreatic polypeptide), and exocrine function (bentiromide PABA test and 72-hour fecal fat) to evaluate outcome (24). Some 30 patients had pancreaticojejunostomy, and 38 were treated medically. No patient with severe disease, defined by abnormalities in at least three of the tests, improved in grade during follow-up; 17 of 24 patients (71%) with mild-to-moderate disease who were treated medically progressed to a severe grade, compared with only 3 of 19 patients (16%) who were treated with pancreaticojejunostomy. These authors suggest that early operation is indicated in chronic pancreatitis to preserve glandular function. As part of a subsequent study using the same grading system, Nealon and Thompson randomized 17 patients with a diagnosis of chronic pancreatitis to either operation or medical therapy (25). Nine of these patients had a pancreaticojejunostomy. Seven of the nine patients who underwent operation retained their status during a follow-up period of 14–16 months, compared with only two of eight patients in the nonoperated group.

While established endocrine and exocrine deficits are not likely to be improved after pancreaticojejunostomy, the operation itself does not seem to impair glandular function. In our experience, only 11 of 53 nondiabetic patients developed diabetes during long-term follow-up after pancreatic ductal drainage (18); 8 of these 11 required insulin. Likewise, only 6 of 24 patients with non-insulin-dependent diabetes required insulin postoperatively. Overall, almost half of our patients never became diabetic, and only 28% required insulin. Pancreatic enzymes were required by 20% of our patients preoperatively, and this increased to 33% during long-term postoperative follow-up. Frey and Amikura reported that only 11% of their patients had progression of diabetes, and none had worsening of exocrine function after local resection of the head of the pancreas combined with longitudinal pancreaticojejunostomy (11). Adams et al. followed 62 patients after pancreaticojejunostomy a mean of 6.3 years and found that only 23% required insulin and only 34% required pancreatic enzymes (26).

Jalleh and Williamson found no significant change in the incidence of diabetes in their 23 patients who were treated with pancreaticojejunostomy (27). Likewise, they found no significant change in the glucose tolerance test in the eight patients who were studied before and after pancreatic duct drainage.

While pancreaticojejunostomy is a safe and effective means of relieving intractable pain in chronic pancreatitis, long-term mortality after this procedure remains a distressing problem because of the patient population on whom it is performed. Almost 40% of our patients survived less than 5 years after pancreaticojejunostomy (18). Continued alcoholism was an important factor contributing to this high mortality. This underscores the importance of getting these patients to abstain from alcohol. Other studies have also found a high late death rate and have attributed this mortality to comorbid conditions and continued alcoholism. Abstinence from alcohol is also important in achieving optimal pain relief with pancreaticojejunostomy. Talamini et al. have shown that cessation of drinking and of smoking both significantly reduce the risks of pain relapses (28).

As parenchymal scarring and fibrosis progress in chronic pancreatitis, increasing external pressure can be exerted on the intrapancreatic portion of the common bile duct and on the peripancreatic duodenum. These structures can then become obstructed. Chronic biliary tract and duodenal obstruction have been present in 30% and 15%, respectively, of patients having lateral pancreaticojejunostomy in our experience (29). Other surgeons have noted a similar concurrence of these conditions in patients requiring operative intervention for chronic pancreatitis. Biliary tract and duodenal obstruction can cause persistent symptoms if they are not dealt with at the initial operation, and they can cause recurrent pain if they develop after pancreaticojejunostomy. In the series reported by Adams et al., 6 of 84 patients required reoperation after lateral pancreaticojejunostomy (26). Two of these operations were to correct biliary stenosis, two to correct duodenal stenosis causing gastric outlet obstruction, and one to correct both of these problems. The remaining patient had a total pancreatectomy for recurrent pain and pancreatitis.

Although some surgeons would favor pancreatic resection when dealing with associated biliary and/or duodenal obstruction, our approach has been to perform combined drainage procedures to deal with these complications (29). Resection substantially increases the likelihood of diabetes, while combined drainage does not. In patients with fixed common bile duct obstruction, the biliary tract may be decompressed by either a choledochoduodenostomy or a choledochojejunostomy using either the Roux loop constructed to drain the pancreas or a second isolated Roux loop (Fig. 35.4). The extent of disease and individual variations in anatomy and body habitus usually dictate which of these alternatives is the most straightforward way of decompressing the biliary tree. Duodenal obstruction can be relieved with a gastrojejunostomy. We have shown that combined biliary drainage and/or gastrojejunostomy does not increase the morbidity and mortality of lateral pancreaticojejunostomy, while achieving the same high likelihood of relief of pain (28). Other surgeons have also found a frequent need to combine biliary bypass with pancreatic ductal decompression. Nealon et al. performed a biliary bypass in 37% of their patients undergoing pancreaticojejunostomy (24).

Pancreatic pseudocysts occur with much greater frequency in chronic pancreatitis than in acute pancreatitis. As many as 35–50% of patients with chronic pancreatitis will develop a pseudocyst (30). Patients with chronic pancreatitis who have only drainage of their pseudocysts are likely to require reoperation for intractable pain or recurrence of pseudocyst. In Frey and Amikura's series of 50 patients undergoing "unroofing"-type resection of the head of the pancreas combined with longitudinal pancreaticojejunostomy, 8 had undergone a prior pseudocyst drainage procedure (11). Of 81 patients we have followed after pseudocyst drainage, 15 needed reoperation (31); the cause for reoperation was unrelenting pain in seven and recurrent pseudocyst in seven.

Since a pseudocyst may indicate underlying chronic pancreatitis, patients with a long history of alcohol abuse, pancreatic calcifications, and exocrine or endocrine insufficiency should have a thorough evaluation of their pancreatic ductal system before operation on the cyst. If the pancreatic duct is noted to be dilated on CT or ERCP, it should be decompressed with a lateral pancreaticojejunostomy at the time that the cyst is drained. Cysts that are primarily intrapancreatic can be drained by extending the incision of the pancreatic duct to include the pseudocyst and incorporating the opening into the overlying Roux limb (Fig. 35.5). Larger extrapancreatic pseudocysts can be drained by opening the cyst in a dependent position and extending the Roux limb over this opening for a separate anastomosis. In our experience, combining pseudocyst drainage with lateral pancreaticojejunostomy has not increased the morbidity or mortality of either procedure. We have yet to identify a patient with chronic pancreatitis who has had a recurrent pseudocyst after undergoing complete pancreatic ductal drainage. Nealon et al. also reported a frequent need to combine lateral pancreaticojejunostomy with pseudocyst drainage. In their series of 41 patients undergoing pancreaticojejunostomy, 8 (20%) also required pseudocyst drainage, and 8 (20%) required both pseudocyst and biliary bypass (24).

When pain persists or recurs after lateral pancreaticojejunostomy, the patient must be reevaluated and other possible causes of the pain must be ruled out. If none is found, some surgeons proceed to pancreatic resection. In our experience and that of others, pancreatic resection has little benefit in patients who have failed pancreatic ductal drainage. On the other hand, evaluation of these patients for undrained segments of pancreatic duct has been worthwhile. Fourteen patients in our series who had continued pain after ductal drainage were treated with a second drainage of the ductal system (15). Seventy-one percent of these patients were pain free or substantially improved after redrainage. As with initial ductal drainage, there was minimal loss of endocrine or exocrine function. During the same period, various

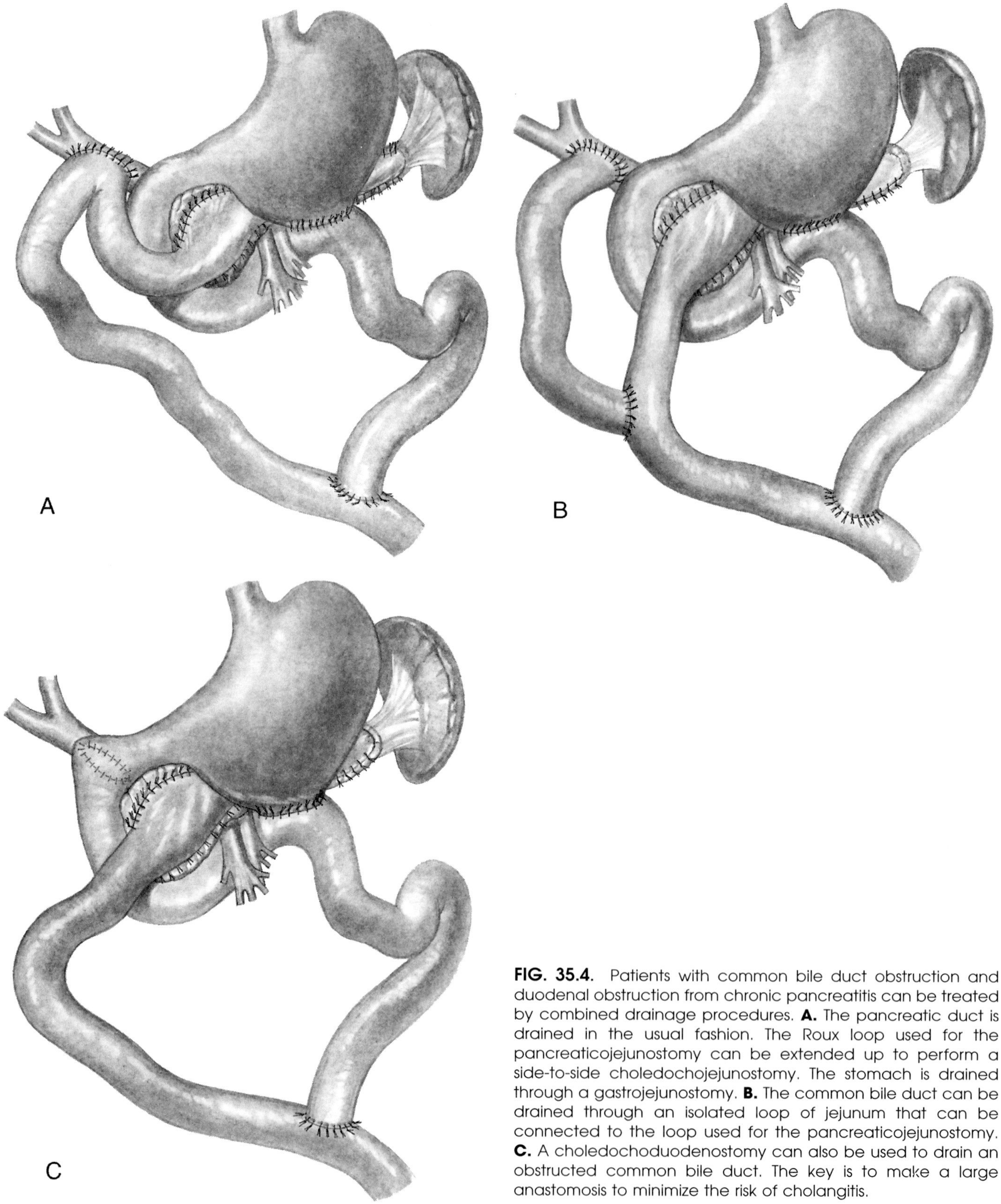


**FIG. 35.4.** Patients with common bile duct obstruction and duodenal obstruction from chronic pancreatitis can be treated by combined drainage procedures. **A.** The pancreatic duct is drained in the usual fashion. The Roux loop used for the pancreaticojejunostomy can be extended up to perform a side-to-side choledochojejunostomy. The stomach is drained through a gastrojejunostomy. **B.** The common bile duct can be drained through an isolated loop of jejunum that can be connected to the loop used for the pancreaticojejunostomy. **C.** A choledochoduodenostomy can also be used to drain an obstructed common bile duct. The key is to make a large anastomosis to minimize the risk of cholangitis.

pancreatic resections were performed on seven patients with pain after ductal drainage. None was rendered free of pain, and three eventually died from complications of diabetes. Other reports have also noted pain relief after more thorough drainage of the pancreatic duct (32).

Once other causes have been ruled out, all patients with persistent or recurrent pain after pancreaticojejunostomy should undergo dynamic CT scanning of the pancreas or ERCP if necessary to delineate the pancreatic duct. If the anastomosis is occluded or if residual undrained segments are identified,

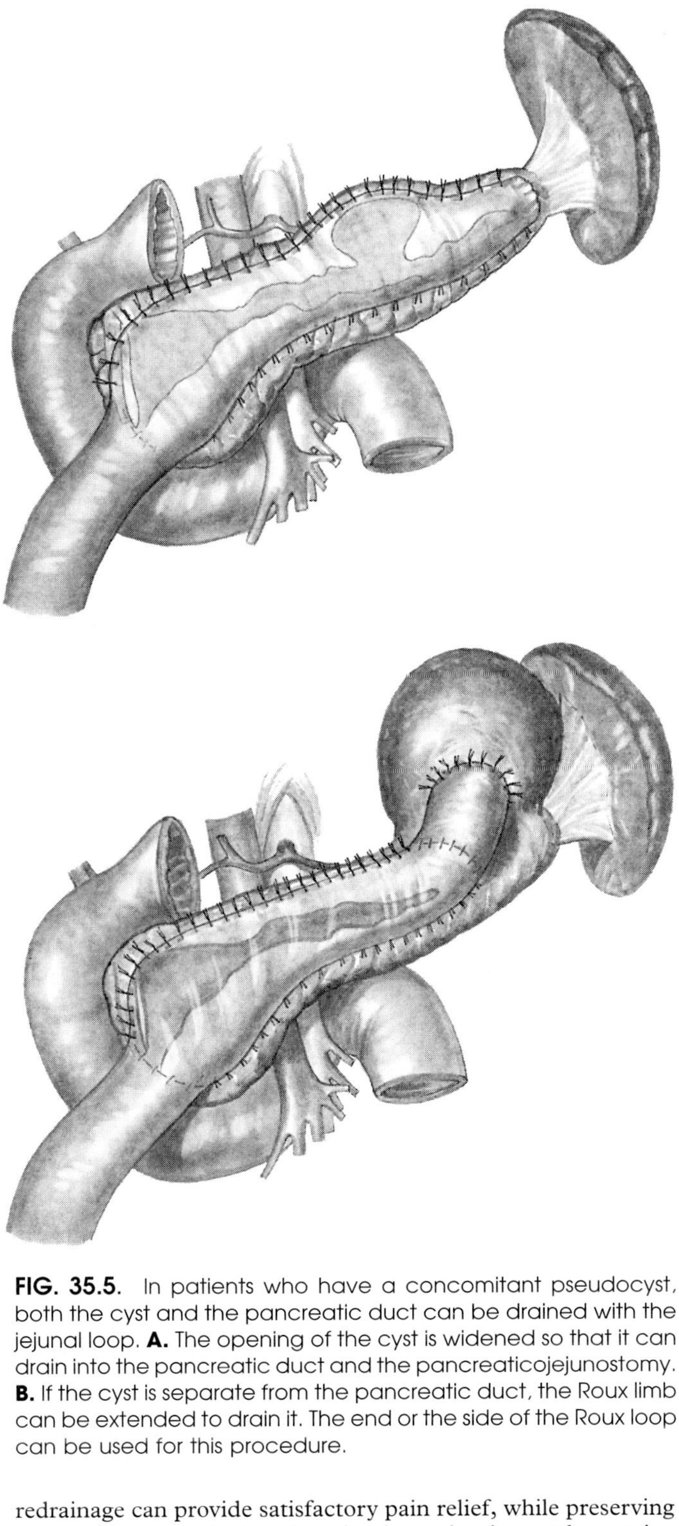


**FIG. 35.5.** In patients who have a concomitant pseudocyst, both the cyst and the pancreatic duct can be drained with the jejunal loop. **A.** The opening of the cyst is widened so that it can drain into the pancreatic duct and the pancreaticojejunostomy. **B.** If the cyst is separate from the pancreatic duct, the Roux limb can be extended to drain it. The end or the side of the Roux loop can be used for this procedure.

redrainage can provide satisfactory pain relief, while preserving pancreatic tissue that will maintain endocrine and exocrine function.

## SUMMARY

Complete drainage of the pancreatic ductal system can be achieved with a side-to-side pancreaticojejunostomy. This procedure is the preferred method of treating intractable pain of chronic pancreatitis in patients who have a dilated duct. Functioning pancreatic tissue is not sacrificed, and the natural tendency to develop endocrine or exocrine insufficiency in chronic pancreatitis is not exacerbated. Common complications of chronic pancreatitis such as obstruction of the biliary tract or duodenum and pseudocysts can be treated concurrently without an increase in morbidity or mortality.

## REFERENCES


1. Klöppel G, Maillet B. The morphological basis for the evolution of acute pancreatitis into chronic pancreatitis. Virchows Arch (A) 1992;420:1–4.
2. Doubilet H, Mulholland JH. Eight year study of pancreatitis and sphincterotomy. JAMA 1956;160:521–528.
3. Link G. The treatment of chronic pancreatitis by pancreatostomy. Ann Surg 1911;53:768–782.
4. Cattell RB. Anastomosis of the duct of Wirsung; its use in palliative operations for cancer in the head of the pancreas. Surg Clin North Am 1947;27:636–643.
5. DuVal MK Jr. Caudal pancreaticojejunostomy for chronic relapsing pancreatitis. Ann Surg 1954;140:775.
6. Zollinger RM, Keith LM, Ellison EH. Pancreatitis. N Engl J Med 1954;251:497–502.
7. Puestow CB, Gillesby WJ, et al. Retrograde surgical drainage of pancreas for chronic relapsing pancreatitis. Arch Surg 1958;76: 898–906.
8. Partington PF, Rochelle REL. Modified Puestow procedure for retrograde drainage of the pancreatic duct. Ann Surg 1960;152: 1037–1043.
9. Frey CF, Smith GJ. Description and rationale of a new operation for chronic pancreatitis. Pancreas 1987;2:701–707.
10. Frey CF, Pitt HA, Yeo CJ, Prinz RA. A plea for uniform reporting of patient outcome in chronic pancreatitis. Arch Surg 1996;131: 233–234.
11. Frey CF, Amikura K. Local resection of the head of the pancreas combined with longitudinal pancreaticojejunostomy in the management of patients with chronic pancreatitis. Ann Surg 1994; 220(4):492–507.
12. Prinz RA. Surgical options in chronic pancreatitis. Int J Pancreatol 1993;14(2):97–105.
13. Delcore R, Rodriguez FJ, Thomas JH, Forster J, Hermreck AS. The role of pancreatojejunostomy in patients without dilated pancreatic ducts. Am J Surg 1994;168:598–602.
14. Machi J, Sigel B, Zaren, HA, Kurhiji T, Yamashit Y. Operative ultrasonography during hepatobiliary and pancreatic surgery. World J Surg 1993;17:640–646.
15. Prinz RA, Aranha GV, Greenlee HB. Redrainage of the pancreatic duct in chronic pancreatitis. Am J Surg 1986;151:150–156.
16. Rao R, Prinz RA. Surgical therapy in chronic pancreatitis. Curr Opinion Gen Surg 1993;287–293.
17. Prinz RA, Greenlee HB. Pancreatic duct drainage in chronic pancreatitis. Hepatogastroenterology 1990;37:295–300.
18. Prinz RA, Greenlee HB. Pancreatic duct drainage in 100 patients with chronic pancreatitis. Ann Surg 1981;194:313–320.
19. Wilson TG, Hollands MJ, Little JM. Pancreaticojejunostomy for chronic pancreatitis. Aust NZ J Surg 1992;62:111–115.
20. Bradley EL III. Long-term results of pancreatojejunostomy in patients with chronic pancreatitis. Am J Surg 1987;153:207–213.
21. Hart MJ, Miyashita H, Morita N, White TT. Pancreaticojejunostomy report of a 25 year experience. Am J Surg 1983;145:567–570.
22. Sarles JC, Nacchiero M, Garani F, Salasc B. Surgical treatment of chronic pancreatitis. Am J Surg 1982;144:317–321.
23. Sato T, Miyashita E, Yamauchi H, Matsuno S. The role of surgical treatment for chronic pancreatitis. Ann Surg 1986;203: 266–271.
24. Nealon WH, Townsend CM, Thompson JC. Operative drainage of the pancreatic duct delays functional impairment in patients with chronic pancreatitis. Ann Surg 1988;208(3):321–329.
25. Nealon WH, Thompson JC. Progressive loss of pancreatic function in chronic pancreatitis is delayed by main pancreatic duct decompression. Ann Surg 1993;217(5):458–468.
26. Adams DV, Ford MC, Anderson MC. Outcome after lateral pancreaticojejunostomy for chronic pancreatitis. Ann Surg 1994; 219(5):481–489.
27. Jalleh RP, Williamson RCN. Pancreatic exocrine and endocrine function after operations for chronic pancreatitis. Ann Surg 1992;216(60):656–662.

28. Talamini G, Bassi C, Falconi M, Sartori N, Salvia R, et al. Pain relapses in the first 10 years of chronic pancreatitis. Am J Surg 1996;171:565–569.
29. Prinz RA, Aranha GV, Greenlee HB. Combined pancreatic duct and upper gastrointestinal and biliary tract drainage in chronic pancreatitis. Arch Surg 1985;120:361–386.
30. Munn JS, Aranha GV, Greenlee HB, Prinz RA. Simultaneous treatment of chronic pancreatitis and pancreative pseudocyst. Arch Surg 1987;122:662–667.
31. Aranha GV, Prinz RA, Freeark RJ, et al. Evaluation of therapeutic options for pancreatic pseudocysts. Arch Surg 1982;177:717–721.
32. Markowitz JS, Rattner DW, Warshaw AL. Failure of symptomatic relief after pancreaticojejunal decompression for chronic pancreatitis. Arch Surg 1994;129:374–380.

# 36

# Pancreaticoduodenectomy for Chronic Pancreatitis

Roger G. Keith

Resective procedures for chronic pancreatitis must be carefully approached by the surgeon with the recognition that ablation leads almost inevitably to reduction of endocrine and exocrine function. Selection of patients for resective surgery must consider the indications for this procedure, the pathologic derangements of the gland and its ductal system, and the consequences of pancreatic insufficiency on the potential rehabilitation of the individual patient. Each patient must be given independent evaluation of all factors; no decisions should be based on pathologic anatomy alone.

Most patients will present for operation as a consequence of the pain associated with chronic pancreatitis. Although other complications such as cyst formation, biliary obstruction, duodenal obstruction, fistula formation, and pancreatic ascites can occur without pain, nonresective surgical procedures will satisfactorily treat most of these complications, occurring either alone or occurring in combination. A pancreatic mass lesion in the head of the gland must be differentiated from a neoplasm in all cases of suspected chronic pancreatitis.

Morbidity and mortality following pancreaticoduodenectomy have improved substantially in the past decade. As a result, with increasing frequency, surgeons feel this resective procedure is indicated for benign and malignant conditions primarily affecting the head of the pancreas. The appeal of a pancreaticoduodenectomy is related to the preservation of endocrine function with salvage of a minimally diseased distal pancreas. This is particularly true for chronic alcoholic pancreatitis, in which subtotal or total pancreatectomy frequently led to insulin-dependent diabetes mellitus. In such patients, resumption of alcohol intake results in major complications in diabetic management. Thus the Whipple operation has become a common resective procedure for chronic pancreatitis.

To assess the outcome of any surgical treatment for chronic pancreatitis, it is necessary to evaluate the immediate outcome of the operation and its complications; its effect on long-term pain relief and analgesic requirements, the degree of pancreatic insufficiency, and the need for replacement therapies including insulin therapy of diabetes and enzyme therapy of steatorrhea. In addition to nutritional rehabilitation, it is necessary to determine the likelihood of socioeconomic rehabilitation of the individual patient following resective surgery. An ideal operation will be completely effective in relieving pain while preserving pancreatic endocrine function. The treated patient should be capable of an unrestricted diet requiring enzyme replacement and vitamin therapies; however, there should be no lingering interference with the patient's ability to return to a previous occupation, and to establish meaningful and productive relationships in the environment.

## INDICATIONS FOR PANCREATICODUODENECTOMY FOR CHRONIC PANCREATITIS

### Pain

Intractable pain is the single most common and disabling feature of chronic pancreatitis. The pain is usually constant, occurring both day and night. It is described as severe, and it requires near narcotic or narcotic analgesia for relief. The pain is located in the epigastrium and upper anterior abdomen, and it is usually felt through to the corresponding position in the back.

Eating typically aggravates the pain, to the extent that patients often markedly reduce intake, resulting in substantial weight loss and nutritional insufficiency. The pain is also aggravated by lying on the back, so many patients will sleep in a sitting posture or with the back flexed, lying on the side. Aside from analgesics, there are no noninvasive ways to relieve the pain, although some alcoholic patients state that alcohol ingestion reduces its severity. The pathophysiology of the pain from chronic pancreatitis has been attributed to perineural inflammation, increased intraductal pressure, increased intracapsular tissue pressure within the gland, peripancreatic inflammation, and ischemia (1–5).

To quantify the disabling nature of the pain, a visual analogue scale can be used, or the analgesic prescription profile for the patient could be obtained from physicians or pharmacists. Through the accuracy of the latter method, it may be feasible to determine the degree of dependency or narcotic addiction for a given patient. Narcotic addiction is not unusual. However, this may not be a contraindication to surgical treatment, as relief of organic causes for pain commonly allows rehabilitation from addiction. Many patients with chronic pancreatitis, who have pain as the dominant symptom complex indicating a need for surgical treatment, have associated symptoms that may compound the indications for surgical treatment, even in the face of less severe and disabling pain.

### Mass Lesion in the Head of the Pancreas

The derangements in the pancreas in chronic pancreatitis are most frequently the long-term result of excessive consumption of alcohol. Such changes affect the entire gland. Usually, the involvement is diffuse, without dominant lesions noted in a single part of the pancreas alone (6, 7). The most common abnormalities of the ductal system are those that result in diffuse ductular dilatation, with or without intervening areas of stricture. Less frequently, the pathology may dominate one portion of the pancreas, resulting in a chronic inflammatory mass. This most commonly affects the head of the gland. It has been proposed that this configuration is a result of the initiation of pathologic changes occurring in the head, the so-called pacemaker theory, in which all disease is initiated and develops from this location (8). Repeated episodes of biliary pancreatitis or complicated acute pancreatitis may result in dominant pathology arising in the head of the gland. Such pathology may even be complicated by prior open or endoscopic intervention.

Carcinoma of the head of the pancreas is always a possibility in dealing with a chronic inflammatory mass from chronic pancreatitis (9, 10). On rare occasions the mass lesion could also be due to lymphoma, a cystic neoplasm, or an islet cell tumor that may be localized to the head. Two features are helpful in the clinical differentiation between chronic pancreatitis and adenocarcinoma of the head of the pancreas. In the latter condition, progressive unremitting biliary obstruction is inevitable, and patients present with unrelenting obstructive jaundice. If the mass lesion is secondary to chronic pancreatitis, there is usually a history of longstanding ingestion of alcohol predating the development of pain and the mass lesion. Endocrine insufficiency may occur in both conditions and is not a reliable distinguishing feature. Similarly, weight loss may be common to both conditions, although the acuity of the loss may be more in keeping with a neoplastic mass.

Diagnostic imaging studies are helpful in differentiating chronic pancreatitis from malignancy. Ultrasound or computed tomographic (CT) imaging may identify calcific changes within the parenchyma of the gland, which is pathognomonic of chronic alcoholic pancreatitis (Fig. 36.1). Distal dilatation of the pancreatic duct is seen in both conditions and cannot distinguish the two entities. Cholangiography by endoscopic or percutaneous methodologies may demonstrate a complete obstruction of the distal bile duct, featuring a typical meniscus at the point of obstruction in carcinoma of the head of the pancreas. Contrary to this is the long, smooth stricture of the distal bile duct typical of chronic pancreatitis. This form of obstruction is rarely complete on cholangiographic study. Pancreatography by the endoscopic route may also show a complete proximal obstruction to the pancreatic duct with neoplasms affecting the head. In chronic pancreatitis, the pancreatic duct on endoscopic retrograde cholangiopancreatogrphy (ERCP) may show irregular stricturing in the head, with areas of dilatation affecting the more distal (upstream) gland, including the secondary and tertiary branches of the ductal system (Fig. 36.2).

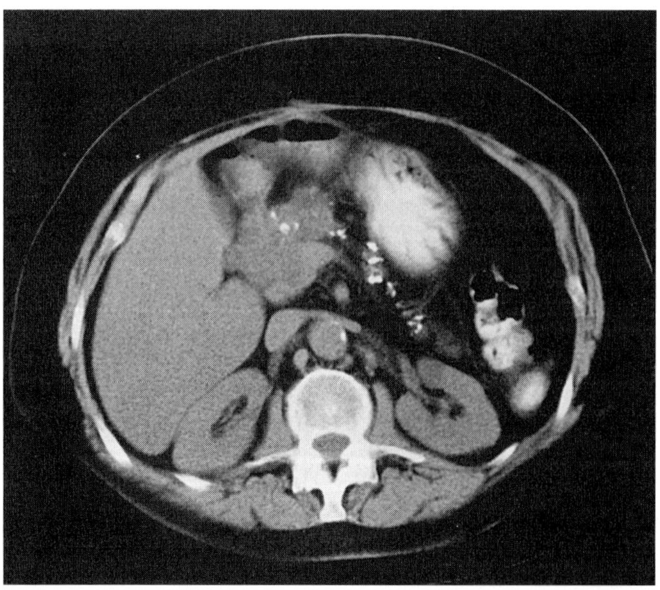

**FIG. 36.1.** CT scan showing calcification along the course of the body of the pancreas and within a dominant mass lesion of the head of the pancreas.

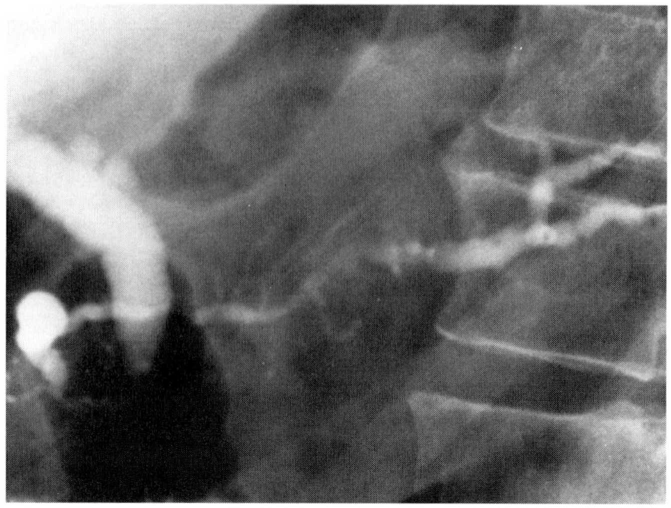

**FIG. 36.2.** ERCP showing a stricture of the distal common bile duct and irregular stricturing and secondary dilation of the pancreatic duct.

With complicated biliary pancreatitis that leads to chronic pancreatitis, the calcific changes are infrequent and may be restricted to the region of the chronic inflammation in the head of the gland alone. In patients with chronic pancreatitis, there may be nonhomogeneous changes in the head of the gland on CT imaging (Fig. 36.3), whereas the typical adenocarcinoma of the head of the pancreas appears as a homogeneous nonenhancing lesion on CT imaging.

A definitive preoperative diagnosis of malignancy may be obtained by percutaneous fine-needle aspiration biopsy of the dominant lesion for cytologic examination. Such a study should be considered when characteristics of chronic pancreatitis are absent and the lesion in the head of the gland is of large diameter or is encroaching on the portal vein, indicating a low probability of curative resection for a neoplasm. Normal cytology does not preclude the diagnosis of carcinoma. The author considers normal biopsy results in the face of other clinical and imaging features of chronic pancreatitis to support a recommendation for resective therapy for chronic pancreatitis.

## Pancreatic Ductal Status

Diffuse dilatation of the pancreatic duct is not necessarily a contraindication to pancreaticoduodenectomy; however, a more appropriate operation for chronic pancreatitis with this type of ductal derangement is usually a longitudinal pancreaticojejunostomy. Bradley and Gregg et al. (11, 12) have clearly demonstrated that pancreatic ductal decompression is effective in relieving the parapancreatic fibrosis that may affect the distal common bile duct and even the duodenum. Only a small selected group of patients may require a secondary biliary tract decompression as described by Aranha et al. (13).

When endoscopic retrograde pancreatography demonstrates disease of the small ducts through the entire pancreas, and indications for surgery are evident, a decompressive procedure is not feasible. Some surgeons will attempt pancreaticojejunostomy for ducts with a diameter less than 1 cm. (14); however, greater success will be achieved with longitudinal pancreaticojejunostomy for patients whose duct is 1.0 cm or more in diameter (15). Resective procedures for chronic pancreatitis should be considered for most patients with small duct disease. If pancreaticoduodenectomy is selected for patients with diffuse ductal dilatation, the surgeon must recognize the increased operative morbidity and long-term changes in quality of life after this resection, compared with pancreatic ductal decompression.

## Biliary Tract Obstruction

Progressive obstructive jaundice is unusual in chronic pancreatitis. Frey et al. reviewed 3274 patients hospitalized with chronic pancreatitis and reported an incidence of bile duct obstruction of 3.2–9.9% (16). Biliary obstruction associated with large pseudocysts involving the region of the head of the pancreas frequently responds to definitive management of the cyst alone and should be excluded from indications for radical pancreaticoduodenectomy in chronic pancreatitis (17).

Episodes of recurrent cholangitis do occur secondary to strictures of the distal common bile duct from chronic pancreatitis (13, 14, 16). Such septic episodes present an acute risk to patients with longstanding chronic pancreatitis (12). Although they usually respond to antibiotic therapy, such episodes should be considered an added indication for pancreaticoduodenectomy. If the biliary obstruction is isolated, without evidence of pain or other features of chronic pancreatitis, the surgeon may consider decompression of the biliary tract alone, rather than pancreaticoduodenectomy (11, 13). Endoscopic stenting of biliary strictures has been common practice in the past decade and can be considered for patients who are not surgical candidates or in whom biliary tract obstruction is the sole clinical feature. However, endoscopic stenting has an ever-increasing incidence of septic complications and may be of only temporary value in the overall management of biliary tract obstruction in chronic pancreatitis.

## Duodenal Stenosis

Duodenal stenosis due to the periduodenal scarring of chronic pancreatitis is a feature of advanced disease, dominant in the head of the gland (9, 11). The radiologic documentation of the obstructing lesion may be difficult to differentiate from an annular carcinoma or Crohn's disease affecting the duodenum. This distinction may be made on endoscopy when normal mucosa is seen throughout the length of the duodenal stricture. This pathology alone is not an indication for pancreaticoduodenectomy. However, when combined with chronic unremitting pain and other complications such as biliary tract strictures, strong consideration should be given to resective procedures involving the duodenum and head of pancreas.

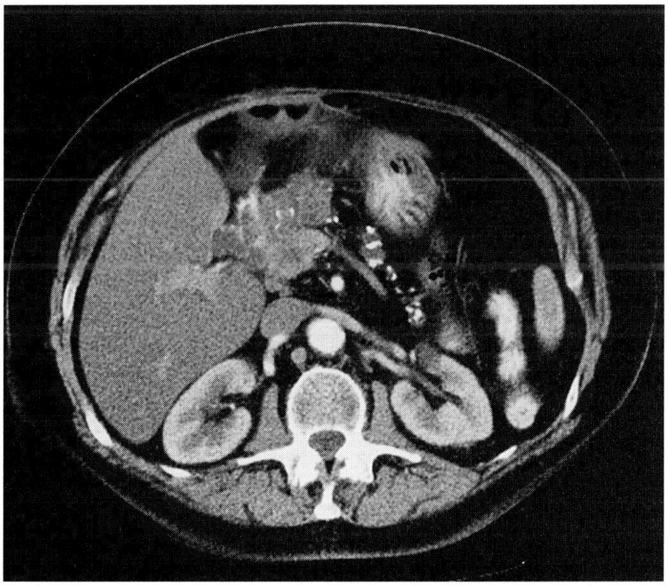

**FIG. 36.3.** CT scan showing a nonhomogeneous mass involving the head of the pancreas in chronic pancreatitis.

If duodenal stenosis is the sole presenting feature of chronic pancreatitis without intractable pain, the treatment should be gastrojejunostomy without pancreaticoduodenectomy. If the duodenal stenosis is associated with distal bile duct obstruction but not the pain of chronic pancreatitis, biliary tract decompression by a biliary enteric anastomosis combined with gastrojejunostomy for the duodenal stricture is advised. When the severe pain of chronic pancreatitis or the presence of a mass lesion component is combined with duodenal obstruction, pancreaticoduodenectomy may be the operation of choice.

## Endocrine Insufficiency

Diabetes mellitus is common in chronic pancreatitis and is present in over one-third of patients. When considering resective therapy for chronic pancreatitis, diabetes mellitus is a major problem that must be considered in patient selection. Established diabetes mellitus is neither an indication nor a contraindication to pancreaticoduodenectomy. Successful resection for management of pain or other compounding indications may not substantially affect the insulin requirements postsurgery. The nutritional intake of such patients may markedly improve, however, and therefore the insulin therapy may require postsurgical modification.

In patients without diabetes mellitus, it is necessary to consider all candidates for resection as potential diabetics postsurgery. Endocrine insufficiency is less likely following pancreaticoduodenectomy than it is following subtotal pancreatectomy (15, 18). Nonetheless, the incidence of endocrine insufficiency increases with time, following resection. Patient selection for pancreaticoduodenectomy must take into consideration the patient's ability to manage insulin therapy and dietary regulation. The potential role of recurrent alcoholism is a very serious consideration for any patient who is or will become diabetic. The long-term complications of diabetic management after resections for chronic pancreatitis are often attributable to recurrent alcoholism, with potentially fatal complications of insulin therapy in this unstable subset of patients (15).

## Exocrine Insufficiency

Most patients with chronic pancreatitis presenting with pain have a history of poor food intake and demonstrate longstanding nutritional insufficiency. Following successful surgery, the increase in dietary intake may unmask exocrine insufficiency. These patients may show evidence of maldigestion as a result of enzymatic insufficiency. This can occur regardless of the surgical procedure, as it is based on longstanding destruction of acinar tissue. Following resective therapy, almost all patients require oral enzymatic therapy and dietary regulation. The dietary changes may be affected by the nature of the reconstruction following pancreaticoduodenectomy.

Nutritional deficiencies should not preclude resection in chronic pancreatitis. However, severely depleted patients may require preoperative therapy with parenteral nutrition. This may be required for up to 3 or 4 weeks prior to surgery in the most severe cases. Endocrine insufficiency is commonly unmasked by parenteral nutritional therapy for chronic pancreatitis because of the large caloric, including glucose, load.

## Abstinence from Alcohol

Although some authorities do not feel that continuing alcohol abuse is a contraindication to surgery, the potential for success in pain relief and ultimate rehabilitation make the social aspects of chronic alcoholic pancreatitis of paramount importance in selecting candidates for resective therapy. Improved results will definitely be obtained if planned resection is restricted to candidates with a documented history of abstinence from alcohol for periods up to 1 year. Adequate family and other social support systems also increase the long-term success of surgical treatment. Postresective therapy should be considered lifelong in all patients with chronic alcoholic pancreatitis. Such patients usually have a dependent personality and will require continuing support to avoid recurrence of alcoholism or other substance dependencies. The support team should include the surgeon as well as nutritional and social therapists. Relapse of chronic pancreatitis following resective therapy is frequently attributed to recurrence of alcoholism. This is preventable by dedicated support systems established for lifelong follow-up.

### Failure of Previous Surgical Procedures

Following previous distal pancreatectomy or subtotal pancreatectomy, a small percentage of patients continue to have unremitting pain and associated disability, with or without other compounding complications. This may also occur with a small group of patients following pancreaticojejunostomy (15, 19). Completion of resective procedures by pancreaticoduodenectomy will convert these patients to total pancreatectomy. The surgeon must be aware of the substantial risks for continuing drug dependency and high morbidity and mortality associated with insulin-dependent diabetes if there is recurrence of alcoholism in patients following total pancreatectomy. Therefore, selection of patients for completion pancreatectomy by pancreaticoduodenectomy must focus on the long-term risks of insulin dependency and rehabilitation.

Following failure of pancreaticojejunostomy, consideration may be given to subtotal pancreatectomy or pancreaticoduodenectomy. In these patients, the inevitability of insulin-dependent diabetes is less likely than with completion pancreatectomy. The pathologic anatomy in the gland must be evaluated after failure of prior pancreatic duct decompression. If areas of undrained pancreatic ducts are evident in the head of the gland, along with parenchymal or ductal calcification and/or biliary obstruction, pancreaticoduodenectomy in combination with revision of the previous decompressive procedure may be the best approach. Sometimes, however, a localized obstruction of the previous pancreaticojejunostomy can be identified and revised. Such revision may require creation of a new Roux en Y as the previously created jejunal segment may have shortened to a significant extent.

## SURGICAL CONSIDERATIONS

Pancreaticoduodenectomy removes the head of the pancreas, distal common bile duct, and duodenum. However, variations in the reconstruction have been used with varying success or morbidity. The standard pancreaticoduodenectomy removes the antrum and pylorus of the stomach along with the duodenum and proximal jejunum. The order and technique of the biliary and pancreatic anastomoses varies between different surgical centers. The anastomosis most responsible for increasing morbidity and mortality following pancreaticoduodenectomy is the pancreatic reconstruction (20). The incidence of anastomotic leakage and the subsequent complications of abscess and hemorrhage are related to the nature of the reconstruction rather than to the sequence of the biliary tract and pancreatic anastomoses.

Pylorus preservation following pancreaticoduodenectomy was pioneered by Traverso and Longmire (8). This form of duodenojejunal reconstruction was designed to eliminate the complications of gastrectomy associated with the standard Whipple procedure. Long-term complications of dumping, hypoglycemia, alkaline reflux gastritis, delayed gastric emptying, and stomal ulceration are all possible sequelae of the gastric resection. Preservation of the antrum and pylorus with an intact vagal innervation should preclude all of these complications except stomal ulceration and delayed gastric emptying.

### Standard Pancreaticoduodenectomy

Following standard pancreaticoduodenectomy, including distal gastric resection, the pancreatic reconstruction is of paramount importance to early postoperative outcome. (Catgut sutures rapidly dissolve in this situation and are to be avoided.) The order of the biliary and pancreatic anastomoses may vary and probably does not have an important impact on the success of the pancreatic anastomosis. In the past, the pancreatic anastomosis has most frequently been end to end. This was most commonly an inverting type of reconstruction, with a second layer of sutures from the seromuscular jejunum to the more distal capsule of the body of the pancreas, which is designed to invert the initial end-to-end anastomosis. Such a reconstruction does not create an anastomosis of the pancreatic ductal epithelium to the jejunal mucosa. Rather, it provides free flow to the lumen of the jejunum. Some surgeons have placed a stent within the lumen of the pancreatic duct. In my opinion, this does not enhance the continuity of this anastomosis in any way and may lead to obstructive pancreatitis. This type of anastomosis is most applicable when the pancreatic duct is not dilated. If it is to be used, this reconstruction is facilitated if it is the first (most proximal) anastomosis, followed in order by the biliary and gastric reconstruction. Modifications of this technique may bring the open end of the jejunum to the epithelium of the pancreatic duct in a purse-string manner followed by a multiple-layer inversion component to complete the anastomosis. This modification may lead to leakage because of the discrepancy between the ductal lumen and the jejunal purse string, or it may fail to preserve the continuity of flow into the jejunal lumen.

A preferable method for the pancreaticojejunal anastomosis features an end-of-pancreas to side-of-jejunum reconstruction that usually employs a temporary stent. [*Editor's note:* see Chapter 55 for depiction of techniques.] Although this anastomosis may precede or follow the biliary reconstruction, it is probably safer to make it the most proximal anastomosis. This anastomosis features a duct-epithelium-to-mucosa anastomosis at a convenient antimesenteric site in the jejunum, where a small enterotomy is made corresponding in size to the diameter of the pancreatic duct. The stent passes from the pancreatic duct through this anastomosis to the lumen of the jejunum. It may then be left internally to pass spontaneously or preferably is exteriorized at a distal point in the jejunal limb. Following the mucosal epithelial anastomosis, the seromuscular layer of the jejunum is buttressed to the previously oversewn remnant of the transected pancreas. This anastomosis is generally favored by the author, particularly when the duct is dilated, for then the two epithelial surfaces can be easily coupled to preserve continuity of pancreatic flow into the jejunum. Colleagues recommend its routine use (20a, 20b). In patients whose pancreas was small or atrophic and whose pancreatic duct was tiny, studies were performed simply oversewing the transected end of the residual pancreas, including the transected duct. This was accomplished by stapling or by suture, with or without occlusion of the ductal lumen by acrylic injections. These techniques were accompanied by high fistula rates (21) and have been largely discontinued. Today, opinion is unanimous or nearly unanimous that restoration of flow of pancreatic juice into the intestine is an important goal of reconstruction.

### Pylorus-Preserving Pancreaticoduodenectomy

Pyloric preservation has become a more frequently used variation of pancreaticoduodenectomy. This is an appropriate operation for patients with chronic pancreatitis whose long-term survival should be the expectation and in whom problems of nutrition are of paramount importance. These factors are also important when this operation is performed for pancreatic malignancy. Long-term survival in the latter group, however, is infrequent, and the nutritional advantages may not be realized.

Reconstruction of the biliary tract, pancreas, and stomach may take two forms with pylorus preservation. Initially, the postpyloric duodenal cuff was anastomosed end to end to the limb of the jejunum. Thereafter, the bile duct and pancreas were respectively anastomosed to the jejunum. In such a variation, the pancreaticojejunal anastomosis is fashioned in an end-of-pancreas to side-of-jejunum manner. Again, the surgeon must make a choice of performing this anastomosis with or without a stent. The preferable mode of reconstruction is to create a Roux limb in which the biliary and pancreatic anastomoses are completed proximal to the duodenojejunal anastomosis. The order of the pancreatic and biliary anastomoses is the preference of the surgeon. Although numerous surgeons have used the end-to-end pancreatojejunostomy, the end-to-side, mucosa-to-mucosa anastomosis, stented, appears to be the preferable method. A lack of unanimity among colleagues is recognized. The pancreas may be anastomosed first, with the biliary jejunal anastomosis to follow, or the order may be reversed, with the pancreaticojejunostomy first. The duodenojejunal anastomosis will then follow the biliary and pancreatic reconstruction, using the end of the duodenal cuff to the side of the jejunum distal to the biliary and pancreatic reconstruction.

In considering the variations in reconstruction for pyloric preservation, the critical feature is again the pancreaticojejunal anastomosis with its risk of leakage and dehiscence. The technique of reconstruction in which the duodenojejunostomy is the first anastomosis, the biliary second, and the pancreatojejunal third (downstream) increases the potential gravity of any dehiscence of the pancreaticojejunal anastomosis, as this order of reconstruction permits bile, as well as gastric contents, to leak in greater volumes than does the Roux limb variant of reconstruction. Adequacy of intraluminal and external drainage of the reconstruction site must be considered in both the pylorus-preservation and the standard Whipple procedures.

### Vagotomy

Truncal vagotomy is not a routine part of a standard Whipple procedure. There are certain advantages, however, to adding truncal vagotomy to this operation, for patients with chronic pancreatitis are likely to be long-term survivors. Although antrectomy effectively reduces acid secretion up to 70% of maximum, the addition of truncal vagotomy will preclude the need for future acid suppression by $H_2$-receptor blockers or proton pump inhibitors. This will effectively eliminate the long-term development of a stomal ulcer. Of greater importance is the role of even minimal residual acidity in the gastric remnant in the inactivation of orally administered pancreatic enzymes in the long-term nutrition management of these patients. If acid inactivation of oral enzymes occurs, then acid-suppression therapy may be a lifelong requirement to maximize the efficiency of the enzymes. Obviously, truncal vagotomy following a pylorus-preserving pancreaticoduodenectomy reverses some of the proposed benefits of this procedure. As acid production is minimally affected with the pylorus-preserving operation, it is likely that some of these patients may require combined acid suppression with oral enzyme therapy to maximize long-term pancreatic exocrine effectiveness. Acid-resistant encapsulation of these enzyme supplements, however, has significantly diminished their inactivation during their passage through the stomach.

### Cholecystectomy

Cholecystectomy should be a routine component of pancreatoduodenectomy regardless of the type of reconstruction. Preserving the gallbladder increases the likely need for early postoperative cholecystectomy because of increased stasis of bile in the gallbladder, secondary to resection of the distal bile duct. Routine cholecystectomy should be considered regardless of the calculous status of the gallbladder. Another advantage to routine cholecystectomy is the technical improvement in exposure of the porta hepatis during bile duct reconstruction.

## RESULTS FOLLOWING PANCREATICODUODENECTOMY FOR CHRONIC PANCREATITIS

The operative mortality for pancreatoduodenectomy for chronic pancreatitis should be equivalent to or *less than* that for carcinoma of the head of the pancreas. That is, the expected mortality in centers with a substantial annual volume of this operation should be under 5%. Several centers have recently reported no hospital mortality in a series of pancreatoduodenectomies exceeding 100 cases (19, 21, 22). Rates will be higher in those centers in which the procedure is done infrequently, the surgeons having had less experience in preventing and managing postoperative complications. Actually, the mortality rate following resection of the head of the pancreas for chronic pancreatitis has usually been lower than that for carcinoma of the pancreas. The major causes of mortality following a pancreatoduodenectomy for chronic pancreatitis are intraabdominal hemorrhage or sepsis related to pancreatic anastomotic dehiscence (20). The incidence of complications will also be affected by associated cardiopulmonary or renal disease. The increased incidence of diabetes mellitus in the pancreatitis population will also increase the risk of postoperative complications. Mortality related to massive intraabdominal hemorrhage will occur early in the postoperative course, whereas deaths related to sepsis will be later and will likely follow other prolonged complications. Preventive measures to avoid morbidity and mortality include adequate prophylactic drainage, precise hemostasis of major vessels in areas of severe fibrosis, and, when indicated, early reoperation or interventional procedures by percutaneous techniques as indicated. Total parenteral nutrition in postoperative support is important and should be instituted at the earliest indication of a prolonged postoperative course.

### Early Postoperative Morbidity

**Leakage of Bile or Biliary Obstruction.** Chronic pancreatitis is occasionally associated with obstructive jaundice, especially in those patients undergoing a Whipple procedure. Even if there is only moderate ductular dilatation noted on cholangiography, the periportal fibrosis characteristic of chronic pancreatitis increases the difficulties related to the biliary reconstruction. Early leakage of bile is uncommon, is usually transient, and can be managed by prophylactic external drainage. Stenting of the biliary anastomosis is controversial. If the luminal diameter of the bile duct is 1 cm or more, it is unnecessary to place an internal stent. However, a smaller diameter with marked fibrosis should suggest stenting in an effort to prevent early stenosis and stricture formation at this anastomosis. The preferable placement of a proximal stent is from above, through the wall of the bile duct, through the anastomosis, and into the jejunum. Evidence of early obstruction at the biliary anastomosis should be confirmed by cholangiography or radionuclide scanning. Although most uncommon, if continued stenting is indicated, consideration should be given to secondary operative reconstruction or possibly placement of expandable metal or other stents to ensure adequacy of the lumen.

Persistent biloma in the region of the biliary anastomosis, despite prophylactic external drainage, should usually be treated by percutaneous placement of drains in the subhepatic area of the leak. Such drainage catheters should be placed under ultrasound or CT guidance. Cholangiographic evidence of complete dehiscence of the biliary anastomoses should be immediately followed

**TABLE 36.1. Incidence of Pancreatic Leak and Delayed Gastric Emptying following Pancreaticoduodenectomy for Chronic Pancreatitis**

| Reference | P.D.[a] | P.P.P.D.[b] | Leak | Delayed Emptying | Follow-Up |
|---|---|---|---|---|---|
| Barnes (1996) | 11 | 48 | 8% | 25% | 2 months |
| Braasch (1986) | — | 28 | — | 50% | 1 month |
| Fernandez-del Costillo (1995) | 22 | 16 | 6.3% | 1% (a)<br>24% (b) | 1 month |
| Fink (1988) | 6 | 6 | — | 2-Fold (a)<br>Normal (b) | 3-4 years |
| Howard (1990) | 28 | — | 0% | 0% | 5 years |
| Trede (1988) | 104 | — | 10% | — | 10 years |
| Warshaw (1985) | 8 | 8 | — | Normal (a)<br>2-Fold (b) | 1 month |

[a]Pancreaticoduodenectomy (a).
[b]Pylorus-preserving pancreaticoduodenectomy (b).

by reoperation for reconstruction. A delay in the reconstruction will lead to progressive fibrosis, necessitating a higher reconstruction of the bile duct at a later date.

**Pancreatic Leakage (Table 36.1).** Because of the exocrine insufficiency characteristic of chronic pancreatitis, the enzymatic content of the pancreatic fluid is often less than that in patients undergoing a Whipple procedure for neoplasia. Nonetheless, if anastomotic leakage occurs, the volume of water and bicarbonate-rich secretions will be adequate to cause persistent internal collection or external drainage of pancreatic fluid. Depending on the sequence of the various anastomoses, the pancreatic leak may be further complicated by leakage of intestinal fluids, including bile. In the past, the incidence of pancreatic leakage has been directly related to the small size of the duct and to a soft friable pancreas (23). Today, the incidence of this complication may be diminishing, and in fact, it may be preventable (20a). Thus, chronic pancreatitis will predispose to a lower rate of leakage than pancreatoduodenectomy for neoplasia (10). Subsequent morbidity and possible mortality following a pancreatic leak will be affected by the adequacy of external drainage and the implementation of total parenteral nutritional support. Stenting of end-to-side anastomoses is a very common practice, and this technique may decrease external pancreatic leakage, although it does not ensure that the dehiscence will heal any more promptly.

Confirmation of pancreatic dehiscence is obtained by chemical analysis of fluid collected from external drains, which will have elevated enzyme content even with chronic pancreatitis. Bicarbonate content can also be analyzed for confirmation. Pancreatic ductal visualization by percutaneous pancreatography (fistulogram) may provide further confirmation.

The mainstay of treatment for a pancreatic leak is the establishment of adequate drainage, parenteral nutrition, and pancreatic suppression by octreotide. Reoperation, except for improving drainage, should be discouraged, since the ability to reconstitute this anastomosis is limited. Pancreatic leaks may persist for some time, with the patient's overall recovery otherwise affected. Long-term management of a pancreatic fistula is discussed below.

**Intraabdominal Bleeding.** Most bleeding in the early postoperative period is self-limiting. This bleeding is of small venous or diffuse capillary origin, from the large, raw retroperitoneal surfaces created during the dissection. The obliterative peripancreatic fibrosis typical of chronic pancreatitis renders this complication less frequent after pancreaticoduodenectomy for neoplasia. Careful intraoperative hemostasis minimizes this minor postoperative bleeding. Adequate external drainage with closed continuous-suction drains in dependent areas of the abdominal cavity will usually evacuate the serosanguinous collections.

Less frequently, intraabdominal hemorrhage is massive and potentially fatal (20). Such bleeding originates from a major branch of the hepatic or superior mesenteric arteries or from the superior mesenteric or portal veins. The longer the time between the day of operation and the onset of bleeding, the more likely it is that local tamponade of such bleeding will occur from postoperative tissue adherence. However, repeated episodes of bleeding are characteristic of major vessel disruption. Massive uncontrolled bleeding presents with sudden onset of hypovolemia and shock associated with severe abdominal pain. External or internal blood loss may not be evident immediately. Successful resuscitation with blood replacement should be followed by emergency angiography with potential embolization if feasible. Otherwise, immediate relaparotomy for operative control of vascular disruption is necessary to prevent death. Cautious exploration of the operative site is dictated by the localization of fresh bleeding after evacuation of hematoma and pooled blood. The surgeon must be careful not to disrupt intact operated areas, to avoid diffuse bleeding that will make localization much more difficult. Direct suture ligation of major blood vessels is appropriate therapy, with the concomitant use of hemostatic agents such as synthetic collagen and fibrin glues. The surgeon must carefully reevaluate all anastomotic lines to ensure that no further disruption has occurred during the surgery to control hemorrhage.

**Intraabdominal Abscess.** Sepsis during the 2nd to 3rd week after pancreaticoduodenectomy is most likely due to an intraabdominal abscess. Earlier sepsis may be due to complicated wound infection. Abdominal abscess formation is a sign of otherwise undetected anastomotic dehiscence or a consequence of undrained fluid accumulation. The sites of abscess formation will usually be perianastomotic and frequently subhepatic. Pelvic collections or suprahepatic abscesses must also be suspected. Effective postoperative external drainage is the mainstay of prophylaxis. Controversies continue regarding the nature of such drainage systems. The important principle is that the drainage must allow egress of any fluid collection.

Suspicion of intraabdominal abscess formation should be followed by diagnostic imaging studies, which may require both ultrasound and CT scanning methodologies. Once an intraabdominal collection is recognized, inadequate drainage should be corrected by image-guided placement of appropriate-sized percutaneous catheters, which should remain in place until the patient is afebrile, drainage is minimal, and sinograms demonstrate a minimal residual cavity at the abscess site. Percutaneous drainage catheters should not be left in place for an extended time, as secondary erosive complications can result. When accessibility for percutaneous drainage is impossible, open surgical drainage is required. The surgical approach should be through the most direct incision that will avoid unnecessary disruption of reconstructions from the original procedure. The surgeon should not hesitate to consider a new incision to achieve more effective drainage.

**Delayed Gastric Emptying (Table 36.1).** Mechanical obstruction of the upper gastrointestinal (GI) tract must be distinguished from prolonged postoperative ileus. Mechanical obstruction is usually related to anastomotic edema or fibrinous adhesions of the small intestine. Such complications are self-limiting and should be treated with GI decompression and parenteral nutritional support. Enteral feeding by prophylactic tube placement at the original operation may be continued so long as there is no evidence of distal obstruction beyond the feeding port.

Warshaw and Torchiana (24) first described the early delay in gastric emptying associated with pylorus-preserving pancreaticoduodenectomy. They noted requirements for prolonged nasogastric drainage up to 14 days before oral feeding could be initiated. This delay was double that with the cohort standard pancreaticoduodenectomy in their study. Braasch et al. described similar early delay in emptying with pylorus preservation (25). In a later review of this subset, Fink et al. noted no delay in the pylorus-preservation patients, but a delay in standard pancreaticoduodenectomy (26). Yeo et al. demonstrated improved emptying after pancreaticoduodenectomy with erythromycin (27).

Persistent GI obstruction beyond the fourth postoperative week must be evaluated for other causes that may not be spontaneously reversible. Upper GI contrast studies with water-soluble agents as well as upper GI endoscopy is valuable in determining the location and nature of such persisting obstruction. Complete obstruction demonstrated by these techniques may require repeat operation for lysis of fibrous adhesions that may result from undetected localized abscess formation.

Although infrequent, early presentation of complete GI obstruction associated with severe pain and toxemia may occur secondary to strangulated internal herniation of the small bowel. Imaging studies are valuable in determining this complication. Urgent reoperation is required to prevent strangulation or to resect small bowel segments if infarction has already occurred.

### Late Postoperative Morbidity

**Pancreatic Fistula.** Persistent pancreatic leakage beyond the first 2 or 3 weeks indicates an established fistula. This may be a long-term complication following pancreaticoduodenectomy. The leak is from the site of the pancreaticojejunal anastomosis and usually results from complete disruption of this anastomosis, with healing of the jejunal defect and persistence of pancreatic leakage from the duct. Leakage at this time beyond operation can be safely documented by a fistulogram. Measuring the enzyme content and recording the daily fluid volumes are mandatory in ongoing management of this complication. Adequate control of drainage will prevent local skin complications. A fistula of pure pancreatic juice with its inactive secretions can be collected in a stomal appliance without irritating the abdominal wall.

A pancreatic fistula can be expected to close under conservative treatment. However, the duration of drainage will be prolonged. Conservative measures that have been used include cessation of oral feeding, long-term total parenteral nutrition, and combined administration of somatostatin analogues. When patients with persisting pancreatic fistulas are not systemically ill, the above-mentioned therapies may be provided on an ambulatory basis in centers with an established home parenteral nutrition program.

Surgical closure of a pancreatic fistula should be delayed until at least 6 months of conservative therapy has been tried. Operative treatment may require direct reconstruction of the pancreaticojejunal anastomosis. A well-established fistula tract may be used to internalize the fistula into a separate segment of jejunum.

In most patients, conservative therapy allows closure of the fistula within the first 3 months. As healing occurs, the fistula may close and reopen on numerous occasions before obliteration of the fistula tract is complete and all drainage permanently stops. Undue recurrence of symptoms of pain or fever during the closure phase must be assessed for possible development of intraabdominal collections of pancreatic juice or abscess formation.

**Stricture of the Pancreatic Duct.** Obliterative fibrosis of the pancreaticojejunal anastomosis is not uncommon when the original chronic pancreatitis is associated with small ductal disease. This complication may occur within the first several months of surgery or be delayed several years after operation. In either case, onset is characterized by the development of clinical evidence of steatorrhea with intake of a normal diet. Early presentation following pancreaticoduodenectomy may be associated with recurrence of pain due to pancreatic ductal obstruction. With later onset, the occlusion may be insidious, with painless onset of steatorrhea. The stenosis may be documented by ultrasound or CT scanning, although dilatation of the duct is not always evident. Endoscopic retrograde pancreatography is not technically feasible in most cases of pancreaticoduodenectomy, regardless of pylorus preservation.

This complication is important largely in the management of the resultant exocrine insufficiency. Oral enzyme therapy is required at the onset of clinical steatorrhea and must be sustained for life, to maintain an adequate nutritional state following pancreaticoduodenectomy complicated by pancreatic ductal stenosis. Attempts at surgical reconstruction are not necessary and likely will be followed by restenosis, eventually requiring further pancreatic enzyme replacement.

**Bile Duct Stricture.** Because the bile duct is involved in the peripancreatic fibrosis of chronic pancreatitis, there may be a slightly increased risk of stricture formation in the late follow-up after pancreaticoduodenectomy. Stricture formation may result from inadequate blood supply of the bile duct at the anastomosis, possibly complicated by previous bile leak. Bile duct stricture presents with an insidious onset of extrahepatic cholestasis. Infrequently, this may be associated with bouts of cholangitis. This stricture can usually be confirmed by ultrasound or CT imaging, nuclear medical biliary scan, or transhepatic cholangiography.

Minimal stenosis at the site of reconstruction of the bile duct may be successfully treated by transhepatic anastomotic balloon dilatation complemented with antibiotic therapy and choloretic therapy using ursodeoxycholic acid. Persistent stricture formation should be treated by reconstruction of the biliary enteric anastomosis. Although short-term results of transhepatic balloon dilatation and stenting of surgical anastomoses are encouraging, the long-term results after pancreaticoduodenectomy are not well documented. Recurring episodes of obstruction with secondary cholangitis eventually result in biliary fibrosis progressing to secondary biliary cirrhosis. This irreversible condition may subsequently require liver transplantation. Avoidance of this unnecessary organ replacement is best achieved through careful reconstruction of the biliary enteric anastomosis.

**Portal Vein Thrombosis.** Most patients in the United States with chronic pancreatitis do not have associated liver disease. Therefore, portal vein thrombosis may progress slowly, during which time collateral venous circulation is established. With normal hepatic venous circulation, transhepatic circulation is unaffected, and extrahepatic collateralization will suffice to prevent sequelae of portal hypertension. However, a more isolated thrombosis in the portal circulation may result in secondary gastrointestinal bleeding. Isolated splenic vein thrombosis secondary to surgery or to the underlying disease in the remnant of the pancreas will result in isolated gastric varices (28) because of the high arterial flow sustained to the stomach and spleen. The resultant collateral venous drainage through the gastroepiploic system to the intact portal vein will create segmental portal hypertension in the submucosal venous plexus of the stomach. Due to operative interruption of the right gastroepiploic venous system at the time of a standard pancreatoduodenectomy, the collateral venous circulation may be somewhat unpredictable. As a result, gastric variceal bleeding will occur in a small number of these patients. This may present as profound iron deficiency anemia or frank upper GI hemorrhage. The diagnosis is best established by selective splenic arteriography and venography. Gastroscopy may reveal enlarged mucosal folds only. Treatment for bleeding from this source requires splenectomy to disrupt the arterial inflow into this portal venous compartment.

**Alkaline Reflux Gastritis.** Alkaline reflux gastritis, a late complication, is related only to standard pancreaticoduodenectomy, but the relationship to symptoms of abdominal pain, dyspepsia, and vomiting after standard reconstruction is controversial. The presence of bile in the gastric remnant is universal after this type of operation. Gastric acidity, in combination with the bile, has been proposed as a cause of disruption of the gastric mucosal barrier with subsequent diffuse erosive gastritis. Successful therapy using antacid and mucosal protective agents may support this diagnosis, especially if initial endoscopic biopsies showing severe erosive gastritis are reversed following such treatment. Reconstructive surgery to create a Roux-en-Y gastrojejunostomy following a previous Whipple procedure is rarely indicated for this complication.

**Stomal Ulceration.** If vagotomy is added to the standard Whipple procedure, a stomal ulcer will be prevented. However, not all surgeons include a vagotomy; so stomal ulcers may occur at the jejunal side of the gastrojejunostomy. The usual presentation is intractable pain in the epigastrium or back, typically relieved by food and aggravated by an empty stomach, often during the night. Endoscopic examination of the gastric remnant and gastrojejunostomy will identify this ulcer. Successful healing will occur with $H_2$-receptor blockers or proton pump inhibitors. Ulcer recurrence or lifelong requirements for oral medications may indicate the need for a thorascopic truncal vagotomy. This approach is least invasive and is the procedure of choice for patients who have had Whipple procedure.

**Dumping Syndrome.** Like any form of subtotal gastrectomy, the standard pancreaticoduodenectomy carries a risk for dumping. This symptom complex is directly related to the rapidity of gastric emptying. Potentially, any patient is at risk for postprandial abdominal distress associated with symptoms of lightheadedness and sweating from autonomic response, splanchnic pooling, and hypoglycemia. Treatment of this complication is strict dietary management. Frequency of meals and meal content must be adjusted to minimize the rapidity of high-volume carbohydrate loading into the proximal small intestine. There is almost no role for surgical reconstruction to correct this postgastrectomy symptom in the standard Whipple patient.

**Gastric Outlet Obstruction.** Following a standard pancreaticoduodenectomy, patients rarely complain of early satiety or vomiting after meals unless from gastric atony. Imaging studies of gastric emptying using a food-contrast admixture as well as radionuclide gastric emptying studies may be required to confirm delays in gastric emptying secondary to motility disturbances. Endoscopic proof of stricture of the gastrojejunostomy causing gastric outlet obstruction indicates a need for surgical revision. This late complication is due to stomal inflammation and recurrent scarring. Endoscopic evaluation must determine the presence or absence of stomal ulceration, as the surgical revision may require vagotomy.

Despite increasing acceptance of pylorus-preserving pancreaticoduodenectomy, there is still controversy regarding the benefits of retaining the antrum and pyloric sphincter (8, 24, 25). Clearly, the gastric reservoir is maintained, and alkaline reflux associated with standard pancreaticoduodenectomy is virtually eliminated. However, physiologic gastric emptying is not always preserved. The delayed gastric emptying associated with pylorus preservation may be due to inadvertent denervation of the vagal fibers or devascularization of the distal gastric remnant and duodenal cuff. Stricture formation at the duodenojejunal anastomosis may also occur with resultant gastric retention. Evaluation of the symptoms of gastric retention following pylorus preservation requires endoscopy and gastric emptying studies as described for the standard pancreaticoduodenectomy. Conversion to subtotal gastrectomy may be required for persistent gastric retention following an initial pylorus-preserving pancreaticoduodenectomy.

## QUALITY-OF-LIFE OUTCOMES FOLLOWING PANCREATICODUODENECTOMY FOR CHRONIC PANCREATITIS

### Freedom from Pain

The ideal outcome following any surgical procedure for painful chronic pancreatitis is total freedom from preexistent pain. The only pancreatic resection certain to achieve this outcome lifelong is total removal of all diseased parenchyma. Because the pathologic process affects the entire pancreas in chronic alcoholic pancreatitis, any resective procedure that preserves portions of the gland may result in residual or recurrent pain if the remnant has preserved innervation. Pancreaticoduodenectomy is the resection of choice for patients with dominant disease in the head of the gland. The pain relief is achieved with preservation of less diseased pancreas in the body and tail, combined with adequate ductal drainage. The best results will be obtained through appropriate patient selection and skilled surgical technique.

Pain relief must be reliable and durable. This implies long-term follow-up of all patients undergoing pancreaticoduodenectomy. Studies must document pain profile, analgesic requirements including addiction withdrawal, and recurrent attacks of acute pain from any relevant cause. Lifelong follow-up of chronic pancreatitis patients has improved their outcomes through the support provided to this dependent population.

Recurrence of alcoholism clearly correlates with recurrent pain following resection, regardless of complicating postsurgical pathology (29). Abstaining patients with recurrence of pain after pancreaticoduodenectomy must be investigated for reversible pathology in the gland (20).

Short-term relief of pain has been clearly documented for most patients undergoing pancreaticoduodenectomy, with or without pylorus preservation (10, 14, 18, 31). Complete freedom of pain has not been universal after such resective procedures. Patients with chronic pancreatitis due to complicated biliary tract disease sustain improvement longer than those with chronic alcoholism. Long-term follow-up of patients having pancreaticoduodenectomy reveals an increasing rate of recurrence of chronic pain. This is usually less severe than in the preoperative state. Usually, there is a strong correlation with recurrent alcoholism (15). Continued use of controlled analgesics for relief of less severe pain after pancreaticoduodenectomy is an accepted outcome in patients with otherwise successful rehabilitation after pancreaticoduodenectomy. Because of the short duration of relief, percutaneous nerve-blocking procedures are of limited value in this postsurgical population.

Overall, pancreaticoduodenectomy, with or without pylorus preservation, has achieved good-to-excellent results for pain relief. Excellent results equate to freedom from pain and cessation of all analgesic use. Good results are interpreted as lesser pain than before operation and minimal analgesic requirements. Poor results equate to no improvement or worsening of pain and occur in 15–30% of patients in long-term follow-up of pancreaticoduodenectomy for chronic pancreatitis (9, 14).

**Diabetes Mellitus.** The diabetes of patients who are insulin-dependent diabetics before pancreaticoduodenectomy is not significantly changed by this operation. The aggravation of diabetes that occurs is in the subset of pancreaticoduodenectomy patients who resume frequent alcohol ingestion. The prognosis for this group of patients is poor. Late mortality is directly related to the complications of diabetes mellitus, not the underlying chronic pancreatitis (9, 14).

Pancreaticoduodenectomy has achieved a favorable reputation as the resection of choice for chronic pancreatitis because of its low incidence of resultant endocrine insufficiency. In most patients, preservation of the body and tail of the pancreas is adequate to sustain insulin synthesis. The operation does not protect the residual parenchyma from the ongoing chronic inflammatory process. Therefore, prolonged follow-up of patients will document a gradual increase in incidence of insulin-dependent diabetes (15, 30).

The incidence of diabetes is less than that for subtotal resections of the distal pancreas, which reaches 80% or more (15). However, the subtotal left-to-right pancreatectomy patient has total sparing of the duodenum with its endocrine and digestive functions.

Complications of diabetes mellitus following pancreaticoduodenectomy are less frequent and less severe than those with juvenile onset or adult diabetes. Because of the high frequency of alcohol dependency in the subset of patients undergoing pancreaticoduodenectomy, the acute complications of insulin therapy are troublesome and may prove fatal. Diabetic management may be stable if a compliant patient can maintain appropriate diabetic dietary protocol. The mainstays of therapy are education, regular use of a glucometer, and supervised adjustment of insulin dosage through an ambulatory diabetes management group. Insulin doses are often lower than those for comparable patients with insidious-onset diabetes (15). Overall, the abstaining nondiabetic patient who has undergone a pancreaticoduodenectomy for chronic pancreatitis will have a low incidence of postsurgery insulin requirements. This is the distinct advantage of this type of resection. Late onset of insulin dependency still occurs secondary to disease progression.

**Nutritional Status.** The hallmark of improved nutritional status following any surgery for chronic pancreatitis is weight gain. Failure to gain weight will result from either inadequate food intake or digestive insufficiency, most frequently related to pancreatic exocrine deficiency. Despite the patency of the pancreaticojejunal anastomosis, pancreatic juice is usually deficient in digestive enzymes in patients with chronic pancreatitis who had disease severe enough to require surgical intervention. Therefore, once food intake has been restored to normal volume and fat and protein content, maldigestion may occur or become more evident because of exocrine insufficiency. Without enzyme replacement therapy, weight gain is unlikely.

Liberal use of high lipase enzyme replacement should achieve weight gain in excess of 10% of the patient's presurgical status. The nutritional recovery of patients following standard pancreatectomy relates to the gastrectomy. The gastric reservoir is reduced slightly, gastric emptying can be excessively rapid, and alkaline reflux can affect appetite. There is a high probability that food intake may be impaired despite the fact that food-precipitated pain has been relieved. To achieve the best results following the standard pancreaticoduodenectomy, a dietary pattern of frequent feeding of up to six small meals should be considered. It may be advisable to restrict carbohydrates and fluids and to consider medication to combat alkaline reflux. Pylorus preservation upholds gastric reservoir function and prevents alkaline reflux. So long as delayed gastric emptying can be avoided, this variation of pancreaticoduodenectomy may result in improved oral intake and has been shown to improve early weight gain (31).

Long-term iron and vitamin deficiency may also occur after standard pancreaticoduodenectomy, because of failure of small intestinal absorption secondary to the pancreaticoduodenectomy. Supplemental therapies should be considered as a prophylactic measure, and monitoring of appropriate serum levels should be maintained. Nutritional benefits following pancreaticoduodenectomy are less predictable than endocrine preservation for many reasons. Failure to gain weight will require individualized investigation. Adequate food intake is more probable with pylorus preservation; however, patients with both forms of pancreaticoduodenectomy may benefit from lifelong administration of pancreatic enzyme supplements.

**Alcohol and Drug Dependency.** Patients whose chronic pancreatitis is caused by chronic alcoholism require lifelong treatment of their dependency. Patient selection prior to surgery is critical in reducing the postsurgical problem of recurrent alcohol dependency. Surgery is inadvisable in a patient with sustained alcohol drinking. Recurrence of alcoholism has been described in 25–35% of patients during the first 3 years after any surgery for chronic alcoholic pancreatitis (9, 14, 15, 31). Recurrence of alcohol intake will affect recurrent pancreatic pathology, which will present as recurring and persisting pain (29). Alcohol is also deleterious in insulin management. Late mortality following surgery for chronic pancreatitis is most frequently associated with recurrent alcoholism in the diabetic (14, 15). Appropriate support systems should be maintained for all patients with a history of chronic alcoholic pancreatitis. Most programs have a multidisciplinary team to manage these patients in the long term.

Analgesic dependency is often difficult to separate from residual organic pain of chronic pancreatitis. Dependency must be suspected in patients who achieve no improvement following pancreaticoduodenectomy and require continued high doses of analgesic. Patients who have been converted to total pancreatectomy by pancreaticoduodenectomy as a second operation should be completely free of pain. Analgesic requirements in this subset clearly must be considered drug dependency. Like alcohol dependency, drug dependency must be treated by a well-organized addiction-management program.

**Return to Work.** Ultimate rehabilitation for patients having pancreaticoduodenectomy includes return to productive work. Reports of full rehabilitation at 3–5 years rarely exceed 65% (15, 31). Many patients recover and maintain normal daily activities but do not return to self-sufficiency through new employment. Failure to achieve self-sufficiency is multifactorial, with relevance to nutritional status, residual pain, and associated depression. Many patients must change jobs to maintain employment. Repeated time loss due to illness often leads to termination of work activities for this patient population.

**Quality-of-Life Measurements.** Studies have attempted to quantify the long-term outcome after surgery for chronic pancreatitis (32, 33). Standardized formulas for evaluation of outcome after specific diseases are not ideally suited for chronic pancreatitis. Therefore, a combination of objective scoring systems will be required to address pain, nutrition, and socioeconomic rehabilitation. Overall outcome will be clearly related to appropriate patient selection and maintenance of lifelong multidisciplinary support systems.

## REFERENCES

1. Bockman DE, Buchler M, Malfertheiner P, Beger HG. Analysis of nerves in chronic pancreatitis. Gastroenterology 1988;94:1459–1469.
2. Keith RG, Keshavjee SH, Kerenyi NR. Neuropathology of chronic

pancreatitis in humans. Can J Surg 1985;28:207–211.
3. Bradley EL 3d. Pancreatic duct pressure in chronic pancreatitis. Am J Surg 1982;144:313–316.
4. Ihse I, Borch K, Larsson J. Chronic pancreatitis: results of operations for relief of pain. World J Surg 1990;14:53–58.
5. Bornman PC, Marks IN, Girdwood AH, Clain JE, Narunsky L, et al. Is pancreatic duct obstruction or stricture a major cause of pain in calcific pancreatitis? Br J Surg 1980;67:425–428.
6. Sarles H, Sahel J. Pathology of chronic calcifying pancreatitis. Am J Gastroenterol 1976;66:117–139.
7. Singh SM, Reber HA. The pathology of chronic pancreatitis. World J Surg 1990;14:2–10.
8. Traverso LW, Longmire WP Jr. Preservation of the pylorus in pancreaticoduodenectomy. Surg Gynecol Obstet 1978;146: 959–962.
9. Izbicki JR, Bloechle C, Knoefel WT, Wilker DK, Dornschneider G, et al. Complications of adjacent organs in chronic pancreatitis managed by duodenum-preserving resection of the head of the pancreas. Br J Surg 1994;81:1351–1355.
10. Barnes SA, Lillemoe KD, Kaufman HS, Sauter PK, Yeo CJ, et al. Pancreaticoduodenectomy for benign disease. Am J Surg 1996;171:131–135.
11. Bradley EL. Parapancreatic biliary and intestinal obstruction in chronic obstructive pancreatitis. Is prophylactic bypass necessary? Am J Surg 1986;151:256–258.
12. Gregg JA, Carr-Locke DL, Gallagher MM. Importance of common bile duct stricture associated with chronic pancreatitis. Diagnosis by endoscopic retrograde cholangiopancreatography. Am J Surg 1981;141:199–203.
13. Aranha GV, Prinz RA, Freeark RJ, Greenlee HB. The spectrum of biliary tract obstruction from chronic pancreatitis. Arch Surg 1984;119:595–600.
14. Frey CF. Current management of chronic pancreatitis. Adv Surg 1995;28:337–370.
15. Keith RG, Saibil FG, Sheppard RH. Treatment of chronic alcoholic pancreatitis by pancreatic resection. Am J Surg 1989;157: 156–162.
16. Frey CF, Suzuki M, Isaji S. Treatment of chronic pancreatitis complicated by obstruction of the common bile duct or duodenum. World J Surg 1990;14:59–69.
17. Bradley EL, Clements JL Jr, Gonzalez AC. The natural history of pancreatic pseudocysts: a unified concept of management. Am J Surg 1979;137:135–141.
18. Howard JM, Zhang Z. Pancreaticoduodenectomy (Whipple resection) in the treatment of chronic pancreatitis. World J Surg 1990;14:77–82.
19. Trede M, Schwall G, Saeger HD. Survival after pancreatoduodenectomy. 118 consecutive resections without an operative mortality. Ann Surg 1990;211:447–458.
20. Trede M, Schwall G. The complications of pancreatectomy. Ann Surg 1988;207:39–47.
20a. Howard JM. Pancreatojejunostomy: leakage is a preventable complication of the Whipple resection. J Am Coll Surg, in press.
20b. Warren K. Discussion of paper. Greene BS, Loubeuq JM, Peoples JD, Elliot DW. Are pancreatoenteric anastomoses improved by mucosa to mucosa sutures. Am J Surg 1991;161:45–49.
21. Cameron JL, Pitt HA, Yeo CJ, Lillemoe KD, Kaufman HS, Coleman J. One hundred and forty-five consecutive pancreaticoduodenectomies without mortality. Ann Surg 1993;217: 430–435.
22. Fernandez-del Castillo C, Rattner DW, Warshaw AL. Standards for pancreatic resection in the 1990's. Arch Surg 1995;130:295–299.
23. Marcus SG, Cohen H, Ranson JH. Optimal management of the pancreatic remnant after pancreaticoduodenectomy. Ann Surg 1995;221:635–645.
24. Warshaw AL, Torchiana DL. Delayed gastric emptying after pylorus-preserving pancreaticoduodenectomy. Surg Gynecol Obstet 1985;160:1–4.
25. Braasch JW, Deziel DJ, Rossi RL, Watkins E Jr, Winter PF. Pyloric and gastric preserving pancreatic resection. Ann Surg 1986;204: 411–418.
26. Fink AS, DeSouza LR, Mayer EA, Hawkins R, Longmire WP Jr. Long term evaluation of pylorus preservation during pancreaticoduodenectomy. A prospective, randomized, placebo-controlled trial. World J Surg 1988;12:663–670.
27. Yeo CJ, Barry MK, Sauter PK, Sostre S, Lillemoe KD, et al. Erythromycin accelerates gastric emptying after pancreaticoduodenectomy. Ann Surg 1993;218:229–238.
28. Keith RG, Mustard RA Jr, Saibil EA. Gastric variceal bleeding due to occlusion of splenic vein in pancreatic disease. Can J Surg 1982;25:301–304.
29. Gullo L, Barbara L, Labo G. Effect of cessation of alcohol use on the course of pancreatic dysfunction in alcoholic pancreatitis. Gastroenterology 1988;95:1063–1068.
30. Gall FP, Gebhardt C, Zirngibl H. Chronic pancreatitis—results in 116 consecutive, partial duodenopancreatectomies combined with pancreatic duct occlusion. Hepatogastroenterology 1982; 29:115–119.
31. Traverso LW, Kozarek RA. The Whipple procedure for severe complications of chronic pancreatitis. Arch Surg 1993;128:1047–1053.
32. Bloechle C, Izbicki JR, Knoefel WT, Kuechler T, Broelsch CE. Quality of life in chronic pancreatitis—results after duodenum-preserving resection of the head of the pancreas. Pancreas 1995;11:77–85.
33. Petrin P, Andreoli A, Antoniutti M, Zaramella D, Da Lio C, et al. Surgery for chronic pancreatitis: what quality of life ahead? World J Surg 1995;19:398–402.

# 37

# Duodenum-Preserving Resection of the Pancreatic Head

H. G. Beger, R. Kunz, and M. Schoenberg

Anatomic, embryologic, and pathomorphologic data exhibit the head of the pancreas to be the pacemaker of chronic pancreatitis. The hypersecretion of acinar cells forms protein plaques within intralobular and interlobular ducts early in the disease, which leads to periductal inflammation and fibrosis. This is thought to be the underlying cause of the disease (1–3). In some instances, chronic pancreatitis results from relapsing acute pancreatitis that causes interstitial acinar and fatty tissue necrosis, inducing perilobular fibrosis. In terms of clinical implications, chronic pancreatitis is a progressive inflammatory disease. In Western countries, it is mainly caused by continuing alcohol abuse. Irreversible morphologic and functional damage to the exo- and endocrine pancreatic tissue compartments is typical (4). After a subclinical phase lasting up to 5 years, recurrent attacks of upper abdominal pain occur, frequently combined with back pain. Signs of malnutrition appear, secondary to the loss of functional exocrine pancreas tissue. In the late clinical phase, one-fourth to one-third of patients with chronic pancreatitis develop an endocrine insufficiency leading to clinical diabetes mellitus.

In 15–30% of patients with chronic pancreatitis accompanied by pain, an inflammatory mass develops in the head of the pancreas. Enlargement of the pancreatic head is the typical radiologic finding in this type of chronic pancreatitis. Differentiating this from a malignancy of the pancreatic head is frequently a diagnostic puzzle (5). Macroscopically, parenchymal calcifications, pancreatic ductal calculi, small cystic cavities, and small areas of necrosis are found within the inflammatory mass in the pancreatic head. Microscopically, atrophy of the exocrine pancreas and a local increase in extracellular matrix are observed. Microscopically, the sensory nerves in the area of chronic pancreatic inflammation are enlarged in diameter, with typical signs of loss of perineurium and infiltration of inflammatory cells between nerve fibers; the nerve network is more widely separated within the enlarged tissue mass (6). This pancreatitis-specific neuritis and the increased tissue pressure, which is caused by the inflammatory process, contribute to the clinical pain syndrome via local liberation of pain hormones (7). In patients with chronic pancreatitis caused by a pancreas divisum, one typically sees an inflammatory process dominant in the head of the pancreas accompanied by narrowing of the main ducts.

## INDICATIONS

Up to one-third of patients with chronic pancreatitis develop an inflammatory mass with enlargement of the pancreatic head. In this subgroup of patients, chronic pancreatitis is caused by long-lasting alcohol abuse; men predominate. Usually the age of patients needing medical treatment is below 35 years; when surgical treatment becomes necessary, most of the patients are younger than 40 years. Severe abdominal pain, either persistent or episodic, predominates in this subgroup of patients; they frequently require increasing analgesic treatment up to the point of nonresponse to medical pain treatment. Besides the pain syndrome, about 50% of patients develop local complications early in the course of chronic pancreatitis, most frequently a common bile duct stenosis in the prepapillary intrapancreatic ductal segment. Specific diagnostic measures reveal a compression or thrombosis of the portal and splenic vein in each fifth patient; in less than 10%, a severe stenosis of the duodenum develops that demands surgical treatment (8).

Surgical treatment of chronic pancreatitis becomes mandatory after failure of medical and endoscopic interventional management, e.g., in the case of nonresponse to extensive analgesic medication, after development of cholestasis or jaundice, or after failure of stenting of the pancreatic duct (Table 37.1). In a small group of patients, "big-duct disease" develops, with a ductal diameter exceeding 7–8 mm. In this group of patients, the Partington-Rochelle ductal drainage procedure has been applied with good short-term results. However, in approximately 40% of patients, the pain syndrome recurs after 5 years (9, 10). Five percent of patients suffer from left-sided pancreatitis, a segmental type of chronic pancreatitis, with a normal ductal system in the head of the pancreas; a spleen-preserving left pancreatic resection is the surgical treatment of choice. However, in most patients, resection of the pancreatic head, using the duodenum-preserving technique is the surgical option of choice (Table 37.2).

## RATIONALE

The inflammatory mass in chronic pancreatitis is predominantly located in the head of the pancreas. The head of the pancreas seems to be the pacemaker of the disease. Pain is mainly a consequence of the inflammatory process in the head, which increases tissue pressure and causes local release of pain hormones. Duodenum-preserving subtotal resection of the head of the pancreas excludes surgery of the stomach, duodenum, and biliary tree, because these peripancreatic organs are not primarily involved in chronic pancreatitis. The surgical procedure preserving the stomach, duodenum, and biliary tree maintains the upper gastrointestinal (GI)-tract physiology within the normal range. The use of the Whipple procedure in chronic pancreatitis seems to be an overtreatment; it results in diabetes mellitus in approximately 20% of patients in the early postoperative period and carries a high level of morbidity and mortality.

After experimental investigations and studies of the blood supply to the duodenum, a duodenum-preserving subtotal resection of the head of the pancreas was first performed in a human in 1972; since then, it has been regularly used in patients with chronic pancreatitis who have an inflammatory mass in the head of the pancreas. Duodenum-preserving pancreatic head resection results in long-lasting pain relief in over 80% of patients

**TABLE 37.1. Indications for Duodenum-Preserving Resection of the Head of the Pancreas in Chronic Pancreatitis**

| Pathomorphology[a] | Radiology, ERCP, CT[b] | Clinical |
|---|---|---|
| Chronic pancreatitis + IMH | Head enlargement<br>CBD stenosis<br>PV-compression/occlusion | Daily abdominal pain<br>Cholestasis/jaundice<br>Portal hypertension, splenomegaly |
| | Duodenal stenosis (<1 cm) | Gastric outlet syndrome |
| Chronic pancreatitis | Small duct disease | Daily abdominal pain |
| Chronic pancreatitis | Pancreas divisum | Daily abdominal pain |

[a]IMH, inflammatory mass in the head of the pancreas.
[b]CBD, common bile duct; PV, portal vein.

(11). In chronic pancreatitis with a common bile duct stenosis caused by inflammatory alterations in the prepapillary intrapancreatic segment of the common bile duct, a biliary anastomosis is also performed, resulting in long-lasting relief of clinical jaundice and biochemical signs of cholestasis (12). In patients with multiple stenosis of the common pancreatic duct and a chain of leaks in the body and tail of the pancreatic main duct, the addition of a ductal drainage procedure increases the incidence of pain-free patients in late follow-up (13). Duodenum-preserving resection of the head maintains, or even improves, the endocrine pancreatic function in chronic pancreatitis (14). Surprisingly, up to 24 years after the duodenum-preserving resection of the pancreatic head, the late mortality is less than 6%, with only about 10% of patients experiencing a further attack of acute pancreatitis (8, 15). Based on a preoperative diagnostic workup that includes contrast-dynamic computed tomography (CT), endoscopic retrograde cholangiopancreatography (ERCP), and angiography, criteria for the application of duodenum-preserving resection of the pancreatic head in 380 consecutive surgically treated patients are given in Table 37.3.

## TECHNIQUES

The duodenum-preserving resection of the head aims at a subtotal resection of the pancreatic head, with removal of the inflammatory mass while preserving the duodenum, the extrahepatic common bile ducts, the gallbladder, and the stomach as well as preserving the pancreatic parenchyma to a large extent. There are three major surgical steps: *(a)* exposure of the head of the pancreas, *(b)* subtotal resection of the head, and *(c)* reconstruction using the upper jejunal loop for interposition. The exposure of the head of the pancreas starts with a Kocher maneuver and division of the gastrocolic and duodenocolic ligaments. After identification and banding of the common hepatic artery and the common bile duct above the entrance into the pancreatic tissue, the neck of the pancreas is mobilized by preparing a tunnel between the portal vein and the dorsal surface of the pancreatic neck. Resection starts with transection of the pancreas along the duodenal level of the portal vein wall (Figs. 37.1 and 37.2). The subtotal resection of the pancreatic head is carried out from the dorsal surface of the pancreatic head toward the intrapancreatic common bile duct and includes the tissue of the uncinate process (Fig. 37.3, *A* and *B*). In most patients, it is not difficult to dissect the pancreatic tissue along the wall of the intrapancreatic common bile duct from the level of the hepatoduodenal ligament toward the papilla. A 5- to 8-mm shell-like segment of the pancreatic head along the duodenal wall is preserved to maintain the blood supply of the third part of the duodenum and to protect the dorsal pancreaticoduodenal arterial arcades (Fig. 37.4). In most patients, the gastroduodenal artery is ligated. The wet weight of operative specimens ranges from 20 to 55 g. Restoration of the pancreatic secretory flow from the left pancreas, including neck, body, and tail of the pancreas to the upper GI tract, is maintained by the use of the first jejunal loop. Two pancreatic anastomoses are needed (Fig. 37.5). In 80% of patients with a narrowing or a stenosis of the intrapancreatic common bile duct, subtotal excision of the inflammatory mass in the head of the pancreas leads to decompression of the common bile duct. In patients whose cholestasis is caused by a stenosis due to intramural inflammation of the common bile duct, a biliary anastomosis with the jejunal loop has to be performed. In patients with multiple stenosis and dilatation of the pancreatic main duct in the corpus and cauda of the pancreas, a Puestow modification of a drainage loop, using side-to-side anastomosis, is performed (Fig. 37.6, *A–C*).

In 380 patients with chronic pancreatitis who had the duodenum-preserving head resection, the following intraoperative pathologic findings were obtained: a single stenosis of the main pancreatic duct in the ductal segment of the head in 39%, a common bile duct stenosis in 48%, a severe duodenal stenosis in 7%, and a portal vein compression due to pancreatic head enlargement in 13%. As a consequence of these local complications, in addition to the duodenum-preserving head resection, an anastomosis of the common bile duct was needed in 23% (Fig. 37.7, *A* and *B*); portal vein decompression was necessary in 13%, and 1.9% required a recanalization procedure of the portal vein because of complete occlusion/thrombosis of the main trunk of the portal vein. A Puestow drainage procedure of the main pancreatic duct in the left pancreas, including the main duct of the body and tail, was performed in 7% (Fig. 37.8), and surgical decompression of the narrowed duodenum as a separate surgical step was performed in 4%.

## EARLY AND LATE POSTOPERATIVE RESULTS

Because of the limited surgical procedure, early postoperative morbidity and mortality were low. In 380 patients after

**TABLE 37.2. Surgery of Chronic Pancreatitis: Ulm Experience (841 Patients[a])**

| Duct Drainage Pseudocyst Drainage | Left resection | Whipple | Head PPPD | Resection[b] DPPHR |
|---|---|---|---|---|
| 211 pts | 197 pts | 20 pts | 40 pts | 380 pts |
| 25% | 23% | 2% | 5% | 45% |

[a]11/1968–4/1982, Department of Surgery, FU Berlin Charlottenburg; 5/1982–9/1995, Department of General Surgery, University of Ulm.
[b]PPPD, pylorus-preserving pancreatic head resection; DPPHR, duodenum-preserving pancreatic head resection.

**TABLE 37.3. Chronic Pancreatitis with Inflammatory Mass in the Head of the Pancreas: Indication for Surgical Treatment (380 Patients[a])**

| | Patients | |
|---|---|---|
| Indication | (n) | (%) |
| Abdominal pain | 354 | 93% |
| IMH[b] (>4 cm) | 302 | 79% |
| CBD-stenosis | 187 | 49% |
| Duodenum stenosis | 23 | 6% |
| Vascular obstruction | 65 | 17% |

[a]11/1972–4/1982, Department of Surgery, FU Berlin; 5/1982–9/1995, Department of General Surgery, University of Ulm.
[b]IMH, inflammatory mass in the pancreatic head.

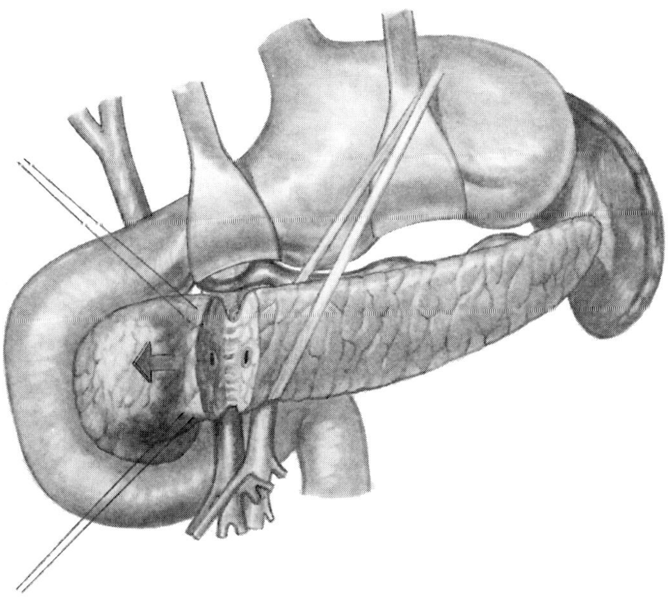

**FIG. 37.1.** Duodenum-preserving resection of the head. First surgical step: transection of the pancreas.

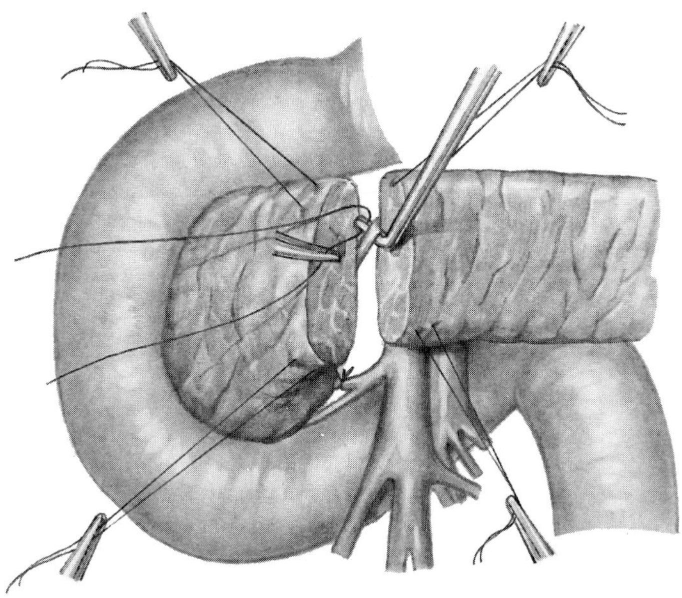

**FIG. 37.2.** Retroportal clearance of the head of the pancreas including dissection of the vessels to the portal vein.

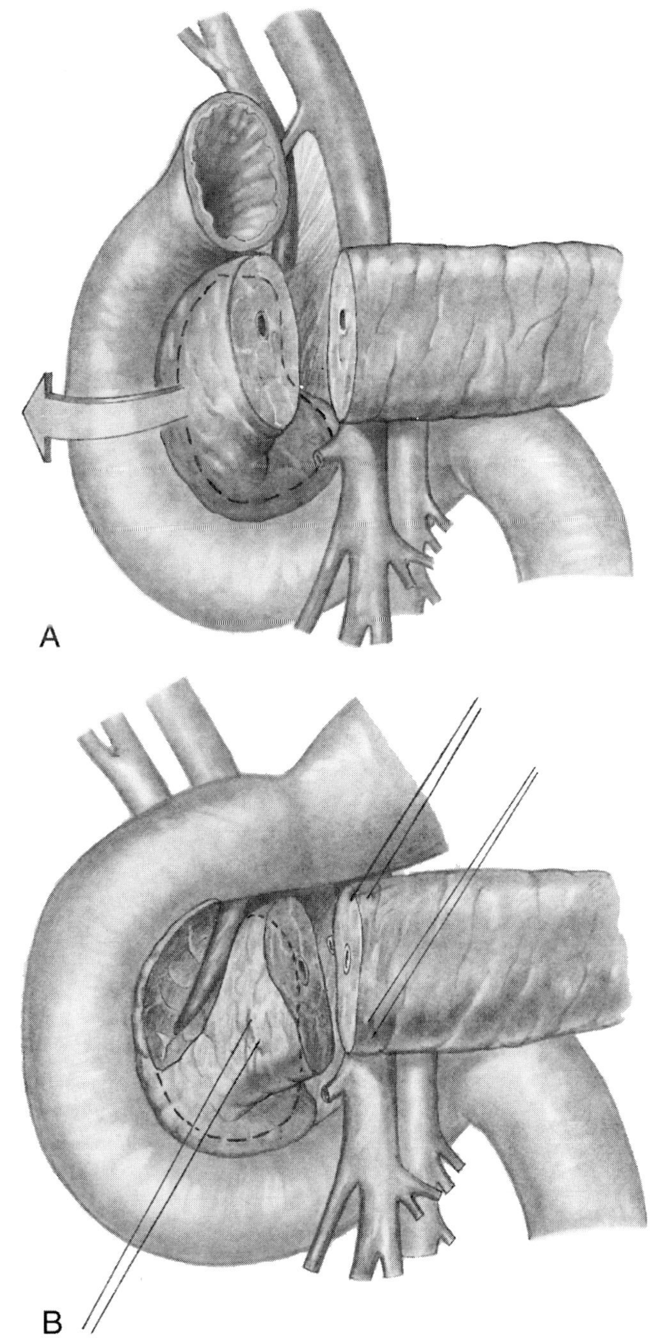

**FIG. 37.3. A.** After transection of the pancreas, the pancreatic head and duodenum are rotated to a ventrodorsal position. **B.** Subtotal resection of the pancreatic head along the intrapancreatic segment of the common bile duct leads in most cases to decompression of the narrowed common bile duct, without incision of the duct. The line of resection is completed through the uncinate process.

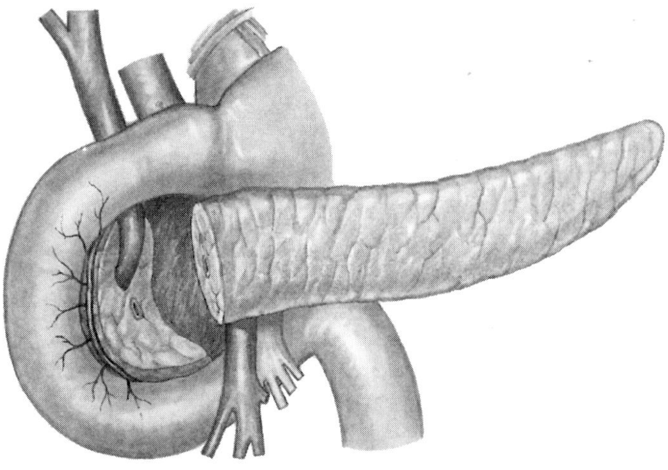

**FIG. 37.4.** After completion of the subtotal resection of the pancreatic head, a shell-like remnant of the pancreatic head along the duodenal C is preserved. The dorsal pancreaticoduodenal arcades are intact, whereas in most cases, the gastroduodenal artery is ligated.

duodenum-preserving resection of the head, hospital mortality was 0.8% (Table 37.4); 5.3% of the patients had to be reoperated. Indications for a reoperation were bleeding from the pancreatic anastomosis, anastomotic leakage, and intraabdominal abscess. Ischemia of the duodenum occurred in two patients; both had to be reoperated for closure of the circumscribed duodenal lesion. The hospital stay of the patients, calculated from the day of surgery until the day of discharge, was a median 13.9 days.

During the follow-up period, ranging from 1 month to 23 years, late morbidity and late mortality after this operation are surprisingly low. Reevaluations of all patients after the duodenum-preserving operation were carried out in 1985, 1989, and 1994 (11, 13, 14, 16). In terms of relief of abdominal complaints, 75–82% of all patients were absolutely pain free, and an additional 7–11% did not need analgesic medication, although they sometimes suffered pain in the upper abdomen. Some 8–11% of patients suffered further pain and needed analgesic treatment at the time of the various reevaluations. More than 60% of all patients were employed. An increase in body weight in the first postoperative months was noted in more than 80% of patients. Full-dose pancreatic enzyme supplementation was obligatory in only one-third of patients; another third needed occasional enzyme supplementation.

Late mortality at the three follow-up periods after duodenum-preserving head resection was 4%, 4.7%, and 8.9%, respectively. Only about 10% had to be hospitalized because of further attacks of pancreatitis. The low hospitalization rate after this operation for advanced chronic pancreatitis provides evidence that surgical excision of the inflammatory process in the head of the pancreas results in nonprogression of the chronic inflammation (Table 37.5).

## ENDOCRINE FUNCTION AFTER RESECTION

Subtotal resection of the head of the pancreas in chronic pancreatitis with an inflammatory mass in the head results in a tissue loss of about 20% of the pancreas. The pancreatic ductal system achieves at least a decompression. The major advantages of this operation for chronic pancreatitis are maintenance of the insulin secretory capacity and avoidance of postoperative deterioration of glucose metabolism (14). Oral glucose tolerance tests showed that glucose metabolism was unchanged in 82% of patients, improved in 9%, and deteriorated in only 2%, compared with preoperative endocrine function.

A series of extensive measurements of hormones and glucose tolerance dynamics in 15 patients, studied in the early and late postoperative periods, revealed that subtotal resection results in improved glucose tolerance 3–6 months after surgery. Preoperative and late postoperative insulin secretion was almost identical. However, basal plasma levels of glucagon, pancreatic polypeptide, and somatostatin postoperatively were significantly lower than the preoperative levels, contributing to the favorable postoperative improvement in glucose metabolism (17). The loss of glucagon- and pancreatic polypeptide–producing endocrine cells of the pancreas, predominantly located in the head of the pancreas, may contribute to the favorable effect after resection of the head. Conservation of the duodenum with maintenance of the enteral insular hormonal axis contributes even more to the metabolic stability early and late postoperatively (Table 37.6).

## ADVANTAGES OF PROCEDURE

The surgical removal of the inflammatory mass in the pancreatic head, preserving the duodenum, extrahepatic biliary tree, and stomach, results in 80–90% of patients having a pain-free life early and late postoperatively; about 90% are free from further attacks of pancreatitis and further hospitalization. The major advantage of using duodenum-preserving head resection in chronic pancreatitis derives from the conservation of the endocrine capacity of the pancreas and duodenum. Results of two prospective clinical trials comparing duodenum-preserving pancreatic head resection with the pylorus-preserving Whipple procedure (18) for chronic pancreatitis revealed the major advantage of the duodenum-preserving technique: 6 months after duodenum-preserving resection, the patients had significantly less pain, greater weight gain, significantly better glucose tolerance, and a higher insulin secretory capacity than patients after pylorus-preserving resection (19). The duodenum-preserving head resection does not lead to complete restoration of the reduced exo- and endocrine function of the pancreas, because the loss of exo- and endocrine function secondary to the inflammatory attacks in chronic pancreatitis cannot be compensated for by any surgical intervention.

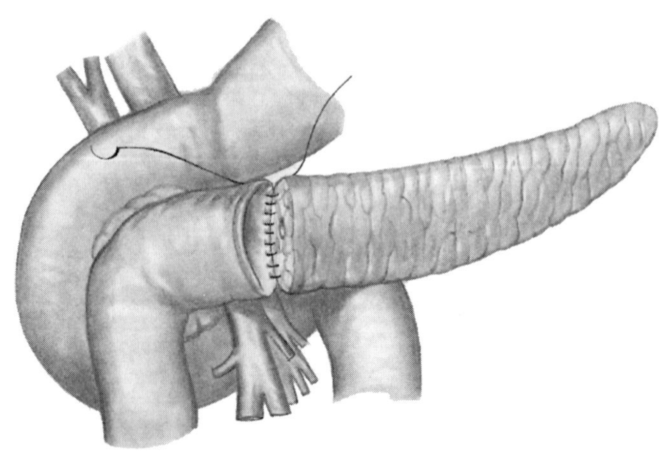

**FIG. 37.5.** To restore the pancreatic secretory flow into the upper intestine, an isolated jejunal loop is interposed. Two pancreatic anastomoses must be performed.

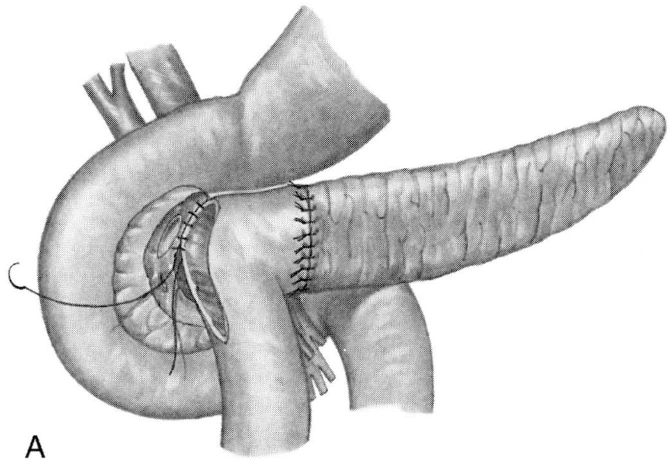

A

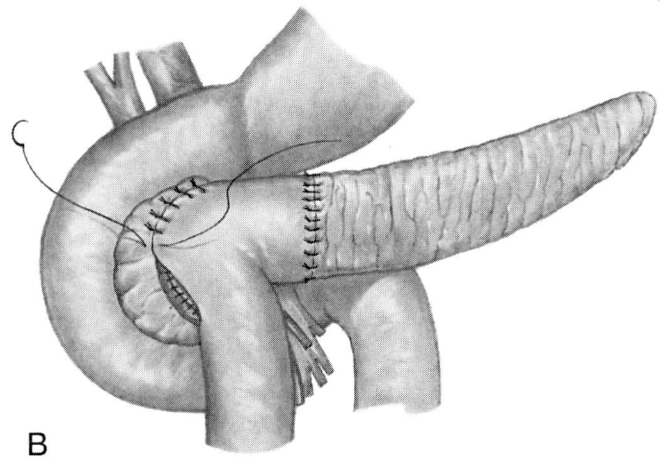

B

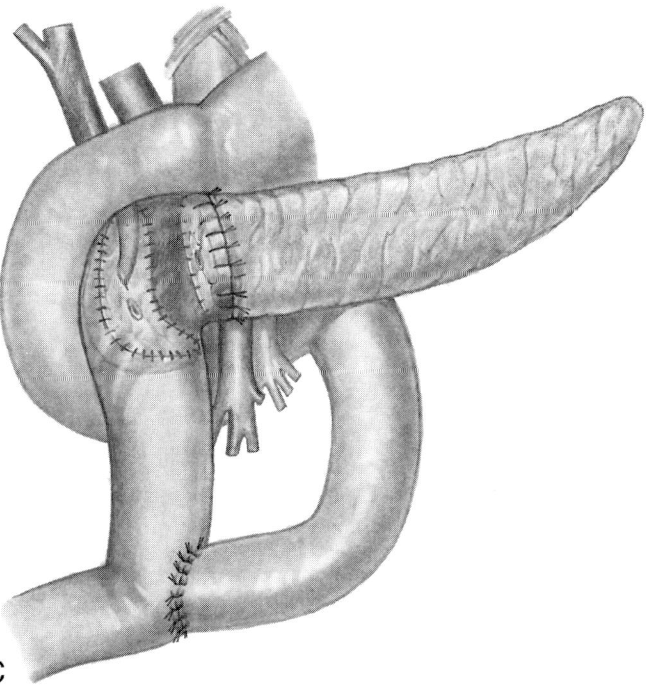

C

**FIG. 37.6.** **A.** A telescopic anastomosis, end-to-end, between the left pancreas and the jejunal loop with single stitches is carried out. **B.** An end-to-side anastomosis, 5–8 cm apart from the pancreatic left anastomosis has to be carried out between the rest of the pancreas head and the interposed jejunal loop. **C.** Two-layer anastomosis, carried out usually with interrupted stitches.

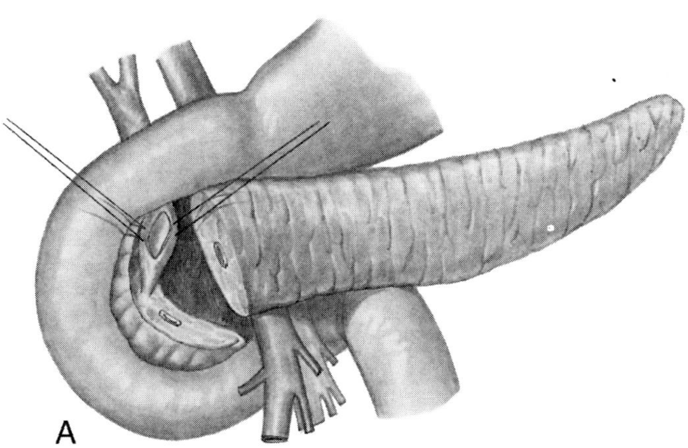

A

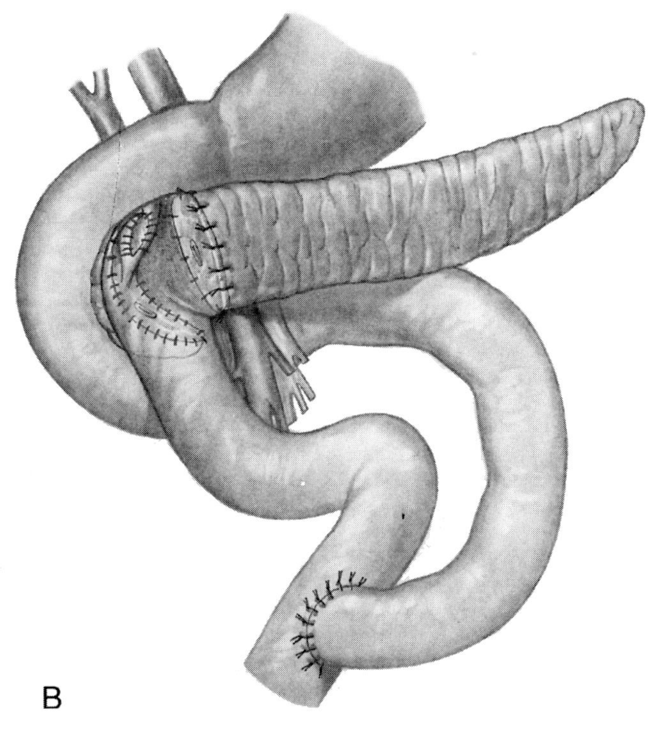

B

**FIG. 37.7.** **A.** In patients with an intramural stenosis due to inflammation of the common bile duct wall, an additional internal biliary anastomosis between common bile duct and the jejunal loop is necessary. **B.** Three anastomoses with the jejunal loop, two pancreatic, one biliary, are completed.

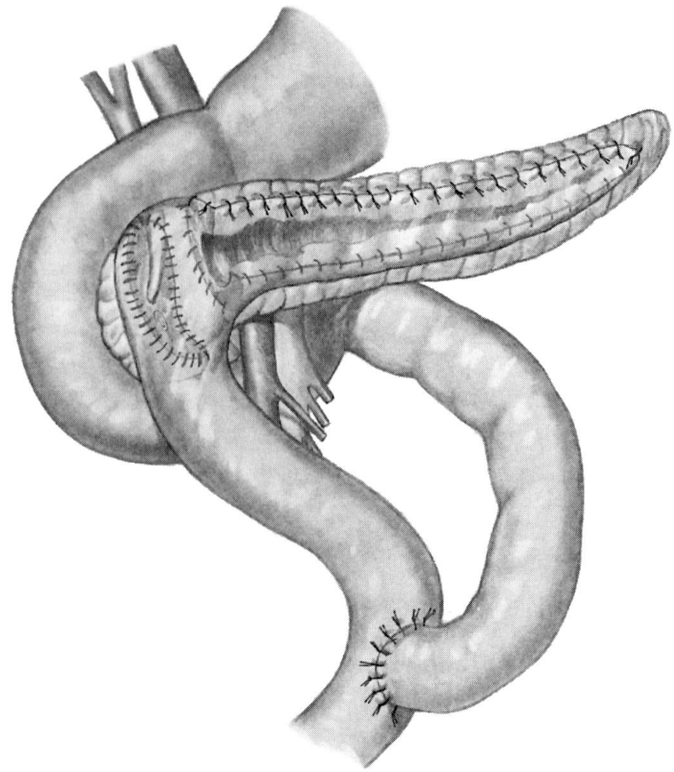

**FIG. 37.8.** In patients with multiple stenosis and dilatations in the ductal system of the left pancreas (chain of leaks), a side-to-side anastomosis including the duct in the neck, body, and tail of the pancreas is performed.

**TABLE 37.4. Duodenum-Preserving Head Resection in Chronic Pancreatitis: Early Postoperative Results (380 Patients[a])**

| | Patients | |
|---|---|---|
| | *(n)* | (%) |
| Relaparotomy | 20 | 5% |
| Postoperatively deteriorated glucose metabolism | 8 | 2% |
| Postoperatively improved glucose metabolism | 33 | 9% |
| Hospital mortality | 3 | 0.8% |

[a]9/1995, Department of General Surgery, University of Ulm.

**TABLE 37.5. Duodenum-Preserving Head Resection in Chronic Pancreatitis: Outcome after DPPHR (298 Patients[a])**

| | |
|---|---|
| Early | |
| Hospital mortality | 1.0% |
| Relaparotomy | 5.7% |
| Postoperative newly developed DM | 2% |
| Postoperative hospitalization | 13.9 days (median) |
| Late outcome after 6-year follow-up (median), 232 patients[b] | |
| Late mortality | 8.9% |
| Pain: none/rare | 88% |
| Professionally rehabilitated | 63% |
| Rehospitalization | 10% |

[a]11/1972–12/1994, Department of General Surgery, University of Ulm.
[b]Büchler M, unpublished data.

**TABLE 37.6. Endocrine Function in Chronic Pancreatitis after Operation**

| | | | Postoperative | | | |
|---|---|---|---|---|---|---|
| | Preoperative[a] | | Early | | Late | |
| **Endocrine Function** | **(128 Patients)** | **%** | **(127 Patients)** | **%** | **(109 Patients)[b]** | **%** |
| Normal | 76 | 59.4 | 77 | 60.6 | 52 | 47.7 |
| Latent diabetes | 27 | 21.1 | 24 | 18.9 | 28 | 25.7 |
| Insulin-dependent | 25 | 19.5 | 26 | 20.5 | 29 | 26.6 |

Beger HG, Büchler M, Bittner R, Oettinger W, Roscher R. Duodenum-preserving resection of the head of the pancreas in severe chronic pancreatitis. Early and late results. Ann Surg 1989;209:273–278.
[a]oGTT in 22 patients; profile of blood glucose in 81 patients.
[b]oGTT in 29 patients; profile of blood glucose in 51 patients; patients with insulin-dependent diabetes mellitus were not tested. Glucose metabolism improved in 5.5%, deteriorated in 13.7%, and was unchanged in 80.7%.

**TABLE 37.7. Chronic Pancreatitis with Inflammatory Mass in the Head: Advantages of the Duodenum-Preserving Operation**

| | |
|---|---|
| Compared with Whipple Resection | |
| Duodenum-preserving resection of the head enables preservation of | stomach |
| | duodenum-jejunum |
| | CBD |
| | duodenal food transit |
| Maintains/improves insulin secretory capacity | |
| Compared with Partington-Rochelle procedure with tissue cored out of the head (FREY): | |
| Duodenum-preserving resection of the head | |
| leads to decompression of the CBD and the portal vein | |
| clears the retroportal inflammatory tissue resulting in a resection of the inflammatory tumor | |
| delays or eradicates progression of chronic pancreatitis in in >70% of patients | |

Unlike the Whipple procedure, the duodenum-preserving pancreatic head resection implies preservation of the stomach, biliary tract, and duodenum. From this point of view, the use of the Whipple procedure is clearly an overtreatment. Results of the most recent series using the Whipple procedure in chronic pancreatitis showed higher early and late postoperative morbidity; approximately 20% of patients after the Whipple procedure were insulin dependent, even in the early postoperative period. Early and late postoperative dumping complaints and attacks of cholangitis in almost half of patients are further disadvantages of the Whipple resection or of the pylorus-preserving Whipple resection (20–24) (Table 37.7).

The technique of coring out pancreatic head tissue, advocated by Frey in 1987, results in operative tissue specimens of about 5 g and is considered a modification of the Partington-Rochelle ductal drainage procedure (25, 26).

## CHRONIC PANCREATITIS CAUSED BY PANCREAS DIVISUM

In pancreas divisum, many patients suffer recurrent attacks of pancreatitis because of the inborn defects of the two pancreatic ducts; these defects result in an outflow stenosis in the prepapillary segment of the duct of Santorini and Wirsung's duct and may lead to progressive chronic pancreatitis (27). In patients with chronic pancreatitis due to pancreas divisum, the leading symptom is upper abdominal pain, which often occurs daily and depends on the food intake. ERCP via the greater and smaller papillae exhibited typical ductal changes, with narrowing of the main duct up to the Santorini knee. CT investigations usually reveal no signs of enlargement of the pancreatic head, ductal and tissue calcifications are rare. After failure of endoscopic and interventional management—e. g., endoscopic sphincterotomy, stenting of the greater and smaller papillae, or multiple stenting—a duodenum-preserving head resection resulted in a complete disappearance of abdominal pain in a small group of patients; no further attacks of pancreatitis were observed in the late postoperative course. In 12 patients with pancreas divisum, endocrine function was maintained after duodenum-preserving head resection. However, exocrine dysfunctions were not improved postoperatively (28).

The use of duodenum-preserving resection in other benign lesions is listed in Table 37.8.

**TABLE 37.8. Duodenum-Preserving Resection of the Head of the Pancreas: Indications[a]**

| Indication | Patients | Hospital Mortality |
|---|---|---|
| Chronic pancreatitis | 380 | 3 0.8% |
| Pancreas divisum | 12 | 0 0% |
| Cystadenoma of the pancreatic head | 10 | 0 0% |
| Endocrine tumor of the pancreatic head (>2cm) | 3 | 0 0% |
| Totals | 405 | 3 0.7% |

[a] 5/1982–9/1995, Department of General Surgery, University of Ulm.

## REFERENCES


1. Pitchumoni CS. Role of nutrition in chronic pancreatitis. In: Beger HG, Büchler M, Ditschuneit H, Malfertheiner P, eds. Chronic pancreatitis: research and clinical management. Berlin: Springer-Verlag 1990:15–25.
2. Durbec JP, Sarles H. Multicenter survey of the etiology of pancreatic diseases: relationship between the relative risk of developing chronic pancreatitis and alcohol, protein and lipid consumption. Digestion 1978;18:337–350.
3. Guy O, Robles-Diaz G, Adrich Z, Sahel J, Sarles H. Protein contents of precipitates present in pancreatic juice of alcoholic subjects and patients with chronic calcifying pancreatitis. Gastroenterology 1983;84:102–107.
4. Singer MV, Gyr KE, Sarles H. Revised classification of pancreatitis: report of the Second International Symposium on the Classification of Pancreatitis in Marseilles, France, March 28–30, 1984. Gastroenterology 1985;89:683–685.
5. Schlosser W, Schoenberg MH, Rhein E, Siech M, Gansauge F, Beger HG. Pankreaskarzinom bei chronischer Pankreatitis mit entzündlichem Pankreaskopftumor. Z Gastroenterol 1996, in press.
6. Bockman D, Büchler M, Malfertheiner P, Beger HG. Analysis of nerves in chronic pancreatitis. Gastroenterology 1988;94:1459–1469.
7. Büchler M, Weihe E, Müller S, Malfertheiner P, Friess H, Beger HG. Neurotransmitter in Pankreasnerven: ein Beitrag zur Schmerzpathogenese bei chronischer Pankreatitis. Langenbecks Arch Chir, Suppl Chir Forum 1989:375–379.
8. Beger HG, Büchler M. Duodenum-preserving resection of the head of the pancreas in chronic pancreatitis with inflammatory mass in the head. World J Surg 1990;14:83–87.
9. Prinz RA, Greenlee HB. Pancreatic duct drainage in chronic pancreatitis. Hepatogastroenterology 1990;37:295–300.
10. Warshaw AL, Popp JW Jr, Schapiro RH. Long-term patency, pancreatic function and pain relief after lateral pancreaticojejunostomy for chronic pancreatitis. Gastroenterology 1980;79:287–293.
11. Beger HG, Witte C, Kraas E, Bittner R. Erfahrung mit einer das Duodenum erhaltenden Pankreaskopfresektion bei chronischer Pankreatitis. Chirurg 1980;51:303–307.
12. Beger HG, Krautzberger W, Gögler H. Résection de la tête du pancréas (pancréatectomie céphalique) avec conservation du duodénum dans les pancréatites chroniques, les tumeurs de la tête du pancréas et les compressions du canal cholédoque. Chirurgie 1981;107:597–604.
13. Beger HG, Krautzberger W, Bittner R, Büchler M, Limmer J. Duodenum-preserving resection of the head of the pancreas in patients with severe chronic pancreatitis. Surgery 1985;98:467–472.
14. Beger HG, Büchler M, Bittner R, Oettinger W, Roscher R. Duodenum-preserving resection of the head of the pancreas in severe chronic pancreatitis. Early and late results. Ann Surg 1989;209:273–278.
15. Beger HG, Bittner R, Büchler M, Block S, Senn T, Malfertheiner P. Die chronische Pankreatitis mit entzündlicher Pankreaskopfvergrösserung. Früh- und Spätergebnisse nach duodenumerhaltender Pankreaskopfresektion. Med Klin 1988;83:548–553.
16. Büchler M, unpublished data.
17. Bittner R, Butters M, Büchler M, Nägele S, Roscher R, Beger HG. Glucose homeostasis and endocrine pancreatic secretion in patients with chronic pancreatitis before and after surgical therapy. Biomed Res 1988;9:28.

18. Büchler MW, Friess H, Müller MM, Beger HG. Randomized trial of duodenum-preserving pancreatic head resection versus pylorus-preserving Whipple in chronic pancreatitis. Am J Surg 1995;169: 65–70.
19. Klempa I, Spatny M, Menzel J, Baca I, Nustede R, et al. Pancreatic function and quality of life after resection of the head of the pancreas in chronic pancreatitis. A prospective, randomized comparative study after duodenum-preserving resection of the head of the pancreas versus Whipple's operation. Chirurg 1995;66:350–359.
20. Gall FP, Mühe E, Gebhardt C. Results of partial and total pancreaticoduodenectomy in 117 patients with chronic pancreatitis. World J Surg 1981;5:269.
21. Leger L, Lenriot JP, Lemaigre G. L'hypertension et la stase portales ségmentaires dans les pancréatites chroniques. J Chir 1980; 95:599.
22. Guillemin G, Cuilleret J, Michael A, Berard P, Foroldi J. Chronic relapsing pancreatitis. Surgical management. Including 63 cases of pancreatico-duodenectomy. Am J Surg 1971; 122:802.
23. Trede M. Therapie der chronischen Pankreatitis—Schlusskommentar. Langenbecks Arch Chir 1987;373:379.
24. Warren KW. Changing patterns in surgery of the pancreas. Surg Clin North Am 1976;56:615.
25. Frey CF, Schmith GJ. Description and rationale of a new operation for chronic pancreatitis. Pancreas 1987;2:701–707.
26. Partington PF, Rochelle REL. Modified Puestow procedure for retrograde drainage of the pancreatic duct. Ann Surg 1960;152: 1037–1043.
27. Blair AJ III, Russell CG, Cotton PB. Resection for pancreatitis in patients with pancreas divisum. Ann Surg 1984;200:590–594.
28. Widmaier U, Schmidt A, Schlosser W, Beger HG. Die duodenumerhaltende Pankreaskopfresektion in der Therapie des Pankreas divisum. Dig Med Week 1996, in press.

# 38

# *Distal Pancreatectomy for Chronic Pancreatitis*

R. C. N. Williamson

## ANATOMIC CONSIDERATIONS

By convention, the distal pancreas is that part of the gland that lies to the left of the midline. Most distal pancreatectomies comprise excision of the tail and body of pancreas with transection through the neck. Sometimes the resection extends across the midline to include all of the neck and a variable portion of the head of the pancreas, depending upon the extent of inflammatory disease.

The neck of the pancreas, which may be slightly narrower than the head and proximal body, overlies the origin of the portal vein from the terminal portions of the splenic vein and superior mesenteric vein. The key to a safe pancreatectomy, whether proximal or distal, lies in the clear identification of this crucial venous nexus and its gentle dissection free from the adjacent pancreatic tissue (1). When this tissue becomes inflamed and scarred in chronic pancreatitis, it frequently adheres to these veins; indeed, venous thrombosis is quite a common complication of severe pancreatitis, especially in the splenic vein. Venous hemorrhage is the main risk of a distal pancreatectomy, and in the context of gross pancreatitis and portal hypertension, the bleeding can occasionally be life threatening. Whereas distal pancreatectomy is a simpler operation than proximal pancreatectomy because there is seldom a need for any anastomosis, the resectional phase of the operation can be just as challenging.

The inferior mesenteric vein either joins the splenic vein 1–2 cm to the left of its termination or it enters at the origin of the portal vein (i.e. there is a venous trifurcation). The middle colic vein usually joins the superior mesenteric vein about 2 cm below its termination, but sometimes it enters very close to the origin of the portal vein. The left gastric (coronary) vein generally runs into the portal vein near the upper border of the neck of the pancreas. In chronic pancreatitis patients with splenic vein thrombosis, the terminal portion of the splenic vein is usually patent, being reconstituted by dilated collaterals running through the pancreas itself or crossing from the left gastric and inferior mesenteric veins. The presence of these collaterals, thin-walled and distended, constitutes a hazard during pancreatectomy for chronic inflammatory disease.

The main arterial supply of the body and tail of the pancreas is from the splenic artery. This substantial vessel runs down from the celiac axis to gain the posterior surface of the upper border of the neck of the pancreas to the left of the midline. When the neck of the pancreas is divided in front of the portal vein, the splenic artery is not seen until dissection continues to the left along the superior border of the gland. Multiple branches of the splenic artery feed the left pancreas, and the parent trunk may deeply groove the gland as it courses toward the spleen in a sinuous fashion. Although one or more of these branches may be larger than its fellows, the concept of an "arteria pancreatica magna" is an exaggeration. The splenic artery breaks up into its terminal splenic branches, including the short gastric and left gastroepiploic arteries, at a variable distance from the splenic hilum. It is sometimes possible to dissect the splenic artery and vein completely free of the pancreas (with ligation and division of the several branches), thereby allowing preservation of the spleen by means of a conservative distal pancreatectomy.

The gastroduodenal artery is closely applied to the pancreas as it runs down from the superior to the inferior border, well to the right of the midline. Its position roughly marks the separation between the head of the pancreas (approximately one-third of the gland) and the remaining two-thirds of the pancreas (neck, body, and tail). In the presence of severe pancreatitis, the vessel may be encased by scar tissue and easier to palpate than to see. The gastroduodenal artery should only need to be secured in those extended distal pancreatectomies that cross the midline. The "watershed" territory of the gland (i.e., the neck) that lies between the gastroduodenal and splenic arteries may receive additional blood supply from the hepatic and superior mesenteric arteries.

## INDICATIONS FOR DISTAL PANCREATECTOMY IN CHRONIC PANCREATITIS

In general terms, distal pancreatectomy is indicated for those patients with intractable pain (2) whose disease is largely confined to the distal pancreas and who have no suitable "target" for a drainage procedure (3, 4). Roux loop drainage of a dilated pancreatic duct and/or pseudocyst has two advantages over a pancreatectomy: *(a)* it is relatively simple and safe because it avoids the need to mobilize the gland and lift it out of its bed of inflammatory scar tissue, and *(b)* it does nothing to cause or exacerbate pancreatic insufficiency, whether endocrine or exocrine (1, 5, 6). Unfortunately, in our experience, barely one-third of patients requiring operation for chronic pancreatitis are suitable for a drainage procedure. In the remaining two-thirds, some form of resection is required.

Although most patients with chronic pancreatitis have generalized disease throughout the gland, it is best to avoid total pancreatectomy as a primary procedure because of the extent and risk of the operation and the inevitable diabetes that results (7). Insulin management can be haphazard in the long-term in this group of predominantly alcoholic patients, and problems of glycemic control underlie many of the late deaths seen in series of total pancreatectomies. In choosing between the two types of partial pancreatectomy, proximal and distal, reliance is placed on the pattern of disease shown by preoperative imaging supplemented by the findings at operation.

The ideal candidate for distal pancreatectomy has clear-cut disease of the body and tail, with calcification and/or pseudocyst formation, and there is an abrupt transition to much more normal tissue at or close to the midline. This situation is seen in the occasional patient who develops left-sided chronic pancreatitis following abdominal trauma with partial disruption of the duct in the neck of the pancreas (complete disruption usually requires an early laparotomy before chronic changes have developed). In most patients with chronic pancreatitis, the choice of resection is more difficult, and the surgeon needs to strike a balance between the advantage of avoiding the anastomoses implicit in a pancreatoduodenectomy (or even a duodenum-preserving resection of the head) and the need to remove the worst foci of disease. Most pancreatectomies for chronic pancreatitis represent a compromise between removing enough tissue to make an impact upon the patient's pain and removing so much tissue that permanent insulin therapy is required. In our experience, removal of the left pancreas is associated with rather more endocrine impairment than an equivalent resection of the right pancreas (8), but the functional outcome of pancreatectomy in this disease is by no means predictable. Our failure rates after left-sided and right-sided resections in terms of recurrent pain are broadly comparable and do not provide any support for Longmire's concept that the head of the pancreas acts as the "pacemaker" of this disease.

Selection for distal pancreatectomy is a relatively straightforward matter in a patient with painful pancreatitis affecting the body and tail of pancreas who is not yet an insulin-dependent diabetic. If the rest of the gland is also severely diseased, and especially if the patient is already on insulin, then one-stage total pancreatectomy must be considered. Progression of chronic pancreatitis following previous resection of the head may be an indication for *completion distal pancreatectomy*. In these patients, the initial benefit of the right-sided resection tends to be short-lived; pain recurs within a year or two and is often accompanied by a further decline in endocrine and exocrine function. In our series of 52 patients receiving proximal pancreatoduodenectomy for chronic pancreatitis, 6 (12%) required completion distal pancreatectomy after a mean interval of 28 months (9).

In the presence of a *chronic pseudocyst* arising within the neck, body, or tail of the pancreas, a choice must be made between internal drainage of the cyst and distal pancreatectomy. In simple terms, the smaller the cyst and the further it lies to the left, the more suitable it is for resection. Resection offers the advantage of removing the part of the gland that gave rise to the cyst, and this is often the site of maximal disease. It is particularly appropriate if there is heavy calcification or diffuse inflammatory swelling of the body and tail. By contrast, large cysts (i.e., >8 cm in diameter) and those lying close to the midline may be treated more safely by means of drainage into a Roux loop of jejunum (10); cysts in the neck of the pancreas contain the portal vein in their posterior wall. The pseudocysts of chronic pancreatitis are mostly intrapancreatic, and as they expand, they destroy the adjacent parenchyma. They seldom resolve spontaneously and are associated with a high complication rate including hemorrhage, infection, splenic vein thrombosis, rupture to cause pancreatic ascites, and persistent fistula if percutaneous drainage is used–up to half of which communicate with the main pancreatic duct (10, 11). Such complications must clearly affect the management. Splenic vein thrombosis causes left-sided portal hypertension and increases the risk of intraoperative bleeding, so drainage of the cyst may be safer. On the other hand, bleeding into the cyst or a fistula is controlled more effectively by resection, even if a portion of the cyst wall is left behind to protect the major vascular structures. Lastly, resection is indicated if there is any suspicion that the swelling is a cystic neoplasm rather than an inflammatory pseudocyst (12). Such suspicion should arise if the cyst has an irregular wall or mixed attenuation on computed tomography (CT) scan and especially if there is no obvious etiologic agent for chronic pancreatitis, with no evidence of calcification and a normal appearance to the rest of the gland on imaging. Biopsy of the cyst wall with frozen-section examination should always be performed if drainage (or subtotal excision) is undertaken.

There is an occasional role for distal pancreatectomy as a *diagnostic procedure*. Some patients are labeled as having chronic pancreatitis on rather tentative grounds. They have chronic abdominal pain of a typical pancreatic distribution, i.e., a constant pain lying deeply within the epigastrium and radiating through to the back. Endoscopic retrograde cholangiopancreatography (ERCP) may be normal or show subtle changes such as minor irregularity of the main duct. Since many of these patients have pancreas divisum, and cannulations of the accessory papilla are technically difficult, radiographs of the main (dorsal) duct may not be available. Alternative diagnoses—esophagitis, gallstones, peptic ulcer disease, irritable bowel syndrome, arthritis of the thoracic spine—should be excluded as far as possible before resorting to pancreatic surgery. If troublesome pain persists, however, and especially if there is exocrine insufficiency on testing and/or some abnormality on ERCP or CT scan, then laparotomy can assist in future management. The operation starts with a thorough search for extrapancreatic disease before the distal pancreas is exposed. If there is clear-cut pancreatitis, an appropriate resection is performed. If the gland appears normal, it may still be reasonable to carry out a limited caudal pancreatectomy to obtain a definitive tissue diagnosis. We have found periductal fibrosis consistent with mild or moderate chronic pancreatitis in some such patients, and this knowledge has been of assistance in their subsequent care (13).

## PREOPERATIVE EVALUATION

### Clinical Assessment

All operations for chronic pancreatitis are major undertakings, so the patient's general health must be assessed in full. In our experience, two in three "surgical" patients with chronic pancreatitis have abused alcohol. Many heavy drinkers are also heavy smokers and therefore at risk of ischemic heart disease and chronic respiratory disease. On the other hand, pancreatitis patients tend to be younger than those requiring pancreatectomy for cancer and therefore more able to withstand a major surgical procedure. The typical patient with chronic pancreatitis is a man in his 40s who has been drinking steadily for 15–20 years. Continuing alcoholism is a relative contraindication to distal pancreatectomy, especially if there is a risk of precipitating diabetes (see Pancreatic Function Tests below), so a determined effort should be made to stop the patient's drinking. Abstinence can be checked by measuring serum ethanol in the clinic and by looking for peripheral macrocytosis and disordered liver enzymes. For reasons that are uncertain (but may include genetic predisposition), alcohol hepatitis and cirrhosis are surprisingly uncommon in patients with severe chronic pancreatitis, irrespective of the cause (14).

Routine laboratory tests comprise full blood count, blood urea and electrolytes, and hepatic function tests, including serum albumin. Serum amylase is normal in chronic pancreatitis except in two circumstances: the presence of a pseudocyst or a recent acute exacerbation of the disease (i.e., acute-on-chronic pancreatitis). If carcinoma enters the differential diagnosis, the estimation of tumor markers, notably CA 19-9, is sometimes of discriminatory value, but normal levels certainly do not exclude the presence of malignancy. Other radiographs are mandatory, and an electrocardiogram should be performed if there is any question of cardiac disease. Pancreatic imaging is discussed below.

### Pancreatic Function Tests

We measure the endocrine and exocrine function of the pancreas both before operation and in the early postoperative period. Diarrhea, steatorrhea, and the need for enzyme replacement therapy are the clinical criteria for abnormal *exocrine* function. Indirect (tubeless) tests of exocrine function are less troublesome to the patient than duodenal intubation studies and less troublesome to the laboratory than fecal analysis for fat or chymotrypsin content. Tubeless tests include the $^{14}C$ triolein breath test, the PABA test (*p*-aminobenzoic acid), and the Pancreolauryl test, which relies on pancreatic secretion of an esterase to hydrolyze fluorescein-dilaurate; fluorescein is absorbed from the gut and excreted in the urine, where its concentration can be measured. Intestinal absorption and renal excretion are "controlled" by giving oral fluorescein alone on the second day of the test, and the result is expressed as a ratio of the test and control studies. Eleven of 42 patients (27%) undergoing distal pancreatectomy for chronic pancreatitis in this department already had either clinical or laboratory evidence of exocrine insufficiency, and this proportion was unchanged postoperatively (8); these figures may be an underestimate since not all patients were fully tested.

The clinical diagnosis of abnormal *endocrine* function is made on the need to treat diabetes mellitus with dietary modification, oral hypoglycemic agents, or insulin. Endocrine function can be measured by means of an oral glucose tolerance test or indirectly by measuring the glycosylated hemoglobin level in the blood. Thirteen of the 42 patients (31%) had preoperative evidence of glucose intolerance (though not all were tested), and this proportion increased to 52% postoperatively (8). There was a significant deterioration in measured endocrine function, and seven patients required treatment for diabetes as a direct consequence of the operation. In summary, patients coming to distal pancreatectomy are unlikely to require insulin thereafter provided their preoperative function is nearly normal and no more than 50–60% of the gland is removed, but the functional outcome is not entirely predictable.

### Pancreatic Imaging

Plain abdominal x-rays are of very limited value except to demonstrate pancreatic calcification. Ultrasound scans may demonstrate enlargement of the gland, pseudocyst formation, calcification, obstruction of the bile duct, and involvement of the portal vein or its tributaries. CT can show all of these features in a manner that is generally easier for the clinician to comprehend. ERCP is important to delineate the anatomy of the pancreatic duct and to exclude any biliary stricture from pancreatitis in the head of the gland. Magnetic resonance (MR) imaging complements the CT scan, and modern MR scanners can also show the pancreatic and biliary duct ductal trees (MR cholangiopancreatography), without the need for injection of contrast material.

The necessity for preoperative visceral angiography has been reduced by the advent of spiral CT scanning with intravenous contrast enhancement. It is valuable to know about occlusion or compression of the splenic or portal veins and the development of left-sided (sinistral) portal hypertension, with or without splenomegaly. Patients with chronic pseudocysts in the body or tail of the pancreas occasionally have pseudoaneurysms of the splenic artery, which may give way and bleed into the gut in the aftermath of an internal drainage procedure (15); such patients may better be served by a distal resection. If other imaging modalities suggest any vascular involvement, then splenic and superior mesenteric angiography remains a useful prelude to distal pancreatectomy. If complete pancreatic ductography cannot be obtained before operation, then consideration should be given to obtaining on-table pancreatograms by one means or another (see Operative Examination of the Pancreas).

## PERIOPERATIVE PRECAUTIONS

Sophisticated modern imaging generally allows the surgeon to determine the most appropriate procedure preoperatively, but the patient should be warned that the final decision can only be made at laparotomy. Sometimes the extent of disease found at operation necessitates a change of plan; for example, from resection to drainage in the case of a large or adherent pseudocyst, from drainage to resection if the pancreatic duct is no longer very dilated, or from distal to proximal (or even total) pancreatectomy if the head of the gland is severely diseased. Patients should also be alerted to the risk of postoperative diabetes or exocrine failure.

Gross anemia should be corrected preoperatively, and cross-matched blood should always be available to counteract hemorrhage during the dissection. Preoperative clues to a difficult distal pancreatectomy are *(a)* splenic vein thrombosis, *(b)* a densely calcified gland, *(c)* a recent attack of acute-on-chronic pancreatitis, *(d)* the presence of a pseudocyst, *(e)* previous celiac plexus blocks, and *(f)* previous pancreatic surgery, especially pseudocyst-gastrostomy. Cessation of smoking, assessment of pulmonary function, and both pre- and post-operative physiotherapy are sensible precautions in a patient with respiratory problems. Nutritional support should be considered in malnourished patients (weight loss is a common feature of severe chronic pancreatitis). All pancreatic operations should be "covered" by broad-spectrum antibiotics (e.g., a cephalosporin or aminoglycoside plus metronidazole) and by some form of thromboprophylaxis (e.g., subcutaneous heparin).

Most patients coming to distal pancreatectomy for chronic pancreatitis need splenectomy as well, so preoperative vaccination against certain encapsulated bacteria is advisable to prevent the outside chance of overwhelming postsplenectomy sepsis (16). If possible, immunization should take place 2–4 weeks before operation, to obtain optimal antibody titers. We currently vaccinate the patient against the pneumococcus, meningococcus, and *Haemophilus influenzae* type B but do not give prophylactic penicillin.

## OPERATIVE EXAMINATION OF THE PANCREAS

The anterior surface of the head of the pancreas can be inspected during *laparoscopy* after cleaning the overlying connective tissue, and the distal gland can be seen by inserting the videocamera into the lesser sac through the lesser omentum. The posterior aspect of the gland is less readily accessible, and the surgeon loses the tactile feel of the gland. Laparoscopic ultrasound can be used to demonstrate the bile duct and pancreatic duct and to display any calculi or dilated segments.

*Laparotomy* for pancreatectomy should generally be performed through a "gable" (bilateral subcostal) incision (17). Before approaching the pancreas, particular attention should be paid to the liver, gallbladder, and bile duct; liver biopsy is a sensible routine in alcoholic patients. Inspection and palpation of the neck, body, and tail of pancreas require creation of a moderately large window in the greater (gastrocolic) omentum so as to enter the lesser sac of the peritoneal cavity. In severe disease, and especially in the presence of a pseudocyst, the lesser sac may be partly obliterated by adhesions between the superior border of the pancreas and the back of the stomach. These adhesions must be released by careful sharp dissection. Incision of the peritoneum along the superior and inferior borders of the pancreas allows exposure of the posterior surface of the gland for thorough inspection and palpation. The normal pancreatic tail extends right out to the hilum of the spleen, but sometimes in end-stage pancreatitis, the distal gland becomes atrophic and "shrinks away" from the spleen. In the presence of established chronic pancreatitis, the gland is indurated, white (as opposed to the normal pale yellow), hyperemic, and scarred. It may be either enlarged or diminished in size, and the surface may be expanded by an intrapancreatic pseudocyst. The early changes of the disease are more subtle and may comprise a slight increase in nodularity and patchy whitening of the parenchyma.

The head of the pancreas should always be examined before deciding upon a distal resection for chronic pancreatitis. An extended Kocher's maneuver is used to mobilize the first, second, and third parts of the duodenum together with the pancreatic head, which is contained within this loop. Following dissection of the peritoneum overlying the front of the pancreas, both aspects of the pancreatic head can be thoroughly examined by means of direct inspection and manual palpation.

There is a limited role for *on-table pancreatography* in patients who are explored with a view to distal pancreatectomy (18). Supplemental information on the pancreatic ductal tree may be needed if the preoperative ERCP is either incomplete, out-of-date, or unobtainable, though CT and MRI plus intraoperative ultrasound scans can also be used to visualize the duct. In a patient with moderate ductal ectasia, an "ambigrade" pancreatogram obtained by direct ductal puncture allows a rational choice between longitudinal pancreaticojejunostomy and distal pancreatectomy. A "butterfly" needle is used to enter the duct, which can sometimes be felt as a softer groove within the indurated pancreas. In patients with an intrapancreatic pseudocyst, on-table cystography will show the presence or absence of a communication with the main pancreatic duct. Depending upon the size of the cyst, contrast can be introduced by a needle or via a catheter inserted through a small incision in the cyst wall and then sutured around the tube. If a dilated duct is found in the neck of pancreas following transection of the gland at this level, then prograde pancreatography can help to determine where to lay open the duct and combine drainage of the head with resection of the body and tail.

## TECHNIQUES OF RESECTION

### Distal Pancreatectomy with Splenectomy (Fig. 38.1)

Many surgeons dissect the pancreas from left to right, starting by mobilizing the spleen and then the tail of the pancreas and proceeding toward the midline. The advantage of this technique is that it establishes the correct posterior plane at an early stage and can allow relatively rapid progress. The disadvantage is that the junction of the splenic and superior mesenteric veins is only displayed toward the end of the procedure, so that a major venous hemorrhage is difficult to control. If the spleen is torn as it is brought up into the wound, then it can be removed after ligation of its major vascular pedicle and before proceeding to elevate the distal pancreas. A crucial part of this *prograde dissection* is the separation of the splenic vein from the posterior aspect of the proximal body of the pancreas, which can be densely adherent. If possible, it is best to ligate the splenic artery before the splenic vein to prevent congestion of the spleen. The artery is identified as it passes from the celiac axis to join the superior border of the proximal body of the pancreas and is doubly ligated on the aortic side. Once the splenic vein has been safely ligated and divided, a safe plane can usually be found between the neck of the pancreas and the portal vein, and the precise site of pancreatic transection is chosen.

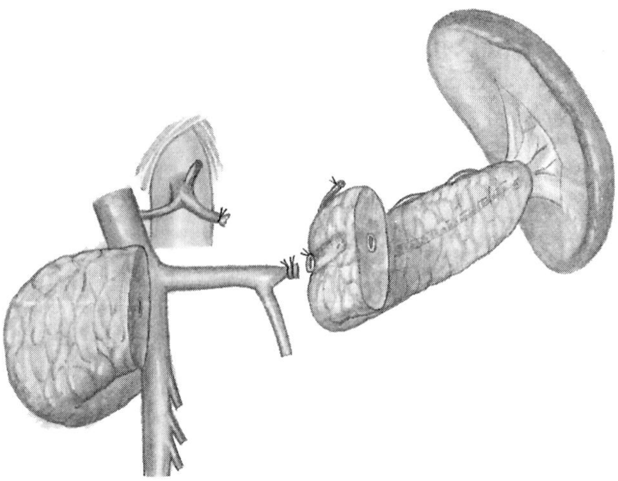

**FIG. 38.1.** A 50% distal pancreatectomy with splenectomy. The neck of the pancreas is divided along the line of the central axis of the portal vein. The splenic artery is ligated as it gains the superior border of the pancreas, and then the splenic vein is ligated behind the pancreatic neck. Although not inevitably true, the inferior mesenteric vein usually enters the splenic vein close to its termination and can therefore be preserved.

It has become our preference when operating for chronic pancreatitis to dissect the pancreas from right to left, i.e. starting in the midline and proceeding toward the left flank (1, 17). The advantage of this technique is that it identifies at an early stage the crucial T-junction between the terminal splenic vein and the portal vein and thus allows precise control of any venous hemorrhage. The disadvantage is that the tunnel behind the neck of the pancreas can be difficult to declare in a patient with severe pancreatitis. In performing this *retrograde dissection*, the neck of the pancreas is held up between stay sutures and is then divided with a scalpel, using a Kocher's dissector to protect the subjacent portal vein. The body of the pancreas is dissected off the terminal portion of the splenic vein, securing the several thin-walled tributaries, until the splenic artery is identified, encircled, ligated, and divided; splenic vein ligation and division then follows. Thereafter, there is no risk of a splenic vein tear extending into the portal vein as the dissection proceeds, either in a completely retrograde fashion or (if the gland is very stuck) by mobilizing the spleen and approaching from the tail as well. Ligation and division of the short gastric vessels (vasa brevia) should be done with care to avoid including a portion of the greater curve of stomach in the ligature, which would otherwise risk a subsequent gastric fistula.

Ideally the pancreas is divided at the junction between relatively normal and clearly abnormal tissue, although in practice there is seldom a sharp transition. The *extent of distal pancreatectomy* can be defined in terms of the approximate percentage of gland removed (Table 38.1). The midpoint of the pancreas is taken as a line drawn down the central axis of the portal vein. Subtotal pancreatectomy is seldom indicated. It renders the patient diabetic but leaves residual tissue with the risk of continuing pain, so a proximal pancreatectomy is generally preferred.

There are several different methods for *managing the amputated stump* of the pancreas, but none is clearly superior. We prefer to identify and underrun the main pancreatic duct by means of an X-suture and then close the parenchyma by means of interrupted nonabsorbable sutures (3/0 silk). Others use a mechanical stapler or an encircling band (19, 20), but these techniques do not readily allow adequate inspection of the main duct and, if necessary, cannulation to obtain an x-ray. If the duct is dilated and especially if there is a proximal stricture, then it can be opened for a few centimeters to allow side-to-side anastomosis to a Roux loop of jejunum (21). Formerly popular on a routine basis, this anastomosis appears to convey little advantage over simple closure of the stump in terms of preventing pancreatic fistula and is probably not worthwhile if the duct is unobstructed and of normal caliber (22).

The incidence of a troublesome pancreatic fistula after distal pancreatectomy is approximately 5%, but the fistula will almost

**TABLE 38.1. Types of Distal Pancreatectomy (According to Percentage of Pancreas Removed)**

| | Percentage of Gland Removed | Point of Transection of Pancreas |
|---|---|---|
| Caudal pancreatectomy | 25–33 | Junction of body and tail (no landmark) |
| Hemipancreatectomy | 50 (40–60) | Directly in front of portal vein (left or right border of vein) |
| Extended distal pancreatectomy | 70 | Junction of head and neck (level of gastroduodenal artery) |
| Subtotal pancreatectomy | 85–95 | To leave a thin rim within duodenal loop |

always close spontaneously. The risk of fistula is one reason for leaving a drain at the end of the operation; otherwise the patient may develop pain and fever and require subsequent percutaneous drainage of a collection under ultrasound control. The more diseased the pancreas, the lower the enzyme content of its juice and the smaller the risk of postoperative fistula.

The amylase content of the pancreatic drain effluent is often surprisingly high in patients who do not develop a "clinical" fistula, i.e., the fluid loss dries up and the drain can safely be removed. Giving prophylactic octreotide (somatostatin analogue) by subcutaneous injection may lower the incidence of postoperative pancreatic fistula (23).

### Spleen-Preserving (Conservative) Distal Pancreatectomy (Fig. 38.2)

It is sometimes possible to separate the body and tail of the pancreas from the splenic artery and vein, dealing with the numerous vascular branches by ligatures or clips, and thus to preserve the spleen (24). An intact spleen plays a useful immunologic role in the opsonization of encapsulated bacteria. It may also reduce the incidence of a subphrenic collection after the operation. Sometimes there are adverse anatomic features such as splenic vessels that deeply groove the pancreas or that divide into their terminal branches away from the splenic hilum and pass in front of the pancreatic tail. Patients should always be immunized in case splenectomy is needed. Severe calcific disease, a distal pseudocyst (especially one on the posterior aspect of the gland), and splenic vein thrombosis usually preclude splenic conservation.

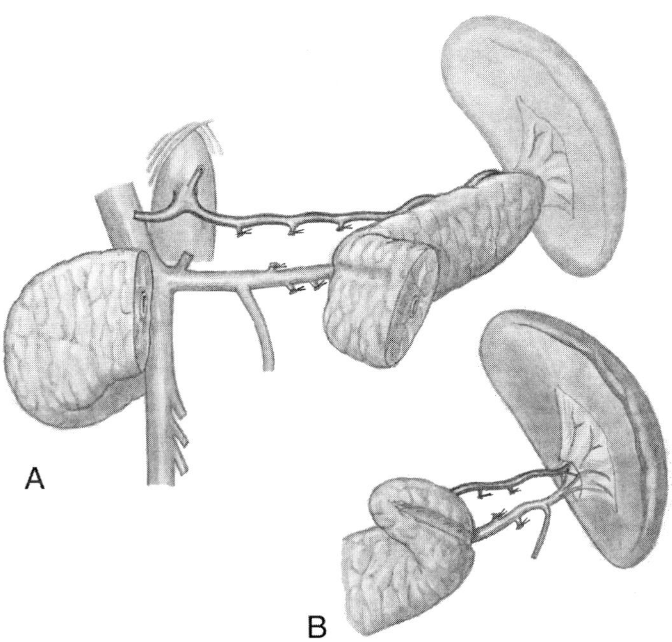


**FIG. 38.2.** Conservative distal pancreatectomy: alternative techniques. **A.** The pancreas is divided in the midline, and the dissection proceeds in a *retrograde* move toward the spleen. **B.** The tail of the pancrease is mobilized, and the dissection proceeds in a *prograde* move toward the portal vein.

As with the conventional resection, the procedure can start either in the flank with elevation of the tail of pancreas or in the midline following mobilization and division of the neck of the pancreas. Again, we favor the retrograde (right to left) approach because the main splenic vessels are exposed and can be clamped if bleeding occurs (22). It is easy to tear small venous branches off the parent vein, and the resultant holes need to be sutured before proceeding. Good retraction within the lesser sac is required as the surgeon approaches the tail of pancreas, and the spleen itself is seldom seen during the dissection. If the splenic artery and vein are ligated either by intent (because of bleeding) or inadvertently, splenectomy may still be avoidable if the point of ligation is well away from the splenic hilum; collateral supply via the short gastric and left gastroepiploic vessels may suffice. Indeed, Warshaw deliberately divides the main splenic vessels during spleen-preserving pancreatectomy (25). If the spleen becomes obviously congested or if its feeding vessels are repeatedly injured, then conservation is abandoned, and the dissection is quickly concluded by means of splenectomy. Lesser bleeding can usually be controlled by accurate sutures placed following removal of the pancreatic specimen. The pancreatic bed should be drained at the end of the procedure.

### Completion Distal Pancreatectomy (Fig. 38.3)

Completion distal pancreatectomy may be indicated in patients who develop recurrent pain following resection of the pancreatic head, with or without duodenectomy (7, 9). In a typical case, the patient has initial pain relief following removal of the right pancreas, but pain returns after 6–12 months, and insulin therapy becomes necessary to supplement deteriorating endocrine function. Further pancreatic imaging usually shows progressive changes of pancreatitis in the body and tail. In a patient who continues to abuse alcohol and/or is not yet on insulin, an attempt should be made to delay reoperation; percutaneous nerve blocks or thoracoscopic splanchnicectomy may provide transient pain relief. Otherwise, completion distal pancreatectomy should be considered to prevent opiate addiction.

The operation starts by identifying and dismantling the pancreaticoenteric anastomosis in front of the portal vein. The jejunal stump is then oversewn, and the pancreatic stump is dissected out in a retrograde (right to left) dissection. Perhaps surprisingly, the operation may present less of a technical challenge than a primary distal pancreatectomy, and a "conservative" technique is sometimes feasible. Patients must be taught to manage their diabetes before being allowed to go home, and exocrine supplements should obviously be given when oral feeding is restarted.

## OUTCOME

### Personal Data

Between 1978 and 1990, 46 patients underwent distal pancreatectomy for chronic pancreatitis, in this unit (22). Of these, 34 had a conventional resection including splenectomy, while 12

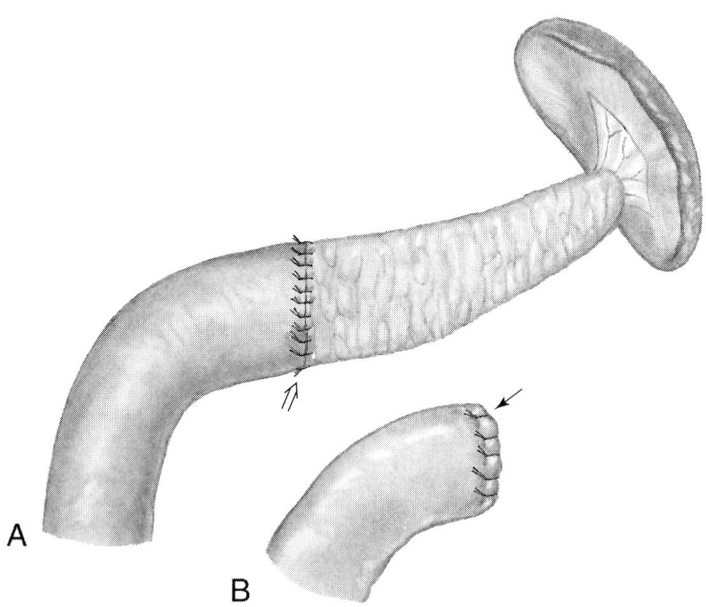


**FIG. 38.3.** Completion distal pancreatectomy following previous resection of the pancreatic head. **A.** The pancreaticojejunal anastomosis *(open arrow)* is identified and taken down. **B.** The jejunal stump *(dark arrow)* is oversewn, and the distal pancreas is resected, with or without the spleen.

had a conservative resection preserving the spleen. There were 31 men and 15 women, with a median age of 38 years (range, 17–75), and alcohol was the predominant cause (63%). In every instance, the indication for operation was severe abdominal pain. Pseudocysts were present in 15 patients (33%), including 4 in whom splenic conservation was still feasible; these were anterior pseudocysts that were not adherent to the splenic vessels. The splenectomy group included 4 patients who required urgent operation for recurrent gastrointestinal bleeding and 5 patients in whom a conservative resection was attempted but abandoned because of technical difficulties. The extent of distal pancreas removed varied from 30 to 80%, with a median of 50%. The pancreatic stump was oversewn in 41 patients, but in 5 with a dilated pancreatic duct, a pancreaticojejunostomy was carried out.

There were no postoperative deaths. Three patients required urgent reoperation for a reactive (early postoperative) hemorrhage. There were two pancreatic fistulas to the skin, which eventually dried up without the need for intervention, and three intraabdominal collections of pancreatic juice that required percutaneous drainage. One gastric fistula closed spontaneously, but a colonic fistula that followed partial devascularization of the transverse colon during a very difficult dissection required reoperation. Pain relief was superior among the patients receiving a conservative resection: 8 of 12 had good pain relief, as opposed to 20 of 34. Likewise, only one completion pancreatectomy was needed after conservative resection, as opposed to five after conventional resection. These data reflect the fact that patients with more severe disease required a splenectomy. The postoperative alteration in pancreatic function has already been described. In brief, endocrine function was impaired, but there was no detectable change in exocrine function. One patient required insulin before the operation, 6 thereafter, and 14 on subsequent follow-up.

### Published Data

Our results are comparable with those from other series of pancreatectomies reported from Europe and North America over the last 10 years (Table 38.2) (26–30). The operation can be carried out with a low mortality rate (5% or less) and with a success rate of approximately 60% in terms of lasting pain relief. It is scarcely surprising that partial pancreatectomy fails to guarantee pain control in what is generally a diffuse disease. Six of our patients (13%) required completion pancreatectomy, mostly within 2 years of the first operation (22). Sawyer and Frey showed that marked pancreatitis at the resection margin could predict the likelihood of further operation (30). Reoperation was needed in 6 of 7 patients with diffuse disease but only 1 of 10 patients with disease limited to the body and tail of the pancreas. The other prognostic criterion is the patient's ability to stop taking alcohol. Progressive pancreatitis is very likely in those who continue to drink. Unfortunately, it can still develop in those who stop, but the risk is almost certainly decreased.

The low incidence of pancreatic fistula (up to 5% in this and other series) probably does not justify the routine use of octreotide injections. However, such treatment is a reasonable precaution in patients with a relatively normal head of the pancreas who are likely to have a high enzyme content in the pancreatic juice. The risk of fistula or a peripancreatic/subphrenic collection indicates that at least one drain should be placed routinely, and we do not remove the drain before the fifth postoperative day.

Marked impairment in glucose tolerance is a feature of all reported series of distal pancreatectomies, but the degree of deterioration is unpredictable. Patients with normal preoperative glucose tolerance may withstand quite an extensive resection (50% or more) without demonstrable change in endocrine function, presumably because the tissue removed was already nonfunctional and the pancreatic remnant is not severely diseased. The fact that distal hemipancreatectomy disturbs endocrine function to a greater extent than proximal hemipancreatectomy may reflect the relative preponderance of islet cells in the body and tail of the pancreas.

## SUMMARY

1. Distal pancreatectomy is indicated for a group of patients with painful chronic pancreatitis in whom there is predominant involvement of the body and tail and relative sparing of the head. Some of these patients will have a pseudocyst and/or splenic vein thrombosis.
2. The pattern of disease should be determined by preoperative imaging—ultrasound, CT, MRI, and ERCP—supplemented by the findings at operation.
3. Distal pancreatectomy usually includes splenectomy, but splenic conservation is sometimes possible in patients with less severe disease; either procedure may be appropriate as a completion pancreatectomy. All patients should be vaccinated against the pneumococcus and other bacteria, preferably before operation.
4. Although the operative mortality rate is less than 5%, these are major operations with a risk of certain complications:

**TABLE 38.2. Results of Distal Pancreatectomy for Chronic Pancreatitis**

| First Author | Year | Reference No. | No. Patients | 30-Day Deaths (%) | Inadequate Pain Relief (%) |
|---|---|---|---|---|---|
| Giannello | 1986 | 26 | 24 | 4 | 20 |
| Morel | 1987 | 27 | 57 | 5 | 33 |
| Kohler | 1987 | 28 | 23 | 4 | 43 |
| Keith | 1989 | 29 | 32 | 3 | 50 |
| Aldridge[a] | 1991 | 22 | 46 | 0 | 39 |
| Sawyer | 1994 | 30 | 17 | 0 | 41 |

[a]Our own series.

reactive hemorrhage, a pancreatic collection or fistula, and occasional fistulas from the stomach or colon.

5. Good long-term pain relief can be anticipated in 60% of patients. The remainder have varying degrees of pain, which may be manageable by simple analgesics but will require a completion (proximal) pancreatectomy in 10–20%.
6. Although pancreatic exocrine function is seldom greatly disturbed, impaired endocrine function is common. A few patients (10–20%) require insulin as a direct consequence of the resection, but several more will drift into insulin dependence over the next few years as a result of progressive pancreatitis (especially if they continue to abuse alcohol).

## REFERENCES


1. Williamson RCN. The pancreas. In: Keen G, Fandon JR, eds. Operative surgery and management. 3rd ed. Oxford: Butterworth-Heinemann, 1994:161–185.
2. Ihse I, Borch K, Larsson J. Chronic pancreatitis: results of operations for relief of pain. World J Surg 1990;14:53–58.
3. Williamson RCN, Cooper MJ. Resection in chronic pancreatitis. Br J Surg 1987;807–812.
4. Cuilleret MD, Guillemin MD. Surgical management of chronic pancreatitis on the continent of Europe. World J Surg 1990;14:11–18.
5. Cooper MJ, Williamson RCN. Drainage operations in chronic pancreatitis. Br J Surg 1984;71:761–766.
6. Bradley EL III. Long-term results of pancreatojejunostomy in patients with chronic pancreatitis. Am J Surg 1987;153:207–213.
7. Fleming WR, Williamson RCN. The role of total pancreatectomy in the treatment of patients with ad-stage chronic pancreatitis. Br J Surg 1995;82:1409–1412.
8. Jalleh RP, Williamson RCN. Pancreatic exocrine and endocrine function after operations for chronic pancreatitis. Ann Surg 1992;216:656–662.
9. Stapleton GN, Williamson RC. Proximal pancreatoduodenectomy for chronic pancreatitis. Br J Surg 1996;83:1433–1440.
10. Grace PA, Williamson RCN. Modern management of pancreatic pseudocysts. Br J Surg 1993;80:573–581.
11. Bradley EL III. Pseudocysts in chronic pancreatitis: development and clinical implications. In: Beger HG, Buchler M, Ditschuneit H, Malfertheiner P, eds. Chronic pancreatitis. Berlin: Springer-Verlag, 1990:260–268.
12. Warshaw A, Rutledge PL. Cystic tumours mistaken for pancreatic pseudocysts Ann Surg 1987;205:393–397.
13. Thompson MH, Williamson RCN, Salmon PR. The clinical relevance of isolated ventral pancreas. Br J Surg. 1980;68:101–104.
14. Fallen RP, Gilbertson SA, Williamson RCN, Foster CS. A morphological and histochemical analysis of the human liver in chronic pancreatitis. GST 1991;32 1386–1391.
15. Breler L, Boissel P, Grosdidier L. Major haemorrhage from pseudocysts and pseudoaneurysms caused by chronic pancreatitis: surgical therapy. World J Surg 1991;15:649–652.
16. Cooper MJ, Williamson RCN. Splenectomy: indications, hazards and alternatives. Br J Surg 1984;71:173–180.
17. Williamson RCN. Pancreas. In: Krik RM, ed. General surgical operations. 3rd ed. Edinburgh: Churchill Livingstone, 1994: 349–373.
18. Desa LA, Williamson RCN. On table pancreatography: the importance in planning operative strategy Br J Surg 1990;77:1145–1150.
19. Scott-Conner CEH, Dawson DL. Technical considerations in distal pancreatectomy with splenic preservation. Surg Gynecol Obstet 1989;168:451–453.
20. Sadek S, Holdsworth R, Cuschierei A. Experience with pancreatic banding: results of a simple technique for dealing with the pancreatic remnant after distal partial pancreatectomy. Br J Surg 1988;75:486–487.
21. Shankar S, Theis B, Russell RCG. Management of the stump of the pancreas after distal pancreatic resection. Br J Surg 1980;77: 541–544.
22. Aldridge MC, Williamson RCN. Distal pancreatectomy with and without splenectomy. Br J Surg 1991;78:976–979.
23. Pederzoli P, Bassi C, Falconi M, Camboni G. Efficacy of octreotide in the prevention of complications of elective pancreatic surgery. Br J Surg 1994;81:265–269.
24. Cooper MJ, Williamson RCN. Conservative pancreatectomy. Br J Surg 1985;72:801–803.
25. Warshaw AL. Conservation of the spleen with distal pancreatectomy. Arch Surg 1988;123:550–553.
26. Giannello P, Lerut J, Guyot JF, Otte JB, Kestens PL. La chirurgie de la pancreatite chrnique. Resections versus drainage. Suivi a long terme de 100 patients operes. Gastroenterol Clin Biol 1985; 10:7–11.
27. Morel PH, Rohner A. Surgery for chronic pancreatitis. Surgery 1987;96(4):599–606.
28. Kohler H, Schafmayer A, Peiper HH. Follow up results of surgical treatment in chronic pancreatitis. Dig Surg 1987;4:67–71.
29. Keith R, Saibil F, Sheppard R. Treatment of alcoholic pancreatitis by pancreatic resection. Am J Surg 1989;157:156–162.
30. Sawyer R, Frey CF. Is there still a role for distal pancreatectomy in surgery for chronic pancreatitis? Am J Surg 1994;168:6–9.

# 39

# Total Pancreatectomy and Its Modifications

R. C. G. Russell

The final procedure in the surgeon's armamentarium for treating chronic pancreatitis is to ablate the whole of the pancreas. The use of this procedure often indicates the failure of previous procedures or indeed their inappropriate use, for an ill-conceived distal pancreatectomy when the major disease is in the head of the gland rarely, if ever, solves the problem and leads inevitably to a total pancreatectomy. Similarly, the idea that the head of the pancreas always drives the disease in chronic pancreatitis is ill conceived when the major stricture formation, often following an episode of acute pancreatitis, has occurred at the neck of the pancreas with distal obstruction. Justifiably, the procedure of total pancreatectomy has a bad reputation. Not only is the operative mortality greater, but the immediate perioperative morbidity is higher, and the late complications considerable. Indeed, there is an excess in early deaths in patients who have had this operation.

The procedure should be used sparingly and only after carefully managed conservative measures have failed to solve the patient's symptoms. The inevitability of diabetes, which is erratic and difficult to manage, ensures that the character of the patient must be assessed preoperatively. Performance of this procedure on a patient who is noncompliant is likely to fail; the patient whose attention to medical detail is limited can find the discipline associated with a balance between food, enzyme replacement, and insulin burdensome. Because many patients who need to have a total pancreatectomy have a history of alcohol abuse and narcotic abuse, it is essential that both these conditions have been adequately controlled and managed preoperatively. The continued use of high doses of narcotic in the postoperative period and particularly in the early posthospital period appears to delay proper patient control of the diabetes or a full appreciation of the type of life to be expected in the postpancreatectomy state. These lessons were learned early in the history of this operation, and despite greater experience, better monitoring of glycemic control, and more convenient insulin preparations, the outcome has not been greatly improved.

## HISTORIC BACKGROUND

In 1943 Rockey described total pancreatectomy in a patient who survived for 15 days before succumbing to a "blow-out" of the ligated end of the common bile duct (1). As always, when history is examined in greater depth, this was not found to be the first report, as Sauve in 1908 described two patients who had had a near total pancreatectomy, the first in reports by Mayo-Robson of an operation by Billroth in 1884, and a second reported by Franke in 1900 (2). The latter operation was undertaken for cancer of the pancreas, but the duodenum was not removed, and some pancreas around the duodenum was preserved, maintaining the arterial arcade and duodenal viability, a forerunner of the Beger procedure. The first successful total pancreatectomy was performed by Priestly on July 14, 1942, at Saint Mary's Hospital, Rochester, in a patient with hypoglycemia in whom no tumor could be palpated. This historic procedure is well described by van Heerden (3), who records that the patient survived for 29 years after the removal of what proved to be an 8 × 5 mm islet adenoma causing hypoglycemia. In 1948, Gaston reported 1 case of total pancreatectomy and reviewed 16 others; 11 had been performed for cancer, with only three survivors; 6 were performed for benign disease, and three had died (4). The next decade saw real advances in the technical aspects of pancreatic surgery, and by 1966, over 150 successful procedures had been reported.

In 1966, Warren et al. reported eight patients who had had a resection for advanced chronic relapsing pancreatitis (5). Characteristically, Warren laid down the principles of managing chronic pancreatitis by total pancreatectomy that are true today. He advised that the procedure was only used for patients with disabling symptoms and in patients who had marked destruction of the pancreatic parenchyma often associated with innumerable points of intraductal obstruction. Of Warren's original patients, six were followed closely, with good results in five. In a report in 1970 by ReMine et al., the drawbacks of performing a total pancreatectomy too late in the disease were emphasized as he pointed out that the debilitation and addiction to drugs and alcohol made useful rehabilitation almost impossible (6). A review of 36 patients from the Mayo Clinic noted that only 3 in this series had undergone total pancreatectomy for benign disease (6). Of the three patients, two died within a year of hypoglycemic problems, and the third died 8 years later, following a massive gastrointestinal hemorrhage. In 1975, Pliam and ReMine found that only two further patients had undergone this operation at the Mayo Clinic for chronic pancreatitis (7). The fact that so few patients were operated on in this center, which had an interest in pancreatic disease, emphasizes the rarity of this procedure and its limited role in the management of pancreatic disease.

By 1978, Braasch et al. from the Lahey Clinic collated the 53 documented cases of total pancreatectomy performed worldwide for pancreatitis and added the Lahey Clinic experience of 26 patients, indicating in that center a changing attitude to the operation and an increased willingness to perform the procedure in specialized centers (8). Their operative mortality was nil, but morbidity both in hospital and delayed was considerable. Diabetic problems were common, and no fewer than 12 late deaths occurred as a result. Interestingly, they reported good relief of epigastric pain, although 3 of their 14 surviving patients still took narcotics. However, in those who survived, there was a failure to normalize life satisfactorily.

The disease in Europe has often apparently presented in a different group of patients from those in America, as a high alcohol intake is socially more acceptable among motivated patients in Europe than those in America. In the decade of 1970–1980, Gall and his colleagues in Erlangen reported 63 total pancreatectomies that were performed between 1972 and 1977 (9). Their operative mortality was high (21%) compared with that of pancreatoduodenectomy (8%). Their morbidity was high, and their late mortality was similar to the American experience. After total pancreatectomy, 11% fewer patients were alive at the end of the follow-up period than after pancreatoduodenectomy. The deaths were accounted for by continued alcohol abuse and hypoglycemia. This late mortality is not entirely surgical. According to Strum and Spiro, the nonoperative treatment of severe pancreatitis is associated with a late mortality rate of 30% (10). This indicates that the complications of the disease and the personality of the patients are associated with a poor outcome. Because of the characteristics of the patient with pancreatitis, many consider that the chance of suitable rehabilitation after surgery is very limited. Much greater care is required by the surgeon in selection of patients, and greater emphasis must be placed on the psychosocial aspects of the disease.

## INDICATIONS

From what has been said, it is necessary to realize that a surgeon must exercise wisdom in preparing a patient with chronic pancreatitis for total pancreatectomy and must acknowledge that the emphasis in surgical practice is on parenchymal-preserving surgery. Thus, before considering this procedure, a full investigation of the pancreas must be performed. A high-quality spiral computed tomography (CT) scan is required to outline the whole pancreas to ensure that an ablative procedure is essential to cure the patient of the disease. The patient's diabetic state must be considered. If the patient is not diabetic, the role of pancreatic transplantation must be considered, particularly the use of islet preservation procedures with implantation into the portal vein. A wide-ranging medical, social, and psychiatric history must be taken to ascertain that all avenues of therapy have been explored prior to this decision.

The indications for total pancreatectomy are as follows:

1. Medical therapy must have failed after an adequate trial. An adequate trial of medical therapy includes a prolonged period of pancreatic rest, with nothing by mouth while on parenteral nutrition. This period (in hospital) also allows assessment of the patient's willingness, compliance, and cooperation with the medical team and their instructions.
2. The pain must be intractable and unrelieved by medical therapy. It is doubtful if total pancreatectomy for this disease is ever indicated in the absence of pain.
3. Operations to preserve the parenchyma must have been considered and shown to have failed or be unlikely to be successful. It is doubtful if total pancreatectomy should ever be performed in a patient with chronic pancreatitis who has neither overt endocrine nor exocrine insufficiency.
4. The complications of pancreatitis may precipitate total excision in a patient who has previously undergone a resection of the head (Fig. 39.1) or the tail of the pancreas. Frequently these patients have had an inappropriate operation because of a lack of appreciation of the lesion causing the pancreatic symptoms.
5. In patients with parenchymatous disease, often related to multiple calculi in the smaller ducts, who are already insulin dependent and enzyme deficient, a total pancreatectomy can be preferable to a partial procedure in that preservation of some pancreas offers no benefit and may be a source of continuing and undermining pancreatic pain.
6. There are a few patients who have minimal-change pancreatitis in which there are diffuse minor changes within the pancreatic ducts that do not respond to partial resection in that if either the head or the tail is preserved, the pain inevitably recurs. These patients are ideal donors for islet cell preservation.

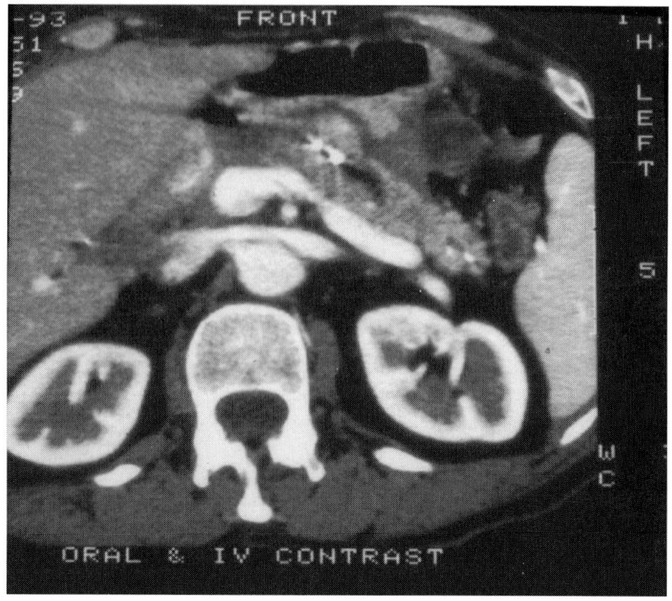


**FIG. 39.1.** CT scan of a patient who had undergone a pancreatoduodenectomy for alcohol-related pancreatitis 8 years previously. Two intraductal calculi can be seen obstructing the pancreatojejunal anastomosis. Inflammatory change can be seen at this anastomosis, between the pancreas and stomach, and in the splenic hilum. The patient is now well 2 years following completion pancreatectomy.

Finally, some authorities have doubted the logic of total pancreatectomy in the sensible management of a benign condition (11), and hence surgeons undertaking this procedure must be prepared to defend their position. It is a useful discipline for the surgeon to outline the reasons for the procedure in detail in the medical notes.

## PREOPERATIVE PREPARATION

Once a decision has been made to offer the patient a total pancreatectomy, the patient must be provided with details of the full implications of the procedure. A nurse practitioner in charge of diabetic patients should discuss the management of the diabetes, and a person with the knowledge of outcome of pancreatic disease, such as an experienced nursing colleague, should outline the need to take the enzyme preparations and control the food intake. A patient who is not diabetic should see a physician specializing in diabetes, preoperatively. Because many of these patients are malnourished, it is preferable to improve their nutrition preoperatively. This is conveniently done by a period of enteral or parenteral feeding, which provides an opportunity for the patient to come to terms with the impending operation and for the staff to assess the patient's willingness to comply with instructions. Many patients decide for themselves at this time whether or not to go ahead with the operation.

A repeat CT scan should be performed preoperatively to determine the current severity of the disease and how it affects the biliary tree. In particular, a decision should be made regarding the feasibility of a duodenum-preserving procedure or a pylorus-preserving procedure. An angiogram is not indicated provided the CT scan is adequately contrast enhanced so that the portal vein is displayed and its patency ascertained. It is most unwise to consider performing this operation in the presence of portal varices or portal hypertension. Infection, a bleeding tendency, and peptic ulceration should be eliminated preoperatively by the appropriate means. Because many patients have coexistent cardiac and respiratory disease as a result of a smoking habit, which often accompanies this disease, a full assessment of their cardiac, pulmonary, and renal function should be undertaken.

## CHOICE OF OPERATION

The approach to surgery is largely dictated by the previous procedures that the patient has undergone. It is rare to undertake this operation in the absence of either previous operations or previous pancreatic surgery. Only 14% of patients in the combined British series had not had a previous procedure (12). Thus, for patients who have had a previous pancreatoduodenectomy, a distal pancreatectomy is all that is required. Preferably, this should preserve the spleen. If the spleen has to be sacrificed, the recommended course of vaccinations should be completed at least 2 weeks before surgery. For those who have initially undergone a distal pancreatectomy or drainage procedure, there is a wider choice in that a duodenum-preserving procedure (13), a pylorus-preserving procedure (14), or the traditional pancreatoduodenectomy including partial gastrectomy can be performed. At present, there is little to recommend one procedure over the other (15); thus technical ease and avoidance of complications are the prime considerations.

## THE OPERATION

If a pancreatoduodenectomy is required, it is carried out as indicated in Chapter 36, Pancreaticoduodenectomy for Chronic Pancreatitis; if a distal pancreatectomy is necessary, it is undertaken as described in Chapter 38, Distal Pancreatectomy, Indications, and Results. For the completion distal pancreatectomy, it is frequently possible to undertake a limited approach through a left transverse incision if the remnant is small, but if the body and tail of the pancreas are inflamed, the procedure invariably turns out to be more difficult than first appreciated. A long transverse midline incision is required with a formal dissection, as chasing the body of the pancreas over the portal vein to the site of the previous pancreatojejunostomy can prove a most difficult dissection. It is essential to ascertain the anatomy of that jejunal anastomosis to perform an appropriate closure. Narrowing the jejunum, which might easily occur, can lead to obstruction of the biliary flow with stasis proximally, leading to cholangitis. After a completion distal pancreatectomy, the patient is expected to do well and respond rapidly to the surgery. Unfortunately, full recovery is frequently delayed because of the management of the diabetes and enzyme deficiency. To allow the patient out of hospital before this is solved can lead to a poor long-term outlook.

### Duodenum-Preserving Total Pancreatectomy

The duodenum-preserving total pancreatectomy was primarily developed to manage the patient with "minimal-change" pancreatitis (16) and those patients who had severe pain in the head of the pancreas with fibrosing pancreatic disease. This procedure is suitable in this case when the head of the pancreas is relatively small, with the inflammatory process being limited to the pancreas and not extending onto the duodenum. It is unwise to perform this procedure in the presence of a large inflammatory mass where the inflammation involves the duodenum.

### Anatomy

The duodenum has a blood supply that is similar to that of the stomach, with multiple mucosal anastomoses that enable blood to pass from the proximal to the distal end (13). The duodenum is supplied by an arcade between the anterior-superior pancreaticoduodenal artery and the anterior-inferior pancreaticoduodenal artery. After departing from the gastroduodenal artery, the anterior-superior pancreatoduodenal artery runs downward to a point 1.5 cm below the ampulla of Vater and then turns to the posterior aspect of the pancreas to anastomose with the anterior-inferior pancreaticoduodenal artery. In 9 of 10 cases, an arcade runs between the posterior-superior pancreaticoduodenal artery and the posterior-inferior pancreaticoduodenal artery. This arcade is located dorsal to the pancreatic head and the common bile duct. Arterial branches to the common bile duct and the papilla of Vater arise from the posterior-superior pancreaticoduodenal artery. In no case are these vessels buried in the pancreatic parenchyma. This anatomic fact enables the preservation of these vessels when the head of the pancreas is removed. In most cases, the pancreas, particularly in relationship to the main papilla and the accessory papilla, is intimately involved with the muscular layer of the duodenum. Some dissection of this layer is necessary during the complete removal of the pancreas from the duodenum. The bile duct can usually be dissected from the pancreas lying in its own protective fascial sheath.

The arcade formation is less clear in the venous anatomy than it is in the arterial anatomy. The posterior-inferior pancreaticoduodenal vein departs from the upper jejunal vein and runs horizontally behind the superior mesenteric vein toward the right on the posterior membrane of the head of the pancreas. It branches to the third portion of the duodenal wall and runs toward the papilla. The posterior-superior pancreaticoduodenal vein joins the posterior side of the portal vein at a point 0–15 mm above the junction of the superior mesenteric vein and the splenic vein. This vessel runs horizontally near the upper edge of the pancreatic head, crosses anterior to the bile duct, and then runs along the right side of the bile duct. Equal care in the preservation of these veins is required, particularly for the first 3–5 cm of their course (17).

### The Procedure

If the body and tail of the pancreas have not been removed, then this should be undertaken. Once the portal vein is exposed, the neck of the pancreas is dissected away from the portal vein onto its right side. The uncinate process of the pancreas is then gently separated from the superior mesenteric vein down to the junction of the vein and the fourth part of the duodenum. In this corner, the pancreas is grasped with tissue-holding forceps and gently lifted upward in a anterosuperior direction. The duodenum and head of the pancreas are not mobilized, a Kocher's maneuver being contraindicated. The dissection along the uncinate process both on the duodenum and portal vein aims at preserving the tributaries of the arteries and veins as much as possible by dividing the vessels in the pancreatic substance. It is essential at this stage to preserve the anterior-inferior pancreatoduodenal vein and artery. It is useful to use bipolar diathermy to cauterize the vessels and ensure a bloodless dissection. Once 2 cm of uncinate process has been dissected away from the portal vein and from the fourth part of the duodenum, the index finger of the left hand can be inserted behind the pancreas into the plane in which the anterior-inferior pancreaticoduodenal artery lies. By carefully lifting the pancreas forward in an anterosuperior direction, the tributaries of the vein and artery can be preserved, and blood flow to the fourth and the third parts of the duodenum maintained. As the dissection approaches the ampulla of Vater, the tethering between the pancreas and the duodenal wall increases such that there is no plane of cleavage. At this point, it is essential to dissect out the bile duct and define its position. If it is not obvious on the posterior part of the mobilized pancreas, then it is wise to extend the dissection up to the junction between the portal vein and the first part of the duodenum. At this point, the bile duct passes beneath the duodenum adjacent to the vein. It is dissected out, and the dissection is continued in the plane between the pancreas and the bile duct down to the ampulla. The blood vessels to the bile duct must be preserved as much as possible. The dissection is now continued to the pancreatic duct at the ampulla, which is divided and oversewn. The bile duct itself is not disturbed, and the pancreatic tissue densely adherent to the wall of the duodenum between the ampulla of Vater and the accessory papilla is dissected out by sharp dissection. If the accessory papilla is found, it is oversewn. The dissection is now continued superiorly to the second and first parts of the duodenum to complete the excision of the pancreas from within the duodenal C-loop. At the end of the procedure, the bile duct is seen preserved on the posterior abdominal wall, and the duodenum is lying free and often flaccid. Occasionally the area of duodenum near the ampulla is slightly cyanosed; use of a hot swab brings about a rapid recovery from this situation, hemostasis is achieved, and the abdomen is closed without drainage.

### Postoperative Care

Changes and advances in pancreatic surgery have led to more careful operative technique and a more controlled operative environment so that after most procedures, the patient has not required an intraoperative blood transfusion, his or her body temperature has remained constant, and all vital parameters have been normalized by the anesthetist throughout the procedure. Intensive care is rarely necessary, and the patient can be well managed in a high-dependency unit. It is essential to have a standardized technique for managing the postoperative diabetes. My routine is to administer a continuous intravenous infusion of 2 L of 5% glucose over 24 hours, concurrently with a half-liter of normal saline over 24 hours plus a continuous intravenous infusion of insulin (1 U/mL). Frequent samples of blood taken by fingerprick are analyzed by use of a portable glucose meter, and the insulin infusion rate is adjusted accordingly to maintain a blood glucose level between 4 and 8 mmol/L (73–145 mg/100 mL). "Sliding-scale" prescriptions should be avoided, as the glycemic control afforded is erratic; the requirement for insulin will vary in the postoperative period as the initial stress of the procedure and hence insulin resistance decreases, or increases if sepsis complicates the recovery. To relieve the immediate postoperative pain, reliance is placed on a bupivacaine nerve block or an epidural anesthetic and the use of nonsteroidal antiinflammatory drugs. Patient-controlled analgesia is to be avoided, as the tolerance of most patients with chronic pancreatitis to narcotics is immense, and the margin between adequate pain relief for these patients and respiratory depression is minimal. Delayed gastric emptying does occur after this procedure, and a nasogastric tube may be required until duodenal motility returns. For simplicity, a jejunostomy tube placed at the time of surgery can be an asset and enable administration of jejunal feeding within 48 hours of the operation. For these patients, it is essential to use predigested feedings to avoid diarrhea. Duodenal motility usually returns around the 5th day but can be delayed for much longer depending on the degree of duodenal ischemia that has occurred. Our experience is that recovery almost invariably occurs. Patience may be required.

Once food is introduced, the patient should start on adequate enzyme replacement therapy. Before going home, the patient must be off narcotics, competent in managing the diabetes and enzyme replacement therapy, and able to live without the support of alcohol.

## RESULTS

The largest recent review is a retrospective study describing collective data on 83 patients from six centers in the United Kingdom (12). Trede and Schwall describe 52 patients who had a total pancreatectomy, but only 17 of these were performed for chronic pancreatitis (18). Smaller experiences of 10 patients (19), 7 patients (20), and 4 patients (21) support the general conclusions reached by larger series. My own series up to the end of 1993 included 63 patients, of whom 15 had a total pancreatectomy as the primary procedure, 15 had undergone a previous proximal pancreatectomy, and 33 a previous distal pancreatectomy. Chronic alcoholic pancreatitis appears to be the commonest indication for total pancreatectomy but accounts for only half the patients. Gallstone pancreatitis, congenital anomalies, trauma, minimal-change pancreatitis, and idiopathic pancreatitis have all led to a total pancreatectomy. The commonest symptom has been pain, with narcotic abuse being frequent. Over 50% of patients were considered to be addicted to narcotics. Most patients are well below their ideal body weight, and much of the weight loss occurs in the period immediately prior to surgery. The length of history prior to operation is approximately 6 years. Between 80 and 90% of patients coming to total pancreatectomy have undergone previous pancreatobiliary procedures, often on more than one occasion. Distal pancreatectomy was the most common procedure, indicating the inappropriate use of this operation in pancreatic disease. Major intraoperative complications appear relatively uncommon, the most notable complication being hemorrhage from the portal vein, with or without associated portal hypertension.

The mortality resulting from this operation is higher than that of pancreatoduodenectomy. In the review by Frey et al., 31 of 324 (9.6%) patients died (22). Other publications (12, 15, 19–21, 23) have shown a lower mortality rate, varying from 0 to 6%. I have lost three patients in 63 operations, and in each instance, the fatality occurred following emergency "salvage" surgery for complications of the disease (two patients) and following prior pancreatic surgery (one patient). The morbidity of the operation is high, with as many as 40% of patients developing complications in the postoperative period (19). Sepsis is the most common complication, followed by biliary or enteric leak. Delayed hemorrhage occurs in a small number. Those who develop complications, particularly sepsis, tend to develop multiple complications with a prolonged inpatient hospital stay and a marked increase in the cost of the procedure. Infection in the pancreatic bed is particularly difficult to eliminate, and a left subphrenic abscess can catch the unwary. Should infection occur or be suspected, immediate CT scanning with contrast is essential. Late complications are rare, but readmission because of the complications of diabetes or weight loss are common.

### Long-Term Results

Flemming and Williamson (23) record detailed late results and note that 6 of their 40 patients required reoperation from 6 weeks to 4 years after total pancreatectomy. For three patients, adhesions required division; for two, an antrectomy was necessary, one for persistent delay in gastric emptying and the other for duodenal ulcer. The other patient had a temporary colostomy that was closed 6 weeks later. Late deaths are a frequent experience in all series. In the series of Flemming and Williamson (23) 15 late deaths were counted during a median follow-up of 42 months. Death occurred at a median age of 47 years (range, 36–59) and at a median of 41 months (2.5–120) after pancreatectomy. There were 11 disease-related deaths, 2 unrelated deaths (myocardial infarction and asthma), and 2 deaths of unknown cause. The related deaths consisted of two patients who had unknown pancreatic cancers that later presented with metastases, two hypoglycemic deaths, and six with pneumonia and uncontrolled diabetes. These patients appear particularly prone to sepsis, either because of the splenectomy or the patient's propensity for drug addiction and alcoholism. This experience is very similar to my own and that of other series. Of the 23 remaining patients in the Flemming and Williamson series (23),

17 were alive and without pain at a median of 45 months, and 4 continued to have pain, 3 of whom were addicted to opiates. It is my experience that after this operation, only 50% of patients have a reasonable result, and the others either die of the complications of the operation or continue to have pain, and as a result of this and diabetic complications, are frequently readmitted to multiple hospitals. Such an outcome emphasizes the need for careful preoperative selection and an accurate psychosocial assessment.

### Diabetes Mellitus

The management of diabetes after total pancreatectomy is said to be troublesome, but once the concept of the variable absorption of food is understood and due attention paid to the exocrine role of the pancreas, then diabetic control becomes straightforward. The essential thing is to train the patient to take adequate enzyme replacement with each meal and with each snack, to avoid malabsorption. After a few months, the enzyme requirement becomes stabilized, and steatorrhea resolves. The failure to appreciate this resulted in the report from Pliam and ReMine (7) that approximately a quarter of their patients who had undergone total pancreatectomy had difficulty managing their diabetes. Some 38% of their patients experienced hypoglycemia, and more than a half of them required hospitalization. McCullaugh et al. (24) and Ihse et al. (25) reported cases of hypoglycemic "shock" that resulted in death. As a consequence of this experience, it became fashionable to restrict the dose of insulin and allow only a relatively low caloric intake, with the consequent risk of malnutrition, hyperosmolar coma, and other diabetic complications. In my experience (26), the dose of insulin required varies from 14 to 96 U/day, with a median at 1, 3, and 5 years of 35.5, 39, and 40 U/day, respectively. Patients who had a duodenum-preserving pancreatectomy required more insulin than those who underwent the standard procedure (at 3 years, 43 U/day vs. 34 U/day). I have interpreted this finding as indicating a more normal dietary intake in those following a duodenum-preserving procedure. This is borne out by the greater weight of that group, compared with their preoperative state. The slight increase in the dose of insulin required after the 1st year indicates a better diet and a more normal lifestyle. The greatest help to the management of the diabetes in these patients is a well-organized joint clinic between the surgeon and diabetologist with the help of liaison nurses dealing with the separate pancreatic and diabetic problems.

## CONCLUSION

Total pancreatectomy is an acceptable operation for correctly selected patients. It can transform their lives from a pain-ridden existence to a normal lifestyle and thus should not be denied to the appropriate patients. Patient care does not end with the operation; the continuing medical care of the surgeon or delegation to the appropriate physician is required. In any salvage procedure, a high mortality in the long-term must be anticipated, but this must be balanced against the natural mortality of 30% in the untreated patient with chronic pancreatitis.

## REFERENCES


1. Rockey EW. Total pancreatectomy for carcinoma: a case report. Ann Surg 1943;118:603–611.
2. Sauve L. Des pancréatectomies et specialement de la pancreatectomie céphalique. Rev Chir 1908;37:113–152.
3. van Heerden JA. The first total pancreatectomy. Am J Surg 1986;151:197–199.
4. Gaston EA. Total pancreatectomy. N Engl J Med 1948;238: 345–354.
5. Warren KW, Poulantzas JK, Kune GA. Life after total pancreatectomy for pancreatitis. Ann Surg 1966;164:830–834.
6. ReMine WH, Priestley JT, Judd ES, King JN. Total pancreatectomy. Ann Surg 1970;172:595–604.
7. Pliam MB, ReMine WH. Further evaluation of total pancreatectomy. Arch Surg 1975;110:506–512.
8. Braasch JW, Vito L, Nugent FW. Total pancreatectomy for end-stage chronic pancreatitis. Ann Surg 1978;188:317–322.
9. Gall FP, Mühe E, Gebhardt C. Results of partial and total pancreaticoduodenectomy in 117 patients with chronic pancreatitis. World J Surg 1981;5:269–275.
10. Strum WB, Spiro HM. Chronic pancreatitis. Ann Intern Med 1971;74:264–277.
11. Imrie CW. Management of recurrent pain following previous surgery for chronic pancreatitis. World J Surg 1990;14:88–93.
12. Cooper MJ, Williamson RCN, Benjamin IS, et al. Total pancreatectomy for chronic pancreatitis. Br J Surg 1988;74:912–915.
13. Lambert MA, Linehan IP, Russell RCG. Duodenum preserving total pancreatectomy for end stage chronic pancreatitis. Br J Surg 1987;74:35–39.
14. Traverso LW, Longmire WP. Preservation of the pylorus in pancreatico-duodenectomy. A follow-up evaluation. Ann Surg 1979;190:312–316.
15. Stone WM, Sarr MG, Nagorney DM, McIlrath DC. Chronic pancreatitis—result of Whipple's resection and total pancreatectomy. Arch Surg 1988;123:815–819.
16. Walsh TN, Theis BA, Rode J, Russell RCG. Minimal change chronic pancreatitis. Gut 1992;33:1566–1571.
17. Kimura W, Nagai H. Study of surgical anatomy for duodenum-preserving resection of the head of the pancreas. Ann Surg 1995;221:359–363.
18. Trede M, Schwall G. The complications of pancreatectomy. Ann Surg 1988;207:39–47.
19. Kiviluotu T, Schröder T, Lempinen M. Total pancreatectomy for chronic pancreatitis. Surg Gynecol Obstet 1985;160:223–227.
20. Keith RG, Saibil FG, Sheppard RH. Treatment of chronic pancreatitis by pancreatic resection. Am J Surg 1989;157:156–162.
21. McAfee MK, van Heerden JA, Adson MA. Is proximal pancreatoduodenectomy with pyloric preservation superior to total pancreatectomy? Surgery 1989;105:347–351.
22. Frey CF, Suzuki M, Isaji S, Zhu Y. Pancreatic resection for chronic pancreatitis. Surg Clin North Am 1989;69:499–528.
23. Flemming WR, Williamson RCN. The role of total pancreatectomy in the treatment of patients with end stage chronic pancreatitis. Br J Surg 1995;82:1409–1412.
24. McCullagh EP, Cook JR, Shirley EK. Diabetes following total pancreatectomy: clinical observations of ten cases. Diabetes 1958;7:298–307.
25. Ihse I, Lilja P, Arnesjo B, Bengmark S. Total pancreatectomy for cancer. An appraisal of 65 cases. Ann Surg 1977;186:675–680.
26. Linehan IP, Lambert MA, Brown DC, Kurtz AB, Cotton PB, Russell RCG. Total pancreatectomy for chronic pancreatitis. Gut 1988; 29:358–365.

# 40

# *Nerve Ablation Procedures*

Ingemar Ihse, Åke Andrén-Sandberg, and Toru Yusa

The principles of surgical treatment of pain in chronic pancreatitis are decompression of intraductal and tissue hypertension, removal of inflamed pancreatic tissue, and blockage or section of sensory nerves. This chapter discusses the current role of percutaneous and surgical approaches to the nervous system in the treatment of pain in chronic pancreatitis.

## PRINCIPAL FEATURES OF PAIN IN CHRONIC PANCREATITIS

Pain is the dominant symptom in chronic pancreatitis. Only 5% of patients with chronic pancreatitis will have a pain-free course dominated by clinical signs of malabsorption. When present, pain is often severe and requires narcotic drugs. It may be either chronic or intermittent. In a study using pain scores, half of the patients reported their pain as severe, and the other half as moderate or slight (1). Pain is often accentuated by food intake, and it is described as gnawing and dull and does not show the paroxysmal pattern of intestinal, biliary, or renal colic. It is generally felt in the epigastrium but may radiate to the back or around the lower chest wall. Studies using electrical stimulation have suggested that pain in the left upper abdomen originates from the pancreatic tail, whereas pain to the right emanates from the pancreatic head (2). Pain located to the thoracolumbar area often has the same features as root pain and augments on movement of the spinal column. However, patients often try to relieve pain by flexing the spine, by sitting forward with the knees flexed against the chest, or by lying on the side with the knees and hips flexed. It has been suggested that pain decreases when the patient with alcoholic pancreatitis stops drinking (3). This assumption is, however, not supported by a recent study (4). Similarly, there is disagreement about whether pain subsides with time and increasing exocrine pancreatic insufficiency (3, 4). Until this controversy is solved, decisions on surgical treatment must not be postponed in the hope that pain will cease with time.

## POSSIBLE CAUSES OF PAIN IN CHRONIC PANCREATITIS

It is generally agreed that the origin of pain in chronic pancreatitis is multifactorial (5). This opinion is supported by the clinical course, in which the features of pain may vary not only between patients but also in the same patient from time to time. Also, the pain pattern not infrequently changes with time, being recurrent and intermittent in the initial stages of the typical case. Later it may become persistent, and in some patients it is said to cease in the long run (see above).

Increased duct-tissue pressure is a common explanation of chronic pancreatic pain, although questioned by some (4). Recent investigations strongly support this hypothesis. At intraoperative measurements, the ductal pressure was found to be higher in patients with chronic pancreatitis and pain than in subjects without pancreatic disease, as studied by endoscopic measurements (6). In another study using the endoscopic route, the ductal pressure was significantly higher in pancreatitis patients with pain than in those who were pain free (7).

Recently, Danish researchers presented a technique for measurement of pancreatic tissue fluid pressure. This method can be used both intraoperatively and percutaneously, the latter being guided by ultrasonography. Patients with painful chronic pancreatitis were found to have elevated pressure in comparison with subjects without known pancreatic disease. The pressure fell to normal values during the laparotomy after the surgical ductal drainage had been completed. The patients were followed postoperatively by the percutaneous technique, and those who continued to be pain free maintained their normal pressure, whereas those who had recurrence of pain had an increase in pressure to the preoperative value (8). Another group used the same technique for intraoperative measurement of tissue fluid pressure and confirmed the presence of increased pressure in pancreatitis patients with pain. They also discussed the possibility of a related compartmental syndrome as a cause of pancreatic pain (9).

Recently, new data were presented on what was called "pancreatitis-associated neuritis." This implies a comparative increase in the number of sensory nerves in inflammatory pancreatic tissue, together with round cell infiltration and a striking disintegration of the perineurium, allowing an unimpeded influx of inflammatory mediators or active pancreatic enzymes (10). It seems reasonable to assume that the two mechanisms discussed above might work together if the increased tissue pressure facilitates the influx of pain transmitters through the damaged perineurium. This could tentatively explain the persistent type of pancreatic pain, whereas acute pain attacks may be associated with acute inflammation and/or autodigestion with ensuing tissue necrosis and pseudocyst formation. One might speculate from this that pancreatic pain is primarily associated with the dynamics of the disorder rather than being a static situation. This would explain the poor correlation between pancreatic pain and morphology, be it by gross inspection, histology, or imaging.

## NERVE SUPPLY OF THE PANCREAS

The pancreas receives nerve fibers from both the sympathetic and parasympathetic nervous systems. The sympathetic nerves reach the pancreas through the greater and lesser splanchnic nerves, and the parasympathetic nerves by way of the vagus nerves (Fig. 40.1). Pain stimuli from the pancreas travel via the celiac ganglion and celiac plexus along the splanchnic nerves to the thoracic sympathetic ganglia (V–XI). It is not clear whether afferent fibers of the vagus are involved in pancreatic pain. All

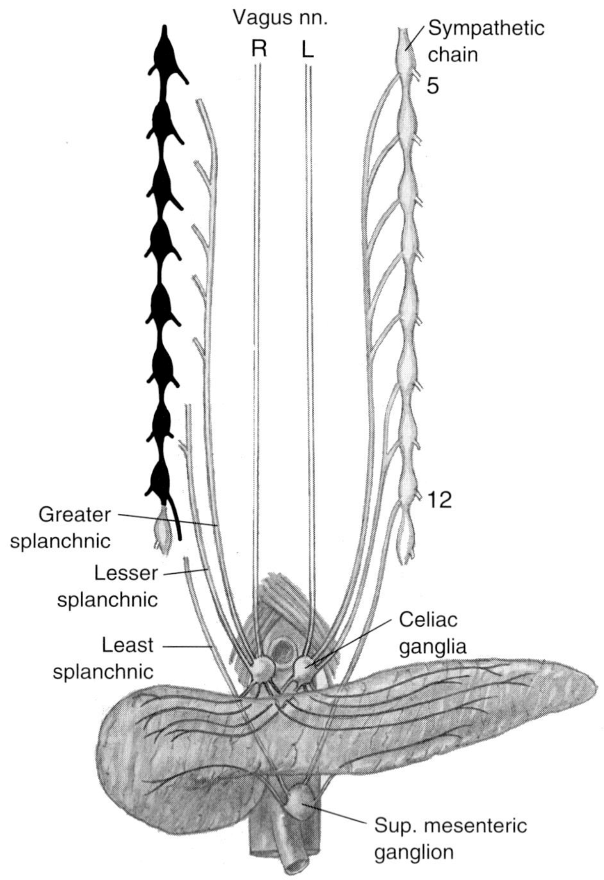


**FIG. 40.1.** Nerve supply of the pancreas.

nerves to and from the pancreas, however, pass through the celiac plexus. Further information on the innervation of the pancreas is given in Chapter 2, Surgical Anatomy.

## CELIAC PLEXUS BLOCK

Celiac blocks can be done either intraoperatively or percutaneously. For long-term effects, injection of alcohol, phenol, or a steroid may be used. As for other nerve block or nerve ablation procedures, celiac plexus block should be considered only for patients with refractory pain that does not have an obvious cause treatable by a different strategy.

Celiac plexus block is done with the patient awake or lightly sedated and placed in a prone position. Two needles are inserted, one from each side, 7–8 cm from the midline at the inferior edge of the 12th rib (11). The lateral body of the first lumbar vertebra (L-1) is located, and the needles are redirected until they slide off the lateral side of the vertebral body. They are then allowed to advance about 2 cm, until the needle tips rest just anterior to the upper part of the body of L-1, behind the aorta and diaphragmatic crura. Ganglia usually lie less than 1.5 cm anterior to the front of the vertebral body, those on the left being lower than those on the right. Proper placement of the needle is essential, and aspiration to rule out leakage of blood, urine, or cerebrospinal fluid, is obligatory. Injection should meet no resistance if the needle is correctly placed. Some 20–25 mL of, for example, 0.25% bupivacaine should be injected on each side. Nerve block with, for example, 25 mL of 50% alcohol is done on each side, 1 or 2 days after the diagnostic block with bupivacaine. The block should be guided by fluoroscopy to ascertain correct spread of the injected contrast medium, and it may be carried out with a catheter, retained for both the diagnostic and therapeutic blocks (11). Celiac block can also be done by transaortic (12) or transcrural approaches (Fig. 40.2). By modifying the technique described above for celiac block, splanchnic nerve block can be obtained if the needles are placed above the diaphragm behind the crura at the anterolateral angle of the middle to upper level of the 12th thoracic vertebral body (T-12), 0.5 cm dorsal to its anterior margin (Fig. 40.3).

A collective study comprising 432 patients with pain due to pancreatic cancer showed good pain relief in 70–100% with a median duration of 3 months. Further blocks also gave good results (11). In a prospective randomized study in patients with pancreatic cancer, which compared intraoperative chemical splanchnicectomy with 50% alcohol ($n$ = 65 patients) with a placebo injection of saline ($n$ = 72), the mean pain score was significantly lower in the alcohol group at 2-, 4-, and 6-month follow-up and at the final assessment (13).

The outcome of celiac blocks is, however, not as good in pancreatitis as in pancreatic cancer. This may reflect the fact that chronic pancreatitis has a tendency to be "centralized," which means that special nociceptive impulses are not needed to experience pain, and if so, a nerve block or nerve ablation cannot be expected to relieve it (11). The questionable value of celiac blocks in chronic pancreatitis is further demonstrated in a prospective randomized study comparing the pain relief after such block and pancreaticogastrostomy, respectively. When evaluated after 6 months, both the pain score and consumption of analgesics were significantly lower after the surgical drainage procedure but unchanged in those who had had the nerve block (14). Side effects after celiac block include orthostatic hypotension, diarrhea, pain at injection site, root pain, and problems with ejaculation. Although the risk of complications is low following

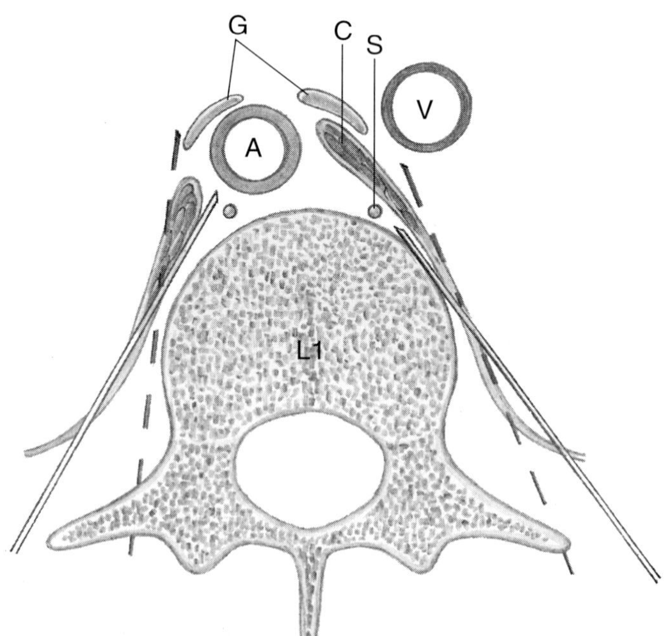


**FIG. 40.2.** Diagram (transverse section) of needle position using classic and transcrural approaches to the coeliac plexus. *A,* aorta; *C,* right diaphragmatic crus; *G,* coeliac ganglia; *L1,* vertebral body of first lumbar vertebra (upper part); *S,* splanchnic nerve(s); *V,* vena cava. (From Bengtsson M, Löfström JB. Nerve block in pancreatic pain. Acta Chir Scand 1990;156:285–291, with permission.)

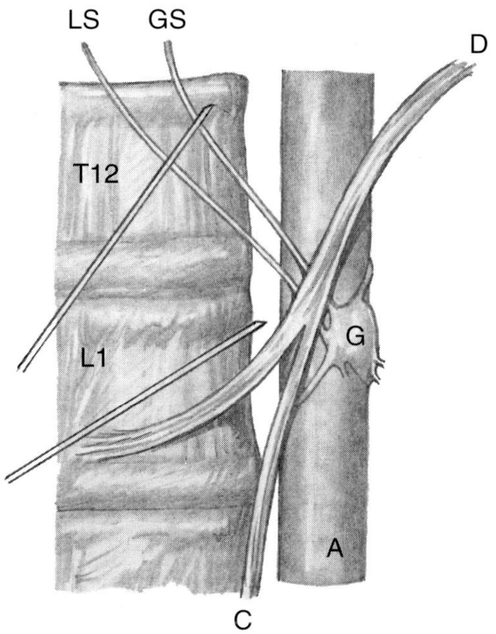


**FIG. 40.3.** Diagram of needle position for classic *(lower needle)* coeliac plexus block and for splanchnic *(upper needle)* nerve block. *A*, aorta; *C*, right crus; *D*, diaphragma; *G*, coeliac ganglia; *GS*, greater splanchnic nerve; *L1*, vertebral body of first lumbar vertebra; *LS*, lesser splanchnic nerve; *T12*, vertebral body of twelfth thoracic vertebra. (From Bengtsson M, Löfström JB. Nerve block in pancreatic pain. Acta Chir Scand 1990;156:285–291, with permission.)

celiac block, we feel that it should be used very restrictively in patients with pain due to chronic pancreatitis.

## SURGICAL NERVE ABLATION PROCEDURES

Several operative procedures have been devised for pain treatment in chronic pancreatitis by nerve ablation: e.g., extraperitoneal left splanchnicectomy using a lumbar approach, intraperitoneal splanchnicectomy using a laterogastric or subpancreatic approach, and bilateral splanchnicectomy using a transhiatal approach (15). However, the results have, in general, been disappointing. The success of surgical splanchnicectomy and celiac ganglionectomy (16), initially reported, has never been confirmed (15). Similarly, the good effect of bilateral vagotomy in combination with left splanchnicectomy via a thoracic surgical approach needs confirmation (17). The same is true for the "complete denervation of the pancreas" (18). It is a general opinion that the results after different neurotomies are unpredictable (15). This may reflect surgical problems related to the deep anatomic location of the splanchnic nerves and celiac ganglia, making them difficult to identify retroperitoneally, a situation that is especially evident in patients with peripancreatic inflammatory changes. Recent interest has been focused on the thoracoscopic route for splanchnicectomy. This new option is discussed below.

## THORACOSCOPIC SPLANCHNICECTOMY

The progress in laparoscopic technique has also entailed development in the field of thoracoscopy. The first report on a case in which thoracoscopic splanchnicectomy was successfully carried out for pancreatic pain was published as late as 1993.

The procedure is done under general anesthesia using double-lumen endotracheal intubation, which makes single-lung ventilation possible. With the patient in a prone position, a trocar is introduced through the fifth intercostal space below the inferior angle of the scapula, and a pneumothorax is induced. If necessary for achieving sufficient working space inside the thoracic cavity, carbon dioxide is insufflated. The trocar is then replaced by an optical cannula, and an operating cannula is inserted through the next, or second next, intercostal space below the optical cannula. The sympathetic chain lying across the neck of the ribs is easily identified, and the splanchnic nerves are visualized. The parietal pleura is incised, and the different nerves grasped with a hook, freed for a distance of about 6 mm and transected by electrocautery. The same procedure is then done on the other side. A small chest tube is placed through the lower port and removed after 6–8 hours, after checking a postoperative chest radiograph and if there are no signs of bleeding. The operating time on each side is 15–20 minutes. In uncomplicated cases, the patient is discharged from the hospital the day after the operation.

We have performed the operation (bilaterally in all cases) in 18 patients with chronic pancreatitis and in 20 with pancreatic cancer. In both groups of patients, obvious pain relief was prospectively registered. Also, the relief has remained unchanged in the patients with chronic pancreatitis who have been followed for as long as 1 year (Fig. 40.4). There was a concomitant reduction in consumption of analgesics. Three patients under-

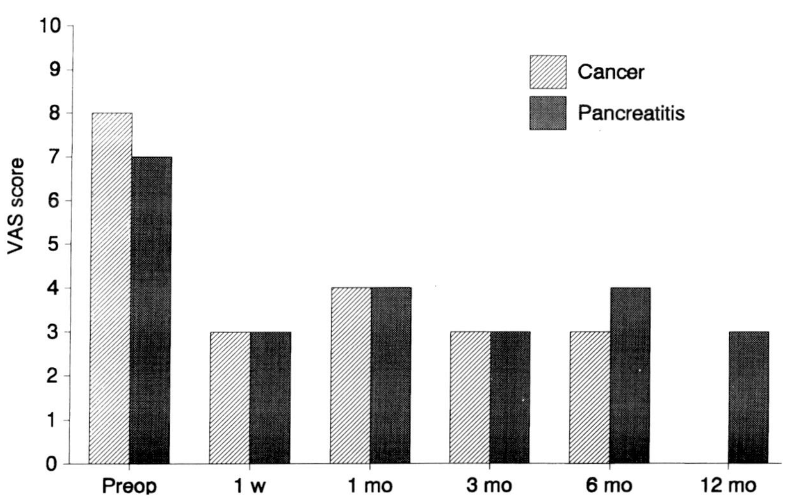


**FIG. 40.4.** Pain relief after thoracoscopic splanchnicectomy as evaluated with the Visual Analogue Scale (VAS). Chronic pancreatitis, $n = 18$; pancreatic cancer, $n = 20$.

went reoperation for intrathoracic bleeding the evening after the operation; in two the bleeding source was at the incision for the larger port, and in one, from an artery close to a splanchnic nerve. These bleeding complications occurred during the first half of the series. One patient had transient pain at a port incision. Otherwise there were no complications.

The experience with thoracoscopic splanchnicectomy is still limited, but the results are promising. More studies are needed, especially for evaluation of the long-term effects, before the future role of the operation can be defined.

## REFERENCES


1. Worning H. Chronic pancreatitis: pathogenesis, natural history and conservative treatment. Clin Gastroenterol 1984;13:871–894.
2. Bliss WR, Burch B, Martin MM, Zollinger RM. Localization of referred pancreatic pain induced by electrical stimulation. Gastroenterology 1950;16:317–323.
3. Ammann RW, Akovbiantz A, Largiader F, Schueler G. Course and outcome of chronic pancreatitis. Longitudinal study of a mixed medical-surgical series of 245 patients. Gastroenterology 1984; 86:820–828.
4. Lankisch PG, Löhr-Happe A, Otto J, Creutzfeldt W. Natural course in chronic pancreatitis. Pain, exocrine and endocrine pancreatic insufficiency, and prognosis of the disease. Digestion 1993;54: 148–155.
5. Ihse I. Pancreatic pain (Leading Article). Br J Surg 1990;77: 121–122.
6. Bradley EL. Pancreatic duct pressure in chronic pancreatitis. Am J Surg 1982;144:313–316.
7. Okazaki K, Yamamoto Y, Kagiyama S, Tamura S, Sakamoto Y, et al. Pressure of papillary zone and pancreatic main duct in patients with chronic pancreatitis in the early stage. Scand J Gastroenterol 1988;23:501–506.
8. Ebbehöj N, Borly L, Bülow J, Rasmussen SG, Madsen P. Evaluation of pancreatic tissue fluid pressure and pain in chronic pancreatitis. A longitudinal study. Scand J Gastroenterol 1990;25: 462–466.
9. Jalleh RP, Aslam M, Williamson RCN. Pancreatic tissue and ductal pressure in chronic pancreatitis. Br J Surg 1991;78:1235–1237.
10. Bockman DE, Büchler M, Malfertheiner P, Beger HG. Analysis of nerves in chronic pancreatitis. Gastroenterology 1988;94:1459–1469.
11. Bengtsson M, Löfström JB. Nerve block in pancreatic pain. Acta Chir Scand 1990;156:285–291.
12. Lieberman RP, Waldman SD. Celiac plexus neurolysis with the modified transaortic approach. Radiology 1990;175:274–276.
13. Lillemoe KD, Cameron JL, Kaufman HS, Yeo CJ, Pitt HA, Sauter PK. Chemical splanchnicectomy in patients with unresectable pancreatic cancer. A prospective randomized trial. Ann Surg 1993; 217:447–457.
14. Madsen P, Hansen E. Coeliac plexus block versus pancreaticogastrostomy for pain in chronic pancreatitis. Scand J Gastroenterol 1985;20:1217–1220.
15. Hollender LF, Laugner B. Pain-relieving procedures in chronic pancreatitis. In: Trede M, Carter DC, eds. Surgery of the pancreas. Edinburgh: Churchill Livingstone, 1993:349–357.
16. Mallet-Guy PA. Late and very late results of resections of the nervous system in the treatment of chronic relapsing pancreatitis. Am J Surg 1983;14:234–238.
17. Stone H, Chauvin E. Pancreatic denervation for pain relief in chronic alcohol associated pancreatitis. Br J Surg 1990;77: 303–305.
18. Hiraoka T, Watanabe E, Katoh T, Hayashida H, Mizutani J, et al. A new surgical approach for control of pain in chronic pancreatitis: complete denervation of the pancreas. Am J Surg 1986;152: 549–551.

# 41

# *Pancreatitis in the Young*[1]

R. C. G. Russell

Pancreatitis in the young is rare; in fact, it is remarkably rare, even in those who have known predisposing factors related to congenital anomalies. The literature related to pediatric pancreatic disease is sparse, and the condition poorly documented. Acute pancreatitis appears exceptionally uncommon, and most patients who present with pancreatitis under the age of 18 years do so with the symptoms of chronic abdominal pain. Indeed, many patients who present in their 20s relate their history back to pain that occurred during childhood and was misdiagnosed as episodes of nonspecific abdominal pain. Children can develop pancreatitis that is unrelated to congenital anomalies. The pancreatitis presents in a similar manner to the disease in the adult, and the investigation profile follows an identical pattern to that in the adult, with history, endoscopic retrograde cholangiopancreatography (ERCP), and computed tomography (CT) providing the baseline information required to define the therapy.

No center has been able to gather a large experience of this disease. In a review of 30 years experience in managing patients under 20 years of age with chronic pancreatitis, Konzen et al. at the Mayo Clinic were only able to review 70 patients (1); 42 of these patients had hereditary pancreatitis, and 28, idiopathic pancreatitis. My own experience over 20 years has included 25 patients, aged 18 years or less, with severe pancreatic disease who had to be admitted to the hospital for definitive therapy. The largest single group was related to trauma, which was very varied, extending from bicycle handlebar injury to surfboard injury to motor vehicle injury. Nine patients presented with hereditary pancreatitis, and three patients had pancreas divisum, two of whom later presented with classical idiopathic calcification, almost certainly unrelated to the pancreas divisum. One patient, a 5-year-old girl with chronic renal failure for which she had had a transplant and was taking cyclosporine had a drug-related pancreatitis; each presentation of the cyclosporine evoked a further episode of pancreatic disease. One patient had hypercalcemia, and another had pancreatitis secondary to a choledochal cyst.

These patients tend to present with their complications and frequently with a long history and at a relatively late stage of their disease. Even trauma patients may have a delayed presentation. In the patients with hereditary pancreatitis, the most common presentation was that of recurrent episodes of severe pain with marked calcification on the x-ray. No fewer than 13 patients presented with a pseudocyst, 3 presented with a transection of the pancreas documented on CT scanning, 4 with an abscess, and 1 each with hemorrhage, a pancreatic fistula, and severe fibrosis. These patients were treated by a Puestow procedure [4], an accessory (Santorini duct) sphincteroplasty [3], a distal pancreatectomy [13], cystogastrostomy [2], a Whipple procedure as the primary procedure in one and as the second procedure in another, and two were managed conservatively.

The variety of presentations necessitates an awareness of this disease in children and the need for skilled investigation. It is now possible to undertake an ERCP with a pediatric videoduodenoscope (10 mm diameter, 3.2 mm channel) (2) and a helical spiral CT scan, which will give clear definition of the pancreas (Fig. 41.1). Therapeutic endoscopic procedures are now possible using a conventional 20-mm biliary sphincterotome. The procedures are safe, with an 8% incidence of postprocedure pancreatitis. The largest series is that of Allendorf, with 110 ERCP procedures in 82 children (3). In all respects, management of these children should mimic that of the adult except that the results tend to be better than in the adult. In my own series, there have been no deaths, minimal postoperative morbidity, and an excellent long-term outcome, with a low incidence of diabetes (3/25) and steatorrhea (5/25) in the long term (range, 2–21 years).

## EMBRYOLOGICALLY RELATED PANCREATITIS

It is difficult to determine the incidence of structural or congenital anomalies associated with pancreatitis. The series of patients studied suggests that the incidence is in the region of 10–15% (Table 41.1). Such a low incidence is surprising considering the embryology of the pancreas.

### Embryology

Two primitive structures are termed the ventral and dorsal anlage because of their original positions with respect to the duodenum (Fig. 41.2). Asymmetric growth enables the ventral anlage to rotate clockwise and fuse with the dorsal bud. This fusion is completed by the 37th day of gestation. The cephalic part of the head, neck, body, and tail is derived from the dorsal anlagen, while the uncinate process and the caudad fourth portion of the head are formed from the ventral anlagen. Each carries its own ductal system, but the final arrangement is a consequence of the

[1]See also Chapters 24 and 19.

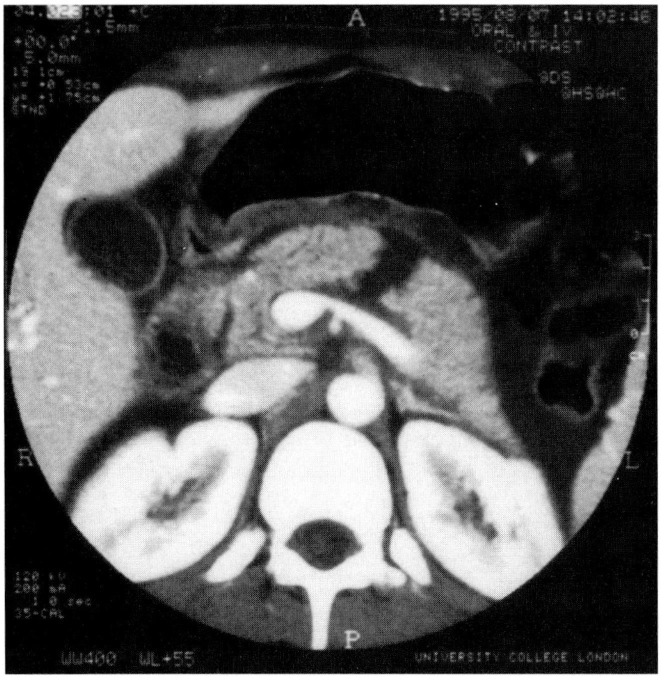


**FIG. 41.1.** CT scan in a young thin girl following a bicycle handlebar injury to the abdomen. The pancreas is completely transected in the midbody.

dorsal duct joining with the ventral duct to form the duct of Wirsung and the dorsal duct, which drains but a small part of the pancreas and enters the duodenum through the accessory papilla, which is situated approximately 1 cm proximal and anterior to the ampulla of Vater (see Chapter 2).

## Congenital Causes of Pancreatitis

Congenital causes of pancreatitis can be subdivided into ductal anomalies, extrinsic ductal obstruction, and the annular pancreas. Ductal anomalies arise from abnormalities of the coalescence of the two primitive ductal systems and are now known as pancreas divisum (Fig. 41.2); the dorsal and ventral ductal systems are completely separate (Fig. 41.3). Variants of pancreas divisum include a filamentous communication between dorsal and ventral ducts and a complete absence of the ventral duct (4). The prevalence of pancreas divisum is variable, depending on whether the data are based on endoscopic findings, in which the reported incidence ranges from 0.3 to 5.8% (5–7), to postmortem series, in which the incidence ranges from 5 to 14% (8–10).

Pancreas divisum rarely presents in children. The reason for this is quite simple; symptoms depend on two anomalies: the presence of the divisum and the obstruction of the outlet. It appears that if the accessory sphincter is functional, no symptoms will accrue. Abnormalities arise because there is an associated obstruction of the accessory sphincter, which appears to arise later in life and has not been a feature of childhood pancreatitis (11–13). Twelve children with pancreas divisum, all of whom were girls with recurrent acute pancreatitis, required exploratory surgery up to 1989 (13). Most of these children had a transduodenal accessory sphincteroplasty to achieve effective pancreatic drainage.

In most reports, this has usually been associated with complete relief of symptoms, and the children, as young as 3 years of age, have responded satisfactorily. In my own experience, a young girl presented at the age of 11 with a 9-year history of pancreatitis and was documented to have pancreas divisum with pancreatic calcification. An accessory sphincteroplasty performed in 1986 was followed by recurrent pain in 1995, associated with calcification. At present no further procedure is necessary, as the symptoms are mild. A second girl, aged 18 at the time of presentation, had a 16-year history of pancreatic pain. An accessory sphincteroplasty performed in 1982 has proven successful to the present time. A third patient, a 15-year-old boy presented with severe episodes of recurrent acute pancreatitis. He had a typical pancreas divisum, and an accessory sphincteroplasty was performed in 1994. Two years later, after repeated attacks of pain, he had a classical calcific pancreatitis of the type seen in the Indian subcontinent. A pancreatoduodenectomy was required to relieve his symptoms. Thus, the two patients with calcification probably had symptoms unrelated to their pancreas divisum, leaving one patient with a true pancreas divisum relieved by an accessory sphincteroplasty. The rarity of this condition in a unit that has specialized in pancreas divisum since 1977 (7, 14) suggests that the diagnosis of pancreas divisum in relationship to abdominal pain should only be made with extreme care and attention to the exclusion of all other causes of abdominal pain.

## Congenital Strictures of the Pancreatic Duct

Congenital strictures of the pancreatic ductal system may occasionally be a cause of pancreatitis (15, 16). Although ductal strictures, particularly in adult patients, are usually secondary to recurrent pancreatic inflammation, a number of cases have been reported in which the symptoms started in childhood and were associated with a single well-defined stricture.

**TABLE 41.1. Prevalence of Congenital Causes of Childhood Pancreatitis**

| | | | Pancreatitis Attributed to Structural Anomalies | |
|---|---|---|---|---|
| Author (Year) | Reference Number | Number of Cases | *(n)* | (%) |
| Synn et al. (1987) | 40 | 48<br>Unselected | 7 | 14 |
| Vane et al. (1989) | 64 | 44<br>Unselected | 6<br>All choledochal cysts | 3 |
| Ziegler et al. (1988) | 60 | 49<br>Unselected | 6<br>2 Choledochal cysts | 15 |
| Tagge (1991) | 15 | 33<br>All surgical | 12 | 36 |
| Weizman and Durie (1988) | 73 | 61<br>Unselected | 5 | 8 |

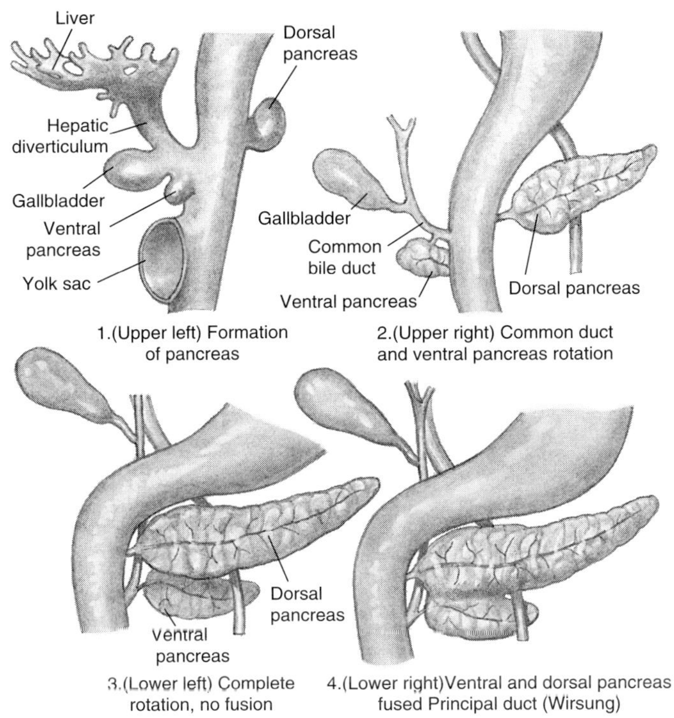


**FIG. 41.2.** Embryology of the developing pancreas, with particular reference to pancreas divisum, showing how the dorsal pancreas is drained into the accessory papilla in this condition, and the ventral pancreas draining via the main papilla is comparatively small.

Leese et al. described a 25-year-old woman with an 11-year history of recurrent pancreatitis in whom a stricture at the site of fusion of the ventral and dorsal ducts was demonstrated at pancreatography (16). There was slight dilatation of the pancreatic duct distal (upstream) to this stenosis. Treatment may be either by a retrograde drainage of the duct (15) or, preferably, a distal pancreatectomy, as the end (retrograde) pancreatojejunostomy rarely remains patent. Similar cases have been described by Turner, with symptomatic improvement following surgery (17). An autopsy study (10) has suggested that congenital ductal strictures may be identified in at least 3% of individuals, although it is likely that only a small proportion of these would have been associated with pancreatitis (17) (Fig. 41.4).

## Common Channel (Anomalous Pancreatobiliary Ductal Union)

The main pancreatic duct and the common bile duct open into the second part of the duodenum, either separately or, more commonly, after joining as a short common channel. The length of the common channel varies from 3–7 mm in adults (18) to less than 2 mm in infants (19). When the common channel exceeds 10 mm, the pancreatobiliary union lies outside the wall of the duodenum and therefore beyond the anatomic sphincter of Oddi. Such an arrangement allows reflux of bile from the bile duct into the pancreatic duct and occurs in approximately 15% of patients, based on data from preoperative cholangiography. The terms common channel syndrome, or anomalous pancreatobiliary ductal union (18), have been used to describe this arrangement, although symptoms rarely arise from it. A common channel is present in more than 70% of patients with choledochal cysts.

Two types of pancreatobiliary union have been identified (20, 21). Either the bile duct appears to join the pancreatic duct or the pancreatic duct appears to join the bile duct. It has been suggested that these variations may be important in determining the subsequent complications. The subsidiary pancreatic duct has been associated with congenital cystic dilation of the bile duct (20), and in those with an angle greater than 40°, the chance of acute pancreatitis is higher (18). The etiologic importance of a long common channel and pancreatitis in children has only been appreciated recently, although a relationship between a common channel and choledochal cysts has been noted since 1969 (22). An additional factor is usually considered a prerequisite to precipitate an attack of pancreatitis. For instance, in Tagge's series of five children with long common channels, only one child had the anomaly as an isolated finding, while two had an annular pancreas and two had common bile duct stones with evidence of ampullary stenosis (15).

The rarity of significant pancreatitis associated with choledochal cysts is borne out by our own experience of finding only one child in our series who had a preceding history of pancreatitis. Nevertheless, when treating choledochal cysts, one must be aware of the relationship between the lower end of the bile duct and the pancreatic duct, to ensure that the pancreatic duct is not damaged at the time of excision of the choledochal cyst. In dealing with dilated ducts, one must also ensure that the pancreatitis is not due to the passage of stones or debris from the choledochal cyst. In a unique experience, Howard at Kings College Hospital, London, has treated 52 type I cases of choledochal cyst, of which 33 were cystic and 19 fusiform dilatation (personal communication). Pancreatitis was the presenting feature at a median age of 4.4 years in 22 children and was seen in both cases of cystic and fusiform dilatation. High levels of amylase were found in the bile in all children who presented with a history of pancreatitis, compared with only 36% of those who presented with jaundice.

Some children with a type Ic choledochal cyst have a high serum amylase level but no evidence of pancreatic inflammation, which has been labeled fictitious pancreatitis by Stringel and Filler (23). The hyperamylasemia has been attributed to either absorption of amylase through denuded epithelium within the choledochal cyst or cholangiovenous reflux at the hepatic sinusoidal level (24). While this phenomenon does occur in some children, true inflammatory pancreatitis is much more common in choledochal cysts than is perhaps realized.

## Choledochoceles (Type III Choledochal Cysts)

Choledochoceles, cystic dilations of the distal bile duct within the wall of the duodenum, were first described and named by

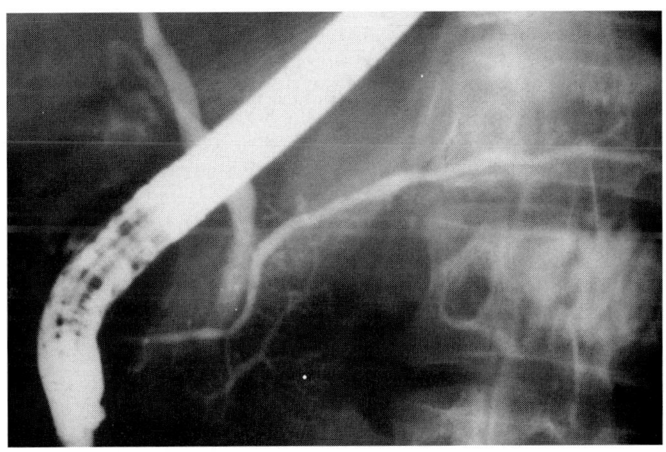

**FIG. 41.3.** ERCP: typical appearance of pancreas divisum. The main pancreatic drainage is via the accessory papilla; the major papilla drains the ventral pancreas alone. The bile duct is also demonstrated.

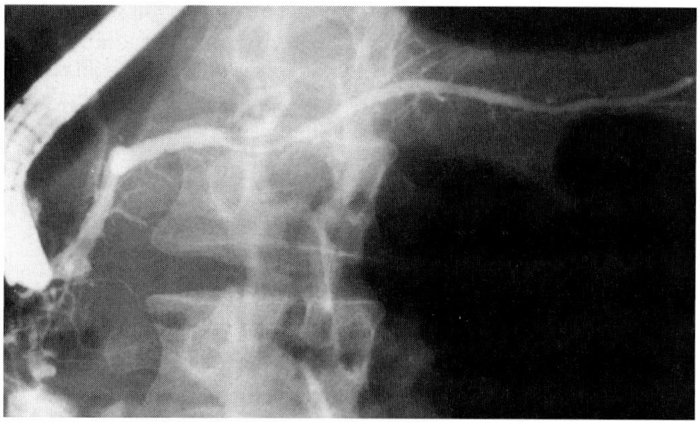

**FIG. 41.4.** ERCP in a young child with chronic pancreatic pain showing a stricture in the pancreatic duct in the body of the pancreas. Eight years following distal pancreatectomy the patient remains pain free.

Wheeler in 1940 (25). A relationship with acute pancreatitis was suggested by Stirling in 1949 (26) and was subsequently confirmed (27–29). The anomaly is usually diagnosed during adult life. An endoscopic sphincteroplasty can achieve adequate drainage and avoid the need for surgical intervention (27).

### Annular Pancreas

Annular pancreas was first described by Tiedmann in 1818 (30) and named by Ecker in 1862 (31). Its incidence is unclear but has been calculated at about 1 in 20,000 (32–35). Its presentation tends to be bimodal, with peaks neonatally and in the 4th and 5th decades. Surprisingly, equal numbers have been reported in adults and children (34). Neonatal presentation has usually been with duodenal obstruction wherein it contributes 15% of all cases (33). The pregnancy may have been associated with polyhydramnios (36). The obstruction is generally classified as intrinsic, as pancreatic tissue is often intimately related to the wall of the duodenum (33). Other congenital anomalies are often associated (36). Adult presentations may be duodenal stenosis, peptic ulceration, chronic pancreatitis, or an incidental finding (34). The etiopathogenesis of annular pancreas is unknown. It may be a component of a more generalized disorder of embryogenesis when associated with trisomy 21, tracheoesophageal fistula, or cardiorenal abnormalities or may occur alone or with local duodenal abnormality only (33). About 80% of neonatal cases and about 20% of adult cases are associated with other congenital anomalies.

The relationship between annular pancreas and pancreatitis was first emphasized in a review of the literature by Drey in 1957 (37). He described features of pancreatitis in 14 of 62 (25%) adult cases of annular pancreas. His patients ranged from 23 to 37 years of age and were mostly male (78%). Kiernan et al. did not mention this relationship in a report and literature review from the Mayo Clinic and rather ascribed symptoms of abdominal pain and vomiting in their patients to peptic ulcer disease, another common association of annular pancreas (34). There have been isolated cases of pancreatitis in children associated with annular pancreas (15, 38). Komura et al. reported a 2-year-old girl with pancreatitis who, at operation, had an annular pancreas and a long pancreatobiliary channel (38). Treatment consisted of a duodenojejunostomy and a hepaticojejunostomy.

Pancreatitis may also occur following curative surgery for both duodenal atresia and annular pancreas. Two cases of annular pancreas have been described by Tagge from his total experience of 12 children with ductal anomalies and pancreatitis (15). Such cases of pancreatitis may be due to the ductal arrangement within the annulus. The entire annulus is of ductal origin, (32) and subsequent episodes of pancreatitis may well be related to a pancreas divisum phenomenon.

### Anomalous Insertion of the Common Bile Duct

Insertion of the common bile duct into the third or fourth part of the duodenum occurs in 1–2% of adults (39). Such positioning of the ampulla appears to predispose to pancreatitis, at least in some children (40, 41). Such an anomaly may be associated with a long common channel, hence the cause of the pancreatitis.

### Stenosis of the Ampulla of Vater

Tagge reported two children with ampullary stenosis and pancreatitis diagnosed at 2 and 4 years (15). Toouli, in his extensive experience of ampullary manometry, did not describe a child with manometrically confirmed ampullary stenosis. However, symptoms had often been present since childhood in these patients presenting with recurrent episodes of pancreatic pain (42).

### Abnormal Biliopancreatic Communication

Rosseland described a 26-year-old woman with intermittent pancreatitis who had an apparently unique abnormality of an accessory connecting duct between the supraduodenal common bile duct and the main pancreatic duct. This was demonstrable on ERCP, and surgical ligation completely relieved her symptoms (43). A number of variants of biliopancreatic communication and pancreatic duct drainage have been described, such as ansa pancreatica (a low looping accessory duct that joins the inferior part of the main duct), although whether they predispose to pancreatitis is debatable (44).

### Congenital Gastrointestinal Duplication Cysts, Pancreatic Cysts, and Duodenal Diverticula

Gastrointestinal and enteric duplication cysts are spherical or tubular structures containing mucosa and a supporting muscularis characteristic of the adjacent gastrointestinal tract. They may be derived from fore-, mid- or hindgut and are invariably located on the mesenteric side of the gastrointestinal tract. Foregut duplications may occur in relationship to the pancreas and be a cause of recurrent pancreatitis (45–48). Williams and Hendren (45) described a 7-year-old child with proven episodes of acute pancreatitis since the age of 2 months. The diagnosis of an intrapancreatic duodenal duplication cyst was made only after three laparotomies and a correct reinterpretation of the operative pancreatogram. Akers described two cases of enteric duplications (46). Gastric duplication cysts communicating with the pancreatic duct have been described, and recurrent acute pancreatitis may occur (49). Congenital pancreatic cysts may also be present with pancreatitis. Such cysts, when large, may obstruct the pancreatic duct, giving rise to pancreatitis in the distal portion of the pancreas. Such anomalies are cured by distal pancreatectomy. If the cyst occurs in the head of the pancreas, an appropriate drainage procedure appears to cure the patient (50).

## HEREDITARY PANCREATITIS

Hereditary pancreatitis is a rare condition of unknown etiology. It was first described in 1952 in a publication from the Mayo Clinic (51). Its inheritance is suggested to be autosomal dominant with variable penetrance; it is the most common cause of pancreatitis in children. The condition may progressively destroy the pancreas, resulting in both exocrine and endocrine pancreatic insufficiency, stones in the duct, and calcification in the parenchyma. Approximately 100 kindreds with 500 cases, mostly among whites, have been described in the English literature (52). In up to 20% of patients, no cause has been identified. It seems that the most common type of recurrent pancreatitis in childhood is familial in which no metabolic or anatomic causal abnormality is recognized. Gross and Jones (53) defined hereditary pancreatitis as inflammation of the pancreas, usually recurrent, with unusual prevalence among blood-related groups of persons. Familial pancreatitis has been observed in at least six different syndromes as described by Howard in 1987 (54).

1. Familial pancreatitis unassociated with any other recognized metabolic abnormality
2. Familial pancreatitis associated with excessive excretion of cystine and lycine in the urine (aminoaciduria)
3. Familial pancreatitis associated with hyperlipidemia
4. Familial hypocalciuric hypercalcemic acute pancreatitis
5. Familial hyperparathyroidism with resultant pancreatitis
6. Familial hypertrophy of the sphincter of Oddi

The onset of pain in hereditary pancreatitis is usually within the first two decades of life (55–57). Pain is often nonspecific and poorly localized (58–59) such that it has been suggested that all children who present with severe recurrent abdominal pain should be suspected of having pancreatitis. However, not all children with pancreatitis present with abdominal pain (56,60). Long periods without clinical manifestations occur (56). As a rule, these attacks are self-limiting, and amelioration of symptoms occurs within several days (61). There are often differences in the age of presentation and the severity of attacks among affected members of a family. Laboratory findings are similar to those seen in other forms of acute pancreatitis: marked elevation of amylase and lipase levels, leukocytosis, and dehydration. The prime investigations are an ERCP with a good quality plain film and a CT scan. Calcification is present in approximately 60% of patients, and the pancreatic ducts are markedly increased in diameter. Pseudocysts are frequently associated.

The treatment of hereditary pancreatitis is similar to that of chronic pancreatitis in the adult. If the attacks are severe and debilitating enough to merit treatment, a full investigation is undertaken to determine if the duct is sufficiently dilated (>8 mm) to merit a drainage procedure of the Partington-Rochelle type. It has been suggested that this should be performed early rather than late, to conserve pancreatic parenchyma and exocrine and endocrine function, but there is little evidence to substantiate these statements. Nevertheless, the outcome of the drainage procedure is invariably good, and the long-term results appear satisfactory. However, over the years, development of diabetes appears almost inevitable. Follow-up in such cases is mandatory, as the onset of diabetes may be many years later.

### Idiopathic Fibrosing Pancreatitis

Idiopathic fibrosing pancreatitis is a rare clinical entity; only 32 cases have been reported (62, 63). In a review of 92 infants and children with pancreatic disorders, Vane et al. did not encounter a single case of fibrosing pancreatitis (64). The mean age at presentation is 10 years (4 months to 20 years), predominately males. The most common symptom is chronic cramping abdominal pain. Jaundice may be a feature. Serum amylase levels are generally normal, except during an attack. Other forms of pancreatitis must be excluded. The etiology of idiopathic fibrosing pancreatitis is unknown. An autoimmune (65) or viral origin (66) has been suggested. Histologically, the acinar structures and islet cells are preserved and there is diffuse infiltration of the pancreas with collagenous bands. Inflammatory cells, both acute and chronic, may or may not be present (65–67).

The macroscopic appearance is of a diffusely enlarged hard gland that is not accompanied by inflammatory changes in the retroperitoneum. The treatment, particularly if jaundice is present, is primarily a bypass procedure; a resection should be undertaken only as a last resort. Idiopathic fibrosing pancreatitis may sometimes resolve in time, and for this reason, a conservative approach should be adopted. As the islet cells are preserved, diabetes is an unusual complication; steatorrhea is frequent.

**TABLE 41.2. Etiology of Pancreatic Pseudocysts**

| | Number of Patients | Percentage |
|---|---|---|
| Trauma | 140 | 65.7 |
| Idiopathic pancreatitis | 55 | 25.8 |
| Hereditary pancreatitis | 3 | 1.4 |
| Anomalies | 3 | 1.4 |
| Biliary disease | 2 | 0.9 |
| Drugs | 1 | 0.6 |
| Total | 213 | |

### Pancreatic Pseudocysts in Children

The pseudocyst is an uncommon disorder in childhood. Most (65%) result from blunt trauma. A total of 213 cases have been reported in the literature (68) (Table 41.2).

The treatment of pediatric pancreatic pseudocyst depends on the etiology and, particularly in trauma, whether or not the pancreatic duct is intact. The most common treatments in the literature are internal drainage (43% of described cases), external drainage (22%), percutaneous drainage (11%), excision (6%) distal pancreatectomy (5%) and a nonoperative approach (14%) (68). The recent trend, particularly in children and where the main duct is intact, is a conservative approach. Octreotide has been successful in association with external drainage. Recent reports suggest that with octreotide complete resolution will occur (69, 70). The evidence is that a primary conservative approach to cysts in childhood is appropriate and the operative approach should be avoided (71, 72).

## CONCLUSION

Childhood pancreatitis is rare. The presentation is confusing in that the child presents with nonspecific abdominal pain. Once the disease is fully established, the treatment should follow the lines of pancreatic disease in the adult. A full investigation is undertaken to determine the site and type of the disease. Cysts should initially be treated conservatively, patients with a large duct should be treated by drainage, and only when all else fails should resection be considered. The eventual outcome is usually good, and long-term complications infrequent. Nevertheless, particularly in hereditary pancreatitis, follow-up is important to treat any exocrine or endocrine insufficiency that may occur. Such patients may be more prone to an increased cancer risk than are those with other forms of chronic pancreatitis.

## REFERENCES

1. Konzen KM, Perrault J, Moir C, Zinsmeister AR. Long-term follow-up of young patients with chronic hereditary or idiopathic pancreatitis. Mayo Clin Proc 1993;68:449–453.
2. Kozarek RA, Christie D, Barclay G. Endoscopic therapy pf pancreatitis in the pediatric population. Gastrointest Endosc 1993;36:665–669.
3. Allendorf M, Werlin SL, Geenen JE, et al. Endoscopic retrograde cholangiopancreatography in children. J Pediatr 1987;110: 206–211.
4. Warshaw AL, Simeone JF, Schapiro RH, Flavin-Warshaw B. Evaluation and treatment of the dominant dorsal duct syndrome (pancreas divisum redefined). Am J Surg 1990;159:59–66.
5. Rosch W, Koch H, Schaffner O, Demling L. The clinical significance of pancreas divisum. Gastrointest Endosc 1976;22:206–207.
6. Gregg JA. Pancreas divisum: its association with pancreatitis. Am J Surg 1977;134:539–543.
7. Cotton PB, Kizu M. Malfusion of dorsal and ventral pancreas. A cause of pancreatitis? Gut 1977;18:A400.

8. Millbourn E. On the excretory ducts of the pancreas in man, with special reference to their relations with each other, to the common duct and to the duodenum. Acta Anat 1950;9:1–34.
9. Millbourn E. Calibre and appearance of the pancreatic ducts and relevant clinical problems. Acta Chir Scand 1959;118: 286–303.
10. Berman LG, Prior JT, Abramow SM, Ziegler DD. A study of the pancreatic duct system in man by the use of vinyl acetate casts of post mortem preparations. Surg Gynecol Obstet 1960;110: 391–403.
11. Wagner CW, Golladay ES. Pancreas divisum and pancreatitis in children. Am Surg 1988;110:206–211.
12. Tuggle DW, Smith E. Pancreas divisum, pancreatic pseudocyst and choledochal cyst in an 8 year old child. J Pediatr Surg 1989;24:52–53.
13. Adzik NS, Shamberger RC, Winter HS, Hendren WH. Surgical treatment of pancreas divisum causing pancreatitis in children. J Pediatr Surg 1989;24:54–58.
14. Cotton PB. Congenital anomaly of pancreas divisum as cause of obstructive pain and pancreatitis. Gut 1980;21:105–114.
15. Tagge EP, Smith SD, Raschbaum GR, Newman B, Weiner ES. Pancreatic ductal abnormalities in children. Surgery 1991;110: 709–717.
16. Leese T, Chiche L, Bismuth H. Pancreatitis caused by congenital anomalies of the pancreatic ducts. Surgery 1989;105:125–130.
17. Turner LJ. Chronic pancreatitis and congenital strictures of the pancreatic duct. Am J Surg 1983;145:582–584.
18. Misra SP, Dwivedi M. Pancreatobiliary ductal union. Gut 1990;31: 1144–1149.
19. Miyano T, Suruga K, Suda K. Abnormal choledochal-pancreatico ductal junction related to the etiology of infantile obstructive jaundice. J Pediatr Surg 1979;14:16–26.
20. Kimura K, Ohto M, Ono T, et al. Congenital cystic dilatation of the common bile duct: relationship to anomalous pancreatobiliary ductal union. Am J Roentgenol 1977;128:571–577.
21. Komi N, Takehara H, Kunimoto M, Miyoshi Y, Yagi T. Does the type of anomalous arrangement of pancreatobiliary ducts influence the surgery and prognosis of choledochal cyst ? J Pediatr Surg 1992;27:728–731.
22. Babbitt DP. Congenital choledochal cysts. New etiological concepts on anomalous relationships of the common bile duct and pancreatic bulb. Ann Radiol (Paris) 1969;19:231–240.
23. Stringel G, Filler RM. Fictitious pancreatitis and choledochal cyst. J Pediatr Surg 1982;17:359–361.
24. Todani T, Urushihara N, Watanabe Y, Toki A, et al. Pseudopancreatitis in choledochal cyst in children: intraoperative study of amylase levels in the serum. J Pediatr Surg 1990;25:203–206.
25. Wheeler WI. An unusual case of obstruction to the common bile duct (choledochocele). Br J Surg 1940;27:446–448.
26. Stirling J. Diverticula in the terminal portion of the common bile duct. Am J Pathol 1949;25:325–337.
27. Goldberg PB, Long WB, Oleaga JA, Mackie JA. Choledochocele as a cause of recurrent pancreatitis. Gastroenterology 1980;78: 1041–1045.
28. Greene FL, Brown JJ, Rubenstein PR, Anderson MC. Choledochocele and recurrent pancreatitis: diagnosis and management. Am J Surg 1985;149:306–309.
29. Gerritsen JJ, Janssens AR, Kroon HM. Choledochocele: treatment by endoscopic sphincterotomy. Br J Surg 1988;75:495–496.
30. Tiedmann F. Über die Verschiedenheiten des Ausführungsganges der Bauchspeicheldrüse bei den Menschen und Säugetieren. Dtsch Arch Physiol 1818;4:403.
31. Ecker A. Bildungsfehler des Pankreas und des Herzens. Z Art Med 1862;14:354.
32. Dowsett JF, Rode J, Russell RCG. Annular pancreas: a clinical, endoscopic, and immunohistochemical study. Gut 1989;30: 130–135.
33. Salonen IS. Congenital duodenal obstruction—a review of the literature and a clinical study of annular pancreas and a follow-up of 36 survivors. Acta Paediatr Scand 1978;272(suppl): 1–87.
34. Kiernan PD, ReMine SG, Kiernen PC, ReMine WH. Annular pancreas—Mayo Clinic experience from 1957–1976 with a review of the literature. Arch Surg 1980;115:46–50.
35. Lehman GA, O Connor KW. Coexistence of annular pancreas and pancreas divisum—ERCP diagnosis. Gastrointest Endosc 1985;31:25–28.
36. Merrill JR, Raffensperger JG. Paediatric annular pancreas—twenty years experience. J Pediatr 1976;11:921–925.
37. Drey NW. Symptomatic annular pancreas in the adult. Ann Intern Med 1957;46:750–772.
38. Komura J, Yano H, Tanaka T, Tsura T. Annular pancreas associated with pancreatobiliary maljunction in an infant. Eur J Pediatr Surg 1993;3:244–247.
39. Auld CD, Thomson JWW. The common bile duct and its anomalies. J R Coll Surg Edinb 1985;30:248–250.
40. Synn A, Mulvihill SJ, Fonkalsrud EW. Surgical disorders of the pancreas in infancy and childhood. Pediatrics 1963;32: 93–102.
41. Doty J, Hassal E, Fonkalsrud EW. Anomalous drainage of the common bile duct into the fourth part of the duodenum. Arch Surg 1985;120:1077–1079.
42. Toouli J, Di Francesco V, Saccone G, Kollias A, Schloithe A, Shanks N. Division of the sphincter of Oddi for treatment of dysfunction associated with recurrent pancreatitis. Br J Surg 1996;83:1205–1210.
43. Rosseland AR, Eltvik LP, Gundersen B, Bakka A. Abnormal connecting duct between the common bile duct and the pancreatic duct. Br J Surg 1988;75:385.
44. Goodman P, Halpert RD, Rabassa AE. Aberrant insertion of the common bile duct into an accessory pancreatic duct: cholangiographic demonstration. Am J Gastroenterol 1991;86:1268–1270.
45. Williams WH, Hendren WH. Intrapancreatic duodenal duplication cyst causing pancreatitis in a child. Surgery 1971;69:708–715.
46. Akers DR, Favara BE, Franciosi RA, Nelson JM. Duplications of the alimentary tract: report of three unusual cases associated with bile and pancreatic ducts. Surgery 1972;71:817–823.
47. Longmire WP, Rose AS. Hemoductal pancreatitis. Surg Gynecol Obstet 1973;136:246–250.
48. Traverso LW, Longmire WP. Pancreatitis of unusual origin. Surg Gynecol Obstet 1975;141:383–386.
49. Johnstone DW, Forde KA, Markowitz D, Green PHR, Farman J, Markowitz M. Gastric duplication cyst communicating with the pancreatic duct: a rare cause of recurrent abdominal pain. Surgery 1991;109:97–100.
50. Athow AC, Wilkinson ML, Saunders AJ, Drake DP. Pancreatic ascites presenting in infancy with review of the literature. Dig Dis Sci 1991;36:245–250.
51. Comfort MW, Steinberg AG. Pedigree of a family with hereditary chronic relapsing pancreatitis. Gastroenterology 1952;21:54–63.
52. Makela P, Aarimaa M. Pancreatography in a family with hereditary pancreatitis. Acta Radiol Diagn 1985;26:63–66.
53. Gross JB, Jones JD. Hereditary pancreatitis: analysis of experience to May 1969. In: Beck IT, Sinclair DG, eds. The exocrine pancreas. London: Churchill, 1962:278–309.
54. Howard JM. Pancreatitis: multiple disease with multiple causes and varying natural history. In: Howard JM, Jordan GL, Reber HA, eds. Surgical disease of the pancreas. Philadelphia: Lea & Febiger, 1987:171–228.
55. Kattwinkel J, Lapey A, di Sant Agnese PA, Edwards WA, Hufty MP. Hereditary pancreatitis: three new kindreds and a critical review of the literature. Pediatrics 1973;51:55–68.
56. Robechek PJ. Hereditary chronic relapsing pancreatitis: a clue to pancreatitis is general ? Am J Surg 1967;113:819–824.
57. Haynes JH, Martin JC, Kurzweg FT. Hereditary pancreatitis. Am Fam Physician 1982;25:153–154.
58. Girard RM, Dubé S, Archambault AP. Hereditary pancreatitis: report of an afflicted Canadian kindred and review of the disease. Can Med Assoc J 1981;125:576–580.
59. Dalton-Clarke HJ, Lewis MH, Levi AJ, Blumgart LH. Familial chronic calcific pancreatitis: a family study. Br J Surg 1985;72:307–308.
60. Ziegler DW, Long JA, Philippart AL, Klein MD. Pancreatitis in childhood: experience with 49 patients. Ann Surg 1988;207: 257–261.
61. Silen W, Steer ML. Pancreas. In: Schwartz SL, ed. Principles of surgery. 5th ed. New York: McGraw-Hill, 1989:1416–1440.
62. Amerson JL, Ricketts RR. Idiopathic fibrosing pancreatitis: a rare cause of obstructive jaundice in children. Am Surg 1996;62: 295–299.

63. Barkin JS, Stollman N, Friedman J, et al. Idiopathic fibrosing pancreatitis causing obstructive jaundice in young adults: two case reports and literature review. Am J Gastroenterol 1994;89: 2063–2065.
64. Vane DW, Grosfield JL, West KW, Rescorla FJ. Pancreatic disorders in infancy and childhood: experience with 92 cases. J Pediatr Surg 1989;24:771–776.
65. Elitsur Y, Siddiqui SY, Sloven D, et al. Chronic pancreatitis with diffuse fibrosis in early childhood. Pancreas 1989;4:504–510.
66. Meneely RL, O'Neill J, Ghishan FK. Fibrosing pancreatitis: an obscure cause of painless obstructive jaundice: a case report and review of the literature. Pediatrics 1981;67:136–139.
67. Atkinson GO Jr, Wyly JB, Gay BB, et al. Idiopathic fibrosing pancreatitis: a cause of obstructive jaundice in childhood. Pediatr Radiol 1988;18:28–31.
68. Mulligan C, Howell C, Hatley R, Martindale R, Clark J. Conservative management of pediatric pseudocyst using octreotide acetate. Am Surg 1995;61:206–209.
69. Morali GA, Braverman DZ, Shemesh D, et al. Successful treatment of pancreatic pseudocyst with a somatostatin analogue and catheter drainage. Am J Gastroenterol 1991;86:515–518.
70. Barkin JS, Reiner DK, Deutsch E. Sandostatin for control of catheter drainage of pancreatic pseudocyst. Pancreas 1991;6: 245–248.
71. Corbally MT, Blake NS, Guiney EJ. Management of pancreatic pseudocyst in childhood: an increasing role for percutaneous external drainage. J R Coll Surg Edinb 1992;37:169–171.
72. Jaffe RB, Arata JA, Matlak ME. Percutaneous drainage of traumatic pancreatic pseudocysts in children. Am J Roentgenol 1989;152:591–595.
73. Weizman Z, Durie PR. Acute pancreatitis in childhood. J Pediatr 1988;113:24–29.

# 42

# Tropical Calculous Pancreatitis

C. S. Pitchumoni and Mathew Varughese

## DEFINITION

A form of nonalcoholic chronic pancreatitis occurring mostly in children and young adults of many developing nations is variously termed tropical pancreatitis, nutritional pancreatitis, Afro-Asian pancreatitis, fibrocalculous pancreatic diabetes (FCPD), tropical calculous pancreatopathy or juvenile pancreatitis syndrome. This syndrome of chronic pancreatitis of the young has been reported from many Afro-Asian countries including Uganda, Nigeria, Congo, Nyasaland (Malawi), Zambia, Ivory Coast, Madagascar, Tunisia, South Africa, Papua New Guinea, Malaysia, Indonesia, Thailand, Sri Lanka, Bangladesh, and India, as well as the Latin American countries of Mexico and Brazil (1–23). This type of chronic pancreatitis, often associated with pancreatic calculi, is limited almost exclusively to regions located 30° north and south of the equator, thus lending support to the use of the descriptive term tropical calculous pancreatitis (TCP). The numerous terms used to describe the disease indicate the uncertainty about the etiology but emphasize the association with malnutrition, the predominant occurrence in children, or the histopathology of the disease. In this chapter, tropical calculous pancreatitis, or TCP, is used to denote the entity.

## EPIDEMIOLOGY

Isolated reports of TCP in the young have been recorded in the surgical literature from India since 1931 (24). The first clear description of the disease, perhaps in its most advanced form, was by Zuidema in 1955 from Indonesia (11). This classic paper described seven undernourished patients with pancreatic lithiasis. The youngest was a 15-year-old girl, markedly undernourished, weighing only 33.5 kg; the oldest was 28 years of age. Zuidema subsequently (1959) reported on 45 patients (1959) between 12 and 45 years of age (12).

Diabetes mellitus dominated the clinical picture, and pancreatic calculi were demonstrated in many. Features of advanced malnutrition such as bilateral parotid gland enlargement and hair and skin changes of kwashiorkor in many of his patients prompted his conclusion that diabetes of the poor in Indonesia resulted from severe protein malnutrition.

Shaper in Uganda in 1960 observed a similar syndrome in the poor populations whose diet was rich in carbohydrate and low in protein and fat (1). The youngest patient was 10 years old. Most patients had a history of epigastric pain indicative of pancreatitis. Shaper felt that the high carbohydrate diet in the presence of protein deficiency led to increased demands on pancreatic enzymes and acinar cell injury. Since Shaper's report, many patients have been documented from India, and indeed the single largest series of patients with TCP reported to date is from the southwestern state of Kerala, in India (15–21). GeeVarghese and Pitchumoni observed this disease in endemic proportions in two major teaching institutions in the state (16). More than 300 cases of TCP were studied in the two hospitals in a period of 5 years. At a recent symposium, it was observed that other states in India are increasingly recognizing this disease as a result of both heightened awareness and routine screening of young diabetics for pancreatic calculi (25). Approximately 2000 patients have been reported in the literature, nearly 1700 of them by GeeVarghese (20).

The true prevalence of the disease is not well established. Most of the data have come from major teaching hospitals in endemic areas. About 10% of the medical inpatients and 12% of all diabetics admitted to one hospital had TCP (17, 20). These data also indicated a male to female ratio in TCP of 1.6:1. Hospital data give an erroneously high prevalence of the disease. A recent epidemiologic study looked at the prevalence of the disease in a village in the state of Kerala in India (26). The survey included 28,567 individuals from 6,079 families; 518 individuals were suspected to have pancreatitis. Using a combination of x-rays, abdominal ultrasound, and a test for exocrine pancreatic function (Chymex), 36 cases were identified. The prevalence of pancreatitis in this highly endemic area was calculated to be 1:793. In contrast to previous hospital-based studies conducted 3 decades ago, this recent community survey showed a female preponderance (male:female ratio, 1:1.8) and onset of the disease at an older age (mean, 23.9) than that reported by other observers.

## CLINICAL FEATURES

### General Features

The cardinal manifestations of TCP are recurrent abdominal pain in childhood, followed by diabetes mellitus and pancreatic calculi before puberty, and death in the prime of life (20). Early detection and recent improvements in the management of diabetes and its complications have resulted in a longer life span (21).

Earlier studies only picked up the late stages of the disease, where extreme emaciation, clinical signs of protein-calorie malnutrition, and bilateral parotid gland enlargement were noted as prominent features (15–20, 27) (Fig. 42.1). The clinical profile of TCP has changed somewhat; in one recent series, severe malnutrition was found in only 25% of patients, although most were underweight (21). A heightened index of suspicion of the disease, early diagnosis, and recent improvements in the management of diabetes and its complications have markedly improved the grim prognosis noted in earlier reports.

### Abdominal Pain

The onset of the disease is insidious in early childhood, with recurrent attacks of upper abdominal or periumbilical pain

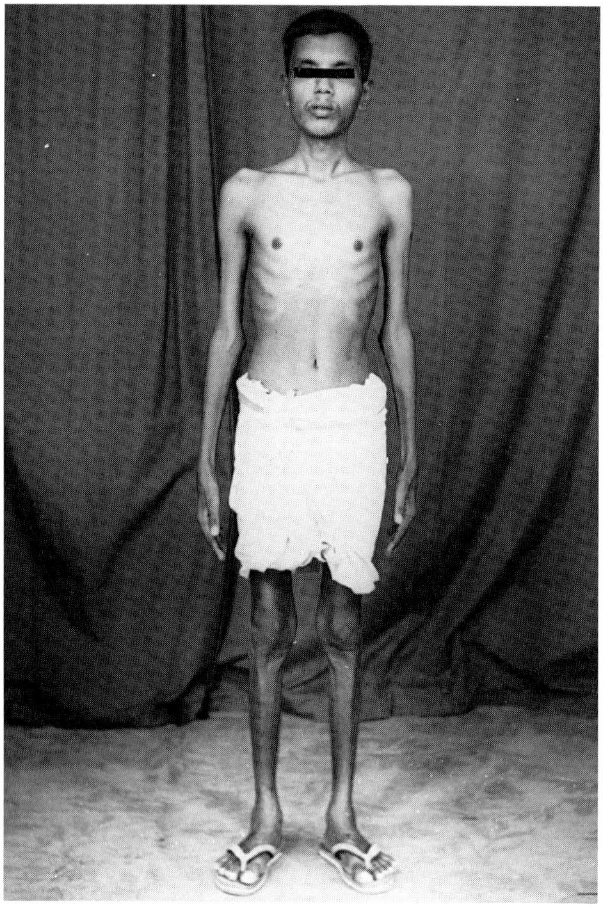

**FIG. 42.1.** A patient with TCP. Note the extreme emaciation. (Courtesy V. Mohan, M.D., Madras)

before the 13th year. About 5% of the juvenile diabetics with pancreatic calculi do not have abdominal pain. The severe pain, which may last for days, may radiate to the lower end of the sternum, the left costal margin and along the left side, or posteriorly to the lumbar spine. It is also associated with retching and vomiting. Even small amounts of food aggravate the abdominal pain, so the patients generally avoid eating.

An interval of several years may pass between the cessation of painful attacks and the onset of diabetes mellitus. Pain totally disappears in a number of patients either before, or some years after, diabetes develops, perhaps because of "burning out of the pancreas" and acinar cell atrophy. It is uncommon for diabetes to precede abdominal pain.

### Exocrine Deficiency

Exocrine pancreatic functional abnormality is the least striking feature of TCP, and the diagnosis of TCP seldom depends on demonstration of pancreatic insufficiency. Serum amylase values are not particularly helpful in the diagnosis. In nearly 70% of cases, a random amylase test may show the level to be below normal, reflecting the extensive destruction of the gland as demonstrated by histologic findings at surgery (17). Measurements of specific pancreatic enzymes and immunoreactive trypsin show a spectrum of exocrine pancreatic insufficiency. In early stages of the disease, serum immunoreactive trypsin is subnormal in only a small number of patients. In those with advanced stages of the disease, both serum immunoreactive trypsin and stool chymotrypsin levels are markedly decreased (28, 29).

Using the Lundh test, the mean tryptic activity was noted to be less than 2 IU/mL in about 90% of those with calculi and only 27% of the patients without calculi. This observation implies that stone formation correlates with a gross reduction of tryptic activity. Secretin-stimulation studies conducted in Indian patients have given conflicting results. In one study of 15 patients, a reduction in the volume of pancreatic secretion was noted, but no change in bicarbonate levels (30) was seen. Recently, a second study from the same center documented a reduction of both volume and bicarbonate levels (31). The results of the latter study are similar to the observations made in alcohol-induced chronic pancreatitis. In a group of patients from Uganda, those with pancreatic lithiasis had consistently abnormal secretory responses; the total volume, bicarbonate output, and maximum bicarbonate concentrations were significantly lower than those in the control group (32). Such discrepancies in the results of secretin-CCK studies are attributed to the stage of the disease and the extent of parenchymal and ductal damage.

Clinical steatorrhea does not become manifest because of the low fat intake in the diet. The daily fat consumption by the patients is only 27 g (19). Less than 20% of patients complain of passing bulky, frothy, or oily stools. However, when the fat intake of the diet is increased to about 100 g/day, over 76% of patients develop demonstrable steatorrhea (33).

### Diabetes

Diabetes is an inevitable consequence of TCP and is usually severe, with fasting blood glucose levels between 200 and 400 mg/dL. One of the characteristic features of this form of diabetes is that despite requiring insulin for control of hyperglycemia, patients rarely become ketotic (21, 35, 36). Patients who have some residual beta cell function as shown by measurable serum C-peptide levels may respond to oral hypoglycemic agents and/or diet (21). At the other end of the spectrum are rare patients with absent or negligible C-peptide levels, who may indeed be prone to ketosis. The vast majority of patients falls somewhere between these two extremes, having enough beta cell reserve to protect against ketosis but not enough to respond to oral agents.

All diabetic complications such as retinopathy, nephropathy, and neuropathy occur on long-term follow-up (21). The frequency of various complications is similar to that seen in primary forms of diabetes. Macrovascular complications (ischemic heart disease and peripheral vascular disease), though rare, do occur (21).

## RADIOLOGIC FEATURES

### Pancreatic Calculi

In contrast to alcoholic pancreatitis, in which the calculi are small, speckled, and ill defined, in TCP the stones tend to be large, dense, and rounded with well-defined edges (34) (Fig. 42.2). Over 90% of patients with TCP eventually develop pancreatic calculi, in contrast to 30–50% of those with alcoholic pancreatitis. In early stages, the calculi may be solitary or few in number and are typically seen to the right of the first or second lumbar vertebrae on a plain abdominal x-ray (17). Often the entire pancreas is studded with calculi. Typically, the larger stones are notable near the head of the pancreas, explained by the fact that they migrate from ductules toward the ampulla, where they become lodged and grow (Fig. 42.3).

## PATHOLOGY

Our knowledge of the pathology of the pancreas in TCP is limited to the late stages of the disease and is based on surgical biopsies or autopsy material (37, 38). The pancreas in advanced stages is fibrotic and small, with an irregular and nodular surface. Occasionally, the gland may be displaced from its normal location as a result of uneven shrinkage and fibrous adhesions. Fat may replace the parenchyma and make the pancreas indistinguishable from surrounding adipose tissue. The pancreas may be firm, soft, or hard, and gritty to touch, varying in consistency from one part to the other, depending on the presence of fibrous tissue, cysts, or calculi. The major pancreatic duct may be eccentrically placed as a result of uneven destruction of glandular tissue. Multiple areas of stenosis and dilatation can be seen. Incomplete obstruction at the ampulla of Vater is seen in the large majority of patients.

Pancreatic calculi vary in size and shape. They range in size from small sand particles to a maximum of almost 4–5 cm in length (34). The location of the stone influences its shape and size. Noncalcified soft stones are also notable. In patients with no radiologically demonstrable calculi on antemortem x-rays of the abdomen, examinations at autopsy show multiple intraductal calculi. Pancreatic calculi are composed almost exclusively of calcium carbonate, mostly in the form of calcite and rarely as vaterite (39). Traces of calcium phosphate, magnesium, urate, and oxalate are also identified. Energy-dispersive x-ray fluorescence studies and scanning electron microscopy of stones have shown an amorphous nidus and a cryptocrystalline periphery (40). The nidus of the stone is rich in iron, chromium, and nickel, and the periphery consists mostly of calcium and small quantities of other trace elements. The calculi in TCP are similar to those from alcoholic pancreatitis in structure and composition (33).

The characteristic microscopic feature of the pancreas is the patchy fibrosis of the entire organ (Fig. 42.4). The ducts and ductules show dilatation or stricture, with periductular fibrosis (37, 38). Denudation of the ductular epithelium and squamous metaplasia are seen. The acinar tissue shows varying degrees of atrophy and destruction of the parenchyma and replacement with fibrous tissue. Interestingly, the islets of Langerhans appear well preserved, in some instances even hypertrophied, giving rise to a true nesidioblastosis (38). As the disease advances, the islets become atrophic, isolated, and surrounded by fibrous tissue. The local nerve bundles are hypertrophic and prominent.

Pancreatic carcinoma has been noted in some surgical as well as postmortem tissues (18, 41, 42). Many reports have emphasized the premalignant nature of the disease. In a series of 220 TCP patients treated surgically by the senior author (M.V.), 15 patients (6.8%) were confirmed to have inoperable pancreatic cancer. A recent international cooperative study has shown that irrespective of etiology, all forms of chronic pancreatitis are associated with a high incidence of pancreatic cancer (43).

The liver in early stages shows glycogen infiltration of cytoplasm and nuclei. Postmortem studies of advanced disease show fatty change and cirrhosis of the liver. Hypertrophy of the parotid gland with varying degrees of round cell infiltration around the normal-appearing ducts has also been noted.

## ETIOLOGIC FACTORS

The etiology for TCP is uncertain. The proposed etiologic factors are all hypothetical, based on epidemiologic data, careful clinical studies, and numerous biochemical evaluations.

### Malnutrition

Based on the observation that TCP almost exclusively affects the poor populations of developing nations, malnutrition is strongly suspected to be a major determinant in the etiology. Since the turnover of protein is quite high in the pancreatic acinar cell, it is quite vulnerable to protein depletion (44).

The pancreas in postmortem examinations of children dying of kwashiorkor (as a result of protein energy malnutrition (PEM)) is shrunken and fibrotic, with marked loss of acinar tissue, quite similar to the findings in TCP (44). The only difference is that pancreatic calculi are not seen in kwashiorkor.

One recent experimental study on bonnet monkeys has further elucidated the relationship between malnutrition and pancreatic injury (45, 46). While studying the new entity of mucoid vasculopathy, the observers were struck by the pancreatic abnormalities in those animals. The monkeys that developed pancreatic changes and vasculopathy were fed a tapioca- or corn starch–based diet that was low in protein (3.5%) but contained unlimited starch. Such a diet is similar in nutritional composition to the diet consumed by poor people in many parts of the developing world. Pancreatic tissue from these experimental animals showed lobular atrophy, accompanied by lipomatous atrophy, and islet cell hyperplasia. The pancreatic ducts showed varying degrees of epithelial hyperplasia. The authors feel that

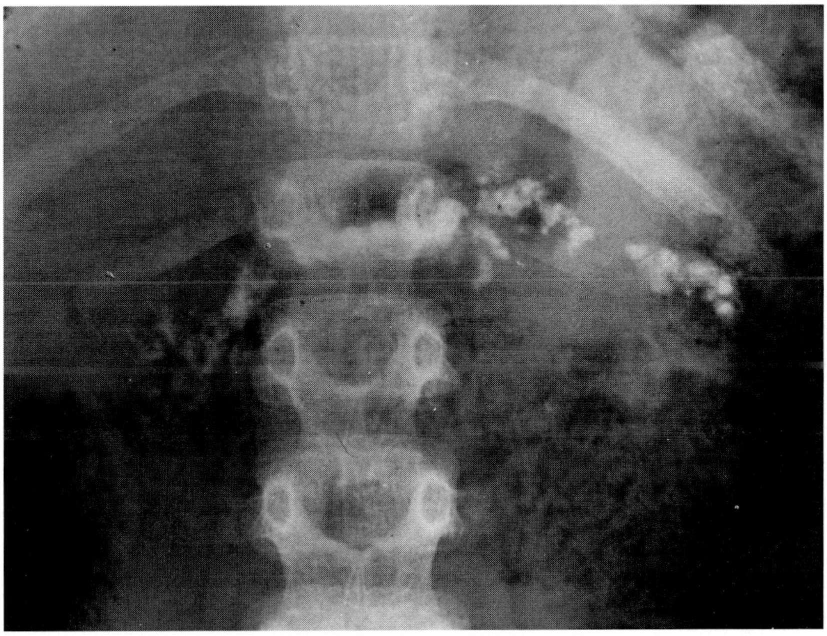

**FIG. 42.2.** Flat plate x-ray of the abdomen showing small and large radiopaque stones distributed along the main pancreatic duct and its side branches.

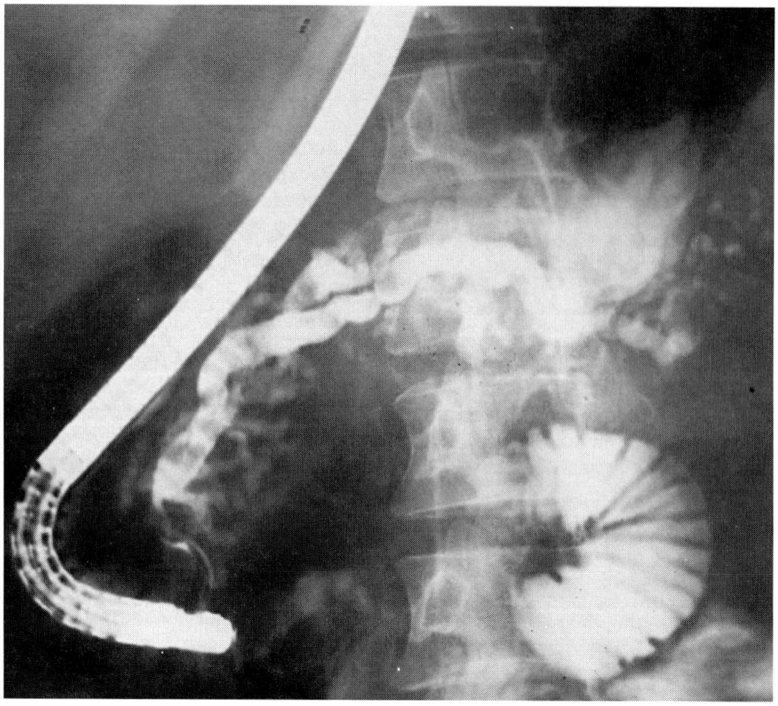

**FIG. 42.3.** ERCP showing a dilated duct and translucent stones.

their recent experiments offer an animal model for TCP; however, pancreatic calculi were not noted, raising a doubt whether the pancreatic changes are indeed those of TCP or only similar to those seen in kwashiorkor.

Since PEM is prevalent in many tropical countries, it is likely to accompany many diseases affecting the poor populations. The existence of large pockets of malnutrition and the relative infrequency of TCP in many parts of the world, indicate that malnutrition by itself is unlikely to be an initiating factor (47). This opinion has been stressed by many observers (18–21).

## Dietary Cyanogen Toxicity

The geographic distribution of TCP overlaps the areas of consumption of cassava (tapioca/manihot esculenta, a root consumed in tropical countries as a source of carbohydrate) (17–20, 48). The root is rich in carbohydrate but poor in protein and the sulfur-containing amino acid methionine. Cyanogen toxicity in the presence of malnutrition and antioxidant deficiency is also proposed as an ideal setting for free radical injury. Cassava is known to contain cyanogenic glycosides such as linamarin and lotaustralin. Cyanide is normally detoxified in the body by conversion to thiocyanate, but this detoxification requires sulfur, which is derived from sulfur-containing amino acids. The results of experimental studies have been quite confusing, and two groups from the same institution during the same period have observed supporting and opposing data for the cassava hypothesis (49–50).

In an experimental study in rats, McMillan and GeeVarghese showed that ingestion of cyanide led to transient hyperglycemia (51). They concluded that their results supported the role of cyanide in the etiopathogenesis of TCP. However, none of the rats in the above experiments developed permanent diabetes. Moreover, the effects were seen only with potassium cyanide and not with cassava. Thus, the relevance of these experiments to the human situation is far from clear. Another experimental study using rats and a cassava diet was interpreted to show no changes in the pancreas. Recent epidemiologic studies also question the cassava hypothesis. TCP is prevalent in many parts of India and Africa where cassava is not consumed. On the contrary, TCP is not seen in a rural West African population that consumes a high cassava diet (52). To date, cassava toxicity in the pathogenesis of TCP remains an unproven hypothesis. It is quite likely that a high cassava diet is equivalent to the high-carbohydrate, low-protein diet used in the experimental studies on bonnet monkeys quoted earlier, in which cyanogen toxicity was apparently not a factor.

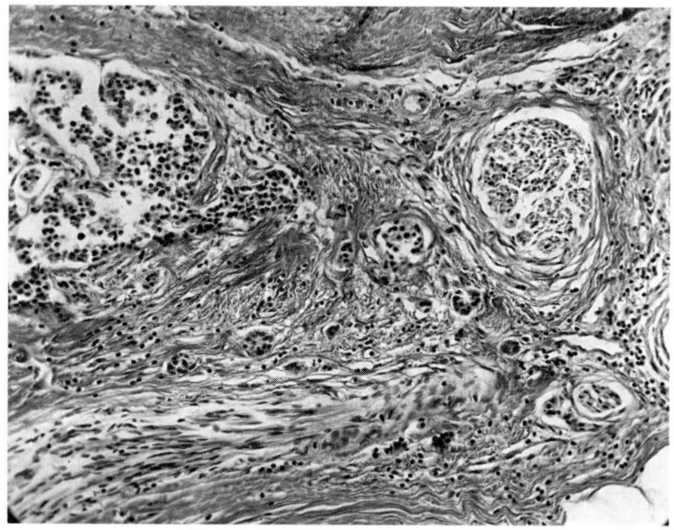

**FIG. 42.4.** Histopathology of TCP. Extensive destruction of parenchyma, replacement by fibrous tissue, well-preserved giant islets.

## Micronutrient Deficiency and Oxidant Stress

Chronic pancreatitis has been linked to "heightened oxidative detoxification reactions" conducted by cytochromes P-450-1 within the pancreas and/or liver. Several factors, including chronic induction of the cytochrome P-450-1 subfamily of monooxygenases by xenobiotics (cigarettes, alcohol, occupational chemicals, dietary corn oil, and so forth), may be involved (53, 54). Certain micronutrient deficiencies are known to induce pancreatic damage. For example, deficiencies of selenium, zinc, and copper induce acinar cell atrophy in experimental animals (44). As components of metalloenzymes, these trace elements also play a role in scavenging free radicals. The theophylline clearance (a measure of cytochrome P-450-1 activity in vivo) is faster in TCP patients than in controls, suggesting that oxidant stress may be involved in the pathogenesis of TCP. A study on the antioxidant status of patients showed low levels of vitamin C and ß-carotene (55), a finding that may tilt the balance in favor of oxidant stress (53, 54). As noted above, malnutrition induces a state of defective ability to scavenge free radicals, while exposure to toxins induces free radical formation, thereby enhancing the susceptibility for free radical damage (55). In spite of the strength of the above observations, free-radical injury to the pancreas is not yet proven and needs further study.

## OTHER FACTORS

### Miscellaneous Factors

Congenital ductal obstruction, viruses, and autoimmune factors have been considered, but the data are not strong enough to incriminate any of them. In a detailed study from India on the dietary intake of TCP patients, the protein intake was found to be 53 g/day, the same as controls. The fat intake of TCP patients and controls was very low (27 g/day) (56). The predisposition of patients to alcoholic pancreatitis, on a very low fat diet noted in some studies, indicates that such a diet somehow enhances the susceptibility to chronic pancreatitis.

### Familial and Genetic Factors

TCP affects many members of some families (18–21, 57, 58). A previous study found 17 families with two or more members having evidence of pancreatitis. Nearly 8% of TCP patients showed evidence of familial aggregation. In some families, there was evidence of vertical transmission of the disease from parents to offspring; in others, there was a horizontal distribution among siblings (19, 58, 59). Familial clustering of cases suggests, but does not necessarily prove, a hereditary etiology for TCP. Several family members could be exposed to the same environmental factors, which could produce the disease in them.

## MANAGEMENT OF PATIENTS WITH TCP

The principles of management of TCP consist of alleviation of abdominal pain, treatment of diabetes and prevention of its complications, and correction of nutritional deficiencies. The treatment of an acute exacerbation of TCP is similar to that of alcoholic pancreatitis. Measures to put the pancreas to rest include no feeding by mouth, nasogastric tube aspiration of the stomach, and appropriate intravenous fluid and electrolyte administration.

The mainstay of diabetes management is insulin administration. In nearly 60% of the patients, the daily dose of insulin required for control is about 60 units. An insulin requirement of more than 200 units per day in the absence of ketosis or infection (true insulin resistance) is notable in some patients. Pancreatic diabetes is brittle, and severe prolonged hypoglycemia resulting in death may occur. Hence, experienced clinicians recommend caution in the administration of insulin if there is a history of hypoglycemia (17–21, 60, 61).

## SURGERY IN TCP

The ductal dilatation characteristic of TCP offers an ideal setting for drainage procedures, and the surgical management of TCP has been previously well reviewed (41, 62–65). The senior author of this chapter (M.V.) has operated on 220 patients with TCP since 1976. The pancreatic duct system in TCP is markedly dilated secondary to obstructions and strictures resulting from calculi at multiple sites. The ideal procedure is a longitudinally split pancreaticojejunostomy after removal of stones. In 34 of the 220 patients, stones were impacted in the ampulla of Vater. These stones were extracted by the transduodenal route, and sphincteroplasty was done in addition to the longitudinal split pancreaticojejunostomy. Although complete relief of abdominal pain was not achieved in all patients, most had satisfactory symptomatic relief. About 25% of patients had recurrence of pain, though less severe. Surgery does not influence the status of diabetes. Resections of the pancreas have not been widely employed as a primary surgical procedure in TCP. The reluctance of most surgeons to perform such a major procedure is based on the young age of patients and the fear of worsening diabetes, which would become extremely difficult to manage.

Extracorporeal shock-wave lithotripsy and stone dissolution, and endoscopic stone removal are procedures that need to be evaluated in the treatment of patients with severe pain. The attractive feature of endoscopic therapy is that it offers an alternative to surgical forms of drainage. The current feeling is that those with a dominant stricture or stone impaction near the head are likely to be the patients of choice for such a therapy (66).

Management of pain in chronic pancreatitis is a frustrating experience. There is no good study evaluating the role of oral pancreatic enzyme therapy of TCP. However, the proponents of enzyme therapy for alcoholic pancreatitis feel that when the ducts are markedly dilated, as in TCP, enzyme therapy will not be beneficial. Therefore, surgical therapy appears to be the logical choice.

## REFERENCES


1. Shaper AG. Chronic pancreatic disease and protein malnutrition. Lancet 1960;2:1223–1224.
2. Kinnear TWG. Patterns of diabetes mellitus in a Nigerian teaching hospital. West Afr Med J 1973;60:228–233.
3. Osuntokun BO, Skinkugbe FM, Francis TI, et al. Diabetes mellitus in Nigerians. A study of 832 patients. West Afr Med J 1971;20: 295–312.
4. Olurin EO, Olurin O. Pancreatic calcification: a report of 45 cases. Br Med J 1969;4:534–539.
5. Sonnet J, Brisbosis P, Bastin JP. Chronic pancreatitis with calcification in Congolese Bantus. Trop Geogr Med 1966;18:97–113.
6. Bourgoignie J, Sonnet J, Dechef G. Clinical study of diabetes mellitus in the Bantu region of Leopoldville. Ann Soc Belg Med Trop 1962;3:261–294.
7. Goodall JWD, Pilbeam STH. Diabetes in Nyasaland (Malawi). Trans R Soc Trop Med Hyg 1964;58:575–578.
8. Chatti N, Chaeb L, Jemni L, et al. Juvenile idiopathic chronic calcifying pancreatitis: report of 10 cases from central Tunisia. Pancreas 1990;5:354–357.
9. Joffe N. Pancreatic calcification in childhood associated with protein malnutrition. Br J Radiol 1963;36:758–761.
10. Richens JE, Wesselingh S. Fibrocalculous pancreatic diabetes in Papua, New Guinea. Trop Geogr Med 1988;40:84–87.
11. Zuidema PJ. Calcification and cirrhosis of the pancreas in patients with deficient nutrition. Doc Med Geogr Trop Amsterdam 1955;5:229–231.
12. Zuidema PJ. Cirrhosis and disseminated calcification of the pancreas in patients with malnutrition. Trop Geogr Med 1959;11: 70–74.
13. Chandraprasert S, Samranvej P, Arthachinta S, Isarena S. Diabetes mellitus and tropical forms of chronic calcific pancreatitis in Thailand. Aust NZ J Med 1976;6:316–320.
14. Nagaratnem N, Gunawardene KRW. Aetiological factors in pancreatic calcification in Ceylon. Digestion 1972;5:9–16.
15. GeeVarghese PJ, Pillai VK, Joseph MP, Pitchumoni CS. The diagnosis of pancreatogenous diabetes mellitus. J Assoc Physicians India 1962;10:713–718.
16. GeeVarghese PJ, Pitchumoni CS. Pancreatic diabetes in Kerala.

Based on a clinicopathological study of 325 diabetic patients with pancreatic calculi. In: Patel JG, Talwalkar NG, eds. Proceedings of the World Congress on Diabetes in the Tropics. Bombay: Diabetic Association of India, 1966:223–229.

17. GeeVarghese PJ. Pancreatic diabetes. Bombay: Popular Parkashan, 1968.
18. Narendranathan M. Chronic calcific pancreatitis of the tropics. Trop Gastroenterol 1981;2:40–45.
19. Balakrishnan V. Chronic calcifying pancreatitis in the tropics. Indian J Gastroenterol 1984;3:65–67.
20. GeeVarghese PJ. Calcific pancreatitis. Bombay: Varghese Publishing, 1985.
21. Mohan V, Chari ST, Viswanathan M, et al. Tropical pancreatitis in southern India. Proc R Coll Physicians Edinb 1990;20:1:34–42.
22. Kar BC, Tripathy BB. Clinical observations on a group of young diabetics. J Assoc Physicians India 1967;15:9–15.
23. Dani R, Nogueira CED. Chronische Kalzifzierende pankreatitris in Brasilien. Eine analysse von 92 allen. Leber Magen Darm 1976;6: 272–275.
24. Kini MG. Multiple pancreatic calculi with chronic pancreatitis. Br J Surg 1938;25:705–706.
25. Balakrishnan V. Chronic pancreatitis in India. Trivandrum: Indian Society of Pancreatology St. Joseph's Press, 1987.
26. Balajl LN, Tandon RK, Tandon BN, Banks PA. Prevalence and clinical features of chronic pancreatitis in southern India. Int J Pancreatol 1994;(1):29–34.
27. Pitchumoni CS. Special problems of tropical pancreatitis. Clin Gastroenterol 1984;13:941–959.
28. Yajnik CS, Katrak A, Kanithar SV, et al. Serum immunoreactive trypsin in tropical pancreatic diabetes syndrome. Ann Clin Biochem 1989;26:69–73.
29. Yajnik CS, Sahasrabudhe RA, Naik SS, et al. Exocrine pancreatic function (serum immunoreactive trypsin fecal chymotrypsin and pancreatic isoamylase) in Indian diabetics. Pancreas 1990;5: 631–638.
30. George PK, Banks PS, Pai KN, et al. Exocrine pancreatic function in calcific pancreatitis in India. Gastroenterology 1971;60: 858–863.
31. Punnose J, Balakrishnan V, Bhadran A. Exocrine pancreatic function in chronic pancreatitis with and without calcification. Indian J Gastroenterol 1987;6:85–86.
32. Banwell JG, Campbell J. Pancreatic exocrine function in African patients. Trans R Soc Trop Med Hyg 1967;61:390–398.
33. Chirayath H. Exocrine pancreas in pancreatic diabetes. In: Pai KN, Soman CR, Varghese R, eds. Pancreatic diabetes. Trivandrum, India: Geo Printers, 1970:16–28.
34. Pitchumoni CS, Mohan AT. Pancreatic stones. Gastroenterol Clin North Am 1990;19:873–893.
35. Mohan V, Ramchandran A, Viswanathan M. Malnutrition related diabetes mellitus. In: Pickup JC, Williams G, eds. Textbook of diabetes. Oxford: Blackwell Scientific Publications, 1991:247–251.
36. Mohan V, Mohan R, Susheela L, et al. Tropical pancreatic diabetes in south India: heterogeneity in clinical and biochemical profile. Diabetologia 1985;28:229–232.
37. Nagalotimath SJ. Pancreatic pathology in pancreatic calcification with diabetes. In: Podolsky S, Viswanathan M, eds. Secondary diabetes: the spectrum of the diabetic syndrome. New York: Raven Press, 1980:117–145.
38. Nair B, Latha P. The pancreas in chronic calcific pancreatitis. In: Balakrishnan V, ed. Chronic pancreatitis in India. Trivandrum, Kerala, India: St. Joseph's Press, 1987:115–120.
39. Schultz AC, Moore PB, Pitchumoni CS. X-ray diffraction studies of pancreatic calculi associated with nutritional pancreatitis. Dig Dis Sci 1986;31:476–480.
40. Pitchumoni CS, Viswanathan KV, GeeVarghese PJ, Banks PA. Ultra-structure and elemental composition of human pancreatic calculi. Pancreas 1987;2:152–158.
41. Thomas PG, Augustine P, Ramesh H, Rangabashyam N. Observations and surgical management of tropical pancreatitis in Kerala and southern India. World J Surg 1990;14:32–42.
42. Chari ST, Mohan V, Pitchumoni CS, Viswanathan M, Madanagopalan N, Lowenfels AB. Risk of pancreatic carcinoma in tropical calcifying pancreatitis: an epidemiological study. Pancreas 1994;9:62–66.
43. Lowenfels AB, Maisonneuve P, Cavallini G, et al. Pancreatitis and the risk of pancreatic cancer. N Engl J Med 1993;328:1433–1437.
44. Pitchumoni CS, Scheele GA. Interdependence of nutrition and exocrine pancreatic function. In: Go VLW, DiMagno EP, Gardner JD, et al., eds. The pancreas: biology, pathology and disease. 2nd ed. New York: Raven Press, 1993:449–473.
45. Sandhyamani S. Vasculopathic and cardiomyopathic changes induced by low protein high carbohydrate tapioca based diet in bonnet monkeys. Am J Cardiovasc Pathol 1992;4:41–50.
46. Sandhyamani S. Pancreatic changes in induced malnutrition: bonnet monkey models for protein malnutrition and tropical chronic calculus pancreatopathy (unpublished).
47. GeeVarghese PJ, Pitchumoni CS, Nair SR. Is protein malnutrition an initiating cause of pancreatic calcification? Assoc Physicians India 1969;14:417–419.
48. GeeVarghese PJ. Cassava diet, tropical calcifying pancreatitis and pancreatic diabetes. In: Delaye F, Ahluwalia R, eds. Cassava toxicity and thyroid research and public health issues. Proceedings of a workshop held in Ottawa, Canada. May 31–June 2, 1982. Ottawa: International Research Center, 1983:77–78.
49. Narendranathan M, Cheriyan A. Lack of association between cassava consumption and tropical pancreatitis syndrome. J Gastroenterol Hepatol 1994;9:282–285.
50. Leena KB, Shenoy KT. Pancreatic ultrastructure in manioz fed animals is similar to chronic pancreatitis (Abstract). Gut 1995; 37(suppl 2):A229.
51. McMillan D, GeeVarghese PJ. Dietary cyanide and tropical malnutrition diabetes. In: Podolsky S, Viswanathan M, eds. Secondary diabetes: the spectrum of the diabetic syndromes. New York: Raven Press, 1980:239–243.
52. Teuscher T, Baillod P, Rosman JB, et al. Absence of diabetes in a rural west African population with a high carbohydrate/cassava diet. Lancet 1987;1:765–768.
53. Chaloner C, Sandle LR, Mohan V, et al. Evidence of induction of cytochrome P450-I in patients with tropical chronic pancreatitis. Int Clin Pharmacol Ther Toxicol 1990;28:235–240.
54. Mohan V, Braganza JM. Xenobiotics in tropical chronic pancreatitis. In: Braganza JM, ed. The pathogenesis of pancreatitis. New York: Manchester University Press, 1991:115–120.
55. Pitchumoni CS, Jain NK, Lowenfels AB, et al. Chronic cyanide poisoning unifying concept for alcoholic and tropical pancreatitis. Pancreas 1988;3:220–222.
56. Balakrishnan V, Sauniere JF, Hariharan M, Sarles H. Diet, pancreatic function and chronic pancreatitis in south India and France. Pancreas 1988;3:30–35.
57. Pitchumoni CS, GeeVarghese PJ. Familial and diabetes mellitus. In: Patel JC, Talwalkar NG, eds. Proceedings of the World Congress on Diabetes in the Tropics. Bombay: Diabetic Association of India, 1970:240.
58. Mohan V, Chari ST, Hitman GA, et al. Familial aggregation in tropical-fibrocalculous pancreatic diabetes. Pancreas 1989;4: 690–693.
59. Kambo PK, Hitman A, Mohan V, et al. The genetic predisposition to fibrocalculous pancreatic diabetes. Diabetologia 1989;32: 45–57.
60. Mohan V, Snehalatha C, Ramachandran A, et al. Pancreatic beta cell function in tropical pancreatic diabetes. Metabolism 1983;32:1091–1092.
61. Mohan V, Snehalatha C, Ramachandran A, et al. Plasma glucagon responses in tropical fibrocalculous pancreatic diabetes. Diabetes Res Clin Prac 1990;9:97–101.
62. Abraham PA. Surgical management of patients with chronic pancreatitis and pancreatic calculi. In: Pai KN, Soman CR, Varghese R, eds. Pancreatic diabetes. Trivandrum, India: Geo Printers, 1970:71–78.
63. Varghese M. Surgery in pancreatic diabetes in secondary diabetes: the spectrum of the diabetic syndromes. In: Podolsky S, Viswanathan M, eds. New York: Raven Press, 1980:231–237.
64. Thomas PG, Augustine P. Surgery in tropical pancreatitis. Br J Surg 1988;75:161–164.
65. Pitchumoni CS, Badiga SM. Chronic pancreatitis. Solving intractable pain and insufficiency. In: Barkin JS, Rogers AI, eds. Different decisions in digestive diseases. St. Louis: CV Mosby, 1994:121–130.

# 43

# Natural History of Pancreatic Pseudocysts

Harry M. Richter, III

All definitions of *pancreatic pseudocyst* concur that the lesion is a collection of fluid within or adjacent to the pancreas, that the surrounding wall of this collection consists of fibrous and granulation tissue, and that this wall specifically lacks an epithelial lining. To this universal description, some would add that the collection contains pancreatic juice or "amylase-rich" fluid. Some require that a patent communication between the collection and the pancreatic duct exists, whether proven or not. Many imply a sense of temporal stability, thus excluding the most evanescent peripancreatic effusions. A causal relationship between the collection and pancreatitis or pancreatic trauma is also routine. Adding the vagaries of the definition of "pseudocyst," frequently used modifiers have no consistent meaning. Thus, to some "chronic pseudocyst" means a pseudocyst that has been in existence for a given length of time; for others it implies that the presenting symptoms are those of a mass lesion, subtle and progressive, rather than those of evolving acute pancreatitis; still others mean only that the pseudocyst arose from the substrate of underlying chronic pancreatitis. The term "acute pseudocyst" is similarly ambiguous. "Infected pseudocyst" denotes to some a grave complication synonymous with "pancreatic abscess," while others use the term for all pseudocysts with fluid yielding a positive bacterial culture. Fortunately, several authors have begun the process of defining a terminology and classification of pseudocysts (1–3). Over time, confusion and miscommunication resulting from ambiguous terminology should disappear (4).

The natural history of pancreatic pseudocysts remains in part speculative and mysterious. Few studies have followed the origin of pseudocysts with serial imaging studies. Many have come to medical attention already fully developed. The natural course of a pseudocyst has traditionally been interrupted by deliberate invasive interference, either surgical or nonsurgical. Few studies present the results of a deliberate expectant approach. The experimental canine model devised by Warren (5) is complex and could easily run afoul of current regulatory guidelines. The aim of this chapter is to synthesize a concept of the natural history of pancreatic pseudocyst. The impact of preexisting chronic pancreatitis, of a discreet antecedent attack of acute pancreatitis, and of the period of elapsed time since such an attack, is explored.

## THE ORIGIN OF PANCREATIC PSEUDOCYSTS

### Pseudocysts following Acute Pancreatitis

Acute pancreatitis of moderate or greater severity is often accompanied by the early development of an acute peripancreatic fluid collection (6). Appearing within 1 or 2 weeks of onset, these collections are considered effusions resulting from the inflammatory process, contained within peripancreatic anatomic spaces by adjacent viscera. Their shape is irregular, they lack a defined wall, and they do not communicate with the main pancreatic duct. As recovery from acute pancreatitis ensues, these collections resorb without sequela.

When an attack of acute pancreatitis results in pancreatic necrosis of limited extent, the potential for direct leakage of pancreatic juice from the gland exists (7). The attack need not be clinically severe; indeed, rarely, the patient does not require medical attention and the acute episode is overlooked. Moreover, acute pancreatitis with limited necrosis may occur in a patient with established chronic pancreatitis (4), and several series document pseudocysts arising from this scenario. Recovery from the acute inflammation is the rule, but pancreatic juice leaking from the duct in the region of necrosis begins to accumulate in the space adjacent to the pancreas. Often, this fluid occupies the potential space of the lesser omenta bursa (lesser sac), limited anteriorly by the stomach, inferiorly by the transverse mesocolon, laterally by the spleen and splenic flexure on the left and the duodenum on the right. These visceral surfaces form an initial restraining boundary of the escaping pancreatic juice. The ensuing inflammatory reaction, stimulated perhaps by pancreatic enzyme action and local fat and pancreatic necrosis, induces the development of a distinct surrounding wall. As the wall matures and thickens, it consists of granulation tissue, blood vessels, and connective tissue with fibrosis. The maturing pseudocyst often assumes a spherical or oval shape, presumably under the influence of biomechanical forces. Necrotic debris may disintegrate and disappear or may persist within the pseudocyst cavity.

The concept that pseudocysts arising after acute pancreatitis always initially communicate with the pancreatic duct is an inference based upon clinical, laboratory, and radiographic observations. First, the measured amylase concentration in pseudocyst fluid is many times greater than the simultaneous serum amylase concentration (8, 9). Second, percutaneous external drainage of such a pseudocyst results in a prolonged (several weeks) period of drainage, strongly suggesting the presence of a pancreatic duct fistula (8, 10). Communication between the duct and the pseudocyst is demonstrated by endoscopic pancreatography in fewer than half of the cases so studied (11). Contrast injection directly into the pseudocyst reveals a duct connection even less frequently (10). Negative radiographic studies do not rule out a connection. Injection pressure during endoscopic pancreatography is deliberately limited to avoid aggravation of pancreatitis, thus reducing the positive yield. Pseudocyst distension during direct contrast injection may temporarily occlude the connection to the main pancreatic duct. A computed tomography (CT) scan obtained following endoscopic pancreatography injection would be a more sensitive means of detecting small amounts of contrast within the pseudocyst (J. Turcotte, in discussion of reference 27). Does the duct connection remain patent for the entire life span of a pseudocyst? One may well assume that a connection between the pancreatic duct and the pseudocyst could close spontaneously with maturation of postinflammatory scar around the ductal leak. Clearly this eventually happens routinely after external pseudocyst drainage and most often after internal drainage as well.

The sequence of events leading to pseudocyst after an apparent acute pancreatitis most commonly occurs in patients with a morphologically normal gland. Acute alcoholic pancreatitis accounts for a very substantial majority of patients reported in North American series. Gallstone pancreatitis, postprocedural pancreatitis, idiopathic pancreatitis, and other assorted causes account for the remainder. This same mechanism of pseudocyst formation may also occur in patients with established chronic pancreatitis. Of 83 patients described by D'Egidio and Schein, 26 developed postnecrotic pseudocysts superimposed upon chronic pancreatitis (3). Warshaw and Rattner (12) studied 42 patients with pancreatic pseudocysts; 22 of these developed following an attack of acute pancreatitis, and 8 in this group had established chronic pancreatitis. In an investigation of the value of preoperative endoscopic retrograde cholangiopancreatography (ERCP) in pseudocyst patients, Nealon et al. (11) identified patients having pseudocysts following an attack of acute pancreatitis who also had ductal changes of chronic pancreatitis. Finally, Crass and Way (13) compared the features of patients with "acute" pseudocysts (developing after an overt attack of pancreatitis) with those with "chronic" pseudocysts developing in the absence of an overt antecedent attack of pancreatitis. The proportion of patients with pancreatic calcification (i.e., chronic pancreatitis) was the same in the acute and the chronic pseudocyst groups. In summary, the presence of underlying chronic pancreatitis does not preclude the occurrence of acute pancreatitis nor the subsequent evolution of an "acute" pseudocyst.

A second putative mechanism for the genesis of pseudocysts in patients with chronic pancreatitis probably accounts for most such pseudocysts. According to this proposed mechanism, a pancreatic duct branch becomes obstructed because of pancreatic ductal stones or inspissated pancreatic proteinaceous material (3, 4, 14). Ongoing secretion of pancreatic juice peripheral to this ductal occlusion leads to progressive dilation of the duct, eventually resulting in the appearance of a cystic mass filled with pancreatic juice. Such pseudocysts, sometimes termed "retention pseudocysts," often appear to be within the parenchyma of the gland itself. Although a connection to the main pancreatic duct may not be evident, such a pseudocyst is clearly in continuity with one or more branch ducts. The pseudocyst may be clinically silent or may cause progressive symptoms of an enlarging mass, but the lesion itself will be of indeterminate age, there being no index attack of acute pancreatitis that initiated the process.

Traumatic pseudocysts may follow either blunt or penetrating abdominal injury, either mechanism of injury causing pancreatic duct disruption. Especially in children, the blunt injury (often a bicycle accident) may escape medical attention until pseudocyst symptoms arise several weeks later. Occasionally, even after exploratory laparotomy for trauma, pancreatic duct injury is unrecognized. A pseudocyst is then likely to develop in the postoperative period. In any event, traumatic pseudocysts presumably develop in a manner analogous to those following ductal disruption during an attack of acute pancreatitis, with leaking pancreatic juice contained by surrounding organs and a distinct wall evolving over time.

## COMPLICATIONS OF PANCREATIC PSEUDOCYSTS

Pseudocysts may remain asymptomatic, they may cause pain alone, or they may cause additional symptoms such as early satiety, nausea, and vomiting due to gastric compression. In addition to these routine clinical features, a pseudocyst may result in more serious or even life-threatening complications. The management of pancreatic pseudocyst depends in part upon an estimate of the risk of such a complication.

**Hemorrhage.** At least two distinct mechanisms of pseudocyst hemorrhage occur. The maturing wall of a pseudocyst in evolution, following acute pancreatitis, is a vascular structure. Local inflammatory conditions, perhaps promoted by the presence of (presumably activated) pancreatic enzymes, cause vessel disruption with resultant bleeding into the pseudocyst cavity. This scenario appears most likely during the first 6–12 weeks of the pseudocyst development. Such bleeding may be subclinical, evidenced by the appearance on CT scan of clot within the cyst or of old blood evacuated at the time of operation. At other times, however, bleeding results in acute worsening of pain, enlargement of the pseudocyst, and signs of hypovolemia. Gastrointestinal hemorrhage soon after elective pseudocyst enteric drainage could also result from bleeding vessels in the cyst wall, although suture-line hemorrhage must also be suspected.

A second mechanism for hemorrhage results from erosion of a pseudocyst into a peripancreatic artery, typically the splenic artery or the gastroduodenal artery (15, 16). The arterial erosion is perhaps as much the result of pressure necrosis from the adjacent pseudocyst as from true enzymatic digestion. Most often, the patient has underlying chronic pancreatitis, and the pseudocyst is chronic as well, having no antecedent symptoms of acute pancreatitis. Arteriography will likely reveal a pseudoaneurysm of the involved artery, suggesting transcatheter control as temporary or even definitive therapy.

**Rupture.** Rupture of a pseudocyst may occur acutely, resulting in symptoms of peritonitis (17). Occasionally, rupture follows an episode of intracystic hemorrhage. Frank perforation most commonly supervenes as an acute pseudocyst evolves, though this complication is described in chronic, asymptomatic cysts as well. A pseudocyst may also slowly leak its content into the peritoneal cavity or a pleural space, resulting in the syndrome of pancreatic ascites or pancreatic pleural fistula. Such "internal fistulae" are clearly sustained by a patent communication with the pancreatic duct, by way of the pseudocyst cavity. The vast majority of such patients have chronic pancreatitis and present without an apparent acute attack of pancreatitis (hence a chronic pseudocyst as well). Finally, a pseudocyst may spontaneously necessitate into an adjacent enteric viscus. Spontaneous cure may result, but often the pseudocyst decompression is inadequate. In that case, the contaminated cavity requires more deliberate drainage. Moreover, enteric erosion has also caused severe gastrointestinal hemorrhage.

**Infection.** The fluid contained in most pancreatic pseudocysts is sterile. Positive bacterial cultures have been reported in a substantial number of patients who have no overt sign of clinical infection (9, 18). In the absence of clinical sepsis, the appearance of such bacteria does not alter the therapeutic strategy. In particular, asymptomatic contamination does not preclude or endanger operative enteric drainage of the pseudocyst (18). The origin of the bacteria is unknown; pancreatic juice itself is not always sterile. Most culture data come from operative series; the incidence of contamination in undrained pseudocysts is unknown. Whether pseudocyst contamination would, if observed indefinitely, invariably lead to pancreatic abscess and sepsis is open to question.

Clinically overt infection of a pseudocyst is now called "pancreatic abscess," this latter term specifically excluding the distinct entity "infected pancreatic necrosis." Infection may occur in acute or chronic pseudocysts, without a clearly established differential probability. In contrast with the entity "infected pancreatic necrosis," pseudocyst infection represents a well-demarcated cavity containing pus and bacteria but little or no solid necrotic debris. Hence, percutaneous catheter drainage accompanied by appropriate antibiotic therapy may be sufficient therapy.

**Obstruction.** Pseudocysts rarely obstruct neighboring regions of the alimentary tract. A pseudocyst in the head of the gland will often displace and may narrow the common bile duct. Such biliary compression can cause obstructive jaundice, proven by resolution of the jaundice and restitution of normal biliary geometry following pseudocyst drainage. More often, however, biliary stricture results from encasement of the distal duct within the fibrotic process of chronic pancreatitis. Pseudocyst drainage alone would then perpetuate the biliary obstruction. Finally, a pancreatic pseudocyst may obstruct, and cause thrombosis of, an adjacent splanchnic vein, usually the splenic vein. Left-sided (sinistral) portal hypertension results, and gastric varices may develop. Gastric variceal hemorrhage could occur, but usually does not.

## NATURAL HISTORY

Prior to the introduction of diagnostic ultrasound in the early 1970s, the diagnosis of pancreatic pseudocyst rested upon clinical criteria and indirect imaging methods, such as upper gastrointestinal contrast radiographs. In these circumstances, asymptomatic or small pseudocysts went unsuspected and undiagnosed, while clinical attention focused on the subset of larger, symptomatic, or complicated pseudocysts (17). The potential for many pseudocysts to disappear or at least remain clinically silent could not be appreciated. Modern diagnostic techniques, including ultrasound, CT, and ERCP, have opened a window on the natural history of peripancreatic fluid collections of all varieties. In spite of these developments, however, most conclusions regarding natural history are inferential, being based largely upon retrospective reviews of surgical series that often failed to distinguish the mode of onset of the pseudocyst or the underlying pancreatic pathology (4).

Probably the most pertinent characteristic determining the outcome of pancreatic pseudocyst is its mode of presentation, and "acute" pseudocyst follows a recognized, proven attack of acute pancreatitis. Depending upon the series, alcoholic pancreatitis or gallstone pancreatitis predominate, with an assortment of other causes contributing the remainder. As noted above, this sequence has been documented in patients with underlying chronic pancreatitis, but most often, the gland is morphologically normal at the outset of the attack. Especially in the past, these patients were frequently observed in the hospital, for subsidence of the acute attack, and maturation of the fluid collection. Because past and current surgical dogma recommends a 6-week period of cyst maturation before surgery, the short-term course of acute pseudocysts is known. Several series document the result of deliberate delay or avoidance of operation for acute pseudocyst. At least 20% of acute pseudocysts resolve spontaneously (19–21). Both Bradley et al. (19) and Aranaha et al. (20) reported further spontaneous resolution with longer periods of observation.

During this same period of observation, many patients undergo urgent drainage of their peripancreatic fluid collection because of documented or suspected infection. Interpretation of this outcome is particularly confusing. Ongoing pancreatitis or pancreatitis with necrosis often simulates infection. Perhaps dependable exclusion of infection would have avoided some urgent interventions (22). On the other hand, clinical deterioration mandates evacuation of fluid and necrotic debris, whether or not infection has been proved. The greatest morbidity and mortality for pseudocyst treatment occurs in this group, in which the severity of the underlying pancreatitis is most likely the true determinant of outcome.

Hemorrhage and acute rupture, if they are to happen, also usually occur within 6 to 12 weeks of the index attack of pancreatitis. Behrman et al. (23) linked both size and outcome of acute pseudocysts directly to the severity of, but not to the cause of, the initiating attack of pancreatitis. Conversely, Imrie's group (20) found that biliary pancreatitis gave rise to acute pseudocysts with a particularly virulent perioperative course. Further, Nguyen et al. (24) demonstrated no resolution of gallstone-induced pseudocysts, compared with a 9% regression rate overall.

Bradley et al., in 1979, published the results of a prospective trial of deliberate nonoperative management of pancreatic pseudocyst (25). Although not clearly established, the vast majority of patients probably had an acute pseudocyst. At least a few had chronic pancreatitis in addition to a pseudocyst. While this study is open to the criticism that a substantial fraction of patients were lost to follow-up (and thus spontaneous regression may be underestimated), the cumulative occurrence of pseudocyst complications and attendant mortality is undeniable. Within the first 6 weeks of pseudocyst documentation, 40% of the pseudocysts resolved, while 20% of patients suffered a pseudocyst complication. Between 6 and 12 weeks' observation, resolution was uncommon but complications predominated. After 12 weeks, additional complications appeared, whereas no further resolution was documented. The conclusions of this carefully conducted study were that spontaneous resolution of acute pseudocysts rarely occurs after 6 weeks; that after 6 weeks, the frequency of serious complications increases dramatically; and consequently, that operation should not be delayed beyond 6 weeks. These conclusions firmly reinforced the impression gained from earlier studies and formed what appeared to be a sound basis for clinical practice.

At about the same time, Crass and Way reported their experience with pancreatic pseudocyst (13). These investigators differentiated their patients by mode of presentation. "Acute" pseudocysts followed an attack of acute pancreatitis; some of these patients had chronic pancreatitis. "Chronic" pseudocysts presented without an overt antecedent attack of pancreatitis. Many of these patients were presumed to have chronic pancreatitis, but the authors specifically suggested that some had merely suffered a mild or subclinical (or perhaps forgotten) acute attack. Many of the patients not needing urgent operation were observed initially, but a deliberate protocol of nonoperative treatment was not explicitly intended. An acute pseudocyst might sometimes regress, but it more frequently gave rise to a complication. Eleven of 46 chronic pseudocysts presented with a complication. Of the remaining 35, neither resolution nor complication was documented, though an aggressive surgical policy precluded long-term observation. Moreover, chronic pseudocysts have a mature wall at the time of presentation; a sutured cyst-enteric anastomosis was universally possible, even without a preoperative delay.

The observations of Bradley et al. and of Crass and Way found support in several subsequent reports. Using a similar definition, Warshaw and Rattner (12) confirmed the relative stability of chronic pseudocysts. These pseudocysts were found to be ripe for surgical internal drainage when they are present, and they are unlikely to regress without operation. Acute pseudocysts had about the same small likelihood of resolution as of complication. Mullins et al. (18) also identified a group of patients with chronic pseudocysts eligible for early operation and described CT criteria for identifying these pseudocysts.

Pseudocysts arising in patients with chronic pancreatitis account for about half of the lesions reported in various series, at least those from North America. Although a few of these are true "acute" pseudocysts, the great majority qualify as "chronic" pseudocysts, and similarly, most "chronic" pseudocysts arise solely from underlying chronic pancreatitis. The usual occurrence of a chronic pseudocyst superimposed upon chronic pancreatitis is considered a particularly stable lesion. Thus, spontaneous resolution of the cyst has been reported to be negligible (12, 14, 21), whereas the need for operative intervention is more likely than for acute pseudocyst (26). In addition to these potential variations in natural history, the outcome of elective surgical enteric drainage over the long term reflects the persistent chronic pancreatic disease. For example, after simple pseudocyst drainage, recurrent pseudocysts are not rare, while persistent or recurrent abdominal pain referable to the pancreas is quite common. Therefore, several authors recommend concomitant pancreatic duct drainage when practical (11, 27). Chronic pseudocyst leakage (internal fistula) and hemorrhage from arterial pseudoaneurysm are both complications most commonly associated with chronic pseudocysts superimposed upon chronic pancreatitis. Therefore, therapeutic nonchalance is never warranted.

The surgical bias favoring planned, early operation for pancreatic pseudocyst had obscured the possibility that a subset of stable, relatively asymptomatic patients with pseudocyst might avoid operation (or other invasive therapy) altogether. Two recent studies have addressed the results of a deliberate nonoperative approach for selected patients with pseudocyst. Yeo et al. (28) followed 75 patients, reserving operation for intractable symptoms, enlargement of the pseudocyst, or complications. Over time, only half of the patients so followed required operation. Serial imaging studies of the remainder demonstrated either pseudocyst resolution, shrinkage, or stable size without symptom or complication. Patients with chronic pancreatitis were equally likely to succeed nonoperative management as those without. Only initial pseudocyst size above 6 cm predicted eventual need for operation, though several patients with larger pseudocysts successfully avoided operation.

Vitas and Sarr (29) reported similar results from a retrospective review of pancreatic pseudocyst at their institution. About half of the patients underwent initial operative treatment, either for acute complication or severe or persistent symptoms. The remainder were treated initially without operation. Over time, about one-third of those under observation underwent subsequent operation, while two-thirds avoided operation altogether. Of those undergoing initial nonoperative treatment, only six developed complications (five requiring operation). Most subsequent operations were elective, often for symptoms attributable to underlying chronic pancreatitis. About half of patients with underlying chronic pancreatitis and pseudocyst managed expectantly succeeded nonoperative therapy. Long-term follow-up was incomplete in the nonoperated group; among those studied, pseudocyst resolution or shrinkage was radiographically documented in about half. Smaller pseudocysts were much more likely to resolve, but even those above 10 cm in diameter occasionally resolved.

Both of these studies challenge the established principle of mandatory drainage of pancreatic pseudocyst. Clearly, selected patients can safely be observed for long periods of time without operation. Resolution of the pseudocyst may occur even if the cyst is large or if that patient has chronic pancreatitis. In both studies, pseudocyst complications did occur, but all patients were salvaged by appropriate treatment. Can the relative safety and success of their expectant treatment be reconciled with the prevalent attitude favoring preventative operation? Perhaps the tertiary referral nature of these surgical practices may have weighted their case mix toward a more chronic and hence stable group. Also, the nature of the patient population under study, in each series, may have added to the confidence with which the authors withheld prophylactic surgical treatment. Nonoperative treatment requires that the patient recognize and immediately respond to symptoms of a potential complication. Notably, half or more of the patients in each series eventually underwent operation. Patients most likely to suffer complications may have been subjected to earlier operation, using standard surgical indications, thus resulting in a group of more stable pseudocysts for observation. In any event, these studies provide clear impetus for further exploration of the safety and outcome of expectant treatment.

Pancreatic pseudocysts have long been the surgeon's domain, and traditionally surgeons have recommended operations for all but the most innocent lesions. Percutaneous pseudocyst drainage and endoscopic pseudocyst drainage have now joined the therapeutic armamentarium. The relative roles of these three invasive methods, together with that of expectant management remain to be determined. It now seems certain that under strictly supervised controlled circumstances, prophylactic or gratuitous pseudocyst drainage may be avoided, and more definite criteria for pseudocyst management alternatives will be learned.

## REFERENCES

1. Bradley EL. A clinically based classification system for acute pancreatitis. Arch Surg 1993;128:586–590.
2. Yeo CJ, Sarr MG. Cystic and pseudocystic diseases of the pancreas. Curr Probl Surg 1994;31:187–243.
3. D'Egidio A, Schein M. Pancreatic pseudocysts: a proposed classification and its management implications. Br J Surg 1991; 78:981–984.
4. Grace PA, Williamson RCN. Modern management of pancreatic pseudocysts. Br J Surg 1993;80:573–581.
5. Warren WD, Marsh WH, Muller WH. Experimental production of pseudocysts of the pancreas with preliminary observation on internal drainage. Surg Gynecol Obstet 1957;105:385–392.
6. Ranson JHC, B.M., B.Ch., Balthazar E, Caccavale R, Cooper M. Computed tomography and the prediction of pancreatic abscess in acute pancreatitis. Ann Surg 1985;201:656–665.
7. Neoptolemos JP, London NJ, Carr-Locket DL. Assessment of main pancreatic duct integrity by endoscopic retrograde pancreatography in patients with acute pancreatitis. Br J Surg 1983;80: 94–99.
8. D'Egidio A, Schein M. Percutaneous drainage of pancreatic pseudocysts: a prospective study. World J Surg 1991;16:141–146.
9. Aranha GV, Prinz RA, Freeark RJ, Kruss DM, Greenlee HB. Evaluation of therapeutic options for pancreatic pseudocysts. Arch Surg 1982;117:717–721.
10. vanSonnenberg E, Wittich GR, Casola G, Brannigan TC, Karnel F, et al. Percutaneous drainage of infected and noninfected

pancreatic pseudocysts: experience in 101 cases. Radiology 1989;170:757–761.

11. Nealon WH, Townsend CM, Thompson JC. Preoperative endoscopic retrograde cholangiopancreatography (ERCP) in patients with pancreatic pseudocyst associated with resolving acute and chronic pancreatitis. Ann Surg 1989;209:532–540.
12. Warshaw AL, Rattner DW. Timing of surgical drainage for pancreatic pseudocysts. Clinical and chemical criteria. Ann Surg 1985;202:720–724.
13. Crass RA, Way LW. Acute and chronic pancreatic pseudocysts are different. Am J Surg 1981;142:660–663.
14. Bourliere M, Sarles H. Pancreatic cysts and pseudocysts associated with acute and chronic pancreatitis. Dig Dis Sci 1989;34: 343–348.
15. El Hamel A, Parc R, Adda G, Bouteloup PY, Huguet C, Malafosse M. Bleeding pseudocysts and pseudoaneurysms in chronic pancreatitis. Br J Surg 1991;78:1059–1063
16. Adams DB, Zellner JL, Anderson MC. Arterial hemorrhage complicating pancreatic pseudocysts: role of angiography. J Surg Res 1993;54:150–156.
17. Sankaran S, Walt AJ. The natural and unnatural history of pancreatic pseudocysts. Br J Surg 1975;62:37–44.
18. Mullins RJ, Malangoni MA, Bergamin TM, Casey JM, Richardson JD. Controversies in the management of pancreatic pseudocysts. Am J Surg 1988;155:165–172.
19. Bradley EL, Gonzales AC, Clements JL. Acute pancreatic pseudocysts. Incidence and implications. Ann Surg 1976;184:734–737.
20. Aranha GV, Prinz RA, Esguerra AC, Greenlee HB. The nature and course of cystic pancreatic lesions diagnosed by ultrasound. Arch Surg 1983;118:484–488.
21. Imrie CW, Buist LJ, Shearer MG. Importance of cause in the outcome of pancreatic pseudocysts. Am J Surg 1988;156:159–162.
22. Hiatt JR, Fink AS, King W, Pitt HA. Percutaneous aspiration of peripancreatic fluid collections: a safe method to detect infection. Surg 1987;101:523–529.
23. Behrman SW, Melvin WS, Ellison EC. Pancreatic pseudocysts following acute pancreatitis. Am J Surg 1996;172:228–231.
24. Nguyen BLT, Thompson JS, Edney JA, Bragg LE, Rikkers LF. Influence of the etiology of pancreatitis on the natural history of pancreatic pseudocysts. Am J Surg 1991;162:527–531.
25. Bradley EL, Clements JL, Gonzalez AC. The natural history of pancreatic pseudocysts: a unified concept of management. Am J Surg 1979;137:135–141.
26. Williams KJ, Fabian TC. Pancreatic pseudocyst. Recommendations for operative and nonoperative management. Am Surg 1992;58:199–205.
27. Munn JS, Aranha GV, Greenlee HB, Prinz RA. Simultaneous treatment of chronic pancreatitis and pancreatic pseudocyst. Arch Surg 1987;122:662–667.
28. Yeo CJ, Bastidas JA, Lynch-Nyhan A, Fishman EK, Zinner MJ, Cameron JL. The natural history of pancreatic pseudocysts documented by computed tomography. Surg Gynecol Obstet 1990;170:411–417.
29. Vitas GJ, Sarr MG. Selected management of pancreatic pseudocysts: operative versus expectant management. Surgery 1992;111:123–130.

# 44

# *Treatment of Pancreatic Pseudocysts*

Harvey L. Bumpers and Edward L. Bradley, III

***The fascination that pseudocysts hold for surgeons is beyond understanding.***
Robert M. Zolinger, Sr.

Surgeons have long held an active interest in the management of pancreatic pseudocysts. In fact, the first recorded attempt at surgical therapy for pseudocysts was in 1865 when LeDentu attempted transcutaneous drainage with a trocar. Unfortunately, this approach resulted in peritonitis and death. Alternative methods of pseudocyst drainage such as cystogastrostomy (Jedlicka, 1921), transduodenal cystoduodenostomy (Kirschner, 1923), cystojejunostomy-in-continuity (Henle and Hahn, 1927), and cystojejunostomy Roux-en-Y (Koenig, 1946) were subsequently introduced (1).

While precise documentation is lacking, it has been estimated that 5000–7000 new cases of pancreatic pseudocysts are discovered each year in America in the clinical setting of acute pancreatitis. In addition, more than half of all patients with an established diagnosis of chronic pancreatitis will develop a pseudocyst at some time during the course of the disease. Thus, it is extremely likely that practicing general surgeons will encounter several such patients during their careers. When this prevalence is combined with the complexities inherent in the subject matter, opportunities for clinical errors in diagnosis and management become apparent. The necessity for maintaining and improving one's database is clear.

While few would question the overall efficacy and safety of surgical cystenteric drainage (see below), opinions and fashions change, fluctuations that often lead to the introduction of alternative methods of treatment. Furthermore, in recent years there has been a truly remarkable evolution in disease definitions, terminology, and technology with respect to the diagnosis and therapy of pancreatic disease. Particularly noteworthy in this regard have been the recent advances in endoscopic therapy. Few observers doubt that endoscopic surgery will become of increasing importance in the future management of pancreatic disease.

As a result of these rapid developments, the optimal method of management for patients with pancreatic pseudocysts is once again in question. It is our intention to address these issues in this chapter and to clarify some of the currently existing confusion in the choice of management options.

## DEFINITIONS, TERMINOLOGY, AND CLINICAL SIGNIFICANCE

It is axiomatic that optimal therapy depends upon precision in diagnosis. In turn, precision in diagnosis requires accurate definitions of disease. The working definitions of peripancreatic fluid collections, acute and chronic pseudocysts, and pancreatic abscess offered by the Atlanta International Symposium represent an important advance in clinical patient management:

> Acute Pseudocyst. A collection of pancreatic juice enclosed by a wall of fibrous or granulation tissue arising as a consequence of acute pancreatitis or pancreatic trauma. On imaging studies they are *round* or *oval*, and have a well defined wall. Their formation requires *four or more weeks* after onset of acute pancreatitis or injury. They are usually rich in pancreatic enzymes, and most often sterile (2)

The series of clinically based definitions from the Atlanta Symposium have attempted to distinguish between acute pseudocysts, acute pancreatic fluid collections (peripancreatic fluid collections of less than 4-weeks duration arising in conjunction with an episode of acute pancreatitis), and chronic pseudocysts (pseudocysts developing in patients with chronic pancreatitis). Since optimal management of these three conditions may differ markedly, these distinctions are not merely academic exercises in taxonomy but, in fact, are critical for optimum patient care. Acute pancreatic fluid collections rarely require any form of therapy, since spontaneous resolution is the rule. Alternatively, acute and chronic pseudocysts may or may not require therapy, depending upon a number of other factors.

The single most common problem encountered in the clinical management of patients with presumed "pancreatic pseudocysts" is that the definitive diagnosis of a pancreatic pseudocyst is confounded by the large number of lesions that can clinically masquerade as pseudocysts (Table 44.1). Ill-advised internal drainage of a cystic neoplasm under the mistaken label of "pseudocyst" results in gross undertreatment of a potential malignancy (3) (Fig. 44.1). Similarly, internal drainage of a localized collection of pancreatic or parapancreatic necrosis under the guise of "pseudocyst" may lead to secondary infection, anastomotic dehiscence, and death (Fig. 44.2).

Since the current state of imaging technology with endoscopic retrograde cholangiopancreatography (ERCP), ultrasound, computed tomography (CT) scanning, and magnetic resonance imaging (MRI) does *not* permit precise distinction between pancreatic pseudocysts and other cystic lesions of the pancreas and since approximately 20% of "pseudocysts" will eventually turn out to be another type of lesion, the wisest therapeutic course is to consider all radiologic diagnoses of "pseudocyst" with great caution. In particular, beware of the imaging diagnosis of "pseudocyst" in a middle-aged female with no antecedent

**TABLE 44.1. Pancreatic and Parapancreatic Cystic Lesions That Have Masqueraded As Pancreatic Pseudocysts**

True cysts
- Enterogenous cyst
- Solitary cyst
- Dermoid cyst
- Lymphoepithelial cyst
- Cystic fibrosis
- Von Hippel-Lindau disease
- Endometrial cyst

Neoplastic cysts
- Serous cystadenoma
- Mucinous cystadenoma
- Cystadenocarcinoma
- Papillary cystic neoplasm
- Solid malignancies with central cavitation (lymphoma, endocrine tumors, adenocarcinoma, choriocarcinoma, sarcomas)

Miscellaneous
- Postpancreatitic necrotic collections
- Hydatid cyst
- Choledochal cyst
- Juxtapancreatic aneurysms

Senior author's personal experience.

history of pancreatitis (cystic neoplasm is a strong possibility). Precise differentiation between a cystic neoplasm and a pseudocyst can often be accomplished by analysis of cyst fluid obtained by transcutaneous aspiration (4) (Table 44.2). Failure to recognize that a "pseudocyst" is in fact a localized collection of necrosis permits the possibility of internal drainage into a loop of bowel, with the subsequent potential for secondary infection and ultimate anastomotic dehiscence. Until you have reason to believe otherwise, in all patients with severe acute pancreatitis it is wisest to consider that a "pseudocyst" may in reality be localized pancreatic necrosis. Localized collections of pancreatic necrosis can often be distinguished from pseudocysts by high CT densities (>15 Hounsfield units (HU)), as opposed to "water densities" (<10 HU), which are commonly seen in pseudocysts.

In brief, an imaging diagnosis of "pancreatic pseudocyst" should always be taken with a grain of salt, and the clinical context in which the "pseudocyst" arises should be carefully integrated into the working diagnosis. Few experienced pancreatic surgeons have not been faced with complications attributable to an improper surgical procedure based upon an erroneous imaging diagnosis of "pseudocyst"—either internally drained malignancies or massive retroperitoneal infections from anastomotic dehiscence and iatrogenic secondary infection of sterile pancreatic necrosis. Clearly, an informed surgeon is the antidote to such misadventures, and close communication with the consulting radiologist is strongly advised.

## ELECTIVE THERAPY OF PANCREATIC PSEUDOCYSTS

In general, the clinician can choose from among four major approaches to the elective therapy of pancreatic pseudocysts:

1. Observation
2. Endoscopic therapy
   a. Transpapillary drainage
   b. Transenteric drainage
   c. Laparoscopic surgical techniques
3. Radiologic therapy
   a. Transcutaneous aspiration
   b. Indwelling catheter drainage
   c. Transenteric prosthetic devices
4. Open surgery
   a. Resection
   b. Internal drainage

How does one select the optimal approach from among these possible options? In actual clinical practice, there are indications for each of these approaches in specific patients, and the accomplished surgical practitioner matches the approach to the patient rather than attempting to apply one particular approach to all patients. Only by learning the relative merits and limitations of each approach, however, can informed treatment decisions be made.

### Observation

The natural history of a disease can markedly affect the indications for therapy. Furthermore, before instituting any form of interventional therapy, one must know whether *any* form of therapy is superior to *no* therapy; i.e., the null treatment option.

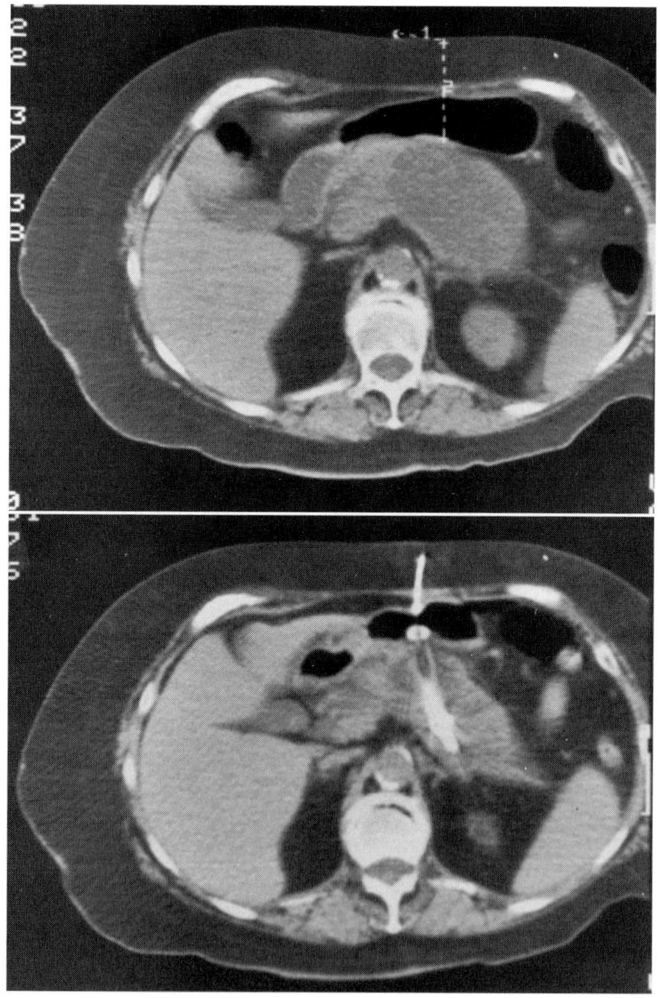

**FIG. 44.1.** Cystic lesion in body and tail of the pancreas, which was assigned a radiologic diagnosis of "pseudocyst" *(top)*. Transcutaneous transgastric placement of double ballooned prosthetic device to effect transgastric drainage. No biopsy was obtained. The "pseudocyst" was subsequently discovered by gastroscopic biopsy to be a cystadenocarcinoma requiring en bloc pancreatectomy, gastrectomy, and resection of the abdominal wall.

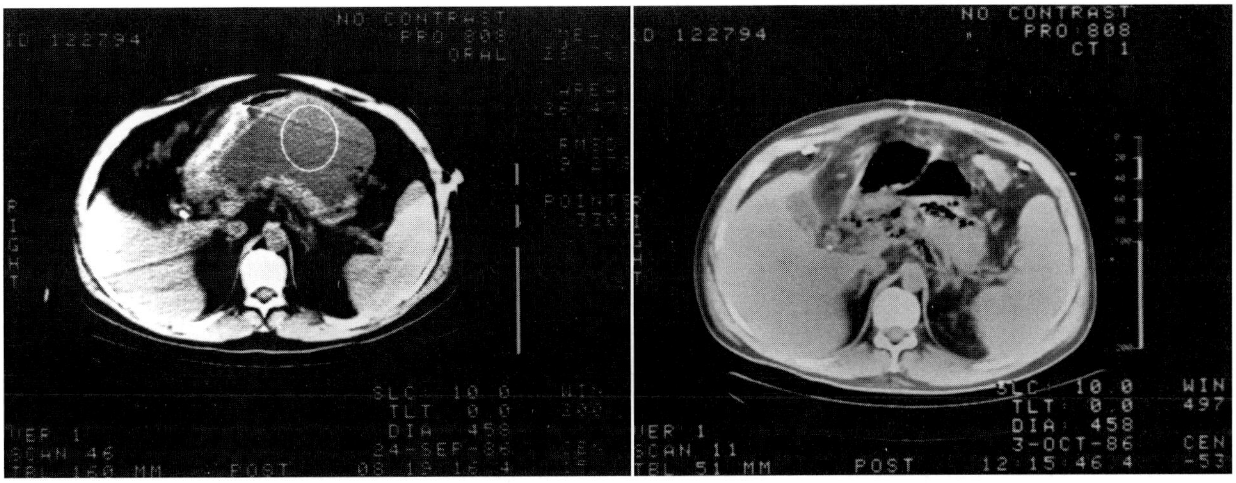

**FIG. 44.2.** CT diagnosis of a "pseudocyst" in a patient with severe acute pancreatitis, despite a tissue density within the cursor of 33 HU and findings compatible with pancreatic necrosis *(left)*. Subsequent "cystogastrostomy" eventuated in dehiscence of the gastric anastomosis and the development of infected pancreatic necrosis (note extensive retroperitoneal infection and air bubbles on the film on the *right*).

Or as one of our surgical forebears once said, "God heals; the doctor takes the money."

In 1979, we reported the first *prospective* series of patients with untreated pancreatic pseudocysts (5). Some 54 patients, diagnosed by sonography, were followed weekly by serial sonograms, from onset to more than 19 weeks. Eleven patients (20%) experienced spontaneous resolution of the "pseudocyst" within the first 6 weeks after formation. With the perspective of today's definitions, these spontaneous fluid resolutions occurred in patients with acute pancreatic fluid collections and lacked the requisite fibrous wall to become pseudocysts. In contrast to these early resolutions, only one spontaneous resolution occurred after 6 weeks of observation (now more properly called an acute pseudocyst). Moreover, the incidence of complications (rupture, abscess, common duct obstruction, and fistulas) seemed to increase with the length of observation.

The observed complication rates were 21% (0–6 weeks), 46% (7–12 weeks), 60% (12–18 weeks), and 67% (>19 weeks). The overall mortality rate was 12%, and 22 patients (41%) experienced a serious complication. It was concluded that the risk of observation exceeded the risk of surgery after 6 weeks of observation.

More recently, two *retrospective* studies have suggested that prolonged observation of pancreatic pseudocysts is not as dangerous as our older study predicted. Yeo et al. (6) retrospectively reviewed 75 patients treated for pancreatic pseudocyst, of whom 36 were treated by observation alone. These observed patients with mature pseudocysts were all asymptomatic and were followed serially with CT scans for a mean of 1 year. The findings indicated that spontaneous resolution occurred in 60% of cases and that the pseudocyst remained stable or decreased in size in 40%. There was only one complication, a case of self-limited intracystic hemorrhage, which could be attributed to long-term observation. However, substantial differences were noted between the operative and nonoperative groups, suggesting treatment selection bias. In particular, pseudocysts were much smaller in the nonoperative group, averaging approximately 5.8 cm. In the second retrospective study, Vitas and Sarr (7) considered operative treatment of "asymptomatic" pancreatic pseudocysts. They reviewed the clinical outcome of 68 patients with asymptomatic pseudocysts and found that 63% remained healthy after a follow-up averaging 51 months. Although the serious complication rate of 9% was higher than that reported in Yeo's study, it was low compared with current expectation. Twenty-four (35%) of their patients were forced to undergo operative therapy for definitive treatment of the pseudocyst or a complication during the period of observation. As in the Baltimore study, most of the pseudocysts that resolved were 5 cm or less, suggesting that patient selection appears crucial to obtaining good results with persistent observation. The data from these recent retrospective studies are summarized in Table 44.3.

How can we reconcile the relative safety of persistent observation in the retrospective studies with the adverse results attributed to nonsurgical treatment in our earlier prospective study? Perhaps the most important determinant of results is that of size; pseudocysts in the retrospective studies were relatively small. It has been known for many years that small pseudocysts rarely cause problems. Secondly, patients in the retrospective series were "asymptomatic," and pseudocysts were often discovered by CT or MRI; in the older study, all patients were symptomatic and were discovered by sonography. Finally, since *all* patients in the two retrospective series were not observed, a

**TABLE 44.2. Biochemical Differentiation of Cystic Pancreatic Neoplasms from Pseudocysts**

| Diagnosis | Viscosity | CEA | CA 125 | Enzyme Levels | Cytology |
|---|---|---|---|---|---|
| Pseudocyst | Low | Low | Low | High | Negative |
| Serous cystadenoma | Low | Low | Variable | Variable | Negative |
| Mucinous cystadenoma | Usually high | High | Variable | Variable | Usually positive |
| Cystadenocarcinoma | High | High | High | Variable | Usually positive |

Adapted from Lewandrowski K, Southern JF, Pins UR, et al. Cyst fluid analysis in the differential diagnosis of pancreatic pseudocysts, cystadenomas, and cystadenocarcinomas. Ann Surg 1993; 217:41–47.

**TABLE 44.3. Asymptomatic Pancreatic Pseudocysts: Results of Recent Retrospective Studies**

| | Yeo et al., 1990 | Vitas and Sarr, 1992 |
|---|---|---|
| Number of patients | 75 | 114 |
| Number treated medically | 36 (48%) | 68 (60%) |
| Number of complications | 1 (3%) | 6 (9%) |
| Number requiring surgery | 0 | 24 (24%) |
| Average follow-up | 12 months | 51 months |
| Average size | 5.8 cm | 4.9 cm |

real possibility exists for treatment selection bias. Were patients with small pseudocysts preferentially chosen for observation? Do asymptomatic patients with pseudocysts have a different clinical course from patients who are symptomatic? Since the answers to these and other questions are presently unknown, the efficacy and safety of persistent observation of pancreatic pseudocysts, compared with operative intervention, cannot be known. Until prospective randomized data are available to address these issues, how should we proceed?

Although observation has been recommended for the asymptomatic pseudocyst, many other factors must be considered before it is adopted as the primary means of managing these lesions. Asymptomatic pancreatic pseudocysts managed by observation alone should probably be under 6 cm. However, since spontaneous resolution is rare after 2 months (8), consideration should be given to intervention after this time. Pseudocysts larger than 6 cm, those increasing in size or failing to resolve, symptomatic pseudocysts, and those associated with common duct obstruction, infection, or hemorrhage, should be managed differently.

Octreotide acetate, a long-acting analogue of somatostatin and inhibitor of pancreatic secretion, has been used in the observational treatment of pancreatic pseudocysts. Since octreotide affects pancreatic exocrine function by decreasing the secretion of gastrointestinal tract hormones that stimulate pancreatic secretion, pancreatic secretory pressure into the pseudocyst may be reduced. Furthermore, it directly binds to somatostatin receptors on acinar cells to reduce their secretions. Although Gullo and Barbara reported a decrease in pseudocyst diameter and symptomatic relief of pain in a small series of pseudocysts after therapeutic dosages of octreotide (9), not enough data exist to allow definitive conclusions regarding the effectiveness of octreotide as a primary method of treating these pancreatic lesions.

In summary, patients in absolute need of interventional therapy can usually be identified by symptoms of pain, gastric outlet obstruction, an inability to tolerate oral feeding, fever, or jaundice due to bile duct obstruction. Acute pancreatic pseudocysts that are symptomatic, larger than 6 cm, or expanding usually necessitate intervention. Because of the severity of complications arising from chronic pseudocysts and relative infrequency of their spontaneous resolution, it is recommended that they be drained shortly after diagnosis.

## Endoscopic Therapy

Endoscopy has engendered multiple techniques for drainage of pancreatic pseudocysts. Through the use of endoscopy, pseudocysts can be drained via the stomach, duodenum, or pancreatic duct. These procedures include transpapillary drainage, transenteric drainage, and laparoscopic surgical techniques. Although these procedures have been employed on an elective basis to treat pseudocysts, principal and persuasive argument for these techniques centers around issues concerning critically ill patients who cannot tolerate a lengthy surgical procedure. Evaluation of the use of laparoscopy as a therapeutic maneuver for draining pancreatic pseudocysts has been limited by the paucity of published information and the anecdotal character of the reports.

***Transpapillary drainage.*** ERCP is necessary prior to any planned drainage of pseudocysts via the pancreatic duct. Pancreatography identifies the ductal anatomy and establishes the existence of any communication between the pancreatic duct and the pseudocyst. Clearly, noncommunicating pseudocysts do not lend themselves to successful transpapillary drainage. Precautions must be taken during the ERCP to prevent complications. It is highly recommended that these patients have antibiotic protection during the procedure and that some form of drainage be carried out within 24 hours after identifying a communication, to decrease the risk of infection and abscess formation.

An internal stent is often used to treat an established communicating pseudocyst. The stent is placed in the duodenum, through the papilla, and across the ductal disruption into the pseudocyst. Though more cumbersome and less desirable from the patient's point of view, a nasopancreatic drain can also be used. Sphincterotomy used in conjunction with stenting allows easier manipulations, but it is often unnecessary. Kozarek et al. treated 18 patients by transpapillary stenting, with initial resolution of 89% of ductal disruptions and 86% of the peripancreatic fluid collections (10). However, after 16 months of follow-up, seven patients (40%) had required open surgical intervention. These findings suggest that widespread use of the transpapillary technique will be unlikely and that indications may become restricted to those too critically ill for surgery. Another potential limitation to this mode of therapy is the rapid development of pancreatic ductal stenosis, thought to be induced by mechanical abrasion of the plastic stent against the ductal mucosa (11).

***Transenteric drainage.*** Endoscopic drainage between the intestinal lumen and the interior of a pseudocyst depends on firm inflammatory adherence between the pseudocyst and the gastrointestinal tract. Unlike the added security provided by suturing during open procedures, endoscopic transenteric cystenterostomies depend entirely on endogenous adhesions to prevent dehiscence. In the senior author's experience with 156 operated patients, firm adherence between the pseudocyst and the intestinal tract was found in only 42% of the patients and usually involved the stomach. In the absence of such adherence, separation of the intestinal tract from the pseudocyst is possible, a complication that would result in uncontrolled pancreatic and intestinal fistulas.

CT scanning or ultrasonography can be used to determine whether the pseudocyst is close enough to the enteric wall to allow transenteric drainage. Once the point of maximal bulging into the gastrointestinal lumen is located, the cyst is punctured with the diathermic needle. This opening can be lengthened with a sphincterotomy wire and functions as a cystenterostomy (12). Cremer et al. have reported excellent success with this procedure in 33 patients, observing only two complications and no mortality (13). Transenteric cystenterostomy was definitive treatment in 80% of his patients. Unfortunately, the experience of others has not been as favorable, with major complication rates of 20% and above (12, 14, 15). Hemorrhage, sepsis, peritonitis, and stent plugging lead the list of complications. Death has been reported on several occasions. While it is apparent that this procedure can provide effective therapy, further studies are necessary to determine if the benefits outweigh the risks.

***Laparoscopy.*** Minimally invasive surgery has been used in the drainage of pancreatic pseudocysts (15, 16). Experience with laparoscopy and these pancreatic lesions is still at a very early stage. Since most of the difficulties encountered in applying laparoscopic approaches to internal drainage of pancreatic pseudocysts are technical, it is likely that the development of new instrumentation and innovative approaches will one day give laparoscopic surgical techniques a prominent place in management.

## Radiologic Therapy

Management of the pancreatic pseudocyst by interventional radiologic techniques has enjoyed comparatively widespread enthusiasm. Radiologic drainage has been the main mode of treatment for poor-risk patients in need of pseudocyst drainage. These are also the procedures of choice for managing acute pancreatic fluid collections that are symptomatic, infected, or expanding. Acute fluid collections that are less than 4 weeks old cannot be confidently expected to hold sutures and allow safe internal drainage by means of cystenteric anastomosis. Drainage can be performed under the guidance of CT scanning, ultrasonography, or fluoroscopy.

***Percutaneous aspiration.*** Simple aspiration has been effective as a diagnostic tool for peripancreatic fluid collections but has proved wholly inadequate as definitive therapy for pancreatic pseudocysts. Despite the attractiveness of simple aspiration, the observed recurrence rate of 70% is unacceptable. Chronic pseudocysts have thick walls and cannot be completely collapsed by simple aspiration. Perhaps another problem hindering the effectiveness of this technique is the fact that 40–60% of pseudocysts have ductal communication. This results in rapid reaccumulation of cystic fluid, usually within 24 hours after simple aspiration (17).

***Percutaneous catheter drainage (PCD).*** PCD has proved much more effective than simple aspiration and in some institutions has become the therapeutic procedure of choice. Since the original description in 1976, the technique of PCD has flourished with the improvements in radiologic instrumentation and catheter designs. A 7- to 12-French pigtail catheter is percutaneously guided into the pseudocyst over a needle-inserted guide wire under the direction of ultrasound, CT scan, or fluoroscopy. Accepted indications for using PCD are symptomatic patients too ill for surgery, symptomatic immature pseudocysts, and infected pseudocysts. However, the presence of necrosis in the infected pseudocyst may severely hamper the success of this procedure, because the content of these pseudocysts is too thick and is accompanied by tissue debris that prevents adequate drainage through the relatively small catheter.

Success rates for PCD over the past 20 years have been reported to average approximately 70% of cases. However, Criado et al. reported a success rate of only 21%, and most (60%) of their patients required subsequent surgery (18). Depending on the complexity of the pseudocyst, indwelling catheter drainage time to resolution ranged from 7 days in a simple pseudocyst to 210 days in a large communicating pseudocyst. The average time of catheter drainage in this series was 48 days, which is similar to results from other studies. Pancreatic pseudocysts resulting from acute alcoholic pancreatitis seem to be a special case in that they are much less responsive to PCD, often requiring as long as 6 months for resolution, if it occurs at all. Problems with PCD are also encountered with multiloculated or multiple pseudocysts. Adams et al. (19) reported two patients in their series with two pseudocysts each. Although the patients received double catheters to drain each pseudocyst, this was unsuccessful in both patients, and subsequent internal drainage was necessary. This observation suggests that an initial open surgical approach is better for multiple and loculated pseudocysts.

Morbidity rates for PCD range as high as 40%, even though mortality rates are low, with most workers reporting no mortality (18–20). In a comparison of internal drainage and PCD (18), overall morbidity was found to be much higher with PCD (39%) than with surgery (17%). Many PCD patients developed persistent pancreatic fistulas, and 50% developed catheter site infections. Thus, the disadvantages that accompany PCD must be considered, including catheter-related site infections, hemorrhage, fistulas, and long-term failures requiring surgery as definitive treatment. Perhaps the major disadvantage of PCD is the creation of pancreatic fistulas that often require 6 weeks or more to close and often lead to catheter-related infections (21). Skin contaminants account for most of these catheter-related infections; *Staphylococcus aureus*, the usual microorganism, responds well to antibiotics. Among other less frequently encountered complications are pneumothorax, sheared-off radiologic guide wire, empyema, and myocardial infarction.

Octreotide has shown some success as an adjunctive treatment in the patient with PCD (22, 23). The addition of octreotide to PCD shows promise in accelerating closure of pancreatic fistulas (24), which often complicate PCD. This potent inhibitor of pancreatic secretion significantly decreases fistula drainage via percutaneous catheters, leading to diminished necessity for long-term catheterization.

PCD has an undisputed role in the primary treatment of pancreatic pseudocysts. Moreover, an interdisciplinary approach between radiologists and surgeons is usually in the best interests of the patient. However, PCD should probably not be used in the following circumstances: whenever a communication has been demonstrated between the pancreatic duct and a pseudocyst (to avoid creation of a long-term pancreatic fistula), whenever a cystic pancreatic neoplasm cannot be reliably excluded (to avoid transcutaneous drainage of a malignancy), in patients with acute pancreatic fluid collections without clinical evidence of infection (most resolve spontaneously), whenever a chronic pseudocyst is associated with common duct obstruction or dilation of the main pancreatic duct (open surgery is required for combined lesions), and in the presence of pancreatic ascites or the suspicion of intracystic hemorrhage (frequent indications for surgery). Final resolution of the role of PCD versus open surgical drainage awaits appropriately designed clinical studies.

## Open Surgery

The indications for open surgery in patients with pancreatic pseudocysts are controversial. In the opinion of the authors, open surgical drainage is preferable to all other forms of management for symptomatic patients with persistent pseudocysts larger than 5 cm. However, as evidenced by the wealth of treatment options listed above, agreement is not uniform. Nevertheless, most surgeons would agree that an open surgical approach is usually chosen for all patients with *recurrent* pseudocysts, pseudocysts combined with *common duct* or *duodenal stenosis,* symptomatic pseudocysts associated with a *dilated pancreatic duct,* or those "pseudocysts" for which a diagnosis of *cystic neoplasm* cannot be excluded.

The role of routine preoperative ERCP is also controversial. Although a few workers have advocated routine preoperative pancreatography to detect unsuspected associated lesions (25), cholangiopancreatography is not without risk. Moreover, a thorough exploration at the time of surgery, which includes evaluation of the duodenum, palpation of the gall bladder and the common duct, and ballottement of the pancreatic duct, can provide the same information as ERCP in the usual pancreatic pseudocyst. Since pancreatography can indeed be helpful in the complicated or recurrent case, we recommend the selective use of endoscopic pancreatography. Because it is possible to introduce bacteria into the pseudocyst by means of the endoscope, we advise broad-spectrum antibiotic coverage during pancreatography and elective surgical drainage within 24 hours after ERCP. Despite some claims to the contrary, the mere presence of bacteria on a gram stain of aspirated pseudocyst fluid is not an indication for abandoning internal drainage. Unless the patient is septic or frank pus is obtained when the pseudocyst is incised, internal drainage can still be safely carried out. It is our practice

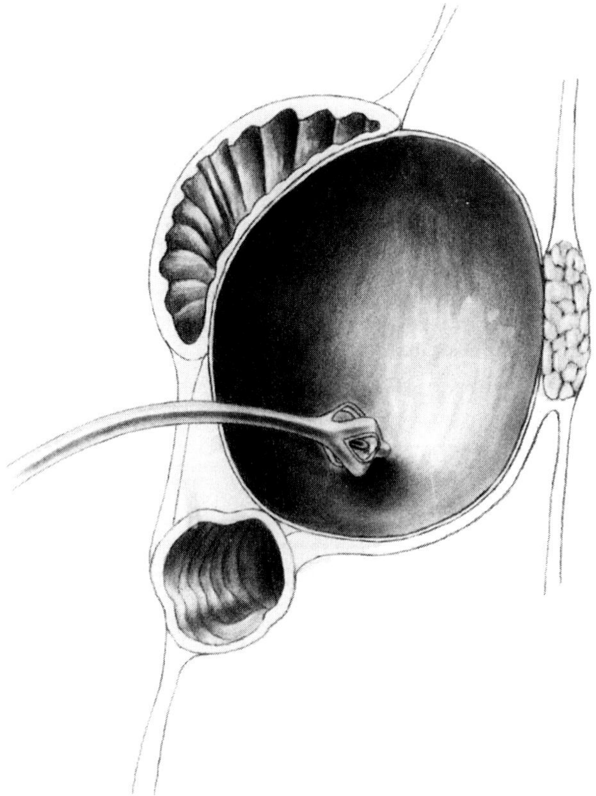

**FIG. 44.3.** Transverse depiction of external drainage of a pseudocyst using a large mushroom catheter. Use of this technique is now largely restricted to thin-walled pseudocysts incapable of holding sutures and frankly infected pseudocysts. (Used with permission from Bradley EL III, Zeppa R. The Pancreas (Chapter 37). Davis-Christopher Textbook of Surgery, 13th ed. DC Sabiston, ed. W.B. Saunders, Philadelphia, PA. 1986.)

to use a hyperosmotic mechanical bowel preparation the night before surgery and systemic antibiotics on call, as the surgical approach to an individual lesion must occasionally be extended beyond cystenteric drainage.

Regardless of the chosen technique of surgical drainage, a biopsy of the cyst wall *must* be obtained. Finding *any* type of endothelium in the wall of the "pseudocyst" means that the lesion is actually a true cyst or a cystic neoplasm, rather than a pseudocyst. In the vast majority of cases, the simple expedient of obtaining a frozen section of the cyst wall will prevent the inadvertent anastomosis of a neoplastic cyst to the uninvolved gastrointestinal tract.

For most uncomplicated pancreatic pseudocysts, a midline incision is satisfactory. For all other situations, we prefer a subcostal incision, which can be extended to bisubcostal if necessary. Complete exposure of the pancreas is one of the major keys to success in pancreatic surgery. Not only is technical performance facilitated, but associated lesions are frequent, and many can be found only with appropriate exposure. It is well to keep in mind that 8–10% of patients harbor multiple pseudocysts, and a thorough exploration is mandatory to prevent "recurrence."

Depending upon individual associated findings, such as gallstones, common duct stricture, main pancreatic duct dilation, duodenal obstruction, or multiple pseudocysts, cyst drainage may need to be combined with another procedure designed to address the associated condition (26). Choledochoduodenostomy is often chosen to relieve common duct obstruction due to chronic pancreatitis in patients undergoing pseudocyst drainage. As an alternative when local duodenal conditions prevent common duct–duodenal anastomosis, choledochojejunostomy can often be performed with the same Roux limb that is used to drain the pseudocyst. Similarly, a dilated pancreatic duct associated with a pseudocyst can often be approached by using the same Roux limb to drain both the pseudocyst and the pancreatic duct. Multiple pseudocysts can be individually drained into the same Roux limb.

Five techniques for pseudocyst drainage are available when elective open surgery is chosen for uncomplicated pseudocysts:

1. External drainage
2. Cystogastrostomy
3. Cystoduodenostomy
4. Cystojejunostomy
5. Resection

The choice of one of the specific forms of internal drainage is usually made on the basis of the anatomic location of the pseudocyst. In general, the pseudocyst should be drained into the closest intestinal segment. External drainage is reserved for unexpectedly complicated lesions, while resection is often chosen for pseudocysts that have recurred.

**External Drainage.** Although frequently used in the past, external drainage has few current adherents (27). The principal disadvantages to external drainage are *(a)* the potential for hemorrhage from mechanical abrasion by the drainage tube, *(b)* the frequent development of secondary infection, and *(c)* creation of a long-term pancreatic fistula. As a result of these deficiencies, today external drainage of pancreatic pseudocysts is used principally when a misdiagnosis has been made, when the risk of anastomotic dehiscence is high because of an unantici-

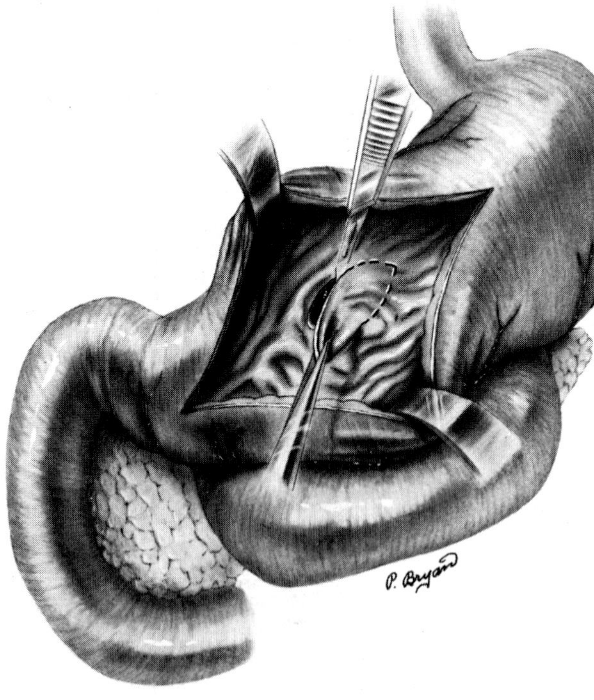


**FIG. 44.4.** Technique of cystogastrostomy demonstrating length of incision through the fused posterior gastric-pseudocyst common wall. In the absence of such inflammatory fusion, Roux-en-Y cystojejunostomy should be done. (Used with permission from Bradley EL III, Zeppa R. The Pancreas (Chapter 37). Davis-Christopher Textbook of Surgery, 13th ed. DC Sabiston, ed. W.B. Saunders, Philadelphia, PA. 1986.)

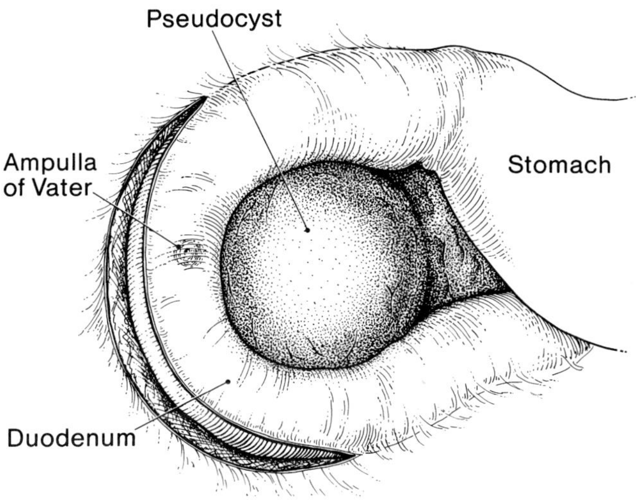


**FIG. 44.5.** An ideal candidate for cystoduodenostomy: a large *pseudocyst* in close proximity to the third portion of the *duodenum*. Note the extensive Kocher maneuver.

pated infected pseudocyst, or when an unexpectedly immature wall is discovered that is judged to be incapable of holding sutures. The technique is best performed by placing a large-bore catheter (20 French or greater) into the pseudocyst cavity through an omental apron (Fig. 44.3). When the pseudocyst has resolved, a smaller catheter may be exchanged for long-term drainage if drainage fluid amylase levels continue to be elevated. In the absence of a demonstrated pancreatic fistula, infection, or a persistent pseudocyst, the tube may be pulled in 2–3 weeks.

**Cystogastrostomy.** Cystogastrostomy is chosen whenever the pseudocyst abuts the posterior gastric wall. In one sense, it is not an anastomosis between the posterior gastric wall and the pseudocyst; the best results are obtained when inflammatory adherence already exists between the stomach and the pseudocyst. To evaluate whether or not the requisite adherence is present, the gastrocolic omentum is opened, and the exploring hand is placed into the lesser sac. In the absence of such adhesion, it is wiser to substitute a retrocolic cystojejunostomy Roux-en-Y. One group (28) recommends against cystojejunostomy for giant pseudocysts (>15 cm), attributing their less desirable results with cystogastrostomy in these cases to nondependent drainage. Others have experienced little difficulty with incomplete drainage in giant cysts managed by cystogastrostomy (29). Our choice with giant pseudocysts is most often Roux-en-Y cystojejunostomy.

It is our opinion that cystogastrostomy should also be abandoned whenever evidence of splenic vein obstruction (dilated gastroepiploic vein, enlarged short gastric veins, marked venous bleeding from anterior gastrotomy) is noted. High pressure in the veins of the gastric wall is a predisposing condition for postoperative hemorrhage. Postoperative bleeding is decidedly more common after cystogastrostomy than after other forms of internal drainage, and efforts must be made to prevent its development.

Once cyst-gastric adherence extending over the length of the proposed cystotomy has been demonstrated, the anterior gastric wall is incised with electrocautery for 5 cm (Fig. 44.4). Two large stay sutures are then placed through the combined posterior gastric-pseudocyst wall to facilitate the proposed incision through the posterior gastric wall into the pseudocyst. Using the electrocautery, a 5–10 cm incision in the long axis of the stomach is made into the pseudocyst. Interrupted figure-of-eight sutures of 2-0 controlled-absorption sutures are used liberally through the combined posterior gastric and pseudocyst wall to control bleeding vessels and prevent postoperative hemorrhage. No pancreatic drainage is required. With effective drainage, pseudocysts are usually undetectable by the 2nd week.

**Cystoduodenostomy.** Cystoduodenostomy is chosen whenever the pseudocyst abuts the medial (mesenteric) wall of the duodenum. In the past, cystoduodenostomy was considered a dangerous operation because of a high incidence of anastomotic dehiscence, hemorrhage, and duodenal obstruction. In an earlier work, we determined that these complications were largely attributable to the relatively high-tension on laterolateral cystoduodenal anastomoses and that transduodenal cystoduodenostomy is a comparatively safe and effective procedure (30).

Transduodenal cystoduodenostomy, although actually a cystotomy, is more technically demanding than the other forms of internal drainage, since both the greater and lesser ampullae, the common bile duct, and the anterior and posterior gastroduodenal arteries must be avoided. Following an extensive Kocher maneuver, the proposed site of cystoduodenotomy is chosen to protect the ampulla (Fig. 44.5). Usually, this will be distal to the ampulla of Vater. The lateral duodenum is opened longitudinally, and the distance between the medial duodenal wall and the interior of the pseudocyst is estimated by the distance a needle must pass through the medial duodenal wall and pancreatic tissue before encountering pseudocyst fluid. If more than 1 cm of pancreatic tissue must be traversed, cystoduodenotomy is abandoned, and cystojejunostomy Roux-en-Y substituted. If the pseudocyst is within the required proximity to the medial duodenal wall, electrocautery is used to enter the pseudocyst cavity through the medial wall of the duodenum. When making the duodenocystotomy, the plane of entry into the pseudocyst must be kept midway between the anterior and posterior surfaces of the head of the pancreas to avoid the pancreatoduodenal arteries (Fig. 44.6). The incision should be 5 cm in length.

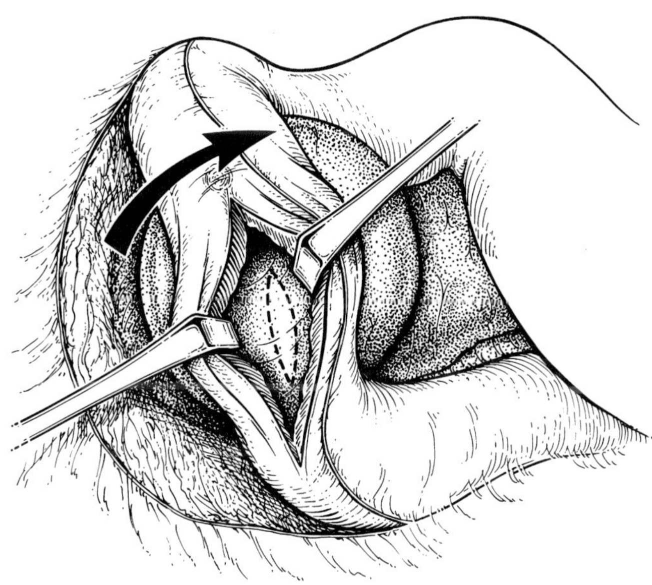

**FIG. 44.6.** Technique of transduodenal cystoduodenostomy. It is important to keep the incision in the medial duodenal wall midway between the anterior and posterior surfaces. Note that the ampulla (just under the *arrow*) is safely out of the way.

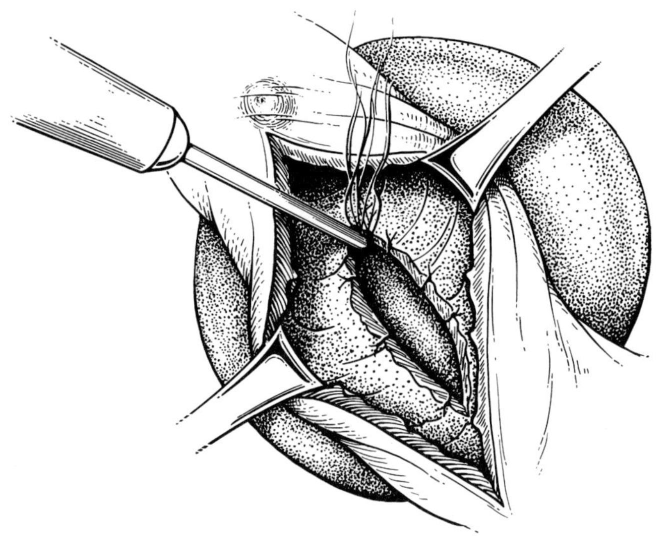

**FIG. 44.7.** Transduodenal cystoduodenostomy. Note the length of the incision through the medial duodenal wall into the pseudocyst and the use of interrupted hemostatic sutures. In contrast to the transduodenal approach, laterolateral cystoduodenostomy is accompanied by markedly increased risk and should rarely be done.

Hemostatic figure-of-eight sutures should be applied to the duodenal and cyst wall as described for cystogastrostomy (Fig. 44.7). Drainage of the duodenal closure is recommended for 3–4 days or until oral feeding is well tolerated.

**Cystojejunostomy.** While cystojejunostomy can be performed by means of an in-continuity anastomosis between the pseudocyst and the jejunum (Braun anastomosis), the preferred anastomotic technique today is a Roux-en-Y, via a subcolic or retrocolic approach. Advocates of in-continuity open surgical or laparoscopic cystojejunostomy cite ease and speed (16). However, the risks associated with dehiscence or leakage of an in-continuity anastomosis (activated pancreatic fistula, intestinal fistula, abscess formation) far exceed the risks of dehiscence or leakage of a properly performed Roux-en-Y (unactivated pancreatic fistula). For this reason, the overwhelming majority of surgeons prefer the Roux anastomosis.

If the pseudocyst is presenting through the base of the mesocolon and if care is taken to avoid the middle colic vessels, the cystotomy can be placed subcolically through the transverse mesocolon. Using the electrocautery, a minimal 5-cm incision is made through the mesocolon into the cyst. If the pseudocyst does not present through the mesocolon, a retrocolic Roux Y limb is carried up to the inferior surface of the cyst by means of a hole in the transverse mesocolon (Fig. 44.8). We prefer to perform the cystojejunostomy in a side-to-side fashion, since this permits a larger anastomosis than end-jejunum to side-pseudocyst. The cystenteric anastomosis is fashioned with a single layer of 2-0 controlled-absorption sutures. The operation is completed with an enteroenterostomy 50 cm downstream from the pancreatic anastomosis, closure of the resultant mesenteric defects, and closed suction drainage. Drainage is continued for 7 days or until oral feeding fails to provoke a pancreatic fistula, announced by an increase in food-stimulated drainage volume.

**Resection.** Since excision of pancreatic pseudocysts results in greater mortality and morbidity than the various forms of internal drainage (Table 44.4), resection is currently reserved for *recurrent* pancreatic pseudocysts located in the body and tail (Fig. 44.9) or for true cystic lesions or cystic neoplasms discovered at the time of operation by frozen section of the wall.

### Comparison of Open Surgical Techniques

As shown in the collected surgical results in Table 44.4, internal surgical drainage of pancreatic pseudocysts is clearly superior to either external drainage or resection in terms of mortality. Accordingly, internal drainage should be routinely chosen over external drainage or resection in the absence of the extenuating circumstances discussed above. Furthermore, the results shown in this table should be considered a time-tested standard against which other putative therapeutic options must be judged. Given the recent development of alternative therapies (endoscopic transenteric drainage, percutaneous catheter drainage, and laparoscopic cystenterostomy) and the limited time for evaluation, it will be a number of years before the optimal form of drainage for pancreatic pseudocysts can be established. In the interim, until comparative results are available, the authors believe that internal surgical drainage represents the only tried-and-true approach to the elective therapy of pancreatic pseudocysts and that no apologies are required for its application. If another therapeutic approach is objectively demonstrated to be superior to open surgery, it can and should be adopted at that time.

## EMERGENCY SURGERY

For all practical purposes, arterial hemorrhage into a pseudocyst represents the only complication that must be regarded as a true

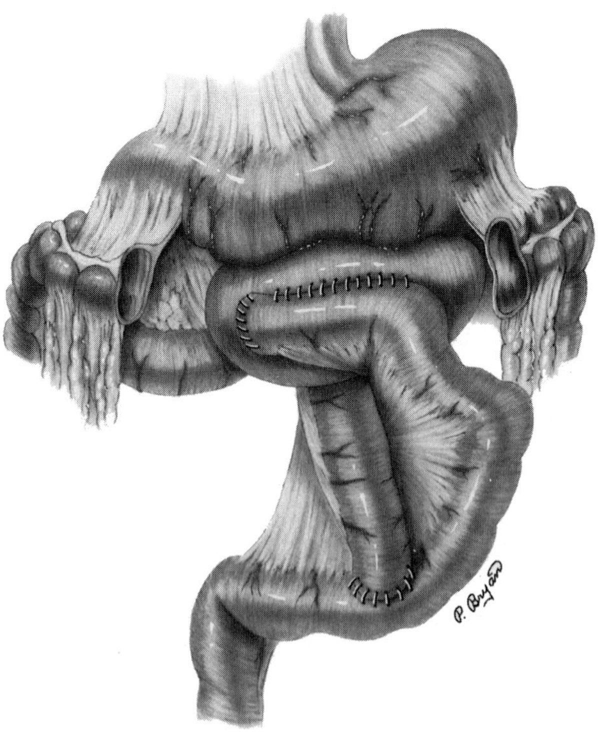

**FIG. 44.8.** Roux-en-Y cystojejunostomy. Note the side-to-side anastomosis. (Used with permission from Bradley EL III, Zeppa R. The Pancreas (Chapter 37). Davis-Christopher Textbook of Surgery, 13th ed. DC Sabiston, ed. WB Saunders, Philadelphia, PA 1986.)

**TABLE 44.4. Collected Mortality Results of Open Surgical Procedures for Pancreatic Pseudocysts**

| | 1969–1983 | | 1984–1992 | |
|---|---|---|---|---|
| | No. | Rate (%) | No. | Rate (%) |
| External drainage | 465 | 11.4 | 85 | 7.1 |
| Resection | 231 | 0.8 | 51 | 1.8 |
| Cystogastrostomy | 435 | 6.8 | 193 | 5.2 |
| Cystojejunostomy | 306 | 4.5 | 306 | 1.9 |
| Cystoduodenostomy[a] | 88 | 2.3 | 30 | 0 |

[a] Transduodenal approach.

emergency. Intracystic hemorrhage into pancreatic pseudocysts occurs infrequently but is attended by prohibitive mortality rates of 50% and more (31). The onset of sudden abdominal pain in a patient previously known to have a pseudocyst, combined with the presence of a pulsatile mass, which is often accompanied with a bruit (Fig. 44.10), is virtually pathognomonic of this complication. Most patients presenting with intracystic pancreatic hemorrhage fit the profile of an alcohol abuser with chronic pancreatitis. Rupture of the pseudocyst with intraabdominal exsanguination is the dreaded endpoint. Most often intracystic hemorrhage results from inflammatory erosion into the splenic artery or its branches (31). On occasion, the hemorrhage may be due to erosion into the gastroduodenal artery or other peripancreatic vessels, such as the anterior or posterior gastroduodenal arteries.

A much rarer presentation of intracystic hemorrhage has been called *hemosuccus pancreaticus*. In this condition, hemorrhage occurs within a *communicating* pseudocyst, with resultant passage of arterial blood into the pancreatic duct and out through the ampulla of Vater. Patients present with gastrointestinal bleeding, but the usual gastric and duodenal sites are normal (Fig. 44.11). Endoscopic visualization of hemorrhage from the ampulla is pathognomonic.

The major role of angiography in intracystic hemorrhage is diagnostic. Attempts at therapeutic transcutaneous embolization of the pseudoaneurysm by means of an arterial catheter are often unsuccessful and may prove to be a waste of valuable time.

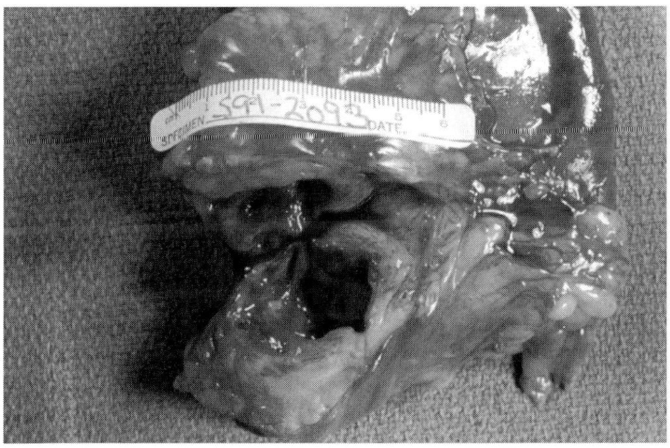

FIG. 44.9. Recurrent pseudocyst after cystojejunostomy treated by distal pancreatectomy. Note the thickened wall.

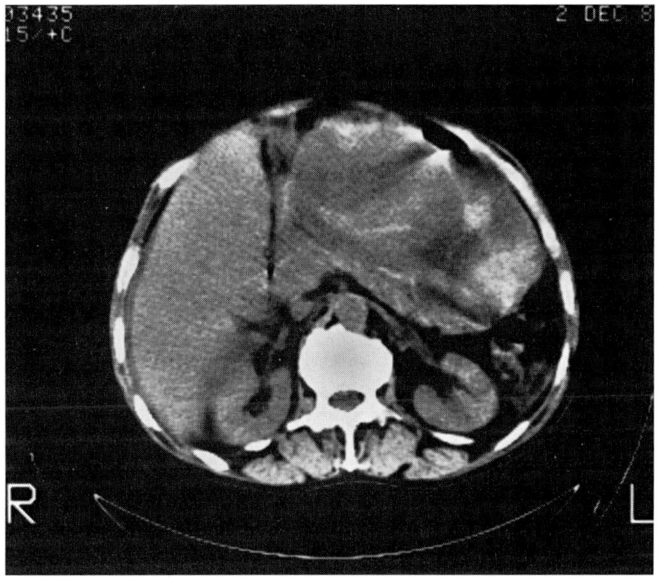


FIG. 44.10. CT scan in a patient with a known pseudocyst being treated by observation, who suddenly developed a painful abdominal mass accompanied by a bruit. Note the large high density mass replacing the pseudocyst. Operative transcystic control of the bleeding splenic artery was successful.

However, angiography to provide therapeutic embolization may be useful in the critically ill patient with prohibitive surgical risk. It is our contention that the open surgical approach should be the procedure of choice for any patient with pancreatic pseudocyst hemorrhage who is judged capable of tolerating major surgery. Dynamic CT scanning is of less value in this situation than arteriography, even though it too can be diagnostic, since tomography cannot often identify the specific bleeding vessel.

At the time of exploration, a direct approach to the bleeding vessel is often best. The aorta is cross-clamped or compressed, and the pseudoaneurysm incised. A finger is placed over the defect in the artery (the splenic artery is most commonly involved) and large nonabsorbable sutures are placed beneath the tamponading finger. When hemostasis is complete, the pseudocyst/pseudoaneursym is partially closed over a large drainage tube, which is brought out as external gravity drainage. Occasionally, a pancreatic fistula will result, but if hemostasis has been achieved, rebleeding is rare. Urgent pancreatoduodenectomy is occasionally necessary for hemorrhagic pseudocysts in the head of the pancreas.

Ruptured and abscessed pancreatic pseudocysts require less urgent treatment. Ruptured pseudocysts result in a chemical peritonitis and pancreatic ascites. Repeated aspiration of the ascites carries a high likelihood for peritoneal contamination. Early surgical intervention is necessary to prevent secondary infection and other comorbidities associated with the intraabdominal chemical burn and tissue digestion. According to the Atlanta definitions, secondary infection occurring in a pancreatic pseudocyst should more properly be termed a pancreatic abscess (2). Percutaneous catheter drainage is often effective treatment for abscessed pseudocysts in the absence of associated pancreatic necrosis, since drainage of purulent material can occur through comparatively small drains. Whenever pancreatic necrosis and infection are demonstrated to coexist, however, open surgical drainage is necessary to provide adequate drainage.

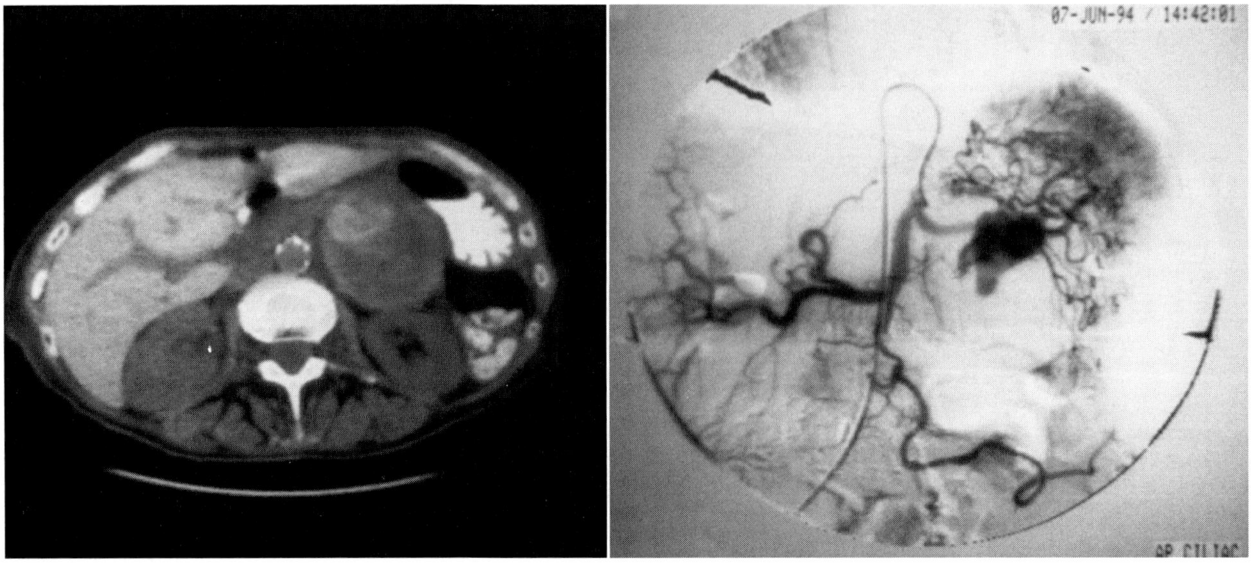


**FIG. 44.11.** On the *left* is a demonstration of a splenic pseudoaneurysm within a pancreatic pseudocyst in a poor-risk patient hemorrhaging from the ampulla of Vater (hemosuccus pancreaticus). Angiogram on *right* confirms the splenic false aneurysm, but therapeutic embolization was unsuccessful, and emergency surgical resection was required.

## REFERENCES


1. Praderi RC. History of pancreatic surgery. In: Trede M, Carter DC, eds. Surgery of the pancreas. London: Churchill Livingstone, 1993:3–15.
2. Bradley EL III. A clinical based classification system for acute pancreatitis. Arch Surg 1993;128:586–590.
3. Lumsden A, Bradley EL III. Pseudocyst or cystic neoplasm? Differential diagnosis and initial management of cystic pancreatic lesions. Hepatogastroenterology 1989;36:462–466.
4. Lewandrowski K, Southem JF, Pins UR, et al. Cyst fluid analysis in the differential diagnosis of pancreatic pseudocysts, cystadenomas, and cystadenocarcinomas. Ann Surg 1993;217:41–47.
5. Bradley EL III, Clements J Jr, Gonzalez A. The natural history of pancreatic pseudocysts: a unified concept of management. Am J Surg 1979;137:135–141.
6. Yeo CJ, Bastidas JA, Lynch-Nyham A, Fischman EK, Zinner MJ, Cameron JL. The natural history of pancreatic pseudocyst documented by computed tomography. Surg Gynecol Obstet 1990;170:411–417.
7. Vitas GJ, Sarr MG. Selected management of pancreatic pseudocysts: operative versus expectant management. Surgery 1992;111:123–130.
8. Imrie CW, Shearer MG. The diagnosis and management of pancreatic pseudocysts. In: Johnson CD, Imrie CW, eds. Pancreatic disease: progress and prospects. London: Springer-Verlag, 1991:299–309.
9. Gullo L, Barbara L. Treatment of pancreatic pseudocysts with octreotide. Lancet 1991;338:540–541.
10. Kozarek RA, Ball TJ, Patterson DJ, Freeny PC, Ryan JA, Traverso WL. Endoscopic transpapillary therapy for disrupted pancreatic duct and peripancretic fluid collections. Gastroenterology 1991;100:1362–1370.
11. Kozarek RA. Pancreatic stent induced ductal changes consistent with chronic pancreatitis. Gastrointest Endosc 1990;36:93–95.
12. Huibregtse K, Smits ME. Endoscopic management of disease of the pancreas. Am J Gastroenterol (suppl) 1994;89:66–77.
13. Cremer M, Devier J, Engelhorn L. Endoscopic management of cysts and pseudocysts in chronic pancreatitis: long term follow up after 7 years of experience. Gastrointest Endosc 1989;35:1–9.
14. Sahel J, Basted C, Pellat B, Schurgers P, Sarles H. Endoscopic cystduodenostomy of cysts of chronic calcifying pancreatitis. A report of 20 cases. Pancreas 1987;2:447–453.
15. Atabek U, Mayer D, Amin A, Camishion RC. Pancreatic cystgastrostomy by combined upper endoscopy and percutaneous transgastric instrumentation. J Laproendosc Surg 1993;3:501–504.
16. Baca I, Klempa I, Götzen V. Laparoskopische pankreatojejunostomie ohne entero-enteroanastomose. Chirurg 1994;65:378–381.
17. Hancke S, Petersen JF. Percutaneous puncture of pancreatic cysts guided by ultrasound. Surg Gynecol Obstet 1976;142:551–552.
18. Criado E, DeStefano AA, Weiner TM, Jaques PF. Long term results of percutaneous catheter drainage of pancreatic pseudocyst. Surg Gynecol Obstet 1992;175(4):293–298.
19. Adams DB, Harvey TS, Anderson MC. Percutaneous catheter drainage of pancreatic pseudocysts. Am Surg 1991;57:29–33.
20. Adams DB, Anderson MC. Percutaneous catheter drainage compared with internal drainage in the management of pancreatic pseudocyst. Ann Surg 1992;215:571–578.
21. Moran B, Rew DA, Johnson CD. Surgical debate. Pancreatic pseudocyst should be treated by surgical drainage. Ann R Coll Surg Engl 1994;76:54–58.
22. D'Agostino HB, VanSonnenberg E, Sanchez RB, Goodacre BW, Villaveiran RG, Lyche K. Treatment of pancreatic pseudocyst with percutaneous drainage and octreotide. Radiology 1993;187:685–688.
23. Morali GA, Braver DZ, Shemesh D, Abramovitz Z, Jacobsohn WZ. Successful treatment of pancreatic pseudocyst with a somatostatin analogue and catheter drainage. Am J Gastroenterol 1991;86:515–518.
24. Prinz RA, Pickleman J, Hoffman JP. Treatment of pancreatic cutaneous fistula with somatostatin analog. Am J Surg 1989;155:36–42.
25. O'Connor M, Kolars J, Ansel H, Silvia S, Vennes J. Pre-operative endoscopic retrograde cholangiopancreatography in the surgical management of pancreatic pseudocysts. Am J Surg 1986;151:18–24.
26. Munn JS, Aranha GS, Greenlee HB, Prinz RA. Simultaneous treatment of chronic pancreatitis and pancreatic pseudocyst. Arch Surg 1987;122:662–667.
27. Elechi EN, Callender CO, Lefall LD Jr, Kurtz LH. The treatment of pancreatic pseudocysts by external drainage. Surg Gynecol Obstet 1979;148:707–710.
28. Johnson LB, Rattner DW, Warshaw AL. The effect of size of giant pancreatic pseudocysts on the outcome of internal drainage procedures. Surg Gynecol Obstet 1991;173:171–174.
29. Newell KA, Liu T, Aranha GV, Prinz RA. Are cystogastrostomy and cystojejunostomy equivalent operations for pancreatic pseudocysts? Surgery 1990;108:635–640.
30. Bradley EL III. Cystoduodenostomy: newer perspectives. Ann Surg 1984;200:698–702.
31. Adams DB, Zellner JL, Andersen MC. Arterial hemorrhage complicating pancreatic pseudocysts: role of angiography. J Surg Res 1993;54:150–156.

# 45

# Epidemiology of Pancreatic Cancer

Albert B. Lowenfels, Patrick Maisonneuve, and Peter Boyle

In earlier decades misdiagnosis and/or underdiagnosis of pancreatic cancer has interfered with an accurate understanding of the epidemiology of this disease. At present, biopsies are more widely employed, and the accuracy of imaging techniques has rapidly improved. About 75% of pancreatic cancers now reported to U.S. cancer registries have histologic verification; the percentage of biopsy-positive cancers in most other countries is lower.

Since mortality rates and incidence rates for this tumor are so similar, either measure can be used to study the epidemiology of pancreatic neoplasms.

## DESCRIPTIVE EPIDEMIOLOGY

In most countries pancreatic cancers are rare, but since it is such a lethal tumor, pancreatic cancer in Western countries is usually listed among the leading causes of death from cancer. For example, in the United States, pancreatic cancer is the fourth most frequent cause of death from cancer in males and the fifth most frequent cause of cancer death in females. As with other digestive tract tumors, the risk of pancreatic cancer increases rapidly with age: approximately 20% of these cancers are seen before age 60, and in the United States, about 1% of the entire population will eventually develop this cancer. Cancer rates are higher in males than females, higher in urban rather than rural populations, and consistently higher in black than in white populations (1). Tables 45.1 and 45.2 list world incidence rates for male and female populations with high and low reported incidence rates of pancreatic cancer (2).

## TIME TRENDS

As pointed out above, some of the apparent increase in the incidence of pancreatic cancer can be explained by more accurate diagnostic methods; nevertheless, increased diagnostic accuracy is unlikely to explain the steady increase in this tumor observed in many countries. Since pancreatic cancer is so strongly related to smoking, some of the temporal changes in the incidence of this tumor are undoubtedly caused by changes in smoking. Increases in pancreatic cancer generally follow increases in tobacco smoking after about a 20-year lag period.

***United States.*** The United States is exceptional in that incidence and mortality rates in males have recently declined. Unfortunately, there has been a simultaneous increase in female pancreatic cancer, as more and more females have become smokers. If these trends continue, the current 25% male excess of pancreatic cancer will disappear in the decades ahead (Fig. 45.1).

***Europe.*** In nearly all European countries except the United Kingdom, the mortality rate for pancreatic cancer is increasing for both males and females (3). Mortality rates are now in the range of 8–12/100,000/year for males and 4–6/100,000/year in females.

## RISK FACTORS FOR PANCREATIC CANCER

### Smoking

Conclusive evidence underscores the importance of smoking as a causal agent for experimental as well as human pancreatic cancer (4–10). In animals, NNK, a tobacco-specific nitrosamine contained in cigarette smoke produces experimental cancer in two organs: the lung and the pancreas (11). In humans, there is a strong international correlation between pancreatic cancer and lung cancer rates, suggesting that these two lethal tumors share the same risk factor. Since the pancreas is exposed only indirectly to inhaled tobacco smoke, the effects of smoking are less pronounced on the pancreas than on the lung. Nevertheless, smoking is the commonest known cause for pancreatic cancer and accounts for approximately 30% of all cases. Most studies report that smokers have at least a twofold increased risk of pancreatic cancer, compared with nonsmokers.

Follow-up studies of large groups of normal individuals provide the strongest evidence linking smoking and pancreatic cancer. An early cohort study of 50,000 college graduates showed that smoking 10 or more cigarettes per day, as recorded on college health records, results in a 2.4-fold increased risk of pancreatic cancer after an interval of 15 or more years (12). A more recent study of over 34,000 British physicians is just as convincing. The overall risk of pancreatic cancer in physicians who smoked 25 or more cigarettes per day was three times greater than that for nonsmokers, and there was a clear dose response (13).

### Diet and Pancreatic Cancer

**Alcohol.** Heavy alcohol consumption damages the pancreas, often producing chronic pancreatitis, but is alcohol related to pancreatic cancer? Early reports suggested that there might be a link between alcohol and pancreatic cancer, but nearly all recent

**TABLE 45.1. Male Incidence Rates for Pancreatic Cancer: High- and Low-Risk Populations**

| Population | Incidence/ 100,000/Year |
|---|---|
| United States, Alameda (black) | 13.7 |
| United States, Bay Area (black) | 13.5 |
| United States, Atlanta (black) | 13.1 |
| United States, Detroit (black) | 12.5 |
| United States, New Orleans (black) | 11.9 |
| United States, Los Angeles (black) | 11.7 |
| Czech Republic, Bohemia and Moravia | 11.7 |
| Latvia | 11.2 |
| New Zealand (Maori) | 11.0 |
| Thailand, Chiang Mai | 2.4 |
| France, Martinique | 2.3 |
| Mali, Bamako | 2.2 |
| Algeria, Setif | 2.0 |
| Thailand, Khon Kaen | 1.4 |
| India, Madras | 1.2 |
| India, Bangalore | 1.0 |
| India, Ahmedabad | 0.7 |

Data from Parkin DM, Muir CS, Whelan SL, Gao YT, Ferlay J, Powell J, eds. Cancer incidence in five continents. Lyon: International Agency for Research on Cancer, 1992:1–1033.

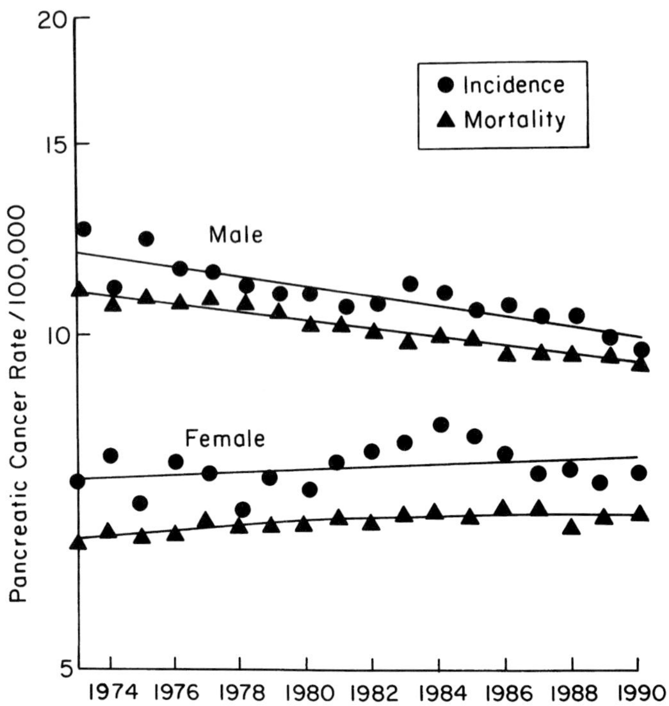


**FIG. 45.1.** Changes in incidence and mortality of pancreatic cancer (log scale) in white males and females, United States: 1974–1990. Male rates are decreasing, but female rates are rising. (From Miller BA, Silverman DT, Kaplan R. Pancreas. In: Miller BA, Ries LAG, Hankey BF, et al., eds. SEER cancer statistics review: 1973–1990, National Cancer Institute. Bethesda, MD: National Institute of Health, 1993:XXI.1–XXI.15.)

**TABLE 45.2. Female Incidence Rates for Pancreatic Cancer: High- and Low-Risk Populations**

| Population | Incidence/ 100,000/Year |
|---|---|
| United States, Alameda (black) | 11.9 |
| United States, Bay Area (black) | 11.6 |
| United States, Detroit (black) | 10.5 |
| New Zealand (Maori) | 9.8 |
| United States, New Orleans (black) | 9.7 |
| United States, Los Angeles (Japanese) | 8.7 |
| United States, Hawaii (Hawaiian) | 7.8 |
| United States, Los Angeles (black) | 7.7 |
| United States, Connecticut (black) | 7.3 |
| United States, Hawaii (Chinese) | 7.2 |
| France, Tarn | 1.4 |
| Algeria, Setif | 1.1 |
| India, Bangalore | 0.7 |
| India, Madras | 0.7 |
| Mali, Bamako | 0.4 |
| India, Ahmedabad | 0.2 |

Data from Parkin DM, Muir CS, Whelan SL, Gao YT, Ferlay J, Powell J, eds. Cancer incidence in five continents. Lyon: International Agency for Research on Cancer, 1992:1–1033.

reports have concluded that alcohol is not a risk factor for pancreatic cancer (5, 14–16).

**Coffee.** In 1981, a report from Massachusetts suggested that coffee was a strong risk factor for pancreatic cancer (17). A second report from the same group and nearly all subsequent reports have concluded that the evidence is insufficient to establish coffee drinking as a risk factor for pancreatic cancer (16, 18–21). Since smoking is a risk factor for pancreatic cancer and since most smokers drink coffee, it is easy to understand why a few centers have found this association, but most have not.

**Other Dietary Items.** Several studies have attempted to find particular dietary items that might increase or decrease the risk of pancreatic cancer. Excess intake of calories, fats, and/or carbohydrates have been linked to pancreatic cancer in a few studies; consumption of fresh fruits and vegetables seems to be protective (22–25).

### Medical Disorders

**Pancreatitis.** Chronic pancreatitis is characterized by widespread cellular dysfunction and glandular destruction. Do patients with chronic pancreatitis have an increased risk of pancreatic cancer? A cohort study of more than 2000 patients in six countries with well-defined chronic pancreatitis revealed a significantly elevated risk of pancreatic cancer: patients with chronic pancreatitis followed for 2 or more years had a 16-fold increased risk of pancreatic cancer; patients with a minimum follow-up period of 5 years had a 14-fold increase in risk (26) (Table 45.3). Similar risks were found in males, in females, and in both alcoholic and idiopathic forms of pancreatitis (Table 45.4). The cumulative 25-year risk of pancreatic cancer in patients with any form of chronic pancreatitis is about 4% (Fig. 45.2).

Additional recent studies have confirmed these findings, so it appears that chronic pancreatitis is a strong risk factor for pancreatic cancer (27–30). However, since pancreatitis is an uncommon disease, only a small fraction of all pancreatic cancers are causally related to pancreatitis.

**Diabetes.** Diabetes afflicts approximately 5% of all adults, and diabetes often accompanies pancreatic cancer. But is this common chronic disorder causally related to pancreatic cancer? To investigate the problem it is necessary to study the duration of diabetes prior to the diagnosis of pancreatic cancer. Reports that look closely at the duration of diabetes suggest that although many patients with pancreatic cancer do have diabetes, the diabetes is usually of recent onset and probably secondary to ductal obstruction from pancreatic cancer. Preexisting diabetes of long duration is not likely to lead to an increased risk of pancreatic cancer (31–33).

**Typhoid.** Typhoid fever is now rare in Western countries, but it can lead to a carrier state in which typhoid bacteria colonize the biliary tract. In an intriguing long-term follow-up study of typhoid carriers, the risk of pancreatic cancer appeared to be increased (34). Reflux of infected bile into the pancreatic ductal system could be the causal mechanism.

**Gallstone Disease.** Gallstones are a common cause of acute pancreatitis, but neither gallstones nor cholecystectomy appears to alter the risk of pancreatic cancer (35). The initial symptoms of pancreatic cancer can mimic biliary tract disease, explaining why some studies have observed an association between onset of biliary tract disease (or cholecystectomy) and pancreatic cancer.

**Peptic Ulcer Disease.** Some studies have shown a link between peptic ulcer disease and pancreatic cancer (10, 36). The most plausible explanation for this finding is that both diseases are linked to a shared risk factor; namely, smoking.

### Genetic Diseases

All the known or suspected causes for pancreatic cancer (smoking, medical diseases, diet) explain only a fraction of the observed cases. Many additional cases are presumably related to genetic disorders. Information about genetic causes of pancreatic cancer is accumulating rapidly and will undoubtedly explain and, one hopes, reduce the burden of this disease in future generations.

**Familial Pancreatic Cancer.** The strongest evidence for a genetic basis for some cases of pancreatic cancer comes from reports of aggregation of this tumor within families. For example, many members of the current French-speaking population of the province of Quebec, Canada, originated from a small group of French settlers who were geographically isolated for several generations. Intermarriage could be the explanation for the frequency of familial pancreatic cancer observed in this region. In one report, patients with pancreatic cancer were 13 times more likely to have a family member with pancreatic cancer than a group of matched controls (37).

During the 1700s, a large group of the original French settlers in northeast Canada were forced to migrate to other regions. Many eventually settled in Louisiana and are now known as Acadians. In a study of pancreatic cancer in Louisiana, Acadians were discovered to be at higher risk for this disease than other groups, suggesting that migrants from Canada carried their genetic susceptibility with them to a new location (38).

Other studies have found aggregations of pancreatic cancer within kindreds. In one report, pancreatic cancer has been traced through three generations, including progeny from two of the progenitor's three marriages (39). In another large pedigree, pancreatic cancer was inherited in an autosomal dominant fashion accompanied by diabetes or pancreatic exocrine insufficiency (40).

**Cystic Fibrosis.** Ninety percent of patients with cystic fibrosis, the commonest recessive genetic disorder of Caucasians, suffer from pancreatic insufficiency which usually begins in early childhood and requires supplemental pancreatic enzyme therapy. There is strong evidence for an increased risk of pancreatic cancer in this group of patients (41, 42). The cause of the observed excess might be the effect of the pathologic alterations in the gland caused by the cystic fibrosis process.

**TABLE 45.3. Country-Specific and Overall Risk of Pancreatic Cancer in 1552 Subjects with Chronic Pancreatitis Who Were Followed for More Than 2 Years (26)**

| Country | Cancers (*N*) | SIR | 95% CI |
|---|---|---|---|
| Italy | 7 | 18 | (7.3–37) |
| Switzerland | 8 | 19.9 | (8.6–39) |
| Germany | 7 | 17.8 | (3.7–52) |
| Denmark | 5 | 15.9 | (5.1–37) |
| United States | 4 | 14.4 | (3.9–37) |
| Sweden | 2 | 9.7 | (1.2–35) |
| Total | 29 | 6.5 | (11.1–24) |

SIR denotes standardized incidence ratio, or the ratio of observed cases of pancreatic cancer to expected cases in background population. CI denotes confidence interval.

**TABLE 45.4. Risk of Pancreatic Cancer in 1198 Subjects with Chronic Alcoholic Pancreatitis and 354 Subjects with Chronic Nonalcoholic Pancreatitis**

| Pancreatitis Type | Duration (years)[a] | Cancers (*N*) | SIR (95% CI)[b] |
|---|---|---|---|
| Alcoholic | 2 | 16 | 15.1 (8.6–24) |
| | 5 | 10 | 13.2 (6.3–24) |
| Nonalcoholic | 2 | 13 | 18.7 (9.9–32) |
| | 5 | 8 | 16.2 (7.0–32) |

Data from Lowenfels AB, Maisonneuve P, Cavallini G, et al. Pancreatitis and the risk of pancreatic cancer. International Pancreatitis Study Group. N Engl J Med 1993;328:1433–1437.

[a]Data analyzed after a minimum follow-up of 2 or 5 years.

[b]SIR denotes standardized incidence ratio, or the ratio of observed cases of pancreatic cancer to expected cases in background population. CI denotes confidence interval.

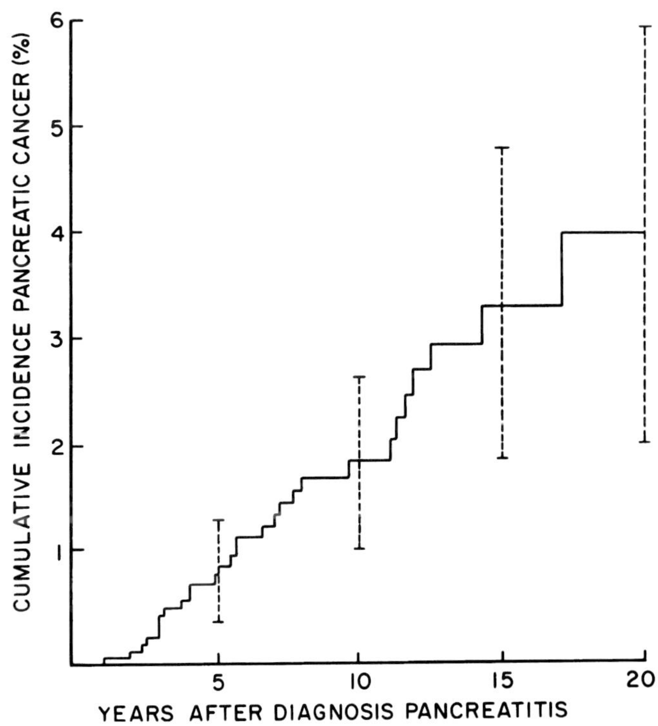


**FIG. 45.2.** Cumulative incidence of pancreatic cancer in 1552 subjects with chronic pancreatitis with a minimum of 2 years of follow-up (26). Vertical lines represent 95% confidence intervals. The numbers in parenthesis are the numbers of subjects at risk. One additional cancer developed after 25 years of follow-up.

**Breast Cancer in Family.** A population-based study performed in Iceland examined the frequency of pancreatic cancer in families in which at least one female member had been diagnosed with breast cancer. Compared with families without a history of breast cancer, there was a 60% increased risk of pancreatic cancer in first-degree male relatives (43).

**Hereditary Pancreatitis.** Hereditary pancreatitis is characterized by *(a)* early age at onset, *(b)* multigenerational involvement, and *(c)* absence of other known causes of pancreatitis such as alcohol and or gallstones. Many of these patients eventually progress to chronic pancreatitis. The limited available data suggest that this rare form of pancreatitis may be associated with about a 5% cumulative risk of cancer—similar to what has been observed in other more common forms of chronic pancreatitis (44).

**K-*ras* Mutations.** K-*ras* mutations are the commonest genetic mutation in patients with pancreatic cancer and are more frequent in patients with pancreatic cancer than in any other tumor (45, 46). In one series, K-*ras* mutations at codon 12 were detected in 16 of 16 patients with confirmed pancreatic cancer (47). K-*ras* alterations can be detected in blood, stool, and pancreatic juice from patients with pancreatic cancer, and mutations can also be found in patients with chronic pancreatitis (48–50). K-*ras* mutations may eventually offer an opportunity for a screening test, but, at present, K-*ras* mutations most likely represent a stage in the formation of pancreatic cancer rather than being a true risk factor.

**Melanoma Kindreds.** Melanomas sometimes appear in several members of the same family; some of these melanoma-prone kindreds have an increased risk of pancreatic cancer. In one report, 7 of 19 nonmelanoma cancers in these kindreds arose in the pancreas (51); in another melanoma kindred, 3 of 12 family members developed pancreatic cancer (52). For the development of this tumor, a *p16M* mutation appears to be necessary.

**Familial Adenomatous Polyposis.** Familial adenomatous polyposis, an autosomal dominant disease, has an unusually high risk of colon cancer. It may also be associated with other, extracolonic tumors. One prospective study of 1391 affected or at-risk patients detected a four- to fivefold increased risk of pancreatic cancer. The lifetime absolute risk was estimated to be 1.7% (53).

## OCCUPATIONAL RISK FACTORS

Despite many studies of occupation and pancreatic cancer, there has been no clear agreement about any specific occupation or industrial exposure as a risk factor for pancreatic cancer. Exposure to ionizing radiation or to DDT may cause pancreatic cancer, but other exposures are more controversial (54, 55). In most studies, it has been difficult to control for smoking, a known risk factor for pancreatic cancer. Occupational exposure does not appear to have a major role as a cause for neoplasms of the pancreas.

## SUMMARY

Smoking is clearly the strongest known risk factor for pancreatic cancer. Although the association between smoking and pancreatic cancer is less dramatic than that for lung cancer, smoking remains the single agent most likely to cause this lethal tumor, and the only etiologic agent for which a population-based prevention strategy can be designed and implemented. For those countries where smoking rates are rising, we can predict a steady increase in the incidence of pancreatic cancer; in contrast, in countries where there has been a reduction in smoking, we can anticipate a decline in pancreatic cancer rates. Diet, some predisposing diseases such as pancreatitis, and certain genetic disorders, although causally linked to pancreatic cancer, currently offer less opportunity for reducing the risk of this lethal cancer than do measures aimed at control of smoking.

**Acknowledgment**

Supported by grants from the C. D. Smithers Foundation.

## REFERENCES

1. Miller BA, Silverman DT, Kaplan R. Pancreas. In: Miller BA, Ries LAG, Hankey BF, et al., eds. SEER cancer statistics review: 1973–1990. National Cancer Institute. Bethesda, MD: National Institute of Health, 1993:XXI.1–XXI.15.
2. Parkin DM, Muir CS, Whelan SL, Gao YT, Ferlay J, Powell J, eds. Cancer incidence in five continents. Lyon: International Agency for Research on Cancer, 1992:1–1033.
3. La Vecchia C, Lucchini F, Negri E, Boyle P, Maisonneuve P, Levi F. Trends of cancer mortality in Europe, 1955–1989. Eur J Cancer 1992;28:132–235.
4. Kalapothaki V, Tzonou A, Hsieh CC, Toupadaki N, Karakatsani A, Trichopoulos D. Tobacco, ethanol, coffee, pancreatitis, diabetes mellitus, and cholelithiasis as risk factors for pancreatic carcinoma. Cancer Causes Control 1993;4:375–382.
5. Zatonski WA, Boyle P, Przewozniak K, Maisonneuve P, Drosik K, Walker AM. Cigarette smoking, alcohol, tea and coffee consumption and pancreas cancer risk: a case-control study from Opole, Poland. Int J Cancer 1993;53:601–607.
6. Bueno de Mesquita HB, Maisonneuve P, Moerman CJ, Runia S, Boyle P. Life-time history of smoking and exocrine carcinoma of the pancreas: a population-based case-control study in the Netherlands. Int J Cancer 1991;49:816–822.
7. Howe GR, Jain M, Burch JD, Miller AB. Cigarette smoking and cancer of the pancreas: evidence from a population-based case-control study in Toronto, Canada. Int J Cancer 1991;47:323–328.
8. Akiba S, Hirayama T. Cigarette smoking and cancer mortality risk in Japanese men and women—results from reanalysis of the six-prefecture cohort study data. Environ Health Perspect 1990;87:19–26.
9. Boyle P, Hsieh CC, Maisonneuve P. Epidemiology of pancreas cancer. Int J Pancreatol 1989;5:327–346.
10. Mack TM, Yu MC, Hanisch R, Henderson BE. Pancreas cancer and smoking, beverage consumption, and past medical history. JNCI 1986;76:49–60.
11. Rivenson A, Hoffmann D, Prokopczyk B, Amin S, Hecht SS. Induction of lung and exocrine pancreas tumors in F344 rats by tobacco-specific and *Areca*-derived *N*-nitrosamines. Cancer Res 1988;48:6912–6917.
12. Whittemore AS, Paffenbarger RS, Anderson K, Halpern J. Early precursors of pancreatic cancer in college men. J Chron Dis 1983;36:251–256.
13. Doll R, Peto R, Wheatley K, Gray R, Sutherland I. Mortality in relation to smoking: 40 years' observations on male British doctors. Br Med J 309;901–911:1994.
14. Velema JP, Walker AM, Gold EB. Alcohol and pancreatic cancer. Insufficient epidemiologic evidence for a causal relationship. Epidemiol Rev 1986;8:28–42.
15. Tonnesen H, Moller H, Andersen JR, Jensen E, Juel K. Cancer morbidity in alcohol abusers. Br J Cancer 1994;69:327–332.
16. Bueno de Mesquita HB, Maisonneuve P, Moerman CJ, Runia S, Boyle P. Lifetime consumption of alcoholic beverages, tea and coffee and exocrine carcinoma of the pancreas: a population-based case-control study in the Netherlands. Int J Cancer 1992;50:514–522.
17. MacMahon B, Yen S, Trichopoulos D, Warren K, Nardi G. Coffee and cancer of the pancreas. N Engl J Med 1981;304:630–633.
18. Hsieh CC, MacMahon B, Yen S, Trichopoulos D, Warren K, Nardi G. Coffee and pancreatic cancer (chapter 2). N Engl J Med 1986;315:587–589.
19. Stensvold I, Jacobsen BK. Coffee and cancer: a prospective study of 43,000 Norwegian men and women. Cancer Causes Control 1994;5:401–408.
20. Ghadirian P, Simard A, Baillargeon J. Tobacco, alcohol, and coffee and cancer of the pancreas: a population-based,

case-control study in Quebec, Canada. Cancer 1991;67:2664–2670.

21. Jain M, Howe GR, St. Louis P, Miller AB. Coffee and alcohol as determinants of risk of pancreas cancer: a case-control study from Toronto. Int J Cancer 1991;47:384–389.
22. Baghurst PA, McMichael AJ, Slavotinek AH, Baghurst KI, Boyle P, Walker AM. A case-control study of diet and cancer of the pancreas. Am J Epidemiol 1991;134:167–179.
23. Kalapothaki V, Tzonou A, Hsieh CC, et al. Nutrient intake and cancer of the pancreas: a case-control study in Athens, Greece. Cancer Causes Control 1993;4:383–389.
24. Bueno de Mesquita HB, Maisonneuve P, Runia S, Moerman CJ. Intake of foods and nutrients and cancer of the exocrine pancreas: a population-based case-control study in the Netherlands. Int J Cancer 1991;48:540–549.
25. Negri E, La Vecchia C, Franceschi S, D'Avanzo B, Parazzini F. Vegetable and fruit consumption and cancer risk. Int J Cancer 1991;48:350–354.
26. Lowenfels AB, Maisonneuve P, Cavallini G, et al. Pancreatitis and the risk of pancreatic cancer. International Pancreatitis Study Group. N Engl J Med 1993;328:1433–1437.
27. Bansal P, Sonnenberg A. Pancreatitis is a risk factor for pancreatic cancer. Gastroenterology 1995;109:247–251.
28. Fernandez E, La Vecchia CL, Pora M, Negri E, D'Avanzo B, Boyle P. Pancreatitis and the risk of pancreatic cancer. Pancreas 1995;11:185–189.
29. Chari ST, Mohan V, Pitchumoni CS, Viswanathan M, Madanagopalan N, Lowenfels AB. Risk of pancreatic carcinoma in tropical calcifying pancreatitis: an epidemiologic study. Pancreas 1994;9:62–66.
30. Ekbom A, McLaughlin JK, Karlsson BM, et al. Pancreatitis and pancreatic cancer: a population-based study. J Natl Cancer Inst 1994;86:625–627.
31. Gullo L, Pezzilli R, Morselli Labate AM. Diabetes and the risk of pancreatic cancer. Italian Pancreatic Cancer Study Group. N Engl J Med 1994;331:81–84.
32. La Vecchia C, Negri E, Franceschi S, D'Avanzo B, Boyle P. A case-control study of diabetes mellitus and cancer risk. Br J Cancer 1994;70:950–953.
33. Adami HO, McLaughlin J, Ekbom A, et al. Cancer risk in patients with diabetes mellitus. Cancer Causes Control 1991;2:307–314.
34. Caygill CP, Hill MJ, Braddick M, Sharp JC. Cancer mortality in chronic typhoid and paratyphoid carriers. Lancet 1994;343:83–84.
35. Bueno de Mesquita HB, Maisonneuve P, Moerman CJ, Walker AM. Aspects of medical history and exocrine carcinoma of the pancreas: a population-based case-control study in the Netherlands. Int J Cancer 1992;52:17–23.
36. Eide TJ, Viste A, Andersen A, Sooreide O. The risk of cancer at all sites following gastric operation for benign disease. A cohort study of 4,224 patients. Int J Cancer 1991;48:333–339.
37. Ghadirian P, Boyle P, Simard A, Baillargeon J, Maisonneuve P, Perret C. Reported family aggregation of pancreatic cancer within a population-based case-control study in the Francophone community in Montreal, Canada. Int J Pancreatol 1991;10:183–196.
38. Falk RT, Pickle LW, Fontham ET, Correa P, Fraumeni JFJ. Life-style risk factors for pancreatic cancer in Louisiana: a case-control study. Am J Epidemiol 1988;128:324–336.
39. Lynch HT, Fusaro L, Lynch JF. Familial pancreatic cancer: a family study. Pancreas 1992;7:511–515.
40. Evans JP, Burke W, Chen R, et al. Familial pancreatic adenocarcinoma: association with diabetes and early molecular diagnosis. J Med Genet 1995;32:330–335.
41. Sheldon CD, Hodson ME, Carpenter LM, Swerdlow AJ. A cohort study of cystic fibrosis and malignancy. Br J Cancer 1993;68:1025–1028.
42. Neglia JP, FitzSimmons SC, Maisonneuve P, et al. The risk of cancer among patients with cystic fibrosis. N Engl J Med 1995;332:336.
43. Tulinius H, Olafsdottir GH, Sigvaldason H, Tryggvadottir L, Bjarnadottir K. Neoplastic diseases in families of breast cancer patients. J Med Genet 1994;31:618–621.
44. Gross JB. Hereditary pancreatitis. In: Go VLW, ed. The exocrine pancreas: biology, pathology, and diseases. New York: Raven Press, 1986:829–839.
45. Caldas C, Kern SE. K-ras mutation and pancreatic adenocarcinoma. Int J Pancreatol 1995;18:1–6.
46. Hruban RH, van Mansfeld AD, Offerhaus GJ, et al. K-ras oncogene activation in adenocarcinoma of the human pancreas. A study of 82 carcinomas using a combination of mutant-enriched polymerase chain reaction analysis and allele-specific oligonucleotide hybridization. Am J Pathol 1993;143:545–554.
47. Trumper LH, Burger B, von Bonin F, et al. Diagnosis of pancreatic adenocarcinoma by polymerase chain reaction from pancreatic secretions. Br J Cancer 1994;70:278–284.
48. Caldas C, Hahn SA, Hruban RH, Redston MS, Yeo CJ, Kern SE. Detection of K-ras mutations in the stool of patients with pancreatic adenocarcinoma and pancreatic ductal hyperplasia. Cancer Res 1994;54:3568–3573.
49. Tada M, Omata M, Kawai S, et al. Detection of ras gene mutations in pancreatic juice and peripheral blood of patients with pancreatic adenocarcinoma. Cancer Res 1993;53:2472–2474.
50. Yanagisawa A, Ohtake K, Ohashi K, et al. Frequent k-ras oncogene activation in mucous cell hyperplasias of pancreas suffering from chronic inflammation. Cancer Res 1993;53:953–956.
51. Goldstein AM, Fraser MC, Struewing JP, et al. Increased risk of pancreatic cancer in melanoma-prone kindreds with p16INK4 mutations. N Engl J Med 1995;333:970–974.
52. Whelan AJ, Bartsch D, Goodfellow PJ. A familial syndrome of pancreatic cancer and melanoma with a mutation in the CDKN2 tumor-suppressor gene. N Engl J Med 1995;333:975–977.
53. Giardiello FM, Offerhaus GJ, Lee DH, et al. Increased risk of thyroid and pancreatic carcinoma in familial adenomatous polyposis. Gut 1993;34:1394–1396.
54. Garabrant DH, Held J, Langholz B, Peters JM, Mack TM. DDT and related compounds and risk of pancreatic cancer. J Natl Cancer Inst 1992;84:764–771.
55. Everhart J, Wright D. Diabetes mellitus as a risk factor for pancreatic cancer. JAMA 1995;273:1605–1609.

# 46

# *Molecular Biology: Diagnostic and Therapeutic Potentials*

C. S. Frances McCormick and Nicholas R. Lemoine

In spite of pancreatic carcinoma being the fifth most common cause of cancer death, relatively little is known of its molecular and cellular basis, though in recent years more intensive studies have begun to identify consistent genetic and chromosomal abnormalities. This aggressive tumor tends to present at a late stage, with extensive local infiltration and/or metastases and has a very poor prognosis. A variety of regulatory mechanisms contribute to the development and growth of pancreatic carcinoma, including overexpression of receptor-ligand systems, oncogene activation, and loss of tumor-suppressor gene function.

A particular genetic profile seems to distinguish pancreatic adenocarcinoma from other epithelial tumors of the gastrointestinal tract, and most show alterations of the p53 and *CDKN2* tumor-suppressor genes and the *KRAS* oncogene.

This chapter reviews the current knowledge of the molecular and cellular biology of pancreatic cancer and indicates how this may be exploited to provide a basis for the development of novel approaches to aid early diagnosis and for therapeutic and screening purposes.

## GROWTH FACTORS AND THEIR RECEPTORS

Pancreatic carcinoma shows an excessive expression of ligands and receptors that participate in aberrant autocrine and paracrine pathways, contributing to pancreatic tumor cell growth. Some of these changes also occur in chronic pancreatitis, suggesting that overexpression of these receptor-ligand systems in itself does not suffice to produce malignant transformation but probably acts in a facultative manner when accompanied by other genetic abnormalities.

### Epidermal Growth Factor Receptor (EGFR) Family

The EGFR is normally expressed at the apical surface of ductal cells, and in the normal pancreas there is expression at low levels (1), which is thought to regulate normal pancreatic exocrine function. Increased expression of both EGFR and several of its ligands (EGF, transforming growth factor alpha (TGF$\alpha$), amphiregulin, and betacellulin) is seen in both chronic pancreatitis and pancreatic adenocarcinoma (2–7). The presence of EGFR with either ligand EGF or TGF$\alpha$ is associated with more aggressive disease and shorter postoperative survival (7). Amphiregulin is present in the nuclei of ductal cells of the normal pancreas, whereas in pancreatic carcinoma, it may be present in either the nucleus and cytoplasm or only the cytoplasm of the malignant ductal cells (4, 5). The significance of this varied localization is uncertain, but it has been shown that cytoplasmic localization of amphiregulin is associated with a significant reduction in postoperative survival (5). Therefore, overexpression of EGFR and one or more of its ligands indicates a poor prognosis, and this has been correlated with enhanced metastatic potential, tumor invasiveness (1, 6), and a shorter postoperative survival period (7).

There are three additional receptors closely related to EGFR: HER2 (also known as c-erbB-2), HER3 (c-erbB-3), and HER4 (c-erbB-4) (8, 9). The ligands of HER2 are unknown; HER3 and HER4 bind to the family of heregulins (neu differentiation factors). There is overexpression of HER2 and HER3 in pancreatic cancer (10). HER2 shows tumor-specific overexpression because of transcriptional up-regulation rather than gene amplification in 20–50% of pancreatic carcinomas (11–15). Enhanced HER2 expression in pancreatic cancer does not appear to be associated with tumor progression, but rather, it is associated with a better-differentiated phenotype (15). In contrast, recently it has been shown that increased HER3 immunoreactivity is associated with tumor progression and reduced postoperative survival (16).

Hepatocyte growth factor (HGF) and MET receptor HGF, also known as scatter factor, are important mediators of epithelial-stromal reactions via a cell surface tyrosine kinase receptor encoded by the *MET* oncogene (17, 18) which, when phosphorylated, stimulates cells to move and proliferate. Until recently, little was known about the role of HGF and MET in pancreatic cancer.

HGF is present in the stromal cells of the normal pancreas, as determined by immunohistochemistry and mRNA detection. There is a tenfold elevation in pancreatic carcinoma, presumably derived from the stromal cells or the islets of Langerhans but not from the malignant epithelial cells (19–21). In vitro, HGF causes the phosphorylation of the MET receptor in human pancreas cell lines and stimulates them to move. In cell lines that overexpress the MET receptor, there is constitutive autophosphorylation, even in the absence of exogenous ligand. It is thought that the up-regulation of this system may stimulate growth and enhance motility and so may enable tumor invasion and metastasis to occur (19, 20).

A recent study (22) has shown the presence of increased MET and HGF expression in hyperplastic, dysplastic, and malignant ductal epithelial cells of the pancreas. This suggests that overexpression of this receptor-ligand system is an important and consistently early molecular event in the development of pancreatic cancer. It is unclear whether the HGF immunoreactivity within the malignant epithelial cells represents epithelial production of this factor or whether it merely represents the internalization of the HGF-MET complex. Even so, these findings show increased HGF-MET interaction within these cells.

### Transforming Growth Factor ß (TGFß) Family

The TGFß family is a superfamily of regulatory polypeptides, including three isoforms (TGFß1, TGFß2, and TGFß3) and three major receptors (TGFßRI, TGFßRII, and TGFßRIII). Of the receptors, TGFßRII shows serine/threonine kinase activity and it depends upon the presence of TGFßRI for functional activity (23, 24). TGFßRIII is not believed to be involved in signal transduction (23, 25). This family is implicated in the regulation of cell growth and differentiation, angiogenesis, and tumorigenesis (26–28). The role of TGFß is complex, since its effect on a wide range of cell types varies with concentration and the surrounding environment, both in vitro and in vivo. In most cells of epithelial origin, TGFß acts as a potent growth inhibitor (26–29). In pancreatic cancer, there is a multifold increase in the expression of isoforms TGFß1, TGFß2, and TGFß3, in particular TGFß1 (30). The expression of the TGFß2 isoform is correlated with advanced tumor stage. However, degenerating nonneoplastic cells adjacent to the invasive tumor also may show increased TGFß expression, and so up-regulation of the TGFß isoforms should not be considered to be tumor specific (31). There is increased expression of TGFßRII in pancreatic cancer in comparison with the low levels found in normal pancreas; levels of TGFRßIII are similar in both normal pancreas and pancreatic cancer (31). Human cancer cells are thought to gain a growth advantage from the loss of responsiveness to the inhibitory actions of the TGFß isoforms, but it is unclear if there is a direct effect on the tumor cells or an indirect effect on the stroma by stimulating angiogenesis, altering expression of adhesion molecules, or by increasing production of extracellular matrix components thereby enhancing the metastatic potential of the tumor cells (32). It has been suggested that immunosuppression also may be implicated through effects of TGFß on lymphocytes, although there is as yet little evidence to support this hypothesis.

### Fibroblast (Heparin-Binding) Growth Factors (FGF) and Receptors (FGFR)

There are nine members of the FGF family (FGF1–9) and four high-affinity growth factor receptors (FGFR1–4) showing tyrosine kinase activity (33–37). FGF1 and FGF2 are closely related prototypes (33) that are seen at low levels in the normal pancreas but show increased production in chronic pancreatitis (34, 35). FGF2 expression is enhanced particularly in areas of degeneration/regeneration with pseudoglandular hyperplasia (35). Overexpression of FGF1 was found to be associated with advanced-stage pancreatic ductal adenocarcinoma (35), but this has not been found by another group (34). Increased expression of FGF2 is found in approximately 50% of pancreatic tumors, with some association with advanced tumor stage (34, 36). FGFs may either bind to low-affinity heparin sulfate proteoglycans where they are stored or they may bind to the high-affinity FGF receptors. The expression of FGFR-1, FGFR-3, and FGFR-4 is seen in the acinar cells of the normal adult pancreas (34). Expression of one or more of these receptors is present in the tumor cell of approximately 60% of pancreatic cancers (34, 37), including a number of different splice variants (37)

## ONCOGENES

### *KRAS*

*KRAS* is one member of a family of three human *RAS* genes that encode for small GTP-binding proteins that are involved in signal transduction from tyrosine kinase receptors, such as the EGF receptor. They are normally activated by binding GTP through interaction with a guanine nucleotide exchange factor triggered by tyrosine kinase receptors and returned to the resting state by intrinsic GTPase activity enhanced by GTPase-activating proteins (GAPs). Point mutations reduce the ability of the *KRAS* gene to respond to GAPs, and hence there is failure to hydrolyze bound GTP, causing the gene to be perpetually locked into the active conformation and thus continuously transmitting a growth signal to the nucleus. Also, signal transduction systems from a variety of growth factor receptors overexpressed in pancreatic carcinoma converge on the RAS protein, producing further growth stimulation.

*KRAS* mutations are the most common genetic event described in pancreatic carcinoma; there is a missense mutation at codon 12 of the *KRAS* oncogene in at least 75% of advanced ductal adenocarcinomas, unlike other tumors, including colorectal adenocarcinomas, which also show mutations at codons 13 and 61 (38–46). Interestingly, a familial form of pancreatic carcinoma has been described that is associated with mutations at codon 13 (47). Another interesting observation is the predominant base change seen at codon 12 within different tumors (48). The most common base change in pancreatic cancer is guanine to adenine (G to A), similar to those in colorectal cancer but different from the guanine to thymine (G to T) transition seen in lung cancers. While cigarette smoking is a common etiologic factor in both pancreatic and lung cancers, different chemical constituents are thought to be involved. The G to T transitions in lung cancer are thought to be caused by benzpyrene forming adducts with guanine residues and causing misrepair; the G to A base change seen in pancreatic cancers may be produced by a different type of carcinogen, such as aromatic amines and *N*-nitrosamines. However, there is a varied spectrum of different *RAS* mutations at codon 12 in human pancreatic carcinoma, and while the commonest (G to A) gives rise to an aspartic acid mutation, others include valine, arginine, and cysteine amino acid substitutions. The heterogeneity of these *KRAS* mutations is more suggestive of the involvement of multiple carcinogens or errors in the DNA repair mechanism rather than specific mutagens. Also, the pattern of *KRAS* mutations has been reported to differ markedly in Japanese and Europeans, and there appear to be regional variations within Europe (49), raising the possibility of ethnic and/or environmental differences. A group of pancreatic cancers do not show *RAS* mutations, which suggests the presence of another genetic pathway for pancreatic tumorigenesis. By correlating all these genetic findings with epidemiology, it may be possible to identify geographic or ethnic differences in the pathogenesis of this disease as well as identifying specific genotoxic substances.

*KRAS* point mutations appear to be an early event in pancreatic tumorigenesis and are found not only in invasive ductal adenocarcinoma but also in severe dysplasia of the ductal epithelium (38–40, 50), as well as in carcinoma in situ (51). Most pancreatic cancers have the same mutant *KRAS* allele in both the primary and the secondary tumor, but some groups have identified a small number of tumors with two different *KRAS* mutations, suggesting the involvement of independent clones (38, 39, 50). Recently there have been reports of *KRAS* mutations in mucous cell hyperplasia without dysplasia (40–42), especially when associated with a familial history of pancreatic carcinoma (42). Interestingly, there is a report of an increased risk of pancreatic carcinoma in those with chronic pancreatitis (43).

*KRAS* mutations may also be found (at lower frequency) in other pancreatic tumors of ductal origin, including cystadenoma, cystadenocarcinoma, (45) and intraductal papillary neoplasia associated with severe dysplasia (46, 52). There is a very low incidence in ampullary or acinar cell carcinomas, (53–57) and none are seen in endocrine tumors (58).

## TUMOR-SUPPRESSOR GENES

### p53

The tumor-suppressor gene p53 encodes a nuclear phosphoprotein with a short half-life. It is implicated in the control of the cell cycle, apoptosis, DNA repair and synthesis, cell differentiation, and genomic plasticity. p53 activity is regulated by several factors, including the cellular environment, interaction with cellular and oncoviral proteins, and the physical conformation of the p53 protein.

Mutations of the p53 tumor-suppressor gene are probably the most common genetic event in human carcinoma. The wild-type p53 acts as a recessive tumor-suppressor gene, but mutant forms can act as dominant oncogenes (59). The p53 gene products with missense mutations interfere with the wild-type p53, providing a double negative effect (60). More than 50% of pancreatic tumors have some type of gene alteration (40, 61–66), and up to 80% show allelic loss (deletion of one copy of the gene) at the p53 locus 17p13 (61). A broad range of mutations are seen in p53, unlike *KRAS,* which shows missense mutations restricted to a single codon. Most p53 mutations are missense point mutations that lie within the coding sequence, particularly in the evolutionarily conserved exons 5–9. Fifty-five percent of point mutations are transitions (change of a pyrimidine to another pyrimidine). Transversions (change of a pyrimidine to a purine or vice versa) are more commonly seen in lung, as well as head and neck tumors that are associated with cigarette smoking, rather than pancreatic cancer. Smoking is a documented risk factor for pancreatic cancer, but it appears to have a weaker association than for other tumors. Also, there are intragenic frameshift mutations, including deletions, microinsertions, and splice-site mutations leading to the formation of truncated proteins that are particularly common in pancreatic carcinoma. These deletions and insertions appear to be a special feature in pancreatic cancer, compared with other tumors, and they tend to occur in homocopolymer tracts. These mutations are unlikely to exert a dominant negative effect, and it is unclear if frameshift mutations give a strong growth advantage to the affected cell lineage.

The range of mutations in p53 has provided clear evidence for carcinogen fingerprinting, and on examination of this spectrum, it may be possible to identify specific mutagens. Exposure to cigarette smoke has been correlated with G:C to T:A transversions in lung cancers (67). The frequency and range of p53 mutations can act as an indicator of carcinogen exposure, which may prove useful in assessing human cancer risk. The heterogeneous spectrum of p53 mutations suggests that p53 mutations may arise not only from exposure to a particular chemical mutagen but also from endogenous mutagenesis. An example of the latter is the deamination of methylated cytosine residues, which occurs most frequently at CpG sites.

### *CDKN2 (p16/CDKN41/MTS1/p16$^{INK4}$)*

*CDKN2* is a tumor-suppressor gene critical to cell-cycle control through the inhibition of cyclin-dependent kinase 4 (CDK4), which complexes with cyclin D1. The locus lies at 9p21, and mutations are rare in most other primary tumors; however, studies have shown the inactivation of *CDKN2* in approximately 80% of pancreatic carcinomas (68, 69). Also, there have been reports of aberrations of the *CDKN2* gene in the germ line of some patients with pancreatic carcinoma associated with familial melanoma (70, 71).

Loss of function usually occurs by mutation of one allele and deletion of the other. The remainder show homozygous deletion of both alleles. The deleted fragment commonly includes the candidate suppressor gene p15, which lies at a closely adjacent locus. It is possible that this gene is also important in the pathogenesis of pancreatic cancer.

### *DCC*

The *DCC* gene is situated on chromosome 18q. Allelic imbalance is frequently seen on the long arm of chromosome 18q, and so initial reports suggested abnormalities in the expression of the *DCC* gene in pancreatic cancer (66, 72), but subsequent studies have shown that deletion of the *DCC* locus is rare (73). The reported abnormalities may not involve the *DCC* gene locus directly but may target the site of a tumor-suppressor gene at a flanking location on chromosome 18q (73).

### *RB1*

The tumor-suppressor gene *RB1* is rarely affected in pancreatic carcinoma (74). Recently, a high prevalence of allelic imbalance around the *RB1* gene locus at chromosome 13q14 has been reported, which may reflect involvement of the *BRCA 2* gene at 13q12 (75, 76).

### *APC*

*APC* is located at chromosome 5q21 and was first identified in patients with familial adenomatous polyposis (77). At present there is a discrepancy of results between Western groups that have found no evidence of gene mutations or loss of protein expression of the *APC* gene (78, 79) and some Japanese authors who reported inactivating mutations in a small number of cases, predicting a truncation of the gene product (80). The significance of this discrepancy has not been explained yet, and whether it represents some form of ethnic variation remains to be seen.

### Microsatellite Instability

Microsatellites are short repetitive sequences of DNA, scattered throughout the genome, which vary between individuals and have a relatively low inherent mutation rate. Microsatellite DNA is affected by a third type of cancer gene (other than oncogenes and tumor-suppressor genes) that has recently gained attention. A family of DNA mismatch-repair genes *(hMSH2, hMLH1, hPMS1* and *hPMS2)* is recognized as involved in an inherited cancer predisposition syndrome (Lynch syndrome type 2) and some types of sporadic cancer. Abnormalities of these genes allow ubiquitous somatic mutations to accumulate throughout the genome, producing microsatellite instability (MSI), which may be visualized by polymerase chain reaction (PCR) analysis. MSI has been seen in several tumors, including colorectal and gastric tumors, but the presence of MSI in pancreatic cancer is controversial. In the literature, Japanese studies tend to support the presence of MSI in pancreatic cancer (81); most Western groups find this to be a rare phenomenon (79). This apparent geographic variation raises the possibility of ethnic differences.

## MATRIX METALLOPROTEINASES (MMP)

Tumor invasion involves local infiltration and distant metastasis and requires the breakdown of the extracellular matrix (ECM). The matrix metalloproteinases are a family of nine zinc-containing proteolytic enzymes that digest at least one of the components of the ECM. They are subdivided into four groups depending upon their substrate specificity, the specific collagenases (MMP1 and MMP8), the gelatinases (MMP2 and MMP9), the stromelysins (MMP3, MMP10, and MMP11) and the putative MMP (MMP7) (82).

MMPs are secreted initially as proenzymes that are activated by cleavage of specific peptide sequences. They play a role in a wide range of normal processes including wound healing, embryonic development, menopausal involution of the uterus, and pathologic conditions such as connective tissue disease as well as tumor invasion and metastasis (83, 84). All are inhibited by specific tissue inhibitors of the metalloproteinases (TIMPs), which consist of a family of three enzymes, TIMP1–3. The activity of MMPs on the ECM depends upon the balance between these enzymes and their inhibitors. A number of studies have correlated malignant potential with MMP activity. MMP9 production by cancer cell lines is associated with increased metastatic potential, while collagenase activity is associated with stromal vascular and lymphatic invasion as well as high tumor grade (83, 85–87). Stromelysin expression also has been correlated with tumor progression (88). Studies have indicated the importance of the epithelial-stromal interaction in the production of degradative enzymes and have suggested the occurrence of differences in MMP production patterns between different tumor types. TIMPs bind noncovalently to the active MMPs (89), and only small increases of either MMPs or TIMPs are required to cause significant net proteolytic activity (90).

Pancreatic cancer cell lines have been shown to exhibit collagenolytic and gelatinolytic activity due to MMP activity (91–94). Features of pancreatic carcinoma such as the intense stromal reaction, the aggressive local behavior, and loss of collagen type 4 in the basement membrane all suggest that MMPs are likely to play an important role in pancreatic cancer. MMP2 and TIMP1 are more strongly expressed in pancreatic carcinoma than in the normal adjacent pancreas, and TIMP1 immunoreactivity is reduced in tumors with lymph node metastases (95), while MMP2 immunoreactivity is increased with tumor dedifferentiation (95).

## CYTOKINE NETWORKS

Presently, only a few of the regulatory mechanisms involved in the development and growth of pancreatic cancer are known. Pancreatic cancer cells appear to be both a source and a target of various cytokines. These factors appear to be involved in both autocrine and paracrine regulation of tumor growth with a complex interaction between stimulatory and inhibitory cytokines. For instance, tumor necrosis factor alpha (TNF-α) is a proinflammatory mediator that is synthesized by macrophages and binds to well-defined receptors. It exhibits a cytotoxic effect that is thought to involve phospholipase $A_2$ and oxidative damage (96). Normal cells are not lysed when treated by TNF-α alone, but TNF-α-mediated cytotoxicity appears to require further inhibition of protein synthesis, and its potency is strengthened by the induction of further cytokines. Interferon-γ (IFN-γ) has a synergistic cytostatic effect with TNF-α on tumor cells (97), which is related to the increased expression of the TNF receptor (98). TNF-α also affects tumor growth by stimulating growth factors and their receptors, particularly EGFR.

Several cytokines are thought to play a role in the development of the desmoplasia associated with pancreatic cancer. Platelet-derived growth factor (PDGF) has a pleiotropic effect on mesenchymal cells and is found to be produced by pancreatic cancer epithelial cells and several cell lines (99). PDGF expression is augmented by several factors, including TGF-ß and interleukin-1 (IL-1). Also, its transcription is up-regulated by TNF-α. Fibroblasts are stimulated by several other factors including granulocyte-macrophage colony-stimulating factor (100), which is produced by the pancreatic cancer cells and is enhanced by TNF-α. Fibroblasts also are stimulated by the production of FGFs by the malignant epithelial cells.

Cytokines also play a role in the recruitment of effector cells in the tumor by altering cell adhesion and chemotaxis. For instance, TNF-α and IL-1 stimulate the expression of several adhesion molecules including E-selectin and ICAM-1 (intercellular adhesion molecule-1), VCAM-1 (vascular cell-adhesion molecule-1), and P-selectin.

## CYTOGENETICS

A recent review of the cytogenetic abnormalities in pancreatic carcinoma indicates a wide variety of karyotypic abnormalities, most of which are complex and include numerical and structural abnormalities (101). The most frequent findings are whole chromosomal gains in chromosomes 20 and 7 and whole chromosomal losses in chromosomes 18, 13, 12, 17, and 6. Structural abnormalities are common; the most frequently affected chromosomal arms are 1p, 6q, 7q, 17p, 1q, 3p, 11p, and 19q, and losses of portions of the long arm of chromosome 6q in approximately 8% of cases. In addition, double minute chromosomes are identified in approximately 8% of tumors, suggesting gene amplification.

## DIAGNOSTIC APPLICATIONS

The detection of pancreatic lesions has become easier with recent advances in diagnostic imaging modalities such as computed tomography, abdominal ultrasonography, and endoscopic cholangiopancreatography (ERCP); however, the definitive diagnosis of pancreatic carcinoma remains elusive in many cases and requires the assistance of cytodiagnosis. Exploitation of the current knowledge of the molecular biology of pancreatic cancer has enabled development of several new approaches to diagnosis, which presently are adjuncts to conventional techniques. These include biochemical and cytologic analysis of pure pancreatic juice and brushings from ERCP, and fine-needle aspirates of pancreas as well as serum, and stool samples. The biochemical studies involve analysis of multiple assays of tumor-associated antigens including oligosaccharides. One of the more important of these is CA 19-9, the elevation of which aids diagnosis of pancreatic cancer (102–104) and acts as an indicator of resectability (105). Changes in the quantity of elastase 1 also appear to be of diagnostic value (106–110).

Mutations of oncogenes and tumor-suppressor genes in material may be detected by simple and sensitive PCR-based assays. Mutations in *KRAS* and p53 genes appear to be the most promising candidates, and several reports indicate good correlation of positive results with a histologically proven diagnosis of pancreatic cancer (111, 112). *KRAS* mutations may not only be detected in body fluids but also in stool samples (113). Recently it has been reported that tumor cells carrying *KRAS* mutations can be detected in the peripheral blood of patients with pancreatic cancer, even when there are no clinically identifiable metastases (114).

Accumulation of mutant p53 can be detected very easily by immunochemical assays that can be used to detect cells in body fluids. Also, detection of anti-p53 antibodies in the blood has been suggested as a potential screening test (115).

Inactivation of the p16 gene appears to occur almost exclusively in pancreatic carcinoma and not in other gastrointestinal tract carcinomas; thus it may be possible to detect mutations of this gene and design multiplex genetic assays that could help to localize the origin of the shed neoplastic cells.

In the future, it is hoped that further advances in our knowledge of the genetic events of pancreatic cancer, including identification of those events associated with the earliest stages of neoplasia and preneoplasia, coupled with the advancement in technology, will enable pancreatic cancer to be diagnosed at an early, treatable stage. Also, identification of the responsible gene(s) should allow counseling and even preventative intervention in families with an inherited site-specific predisposition to pancreatic cancer.

## THERAPEUTIC POTENTIALS

The current knowledge of consistent genetic abnormalities coupled with improved gene transfer technology has enabled certain molecular changes to become targets for gene therapy. Molecular mimics may be used to modulate or restore function of cancer gene products, or alternatively, genetic intervention strategies may be developed to destroy cancer cells. In the future, it is envisaged that more sophisticated gene therapies will enable effective somatic therapy for cancer, initially for localized disease, but ultimately by systemic delivery for widespread micrometastatic disease.

Some of the therapeutic stratagems may be directed against tumor-modulating stromal components. As discussed above, the MMP enzyme system is important in pancreatic cancer invasion and metastasis. Matrix breakdown only occurs when the levels of activated enzymes exceed those of the inhibitors. In vitro invasion and metastatic lung colonization by human tumor xenografts are reduced by treatment with exogenous human recombinant TIMP1 (116, 117). TIMP2 inhibits the invasion of smooth muscle cell monolayers by HT1080 cells and *RAS*-transformed rat embryo fibroblasts, and it appears to prevent collagen breakdown and invasion by the tumor cells (118, 119). Several low-molecular-weight inhibitors of MMPs have been developed for therapeutic use; the first synthetic one to enter clinical trials in cancer patients was BB94, developed by British Biotech Pharmaceuticals Limited (Oxford, UK). This appears to have inhibitory effects against all the MMPs and has been shown to decrease the tumor burden of human ovarian carcinoma xenografts (120). One disadvantage of this compound is its low solubility, though an analogue with greater solubility has been developed. Currently, alternative synthetic compounds are being developed by other biotechnology companies.

## Germ Line Gene Therapy

In theory, gene therapy could be applied to germ cells; this has been deemed ethically unacceptable, and so permanent correction of familial cancer predisposition syndromes by gene transfer into germ cells (usually ova) cannot be contemplated presently (121, 122). However, genetic intervention in the form of in vitro fertilization and preimplantation diagnosis is routinely carried out for familial genetic diseases such as cystic fibrosis (123), and now this has also been applied to the prevention of site-specific cancer predisposition syndromes, such as familial adenomatous polyposis. With the recognition that pancreatic cancer may occur as part of multisite syndromes such as familial atypical multiple mole melanoma syndrome (124), similar strategies could be applied.

## Somatic Gene Therapy

Somatic gene therapy, the introduction of genetic material into the diploid cells of an individual, could be used to treat many different diseases, including established cancer. It could also be used in the prevention of cancer in cases of inherited cancer predisposition syndromes at an intermediate stage when the disease still involves only a single genetic abnormality rather than at the multigene stage seen in established cancer. For example, in patients with familial adenomatous polyposis caused by "loss of function" mutations in the *APC* gene, the introduction of a normal gene into the intestinal epithelial cells by intraluminal delivery of liposome-complexed DNA has led to temporary restoration of functional gene expression (125). It is envisaged that stratagems including vascular delivery of viral constructs could allow permanent reconstruction through stable integration into intestinal stem cells. In the future, similar approaches could be applied to treat those individuals known to carry a genetic abnormality predisposing to pancreatic cancer.

There are four approaches to genetic intervention for cancer therapy:

1. Replacement or augmentation of tumor-suppressor gene function
2. Blockade of dominant gene expression
3. Genetically directed enzyme producing therapy (GDEPT)
4. Genetic immunodulation

They are outlined below.

**Replacement or Augmentation of Tumor-Suppressor Gene Function.** Mutational inactivation of several tumor-suppressor genes, namely p53 and p16, frequently occurs in pancreatic carcinoma, and these are potential targets for genetic intervention to replace their tumor-suppressor function. *TP53* is one of the most important tumor-suppressor genes (65, 126–130) involved in the early stage of tumorigenesis, and restoration of its function can cause phenotypic reversion of transformed cells in vivo and in vitro. However, in approximately 35% of cases, no *TP53* gene abnormalities are detected, and even in those cases with mutations, there can be significant intratumoral heterogeneity of expression. Also, some evidence of an alternative mechanism of p53 inactivation has been found in the up-regulated expression of the MDM2 gene product in about 60% of pancreatic cancers and cell lines (131).

Many of the missense mutations that affect the suppressor function may simultaneously activate a transdominant transforming function that can complicate simple gene addition therapy. The restoration of *TP53* function, though complicated, remains an attractive target, and a clinical trial for the delivery of wild-type (normal) *TP53* to the operative site of resected bronchial carcinoma has been approved (132).

p16 is another tumor-suppressor gene that is abnormal in approximately 80% of pancreatic cancer cases. It has recently been shown that ectopic expression of $p16^{INK4}$ can block entry into the S phase of the cell cycle induced by a *RAS* oncogene and/or the *c-myc* oncogene, provided there is functional retinoblastoma protein (133). Most pancreatic cancers have normal *RB1* genes, and so there is potential for a $p16^{INK4}$ replacement strategy in this disease.

As indicated above, pancreatic cancer does not appear to involve other tumor-suppressor genes; therefore, these genes tend not to be considered as targets for therapy.

**Blockade of Dominant Gene Expression.** Dominant gene expression may be inhibited by several means, one of which is the antisense oligonucleotide approach. This involves the use of exogenous short, synthetic single-stranded oligonucleotide sequences, which are mostly DNA based. There is inefficient cellular uptake of these proteins, and they are released into the cytoplasm where they are thought to block translation of mRNA, by a variety of mechanisms. Most work has used modified oligonucleotides that have increased stability and lipid solubility. Chimeric oligonucleotides have the modified linkage for only part of the model, either at the 5′ or 3′ end, as intracellular degradation is usually due to exonuclease activity (134). Candidates for potential antisense therapies include the p53 and *KRAS* genes.

Phosphorothiate oligonucleotides have been given systemically to humans (134, 135). A phase I clinical trial used a phosphorothiate oligonucleotide directed against p53 exon 10, OL(1)p53. It was given by continous infusion for 10 days and was well tolerated, with few side effects. This oligopeptide has been reported to have a significant antiproliferative effect on acute myelogenous leukemia, both in vitro and when given by systemic infusion to patients, to inhibit the growth of their leukemic blasts in vitro (136, 137). However, there is no evidence that the effect of this oligonucleotide involves either an antisense interaction or regulation of p53 expression. Results from in vitro transcription/translation experiments strongly suggest that the encouraging antiproliferative effects of OL(1)p53 are not due to a specific antisense interaction leading to modulation of p53 expression (138). Fully phosphorothiate-substituted oligonucleotides are known to have undesirable features such as non-sequence-specific protein binding, slow cellular uptake, and activation of RNase H at sites other than the main target sequence (139). Even if the perfect oligonucleotide could be developed, problems would still remain. Even in malignancies showing expression of mutant p53 with loss of the wild-type allele, effective suppression of the mutant p53 may be hazardous, as certain mutant proteins will retain important wild-type functions. Indeed, reduction in the expression of a mutant p53 protein by antisense interaction has been reported to enhance tumor-cell proliferation and tumorigenicity of lung cancer cell lines (140).

The *KRAS* oncogene is activated in approximately 75% of pancreatic carcinomas by mutation at codon 12, and it is a compelling target for therapeutic intervention. Inhibition of the *RAS*-signaling pathway via several independent methodologies has been shown to modulate critical aspects of *RAS*-mediated transformation in whole cells (141–143). One genetic approach uses the expression of a segment of the *KRAS* cDNA in an antisense orientation to reduce the growth of human lung adenocarcinoma cells in vitro and as orthotopic tumors in mice (144, 145). Three regions of the *KRAS* mRNA have been targeted in the design of antisense oligopeptides (146). These were able to produce dose-dependent antiproliferative effects in human pancreatic cancer cell lines, though there was generally poor discrimination between the antisense and the control (either sense, mismatched, or randomized) oligonucleotides. There was little evidence for reduced KRAS protein levels, using western blot analysis, in any of the tested cell lines from the oligonucleotide-treated cells.

The use of a given oligopeptide in different cell lines appears to produce variable responses. A subline of DHL-4 lymphoma cells developed resistance to an antisense oligonucleotide by the emergence of intracellular degradation that was absent in the parental line (147).

Alternative therapies utilize other means to inactivate the mutant gene. By specific targeting, a mutant *KRAS* gene was genetically disrupted in two human colon cancer cell lines, and this produced loss of anchorage-independent growth (148). Mutant RAS proteins have also been produced that do not transmit growth signals themselves and also block signal transduction from other (wild-type or mutant) RAS proteins in the cell in a dominant manner.

Interference with the localizaton of the mutant gene product may alter its functioning. The RAS protein must be localized to the cell membrane, a process that requires lipid modification of its carboxy terminals. This can be inhibited by drugs that interfere with HMG CoA reductase or other enzymes involved in the metabolism of cholesterol. Drugs such as lovastatin have been shown to inhibit growth and tumorigenicity of pancreatic cancer cells (149, 150).

**Genetically Directed Enzyme Producing Therapy (GDEPT).** The principle is to take advantage of the transcriptional differences between normal and tumor cells or between tumor cells of one tissue and the rest of the individual. Gene transfer into the target cells enables the expression of a gene encoding for a prodrug-activating enzyme whose expression is directed by a tumor/tissue-specific gene promoter. These enzymes are themselves innocuous, but they produce cellular susceptibility of the target cells to the toxin metabolized from the subsequently administered prodrug. A variety of gene promoters might be exploited for GDEPT in pancreatic carcinoma, and already there have been encouraging results reported with the human HER2 promoter (151) and the CEA promoter (152). When the HER2 promoter is fused to the cytosine deaminase gene or HSV thymidine kinase gene and introduced into pancreatic cells in vitro or in vivo using plasmid and viral vectors, expression of the insert occurs only in the HER2-expressing cancer cells (151). This is very encouraging evidence for the specificity of targeting gene expression to minimize potential toxicity in clinical trials.

The *CEA* gene is expressed in a variety of adenocarcinomas, as well as normal intestinal cells, and is a candidate for the tissue-selective targeting of gene expression. The *CEA* promoter was fused to the *HSV-tk* gene and introduced to the *CEA*-positive pancreatic cell line BxPc3 by use of an amphotropic retrovirus (152). When treated with the prodrug ganciclovir, the tumor cells were killed, and the fact that not all the target cells needed to be transduced for significant cytotoxicity to be observed suggested a bystander effect.

Other candidate promoter systems include those of the *MUC1, MUC2, MUC4,* and *MUC5* genes (153, 154) and those of other up-regulated receptor-ligand systems, especially FGFs and FGFRs (34–37, 155).

**Genetic Immunodulation.** Genetic immunodulation involves stratagems to induce a systemic cytotoxic immune response directed specifically against tumor cells (156). Local expression or delivery of exogenous cytokines at the site of a tumor can produce impressive antitumor responses (157) both against the transduced tumor cells and against subsequent challenge with parental cells (158–161), though the effects vary depending upon the cytokine chosen and the tumor model. However, no significant advantage has been achieved to date by the use of systemic cytokines in the treatment of pancreatic cancer, and indeed, using such agents may be associated with serious side effects (162, 163). Newer studies have shown the temporary arrest of tumor progression after injection of TNF-α into solid neoplasms (164). Areas of interest include the enhancement of local cytokine secretion by either transfected tumor infiltrating lymphocytes or transfected tumor cells; another area is the use of monoclonal antibodies to produce cytokine-modulated antigen expression. TNF-α stimulates the expression of EGFR in vitro (165), which favors EGFR-specific monoclonal antibodies of the isotope IgG2a. In one study, monoclonal antibody IgG2a used in tumor and melanoma cell lines produced antibody-dependent cytotoxicity of the tumor cells (166).

Inoculation of experimental animals with plasmids encoding a variety of proteins has been shown to stimulate both antibody and T-cell immune responses that are specific and sometimes long-lived (167, 168). Some tumors such as malignant melanoma show more convincing evidence of specific tumor-associated antigens. Possible candidate antigens for pancreatic carcinoma include underglycosylated mucins, which can be recognized by MHC-unrestricted T cells (169). Mutated tumor-suppressor genes and oncogenes such as *RAS* and *TP53* represent potential targets for immune recognition and attack stimulated by using constructs that direct expression of fragments of these genes that contain T-cell epitopes (170). Recently, a study using mutant RAS peptides as a vaccine for specific immunotherapy in a small number of pancreatic carcinoma patients produced a transient RAS-specific T-cell response in several patients, though no major therapeutic response was seen (171).

Other potential targets may include normal proteins that show elevated expression in pancreatic carcinoma and so act as a tumor antigen for an immune response (172 173), such as up-regulation of growth factor receptors. Also, in pancreatic cancer there is reexpression of embryonic antigens, in particular CEA, and this has been used for active adoptive immunotherapy (174).

In summary, there have been dramatic advances, led by the laboratory, in our understanding of the cellular and molecular genetic basis of pancreatic cancer over the last decade. The challenge now is to harness and translate this knowledge into stratagems for screening and for diagnostic and therapeutic purposes to benefit those in the clinic who are affected or at risk of the disease.

## REFERENCES

1. Korc M, Chandrasekar B, Yamanaka Y, Friess H, Buchler M, Beger HG. Overexpression of the epidermal growth-factor receptor in human pancreatic cancer is associated with concomitant increases in the levels of epidermal growth-factor and transforming growth-factor-alpha. J Clin Invest 1992;90:1352–1360.
2. Shing Y, Christofori G, Hanahan D, et al. Betacellulin: a mitogen from pancreatic beta cell tumours. Science 1993;259:125–133.

3. Barton CM, Hall PA, Hughes CM, Gullick WJ, Lemoine NR. Transforming growth factor alpha and epidermal growth factor in human pancreatic cancer. J Pathol 1991;163:111–116.
4. Ebert M, Yokoyama M, Kobrin MS, et al. Induction and expression of amphiregulin in human pancreatic cancer. Cancer Res 1994;54:3959–3962.
5. Yokoyama M, Ebert M, Funatomi H, et al. Amphiregulin is a potent mitogen in human pancreatic cancer cells: correlation with patient survival. Int J Oncol 1995;6:625–663.
6. Lemoine NR, Hughes CM, Barton CM, et al. The epidermal growth factor receptor in human pancreatic cancer. J Pathol 1992;166:7–12.
7. Yamanaka Y, Friess H, Kobrin MS, Buchler M, Beger HG, Korc M. Coexpression of epidermal growth factor receptor and ligands in human pancreatic cancer is associated with enhanced tumor aggressiveness. Anticancer Res 1993;13:565–570.
8. Kraus MH, Issing W, Miki T, Popescu NC, Aaronson SA. Isolation and characterization of ERBB3, a third member of the ERBB/epidermal growth factor receptor family, evidence for overexpression in a subset of human mammary tumours. Proc Natl Acad Sci USA 1989;86:9193–9197.
9. Plowman GD, Culouscou JM, Whitney GS, et al. Ligand-specific activation of HER4/p180erbB4, a fourth member of the epidermal growth factor receptor family. Proc Natl Acad Sci USA 1993;90:1746–1750.
10. Lemoine NR, Lobresco M, Leung H, et al. The erbB-3 gene in human pancreatic cancer. J Pathol 1992;168:269–273.
11. Hall PA, Hughes CM, Staddon SL, Richman PI, Gullick WJ, Lemoine NR. The c-erbB-2 proto-oncogene in human pancreatic cancer. J Pathol 1990;161:195–200.
12. Lei S, Appert HE, Nakata B, Domenico DR, Kim K, Howard JM. Overexpression of HER-2/neu oncogene in pancreatic cancer correlates with shortened survival. Int J Pancreatol 1995;17: 15–21.
13. Williams TM, Weiner D, Greene MI, Maguire HC. Expression of c-erbB-2 in human pancreatic adenocarcinomas. Pathobiology 1991;59:46–52.
14. Yamanaka Y. The immunohistochemical expressions of epidermal growth factors, epidermal growth factor receptors and c-erbB-2 oncoprotein in human pancreatic cancer. Nippon Ika Daigaku Zasshi 1992;59:51–61.
15. Yamanaka Y, Friess H, Kobrin MS, et al. Overexpression of the HER/neu oncogene in human pancreatic cancer. Hum Pathol 1993;24:1127–1134.
16. Friess H, Yamanaka Y, Kobrin MS, Do DA, Buchler MW, Korc M. Enhanced erbB-3 expression in human pancreatic cancer correlates with tumour progression. 1995;1:1413–1420.
17. Naldini L, Weidner M, Vigna E, et al. Scatter factor and hepatocyte growth factor are indistinguishable ligands for the Met receptor. EMBO J 1991;10:2867–2878.
18. Weidner KM, Sachs M, Birchmeier W. The Met receptor tyrosine kinase transduces motility, proliferation, and morphogenic signals of scatter factor/hepatocyte growth factor. J Cell Biol 1993;121:145–154.
19. Ebert M, Yokoyama M, Friess H, Buchler MW, Korc M. Coexpression of the c-met protooncogene and hepatocyte growth-factor in human pancreatic-cancer. Cancer Res 1994;54:5775–5778.
20. DiRenzo MF, Poulsom R, Olivero M, Comoglio PM, Lemoine NR. Expression of the met hepatocyte growth factor receptor in human pancreatic cancer. Cancer Res 1995;55:1129–1138.
21. Tsuda H, Iwase T, Matsumoto K, et al. Immunohistochemical localization of hepatocyte growth factor protein in pancreas islet A-cells of man and rats. Jpn J Cancer Res 1992;83:1262–1266.
22. Furukawa T, Duguid WP, Kobari M, Matsuno S, Tsao M-S. Hepatocyte growth factor and Met receptor expression in human pancreatic carcinogenesis. Am J Pathol 1995;147: 889–895.
23. Wrana JL, Attisano L, Carcamo J, et al. TGF beta signals through a heterodimer protein kinase receptor complex. Cell 1992;71: 1003–1014.
24. Lin HY, Wang XF, Ng-Eaton E, Weinberg RA, Lodish HF. Expression cloning of the TGF-beta type II receptor, a functional transmembrane serine/threonine kinase. Cell 1992;68:775–785.
25. Wang X-F, Lin HY, Ng-Eaton E, Downward J, Lodish HF, Weinberg RA. Expression cloning and characterization of the TGF-beta type III receptor. Cell 1991;67:797–805.
26. Massague J. The transforming growth factor-ß family. Annu Rev Cell Biol 1990;6:597–641.
27. Massague J, Cheifetz Z, Laiho M, Ralph DA, Weis FMB, Zentella A. Transforming growth factor-ß. Cancer Surv 1992;12:81–103.
28. Sporn MB, Roberts AB. Transforming growth factor-ß: recent progress and new changes. J Cell Biol 1992;119:1017–1021.
29. Baldwin RL, Korc M. Growth inhibition of human pancreatic carcinoma cells by transforming growth factor beta-1. Growth Factors 1993;8:23–34.
30. Friess H, Yamanaka Y, Buchler M, et al. Enhanced expression of transforming growth-factor-beta isoforms in pancreatic-cancer correlates with decreased survival. Gastroenterology 1993;105: 1846–1856.
31. Friess H, Yamanaka Y, Buchler M, et al. Enhanced expression of the type II transforming growth factor beta receptor in human pancreatic cancer cells without alteration of type III receptor expression. Cancer Res 1993;53:2704–2707.
32. Roberts AB, Sporn MB, Assoian RK, Smith JM, Roche NS. Transforming growth factor type beta: rapid induction of fibrosis and angiogenesis in vivo and stimulation of collagen formation in vitro. Proc Natl Acad Sci USA 1986;83:4167–4171.
33. Klagsbrun M. The fibroblast growth factor family: structural and biological properties. Prog Growth Factor Res 1989;1:207–235.
34. Leung HY, Hughes CM, Kloppel G, Williamson RCN, Lemoine NR. Localization of expression of fibroblast growth factors and their receptors in pancreatic adenocarcinoma by in-situ hybridization. Int J Oncol 1994;4:1219–1223.
35. Friess H, Yamanaka Y, Buchler M, et al. Increased expression of acidic and basic fibroblast growth-factors in chronic-pancreatitis. Am J Pathol 1994;144:117–128.
36. Yamanaka Y, Friess H, Buchler M, et al. Overexpression of acidic and basic fibroblast growth-factors in human pancreatic-cancer correlates with advanced tumor stage. Cancer Res 1993;53:5289–5296.
37. Kobrin MS, Yamanaka Y, Friess H, Lopez ME, Korc M. Aberrant expression of type I fibroblast growth factor receptor in human pancreatic adenocarcinomas. Cancer Res 1993;53:4741–4744.
38. Motojima K, Urano T, Nagata Y, Shiku H, Tsurifune T, Kanematsu T. Detection of point mutations in the Kirsten-ras oncogene provides evidence for the multicentricity of pancreatic carcinoma. Ann Surg 1993;217:138–143.
39. Grunewald R, Lyons J, Frohlich A, et al. High frequency of Ki-ras codon 12 mutation in pancreatic adenocarcinomas. Int J Cancer 1989;43:1037–1041.
40. Yanagisawa A, Ohtake K, Ohashi K, et al. Frequent c-Ki-ras oncogene activation in mucous cell hyperplasias of pancreas suffering from chronic inflammation. Cancer Res 1993;53: 953–956.
41. Caldas C, Hahn SA, da Costa LT, et al. Frequent somatic mutations and homozygous deletions of the p16 (MTS1) gene in pancreatic adenocarcinoma. Nature Genet 1994;8:27–31.
42. DiGiuseppe JA, Hruban RH, Offerhaus GJA, et al. Detection of K-ras mutations in mucinous pancreatic duct hyperplasia from a patient with a family history of pancreatic cancer. Am J Pathol 1994;144:889–895.
43. Lowenfels AB, Maisonneuve P, Cavallini G, et al. Pancreatitis and the risk of pancreatic cancer. International Pancreatitis Study Group. N Engl J Med 1993;328:1433–1437.
44. Gonzales-Cadavid NF, Zhou D, Battifora H, Bar-Eli M, Cline MJ. Direct sequencing analysis of exon 1 of the c-K-ras gene shows a low frequency of mutations in human pancreatic adenocarcinomas. Oncogene 1989;4:1137–1140.
45. Yanagisawa A, Kato Y, Ohtake K, et al. c-Ki-ras point mutations in ductectatic-type mucinous cystic neoplasms of the pancreas. Jpn J Cancer Res 1993;82:1057–1060.
46. Tada M, Omata M, Ohto M. Ras gene mutations in intraductal papillary neoplasms of the pancreas. Analysis in five cases. Cancer 1991;67:634–637.
47. Evans JP, Burke W, Chen R, et al. Familial pancreatic adenocarcinoma: association with diabetes and early molecular diagnosis. J Med Genet 1995;32:330–335.
48. Capella G, Villanueva A, Erill N, Lluis F. Molecular epidemiology of protooncogene and tumour-suppressor gene mutations. In: Neoptolemos JP, Lemoine NR, eds. Pancreatic cancer:

molecular and clinical advances. Oxford: Blackwell Science, 1996:171–173.
49. Scarpa A, Capelli P, Villanueva A, et al. Pancreatic cancer in Europe: Ki-ras gene mutation pattern shows geographical differences. Int J Cancer 1994;57:167–171.
50. Pellegata NS, Sessa F, Renault B, et al. K-ras and p53 gene mutations in pancreatic cancer: ductal and non-ductal tumors progress through different genetic lesions. Cancer Res 1994;54: 1556–1560.
51. Lemoine NR, Jain S, Hughes CM, et al. Ki-ras oncogene activation in preinvasive pancreatic cancer. Gastroenterology 1992;102:230–236.
52. Hoshi T, Imai M, Ogawa K. Frequent K-ras mutations and absence of p53 mutations in mucin-producing tumors of the pancreas. J Surg Oncol 1994;55:84–91.
53. Miki H, Matsumoto S, Harada H, et al. Detection of c-Ki-ras point mutation from pancreatic juice. A useful diagnostic approach for pancreatic carcinoma. Int J Pancreatol 1993;14:145–148.
54. Motojima K, Tsunoda T, Kanematsu T, Nagata Y, Urano T, Shiku H. Distinguishing pancreatic carcinoma from other periampullary carcinomas by analysis of mutations in the Kirsten-ras oncogene. Ann Surg 1991;214:657–662.
55. Stork P, Loda M, Bosari S, Wiley B, Poppenhusen K, Wolfe H. Detection of K-ras mutations in pancreatic and hepatic neoplasms by non-isotopic mismatched polymerase chain reaction. Oncogene 1991;6:857–862.
56. Masson P, Andren-Sandberg A. Crude isolation of DNA from unselected human pancreatic tissue and amplification by the polymerase chain reaction of Ki-ras oncogene to detect point mutations in pancreatic cancer. Acta Oncol 1992;31: 421–424.
57. Urban T, Ricci S, Grange J-D, et al. Detection of c-Ki-ras mutation by PCR/RFLP analysis and diagnosis of pancreatic adenocarcinomas. J Natl Cancer Inst 1993;85:2008–2012.
58. Yashiro T, Fulton N, Hara H, et al. Comparison of mutations of ras oncogene in human pancreatic exocrine and endocrine tumors. Surgery 1993;114:758–763.
59. Lane D, Benchimol S. p53: oncogene or anti-oncogene? Genes Dev 1990;4:1–8.
60. Vogelstein B, Kinzler K. p53 function and dysfunction. Cell 1992;70:523–526.
61. Redston MS, Caldas C, Seymour AB, et al. p53 mutations in pancreatic carcinoma and evidence of common homocopolymer tracts in DNA microdeletions. Cancer Res 1994;54:3025–3033.
62. Berrozpe G, Schaeffer J, Peinado MA, Real FX, Perucho M. Comparative analysis of mutations in the p53 and K-ras genes in pancreas cancer. Int J Cancer 1994;58:185–191.
63. Kalthoff H, Schmiegel W, Roeder C, et al. p53 and K-RAS alterations in pancreatic epithelial cell lesions. Oncogene 1993;8:289–298.
64. Ruggeri BA, Klein-Szanto AJP, Huang LY, Lang D. P53 and RB-1 tumor suppressor gene expression and alterations in human pancreatic cancer. Int J Pancreatol 1994;16:193–196.
65. Scarpa A, Capelli P, Mukai K, et al. Pancreatic adenocarcinomas frequently show p53 gene mutations. Am J Pathol 1993; 142:1534–1543.
66. Simon B, Weinel R, Hohne M, et al. Frequent alterations of the tumor suppressor genes p53 and DCC in human pancreatic cancer. Gastroenterology 1994;106:1645–1651.
67. Greenblat MS, Bennet WP, Hollstein M, Harris CC. Mutations in the p53 tumour suppressor gene; clues to cancer aetiology and molecular pathogenesis. Cancer Res 1994;54:4855–4878.
68. Kamb A, Gruis NA, Weaver-Feldhaus J, et al. A cell cycle regulator potentially involved in the genesis of many tumor types. Science 1994;264:436–440.
69. Lui Q, Yan Y-X, McClure M, Nakagawa H, Fujimura F, Rustgi AK. MTS-1 (CDKN2) tumour suppressor gene deletions are a frequent event in esophagus squamous cancer and pancreatic adenocarcinoma cell lines. Oncogene 1995;10:619–622.
70. Hussussian CJ, Struewing JP, Goldstein AM, et al. Germline p16 mutations in familial melanoma. Nature Genet 1994;8:15–21.
71. Kamb A, Shattuck-Eidens D, Eeles R, et al. Analysis of the p16 gene (CDNK2) as a candidate for the chromosome 9p melanoma susceptibility locus. Nature Genet 1994;8:23–26.
72. Hohne MW, Halatsch M-E, Kahl GF, Weinel RJ. Frequent loss of expression of the potential tumor suppressor gene DCC in ductal pancreatic adenocarcinoma. Cancer Res 1992;52: 2616–2619.
73. Barton CM, McKie AB, Hogg A, et al. Abnormalities of the RB1 and DCC tumor suppressor genes: uncommon in human pancreatic adenocarcinoma. Mol Carcinogen 1995;13:61–69.
74. Seymour AB, Hruban RH, Redston M, et al. Allelotype of pancreatic adenocarcinoma. Cancer Res 1994;54:2761–2764.
75. Wooster R, Neuhausen SL, Mangion J, et al. Localization of a breast cancer susceptibility gene BRCA 2, to chromosome 13q12–13. Science 1994;265:2088–2090.
76. Schutte M, da Costa LT, Hahn SA, et al. Identification by representational difference analysis of a homozygous deletion in pancreatic carcinoma that lies within the BRCA2 region. Proc Natl Acad Sci USA 1995;92:5950–5954.
77. Kinzler K, Nilbert M, Vogelstein B, et al. Identification of a gene located at chromosome 5q21 that is mutated in colorectal cancers. Science 1991;251:1366–1370.
78. Smith KJ, Johnson KA, Bryan TM, et al. The APC gene product in normal and tumor cells. Proc Natl Acad Sci USA 1993;90:2846–2850.
79. McKie AB, Filipe MI, Lemoine NR. Abnormalities affecting the APC and MCC tumour suppressor gene loci on chromosome 5q occur frequently in gastric cancer but not in pancreatic cancer. Int J Cancer 1993;55:598–603.
80. Horii A, Nakatsuru S, Miyoshi Y, et al. Frequent somatic mutations of the APC gene in human pancreatic cancer. Cancer Res 1992;52:6696–6698.
81. Han H-J, Yanagisawa A, Kato Y, Park J-G, Nakamura Y. Genetic instability in pancreatic cancer and poorly differentiated type of gastric cancer. Cancer Res 1993;53:5087–5089.
82. Murphy GJP, Murphy G, Reynolds JJ. The origin of matrix metalloproteinases and their familial relationships. FEBS Lett 1991;289:4–7.
83. Liotta LA, Tryggvason K, Garbisa S, Hart I, Foltz CM, Shafie S. Metastatic potential correlates with enzymatic degradation of the basement membrane collagen. Nature 1980;284:67–68.
84. Docherty AJ, Murphy G. The metalloproteinase family and the inhibitor TIMP: a study using cDNAs and recombinant proteins. Ann Rheum Dis 1990;49:469–479.
85. Yamagata S, Tanaka R, Ito Y, Shimizu S. Gelatinases of metastatic cell lines of murine colonic carcinoma as detected by substrate gel-electrophoresis. Biochem Biophys Res Comm 1988;151: 158–162.
86. Yamagata S, Tanaka R, Ito Y, Shimizu S. Gelatinases of murine metastatic tumour cells. Biochem Biophys Res Comm 1989;158: 228–234.
87. Nakajima M, Welch DR, Belloni PN, Nicholson GL. Degradation of basement membrane type 4 collagen and lung subepithelial matrix by rat mammary adenocarcinoma cell clones of differing metastatic potentials. Cancer Res 1987;47:4869–4876.
88. Matrisian LM, Bowden GT. Stromelysin/transin and tumour progression. Semin Cancer Biol 1990;1:107–115.
89. Cawston TE, Galloway WA, Mercer E, Murphy G, Reynolds JJ. Purification of rabbit bone inhibitor of collagenase. Biochem J 1981;195:159–165.
90. Ponton A, Coulombe B, Skup D. Decreased expression of tissue inhibitor of metalloproteinases in metastatic tumour cells leading to increased collagenase activity. Cancer Res 1991;51:2138–2143.
91. Zucker S, Lysik RM, Wieman J, Wilkie DP, Lane B. Diversity of human pancreatic cancer cell proteinases: role of cell membrane metalloproteinases in collagenolysis and cytolysis. Cancer Res 1985;45:6168–6178.
92. Zucker S, Wieman JM, Lysik RM, et al. Enrichment of collagen and gelatin degrading activities in the plasma membranes of human cancer cells. Cancer Res 1987;47:1608–1614.
93. Zucker S, Moll UM, Lysik RM, et al. Extraction of type-IV collagenase/gelatinase from plasma membranes of human cancer cells. Int J Cancer 1990;45:1137–1142.
94. Zucker S, Moll UM, Lysik RM, DiMassimo EI, Schwedes JW, Liotta LA. Extraction of type IV collagenase/gelatinase from plasma membranes of human pancreatic cancer cells. Matrix (Suppl) 1992;1:411.
95. Bramhall S, Lemoine N, Stamp G, Donovan I, Dunn J, Neoptolemos J. 72 kDa collagenase, stromelysin-1 and tissue inhibitor of

metalloproteinase-1 expression in pancreatic cancer (Abstract). Digestion 1994;55:286.
96. Vilchek J, Lee TH. Tumour necrosis factor. J Biol Chem 1991;266: 1338–1344.
97. Sugarman BJ, Aggarwal BB, Hass PE, Figari IS, Palladino MA, Shephard HM. Recombinant human tumour necrosis factor-α: effects on proliferation of normal and transformed cells in vitro. Science 1985;230:943–945.
98. Folkman J, Klasbrun M. Angiogenic factors. Science 1987;235: 442–447.
99. Kalthoff H, Roeder C, Humburg I, Thiele H-G, Greten H, Schmiegel W. Modulation of platelet-derived growth factor A- and B-chain/c-sis mRNA by tumour necrosis factor and other agents in adenocarcinoma cells. Oncogene 1991;6:1015–1021.
100. Dedhar S, Gaboury L, Galloway P, Eaves C. Human granulocyte-macrophage colony-stimulating factor is a growth factor active on a variety of cell types of nonhemopoietic origin. Proc Natl Acad Sci USA 1988;85:9253–9257.
101. Griffin CA, Hruban RH, Morsberger LA, et al. Consistent chromosome abnormalities in adenocarcinoma of the pancreas. Cancer Res 1995;55:2394–2399.
102. Satake K, Takeuchi T, Homma T, Ozaki H. CA 19-9 as a screening and diagnostic tool in symptomatic patients: the Japanese experience. Pancreas 1994;9:703–706.
103. Frebourg T, Bercoff E, Manchon N, et al. The evaluation of CA 19-9 antigen level in the early detection of pancreatic cancer. A prospective study of 866 patients. Cancer 1988;62:2287–2290.
104. Sakate K, Takeuchi T. Comparison of CA 19-9 with other tumour markers in the diagnosis of cancer of the pancreas. Pancreas 1994;9:720–724.
105. Forsmark CE, Lambiase L, Vogel SB. Diagnosis of pancreatic cancer and prediction of unresectability using the tumour-associated antigen CA 19-9. Pancreas 1994;9:731–734.
106. Nakaizumi A, Tatsuta M, Uehara H, et al. A prospective trial of early detection of pancreatic cancer by ultrasonographic examination combined with measurement of serum elastase 1. Cancer 1992;69:936–940.
107. Satake K, Chung YS, Umeyama K, Takeuchi T, Kim YS. The possibility of diagnosing small pancreatic cancer (less than 4.0 cm) by measuring various serum tumor markers. A retrospective study. Cancer 1991;68:149–152.
108. Ito T, Kimura T, Nawata H. Serum elastase 1 appears specific for cancer of the pancreatic head. Am J Gastroenterol 1991;86: 1778–1783.
109. Gentiloni N, Caradonna P, Costamagna G, et al. Pancreatic juice 90K and serum CA 19-9 combined determination can discriminate between pancreatic cancer and chronic pancreatitis. Am J Gastroenterol 1995;90:1069–1072.
110. Nakaizumi A, Tatsuta M, Uehara H, et al. A prospective trial of early detection of pancreatic cancer by ultrasonographic examination combined with measurement of serum elastase 1. Cancer 1992;69:936–940.
111. van Es JM, Polak MM, van den Berg FM, et al. Molecular markers for the diagnostic cytology of neoplasms in the head region of the pancreas: mutation of K-ras and overexpression of the p53 protein product. J Clin Pathol 1995;48:218–222.
112. Van Laethem J-L, Vertongen P, Deviere J, et al. Detection of C-Ki-ras gene codon 12 mutations from pancreatic duct brushings in the diagnosis of pancreatic tumours. Gut 1995;36: 781–787.
113. Caldas C, Hahn SA, Hruban RH, Redston MS, Yeo CJ, Kern SE. Detection of K-ras mutations in the stool of patients with pancreatic adenocarcinoma and pancreatic ductal hyperplasia. Cancer Res 1994;54:3568–3573.
114. Tada M, Omata M, Kawai S, et al. Detection of ras gene mutations in pancreatic juice and peripheral blood of patients with pancreatic adenocarcinoma. Cancer Res 1993;53:2472–2474.
115. Marxsen J, Schmiegel W, Roder C, et al. Detection of the anti-p53 antibody-response in malignant and benign pancreatic disease. Br J Cancer 1994;70:1031–1034.
116. Alvarez OA, Carmichael DF, DeClerck YA. Inhibition of collagenolytic activity and metastasis of tumour cells by a recombinant human tissue inhibitor of metalloproteinases. J Natl Cancer Inst 1990;82:589–595.
117. Schultz RM, Silberman S, Persky B, Bajkowski AS, Carmichael DF. Inhibition by human recombinant tissue inhibitor of metalloproteinases of human amnion invasion and lung colonisation by murine B16-F10 melanoma cells. Cancer Res 1988;48:5539–5545.
118. De Clerk YA, Yean T-D, Lu HS, Ting J, Langley KE. Inhibition of autoproteolytic activation of interstitial procollagenase by recombinant metalloproteinase inhibitor MI/TIMP2. J Biol Chem 1991;266:3893–3899.
119. Albini A, Melchiori A, Santi L, Liotta LA, Brown PD, Stetler-Stevenson WG. Tumour cell invasion inhibited by TIMP2. J Natl Cancer Inst 1991;83:775–779.
120. Davis B, Brown PD, East N, Crimmin MJ, Balkwill FR. A synthetic metalloproteinase inhibitor decreases tumour burden and prolongs survival of mice bearing human ovarian carcinoma xenografts. Cancer Res 1993;53:2087–2091.
121. Harris JD, Sikora K. Human genetic therapy. Mol Aspects Med 1993;14:455–546.
122. Wivel NA, Walters L. Germline gene modification and disease prevention: some medical and ethical perspectives. Science 1993;262:533–538.
123. Gullick WJ, Handyside A. Pre-implantation diagnosis of inherited predisposition to cancer. Eur J Cancer 1994;30A:2030–2032.
124. Lynch HT, Fusaro L, Furaso R, Lynch J, Smyrk T. Hereditary pancreatic cancer. Pedigree analysis of pancreatic cancer families. Int J Pancreatol 1994;16:210–214.
125. Westbrook CA, Chamura SJ, Arenas RB, Kim SY, Otto G. Human APC expression in rodent colonic epithelium in vivo using liposomal gene delivery. Hum Mol Genet 1994;3:2005–2010.
126. Barton CM, Staddon SL, Hughes CM, et al. Abnormalities of the p53 tumour suppressor gene in human pancreatic cancer. Br J Cancer 1991;64:1076–1082.
127. Casey G, Yamanaka Y, Friess H, et al. p53 mutations are common in pancreatic cancer and are absent in chronic pancreatitis. Cancer Lett 1993;69:151–160.
128. Boschman CR, Stryker S, Reddy JK, Ras MS. Expression of p53 protein in precursor lesions and adenocarcinoma of human pancreas. Am J Pathol 1994;145:1291–1295.
129. Ruggeri B, Zhang SY, Caamano J, DiRado M, Flynn SD, Klein-Szanto AJ. Human pancreatic carcinomas and cell lines reveal frequent and multiple alterations in the p53 and Rb-1 tumor-suppressor genes. Oncogene 1992;7:1503–1511.
130. Zhang SY, Ruggeri B, Agarwal P. Immunohistochemical analysis of p53 expression in human pancreatic carcinomas. Arch Pathol 1994;118:150–154.
131. Ebert M, Yokoyama M, Kobrin MS, Friess H, Buchler MW, Korc K. Increased MDM2 expression and immunoreactivity in human pancreatic adenocarcinoma. Int J Oncol 1994;5:1279–1284.
132. Roth JA, Muthopadhyay T, Zhang WW, Fujiwara T, Georges R. Gene replacement strategies for the prevention and treatment of cancer. Eur J Cancer 1994;30a:2032–2037.
133. Serrano M, Gomez-Lahoz E, DePintro RA, Beach D, Bar-Sagi D. Inhibition of ras-induced proliferation and cellular transformation by $p16^{ink4}$. Science 1995;267:249–252.
134. Spinolo J, Iversen P, Smith L, et al. Antisense p53 oligodeoxynucleotide for systemic human anti-leukemic therapy. Hum Gene Ther 1992;3:2A.
135. Giles R, Tidd D. Increased specificity for antisense oligodeoxynucleotide targeting of RNA cleavage by RNase H using chimeric methylphosphonodiester/phosphodiester structures. Nucleic Acids Res 1992;20:763–770.
136. Bayever E, Iversen P, Bishop M, et al. Systemic administration of a phosphorothioate oligonucleotide complementary to p53 in acute myelogenous leukemia and myelodysplastic syndrome: phase I clinical trial. Cancer Gene Ther 1993;1(suppl):11A.
137. Bishop M, Bayever E, Iversen P, et al. Phase I trial of systemic administration of OL(1)p53 oligonucleotide in refractory acute myelogenous leukemia and advanced myelodysplastic syndrome. Blood 1993;82(10)(suppl):1757A.
138. Barton CM, Lemoine NR. Antisense oligonucleotides directed against TP53 have antiproliferative effects unrelated to effects on p53 expression. Br J Cancer 1995;71:429–437.
139. Stein C, Kreig A. Problems in the interpretation of data derived from the in vitro and in vivo use of antisense oligonucleotides. Antisense Res Dev 1994;4:67–69.
140. Mukhopadhyay T, Roth J. A codon 248 p53 mutation retains tumour suppressor function as shown by enhancement of

tumour growth by antisense p53. Cancer Res 1993;53:4362–4366.
141. James G, Goldstein J, Brown M, et al. Benzodiazepine peptidomimetics: potent inhibitors of ras farnesylation in animal cells. Science 1993;260:1937–1942.
142. Kohl N, Mosser S, deSolms S, et al. Selective inhibition of ras-dependent transformation by a farnesyltransferase inhibitor. Science 1993;260:1934–1937.
143. Kohl NE, Wilson FR, Mosser SD, et al. Protein farnesyltransferase inhibitors block the growth of ras-dependent tumours in nude mice. Proc Natl Acad Sci USA 1994;91:9141–9145.
144. Mukhopadhyay T, Tainsky M, Cavender A, Roth J. Specific inhibition of K-ras expression and tumourigenicity on lung cancer cells by antisense RNA. Cancer Res 1991;51:1744–1748.
145. Georges R, Mukhopadhyay T, Zhang Y, Yen N, Roth J. Prevention of orthotopic human lung cancer growth by intratracheal instillation of a retroviral antisense K-ras construct. Cancer Res 1993;53:1743–1746.
146. Carter G, Gilbert C, Lemoine NR. Effects of antisense oligonucleotides targeting the KRAS oncogene in pancreatic cancer cell lines. Int J Oncol 1995;6:1105–1112.
147. Ryte A, Morelli S, Mazzei M, et al. Oligonucleotide degradation contributes to resistance to antisense compounds. Anticancer Drugs 1993;4:197–200.
148. Shirasawa S, Furuse M, Yokoyama N, Sasazuki T. Altered growth of human colon cancer cell lines disrupted at activated Ki-ras. Science 1993;260:85–88.
149. Mikulski SM, Viera A, Darzynkiewicz Z, Shogen K. Synergism between a novel amphibian oocyte ribonuclease and lovastatin in inducing cytostatic and cytotoxic effects in human lung and pancreatic carcinoma cell lines. Br J Cancer 1992;66: 304–310.
150. Sumi S, Beauchamp RD, Townsend CM, et al. Inhibition of pancreatic adenocarcinoma cell growth by lovastatin. Gastroenterology 1992;103:982–989.
151. Harris JD, Gutierrez AA, Hurst HC, Sikora K, Lemoine NR. Gene therapy for cancer using tumour-specific prodrug activation. Gene Ther 1994;1:170–175.
152. Di Maio JM, Clary BM, Via DF, Coveney E, Pappas TN, Lyerly HK. Directed enzyme prodrug gene therapy for pancreatic cancer in vivo. Surgery 1994;116:205–213.
153. Balague C, Gambus G, Carrato C, et al. Altered expression of MUC2, MUC4 and MUC5 mucin genes in pancreas tissue and cancer cell lines. Gastroenterology 1994;106:1054–1061.
154. Hollingsworth MA, Strawhecker JM, Caffrey TC, Mack DR. Expression of MUC1, MUC3 and MUC4 mucin mRNAs in human pancreatic and intestinal tumour cell lines. Int J Cancer 1994;57: 198–203.
155. Leung HY, Gullick WJ, Lemoine NR. Expression and functional-activity of fibroblast growth-factors and their receptors in human pancreatic-cancer. Int J Cancer 1994;59:667–675.
156. Pardoll DM. Cancer vaccines. Immunol Today 1993;14:310–316.
157. Colombo MP, Modesti A, Parmiani G, Forni G. Perspectives in cancer research: local cytokine availability elicits tumour rejection and systemic immunity through granulocyte-T-lymphocyte cross-talk. Cancer Res 1992;52:1–5.
158. Cavallo F, Giovarelli M, Gulino A, et al. Role of neutrophils and CD4+ T lymphocytes in the primary and memory response to nonimmunogenic murine mammary adenocarcinoma made immunogenic by IL-2 gene. J Immunol 1992;149:3627–3635.
159. Dranoff G, Jaffee E, Lazenby A, et al. Vaccination with irradiated tumour cells engineered to secrete murine granulocyte-macrophage colony stimulating factor, stimulates potent, specific and long-lasting anti-tumour immunity. Proc Natl Acad Sci USA 1992;90:3539–3543.
160. Hock H, Dorsch M, Diamantstein T, Blankenstein T. Interleukin-7 induces CD4+ T cell-dependent tumour rejection. J Exp Med 1991;74:1291–1298.
161. Pardoll D. New strategies for active immunotherapy with genetically engineered tumour cells. Curr Opin Immunol 1992; 4:6219–6222.
162. Brown TD, Goodman P, Flemming T, MacDonald JS, Hersh EM, Braun TJ. A phase II trial of recominant tumour necrosis factor in patient with adenocarcinoma of the pancreas. J Immunother 1991;10:376–378.
163. Abbruzzese JL, Levin B, Ajani JA, et al. A phase II trial of recombinant interferon-gamma and recombinant tumour necrosis factor in patients with advanced gastrointestinal malignancies: results of a trial terminated by excessive toxicity. J Biol Response Mod 1990;9:522–527.
164. Watanabe N, Yamauchi N, Maeda M, et al. Recombinant human tumour necrosis factor causes regression in patients with advanced malignancies. Oncology 1994;51:360–365.
165. Schmiegel W, Roeder C, Schmielau J, Rodeck U, Kalthoff H. Tumor necrosis factor alpha induces the expression of transforming growth factor alpha and the epidermal growth factor receptor in human pancreatic cancer cells. Proc Natl Acad Sci USA 1993;90:863–867.
166. Herlyn D, Powe J, Ross AH, Herlyn M, Koprowski H. Inhibition of tumour growth by IgG2a monoclonal antibodies correlates with the antibody density on tumour cells. J Immunol 1985;134:1300–1304.
167. Ulmer JB, Donnelly JJ, Parker SE, et al. Heterologous protection against influenza by injection of DNA encoding a viral protein. Science 1993;54:1745–1749.
168. Hawkins RE, Winter G, Hamblin TJ, Stevenson FK, Russel SJ. A genetic approach to idiotypic vaccination. J Immunother 1993;4:273–278.
169. Barnd DL, Lan MS, Metzger RS, Finn OJ. Specific tumour histocompatibility complex-unrestricted recognition of tumour-associated mucins by human cytotoxic cells. Proc Natl Acad Sci USA 1989;86:7159–7163.
170. Schlichtholz B, Legros Y, Gillet D, et al. The immune response to p53 in breast cancer patients is directed against immunodominant epitopes unrelated to the mutational hotspot. Cancer Res 1992;52:6380–6384.
171. Gjertsen MK, Bakka A, Breivik J, et al. Vaccination with mutant ras peptides and induction of T-cell responsiveness in pancreatic carcinoma patients carrying the corresponding RAS mutation. Lancet 1995;346:1399–1400.
172. Kawakami Y, Eliyahu S, Delgade CH. Identification of a human melanoma antigen recognized by tumour-infiltrating lymphocytes associated with in vivo tumour rejection. Proc Natl Acad Sci USA 1994;91:6458–6462.
173. Coulie PG, Brichard VA, Van Pel A, et al. A new gene coding for a differentiation antigen recognised by autologous cytolytic T lymphocytes on HLA-A2 melanomas. J Exp Med 1994;180:35–42.
174. Conry RM, Lobuglio AF, Loechel F, et al. A carcinoembryonic antigen polynucleotide vaccine has in vivo antitumour activity. Gene Ther 1995;2:59–65.

# 47

# *Tumor Markers for Pancreatic Cancer*

Katsusuke Satake

The incidence of pancreatic cancer is increasing worldwide. Extremely low 5-year survival of pancreatic cancer in general reflects the fact that this neoplasm is usually diagnosed in an incurable stage despite the availability of a variety of diagnostic methods. Thus, there is a great need for new approaches that may prove useful in the early diagnosis and treatment of pancreatic cancer. Since tumor cells may express or secrete abnormal antigens, many laboratories have focused their efforts on producing specific antibodies to them, and a number of tumor antigenic markers have been successfully identified as a result.

Tumor markers can be defined as biochemical substances produced by tumors which when present in the circulation in measurable amounts may provide evidence of the presence of neoplastic disease (1). Tumor markers produced within tumors, whether by malignant cells or stromal cells, are said to be "tumor derived," whereas markers produced by nonmalignant cells as a result of being affected by the tumor are said to be "tumor associated." Increased circulating levels of tumor markers can be attributed to several causes including inappropriate production, as in the expression of oncofetal antigens (e.g., carcinoembryonic antigen [CEA] and α-fetoprotein [AFP]), ectopic production (e.g., human chorionic gonadotropin-beta subunit [hCGß] and adrenocorticotrophic hormone [ACTH]), increased accessibility to the circulation (e.g., prostatic acid phosphatase [PAP]), and cellular necrosis and release of tumor cell contents into the circulation (e.g., tissue polypeptide antigen [TPA]).

Attempts have been made to use tumor markers in blood and tissue *(a)* to monitor the course of disease during therapy, *(b)* to assess therapeutic efficacy, *(c)* to differentiate between stages of malignant disease, *(d)* to assist diagnosis in symptomatic patients, and possibly *(e)* to serve as a clue in early diagnosis. As shown in Table 47.1, many tumor markers have been widely used to detect pancreatic cancer, and some of the markers assessed to date are discussed in this chapter.

## CLINICAL APPLICABILITY OF SERUM TUMOR MARKERS TO PANCREATIC CANCER

It is very important to understand the meaning of measurements of tumor markers when using them to detect pancreatic cancer. Tumor markers possess varying degrees of sensitivity with regard to pancreatic cancer, but none of the assays are sensitive or specific enough to be used as a screening test for it; thus, it is not recommended that they be used independently to establish a diagnosis of pancreatic cancer. Elevated levels in patients can be thought of as meaningful. In such instances, further diagnostic efforts are required to definitely establish the presence or absence of pancreatic cancer, and it is important to select markers that are highly sensitive and specific for pancreatic cancer.

Most of the tumor markers described in this chapter can be used to monitor the response of patients after either medical or surgical treatment. Usually, a rise in serum tumor marker levels enables detection of a recurrence before it is evident clinically. However, sensitivity and specificity differ from marker to marker. Serum tumor markers, accurately measured and properly interpreted, can serve as useful adjuncts in the diagnosis of pancreatic cancer and in monitoring patients after treatment.

### Pancreatic Enzymes

Serum pancreatic enzymes are widely measured as tumor markers of pancreatic cancer. Patients with pancreatic cancer, especially cancer of the head of the pancreas, have elevated levels of pancreatic enzymes. Obstruction of the pancreatic duct by the tumor may lead to their release into the circulation because of pancreatic juice congestion and associated pancreatitis. They are usually increased in acute and relapsing chronic pancreatitis but are also increased in some cases of pancreatic cancer.

The Japanese Pancreatic Cancer Registry (1994) (2) reported elevated serum amylase levels in 309 of 1100 cases of pancreatic cancer (28.1%), elevated serum lipase levels in 125 of 1100 cases (11.4%), and elevated serum elastase 1 levels in 784 of 1100 cases (71.2%). Of these enzymes, serum elastase 1 showed the highest sensitivity for pancreatic cancer, and 341 of the 784 patients (43.4%) with elevated serum elastase 1 levels were treated by resection.

Serum elastase 1 has been used as a marker in the most extensive diagnostic studies, and the levels were found to be higher for longer periods than serum amylase levels, which made it possible to diagnose pancreatic cancer. About 70% of patients with pancreatic cancer have elevated serum elastase 1 (3). Suzuki et al. (4) found that 75% of patients with pancreatic cancer smaller than 2.0 cm in diameter had elevated serum elastase 1 levels, only 4% had elevated serum amylase levels, and none had elevated carbohydrate antigen (CA) 19-9 levels. Recently, Hayakawa et al. (5) performed a prospective study on the early detection of pancreatic cancer on the basis of serum elastase 1 measurement. The study involved 722 patients over 40 years of age with symptoms suggesting pancreatic disease, such as upper abdominal pain, discomfort, mass, jaundice, weight loss, or diabetes. Elevated serum elastase 1 levels were found in 171 of the 722 patients (23.8%); a diagnosis of pancreatic cancer subsequently was made in 22, 17 of whom had elevated serum elastase 1 levels, and 10 underwent radical surgery. Three of the 10 patients had a pancreatic cancer smaller than 2.0 cm in diameter, and 2 of the 3 survived more than 3 years.

Our own comparative study showed that 51.1% of the pancreatic cancer patients had elevated serum elastase 1 levels (Table 47.2), and the proportions with T1 cancer (tumor size

**TABLE 47.1. Serum Tumor Markers to Pancreatic Cancer**

Pancreatic enzymes
Pancreatic secretory trypsin inhibitor (PSTI)
  Tumor-associated trypsin inhibitor (TATI)
Pancreatic hormone
  Islet amyloid polypeptide (IAPP)
Cancer-associated antigens
  α-Fetoprotein
  Carcinoembryonic antigen (CEA)
  Pancreatic oncofetal antigen (POA)
  Tissue polypeptide antigen (TPA)
  Tissue polypeptide-specific antigen (TPS)
Pancreatic cancer–associated antigen with monoclonal antibody
  Carbohydrate antigen 19-9 (CA 19-9)
  Carbohydrate antigen 50 (CA 50)
  SPan-1
  DU-PAN-2
  SLEX (FH 6)
  Carbohydrate antigen 242 (CA 242)
  TAG-72 (CA 72.4)

<2.0 cm) and T2 cancer (tumor size, 2.1–4.0 cm) were 28.6 and 52.6%, respectively. Chang and Takeuchi also found elastase 1 to have high sensitivity: 62.0% in T1 lesions and 72.0% in T2 (6) (Table 47.3).

These results demonstrate that careful measurement of serum elastase 1 makes it possible to detect small pancreatic cancers.

## PANCREATIC SECRETORY TRYPSIN INHIBITOR (PSTI)

Increased proteolytic activity has been demonstrated in association with malignant transformation and tumor invasion (7). Increased synthesis and release of protease inhibitors have been found as a response to the proteolytic activity of the tumor (8). PSTI is a polypeptide (6 kDa) secreted by pancreatic acinar cells together with zymogens (9). PSTI is a specific trypsin inhibitor that reacts with trypsin in a 1:1 molar ratio and has been reported to protect pancreatic cells from inadvertent activation of trypsinogen to trypsin, thereby preventing autodigestion. In addition to pancreas, PSTI has been demonstrated in various other fetal and adult normal tissues (10). Radioimmunoassays have revealed PSTI in the serum and urine of healthy persons (11). Increased serum PSTI concentrations are found in a variety

**TABLE 47.2. Usefulness of Various Tumor Markers in the Diagnosis of Pancreatic Cancer[a]**

| | SPan-1 | CA19-9 | DU-PAN-2 | CA50 | CEA | Elastase 1 |
|---|---|---|---|---|---|---|
| Sensitivity | | | | | | |
| % | 81.4 | 79.4 | 47.7 | 64.9 | 59.0 | 51.1 |
| *N* | 522/641 | 454/572 | 114/239 | 48/94 | 121/205 | 70/137 |
| Specificity | | | | | | |
| % | 67.5 | 72.5 | 85.3 | 73.2 | 63.9 | 75.6 |
| *N* | 1231/1825 | 1014/1394 | 481/564 | 71/97 | 248/388 | 93/123 |
| Positive predictive value | | | | | | |
| % | 46.8 | 54.2 | 57.9 | 64.9 | 46.6 | 70.0 |
| *N* | 522/1116 | 454/838 | 114/197 | 48/74 | 121/261 | 70/100 |
| Negative predictive value | | | | | | |
| % | 91.2 | 89.5 | 79.4 | 73.2 | 74.7 | 58.0 |
| *N* | 1231/1350 | 1010/1128 | 481/606 | 71/97 | 248/332 | 93/160 |
| Diagnostic accuracy | | | | | | |
| % | 71.1 | 74.5 | 74.1 | 69.9 | 62.2 | 62.7 |
| *N* | 1753/2466 | 1464/1966 | 595/803 | 114/171 | 369/593 | 163/260 |

[a]*Sensitivity*, (patients with pancreatic cancer with positive tests/all patients with pancreatic cancer tested) × 100; *Specificity*, (patients without pancreatic cancer with negative tests/all patients without pancreatic cancer tested) × 100; *Positive predictive value*, (patients with pancreatic cancer with positive tests/all patients with positive tests) × 100; *Negative predictive value*, (patients without pancreatic cancer with negative tests/all patients with negative tests) × 100; *Diagnostic accuracy*, ((patients with pancreatic cancer with positive tests + patients without pancreatic cancer with negative tests)/all patients tested) × 100.

**TABLE 47.3. Sensitivity of Various Tumor Markers in T1 and T2 Pancreatic Cancer**

| | CA19-9 | | SPan-1 | | CEA | | DU-PAN-2 | | CA50 | | Elastase 1 | |
|---|---|---|---|---|---|---|---|---|---|---|---|---|
| | T1 | T2 | T1 | T2 | T1 | T2 | T1 | T2 | T1 | T2 | T1 | T2 |
| Current study | | | | | | | | | | | | |
| % | 62.5 | 77.7 | 58.3 | 79.6 | 30.8 | 46.9 | 22.2 | 40.0 | 60.0 | NT[a] | 28.6 | 52.6 |
| *N* | 15/24 | 42/54 | 14/24 | 43/54 | 4/13 | 23/49 | 2/9 | 12/30 | 3/5 | | 2/7 | 20/38 |
| Chang and Takeuchi (6) | | | | | | | | | | | | |
| % | 37.5 | 88.9 | 25.0 | 82.2 | NT | NT | 25.0 | 62.1 | NT | NT | 62.5 | 72.0 |
| *N* | 3/8 | 40/45 | 2/8 | 37/45 | | | 2/8 | 18/29 | | | 5/8 | 13/18 |

[a]*NT*, not tested.

of cancers, especially pancreatic cancer (74%) (12, 13). However, elevated levels have also been observed in the serum and urine of most patients with acute and chronic relapsing pancreatitis and have been claimed to reflect the severity of the pancreatitis (11, 14). We used a radioimmunoassay to measure serum PSTI levels in our previous study and found that they were elevated in only 33% of 41 patients with pancreatic cancer, as opposed to 77% of 45 patients with acute pancreatitis and 60% of 10 patients with chronic relapsing pancreatitis (15).

Stenman et al. (16) isolated a trypsin inhibitor, referred to as tumor-associated trypsin inhibitor (TATI), from the urine of a patient with ovarian cancer. The amino acid sequence and the immunologic properties of the molecule showed TATI to be identical to, or at least closely related to, PSTI (17). A radioimmunoassay for the measurement of TATI in serum and urine has been developed. It has revealed that most patients with pancreatic cancer have increased serum concentrations of TATI (85%) (17). An even higher proportion of these patients had elevated values (90%) in the urine. TATI was expressed immunohistochemically in half of the specimens from pancreatic carcinomas, but staining intensity was weaker than in adjacent normal pancreas. The TATI in serum and urine seems to originate in normal pancreatic acini rather than in the carcinoma itself. Elevated TATI levels are also found in various benign and malignant disorders of other organs. The TATI concentrations in serum and urine in pancreatic diseases were similar to those of PSTI. Many other pancreatic enzymes such as trypsin, lipase, and ribonuclease have been used, but no definitive data have been obtained.

## PANCREATIC HORMONE

### Islet Amyloid Polypeptide (IAPP)

IAPP contains 37 amino acids and is produced by the ß cells of the pancreas. IAPP, found in the pancreas of 90% of patients with non-insulin-dependent diabetes mellitus (18), produced glucose intolerance (19), reduced food intake (20), and induced cachexia (21). Disturbed glucose metabolism is present in up to 80% of patients with pancreatic cancer. Diabetes was previously thought to be a factor predisposing patients to pancreatic cancer. Furthermore, metabolic disorders occur frequently in patients with pancreatic cancer, a disease characterized by weight loss and severe cachexia. Diabetes and weight loss are early signs of pancreatic cancer. Thus, the measurement of plasma IAPP levels may detect early pancreatic cancer.

Permert et al. (22) found elevated plasma IAPP levels in pancreatic cancer and non-insulin-dependent diabetes. After removal of pancreatic cancer, the levels normalized, indicating that the remaining ß cells secrete IAPP normally. They suggested that measurement of plasma IAPP levels could prove valuable in the diagnosis of pancreatic cancer in the small subgroup of patients with newly diagnosed non-insulin-dependent diabetes who present with weight loss rather than obesity.

Approximately 60–80% of patients developed glucose intolerance within 2 years preceding the diagnosis of pancreatic cancer (22, 23). The measurement of plasma IAPP may become a useful adjunct method to detect early pancreatic cancer in those patients.

## CANCER-ASSOCIATED ANTIGENS

A vigorous attempt has been made to identify a pancreatic cancer–associated antigen that might be helpful in diagnosis. Attention has focused on AFP, CEA, pancreatic oncofetal antigen (POA), TPA, and tissue polypeptide specific antigen (TPS).

### α-Fetoprotein

AFP is clearly of no value in the diagnosis of pancreatic cancer.

### Carcinoembryonic Antigen

CEA, first detected in 1965 by Gold and Freedman (24), is probably the most extensively studied tumor marker and can be regarded as a clinical reference marker for gastrointestinal (GI) cancer. CEA is a 180-kDa glycoprotein mainly associated with the surface of tumor cells. It consists of a large number of branched oligosaccharide chains linked to a polypeptide chain (25). The antibodies to CEA used in most studies are polyclonal antibodies directed at the peptide moiety of the molecule. In recent years, several groups have produced monoclonal antibodies that react with different epitopes on the CEA molecules (26, 27).

Elevated CEA serum levels are found in patients with a variety of cancers, particularly cancers of the GI tract, ovary, lung, and breast. However, a wide variety of benign conditions may also cause moderate increases in the serum CEA concentration. A large proportion of patients with pancreatic cancer have elevated CEA levels, but most of the patients have advanced disease. Data on the potential value of CEA as an indicator of the stage, differentiation, and prognosis of pancreatic cancer are limited. Poorly differentiated carcinomas have been claimed to be associated with higher CEA levels than well-differentiated carcinomas, and tumors that have metastasized, with higher levels than local tumors (28). A positive correlation between low initial levels of CEA and survival has been demonstrated (28). Although CEA serum levels in pancreatic cancer patients have been found to be higher than in control patients, the CEA assay is of limited value in the differential diagnosis between malignant and benign disease (23). Elevated CEA levels have been demonstrated in as many as 43–64% of benign pancreatic disorders, including both acute and chronic pancreatitis.

Liver insufficiency and severe benign liver disease such as cirrhosis, chronic active hepatitis, and liver abscess are frequent causes of elevated CEA values (30, 31). Benign extrahepatic biliary obstruction, especially if associated with cholangitis, often causes markedly elevated CEA levels, which decrease after decompression of the cholestasis (32). The effect of extrahepatic biliary obstruction must be considered when interpreting CEA values in patients with pancreatic cancer. Biliary decompression without tumor resection results in a decrease in CEA levels but not to within normal limits (32). In our study, 121 of 205 patients with pancreatic cancer (59%) had elevated CEA levels. The specificity of CEA in these patients was 63.9%.

CEA has been used to monitor the regression of pancreatic cancer in response to chemotherapy and radiotherapy and for postoperative follow-up.

### Pancreatic Oncofetal Antigen

POA is a glycoprotein detected by raising antisera in rabbits to extracts of human fetal pancreas (33, 34). POA has been demonstrated by immunohistochemistry in most pancreatic ductal adenocarcinomas (97%), as well as in normal adult pancreas, in other GI carcinomas, and in normal adult tissues (35). Increased serum concentrations of POA have been reported in patients with pancreatic cancer. The reported sensitivity of POA for pancreatic cancer has ranged between 17 and 81%. However, elevated POA values are also found in a variety of other cancers (14–36%), in benign conditions including pancreatitis (13–18%) and hepatobiliary disorders (27%), and during pregnancy (33, 35, 36). Schmiegel et al. (37) have shown that POA is poorer than CA 19-9 and CEA as a marker for pancreatic cancer. This test appears to lack the diagnostic accuracy needed for either a screening test or an independent test in symptomatic patients.

### Tissue Polypeptide Antigen and Tissue Polypeptide-Specific Antigen

TPA, an epitope of a glycoprotein with a keratin-like structure (37), has been reported to have good sensitivity in diagnosing pancreatic cancer, even if its specificity is less satisfactory (38, 39). This limited specificity is mainly attributable to jaundice, which alters TPA levels in the circulation the same as CA 19-9 levels (40–45). Jaundice, in fact, may reduce glycoprotein metabolism, which occurs mainly in the liver (46, 47).

Recently, TPS, a new monoclonal antibody used to identify an epitope on the TPA molecule, has been proposed for the detection of malignant growth (48), but few data on its behavior in patients with pancreatic cancer are available in the literature. Plebani et al. (49) compared the clinical usefulness of TPS, TPA, and CA 19-9 measurements in pancreatic cancer and concluded that CA 19-9 is the best serologic indicator of pancreatic cancer, with TPA and TPS lacking both sensitivity and specificity.

### Pancreatic Cancer-Associated Antigens with Monoclonal Antibody

Monoclonal antibodies, which represent immunoreagents with defined specificity and affinity, have made it possible to identify and characterize new markers of tumors of the GI tract, such as CA 19-9, etc. Monoclonal antibodies to GI cancer-associated antigens have also been used in diagnostic and therapeutic applications. Monoclonal antibodies to the following pancreatic cancer-associated antigens have been used to detect pancreatic cancer: CA 19-9, SPan-1, DU-PAN 2, sialosylated Lewis X, and carbohydrate antigen 50 (CA 50).

### Carbohydrate Antigen 19-9

CA 19-9 was originally raised against a human cell line, SW 1116, which was derived from a colorectal carcinoma (50). CA 19-9 antigen is also referred to as GI cancer–associated antigen (GICA). Its antigenic determinant, sialosylfucosyllactoteraose, corresponds to a sialylated Lewis$^a$ blood group substance (51). The CA 19-9 antigen occurs mainly as a monosialoganglioside in adenocarcinoma tissues and as a high-molecular-weight carbohydrate-rich glycoprotein, the mucin fraction, in the serum of adenocarcinoma patients. The antigenic determinant residues, the carbohydrate side chains of these molecules, and the sialyl and fucosyl residues are essential for binding to the 19-9 antibody (52, 53). The fucosyltransferase enzyme responsible for adding an α-1-γ linkage to the *N*-acetylglucosamine of blood group oligosaccharides is encoded by the Lewis gene (54). Thus, approximately 5% of the population who lack the Lewis gene are unable to synthesize the complete CA 19-9 antigen (55).

Immunohistochemical studies show that CA 19-9 is often expressed in various carcinomas (50–53). However, it is also a normal constituent of many tissues (e.g., pancreatic ductal epithelium). Most healthy individuals have low serum CA 19-9 concentrations, and only 0.6% of normal subjects have values above 37 U/mL, which has been used as the cutoff value for the test (60). Smoking does not affect CA 19-9 levels.

Early studies reported the presence of CA 19-9 antigen in the serum of patients with GI carcinoma. Using the improved CA 19-9 radioimmunoassay developed by Del Villano et al. (60), numerous investigators have established its great value. In their reports, the sensitivity and the specificity of the assay for pancreatic cancer ranged from 69 to 93%, and from 78 to 98.5%, respectively. Nevertheless, most of the pancreatic cancer in these studies was diagnosed in advanced stages.

Jalanko et al. (61) reported that 71 of 91 patients with pancreatic cancer had elevated serum levels. High levels were found especially in advanced cases, but five of eight patients with resectable pancreatic cancer also had elevated levels. Similar results have been reported by many investigators. High specificity with moderate sensitivity was also found in gastric cancer, especially in advanced cases. In addition, high serum CA 19-9 concentrations were found in a high proportion of cholangiocarcinoma patients, whereas patients with liver cell cancer rarely have elevated levels.

Recently, Pleskow et al. (62) assessed the usefulness of serum CA 19-9 in the diagnosis of pancreatic cancer in 261 patients suspected of having pancreatic disorders. In the 54 of those patients ultimately shown to have pancreatic cancer, the CA 19-9 assay was found to have a sensitivity of 70% and a specificity of 87%. The positive predictive value was 59%; the negative predictive value was 92%. They were unable to find any significant difference between its sensitivity in local/regional disease ($N$ = 6) and distant metastasis ($N$ = 14) (50% vs. 71%). However, they concluded that CA 19-9 is a more sensitive and specific marker for pancreatic cancer than other tumor markers and that it should be useful in testing patients with suspected pancreatic cancer. In one series (63), serum CA 19-9 levels exceeded normal values in only one of eight patients with cancers smaller than 3.0 cm in diameter; in another report, a combination of ultrasound and CA 19-9 measurements resulted in diagnosing 13 of 14 cancers (93%) of the same small size (<3.0 cm in diameter) (64).

In our studies (Table 47.2), 79.4% of patients (454 of 542) with pancreatic cancer had values above the cutoff level. This was the highest sensitivity among malignant diseases, including gastric cancer (26%, 39 of 304) and colorectal cancer (31.7%, 33 of 104). It was also highly sensitive in liver cell cancer and biliary tract cancer (35.4%, 58 of 164, and 64.4%, 65 of 101, respectively), while sensitivity in other cancers was 23.8% (24 of 101). Among the benign diseases, sensitivity was relatively low in chronic pancreatitis and other benign pancreatic diseases (18.7%, 58 of 164, and 24.4%, 11 of 45, respectively), although sensitivity was high in benign hepatobiliary disease (chronic hepatitis, 29.6%, 16 of 54; liver cirrhosis, 19.5%, 17 of 87; biliary calculus, 26.2%, 10 of 38). Sensitivity in other benign diseases was low. Specificity and diagnostic accuracy were 72.5 and 74.5%, respectively.

The major problem with CA 19-9 measurements in the detection of pancreatic cancer has been that biliary tract diseases causing obstructive jaundice are usually associated with elevated levels (65, 66). Furthermore, as mentioned above, CA 19-9 is thought to be a sialylated Lewis$^a$ blood group antigen. Thus, Lewis a-negative, b-negative pancreatic cancer patients cannot produce CA 19-9.

Although the measurement of serum CA 19-9 has disadvantages as described above, CA 19-9 is still the most valuable tumor marker for detecting pancreatic cancer and monitoring patients' response to chemotherapy and surgical treatment.

### Carbohydrate Antigen 50

CA 50 antigen is defined by monoclonal antibody C50 (IgM) obtained by immunizing mice with human colonic adenocarcinoma cell line COLO 205 (67). Like CA 19-9, CA 50 reacts with sialosylfucosyllactotetraose (sialylated Lewis$^a$) (68). In addition, CA 50 reacts with at least one other carbohydrate structure, sialosyllactotetraose, lacking the fucose molecule of the sialylated Lewis$^a$ blood group structure (69). CA 50 is expected to have broader reactivity than CA 19-9, because CA 50 can react in Lewis$^a$-negative subjects, who lack the appropriate fucosyltransferase enzyme and cannot express Lewis$^a$ as CA 19-9, but who can synthesize sialosyllactoterase.

Immunohistochemically, CA 50, like CA 19-9, has been found to be expressed in most pancreatic carcinomas, and the level of expression is correlated with the degree of differentiation, being greatest in well-differentiated carcinomas (70). However, both CA 19-9 and CA 50 are also expressed in normal pancreas and in pancreatitis; consequently, immunohistochemical staining for CA 19-9 and CA 50 cannot be used to distinguish between benign and malignant pancreatic lesions (70).

Healthy individuals have low CA 50 concentrations. High serum concentrations of CA 50 measured by radioimmunoassay have been reported in patients with various GI cancers and have been found in 58–91% of patients with pancreatic cancer (71, 72). Increased serum concentrations of CA 50 have also been detected in patients with benign pancreatic disease (12–32%), biliary disease (35–38%), and liver disease (22–59%).

The sensitivity of CA 50 for pancreatic cancer in our studies (Table 47.2), was 64.9% (48 of 74). Although the number of patients was small, 50% of the patients with malignant hepatobiliary disease and 40% of those with colorectal disease were positive. Even in benign diseases, the false-positive rate was high. In a study in Sweden (73), elevated serum CA 50 levels were found in 22 of 24 patients with pancreatic cancer, in 1 of 8 patients with chronic pancreatitis, and in 6 of 14 patients with acute pancreatitis. Its low positive predictive value, however, makes it unsuitable for the detection of pancreatic cancer. Since a good correlation exists between CA 50 and CA 19-9 values, there is no advantage to measuring both markers as a means of detecting pancreatic cancer.

## SPan-1

SPan-1 monoclonal antibody was produced by immunizing Balb/c mice with a mucin-producing human pancreatic cancer cell line, SW 1990 (74). A radioimmunoassay for this antigen was developed, and serum SPan-1 measurements by this method showed high sensitivity (92.5%) and high specificity (82.9%) for the diagnosis of pancreatic cancer. The positive predictive value was 51.2%; the negative predictive value was 98.3%. However, the proportion of false-positive findings with this assay was 59% in hepatobiliary cancer, 23% in gastric cancer, 13% in colorectal cancer, and 14% in other cancers and benign GI disease. Sensitivity in chronic pancreatitis and acute pancreatitis was 5% and 10%, respectively (75).

SPan-1 reacts with sialylated blood group Lewis$^{a}$ antigen as does CA 19-9, and it also reacts with at least one other as yet unidentified carbohydrate structure. Thus, SPan-1 is suspected of having broader reactivity than CA 19-9, the same as CA 50. SPan-1 was positive in four of six tissue samples of colon cancer from patients with the Lewis a-negative, b-negative phenotype, whereas CA 19-9 was negative in all six (75).

In our series (Table 47.2), SPan-1 had the highest sensitivity for pancreatic cancer (81.4%), and its sensitivity in hepatic and biliary disease was also high (liver cell cancer, 56.0%, 131 of 234; biliary tract cancer, 70.3%, 111 of 153)—higher than CA 19-9. Its sensitivity was 31.4% (112 of 153) in gastric cancer, 28.7% (43 of 150) in colorectal cancer, and 22.8% (26 of 114) in other GI cancers. Although the sensitivity of SPan-1 in chronic pancreatitis (13.6%, 45 of 330) and other benign pancreatic diseases (13.0%, 7 of 54) is lower than that of CA 19-9, its sensitivity in benign hepatobiliary diseases, including chronic hepatitis (31.5%, 29 of 92) and cirrhosis of the liver (45.0%, 62 of 135), was, with the exception of biliary calculus (5.3%, 3 of 57), higher than that of CA 19-9. Sensitivity in other benign diseases was found to be 11.0% (9 of 82). The specificity and diagnostic accuracy of SPan-1 for pancreatic cancer were 67.5% and 71.1%, respectively, also lower than the corresponding values for CA 19-9 (76).

SPan-1 is a tumor-associated glycoprotein. Thus, SPan-1 measurements had the same disadvantage of CA 19-9 and CA 50 in jaundiced patients. Since a good correlation exists between SPan-1, CA 19-9, and CA 50 values, simultaneously measuring all three markers to detect pancreatic cancer is not worthwhile.

## DU-PAN-2

DU-PAN-2 monoclonal antibody was produced by immunizing mice with a pancreatic ductal adenocarcinoma cell line (HPAF). The DU-PAN-2 epitope has not been determined yet, but it is expressed on a mucinlike glycoprotein and is distinct from that of CEA and CA 19-9 (77). The antigen is present in the ductal epithelium of fetal pancreas, normal adult pancreas, and in pancreatic adenocarcinomas, as well as in some other benign and malignant tissues such as normal gallbladder and bile duct (78).

Metzgar et al. (79) developed a competitive radioimmunoassay for DU-PAN-2 and found values above the cutoff value (400 U/mL) in the serum of 8 of 20 patients with gastric cancers (40%), 8 of 76 with colorectal cancers (10.5%), and 3 of 58 patients (5.1%) with benign GI disease. Serum from 68% of 89 pancreatic cancer patients had DU-PAN-2 levels above normal. Their group (80) later demonstrated above-normal serum DU-PAN-2 levels in 94% (31 of 33) of pancreatic cancer patients, although a different cutoff value (300 U/mL) was used. Further, serial determinations of serum DU-PAN-2 antigen provided a sensitive means of monitoring the progression of pancreatic cancer.

Extensive studies to assess serum DU-PAN-2 in various diseases have been performed in Japan using either sandwich or enzymatic immunoassays. Sawabu et al. (81), who used an enzymatic immunoassay, reported finding serum DU-PAN-2 levels above 400 U/mL (normal cutoff value) in 50% of pancreatic cancer patients, 55% of liver cell carcinoma patients, and 43% of biliary tract cancer patients; Cho et al. (82) obtained similar results.

In our studies (Table 47.2), 42.7% of pancreatic cancers (114 of 236) were associated with serum DU-PAN-2 levels above 400 U/mL, 27.5% (25 of 91) of liver cell carcinomas, and 41.0% (25 of 61) of biliary tract cancers. Using a cutoff level of 300 U/mL, Ichihara et al. (83) demonstrated serum DU-PAN-2 sensitivities in pancreatic cancer, biliary tract cancer, and liver cell cancer of 54, 47, and 44%, respectively. These results indicate that elevated serum DU-PAN-2 levels are usually observed in hepatobiliary malignancies. Okura and Tajiri (84) demonstrated a good correlation between GOT and serum DU-PAN-2, suggesting that elevated serum DU-PAN-2 levels may be influenced by liver function.

## SLEX (FH 6)

The monoclonal antibody SLEX was produced by immunizing mice with a fucoganglioside, 6B, which accumulates in human colonic adenocarcinoma but is absent in normal colonic mucosa, and was isolated from a monosialoganglioside fraction of colonic adenocarcinoma. SLEX has been shown to be highly reactive with many human cancer cells but less reactive or unreactive with a variety of normal cells. The epitope is sialylated Lewis blood group antigen (79, 85).

An SLEX immunoassay has been developed, and extensive studies to measure serum SLEX in various diseases have been performed in Japan. Imura et al. of the SLEX Study Group (86) used an SLEX radioimmunoassay kit to measure serum SLEX in 1261 patients with malignant tumors and 717 with nonmalignant diseases. They found this kit to be reliable; the mean value in 1106 healthy controls was 21.5 U/mL (±6.3 SD). When a cutoff value of 38 U/mL was used, its sensitivity in malignant disease was 4.7%. Among malignant diseases, the sensitivity of the assay was 45% in lung cancer, 64% in pancreatic cancer, and 57% in ovarian cancer.

In our experience, SLEX sensitivity for various GI malignancies was 42.2% in pancreatic cancer and 22.2% in biliary tract cancer, but less than 10% in others. The SLEX Study Group found no correlation with other tumor markers. They concluded that diagnostic efficiency was increased significantly by use of a combination of SLEX assay with other markers and that serial determinations had clinical applicability in monitoring patients after medical or surgical treatment. However, the sensitivity of this assay is very low in malignant disease, which is a disadvantage from the standpoint of clinical application.

### Carbohydrate Antigen 242

CA 242 was isolated in 1985 by Lindholm et al. and obtained by immunizing mice with the human adenocarcinoma cell line COLO 205 and fusion with mouse myeloma cell line Sp 2/0. The epitope, recognized by CA 242, is a sialylated carbohydrate structure related to the type 1 chain. It is situated on the same macromolecule as CA 50 but is completely different from it (87).

Immunoperoxidase staining revealed expression of CA 242 by 93% (38 of 41) of well- to moderately differentiated ductal adenocarcinomas of the pancreas and all cystadenocarcinomas. Only two of seven poorly differentiated adenocarcinomas stained, and the proportion of positive cells was smaller than in well-differentiated carcinomas. Only occasional cells stained in one of five anaplastic carcinomas. In normal pancreas, only a few small terminal ducts were CA 242 positive. Carcinomas always stained more strongly for CA 242 than normal pancreas (88). Haglund et al. (88) also compared the expression of CA 242 in pancreatic tissue with that of CA 19-9 and CA 50 and found that the expression of CA 242 resembles that of CA 50 and is similar to CA 19-9. Serum CA 242 levels determined by fluoroimmunoassay (DELFIA research kit; Pharmacia Diagnostics) were elevated in 15 of 23 patients with pancreatic carcinoma (65%). They concluded that this antigen is expressed in the serum of many patients with pancreatic cancer and thus is a potential candidate for a new serum tumor marker. Recently, Rothlin et al. (87) used the same method to measure serum CA 242 in pancreatic cancer and compared it with CA 19-9 and CA 50. They found sensitivity for pancreatic cancer of 66.2, 70.6, and 70.6% for CA 242, CA 19-9, and CA 50, respectively. The differential diagnosis between pancreatic cancer and chronic pancreatitis could be made with a sensitivity of 64.7, 79.4, and 77.9%, respectively. They concluded that on its own, CA 242 does not improve the sensitivity achieved with CA 19-9 and CA 50. Furthermore, Plebani et al. (89) demonstrated that the antibody raised against CA 19-9 or CA 242 reacts very similarly with CA 242 and concluded that CA 242 does not offer a significant advantage over CA 19-9 in pancreatic cancer diagnosis because of its remarkably similar behavior.

### TAG-72 (CA 72.4)

TAG-72 is a human tumor-associated antigen defined by the murine monoclonal antibody B 72.3 and prepared from a membrane-enriched fraction of a human metastatic breast carcinoma. It is a high-molecular-weight ($10^8$) glycoprotein with the characteristics of a mucin (90).

B 72.3 appears to react with the *o*-linked disaccharide, *N*-acetyl-neuraminic acid-alpha 2→6-*N*-acetylgalactosamine alpha 1→0-Ser/Thr (sialosyl-TN structure) (91). TAG-72 has been shown to differ from CEA, CA 19-9, CA-125, and CA 15-3 (92). Several reports on serum TAG-72 or CA 72.4 in colonic (93), ovarian (94), and gastric cancer (95) have been published. The clinical value of TAG-72 in pancreatic cancer has also been reported (96–100). High TAG-72 serum levels were found in 34% of patients with pancreatic cancer (46 of 138) but in only 1 of 61 patients with chronic pancreatitis (6.1%). Recently, Pasquali et al. (100) found that the sensitivity of serum TAG-72 levels in patients with pancreatic cancer was 44.8%, with a positive predictive value of 92.8%. Its specificity for chronic pancreatitis was as high as that of CA 19-9 (95.5%). Despite differences between the chemical structures of the two antigens, they found a large overlap in patients expressing both antigens, since only one of the patients with high TAG-72 levels had a CA 19-9 level in the normal range. They concluded that the clinical value of TAG-72 as serodiagnostic test for detecting pancreatic carcinoma is poorer than that of CA 19-9; nor can any advantage be expected of determining both serum CA 19-9 and TAG-72 in pancreatic cancer.

## POSSIBILITY OF DIAGNOSING SMALL PANCREATIC CANCERS WITH DIFFERENT SERUM TUMOR MARKERS

According to the report of the Japanese Pancreatic Cancer Registry in 1994, serum CA 19-9 levels were found to be elevated in 813 of 1100 (73.9%) pancreatic cancer patients at the time of their first visit to the hospital, with 329 of them (40%) treated by resection. The resectabilities of histologically proven T1 tumors (<2 cm) and T2 tumors (2.1–4.0 cm) were 96 and 78.5%, respectively, whereas the resectabilities of T3 tumors (4.1–6.0 cm) and T4 tumors (>6 cm) were only 51 and 31%, respectively. These findings indicate that measurement of CA 19-9 levels may provide us with information that will facilitate the detection of resectable pancreatic cancers, which are usually small, although small does not necessarily mean early cancer.

The same report also stated that the survival rate for resected pancreatic cancer was much higher than that for conservative treatment. Furthermore, the 5-year survival rates of resected T1 and T2 tumors were 37.8 and 16.2%, respectively, but for resected T3 and T4 tumors were only 13.5 and 8.3%, respectively. It is important to detect resectable pancreatic cancers, especially small pancreatic cancers to improve the prognosis.

As shown in Table 47.3, CA 19-9 assay had sensitivities of 62.5 and 77.7% in T1 tumors and T2 tumors, respectively, while SPan-1 assay had sensitivities of 58.1% in T1 tumors and 79.6% in T2 tumors in the same blood samples. Other serum markers were less sensitive. Chang and Takeuchi (6) reported similar results, but they found elastase 1 to have high sensitivity, as previously described. These results suggest that nearly 70% of small pancreatic cancers (<4 cm) release pancreatic cancer–associated antigens and are accompanied by high serum elastase 1 levels.

#### Case Report

A 66-year-old female had a 1-year history of epigastric discomfort and diarrhea after ingestion of fatty foods. A diagnosis of chronic pancreatitis was made, and the patient was treated medically. She improved. A routine examination on May 2, 1988, at her first visit, showed an elevated serum CA 19-9 level, but ultrasonography showed negative findings. Her serum CA 19-9 levels gradually increased thereafter, but no abnormal imaging findings were detected until December 1, 1988, at which time the serum CA 19-9 level was 496 U/mL (Fig. 47.1). Ultrasonography on the same day revealed a slight dilation of the pancreatic and bile ducts (Fig. 47.2). Endoscopic pancreatocholangiography showed partial stenosis of the pancreatic and bile ducts due to a small pancreatic cancer (Fig. 47.3). At surgery, a T2 tumor (2.2 × 2.3 cm) was identified in the head of the pancreas, with retroperitoneal and portal vein invasion (stage III). Pancreatoduodenectomy with partial resection of the portal vein was performed, and the patient survived for nearly 4 years.

As previously stated, no serum tumor marker assay used alone is sensitive or specific enough to be a pancreatic cancer screening test. While elevated tumor marker levels can be considered significant in patients with symptoms of pancreatic disease, further diagnostic efforts to verify the presence of pancreatic cancer are required, as shown in this case report. Tumor marker

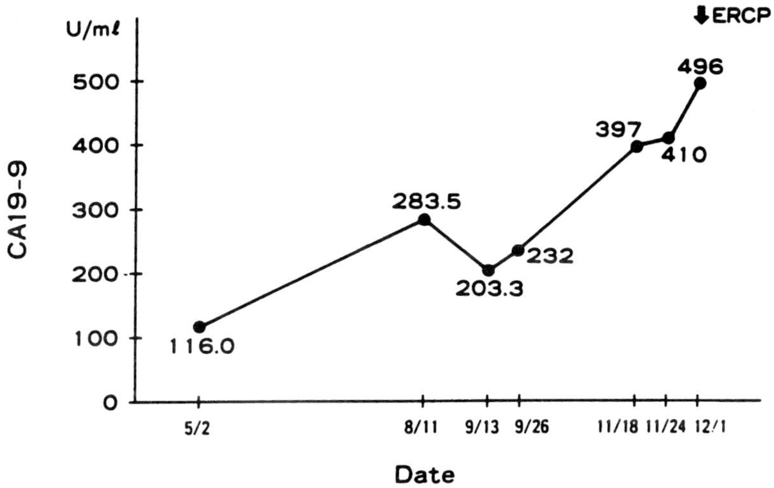


**FIG. 47.1.** Serial changes of serum CA 19-9 levels.

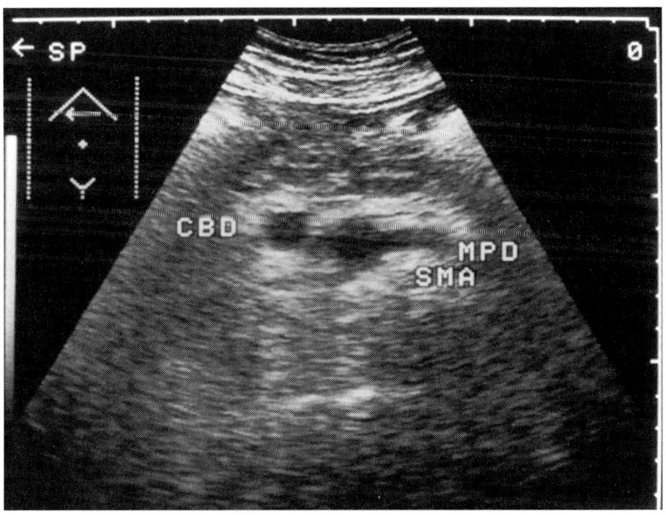


**FIG. 47.2.** Ultrasonography shows a slight dilatation of the main pancreatic duct *(MPD).*

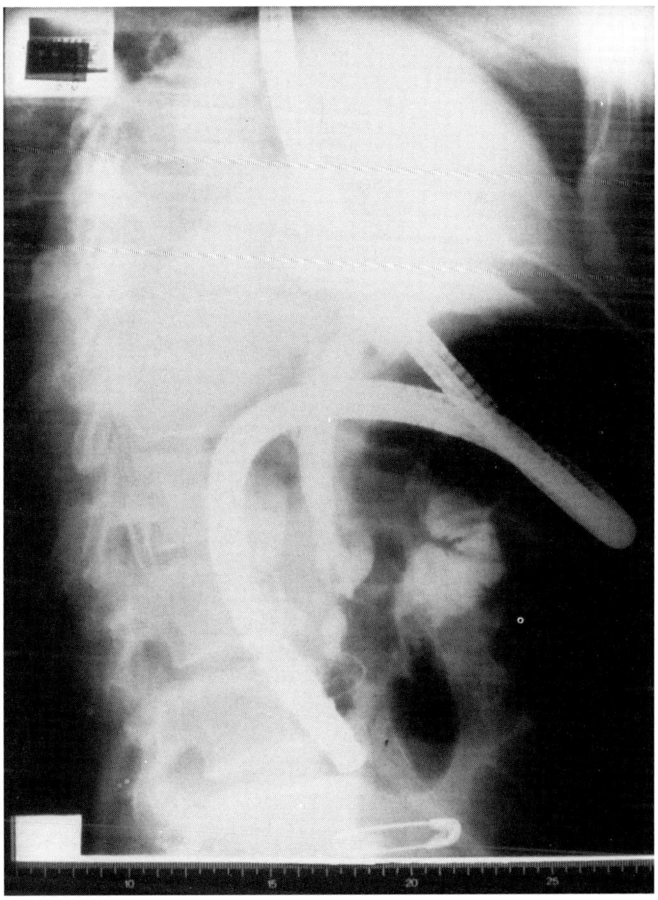

**FIG. 47.3.** ERCP shows a partial obstruction of the main pancreatic duct and the bile duct, due to pancreatic tumor.

measurement can serve as a very useful adjunct to the diagnosis of pancreatic cancer, including small pancreatic cancers.

### Combinations of Different Tumor Markers

A strong positive correlation exists between CA 19-9, SPan-1, CA 50, and CA 242. Combinations of these markers have failed to provide any advantage because of the similarity of the antigens. Even in T1 and T2 tumors, various combinations of tumor markers only slightly improve the detection of small pancreatic cancers (Figs. 47.4, 47.5, and 47.6). (101). Kuno et al. (102) examined 403 patients suspected of having pancreatic cancer by using a combination assay of various tumor markers (CA 19-9, DU-PAN-2, TPA, elastase 1, $\gamma$-glutamyltranspeptidase, lactate dehydrogenase, lipase, amylase, and alkaline phosphatase). The diagnostic value of these markers was compared by multivariate analysis (computeraid multivariate and pattern analysis system for examine-1: CAMPAS-PX1), and they diagnosed 47 of 403 patients with pancreatic cancer by this method. Although they did not mention the resectability of the 47 pancreatic cancers, they concluded that CAMPAS-PX1 provided the most effective markers for diagnosing pancreatic cancer; but in terms of its cost-benefit ratio, CAMPAS-PX1 was no better than the CA 19-9 assay used alone. Pasanen et al. (103) assessed the combined use of CA 19-9, CA 242, and proton nuclear magnetic resonance $^{1}$H NMR spectroscopy of plasma to detect pancreatic cancer, and found that it yielded only slightly better accuracy in the diagnosis of pancreatic cancer. Combination of CA 19-9 with growth-related antigens (alkaline phosphatase, isoenzymes, ribonuclease) and tumor-associated markers (ferritin, ratio of ferritin to serum iron, sialic acid), however, has been reported to improve its usefulness in early tumor detection (104). Combination of CA 19-9 with imaging procedures, such as ultrasonography, endoscopic pancreatocholangiography, or computed tomography, is another means of improving sensitivity (105).

### Mass Screening for Pancreatic Cancer in Asymptomatic and Symptomatic Subjects by Using Serum Tumor Markers and Imaging Studies

As described above, it is important to determine whether combining measurements of serum tumor markers and imaging procedures is a valuable method of mass screening to detect pancreatic cancer. The Japan Pancreatic Cancer Study Group conducted mass screening to detect pancreatic cancer in subjects with and without abdominal complaints during two different periods, 1984–1985 and 1987–1988 (106, 107). All patients were over age 40, and screening was conducted at 17 hospitals throughout Japan. All of the subjects underwent either ultrasonography or serum CA 19-9 and elastase 1 determinations as the initial screening test. Whenever abnormal results were obtained, additional studies were carried out, including either repeat ultrasonography or endoscopic retrograde pancreatocholangiography (ERCP), with cytology, angiography, percutaneous transhepatic cholangiography (PTC), or abdominal computed tomography (CT). The final diagnosis was made either clinically or histologically.

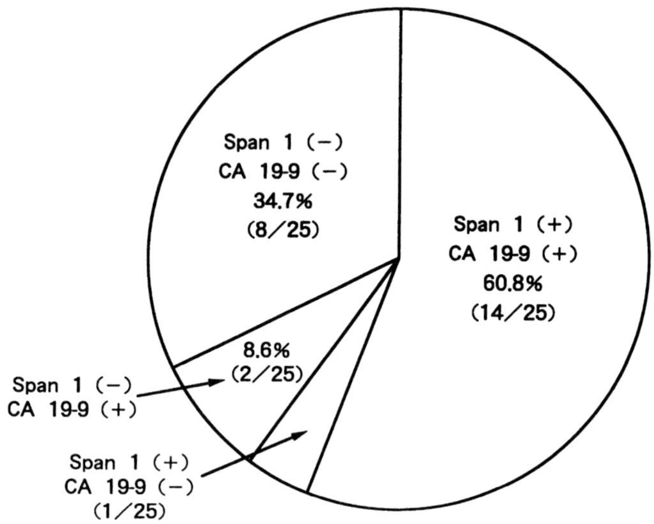


**FIG. 47.4.** The combination assay of serum SPan-1 and CA 19-9 in the diagnosis of T1 pancreatic cancer.

A total of 8,756 symptomatic patients and 12,840 asymptomatic subjects were examined by this method during these two periods. A final diagnosis of pancreatic cancer was made in 141 of the 8756 symptomatic patients (1.6%), and 47 of them underwent resection. Only 40 of the 12,840 asymptomatic persons (0.03%) were diagnosed as having pancreatic cancer, and only 1 of them was treated by resection. In addition, during the earlier period of the study (1984–1985), 73 carcinomas of other digestive organs (1.6%), including 15 hepatomas, 25 biliary tract cancers, and 32 GI cancers were detected in 2037 symptomatic patients, indicating that outpatient clinic screening by the serum tests and ultrasonography is very effective in detecting both resectable pancreatic cancer and other digestive cancers.

For mass screening for any type of cancer to be cost-effective, the mortality rate must be greater than 40 per 100,000 population. The mortality rate of pancreatic cancer per person over age 40 in Japan is about 23 per 100,000. Thus, these results led to the conclusion that mass screening, based on detection of elastase 1, CA 19-9 assay, and ultrasonography is not worthwhile as a means of detecting pancreatic cancer in asymptomatic persons from the standpoint of cost-effectiveness. However, using the same tools to screen symptomatic patients in outpatient clinics is very effective in finding resectable pancreatic cancers.

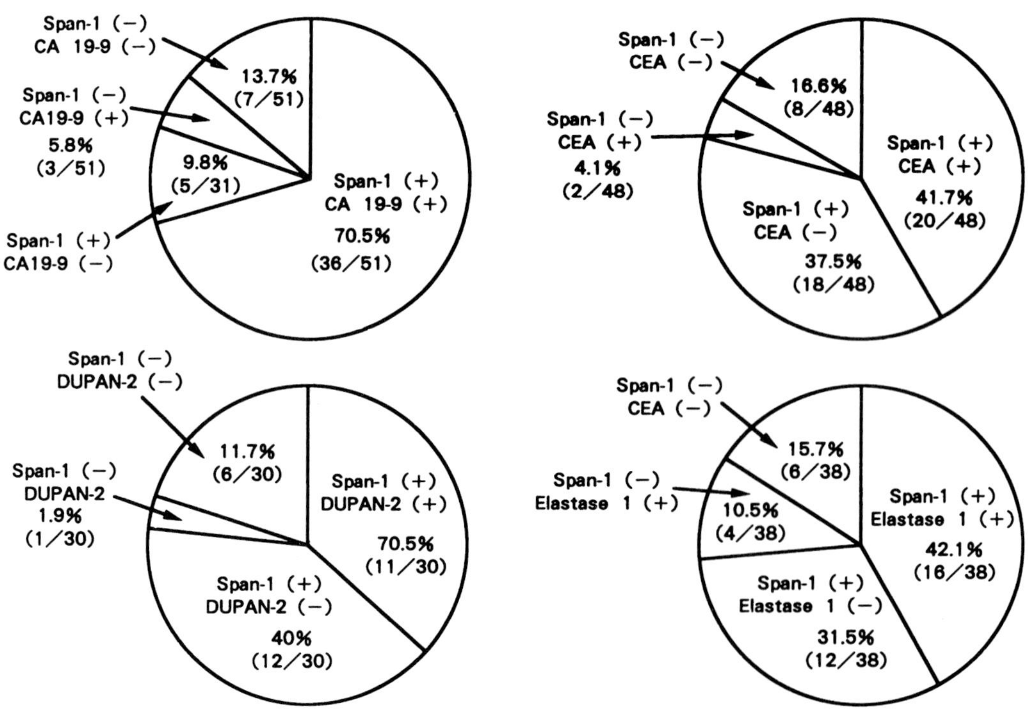


**FIG. 47.5.** The combination assay of serum SPan-1 and other tumor markers in the diagnosis of T2 pancreatic cancer.

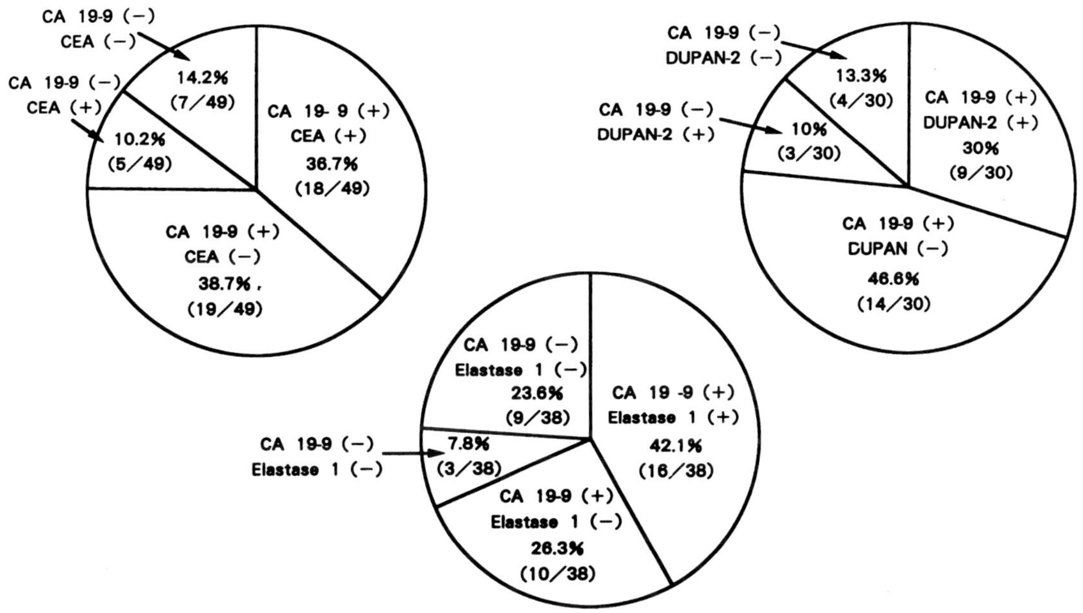


**FIG. 47.6.** The combination assay of serum CA 19-9 and other tumor markers in the diagnosis of T2 pancreatic cancer.

## Possibility of Using Oncogenes and Tumor Suppressor Genes as Tumor Markers of Pancreatic Cancer

The study of oncogenes and tumor-suppressor genes provides us with knowledge of the genetic basis of cancer. There is increasing evidence that cancer results from an accumulation of dominant and recessive mutations among these oncogenes and tumor-suppressor genes. Experimental studies suggest that multiple mutations are required to transform cells. Identification of the genetic changes in pancreatic cancer may yield specific markers for this disease. Identifying the mutations that occur in pancreatic cancer may provide important information on the early stage of pancreatic cancer. Although no methods of detecting the premalignant stages of pancreatic cancer are currently available, the study of genetic markers may play a central role in the development of techniques for early detection of pancreatic cancer.

The frequencies with which specific mutations occur need to be known for genetic markers to become diagnostically useful. Specificity is also important to enable differentiation of pancreatic ductal cell adenocarcinoma from hyperplastic nonmalignant conditions and from other periampullary carcinomas that have a better prognosis. It would also be valuable to know which mutations are early events and which are late events and if they are related to the malignant potential of the tumor (see Chapter 46, Molecular Biology: Diagnostic and Therapeutic Potentials).

## REFERENCES

1. Helbert AF. Tumor marker tests in patients monitoring. Lab Med 1982;13:528–533.
2. The Japanese Pancreatic Cancer Registry. J Jpn Pancreas Soc 1994;9:499–527 (in Japanese).
3. Satake K, Kanazawa G, Koh I, Chung YS, Umeyama K. Evaluation of serum pancreatic enzymes, carbohydrate antigen 19-9, and carcinoembryonic antigen in various pancreatic diseases. Am J Gastroenterol 1985;80:630–636.
4. Suzuki T, Naito A, Manabe T, et al. Clinic of the pancreatic cancer. Naika 1984;53:675–682 (in Japanese).
5. Hayakawa T, Kondoh T, Shibata T, et al. Prospective trial for early detection of pancreatic cancer by elevated serum immunoreactive elastase. Gastroenterol Jpn 1990;25:727–731.
6. Chang JH, Takeuchi T. Clinical significance of measurement of serum SPan-1 antigen in the diagnosis of pancreatic cancer. J Jpn Pancreas Soc 1990;5:80–88.
7. Mullins DE, Rohrlich ST. The role of proteinases in cellular invasiveness. Biochim Biophys Acta 1983;695:177–214.
8. Strauli P. A concept of tumor invasion. In: Strauli P, Barrett AJ, Baici A, eds. Proteinase and tumor invasion. New York: Raven Press, 1980:1–5.
9. von Fritz H, Woitinas F. Uber proteinaseinhibitoren. 11. Isolierung and Charakterisiering von Proteinaseinhibitoren aus den Bauchspeicheldruzen verschiedener Wirbeltiere und des Menschen. Hoppe-Seyler's Z Physiol Chem 1966;348:168–180.
10. Fukayama M, Hayashi Y, Koike M, Ogawa M, Kosaki G. Immunohistochemical localization of pancreatic secretory trypsin inhibitor in fetal and adult pancreatic and extrapancreatic tissues. J Histochem Cytochem 1986;34:227–235.
11. Eddeland A, Ohlsson K. A radioimmunoassay for measurement of human pancreatic secretory trypsin inhibitor in different body fluid. Hoppe-Seyler's Z Physiol Chem 1978;359:671–675.
12. Matsuda K, Ogawa M, Murata A, Kitahara T, Kosaki G. Elevation of serum immunoreactive pancreatic secretory trypsin inhibitor contents in various malignant disease. Res Commun Chem Pathol Pharmacol 1983;40:301–305.
13. Murata A, Ogawa M, Matsuda K, Matsuura N, Kosaki G. Immunoreactive pancreatic secretory trypsin inhibitor in gynecological diseases. Res Commun Chem Pathol Pharmacol 1983;41:493–499.
14. Ogawa M, Matsuda K, Matsuda Y, et al. Evaluation of immunological assays of serum pancreatic enzymes and secretory trypsin inhibitor for diagnosis and management of acute pancreatitis. In: Sato T, Yamauchi H, eds. Pancreatitis. Tokyo: University of Tokyo Press, 1985:107–115.
15. Satake K, Inui A, Sogabe T, et al. The measurement of serum immunoreactive pancreatic secretory trypsin inhibitor in gastrointestinal cancer and pancreatic disease. Int J Pancreatol 1988;3:323–332.

16. Stenman UH, Huhtala ML, Koistinen R, Seppala M. Immunochemical demonstration of an ovarian cancer-associated urinary peptide. Int J Cancer 1982;30:53–57.
17. Huhtala ML, Pesonen K, Kalkkinen N, Stenman UH. Purification and characterization of a tumor associated trypsin inhibitor from the urine of a patient with ovarian cancer. J Biol Chem 1982;257:13713–13717.
18. Westermark P, Wilander E, Westermark GT, Johnson KH. Islet amyloid polypeptide-like immunoreactivity in the islet B cells of type 2 (non-insulin-dependent) diabetes and non-diabetic individuals. Diabetologica 1987;32:887–892.
19. Sowa R, Sanke T, Hirayama J, et al. Islet amyloid polypeptide amide causes peripheral insulin resistance in vivo in dogs. Diabetologica 1990;33:118–120.
20. Chance WT, Balasubramaniam A, Zhang FS, Wimalawanse SJ, Fisher JE. Anorexia following the intrahypothalamic administration of amylin. Brain Res 1991;539:352–354.
21. Arnelo U, Reidelberger R, Permert J, Westermark P, Adrian TE, Larsson J. Islet amyloid polypeptide: an anorectic factor in patients with pancreatic cancer. Pancreas 1995;18:288–289.
22. Permart J, Larsson J, Westermark GT, et al. Islet amyloid polypeptide in patients with pancreatic cancer and diabetes. N Engl J Med 1994;330:313–318.
23. Schwats SS, Zeidler A, Moossa AR, Kuku SF, Rubenstein AH. A prospective study of glucose intolerance, insulin, C-peptide, and glucagon in patients with pancreatic cancer. Am J Dig Dis 1978;23:1107–1114.
24. Gold P, Freedman SO. Demonstration of tumor-specific antigens in human colonic carcinomata by immunological tolerance and adsorption technique. J Exp Med 1965;121:439–462.
25. Hammarstrom S, Engvall E, Johansson BG, Svensson S, Sundblad G, Goldstein IJ. Nature of the tumor-associated determinant(s) of carcino-embryonic antigen. Proc Natl Acad Sci USA 1975;72:1528–1532.
26. Hedin A, Carlsson L, Berglund A, Hammarstrom S. A monoclonal antibody-enzyme immunoassay for serum carcinoembryonic antigen with increased specificity for carcinomas. Proc Natl Acad Sci USA 1983;80:3470–3474.
27. Lindgren J, Bang B, Hurme M, Makela O. Monoclonal antibodies to carcino-embryonic antigen (CEA): characterization and use in a radioimmunoassay for CEA. Acta Pathol Microbiol Immunol Scand 1982;90:159–165.
28. Klapdor R, Lehmann U, Bahlo M, et al. CA 19-9 and CEA in the follow-up of exocrine pancreatic cancer disease. Gastroenterology 1984;86:1137.
29. Kalser MH, Barkin JS, Redlhammer D, Heal A. Circulating carcinoembryonic antigen in pancreatic cancer. Cancer 1978; 42:1468–1471.
30. Begent RHJ. The value of carcinoembryonic antigen measurement in clinical practice. Ann Clin Biochem 1984;21:231–238.
31. Hansen HJ, Sydney JJ, Miller E, et al. Carcinoembryonic antigen (CEA) assay. A laboratory adjunct in the diagnosis and management of cancer. Hum Pathol 1974;5:139–147.
32. Carr-Locke DL. Serum and pancreatic juice carcinoembryonic antigen in pancreatic and biliary disease. Gut 1980;21: 656–661.
33. Banwo O, Versey J, Hobbs JR. New oncofetal antigen for human pancreas. Lancet 1974;i:643–645.
34. Gelder FB, Reese CJ, Moosa AR, Hall T, Hunter R. Purification, partial characterization, and clinical evaluation of a pancreatic oncofetal antigen. Cancer Res 1978;38:313–324.
35. Kawa S. Immunoperoxidase detection of pancreatic oncofetal antigen in human tissues. Gastroenterol Jpn 1985;20:361–367.
36. Nishida K, Sugiura M, Yoshikawa T, Kondo M. Enzyme immunoassay of pancreatic oncofetal antigen (POA) as a marker of pancreatic cancer. Gut 1985;26:450–455.
37. Schmiegel WH, Eberl W, Kreiker C, et al. Multiparametric tumor marker (CA 19-9, CEA, AFP, POA) analyses of pancreatic juice and sera in pancreatic disease. Hepatogastroenterology 1985; 32:141–145.
38. Ochi Y, Ura Y, Hamazu M, Ishida M, Kajita Y, Nakajima Y. Immunological study of tissue polypeptide antigen (TPA)—demonstration of keratin-like sites and blood group antigen-like sites on TPA molecules. Clin Chem Acta 1985;151:157–167.
39. Panucci A, Fabris C, Del Favero G, et al. Tissue polypeptide antigen (TPA) in pancreatic cancer diagnosis. Br J Cancer 1985;52:801–803.
40. Basso D, Fabris C, Del Favero G, et al. Combined determination of serum CA 19-9 and tissue polypeptide antigen: why no improvement in pancreatic cancer diagnosis? Oncology 1988; 45:24–29.
41. Paganuzzi M, Onetto M, Marroni P, et al. CA 19-9 and CA 50 in benign and malignant pancreatic and biliary disease. Cancer 1988;61:2100–2108.
42. Oshio G, Manabe T, Watanabe Y, et al. Comparative studies of DU-PAN-2, carcinoembryonic antigen, and CA 19-9 in the serum and bile of patients with pancreatic and biliary tract diseases: evaluation of the influence of obstructive jaundice. Am J Gastroenterol 1990;85:1370–1376.
43. Basso D, Fabris C, Meggiato T, et al. Serum levels of CA 19-9 and tissue polypeptide antigen (TPA) are related to the presence of a benign extrahepatic cholestasis. Med Sci Res 1989;17:13–14.
44. Basso D, Fabris C, Piccoli A, Plebani M, Del Favero G. Serum tissue polypeptide antigen in pancreatic cancer and other gastrointestinal cancer. J Clin Pathol 1989;42:555.
45. Basso D, Fabris C, Del Favero G, et el. How does liver dysfunction influence serum CA 19-9 in pancreatic cancer?. Ital J Gastroenterol 1990;22:1–6.
46. Thomas P. Studies on the mechanisms of biliary excretion of circulating glycoproteins. The carcinoembryonic antigen. Biochem J 1980;192:837–843.
47. Mcfarlane IG. Hepatic clearance of serum glycoprotein. Clin Sci 1983;64:127–135.
48. Matino P, Buccheri G, Preatoni A, Ferrigno D, Luporini AC, Pravettoni G. Tissue polypeptide specific antigen (TPS) and objective response to treatment in solid tumor. Int J Biol Markers 1992;7:65–67.
49. Plebani M, Basso D, Del Favero G, et al. Clinical utility of TPS, TPA and CA19-9 measurement in pancreatic cancer. Oncology 1993;50:436–440.
50. Koprowski H, Steplewski Z, Mitchell K, Herlyn M, Herlyn D, Fuhrer P. Colorectal carcinoma antigens detected by hybridoma antibodies. Somatic Cell Genet 1979;5:957–971.
51. Tempero MA, Uchida E, Takasaki H, Burnett DA, Steplewski Z, Pour PM. Relationship of carbohydrate antigen 19-9 and Lewis antigens in pancreatic cancer. Cancer 1987;47:5501–5503.
52. Magnani JL, Nilsson B, Brockhous M, et al. A monoclonal antibody-defined antigen associated with gastrointestinal cancer is a ganglioside containing sialylated lacto-*N*-fucopentaose 11. J Biol Chem 1982;247:14365–14369.
53. Magnani JL, Steplewski Z, Koprowski H, Ginsburg V. Identification of the gastrointestinal and pancreatic cancer-associated antigen detected by monoclonal antibody 19-9 in the sera of patients as mucin. Cancer Res 1983;43:5489–5492.
54. Watkins WM. Biochemistry and genetics of the ABO, Lewis, and P blood group systems. Adv Hum Genet 1980;10:1–136.
55. Koprowski H, Blaszezyk M, Steplewski Z, Brockhaus M, Magnani J, Ginsburg V. Lewis blood-type may affect the incidence of gastrointestinal cancer. Lancet 1982;1:1332–1333.
56. Atkinson BF, Ernst CS, Herlyn M, Steplewski Z, Sears HF, Koprowski H. Gastrointestinal cancer-associated antigen in immunoperoxidase assay. Cancer Res 1982;42:4820–4823.
57. Dietel M, Arps H, Klapdor R, Muller-Hagen S, Sieck M, Hoffmann L. Antigen detection by the monoclonal antibodies CA 19-9 and CA 125 in normal and tumor tissue and patients' sera. J Cancer Res Clin Oncol 1986;111:257–265.
58. Haglund C, Lindgren J, Roberts PJ, Nording S. Gastrointestinal cancer-associated antigen CA 19-9 in histological specimens of pancreatic tumours and pancreatitis. Br J Cancer 1986;53: 189–195.
59. Sipponen J, Lindgren J. sialylated Lewis$^a$ determinant CA 19-9 in benign and malignant gastric tissue. Acta Pathol Microbiol Immunol Scand (A) 1986;94:305–311.
60. Del Villano BC, Bremnen S, Block P, et al. Radioimmunometric assay for a monoclonal antibody defined tumor marker, CA 19-9. Clin Chem 1983;29:549–552.
61. Jalanko H, Hagluund C, Roberts PJ, Kuusela P. Tumor markers in gastrointestinal cancer. In: Holmgren J, ed. Tumor marker antigens. Stockholm: Studentlitterature, 1985;114–122.

62. Pleskow DK, Berger HJ, Gyves J, Allen E, Mclean A, Podolsky DK. Evaluation of a serologic marker CA 19-9 in the diagnosis of pancreatic cancer. Ann Intern Med 1989;110:704–709.
63. Sakahara H, Endo K, Nakajima K, et al. Serum CA 19-9 concentration and computed tomography finding in patients with pancreatic cancer. Cancer 1986;57:1324–1326.
64. Ishii H, Yamamura H, Tatsuta M, Okuda S, Kitamura T. Value of ultrasonography combined with measurement of serum tumor markers in the diagnosis of pancreatic cancer of less than 3 cm in diameter. Cancer 1986;57:1947–1951.
65. Albert MB, Steinberg WM, Henry JP. Elevated serum levels of tumor marker CA 19-9 in acute cholangitis. Dig Dis Sci 1988;33: 1223–1225.
66. Basso D, Meggiato T, Fabris C, et al. Extra-hepatic cholestasis determines a reversible increase of glycoprotein tumor markers in benign and malignant diseases. Eur J Clin Invest 1992;22: 800–804.
67. Lindholm L, Holmgren J, Svennerholm L, et al. Monoclonal antibodies against gastrointestinal tumor associated antigen isolated as monosialogangliosides. Int Arch Allergy Appl Immunol 1983;71:178–181.
68. Mansson JE, Fredman P, Nilsson O, Lindholm L, Holmgren J, Svennerholm L. Chemical structure of carcinoma ganglioside antigens defined by monoclonal antibody C 50 and some allied gangliosides of human pancreatic adenocarcinoma. Biochim Biophys Acta 1985;834:110–117.
69. Nilsson O, Mansson JE, Lindholm L, Svennerholm L. Sialosyllactotetraosylceramine, a novel ganglioside antigen detected in human carcinoma by a monoclonal antibody. FEBS Lett 1985; 182:398–402.
70. Hagland C, Lindgren J, Roberts PJ, Nordling S. Tissue expression of the tumor marker CA 50 in benign and malignant pancreatic lesions. Int J Cancer 1986;38:841–846.
71. Ishii M, Abe A, Ohkura A. Fundamental evaluation and clinical usefulness of CA 50 EIA kit. Jpn J Cancer Res 1987;14:2548–2555 (in Japanese).
72. Watanabe H, Kotani H, Satomura Y. Clinical usefulness of the measurement of serum CA 50 levels in various gastrointestinal cancer. Igaku No Ayumi 1981;141:861–822 (in Japanese).
73. Blind PJ, Dahgren ST. Serum levels of the carbohydrate antigen CA 50 in pancreatic disease. Acta Chir Scand 1987;153: 45–49.
74. Chung YS, Satake K, Umeyama K, Kim YS. Monoclonal antibody SPan-1 against pancreatic cancer cell and characterization of antigen. J Jpn Surg Soc 1989;87:236 (in Japanese).
75. Chung YS, Ho JJL, Kim YS, et al. The detection of human pancreatic cancer-associated antigen in the serum of cancer patients. Cancer 1987;60:1636–1643.
76. Umeyama K, et al. and the Japan SPan-1 Study Group. Clinical evaluation of measurement of pancreatic cancer associated antigen SPan-1. J Jpn Pancreas Soc 1988;3:528–529.
77. Metzgar RS, Gaillard MT, Levine SJ, Tuck FL, Bossen EH, Borowitz MJ. Antigens of human pancreatic adenocarcinoma cell defined by murine monoclonal antibodies. Cancer Res 1982; 42:601–608.
78. Borowitz MJ, Tuck FL, Sindelar WF, Fernsten PD, Metzgar RS. Monoclonal antibodies against human adenocarcinoma: distribution of DU-PAN-2 antigen on glandular epithelia and carcinomas. J Natl Cancer Inst 1984;72:999–1003.
79. Metzgar RS, Rodorigerez N, Finn OJ, et al. Detection of a pancreatic cancer-associated antigen (Dupan-2 antigen) in serum and ascites of patients with adenocarcinomas. Proc Natl Acad Sci USA 1984;81:5242–5246.
80. Mahvi DM, Meyers WC, Bast RC, Seigler HF, Metzgar RS. Carcinoma of pancreatic cancer. Therapeutic efficacy as defined by a serodiagnostic test utilizing a monoclonal antibody. Ann Surg 1985;202:440–445.
81. Takemori Y, Sawabu N, Satomura Y, et al. The measurement of serum DUPAN-2 levels utilizing EIA kit. Jpn J Cancer Res 1987;14: 119–126 (in Japanese).
82. Cho M, Watanabe S, Takeuchi T. Clinical evaluation of serum DUPAN-2 measurement: pancreatic cancer. Jpn J Pancreas Soc 1986;1:69–77 (in Japanese).
83. Ichihara T, Nakao S, Sakamoto J, et al. CA 50, CA 19-9, DUPAN-2 in pancreatic cancer. Jpn J Pancreas Soc 1987;2:13–23 (in Japanese).
84. Okura H, Tajiri H. Tumor markers in pancreatic cancer. Pharma Medica 1987;5:21–27 (in Japanese).
85. Fukushi Y, Nudelman E, Levery SB, Hakomori S, Rauvala H. Novel fucolipid accumulating in human adenocarcinoma. 111. A hybridoma antibody (FH 6) defining a human cancer-associated difucoganglioside. J Biol Chem 1984;259:10511–10517.
86. Imura H, et al. and the Japan SLEX Study Group. Initial basic and clinical evaluation of a solid-phase immunoradiometric assay sialy SSEA-1 antigen. Jpn J Cancer Chemother 1987;14:1322–1331 (in Japanese).
87. Rothlin MA, Joller H, Largiader F. CA 242 is a new tumor marker for pancreatic cancer. Cancer 1993;71:701–707.
88. Haglund C, Lindgren J, Roberts PJ, Kuusela P, Nording S. Tissue expression of the tumour associated antigen CA 242 in benign and malignant pancreatic lesions. A comparison with CA 50 and CA 19-9. Br J Cancer 1989;60:845–851.
89. Plebani M, Basso D, Navagalia F, et al. Is CA 242 really a new tumour marker for pancreatic adenocarcinoma? Oncology 1995;52:19–23.
90. Johnson VG, Schlom J, Paterson AJ, Bennet J, Magnani JL, Clocher D. Analysis of a tumor-associated glycoprotein (TAG-72) identified by monoclonal antibody B 72.3. Cancer Res 1986;46: 850–857.
91. Kjeldsen T, Clausen H, Hirohashi S, Ogawa T, Lijima H, Hakomori S. Preparation and characterization of monoclonal antibody directed to the tumor associated *o*-linked sialosyl-2→6 alpha-*N*-acetylgalactosaminyl (sialosyl-Tn) epitope. Cancer Res 1988; 48:2214–2220.
92. Gero EJ, Colcher D, Ferroni P, et al. CA 72-4 radioimmunoassay for the detection of the TAG-72 carcinoma-associated antigen in serum of patients. J Clin Lab Anal 1989;3:360–363.
93. Thor A, Gorstein F, Ohuchi N, Szpak CA, Johnston WW, Scholm J. Tumor-associated glycoprotein (TAG-72) in ovarian carcinomas defined by monoclonal antibody B 72.3. J Natl Cancer Inst 1986;76:995–1006.
94. Hamazoe R, Maeta M, Matsui T, Shibata S, Shirota S, Kaibara N. CA 72-4 compared with carcinoembryonic antigen as a tumour marker for gastric cancer. Eur J Cancer 1992;28A: 1351–1354.
95. Paterson AJ, Scholm J, Sears HF, Bennet J, Colcher D. A radioimmunoassay for the detection of a human tumor-associated glycoprotein (TAG-72) using monoclonal antibody B 72.3. Int J Cancer 1986;37:659–666.
96. Klug TL, Sattler MA, Cocher D, Scholm J. Monoclonal antibody immunoradiometric assay for an antigenic determinant (CA 72) on a novel pancarcinoma antigen (TAG-72). Int J Cancer 1989;38:661–669.
97. Heptner G, Domschke S, Domschke W. Comparison of CA 72-4 with CA 19-9 and carcinoembryonic antigen in the serodiagnostis of gastrointestinal malignancies. Scand J Gastroenterol 1989;24:745–750.
98. Piatino P, Fusaro A, Daziano E, Polloni R, Mosso R, Cacace G. TAG 72: un nuovo antigene tumore associatoriconosciuto da un anticorpo monoclonale. Minerva Med 1990;81:756–757.
99. Kornek GV, Depisch D, Rosen HR, Temsch EM, Scheithauser W. Comparative analysis of CA 72-4, CA 195 and carcinoembryonic antigen in patient with gastrointestinal malignancies. J Cancer Res Clin Oncol 1992;118:318–320.
100. Pasquali C, Sperti C, D'Andrea AA, Costatino V, Filipponi C, Pedrazzoli S. Clinical value of serum TAG-72 as a tumor marker for pancreatic carcinoma. Int J Pancreatol 1994;15: 171–177.
101. Satake K, Chung YS, Yokomatsu H, et al. Various tumor markers for small pancreatic cancer with special reference to the present status of pancreatic cancer in Japan and our experience over the past 2 years. Pancreas 1991;6:234–241.
102. Kuno N, Kurimoto K, Fukushima M, et al. Effectiveness of multivariate analysis of tumor markers in diagnosis of pancreatic carcinoma: a prospective study in multiinstitutions. Pancreas 1994;9:725–730.
103. Pasanen PA, Kauppinen R, Eskelinen M, Partanen K, Pikkarainen P, Alhava E. The value of combined use of serum tumor markers and nuclear magnetic spectroscopy of plasma in the detection

of pancreatic cancer among patients with jaundice or cholestasis: results from a prospective study. Anticancer Res 1993;13:763–768.

104. Kobayashi T, Kawakubo T. Prospective investigation of tumor markers and risk assessment in early cancer screening. Cancer 1994;73:1946–1953.

105. Niederau C, Grendell JH. Diagnosis of pancreatic carcinoma. Imaging technique and tumor markers. Pancreas 1992;7:66–86.

106. Homma T, Tsuchiya R. The study of the mass screening of persons without symptoms and of screening of out-patients with gastrointestinal complaints or icterus for pancreatic cancer in Japan, using CA 19-9, and elastase 1 or ultrasonography. Int J Pancreatol 1991;9:119–124.

107. Satake K, Takeuchi T, Homma T, Ozaki H. CA 19-9 as a screening and diagnostic tool in symptomatic patients: the Japanese experience. Pancreas 1994;9:703–706.

# 48

# *Benign and Premalignant Lesions*

Parviz M. Pour

Through international collaboration, advances have been made in the diagnosis and classification of pancreatic cancer. The previous large list of tumors that was based purely on their morphologic patterns has now been modified and has become more clinically oriented (1). The use of molecular biologic and immunohistochemical techniques has contributed to better understanding of the tumor type. Moreover, a new tumor entity, intraductal tumor, has been recognized, and advances in tumor registry and tissue workups have narrowed the spectrum of benign tumors. These advances have benefited some groups of patients and prolonged their survival by early surgery. Despite this progress, tumor histogenesis has remained a problem, although sporadic observation of early cancer (2–4) has favored the origin of tumors from ductal epithelium.

Much work has been concentrated on the recognition of cancer precursor lesions and in the definition of malignancy by molecular biology. These studies, however, have led to disappointing results, as the mutation of the *c-Ki-ras* oncogene that initially seemed to be a hallmark of pancreatic malignancy (5, 6), has been found in benign-appearing lesions (7, 8). These findings have been interpreted as either a reflection of the initiation of carcinogenesis, one of the many events associated with malignancy, or an indication that hyperplastic lesions are precursors of tumors. Certainly much work is needed for clarification and detection of other more specific tumor markers.

In this chapter the current knowledge of benign and premalignant exocrine pancreatic lesions is described.

## BENIGN EXOCRINE PANCREATIC LESIONS

Benign lesions of the exocrine pancreas include hyperplastic ductal epithelium, focal hyperplasia of acinar cells, and diffuse or focal hyperplasia of ductal/ductular cells.

### Benign Ductal Lesions

**Ductal Cell Hyperplasia.** Ductal cell hyperplasia, the most common benign lesion of the pancreas, is seen in many normal pancreata, especially in aged individuals. The term *hyperplasia* should be reserved for lesions that show multiplication of the epithelium and should be distinguished from cell *hypertrophy,* which may or may not accompany hyperplasia (Fig. 48.1). Whether this hyperplasia is reactive or premalignant has not been resolved. Molecular biologic studies have not settled the problem because mutation of the *c-Ki-ras* gene has been detected in some simple ductal cell hyperplasia. Consequently, nothing has changed the microscopic diagnostic criteria.

**Cystic Ductal Lesions.** Focal duplication and distension of ducts or ductules can be seen in some normal pancreata. These lesions may or may not be associated with fibrosis. The cystic ducts are lined by atrophic epithelium and may show focal or extended epithelial denudation and contain mucin. Whether they develop because of a block in the proximal ductal lumen or by retraction by scars is not always clear.

**Serous Cystadenoma.** Serous cystadenoma, previously called microcystic adenoma, was once considered a benign pancreatic tumor. However, recent observations point to their malignant potential. Therefore, these tumors, despite their benign appearance, should be carefully sampled and examined, as focal invasion or even vascular invasion may escape recognition (9). Typically, these lesions occur predominantly in women and are characterized by slow growth and the absence of symptoms until they become large enough to obstruct the surrounding structures. A reticulum septumlike appearance, calcification, and a central stellate scar are among the findings by ultrasonography (US) and computed tomography (CT). Histologically, the tumor shows small cysts lined by usually uniform epithelium, typically containing glycogen. DNA ploidy and argyrophilic nuclear organizer counts may be the only criteria for distinguishing between a benign and a malignant tumor (9). These lesions may be composed of large cysts, as a macrocystic or lymphangiomatoid variant, and therefore, the term serous cystadenoma should be given to these lesions (10).

**Mucinous Cystadenoma.** Usually a unilocular tumor, mucinous cystadenoma also occurs predominantly in the body and tail of the pancreas and is seen predominantly in women. The cyst is lined by a columnar mucin-producing epithelium surrounded by "ovarian-type" stroma. As with serous cystadenoma, these tumors tend to malignancy and may show focal atypia of the epithelium upon careful sampling (Fig. 48.2).

**Intraductal (Papillary-Mucinous) Adenoma.** Intraductal papillary-mucinous) adenoma usually shows distension of a short or long segment of the main duct or duct branches, with papillary protrusion of usually uniform epithelium. Mucin, in different amounts, can be produced. Step-sectioning may show continuous or discontinuous growth of the tumor and focal atypia. The *c-Ki-ras* mutation may be found, and accumulating experience suggests that these lesions generally show potential for malignancy. Careful examination of the specimens is necessary to rule out malignancy. The "adenoma-like" structures can be found in a clearly invasive tumor, indicating that the transformation of benign to malignant epithelium can occur at any time.

### Acinar Cell Hyperplasia

Focal enlargement of acinar cells has been termed *acinar cell foci, hyperplastic acinar cell nodules,* or *atypical acinar cell nodules* and has been observed in the normal and diseased pancreas. The remarkably wide variation in the reported incidence of these lesions is based largely on the pathologists' awareness of them and on the extent of screening. The opinion about their biology

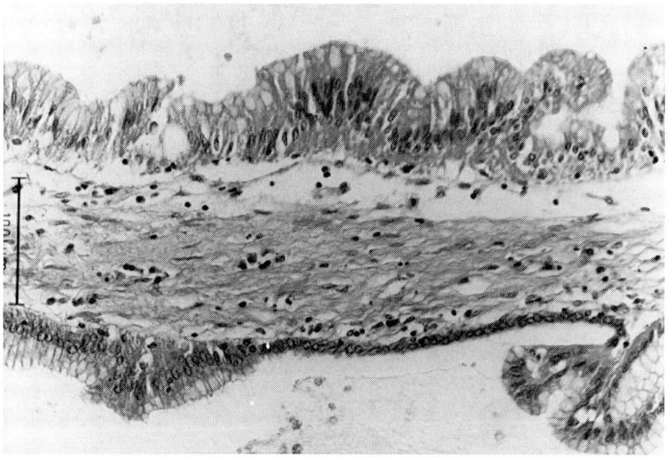

**FIG. 48.1.** Normal, hypertrophy, hypertrophy and hyperplasia of ductal epithelium in a multilocular cyst. Note the polar arrangement of uniform nuclei. Bar = 100 μm; H & E.

differs from premalignant (11) to reparative regenerative (12). Considering the incidence of acinar cell carcinoma, it is difficult to assume that they represent a tumor precursor lesion.

### Ductular Hyperplasia

Diffuse proliferation of centroacinar cells is seen in the pancreas of one with infantile hyperinsulinemic hypoglycemia syndrome. The proliferation affects almost the entire pancreas and in the H & E stained slides is characterized by disruption of the normal architecture of acini by light, irregularly large areas composed of light centroacinar cells (Fig. 48.3). The centroacinar proliferation is usually associated with nesidioblastosis and formation of acinar cell foci. Because small ducts also show cell hyperplasia (Fig. 48.3), one can term the condition pancreatic panhyperplasia. Hyperplastic ductular cells may appear abnormal, and the concomitant presence of fibrosis and inflammation may create suspicion of malignancy. However, unlike the malignant cells, with H & E staining, hyperplastic ductular cells have abundant, usually metachromatic cytoplasm and normochromatic or hypochromatic regular nuclei (Fig. 48.4).

Distorted ductular structures embedded in fibrous tissue found in some cases of chronic pancreatitis may also lead to misdiagnosis (Fig. 48.5). Here again, the cytologic characteristics and the experience of the pathologist are imperative for correct diagnosis. Extreme care is advised in the evaluation of the lesions. Careless evaluations may have contributed to the controversial opinion about the association between chronic pancreatitis and pancreatic cancer (13).

### Ductular Cell Adenoma

According to some reports, serous cystadenoma arises from centroacinar cells. This conclusion is based on the surplus of glycogen that is present embryonically in centroacinar cells.

## PREMALIGNANT EXOCRINE PANCREATIC LESIONS

### Premalignant Ductal Epithelium

The terms *atypical ductal hyperplasia* and *ductal dysplasia* have been used interchangeably, although no clear definitions exist for their diagnosis. Some consider dysplasia a more advanced change with malignant potential, whereas others feel that atypia may be a premalignant stage. Some ducts in chronic pancreatitis patients could show an atypical pattern, especially when there are ongoing regenerative, degenerative, and reparative processes. These changes have led to the assumption that chronic pancreatitis presents a predisposing factor for pancreatic cancer. The finding of the *c-Ki-ras* mutation in such lesions lends no support, because this mutation has also been observed in histologically normal epithelium. In fact, every change of ductal epithelium associated with irregular cell size and cell arrangement, whether multilayered or not, deserves the description atypical. These lesions could occur sporadically in a duct or be associated with hyperplasia and lesions consistent with *carcinoma (ca) in situ* or frank carcinoma (Fig. 48.6). Hence, atypical changes may represent an early step in malignancy. Consequently, the presence of such lesions in a specimen indicates careful screening of the specimens, eventually by serial sectioning, because (as stated below) more advanced stages of malignancy can be present in other sectors of the same duct.

Diagnosis of ca in situ presents no problem to an experienced pathologist. Cellular atypia, loss of cell polarity, irregular nuclei and cell size, formation of epithelial bridging, and glands-within-gland formation or irregular papillary configuration without a vascular core are among the characteristics of this epithelium. However, this cancer precursor lesion can present as a single epithelial cell layer and may escape detection. The lesions could be local but are usually multifocal and may extend in a continuous or broken pattern along the duct and ductal branches. Special staining and immunohistochemistry may show scattered endocrine cells within epithelium. Based on their presence also in the early malignant lesions and in their metastases, these endocrine cells seem to be malignant.

In our series, two patients with lesions that were found incidentally and diagnosed as ca in situ, were rediagnosed as early cancers after serial sectioning. In one case, the altered epithelium extended into a side branch, where it broke the duct wall and invaded the stroma. In the other case, found in a patient with gastric cancer, ductal epithelium showed atypical epithelia interchanged with ca in situ lesions that again extended into a side branch and broke into the surrounding tissue. Despite their small size (2 mm and 6 mm), the tumors had invaded the nerves. These cases illustrate the importance of

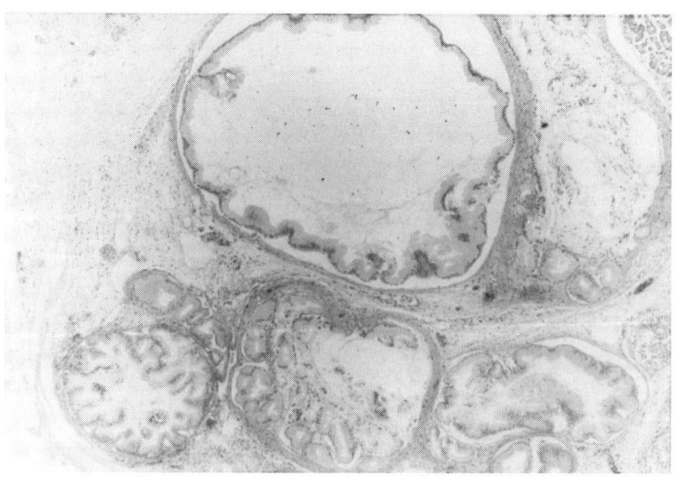

**FIG. 48.2.** Mucinous multilocular cystic lesions found incidentally at autopsy. The cysts are lined by simple mucous cell hyperplasia. The apparent papillary formation is probably due to the contraction of the cyst wall by formalin fixation. Some of the cysts contain a conspicuous amount of mucin and shedding of the epithelium. H & E, ×100.

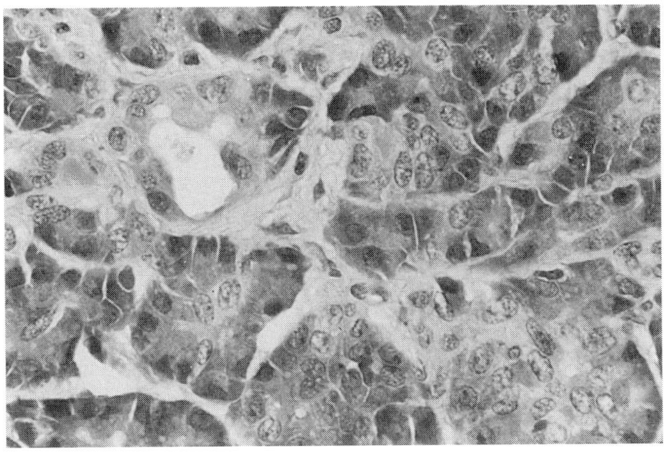

**FIG. 48.3.** Diffuse proliferation of centroacinar cells in the pancreas of a 4-year-old boy with hyperinsulinemic hypoglycemia. Note enlargement of cells in a ductule with abundant metachromatic cytoplasm and nuclei identical to those of the centroacinar cells. H & E, ×50. See color insert.

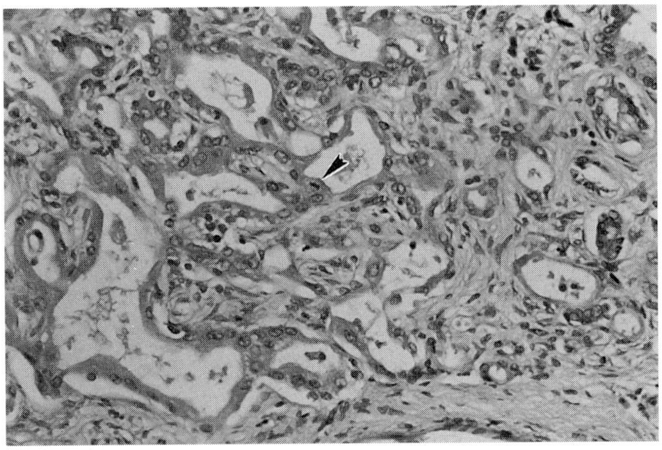

**FIG. 48.5.** Proliferation and ramification of ductules in a patient with florid chronic pancreatitis. Despite the irregular ductular arrangements and occasional mitosis *(arrow)*, the epithelium is single layered, and the cell nuclei are uniform, lying parallel to the lumen. H & E ×650. See color insert.

careful screening of specimens in patients with atypia or ca in situ changes.

### Serous Cystadenoma (Carcinoma)

As stated above, serous cystadenomas show a tendency for malignant transformation. Consequently, these lesions should be considered benign only after careful sampling and histologic diagnosis. Metastases of these tumors can have the same benign appearance as the primary tumor (9).

### Mucinous Cystic Tumors

As with serous cystadenoma, mucinous cystic tumors can show focal microscopic or grossly visible malignant patterns. Therefore, these lesions also must be considered potentially malignant and be treated as such.

### Intraductal "Papillary-Mucinous" Tumors

Intraductal tumors are histologically diverse lesions in terms of intraductal localization and epithelial configuration. Although part of the lesion may lack any abnormalities, another part a short distance away can show atypia, in situ ca, or even microinvasion. Although part of the usually distended duct can show normal epithelium, the next section can present convincing criteria for malignancy. Therefore, most pathologists today spend considerable time dissecting and examining these lesions meticulously.

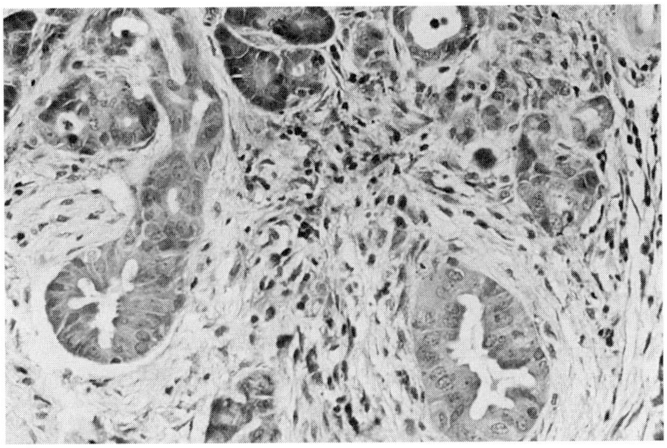

**FIG. 48.4.** Another area of the pancreas from the patient in Figure 48.3. There is a striking hypertrophy and hyperplasia of ductular cells with large metachromatic cytoplasm. The nuclei are crowded in some areas but are regular. There is a focal chronic inflammation, fibrosis, and atrophy. H & E, ×650. See color insert.

### Solid Papillary Tumor

Solid papillary tumor occurs mainly in the tail of the pancreas of predominantly young fertile women and is characterized by the presence of a pseudopapillary configuration of uniform cells and frequent hemorrhage, fibrosis, calcification, or ossification. Although this tumor is usually resectable with favorable prognosis, local recurrence or distant metastases (mainly in the liver or lung) may occur (14). Therefore, these lesions should also be considered potentially malignant. Complete removal of the tumor by either distal pancreatectomy or pancreatoduodenostomy is recommended (14).

## PREMALIGNANT ACINAR CELL LESIONS

Premalignant acinar cell lesions are extremely rare, and as stated above, some pathologists consider the focal hyperplasia or foci of acinar cells as possible malignant precursor lesions. In a large series from Japanese and European institutions, no such lesions have been observed.

## PREMALIGNANT DUCTULAR LESIONS

In some cases of chronic pancreatitis associated with perpetual degenerative and reparative processes, ductal and ductular cells may show patterns that are consistent with atypia but lack definite signs of malignancy (Fig. 48.7). Early premalignant or malignant ductular changes in an otherwise normal tissue have been observed rarely (15) and incidentally. In such cases, ductular changes represent a miniature of premalignant ductal changes, except that the epithelium is rarely multilayered (Fig. 48.7).

The malignant potential of serous cystadenoma was discussed above.

In summary, it appears that benign lesions are not common in the pancreas. Why they tend to become malignant is obscure.

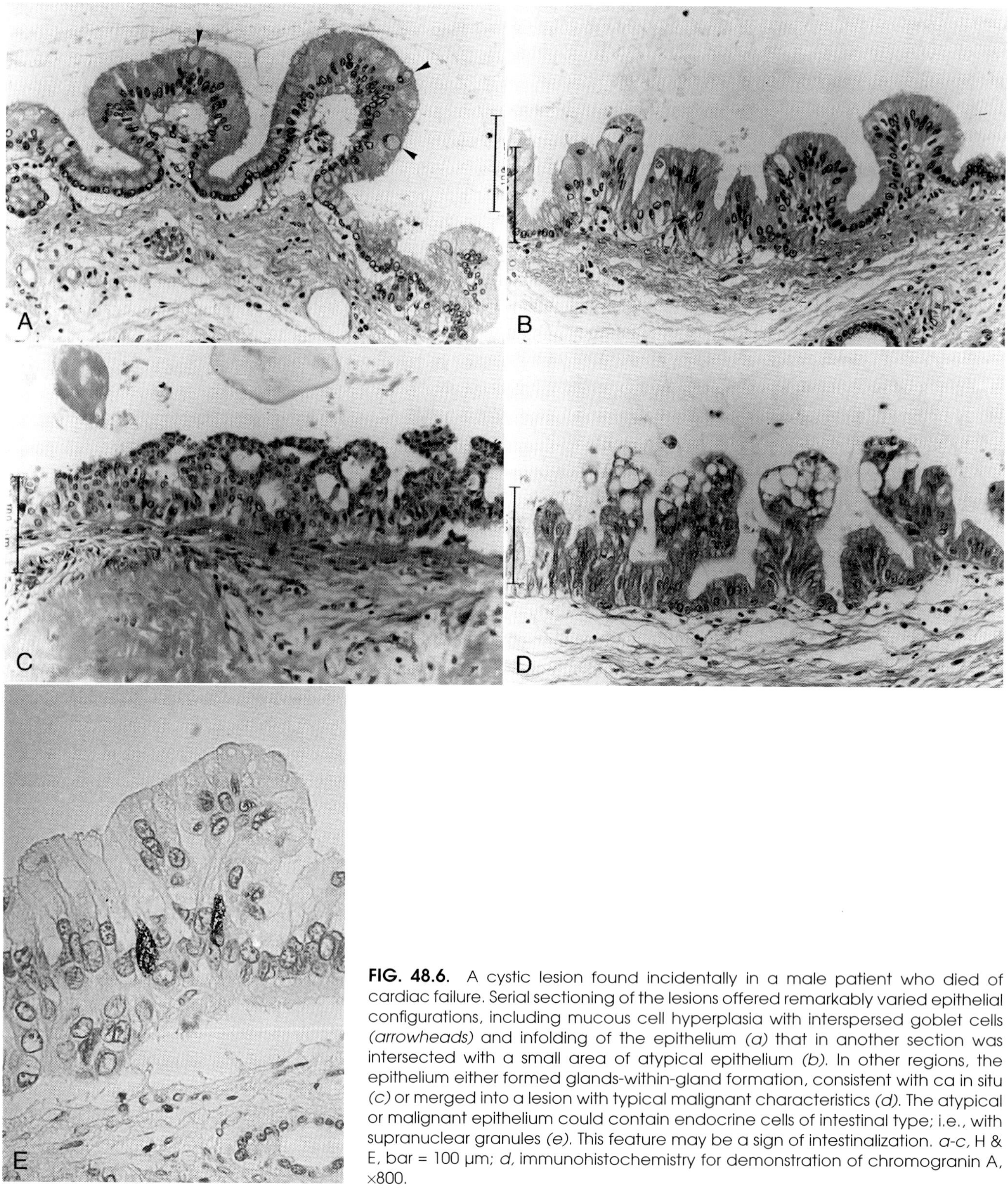


**FIG. 48.6.** A cystic lesion found incidentally in a male patient who died of cardiac failure. Serial sectioning of the lesions offered remarkably varied epithelial configurations, including mucous cell hyperplasia with interspersed goblet cells *(arrowheads)* and infolding of the epithelium *(a)* that in another section was intersected with a small area of atypical epithelium *(b)*. In other regions, the epithelium either formed glands-within-gland formation, consistent with ca in situ *(c)* or merged into a lesion with typical malignant characteristics *(d)*. The atypical or malignant epithelium could contain endocrine cells of intestinal type; i.e., with supranuclear granules *(e)*. This feature may be a sign of intestinalization. *a-c*, H & E, bar = 100 μm; *d*, immunohistochemistry for demonstration of chromogranin A, ×800.

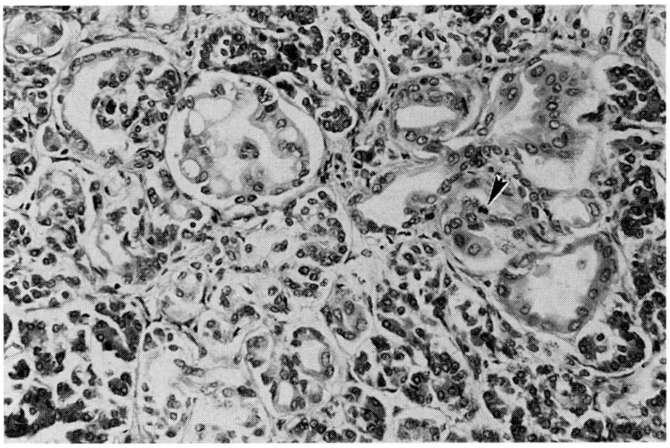

**FIG. 48.7.** Lesion found at autopsy of a patient with no known pancreatic disease. A small area shows abnormal ductular structures, focal epithelial multilayering, a few mitoses *(arrowhead)*, and goblet cell metaplasia *(top left)*. The term *atypia* can be applied to this lesion. Because we have observed a similar pattern in an early ductular cancer (see reference 14), we believe that such lesions have malignant potential. H & E, ×400. See color insert.

## REFERENCES


1. Pour PM, Konishi Y, Klöppel G, Longnecker DS, eds. Atlas of exocrine pancreatic tumors: morphology, biology, and diagnosis with international guide for tumor classification. Heidelberg: Springer-Verlag, 1994.
2. Mizumoto K, Inagaki T, Koizumi M, Uemura M, Ogawa M, et al. Early pancreatic duct adenocarcinoma. Hum Pathol 1988;19:242–244.
3. Mizumoto K, Tsutsumi M, Kitazawa S, Tsujita S, Nakayama M, et al. Intraductal carcinoma in a surgically resected pancreas with chronic pancreatitis. Int J Pancreatol 1990;7:279–285.
4. Obara T, Saitoh Y, Maguchi H, Ura H, Kitazawa S, et al. Multicentric development of intraductal carcinoma through atypical papillary hyperplasia. Hum Pathol 1992;23:82–85.
5. van Laethem JL, Vertongen P, Deviere J, van Rampelbergh J, Rickaert F, et al. Detection of c-Ki-ras gene codon 12 mutations from pancreatic duct brushing in the diagnosis of pancreatic tumors. Gut 1995;36:781–787.
6. DiGiuseppe JA, Hruban RH, Offerhaus GJ, Clement MJ, van den Berg FM, et al. Detection of K-ras mutations in mucinous pancreatic duct hyperplasia from patient with a family history of pancreatic carcinoma. Am J Pathol 1994;144:889–895.
7. Tada M, Ohashi M, Shiratori Y, Okudaira T, Komatsu Y, et al. Analysis of K-ras mutation in hyperplastic duct cells of the pancreas without pancreatic disease. Gastroenterology 1996;110:227–231.
8. Yanagisawa A, Ohtake K, Ohashi K, Hori M, Kitagawa T, et al. Frequent c-Ki-ras oncogene activation in mucous cell hyperplasias of pancreas suffering from chronic inflammation. Cancer Res 1993;53:953–956.
9. Funabiki T, Kamei K. Serous cystadenocarcinoma. In: Pour PM, Konishi Y, Klöppel G, Longnecker DS, eds. Atlas of exocrine pancreatic tumors: morphology, biology and diagnosis with international guide for tumor classification. Heidelberg: Springer-Verlag, 1994:101–106.
10. Funabiki T, Kamei K, Lewandrowski KB. Serous cystadenoma. In: Pour PM, Konishi Y, Klöppel G, Longnecker DS, eds. Atlas of exocrine pancreatic tumors: morphology, biology and diagnosis with international guide for tumor classification. Heidelberg: Springer-Verlag, 1994:31–43.
11. Longnecker DS, Shinozuka H, Dekker A. Focal acinar cell dysplasia in human pancreas. Cancer 1980;45:534–540.
12. Kodama T, Mori W. Atypical acinar cell nodules of the human pancreas. Acta Pathol Jpn 1983;33:701–714.
13. Pour PM. Is there a link between chronic pancreatitis and pancreatic cancer. In: Beger H, Büchler M, eds. Chronic pancreatitis. Heidelberg: Springer-Verlag, 1990:106–112.
14. Yamaguchi K, Morohoshi T, Zamboni G. Solid cystic tumors. In: Pour PM, Konishi Y, Klöppel G, Longnecker DS, eds. Atlas of exocrine pancreatic tumors: morphology, biology and diagnosis with international guide for tumor classification. Heidelberg: Springer-Verlag, 1994:83–101.
15. Pour PM, Sayed S, Sayed G, Wolf GL. Hyperplastic preneoplastic and neoplastic lesions found in 83 human pancreas. Am J Clin Pathol 1982;77:137–152.

# 49

# Clinical Pathology of Exocrine Tumors

Günter Klöppel

Most exocrine pancreatic tumors are malignant. They comprise ductal adenocarcinoma and its variants, which are the carcinomas that are meant whenever pancreatic cancer is discussed. Non-duct-type tumors are infrequent, but they include a number of neoplasms with special morphologic and biologic features: acinar cell carcinoma, pancreatoblastoma, solid-cystic tumors, and the functionally active and inactive endocrine neoplasms. Nonepithelial tumors of and metastases to the pancreas are exceedingly rare (cf. Chapters 66 and 67).

## PHENOTYPIC DIFFERENTIATION

The phenotype of most epithelial tumors of the pancreas reflects more or less the morphology of either of the three main cell types of the gland: the duct cell, the acinar cell, or the endocrine cell (Table 49.1).

More than 90% of pancreatic tumors are carcinomas of the ductal phenotype. Histologically and ultrastructurally they imitate the structure of the mucin-producing cuboidal cells that line the interlobular ducts (1–3) (Fig. 49.1). This resemblance is still evident in poorly differentiated carcinomas (4). In contrast to acinar cell carcinomas, the ductal carcinomas are immunocytochemically usually negative for pancreatic enzymes such as amylase, lipase, trypsin, and chymotrypsin (5, 6). Furthermore, these tumors express the same set of intracellular markers as the normal pancreatic and biliary duct cells, i.e., villin and keratins 7, 8, 18, and 19 (4, 7–9). Acinar cells lack keratins 7 and 19 as well as villin. Acinar cell carcinoma fails to show the K-*ras* point mutation at codon 12, nor is the p53 protein overexpressed at the high frequency known to occur in ductal adenocarcinomas (6, 10). Ductal adenocarcinomas, especially if they are well differentiated, may contain some scattered neuroendocrine cells (11, 12), but these are only occasionally retained in the respective metastases (13, 14).

The acinar cell phenotype of pancreatic tumors is characterized by the expression of pancreatic enzymes, which can be immunocytochemically identified (5, 6, 15, 16). In addition, the tumor cells may show electron-dense granules with tightly fitting membranes, imitating the ultrastructural features of zymogen granules. The neoplasms displaying these characteristics are acinar cell carcinoma and pancreatoblastoma. Some of these tumors may also contain scattered neuroendocrine cells (5, 6, 17) or may even be classified as truly mixed tumors (17).

Tumors arising from the endocrine cell compartment display all the features of the neuroendocrine cell system and express hormones, usually of pancreatic origin (14, 18).

On the basis of the outlined phenotypic criteria, the epithelial tumors of the pancreas may be classified as ductal, acinar, and endocrine neoplasms (Table 49.1). These tumors also differ in their biologic features; ductal adenocarcinomas have the worst prognosis, and endocrine tumors the best. True mixed tumors, in which the different epithelial components are intimately admixed in both the primary tumor and the metastases, appear to be exceptionally rare in the pancreas (13). Also rare are neoplasms (e.g., solid-pseudopapillary tumors) in which the phenotypic relationship to the known cellular elements of the pancreas is still unclear.

## WHO CLASSIFICATION

The recently published WHO classification (19) (Table 49.2), like other classifications that were developed earlier (16, 20) or are still to appear (14), is based primarily on standard microscopic observations. However, it also incorporates diagnostically valuable immunocytochemical findings that allow the classification into benign tumors (adenoma), borderline tumors (tumors with uncertain malignant potential), and malignant tumors. Also incorporated are immunocytochemical findings that help to identify the tumor and determine its phenotype precisely.

### Ductal Adenocarcinoma

**General Features.** Ductal adenocarcinoma of the pancreas is characterized by its preferential localization in the head of the pancreas, by marked desmoplasia associated with the growth of usually well-differentiated ductlike glands, and by production of mucin, expression of carbohydrate antigens such as CEA, CA 19-9, DU-PAN-2, and SPan-1, and expression of the keratins 7, 8, 18, and 19 (14, 21, 22).

Ductal adenocarcinoma increases in incidence with age and is very rare in the first 3 decades of life (23, 24). Men are affected slightly more often than women. Tumors in the head of the pancreas usually cause jaundice, because they obstruct the common bile duct. Tumors in the body and tail of the pancreas only produce symptoms when they are advanced and have invaded the peritoneum or the stomach and intestines or metastasized to the liver.

**Gross Pathology.** Sixty to 70% of the carcinomas are found in the head of the pancreas; the remainder occur in the pancreas body and/or tail or rarely in the uncinate process. It is not known why ductal adenocarcinomas originate so commonly from the head of the gland. One hypothesis suggests that reflux of carcinogen-containing bile into the main pancreatic duct induces the head carcinomas. Another possibility is that carcinogens conveyed in the blood are released into the pancreatic ducts and attain their highest concentration and greatest effect in the main duct of the pancreatic head. These concepts are weakened somewhat, however, by the observation that almost 50% of the head carcinomas occur in the upper dorsal part of the head of the pancreas, adjacent to or around the common bile duct and distant from the main duct. These carcinomas do not seem to originate from the main pancreatic duct but instead may arise

**TABLE 49.1. Classification of Pancreatic Epithelial Tumors According to Their Phenotype**

Duct cell phenotype
- Serous cystic adenoma
- Intraductal papillary-mucinous tumor
- Mucinous cystic tumor
- Ductal adenocarcinoma
  - Mucinous noncystic carcinoma
  - Adenosquamous carcinoma
  - Anaplastic carcinoma

Acinar cell phenotype
- Acinar cell carcinoma
- Acinar cystadenocarcinoma
- Pancreatoblastoma

Endocrine cell phenotype
- Endocrine tumor

Mixed phenotype
- Mixed exocrine-endocrine tumor

Undefined phenotype
- Solid-pseudopapillary tumor

**TABLE 49.2. Histologic Classification of Epithelial Tumors of the Exocrine Pancreas**

Benign tumors
- Serous cystadenoma
- Mucinous cystadenoma
- Intraductal papillary-mucinous adenoma
- Mature teratoma

Borderline tumors (uncertain malignant potential)
- Mucinous cystic tumor with moderate dysplasia
- Intraductal papillary-mucinous tumor with moderate dysplasia
- Solid-pseudopapillary tumor

Malignant
- Severe ductal dysplasia—carcinoma in situ
- Ductal adenocarcinoma
  - Mucinous noncystic carcinoma
  - Signet ring cell carcinoma
  - Adenosquamous carcinoma
  - Undifferentiated (anaplastic) carcinoma
  - Mixed ductal-endocrine carcinoma
- Osteoclast-like giant cell tumor
- Serous cystadenocarcinoma
- Mucinous cystadenocarcinoma
  - Noninvasive
  - Invasive
- Intraductal papillary-mucinous carcinoma
  - Noninvasive
  - Invasive (papillary-mucinous carcinoma)
- Acinar cell carcinoma
  - Acinar cell cystadenocarcinoma
  - Mixed acinar-endocrine carcinoma
- Pancreatoblastoma
- Solid-pseudopapillary carcinoma
- Miscellaneous carcinomas

from the duct of Santorini, one of its small branches, or, possibly, the distal common bile duct.

The tumors are hard, pale, and poorly demarcated (Fig. 49.2). Hemorrhage and necrosis are usually absent. Microcystic structures may be present and indicate a well-differentiated ductal adenocarcinoma. The size of pancreas head carcinomas in resected specimens usually ranges from 2 to 3 cm. Tumors smaller than 2 cm are infrequent (25). In autopsy series, the average size is 4–6 cm (22, 26, 27). Carcinomas of the body and/or tail are generally larger than carcinomas of the head (22). At diagnosis, their size averages between 5 and 7 cm, and some of them occupy the total body-tail region. The tumor sizes noted in recently compiled series tend to be smaller, probably due to earlier diagnosis.

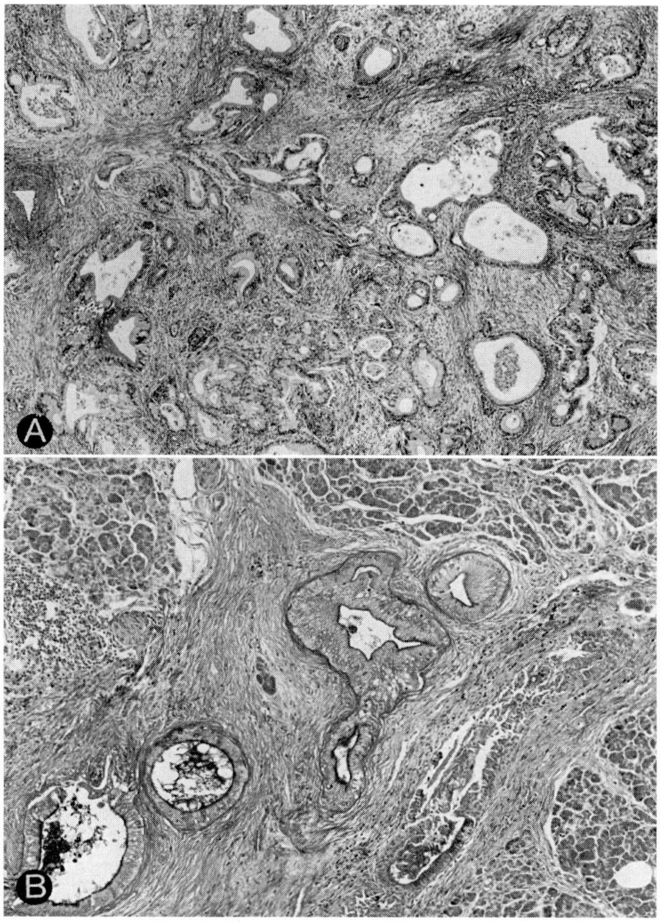


**FIG. 49.1.** Well-differentiated ductal adenocarcinoma. **A.** Imitation of ductlike structures. H & E, ×60. **B.** Mucin-producing tumor cells with apical PAS positivity. PAS, ×120.

**Microscopy.** Histologically, most ductal adenocarcinomas are characterized by well-developed glandular structures, which more or less imitate normal pancreatic ducts (Fig. 49.1). In their arrangement and distribution, the neoplastic glands disregard the lobular architecture of the gland and replace the normal pancreatic tissue. They are usually embedded in a dense fibrous stroma, which contains type I and V collagen and fibronectin, but rarely type III collagen. The columnar to cuboidal tumor cells often form a basement membrane, which can be identified by its laminin content (28). Basal membrane loss and decrease in collagen content correlate with increasing disorganization of the neoplastic glands and discontinuous laminin deposition (29). These findings indicate a close relationship between the neoplastic epithelium and the formation and production of basal membrane material and stromal components. This interaction is most likely regulated by the more or less preserved capability of the tumor cells to produce basal membrane proteins (30, 31), collagens, and receptors that can anchor the cell on the basal membrane (32).

Extension into the adjoining pancreatic tissue occurs mainly

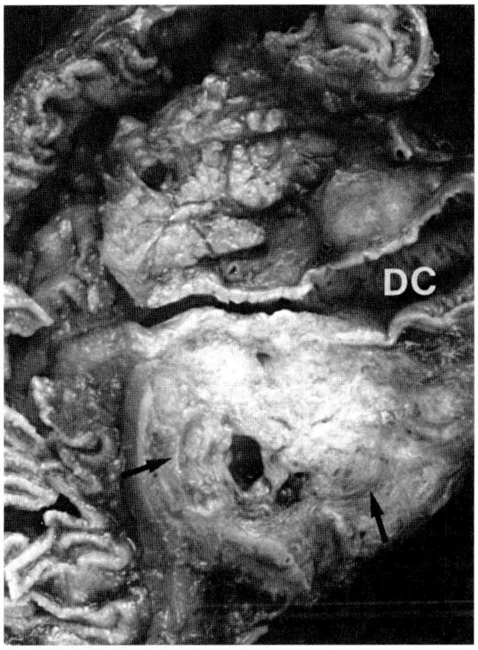


**FIG. 49.2.** Ductal adenocarcinoma in the head of the pancreas. Note stenosis of the bile duct *(DC)* and the blurred margin of the tumor *(arrows).*

via the interlobular septa and by infiltration and replacement of the acinar tissue. Another route of intrapancreatic spread is via the interlobular ducts. Foci of intraductal carcinoma *(carcinoma in situ)* in the presence and immediate vicinity of an invasive ductal carcinoma (Fig. 49.3) were found in up to 24% of resection specimens (33, 34) (cf. also Chapter 48).

Multicentric foci of carcinoma in situ distant from an invasive ductal carcinoma in the head of the pancreas have been reported in 15–40% of cases (35–38). In a study by our group, we found no skip lesions in 37 total pancreatectomy specimens with a pancreas head carcinoma (39). However, there were three cases (8%) with continuous intraductal spread along the main pancreatic duct from the head to the tail. On the basis of this study, it appears that multicentricity may be less frequent than has been thought (37, 38).

Tumor growth into the peripancreatic retroperitoneal fatty tissue is common and occurs early during the course of the disease. Apart from direct invasion of the fatty tissue, the tumor extends along nerves (perineural invasion) and within lymphatic channels.

**Microscopic Grading.** The tumors may be graded on the basis of their histologic and cytologic appearance and their mitotic activity (Table 49.3) (19, 27). Well-differentiated carcinomas (G1) are composed of ductlike tubular glands with prominent mucin secretion. They are embedded in dense stroma (Fig. 49.4, *a*) and lined by columnar cells showing little nuclear polymorphism. Between and at the bases of the neoplastic cells there are often endocrine cells. The mitotic activity is low (up to 5 mitoses/10 HPF). Well-differentiated carcinomas commonly show intrapancreatic extension as an in situ component via large ducts.

In moderately differentiated carcinomas (G2), the glands are more irregular and smaller. These glands are lined by cylindrical to cuboidal cells that produce mucin in variable amounts and have irregularly sized nuclei (Fig. 49.4, *b*). The mitotic activity ranges between 6 and 10 figures/10 HPF.

In poorly differentiated tumors (G3), the glandular pattern is

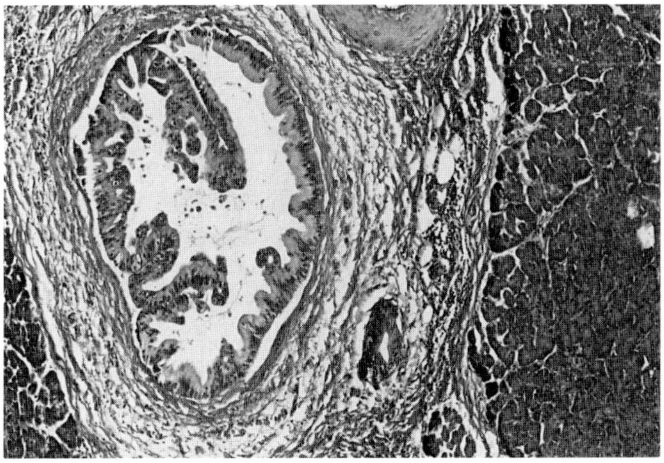

**FIG. 49.3.** Intraductal tumor extension (carcinoma in situ component) of ductal adenocarcinoma. H & E, ×120.

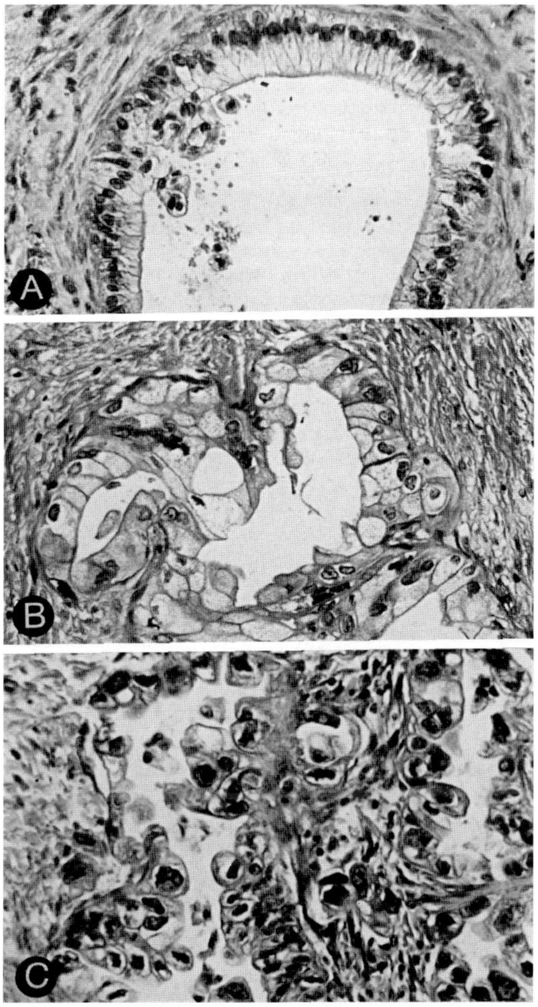


**FIG. 49.4.** Histologic differentiation in ductal adenocarcinoma. **A** Well-differentiated (G1) tumor, **B** moderately differentiated (G2) tumor, **C** poorly differentiated (G3) tumor. H & E, ×250). (From Klöppel G, Maillet B. Pathology of the pancreas. In: Baert AL, Delorme G, eds. Radiology of the pancreas. Berlin: Springer, 1994, with permission of the publisher).

**TABLE 49.3. Histologic Grading of Pancreatic Duct Cell Adenocarcinoma**

| Tumor Grade | Glandular Differentiation | Mucin Production | Mitoses (per 10 HPF) | Nuclear Anaplasia |
|---|---|---|---|---|
| 1 | Well-differentiated ductlike glands | Intensive | 1–5 | Little polymorphism, polar arrangement |
| 2 | Moderately differentiated ductlike and tubular glands | Irregular | 6–10 | Some polymorphism |
| 3 | Poorly differentiated glands, mucoepidermoid and pleomorphic structures | Abortive | >10 | Marked polymorphism and increased nuclear size |

usually bizarre or abolished, the epithelial anaplasia prominent, the mucin production reduced, and the desmoplastic response minimal (Fig. 49.4, *c*). There are more than 10 mitoses per 10 HPF. When grading is done carefully, survival has been found to correlate with grade (27).

**Immunocytochemical Markers.** Among the markers for ductal adenocarcinoma, CA 19-9 (which recognizes a carbohydrate structure shared by a monosialoganglioside and a mucin) and CEA are used most often. For unknown reasons, CA 19-9 proves to be superior to CEA in the serologic recognition of pancreatic carcinoma. CA 19-9 has been found to be markedly increased in the serum of 70–80% of patients with pancreatic carcinoma (40, 41), though at the tissue level this antibody does not discriminate between normal pancreatic ducts and neoplastic glands (42–44). In contrast, monoclonal antibodies directed against epitopes present on either CEA or the CEA-related antigen, nonspecific cross-reacting antigen 95 (NCA 95), are capable of discriminating between nonneoplastic duct changes and carcinoma structures as well as duct-type adenocarcinomas and non-duct-type neoplasms, such as acinar cell carcinoma and endocrine tumors (45) (Fig. 49.5).

Apart from CA 19-9 and CEA, there are several other markers, for instance DU-PAN 2 (46, 47) or the mucin markers M1 (48) and MUC1 (49–51), which were shown to be commonly expressed in pancreatic carcinoma. However, none of the markers so far known is specific for pancreatic carcinoma.

Recent studies have shown that 40–50% of ductal adenocarcinomas may express metallothionein (52), CD44v6 (a splice variant of standard CD44) (53, 54), or membranous E-cadherin (55). Since these molecules may play a role in tumor invasiveness or in the metastatic process, their gain or loss might have prognostic value (cf. also Chapter 52).

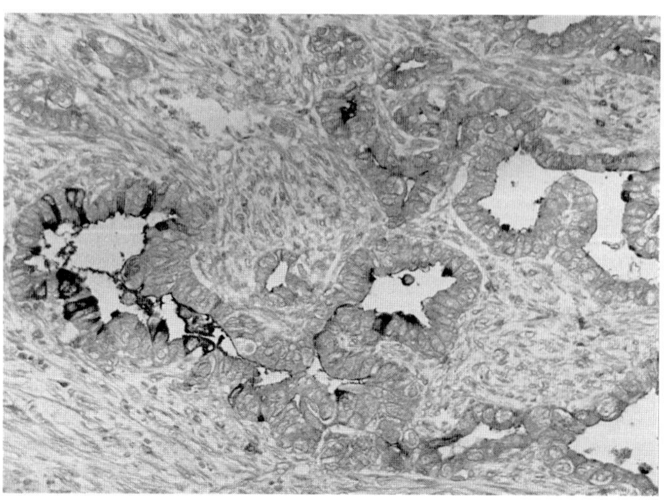

**FIG. 49.5.** Well-differentiated ductal adenocarcinoma extensively expressing CEA, ×60. (From Klöppel G, Maillet B. Pathology of the pancreas. In: Radiology of the pancreas. Berlin: Springer, 1994, with permission of the publisher).

**Extension and Metastasis.** Direct tumor extension beyond the gland is common (Fig. 49.6), even when the primary carcinoma is small (56). It is therefore an exception to find a resected carcinoma that is still limited to the pancreas (57). In head carcinomas, peripancreatic tumor invasion primarily involves the retroperitoneal fatty tissue behind the pancreas head, surrounding the large mesenteric vessels and the nerve plexus. In advanced cases, the walls of veins, neighboring organs, and/or the peritoneum are invaded. In carcinomas of the body and tail, local extension is usually greater, because of delayed tumor detection, and includes involvement of the spleen, stomach, left adrenal gland, colon, and peritoneum (21, 22).

Lymphatic spread usually precedes hematogenous spread. The lymph nodes most commonly involved in pancreas head carcinoma are, in descending order of frequency, the retroduodenal (posterior pancreaticoduodenal) and the superior pancreatic head groups, the inferior head and the superior body groups, and the anterior pancreaticoduodenal and the inferior body groups (58). This lymph node compartment is usually resected together with the head of the pancreas, using a standard Whipple procedure (59). More distal nodal metastases may occur in two other compartments. The first includes the hepatoduodenal ligament, the celiac trunk, and the root of the superior mesenteric artery. The second lies below the left renal vein on both sides of the aorta at the level of the renal arteries (60). These lymph node compartments are only removed if an extended Whipple procedure is performed (61). Hematogenous metastases occur, in approximate order of frequency, in the liver, lungs, adrenals, kidneys, bones, brain, and skin (21, 22, 62).

Carcinomas of the body and tail metastasize especially to the superior and inferior body and head lymph node groups and the splenic hilus lymph nodes. They may also spread via lymphatic channels to pleura and lung. Distant metastases occur primarily in the liver.

**Recurrence.** The vast majority of patients operated on for a pancreatic carcinoma die of tumor recurrence within 1 or 2 years (63, 64). The origin of the recurrent tumor may lie in either *(a)* the remainder of the gland (in the case of a Whipple resection), *(b)* tumor nests remaining in the retroperitoneal spaces behind the pancreatic head and the large mesenteric vessels, or *(c)* lymph node or liver metastases too small to be detected during operation.

In view of the problem of tumor recurrence from remaining multicentric tumor foci in the pancreatic remnant after removal of a tumor in the head of the pancreas, we examined 37 total pancreatectomy specimens of head carcinoma (39). In three patients, microscopic tumor tissue was detected beyond the usual Whipple resection line in the body and tail of the pancreas. In each of these patients, the tumor tissue was found to spread continuously, either intraductally or invasively, from the grossly visible tumor in the head of the pancreas into the body and the tail. Tumor multicentricity was not observed in this study. According to these results, we conclude that in ductal adenocarcinoma of the head of the pancreas, microscopic tumor extension

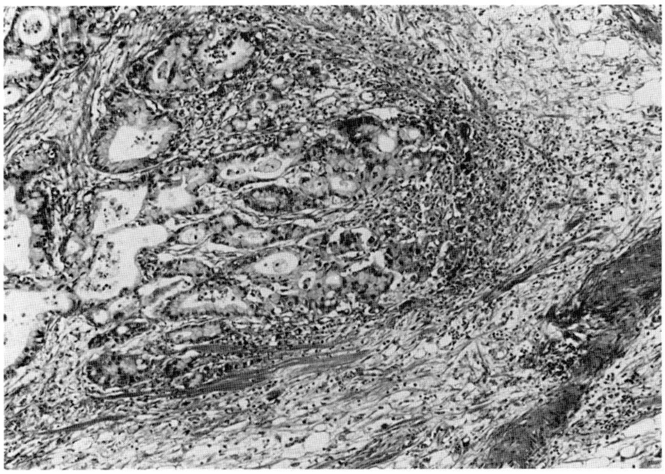

**FIG. 49.6.** Ductal adenocarcinoma: direct tumor extension into the retroperitoneal tissue. H & E, ×60.

beyond the Whipple resection line may not be as common as has been reported in the literature (25–38%, reviewed in (39)). According to our data, it can be expected in only 5–10% of cases. Thus, a Whipple procedure appears to be adequate treatment for most patients with pancreatic carcinoma in the head of the gland.

The most important source of recurrent tumor seems to be tumor cell clusters left behind in the retroperitoneal tissue, even after so-called curative resections. Follow-up examinations of 24 operated patients (Whipple procedure) at 4- to 8-week intervals by use of ultrasonography, computed tomography (CT), and tumor marker analysis (CEA and CA 19-9) were reported by Guthoff et al. (65). In 20 patients, the first visible indication of recurrence was the growth of tumor tissue in the area dorsal to the portal vein, close to the superior mesenteric artery. The growth pattern was either relatively circumscribed or, more frequently, diffuse. In all of these patients, lymph node or liver metastases developed later in the course of the disease. Only two recurrences were clearly of lymph node origin, and in one patient, small liver metastases preceded the diagnosis of local recurrence. In 20 of 24 patients, tumor recurrence occurred 3–8 months postoperatively. Approximately half of the recurrences were discovered by all three methods at the same time. In one-quarter of the patients, ultrasonography and CT were superior to the tumor markers; in the remaining patients, the continuous increase in tumor markers was the first indication of tumor recurrence. These results suggest that in most patients resected for pancreatic ductal carcinoma, tumor cells left behind in perineural spaces or lymphatic channels of the retroperitoneal fatty tissue dorsal to the pancreas and the adjacent large vessels (56) may later give rise to tumor recurrence.

The peritoneum and the bone marrow are also rare sites of recurrence, although malignant cells are detected cytologically in one-quarter of the patients during laparoscopy (66) and one-half of the patients when bone marrow trepanation is performed during a Whipple procedure (67) (for prognosis, cf. also Chapter 52).

## Variants of Ductal Adenocarcinoma

Mucinous noncystic carcinoma (colloid carcinoma), signet ring cell carcinoma, adenosquamous carcinoma (mucoepidermoid carcinoma, squamous carcinoma), undifferentiated (anaplastic) carcinoma, and mixed ductal-endocrine carcinoma are considered varieties of ductal adenocarcinoma (14, 21, 22).

In *mucinous noncystic carcinoma,* excessive mucin production results in a gelatinous cut surface ("colloid" or gelatinous carcinoma) (Fig. 49.7). These tumors show well to moderately differentiated cuboidal cells lining lakes of mucin or floating free in mucin. Mucinous noncystic carcinomas and ductal adenocarcinomas occur in similar locations and in patients of similar age. Mucinous noncystic carcinoma patients might have a better prognosis, possibly roughly proportional to the amount of mucin produced, than ductal adenocarcinoma patients (22).

In the very rare *signet ring cell carcinoma,* the pancreatic tissue is more or less diffusely invaded by signet ring cells.

In *adenosquamous carcinoma,* the glandular and squamous cell carcinoma components are mixed and variably distributed in the tumor (Fig. 49.8). Pure squamous cell carcinomas seem to be very rare, since an intensive workup of these tumors usually reveals some foci of glandular differentiation (68). In addition, there may be anaplastic and spindle cell foci. In gross appearance, male:female ratio, and localization, adenosquamous carcinoma resembles ductal adenocarcinoma. As almost all of these carcinomas are poorly differentiated, they usually have a poor prognosis.

In *undifferentiated (anaplastic) carcinoma,* a pattern of extreme anaplasia with bizarre cellular pleomorphism and numerous mitoses is found (69) (Fig. 49.9). However, focal ductlike or small glandular elements are also a common component of this tumor type, providing evidence of its duct cell origin (21, 22). The epithelial nature of the pleomorphic and occasionally spindle-shaped cells is revealed by the immunocytochemical demonstration of cytokeratin. In addition, the tumor cells may stain for vimentin. At the time of diagnosis, these tumors are usually large and relatively soft, often with central necrosis and hemorrhage. The tumors occur with equal frequency in the head and body/tail. There is no age or sex predilection. Their prognosis is poor. This is most likely also true of the *giant cell tumor with osteoclast-like cells* (70), although some reports suggest that this tumor type behaves less aggressively than ordinary duct cell carcinoma (71). The role of the osteoclast-like cells, which are nonneoplastic in origin, is obscure (72–74).

In the very rare *mixed ductal-endocrine carcinoma,* there is an intimate intermingling of cells of neuroendocrine nature and those showing ductal features (13, 14).

Among the carcinomas of the pancreas that do not totally fit into one of the above-mentioned categories are such tumors as *ciliated cell carcinoma* (75), and *clear cell carcinoma* (22). *Small cell carcinoma* is a neuroendocrine tumor and should no longer be discussed with the exocrine tumors.

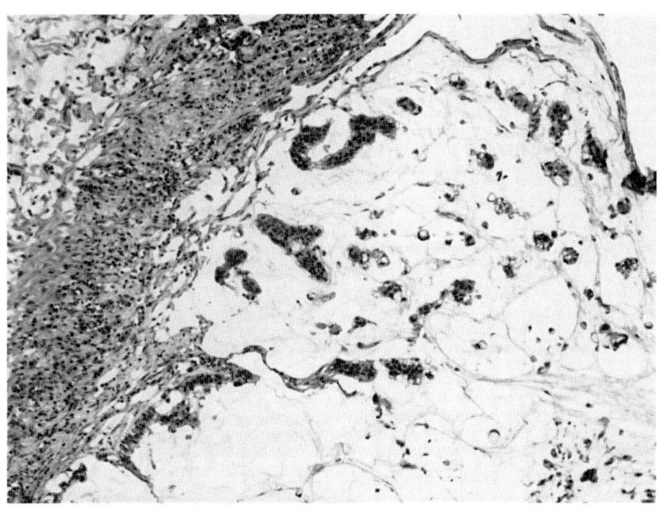

**FIG. 49.7.** Mucinous noncystic carcinoma. Neoplastic cuboidal cells floating in a lake of mucin. H & E, ×220.

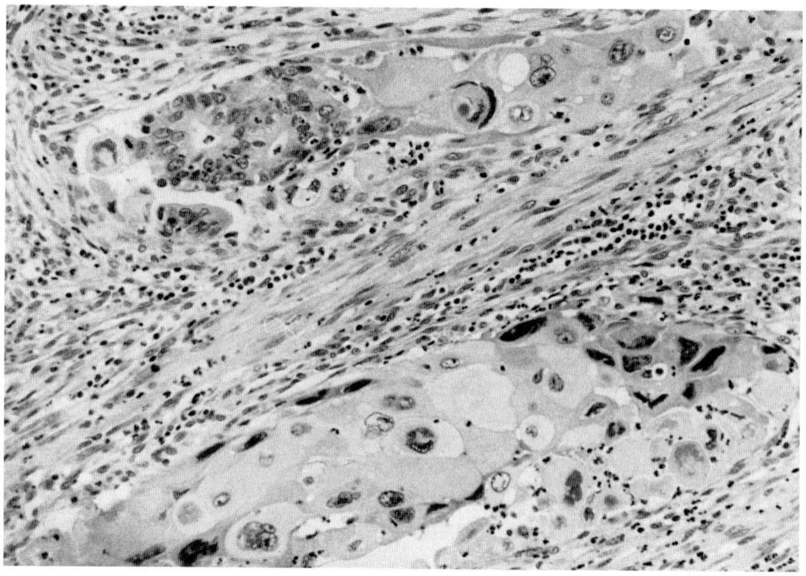

**FIG. 49.8.** Adenosquamous carcinoma. H & E, ×250.

## Serous Cystic Tumors

Serous cystic tumor is a cystic neoplasm composed of multiple, usually small cysts (1 mm to 2 cm), which are lined by cuboidal epithelium with clear, glycogen-rich cytoplasm. Most serous cystic tumors are benign. Malignant tumors (serous cystadenocarcinoma) are very rare (76, 77). Serous cystadenoma can be separated into microcystic and oligocystic types. Recently, a solid variant has also been described (78). The serous microcystic type occurs almost exclusively in elderly women in their 6th or 7th decade of life (79, 80). Usually it is found incidentally, either at laparotomy or at autopsy. It accounts for 1% or less of pancreatic exocrine tumors and comprises 4–10% of all cystic lesions of the pancreas (81). The oligocystic type affects both sexes equally and is usually also an incidental finding, but it may occasionally compress the common bile duct (82).

Macroscopically, *serous microcystic adenoma* is a large, spherical and multiloculated cystic tumor (size range, 6–11 cm) containing watery fluid and displaying a central stellate scar (83) (Fig. 49.10). The fibrous stroma occasionally shows a sunburst-like calcification. The tumors are well demarcated, and two-thirds occur in the body/tail portion of the gland (82, 84).

*Serous oligocystic adenoma* seems to correspond to the macrocystic type of serous cystic adenoma described by Lewandrowski et al. (85). It is poorly demarcated and shows no central stellate scar.

Histologically, the two types are indistinguishable. The cysts are lined by flattened epithelium with clear (glycogen-rich) cytoplasm that fails to stain for mucin and CEA (82). Intracystic micropapillae are common.

## Mucinous Cystic Tumor

Mucinous cystic tumor (MCT) is a cystic neoplasm with a dense fibrous wall lined by highly differentiated, columnar, mucin-secreting epithelium that shows benign, borderline, or malignant features. Mucinous cystadenomas are potentially malignant and may transform into cystadenocarcinomas, particularly if treated by drainage; thus MCT, whether benign or malignant, has also been collectively termed mucinous cystic neoplasm (86).

MCT accounts for approximately 1–2% of pancreatic exocrine tumors. They occur in middle-aged women (age range, 20–70 years) and are usually found in the tail of the pancreas. Symptoms are often those of an expanding abdominal mass.

Macroscopically, the tumors are usually large (size range, 2–30 cm; average, 6 cm) and consist of a unilocular cyst or

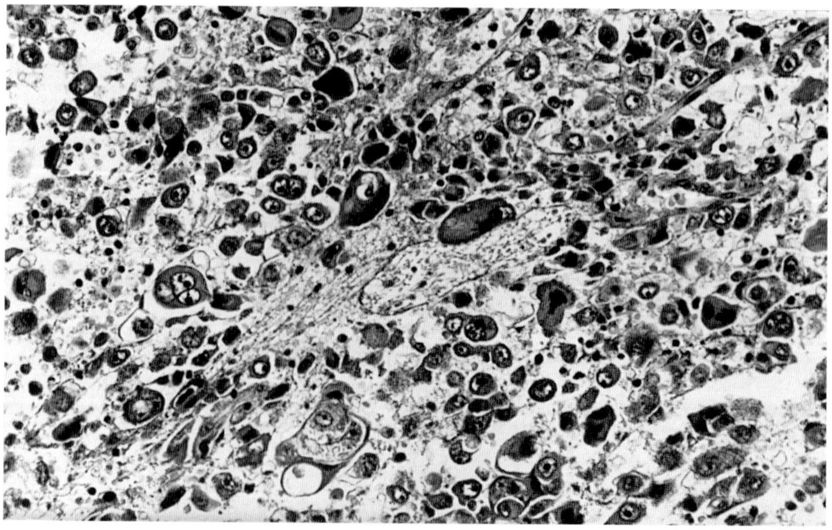

**FIG. 49.9.** Undifferentiated (anaplastic) carcinoma. H & E, ×250.

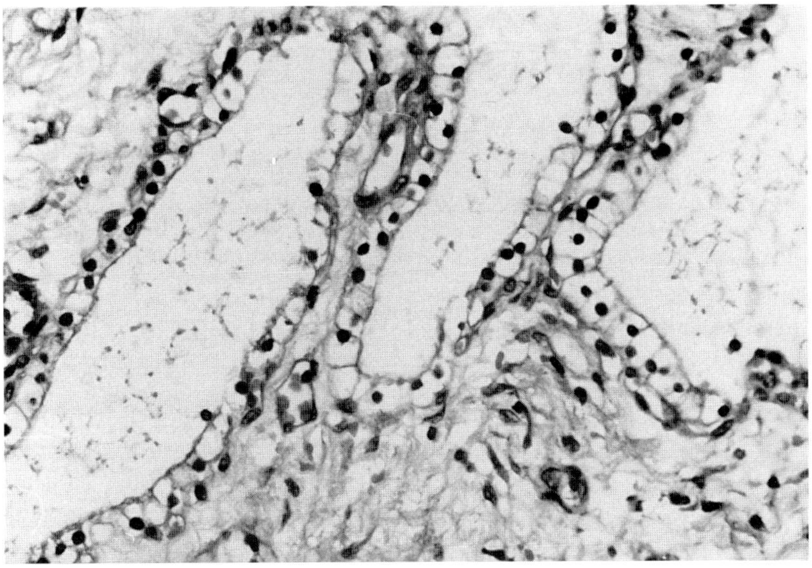

**FIG. 49.10.** Serous cystic adenoma. Cuboidal cells with water clear cytoplasm. H & E, ×250.

multiple separate cysts filled with viscous mucin. The thick fibrous capsule occasionally contains some small cysts or calcifications. The inner surface of the cysts may display papillary excrescences and solid tissue. The cysts usually do not communicate with the pancreatic duct (85, 87, 88).

Histologically, the cysts are lined by columnar mucin-producing and often papillary epithelium that may show an intestinal phenotype (Fig. 49.11) and contain single neuroendocrine cells (89). The connective tissue supporting the epithelium is densely cellular ("ovarian like"). In mucinous cystic tumors classified as adenomas, the epithelium does not show any significant atypia. Mucinous cystadenocarcinomas, in contrast, have a severely atypical epithelium. Tumors that show a higher degree of atypia than adenomas but still lack severely dysplastic changes in the epithelium are called borderline tumors. Since the severely dysplastic changes may only be focal, it is necessary to obtain as many samples as possible. Immunocytochemically, the tumors are positive for CEA and CA 19-9, both of which can also be found in the cyst fluid, sometimes at high levels (90).

If these lesions are recognized early enough (i.e., when the tumor does not show an invasive component or shows only a microinvasive component) and the tumor can be completely excised, it is possible to cure the patient. If the patient presents with macroinvasion or metastasis, the prognosis is similar to that of ductal adenocarcinoma (86, 87).

### Intraductal Papillary-Mucinous Tumor

Intraductal papillary-mucinous tumor (IPMT) is an intraductal, occasionally cystic, neoplasm composed of papillary proliferations of columnar, mucin-secreting cells that may show benign, borderline, or clearly malignant features. Because papillary proliferations are prominent in some of the tumors, while others are distinguished by mucin hypersecretion, two variants of IPMT (i.e., an intraductal papillary neoplasm and an intraductal mucin-hypersecreting neoplasm) have been distinguished (91, 92). These tumors have also become known under a number of other names, such as intraductal papilloma, villous adenoma of the pancreatic duct, intraductal papillary adenocarcinoma, intraductal carcinoma, early pancreatic duct carcinoma, intraductal mucin-hypersecreting tumor, mucin-producing tumor, and mucinous ductal ectasia (21, 93–99). The new WHO classification uses the term intraductal papillary-mucinous tumor (IPMT) (100) to cover the totality of these tumors (19).

IPMT account for approximately 1–2% of the exocrine pancreatic tumors. They affect men more frequently than women, and most patients are older than 50 years of age. IPMT usually cause pancreatitis-like symptoms that may be present for years (91, 92, 101, 102).

Macroscopically, IPMT is either a focal lesion (usually involving a part of the main pancreatic duct and only rarely a secondary duct) or a diffuse lesion that spreads over the pancreatic duct system and may even extend to the ampulla. In two-thirds of cases, the head portion of the main pancreatic duct is affected (101). Due to intensive papillary growths and/or massive discharge of mucin, the main duct is ectatic or even cystic (average diameter, 2 cm), and the remaining pancreas shows obstructive chronic pancreatitis (91, 92).

Histologically, IPMT show arborizing papillary proliferations of columnar mucin-producing cells originating from the duct epithelium (Fig. 49.12). Occasionally, the tumor cells display oncocytic differentiation (103). Like mucinous cystic tumors, IMPT also seem to follow an adenoma-carcinoma sequence. They are therefore typed on the basis of their epithelial differen-

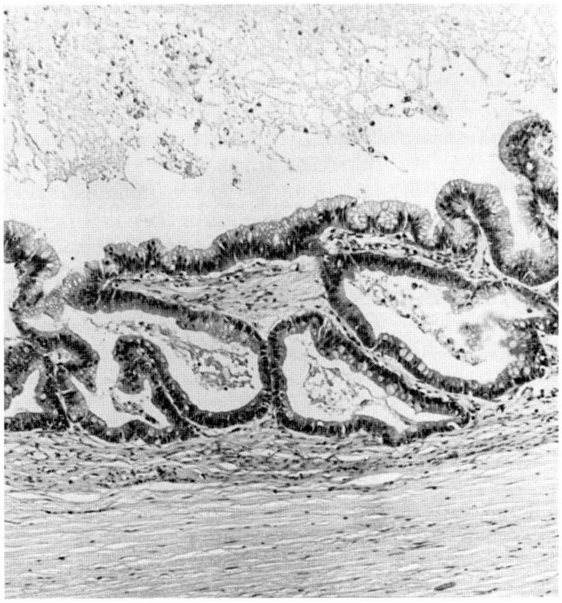

**FIG. 49.11.** Mucinous cystic tumor. Tumor wall lined by partly atypical columnar cells. H & E, ×120.

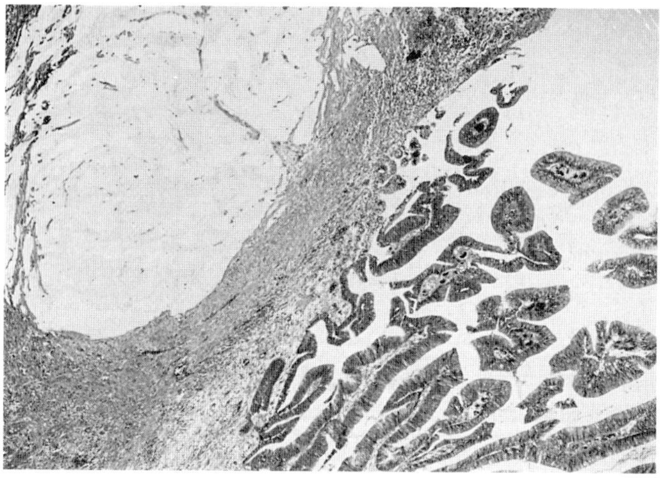

**FIG. 49.12.** Intraductal papillary-mucinous tumor. Intraductal proliferations with excessive mucin production. H & E, ×120.

tiation as adenoma, borderline tumor, and carcinoma (100). Adenoma is defined as a tumor showing only mild epithelial dysplasia, while a borderline tumor is characterized by moderate dysplasia, and an intraductal carcinoma by severe dysplasia–carcinoma in situ changes (62, 88, 91, 93, 96, 99). True invasive growth with or without metastatic spread is observed in approximately 10–20% of the tumors (88, 96, 101). In their invasive part, papillary-mucinous carcinomas often have the appearance of mucinous noncystic carcinoma. Immunocytochemically, the tumors stain for CEA and CA 19-9 as well as gastroenteropancreatic markers (100). Occasionally, the tumors may also contain neuroendocrine cells producing hormones such as serotonin or gastrin (104). Mutated K-*ras* oncogene is present in 30% and more of the tumors (100).

If tumor growth remains intraductal, the overall prognosis is good for most patients after complete tumor resection. Disease-free survival for more than 10 years has been reported (92, 101, 102). Even if a patient is inoperable, long-term survival seems to be possible (101). However, once a deeply invasive tumor has developed, the prognosis is usually poor.

## Solid-Pseudopapillary Tumor

Solid-pseudopapillary tumor is a benign or low-grade malignant tumor that is composed of monomorphous cells variably expressing epithelial, mesenchymal, and neuroendocrine markers. This tumor has also been referred to as solid-cystic (105), papillary-cystic (106), or solid and papillary epithelial neoplasm (107). The new WHO classification (19) proposes the term solid-pseudopapillary tumor (SPT), because this name encompasses the two most conspicuous histologic features, the solid and the pseudopapillary patterns.

Biologically, SPT shows two peculiarities: most tumors behave benignly and occur in young women of various races (5, 107, 108). Local recurrence is rare and usually only occurs in patients with incomplete resection (109). Frankly malignant tumors (solid-pseudopapillary carcinoma) with metastases to the liver are rare (110). Despite the striking predilection for young women, there is no associated endocrine abnormality that might explain this condition. Clinically, the patients are asymptomatic or complain of upper abdominal discomfort, occasionally of sudden onset.

Macroscopically, SPT presents as a large, round, soft mass (size range, 3–20 cm in diameter; average, 8 cm), which is well demarcated and may occur anywhere in the pancreas or attached to it (108). The cut surface reveals lobulated, light-brown solid tissue admixed with pseudocystic areas filled with hemorrhagic and necrotic debris.

Histologically, the solid parts consist of monomorphous eosinophilic and/or clear cells that are supported by hyalinized fibrovascular stalks. In addition, there are pseudopapillary areas with variable sclerosis and other degenerative changes. Finally, the tumor tissue shows hemorrhage, calcification, and foreign body reactions to cholesterol crystals (Fig. 49.13). The malignant tumors (solid-pseudopapillary carcinoma) are characterized by nerve sheath and vascular invasion and/or metastasis. Immunocytochemically, the tumor cells stain for $\alpha$-1-antitrypsin, vimentin, neuron-specific enolase, nuclear progesterone receptor, and, rarely, cytokeratin (5, 105, 109, 111, 112). Recently, a case of SPT with an unbalanced chromosomal translocation, der(17)t(13;17)(q14;p11), has been described (113).

## Acinar Cell Carcinoma

Acinar cell carcinoma (ACC) is a rare malignant epithelial neoplasm showing acinar cell differentiation. Unequivocal cases of acinar cell adenoma have not yet been published.

ACC occurs mostly in the 5th to 7th decade of life, but some rare examples have been reported in children (5, 6, 15, 114). Males predominate over females by a ratio of 2:1. Many patients present clinically with distant metastases from an occult carcinoma (62). Individual patients may show disseminated subcutaneous fat necrosis, polyarthralgia, and blood eosinophilia (114, 115). These lesions presumably result from the release of lipase by the tumor.

Macroscopically, ACC appears as a fleshy, lobulated mass that is fairly well demarcated, but shows invasive growth into the surrounding tissues. ACC ranges in size from 2 to 16 cm and is equally distributed in the pancreas. The tumor tissue is brown to yellow, with soft consistency and areas of necrosis. A cystic variant also exists (116, 117). Metastases are mainly found in the regional lymph nodes, the liver, and the lungs.

Histologically, the tumors show an acinar pattern, supported by scanty stroma (Fig. 49.14). However, tumors with solid patterns also occur, and these are reminiscent of an endocrine tumor. On immunocytochemistry and electron microscopy, pancreatic enzymes and zymogen granules (some with a fibrillary structure (118)) can be demonstrated (5, 119). In addition, some tumors also contain scattered neuroendocrine cells (positive for chromogranin A and/or synaptophysin and pancreatic hormones such as somatostatin) (6, 15). A few of these tumors may be considered true mixed acinar-endocrine carcinomas (120).

The survival of patients with ACC may be better than that of patients with ductal adenocarcinoma (15). However, in general it is unfavorable. Some patients seem to respond to chemotherapy (115).

## Pancreatoblastoma

Pancreatoblastoma is a rare malignant neoplasm composed of epithelial tissue with acinar differentiation, squamoid cell nests, and occasional endocrine cells. Pancreatoblastomas are very rare and occur predominantly in young children between 1 and 8 years of age (17, 121). Boys are more frequently affected than girls. Recently such tumors have also been observed in adults (17, 122–124).

Macroscopically, the large, soft, rounded tumors (size range, 7–12 cm) disclose a lobulated yellowish brown cut surface, with central pseudocystic foci of necrosis. The tumors occur in the pancreas or are attached to it.

Histologically, there is usually an acinar cell pattern (5, 121) with squamoid nests and occasional mesenchymal components (62). Ultrastructurally, zymogen granules can be identified. Some tumors produce $\alpha$-fetoprotein (125) and contain single endocrine cells.

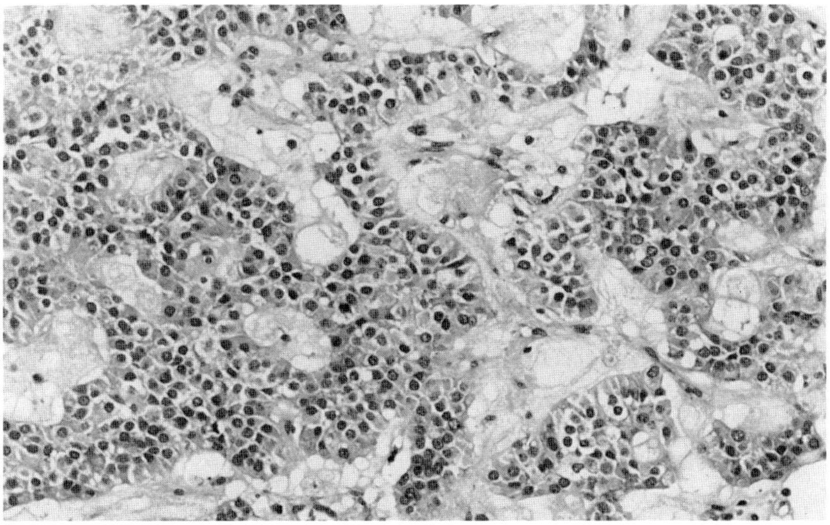

**FIG. 49.13.** Solid-pseudopapillary tumor. Solid component with hyalinized vascular structures. H & E, ×120.

If pancreatoblastoma is well encapsulated, complete surgical removal seems to be associated with a fairly good prognosis in children. Other pancreatoblastomas may respond to chemotherapy (17). The prognosis of adults with pancreatoblastoma is unfavorable (17).

## Miscellaneous Carcinomas

Among the carcinomas of the pancreas that do not fit totally into one of the above-mentioned categories are such tumors as small cell carcinoma (126), ciliated cell carcinoma, oncocytic carcinoma (127), clear cell carcinoma (62), and clear cell sugar tumor (128). Since small cell carcinoma stains for neuroendocrine markers, it is part of the spectrum of neuroendocrine tumors (14). The so-called microadenocarcinoma (62) probably does not form an entity of its own but belongs to either the ductal, endocrine, or acinar tumors (17).

## Nonepithelial Tumors

Primary nonepithelial malignant tumors of the pancreas are extremely uncommon. Those that have been reported include examples of almost all known histologic types of malignant soft tissue tumors (14, 129). The tumor that has been observed most frequently is leiomyosarcoma (130, 131). Recently, peripheral neuroectodermal tumors (PNET) involving the pancreas have been described. They responded well to chemotherapy (132).

Malignant lymphomas and plasmacytomas only rarely arise in the pancreas, whereas secondary involvement of the pancreas by advanced lymphomas is not infrequent (14).

## Secondary Tumors

The pancreas is uncommonly the site of metastases from primary carcinomas in other organs such as the breast, the lung (small cell carcinoma), the skin (melanoma), and the kidney (clear cell carcinoma) (14).

## Differential Diagnosis of Pancreatic Tumors

The differential diagnosis of the most important tumors of the exocrine pancreas includes *(a)* ductal adenocarcinoma versus chronic pancreatitis, *(b)* ductal adenocarcinoma versus other tumors of the pancreas or the gastrointestinal (GI) tract, and *(c)* cystic tumors of the pancreas versus pseudocyst.

### Ductal Adenocarcinoma versus Chronic Pancreatitis

***Clinical criteria.*** Patients younger than 40 years are more likely to have chronic pancreatitis than carcinoma. The opposite is true of patients older than 50 years with painless jaundice of relatively short duration.

***Macroscopic criteria.*** Irregular scarring of the parenchyma with calculi in the ducts and duct dilations alternating with strictures are characteristic of chronic pancreatitis. In addition, there may be pseudocysts. Most carcinomas, on the contrary, are distinguished by a poorly demarcated mass in the head of the pancreas, which causes stenosis of the common bile duct and usually also of the pancreatic duct. The ducts then show severe prestenotic dilation.

***Microscopic criteria.*** In chronic pancreatitis, even in cases with severe fibrosis, the lobular architecture is preserved. This implies that after the loss of the acinar tissue the remaining small ducts and distorted islets are still arranged in a lobular pattern, but the islets may accumulate in large aggregates that may be confused with solid (endocrine) tumors. The ducts, though irregularly formed and sometimes displaying mucinous hypertrophy and papillary hyperplasia, show uniform nuclei and almost no nucleoli. Mucin production is minimal. In ductal adenocarcinoma, the neoplastic duct structures and glands are distributed unevenly in the pancreatic tissue; their arrangement is disorderly, and they are sometimes ruptured. In addition, they may invade perineural spaces. The neoplastic ducts are formed by slightly to severely atypical columnar to cuboidal cells that contain enlarged nuclei, most of which display conspicuous nucleoli. Mitoses may also be seen, as well as variable degrees of mucin production. The pancreatitis-like changes caused by

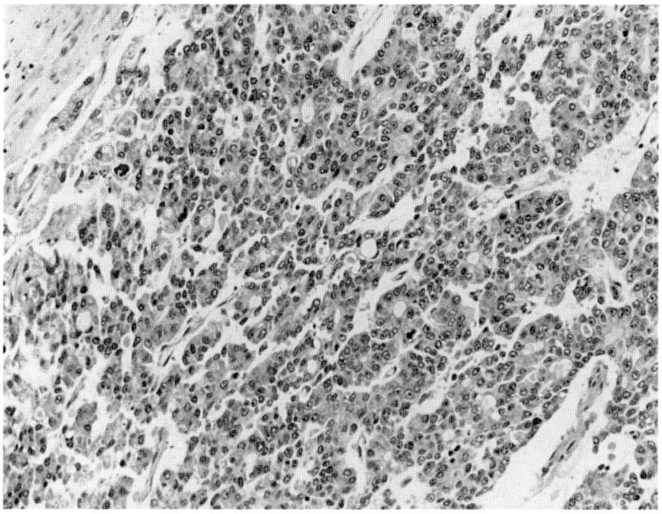

**FIG. 49.14.** Acinar cell carcinoma. H & E, ×120.

tumorous duct obstruction usually surround large parts of the tumor and are indistinguishable from chronic pancreatitis.

***Immunocytochemical Criteria.*** In chronic pancreatitis, the ducts do not stain for CEA (with very few exceptions) when monospecific monoclonal antisera are used that do not recognize the nonspecific cross-reacting antigens. In ductal adenocarcinoma, most neoplastic ducts stain for CEA. CA 19-9 or B 72.3 staining does not discriminate between ductal adenocarcinoma and chronic pancreatitis.

### Ductal Adenocarcinoma versus Other Tumors of the Pancreas and the Gastrointestinal Tract

***Ampullary Adenocarcinoma.*** Ampullary adenocarcinomas need to be distinguished from ductal adenocarcinoma because of their generally better prognosis. This distinction is not possible by means of histology or immunocytochemistry, because these tumors share the same microscopic features. The only way to distinguish between the two is by carefully assessing the macroscopic and microscopic localization of the lesion. The same is true for carcinomas of the intrapancreatic segment of the common bile duct. However, if such tumors are advanced, even careful macroscopic examination may not allow the pathologist to distinguish clearly between adenocarcinomas of the distal bile duct and those of the head of the pancreas. Periampullary carcinomas of duodenal origin that invade the pancreas may be recognized on the basis of tubulopapillary glands lined predominantly by cells with an intestinal phenotype.

The differential diagnosis of ductal adenocarcinoma versus acinar cell carcinoma, pancreatoblastoma, solid-pseudopapillary tumor, neuroendocrine tumor, and the various cystic and intraductal neoplasms relies on the distinctive histologic pattern, the immunocytochemical marker constellation, and the biology of the respective tumors:

***Acinar Cell Carcinoma.*** Acinar cell carcinomas commonly show a solid pattern with mixed acinar (slightly PAS positive), trabecular, and endocrine-like components. They stain for pancreatic enzymes and are usually negative for CEA but may show single neuroendocrine cells.

***Pancreatoblastoma.*** Pancreatoblastomas are rare tumors in small children (1–10 years), which may, however, also occur in adults. Histologically, these tumors are characterized by acinar cell differentiation and the presence of so-called squamoid nests.

***Solid-Pseudopapillary (Solid-Cystic, Papillary Cystic or Solid and Papillary) Tumors.*** These tumors consist of monomorphic cells arranged in a solid and/or pseudopapillary pattern with large areas of hemorrhage. The large, well-demarcated tumors stain focally for α-1-antitrypsin, occur predominantly in adolescent girls and young women (10–45 years), and usually are benign.

***Neuroendocrine Tumors.*** Neuroendocrine tumors exhibit solid and/or trabecular structures with occasional true glandular formations but without mucin production. They stain for neuroendocrine markers and usually one or more pancreatic hormones. Endocrine tumors occur in all age classes, can be associated with distinct hormonal syndromes, and, even if malignant, have a much more favorable prognosis than ductal adenocarcinoma.

***Anaplastic Carcinoma.*** Anaplastic carcinomas have to be differentiated from metastases of amelanotic melanoma (S-100 positivity), pleomorphic rhabdomyosarcomas (desmin and/or actin positivity), undifferentiated sarcomas (vimentin positivity), choriocarcinoma (human choriogonadotropin-ß positivity). It may be very difficult or even impossible to distinguish anaplastic carcinoma from a metastasis of a large cell lung carcinoma. Signet ring cell carcinomas of the stomach infiltrating the pancreas are also indistinguishable from those arising in the pancreas. Metastases of renal cell carcinoma, which can occur in the pancreas years after the resection of the primary tumor, may be differentiated from clear cell carcinoma on the basis of their frequent vimentin positivity and mucin negativity. Metastases of carcinomas of the pancreas to the ovary or the lung may simulate primary mucinous tumor of the ovary or primary lung adenocarcinoma, respectively.

***Liver Metastases.*** The distinction between liver metastases of pancreatic ductal adenocarcinoma and those of other mucin-producing adenocarcinomas of the GI tract is impossible on the basis of histology alone. The only hint may be that metastases of pancreatic carcinomas often display small glands embedded in marked desmoplastic stroma and are accompanied by cholestasis—features they share, however, with bile duct carcinomas. If frozen tissue is available, ductal adenocarcinomas may be distinguished from most gastrointestinal carcinomas on the basis of their keratin pattern (keratins 7, 8, 18, 19), because the latter tumors express only keratins 8, 18, and 19 (133). However, so far most of the monospecific keratin antibodies available require frozen tissue; hence, this differentiation is not possible in paraffin material. Moreover, ductal adenocarcinomas share the expression of CEA, CA 19-9, and other tumor markers with the mucin-producing adenocarcinomas of gastrointestinal, biliary, or pulmonary origin, so there is no specific marker for pancreatic carcinoma.

### Cystic Tumors of the Pancreas versus Pseudocyst

***Pseudocyst.*** Pseudocysts account for 75% of all cystic lesions of the pancreas. They are sequelae of acute or chronic pancreatitis and result from extensive autodigestive tissue necrosis. Their wall is composed of hemosiderin-containing granulation tissue (inner layer) and usually a fibrotic outer layer. There is no epithelial lining. The cyst contains necrotic debris and pancreatic enzymes.

The most important neoplastic cystic lesions are microcystic serous adenoma, mucinous cystic neoplasm, solid-pseudopapillary tumor, and intraductal papillary and mucinous tumor. Very rare are lymphoepithelial cysts and congenital cysts. Cystic changes are occasionally seen in endocrine or vascular tumors.

***Microcystic Serous Adenoma.*** Microcystic serous adenoma is a large and well-demarcated multilocular cystic tumor. It stains negative for mucin and occurs in old women.

***Mucinous Cystic Neoplasms.*** Mucinous cystic neoplasms are usually unilocular tumors that occur in the tail of the pancreas in women aged 20–60 years. The cyst-lining cells stain for mucin and may become malignant.

***Solid-Pseudopapillary Tumors.*** The features of these peculiar tumors have already been discussed (cf. Ductal Adenocarcinoma versus Other Tumors of the Pancreas and the GI Tract).

***Intraductal Papillary and Mucinous Tumors.*** Intraductal papillary and mucinous tumors show papillary structures composed of columnar cells. They are confined to the duct system. Some of them show severe cellular atypia, but they rarely become malignant. The patients are usually rather old (50–70 years) and often present with a long history of chronic pancreatitis.

## REFERENCES


1. Cubilla AL, Fitzgerald PJ. Morphological patterns of primary nonendocrine human pancreas carcinoma. Cancer Res 1975; 35:2234–2248.
2. Kodama T. A light and electron microscopic study on the pancreatic ductal system. Acta Pathol Jpn 1983;33:297–321.
3. Kern HF. Fine structure of the human exocrine pancreas. In: Go VLW, Gardner JD, Brooks FP, Lebenthal E, DiMagno EP, Scheele GA, eds. The exocrine pancreas: biology, pathobiology, and diseases. New York: Raven Press, 1986:9–19.
4. Kern HF, Röher HD, von Bülow M, Klöppel G. Fine structure of three major grades of malignancy of human pancreatic adenocarcinoma. Pancreas 1987;2:2–13.
5. Morohoshi T, Kanda M, Horie A, et al. Immunocytochemical markers of uncommon pancreatic tumors. Acinar cell carci-

noma, pancreatoblastoma, and solid cystic (papillary-cystic) tumor. Cancer 1987;59:739–747.
6. Hoorens A, Lemoine NR, McLellan E, et al. Pancreatic acinar cell carcinoma. An analysis of cell lineage markers, p53 expression, and Ki-*ras* mutation. Am J Pathol 1993;143:685–698.
7. Moll R, Robine S, Dudouet B, Louvard D. Villin: a cytoskeletal protein and a differentiation marker expressed in some human adenocarcinomas. Virchows Arch (B) Cell Pathol 1987;54: 155–169.
8. Kim JH, Ho SB, Montgomery CK, Kim YS. Cell lineage markers in human pancreatic cancer. Cancer 1990;66:2134–2143.
9. Elsässer HP, Klöppel G, Mannherz HG, Flocke K, Kern HF. Immunohistochemical demonstration of villin in the normal human pancreas and in chronic pancreatitis. Histochemistry 1991;95:383–390.
10. Klöppel G. Gene changes and pancreatic carcinoma: the significance of K-*ras*. Dig Surg 1994;11:164–169.
11. Bommer G, Friedel U, Heitz PU, Klöppel G. PP cell distribution and hyperplasia: immunocytochemical morphology in normal pancreas, chronic pancreatitis and pancreatic carcinoma. Virchows Arch (A) Pathol Anat 1980;387:319–331.
12. Permert J, Mogaki M, Andrén-Sandberg A, Kazakoff K, Pour PM. Pancreatic mixed ductal-islet tumors. Is this an entity? Int J Pancreatol 1992;11:23–29.
13. Eusebi V, Capella C, Bondi A, Sessa F, Vezzadini P, Mancini AM. Endocrine-paracrine cells in pancreatic exocrine carcinomas. Histopathology 1981;5:599–613.
14. Solcia E, Capella C, Klöppel G. Tumors of the pancreas. Washington, DC: Armed Forces Institute of Pathology, 1997.
15. Klimstra DS, Heffess CS, Oertel JE, Rosai J. Acinar cell carcinoma of the pancreas: a clinicopathologic study of 28 cases. Am J Surg Pathol 1992;16:815–837.
16. Klöppel G. Pathology of nonendocrine pancreatic tumors. In: Go VLW, DiMagno EP, Gardner JD, Lebenthal E, Reber HA, Scheele GA, eds. The pancreas: biology, pathobiology, and disease. New York: Raven Press, 1993:871–897.
17. Klimstra DS, Wenig BM, Adair CF, Heffess CS. Pancreatoblastoma. A clinicopathologic study and review of the literature. Am J Surg Pathol 1995;19:1371–1389.
18. Klöppel G, Höfler H, Heitz PU. Pancreatic endocrine tumours in man. In: Polak JM, ed. Diagnostic histopathology of neuroendocrine tumours. Edinburgh: Churchill Livingstone, 1993:91–121.
19. Klöppel G, Solcia E, Longnecker DS, Capella C, Sobin LH. Histologic typing of tumours of the exocrine pancreas. Berlin: Springer, 1996.
20. Pour PM, Konishi Y, Klöppel G, Longnecker DS. Atlas of exocrine pancreatic tumours: morphology, biology, and diagnosis with an international guide for tumour classification. Tokyo: Springer, 1994.
21. Klöppel G. Pancreatic, non-endocrine tumours. In: Klöppel G, Heitz PU, eds. Pancreatic pathology. Edinburgh: Churchill Livingstone, 1984:79–113.
22. Cubilla AL, Fitzgerald PJ. Tumors of the exocrine pancreas. Washington, DC: Armed Forces Institute of Pathology, 1984.
23. Ivy EJ, Sarr MG, Reiman HM. Nonendocrine cancer of the pancreas in patients under age forty years. Surgery 1990;108: 481–487.
24. De Vuyst M, Rickaert F, De Roy G, Klöppel G. The spectrum of ductal adenocarcinomas and other tumors of the pancreas in patients younger than 40 years of age (Abstract). Pathol Res Pract 1993;189:681.
25. Hermanek P. Staging of exocrine pancreatic carcinoma. Eur J Surg Oncol 1991;17:167–172.
26. Morohoshi T, Held G, Klöppel G. Exocrine pancreatic tumours and their histological classification. A study based on 167 autopsy and 97 surgical cases. Histopathology 1983;7:645–661.
27. Klöppel G, Lingenthal G, von Bülow M, Kern HF. Histological and fine structural features of pancreatic ductal adenocarcinomas in relation to growth and prognosis: studies in xenografted tumours and clinicohistopathologic correlation in a series of 75 cases. Histopathology 1985;9:841–856.
28. Haglund C, Nordling S, Roberts P, Ekblom P. Expression of laminin in pancreatic neoplasms and in chronic pancreatitis. Am J Surg Pathol 1984;8:669–676.
29. Mollenhauer J, Roether I, Kern HF. Distribution of extracellular matrix proteins in pancreatic ductal adenocarcinoma and its influence on tumor cell proliferation in vitro. Pancreas 1987;2: 14–24.
30. Haberern-Blood C, Liotta LA, Rao CN, Kupchik HZ. Laminin expression by human pancreatic carcinoma cells in the nude mouse and in culture. J Natl Cancer Inst 1987;79:891–898.
31. Löhr M, Trautmann B, Göttler M, et al. Human ductal adenocarcinomas of the pancreas express extracellular matrix proteins. Br J Cancer 1994;69:144–151.
32. Ingber DE, Madri JA, Jamieson JD. Basement membrane as a spatial organizer of polarized epithelia. Exogenous basement membrane reorients pancreatic epithelial tumor cells in vitro. Am J Pathol 1986;122:129–139.
33. Cubilla AL, Fitzgerald PJ. Morphological lesions associated with human primary invasive nonendocrine pancreas cancer. Cancer Res 1976;36:2690–2698.
34. Klöppel G, Bommer G, Rückert K, Seifert G. Intraductal proliferation in the pancreas and its relationship to human and experimental carcinogenesis. Virchows Arch (A) Pathol Anat 1980;387:221–233.
35. Pliam MB, ReMine WH. Further evaluation of total pancreatectomy. Arch Surg 1975;110:506–512.
36. Ihse I, Lilja P, Arnesjö B, Bengmark S. Total pancreatectomy for cancer: an appraisal of 65 cases. Ann Surg 1977;186:675–680.
37. Tryka AF, Brooks JR. Histopathology in the evaluation of total pancreatectomy for ductal carcinoma. Ann Surg 1979;190: 373–379.
38. van Heerden JA. Pancreatic resection for carcinoma of the pancreas: Whipple versus total pancreatectomy—an institutional perspective. World J Surg 1984;8:88
39. Klöppel G, Lohse T, Bosslet K, Rückert K. Ductal adenocarcinoma of the head of the pancreas: incidence of tumour involvement beyond the Whipple resection line. Histological and immunocytochemical analysis of 37 total pancreatectomy specimens. Pancreas 1987;2:170–175.
40. Malfertheiner P, Ditschuneit H. Diagnostic procedures in pancreatic disease. Berlin: Springer, 1986.
41. Schmiegel WH, Kreiker C, Eberl W, et al. Monoclonal antibody defines CA 19-9 in pancreatic juices and sera. Gut 1985;26: 456–460.
42. Atkinson BF, Ernst C, Herlyn M, Steplewski Z, Sears HF, Koprowski H. Gastrointestinal cancer-associated antigen in immunoperoxidase assay. Cancer Res 1982;42:4820–4823.
43. Iwase K, Kato K, Nagasaka A, et al. Immunohistochemical study of neuron-specific enolase and CA 19-9 in pancreatic disorders. The value of neuron-specific enolase as a marker for islet cell and nerve tissue. Gastroenterology 1986;91:576–580.
44. Itai S, Arii S, Tobe R, et al. Significance of 2–3 and 2–6 sialylation of Lewis A antigen in pancreas cancer. Cancer 1988;61:775–787.
45. Bätge B, Bosslet K, Sedlacek HH, Kern HF, Klöppel G. Monoclonal antibodies against CEA-related components discriminate between pancreatic duct type carcinomas and nonneoplastic duct lesions as well as nonduct type neoplasias. Virchows Arch (A) Pathol Anat 1986;408:361–374.
46. Metzgar RS, Gaillard MT, Levine SJ, Tuck FL, Bossen EH, Borowitz MJ. Antigens of human pancreatic adenocarcinoma cells defined by murine monoclonal antibodies. Cancer Res 1982; 42:601–608.
47. Tempero M, Takasaki H, Uchida E, et al. Co-expression of CA 19-9, DU-PAN-2, CA 125, and TAG-72 in pancreatic adenocarcinoma. Am J Surg Pathol 1989;13:89–95.
48. Sessa F, Bonato M, Frigerio B, et al. Ductal cancers of the pancreas frequently express markers of gastrointestinal epithelial cells. Gastroenterology 1990;98:1655–1665.
49. Ho SB, Niehans GA, Lyftogt C, et al. Heterogeneity of mucin gene expression in normal and neoplastic tissues. Cancer Res 1993;53:641–651.
50. Osako M, Yonezawa S, Siddiki B, et al. Immunohistochemical study of mucin carbohydrates and core proteins in human pancreatic tumors. Cancer 1993;71:2191–2199.
51. Ho JJL, Kim YS. Serological pancreatic markers and the MUC1 apomucin. Pancreas 1994;9:674–691.
52. Ohshio G, Imamura T, Okada N, et al. Immunohistochemical study of metallothionein in pancreatic carcinomas. J Cancer Res Clin Oncol 1996;122:351–355.

53. Takada M, Yamamoto M, Saitoh Y. The significance of CD44 in human pancreatic cancer: II. The role of CD44 in human pancreatic adenocarcinoma invasion. Pancreas 1994;9:753–757.
54. Castellà EM, Ariza A, Ojanguren I, et al. Differential expression of CD44v6 in adenocarcinoma of the pancreas: an immunohistochemical study. Virchows Arch 1996;429:191–195.
55. Pignatelli M, Ansari TW, Gunter P, et al. Loss of membranous E-cadherin expression in pancreatic cancer: correlation with lymph node metastasis, high grade, and advanced stage. J Pathol 1994;174:243–248.
56. Nagai H, Kuroda A, Morioka Y. Lymphatic and local spread of T1 and T2 pancreatic cancer. A study of autopsy material. Ann Surg 1986;204:65–71.
57. Ohta T, Nagakawa T, Ueno K, et al. The mode of lymphatic and local spread of pancreatic carcinomas less than 4.0 in size. Int Surg 1993;78:208–212.
58. Cubilla AL, Fortner JG, Fitzgerald PJ. Lymph node involvement in carcinoma of the head of the pancreas area. Cancer 1978;41: 880–887.
59. Trede M, Schwall G, Saeger HD. Survival after pancreatoduodenectomy. 118 consecutive resections without an operative mortality. Ann Surg 1990;211:447–458.
60. Nagakawa T, Kobayashi H, Ueno K, Ohta T, Kayahara M, Miyazaki I. Clinical study of lymphatic flow to the paraaortic lymph nodes in carcinoma of the head of the pancreas. Cancer 1994;73:1155–1162.
61. Nagakawa T, Nagamori M, Futakami F, et al. Results of extensive surgery for pancreatic carcinoma. Cancer 1996;77:640–645.
62. Mikal S, Campbell AJA. Carcinoma of the pancreas. Diagnostic and operative criteria based on one hundred consecutive autopsies. Surgery 1950;28:963–969.
63. Connoly MM, Dawson PJ, Michelassi F, Moossa AR, Lowenstein F. Survival in 1001 patients with carcinoma of the pancreas. Ann Surg 1987;206:366–373.
64. Gudjonsson B. Cancer of the pancreas. Cancer 1987;60:2284–2303.
65. Guthoff A, Rothe B, Klapdor R, Klöppel G, Greten H. Site of recurrence after resection for pancreatic carcinoma. Dig Dis Sci 1987;32:1168.
66. Del Castillo CF, Warshaw L. Peritoneal metastases in pancreatic cancer. Hepatogastroenterology 1993;40:430–432.
67. Juhl H, Stritzel M, Wroblewski A, et al. Immunocytological detection of micrometastatic cells: comparative evaluation of findings in the peritoneal cavity and the bone marrow of gastric, colorectal and pancreatic cancer patients. Int J Cancer 1994;57:330–335.
68. Ishikawa O, Matsui Y, Aoki I, Iwanaga T, Terasawa T, Wada A. Adenosquamous carcinoma of the pancreas. Cancer 1980;46: 1192–1196.
69. Tschang TP, Garza-Garza R, Kissane JM. Pleomorphic carcinoma of the pancreas: an analysis of 15 cases. Cancer 1977;39:2114–2126.
70. Dworak O, Wittekind C. Osteoclastic giant cell tumour of the pancreas. An immunohistological study and review of the literature. Pathol Res Pract 1993;189:228–231.
71. Rosai J. Carcinoma of pancreas simulating giant cell tumor of bone. Electron-microscopic evidence of its acinar cell origin. Cancer 1968;22:333–344.
72. Fischer HP, Altmannsberger M, Kracht J. Osteoclast-type giant cell tumour of the pancreas. Virchows Arch (A) Pathol Anat 1988;412:247–253.
73. Goldberg RD, Michelassi F, Montag AG. Osteoclast-like giant cell tumour of the pancreas: immunophenotypic similarity to giant cell tumour of bone. Hum Pathol 1991;22:618–622.
74. Dizon MA, Multhaupt HAB, Paskin DL, Warhol MJ. Osteoclastic giant cell tumor of the pancreas. An immunohistochemical study. Arch Pathol Lab Med 1996;120:306–309.
75. Morinaga S, Tsumuraya M, Nakajima T, Shimosato Y, Okazaki N. Ciliated-cell adenocarcinoma of the pancreas. Acta Pathol Jpn 1986;36:1905–1910.
76. George DH, Murphy F, Michalski R, Ulmer BG. Serous cystadenocarcinoma of the pancreas: a new entity? Am J Surg Pathol 1989;13:61–66.
77. Yoshimi N, Sugie S, Tanaka T, et al. A rare case of serous cystadenocarcinoma of the pancreas. Cancer 1992;69:2449–2453.
78. Perez-Ordonez B, Naseem A, Lieberman PH, Klimstra DS. Solid serous adenoma of the pancreas. The solid variant of serous cystadenoma? Am J Surg Pathol 1996;20:1401–1405.
79. Becker WF, Welsh RA, Pratt HS. Cystadenoma and cystadenocarcinoma of the pancreas. Ann Surg 1965;161:845–860.
80. Bogomoletz WV, Adnet JJ, Widgren S, Stavrrou M, McLaughlin JE. Cystadenoma of the pancreas: a histological, histochemical and ultrastructural study of seven cases. Histopathology 1980; 4:309–320.
81. Didolkar MSD, Malhotra Y, Holyoke ED, Elias G. Cystadenoma of the pancreas. Surg Gynecol Obstet 1975;140:925–928.
82. Egawa N, Maillet B, Schröder S, Foulis A, Mukai K, Klöppel G. Serous oligocystic and ill-demarcated adenoma of the pancreas: a variant of serous cystic adenoma. Virchows Arch 1994;424:13–17.
83. Compagno J, Oertel JE. Microcystic adenomas of the pancreas (glycogen-rich cystadenomas): a clinicopathologic study of 34 cases. Am J Clin Pathol 1978;69:289–298.
84. Pyke CM, van Heerden JA, Colby TV, Sarr MG, Weaver AL. The spectrum of serous cystadenoma of the pancreas. Clinical, pathologic, and surgical aspects. Ann Surg 1992;215: 132–139.
85. Yamaguchi K, Enjoji M. Cystic neoplasm of the pancreas. Gastroenterology 1987;92:1934–1943.
86. Compagno J, Oertel JE. Mucinous cystic neoplasms of the pancreas with overt and latent malignancy (cystadenocarcinoma and cystadenoma). A clinicopathologic study of 41 cases. Am J Clin Pathol 1978;69:573–580.
87. Warshaw AL, Compton CC, Lewandrowski K, Cardenosa G, Mueller PR. Cystic tumors of the pancreas. New clinical, radiologic, and pathologic observations in 67 patients. Ann Surg 1990;212:432–443.
88. Yamada M, Kozuka S, Yamao K, Nakazawa S, Naitoh Y, Tsukamoto Y. Mucin-producing tumour of the pancreas. Cancer 1991;68:159–168.
89. Albores-Saavedra J, Nadji M, Henson DE, Angeles-Angeles A. Enteroendocrine cell differentiation in carcinomas of the gallbladder and mucinous cystadenocarcinoma of the pancreas. Pathol Res Pract 1988;183:169–175.
90. Warshaw AL. Implications of peritoneal cytology for staging of early pancreatic cancer (Abstract). Proceedings of the 4th Meeting of the International Association for Pancreatology, and the 3rd Symposium of the International Pancreatic Cancer Study Group 1990;1:622.
91. Morohoshi T, Kanda M, Asanuma K, Klöppel G. Intraductal papillary neoplasms of the pancreas. A clinicopathologic study of six patients. Cancer 1989;64:1329–1335.
92. Rickaert F, Cremer M, Devière J, et al. Intraductal mucin-hypersecreting neoplasms of the pancreas. A clinicopathologic study of eight patients. Gastroenterology 1991;101: 512–519.
93. Conley CR, Scheithauer BW, Weiland LH, van Heerden JA. Diffuse intraductal papillary adenocarcinoma of the pancreas. Ann Surg 1987;205:246–249.
94. Itai Y, Kokubo T, Terano A. Mucin-hypersecreting carcinoma of the pancreas. Radiology 1987;165:51–55.
95. Warshaw AL, Berry J, Gang DL. Villous adenoma of the duct of Wirsung. Dig Dis Sci 1987;32:1311–1313.
96. Mizumoto K, Inagaki T, Koizumi M, et al. Early pancreatic duct adenocarcinoma. Hum Pathol 1988;19:242–244.
97. Bastid C, Bernard JP, Sarles H, Payan MJ, Sahel J. Mucinous ductal ectasia of the pancreas: a premalignant disease and a cause of obstructive pancreatitis. Pancreas 1991;6:15–22.
98. Obara T, Maguchi H, Saitoh Y, et al. Mucin-producing tumour of the pancreas: a unique clinical entity. Am J Gastroenterol 1991;86:1619–1625.
99. Milchgrub, Campuzano M, Casillas J, Albores-Saavedra J. Intraductal carcinoma of the pancreas. Cancer 1992;69: 651–656.
100. Sessa F, Solcia E, Capella C, et al. Intraductal papillary-mucinous tumours represent a distinct group of pancreatic neoplasms: an investigation of tumour cell differentiation and K-*ras*, p53, and *c-erb*B-2 abnormalities in 26 patients. Virchows Arch 1994;425: 357–367.
101. Azar C, Van de Stadt J, Rickaert F, et al. Intraductal papillary

mucinous tumours of the pancreas. Clinical and therapeutic issues in 32 patients. Gut 1996;39:457–464.

102. Loftus EV, Jr., Olivares-Pakzad BA, Batts KP, et al. Intraductal papillary-mucinous tumors of the pancreas: clinicopathologic features, outcome, and nomenclature. Gastroenterology 1996; 110:1909–1918.
103. Adsay NV, Adair CF, Heffess CS, Klimstra DS. Intraductal oncocytic papillary neoplasms of the pancreas. Am J Surg Pathol 1996;20:980–994.
104. Nishihara K, Fukuda T, Tsuneyoshi M, Kominami T, Maeda S, Saku M. Intraductal papillary neoplasm of the pancreas. Cancer 1993;72:689–696.
105. Klöppel G, Morohoshi T, John HD, et al. Solid and cystic acinar cell tumour of the pancreas. A tumour in young women with favourable prognosis. Virchows Arch (A) Pathol Anat 1981;392: 171–183.
106. Boor PJ, Swanson MR. Papillary-cystic neoplasm of the pancreas. Am J Surg Pathol 1979;3:69–75.
107. Oertel JE, Mendelsohn G, Compagno J. Solid and papillary epithelial neoplasms of the pancreas. In: Humphrey GB, Grindey GB, Dehner LP, Acton RT, Pysher TJ, eds. Pancreatic tumours in children. Den Haag: Martinus Nijhoff, 1982:167–171.
108. Klöppel G, Maurer R, Hofmann E, et al. Solid-cystic (papillary-cystic) tumours within and outside the pancreas in men: report of two patients. Virchows Arch (A) Pathol Anat 1991;418: 179–183.
109. Lieber MR, Lack EE, Roberts JR, et al. Solid and papillary epithelial neoplasm of the pancreas. Am J Surg Pathol 1987;11:85–93.
110. Matsunou H, Konishi F. Papillary-cystic neoplasm of the pancreas. A clinicopathologic study concerning the tumor aging and malignancy of nine cases. Cancer 1990;65:283–291.
111. Chott A, Klöppel G, Buxbaum P, Heitz PU. Neuron specific enolase demonstration in the diagnosis of a solid-cystic (papillary cystic) tumour of the pancreas. Virchows Arch (A) Pathol Anat 1987;410:397–402.
112. Zamboni G, Bonetti F, Scarpa A, et al. Expression of progesterone receptor in solid cystic tumour of the pancreas. A clinicopathological, immunohistochemical and ultrastructural study of ten cases. Virchows Arch (A) Pathol Anat 1993;423:425–431.
113. Grant LD, Lauwers GY, Meloni AM, et al. Unbalanced chromosomal translocation, der(17)t(13;17)(q14;p11) in a solid and cystic papillary epithelial neoplasm of the pancreas. Am J Surg Pathol 1996;20:339–345.
114. Burns WA, Matthews MJ, Hamosh M, VanderWeide G, Blum R, Johnson FB. Lipase secreting acinar cell carcinoma of the pancreas with polyarthropathy—a light and electron microscopic, histochemical and biochemical study. Cancer 1974;33: 1002–1009.
115. van Klaveren RJ, de Mulder PHM, Boerbooms AMT, et al. Pancreatic carcinoma with polyarthritis, fat necrosis, and high serum lipase and trypsin activity. Gut 1990;31:953–955.
116. Cantrell BB, Cubilla AL, Erlandson RA, Fortner J, Fitzgerald PJ. Acinar cell cystadenocarcinoma of human pancreas. Cancer 1981;47:410–416.
117. Stamm B, Burger H, Hollinger A. Acinar cell cystadenocarcinoma of the pancreas. Cancer 1987;60:2542–2547.
118. Chong JM, Fukuyama M, Shiozawa Y, et al. Fibrillary inclusions in neoplastic and fetal acinar cells of the pancreas. Virchows Arch 1996;428:261–266.
119. Kuopio T, Ekfors TO, Nikkanen V, Nevalainen TJ. Acinar cell carcinoma of the pancreas. Report of three cases. APMIS 1995;103:69–78.
120. Klimstra DS, Rosai J, Heffess CS. Mixed acinar-endocrine carcinomas of the pancreas. Am J Surg Pathol 1994;18:765–778.
121. Horie A, Haratake J, Jimi A, Matsumoto M, Ishii N, Tsutsumi Y. Pancreatoblastoma in Japan, with differential diagnosis from papillary cystic tumour (ductuloacinar adenoma) of the pancreas. Acta Pathol Jpn 1987;37:47–63.
122. Palosaari D, Clayton F, Seaman J. Pancreatoblastoma in an adult. Arch Pathol Lab Med 1986;110:650–652.
123. Hoorens A, Gebhard F, Kraft K, Lemoine NR, Klöppel G. Pancreatoblastoma in an adult: its separation from acinar cell carcinoma. Virchows Arch 1994;424:485–490.
124. Klimstra DS, Wenig D, Heffess CS. Pancreatoblastoma: a clinicopathologic study (Abstract 773). Mod Pathol 1994;7: 133A.
125. Morohoshi T, Sagawa F, Mitsuya T. Pancreatoblastoma with marked elevation of serum alpha-fetoprotein. An autopsy case report with immunocytochemical study. Virchows Arch (A) Pathol Anat 1990;416:265–270.
126. Reyes CV, Wang T. Undifferentiated small cell carcinoma of the pancreas: a report of five cases. Cancer 1981;47:2500–2502.
127. Huntrakoon M. Oncocytic carcinoma of the pancreas. Cancer 1983;51:332–336.
128. Zamboni G, Pea M, Martignoni G, et al. Clear cell ''sugar'' tumor of the pancreas. A novel member of the family of lesions characterized by the presence of perivascular epithelioid cells. Am J Surg Pathol 1996;20:722–730.
129. Bardaxogou E, Manganas D, Landen S, et al. Hemangiopericytoma of the pancreas: report of a case and review of the literature. Hepatogastroenterology 1995;42:172–174.
130. Ishikawa O, Matsui Y, Aoki Y, Iwanaga T, Terasawa T, Wada A. Leiomyosarcoma of the pancreas. Am J Surg Pathol 1981;5: 597–602.
131. de Alva E, Torramadé J, Vazquez JJ. Leiomyosarcoma of the pancreas. Virchows Arch (A) Pathol Anat 1993;422:419–422.
132. Lüttges J, Pierré E, Zamboni G, et al. Maligne nicht-epitheliale Tumoren des Pankreas. Pathologe 1997;in press.
133. Osborne M, van Essen G, Weber K, Klöppel G, Altmannsberger M. Differential diagnosis of gastrointestinal carcinomas by using monoclonal antibodies specific for individual keratin polypeptides. Lab Invest 1986;55:497–594.

# 50

# *Staging of Pancreatic Cancer*

Tsukasa Tsunoda and Toshifumi Eto

The stage of cancer should accurately reflect both the prognosis of patients suffering from the disease and the resectability of tumors. There have been a number of proposals in the past for staging of pancreatic carcinoma (Biometry Branch, National Cancer Institute 1972 (1, 2), Hermreck et al. 1974 (3), Leadbetter et al. 1975 (4), Klöppel et al. 1979 (5, 6), Cubilla et al. 1979 (7), Cancer of the Pancreas Task Force 1981 (8), Fortner 1984 (9), Deixonne et al. 1986 (10)). The Union Internationale Contre le Cancer (UICC) recommended a stage classification for pancreatic cancer based on TNM factors (UICC stage classification, UICC-SC) (11, 12). Meanwhile, the Japan Pancreas Society proposed a more complex stage classification plan that included tumor size (T factor), serosal invasion (s factor), retroperitoneal invasion (RP factor), and invasion to the portal venous systems (PV factor) (JPN stage classification, JPN-SC) (13). The differences between UICC-SC and JPN-SC have been evaluated by a few authors, including the present authors. In 1993, the Japan Pancreas Society proposed a new stage classification based on TNM factors, incorporating the concept of UICC T factor, that is, a new T factor including the local extent of the primary tumor (14).

The purpose of this chapter is to describe the differences between UICC-SC and JPN-SC, to introduce the newly proposed Japanese stage classification (new JPN-SC) (14), and to discuss which staging system is the most efficient on the basis of our analysis of a large series of cases of carcinoma of the head of the pancreas (15, 16).

## UICC STAGE CLASSIFICATION

The UICC-SC described *TNM classification of malignant tumors* is composed of three staging factors: primary tumor (T factor), regional lymph nodes (N factor), and distant metastasis (M factor). In UICC-SC, T factor (T1a, b, T2, T3; tumor size and/or local extent of the primary tumor), N factor (N0, N1; the absence or presence of regional lymph node metastasis (Fig. 50.1, *A* and *B*), and M factor (M0, M1; the absence or presence of distant metastasis) are used for staging of the disease (Table 50.1). Local extent of the tumor is expressed as either a tumor limited to the pancreas (T1) or invasion to the duodenum (T2), bile duct (T2), peripancreatic tissues (T2), stomach (T3), spleen (T3), colon (T3), and adjacent large vessels (T3). Tumors limited to the pancreas are further subdivided according to size (smaller than 2 cm, T1a; larger than 2 cm, T1b).

## JAPANESE STAGE CLASSIFICATION

The Japanese stage classification described in *General Rules for Cancer of the Pancreas* (1986) (13) is composed of six staging factors: T factor, S factor, RP factor, PV factor, lymph node metastasis (N factor), and distant metastasis (M factor), including hepatic metastasis or peritoneal dissemination (Table 50.2). The severity of the S, RP, and PV factors is graded as 0 (no invasion), 1 (suspected invasion), 2 (definite invasion), or 3 (severe invasion). The JPN T factor refers only to tumor size. The JPN S, RP, and PV factors correspond to the local extent of the tumor in UICC T factor. Thus, the JPN N factor is divided into 4 grades, while UICC-SC takes an all-or-nothing approach (Tables 50.3, 50.4, and Fig. 50.2, *A* and *B*).

## THE NEW JAPANESE STAGE CLASSIFICATION BASED ON TNM FACTORS

The National Pancreatic Cancer Registry of Japan registered cases of ductal carcinoma of the pancreas (excluding cystadenocarcinoma and islet cell carcinoma) from 334 institutions during the 10-year period from 1981 to 1990 and analyzed the data using JPN-SC. The results, which have been reported in detail by the Pancreatic Cancer Registration Committee of the Japan Pancreas Society (17), Yamamoto et al. (18, 19), and these authors (15, 16), show that JPN-SC reflected the prognosis of the disease more accurately than UICC-SC. However, UICC-SC is familiar to pancreatologists all over the world. In September 1993, the Japan Pancreas Society proposed a new staging system using TNM factors in which each factor is delineated by definition of JPN-SC factors (14) (Table 50.5).

### T Factor in the New JPN-SC

The new T factor includes not only tumor size (TS factor), but also S factor, PV factor, RP factor, DU factor (invasion to the duodenal wall), CH factor (invasion to the intrapancreatic bile duct) and *A* factor (invasion to the arterial vessels). DU and CH factors are newly employed as prognostic factors because UICC T factor includes DU and CH factors. *A* factor becomes independent from RP factor. T factor is divided into four grades (T1a, T1b, T2, T3).

### N Factor in the New JPN-SC

The new N factor is classified into four grades because the grading of N factor in JPN-SC reflected the prognosis of the diseases more accurately than that in UICC-SC (Table 50.6).

### M Factor in the New JPN-SC

Positive distant metastasis (M1), including JPN H (liver metastasis, H1, 2, 3) and JPN P (peritoneal dissemination, P1, 2, 3), is a factor in the poorest prognosis group. Metastasis in any lymph

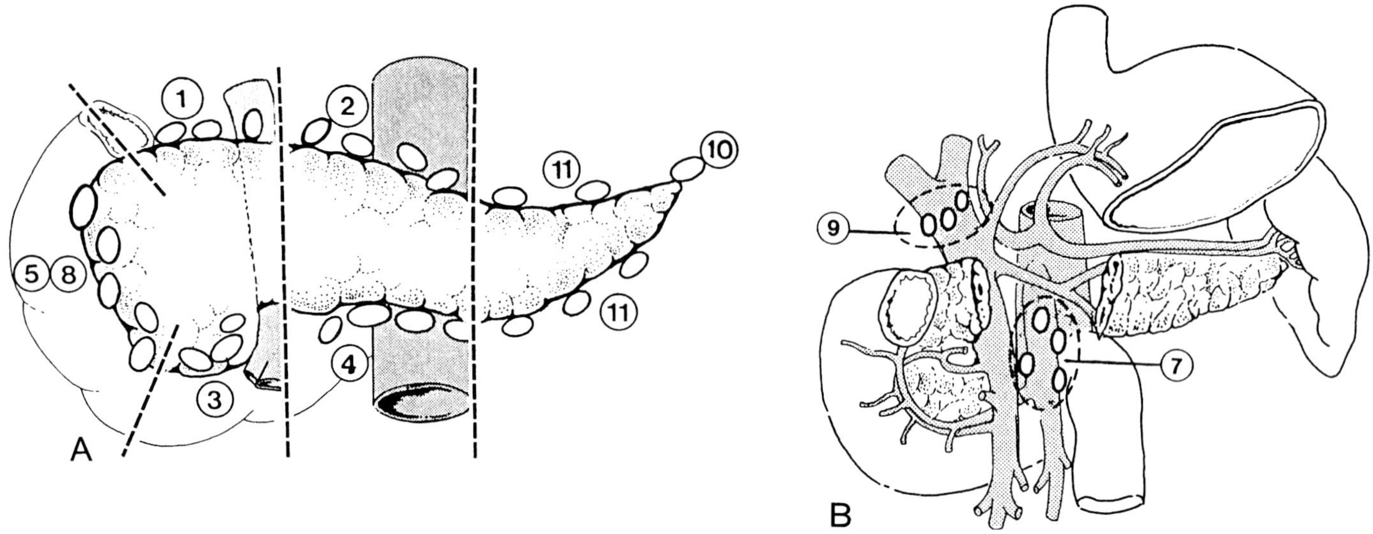


**FIG. 50.1.** **A** and **B.** Regional lymph nodes in UICC-SC are peripancreatic nodes and can be subdivided as follows. Superior: superior to head *(1)* and body *(2)*; inferior: inferior to head *(3)* and body *(4)*; anterior: anterior pancreaticoduodenal *(5)*, pyloric *(6)* (not shown), and proximal mesenteric *(7)*; posterior: posterior pancreaticoduodenal *(8)*, common bile duct *(9)* and proximal mesenteric *(7)*; splenic: hilum of spleen *(10)*, and tail of pancreas *(11)*.

node other than regional lymph nodes is classified as distant metastasis.

## THE MOST EFFICIENT STAGING SYSTEM

Our investigation on a large series of resected pancreatic cancer cases (15, 16) demonstrated that JPN-SC reflected the postoperative prognosis much better than UICC-SC (Figs. 50.3 and 50.4). In UICC-SC, the postoperative cumulative survival (PCS) rates were lower in stage II than in stage III, and there were no significant differences between the two stages. UICC-SC tends to classify patients in a less advanced stage (20). To decide which stage classification best reflects the prognosis of pancreatic carcinoma, it is necessary to evaluate the staging criteria separately.

**TABLE 50.1. UICC Stage Classification**

| | | | |
|---|---|---|---|
| Primary tumor (T) | | | |
| TX | Primary tumor cannot be assessed | | |
| T0 | No evidence of primary tumor | | |
| T1 | Tumor limited to the pancreas | | |
| | T1a Tumor 2 cm or less in greatest dimension | | |
| | T1b Tumor more than 2 cm in greatest dimension | | |
| T2 | Tumor extends directly to the duodenum, bile duct, or peripancreatic tissues | | |
| T3 | Tumor extends directly to the stomach, spleen, colon, or adjacent large vessels | | |
| Regional lymph nodes (N) | | | |
| NX | Regional lymph nodes cannot be assessed | | |
| N0 | No regional lymph node metastasis | | |
| N1 | Regional lymph node metastasis | | |
| Distant metastasis (M) | | | |
| MX | Presence of distant metastasis cannot be assessed | | |
| M0 | No distant metastasis | | |
| M1 | Distant metastasis | | |
| Stage grouping | | | |
| Stage I | T1 | N0 | M0 |
| | T2 | N0 | M0 |
| Stage II | T3 | N0 | M0 |
| Stage III | Any T | N1 | M0 |
| Stage IV | Any T | Any N | M1 |

### T Factor

UICC T factor includes both tumor size and local extent of the primary tumor, while Japanese T factor refers to tumor size alone. Our investigation showed that UICC T factor reflected the postoperative prognosis much better than JPN T factor (15, 16).

In UICC, as shown in Figure 50.5, significant differences were observed in the 1-, 3-, and 5-year PCS rates between T1a and T1b, T1a and T2, T1a and T3, T1b and T2, T1b and T3, and T2 and T3. However in JPN, the 3-year and 5-year PCS rates of T2 and T3 were lower than those of T4 (Fig. 50.6). Only in cases with a tumor smaller than 2 cm (JPN T1) were 1-, 3-, and 5-year survival rates also significantly better than those of cases with cancers larger than 2 cm (JPN T2, T3, T4) in the studies of Tsuchiya et al. (21) and Yamamoto et al. (18). Therefore, it is reasonable to divide tumor size into two grades, namely, one smaller than and one larger than 2 cm. However, Tsuchiya et al. (22) reported that even among 106 patients with tumors smaller than 2 cm, only 44% belonged to stage I, which means no local extension of the tumor; 14% belonged to stage III or IV because of lymph node metastases (30%), capsular invasion (20%), or retroperitoneal invasion (12%) in JPN-SC; and 13 (28.8%) of 45 stage I patients died of tumor recurrence after operation. This fact and the superiority of UICC T factor suggest that tumor size and local extent of the primary tumor should be evaluated as one staging factor (T factor).

Table 50.7 shows the PCS rates by S, RP, and PV factors in JPN-SC (16). There were significant differences in the PCS rates between S0 and the other grades of S factor. However, no significant differences were observed in 3-year and 5-year PCS rates between S1 and S2, or S2 and S3. Significant differences were observed in the 1-, 3-, and 5-year PCS rates between RP0

**TABLE 50.2. JPN Stage Classification**[a]

| | | | | | | |
|---|---|---|---|---|---|---|
| Stage I | T1 (0–2 cm) | S0 | RP0 | PV0 | N0 | M0 |
| Stage II | T2 (2.1–4.0 cm) | S1 | RP1 | PV1 | N1 | M0 |
| Stage III | T3 (4.1–6.0 cm) | S2 | RP2 | PV2 | N2 | M0 |
| Stage IV | T4 (>6.1 cm) | S3 | RP3 | PV3 | N3 | M1 |

[a]T, size of tumor; S, serosal invasion; RP, retroperitoneal invasion; PV, invasion to portal venous sytem; S0, RP0, PV0, absence of invasion; S1, RP1, PV1, suspected invasion; S2, RP2, PV2, definite invasion; S3, RP3, PV3, severe invasion; N, lymph node metastasis (N0: no lymph node involvement; N1, involvement of primary group of lymph nodes situated closely to the tumor; N2, involvement of secondary group of lymph nodes between N1 and N3; N3, involvement of tertiary group of lymph nodes regarded as juxtaregional lymph nodes); M0, no distant metastasis; M1, distant metastasis including hepatic metastasis or peritoneal dissemination.

and the other grades of RP factor, and between RP1 and RP3, and RP2 and RP3. Only between RP1 and RP2 was no significant difference observed. There were significant differences in 1-, 3-, and 5-year PCS rates between PV0 and the other levels of PV factor, in 1-year and 5-year PCS rates between PV1 and PV3, and in 1-year PCS rates between PV2 and PV3. However, no significant differences were observed between PV1 and PV2. These results indicate that RP and PV factors are extremely

**TABLE 50.3. Regional Lymph Nodes and Their Station Numbers**

| | |
|---|---|
| 1 | Right cardial lymph nodes |
| 2 | Left cardial lymph nodes |
| 3 | Lymph nodes along the lesser curvature of the stomach |
| 4 | Lymph nodes along the greater curvature of the stomach |
| 5 | Suprapyloric lymph nodes |
| 6 | Infrapyloric lymph nodes |
| 7 | Lymph nodes along the left gastric artery |
| 8 | Lymph nodes along the common hepatic artery |
| 8a | Anterosuperior group |
| 8p | Posterior group |
| 9 | Lymph nodes around the celiac artery |
| 10 | Lymph nodes at the splenic hilum |
| 11 | Lymph nodes along the splenic artery |
| 12 | Lymph nodes in the hepatoduodenal ligament |
| 12h | Lymph nodes of the hepatic hilum (porta hepatis) |
| 12a | Lymph nodes along the hepatic artery |
| 12a1 | Upper-half group |
| 12a2 | Lower-half group |
| 12p | Lymph nodes behind the portal vein |
| 12p1 | Upper-half group |
| 12p2 | Lower-half group |
| 12b | Lymph nodes along the bile duct |
| 12b1 | Upper-half group |
| 12b2 | Lower-half group |
| 12c | Lymph nodes at the cystic duct |
| 13 | Lymph nodes on the posterior surface of the pancreatic head |
| 13a | Upper-half group |
| 13b | Lower-half group |
| 14 | Lymph nodes at the root of the mesentery |
| 14A | Lymph nodes along the superior mesenteric artery |
| 14a | Lymph nodes at the origin of the superior mesenteric artery |
| 14b | Lymph nodes at the origin of the inferior pancreaticoduodenal artery |
| 14c | Lymph nodes at the origin of the middle colic artery |
| 14d | Lymph nodes at the origin of the first jejunal branch of the superior mesenteric artery |
| 14V | Lymph nodes along the superior mesenteric vein |
| 15 | Lymph nodes along the middle colic vessels |
| 16 | Lymph nodes around the abdominal aorta |
| 16a1 | Lymph nodes around the abdominal aorta in the esophageal hiatus of the diaphragm |
| 16a2 | Lymph nodes around the abdominal aorta (from the upper margin of the celiac trunk to the lower margin of the left renal vein) |
| 16b1 | Lymph nodes around the abdominal aorta (from the lower margin of the left renal vein to the upper margin of the inferior mesenteric artery) |
| 16b2 | Lymph nodes around the abdominal aorta (from the upper margin of the inferior mesenteric artery to the aortic bifurcation) |
| 17 | Lymph nodes on the anterior surface of the pancreatic head |
| 17a | Upper-half group |
| 17b | Lower-half group |
| 18 | Lymph nodes along the inferior margin of the pancreas |

**TABLE 50.4. Grouping and Lymph Node Designations According to Tumor Location**

| | Tumor Location | |
|---|---|---|
| **Group** | **Head of the Pancreas** | **Body and Tail of the Pancreas** |
| Primary group (N1) | 6, 8a, 8p, 12a2, 12b2, 12p2, 13a, 13b, 14a, 14b, 14c, 14d, 14V, 17a, 17b | 8a, 8p, 9, 10, 11, 14a, 14b, 14c, 14d, 14V, 18 |
| Secondary group (N2) | 9, 11, 12a1, 12b1, 12p1, 12c, 15, 16a1, 16a2, 16b1, 16b2, 18 | 7, 12a2, 12b2, 12p2, 13a, 13b, 15, 16a1, 16a2, 16b1, 16b2, 17a |
| Tertiary group (N3) | 1, 2, 3, 4, 5, 7, 10, 12h, and others more distant | 1, 2, 3, 4, 5, 6, 12a1, 12b1, 12p1, 12c, 12h, and others more distant |

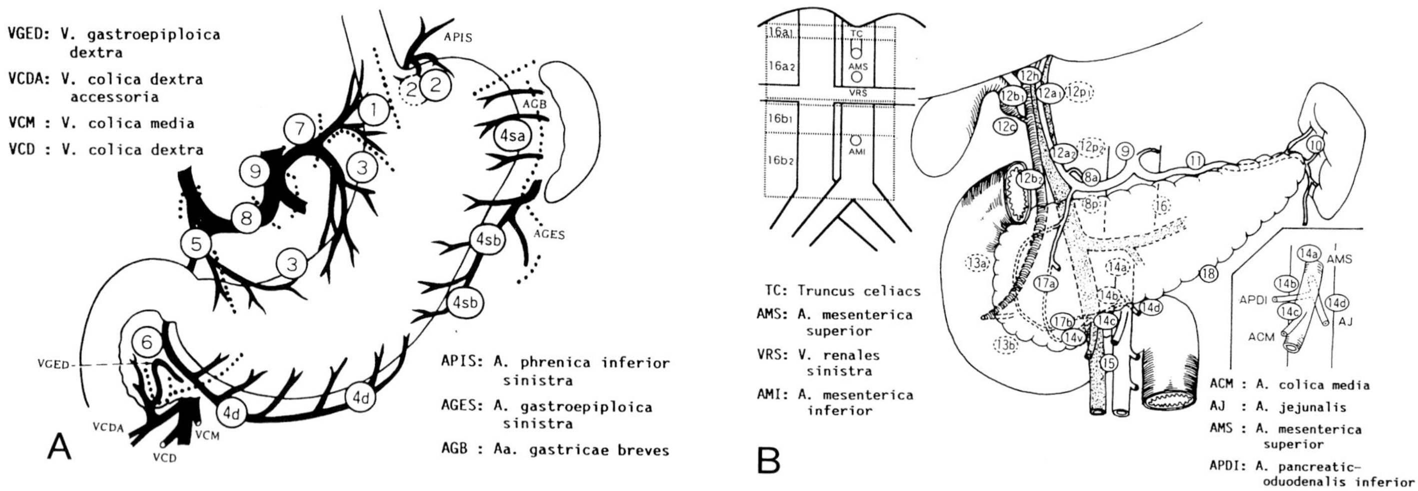


**FIG. 50.2.** **A** and **B.** Regional lymph nodes and their station numbers in JPN-SC. Table 50.3 provides an explanation.

**TABLE 50.5. New JPN Stage Classification**

Primary tumor (T)

| | |
|---|---|
| T1a | TS1 & S0 & RP0 & PV0 & A0 & DU0 & CH0, 1 |
| T1b | TS2, 3, 4 & S0 & RP0 & PV0 & A0 & DU0 & CH0, 1 |
| T2 | Any TS &/or S1 &/or RP1 &/or PV1 &/or A1 &/or DU1, 2, 3 &/or CH2, 3 |
| T3 | Any TS &/or S2, 3 &/or RP2, 3 &/or PV2, 3 &/or A2, 3 |

Regional lymph nodes (N)

| | |
|---|---|
| N0 | No lymph node metastasis |
| N1 | Metastasis to primary group of lymph nodes situated closely to the tumor |
| N2 | Metastasis to secondary group of lymph nodes between N1 and N3 |
| N3 | Metastasis to tertiary group of lymph nodes regarded as juxtaregional lymph nodes |

Distant metastasis (M)

| | |
|---|---|
| M0 | No distant metastasis |
| M1 | Positive distant metastasis including peritoneal dissemination (P) or hepatic metastasis (H) |

New stage grouping

| | | | |
|---|---|---|---|
| Stage I | T1a | N0 | M0 |
| Stage II | T1a | N1 | M0 |
| | T1b, | N0, N1 | M0 |
| Stage III | T1a, T1b | N2 | M0 |
| | T2 | N0, N1, | M0 |
| Stage IVa | T1a, T1b | N3 | M0 |
| | T2 | N2 | M0 |
| | T3 | N0, N1 | M0 |
| Stage IVb | T2 | N3 | M0 |
| | T3 | N2, N3 | M0 |
| | Any T | Any N | M1 |

<table>
<tr><td rowspan="2"></td><td colspan="4">M0, P0, H0</td><td rowspan="2">M1 or P1,2,3 or H1,2,3</td></tr>
<tr><td>N0</td><td>N1</td><td>N2</td><td>N3</td></tr>
<tr><td>T1a</td><td>I</td><td>II</td><td>III</td><td rowspan="2">IVa</td><td rowspan="4">IVb</td></tr>
<tr><td>T1b</td><td>II</td><td>II</td><td>III</td></tr>
<tr><td>T2</td><td>III</td><td>III</td><td>IVa</td><td rowspan="2">IVb</td></tr>
<tr><td>T3</td><td colspan="2">IVa</td><td>IVb</td></tr>
</table>

**TABLE 50.6. New Grouping and Lymph Node Designations According to Tumor Location**

| Group/Tumor Site | Head of the Pancreas | Body and Tail of the Pancreas |
|---|---|---|
| Primary group (N1) | 6, 8a, 8p, 12a2, 12b2, 12p2, 13a, 13b, 14b, 14c, 14d, 14V, 17a, 17b | 8a, 8p, 9, 10, 11, 18 |
| Secondary group (N2) | 9, 11, 12a1, 12b1, 12c, 12p1, 14a, 15, 16a2, 16b1, 18 | 7, 12a2, 12b2, 13a, 13b, 14a, 14b, 14c, 14d, 14V, 15, 16a2, 16b1, 17a, 17b |
| Tertiary group (N3) | 1, 2, 3, 4, 5, 7, 10, 12h, 16a1, 16b2 | 1, 2, 3, 4, 5, 6, 12a1, 12b1, 12c, 12h, 12p1, 16a1, 16b2 |

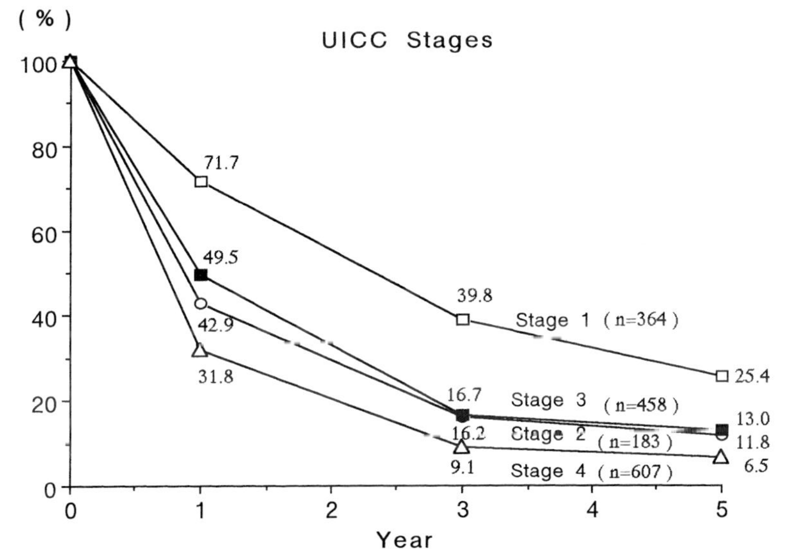


**FIG. 50.3.** Cumulative survival after resectional surgery according to the UICC-stage classification. No significant differences are present in the PCS rates between stages II and III. (Data adapted from Tsunoda T, Eto T, Tsuchiya R. Clinical comparison of UICC and Japanese classifications. Japanese experience. Int J Pancreatol 1994;16(1):105–108.)

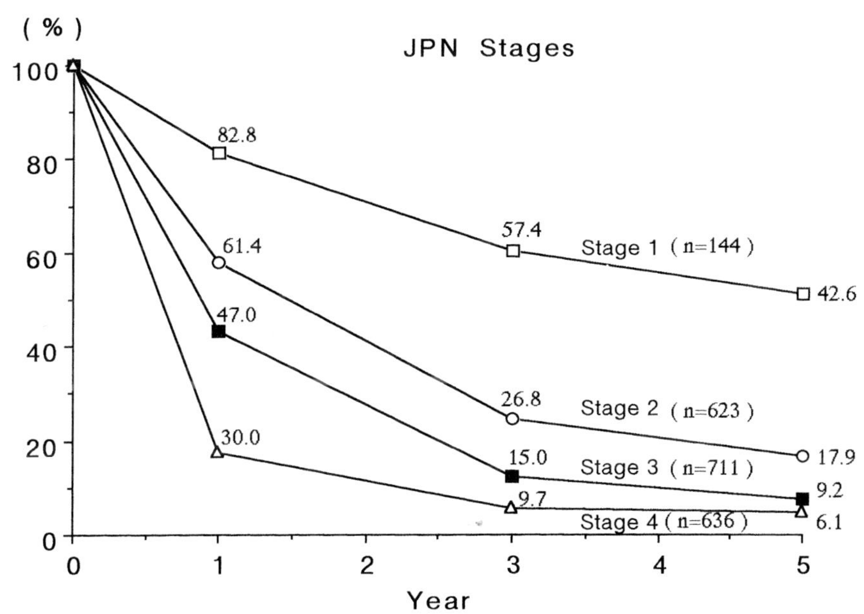


**FIG. 50.4.** Cumulative survival after resectional surgery according to the Japanese stage classification. There are significant differences in the 1-, 3-, and 5-year PCS rates between stages I and II, between I and III, between I and IV, between II and III, and between II and IV ($p < .01$), and in the 1-year and 3-year PCS rates between stages III and IV ($p < .05$). (Data adapted from Tsundoa T, Eto T, Tsuchiya R. Clinical comparison of UICC and Japanese classifications. Japanese experience. Int J Pancreatol 1994;16(1): 105–108.

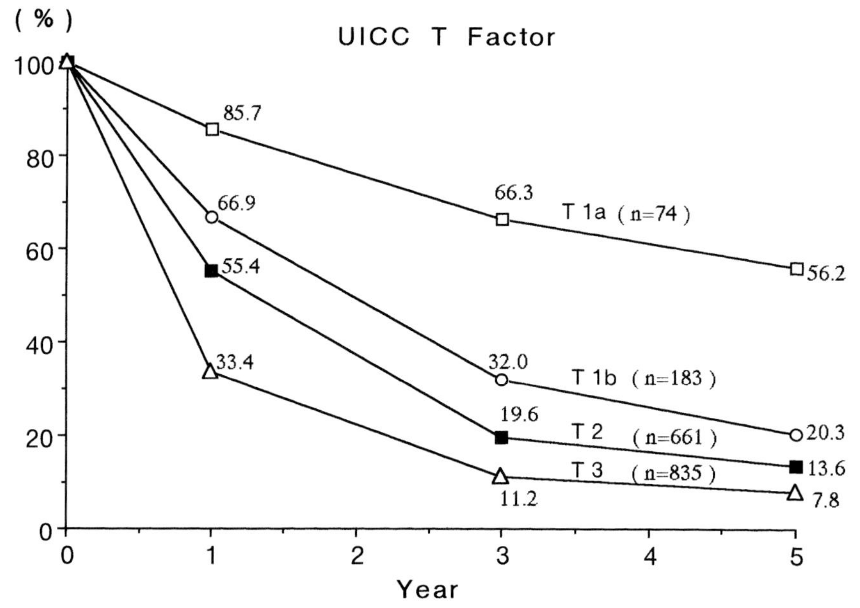


**FIG. 50.5.** Cumulative survival after resectional surgery according to T factor by UICC-SC. Significant differences are observed in the 1-, 3-, and 5-year PCS rates between *T1a* and *T1b*, between *T1a* and *T2*, between *T1a* and *T3*, between *T1b* and *T2*, between *T1b* and *T3*, and between *T2* and *T3* ($p < .01$). (Data adapted from Tsun oda T, Eto T, Tsuchiya R. Staging of pancreatic cancer. A new Japanese stage classification based on TNM factors. In: Beger HG, Warshaw AL, Carr-Locke D, Russell C, Büchler M, et al., eds. The pancreas: a clinical textbook. Oxford, England: Blackwell Scientific Publications, 1996 (in press).)

important for the evaluation of the local extent of the primary tumor, a fact already shown in earlier reports (20, 23).

To evaluate tumor size and local extent factors as one staging factor, as in UICC-SC, we examined the combination of gradings of both tumor size (JPN T factor) and S, RP, and PV factors in the cases without lymph node metastasis (16), because lymph node metastasis may exert an influence on the results of S, RP, and PV factors as an independent prognostic factor. The combination was constructed as shown in Figure 50.7. Except between D and E, each group was clearly separated from the others. In other words, the distinctions among tumors smaller than 2 cm with no invasion (A), tumors larger than 2 cm with no invasion (B), tumors of all sizes with suspected invasion (C), and tumors of all sizes with definite invasion (D) are useful for staging the disease, while the distinction between definite invasion (D) and severe invasion (E) is not useful for staging the disease. The results indicate, therefore, that it is appropriate to arrange the grading of local extent factors into three grades: no invasion, suspected invasion, and positive invasion; also a tumor 2 cm or smaller has a significantly better prognosis after resection than a tumor larger than 2 cm, as long as the tumor does not invade the serosa, the retroperitoneum, or the portal venous system. The

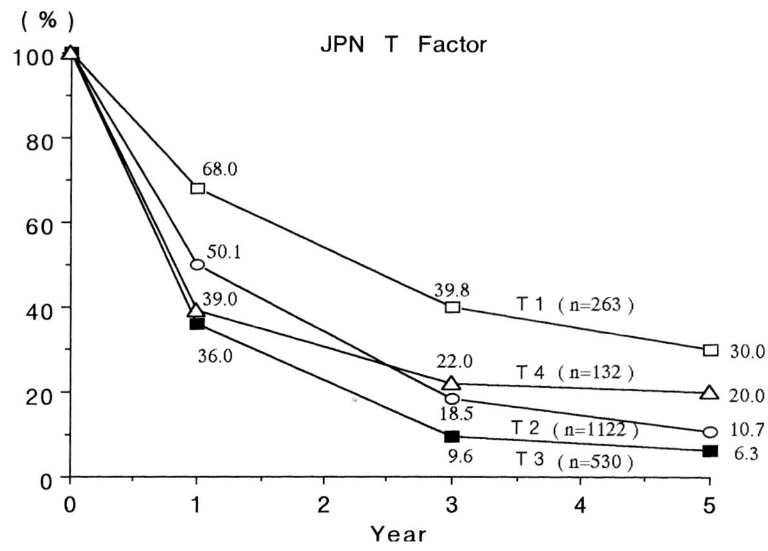


**FIG. 50.6.** Cumulative survival after resectional surgery according to T factor (tumor size) by JPN-SC. The 3-year and 5-year PCS rates of *T2* and *T3* were lower than those of *T4*. (Data adapted from Tsunoda T, Eto T, Tsuchiya R. Clinical comparison of UICC and Japanese classifications. Japanese experience. Int J Pancreatol;1994;16(1):105–108.)

**TABLE 50.7. PCS Rates by Local Extent Factors in JPN-SC**

| Local Extent Factors | | Number of Cases | PCS Rates (%) 1-year | 3-year | 5-year |
|---|---|---|---|---|---|
| S factor | S0 | 1017 | 60.3 | 29.9 | 20.7 |
| | S1 | 432 | 42.2 | 9.9 | 4.9 |
| | S2 | 450 | 35.0 | 8.2 | 4.7 |
| | S3 | 172 | 30.0 | 9.7 | 6.1 |
| RP factor | RP0 | 973 | 59.8 | 28.0 | 18.7 |
| | RP1 | 431 | 43.2 | 15.2 | 10.7 |
| | RP2 | 383 | 38.0 | 14.0 | 9.5 |
| | RP3 | 149 | 26.0 | 5.2 | 2.6 |
| PV factor | PV0 | 1130 | 58.5 | 26.6 | 18.2 |
| | PV1 | 339 | 40.8 | 11.0 | 8.6 |
| | PV2 | 396 | 38.0 * | 13.0 | 7.1 * |
| | PV3 | 223 | 29.0 | 9.4 | 2.7 |

From Tsunoda T, Eto T, Tsuchiya R. Staging of pancreatic cancer. A new Japanese stage classification based on TNM factors. In: Beger HG, Warshaw AL, Carr-Locke D, Russell C, Büchler M, et al., eds. The pancreas: a clinical textbook. Oxford, England: Blackwell Scientific Publications, 1996 (in press).

⊐ $p < .01$

⊐* $p < .05$

category of "suspected invasion" should be evaluated macro- and microscopically in the future.

The DU and CH factors used in the new JPN T factor were evaluated, and the PCS rates are shown in Table 50.8. The 1-, 3-, and 5-year PCS rates of DU0 and CH0, CH1 were similar to those of S0, RP0, and PV0, and those of DU1, DU2, DU3, and CH2, CH3 were similar to those of S1, RP1, and PV1. DU and CH factors were not always superior to S, RP, PV factors.

## N Factors

Lymph node metastasis is considered to be an independent prognostic factor. Figure 50.8 shows the PCS curves and rates by UICC N factor (16). Significant differences were observed between N0 and N1. Figure 50.9 shows the PCS curves and rates by JPN N factor (16). Significant differences were observed in the 1-, 3-, and 5-year PCS rates between N0 and the other grades of N factor and between N1 and N3, and in the 1-year and 3-year PCS rates between N1 and N2, and N2 and N3. As shown in Table 50.9, the rates of pathologic metastasis to the lymph nodes according to Japanese staging of regional lymph nodes ranges from 4.4% to 36% in the primary group (N1), 2.2% to 18% in the secondary group (N2), and 1.1% to 2.9% in the tertiary group (N3). In the secondary group, a high metastatic rate (18.7%) was found in the 16th lymph node (paraaortic node)

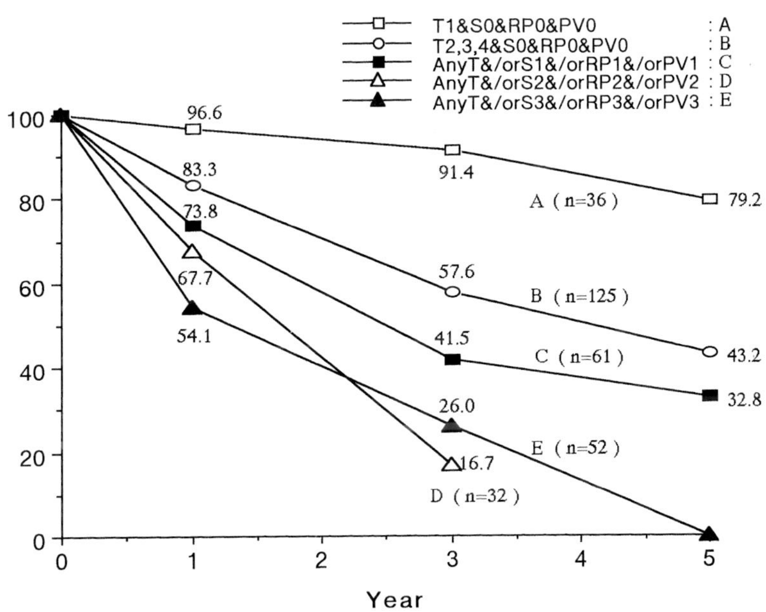


**FIG. 50.7.** Cumulative survival after resectional surgery according to the combination of gradings of both tumor size and local extent factors by JPN-SC. There are significant differences in the 1-, 3-, and 5-year PCS rates between *A* and *B*, between *A* and *C*, between *A* and *D*, between *A* and *E*, between *B* and *C*, between *B* and *D*, between *B* and *E*, between *C* and *D*, and between *C* and *E* ($p < .01$), but no signigficant diferences in the PCS rates between *D* and *E*. (Data adapted from Tsunoda T, Eto T, Tsuchiya R. Staging of pancreatic cancer. A new Japanese stage classification based on TNM factors. In: Beger HG, Warshaw AL, Carr-Locke D, Russell C, Büchler M, et al., eds. The pancreas: a clinical textbook. Oxford, England: Blackwell Scientific Publications, 1996 (in press).)

**TABLE 50.8. PCS Rates by JPN DU and CH Factors**

| Local Extent Factors | | Number of Cases | PCS Rates (%) 1-year | 3-year | 5-year |
|---|---|---|---|---|---|
| DU factor | DU0 | 1117 | 54.0 | 24.0 | 18.7 |
| | DU1 | 292 | 44.3 | 14.7 | 7.6 |
| | DU2 | 342 | 45.3 | 15.3 | 11.2 |
| | DU3 | 445 | 40.6 | 15.0 | 7.2 |
| CH factor | CH0 | 1160 | 57.6 | 31.7 | 23.7 |
| | CH1 | 390 | 57.0 | 20.0 | 11.4 |
| | CH2 | 422 | 49.4 | 16.3 | 11.6 |
| | CH3 | 627 | 46.5 | 12.9 | 7.1 |

From Tsunoda T, Eto T, Tsuchiya R. Staging of pancreatic cancer. A new Japanese stage classification based on TNM factors. In: Beger HG, Warshaw AL, Carr-Locke D, Russell C, Büchler M, et al., eds. The pancreas: a clinical textbook. Oxford, England: Blackwell Scientific Publications, 1996 (in press).
⊐ $p < .01$
⊐* $p < .05$

(16). In terms of N factors, the four grades of JPN factor reflected the prognosis much more accurately than the all-or-nothing approach of UICC N factor.

The grading of lymph node involvement was also extremely important from the standpoint of surgical treatment of the disease. Even when nodal involvement is observed in the primary group (N1) macro- and microscopically, complete clearance of both the primary (N1) and secondary (N2) groups (R2 operations) has contributed greatly to long-term survival after surgery (24–26).

## M Factor

Carcinomas with distant metastases have a poorer prognosis than those with severe local extension; that is, M factor is an independent prognostic factor (17, 18, 20). Saitoh analyzed the data of the Japan Pancreatic Cancer Registry over a period of 10 years and reported that the prognosis of 5648 patients without distant metastasis was better than that of 912 patients with distant metastasis in JPN-SC (17). Yamamoto et al. also analyzed the PCS rates of patients who underwent resection according to M factor, as proposed by UICC, and found a significant difference between M0 and M1 (18). In our small series of resected cases, no M1 patient survived longer than 7 months (20).

Tsuchiya et al. (25) reported with regard to postoperative cumulative survival in patients undergoing R2 operation with and without portal vein resection according to the extent of lymph node metastasis; no patient survived longer than 2 years in the tertiary group (N3). The metastasis in the tertiary group (N3) may be considered distant metastasis (M1).

## Stage Grouping

The evaluation of the local extent of tumor is one of the major differences between UICC-SC and JPN-SC. In UICC-SC, even if a primary tumor involves adjacent organs or large vessels, the tumor is allocated to stage I or II when nodal and distant metastases are absent. In JPN-SC, the patients with these local conditions (RP2, RP3, PV2, PV3, and/or S2, S3) are assigned to stage II or IV. When definite and extensive portal vein invasion is present, for example, the tumor is usually unresectable unless the portal vein is also resected. Definite local spreading such as PV2, PV3, RP2, RP3, and S2, S3, therefore, should be classified into

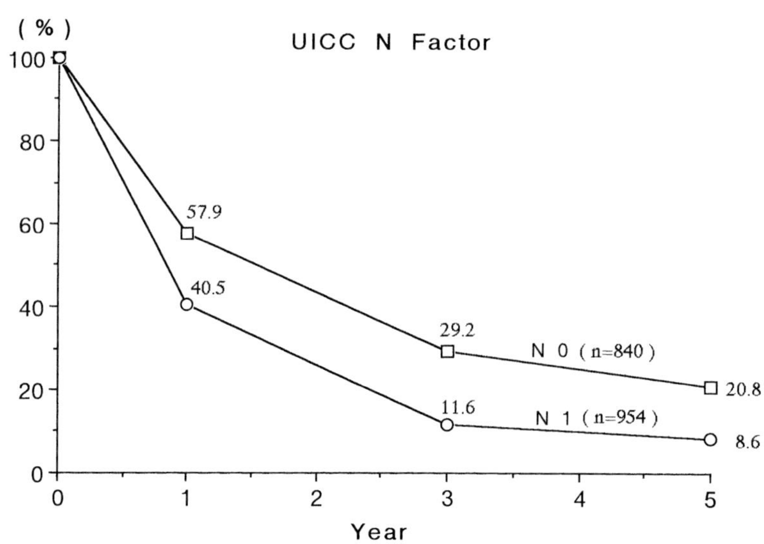


**FIG. 50.8.** Cumulative survival after resectional surgery according to N factor by UICC-SC. Significant differences are observed between *N0* and *N1*. (Data adapted from Tsunoda T, Eto T, Tsuchiya R. Staging of pancreatic cancer. A new Japanese stage classification based on TNM factors. In: Beger HG, Warshaw AL, Carr-Locke D, Russell C, Büchler M, et al., eds. The pancreas: a clinical textbook. Oxford, England: Blackwell Scientific Publications, 1996 (in press).)

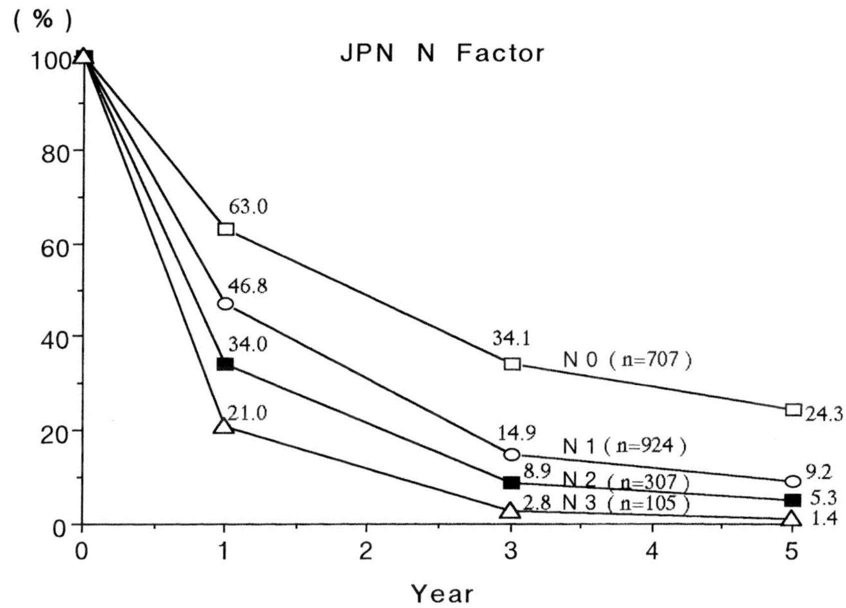


**FIG. 50.9.** Cumulative survival after resectional surgery according to N factor by JPN-SC. There are significant differences in the 1-, 3-, and 5-year PCS rates between N0 and N1, between N0 and N2, between *N0* and *N3* and between *N1* and *N3* ($p < .01$), and in the 1-year and 3 -year PCS rates between *N1* and *N2*, and *N2* and *N3* ($p < .05$). (Data adapted from Tsunoda T, Eto T, Tsuchiya R. Staging of pancreatic cancer. A new Japanese stage classification based on TNM factors. In: Beger HG, Warshaw AL, Carr-Locke D, Russell C, Büchler M, et al., eds. The pancreas: a clinical textbook. Oxford, England: Blackwell Scientific Publications, 1996 (in press).)

the most advanced stage. In JPN-SC, the local extent of tumor, is divided into three grades: no invasion, suspected invasion, and positive invasion.

Lymph node metastasis is as important as local extent of the tumor, and the Japanese grading system was shown to provide a more exact classification. With regard to stage grouping in UICC-SC, positive regional lymph node metastasis is the most important factor in the definition of stage II, regardless of local tumor growth. In UICC-SC, the underestimation of local tumor growth (T factor) and the overestimation of lymph node metastasis (N factor) resulted in the reversal of the results in stage II and III.

The Japan Pancreas Society has proposed a new JPN-SC based on TNM factors defined from the detailed analysis of a large series of resected pancreatic cancer cases (Table 50.5).

## IMPROVEMENT OF STAGE CLASSIFICATION

Since the JPN-SC and the new JPN-SC are more complex than the UICC-SC, the seven parameters (TS, S, RP, PV, *A*, CH, and

**TABLE 50.9. Rates of Pathologic Metastasis to Regional Lymph Nodes in Resected Cases of Carcinoma of the Head of the Pancreas**

| Primary Group (N1) | | | Secondary Group (N2) | | | Tertiary Group (N3) | | |
|---|---|---|---|---|---|---|---|---|
| No.[a] | % | Metastatic Cases/ Examined Cases | No. | % | Metastatic Cases/ Examined Cases | No. | % | Metastatic Cases/ Examined Cases |
| 6 | 7.7 | 126/1633 | 9 | 5.0 | 54/1073 | 1 | 1.6 | 6/383 |
| 8a | 9.6 | 97/1006 | 11 | 7.1 | 65/912 | 2 | 2.4 | 4/168 |
| 8p | 9.6 | 49/816 | 12a1 | 2.7 | 29/1086 | 3 | 2.2 | 28/1261 |
| 12a2 | 4.4 | 60/1353 | 12b1 | 3.7 | 41/1111 | 4 | 1.1 | 15/1402 |
| 12b2 | 10.5 | 163/1559 | 12p1 | 2.2 | 23/1257 | 5 | 2.0 | 26/1314 |
| 12p2 | 6.0 | 84/1404 | 12c | 2.2 | 27/1257 | 7 | 2.8 | 32/1144 |
| 13a | 36.0 | 664/1846 | 15 | 6.5 | 45/694 | 10 | 2.1 | 8/389 |
| 13b | 28.1 | 472/1678 | 16 | 18.7 | 70/909 | 12h | 2.9 | 20/690 |
| 14a | 15.8 | 217/1373 | 18 | 4.6 | 34/747 | | | |
| 14b | 14.8 | 190/1283 | | | | | | |
| 14c | 9.4 | 106/1131 | | | | | | |
| 14d | 11.0 | 127/1156 | | | | | | |
| 14v | 7.7 | 47/607 | | | | | | |
| 17a | 21.5 | 326/1513 | | | | | | |
| 17b | 19.8 | 279/1468 | | | | | | |

From Tsunoda T, Eto T, Tsuchiya R. Staging of pancreatic cancer. A new Japanese stage classification based on TNM factors. In: Beger HG, Warshaw AL, Carr-Locke D, Russell C, Büchler M, et al., eds. The pancreas: a clinical textbook. Oxford, England: Blackwell Scientific Publications, 1996 (in press).
[a]The lymph node number is described in Table 50.3 and Fig. 50.2, *A* and *B*.

DU) used in the new JPN-SC T factor should be reduced to two or three in the near future. CH and DU factors should be excluded as stated above, and PV and *A* factors may be included in the RP factor and/or S factor.

Among the gradings of N factor in the new JPN-SC, N3 (juxtaregional lymph node metastasis) may be dealt with as distant metastasis (M1); that is, the lymph nodes in the primary (N1) and secondary (N2) groups may be the regional lymph nodes. Continuing efforts are necessary to establish a practical, simple, and universal staging system for the disease.

### Acknowledgments

The authors deeply appreciate the cooperation of Dr. Y. Saitoh, chairman of the Committee on the Pancreatic Cancer Registry, and Dr. M. Yamamoto.

## REFERENCES

1. Axtell LM, Culter SJ, Myers MH, eds. Biometry Branch, National Cancer Institute. End results in cancer. Report no. 4, publ. no. 73-272. U.S. Department of Health, Education and Welfare, End Results Section, 1972:81–84.
2. Cubilla AL, Fitzgerald PJ, Fortner JG. Pancreas cancer–duct cell adenocarcinoma: survival in relation to site, size, stage, and type of therapy. J Surg Oncol 1978;10:465–482.
3. Hermreck AS, Thomas CY, Friesen SR. Importance of pathologic staging in the surgical management of adenocarcinoma of the exocrine pancreas. Am J Surg 1974;127:653–657.
4. Leadbetter A, Foster RS Jr, Haines, CR. Carcinoma of the pancreas, results from the Vermont Tumor Registry. Am J Surg 1975;129:356–360.
5. Klöppel G, Sosnowski J, Eichfuss HP, Rückert K, Klapdor R. Akutuelle Aspecte des Pankreas Karzinoms, klinische und Morphologische Andlysen zur Diagnostik und Therapie. Dtsch Med Wochenschr 1979;104:1801–1805.
6. Klöppel G, Lingenthal G, Vorbülow M, Kern HF. Histological and fine structural features of pancreatic ductal adenocarcinomas in relation to growth and prognosis: studies in xenografted tumours and clinico-histological correlation in a series of 75 cases. Histopathology 1985;9:841–856.
7. Cubilla AL, Fitzgerald PJ. Classification of pancreatic cancer (non endocrine). Mayo Clin Proc 1989;54:449–458.
8. Cubilla AL, Fortner J, Fitzgerald PJ. Lymph node involvement in carcinoma of the head of the pancreas area. Cancer 1978;41: 880–887.
9. Fortner JG. Regional pancreatectomy for cancer of the pancreas, ampulla, and other related sites. Tumor staging and results. Ann Surg 1984;199:418–425.
10. Deixonne B, Marty-Duble C, Rignodel C. Pathological anatomy. In: Baumel H, Deixonne B, eds. Exocrine pancreatic cancer. New York: Springer-Verlag, 1986:11–45.
11. UICC. TNM classification of malignant tumours. 4th ed. New York: Springer-Verlag, 1987.
12. UICC. TNM atlas. Illustrated guide to the TNM/pTNM classification of malignant tumours. 3rd ed. New York: 1989.
13. Japan Pancreas Society. General rules for surgical and pathological studies on cancer of the pancreas. 3rd ed. Tokyo: Kanehara & Company, 1987 (in Japanese).
14. Japan Pancreas Society. General rules for the study of pancreatic cancer. 4th ed. Tokyo: Kanehara & Company, 1993 (in Japanese).
15. Tsunoda T, Eto T, Tsuchiya R. Clinical comparison of UICC and Japanese classifications. Japanese experience. Int J Pancreatol 1994;16(1):105–108.
16. Tsunoda T, Eto T, Tsuchiya R. Staging of pancreatic cancer. A new Japanese stage classification based on TNM factors. In: Beger HG, Warshaw AL, Carr-Locke D, Russell C, Büchler M, et al. eds. The pancreas: a clinical textbook. Oxford, England: Blackwell Scientific Publications, 1996, in press.
17. Pancreatic Cancer Registration Committee of the Japan Pancreatic Society. Report of nationwide registration of pancreatic cancer patients in 1981–1990; 1991 (in Japanese).
18. Yamamoto M, Saitoh Y. Tumor spread and the factors influencing prognosis in patients with resected pancreatic carcinoma. In: Pour PM, Konishi Y, Klöppel G, Longnecker DS, eds. Atlas of exocrine pancreatic tumors. New York: Springer-Verlag, 1994: 237–246.
19. Yamamoto M, Ohashi O, Ishida H, Kamigaki T, Onoyama H, Saitoh Y. Relationship between survival and cancer extension. Int J Pancreatol 1994;16(1):118–120.
20. Tsunoda T, Ura K, Eto T, Matsumoto T, Tsuchiya R. UICC and Japanese stage classifications for carcinoma of the pancreas. Int J Pancreatol 1991;8(3):205–214.
21. Tsuchiya R, Tsunoda T. Tumor size as a predictive factor, Int J Pancreatol 1990;7(1–3):117–123.
22. Tsuchiya R, Noda T, Harada N, Miyamoto T, Tomioka T, et al. Collective review of small carcinomas of the pancreas. Ann Surg 1986;203(1):77–81.
23. Zerbi A, Balzano G, Bottura R, Di Carlo V. Reliability of pancreatic cancer staging classifications. Int J Pancreatol 1994;15(1): 13–18.
24. Ishikawa O, Ohhigashi H, Sasaki Y, Kabut T, Fukuda I, et al. Practical usefulness of lymphatic and connective tissue clearance of the carcinoma of the pancreas head. Ann Surg 1988;208(2):215–220.
25. Tsuchiya R, Eto T, Tsunoda T. Radical resection of pancreatic and periampullary neoplasms: pancreatoduodenectomy. In: Braasch JW, Tompkins RK, eds. Surgical disease of the biliary tract and pancreas. St. Louis: CV Mosby, 1994:570–587.
26. Ishikawa O, Ohhigashi H, Nakamori S, Imaoka S. Mode of pancreatic cancer extension and operative curability. Int J Pancreatol 1994;16(1):108–109.

# 51

# *Other Prognostic Factors*

William H. Smith-Mensah and David C. Allison

***Mortality can be defined as one per person.***
G. E. Block, M.D.

Professor Block's comment should be weighed carefully when one considers the use of "prognostic factors" to guide the therapy of patients with pancreatic carcinoma, because the presently available tests provide only statistical inferences and not an absolute prognosis for a given patient. We believe that the possible merits of any new prognostic factors for improving the care of pancreatic cancer patients should be evaluated carefully in prospective clinical protocols before widespread use.

Pancreatic carcinomas often have abnormalities in tumor suppressor genes and oncogenes that are commonly altered in other cancers. For example, the K-*ras* gene is mutated in ≈80% of pancreatic adenocarcinomas, and K-*ras* mutations are thought to be an important early step in pancreatic carcinogenesis (1, 2). Because most pancreatic carcinomas have K-*ras* mutations, this genetic abnormality does not provide independent prognostic information when compared with tumor size, DNA content, and lymph node metastases (2) (Allison et al., unpublished data). However, K-*ras* mutations can be screened with relatively inexpensive assays of DNA fragments from exfoliated cells in stool specimens, and this assay may be of value in the differentiation of chronic pancreatitis from pancreatic carcinoma and in the detection of early-stage pancreatic carcinomas (3).

Other oncogenes and tumor suppressor genes are commonly altered in pancreatic carcinoma: 40–70% of pancreatic carcinomas have abnormalities in the p53 gene (4–6), ≈48% in the *HER-2/neu* gene (7), ≈38% in the *EGF/EGFR* genes (8), 50% in the *DDC* gene (9, 10), 85% in the *MTSI* gene (11), 40% in the *APC* gene (12), and 20% in the *erb B-2* gene (13). Mutations or losses in some of these genes may be specific prognostic determinants for pancreatic cancer patients, although relatively few studies have been carried out to date to evaluate this possibility. This field is evolving rapidly, and it is probable that combinations of specific mutations or losses of certain oncogenes and/or tumor suppressor genes will eventually prove to be useful both in screening tests and as prognostic factors for pancreatic carcinoma.

Assays of tumor genetic heterogeneity are based upon the theory that cancers with substantial variability in their DNA from cell to cell are farther along a genetic evolution toward incurable disease than are tumors with more ordered genomes. In one assay of genetic heterogeneity, tumor DNA is treated with restriction enzymes to allow an estimate of the fraction of each of the chromosomal arms that have lost, or altered, DNA ("fraction of allelic loss," FAL). The FAL assay has been shown to provide independent prognostic information for colorectal carcinomas (14), and a preliminary study suggests that pancreatic cancer patients whose tumors had low FALs had prolonged survivals, compared with patients with high-FAL pancreatic carcinomas (15).

Measurements of DNA content also give estimates of tumor genetic heterogeneity (16–18). Nonproliferating cells rest in the $G_0$ phase of the cell cycle and begin preparation for DNA synthesis in the $G_1$ phase, after receipt of the appropriate molecular signals from the microenvironment. $G_0$- and $G_1$-phase cells have identical DNA contents and appear as a single "$G_0/G_1$ peak" in a standard DNA distribution (Fig. 51.1*A*). The DNA content of a tumor's $G_0/G_1$ peak determines whether it has diploid or aneuploid DNA content. The term *diploid* describes the DNA content of noncancerous $G_0/G_1$ cells. Each of these cells contains a pair of the normal 23 human chromosomes, having received a complete haploid chromosome set from both parents. Diploid $G_0/G_1$ cells have 7 pg of DNA per cell and are assigned a *DNA index* value of 1. Cancers often have *aneuploid* DNA contents, which means that such tumors have abnormal numbers and types of chromosomes in their $G_0/G_1$ cells. The DNA indices of aneuploid cancers are calculated by dividing the DNA contents of the $G_0/G_1$ cancer cells by the DNA contents of the diploid, noncancerous $G_0/G_1$ cells in the tumor stroma (Fig. 51.1*B*). By definition, aneuploid cancers have DNA indices other than 1, usually ranging between 1 and 2.

It has been postulated that aneuploid cancers are more aggressive than diploid cancers because their unbalanced chromosome numbers cause uneven chromosomal segregations into postmitotic daughter cells, leading to increased heterogeneity of chromosome type and number in aneuploid tumor cell populations. It is postulated that more aggressive cancer cells will rapidly appear in dividing aneuploid cells because of the random combinations of different genetic elements produced with each division. These more aggressive aneuploid cells will be, in turn, positively selected for their increased growth rates, abilities to invade and metastasize, etc.

This theory is, however, only partially correct. The behavior of a given cancer is not governed completely by its DNA content. In the case of pancreatic carcinomas, some patients with diploid tumors rapidly die of progressive disease. Also, a few patients with small aneuploid cancers have been observed to survive for more than 5 years after resection, although all patients with aneuploid pancreatic cancers observed to date in our series of 96 patients have eventually succumbed to recurrent cancer (Allison et al., unpublished data). Recent evidence suggests that the

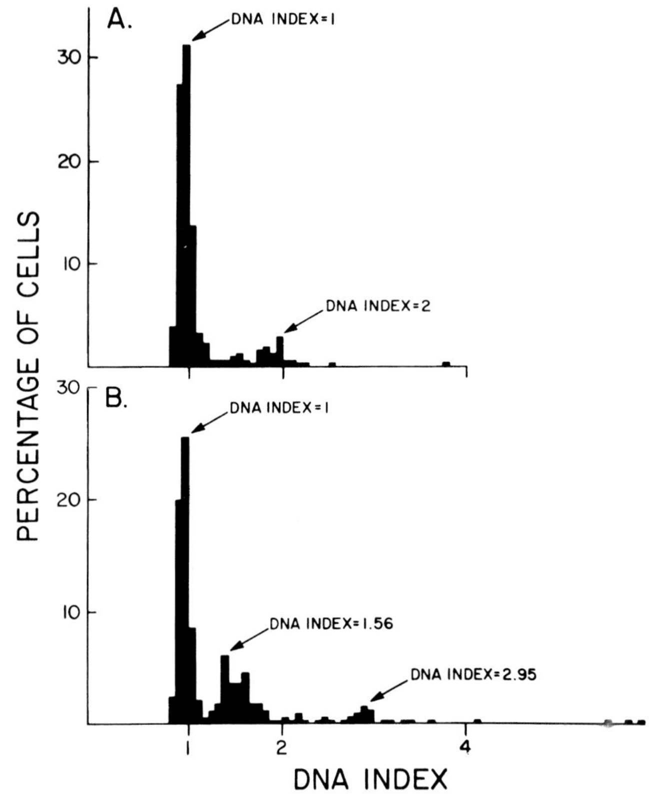


**FIG. 51.1.** DNA distributions of two pancreatic tumors. **A.** This tumor was diploid (DNA index = 1), with a PI of 16%. **B.** This tumor contains both diploid cells (DNA index = 1) and an aneuploid tumor stem line (DNA index = 1.56), with a PI of 27%. Patient B died of progressive pancreatic cancer 12 months after resection, whereas patient A, the patient with the diploid cancer, remains tumor free 4 years after resection. (From Allison DC, Bose KK, Hruban RH, et al. Pancreatic cancer cell DNA content correlates with long-term survival after pancreatoduodenectomy. Ann Surg 1991;214:648. Reproduced with permission.)

genetic stability of cancers may also be governed by mutations, or losses, of p53 and other genes (4, 6).

DNA measurements also provide estimates of a cancer's cell cycle distribution, or the percentages of tumor cells in the $G_0/G_1$, S, and $G_2/M$ phases of the cell cycle. Following the $G_0/G_1$ phase, DNA synthesis occurs in S phase. After S phase, chromosome condensation occurs in the $G_2$ phase, followed by mitosis (M). $G_2/M$ cells have exactly twice the DNA content of $G_0/G_1$ cells (Fig. 51.1). For example, the $G_2/M$ DNA peak of diploid cells with a $G_0/G_1$ DNA index of 1 would have a DNA index of 2 (Fig. 51.1*A*). Figure 51.1*B* shows the DNA distribution of an aneuploid pancreatic cancer with a $G_0/G_1$ DNA index of 1.5; it can also be seen that the $G_2/M$ cancer cells have a DNA index of 3.0. The DNA contents of S-phase cells range from the beginning of the $G_0/G_1$ peak to the end of the $G_2/M$ peak. Thus, the DNA content of the diploid S-phase cells is always between 1 and 2 (Fig. 51.1*A*). Similarly, the DNA indices of the S-phase cells of the aneuploid cancer shown in Figure 51.1*B* are between 1.5 and 3.0. Tumors with a high percentage of S-phase and $G_2/M$-phase cells (or tumors with a "high proliferative index," PI) are considered to be growing more rapidly and generally do behave more aggressively than cancers in which relatively more cells are "resting" in the $G_0/G_1$-phase of the cell cycle.

Most DNA measurements are currently made by flow cytometry, an automated method that requires a suspension of single nuclei prepared from solid cancers to be run through a flow cytometer. DNA content can also be measured by image analysis, a method of measuring the Feulgen stain content of individual nuclei fixed onto slides. The Feulgen stain content of each nucleus is directly proportional to its DNA content. Image analysis allows the morphologic selection of cancer cells for DNA measurements and is especially well suited for measuring the DNA content of pancreatic carcinomas (19). This is because pancreatic carcinomas often elicit a dense stroma made up of host fibroblasts, tumor vascular cells, and inflammatory cells. These diploid host cells often outnumber the cancer cells in a given pancreatic carcinoma (Fig. 51.2). Thus, when such cancers are disaggregated for flow cytometry, the flow-cytometric DNA measurements often completely miss the DNA contents of the aneuploid pancreatic cancer cells because of overlap with the more abundant fluorescent signals from the host stromal cells and the debris of tissue disaggregation. For example, Figure 51.3 shows the flow-cytometric (Fig. 51.3*A*) and the image-analysis (Fig. 51.3*B*) DNA distributions of the pancreatic carcinoma depicted in Figure 51.2. The image-analysis DNA distribution clearly shows that there are relatively rare aneuploid cancer cells in this tumor, with a DNA index of 1.7 (Fig. 51.3*B*), whereas the flow-cytometric DNA measurements (Fig. 51.3*A*) completely missed these aneuploid cancer cells because of overlap with more numerous fluorescent signals from stromal cells and debris. Figure 51.4 shows that what clearly seems to be a diploid pancreatic carcinoma by flow cytometry (Fig. 51.4*A*) is actually an aneuploid cancer with a DNA index of 2.3 when measured by image analysis (Fig. 51.4*B*).

In a direct study of the same 30 pancreatic cancers, only 1 cancer was found to be aneuploid by flow cytometry, whereas 21 of the same 30 cancers were found to be aneuploid by image analysis ($p < 1$) (19). The flow-cytometric DNA measurements provided no independent prognostic information, when compared with the image-analysis DNA measurements by multivariate analysis (19). The superiority of image-analysis DNA measurements over flow cytometry for measuring the DNA contents of pancreatic carcinomas and other scirrhous cancers has been

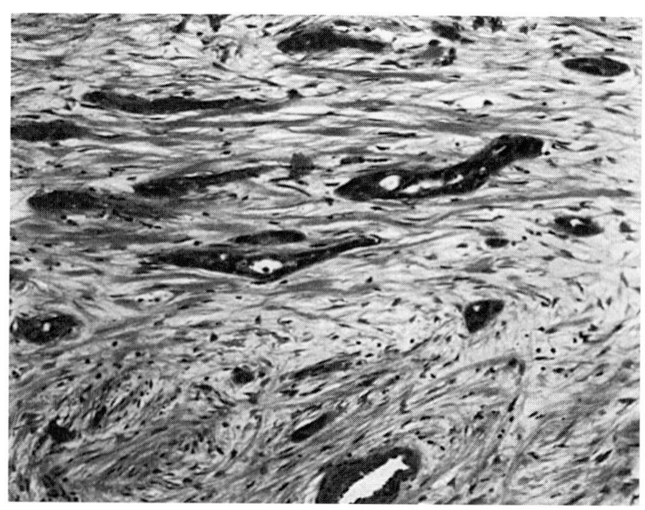

**FIG. 51.2.** Photomicrograph of a pancreatic carcinoma, showing a scirrhous stroma and relatively rare clusters of malignant glands (H & E, original magnification ×200). (From Bose KK, Allison DC, Hruban RH, et al. A comparison of flow cytometric and absorption cytometric DNA values as prognostic indicators for pancreatic carcinoma. Cancer 1993;71:690. Reproduced with permission.)

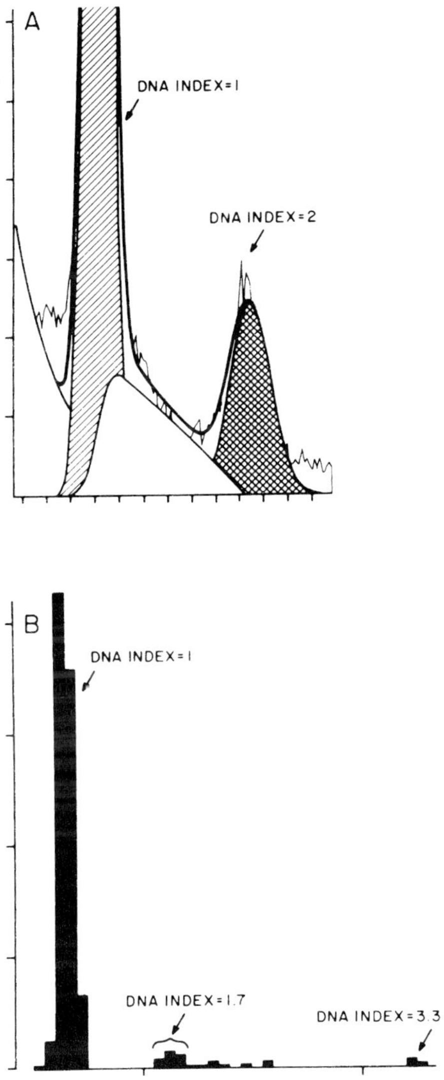


**FIG. 51.3.** Flow- and absorption-cytometric DNA distributions of the pancreatic carcinoma shown in Figure 51.2. **A.** The flow-cytometric DNA distribution shows a relatively elevated S-phase compartment that may have resulted in part from a significant debris artifact. The finding of a large number of counts to the left of the $G_0/G_1$ peak is also consistent with a debris artifact. **B.** The absorption cytometric DNA distribution of this tumor shows small $G_0/G_1$ and $G_2/M$ peaks of morphologically distinct tumor cells, with DNA indices of 1.7 and 3.3, respectively. (From Bose KK, Allison DC, Hruban RH, et al. A comparison of flow-cytometric and absorption-cytometric DNA values as prognostic indicators for pancreatic carcinoma. Cancer 1993;71:690. Reproduced with permission.)

confirmed in several studies (17, 19–22). This work has shown that image-analysis DNA measurements, pathologic tumor size, and the presence of lymph node metastases are the most important, statistically independent, prognostic determinants for patient survival after pancreaticoduodenectomy performed for pancreatic carcinoma (Tables 51.1 and 51.2) (16, 20). Figure 51.5 is a Kaplan-Meier survival plot of the postresection survival rates of pancreatic carcinoma patients with diploid and aneuploid pancreatic cancers after potentially curative Whipple resections. The independence of tumor size from DNA content is illustrated in Figure 51.6, which shows the postresection survival rates of patients with large (>2.5 cm) and small (≤2.5 cm) diploid and aneuploid pancreatic cancers.

Although measured tumor DNA content, lymph node status, and tumor size are each strong predictors of survival for pancreatic carcinoma patients, currently this information has very limited usefulness for improving the care of the patients. These prognostic indicators could be used as stratification variables in studies evaluating different adjuvant therapies for pancreatic carcinoma, but even this application will have minimal impact on the overall treatment and outcome for this disease until more effective adjuvant therapies are found.

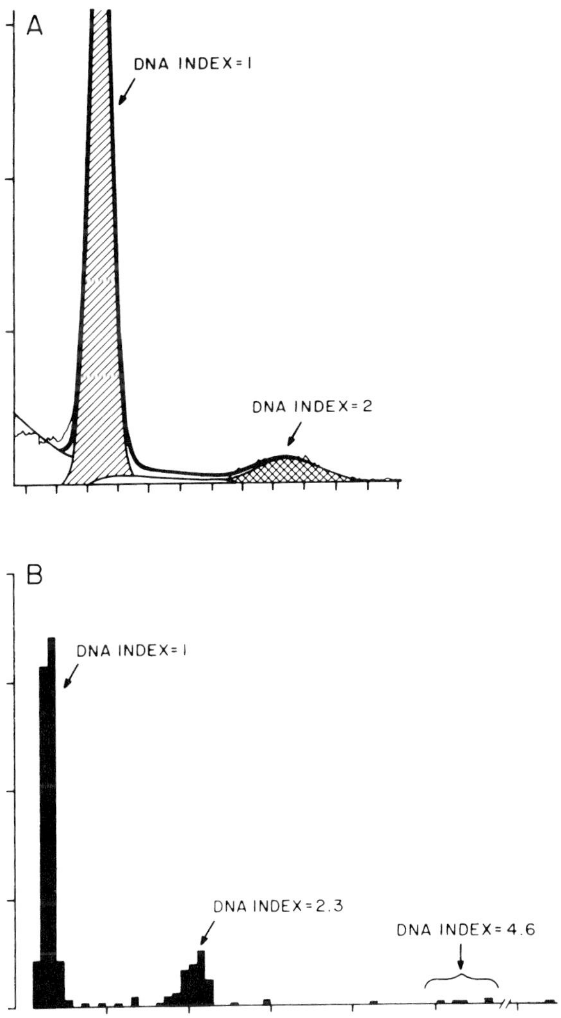


**FIG. 51.4.** Flow- and absorption-cytometric DNA distributions of cells disaggregated from the same pancreatic carcinoma. **A.** The flow-cytometric DNA distribution shows less debris artifact (counts to the left of the $G_0/G_1$ peak) than does the flow-cytometric DNA distribution of the tumor in Figure 51.3*A*, but only nuclei with $G_0/G_1$ and $G_2/M$ DNA indices of 1 and 2, respectively, were detected. **B.** The absorption-cytometric DNA distribution also shows the diploid $G_0/G_1$ peak with a DNA index of 1, but also reveals additional aneuploid $G_0/G_1$ and $G_2/M$ tumor cell peaks with DNA indices of 2.3 and 4.6, respectively. (From Bose KK, Allison DC, Hruban RH, et al. A comparison of flow-cytometric and absorption-cytometric DNA values as prognostic indicators for pancreatic carcinoma. Cancer 1993;71:690. Reproduced with permission.)

**TABLE 51.1. Estimated Hazard Ratios for Death, with Significance Levels, When Prognostic Factors are Considered Individually**

| Variable | Hazard Ratio | 95% Confidence Limits | $p^a$ |
|---|---|---|---|
| Aneuploid vs. diploid | 3.28 | 1.48–7.24 | .003 |
| % $G_0/G_1$ | 0.93 | 0.89–0.96 | <.001 |
| % S | 1.11 | 1.05–1.16 | <.001 |
| % $G_2$/M | 1.05 | 0.98–1.13 | .14 |
| % > $G_2$/M | 1.46 | 1.12–1.89 | .004 |
| $\Sigma$ (S + $G_2$/M + >$G_2$/M)[b] | 1.08 | 1.04–1.12 | <.001 |
| PI[e] (S + $G_2$/M)[b] | 1.08 | 1.04–1.12 | <.001 |
| Tumor size (cm)[c] | 1.28 | 1.04–1.56 | .02 |
| >2.5 cm vs. ≤2.5 cm | 2.75 | 1.36–5.60 | .005 |
| Positive nodes/nodes | 1.15 | 1.02–1.28 | .02 |
| Nodes, positive vs. negative[d] | 3.26 | 1.42–7.62 | .006 |
| Age (years) | 0.99 | 0.95–1.02 | .49 |
| White vs. nonwhite | 0.50 | 0.23–1.08 | .08 |
| F vs. M | 0.86 | 0.44–1.71 | .67 |
| Year of diagnosis | 1.02 | 0.92–1.13 | .69 |

From Allison DC, Bose KK, Hruban RH, et al. Pancreatic cancer cell DNA content correlates with long-term survival after pancreatoduodenectomy. Ann Surg 1991;214:648. Reproduced with permission.
[a] *p* value for hypothesis that the hazard ratio equals 1.0
[b] Hazard ratio for each 1% of PI or $\Sigma$(S + $G_2$/M + >$G_2$/M).
[c] Hazard ratio for each centimeter of tumor diameter.
[d] Hazard ratio for each positive lymph node.
[e] PI, proliferative index.

One potential application of these prognostic variables would be the preoperative identification of those pancreatic carcinoma patients who do not receive sufficient benefit from pancreatoduodenectomy to justify its expense, morbidity, and mortality, because it is possible to measure the DNA contents of pancreatic carcinomas by image analysis on pancreatic carcinoma cells obtained by fine-needle aspiration performed prior to surgical exploration (22, 23). A possible rationale for using this information to select therapy preoperatively is based on the results of a series of 96 pancreaticoduodenectomies for pancreatic carcinomas, in which all of the cancers had image-analysis DNA measurements performed, and the surviving patients were followed for 3–15 years (Allison et al. unpublished results). In this series, 27 tumors had pathologically measured tumor diameters of 4 cm or more. Sixteen of these large cancers had aneuploid DNA contents, and the median survival time of these patients was only 7 months, with the longest survivors dying of recurrent cancer at 12, 16, and 23 months. The benefits of surgical resection, if any, could be questioned for these patients. In contrast, among the 11 patients with diploid pancreatic cancers 4 cm or larger, there are currently 5 survivors, 2 of whom are 5-year survivors (Allison et al. unpublished results). Thus, if improved imaging modalities become available so that one can reliably identify pancreatic carcinomas 4 cm or more in diameter (24), then fine-needle aspiration DNA measurements might allow identification of the patients with the large aneuploid cancers, and such patients might reasonably be randomized among neoadjuvant therapy prior to surgical exploration, immediate exploration, or nonoperative means of palliation.

The enthusiasm for employing preoperative DNA measurements to guide therapy for pancreatic carcinoma patients is tempered by the fear of certain authorities that fine-needle aspiration may dislodge tumor cells and preclude surgical "cure" (25), although real "surgical cures" for pancreatic carcinoma patients are quite rare, with only an approximately 3% 10-year survival rate being reported after resection in even the most favorable series (26, Allison et al., unpublished results). From the viewpoint of cell biology, the fear that fine-needle aspiration will cause tumor cells to disseminate may be unfounded, because it is possible that only tumor cells producing specific enzymes, growth factors, etc. can actually implant, invade, and metastasize. In a study of preoperative fine-needle aspiration for pancreatic cancer patients, it was found that 6% (3/49) of the patients who had this procedure had cancer cells in their peritoneal washings, compared with 9% (1/11) of positive peritoneal washings found for patients not undergoing aspiration (*p* N.S.) (27). This result lends some support for the safety of this procedure.

Future work with new prognostic indicators and the molecular changes associated with pancreatic cancer may eventually clarify which regulatory pathways are mutated or otherwise altered in the genesis of this disease. The initial step in the evaluation of the genetic changes specific for any cancer, including pancreatic carcinoma, is to determine which chromosomal abnormalities are specifically associated with that cancer. The results of such chromosome studies can then be used to guide the exploration of the specific areas of the genome for disease-specific molecular defects using restriction fragment length polymorphism (RFLP) technology and/or polymerase chain reaction (PCR) amplification and sequence analysis (10, 15, 29). Specifically, the loss of a given chromosome in a tumor, especially when combined with the allelic loss of the normal-appearing remaining chromosome, implies the presence of a tumor suppressor gene in that chromosome. Similarly, the consistent gain of a specific chromosome in a cancer implies the presence of tumor-activating oncogenes in that chromosome. Consistent chromosomal structural abnormalities imply a role for an abnormal "fusion protein" in tumorigenesis, or up-regulation of a normally dormant oncogene caused by the crossover. In the standard nomenclature of chromosome studies, "p" refers to the short arm and "q" refers to the long arm of a chromosome.

Chromosome studies of pancreatic carcinomas are in a rapidly expanding and exciting phase of development. Griffin et al. recently noted clonally abnormal karyotypes in 44 of 62

**TABLE 51.2. Estimated Hazard Ratios for Death, with Significance Levels, for Multivariate Proportional Hazards Regression Models[a]**

| Term | Hazard Ratio | 95% Confidence Limits | $p^b$ |
|---|---|---|---|
| Aneuploid | 2.85 | 1.10–7.34 | .03 |
| PI[c] | 1.05 | 1.00–1.10 | .07 |
| Tumor >2.5 cm | 2.98 | 1.40–6.33 | .01 |
| Aneuploid | 4.88 | 1.96–12.16 | <.001 |
| Year of diagnosis | 0.95 | 0.84–1.08 | .44 |
| Tumor size (cm) | 1.38 | 1.11–1.70 | .004 |
| Nodes, positive vs. negative | 2.44 | 1.01–5.87 | .05 |
| Aneuploid | 2.48 | 1.00–6.27 | .05 |
| Tumor >2.5 cm | 2.47 | 1.14–5.35 | .02 |
| PI[c] | 1.05 | 1.00–1.10 | .03 |
| Aneuploid | 4.18 | 1.83–9.54 | <.001 |
| Tumor >2.5 cm | 3.47 | 1.66–7.24 | <.001 |

From Allison DC, Bose KK, Hruban RH, et al. Pancreatic cancer cell DNA content correlates with long-term survival after pancreatoduodenectomy. Ann Surg 1991;214:648. Reproduced with permission.
[a] Each panel represents a separate multivariate model.
[b] *p* value for hypothesis that the hazard ratio equals 1.0.
[c] PI, proliferative index.

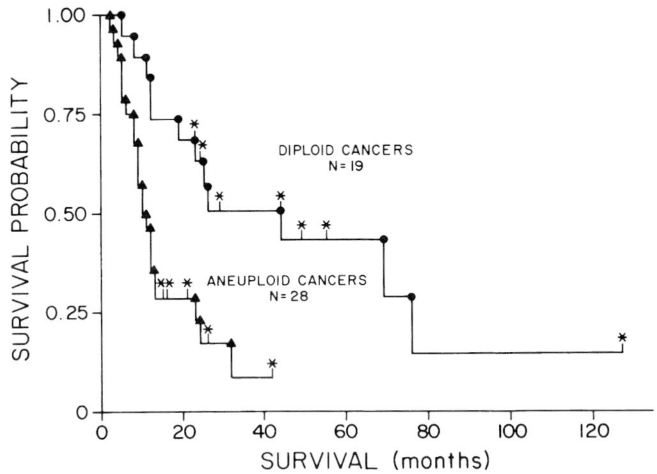


**FIG. 51.5.** Kaplan-Meier survival curves for the 19 patients with diploid *(circles)* and the 28 patients with aneuploid pancreatic carcinoma *(triangles)* who survived pancreatoduodenectomy. *(*)* Time of last follow-up of surviving patients. (From Allison DC, Bose KK, Hruban RH, et al. Pancreatic cancer cell DNA content correlates with long-term survival after pancreatoduodenectomy. Ann Surg 1991;214:648. Reproduced with permission.)

primary pancreatic adenocarcinomas (30, 31). The most frequent whole-chromosome gains were found for chromosomes 20 (8/44) and 7 (7/44). The most frequent whole-chromosome losses were those for 18 (22/44), 13 (16/44), 12 (13/44), and 6 (12/44). Some 209 chromosome break points were identified, and the chromosomal arms most frequently involved were 1p (12 tumors), 6q (22 tumors), 7q, 17p, 1q, 3p, 1p, and 19q (9 tumors each). Also, a portion of the long arm of chromosome 6 appeared to be lost in 9 tumors, and this loss was verified by molecular hybridization studies. Eight of 44 cancers had double minute chromosomes, providing the first in situ genetic evidence for gene amplification in pancreatic adenocarcinoma (31).

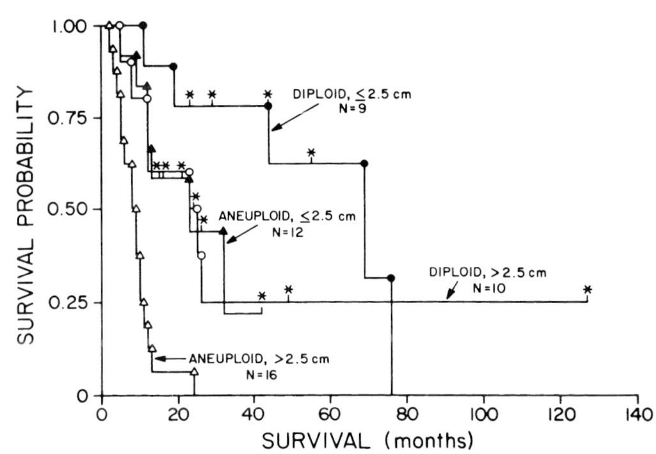


**FIG. 51.6.** Kaplan-Meier survival curves for the 9 patients with small (≤2.5 cm) diploid pancreatic tumors *(closed circles);* the 12 patients with small aneuploid carcinomas *(triangles);* the 10 patients with large (>2.5 cm) diploid cancers *(open circles);* and the 16 patients with large aneuploid cancers *(open triangles).* *(*)* Time of last follow-up of surviving patients. (From Allison DC, Bose KK, Hruban RH, et al. Pancreatic cancer cell DNA content correlates with long-term survival after pancreatoduodenectomy. Ann Surg 1991;214:648. Reproduced with permission.)

In a study of 34 pancreatic adenocarcinomas, Johansson et al. found that 36% had no detectable cytogenetic abnormalities, 24% had relatively "simple" abnormalities, and the remaining 40% had markedly abnormal karyotypes with triploid and near-triploid modal chromosome complements (32, 33). Their findings suggested that structural rearrangements, or loss, of genes located on 1p, 3p, 6q, 8p, and 17p are involved in the pathogenesis of pancreatic carcinoma. Similarly, Seymour has used RFLP analyses to confirm allelic losses for many of the normal-appearing 17p and 18q chromosome arms in pancreatic carcinomas (15). It is of interest that the p53 gene is located on chromosome arm 17p and is lost or mutated in 48% of pancreatic carcinomas (4–6). These and other ongoing studies are just the beginning of the use of the chromosome data for identification of the specific molecular pathways that are deranged in pancreatic cancer. This work will lead to insights into the mechanisms of action of the tumor suppressor genes and oncogenes that are fundamentally important to this disease. Once this knowledge is available, it is hoped that it will provide firm prognostic indicators to guide clinical treatment decisions, as well as to allow the development of specific molecular therapies for pancreatic carcinomas.

## REFERENCES


1. Grünewald K, Lyons J, Frohlich A, et al. High frequency of Ki-ras codon 12 mutations in pancreatic adenocarcinomas. Int J Cancer 1989;43:1037.
2. Hruban RH, van Mansfeld AOM, Offerhaus GJ, et al. K-ras oncogene activation in adenocarcinoma of the human pancreas. A study of 82 carcinomas using a combination of mutant-enriched polymerase chain reaction analysis and allele-specific oligonucleotide hybridization. Am J Pathol 1993;143:545.
3. Caldas C, Hahn SA, Hruban RH, et al. Detection of K-ras mutations in the stool of patients with pancreatic adenocarcinoma and pancreatic ductal hyperplasia. Cancer Res 1994;54:3568.
4. Redston MS, Caldas C, Seymour AB, et al. p53 mutations in pancreatic Ca and evidence of common involvement of homocopolymer tracts in DNA microdeletions. Cancer Res 1994;54:3025.
5. Kalthoff H, Schmiegel W, Roeder C, Kasche D, et al. p53 and K-ras alterations in pancreatic epithelial cell lesions. Oncogene 1993; 8:289.
6. Pellegata NS, Sessa F, Renault B, Bonato M, et al. K-ras and p53 gene mutations in pancreatic cancer: ductal and nonductal tumors progress through different genetic lesions. Cancer Res 1994;54:1556.
7. Lei S, Appert HE, Nakata B, Domenico DR, Howard JM. Overexpression of HER2/neu oncogene in pancreatic cancer correlates with shortened survival. Int J Pancreatol 1995;17:15.
8. Yamanaka Y, Friess H, Kobrin MS, Buchler M, et al. Coexpression of epidermal growth factor receptor and ligands in human pancreatic cancer is associated with enhanced tumor aggressiveness. Anticancer Res 1993;13:565.
9. Simon B, Weinel R, Höhne M, Watz J, et al. Frequent alterations of the tumor suppressor genes p53 and DCC in human pancreatic carcinoma. Gastroenterology 1994;106:1645.
10. Höhne MW, Halatsch ME, Kahl GF, et al. Frequent loss of expression of the potential tumor suppressor gene DCC in ductal pancreatic adenocarcinoma. Cancer Res 1992;52:2616.
11. Caldas C, Hahn SA, da Costa LT, et al. Frequent somatic mutations and homozygous deletions of the p16 (MTSI) gene in pancreatic adenocarcinoma. Nat Genet 1994;8:27.
12. Horii A, Nakatsuru S, Miyoshi Y, Ichii S, et al. Frequent somatic mutations of the APC gene in human pancreatic cancer. Cancer Res 1992;52:6696.
13. Sakorafas GH, Lazaris A, Tsiotou AG, et al. Oncogenes in cancer of the pancreas. Eur J Surg Oncol 1995;21:251.
14. Kern SE, Fearon ER, Tersmette KW, et al. Clinical and pathological associations with allelic loss in colorectal carcinoma. JAMA 1989;261:3099.
15. Seymour AB, Hruban RH, Redston M, et al. Allelotype of pancreatic adenocarcinoma. Cancer Res 1994;54:2761.

16. Allison DC, Bose KK, Hruban RH, et al. Pancreatic cancer cell DNA content correlates with long-term survival after pancreatoduodenectomy. Ann Surg 1991;214:648.
17. Böttger TC, Storkel S, et al. Factors influencing survival after resection of pancreatic cancer: a DNA analysis and histomorphologic study. Cancer 1994;73:63.
18. Porschen R, Remy U, Bevers G, et al. Prognostic significance of DNA ploidy in adenocarcinoma of the pancreas. Cancer 1993;71:3846.
19. Bose KK, Allison DC, Hruban RH, et al. A comparison of flow cytometric and absorption cytometric DNA values as prognostic indicators for pancreatic carcinoma. Cancer 1993;71:690.
20. Yeo CJ, Cameron JC, Lillemoe KD, Sitzman JV, et al. Pancreaticoduodenectomy for cancer of the head of the pancreas. 201 patients. Ann Surg 1995;221:721.
21. Herrera MF, VanHeerden VA, Katzmann JA, et al. Evaluation of DNA nuclear pattern as a prognostic determinant in resected pancreatic ductal adenocarcinoma. Ann Surg 1992;215:120.
22. Bose KK, Curley S, Smith WJ, Allison DC. Differences in the flow and absorption cytometric DNA distributions of mouse hepatocytes and tumor cells. Cytometry 1989;10:388.
23. Evans DB, Frazier ML, Charnsangavej C, Katz RL, et al. Molecular diagnosis of exocrine pancreatic cancer using a percutaneous technique. Ann Surg Oncol 1996;3:241.
24. Ballard RB, Hoffman JP, Gultman MC, Barber L, et al. How accurate is size measurement of pancreas cancer masses by computed axial tomography (CT) scanning? Am Surg 1995;61:686.
25. Warshaw AL. Implications of peritoneal cytology for staging of early pancreatic cancer. Am J Surg 1991;161:26.
26. Conlon KC, Kimstra DS, Brennan MF. Long-term survival after curative resection for pancreatic ductal adenocarcinoma. Ann Surg 1996;223:273.
27. Leach SD, Rose JA, Lowy AM, Evans DB, et al. Significance of peritoneal cytology in patients with potentially resectable adenocarcinoma of the pancreatic head. Surgery 1995;118:472.
28. Barton CM, Staddon SL, Hughes CM, et al. Abnormalities of the p53 tumour suppressor gene in human pancreatic cancer. Br J Cancer 1991;64:1076.
29. Cairns P, Li M, Merlo A, et al. Rates of p16 (MTSI) mutations in primary tumor with 9p loss. Science 1994;265:415.
30. Griffin CA, Hruban RH, Long PP, et al. Chromosome abnormalities in pancreatic adenocarcinomas. Genes Chromosomes Cancer 1994;9:93.
31. Griffin CA, Hruban RH, Morsberger LA, et al. Consistent chromosome abnormalities in adenocarcinoma of the pancreas. Cancer Res 1995;55:2394.
32. Johansson B, Bardi G, Heim S, et al. Nonrandom chromosomal rearrangements in pancreatic carcinomas. Cancer 1992;69:1674.
33. Bardi G, Johansson B, Panelis N, et al. Karyotypic abnormalities in tumours of the pancreas. Br J Cancer 1993;67:1106.

SECTION X

CLINICAL MANAGEMENT OF CARCINOMA OF THE EXOCRINE PANCREAS

# 52

# *Diagnosis and Clinical Staging of Pancreatic Cancer*

Gregory G. Tsiotos and Michael G. Sarr

Pancreatic ductal adenocarcinoma is the most common malignancy of the exocrine pancreas. Its incidence in the western world has increased in the last 4 to 5 decades for unknown reasons, and, for equally unknown reasons, now appears to be leveling off (1). Twenty-eight to 30 thousand new patients will be diagnosed with this disease in the United States next year, and an almost equal number will eventually succumb to it. Of these newly diagnosed patients, only 10–15% will be determined to have "clinically" resectable disease preoperatively, but only half (or less) of this subgroup will actually undergo a curative resection. Unfortunately, the very aggressive behavior of this neoplasm is reflected in the fact that it represents the fourth and fifth most common cause of cancer-related deaths in men and women, respectively, and the second most common cause of death due to gastrointestinal malignancy.

During the last decade, improvements in patient care, surgical technique, possibly earlier diagnosis, and concentration of patients in centers of excellence with a major interest in pancreatic surgery have led to a marked decrease in the operative morbidity and mortality of major pancreatic resections. Currently, the operative mortality of pancreatic resections in major, high-volume, experienced centers with an interest in pancreatic surgery is consistently under 5%. There is also evidence to suggest an improvement in the 5-year survival after resection at such institutions, with reports of actuarial or actual survivals in the neighborhood of 12–24% (2–6) that may be even higher in certain subgroups of patients (4, 5, 7). Despite past nihilistic views and even some current pessimistic views that may involve a cost awareness in the modern era of cost containment (8), it remains unequivocal that surgery offers the only possibility for cure of this dread disease.

As operative resection reaches its limit in the management of this disease, attention has turned to earlier diagnosis and accurate preoperative determination of resectability. With the current explosion of new "star wars" technology, a great array of sophisticated, interventional, and expensive tests have been suggested for diagnosis and clinical staging; their roles are currently under evaluation, but much remains to be defined before they are applied appropriately and rationally.

This chapter *(a)* discusses the clinical characteristics and presentation of pancreatic cancer; *(b)* analyzes the roles of the various imaging and laboratory modalities currently available or under investigation, as they relate to both diagnosis and staging; and *(c)* outlines the authors suggested approach to this challenging problem, based on current information. The chapter focuses on ductal adenocarcinoma of the exocrine pancreas. Neoplasms arising from other cells of origin (cystadenocarcinoma, islet cell neoplasms, etc.) may be referred to, but ductal adenocarcinoma is emphasized, with concentration on the recent literature dealing with its diagnosis and clinical staging. Diagnosis and staging are discussed separately in an attempt to separate the two concepts rationally and to emphasize the different roles of the imaging and invasive procedures in the workup of the patient. The final section presents a diagnostic and staging algorithm based on cost, efficacy, safety, and currently accepted concepts of management.

## DIAGNOSIS OF PANCREATIC CANCER

Most patients with pancreatic cancer have the diagnosis made when they develop jaundice. This means that the pancreatic neoplasm arising in the main pancreatic duct has become large enough to involve (and obstruct) the intrapancreatic portion of the common bile duct. In retrospect, many or most of these patients will have had vague symptoms for several weeks to months prior to the development of jaundice. To have an impact on the natural history of this disease (and there is solid reason to believe that earlier diagnosis at a smaller size does lead to an increased 5-year survival), we must make inroads into recognizing patients with these vague symptoms weeks prior to the onset of biliary obstruction. The physician must maintain a high index of suspicion for the diagnosis of pancreatic cancer in patients with these vague, nonspecific symptoms prior to the onset of jaundice. A heightened awareness of this neoplasm and its symptoms is imperative, not so much in the surgical arena, but more importantly, in the primary care environment where these patients enter the health care field.

### Clinical Presentation

Although many patients with pancreatic cancer first present with painless jaundice, the earliest and most common clinical features are a vague, poorly localized, abdominal discomfort often associated with an inconsequential weight loss, anorexia, and fatigue. The latter complaint can be especially insidious because most patients are over 60 years of age and attribute these symptoms to getting older. Because they are nonspecific, these vague, nonlocalizing symptoms are usually either overlooked by both patient and physician or attributed to another cause that may in fact coexist.

More alarming, but later, symptoms are jaundice and back pain indicating tumor growth extending to surrounding structures. Jaundice is present at the time of diagnosis in about 60–70% of patients and is the symptom that unquestionably alerts the patient or family to seek medical attention. Except for ampullary cancer, which may intermittently obstruct the bile duct but then, presumably by outstripping its blood supply, undergoes necrosis which thereby relieves the obstruction, the jaundice of pancreatic cancer is progressive and unrelenting. Without intervention, the serum bilirubin level continuously increases, to peak at about 18–25 mg/dL. Values above this suggest an underlying hepatic dysfunction. Unlike choledocholithiasis, cholangitis is rarely, if ever, a component in the presentation unless the biliary tree has been instrumented. Pruritus develops later, when the extrahepatic biliary obstruction has become further established.

Back or deep abdominal pain, relieved by sitting forward, so-called pancreatic pain, is also characteristic and is attributed to either direct growth into, or mechanical compression of, the posteriorly located celiac plexus or dilation of an obstructed pancreatic duct. This pain is often most pronounced at night. The recently identified neurotropic growth factors secreted by pancreatic cancer cells may explain this predilection of pancreatic cancer to invade and extend along the neural plexuses of the gland (9). Although jaundice, back pain, or both are present in 90% of patients (10), the term *painless jaundice* with a palpable gallbladder (Courvoisier's sign) has been historically associated with pancreatic cancer. This classic presentation refers to the absence of overt right upper quadrant pain (as seen in patients with gallstone disease) and the enlargement of the gallbladder because of outflow obstruction. Many patients with "painless jaundice," when questioned more closely, will describe other symptoms they have ignored or not fully recognized that long preceded the jaundice.

On occasion, pancreatic cancer presents in an unusual manner. Acute pancreatitis is an unusual mode of presentation allegedly related to partial obstruction of the pancreatic duct. One's clinical suspicion must be very high in the patient without an obvious cause of the acute pancreatitis (e.g., gallstones, alcohol abuse, certain medications, lipid abnormalities). When the episode has resolved, many clinicians recommend an aggressive evaluation, even including a diagnostic endoscopic retrograde cholangiopancreatography (ERCP). Whether this approach is warranted in all patients with acute pancreatitis without obvious cause is unknown. Within this select group of patients, pancreatic cancer still remains a very infrequent etiologic factor. Another unusual presentation is that of a pancreatic pseudocyst, allegedly developing distal to an obstructing neoplasm. This presentation is equally rare but may be more common in patients with preexistent chronic pancreatitis.

Newly developed glucose intolerance or new-onset overt diabetes mellitus may be the first clinical feature in 7–13% of patients (11). Indeed, new-onset glucose intolerance of 1-year's duration or less is associated with an increased relative risk for development or presence of pancreatic cancer (12). An abnormal glucose tolerance test (often with no diabetic symptoms) is present in up to 68% of patients at some stage of their disease. This nonspecific feature has been attributed to the secretion of a diabetogenic factor(s) elaborated by the tumor, especially because of the observation of decreased insulin resistance after tumor resection (13). Recently, interest has centered on the identification of an islet amyloid pancreatic protein (IAPP) that confers a relative glucose resistance in the host (14, 15). It appears that pancreatic cancer cells elaborate a humoral substance that induces ß cells to synthesize IAPP (16). This strong association between new-onset diabetes mellitus and pancreatic cancer represents a viable avenue for further study. Our ability to measure IAPP may also serve as a test to screen patients at increased risk of developing pancreatic cancer (e.g., hereditary pancreatitis, familial pancreatic cancer, chronic pancreatitis).

Symptoms of advanced disease include nausea and vomiting related to gastric outlet obstruction. Mechanical obstruction of the second portion of the duodenum by neoplasms in the head of the gland and the fourth portion of the duodenum by cancers in the midbody of the pancreas are unusual *presenting* problems that suggest advanced disease. Usually, other prominent symptoms have preceded the mechanical duodenal obstruction. In contrast, nausea, vomiting, and early satiety are relatively common symptoms at the time of presentation and diagnosis. The pathogenesis of these symptoms is poorly understood, because most patients lack a mechanical element of duodenal obstruction. Many investigators believe that these symptoms are related to invasion of the neural plexuses by the neoplasm, with a *functional* gastric outlet obstruction secondary to an abnormality in gastric emptying. This is an important concept because "palliation" by a gastrojejunostomy may offer little if any benefit to these patients.

The nonspecific nature of the symptomatology described above explains why there is often so much delay until the patient reaches an experienced surgeon (2 weeks to 2 months). Vague abdominal or back pain is overlooked by both the patient and the primary care physician or attributed to musculoskeletal disorders, gastroesophageal reflux, cholelithiasis, or peptic ulcer disease that may in fact coexist. Valuable time elapses, during which various treatments prove fruitless, symptoms worsen, and the tumor grows. Even the herald symptom of jaundice does not always lead the unwary physician to suspect a periampullary tumor, and quite commonly, patients are worked up or treated for hepatitis for some time before the appropriate diagnosis is entertained. The lesson here is that jaundice developing in anyone over age 40 years should be assumed to be extrahepatic biliary obstruction until proven otherwise. Gallstone disease (which may very well coexist in this older population) is often assumed to be the cause of the biliary obstruction, and many patients undergo other surgical procedures (laparoscopic cholecystectomy, common bile duct exploration, T-tube placement) that only prolong the time to diagnosis and quite possibly complicate subsequent definitive surgery.

## Suspected Pancreatic Cancer—Objective Evaluation

Once a pancreatic cancer is suspected, a well-organized algorithm is needed to make the diagnosis. The choice among the various diagnostic modalities should be based on the efficacy of each test (sensitivity, specificity, positive and negative predictive values, and accuracy), its local availability, its risk, and whether it will yield information that will directly affect the management of the patient or otherwise affect the evaluation plan.

**Laboratory Findings.** In general, routine serum laboratory profiles lack specificity. Nonmicrocytic anemia and hypoalbuminemia reflect the chronic nature of the neoplastic process and its nutritional sequelae, but they are not always present, and they only indicate a chronic disease. More helpful for screening evaluation are the liver function tests. A cholestatic pattern manifested by increases in serum alkaline phosphatase, bilirubin, and α-glutamyl transferase (GGT) levels is highly suggestive of biliary tract obstruction but is in no way specific for pancreatic carcinoma. This profile in the patient over 40 years of age should, however, immediately prompt an aggressive search for a cause of biliary obstruction. Mild increases in serum aspartate aminotransferase (AST), alanine aminotransferase (ALT), and lactate dehydrogenase (LDH) levels are not uncommon with biliary obstruction but are of little or no diagnostic help. Clinical or even biochemical cholestasis in patients with cancer of the body and tail of the gland is usually absent early in the disease and, when present, indicates severe metastatic involvement of the liver and/or the hilum. Increases in serum amylase or lipase levels are uncommon and nondiagnostic. Consideration should be given to checking the prothrombin time in the deeply jaundiced patient, because prolonged exclusion of bile from the gut leads to a malabsorption of vitamin K and decreased hepatic production of clotting factors. Replacement therapy may be needed before proceeding further with some of the invasive procedures needed to objectively secure the diagnosis or to treat the pancreatic cancer.

**Tumor Markers.** Multiple different tumor markers have been identified and studied systematically in an attempt to facilitate an earlier diagnosis of pancreatic cancer or to select high-risk patients for further evaluation. In addition, these tests have been evaluated as staging markers of resectability, prognosis, and postoperative recurrence. The use of tumor markers in the diagnosis of pancreatic neoplasms is very controversial, and the arguments for and against their use are multifactorial. Previous studies examining their use are outlined below.

The carbohydrate antigen 19-9 (CA 19-9) has been evaluated and validated in multiple studies. Using the upper limit of normal (37 u/mL) as a cutoff, the mean sensitivity of the assay for identifying patients with known pancreatic cancer approaches 80% (17). Because the specificity may vary from as low as 73% to more than 95% (17, 18), its true role as a pure screening tool remains unproven. False-negative results are frequent in patients with a Lewis blood group negative phenotype; in addition, false-positive assays can occur in patients with chronic pancreatitis, hepatitis, and cirrhosis, making the use of this "marker" of less (positive or negative) predictive value. Using a higher cutoff (i.e., 90 or 200 u/mL), the specificity increases to almost 100%, but the sensitivity decreases markedly.

CA 19-9 has also been evaluated as a prognostic tool. A CA 19-9 level above 300 u/mL has been associated with very low resectability rates (19), even in the absence of radiographic signs of unresectability. Similarly, when the CA 19-9 level decreases to normal values after resection, any subsequent increase of CA 19-9 is an early indicator of recurrence, serving thus as a very good marker for postoperative surveillance (20) and a potential prognostic factor for long-term survival (17, 21). Unfortunately, without any clear-cut therapeutic option in patients with presumed recurrent disease, the usefulness and cost-effectiveness of such a surveillance program must be questioned.

Because of the low specificity of CA 19-9 alone, a number of other potential tumor markers have been evaluated recently, both alone or in combination. CA 242, another carbohydrate antigen, has a similar sensitivity, but in at least one study (22), this marker had a somewhat higher specificity because many confounding benign hepatobiliary and pancreatic conditions did not appear to lead to false-positive results. Satake and Takeuchi (18) prospectively evaluated several other putative tumor markers simultaneously; the sensitivity, specificity, and accuracy, respectively, of each of the following markers were less than those of CA 19-9: Span-1 (81, 68, 71%), CA-50 (65, 73, 70%), DuPAN-2 (48, 85, 74%), and elastase-1 (51, 76, 63%). Similarly, tissue polypeptide antigen (TPA), and tissue polypeptide specific antigen (TPSA) have been found to add little or nothing to diagnosis or differentiation of pancreatic malignancy from other conditions (23). A ratio of testosterone to dihydrotestosterone of 5 or less appears to add more specificity but at the expense of sensitivity (24) and, while interesting, still adds little improvement in the diagnosis of pancreatic cancer. Another approach with these and other tumor markers has been to combine them in an attempt to improve sensitivity/specificity. Increases in both CA 19-9 and CEA improve specificity to more than 95%, but again, sensitivity falls off (25). One group (26) suggested a complicated mathematical formula based on the sensitivity and specificity of multiple individual tumor markers and claimed a marked improvement in diagnostic accuracy.

The primary argument against the routine use of these tumor markers is that although they may have "statistically significant" differences in a large patient population, their practical use in individual patients remains questionable. Use of CA 19-9 has been marketed quite successfully by laboratories offering this assay, yet its actual usefulness in day-to-day practice is unproven. For such a tumor marker to be of use, it would have to identify patients at high risk before the neoplasm became evident clinically or would have to be able to differentiate a pancreatic cancer from other conditions either mimicking cancer clinically or leading to an apparent mass on an objective imaging test (e.g., chronic localized pancreatitis). With the current sensitivity, specificity, and predictive values of CA 19-9, CEA, CA 242, etc., few if any pancreatologists would use the results of any of these tumor markers to dictate the need for or against any definitive invasive procedure except under very specific, select conditions.

**Molecular Biologic Techniques.** The lessons learned from the association of colon cancer with specific genetic mutations (27) has led to an explosion of research centered on the relationship between alterations in the genetic profile and the development of neoplastic disorders. Two basic groups of genes (oncogenes and tumor suppressor genes), each with different functions, have been identified as having a pivotal role in tumorigenesis. Oncogenes, which are mutated forms of normal cellular "protooncogenes," code for proteins that allow the cell to "gain" a function, thus altering its normal characteristics. Tumor suppressor genes code for proteins that appear to inhibit cellular proliferation. Their loss eliminates one normal (and apparently quite important) defense mechanism within the cell. Both, independently or synergistically, may contribute to tumorigenesis, the former by allowing an abnormal cell clone to develop and multiply and the lack of the latter by preventing the elimination of this abnormal clone by the cell's intrinsic defense mechanisms.

Mutations of the *ras* oncogene are common in several different human and animal cancers (28). Kirsten (K)-*ras* oncogene, one member of the *ras* oncogene family, has been found in human lung, gastric, colonic, and pancreatic cancers. Pancreatic cancer is unique in that it appears to have the highest rate of K-*ras* mutations among many other malignant neoplasms. Several recent studies have confirmed that the rate of K-*ras* mutations in pancreatic ductal adenocarcinomas is between 71 and 96% (29–31). These mutations were found almost exclusively in the second position of codon 12 and less commonly in codons 13 or 61. Unlike cancers in rodent models, mutations in the other *ras* family members, N-*ras* and H-*ras*, are uncommon.

This prevalence of *codon-specific* K-*ras* mutation has allowed the development of a putative, but readily applicable, diagnostic test for the presence of K-*ras* mutations in pancreatic biopsies in patients with presumed pancreatic cancer. After amplification of specific *ras* sequences by the polymerase chain reaction (PCR) technique, three methods (in order of increasing sensitivity) have been used for the detection of K-*ras* mutations: direct sequencing of the PCR product (32), hybridization of allele-specific oligonucleotides to either Southern or dot blots (33), and a modified allele-specific ligation assay (34).

While the presence of K-*ras* mutations in neoplastic pancreatic tissue is not disputed, it would be much more useful in diagnosis to detect this mutation in more readily available samples from patients with suspected pancreatic cancer. K-*ras* mutations have been detected in ERCP-obtained pancreatic juice in 55–77% of patients with pancreatic cancer (35–38), in duodenal juice in 63% (39), in bile obtained from endobiliary drainage tubes despite negative cytology (40), and recently in stool in 55% of patients with proven pancreatic cancer (41). Specimens from mucinous ductal ectasia (intraductal papillary mucinous tumors) of the pancreas (a known premalignant condition) also show K-*ras* mutations frequently (42). In one series, this mutation approached 90% (43). K-*ras* mutations have also been detected in pancreatic resection specimens from patients with ductal carcinoma in situ (44), from a patient with a strong family history of pancreatic cancer (45), and in the pancreatic juice of two patients without any evidence of cancer but who subsequently (18 and 40 months later) developed pancreatic malignancy (38). K-*ras* mutations are also more prevalent among patients with a history of smoking and with hyperplasia of the pancreatic duct. Whether K-*ras* mutations can be a clinically useful diagnostic or even screening tool for pancreatic cancer has yet to be seen. More studies are needed to determine its true sensitivity and specificity, especially in tissue or fluid sampled in a large population of patients with diverse malignant and nonmalignant pancreatic and other nonpancreatic gastrointestinal disorders (30).

From the diverse group of tumor suppressor genes, p53 has been studied extensively. This gene codes for proteins that send inhibitory signals involved in cell division, which functionally select which cells replicate their DNA and undergo mitosis. Mutations of p53 have been demonstrated in up to 50–70% of patients with pancreatic ductal carcinoma (29, 31, 46) but apparently not in patients with intraductal papillary mucinous tumors or other ductal dysplastic lesions (43). Interestingly, mutations of K-*ras* or p53 have not been detected in either exocrine nonductal or endocrine pancreatic carcinomas (29). Since mutations of the K-*ras* oncogene have been seen in both malignant and premalignant pancreatic lesions, whereas p53 mutations appear to occur only in malignant ones, some investigators have postulated that K-*ras* mutations are markers of the pancreatic ductal dysplasia, while the coexistence of the latter (accumulation of events) may be a second hit that allows the dysplastic epithelium to progress to malignancy (29, 47).

In addition to mutations in K-*ras* and p53, other genes have been implicated in the genesis of pancreatic carcinomas. Mutations of the DCC (deleted in colon cancer) gene were found in 50–66% of ductal cancer cells (47, 48) and of the MTS1 gene in 50–85% (49, 50). However, these latter mutations have not yet been studied in depth.

All the aforementioned observations suggest a potential role for the detection of K-*ras*, p53, and other mutations in pancreatic secretions, duodenal aspirates, or even stool as potential clinical tools for screening and early diagnosis of pancreatic cancer. The use of K-*ras* is particularly attractive because of its high prevalence in all stages of this disease and the relative ease of detection (51). Factors that have limited the clinical use of these markers of dysplasia and/or malignancy are the unverified sensitivity from the more easily obtained specimens (duodenal juice, bile, stool) and the unproven specificity (mutations can be present in clinically trivial colonic or pancreatic lesions). However, application of these methods in high-risk subsets of patients with conditions known to be associated with pancreatic cancer (chronic pancreatitis, familial pancreatitis, hereditary pancreatic cancer, intraductal papillary mucinous tumors, late-onset diabetes mellitus in nonobese patients) may, in the near future, help to identify patients who should undergo sophisticated invasive imaging modalities, such as endoluminal ultrasonography and pancreatoscopy (see below). Earlier diagnosis might be achieved, so that intervention could be made at a stage when the disease is still curable.

## Diagnostic Pancreatic Imaging

**Ultrasonography.** Transabdominal ultrasonography offers a relatively cheap, rapid, and quite sensitive screening test for patients with presumed extrahepatic biliary obstruction. Currently it is the most sensitive test for detecting gallstones, an ever-present question in the elderly jaundiced patient. In addition to being able to demonstrate a dilated intra- and extrahepatic biliary tree, other helpful findings of a pancreatic or periampullary mass, liver metastases, ascites, and occasionally peripancreatic lymph nodes may be seen in many patients.

Pancreatic cancer usually appears as a hyperechoic mass, differing in consistency from the normal surrounding pancreatic parenchyma (Fig. 52.1). One theoretical advantage of ultra-

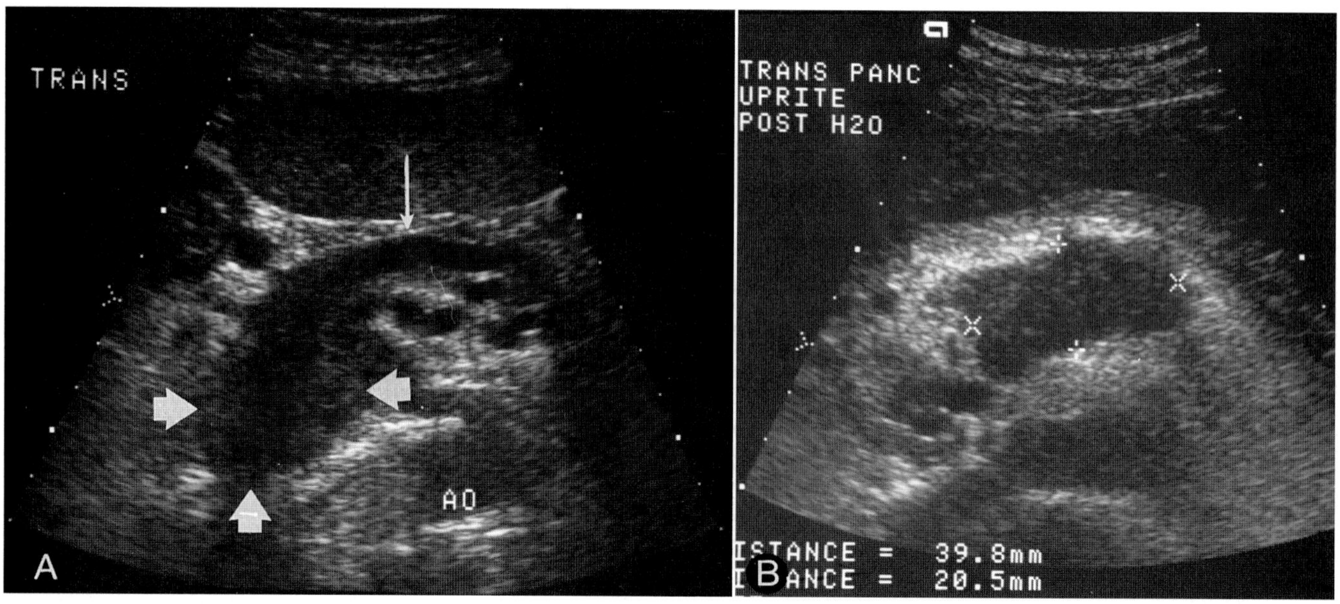


**FIG. 52.1.** Ultrasonography of pancreatic cancer. **A.** Transverse sonogram of the head and body of the pancreas showing a 4-cm hypoechoic, solid mass within the head region consistent with adenocarcinoma *(thick arrows)*. Secondary atrophy of the body of the gland with a dilated pancreatic duct *(thin arrow)*. **B.** Transverse sonogram of the body of the pancreas showing a 3.9 × 2.0 cm hypoechoic solid mass *(stars)* consistent with adenocarcinoma.

sonography is that because of the different echoic density of the neoplasm, the diagnosis of cancer may be evident at an earlier stage (≈1 cm) than with other imaging tests such as computerized tomography (CT) (52). With ultrasonography, provided bowel gas from the duodenum and/or transverse colon does not interfere, one can follow the dilated common bile duct down to its distal point of obstruction, the important piece of information for the hepatobiliary-pancreatic surgeon. In addition, the pancreatic duct can be visualized to determine the presence of obstruction—an expected finding with a pancreatic cancer large enough to obstruct the bile duct.

Ultrasonography may also be useful for neoplasms in the body/tail region. When adequately visualized, the proximity of the neoplasm to the celiac artery (celiac plexus) may be determined, information that may alter the surgeon's decision concerning the advisability of abdominal exploration for potential curative resection.

Although ultrasonography offers a rapid, relatively cheap, and quite sensitive test for screening jaundiced patients for the presence of extrahepatic biliary obstruction, it does have its disadvantages. Its efficacy is often limited by the body habitus of the patient or the presence of bowel gas that obscures the underlying structures. Most importantly, this technique is extremely operator/interpreter dependent (53). In some institutions with exceptional expertise in ultrasonography and pancreatic disease, it plays an important role in the evaluation of pancreatic cancer; however, in most centers, ultrasonographic examination serves as a screening test, primarily for the presence of extrahepatic biliary obstruction.

Ultrasonography has been suggested as the first imaging modality of choice in evaluating the patient with presumed extrahepatic biliary obstruction because it can document intra/extrahepatic dilation of the biliary tree. Other arguments in support of initial ultrasonography are its lack of ionizing radiation, ready access in most hospitals, and allegedly decreased cost. Unfortunately, this myth has been difficult to dispel. While ultrasonography is quite sensitive in detecting extrahepatic biliary obstruction, usually a CT scan is required anyway for complete staging of pancreatic cancer (see below). Because CT is virtually just as sensitive as ultrasonography for detecting biliary obstruction *and* offers better and more complete information about surrounding structures in staging the local and distant extent of the disease, this practice of using ultrasonography as the initial screening procedure is outdated and should be abandoned. Currently, in the older, jaundiced patient in whom a pancreatic cancer is highly suspected, CT should be the initial diagnostic (and staging) procedure employed.

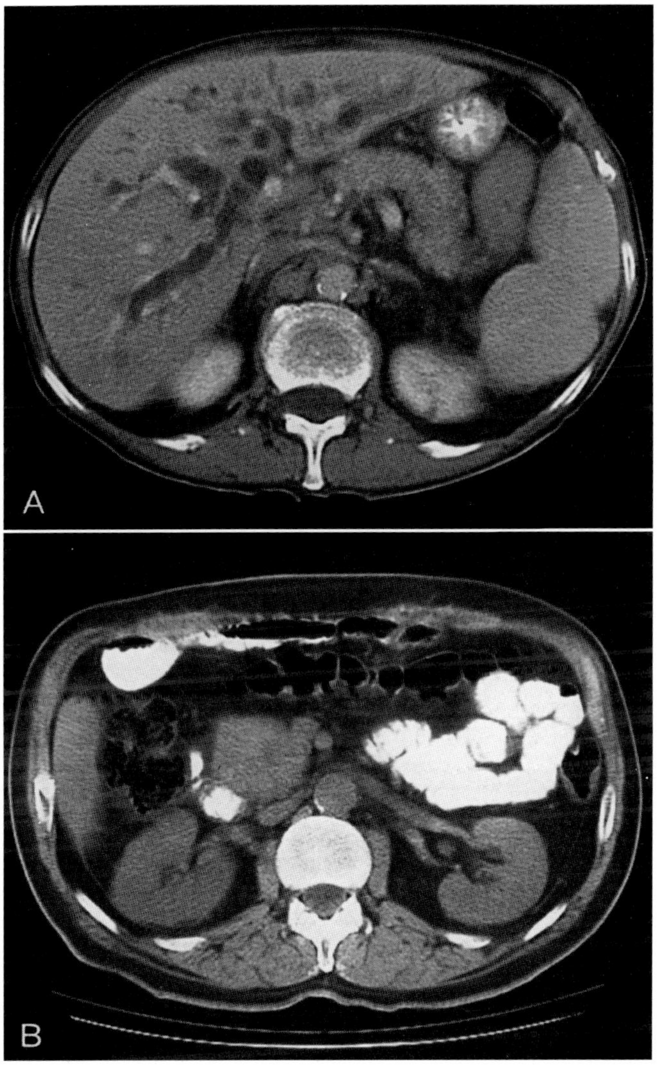


**FIG. 52.2.** CT of pancreatic adenocarcinoma of the head of the pancreas. **A.** Intrahepatic and extrahepatic biliary dilation. **B.** Large mass in head of pancreas; note distance between contrast in duodenum and the superior mesenteric vessels.

**Computerized Tomography (CT).** CT with intravenous contrast is the initial diagnostic imaging procedure of choice currently for patients with a suspected pancreatic cancer—*not ultrasonography*. CT offers more information than ultrasonography and speeds the workup. This imaging technique is of use both for diagnosis and for preoperative clinical staging. Not only does it demonstrate extrahepatic/intrahepatic biliary dilation (Fig. 52.2*A*) as well as ultrasonography, but it also delineates the presence of a pancreatic mass and provides information about liver metastases, peripancreatic nodal spread, ascites, and involvement/obstruction of the superior mesenteric/portal vein confluence (53, 54). "Spiral" or "helical" CT has emerged currently as the gold standard (55).

Pancreatic cancer usually appears as an area of pancreatic enlargement, often as a hypodense, focal lesion (Fig. 52.2*B*). Areas of "fullness" or "enlargement," even in the absence of a discrete mass, should raise the level of suspicion and prompt aggressive investigation. The neoplasm may have areas of cystic necrosis that are usually eccentrically located with irregular borders; confusion with pancreatic pseudocysts or cystic neoplasms of the pancreas should be unusual. Calcification of the neoplasm, while possible, is also quite unusual and, if present, should suggest another diagnosis unless associated with chronic calcific pancreatitis. The size of the tumor mass on CT, however, is often overestimated because of the inflammatory reaction surrounding the neoplasm. The reaction may also be related to a distal, obstructive pancreatitis and thereby falsely confound the clinical impression of the extent of local involvement. This reaction can be especially prominent and worrisome with periampullary lesions that lead to "pancreatitis" of the uncinate process thereby raising the question of resectability because of the proximity of the medial extent of the uncinate enlargement to the superior mesenteric artery.

Unless there are obvious liver lesions suggesting metastases, the CT is not truly diagnostic of pancreatic cancer, but in the absence of tissue histopathology, it can be highly suggestive. CT may reveal an apparent "enlargement" of the head of the pancreas in individuals in whom the anatomic orientation of the gland may be at a different angle to the sagittal plane. Because CT takes sagittal "cuts," if the head-neck region of the pancreas lies a bit more anterior/posterior than is usual, CT cuts through the head region may suggest enlargement. The lack of any

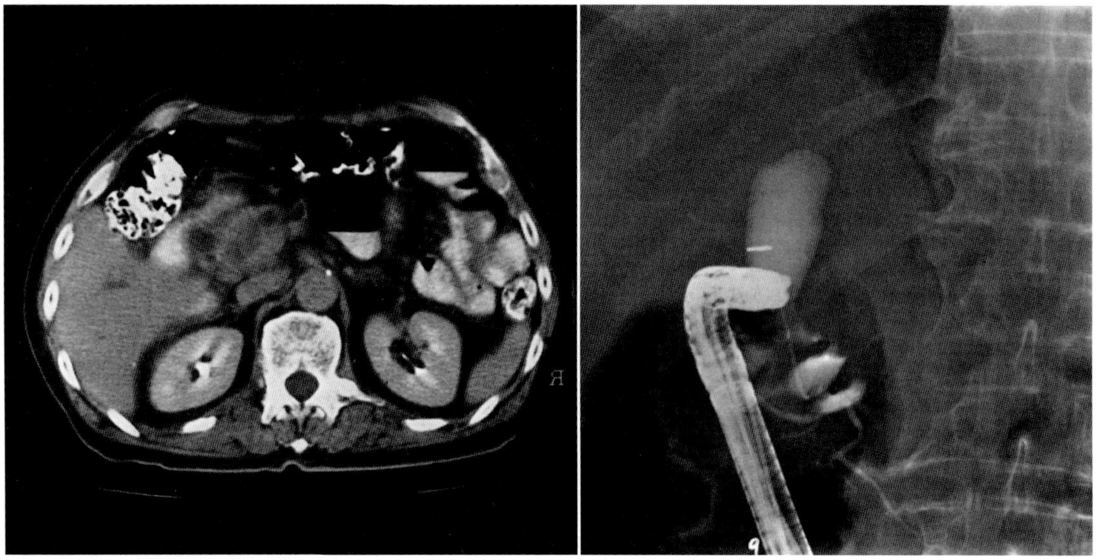

**FIG. 52.3.** CT showing the double duct sign with a dilated intrapancreatic bile duct and pancreatic duct. ERCP showing a stricture in the intrapancreatic portion of the common bile duct and complete occlusion of the proximal pancreatic duct.

density differences, biliary or pancreatic ductal obstruction, or clinical suspicion should dissuade further investigation in most patients. However, this finding can be confusing in patients with vague symptoms suggesting an underlying malignancy. Even more confusing are patients with known chronic pancreatitis who very often will have localized regional enlargement of the pancreas, especially the head region. Differentiation of chronic pancreatitis from a superimposed neoplasm can be difficult or impossible, especially since this patient group is at increased risk of developing pancreatic cancer. As discussed below, biopsy is not completely reliable to differentiate the two entities, and resection may be necessary in selected patients (56). (The use of CT in the staging of patients with pancreatic cancer is discussed below (Staging).)

**Magnetic Resonance Imaging (MRI).** MRI offers no advantage over CT (57) because of low signal-to-noise ratio, motion artifacts, lack of bowel opacification, and low spatial resolution. For the diagnosis of smaller, non-contour-deforming neoplasms, the newer technique of T1-weighted, fat-suppression, spin-echo MRI with gadopentetate dimeglumine (58) may be more sensitive than dynamic CT (59, 60), but no study has compared this technique with the newer technique of spiral CT. In theory, MRI has the potential advantage of lacking ionizing radiation, but MRI machines are less universally available, more expensive to maintain, and require a different, more specialized expertise. Currently, MRI should not be part of the routine diagnostic evaluation of the patient with suspected pancreatic cancer.

**Endoscopic Retrograde Cholangiopancreatography.** Because most pancreatic ductal cancers arise from the main pancreatic duct, direct imaging of the pancreatic duct by ERCP is currently the most sensitive diagnostic test for pancreatic cancer and, in this respect, represents the current gold standard. The sensitivity of ERCP for the diagnosis of ductal cancer approaches 95% (61, 62). Long (>1 cm), irregular strictures of the pancreatic duct are virtually pathognomonic in the appropriate clinical situation (Fig. 52.3). When an intramural process involving the proximal pancreatic duct also extrinsically obstructs the intrapancreatic portion of the common bile duct, the appearance is that of the "double duct" sign; in this situation, one can be almost certain of the diagnosis of pancreatic cancer. Much more difficult to interpret are the short, isolated pancreatic ductal strictures that may occur after trauma or chronic pancreatitis and can masquerade as pancreatic cancer (Fig. 52.4).

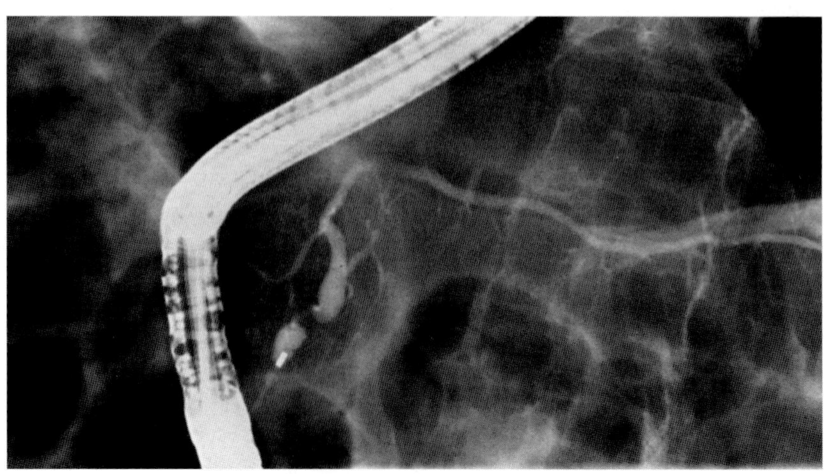

**FIG. 52.4.** ERCP with an isolated, short stricture of the proximal pancreatic duct; this was secondary to an area of isolated chronic pancreatitis.

Differentiation of benign from malignant strictures in the setting of known suspected chronic pancreatitis can be especially difficult or impossible and may require exploration and resection for the final differentiation.

While none would argue with the *reliability* of ERCP in confirming a clinical suspicion of pancreatic cancer in the patient with appropriate clinical findings and a pancreatic mass on CT, *the question of the necessity* for this invasive study routinely is quite controversial. In some centers, ERCP is used as the "next test" after CT to confirm the diagnosis. With the current sophistication of spiral CT, this routine practice is highly questionable. ERCP, being an invasive procedure, is associated with a small but significant risk (≈2–5%) of pancreatitis, cholangitis (when biliary obstruction exists), and even duodenal perforation (≈1–2%). These complications can delay or, if severe enough, even prevent potentially curative therapy of the pancreatic cancer (63). For these reasons, most pancreatologists reserve the use of ERCP for patients in whom the diagnosis is equivocal.

The primary indications for ERCP in the diagnostic evaluation of patients suspected of having pancreatic cancer include the patient with obstructive jaundice in whom no mass is evident on CT, the symptomatic but nonjaundiced patient without an obvious pancreatic mass, or occasionally the patient with known chronic pancreatitis in whom development of a pancreatic neoplasm is suspected. Similarly, ERCP may be the procedure of choice when other noninvasive tests demonstrate biliary and/or pancreatic ductal strictures but no evidence of a neoplasm (64). Other less common indications may include high-risk patients, such as those in a pedigree of familial pancreatic cancer, in whom some other screening test (e.g., serum tumor markers, CT imaging, molecular biologic tests) is abnormal. An additional benefit of ERCP is that the endoscopist gets a direct view of the ampulla. In the *high-risk* patient with a presumed periampullary neoplasm, the observation of an ampullary cancer (as opposed to a periampullary pancreatic ductal cancer) may sway the surgeon into being more aggressive surgically, because the ability to affect survival is so much better with ampullary than with pancreatic ductal cancer. One might also consider a less extensive periampullary resection of an ampullary cancer in the patient who, because of comorbid conditions, is not a candidate for a major pancreatic resection. However, for the good-risk patient who presents with new-onset jaundice and a clinical picture consistent with an underlying pancreatic malignancy, in whom an imaging test clearly shows both a pancreatic mass and the proximal (hepatic) extent of the biliary obstruction, an ERCP offers no further therapeutically useful information concerning staging (65) and subjects the patient to a small risk of the invasive procedure. Since ERCP is a diagnostic procedure and does not usually alter the therapeutic approach, most pancreatic surgeons believe ERCP is unnecessary in most patients with clinically evident pancreatic cancer (see below, staging, endobiliary stents).

### Other Imaging Studies

***Positron Emission Tomography.*** The increased metabolism of glucose by pancreatic adenocarcinoma is the basis of the technique of positron emission tomography (PET). By infusing fluorine-18-labeled fluorodeoxyglucose (FDG), PET can (88–90%) distinguish accurately between cancer and mass-forming chronic pancreatitis (66, 67) by means of increased uptake of radioactive material by the former. FDG-PET appears to be more sensitive than CT for the diagnosis of lymph node metastases (67) and also more sensitive than the previously used single positron emission CT (68). C-11 acetate PET has also been used with some reported success to differentiate cancer from chronic pancreatitis (69). The application of PET is currently limited because of the very expensive, highly sophisticated technology needed (cyclotron and PET scanner). Its place in the diagnostic armamentarium is yet to be fully defined.

***Radionuclide Imaging.*** Use of monoclonal antibodies labeled with a radionuclide that will specifically traffic to pancreatic cancer cells for the diagnosis of pancreatic cancer, similar in principle to octreotide scanning for islet cell neoplasms, prompted some early enthusiasm (see Chapter 76) (70, 71). Unfortunately, this concept has not proven to offer any advantages or increased sensitivity (72). Immunoscintigraphy requires a universal antigen for ductal cancer specific enough for multiple genetically diverse populations. It is neither sensitive nor specific enough to allow early detection of pancreatic cancer or to screen for early cancer in asymptomatic patients at high risk (73).

***Pancreatoscopy.*** Despite improvements in CT, ERCP, endoscopic ultrasonography, and other imaging modalities, a small subgroup of patients remains with a documented pancreatic ductal abnormality (usually a stricture) that cannot be further clarified with the aforementioned methods and in whom a precise histopathologic or other objective diagnosis will have a decisive impact on the choice of further management (i.e., resection, drainage, or observation). In this subgroup, direct visualization of the ductal abnormality might prove diagnostic. Currently, the technology of small-piece endoscopes is such that pancreatoscopy is an expensive, highly specialized technique.

Using a modified endoscope with an additional specialized side port, a guide wire is passed into the main pancreatic duct, over which a small-diameter pancreatic endoscope is carefully passed. Two prototypes of pancreatoscopes have been used. One has a diameter of 3.1 mm and requires both a sphincterotomy for insertion and a dilated pancreatic duct. This endoscope has several advantages including two-way tip deflection, allowing better and wider visualization, and a 1.2-mm channel for a biopsy forceps. The second pancreatoscope has a diameter of 0.8 mm, can be introduced without a prior sphincterotomy, and does not require a dilated pancreatic ductal system. Although less traumatic, this small-diameter, fragile pancreatoscope has three disadvantages: its tip cannot be deflected, it does not provide as good a view, and it cannot obtain tissue for diagnosis (74).

Pancreatoscopy has been reported to be associated with high success rates (70–95%) in experienced hands (75–77) and relatively low risk (0–4%) of postprocedure pancreatitis (75, 76, 78). In addition to its role in the diagnosis of conditions such as intraductal papillary mucinous tumors, proponents of this technique claim that it can accurately distinguish between chronic pancreatitis and cancer, because the ductal system in the former has a smooth surface with mucosal atrophy and a fine, prominent vascular network, whereas in the latter there is tumor infiltration and ductal disruption (74, 79). When performed under appropriate indications, pancreatoscopy may offer "diagnostic gain" in 80–100% of patients (76, 77, 80). Although more experience is needed, pancreatoscopy appears to have a potential role in some patients with suspected ductal abnormalities. Another potential application of this technique might be screening and early diagnosis of pancreatic cancer in patients at increased risk, but no data exist to support such practice at the present time.

## Histopathologic Diagnosis

**Percutaneous Biopsy.** With increased ability to image pancreatic masses under CT or ultrasonography, techniques for obtaining percutaneous core biopsies or fine-needle aspiration (FNA) cytology have been evaluated. While highly specific (99%) and having a high positive predictive value, reported sensitivities and negative predictive values for pancreatic cancer are generally lower, ranging from 60 to 70%. The sensitivity probably varies with the extent of surrounding glandular reaction and pancreatitis in response to the neoplasm. Obviously, the efficacy of the biopsy depends on appropriate positioning of the biopsy needle. This problem is important because CT often overestimates the size of the neoplasm, and biopsies taken from just outside the extent of the direct tumor infiltration will yield only a histologic diagnosis of chronic pancreatitis. While a histologic diagnosis of adenocarcinoma is very reliable (Fig. 52.5), malignancy cannot be excluded with certainty when the pathologist cannot find malignant cells in the specimen. Because of this uncertainty, the use of percutaneous biopsy in the diagnostic algorithm in the patient with a suspected pancreatic cancer has been challenged by pancreatic surgeons for several reasons (63, 81). While percutaneous biopsy is generally quite safe, several potentially serious complications can occur (≈1%), including hemorrhage, pancreatitis, fistula, abscess, and rarely death. While these serious complications are rare, of equal concern are several reports of tumor seeding along the subcutaneous track of the needle (82) or intraperitoneally (83).

Because of its low sensitivity, negative predictive value, potential complications, and risk of seeding of tumor cells, most pancreatologists believe that percutaneous biopsy has little or no role in the evaluation of the good-risk patient with a clinically resectable pancreatic mass (84). A negative percutaneous biopsy would not prevent operative exploration and resection (just as a negative intraoperative biopsy does not absolutely exclude the diagnosis of pancreatic cancer in a patient with a highly suspicious mass). If the results of the percutaneous biopsy will not alter patient management, there seems no reason to perform it, especially with its associated cost, patient discomfort, and potential risks.

There is a definite role for percutaneous pancreatic biopsy in poor-risk patients in whom a major pancreatic resection is not possible, but who are candidates for palliative chemoradiation therapy. They should have a tissue diagnosis before this therapy is started. Percutaneous biopsy avoids an open or laparoscopic biopsy. With an unresectable pancreatic cancer (local extension, liver metastases), a percutaneous biopsy can confirm the diagnosis and allow a nonoperative approach of endoscopic placement of a biliary endoprosthesis and/or palliative chemoradiation therapy.

One other potential role for percutaneous biopsy is in the patient in whom there is a high clinical or radiographic suspicion that the pancreatic mass might *not* be a ductal adenocarcinoma but rather a lymphoma, islet cell neoplasm, or other unusual condition that would either obviate potential exploration or warrant a more aggressive operative approach (85, 86). An example of the latter situation is the patient with back pain and a large mass in the body of the pancreas. Tissue confirmation of a ductal adenocarcinoma would stop most surgeons from exploring this patient, but if the biopsy showed an islet cell neoplasm, resection would be warranted, despite the large size of the neoplasm.

**Pancreatic Ductal Cytology.** There is increasing interest in sampling pancreatic ductal or duodenal luminal secretions to aid in diagnosis. As discussed above (Molecular Biology Techniques), the pancreatic juice can be evaluated for tumor markers such as the K-*ras* mutation and probably more markers in the future. Cytologic evaluation of endoscopic brushings of the pancreatic duct (87) or of pure pancreatic juice obtained at the time of ERCP has been reported (88). Experience is as yet limited, and the sensitivity remains unknown. Arguments for and against this invasive technique are similar to those of percutaneous biopsy and ERCP in the routine diagnostic algorithm. Nevertheless, in the patient in whom the diagnosis is not clinically secure or in the screening of high-risk patients who will be undergoing ERCP, cytologic examination of the pancreatic juice may offer additional information that will directly affect management decisions.

## PREOPERATIVE STAGING OF PANCREATIC CANCER

*Diagnosis* and clinical *staging* of pancreatic cancer are two separate steps in the workup of a patient with suspected pancreatic cancer. Once a diagnosis has been made, the appropriate management options ultimately depend on the clinical staging of the patient. The presence of unresectable disease precipitates a much different management algorithm than when the presumed neoplasm appears resectable "for cure." Thus, it becomes important preoperatively to exclude the factors that define unresectability for cure: *(a)* distant metastases to liver, peritoneal surfaces, or lymph nodes outside the margins of resection; *(b)* invasion of certain peripancreatic blood vessels—superior mesenteric vein/portal vein and common hepatic/proper hepatic artery; and *(c)* invasion of the neural plexuses around the celiac axis or the superior mesenteric artery.

With the explosion of direct and indirect imaging procedures now available, the clinician must choose carefully from the options on the basis of efficacy, cost-effectiveness, risk, and most importantly whether or not the staging procedure will alter management. If the staging procedure will not directly affect the

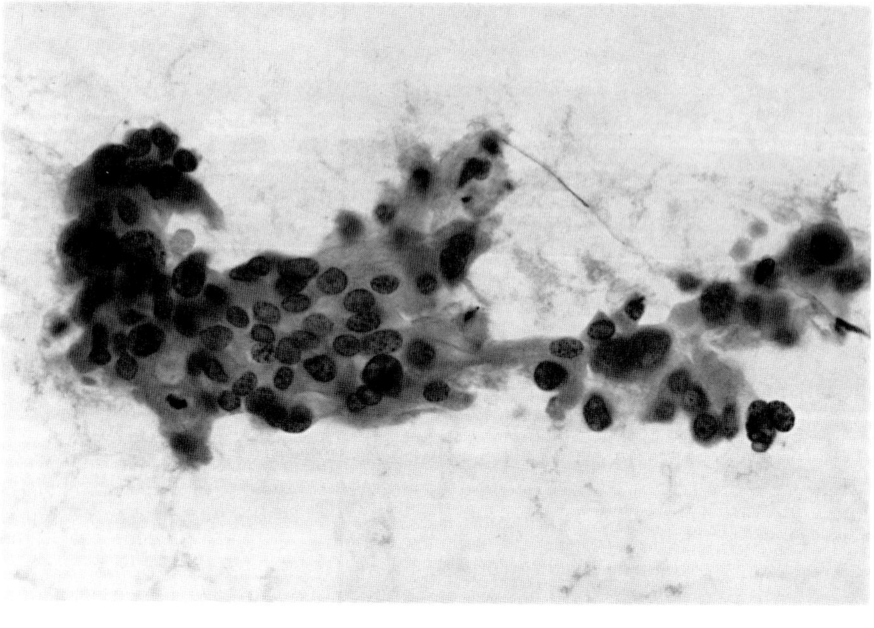

**FIG. 52.5.** A representative cluster of malignant cells from an FNA of pancreatic adenocarcinoma. These cells demonstrate the coarse nuclear chromatin, variability in nuclear size and shape, and disorderly nuclear crowding typical of pancreatic adenocarcinoma cells. Prominent nucleoli often seen in pancreatic adenocarcinoma are not present in this example. (Pap, ×400).

management strategy, it is not justified. The availability of these new procedures does not justify their use. Numerous studies have evaluated the use of CT, angiography, endoscopic ultrasonography, laparoscopy, and biliary stents—each has their own advocates, but all these techniques remain controversial. Each is discussed below by addressing their inherent advantages and disadvantages.

## Computerized Tomography

The development of spiral CT (thin-section, contrast-enhanced helical CT) has proved to be a major advance in pancreatic imaging. The use of thin (1.5 cm) sections in 5-mm intervals rapidly scanned during the phase of peak vascular enhancement has helped to delineate accurately the relationship between the neoplasm and the peripancreatic blood vessels. Computerized three-dimensional vascular reconstruction may be achieved to better determine the crucial issue of the proximity of the neoplasm to the peripancreatic vessels. In addition, less contrast is required, and liver metastases appear to be detected with improved sensitivity (89, 90). Preoperative prediction of resectability with CT has improved from ≈50% to ≈90% in some reports (54, 91, 92). Recently, spiral CT has been reported to be highly sensitive (91%), specific (94%), and accurate (93%) compared with operative findings (93). Whether these possibly overly optimistic results can be reproduced in other centers has yet to be proven.

**Distant Disease.** Sensitivity of CT in demonstrating *liver metastases* depends primarily on their size. Most lesions (≈90%) of 2 cm or larger are evident as less dense defects in the hepatic parenchyma; metastases smaller than 1 cm are usually not evident and are missed if present. This has been one of the strong arguments in support of preoperative staging laparoscopy (see below). Detection of *nodal metastases* is much less accurate. While enlarged peripancreatic lymph nodes, especially along the common hepatic artery, are often evident, it is virtually impossible to determine whether they are nodal metastases or just enlarged reactive nodes so commonly seen with established extrahepatic biliary obstruction. While the presence of these enlarged nodes must be acknowledged by the surgeon, it remains difficult or impossible to alter the management strategy (explore for resection vs. nonoperative palliation) solely on the basis of the presence of enlarged peripancreatic nodes unless they are widespread, located outside the field of reasonable resection, and amenable to percutaneous biopsy.

*Peritoneal metastases* are rarely imaged directly, but their presence may be inferred by the presence of ascites. Ascites in the patient with a suspected pancreatic cancer should precipitate percutaneous aspiration cytology and, if negative, a laparoscopic examination in an attempt to confirm peritoneal metastases and thereby avoid a nontherapeutic celiotomy.

**Vascular Involvement.** A critical role of preoperative staging is to determine the proximity of the primary neoplasm to the major peripancreatic vascular structures—superior mesenteric vein, portal vein, superior mesenteric artery, and on occasion the common hepatic artery. This has stimulated interest in the timing of rapid scanning during bolus intravenous contrast injection to maximize the intravenous uptake versus the pancreatic enhancement in an attempt to evaluate the normally present "fat" plane between the posterolateral superior mesenteric artery/portal vein and the head/uncinate region of the pancreas. Preservation of this plane strongly suggests lack of direct invasion or abutment of the primary neoplasm with these veins. Preservation of the superior mesenteric vein/portal vein contour throughout its extent but loss of the fat plane is an indeterminate finding that also suggests unresectability. However, this finding is less accurate because the primary neoplasm may incite a distal "obstructive" pancreatitis, especially in the uncinate process, which masquerades as local tumor extension. Occlusion of the superior mesenteric vein/portal vein junction, especially with the presence of collateral vessels, is an absolute sign of unresectability and should preclude abdominal exploration and attempts at resection. Compression of these veins with loss of the smooth contrast column within is consistent with, *but not necessarily* diagnostic of, tumor involvement. (The controversial concept of superior mesenteric vein/portal vein resection in curative resection is discussed elsewhere.)

Because neoplasms of the uncinate process are especially difficult to evaluate intraoperatively, their preoperative staging becomes very important. Uncinate lesions arise posterolateral to the superior mesenteric vein, so venous involvement cannot be determined accurately by intraoperative maneuvers until the neck of the pancreas has been transected (thus committing the surgeon to a proximal pancreatectomy). CT imaging is an especially crucial technique but can be difficult to interpret for accurate staging. Proximity to *both* the posterior superior mesenteric vein and the right lateral aspect of the superior mesenteric artery becomes important. Concomitant pancreatitis may provide a false-positive sign of superior mesenteric vein/superior mesenteric artery encroachment but usually not of direct vascular involvement. Correlation of clinical signs (back pain, severe weight loss) and these CT findings is important in patients with uncinate neoplasms, to prevent nontherapeutic celiotomies or noncurative major pancreatic resections.

Pancreatic cancers arising in the neck or proximal body of the gland are rarely resectable because by the time symptoms arise, they have extended through the pancreatic capsule to involve the common hepatic artery and/or the celiac plexus. CT can provide valuable information about tumor extension to these structures and thereby preclude a nontherapeutic celiotomy. Indeed, resectability is unusual with these lesions (94), but when feasible, extended survival is possible. Thus no pancreatic surgeon wishes to deny these patients the possibility of resection unless there are pathognomonic signs of unresectability. Extracapsular extension in itself does not preclude resection *unless* it involves the celiac axis or the very proximal splenic artery. Most pancreatic surgeons consider splenic vein thrombosis/occlusion a sign of locally advanced disease that precludes exploration. Correlation with clinical presentation (back pain, severe weight loss, etc.) is especially crucial and may warrant the use of other, more invasive staging procedures (laparoscopy, angiography) in an attempt to prevent nontherapeutic celiotomy.

## Angiography

One of the primary reasons for the low resectability rates (25–50%) in patients with "clinically resectable" pancreatic cancer is unexpected vascular involvement of the superior mesenteric or portal vein and/or the superior mesenteric artery despite a CT scan, which failed to demonstrate this direct extension. To avoid an unnecessary operation, several groups proposed preoperative imaging of the major peripancreatic vessels as a staging procedure. It was presumed that the venous phase of the celiac and superior mesenteric arteriograms, by depicting the contour of the vessels in the vicinity of the tumor, would be a more specific indicator for vascular involvement and thereby provide a better means of assessing resectability than CT alone.

Preoperative angiography became very popular as a staging procedure in the last decade. Some pancreatic surgeons continue to perform angiography routinely whenever operation with curative intent is contemplated. Warshaw et al. (95) claimed that a negative arteriogram was associated with high (78%) resectability rates when used as a part of a multimodality workup. However, it was not clear in that study just how angiography decreased the number of unnecessary operations. More recently, the same group (96) reported that routine angiography demonstrated vascular encasement in 48% of the patients with no

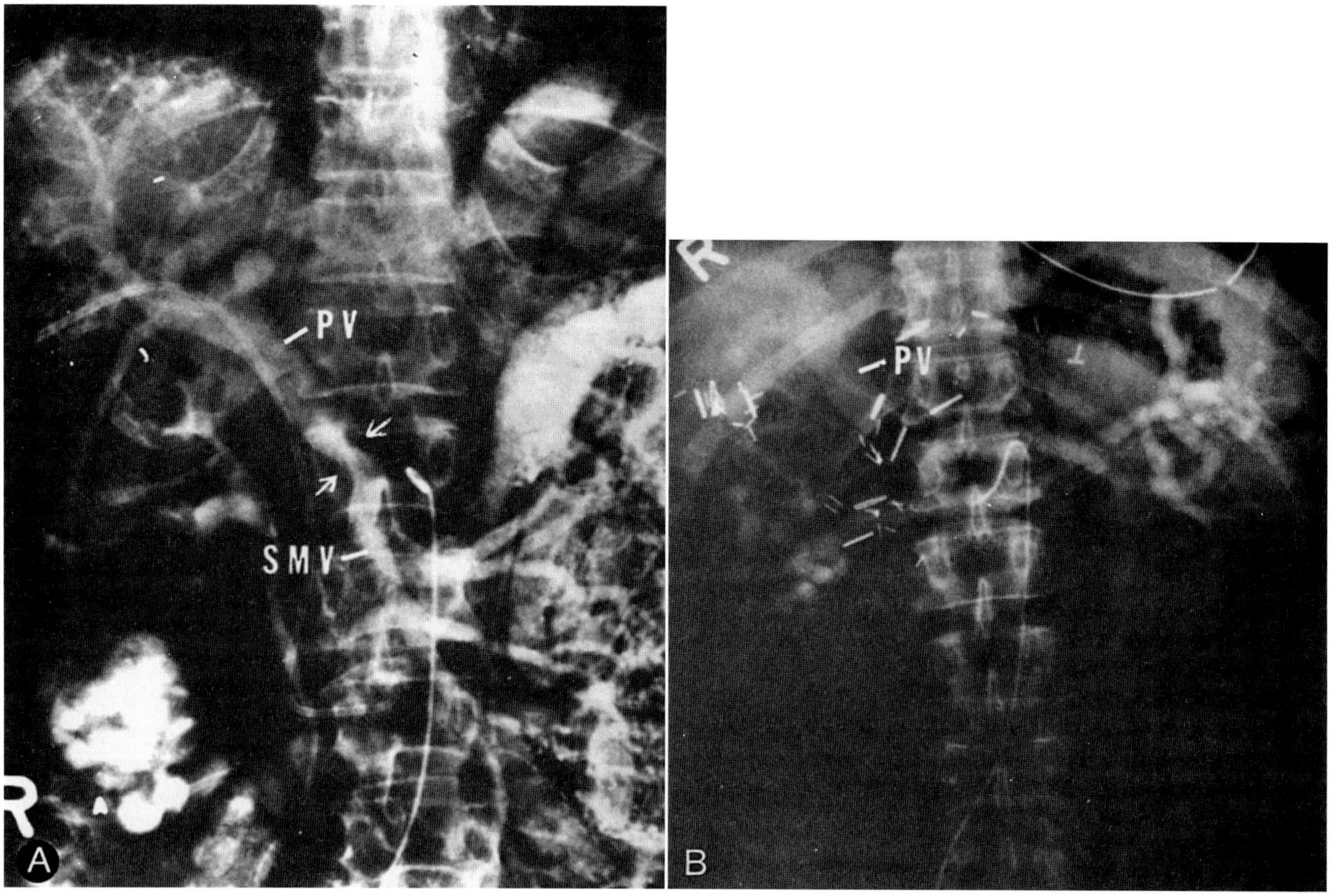


**FIG. 52.6. A.** Venous phase of this superior mesenteric artery injection demonstrates notching of the right wall of the portal vein–superior mesenteric vein junction. This is a normal variant. The defect in the portal vein–superior mesenteric vein junction *(arrow)* is secondary to the inflow of noncontrast media containing splenic venous blood. These phenomena can account for false-positive venograms in the evaluation of periampullary neoplasms. **B.** Venous phase of this celiac axis injection demonstrates drainage of the spleen is by collaterals because the splenic vein is occluded. The superior mesenteric vein was not visualized after superior mesenteric artery injection and was believed to be occluded. These findings were documented at laparotomy. The patient was unresectable. (Reprinted with permission from Dooley WC, Cameron JL, Pitt HA, et al. Is preoperative angiography useful in patients with periampullary tumors? Ann Surg 1990;211:649–655.)

evidence of unresectability by CT and preoperative laparoscopy; these patients were subjected to radiotherapy, but unresectability was not confirmed surgically.

As pancreatic adenocarcinoma infiltrates and invades surrounding tissues, it causes a desmoplastic inflammatory reaction such that the pancreatic "mass" is larger than the cancer itself. This mass effect may indent the vessels and appear as a segmental stenosis (Fig. 52.6*A*). Some carcinomas behave as "pushers" and not as "invaders," resulting in a false-positive angiogram. In such circumstances, the pancreatic mass will compress the vessel, but a clear plane between the two will still exist, permitting a curative resection. Conversely, carcinomas that have infiltrated the adventitia, but not into the wall of the vessel, may produce no discernible abnormality in the contrast column within the vascular lumen, resulting in a false-negative angiogram. In this situation, the surgeon will find the pancreatic mass intimately adherent to the vessel wall without an intervening plane of normal tissue. Most pancreatic surgeons would consider this a contraindication for resection. If a major peripancreatic vessel appears occluded on angiogram (Fig. 52.6*B*), it is highly likely that this represents direct invasion by the malignant process and thereby unresectability. This finding is usually recognizable on a good quality, contrast-enhanced CT.

Dooley et al. (97) carried out angiographic staging in all patients with clinically "resectable" tumors on CT; all were explored on the basis of CT findings regardless of the angiographic diagnosis. Major vessel occlusion was present in 12% of patients and precluded resection in all. Interestingly though, more than one-third of the patients (35%) with vessel "encasement" on angiography proved to have resectable disease (Fig. 52.6*A*), whereas in one-fourth of the patients with normal angiograms, the tumor proved unresectable. Similarly, others have been unable to demonstrate a significant difference in predictive value of angiography over CT for resectability or unresectability (98). One prospective study showed that dynamic CT could predict unresectability better than angiography (97 vs. 88%), and the positive predictive value of angiography for resectable disease was only 44% (99).

The data currently available suggest that preoperative angiography for staging is not justified in patients with pancreatic cancer. In addition to its false-positive and false-negative results, angiography carries a small risk, is expensive, and delays definitive therapy. For these reasons, angiography is an unreliable test upon which to base the decision to operate or not. Angiography adds little useful data to good quality, contrast-enhanced CT, especially since the advent of the more sensitive spiral CT.

The combination of CT with simultaneous arterial portography after catheterization of the celiac and superior mesenteric arteries, so-called CT angiography, has been recently evaluated. Preliminary results suggest this technique is more sensitive and specific than angiography in revealing vascular involvement (92). In theory, the same limitations of peripancreatic vascular imaging apply to CT angiography. The author's conclusion that this is the single most important test in patients with pancreatic cancer has been disputed by a prospective study that showed no benefit of this more invasive test, compared with dynamic CT (100).

Another argument in support of routine preoperative angiography has been that it can demonstrate important vascular anomalies in 30–34% of patients, so that injury to these vessels or ischemia to the organ they supply may be prevented, reconstruction may be planned (101), or the operative technique may be modified (102). The more common vascular anomalies relevant to pancreatic surgery are an aberrant (replaced) right hepatic artery originating from the superior mesenteric artery, an aberrant (replaced) left hepatic artery, originating from the left gastric artery, and a stenotic celiac artery. However, these anomalies should be readily apparent to an experienced pancreatic surgeon. The replaced right hepatic artery should be appreciated as an arterial pulse that lies in the posterior aspect of the hepatoduodenal ligament; the replaced left hepatic artery as an arterial vessel in the lesser omentum; and the clinically relevant stenotic celiac artery by a very large gastroduodenal artery that, when occluded, leads to the loss of a pulse in the common hepatic artery. These anatomic variations, while not uncommon, should be easy to recognize intraoperatively if one looks systematically for them. The surgeon exploring patients with presumed pancreatic cancer with intent to resect should be familiar with the normal anatomy of the region as well as its variations and should not need to depend on an angiogram to identify the individual patient's peripancreatic vascular anatomy. The concept that visceral angiography should be considered a "road map" for exploration comes from inexperience and does not justify this approach.

### Endoscopic Ultrasonography (EUS)

EUS appears quite promising as a staging procedure to decrease the number of patients who undergo exploration for resection only to find unresectable disease secondary to vascular involvement. A specially designed endoscope loaded with a side-oriented, high-frequency transducer is advanced into the third or fourth portion of the duodenum and slowly pulled back. EUS can examine the body, neck, head, and uncinate process of the pancreas; visualize the superior mesenteric artery, superior mesenteric vein, and portal vein; and determine the anatomic relationship of the tumor to these vessels. The tail of the pancreas is a relative blind area for EUS. EUS is thus ideally suited to assess pancreatic masses, by essentially "palpating" the entire pancreas through the lumen of the stomach and duodenum (103).

EUS can accurately determine the size and local extent of a pancreatic cancer (62) (Fig. 52.7*A*), but it cannot reliably assess metastatic involvement of the liver or the lymph nodes (104). Its major role is as an adjunct to CT in assessing peripancreatic vascular involvement (Fig. 52.7*B*). This proposed role has been investigated in four prospective studies. Each used a similar number of patients and reached contradictory results. One showed that EUS and dynamic CT were equally ineffective (29%) in assessing portal vein involvement (105), the second failed to demonstrate any significant advantage to EUS (106), and the third suggested that EUS was significantly more accurate than CT or angiography in achieving this task (62). The authors of the fourth study (107) established three criteria for vascular invasion: *(a)* tumor within the vessel lumen, *(b)* an abnormal contour of the vessel with loss of the hyperechoic vessel-parenchyma interface; and *(c)* presence of venous collaterals in the area of a mass that obliterates the normal anatomic location of a major vessel. At least one of these signs was present in all patients with vascular involvement, and all these findings were absent in all patients without vascular involvement. The diagnostic accuracy of EUS in their hands approached 100%. Although EUS appears promising, it is highly operator dependent and not yet widely available. More experience needs to be gained, and EUS needs to be compared with spiral CT.

In addition to its proposed use in staging, EUS has also been used for diagnosis of pancreatic cancer. Because of the proximity of the ultrasound probe to the tissue under examination and its ability to visualize almost the entire gland, EUS should be an

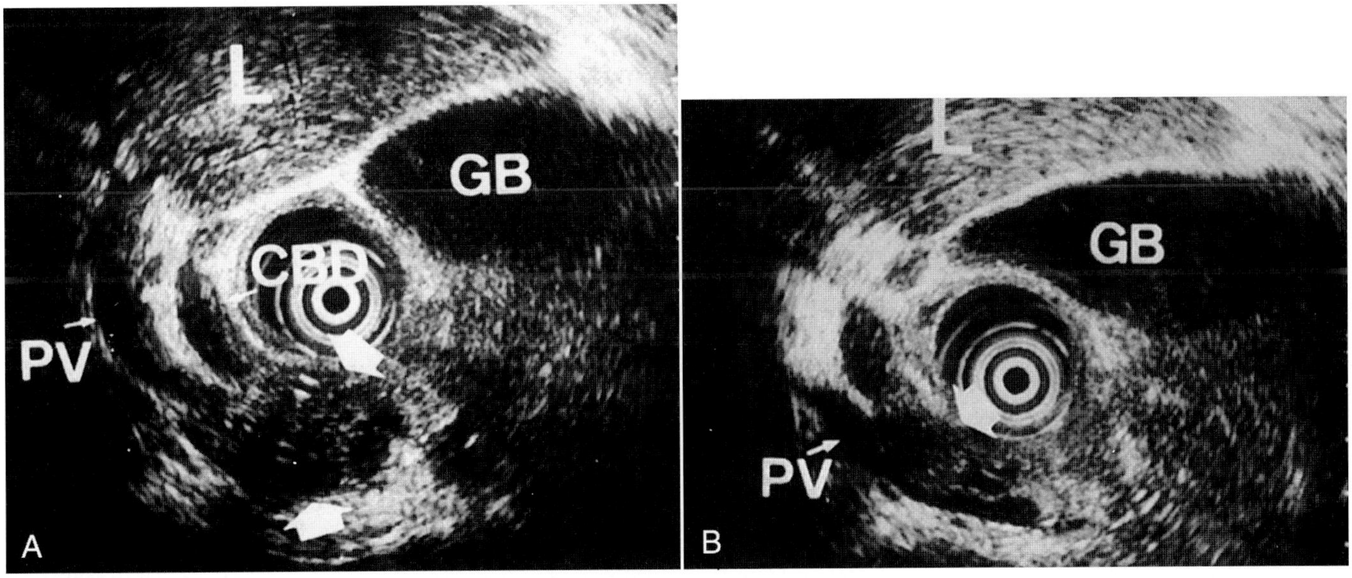


**FIG. 52.7.** **A.** EUS picture from the duodenum shows the hypoechoic round mass *(arrows)* with neighboring organs. **B.** By the serial EUS scanning, involvement of the portal vein is detectable *(arrow)*. (Reprinted with permission from Yasuda K, et al. Endoscopic ultrasonography: diagnosis of pancreatic cancer. Gastrointest Endosc Clin North Am 1995;5:699–712.)

excellent diagnostic modality with experienced endoscopists. Indeed, EUS has shown significantly higher sensitivity, specificity, and accuracy in diagnosing pancreatic neoplasms than dynamic CT, transcutaneous ultrasonography, MRI, and ERCP, especially in neoplasms smaller than 2 cm (105, 108). This advantage of EUS may prove particularly useful in the future as a screening test in subgroups of patients who are at increased risk of developing pancreatic cancer (e.g., patients with chronic pancreatitis, nonobese patients less than 60 years of age with new-onset of diabetes) (109–111).

A further refinement of this technique is the recently introduced intraductal ultrasound probe (112). This thin probe is inserted into the main pancreatic duct to examine the pancreatic parenchyma directly. Initial experience has shown that it may offer even greater sensitivity and specificity than EUS, and it may be more accurate in differentiating benign from malignant masses (61). One study, however, has suggested that it may understage periampullary cancer (113). The ultimate place of intraductal ultrasonography in diagnosis and staging of pancreatic cancer has yet to be determined.

Endovascular intraportal ultrasonography is a very new, invasive procedure that can be performed either via the percutaneous transhepatic approach preoperatively or by cannulation of the superior mesenteric vein/portal vein intraoperatively. Using small-diameter transducers (6 or 8 Fr), several groups have suggested an improved sensitivity to detect or exclude portal venous involvement by neoplasm. The anterior wall of the portal vein appears as an echogenic band 0.5- to 1.0-mm thick; any destruction of this echogenic band is considered a very accurate criterion of direct portal vein invasion by neoplasm (114). Encouraging preliminary results (115) have been confirmed by a recent study that showed 100% sensitivity, 93% specificity, and 97% accuracy of intraportal ultrasonography in diagnosing portal venous involvement and superiority of this technique to CT or arterial portography (114). Other investigators are pursuing this method with similar encouraging preliminary results (116). Although this technique seems impressively accurate, its role has to be questioned and further investigated because of its invasive nature when performed preoperatively and its necessity when performed intraoperatively, because vascular involvement can be directly assessed.

### Laparoscopy

Peritoneal and small liver metastases are features of unresectability often not evident even on the best of preoperative staging spiral CTs. Metastases to the peritoneal surfaces and omentum are usually multiple, widespread, and almost uniformly quite small (1–3 mm). Metastatic lesions to the liver can also be small (1–2 mm) in about 30% of the patients (117) and thus are not evident on CT. In such cases, resection of the primary tumor offers no apparent survival benefit and only subjects the patient to the potential morbidity and mortality of a formal pancreatectomy. Proponents of preoperative staging laparoscopy have shown that these metastases can be recognized by laparoscopic examination, thereby preventing these patients from undergoing a noncurative abdominal operation. An inherent assumption of this approach is that the patient with technically unresectable disease for cure is better palliated by an endobiliary stent than by operative biliary bypass with or without gastroenterostomy. When evaluating the use of diagnostic staging laparoscopy, this inherent bias must be kept in mind.

Diagnostic staging laparoscopy can be performed with minimal morbidity and mortality on an outpatient basis. Using a 30°-angled laparoscope, the entire peritoneal surface is carefully inspected. In addition, care should be taken to examine the paracolic gutters, the hemidiaphragms, and the pelvis. The mesentery should be exposed and explored systematically. The surfaces of the left lobe and most of the right lobe of the liver are amenable to inspection with the exception of segment 7, which may not be able to be well visualized even with an angled scope. Suspicious lesions should be "palpated" laparoscopically and a biopsy specimen taken.

Initial reports claimed an impressive role for laparoscopy. Its pioneers were able to identify peritoneal, omental, or micrometastases of the liver surface, thus proving unresectability in 40% of patients who were thought to have locally resectable disease by all other diagnostic means (118). Another older report claimed an incidence of 82% of metastatic disease precluding resection (119), but not all patients had been screened with CT. In an often-quoted study by Warshaw et al. (95), routine laparoscopy, as a part of multimodality preoperative workup, improved the resectability rate to 78%. Laparoscopy was able to identify distant metastases in 25% of the patients without CT evidence of extrapancreatic involvement, which remained unchanged (25%) in a recent update of this group's experience (96). A very important finding was that staging laparoscopy was more helpful in preventing nontherapeutic celiotomies in patients with cancers of the distal rather than the proximal pancreas (44 vs. 18%). Similar rates (35%) of detection of micrometastases were reported by others as well (120).

To define the role of routine preoperative staging laparoscopy, the following question should be answered: What is the optimal management and palliation of the patient with an unresectable pancreatic cancer? If a mechanical gastric outlet obstruction is one of the presenting features, laparoscopy will not alter the need for a palliative gastroenterostomy. In contrast, if extrahepatic biliary tract obstruction is the main symptom and the patient has a good enough performance status to be considered for a major pancreatic resection, one would expect this patient to have a longer life expectancy than the average patient with a clinically unresectable pancreatic cancer (4–5 months). Many pancreatic surgeons believe that these patients may be better palliated by a surgical procedure (biliary bypass, gastroenterostomy, and celiac plexus block) than by an endoscopically placed endobiliary stent. However, this question remains unanswered. All the previously reported studies comparing survival, cost, total hospitalization until death, and quality of life have compared operative palliation with endobiliary stent in patients deemed to have unresectable disease on clinical grounds (121–123).

The role of staging laparoscopy becomes pivotal in patients with cancers that do not cause biliary or gastric outlet obstruction. This clinical presentation can be encountered occasionally in cancers of the head-neck region, but it is much more common with cancers of the body and tail of the pancreas. Such patients usually do not need palliation of biliary or gastric obstruction, and the only reason they should be submitted to a laparotomy is to have the tumor resected with curative intent. In this subgroup of patients laparoscopy can spare the patient an unnecessary operation with its existing morbidity and time for recuperation. This is the same subgroup in which laparoscopy has its highest yield (44%) (96).

Laparoscopy also has the potential ability to stage nodal disease. In theory, biopsies can be done on suprapancreatic nodes surrounding the common hepatic artery and even the celiac plexus nodes. In addition, an intraoperative, laparoscopically inserted ultrasound probe may prove helpful in evaluating the superior mesenteric/portal venous structures as well as the liver. Further results await technical advances and wider experience with these techniques.

In summary, no one argues with the ability of laparoscopy to recognize small liver and/or peritoneal metastases. However, to adopt the routine use of preoperative diagnostic laparoscopy, the physician must agree that palliation of biliary obstruction is better provided by an endobiliary stent than by an operative biliary bypass. This question, however, is not yet fully answered.

Therefore, if the physician feels that operative biliary bypass is better palliation than an endobiliary stent, there is no role for preoperative staging laparoscopy.

One situation in which laparoscopy may be the diagnostic and staging procedure of choice is in centers that are evaluating neoadjuvant chemotherapy and/or radiotherapy. Patients to be considered for this treatment modality require a tissue diagnosis and assurance of the lack of distant disease. Laparoscopy is the ideal procedure for this new and novel approach.

### Peritoneal Cytology

Positive peritoneal cytology in patients with intraabdominal cancer is a well-recognized phenomenon (124). Although there is some evidence that positive peritoneal cytology is present in only a small number (8%) of patients with pancreatic cancer and is associated with peritoneal carcinomatosis (125), many authors believe it to be more common, ranging between 17 and 30% (83, 96, 124). The presence of malignant cells in peritoneal washings can predict not only tumor unresectability (96) but also a shorter survival, even when the tumor is resected (83). Currently, although most pancreatic surgeons believe that a positive peritoneal washing predicts a poor prognosis and a higher chance of advanced unresectable disease, they would not yet deny the patient with an otherwise "clinically resectable" neoplasm abdominal exploration and the chance for increased survival by resection.

### Endobiliary Stents for Preoperative Biliary Decompression

Endoscopic placement of endobiliary stents for pancreatic carcinoma has become common practice by many physicians and too often occurs before consultation with a surgeon. This is especially true with the wide availability of ERCP in many nonreferral institutions, where the diagnosis of a periampullary tumor is followed by stent placement almost as a knee-jerk response. This invasive procedure usually takes place without a pathologic diagnosis and, more importantly, prior to having assessed whether the tumor is resectable. While not truly a "staging" procedure, this concept of preoperative biliary decompression has been adopted by many as part of the diagnosis, staging, and preparation of the patient with a presumed malignant stricture of the extrahepatic biliary tree.

The purported rationale behind preoperative endoscopic endobiliary stent placement is that it offers a quick and relatively safe way to improve the patient's jaundice and thereby decrease the incidence of postoperative morbidity related to the immunosuppression of jaundice. This practice may also reflect an element of pessimism by the treating physician regarding the availability and feasibility of definitive treatment options. It is a common belief that this palliative measure may be the only procedure that most patients will ever need, and for the minority who will undergo exploration for palliation or resection, placement of a biliary stent "does not burn any bridges" and decreases postoperative morbidity and operative mortality.

This approach, when applied indiscriminately to all patients with pancreatic carcinoma, especially at the initial stages of management, is associated with several problems. First, there is always a small but not insignificant risk of complications (bile duct or duodenal perforation, hemorrhage, pancreatitis) that may delay definitive therapy and compromise the final outcome (63). Second, it converts a sterile biliary system to a colonized one with bacterobilia, increasing the risk for cholangitis and possibly for postoperative infective complications. For these reasons, before an endobiliary stent is placed, patients with presumed or proven pancreatic cancer should be thoroughly staged, and the question of tumor resectability decided first.

In the good-risk patient in whom the pancreatic mass is deemed resectable on the basis of appropriate staging, preoperative biliary decompression by *placement of an endoprosthesis has no place*. Some surgeons have suggested that a stent can be helpful during exploration and bile duct dissection, serving as a guide intraoperatively. It is doubtful, though, whether an experienced pancreatic surgeon needs a biliary stent to identify and safely dissect the bile duct. Moreover, the intraluminal foreign body incites an inflammatory reaction in the hepatoduodenal ligament, making dissection more difficult. A dilated bile duct makes for an easier biliary-enteric anastomosis, a finding not as prominent after decompression.

Several groups have postulated that preoperative biliary decompression may decrease perioperative morbidity and mortality (126). Most of this argument has been based on old retrospective studies. There is evidence that patients with obstructive jaundice may be more prone to develop portal and peripheral endotoxemia with compromise of renal function (127). This latter finding may hold true in patients with profound jaundice due to proximal cholangiocarcinomas, especially when a liver resection is anticipated; preoperative biliary decompression may improve the function of the remaining hepatic parenchyma and decrease the risk of postoperative hepatic and renal failure and sepsis (128). In clinical practice, however, the routine use of endobiliary stents preoperatively in the vast majority of patients with pancreatic cancer has led to mixed results (126, 129). Preoperative placement of a biliary endoprosthesis can delay definitive treatment and may in fact prolong hospital stay without decreasing morbidity and mortality (130, 131). Indeed, three prospective studies have failed to show any significant benefit of preoperative biliary decompression (121–123).

In patients with unresectable tumors, other parameters should be considered prior to making the decision for stent placement; e.g., presence of gastric outlet obstruction and life expectancy. If the former is a presenting feature of the disease, endoscopic palliation of the jaundice will not alleviate the need for operative gastrojejunostomy. In this situation and when the patient is expected to live longer than 6 months, the long-term results of surgical versus endoscopic biliary decompression should be weighed. Prospective randomized trials of patients with known, clinically unresectable pancreatic cancer (estimated mean life expectancy, 4–5 months) (121–123, 132) have shown that biliary endoprostheses have success comparable to that of surgery in palliating jaundice and have the additional benefit of lower procedure-related morbidity and hospitalization. However, this benefit occurs at the expense of a greater incidence of recurrent jaundice and cholangitis, as high as 30–38% (121, 122), requiring readmission and stent change and offsetting the initial advantage of shorter hospital stay (121, 133). Furthermore, stented patients, if they live long enough, are at risk (at least 9–14%, if not greater) (121–123) of developing gastric outlet obstruction, which would necessitate an operation at a later stage of the disease, when they would be more incapacitated and more prone to complications. The introduction of the self-expanding metal stents appears to have decreased the incidence of stent occlusion, and although expensive, they may alter recommendations concerning endoscopic versus operative palliation.

Biliary stent placement becomes the ideal palliative measure for patients with serious comorbid conditions that make them unsatisfactory candidates for potential pancreatic resection or for patients with clinically unresectable tumors, a short life expectancy, and no duodenal obstruction. This subgroup will have the best quality of life with endoscopic palliation. In summary, preoperative biliary decompression should be used selectively, not routinely, in patients with extrahepatic biliary obstruction. A lot of thought is needed in selecting the subgroup of patients who

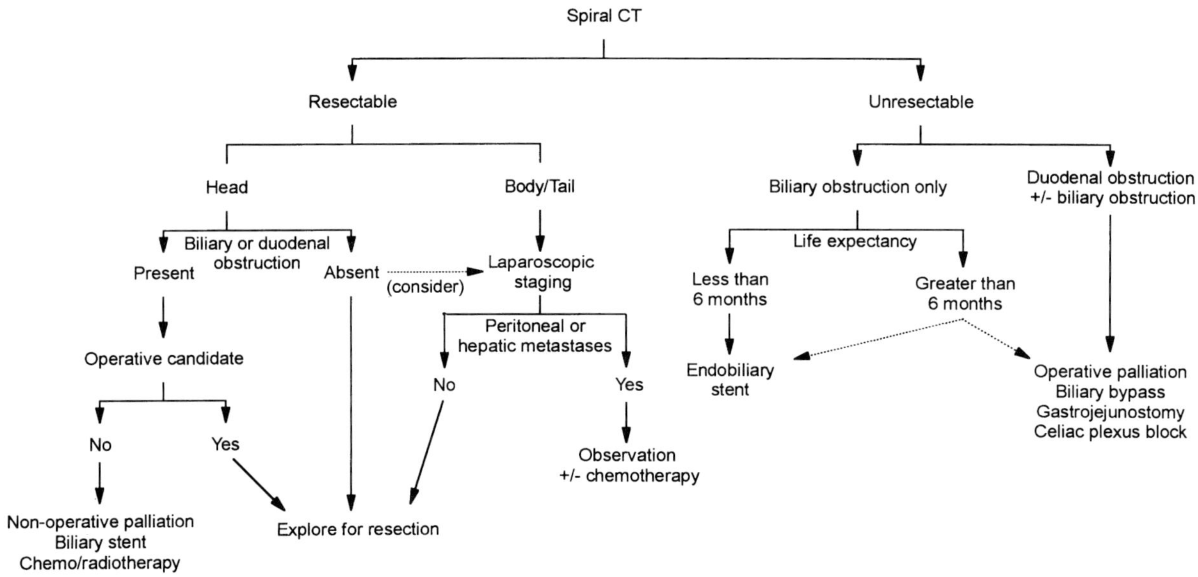


**FIG. 52.8.** Algorithm to use when there is clinical suspicion of pancreatic cancer.

would benefit from this invasive procedure. This decision often requires the experience and judgment of a referral center with a special interest in pancreatic disease.

## OUR APPROACH TO DIAGNOSIS AND STAGING

When a good-quality CT demonstrates a clinically resectable mass in the proximal gland (head or uncinate process), which is causing biliary obstruction, and there is no evidence of regional or distant metastases in a good-risk patient, we believe that operative exploration for potential resection is usually warranted without further investigation (Fig. 52.8). This continues to be our approach, even if the tumor proves unresectable, because we believe that this subgroup of patients is better served by surgical than by endoscopic palliation. For pancreatic cancers of the body and tail, laparoscopy is probably the procedure of choice because it may prevent an unnecessary celiotomy if intraperitoneal micrometastases are present. These patients will need only pain management, and in this context, a transcutaneous celiac plexus block is generally very successful. For masses in the head of the gland that do not cause biliary obstruction but look resectable on a good-quality CT, the decision is more difficult. One would question the diagnosis of ductal cancer of the pancreas because of the lack of biliary obstruction. One might consider a "staging" or diagnostic laparoscopy to see if evidence can be obtained to support or confirm a different diagnosis. If not, resection seems warranted. We believe that patients with biliary obstruction due to unresectable disease who are in excellent general condition and are expected to live more than 6 months will enjoy a better quality of life if they undergo surgical, rather than endoscopic, palliation. We usually reserve endoscopic palliation with endobiliary stents for the poor-risk surgical candidate (regardless of local resectability of the tumor) and for patients with jaundice due to clinically unresectable tumors and a presumed life expectancy under 6 months.

These general guidelines are based on the available knowledge of the efficacy, risks, and cost-effectiveness of the various diagnostic and staging modalities and represent a rational, realistic approach to the evaluation of the patient with a suspected pancreatic cancer. The principles outlined above may, of course, be subject to modification if new treatment modalities prove successful. For instance, if neoadjuvant chemotherapy and/or radiotherapy protocols prove beneficial, then preoperative, pretherapeutic biopsy confirmation and staging of the tumor will be necessary before starting the neoadjuvant treatment. Under these conditions, diagnostic and staging laparoscopy would seem more important.

## SUMMARY

The role of the primary care physician is crucial in the optimal management of patients with pancreatic cancer. Increased awareness and a low threshold of suspicion are probably the most important means of decreasing the delay in diagnosis of pancreatic cancer. Triage is equally important. It cannot be overemphasized that patients with suspected cancer of the pancreas should undergo the final evaluation and operation in large-volume centers with a proven record of low morbidity and mortality in pancreatic surgery.

Vague abdominal complaints or back pain associated with constitutional symptoms (weight loss, fatigue, anorexia) in an elderly patient should raise suspicion for malignancy and prompt further investigation. Obstructive jaundice in a patient older than 50 years with no history of hepatic or gallstone disease should be an indication for a diagnostic and screening CT scan (preferably spiral CT), thereby avoiding the cost, time, and less helpful results of ultrasound. With current techniques of resection reaching limits in the management of pancreatic cancer, further improvement in final outcome will depend upon earlier diagnosis and new adjuvant treatment modalities. When subgroups of the population at increased risk for development of this disease are identified and submitted to refined, sophisticated imaging modalities, pancreatic adenocarcinoma might be diagnosed at an early stage (134). Under these circumstances, the treatment of this disease may prove more successful, with an increase in survival and cure rate.

## REFERENCES

1. Riela A, Zinsmeister AR, Melton LJ, Weiland LH, DiMagno EP. Increasing pancreatic cancer incidence in women over five decades in Olmsted County. Mayo Clin Proc 1992;67: 839–845.
2. Nitecki SS, Sarr MG, Colby TV, et al. Long term survival after resection for ductal adenocarcinoma of the pancreas: is it really improving? Ann Surg 1995;221:59–66.

3. Trede M, Schwall G, Seager H. Survival after pancreaticoduodenectomy. Ann Surg 1990;211:447–458.
4. Geer RJ, Brennan MF. Prognostic indicators for survival after resection of pancreatic adenocarcinoma. Am J Surg 1993;165: 68–73.
5. Cameron JL, Crist DW, Sitzman JV, et al. Factors influencing survival after pancreatoduodenectomy for pancreatic cancer. Am J Surg 1991;161:120–125.
6. Yeo CJ, Cameron JL, Lillemoe KD, et al. Pancreaticoduodenectomy for cancer of the head of the pancreas: 201 patients. Ann Surg 1995;221:721–733.
7. Tsuchiya R, Tsunoda T, Ishida T, Saitoh Y. Resection for cancer of the pancreas—the Japanese experience. Ballieres Clin Gastroenterol 1990;4:931–939.
8. Gudjonsson B. Carcinoma of the pancreas: critical analysis of costs, results of resections and the need for standardized reporting. J Am Coll Surg 1995;181:483–503.
9. Bockman DE, Buchker M, Beger HG. Interaction of pancreatic ductal carcinoma with nerves leads to nerve damage. Gastroenterology 1994;107:219–230.
10. Kalser MH, Barkin J, MacIntyre JM. Pancreatic cancer: assessment of prognosis by clinical presentation. Cancer 1985;56: 397–402.
11. Cujick J, Babiker AG. Pancreatic cancer, diabetes mellitus and gallbladder disease. Int J Cancer 1989;43:415–421.
12. La Vecchia C, Negri E, Franceschi S, D'Avanzo B, Boyle P. A case-control study of diabetes mellitus and cancer risk. Br J Cancer 1994;70:950–953.
13. Permert J, Ihse I, Jorfeldt I, Von Schenck H, Arnquist HJ, Larsson J. Improved glucose metabolism after subtotal pancreatectomy for pancreatic cancer. Br J Surg 1993;80:1047–1050.
14. Oosterwijk C, Hoppener JWM, van Hulst KL, Lips CJM. Pancreatic islet amyloid formation in patients with noninsulin-dependent diabetes mellitus. Int J Pancreatol 1995;18:7–14.
15. Sowa S, Sanke T, Hirayama J, et al. Islet amyloid polypeptide amide causes insulin resistance in vivo in dogs. Diabetologia 1990;33:118–120.
16. Pemert J, Larsson J, Westermark GT, et al. Islet amyloid polypeptide in patients with pancreatic cancer and diabetes. N Engl J Med 1994;330:313–318.
17. Steinberg W. The clinical utility of CA 19-9 tumor-associated antigen. Am J Gastroenterol 1990;85:350–355.
18. Satake K, Takeuchi T. Comparison of CA 19-9 with other tumor markers in the diagnosis of the cancer of the pancreas. Pancreas 1994;9:720–724.
19. Forsmark CE, Lambiase L, Vogel SB. Diagnosis of pancreatic cancer and prediction of unresectability using the tumor-associated antigen CA 19. Pancreas 1994;9:731–734.
20. Glenn J, Steinberg WM, Kurtzman SH, Steinberg SM, Sindelar WF. Evaluation of the utility of a radioimmunoassay for serum CA 19-9 levels before and after treatment of carcinoma of the pancreas. J Clin Oncol 1988;6:462–468.
21. Yasue M, Sakamoto J, Teramukai S, et al. Prognostic values of postoperative CEA and CA 19-9 levels in pancreatic cancer. Pancreas 1994;9:735–740.
22. Kawa S, Tokoo M, Hasebe O, et al. Comparative study of CA 242 and CA 19-9 for the diagnosis of pancreatic cancer. Br J Cancer 1994;70:481–486.
23. Pasanen PA, Eskelinen M, Partanen, et al. A prospective study of serum tumor markers CEA, CA 50, CA 242, tissue polypeptide antigen and tissue polypeptide specific antigen in the diagnosis of pancreatic cancer with special reference to multivariate diagnostic score. Br J Cancer 1994;69:562–565.
24. Robles-Diaz G, Diaz-Sanchez V, Fernandez-del Castillo C, et al. Serum testosterone: dihydrotestosterone ratio and CA 19-9 in the diagnosis of pancreatic cancer. Am J Gastroenterol 1991; 86:591–594.
25. Steinberg WM, Gelfand R, Anderson KK, et al. Comparison of the sensitivity and specificity of the CA 19-9 and carcinoembryonic antigen assays in detecting cancer of the pancreas. Gastroenterology 1986;90:343–349.
26. Kuno N, Kurimoto K, Fukushima M, et al. Effectiveness of multivariate analysis of tumor markers in diagnosis of pancreatic carcinoma: a prospective study in multiinstitutions. Pancreas 1994;9:725–730.
27. Fearon E, Vogelstein B. A genetic model for colorectal tumorigenesis. Cell 1990;61:759–767.
28. Bos JL. ras oncogenes in human cancer: a review. Cancer Res 1989;49:4682–4689.
29. Pellagata NS, Sessa F, Renault B, et al. K-ras and p-53 gene mutations in pancreatic cancers: ductal and nonductal tumors progress through different lesions. Cancer Res 1994;54:1556–1560.
30. Hruban RH, van Mansfeld ADM, Offerhaus GJA, et al. K-ras oncogene activation in adenocarcinoma of the human pancreas. A study of 82 carcinomas using a combination of mutant-enriched polymerase chain reaction analysis and allele-specific oligonucleotide hybridization. Am J Pathol 1993; 143:545–554.
31. Redston MS, Caldas C, Seymour AB, et al. p-53 mutations in pancreatic adenocarcinoma and evidence of common involvement of homocopolymer tracts in DNA microdeletions. Cancer Res 1994;54:3025–3033.
32. Gonzalez-Cavadid NF, Zhou D, Battifora H, et al. Direct sequencing analysis of exon 1 of the c-K-ras gene shows a low frequency of mutations in human pancreatic adenocarcinomas. Oncogene 1989;4:1137–1140.
33. Verlaan-de-Vries M, Bogaard ME, van den Elst H, et al. A dot-blot screening procedure for mutated ras oncogenes using synthetic oligodesoxynucleotides. Gene 1986;50:3130–3120.
34. Jen J, Powell SM, Papadopoulos N, et al. Molecular determinants of dysplasia in colorectal lesions. Cancer Res 1994;54: 5523–5526.
35. Watanabe H, Sawabu N, Ohta H, et al. Identification of K-ras oncogene mutations in pure pancreatic juice of patients with ductal pancreatic cancers. Jap J Cancer Res 1993;84: 961–965.
36. Tada M, Omata M, Kawai S, et al. Detection of ras gene in pancreatic juice and peripheral blood of patients with pancreatic adenocarcinoma. Cancer Res 1993;53:2472–2474.
37. Kondo H, Sugano K, Fukayama N, et al. Detection of point mutations in the K-ras oncogene at codon 12 in pure pancreatic juice for diagnosis of pancreatic carcinoma. Cancer 1994;73: 1589–1594.
38. Berthelemy P, Bouisson M, Escourrou J, et al. Identification of K-ras mutations in pancreatic juice in the early diagnosis of pancreatic cancer. Ann Int Med 1995;123:188–191.
39. Iguchi H, Sugano K, Fukayama N, et al. Analysis of Ki-ras codon 12 mutations in the duodenal juice of patients with pancreatic cancer. Gastroenterology 1996;110:221–226.
40. Ajiki T, Onoyama H, Yamamoto M, et al. Detection of point mutations in K-ras gene at codon 12 in bile from percutaneous transhepatic choledochal drainage tubes for diagnosis of biliary strictures. Int J Pancreatol 1995;18:215–220.
41. Caldas C, Hahn SA, Hruban RH, et al. Detection of K-ras mutation in stool of patients with pancreatic adenocarcinoma and pancreatic ductal hyperplasia. Cancer Res 1994;54:3568–3573.
42. Tada M, Omata M, Ohto M. ras gene mutations in intraductal papillary neoplasms of the pancreas. Cancer 1991;67:643–647.
43. Hoshi T, Ikai M, Ogawa K. Frequent K-ras mutations and absence of p53 mutations in mucin-producing tumors of the pancreas. J Surg Oncol 1994;55:84–91.
44. Lemoine NR, Jain S, Hughes CH, et al. Ki-ras oncogene activation in preinvasive pancreatic cancer. Gastroenterology 1992; 102:230–236.
45. Digiuseppe JA, Hruban RH, Offerhaus GJA, et al. Detection of K-ras mutations in mucinous pancreatic duct hyperplasia from a patient with family history of pancreatic carcinoma. Am J Physiol 1994;144:889–895.
46. Kalthoff H, Schmiegel W, Roeder C, et al. p53 and K-ras alterations in pancreatic epithelial cell lesions. Oncogene 1993;8:289–298.
47. Simon B, Weinel R, Hohne M, et al. Frequent alterations of the tumor suppressor genes p53 and DCC in human pancreatic carcinoma. Gastroenterology 1994;106:1645–1651.
48. Hohne MW, Halatsch ME, Dahl GF, Weinel RJ. Frequent loss of expression of the potential tumor-suppressor gene DCC in ductal pancreatic adenocarcinoma. Cancer Res 1992;52: 2616–2619.
49. Liu Q, Yan YX, McClure M, et al. MTS-1 (CDKN2) tumor suppressor

gene deletions are a frequent event in esophagus squamous cancer and pancreatic adenocarcinoma cell lines. Oncogene 1995;10:619–622.
50. Caldas C, Hahn SA, da Costa LT, et al. Frequent somatic mutations and homozygous deletions of the MTS1 gene in pancreatic adenocarcinoma. Nature Genet 1994;8:27–32.
51. Caldas C, Kern SE. K-ras mutation and pancreatic adenocarcinoma. Int J Pancreatol 1995;18:1–6.
52. Lees WR. Pancreatic ultrasonography. Clin Gastroenterol 1984; 13:763–789.
53. Balthazar EJ, Chako AC. Computed tomography of pancreatic masses. Am J Gastroenterol 1990;85:343–349.
54. Freeny PC, Marks WM, Ryan JA, Traverso LW. Pancreatic ductal adenocarcinoma: diagnosis and staging with dynamic CT. Radiology 1988;166:125–133.
55. Stephens DH. Neoplastic lesions. In: Margulis AR, Burhenne HJ, eds. Alimentary tract roentgenology. St. Louis: CV Mosby, 1989:1167–1194.
56. Smith CD, Behrns KE, van Heerden JA, Sarr MG. Radical pancreatoduodenectomy for misdiagnosed pancreatic mass. Br J Surg 1994;81:585–589.
57. Steiner E, Stark DD, Hahn PF, et al. Imaging of pancreatic neoplasms: comparison of MR and CT. AJR 1989;152: 487–491.
58. Semelka RC, Ascher SM. MR imaging of the pancreas. Radiology 1993;188:593–602.
59. Vellet AD, Romano W, Bach DB, et al. Adenocarcinoma of the pancreatic ducts: comparative evaluation with CT and MR imaging at 1.5T. Radiology 1992;183:87–95.
60. Gabata T, Matsui O, Kadoya M, et al. Small pancreatic adenocarcinomas: efficacy of MRI with fat suppression and gadolinium enhancement. Radiology 1994:193:683–688.
61. Furukawa T, Tsukamoto Y, Naitoh Y, et al. Differential diagnosis between benign and malignant localized stenosis of the main pancreatic duct by intraductal ultrasound of the pancreas. Am J Gastroenterol 1994;89:2038–2041.
62. Rosch T, Braig C, Gain T, et al. Staging of pancreatic and ampullary carcinoma by endoscopic ultrasonography: comparison with conventional sonography, computed tomography and angiography. Gastroenterology 1992;102:188–199.
63. Temudom T, Sarr MG, Douglas MG, Farnell MB. An argument against routine percutaneous biopsy, ERCP, or biliary stent placement in patients with clinically resectable periampullary masses: a surgical perspective. Pancreas 1995;11:283–288.
64. Jowell PS. Assessment of pancreatic duct strictures. Gastrointest Endosc Clin North Am 1995;5:125–143.
65. Alvarez C, Livingston EH, Ashley SW, et al. Cost-benefit analysis of the work-up for pancreatic cancer. Am J Surg 1993;165:53–58.
66. Kato T, Fukatsu H, Kengo I, et al. Fluorodeoxyglucose positron emission tomography in pancreatic cancer: an unsolved problem. Eur J Nucl Med 1995;22:32–39.
67. Bares R, Klever P, Hauptmann S, et al. F-18 fluorodeoxyglucose PET in vivo evaluation of pancreatic glucose metabolism for detection of pancreatic cancer. Radiology 1994;192:79–86.
68. Inokuma T, Tamaki N, Torizuka T, et al. Value of fluorine-18-fluorodeoxyglucose and thallium-201 in the detection of pancreatic cancer. J Nucl Med 1995;36:229–235.
69. Carpenter S, Wiley J, Owyzang C, Shreve P. C-11 acetate positron emission tomography of the pancreas: a study of the normal pancreas, chronic pancreatitis and neoplasm. Gastroenterology 1995;108:A346.
70. Worlock AJ, Zalutsky MR, Metzgar RS. Radiolocalization of human pancreatic tumors in athymic mice by monoclonal antibody DU-PAN 1. Cancer Res 1990;50:7246–7251.
71. Tsuda T, Koshiba H, Usui T, et al. Radioimmunoscintigraphy of human pancreatic carcinoma xenografts in nude mice with $^{131}$I-labeled monoclonal antibody. Ann Nucl Med 1990;4:71–74.
72. Ho JJ, Bi N, Yan PS, et al. Characterization of new pancreatic cancer-reactive monoclonal antibodies directed against purified mucin. Cancer Res 1991;51:372–380.
73. Klapdor R, Montz R. Radioimmunodiagnosis of pancreatic cancer disease. Int J Pancreatol 1991;9:99–111.
74. Kozarek RA. Direct pancreatoscopy. Gastrointest Endosc Clin North Am 1995;5:259–267.
75. Tajiri H, Kobayashi M, Niwa H, et al. Clinical application of an ultra-thin pancreatoscope using a sequential video converter. Gastrointest Endosc 1993;39:371–374.
76. Riemann JF, Kohler B. Endoscopy of the pancreatic duct: value of different endoscope types. Gastrointest Endosc 1993;39: 367–370.
77. Jung M, Zipf A, Schoonbroodt G, et al. Pancreatoscopy for differential diagnosis of pancreatic duct stenosis. Gastroenterology 1994;106:A299.
78. Jung M, Zipf A, Schoonbroodt G, et al. Mucinous cystadenomas of the pancreas are best diagnosed by pancreatoscopy. Gastroenterology 1995;108:A363.
79. Mizuno S, Nakajima M, Yasuda K, et al. Shape memory alloy catheter system for peroral pancreatoscopy using an ultrathin-caliber endoscope. Endoscopy 1994;26(8):676–680.
80. Zimmer B, Brune I, Kohler B, et al. Muzinose Zystadenome und Zystadenokarzinome des Pankreas—die Pankreatikoskopie als neues Instrument der endoskopischen und feingeweblichen Diagnosesicherung. Z Gastroenterol 1994;32:165–169.
81. Moosa AR, Camagami RA. Diagnosis and staging of pancreatic neoplasms. Surg Clin North Am 1995;75:871–890.
82. Raskleigh-Belcher HJC, Russell RCG, Lees WR. Cutaneous seeding of pancreatic carcinoma by fine-needle aspiration biopsy. Br J Radiol 1986;59:182–183.
83. Warshaw AL. Implications of peritoneal cytology for staging of early pancreatic cancer. Am J Surg 1991;161:26–30.
84. Nakamura R, Machado R, Amikura K, et al. Role of fine needle aspiration cytology and endoscopic biopsy in the preoperative assessment of pancreatic and peripancreatic malignancies. Int J Pancreatol 1994;16:17–21.
85. Webb TH, Lillemoe KD, Pitt HA, et al. Pancreatic lymphoma: is surgery mandatory for diagnosis and treatment? Ann Surg 1989:209:25–30.
86. Essop AR, Posen J, Path FF, et al. Isolated granulomatous pancreatitis. J Clin Gastroenterol 1984:6:61–64.
87. Venu RP, Geenen JE, Kini M, et al. Endoscopic retrograde brush cytology: a new technique. Gastroenterology 1990;99:1 475–1479.
88. Nakaizumi A, Tatsuta M, Uehara H, et al. Cytologic examination of pure pancreatic juice in the diagnosis of pancreatic carcinoma. Cancer 1992;70:2610–2614.
89. Dupuy DE, Costello P, Ecker CP. Spiral CT of the pancreas. Radiology 1992;183:815–818.
90. Wyatt SH, Fishman EK. Spiral CT of the pancreas. Semin Ultrasound CT MRI 1994;15:122–132.
91. Fuhrman GM, Chrnsangavej C, Abbruzzese JL, et al. Thin-section contrast-enhanced computed tomography accurately predicts the resectability of malignant pancreatic neoplasms. Am J Surg 1994;167:104–113.
92. Savader BL, Fishman EK, Savader SJ, Cameron JL. CT arterial portography vs pancreatic angiography in the assessment of vascular involvement in pancreatic and periampullary tumors. J Comput Assist Tomogr 1994;18:916–920.
93. Gmeinwieser J, Feuerbach S, Hohenberger W, et al. Spiral-CT in diagnosis of vascular involvement in pancreatic cancer. Hepatogastroenterology 1995;42:418–422.
94. Dalton RR, Sarr MG, van Heerden JA, Colby TV. Carcinoma of the body and tail of the pancreas: is curative resection justified? Surgery 1992;111:489–494.
95. Warshaw AL, Gu Z-Y, Wittenberg J, Waltman AC. Preoperative staging and assessment of resectability of pancreatic cancer. Arch Surg 1990;125:230–233.
96. Fernandez-del Castillo C, Rattner DW, Warshaw AL. Further experience with laparoscopy and peritoneal cytology in the staging of pancreatic cancer. Br J Surg 1995;82:1127–1129.
97. Dooley WC, Cameron JL, Pitt HA, et al. Is preoperative angiography useful in patients with periampullary tumors? Ann Surg 1990;211:649–655.
98. Murugiah M, Windsor JA, Redhead DN, et al. The role of visceral angiography in the management of pancreatic and periampullary cancer. World J Surg 1993;17:796–800.
99. Bakkevold KE, Arnesjo B, Kambestad B. Carcinoma of the pancreas and papilla of Vater: assessment of resectability and factors influencing resectability in stage 1 carcinomas. A

prospective multicenter trial in 472 patients. Eur J Surg Oncol 1992;18:494–507.
100. Soyer P, Lacheheb D, Belkacem A, Levesque M. Involvement of superior mesenteric vessels and portal vein in pancreatic adenocarcinoma: detection with CT during arterial portography. Abdom Imag 1994;19:413–416.
101. Rong GH, Sindelar WF. Aberrant peripancreatic arterial anatomy: considerations in performing pancreatectomy for malignant neoplasms. Am Surg 1987;53:726–729.
102. Biehl TR, Traverso LW, Hauptmann E, Ryan JA Jr. Preoperative visceral angiography alters intraoperative strategy during the Whipple procedure. Am J Surg 1993;165:607–612.
103. Kaufman AR, Sivak MV Jr. Endoscopic ultrasonography in the differential diagnosis of pancreatic disease. Gastrointest Endosc 1989;35:214–219.
104. Yasuda K, Mukai H, Nakajima M, Kawai K. Staging of pancreatic carcinoma by endoscopic ultrasonography. Endoscopy 1993; 25:151–155.
105. Muller MF, Meyenberger C, Bertschinger P, et al. Pancreatic tumors: evaluation with endoscopic US, CT and MR imaging. Radiology 1994;190:745–751.
106. Kato T, Tsukamoto Y, Naitoh Y, et al. Ultrasonographic and endoscopic ultrasonographic angiography in pancreatic mass lesions. Acta Radiol 1995;36:381–387.
107. Snady H, Bruckner H, Siegel J, et al. Endoscopic ultrasonographic criteria of vascular invasion by potentially resectable pancreatic tumors. Gastrointest Endosc 1994;40:326–333.
108. Rosch T, Lorenz R, Braig C, et al. Endoscopic ultrasound in pancreatic tumor diagnosis. Gastrointest Endosc 1991;37: 347–352.
109. Lowenfels AB, Maissonneuve P, Cavallini G, et al. Pancreatitis and the risk of pancreatic cancer. N Engl J Med 1993;328:1433–1437.
110. Gullo L, Pezilli R, Morselli Labate AM and Italian Pancreatic Cancer Study Group. Diabetes and the risk of pancreatic cancer. N Engl J Med 1994;331:81–84.
111. Everhart J, Wright D. Diabetes mellitus as a risk factor for pancreatic cancer. JAMA 1995;273:1605–1609.
112. Mukai H, Mizuno S, Hayakumo T, et al. Clinical evaluation of an ultrasonic probe in the diagnosis of biliary and pancreatic tumors (Abstract). Gastrointest Endosc 1991;37:275.
113. Tamada K, Ido K, Ueno N, et al. Preoperative staging of extrahepatic bile duct cancer with intraductal ultrasonography. Am J Gastroenterol 1995;90:239–246.
114. Kaneko T, Nakao A, Inoue S, et al. Intraportal endovascular ultrasonography in the diagnosis of portal vein invasion by pancreatobiliary carcinoma. Ann Surg 1995;222:711–718.
115. Noguchi T, Makuuchi M, Maruta F, et al. Intraportal US with 20 Mhz and 30 Mhz scanning catheters. Work in progress. Radiology 1993;186:203–205.
116. Lundstedt C, University of Lund, Sweden, personal communication, 1995.
117. Ward EM, Stephens DH, Sheedy PF. Computed tomographic characteristics of pancreatic carcinoma: an analysis of 100 cases. Radiographics 1983;3:547–565.
118. Warshaw AL, Tepper JE, Shipley WU. Laparoscopy in the staging and planning of therapy for pancreatic cancer. Am J Surg 1986;151:76–80.
119. Cuschieri A. Laparoscopy for pancreatic cancer: does it benefit the patient? Eur J Surg Oncol 1988;14:41–44.
120. John TG, Greig JD, Carter DC, Garden OJ. Carcinoma of the pancreatic head and periampullary region: tumor staging with laparoscopy and laparoscopic ultrasonography. Ann Surg 1995;221:156–164.
121. Bornman PC, Harries-Jones EP, Tobias R, et al. Prospective controlled trial of transhepatic biliary endoprostheses versus biliary surgery for incurable carcinoma of the head of the pancreas. Lancet 1986;1:69–71.
122. Sheperd HA, Royle G, Ross APR, et al. Endoscopic biliary endoprosthesis in the palliation of malignant obstruction of the distal common bile duct. Br J Surg 1988;75:1166–1168.
123. Smith AC, Dowsett JF, Russell RCG, Hatfield ARW, Cotton PB. Randomized trial of endoscopic stenting versus surgical bypass in malignant low bile duct obstruction. Lancet 1994;344:1655–1659.
124. Martin JK Jr, Goellner JR. Abdominal fluid cytology in patients with gastrointestinal malignant lesions. Mayo Clin Proc 1986;61: 467–471.
125. Lei S, Kini J, Kim K, Howard JM. Pancreatic cancer: cytologic study of peritoneal washings. Arch Surg 1994;129:639–642.
126. Lygidakis NJ, van der Heyde MN, Lubler MJ. An evaluation of preoperative biliary drainage in the surgical management of pancreatic head carcinoma. Acta Chir Scand 1987;153: 665–668.
127. Bailey MF. Endotoxin, bile salts and renal function in obstructive jaundice. Br J Surg 1976;63:774–778.
128. Ido M, Higashiguchi T, Tanigawa K, Kawarada Y. Cell biological evaluation of biliary drainage prior to hepatectomy in obstructive jaundice. Hepatogastroenterology 1995;42: 308–316.
129. Smith RC, Pooley M, George CR, Faithful GR. Preoperative percutaneous transhepatic internal drainage in obstructive jaundice: a randomized controlled trial examining renal function. Surgery 1985;97:641–648.
130. Pitt HA, Gomes AS, Lois JF, et al. Does preoperative percutaneous biliary drainage reduce operative risk or increase hospital cost? Ann Surg 1985;201:545–553.
131. Nakeeb A, Pitt HA. The role of preoperative biliary decompression in obstructive jaundice. Hepatogastroenterology 1995;42: 332–337.
132. Anderson JR, Sorenson SM, Kruse A, et al. Randomized trial of endoscopic endoprosthesis versus operative bypass in malignant obstructive jaundice. Gut 1989;30:1132–1135.
133. van den Bosch RP, van den Schelling GP, Klinkebijl JH, et al. Guidelines for the application of surgery and endoprostheses in the palliation of obstructive jaundice in advanced cancer of the pancreas. Ann Surg 1994;219:18–24.
134. Urrutia R, DiMagno EP. Genetic markers: the key to early diagnosis and improved survival in pancreatic cancer? Gastroenterology 1996;110(1):306–310.

# 53

# *Endoscopic Management*

David R. Fletcher

Cancer of the pancreas was formerly the sole province of the surgeon, occasionally to resect for possible cure, but usually to alleviate biliary or duodenal obstruction (1). Technology, however, has led to other therapeutic options. Radiologically placed percutaneous transhepatic drainage tubes or stents were used in those with advanced disease (2). Complications remained a problem and the development of endoscopic retrograde cholangiopancreatography (ERCP) with associated plastic luminal stents rapidly replaced the percutaneous technique (3). Finally, there has been the development of laparoscopic biliary bypass (4, 5), which is discussed in more detail in Chapter 13. With these multiple options, how do we choose the most appropriate strategy for the individual patient?

Because carcinoma of the pancreas is rarely resectable or curable (6, 7), palliation is usually all that can be offered. The *principles of palliation* are as follows: *(a)* to rapidly relieve symptoms, i.e., restore bile flow to the intestine, with relief of duodenal obstruction, if required; *(b)* to maintain the patient symptom free, until the inevitable death, usually within 6 months (6, 7); *(c)* to achieve this at the least cost to the patient in terms of morbidity and hospital stay; and *(d)* to accomplish palliation without compromising the potential for cure by surgical resection. The problem, however, is that many patients do not have these principles fulfilled. When the patient is referred for diagnostic ERCP, some enthusiasts believe that endoscopic stent is the only therapeutic option (8), and the patient never gets the opportunity to see a surgeon.

## BENEFITS OF ALTERNATE STRATEGIES

The treatment options differ in terms of benefits in both the early and late phases, as well as in terms of costs, i.e., complications. The differences between the traditional choices, *surgery* and *endoscopic stent*, have been clearly demonstrated in a controlled clinical trial from Middlesex, London. Surgery has the immediate disadvantage of having a higher initial mortality than stent (14 vs. 3%) as well as a higher major complication rate (29 vs. 11%) and a longer hospital stay (26 days vs. 20 days) (9). In the longer term, however, surgery has the advantage, as failure of palliation (i.e., need for retreatment) is far more frequent with stents. Recurrent jaundice was far more frequent with the stent than with surgery (36 vs. 2%), as was late gastric outlet obstruction (17 vs. 7%).

The high long-term failure rate of stents, has been improved with the development of expandable metal stents (10–12). The stents can expand up to 1 cm in diameter. Because they are mesh rather than solid plastic and thus have a small surface area, they are not affected by bacterial biofilm, the cause of plastic stent obstruction and failure. A further advantage of the mesh stents, not related to pancreatic tumors, is that when placed at the hilus, uninvolved ducts or branches can drain between the wire mesh and not obstruct as do plastic stents. In the case of the cystic duct, plastic stent obstruction was a cause of acute cholecystitis (13) a further mechanism for failure of palliation. The disadvantage of the metal stents, however, is that tumor ingrowth can occur through the mesh, a problem more likely with intrinsic tumors such as cholangiocarcinoma than with extrinsic tumors such as pancreatic cancer. This problem may be reduced with a new type of coil metal stent (14).

Controlled clinical trials have shown that the metal stents are superior to plastic ones. Stent obstruction and the need for reintervention are reduced by approximately 50% as a result of the duration of stent patency being doubled (15, 16). Stent failure and therefore palliative failure still occur, however, in 20–30% (15, 16).

To summarize, the *difference between surgery and a stent* is that with surgery the patient buys the treatment and pays with an immediate higher rate of complication and possible operative death, but later is free of symptoms from obstruction. The alternate option is to rent the treatment with a stent, which carries a lower initial morbidity but has recurrent installments to pay as a result of recurrent obstruction, though these installments are lower with a metal stent than with a plastic one.

By contrast, the *laparoscopic bypass* potentially has the advantages of both approaches: the benefits of a minimal access approach of the stent, but the potential long-term patency of a surgical bypass. An added advantage of the technique is that laparoscopy can be used prior to laparotomy to confirm resectability. If hepatic or small peritoneal metastases are identified, or if laparoscopic intraoperative ultrasound shows nonresectability (see Chapter 13), laparoscopic biliary bypass can be performed without unnecessary laparotomy. At the same time, the opportunity to cure the few with surgery, where this is possible, is not compromised. However, because the bypass is to the gallbladder, case selection is of critical importance for long-term success (4, 5). The gallbladder must be present and contain no stones, and the cystic duct should enter the common duct at least 2 cm above the tumor, so that it is not obstructed by later tumor growth, leading to recurrent jaundice.

## SELECTION FOR THERAPY

To obtain the maximum benefit and minimize potential disadvantages of each technique, therapy has to be tailored for each individual patient. First, nonresectability has to be confirmed, preferably preoperatively. Second, surgical risk and probable survival time need to be determined.

First, the question of resectability should be settled, preferably preoperatively to avoid unnecessary laparotomy for the patient. The subject is discussed in Chapters 10, 51, and 52. Nonresectability may be determined when ultrasound shows liver metastases or extra pancreatic nodes. Similarly, computed tomography (CT) scanning may demonstrate this and also may show tumor encasement of superior mesenteric vessels. A recent addition is endoscopic ultrasound (Chapter 9) (17), which the author is finding useful. Its potential is to show, preoperatively and relatively noninvasively, tumor size, nodal involvement, and vascular involvement. The alternative to endoscopic ultrasound is laparoscopic ultrasound, but the latter commits the patient to general anesthesia and laparoscopy before the determination is made that the patient is inoperable. For the fitter patient, however, this is not a major disadvantage, because laparoscopic ultrasound allows laparoscopic bypass, as indicated above, and even if this is not appropriate, it allows surgical biliary bypass with or without gastrointestinal bypass, which gives superb palliation with minimal risk to the fitter patient.

Once nonresectability has been confirmed, the patient's surgical risk should be determined. The relationship between the number of risk factors and operative morbidity and mortality has been well documented, for example, by Pitt et al. (18). The high-risk patient clearly should be offered a nonoperative approach when possible.

The final selection is based on probable survival time. This is harder to predict. It is partly determined by risk factors for surgery, as indicated above (i.e., presence of complications). However, the two factors correlating best with poor survival are presence of liver metastases on ultrasound and primary tumor size exceeding 4 cm (9). Patients whose survival is going to be short (i.e., who will not live long enough to develop late complications of stent obstruction) are particularly best managed by a nonoperative approach.

The author's criteria for selecting therapy for patients are seen in Table 53.1 (19). Surgery is used for those potentially resectable (i.e., low-risk, longer survival) plus those in whom it is the only option (i.e., salvage after failure of other techniques). Percutaneous stents are used as an adjunct; for example, in assisting in the placement of an endoscopic stent or when it is the only option in a terminal patient. Endoscopic stents and laparoscopic bypass are used for the same patients, those with nonresectable disease and those at high risk for surgery. They are also both used for patients with shorter survival, but those whose survival is likely to be less than 6 months are managed by an endoscopic stent and those whose survival is likely to be more than 6 months are managed by laparoscopic bypass, provided that the gallbladder is suitable.

**TABLE 53.1. Author's Criteria for Selecting Patients for Alternative Therapies**

- Surgery
  - Potentially resectable
  - Low risk
  - Longer survival
  - Only option
- Percutaneous stent
  - Adjunct
  - Only option
- Endoscopic stent
  - Non-resectable
  - High risk
  - Survival <6 months
- Laparoscopic bypass
  - Non-resectable
  - High risk
  - Survival >6 months
  - Gallbladder suitable

Derived from Rhodes M, Nathanson L, Fielding G. Laparoscopic biliary and gastric bypass: a useful adjunct in the treatment of carcinoma of the pancreas. Gut 1995;36:778–780, with permission.

A *management algorithm* is seen in Figure 53.1. In the patient with obstructive jaundice, if the ultrasound shows a pancreatic mass and the patient is high risk, unresectable, and likely to have a short survival, then an ERCP is immediately performed, and a plastic stent inserted as definitive treatment. For patients who are better risks and possibly resectable, with longer survival (unless they have had prolonged jaundice and cholangitis, for which an ERCP plastic stent is placed as a temporary maneuver), the next step is a CT scan and endoscopic ultrasound, if available. If the lesion is unresectable (most), but the gallbladder is unsuitable for bypass (stones, previous removal), then the patient has an ERCP and placement of a metal stent. If the tumor is unresectable and the gallbladder still appears suitable, then a laparoscopy is performed with on-table cholangiography. Fine-needle aspiration cytology should be performed to confirm the diagnosis. If the gallbladder is suitable, laparoscopic cholecystenterotomy is performed; if not, the patient either goes to laparotomy and operative bypass or the more technically competent might perform a laparoscopic bypass to the common hepatic duct.

If the CT scan and/or endoscopic ultrasound show that the lesion is still potentially resectable, then an ERCP is next performed. Those patients who are the best risk and highly likely to be resectable then have a laparotomy where, one hopes, resection will be performed. The small proportion in whom this remains technically impossible will have a palliative bypass. Those patients who, after ERCP, are thought to be at intermediate surgical risk or in whom there is some doubt about resectability, go to laparoscopy with on-table ultrasound, if it is available. Those who are confirmed to be resectable can go onto laparotomy; those who are unresectable go to either laparoscopic cholecystenterostomy or bypass surgery, depending upon the suitability of the gallbladder for laparoscopic bypass. If ERCP suggested duodenal invasion or CT shows bulky disease at the time of laparotomy, gastric bypass by gastroenterostomy should also be performed. This is less of an issue, however, now that laparoscopic gastroenterostomy is also available (20).

## ENDOSCOPIC STENTS

### Plastic Stents

Originally designed as a double pigtail stent, delivered straightened over a guide wire with the pigtails preventing dislodgment, plastic stents have been replaced by the straight Amsterdam-type stent, with flaps cut in the proximal and distal ends to help prevent dislodgment (Fig. 53.2). They come in various sizes, the commonest used are 10 French and 11.5 French, the latter the preference of the author. This latter size is the largest that can be pushed through the working channel of the standard wide-channel duodenoscopes. The wider the diameter of the stent, the longer the delay before stent occlusion occurs (one hopes). The standard stents are made of polyethylene, though newer smoother materials are being developed in the hope that they will reduce the development of bacterial biofilm and occlusion. Soehendra has reported prolongation of stent patency (approximately 40%) by using a Teflon stent without side holes, which are thought to contribute to early bacterial clogging (21).

### Metal Stent

There are two basic types of metal stents, the balloon-mounted stent (Strecker) and the self-expanding stents (Wallstent, Gianturco, InStent). The Strecker stent (Microvasive, Boston Scientific Corporation) is made from a single tantalum thread that interlocks in a woven meshwork and is delivered on a balloon; the system is 7 Fr in diameter. The stent expands to 8 mm and is available in lengths of 4, 6, and 8 cm (16). The stent is expanded

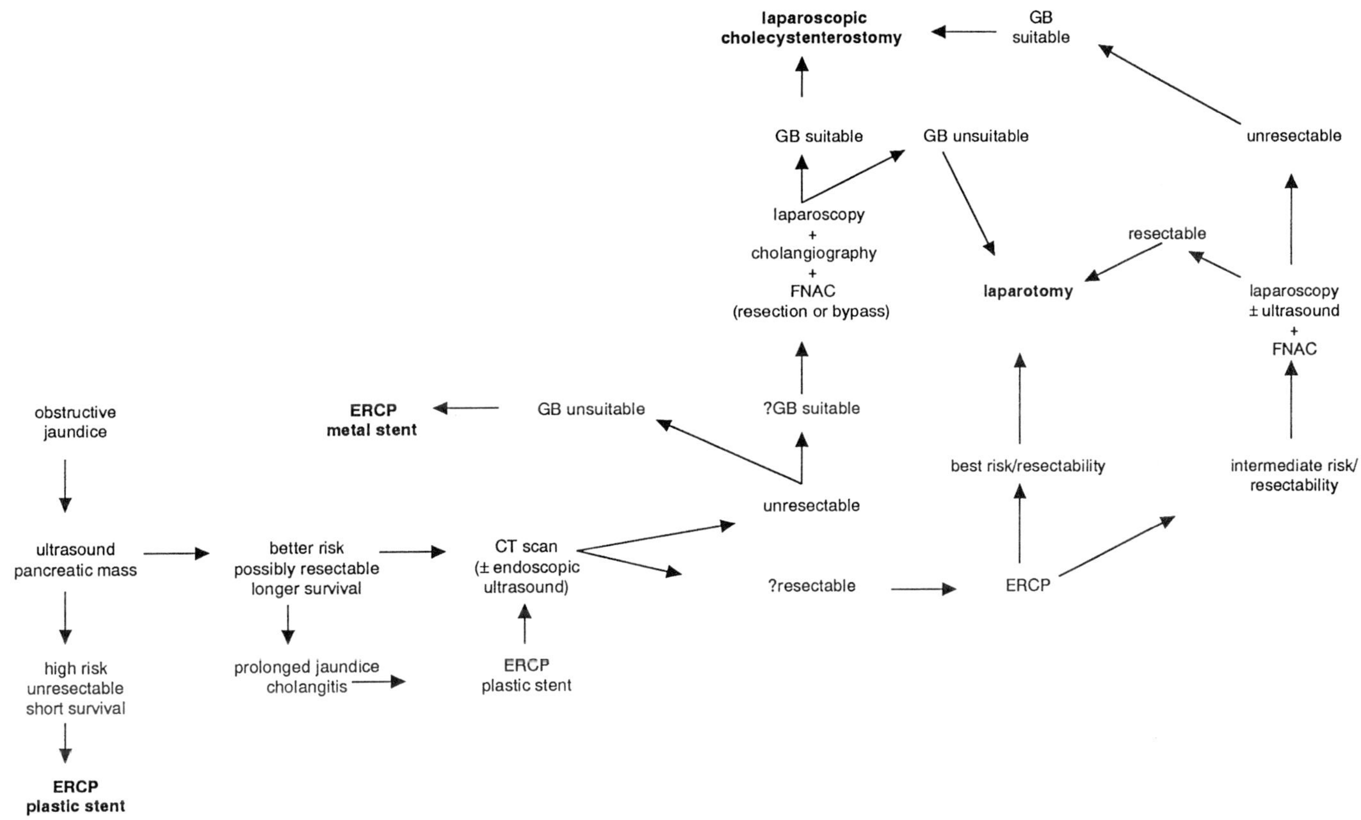


**FIG. 53.1.** Management algorithm for a patient presenting with obstructive jaundice. The approach depends on whether endoscopic or laparoscopic ultrasound is available for staging. The former is advantageous, as it allows choice of therapy prior to general anesthesia.

by the balloon fluoroscopically when it is placed across the stricture, after which there is no further expansion. A potential disadvantage is balloon rupture or difficulty in retracting the balloon once the stent is expanded (22).

The *Gianturco Z Stent* (Wilson Cook) is constructed like a cylindrical cage, which is expanded by withdrawing an outer retaining catheter to measure 8 mm in diameter and 3 cm long (11). This means that multiple stents may need to be inserted for longer strictures; the second disadvantage is that because the mesh is wide, it theoretically allows tumor ingrowth. Placement of a membrane over the wire cage to prevent this ingrowth is being explored, but membrane-enclosed stents have the potential disadvantages of cystic duct occlusion and cholecystitis (13).

The *InStent* (Eden Prairie, Minnesota) is a flat coiled spring made of nickel-titanium alloy locked onto a 12 French delivery catheter. When released (i.e., unlocked first from the distal end and then the proximal end) it unwinds, shortens, and expands to approximately 8 mm in diameter (14). Because it shortens from both ends (Fig. 53.3), care must be taken in calculating the length of stent required, to be sure the stricture is bypassed. To assist in this process, stents come in either 5-, 6-, or 7-cm lengths. The advantages of the stent are that *(a)* it has a strong radial force and is probably the most efficient in expanding the stricture, *(b)* it is less likely to get tumor ingrowth because of the nature of the flat ribbon of the coil, and *(c)* because it is in one length, it is the only stent that potentially can be removed after deployment.

The *Wallstent* (Schneider, Switzerland) is the stent with which most clinical experience has been obtained, including that by the author. It is made of stainless steel alloy filaments, which are braided into a tube (Fig. 53.4) (15, 16). The stent is mounted on a 9 French delivery catheter and held in place by a retractable membrane (Fig. 53.5).

Like the InStent, in expanding to its maximum diameter of 10 mm, the stent shortens, principally from the distal end. For this reason, the stents are made in variable lengths from 39 to 116 mm, which will be 2–5 mm shorter when implanted. The advantages of the stent are that *(a)* it is relatively simply deployed; *(b)* it has a finer mesh, which theoretically reduces tumor ingrowth; and *(c)* it comes in variable lengths. Its disadvantage is that it is relatively rigid and can kink and obstruct the bile duct at its upper end (15). Also, like any other metal stent, it can be obstructed by tumor ingrowth or overgrowth of the ends. Its final disadvantage is its considerable cost ($900.00, Australian, compared with $20.00 for a plastic stent) (15). For this reason, the author reserves metal stents for patients who will survive long enough to make the expense worthwhile.

## TECHNIQUE

### Plastic Stent

As the patient has obstructive jaundice, prophylactic intravenous antibiotics will have been used. Both a pancreatogram and a cholangiogram ideally are obtained, and brush cytology of the pancreatic duct can be performed, though the author has found the technique disappointing. The common duct is selectively cannulated, and a small sphincterotomy performed so that the stent does not occlude the pancreatic duct when finally placed. An 035 guide wire is passed across the stricture, and if it is felt to be tight, a Soehendra (9 French) stricture-dilating catheter (or stricture-dilating balloon if it is particularly tight) is passed over the guide wire to make stent insertion easier. If the stent jams in the stricture and the stent delivery system bows between the endoscope and the papilla, then control of the stent is lost. It has

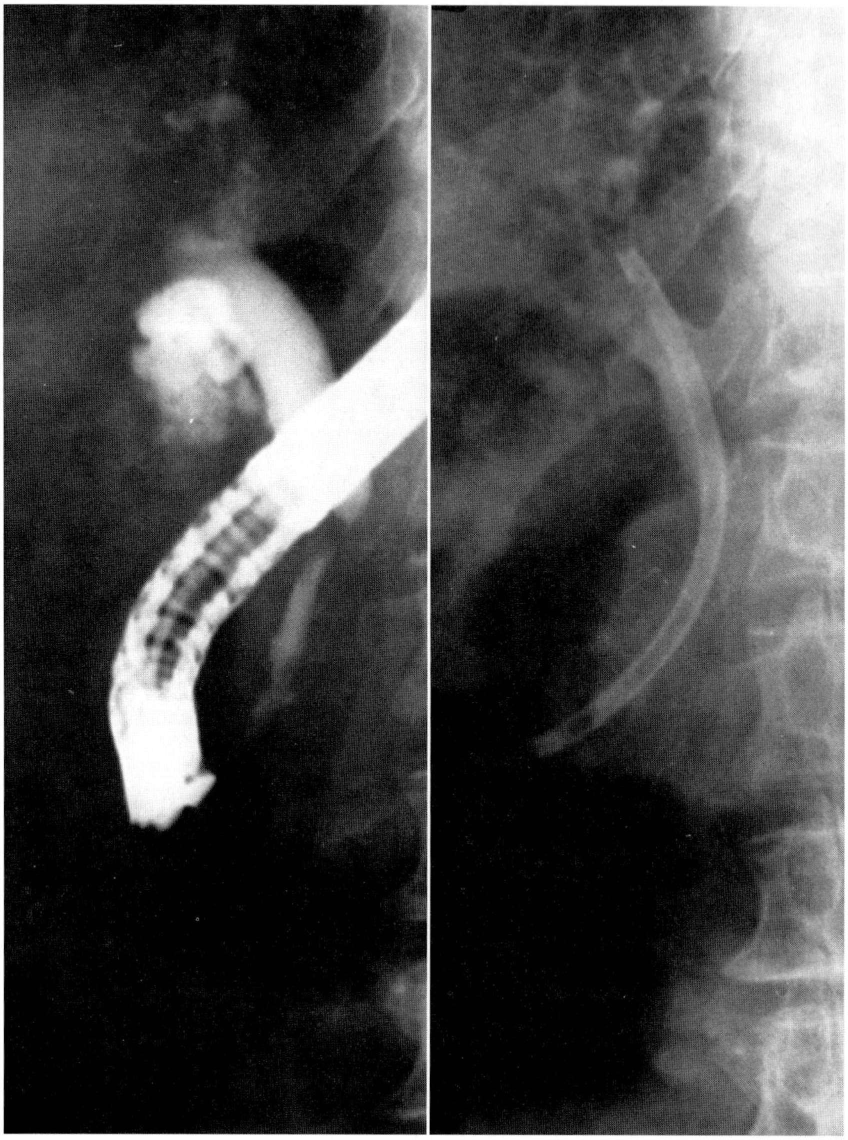

**FIG. 53.2.** Cachectic 82-year-old male with large pancreatic head lesion invading the common bile duct in its midportion *(left)* and immediately following placement of a 9-cm 11.5 Fr straight plastic stent *(right).*

to be withdrawn, and the whole process restarted. However, this is uncommon with pancreatic cancer, the easiest condition to stent by far.

A stiff stenting catheter is then passed over the guide wire, and contrast is injected into the proximal ductal system so that the stricture can be clearly identified and accurate stent placement performed. An appropriate length, 11.5 Fr (preferable) straight stent is passed onto the guide wire and pushed into and down the endoscope by a pushing catheter while an assistant holds the guide wire and stenting catheter taut. The stent is lifted up into the stricture by use of a combination of the pushing catheter and the endoscope bridge. After accurate placement, with the stent just protruding from the papilla, the stenting catheter is withdrawn along with the guide wire, and bile flow is visually confirmed. The stent should be left just protruding from the papilla for easy removal and replacement at a later date. If the stent passes up into the bile duct, it is very difficult to retrieve, and if it slides out and the tip jams against the adjacent duodenal wall, it is difficult to get a snare around it to remove it.

### Metal Stent

Insertion of a Wallstent is described, because this is the stent with which most experience has been obtained, though it is likely the InStent will attract many users. Prophylactic antibiotics, imaging of both ductal systems, and cytology are as described above. After identifying the stricture in the bile duct, contrast is injected so that radiologic placement of the stent can be accurately performed. A guide wire is passed well into the ductal system, (035 or 038) and the ERCP catheter is withdrawn. If the stricture appears tight, a Soehendra 9 French dilating catheter is passed. A stent of the appropriate length, taking into consideration shortening, is prepared. The stent consists of a mesh constrained on the catheter by a retractable membrane (Fig. 53.5). A vacuum is created between the membrane and the stent, by use of a syringe attached to the delivery system, following which the control tap is closed. A syringe of contrast is attached to the tap, and when it is opened, contrast fills the space between the stent and membrane. Holding the guide wire rigid, the delivery system is passed over the guide wire and positioned so that the lower and middle radiopaque marks (Fig. 53.5) are well below and above the stricture, respectively. As the stent enters the bile duct, care is required in using the bridge elevator of the scope when the membrane section is exiting the endoscope, because of the risk of disruption of the membrane.

Using a screw device on a syringe and a pressure transducer, the space between the membrane and stent is pressurized to 5

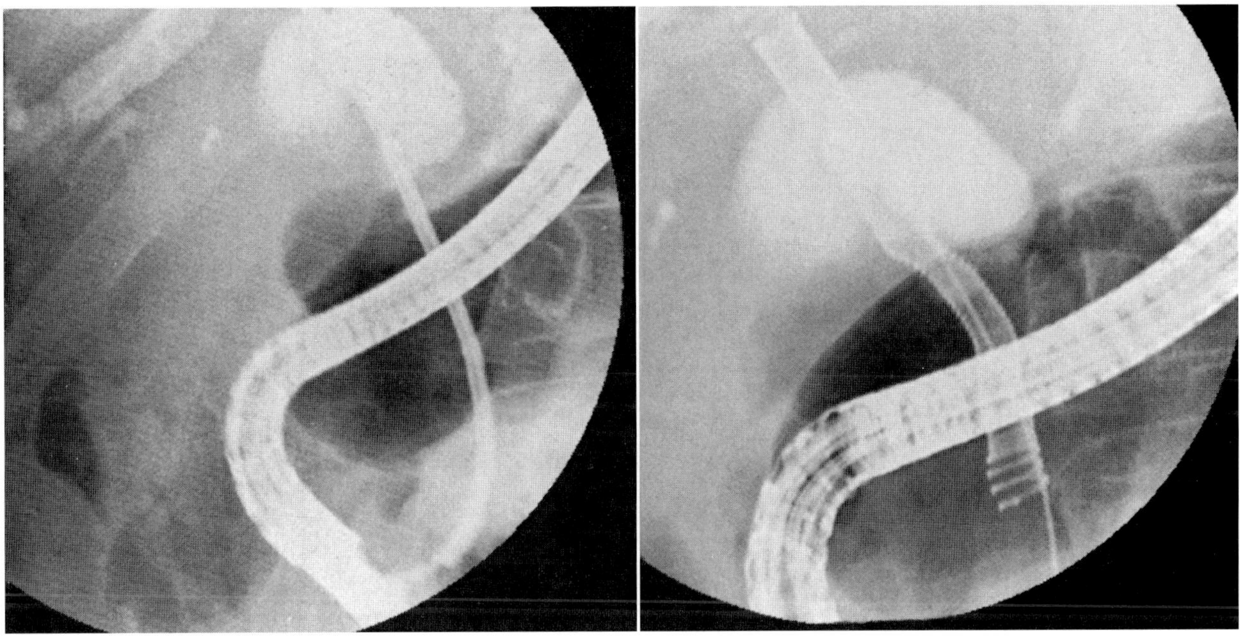

**FIG. 53.3.** An InStent contained on its delivery system *(left)* and immediately following deployment *(right)*, showing expansion in diameter, but shortening at both ends. (Courtesy InStent, Inc. Eden Prairie, Mn)

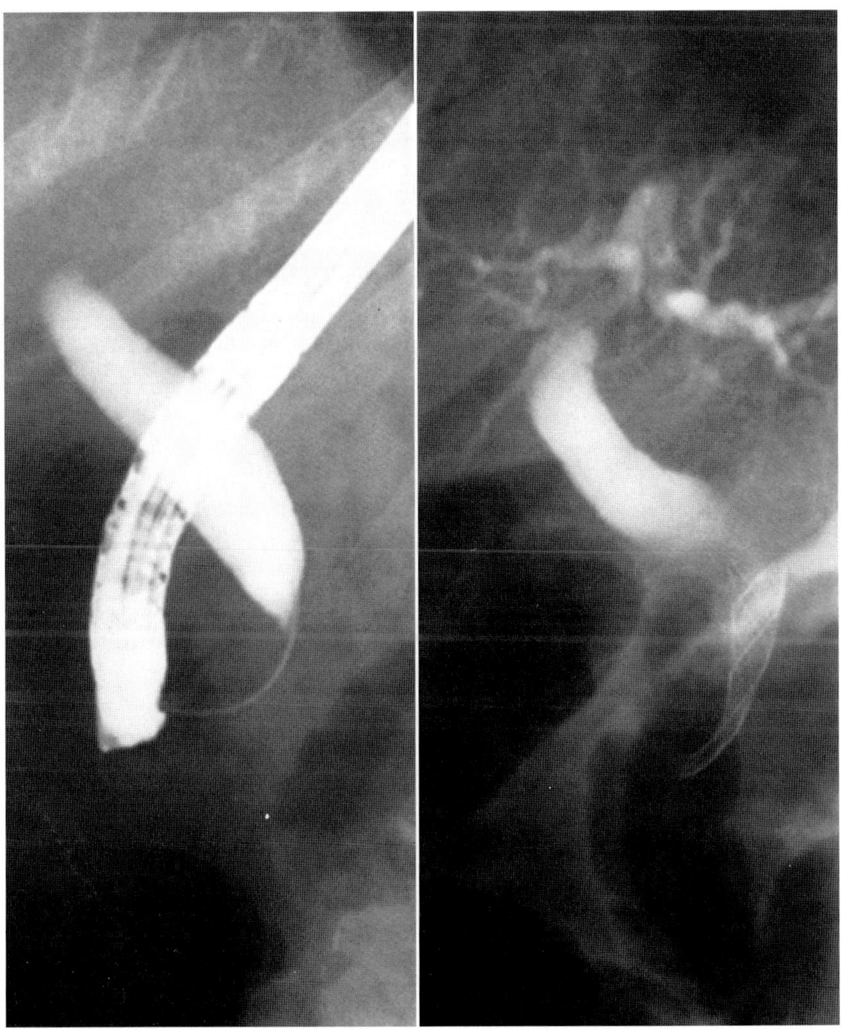

**FIG. 53.4.** A 78-year-old male with carcinoma of the head of the pancreas, nonresectable on CT, showing low common duct obstruction before *(left)* and immediately after insertion of a Wallstent *(right)*. The upper end is fully expanded in the dilated bile duct, and the lower end extending across the papilla into the duodenum is not yet fully expanded.

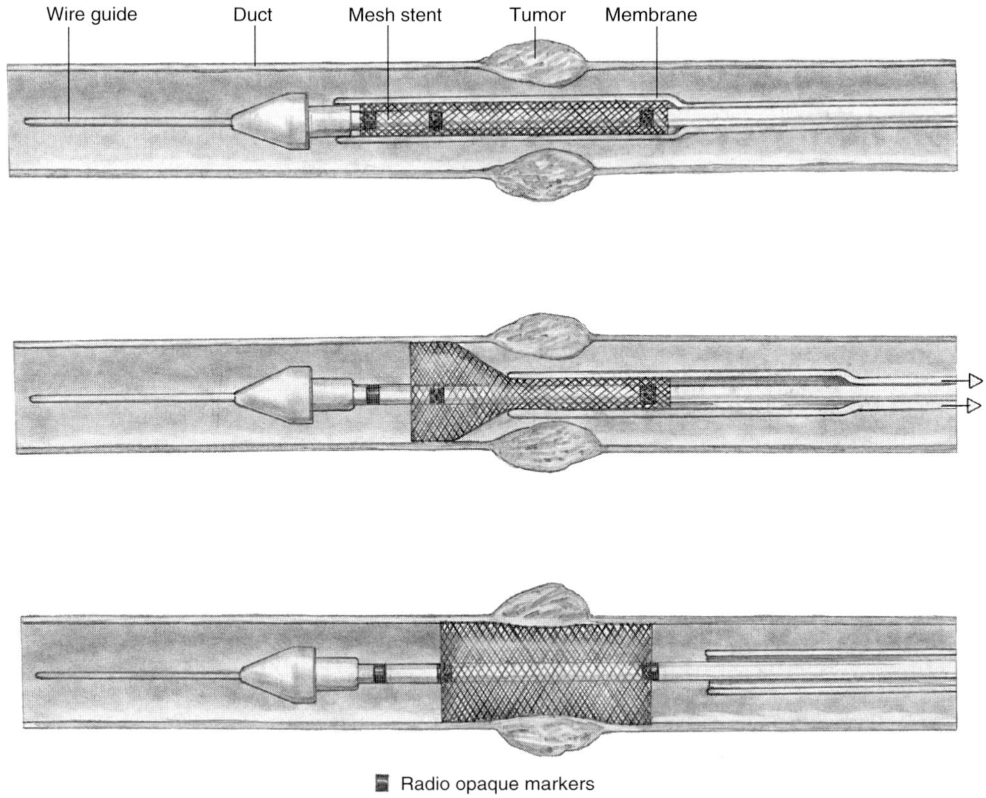


**FIG. 53.5.** Diagrammatic representation of placement of a Wallstent. The mid and lower markers are placed above and below the tumor, and as the membrane is withdrawn, the stent expands from the upper end, shortening as it does, to finally lie across the malignant stricture.

**TABLE 53.2. Survival and Late Complications of Metal versus Plastic Stents**

| | Treatment | |
|---|---|---|
| | **Metal Stent (*N* = 49)** | **Polyethylene Stent (*N* = 56)** |
| Survival median (range) (days) | 175 (1–450) | 147 (14–423) |
| Stent obstruction | 16 (33%) | 30 (54%) |
| Presentation | | |
| Cholangitis | 12 | 23 |
| Jaundice | 4 | 5 |
| ``Flulike''/cholestasis | 0 | 2 |
| Cause | | |
| Sludge | 4 | 29 |
| Tumor ingrowth | 10 | — |
| Kinking bile duct | 2 | 0 |
| Dislocation | 0 | 1 |
| Patency, median (range) (days) | 273 (14–363) | 126 (7–482) |
| Total number of ERCPs | 64 | 102 |
| Total number of stent exchanges | | |
| 0 | 35 | 33 |
| 1 | 14 | 12 |
| ≥2 | 0 | 11 |
| Duodenal stenosis | 2 | 5 |

Derived from Davids PH, Groen AK, Rauws EAJ, Tytgat GNJ, Huibregtse K. Randomised trial of self expanding metal stents versus polyethylene stents for distal malignant biliary obstruction. Lancet 1992;340;1488–1492, with permission.

atm, following which the membrane is pulled back, freeing the upper end of the stent. With the stent half deployed, its position can finally be adjusted, particularly pulling it back. It is much more difficult to push the stent in with the end flared. When position is absolutely certain, the membrane is fully withdrawn and the stent liberated and deployed. With pancreatic cancer, it is preferable to have the stent protruding into the duodenum, so tumor growth does not occur over the lower end. The immediate position of the stent can be seen in Figure 53.4. It will expand further over the next 24 hours.

## ENDOSCOPIC STENT RESULTS

The results of the two types of stent, plastic and metal, are best seen in two controlled clinical trials. Although both trials contain primarily patients who had pancreatic cancer, they both contain a few patients with a better prognosis, periampullary carcinoma (15, 16).

Immediate results are similar for both plastic and metal stents. Success rates were the same at 95% or greater, cholangitis occurred with both stents (10–12%), and mortality was similar in one trial (10% plastic vs. 13% metal) (16) but was greater in the metal stent group in the second trial (14 vs. 4%) (15). This is unlikely to be clinically significant; only one patient died of sepsis from recurrent cholangitis—the rest of the deaths were due to cardiac failure or cachexia.

The real difference between the stents can be seen in the longer term (Table 53.2, Fig. 53.6). The later results show the median patency of metal stents is almost double that of plastic. Further, not only was the original number of ERCPs required to place the stent reduced (by approximately one-third), but the number requiring multiple stent exchanges was reduced. In particular, note that the proportion with an obstructed stent and cholangitis was halved. When obstruction did occur, the mechanism was different, either tumor ingrowth or kinking, rather than dislocation or sludge (Table 53.2). In all patients, when obstruction occurred, placement of a second plastic stent across the obstructed metal stent provided palliation until death (Table 53.2).

Though the plastic stents are far cheaper than the metal stents, in the longer term, management using the latter is cheaper. With the reduction in the number of ERCPs required in the first place and in the need for reintervention, time in hospital for stent failure was reduced by two-thirds (11.8 days, plastic vs. 4 days, metal). As a result, the overall cost for stent insertion and management of complications was reduced by one-third (Deutsche marks, 6000, plastic vs. 4000, metal) (16).

Though the metal stent is clearly an improvement over the plastic stent in terms of palliation, late failure and therefore failure of palliation still occur in 22–33% (15, 16), to which must be added those who fail because of duodenal stenosis. For this reason, the author still recommends laparoscopic bypass, where possible, for pancreatic cancer. All seven laparoscopic cholecystenterostomies performed by the author (19) were for pancreatic cancer, and only one patient was readmitted for recurrent obstructive jaundice. Similarly, the experience of Rhodes et al. included only patients with pancreatic cancer and likewise included those who had failed alternate forms of therapy or who had either presented with, or re-presented with, gastric outlet obstruction (20). None of their patients returned for further intervention, an example of ideal palliation. These results suggest that in palliating pancreatic cancer, the laparoscopic biliary bypass, with or without gastric bypass, should be the first option, when technically possible. Further, it shows that when a stent is used by necessity, if duodenal obstruction occurs later, gastric bypass can still be achieved laparoscopically and is probably preferable to the option of duodenal stenting with a metal stent, which has been described (23).

## CONCLUSION

Endoscopic stenting has made a substantial contribution in palliating symptoms of patients with pancreatic cancer. The development of metal stents has substantially improved the ability of the endoscope to palliate this condition. Management algorithms for obstructive jaundice, however, have to be developed to allow the patient to receive the best therapeutic option. As each therapeutic modality has advantages and disadvantages, the patient should be selected for the option that gives maximum advantage and minimum disadvantage. Plastic endoscopic stents should be used for obstructive jaundice only in patients whose survival is likely to be 1–3 months or in those in whom symptoms are severe or cholangitis has occurred while staging investigations are performed. Because of their cost, metal endoscopic stents should be used in patients with longer survival in whom nonresectability has been confirmed. Before a metal stent is placed, however, it should be confirmed that the patient is not appropriate for laparoscopic biliary bypass, with or without gastric bypass.

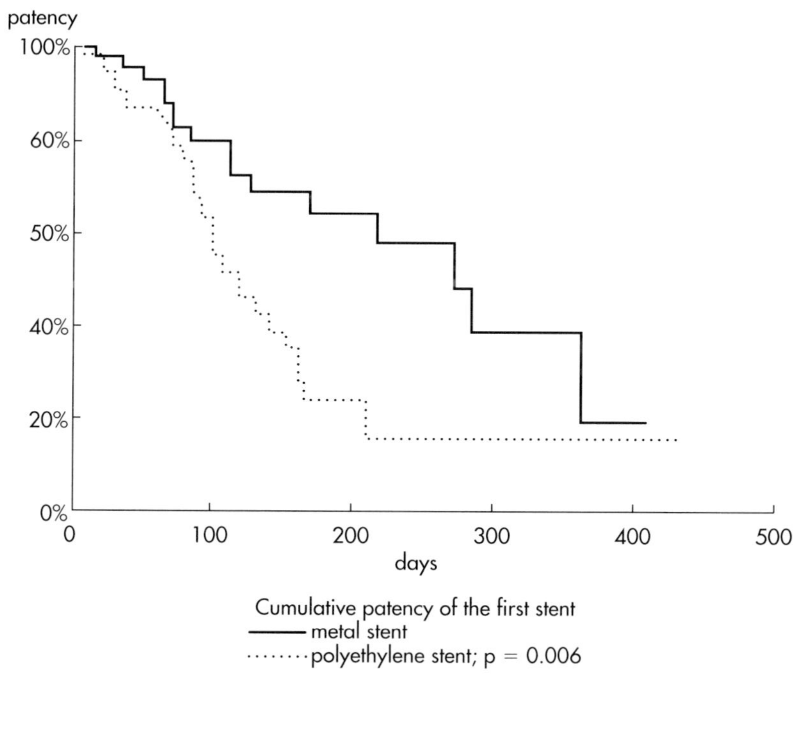


**FIG. 53.6.** Cumulative patency of plastic versus metal stents over time. (From Davids PH, Groen AK, Rauws EAJ, Tytgat GNJ, Huibregtse K. Randomised trial of self expanding metal stents versus polyethylene stents for distal malignant biliary obstruction. Lancet 1992;340;1488–1492. Reproduced with permission.)

**Acknowledgments**
Mrs Margaret Clarey is thanked for preparation of the manuscript.

## REFERENCES

1. Huang JF, Little JM. Malignant jaundice. Aust NZ J Surg 1987;57: 905–909.
2. Bornman PC, Harries-Jones EP, Tibias R. Prospective controlled trial of transhepatic biliary endoprosthesis versus bypass surgery for incurable carcinoma of head of pancreas. Lancet 1986; 69–71.
3. Speer AG, Cotton PB, Russell RCG, et al. Randomised trial of endoscopic versus percutaneous stent insertion in malignant obstructive jaundice. Lancet 1987;2:57–62.
4. Fletcher DR, Jones RM. Laparoscopic cholecystojejunostomy as palliation for obstructive jaundice in in-operable carcinoma of pancreas. Surg Endosc 1992;6:147–149.
5. Shimi S, Banting S, Cuschieri A. Laparoscopy in the management of pancreatic cancer; endoscopic cholecystojejunostomy for advanced disease. Br J Surg 1992;79:317–319.
6. Fletcher DR, Hurley RA, Hardy KJ. The effect of selective therapy on malignant obstructive jaundice. Med J Aust 1989;51:560–564.
7. Little JM, Wong KP. Palliation of malignant jaundice. Aust NZ J Surg 1991;61:501–504.
8. Summerfield JA. Biliary obstruction is best managed by endoscopists. Gut 1988;29:741–745.
9. Smith AC, Dowsett JF, Russell RCG, et al. Randomised trial of endoscopic stenting versus surgical bypass in malignant low bile duct obstruction. Lancet 1994;344:1655–1660.
10. Domschke W, Foerster EC. Endoscopic implantation of large bore self expanding biliary mesh stent. Gastrointest Endosc 1990;36: 55–57.
11. Irving JD, Adam A, Dick R, et al. Gianturco expandable metallic stents: results of a clinical trial. Radiology 1989;1172:321–326.
12. Neuhaus H, Hagenmuller F, Classen M. Self-expanding biliary stents: preliminary clinical experience. Endoscopy 1989;21: 225–228.
13. Dolan R, Pinkas H, Brady PG. Acute cholecystitis after palliative stenting malignant obstruction of the biliary tree. Gastrointest Endosc 1993;39:447–449.
14. Goldin E, Meyar M, Safra T, et al. A new self expandable and removable metal stent for biliary obstruction: a preliminary report. Endoscopy 1993;25:597–599.
15. Davids PH, Groen AK, Rauws EAJ, Tytgat GNJ, Huibregtse K. Randomised trial of self expanding metal stents versus polyethylene stents for distal malignant biliary obstruction. Lancet 1992;340;1488–1492.
16. Knyrim K, Wagner HJ, Pausch J, Vakil N. A prospective, randomised controlled trial of metal stents for malignant obstruction of the common bile duct. Endoscopy 1993;25:207–212.
17. Hawes RH, Zaidi S. Endoscopic ultrasound of the pancreas. Gastrointest Endosc Clin North Am 1995;1:61–80.
18. Pitt HA, Cameron JL, Postier RG, Gadacz TR. Factors affecting mortality in biliary tract surgery. Am J Surg 1981;41:66–71.
19. Fletcher DR. Malignant biliary obstruction—laparoscopic management. In: Toouli J, Gossett D, Hunter J, ed. Endosurgery. London: Churchill Livingstone, in press.
20. Rhodes M, Nathanson L, Fielding G. Laparoscopic biliary and gastric bypass: a useful adjunct in the treatment of carcinoma of the pancreas. Gut 1995;36:778–780.
21. Seitz U, Vadeyar H, Soehendra N. Prolonged patency with a new designed Teflon biliary prosthesis. Endoscopy 1994;24: 478–482.
22. Bethge N, Wagner HJ, Knyrim K, et al. Technical failure of biliary metal stent deployment in a series of 116 applications. Endoscopy 1992;24;395–400.
23. Maetaine I, Ogawa S, Hoshi H, et al. Self expanding metal stents for palliative treatment of malignant biliary and duodenal stenosis. Endoscopy 1994;26:701–704.

# 54

# *Basis of Operative Decisions*

A.R. Moossa and Marquis Hart

Operative decisions in cancer of the pancreas are based on the result of a mental computation of several factors, including *(a)* the unique anatomy and physiology of the pancreas; *(b)* the preoperative information available from imaging techniques; *(c)* the stage, exact location, and histologic type of the cancer; *(d)* the patient's general condition; and *(e)* the surgeon's experience, expertise, and philosophy regarding the disease.

## ANATOMIC AND PHYSIOLOGIC FACTORS

The pancreas is in many ways more difficult to manage surgically than other abdominal viscera. It is a retroperitoneal organ that has to be approached anteriorly, and access to it must be obtained after thorough mobilization of the stomach, greater omentum, transverse colon, spleen, and various parts of the gland (1).

The organ is situated at a complex anatomic crossroad where its central position provides lymphatic drainage radially along several major routes (the splenic, celiac, hepatic, and superior mesenteric vessels). This makes it hard to design an adequate cancer operation to fulfill Halsted's original oncologic criteria and to remove in an orderly fashion the primary, secondary, and tertiary nodal basins. Moreover, the intimate anatomic association of the pancreas with major vessels of the epigastrium at once limits the extirpative extent of the procedure and dictates what must be removed. Thus, when the tumor spreads a short distance to involve the portal vein–superior mesenteric vein (PV-SMV) axis, the superior mesenteric artery, or the celiac axis, it usually becomes incurable. Similarly, if the gland is removed in a radical fashion, the need to excise the vessels and lymph nodes that go with it makes removal of the duodenum, gallbladder, common bile duct, upper jejunum, distal stomach, and sometimes the spleen necessary (Fig. 54.1).

When only part of the pancreas is removed or even if the gland is incised, safe management of any draining pancreatic juice is important, since the enzymes, if allowed to remain in the peritoneal cavity or retroperitoneum, may wreak havoc. The first principle of pancreatic surgery is, therefore, provision of adequate external drainage. Similarly, the accumulation of serum, lymph, and blood following major pancreatic or pancreatoduodenal resection needs to be drained. Further, since catgut is a protein substance that is readily digested by trypsin, it cannot be trusted as a ligature on major vessels or as suture material for anastomosis or for closing the abdomen. Silk, cotton, nylon, or prolene are much safer.

## PREOPERATIVE INVESTIGATIONS

### How Much Information Is Essential for the Surgeon?

Over the past 2 decades, several investigative tools have come to the forefront of pancreatic imaging (2). They provide the surgeon with vital preoperative information that helps in planning surgical strategy and often obviates the need for many time-consuming ancillary procedures on the operating table. Ultrasonography and/or computed tomography (CT) of the pancreas provide clues to the presence of any mass in the gland, dilation of the extrahepatic biliary tree, and any liver metastases. Endoscopic retrograde cannulation of the papilla (ERCP) delineates the state of the main pancreatic duct and/or the common bile duct and establishes the degree of obstruction and proximal dilation of the two main ducts. Most importantly, positive cytology results from the papillary aspirate confirms suspicion of cancer. This technique, however, is grossly overused and is not essential in every case. It introduces infection in an obstructed ductal system and may lead to severe suppurative cholangitis and pancreatitis, especially if surgery is delayed.

Endoscopic ultrasonography is another modality in its early stage of development (3). It uses direct surface contact to establish the presence and size of a pancreatic head mass, its extension into adjacent structures, the locoregional lymphadenopathy, and the possibility of vascular involvement. The technique requires a well-trained endoscopist who is knowledgeable in ultrasonography. Experience is necessary before accurate and reliable conclusions can be drawn.

A celiac and superior mesenteric arteriogram outlines variations in the foregut vasculature and can warn the surgeon about portal and splenic vein involvement and the presence of subclinical portal hypertension that will intensify intraoperative hemorrhage. Encasement of the major arteries (hepatic, splenic, or superior mesenteric) usually indicates unresectability of the cancer.

Major anatomic variation of the foregut vasculature is demonstrated in at least 25% of angiographic studies. Damage to the hepatic arterial supply is especially likely when it originates from the superior mesenteric artery and is not easily palpable behind and to the right of the common bile duct; this can lead to fatal hepatic necrosis in the jaundiced patient.

On the basis of our early experience, we previously advocated routine preoperative angiography in all cases. We no longer do. We now selectively perform preoperative angiography only in rare instances in which unusual technical difficulties are anticipated, such as *(a)* previous major abdominal operations, *(b)* preoperative radiotherapy, *(c)* a morbidly obese patient, or *(d)* an anticipated need to excise major vessels.

## PREOPERATIVE BILIARY DECOMPRESSION

Percutaneous transhepatic biliary decompression or endoscopic drainage is often routinely performed as a "knee-jerk reflex." Several prospective randomized trials have shown no benefit from relieving the jaundice preoperatively. These procedures introduce infection in an obstructed biliary tree and are often associated with postoperative septic complications (4).

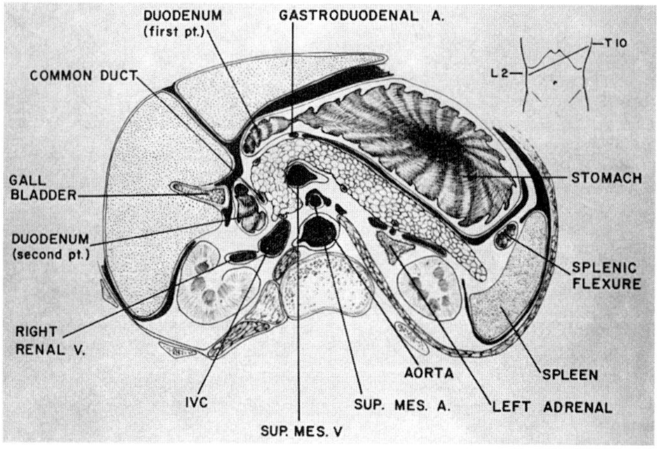


**FIG. 54.1.** Oblique transverse cross-section of the upper abdomen viewed from below. Section passes through the long axis of the pancreas at approximately the level indicated in the inset figure. (Reprinted with permission from Mackie CR, Moossa AR. Surgical anatomy of the pancreas. In: Moossa AR, ed. Tumor of the pancreas. Baltimore: Williams & Wilkins, 1980:2.)

## THE NEED FOR PREOPERATIVE TISSUE DIAGNOSIS

Surgical attitudes regarding cancer of the head of the pancreas have altered considerably over the past decade for two main reasons: *(a)* the mortality rate of pancreatoduodenal resections has declined dramatically and is in the region of 1–2% in expert hands and *(b)* patient survival following resection has also shown a distinct improvement. Five-year survival rates of 20–40% are reported from various centers (5).

The need to obtain a tissue diagnosis by percutaneous fine-needle aspiration or core needle biopsy under ultrasonic or CT guidance has become an irrational obsession (6). *Sampling error* is the major problem, because all pancreatic cancers are associated with varying degrees of histologic pancreatitis. Interpretative errors are also not rare, even when the pathologist is very experienced in the field. Thus, normal biopsy results do not exclude cancer and do not affect the decision to resect any pancreatic mass. Injudicious needling of the pancreas invariably induces some traumatic pancreatitis that later makes mobilization and dissection of the pancreas from the adjacent tissues exceedingly difficult, even for the most experienced surgeon. Finally, the pancreas is a very vascular organ with a rich lymphatic network and without a true glandular capsule. Standard oncologic principles therefore dictate that unnecessary needling of any tumor in the gland is likely to encourage metastatic spread.

## CONTRAINDICATIONS FOR ABDOMINAL EXPLORATIONS

One should avoid a purely diagnostic laparotomy in patients who, clinically and on imaging studies, have metastatic disease and/or unresectable disease, especially if the patient is frail and elderly, unless surgical palliation is contemplated. In such cases, percutaneous biopsy of an appropriate metastasis and/or the primary tumor is advisable to confirm the diagnosis, especially if the patient is a possible candidate for treatment with radiotherapy and/or chemotherapy. The patient with metastatic and/or unresectable disease can be easily palliated nonoperatively. On the other hand, one must never hesitate to explore a relatively fit and young patient in whom a histologic diagnosis is essential and miss the opportunity of being able to debulk a more favorable tumor such as an apudoma. Every effort must be made to obtain an exact tissue diagnosis nonoperatively or, if indicated, by laparoscopy or laparotomy.

The role of laparoscopy in staging pancreatic cancer is relatively new and its exact place is being explored in various centers (7). It is perfectly reasonable to advocate laparoscopy as the preliminary procedure to laparotomy. If liver metastases, peritoneal seeding, or gross invasion of the mesenteric vessels is established at laparoscopy, and tissue diagnosis is obtained by laparoscopic biopsy, the patient can be spared a laparotomy. Nonoperative palliation (i.e., *endoscopic stenting*) for the relief of obstructive jaundice can be performed later. Alternatively, if the surgeon is competent with laparoscopic surgery, both a biliary-enteric anastomosis and a gastrojejunostomy can be performed laparoscopically at the same sitting. If the surgeon plans to explore the abdomen for "open" palliative bypasses, then the preliminary laparoscopic procedure is not warranted. The advent of laparoscopic contact ultrasonography will no doubt further enhance the diagnostic and staging potential of laparoscopy.

## PREOPERATIVE EVALUATION AND PREPARATION

While specific investigative procedures should be kept to a minimum, general clinical assessment of the patient must be thorough to evaluate any concomitant comorbid factors. The patient with a cancer in the head of the pancreas is usually jaundiced and must be kept well hydrated, with intravenous fluids if necessary, to maintain diuresis and prevent the risk of renal failure. Vitamin K should be administered routinely to all jaundiced patients. Anemia is corrected by transfusion of packed red blood cells as deemed necessary, depending on its severity. While a substantial number of patients can undergo major pancreatoduodenal resection without any blood transfusion, six units of packed red blood cells, fresh frozen plasma, and platelets should be made available in case they are required. The patient should undergo some form of bowel preparation, using a combination of mild laxatives, enemas, and, if indicated, nonabsorbable antibiotics. Broad-spectrum systemic antibiotics must be administered prophylactically in the perioperative period.

## ABDOMINAL EXPLORATION

The three key words to the success of major pancreatic procedures are *access, exposure,* and *assistance.*

The incision chosen depends upon the patient's body habitus and the surgeon's personal preference. In an individual with an unusually narrow subcostal angle, a long midline incision starting at the xiphisternum and ending well below the umbilicus is appropriate. If the patient has a wide subcostal angle, an oblique-transverse upper abdominal incision over the long axis of the pancreas is preferred. Alternatively, a bilateral subcostal incision with a vertical extension toward the xiphisternum, if necessary, will provide ample access.

A thorough abdominal exploration with visualization and palpation of all abdominal and pelvic structures is an essential first step. Special attention should be paid to the liver surfaces, the transverse mesocolon, the root of the mesentery, and the ligament of Treitz.

A lesion in the head of the pancreas is considered unresectable if there are distant metastases, involvement of major vessels (hepatic artery or the superior mesenteric vessels), or extension beyond the usual pancreatoduodenectomy specimen (i.e., *peritoneal or omental seeding*). PV-SMV involvement per se does not always indicate unresectability, because a localized excision of the major vein with the pancreatic specimen can be done with subsequent vascular reanastomosis. The same applies if there is minimal puckering of the transverse mesocolon, because it can be excised with the whole specimen and, if necessary, the transverse colon can also be removed and anastamosed in an end-to-end manner. Biopsy of peripancreatic lymph nodes is not performed because abnormal biopsy results are not necessarily a contraindication to resection.

## INTRAOPERATIVE BIOPSY?

Obtaining a tissue diagnosis in the operating room to differentiate between carcinoma of the head of the pancreas and chronic pancreatitis before proceeding with a major resection has been one of the most discussed dilemmas in pancreatic surgery. This problem rarely occurs when the patient is jaundiced. We perform, on average, about 60 pancreatoduodenal resections annually for suspected periampullary malignancy, and it is unusual for us to resect a lesion that turns out to be benign more than once every 2 years. Occasionally, a tumor is small and hidden in the midst of a virtually ligneous gland that is totally involved in fibrotic and calcific pancreatitis. In such instances, the diagnosis may elude discovery until the whole excision specimen reaches the surgical pathology laboratory or the autopsy table, no matter how great an effort is made to obtain representative biopsy material at operation. Apart from the sampling problem, some pancreatic tumors, especially the diffuse infiltrating and sclerosing type, present the pathologist with a very difficult problem of identification on frozen section histology.

It is helpful to remember two old adages: *(a)* in the absence of acute inflammation, hard, solid (noncystic) masses in the head of the pancreas associated with obstructive jaundice and proximal bile duct dilation are usually *carcinoma,* not chronic pancreatitis; and *(b)* the presence of gallstones in this setting is usually incidental, and choledocholithiasis is rarely the cause of the biliary obstruction. Obviously, such generalizations, although helpful, will not serve to differentiate all carcinomas from chronic pancreatitis or choledocholithiasis. An operative cholangiogram through the cystic duct will eliminate all doubts about choledocholithiasis.

The decision to perform an intraoperative pancreatic biopsy is based on numerous factors including the overall clinical picture, the suspected diagnosis, the results of any preoperative examination, the resectability of the mass, the pathologist's experience with frozen section histologic examination of the gland, and the surgeon's philosophy. As mentioned above, a *pancreatic biopsy result negative for cancer does not rule out malignant disease.* Under favorable conditions, we carry out a resection without any preliminary biopsy, provided informed consent has been obtained. All unresectable or metastatic pancreatic tumors are diagnosed by biopsy and frozen section histology before the patient leaves the operating room, even if the job is time consuming. This removes doubt—an especially important point when a palliative procedure restores the patient to relative health for a long period and doubt is raised about the diagnosis. A known positive biopsy for ductal adenocarcinoma will then prevent a fruitless second laparotomy.

The first essential step in evaluation of a mass in the head of the pancreas is a Kocher maneuver. The peritoneal reflection lateral to the second portion of the duodenum is incised in front of the right kidney, and the duodenum and pancreatic head are elevated anteriorly and to the left of the patient. This exposes, in turn, the right kidney, right renal vein, inferior vena cava and gonadal vessels, left renal vein, and the abdominal aorta. The anterior perinephric fat, Gerota's fascia, aortocaval nodes, and soft tissues are freed from the adventitia of these vessels and are mobilized anteriorly to the left of the patient. This is done in all instances of proven or suspected cancer of the periampullary region.

A properly executed extensive Kocher maneuver reveals any possible invasion of the right lumbar gutter structures and facilitates examination of the portal vein and superior mesenteric artery, thus identifying their relationship to the tumor. The artery can be felt with the fingers behind the head of the gland. If the uncinate process as palpated behind the gland appears to be fixed to the right wall of the superior mesenteric artery or PV-SMV axis, the tumor is probably incurable. The PV-SMV axis lies anterior and to the right of the superior mesenteric artery; that is, it is closer to the operator and is not normally palpable. The next step is to check this major vein from the anterior aspect of the gland by opening the lesser sac widely. This is achieved by dividing the relatively avascular portion of the gastrocolic omentum close to the transverse colon along its whole length. The greater curvature of the stomach and attached omentum are elevated anteriorly and superiorly while the transverse colon and its mesocolon are retracted inferiorly. The leaf of the transverse mesocolon is followed posteriorly down to the pancreas. The middle colic vein is easily identified and traced to where it enters the superior mesenteric vein just below and behind the neck of the pancreas. As soon as the superior mesenteric vein goes behind the neck of the gland, it is joined by the splenic vein to form the portal vein. At this stage, anatomic variations must be carefully noted. Often the inferior mesenteric vein joins the right angle bifurcation of the superior mesenteric and splenic veins to form the tripod vein of Douglas.

There is seldom any tributary to the anterior surface of these two major veins behind the neck of the pancreas, and instruments or fingers can be gently inserted from below, anterior to the PV-SMV axis, to assess tumor invasion. Some surgeons prefer to enter this space from above; if this is done, ligation and division of the gastroduodenal artery at its origin from the hepatic artery should be done to facilitate the approach. If the PV-SMV axis is invaded in this anterior location, the patient is not curable. When obvious invasion at this site is encountered, the surgeon must give serious consideration to refraining from a major resection. If the neck of the pancreas can be freely elevated off these major veins, pancreatic transection at this site can be achieved to proceed with a standard pancreatoduodenectomy. If the tumor appears resectable at this point, we prefer to take down the gallbladder from its bed and transect the common hepatic duct just below the bifurcation. The porta hepatis and all its vessels are skeletonized, removing all possible lymph nodes and connective tissues, down to the celiac axis. The stomach is next transected at the junction of the gastric body and antrum to facilitate exposure, and the origins of the superior mesenteric artery and vein are also carefully cleared of attached nodes and connective tissue.

Occasionally, at the stage of the dissection when there is no turning back, the posterior aspect of the PV-SMV axis is found to be invaded. If the invasion is minimal, we would resect no more than about 1–1.5 cm of the major vein if this helps to get soft tissue clearance (8). Otherwise, we cut through the tumor to shave the uncinate process off the vein, such cases being considered incurable. Resection of the major *arteries* is no longer advocated because it does not improve survival and it increases the operative mortality and morbidity.

Following the resection, all the major vessels are carefully scrutinized, and all the remaining soft tissues and lymph nodes are carefully excised and sent separately for pathologic examination. After the major vessels have been totally skeletonized, the margins of the resection are carefully outlined with hemoclips, as this will help in planning a radiation port if radiation therapy is considered postoperatively.

Data supporting the advisability and benefit of regional lymphadenectomy and excision of surrounding connective tissue to skeletonize the major vessels have come from several sources, especially Japan (9). However, many surgeons do not consider this time-consuming and tedious task essential to improve survival and decrease local recurrence. Others believe that the pylorus-preserving pancreatoduodenal (PPPD) resection is equally applicable to cancer in the periampullary region. Although the PPPD has clear theoretical advantages in benign disease, we do not espouse it for cancer, since it further reduces the already small surgical margins and may well short-change the patient by compromising an already small chance of cure (10, 11).

## RECONSTRUCTION

The sequence of the anastomoses from proximal to distal varies according to the surgeon's personal preference and to anatomic factors. The Achilles' heel of a pancreatoduodenal resection is the pancreatojejunal anastomosis, and we prefer to tackle this first. If the pancreatic duct is dilated, we perform a duct-to-mucosa anastomosis. Whether the anastomosis should be stented or not is debatable and depends on how satisfied, emotionally and psychologically, the surgeon is with the completed product.

If the pancreatic duct is not dilated and the pancreas parenchyma is very soft, we prefer to invaginate the cut end of the pancreas into the open jejunum, according to the method of Hunt. A few inches distal along the jejunum, the hepaticojejunostomy is performed in end-to-side fashion, and the gastrojejunostomy is performed further downstream. We often buttress the pancreatojejunal anastomosis posteriorly by interposing the mobilized round ligament and falciform ligament of the liver between the anastomosis and the major veins. We routinely decompress the afferent jejunal limb by passing a sump NG tube through the gastrojejunostomy into that blind limb. Continuous low-grade suction is applied to the NG tube for 4–5 days postoperatively. We routinely advocate the placement of closed suction (Jackson-Pratt type) drains to the subhepatic space a few centimeters *away* from the anastomosis.

In some instances, a total pancreatectomy must be seriously considered. This should be performed only in good-risk patients who are already insulin-requiring diabetics whenever the tumor appears to extend beyond the neck of the gland or if the pancreatic parenchyma is exceedingly soft, friable, and so inflamed that it does not hold sutures safely.

## SURGICAL PALLIATION IN CANCER OF THE PANCREAS

Surgeons who explore the abdomen of a patient with pancreatic cancer have major responsibilities to the patient and to colleagues who are eventually going to treat the patient. When they consider the patient incurable, they must always obtain a tissue diagnosis and adequately stage the disease to delineate its extent, because these are important determinants in planning and assessing any type of treatment postoperatively. A biopsy of masses in the pancreas that have metastasized or are locally unresectable is always done until a definite histologic diagnosis is made on frozen section study. This removes all doubt about the exact diagnosis, especially if the patient happens to survive longer than predicted, and it can prevent a fruitless second laparotomy. All locally unresectable masses are then outlined with silver clips to help in the planning of a possible radiation port later on.

There is long-held belief that pancreatic resection is too formidable a procedure to be used for palliative purposes. Hence, most surgeons never knowingly perform a total pancreatectomy or pancreatoduodenectomy for palliation, although this is often all they may achieve. Recently, this view has been challenged by the Hopkins' group (12). Pancreatoduodenectomy has been performed for locally unresectable cancer as defined previously, leaving behind microscopically positive margins for tumor. They showed acceptably low mortality and morbidity that compared with those of conventional bypass procedures. This more aggressive approach, therefore, has to be considered in individual cases, especially if the patient is relatively young and in good functional status that will permit postoperative radiotherapy and chemotherapy.

The symptoms that the surgeon must think of palliating in all instances are *jaundice, intractable pruritus,* and *impending cholangitis.* This can be palliated by cholecystojejunostomy, provided that the gallbladder is dilated and the cystic duct is patent. If the cystic duct is long and thin and is close to where the tumor obstructs the common bile duct, it is much safer to perform a cholecystectomy, transect the common hepatic duct higher up, and perform a hepaticojejunostomy.

## DUODENAL OBSTRUCTION

It is tragic when, several weeks or months after decompressing the biliary tree by a biliary-enteric anastomosis, it becomes necessary to reoperate on the patient for duodenal obstruction. The site of obstruction is always in the third and fourth part of the duodenum when the tumor invades the root of the mesentery inferiorly. In patients who are anticipated to survive more than a few months, it is much wiser to avoid the complication and provide the solution at the first operation by performing a gastrojejunostomy. The gastrojejunostomy has to be performed in a mechanically sound manner and should be placed well to the left of the tumor mass on the posterior and most dependent part of the stomach. The addition of bilateral truncal vagotomy to prevent marginal ulceration is now considered optional with the advent of $H_2$-receptor antagonists and proton-pump inhibitors.

The biliary-enteric anastomosis is performed distal to the gastrojejunostomy. Whether a Roux-en-Y or a loop of jejunum is brought up to the biliary tree, with or without a distal side-to-side jejunostomy, is largely a matter of personal preference and sometimes depends on how easily the jejunum can be mobilized to the subhepatic space.

## PAIN

Pain is a distressing symptom in the terminal phase of a patient's life. The characteristic backache of advanced pancreatic cancer can be substantially alleviated by open chemical splanchnicectomy using a 20-gauge spinal needle and a syringe containing 15–20 mL of 6% phenol. The abdominal aorta is identified by palpation with the left index finger and the phenol is then injected into the region between the splanchnic nerves and the celiac ganglion. The site of the injection is retroperitoneal and slightly lateral, posterior, and superior to the origin of the celiac artery. Intermittent aspiration prevents inadvertent injection of the chemical into the vascular system.

## CANCER OF THE BODY AND TAIL OF THE PANCREAS

One is rarely called upon to resect a carcinoma that has arisen in the body and tail of the gland, since such tumors are almost always incurable by the time they reach the surgeon. However, in good-risk patients, unless there is risk of distant metastases by imaging techniques or at laparoscopy, it is worth exploring the abdomen with a view to performing a distal pancreatectomy and splenectomy. Often, the operative recognition of the exact cellular origin of a cancer at this site is not precise, even if it is substantiated by frozen section histology. For these reasons, such lesions should always be resected, since occasionally the patient and the surgeon will have the pleasant surprise of finding that the tumor is less virulent, its cellular origin is not from the exocrine pancreas, and the lesion is in fact an islet cell tumor, lymphoma, or sarcoma.

## CYSTIC TUMORS OF THE PANCREAS

The above discussion dealt exclusively with solid tumors of the pancreas. The surgical philosophy and approach to cystic tumors has to be much more aggressive. All cystic neoplasms, especially the mucinous type, are deemed malignant and need to be excised without any attempt at sampling biopsy. Depending on the location of the tumor, a Whipple procedure or a distal pancreatectomy and splenectomy is indicated. If metastases are present and resectable, they should be excised with the primary lesion, since long-term survival can still be achieved. Even when the tumor has invaded extensively into adjacent structures, careful debulking has a definite place, especially if it is supplemented postoperatively by external radiotherapy with 5-fluorouracil as a radiosensitizer.

## REFERENCES


1. Moossa AR, Mulholland MW. Pancreas—anatomy and structure anomalies. In: Yamada T, ed. Textbook of gastroenterology, vol. 2. Philadelphia: JB Lippincott, 1991:1851.
2. Moossa AR, Gamagami RA. Diagnosis and staging of pancreatic neoplasms. Surg Clin North Am 1995;75:871.
3. Yasuda K, Mukai H, Nakajima M, et al. Staging of pancreatic carcinoma by endoscopic ultrasonography. Endoscopy 1993; 25:151.
4. Matthews JB, Blumgart LH. Percutaneous and endoscopic drainage and endoprosthesis—surgical relevance. In: Blumgart LH, ed. Surgery of the liver and biliary tract. 2nd ed. Edinburgh: Churchill Livingstone, 1994:539–545.
5. Pitt HA. Curative treatment for pancreatic neoplasms. Surg Clin North Am 1995;75:891.
6. Moossa AR. Biopsy of pancreatic masses. In: Burns GP, Bank SS, eds. Disorders of the pancreas. New York: Health Professions Division, McGraw-Hill, 1992:345–356.
7. Chuschieri A. Laparoscopic surgery of the pancreas. J R Coll Surg Edinb 1994;39:178.
8. Ishikawa O, Ohigashi H, Imaoka S, et al. Perioperative indications for extended pancreatectomy for locally advanced cancer involving the portal vein. Ann Surg 1992;215:231.
9. Ishikawa O, Ohigashi H, Sasaki K, et al. Practical usefulness of lymphatic and connective tissue clearance for carcinoma of the pancreatic head. Ann Surg 1988;208:215.
10. Roder JD, Stein JH, Huttl W, et al. Pylorus-preserving vs. standard pancreaticoduodenectomy. An analysis of 110 pancreatic and periampullary carcinomas. Br J Surg 1992;79:152.
11. Moossa AR, Veergandham R. Preservation of the pylorus in resection of the head of the pancreas. J Hepato-Biliary-Pancreat Surg 1994;1(4):349.
12. Lillemoe KD, Cameron JL, Yeo CJ, et al. Pancreaticoduodenectomy: does it have a role in the palliation of pancreatic cancer? Ann Surg 1996;223:718.

# 55

# *Pancreatoduodenectomy (Whipple Resection) with Skeletonization of Vessels for Cancers of the Pancreas and Adjacent Organs*

John M. Howard

## HISTORIC NOTES

The first pancreatoduodenectomy is attributed by Suavé to Alessandro Codivilla who performed a resection of part of the head of the pancreas and duodenum for carcinoma of the pancreas in 1898 (1). Berns (2) performed an earlier resection of the head of the pancreas in 1881; an operation done for cancer of the gastric antrum. Walter Kausch of Berlin in 1909–1912 resected (two stage) the head of the pancreas and duodenum for carcinoma of the ampulla of Vater in three patients (3, 4). Allen Whipple, however, is generally credited for development of the operative procedure that came to bear his name. In 1934 and 1935, he and colleagues performed two-stage resections of carcinoma of the ampulla of Vater in three patients. The first patient died of early disintegration of the anastomotic catgut sutures. The other two patients survived (5). Whipple then developed the one-stage resection. He wrote: "In March of 1940 the writer performed the first recorded one stage removal of the entire head of the pancreas, the entire duodenum with occlusion of the pancreas" (6). This patient had a clinically "nonfunctioning" islet cell carcinoma (alpha cell) of the head of the pancreas. After 5 years, she showed nodules in the liver; she lived for 9 years after the operation before succumbing to the hepatic metastases. Included in Whipple's contributions was the recognition that catgut dissolved rapidly in the milieu of a pancreatoenteric anastomosis.

## DIAGNOSIS AND PREOPERATIVE MANAGEMENT

The diagnosis of carcinoma of the head of the pancreas, discussed in Chapter 52, can be tentatively made at the bedside. It is hoped that in the future, as earlier diagnosis is achieved, these "initial" manifestations will be recognized as late manifestations. Discomfort in the abdomen or back, jaundice, and a history of weight loss in an older patient with acholic stools and no history of biliary colic is typical, particularly if he or she has a prolonged history of cigarette smoking. Ultrasonography is useful to demonstrate the presence or absence of gallstones, but a computed tomography (CT) scan of the abdomen provides better imaging of the pancreas and is helpful in demonstrating metastases, particularly in the liver. Current advances in magnetic resonance imaging may displace other imaging techniques. Gastroduodenoscopy can identify tumors or obstructing lesions at the ampulla of Vater or duodenum. Endoscopic retrograde cholangiopancreatography (ERCP) was helpful in the past in demonstrating carcinoma of the distal common bile duct, but as experience increases, the surgeon finds ERCP less essential.

Arteriography was used earlier to outline the celiac axis and its branches, but with increased experience, most anomalous branches of the arterial system can be recognized at the time of operation. The information sought is thus largely whether any of the large veins are partially or completely occluded or whether there is a suggestion of invasion of the venous wall. A baseline serum CA19-9 level, along with the determination of the Lewis blood types, is valuable primarily in providing a baseline for postoperative follow-up, as the assay is not diagnostic (7). Remeasurement of the CA19-9 level 14–21 days after resection provides a prognostic guide as to whether the tumor has been "completely" resected (i.e., whether or not the serum CA19-9 level has returned to normal (8, 9)). Approximately 10% of patients are Lewis blood type–negative and apparently cannot produce the CA19-9 antigen.

Preoperative percutaneous needle biopsy has been used when liver metastases were suggested by CT scan, but the author discontinued its use for pancreatic biopsy on good-risk patients following a major intraabdominal hemorrhage in one patient, resulting in multiple blood transfusions and a delay in operation. In a second patient, a small peripancreatic abscess found at the point of the needle biopsy resulted in the resection being aborted. Although recommended by others (10), laparoscopy has not been used, as it adds another procedure. The author's approach is to evaluate the cancer in most patients by "seeing and feeling it, and, when feasible, removing it," and if not, bypassing it in most reasonable-risk patients. There have obviously been numerous exceptions, especially in nonjaundiced or poor-risk patients or those with widespread disease.

## EVALUATION AND PREPARATION OF THE PATIENT FOR OPERATION

The patients considered for laparotomy have been evaluated primarily for their cardiovascular, respiratory, and renal reserve as a measure of their ability to survive operation. The author approaches each patient with the intention of resecting the tumor: to perform a "curative" resection if possible or a palliative resection if achievable. The presence of limited ascites is not a contraindication to operation, since in the author's experience, most patients with ascites have not had peritoneal carcinomatosis (11). The presence of obstructive jaundice in a patient believed capable of surviving operation has been accepted as an indication for laparotomy, even in the presence of limited metastases. Endoscopic stenting of the common bile duct is avoided if laparotomy is planned. Unlike the patient with a common bile duct stone, the patient with obstructive jaundice secondary to carcinoma of the head of the pancreas is usually free of cholangitis. Endoscopic stenting may result in cholangitis and may reduce the caliber of the common bile duct. Its advantages in the poor-risk patient, especially one with a long standing biliary obstruction, are recognized.

Preparation of the patient for surgery includes bowel "cleansing and sterilization" the day before operation. Prior to arrival in the operating room, or in the operating room, pneumatic compression cuffs are applied and an initial dose of a broad-spectrum antibiotic is administered intravenously. The jaundiced patient is given parenteral vitamin K preoperatively while the prothrombin level is monitored. Control of diabetes is seldom a problem, but correction of malnutrition has proved difficult. A urinary Foley catheter and a nasogastric catheter are inserted. Central venous catheters and occasionally Swan-Ganz catheters are used.

Arrangements include ensuring a first assistant who can, preferably, perform many of the operative maneuvers including venous repair, if the surgeon's hands are engaged in hemostasis. The pancreatic surgeon should be capable in vascular techniques. Pancreatic bleeding is predominantly venous, and vascular repair and resection are largely venous. Vascular instruments must always be available. Multiple-sized T tubes should be available as well as multiple-sized pliable catheters for intubation of the pancreatojejunostomy. In addition, secretin should be available in case of difficulty in identifying a small transected pancreatic duct.

**Resectabilty Rate.** The rate of resectability for pancreatic carcinoma today varies widely from clinic to clinic, depending on the local preference for shunting of patients for palliation of obstructive jaundice, percutaneous needle biopsy for definitive diagnosis, and the surgeon's aggressiveness in resection. Watanapa and Williamson (1992), in a review of 37 reports in the English language literature over the preceding 20 years, found the *mean* resectability rate for pancreatic exocrine carcinoma prior to 1980 to be 10% (12); the rate rose to 15% in the 1980s, and by 1992, in selected centers it had approached 20%.

Ashton and Longmire (1973) reported a resectability rate of 26% (13). Gall and Köckerling in 1988 (14) estimated the resectability rate at that time as 15–20%. Kümmerle and Ruckert (1984) reported a rate of 22% (15). Allema et al. (1995) estimated a similar rate (16). Each of these reports related to the use of the standard Whipple resection. Hanyu et al. (1993) (17), however, after extending the scope of operation to skeletonization of the vessels and more frequent use of resection of the portal-mesenteric veins, reported their resectability rate as 53%. There is little evidence that the stage of disease at the time of diagnosis has changed appreciably in the past few decades. Resectability rates of cancers of the body and tail of the pancreas remain lower than those for the pancreatic head.

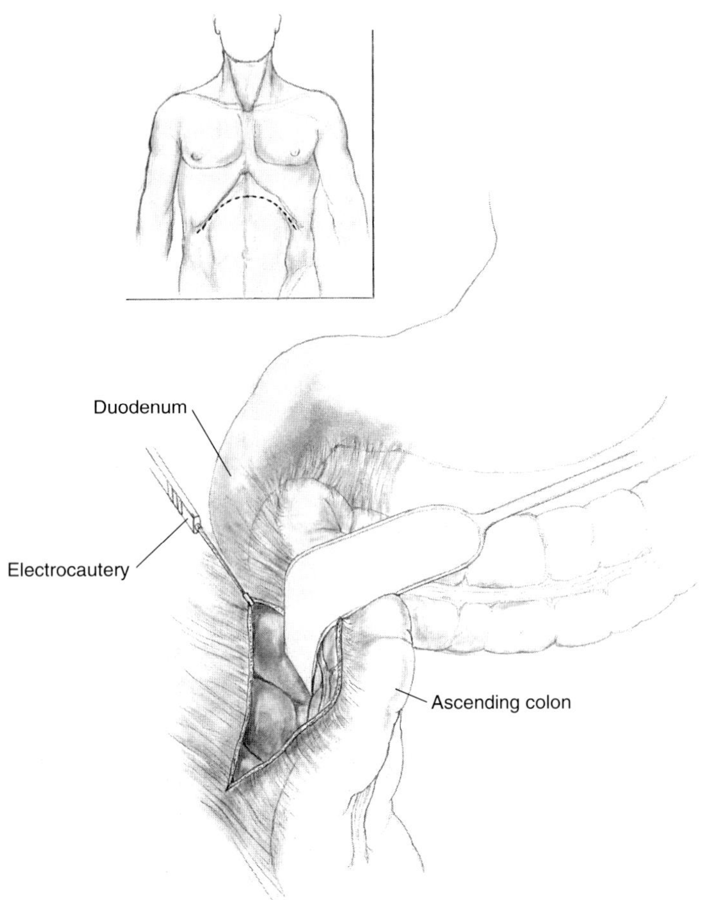


**FIG. 55.1.** Laparotomy is performed via a bilateral subcostal incision *(inset).* With *electrocautery*, the hepatic flexure is mobilized medially to expose the *duodenum.*

## OPERATION

### Exploration and Evaluation of Findings

Laparotomy is performed routinely through a bilateral subcostal incision, beginning on the right side (Fig. 55.1 inset). A vertical incision is usually avoided. If, upon opening the abdomen, the cancer is found to be clearly unresectable, the complete extension of the incision to the left side may not be necessary. Exploration of the liver and peritoneal cavity is initially performed; any ascitic fluid is sampled for cytologic examination. Tissue is taken for frozen and permanent histologic study. (Identification of any unexpected islet cell carcinoma is particularly important).

In exploring the free peritoneal cavity, attention is paid to the inferior surface of the transverse mesocolon, as this is a frequent site of invasion. Electrocautery is used to divide the lateral peritoneum along the hepatic flexure of the colon (Fig. 55.1), which is mobilized medially and inferiorly away from the duodenum. Next, electrocautery is used to incise the thickened peritoneum lateral to the duodenal loop (Fig. 55.2). This is not an entirely avascular area, especially in the patient with obstructive jaundice. The right kidney and its ureter are identified and protected. A Kocher maneuver is then performed, with the pancreas freed retroperitoneally to permit palpation to and behind the superior mesenteric artery (Fig. 55.3 and inset). The mass in the head of the pancreas can thus be localized, and its extent estimated. Direct tumor invasion of the inferior vena cava at the time of exploration has not been encountered by the author, and vena caval hemorrhage, caused by tumor invasion, has not been a problem. Care must be taken, however, to avoid injury to the right ovarian or testicular vein as it empties into the vena cava. Further mobilization of the duodenum and head of the pancreas permits retroperitoneal exposure (Fig. 55.4, *A* and *B*), including the posterior wall of the duodenum and head of the pancreas.

Biopsy of the tumor prior to resection was historically a principle of this operation. With increased experience, this is no longer essential, as an experienced surgeon can usually achieve the diagnosis with near-certainty by palpation. Most benign hard masses in this area are usually best treated by resection. If biopsy is elected, and it usually has been, a wedge biopsy may be done if the tumor is on the anterior or posterior surface of the gland (see Chapter 14). If a wedge biopsy is impractical, a core needle biopsy or fine-needle aspiration is performed. The latter two are

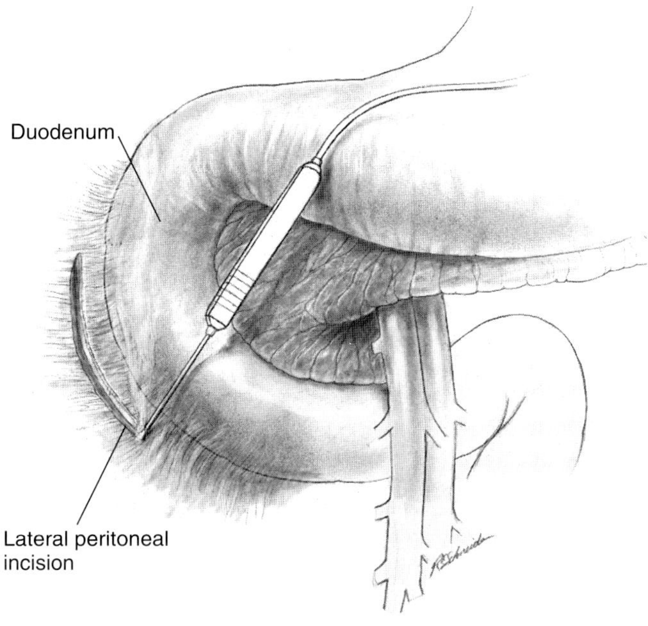


**FIG. 55.2.** Division of the peritoneum lateral to the descending duodenum prior to the Kocher maneuver. The hepatic flexure of the colon has been mobilized medially.

performed with the fingers of the left hand, behind the pancreas; the needle is inserted with the right hand. The left hand is used as a guard to prevent the needle from penetrating the vena cava or aorta, as the needle may penetrate the posterior wall of the tumor. The needle may be inserted transduodenally or directly through the pancreas. Depending on the immediate availability of an expert cytologist, fine-needle biopsy is usually adequate for diagnosis. The resultant specimen is tiny, and if the tumor is unresectable, it may not permit optimal studies for grading, determination of ploidy, and immunohistochemical and molecular biologic determinations. If wedge biopsy is performed, care is taken to minimize the possible spread of cancer cells from the surface of the transected cancer. Suction drainage is maintained at the point of incision, and electrocautery is used to "scorch" the surface of the tumor to minimize the shedding of viable cancer cells, as well as to control any vascular ooze. When a core needle is inserted for biopsy, it is important to pass the needle directly into the tumor to avoid laceration of the pancreatic duct upstream from the tumor, which might lead to a pancreatic fistula if the tumor is not resected. To reiterate, the experienced pancreatic surgeon prefers, but no longer requires, histologic proof of cancer to proceed with resection. No postoperative death has resulted in the author's experience from this decision, and in retrospect, the errors that have been recognized involved failure to resect a suspicious mass at an early stage because of negative biopsies, only to reexplore an advanced cancer at a later date.

Meanwhile, the gastrocolic ligament is divided, usually beginning on the left side at the greater curvature of the stomach where the lesser cavity may be more easily entered (Fig. 55.5). Others preserve the omental vessels. The gastroepiploic vessels along the greater curvature are protected.

Through the resulting gastrocolic space, the anterior surface of the pancreas can be examined along with the lymph nodes and vessels cephalad to the pancreas (Fig. 55.6). It may be helpful to again palpate the anterior surface of the pancreas in association with the Kocher maneuver.

In general, the author elects resection of cancers of the head of the pancreas, whether for cure or for palliation, regardless of the size of the tumor. The operation has been modified to include systematic resection of the retropancreatic and perivascular lymphatics and other soft tissues. Resection of the superior mesenteric or portal veins is an option more frequently adopted. If multiple metastases are present in the liver, the prognosis seems so bad that palliative resection of the pancreas is seldom undertaken. The author no longer considers the presence of one

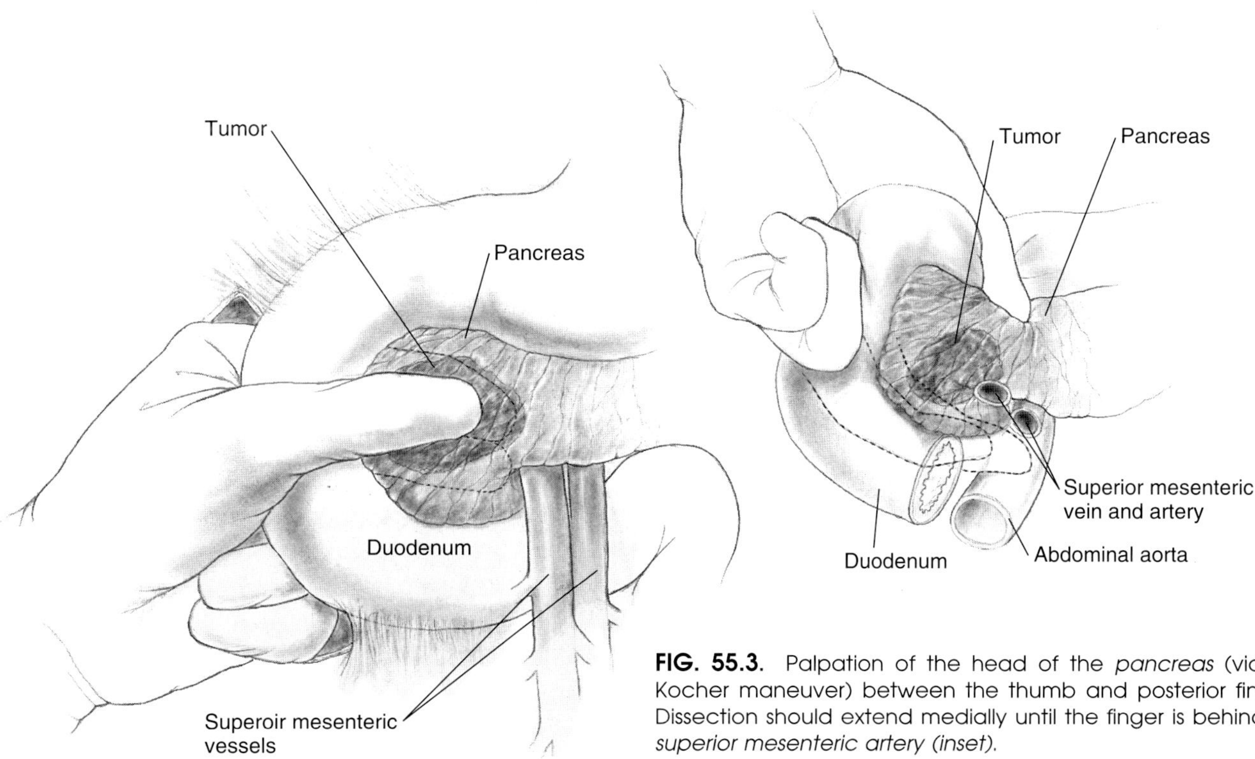


**FIG. 55.3.** Palpation of the head of the *pancreas* (via the Kocher maneuver) between the thumb and posterior fingers. Dissection should extend medially until the finger is behind the *superior mesenteric artery (inset).*

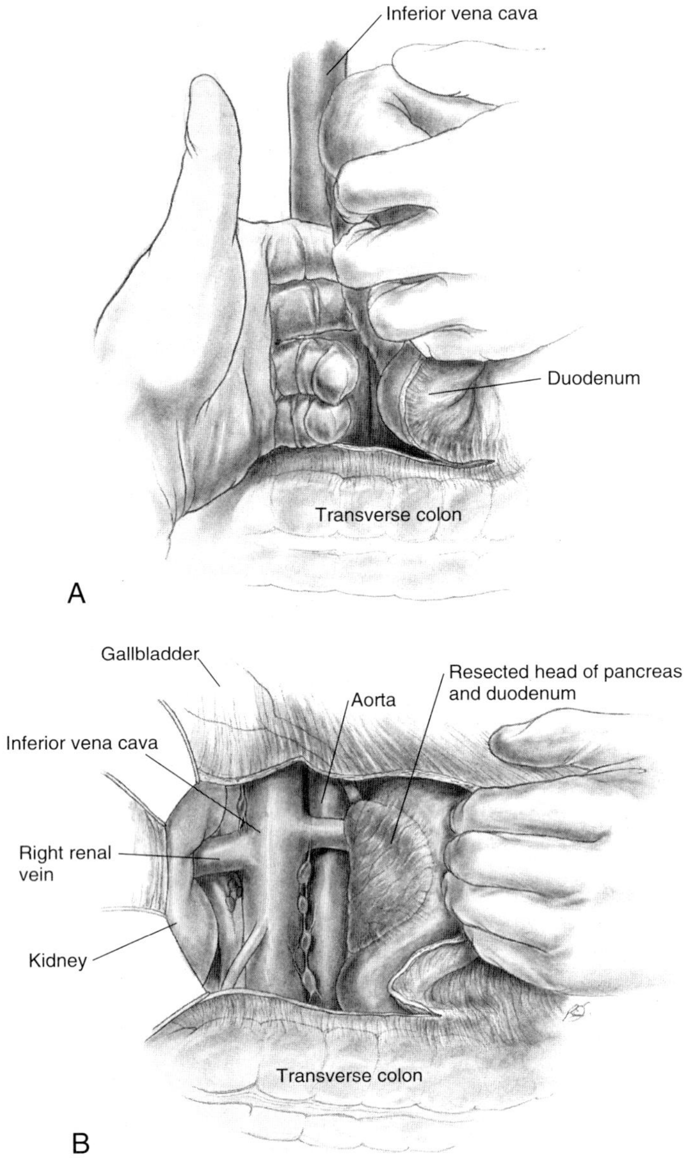


**FIG. 55.4.** **A.** Mobilization of the *duodenum* and head of the pancreas permits retroperitoneal exposure. The posterior wall of the duodenum and head of pancreas are exposed. **B.** The *inferior vena cava* is exposed, as are both renal veins.

or two easily resected metastases to be an *absolute* contraindication to palliative resection in the good-risk patient. Although not currently practiced by his peers, hepatic resection may prove more advantageous as adjuvant therapy improves.

The decision regarding resectability can sometimes not be made at a given moment: the goal remains under consideration as the dissection progresses. *Complete* obstruction of the portal or the superior mesenteric veins used to be an absolute or near absolute contraindication to the Whipple resection, as resection involves division of the essential venous collateral channels, which leads to acute splanchnic hypertension. In 1958, portacaval shunt in association with pancreatoduodenectomy (Whipple resection for carcinoma) was reported to lead to death from hepatic failure (18). There are two issues involved: *(a)* the management of portal hypertension when the collateral venous channels are destroyed and *(b)* whether the coincident shunting of an incompletely identified hepatotrophic factor away from the liver is compatible with health. It is possible that a bypass portacaval-type shunt or vein graft replacement prior to resection might circumvent the hemodynamic problem, although the author does not recommend it. Currently I consider complete obstruction of the portal vein to be a contraindication to pancreatoduodenectomy.

## Resection (the Classical Whipple with Skeletonization of Vessels)

Skeletonization of vessels is not indicated in benign disease. Having ascertained that there is a tumor in or adjacent to the head of the pancreas that appears resectable, the next step in the classical Whipple resection is to divide the stomach between staples, approximately 2 inches proximal to the pylorus (Fig. 55.7) (see the description of the pylorus-preserving procedure below). Others defer gastric division until later in the dissection, but gastric division permits better exposure along the superior border and anterior surface of the pancreas. An early decision is made as to whether the tumor is clearly resectable or whether doubt exists. If resectability seems ensured, the surgeon can first approach either the biliary tract dissection or the pancreatic resection. Either is quite acceptable. Operation may thus be directed to cholecystectomy and transection of the *common bile* duct or the *common hepatic* duct. It is customary to perform cholecystectomy and to transect the bile duct above the cystic duct, but the level of this transection is probably not important with benign lesions or with most *pancreatic cancers, per se*, as a positive margin of the transected duct, above or below the cystic junction, is seldom encountered with pancreatic cancer (4–5%). The presence of a better arterial supply at the level of the common *hepatic* duct seems equivocal.

An aberrant right hepatic artery originates from the superior mesenteric artery in 20% of patients and usually ascends along the right side of the portal vein and common bile duct; it must be detected (Fig. 55.8). Early in the operation, the vessels of the hepatic hilum are isolated, and umbilical tapes are passed around each for control and retraction. Using the pulsation of the common hepatic artery as a guide, the hepatic artery is localized, and a right-angle clamp is passed behind it to grasp an encircling umbilical tape. The common duct is isolated next, and its encircling tape is initially placed above the duodenum, but not necessarily above the cystic duct. Using a right angle clamp for

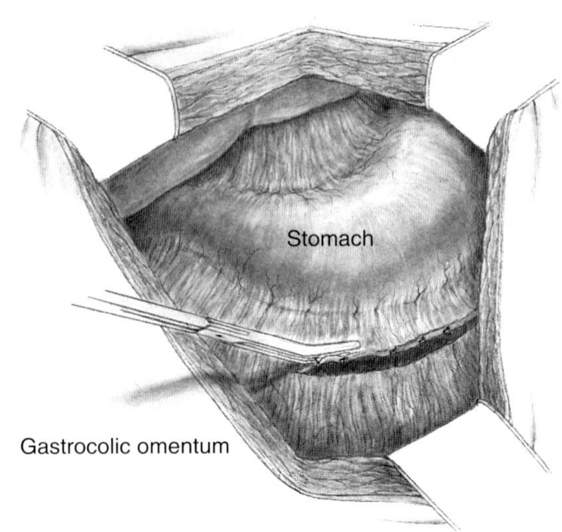


**FIG. 55.5.** Division of the *gastrocolic omentum* to permit anterior exposure of the pancreas and exploration of the lesser peritoneal cavity.

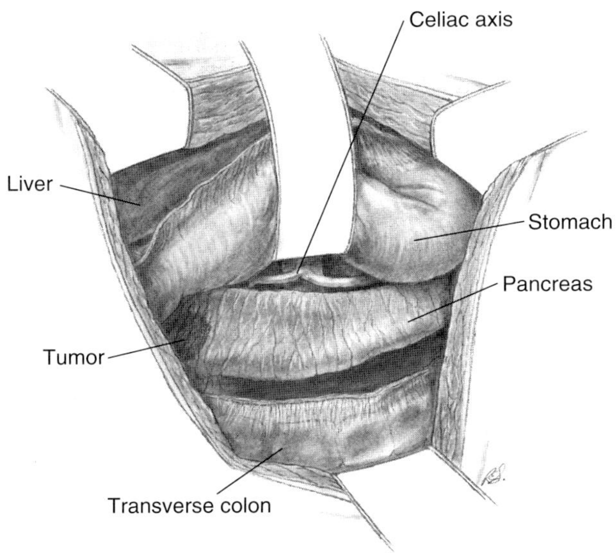


**FIG. 55.6.** Exposure of the anterior surface of the *pancreas* permits initial inspection of vessels and lymph nodes superior to the pancreas.

dissection (Fig. 55.9), the index finger of the left hand is placed behind the common bile duct, which is carefully dissected from the portal vein enough to allow the clamp to be passed posterior to the common duct and thus to grasp an umbilical tape. Next, the portal vein is encircled by approaching it between the artery and the duct, with additional dissection posteriorly behind the vein (Fig. 55.10). Sometimes it is easier to pass an encircling umbilical tape behind all three of the hilar structures (Fig. 55.11*A*) and then bring the separate ends of the tape between the vein and artery and between the vein and common duct, respectively (Fig. 55.11*B*); thus selectively encircling the portal vein. Tears in the portal vein or its tributaries during this procedure can result in vigorous bleeding. Pressure applied by a small sponge beneath the finger can usually control this bleeding, permitting its localization and suture repair. Not infrequently, the application of pressure results in complete and permanent cessation of bleeding. Meanwhile, if needed, the Pringle maneuver is available, in which the surgeon places the left index finger into the foramen of Winslow and uses it and the overlying thumb to compress the portal triad while the vein is repaired. During the hilar dissection, a large lymph node is found behind the common duct and the first part of the duodenum. It actually consists of one or more large soft nodes with a rich blood supply. Its excision for biopsy results in troublesome bleeding and is usually avoided, but subsequently, it is removed en bloc with the pancreas.

Throughout the manipulation of the distal common duct and the adjacent duodenum, the surgeon remains alert to the possibility of encountering a periampullary duodenal diverticulum. Meanwhile, needle aspiration of the distal common duct permits collection of bile for bacterial culture and gross inspection. "White bile," sometimes almost water clear, implies a more longstanding obstruction and greater impairment of hepatic function than does stagnant bile of the thick "motor oil" type.

The common bile duct can be divided at this stage as it expedites dissection and (if there is no evidence of distant spread) choledochojejunostomy is anticipated, which provides drainage whether the ultimate outcome of operation is resection of the pancreas or biliary bypass only. The transection of the duct is done with angled Potts scissors. A narrow cross-section of the duct is excised for frozen section to ascertain that the line of transection is free of cancer. If the line of transection is positive for malignancy, a higher resection with repetition of the biopsy sequence is necessary, and the possibility of *primary carcinoma of the bile duct* is reconsidered. The transected duct on its ampullary side is oversewn for hemostasis and to prevent reflux of its contents into the wound. Hemostasis on the hepatic side of the line of transection is obtained by use of fine absorbable sutures. To minimize necrosis of the duct and fistula formation, electrocautery is used sparingly, if at all. The author characteristically selects the point of transection of the common duct at a point of relative convenience, sometimes below the cystic duct.

Cholecystectomy may be performed at this stage. It is not a simple procedure in spite of the ample exposure, because the gallbladder is frequently large, and bleeding from its hepatic bed is increased. Obstructed, dilated bile ducts result in a low degree of portal hypertension. Bleeding (ooze) decreases after ductal

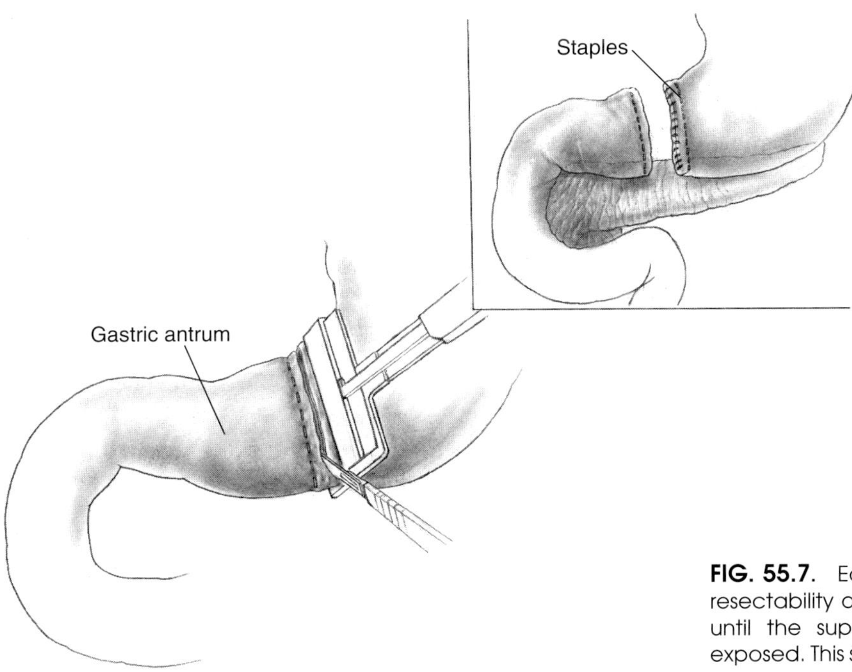


**FIG. 55.7.** Early division of the stomach improves exposure. If resectability of the tumor is in doubt, this step may be delayed until the superior mesenteric and portal veins have been exposed. This step is avoided in the pylorus-preserving operation.

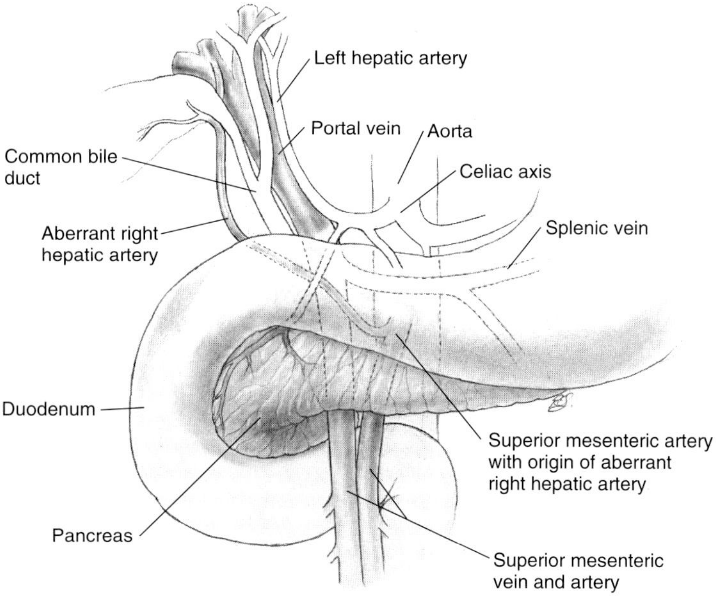


**FIG. 55.8.** The *aberrant right hepatic artery* off the *superior mesenteric artery* is a frequent anomaly, usually running along the right side of the *portal vein* and *common bile duct*. It should be identified early in the dissection.

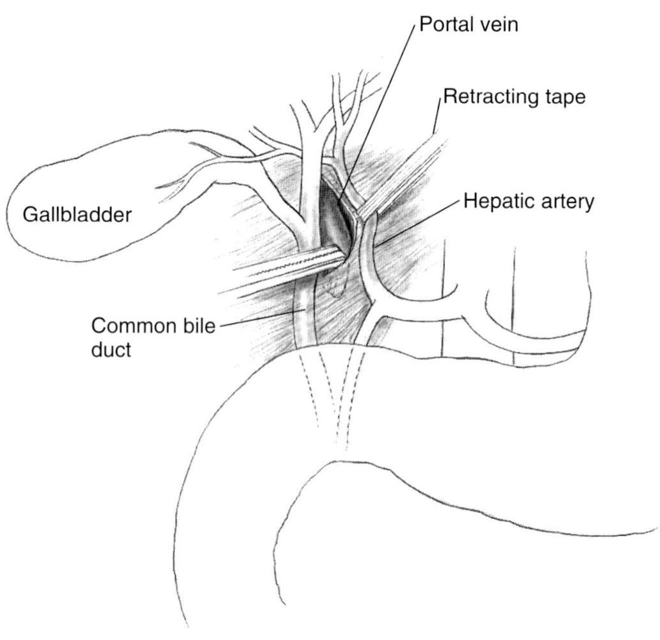


**FIG. 55.9.** The *hepatic artery* is isolated first, then the *common bile duct*. Umbilical tapes are used to retract each. Bleeding from the anterior wall of the *portal vein* is the hazard at this stage.

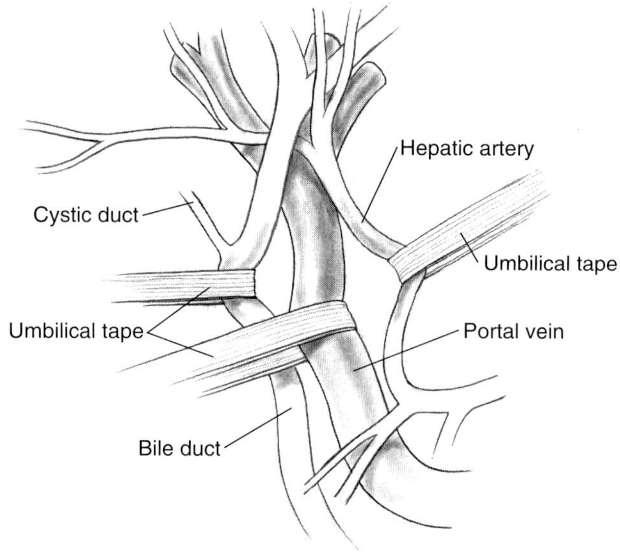


**FIG. 55.10.** The *portal vein* is usually approached between the artery and *bile duct*, thus gaining control of the hepatic hilum.

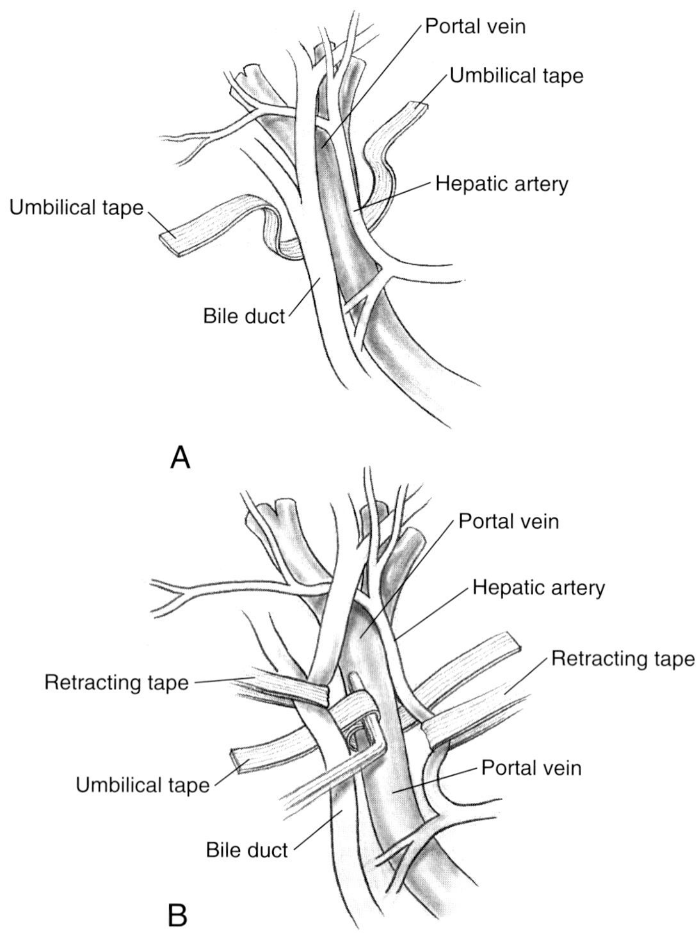


**FIG. 55.11.** Sometimes isolation of the *portal vein* is difficult. It may then be easier to pass a tape behind all three hilar structures (**A**) and then bring its ends up separately between the respective vessels (**B**), thus isolating the *portal vein*. The final maneuver of bringing the tape up between the *hepatic artery* and *portal vein* is not shown.

decompression. A bulldog clamp may be placed across the transected bile duct, but in the absence of cholangitis, the bile duct is usually left unoccluded and observed for the return flow of normal-colored bile from its transected end. Failure of bile flow during the period of observation is of concern, possibly indicating significant hepatic damage. Not infrequently, supraduodenal transection of the bile duct reveals a "double barrel" lumen (Fig. 55.12), usually reflecting a low junction of the cystic and common bile ducts. When this is recognized and proved by passing a probe through the open cystic duct from below, one option is to divide the cystic duct longitudinally and superficially excise its wall, taking care to preserve the blood supply to the common duct. Another option, once the cystic duct transection is proved, is to transect the common duct higher. Occasionally the option of having the choledochojejunal anastomosis encompass both ducts is used. Each has proved satisfactory. (Should the double lumen be the result of transection of both hepatic ducts because of their low junction, each duct must be anastomosed to the jejunum).

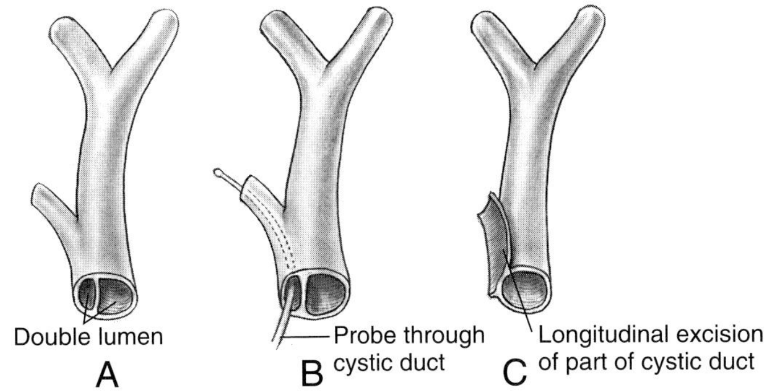


**FIG. 55.12.** The "double barrel" line of transection of the bile duct. The danger is that the *double lumen* (**A**) might reflect a low junction of right and left hepatic ducts. It usually reflects a low junction of cystic and common hepatic ducts. The latter can be proved by passing a probe from below through the open end of the cystic duct (**B**). One option is to excise the outer wall of the cystic duct longitudinally to prevent formation of a mucocele while still protecting the blood supply to the common duct (**C**). Reexcision of the common duct at a higher level may be a better option.

Next, the pancreas is dissected from the superior mesenteric vein and superior mesenteric artery. If preoperative imaging suggests the possibility of venous invasion, exploration of the body of the pancreas and the portal and mesenteric vessels prior to cholecystectomy and division of the stomach is preferable, as invasion in this area is more likely to prevent resection than is invasion in the biliary area. Working from the right side of the operating table and being right-handed, the author approaches the dissection of the neck of the pancreas from the inferior border of the gland, although others approach it from its superior border. The inferior border of the pancreas is dissected from the adjacent adipose tissue of the transverse mesocolon for 2–3 cm (Fig. 55.13), seeking not only to trace the tributaries of the superior mesenteric vein toward their confluence adjacent or behind the pancreas, but also to avoid possible injury to the inferior mesenteric vein, whose relation to the superior mesenteric and splenic veins remains uncertain (Fig. 55.14). The inferior mesenteric vein *may occasionally empty into the superior mesenteric* vein immediately inferior to the pancreas in the transverse mesocolon or behind the pancreas. Small tributary vessels of the superior mesenteric vein immediately inferior to the pancreas are suture ligated and divided (Fig. 55.15*A*). Relying on the relative absence of tributary vessels on the anterior surface of the superior mesenteric vein in its retropancreatic passage, dissection is made with a "peanut" pusher (Fig. 55.15*B*) and the index finger immediately anterior to the superior mesentery vein and behind the overlying pancreas (Fig. 55.15*C*). The dissection is performed with care, because in most patients, the superior mesenteric vein has not been controlled by encircling umbilical tapes. Tumor invasion of the vein increases the risk of venous bleeding. The exploring finger (behind the pancreas) may find minor difficulty in egressing superiorly at the level of the splenic and portal veins. Using a right-angle clamp, dissection craniad to the pancreas is used to expose the tip of the (retropancreatic)

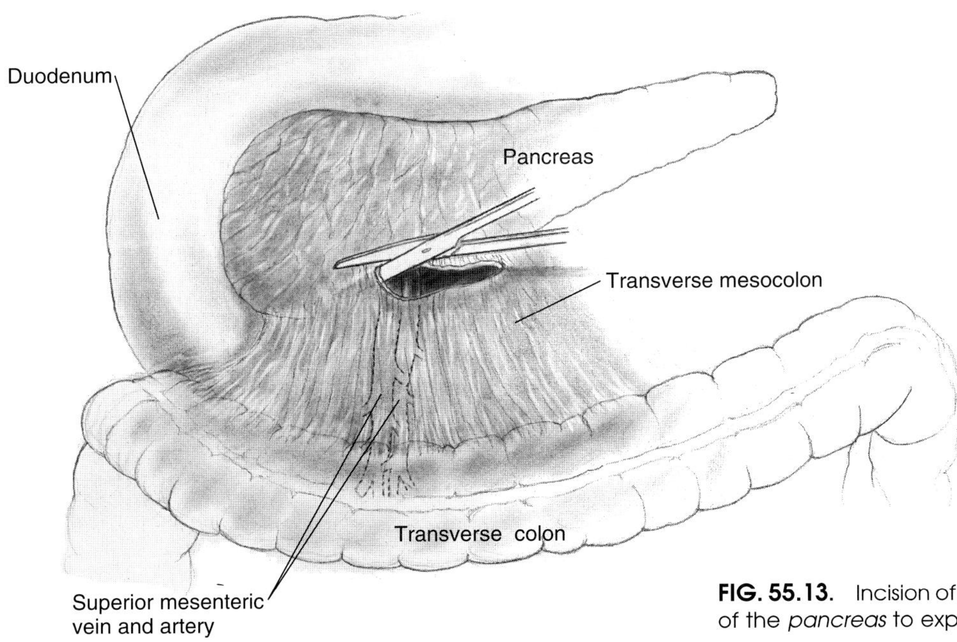


**FIG. 55.13.** Incision of the peritoneum along the inferior border of the *pancreas* to expose the *superior mesenteric vein.*

index finger of the surgeon's left hand, or of a dissector lying behind the pancreas.

An encircling umbilical tape may be passed around the pancreas. The next step is the transection of the pancreas at the level of the superior mesenteric vein or 2–3 cm toward the tail of the pancreas. Although the plan is to resect the pancreas to the splenic side of the superior mesenteric vessels, added exposure can be achieved by transecting the pancreas at the level of the superior mesenteric vein before extending its dissection toward the tail. The pancreas is transected with a scapel while the superior mesenteric vein is protected with a curved clamp or the index finger of the left hand inserted behind the pancreas (Fig. 55.16, *A* and *B*). The main pancreatic duct is identified on the caudal (tail) side of the transection and *protected.* Arterial bleeding from the transected pancreas is brisk. Bleeding from the transected surface of the pancreas (toward the ampulla) is controlled by suture as necessary; often a continuous suture is sufficient to occlude both the bleeders and the pancreatic duct. On the transected side toward the spleen, the arteries are individually suture ligated. *Care is taken to avoid suture occlusion of the duct of Wirsung.* Identification of the duct of Wirsung may occasionally be uncertain if the gland is soft and the duct small. Meanwhile, a full-width biopsy specimen at the line of transection of the pancreas is taken for frozen section, seeking evidence of cancer invasion at this level. If frozen section is positive, further resection is required.

The hepatic artery is dissected from the pancreas, beginning at the celiac axis. The gastroduodenal and, when present, the right gastric artery, (Fig. 55.17) are identified. In the classical Whipple resection (but not in the pylorus-preserving technique), both vessels are transected, and each side is *suture ligated* with vascular sutures. This permits better exposure of the portal vein.

Returning to the line of pancreatic transection, the head of the pancreas is rotated to the patient's right, and the dissection is extended to completely free the superior mesenteric vein from the uncinate lobe. Care is taken inferiorly to prevent avulsing any remaining small venous tributaries passing from the mesocolon to the middle colic and superior mesentery veins. Additional small tributary vessels (Fig. 55.15*A*) inferior to the head of the pancreas are ligated and divided, as their avulsion results in troublesome bleeding. Using "peanut"-type blunt dissection, separation of the uncinate process is the most tedious part of the resection (Fig. 55.18). To complete the dissection of the uncinate process, the two inferior pancreaticoduodenal arteries are identified, *suture ligated* at their points of origin from the superior mesenteric artery, and transected (Fig. 55.19). If the superior mesenteric vein is invaded and its resection is elected, controlling tapes are placed around the vein as it is mobilized. A decision is then made whether to perform a tangential or segmental resection. If the latter is elected, a bulldog clamp may be applied to the superior mesenteric artery prior to occlusion of the vein, but this is not usually necessary. The repair technique (Fig. 55.20) is the same as described below for portal vein reconstruction.

The dissection of the portal vein from the pancreas is now continued. Bleeding from tears in the portal vein can usually be controlled with finger pressure, followed by repair with 5-0 vascular sutures. As the dissection of the vein off the pancreas proceeds, tumor invasion of the vein may be recognized by a small, narrow, longitudinal area on the vein, which may appear firm and white. This is suggestive of invasion. If invasion is present, dissection may be more hazardous, lest the vein be torn. The vein is further freed from the hepatic artery; the posterior surface of the vein is dissected free. If invasion is suspected, encircling tapes are placed around the portal vein, proximal and distal to the point of suspected invasion, and vascular clamps are applied to permit tangential or segmental portal resection (Fig. 55.21*A*). The involved portion of the vein is excised with angled Potts scissors, and a single-layer repair with continuous triangulated 5-0 vascular sutures restores continuity (Fig. 55.21, *B* and *C*).

Having completed the dissection of the uncinate process and the portal vein, the surgeon turns his or her attention to the duodenum. From above the colon, the third and fourth portions of the duodenum are freed along their greater (inferior) curvature with little or no resultant bleeding, as the blood supply enters from the cephalic aspect of the duodenum. Retracting the transverse colon cephalically, a point for transection of the jejunum is selected 10–15 cm distal to the ligament of Treitz. Before dividing the jejunum, it is rotated (antecolic) to the transected pancreas and common bile duct to ensure that an adequate tension-free length of jejunum is achievable. The jejunal mesentery is then incised at the identified point of transection, and the jejunum is divided by use of a GIA stapler or scalpel. The short proximal segment of the jejunum with its mesentery is next dissected proximally, involving the tedious ligation of its mesenteric vessels. After identifying the inferior mesenteric vein lateral to the ligament of Trietz (Fig. 55.22), the ligament is divided, and the dissection is carried behind the transverse mesocolon from both the proximal and distal aspects of the retrocolic duodenum. As the vessels entering the distal duodenum are divided, the distal duodenum and adjacent jejunum may be brought (retrocolic) behind the superior mes-

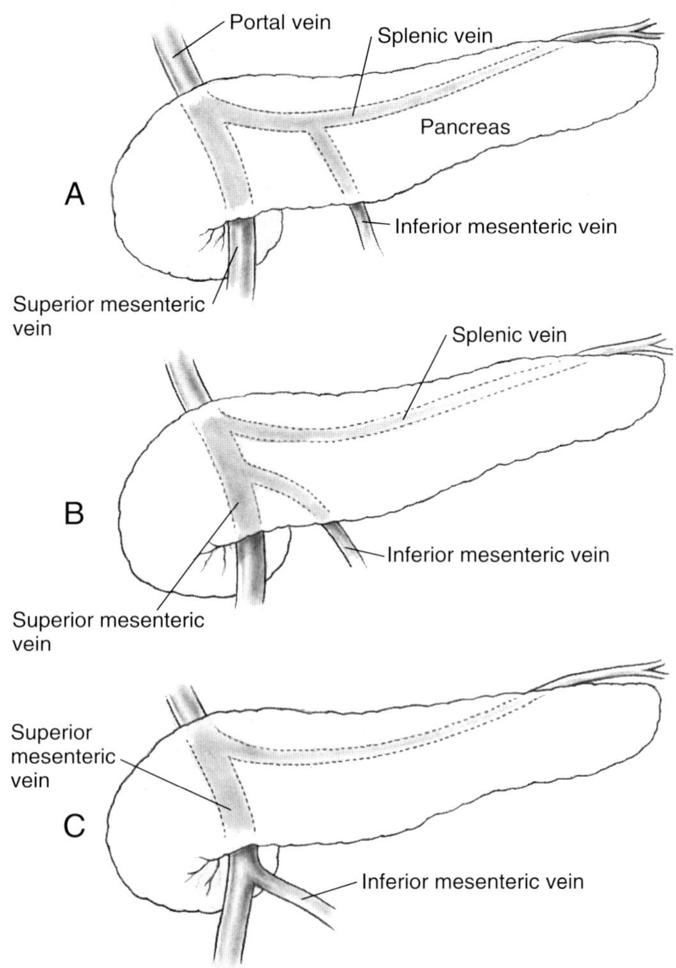


**FIG. 55.14.** The inferior mesenteric vein usually drains into the splenic vein (**A**). When it empties into the *superior mesenteric* behind the *pancreas* (**B**) or within the base of the transverse mesocolon (**C**), it is subject to possible injury.

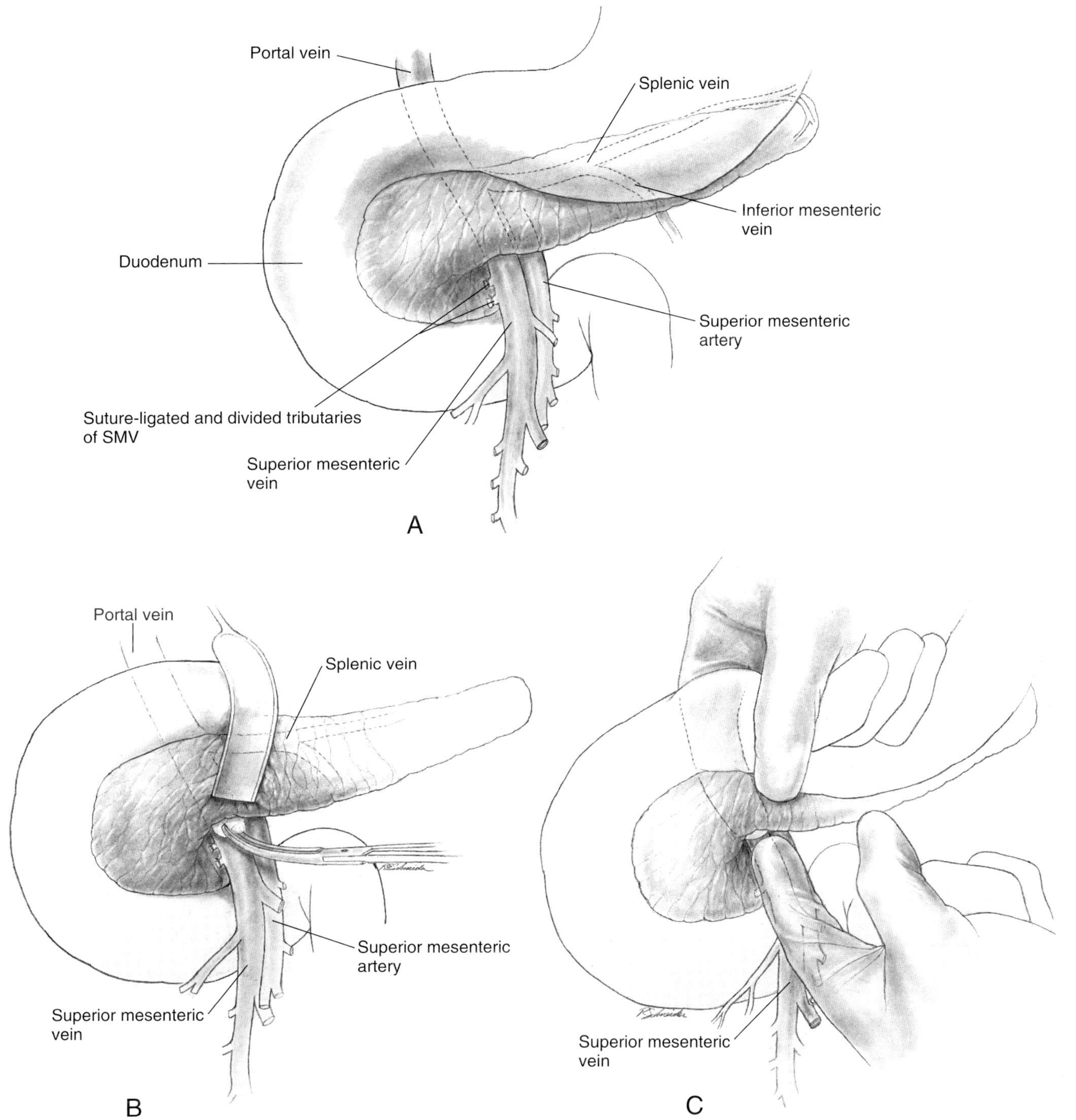


**FIG. 55.15.** **A.** Small tributaries of the *superior mesenteric vein*, inferior to the border of the pancreas are suture ligated and divided. **B.** "Peanut" pushers are used to dissect behind the pancreas along the anterior surface of the *superior mesenteric vein*, beginning along the inferior border of the pancreas. **C.** The index fingers enlarge the retropancreatic tunnel.

enteric vessels (Fig. 55.23 *A* and *B*), facilitating the final dissection. *The superior mesenteric vessels in their passage anterior to the duodenum must be identified and protected.* The head of the pancreas, the gastric antrum, and the entire duodenum are thus removed. The area of dissection is then thoroughly irrigated with warm saline.

In dealing with malignancies, but not benign lesions, attention is next turned toward extending the lymphatic and soft tissue dissection. If not previously done, the residual pancreas is mobilized to permit resection of 2–3 cm of additional pancreas toward the tail. Resection of the pancreas toward the tail may provide safer cancer-free pancreatic margins and also permits resection of additional lymphatics around the terminal portion of the splenic vein, the adjacent celiac axis, and the superior mesentery artery. The celiac ganglia surround the celiac axis and the superior mesenteric artery. Their excision results in disabling diarrhea and is to be avoided in the Whipple operation. The cisterna chyli, occasionally lying anterior to the aorta, is also to be

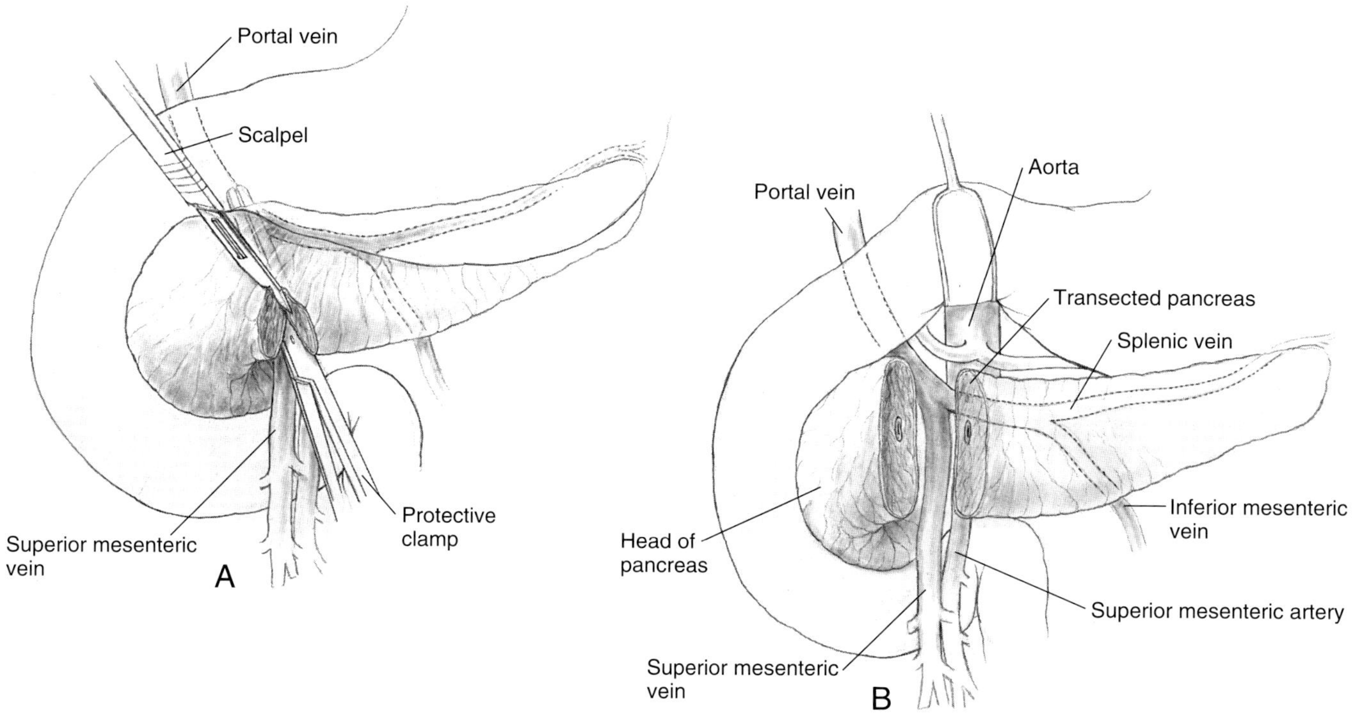


**FIG. 55.16.** **A** and **B.** A *protective clamp* is placed over the anterior surface of the *superior mesenteric vein,* behind the pancreas, and the overlying pancreas is transected with a *scalpel.*

protected, as injury may result in a lymph fistula. Beginning at the celiac axis, the hepatic artery is skeletonized to the base of the liver (Fig. 55.24). Similarly, the terminal splenic vein and superior mesenteric and portal veins are skeletonized in their entirety; care is taken to remove the lymph nodes behind the portal vein. Lymphatics paralleling the common bile duct are excised, but the adventitia of the duct is not removed lest the blood supply to the duct be jeopardized. Lymph nodes around the origin of the superior mesenteric artery are excised, but the author does not skeletonize it in the manner of many Japanese surgeons (see Chapter 56), as this results in resection of the celiac ganglia and subsequent severe diarrhea. If not previously done, cholecystectomy is performed. The lymphatics are then removed from the adventitia of the exposed portion of the inferior vena cava, *including lymph nodes lying between* the vena cava and the aorta and above and below the right renal vein together with overlying adipose tissue (Fig. 55.25). To reiterate, one of the problems in dissection around the celiac axis is minimizing

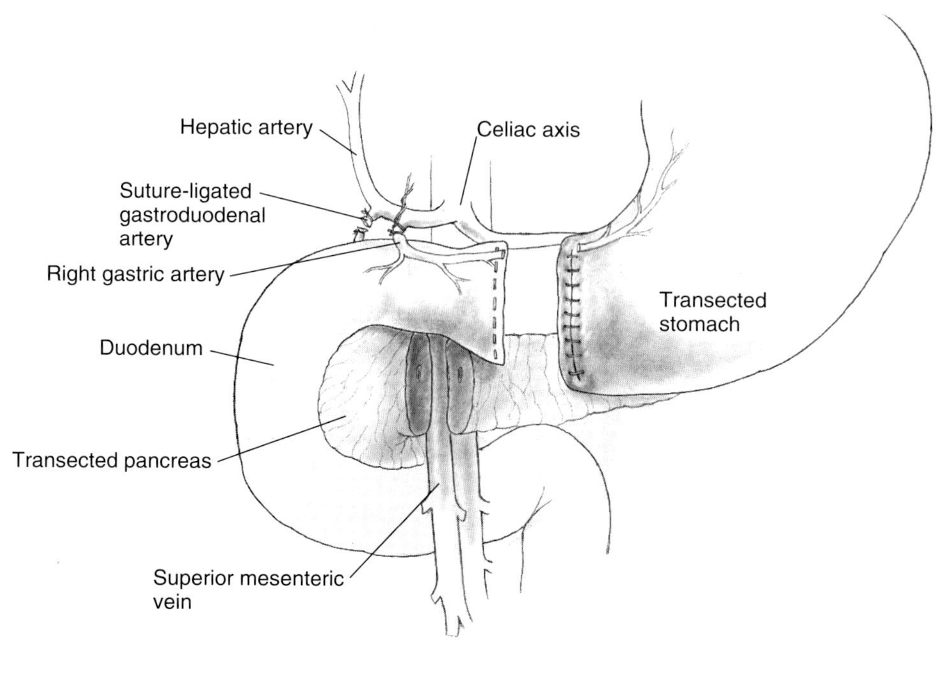


**FIG. 55.17.** Dissection of the *hepatic artery* and the *gastroduodenal and right gastric arteries.* The latter two are suture ligated and divided in the classical Whipple operation, but the *right gastric* is preserved in the pyloric preservation procedure.

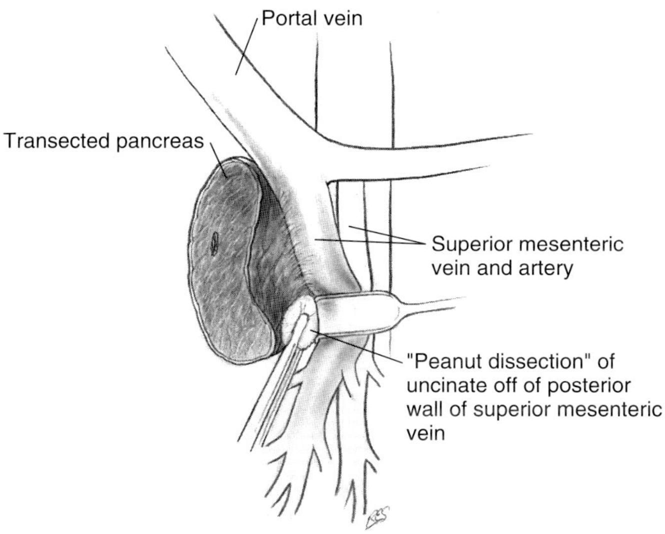


**FIG. 55.18.** Dissection of the uncinate process off the posterior wall of the *superior mesenteric vein.*

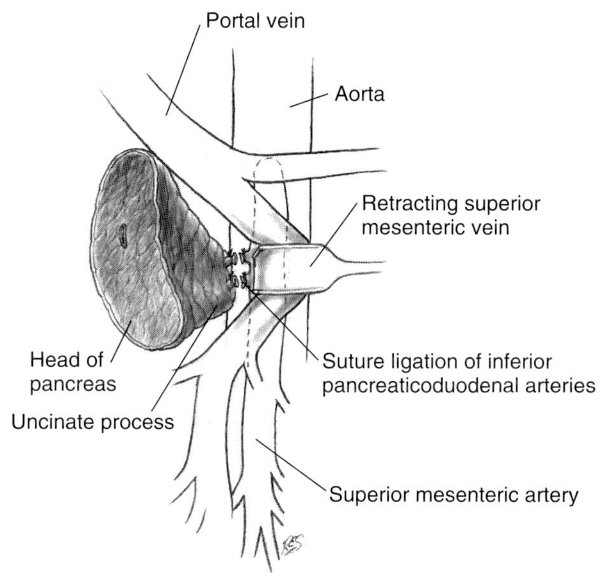


**FIG. 55.19.** *Suture ligation* and division of the *inferior pancreaticoduodenal arteries* at their origin from the *superior mesenteric artery.*

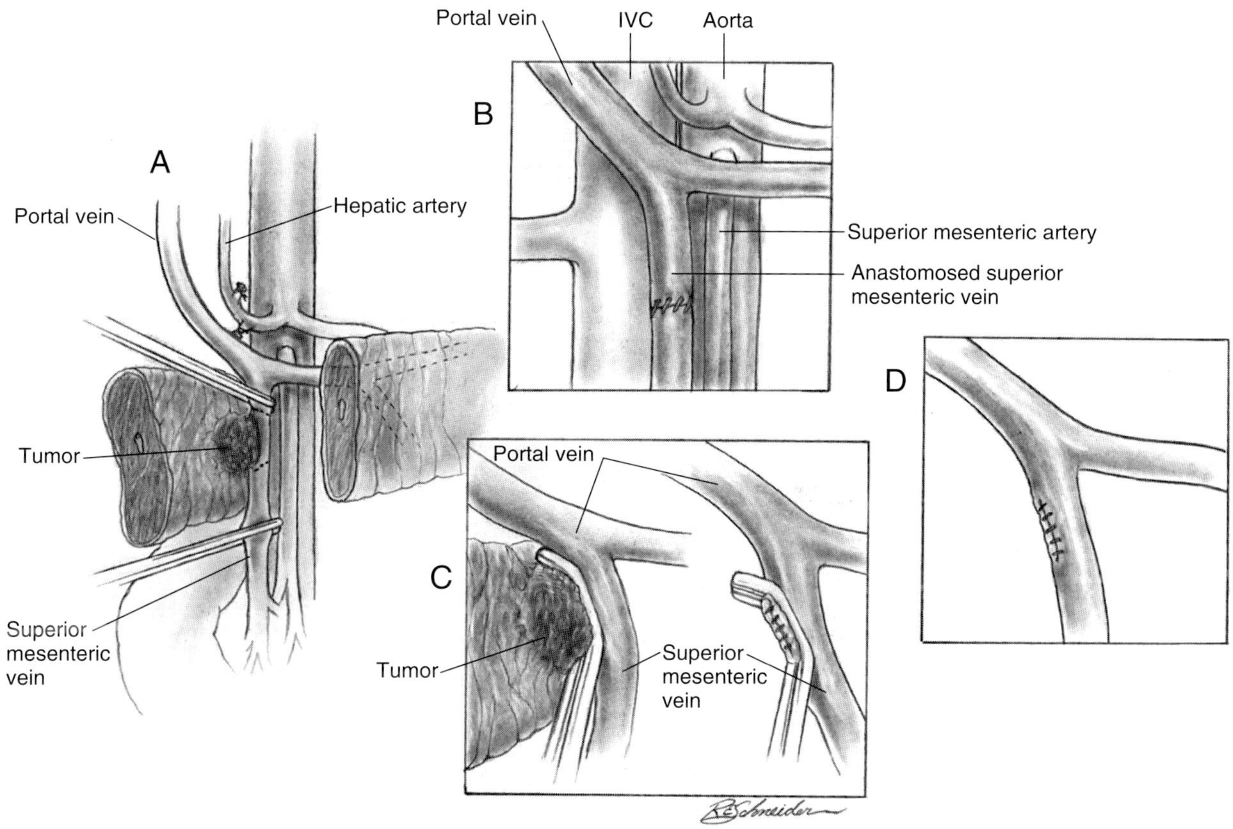


**FIG. 55.20.** Resection of the *superior mesenteric vein* for tumor invasion. A segment of the vein may be resected (**A** and **B**) and reanastomosed end to end, or a tangential resection with lateral repair may be performed (**C** and **D**). Vein graft interposition can be used.

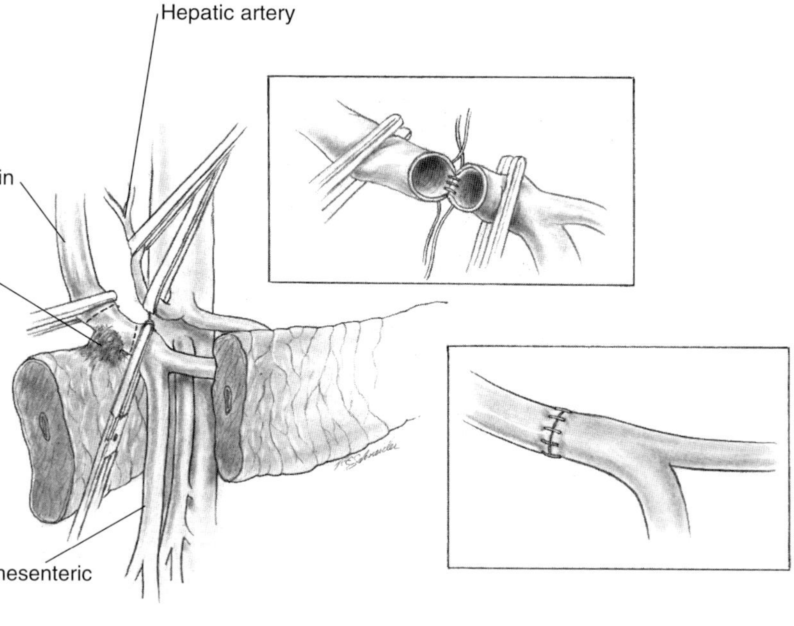


**FIG. 55.21.** Resection of the *portal vein* for tumor invasion. Resultant anastomotic tension is seldom a problem, as the *portal vein* is relatively mobile. A triangulation technique (not shown) of venous repair is often easier. If indicated, a tangential excision may be performed (Fig. 55.20, **C** and **D**).

damage to the celiac ganglia and any anomalous cisterna chyli, as their distinction from lymph vessels and nodes is often difficult.

*Throughout the operation* all resected tissues, including lymph nodes, should be individually located by a predetermined protocol. The bed of the resected pancreas is then outlined with hemoclip markers if postoperative radiotherapy to this area is anticipated. Finally, the area of dissection is thoroughly irrigated for identification and control of any bleeding points.

The literature denotes a significant risk of postoperative intraabdominal hemorrhage following the Whipple resection. This is usually arterial in origin. Although it prolongs operation, the author relies primarily on prevention or control of bleeding by suture ligature rather than by use of hemoclips, electrocautery, or simple ligation for most individual vessels.

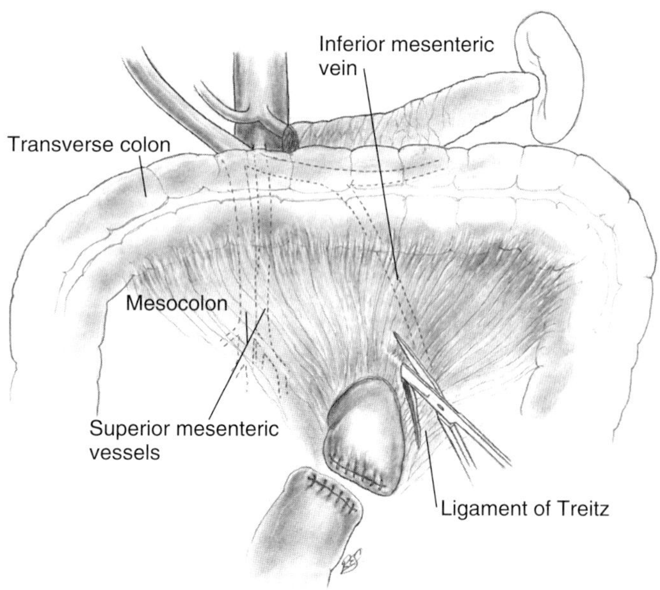


**FIG. 55.22.** Division of the *ligament of Treitz* to expose the retrocolic duodenum. Note the proximity of the *inferior mesenteric vein* in the *mesocolon.*

Management of the omentum is seldom discussed. Its defensive value after such a major operation has led to efforts to protect the vascular supply of at least its left half. Venous stasis and thrombosis may sometimes be noted within the omentum at the end of operation and may occasionally lead to omental gangrene following division of the gastrocolic omentum. Omental recurrence of cancer, as an isolated finding following pancreatic resection, is unusual. As a result, any part of the omentum that appears to have adequate venous drainage at the end of operation is preserved. Tsuchiya et al. (19) have preserved the omentum by lifting it off (separating it from) the transverse colon, thus avoiding division of the gastrocolic omentum.

Vagotomy has not been used. Meanwhile, the pathologist is requested to obtain studies of ploidy, P-51 and K-*ras* mutations, and *neu* oncogene expression and to freeze cancer tissue for additional studies that may be needed later.

## Reconstruction

Whereas the long-term welfare of the patient may depend on the principles of resection, immediate postoperative survival depends to a large extent on the techniques of reconstruction. The jejunum distal to its line of transection is tentatively passed anterior to the colon to again verify that it will permit tension-free anastomoses. If tension cannot otherwise be avoided, the jejunal segment can be taken through either the right or left side of the transverse mesocolon, but subsequent recurrence of cancer may cause jejunal obstruction at the point at which the "Roux-en-Y" passes behind the colon. As a result, the author has changed his technique, preferring now the antecolic approach in operations for carcinoma of the pancreas (Fig. 55.26*A*) and most other malignancies and the retrocolic approach (Fig. 55.26*B*) for benign diseases, as the latter approach may permit better gastric emptying.

The staples at the distal line of transection of the jejunum are inverted with a continuous suture of 4-0 polyglycolic acid–type suture (Vicryl or Dexon), and the hole in the transverse mesocolon at the ligament of Treitz is closed with chromic catgut.

### Choledochojejunostomy

Choledochojejunostomy is selected as the first step in reconstruction. If done prior to pancreaticojejunostomy; the trans-anastomotic catheter to be used with the pancreatojejunostomy is less likely to be inadvertently displaced later in the operation. Although the choledochojejunostomy is the first anastomosis performed, it is downstream from the pancreatojejunostomy. The pancreatic duct will subsequently be anastomosed to the side of the jejunum at a convenient spot, approximately 4–5 cm distal to the closure of the transected jejunum (Fig. 55.26). The common duct is now anastomosed to the jejunum, 5–7 cm distal to the anticipated point of pancreatojejunostomy. One may be surprised that the distance between the pancreatic and choledochal anastomoses is only a few centimeters; a greater length can seldom be used without accordion-like enfolding of the intervening segment of jejunum. As in all gastrointestinal anastomoses, the mucosa-to-mucosa principle is applied.

After identifying the anticipated point of choledochojejunostomy, a short longitudinal slit is made in the antimesenteric border of the jejunum. Care must be taken or this incision will be too long. A single-layered anastomosis, end of the bile duct to the side of jejunum, is performed. Interrupted sutures of 4-0 polyglycolic acid are used; catgut is not used. The first sutures are placed at the medial and lateral angles, respectively, of the anastomosis, and the posterior wall is anastomized first (Fig. 55.27*A*). The slender curved suture needle penetrates first the

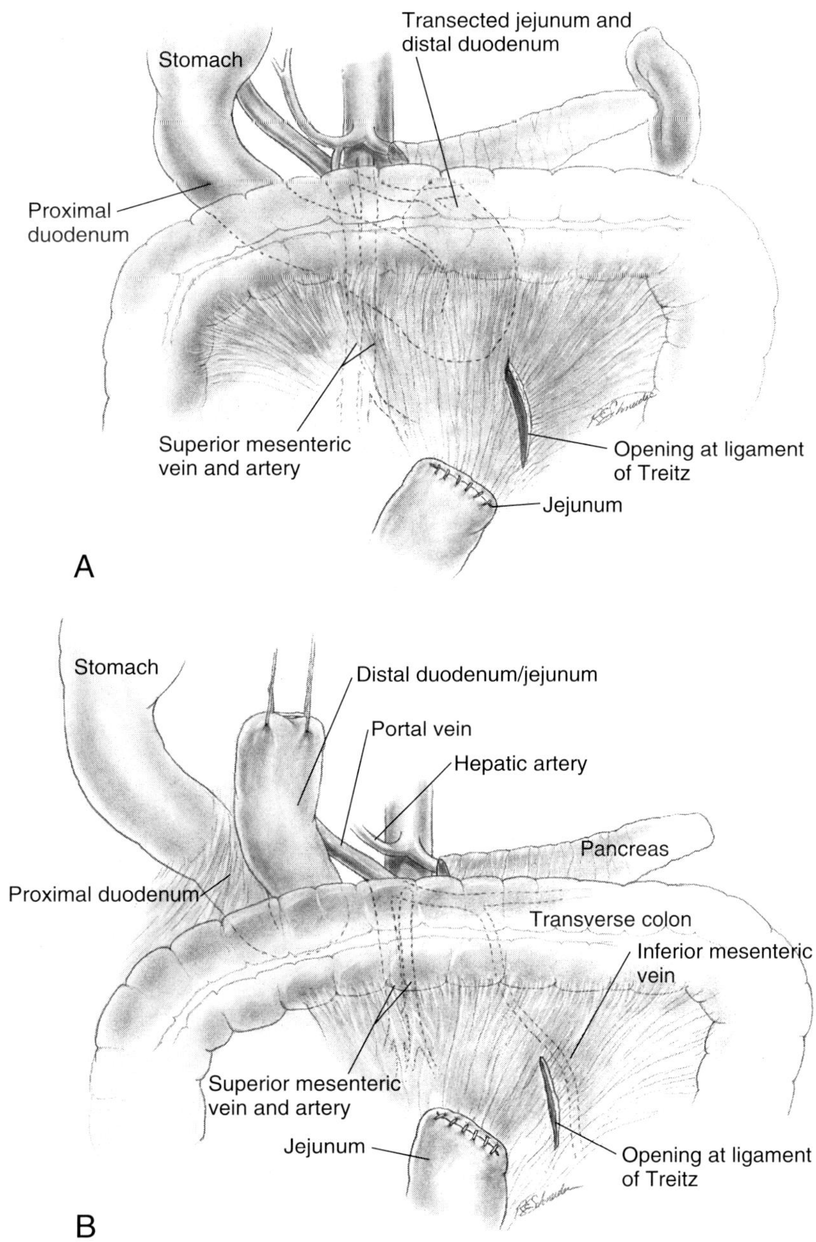


**FIG. 55.23. A** and **B.** The *distal duodenum* and the proximal jejunal segment are brought retrocolically behind the *superior mesenteric vessels* toward the right side, thus completing the resection of the antrum, duodenum, and head of the pancreas.

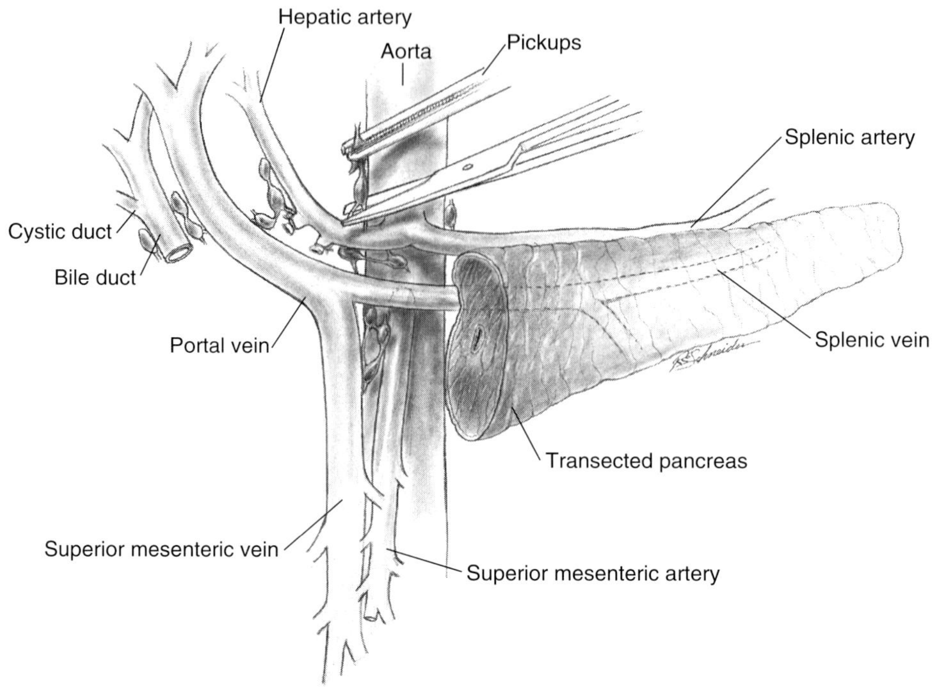


**FIG. 55.24.** Lymph nodes together with adventitia and intervening adipose tissue are resected along the vessels of the hepatic hilum from the terminal *splenic vein* and origin of the *superior mesenteric artery* and celiac axis to the liver.

jejunum from its serosal surface and then the common duct from its mucosal side. The author prefers to begin placing the sutures on the medial side of the anastomosis. Care is required to avoid crossing the sutures and to maintain them in sequential order—feats that are not easy. All of the posterior sutures are placed before any are tied. As they are lifted ventrally and an assistant manually approximates the open jejunum to the bile duct, either the surgeon or an experienced assistant ties the sutures. Care must be taken to prevent the sutures from cutting through the bile duct. If this occurs, all of the sutures may have to be removed and the duct reamputated; with the anastomosis redone.

When all posterior anastomotic sutures are secured, a Cattell-type long-arm T tube is inserted. With a *large dilated* common duct, it may not be essential, *although the author utilizes it routinely*. With a small common duct, it is needed to ensure anastomotic patency. To insert the T tube *in a small duct*, a right-angle clamp is inserted through the transected end of the duct and spread slightly to permit a short longitudinal incision in the anterior wall of the duct; the tips of the clamp provide a protective guide (Fig. 55.27*B*). Next, the tip of the right-angle clamp is pushed through the incision from within the duct to grasp a #1 silk ligature, which is drawn down through the open end of the common duct (Fig. 55.27, *C* and *D*). The tip of the cutaneous arm of the tube is tangentially amputated for a few millimeters to allow it to be passed more easily through the small incision in the anterior wall of the duct. The silk ligature is threaded on a needle to penetrate

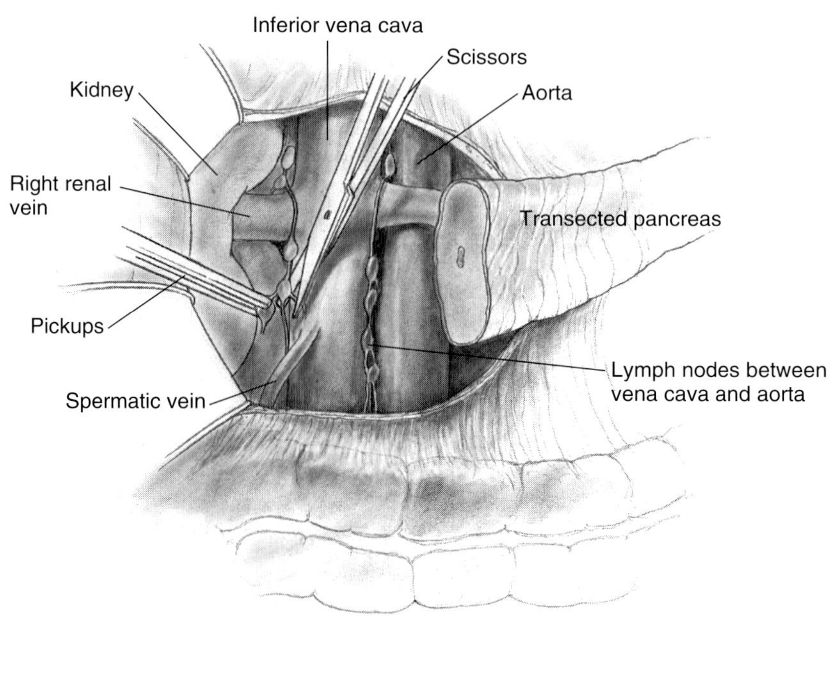


**FIG. 55.25.** The *lymph nodes* above and below the *right renal vein* and between the *vena cava* and *aorta,* along with overlying adipose tissue and adventitia of the *vena cava,* are resected. Dissection is not extended to the left side of the *aorta.*

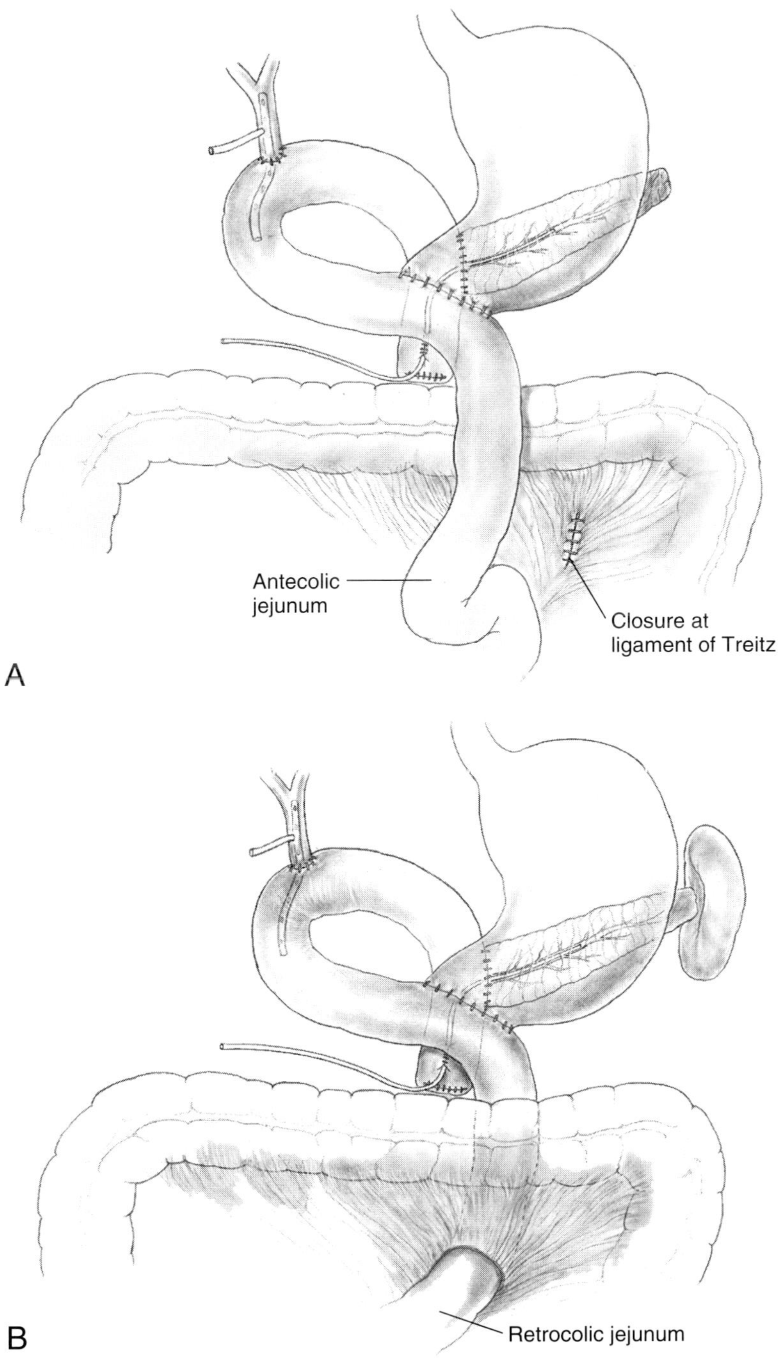


**FIG. 55.26.** **A.** Overview of planned reconstruction with antecolic position of jejunum. Note closure of mesocolon at ligament of Treitz. **B.** Inset shows retrocolic passage of jejunum. The antecolic technique is preferred in patients with cancer, as recurrent cancer is less likely to obstruct the jejunum. The retrocolic approach is preferred with benign diseases, as it probably provides better gastric emptying.

both walls of the end of the cutaneous arm of the T tube and then tied to itself (Fig. 55.27*D*). The opening in the duct will often, of necessity, be rather close to the transected end of the bile duct. This is of concern lest the remaining bridge of the duct between the longitudinal and transverse incisions have an impaired blood supply. This bridge must not be torn. In pulling the silk ligature and guiding the cutaneous arm of the T tube up the common duct and through its anterior wall, minimal tension must be applied on this remaining bridge of tissue. The T tube is thus pushed more than pulled; the silk ligature is a guide, not a tow line (Fig. 55.27*E*). The hepatic arm of the T tube is pushed up the common duct past the anterior choledochotomy, to lie unkinked in the hepatic segment. If the surgeon is unsure about whether the tube is kinked, a small blunt probe may be inserted through the jejunal end of the T tube upward into the hepatic segment. The T tube should be small enough to pass through the choledochojejunostomy without applying lateral pressure on the anastomosis. The distal end of the T tube, preferably 8–10 cm long, with several openings made in its side, is inserted distally into the jejunum. Earlier, preference was given to insertion of this end of the T tube upstream in the direction of the pancreatojejunostomy, to decompress the bowel near the pancreatic anastomosis, but since the pancreatic anastomosis is to be decompressed separately, it is preferable to insert the T tube into the jejunal limb distally.

Using the same interrupted suture technique, the anterior wall of the choledochojejunostomy is completed (Fig. 55.27*F*). This is simpler than the posterior wall. The T tube is then

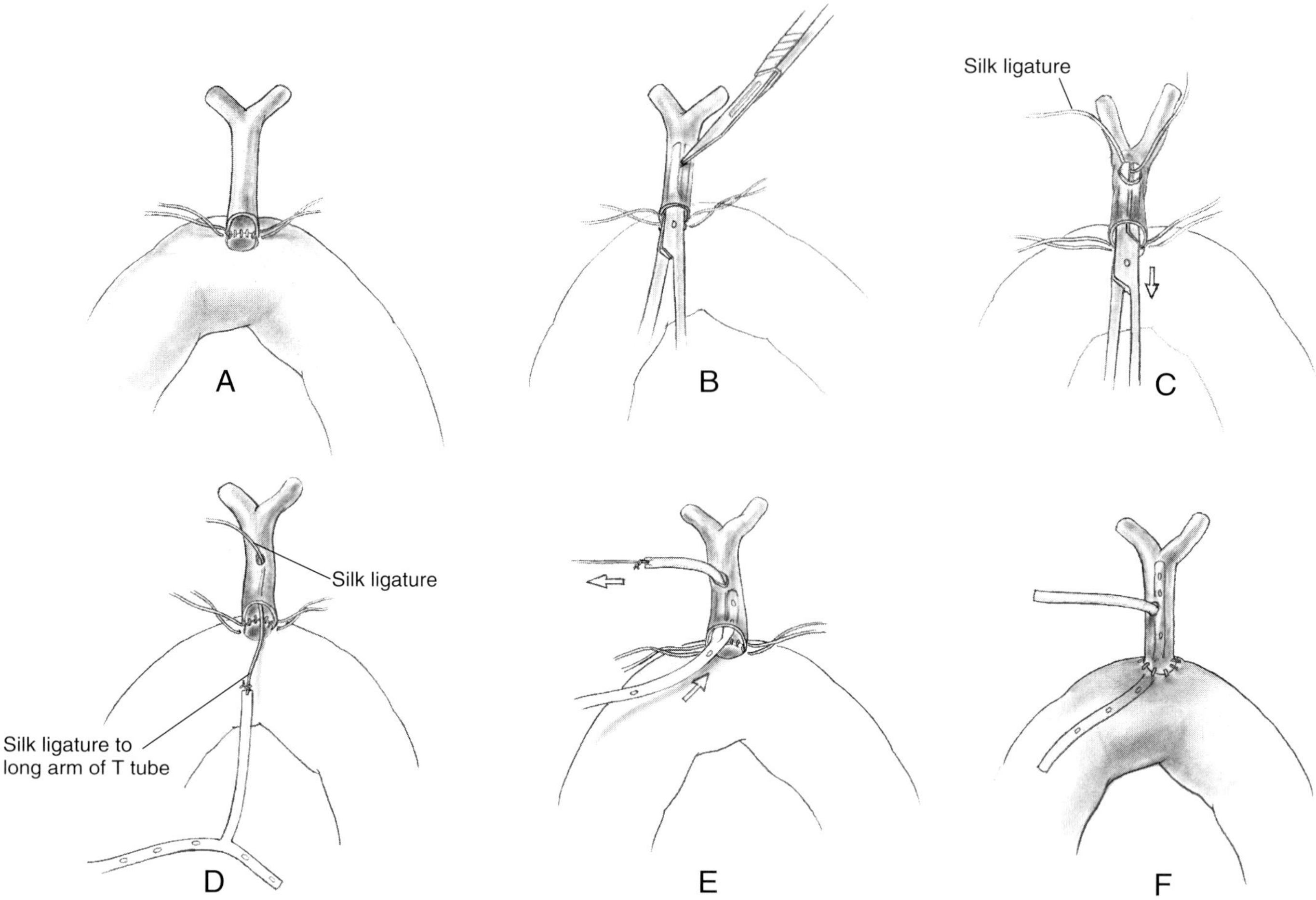


**FIG. 55.27.** Choledochojejunostomy. The steps shown in **C**, **D**, and **E** are useful when the common bile duct is small. **A.** The posterior half of the anastomosis is done first, using interrupted 4-0 polyglycolic acid–type sutures. **B.** Over an intraductal clamp, a short incision is made in the anterior wall of the common bile duct. **C.** A right-angle clamp is inserted through the transected bile duct and through the choledochotomy to grasp a heavy *silk ligature*. **D.** The *silk ligature* is drawn through the bile duct, threaded on a needle, passed through the end of the cutaneous arm of the T tube and tied to itself. **E.** The cutaneous arm of the T tube is guided through the choledochotomy as the hepatic limb of the tube is pushed upward into place. **F.** The completed choledochojejunostomy.

irrigated. Occasionally, one or two fine polyglycolic acid sutures are needed to repair the bile duct around the point of exit of the T tube, but often no sutures are required to make the small opening "water tight."

## Pancreatojejunostomy

With the choledochojejunostomy completed, the upstream pancreaticojejunostomy is next performed. Technically, this may be the most exacting part of the reconstruction, and *the patient's life may depend on the details of this procedure*. In the author's experience, the end-to-side, "mucosa-to-mucosa" anastomosis, intubated, is distinctly superior to the end-to-end anastomosis, which does not adhere to basic surgical principles (20). The main pancreatic duct is again identified. If a small duct is difficult to identify, secretin, 1 unit per kilogram of body weight, can be slowly given intravenously by the anesthesiologist. No definite reaction under anesthesia has been recognized by the author; a single patient experienced a mild, transient tachycardia. Pancreatic juice appears promptly, aiding identification of the duct. If the duct is small, a small, blunt, malleable probe is inserted through its transected end to determine the intrapancreatic angle of the passage of the duct toward the spleen.

Although creating a V-shaped "fish-mouth" line of transection of the pancreas is theoretically advantageous, it is impractical. The cut end of the pancreas is oversewn with interrupted 4-0 Vicryl-type sutures to occlude the transected small ducts and other blood vessels (Fig. 55.28). The main pancreatic duct must not be obstructed by these sutures. As indicated, arteries are oversewn separately, using small polyglycolic acid–type sutures.

The Roux-en-Y jejunal limb is then tentatively approximated to the pancreatic duct to identify the point on the circumference of the bowel that can most readily be approximated to the transected end of the pancreatic duct. With a scalpel, a small opening is made in the antimesenteric segment of the jejunum at this point. Again, *do not make this incision too long.* Before beginning the anastomosis, it is advantageous to select the catheter to be used to intubate this anastomosis. Many types have been evaluated, but among the available choices, a small pediatric feeding tube is preferred. A greater selection of catheters would be desirable, including catheters that had radiopaque markers along their length. (Colleagues have recommended the Teflon catheter used by neurosurgeons for hydrocephalic drainage. Attention is also called to a small silastic catheter described by Tsunoda et al. (21) in Nagasaki, not yet available for use in the United States.) Before introducing the catheter through the

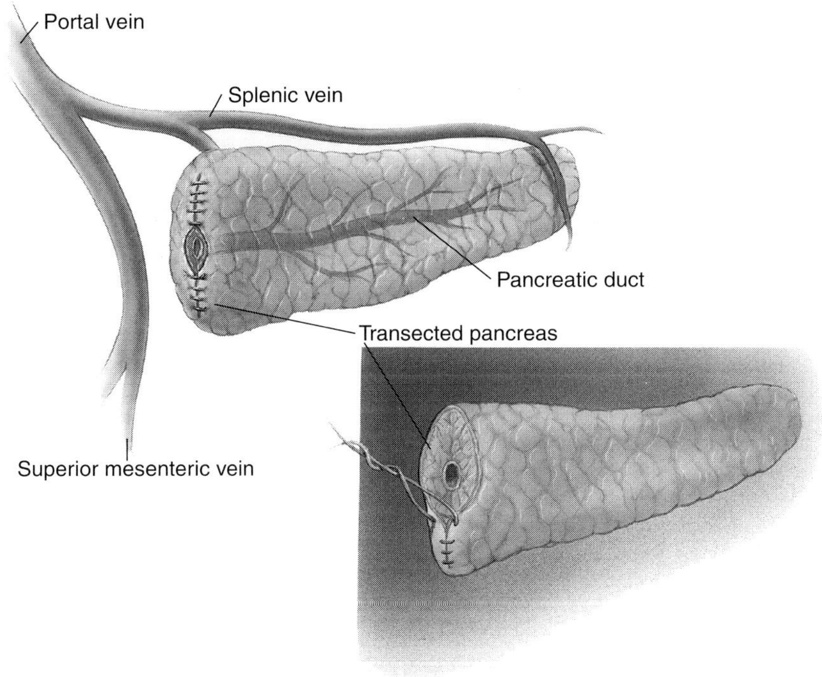


**FIG. 55.28.** End-to-side, mucosa-to-mucosa pancreatojejunostomy. The transected end of the pancreas is oversewn to augment hemostasis and minimize leakage of pancreatic juice from small ductules. The *pancreatic duct* must be protected. (Reproduced, with permission, from Howard JM. Pancreatojejunostomy: leakage is a preventable complication of the Whipple resection. J Am Coll Surg, in press.)

abdominal wall, it is tentatively inserted into the pancreatic duct to ensure that it is not too large and will pass, preferably several centimeters, toward the tail of the gland. The catheter is then inserted through the anterior abdominal wall, inferior to the subcostal incision and away from the superior epigastric artery. A scalpel is used to nick the anterior wall of the jejunal (Roux-Y) segment, to pass the catheter into and down the lumen of the jejunum to the point of anastomosis.

Next, the pancreaticojejunostomy is created; 4-0 polyglycolic acid sutures are selected, as they will withstand digestion by pancreatic secretions for approximately 2 weeks (22). The sutures must be carefully placed, lest they rip through the pancreas, requiring reamputation of the pancreas to maintain an intact anastomotic site. All sutures are placed before any are tied. Again, the suture is inserted by penetrating the jejunum from its serosa to mucosa, bringing the needle out through the jejunal opening, then introducing the point of the needle into the lumen of the pancreatic duct to penetrate the wall of the duct and the parenchyma of the gland, to egress on the surface of the pancreas (Fig. 55.29). Five or more such sutures are usually practical;

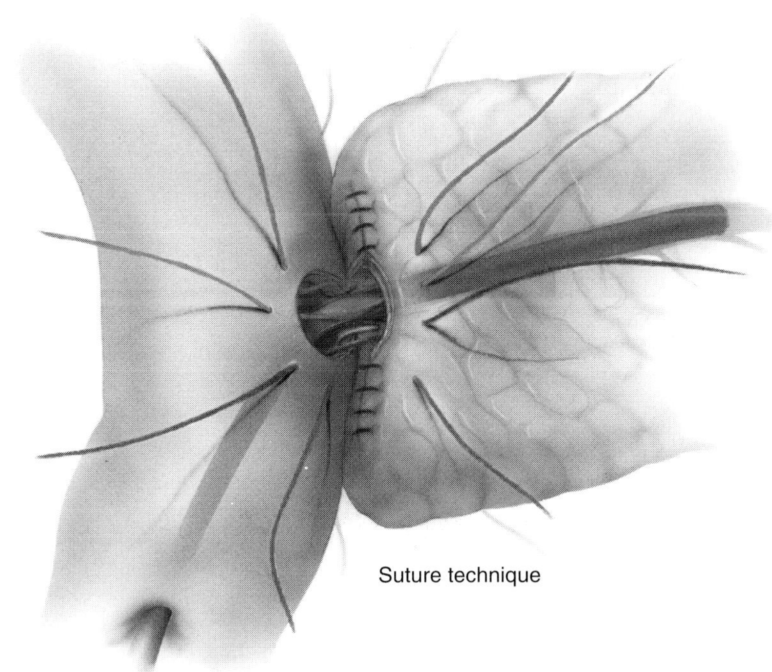


**FIG. 55.29.** See text for details of suture placement. All sutures have been placed, and the posterior sutures have been tied. The transanastomotic catheter is shown in place. (Reproduced, with permission, from Howard JM. Pancreatojejunostomy: leakage is a preventable complication of the Whipple resection. J Am Coll Surg, in press.)

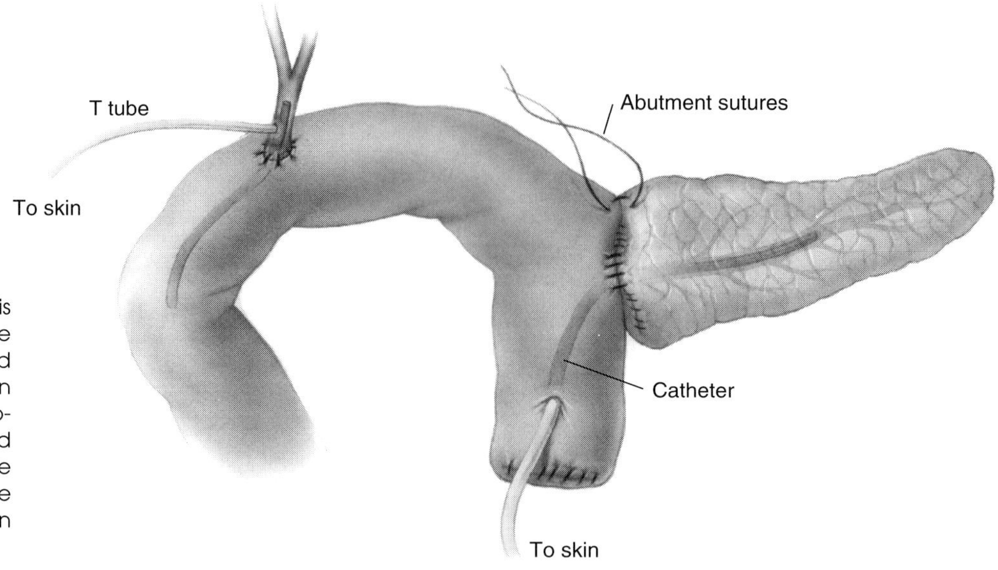


**FIG. 55.30.** With the anastomosis completed, *abutment sutures* are placed between the jejunal wall and the pancreas to minimize tension on the ductal anastomosis. (Reproduced, with permission, from Howard JM. Pancreatojejunostomy: leakage is a preventable complication of the Whipple resection. J Am Coll Surg, in press.)

additional sutures are required with a large pancreatic duct. Again slight tension is placed on all of the untied sutures while the surgeon ties the posterior ones. *The sutures must not cut through the transected pancreas.* When the posterior sutures are tied, the catheter is inserted through the open end of the pancreatic duct to pass toward the tail of the pancreas (Fig. 55.29). The catheter is passed until it meets an obstruction, then withdrawn a short distance to prevent impaction. The tip of the catheter will have been amputated. Several additional side openings would be desirable, but this weakens the catheter and may result in kinking. Irrigation of the catheter indicates its patency. The anterior anastomotic sutures are then tied.

Additional sutures are then placed through the transected pancreas and the adjacent jejunal wall (Fig. 55.30) to abut the transected pancreas to the wall, thereby minimizing any tension on the ductal anastomosis per se. A Witzel tunnel (Fig. 55.31) is created in the jejunum at the point of entrance of the catheter into the Roux-en-Y. After completion of the operation, the catheter is secured to the abdominal wall as shown in Fig. 55.31.

Although the pancreas may be normally soft and its duct may be quite small, there has been no instance in which an effective end-to-side, mucosa-to-mucosa, intubated, pancreatojejunostomy could not be effectively achieved. It is the technique of choice.

The pancreatic anastomotic catheter is used for several reasons. Perhaps its most useful role is preventing occlusion of the pancreatic duct as the surgeon fashions the pancreatojejunostomy. It also decompresses the pancreatic duct in an effort to minimize the chances of fistula formation. Prevention of a late stenosis of the pancreatic duct is a lesser consideration.

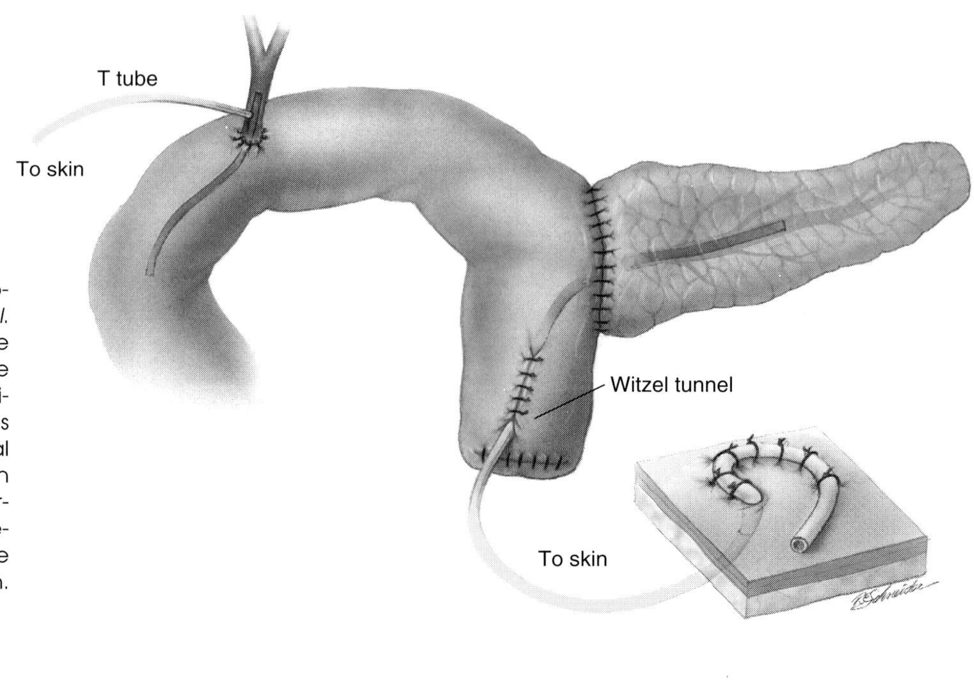


**FIG. 55.31.** The completed anastomosis and creation of a *Witzel tunnel.* Note the technique of fixation of the drainage catheter at the level of the skin, using 3-0 nylon sutures. The semicircular configuration of the sutures minimizes transmission of accidental tension to the intrapancreatic portion of the catheter. (Reproduced, with permission, from Howard JM. Pancreatojejunostomy: leakage is a preventable complication of the Whipple resection. J Am Coll Surg, in press.)

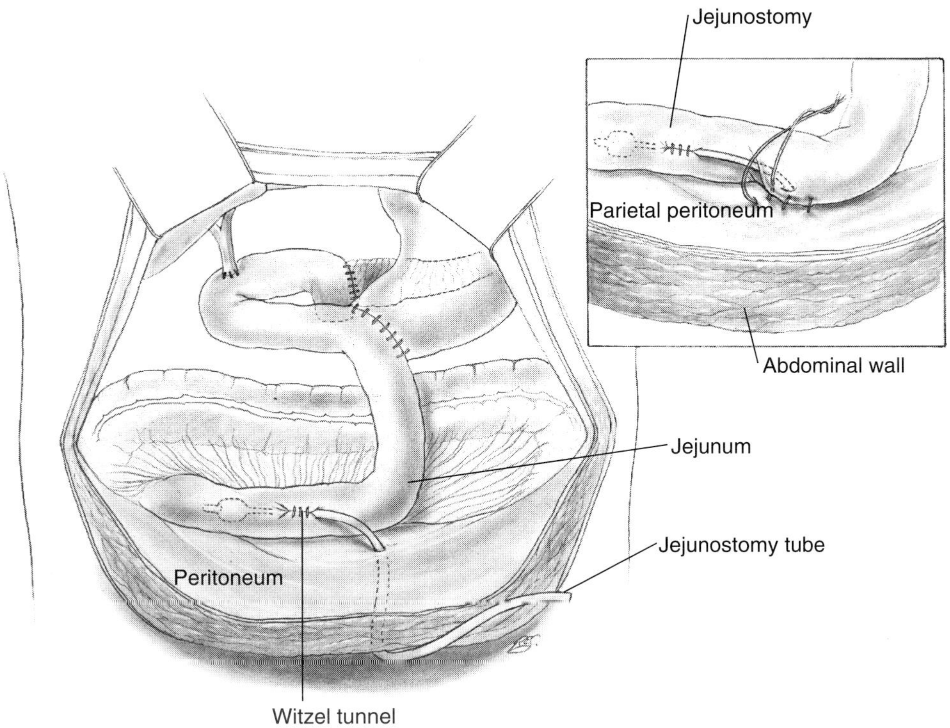


**FIG. 55.32.** The completed reconstruction with the insertion of a feeding *jejunostomy tube*. The catheters intubating the pancreatic, biliary, and gastric anastomoses are not shown. A *jejunostomy tube* has been inserted and secured by a *Witzel tunnel*. Before closing, the *jejunum* is sutured to the anterior *parietal peritoneum* around the jejunostomy catheter (Fig. 55.32 *inset*), and two soft drains are placed near, but not touching, the biliary and pancreatic anastomoses.

### Gastrojejunostomy

Gastrojejunostomy is next performed, using the full width of the stomach for a two-layered anastomosis (Fig. 55.32). One might prefer having the efferent limb of the jejunum at the lesser curvature of the stomach to promote gastric emptying into the efferent limb. The technical problem is that this requires rotation of the "Roux-en-Y," with a tendency to kink at the greater curvature of the stomach. The author therefore usually places the afferent limb on the lesser curvature, although an occasional late problem results from preferential gastric emptying into the afferent loop.

The nasogastric catheter is guided through the gastrojejunostomy into the efferent limb of the jejunum. Since both the pancreatic and the biliary anastomoses are decompressed by their respective catheters, the nasogastric catheter is directed into the efferent limb to promote gastric emptying. Extra holes are cut into the catheter, both proximal and distal to the anastomosis.

Vagotomy has not been used, a decision that requires continued evaluation in patients with benign disease and others whose prospects for longevity are good.

In most patients, especially those who are malnourished or who will receive radiation therapy, a jejunostomy feeding tube is inserted: a small Foley catheter with a 5-mL balloon. The tip of the catheter is amputated to minimize encrustation of feedings with resultant catheter obstruction. The catheter is then inserted through the abdominal wall and into the jejunum at a convenient spot distal to the gastrojejunostomy. Again, a Witzel tunnel is created (Fig. 55.32) with polyglycolic acid sutures. Four or five chromic catgut sutures are used to secure the jejunum to the parietal peritoneum at the point where the jejunostomy tube enters the peritoneal cavity (Fig.32*B*, inset).

The peritoneal cavity is thoroughly lavaged, and any bleeding points identified. Two Jackson Pratt or Penrose drains are inserted through the anterior abdominal wall. One drain is placed posteriorly but not touching the pancreatic and biliary anastomoses. The second is placed behind the stomach, with its tip lying a few centimeters anteriorly, away from the pancreatojejunostomy.

The abdominal wall is then closed with continuous absorbable monofilament sutures on the peritoneum, muscles, and posterior rectus sheath and interrupted 2-0 monofilament nonabsorbable sutures on the anterior rectus sheath. The subcutaneous tissues are irrigated, and the skin and subcutaneous tissues are often left open.

Of importance is the suturing of the T tube and the pancreatic catheter to the anterior abdominal wall. As shown in Fig. 55.31, using 3-0 nylon, each catheter is separately sutured to the anterior abdominal wall, with multiple sutures placed in such a manner that each catheter is secured in the configuration of a circle. This reduces the risk of inadvertent displacement of the catheter in the postoperative period. Both the T tube and the pancreatic catheter are arranged for gravity drainage.

## MODIFICATION OF PYLORUS-PRESERVING PANCREATODUODENECTOMY

Preservation of the pylorus appears to be a reasonable and sometimes preferable modification of the Whipple operation. Introduced by Traverso and Longmire in 1978 (23), the results are difficult to evaluate for patients with pancreatic cancer, as most reports have included multiple disease entities, and some have estimated survival by the Kaplan-Meier method. Delayed gastric emptying has been a problem after both the classical Whipple resection and its pylorus-preserving modification. Patients with pancreatic cancer seldom have problems with mar-

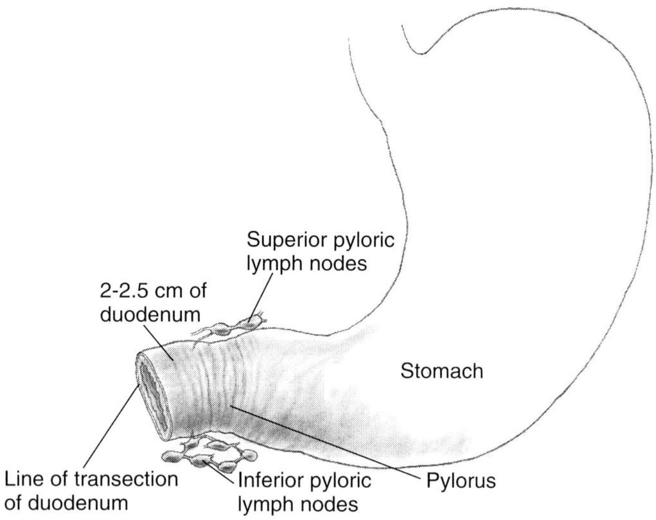


**FIG. 55.33.** Pylorus-preserving resection preserves *2–2.5 cm of proximal duodenum.* Note location of the *superior* and *inferior pyloric nodes,* which remain in situ adjacent to the right gastric artery and to the bifurcation of the gastroduodenal artery, respectively.

ginal ulcer or dumping after either the standard or modified resection. The pylorus-preserving operation appears advantageous in resections for benign disease and perhaps for several of the cancers that are less malignant than exocrine pancreatic cancer. Its ultimate role in the treatment of cancer of the exocrine pancreas is uncertain; it depends on whether or not its potential for a shorter operation and a better nutritional status are consistently achieved (24) versus whether or not cancer in the area of the pyloroduodenal remnant is missed or recurs as a result of the modification (25). If resection for palliation of exocrine cancer of the pancreatic head proves worthwhile, pyloric preservation may be the procedure of choice. The modification has been reported to shorten the duration of operation (26) and is currently the technique of choice in several centers. It is a technique that should be in the armamentarium of all pancreatic surgeons.

The specific goal of the modified operation is to preserve the gastric pylorus along with approximately 2 cm of the proximal duodenum. Safety requires that an adequate vascular supply to the duodenal line of transection be maintained, and functional advantage apparently requires that the vagal innervation of the pylorus and antrum be preserved. These restrictions limit lymph node resections in the area of the pylorus (Fig. 55.33). Thus, in "curative" operations for pancreatic cancer, it seems advisable to limit the procedures to tumors that do not involve the tissues adjacent to the pylorus or proximal duodenal and that are without evidence of metastases to the pyloric lymph nodes (i.e., small cancers in the inferior or caudate segments of the pancreatic head). Using the more radical lymph node dissection being evaluated in Japan, Takada (27) found the 5-year survival in patients with pancreatic cancer treated by the pylorus-preserving operation to equal that of the classical (extended) resection.

### Modifications of Technique of Resection

Following the Kocher maneuver and determination of the relationship of the cancer to the pylorus, resection is performed in a manner similar to that described above for the classical pancreatoduodenectomy. The stomach, however, is not divided. In dissecting the hepatic artery and its branches, the right gastric artery, if present, is identified and preserved (Fig. 55.34). It may arise proximal or distal to the gastroduodenal artery. The gastroduodenal artery is identified, divided, and suture ligated at its origin from the hepatic artery (Fig. 55.34). Braasch et al. (26) and others designate an artery as "right gastric" if it arises from the hepatic proximal to the origin of the gastroduodenal and "supraduodenal" if a variant arises distal to the gastroduodenal (Fig. 55.35, inset). The latter must be preserved. A branch directly from the hepatic artery to the stomach (by any name) does not always exist. As a result, the surgeon must always maintain the option of reverting to the classical Whipple resection should an impaired blood supply to the proximal duodenum result from the pancreatic resection. The superior and inferior

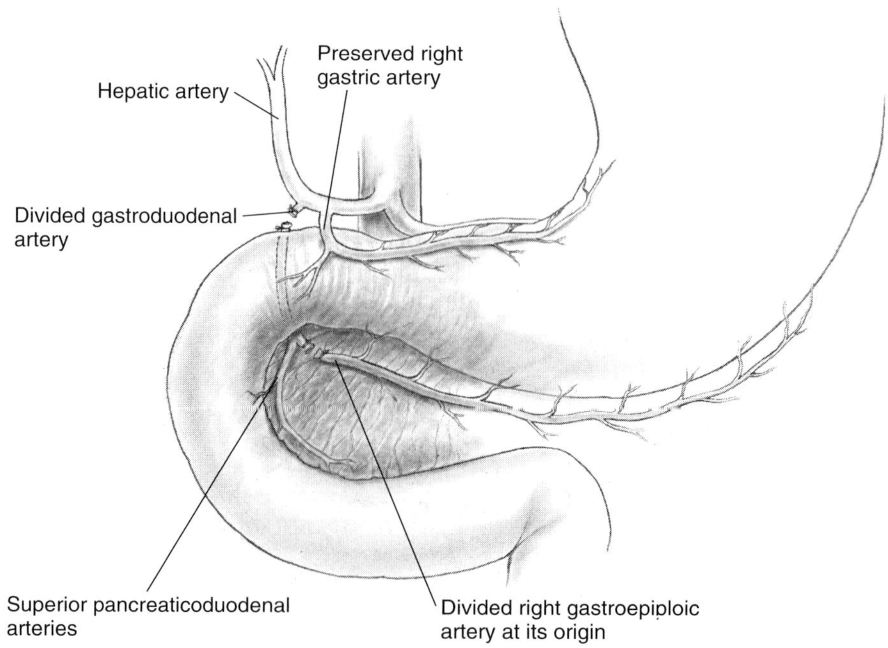


**FIG. 55.34.** The right gastric artery, if present, must be preserved. The gastroduodenal artery is divided at its origin, as is the right gastroepiploic artery.

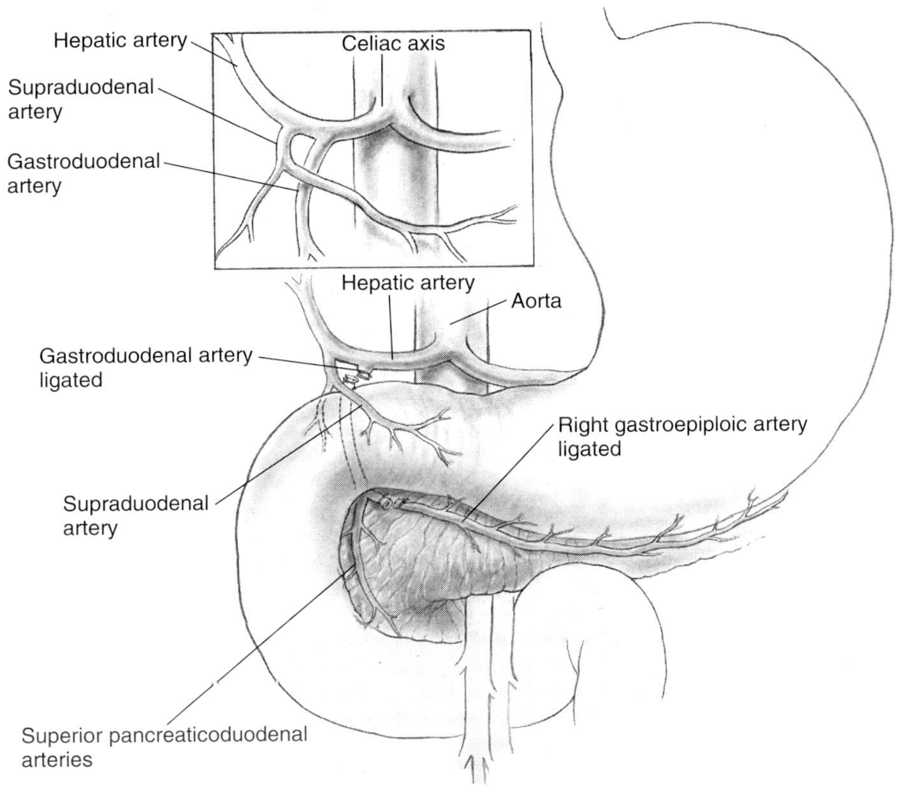


**FIG. 55.35.** The *supraduodenal artery*, distal to the gastroduodenal branch, may be the source of blood flow to the pylorus and proximal duodenum. If present it must be preserved.

pyloric lymph nodes (Fig. 55.33) should be identified and preferably sampled. These include one to three lymph nodes above the duodenum along the right gastric artery and three to five pyloric nodes inferior to the pylorus at the bifurcation of the gastroduodenal artery near the origin of the right gastroepiploic. The right gastroepiploic artery is ligated and divided at its origin with the anterior superior pancreatic artery as they egress from behind the duodenum (Figs. 55.34 and 55.35). Transection of the duodenum, 2–2.5 cm distal to the pylorus, is performed without application of a proximal clamp. Circumferential biopsy of the duodenum at its line of transection is done for frozen section. *An adequate vascular supply to the transected stump must be ensured.* It is probably safer to use fine suture ligatures to control bleeding from the transected duodenum in this critical area than to use electrocautery.

### Reconstruction after Pyloric Preservation

Reconstruction is performed as previously described with pancreatojejunostomy (end to side, mucosa to mucosa, intubated) as the most proximal anastomosis; choledochojejunostomy, (end to side, intubated), as the second; and duodenojejunostomy (end to side) as the third (Fig. 55.36). This maintains the Roux-en-Y principle and permits neutralization of the acid gastric influx by the alkaline pancreatic and hepatic secretions. The duodenojejunostomy is performed as a standard two-layer anastomosis. Considerations as to the antecolic or retrocolic passage of the jejunum are the same as with the classical Whipple resection.

## POSTOPERATIVE CARE FOLLOWING PANCREATODUODENECTOMY

Patients have been initially treated in an intensive care setting. They extravasate plasma and fluid during the operation and the ensuing 48 hours. In the author's experience, patients who have received colloid and red cells as needed during operation are more stable after operation than those who have been given large volumes of crystalloid; 25 g albumin are given every 8–12 hours for the first 24–48 hours after operation. An effort is made to maintain urinary output above 40 mL/hour; a urinary Foley catheter is routinely used.

Earlier, epidural anesthesia was used for postoperative pain control, but it resulted in reduced urinary output, which lessened the reliability of the output as a guide to fluid administration. As a result, the author prefers the more traditional use of narcotics. Electrocardiographic monitoring, EPC cuffs, and pulse oximetry are routinely used. Intravenous hyperalimentation has been used almost routinely. Glucose is poorly tolerated immediately after pancreatic resection; as a result, the glucose concentration in the hyperalimentation fluid has been reduced, and blood levels are initially monitored at bedside at 6- to 8-hour intervals. A hydrogen ion–blocking agent and a broad-spectrum antibiotic are administered intravenously. Early ambulation is achieved; the patient is out of bed on the first postoperative day.

Drainage of pancreatic juice through the pancreatic catheter is anticipated in a volume of approximately 50 mL or more per 24 hours. This volume varies widely, with some patients having no drainage, particularly before enteric feeding is initiated. If occlusion of the tube is suspected, gentle low-pressure irrigation with 2–3 mL of sterile saline has been performed without complication, but the lack of external drainage after the first few days is apparently the result of the juice draining around the anastomotic catheter directly into the jejunum. No problem has resulted.

Feeding through the jejunostomy tube is initiated after the return of peristaltic activity, beginning with tube irrigation with water and followed by small amounts of dilute elemental nutrients. Oral feeding is tested as the nasogastric volume diminishes.

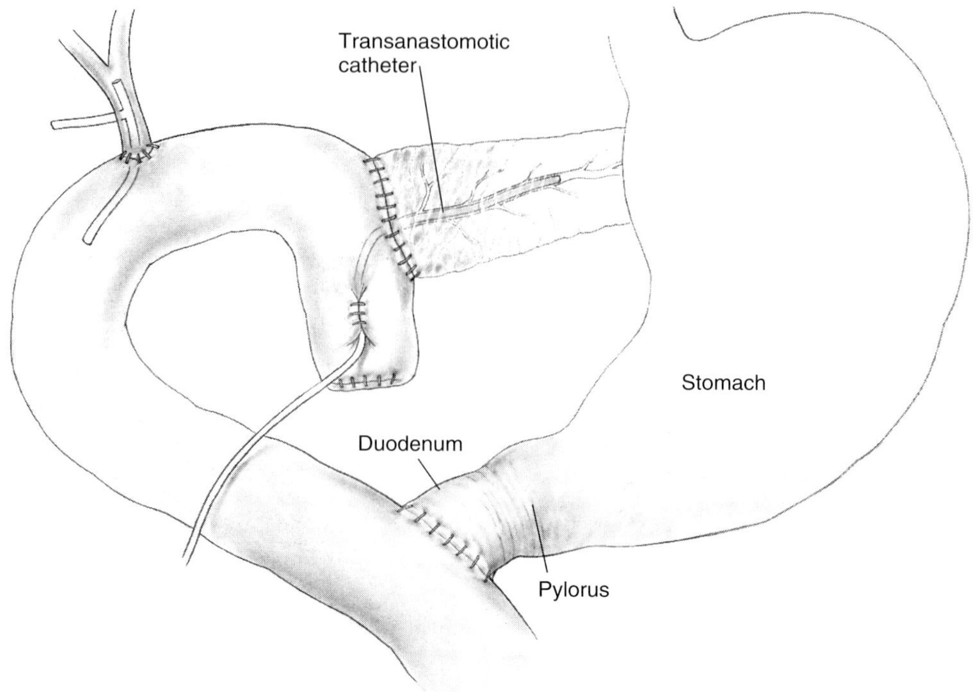


**FIG. 55.36.** Reconstruction after the pylorus-preserving pancreatoduodenectomy. Techniques of anastomosis are identical to those described for the classical Whipple resection. A feeding jejunostomy tube is inserted as shown in Figure 55.32.

**TABLE 55.1. Complications of Pancreatoduodenectomy**

**Postoperative Intraabdominal Complications after 87 Pyloric and Gastric Preserving Pancreatectomies[a]**

| Complication | No. of Patients | No. of Reoperations |
|---|---|---|
| Delayed gastric emptying[b] | 45 | 1 |
| Abdominal abscess | 7 | 6 |
| Pancreatic leak | 7 | 2 |
| Biliary fistula | 6 | 0 |
| Wounds with major sepsis | 2 | 0 |
| Wound with dehiscence | 1 | 1 |
| Intraperitoneal bleeding | 1 | 1 |
| Gastric bleeding | 1 | 1 |
| Hepatic abscess | 1 | 0 |
| Total | 71 | 12 |

**Intraabdominal Complications of 118 Pancreatoduodenectomies[c]**

| Complication | No. of Patients | No. of Reoperations |
|---|---|---|
| Pancreatic leak | 9 | 1 |
| Hemorrhage | | |
| Gastrointestinal | 4 | 1 |
| Intraperitoneal | 2 | 2 |
| Biliary fistula | 3 | — |
| Abscess | 2 | 2 |
| Jejunal torsion | 1 | 1 |
| Total | 21 | 7 |

**Complications after 279 Pancreaticoduodenectomies[d]**

| Complication | No. of Patients | % of Total | Mortality (%) |
|---|---|---|---|
| Delayed gastric emptying | 65 | 23 | 6 |
| Pancreatic anastomotic leakage | 48 | 17 | 8 |
| Abscess | 29 | 10 | 17 |
| Biliary leakage | 24 | 9 | 13 |
| Bleeding | | | |
| Gastrointestinal | 14 | 5 | 14 |
| Intraperitoneal | 8 | 3 | 38 |

[a]Modified from Braasch et al. (26); includes 16 total pancreatectomies.
[b]Gastric suction required for more than 7 days.
[c]Modified from Trede et al. (29); includes 11 total pancreatectomies.
[d]Modified from Miedema et al. (30).

**TABLE 55.2. Pancreatojejunal Leakage (Fistula) Post–Whipple Resection for Multiple Diseases (Selected Reports)**

| Author | Year of Report | Resections | Fistulas | Deaths from Fistula[a] |
|---|---|---|---|---|
| Johnson (32, 39) (collected) | 1993 | 1828 | 248 (13.6%) | 31 (12.5%) |
| Baumel et al. (40) (collected) | 1994 | 366[b] | 32 (9%) | 10 (31%) |
| Braasch et al. (26) | 1986 | 71 | 7 (9.9%) | 2 (29%) |
| Trede & Schwall (41) | 1988 | 233 | 25 (107%) | 5 (20%) |
| Greer & Brennan (42) | 1993 | 114[b] | 2 (2%) | — |
| Cameron et al. (43) | 1993 | 145 | 28 (19%) | 0 |
| Howard (20) | 1997 | 208 | 5 (2.4%) | |
| End to end | 1954–1984 | 152 | 5 (3%) | 1 (20%) |
| End to side | 1984–1996 | 56 | 0 | — |

[a]Percentages in this column refer to the percentage of those with fistula who died.
[b]Cancer of the pancreas.

## COMPLICATIONS

Although frequently mentioned in the literature, *postoperative pancreatitis* is not currently a problem. Earlier in our experience, a major rise in serum amylase was noted to herald the development of a pancreatic fistula rather than pancreatitis. Pancreatitis, per se, if it occurs, suggests the likelihood of iatrogenic occlusion of the pancreatic duct. With the intubated end to side pancreatojejunostomy, this has not been a problem.

*Postoperative bleeding* may be either intraperitoneal or gastrointestinal (Table 55.1). The former may be immediate or delayed and is usually arterial in source; the latter is usually anastomotic (28). Except in the earlier years, when bleeding heralded onset of pancreatojejunal anastomotic leakage, major postoperative bleeding has been a problem in only 2 of the author's last 56 patients. On the fifth postoperative day after resection of a carcinoma of the ampulla of Vater, a patient vomited blood and repeatedly passed blood by rectum. *Careful* upper endoscopy permitted visualization of the choledochojejunostomy. Blood was seen dripping from the T tube into the jejunum. With the suspicion that the site of egress of the T tube through the anterior wall of the common duct might be the point of bleeding, the T tube was withdrawn, and the bleeding stopped. No further therapy was required. A second patient had a pancreatoduodenectomy for a malignant carcinoid tumor of the head of the pancreas. Intraabdominal bleeding occurred within the first few hours. At emergency reoperation, when the subcostal wound was reopened, blood was found in the peritoneal cavity. At first, no bleeding site could be identified, but before reclosing the wound, the wound retractors were relaxed and blood was noted refluxing into the peritoneal cavity from a stab wound in the anterior abdominal wall, the site of a Penrose drain. Further exploration revealed a laceration of a tributary of the superior epigastric artery. The bleeding had been intraperitoneal. When the wound was spread during reexploration, the resultant compression stopped the bleeding, delaying identification of the bleeding site. As a result, drains are now placed away from the superior epigastric artery, and the drain site is inspected from within the peritoneal cavity prior to wound closure. Excluded from the above series is a patient with portal vein occlusion by cancer, in whom pancreatoduodenectomy could not be achieved but who died of acute portasplanchnic venous hypertension with bleeding after vital collateral veins were divided.

*Line sepsis* has been a significant problem, so the central venous catheters are removed as soon as enteric feeding becomes practical. Varying combinations of *atelectasis, pneumonia, and fluid overload* have been encountered but have seldom constituted major postoperative problems. Except for a patient with total pancreatectomy, hemodialysis has not been required, in spite of periods of transient oliguria. *Clostridium difficule* enteritis has occurred several times but has not resulted in major problems. In the absence of a leaking anastomosis, *intraabdominal abscess* is now rare, localized collections of blood or lymph probably being the background factor most frequently involved. With localization of such collections by CT scan, percutaneous drainage is increasingly successful. Operative drainage is now seldom required.

*Leakage of the choledochojejunal anastomosis* (Table 55.1) may occur but seldom constitutes a major problem. Its anatomic diagnosis may require a cholangiogram or fistulogram, as either the pancreatic or biliary fistula may leak amylase-rich fluid and bile. A small amount of bile leakage along drains often stops spontaneously. If it persists beyond 3–5 days, the assumption is often made that the drain is touching the suture line, and the drain is withdrawn a few millimeters. Drainage usually stops. In the author's experience, no recent patient has required reoperation for choledochojejunal fistula.

Often, if supplemental feeding is administered via jejunostomy tube, the catheter becomes obstructed even if frequently irrigated. If it cannot be unplugged by irrigation, a flexible arteriographic catheter can be passed through the tube. The catheter can be maintained, clean but nonsterile, at the bedside for that purpose.

The above problems are not specific for pancreatoduodenectomy. However, three problems have been relatively specific for this operation: Leakage of the pancreatojejunal anastomosis, delayed gastric emptying, and cholestasis.

*Pancreatojejunal anastomotic fistula,* occurring between the 3rd and 12th postoperative days, has often been termed the "Achilles' heel" of this operation—the dreaded complication often resulting in fatality (Table 55.2). Earlier, the fear of this complication led investigators to total pancreatectomy or to occlusion of the duct by suture or by an intraductal injection of an acrylic "glue" (31). In a 1993 review of the literature, Johnson (32) observed an incidence of pancreatic fistula among 1828 patients of 13.6% (Table 55.2). Since this author adopted the end-to-side, "mucosa-to-mucosa" intubated technique, pancreatic fistula has not occurred with the last 56 patients (20) (Figs. 55.28 to 55.31). In my opinion, this technique, modified from that originally described by Cattell (33) and subsequently advocated by Warren (34) and others (35, 36), may largely abolish this complication. Two multicenter studies in Europe (37, 38) demonstrated a reduction in the incidence of pancreaticoenteric fistula when octreotide was given during the early postoperative course. The complication, however, appears to be the result of a technical error and thus to be technically preventable. If such a fistula occurs, it may be heralded by "sentinel bleeding" along the peritoneal drains and/or a rise in amylase concentration in the serum and peritoneal fluid drainage. If there is adequate initial drainage, supportive care including transfusion and intravenous hyperalimentation as needed should be provided, and reopera-

**TABLE 55.3. Reported Incidence of Delayed Gastric Emptying after Whipple Resection (Selected Reports)**

| First Author and Year of Report | Type[a] | No. of Patients | Percentage with Delayed Emptying |
|---|---|---|---|
| Miedema (30) 1992 | C | 279 | 23% |
| Yeo (44) 1993 | C | 118 | 25% |
| Williamson (45) 1993 | C | 12 | 25% |
| Rothmund (46) 1994 | C, PP | 54[b] | 24% |
| Ihse (47) 1996 | C | 36 | 14% |
| | Whipple Resection (Pyloric Preserving) | | |
| Itani (48) 1986 (collected) | PP | 252 | 30% |
| Braasch (26) 1983 | PP | 87[c] | 52% |
| Williamson (45) 1993 | PP | 24 | 8% |
| Ozenc (49) 1993 | PP | 9 | 11% |
| Olah (50) 1993 | PP | 18 | 39% |
| Kingsnorth (51) 1993 | PP | 30 | 3% |
| Zhao (52) 1994 | PP | 65 | 21% |
| Heise (53) 1994 | PP | 18 | 50% |

[a]C, classical; PP, pylor preserving.
[b]18 were pyloric preserving operations.
[c]71 were Whipple, 16 total pancreatectomies.

tion usually avoided. Prevention of anastomotic leakage is extremely important. In a series of 146 patients undergoing Whipple resection for various malignancies, Allema et al. in 1995 (16) reported 7 postoperative deaths; 6 were the result of this anastomotic leakage.

*Delayed gastric emptying* is a frequent and significant postoperative problem (Table 55.3), which appears to be the result of gastric atony. Metoclopramide (Reglan) has been used almost routinely by the author, without apparent benefit. Although apparently not yet studied in the pancreatic cancer patient, the basic defect has been postulated to be a deficit in motilin, a motor hormone. Erythromycin was noted to have motilin-like characteristics, and its use was recommended (44). Its postoperative use to promote gastric emptying in patients with other problems met with limited success, and its usefulness deserves continued evaluation. A dose of 200 mg of erythromycin lactobionate in 50 mL of saline, intravenously, every 6 hours beginning on the third postoperative day, is suggested (44). Motilin has not been available clinically for intravenous evaluation. Earlier, especially after palliative gastrojejunostomy for unresectable pancreatic cancer, gastroscopy was performed, and at no time did the author find mechanical obstruction of the gastrojejunostomy. Reexploration after palliative anastomoses revealed no evidence of anastomotic obstruction. Gastrografin has been noted to pass from the stomach when barium or food does not. With conservative support, including jejunostomy feeding or parenteral nutrition, gastric emptying resumes; *reoperation for this problem should usually be avoided.*

*Cholestasis* is an infrequent complication that is incompletely understood and, perhaps, underreported, as it may be confused early with incomplete relief of biliary obstruction and merges later into the confusing category of "multiple organ failure." It consists of a secondary or continuing rise in serum bilirubin in the absence of any obstruction in the major biliary ducts. A T tube, permitting cholangiography, is helpful in excluding anastomotic obstruction. Cholestasis was associated with late hospital deaths of two of the author's patients. The cause of cholestasis is unknown; it is sometimes attributed to sepsis or to severe preoperative hepatic damage from prolonged obstruction. Delayed enteric feeding and associated excessive intravenous glucose may be factors. There is apparently no evidence that intravenous administration of lipid contributes.

### Extraabdominal Complications

A few significant extraabdominal complications are almost inevitable. In their series of 84 pylorus-preserving resections, 71 of the Whipple type, Braasch et al. (26) noted myocardial infarction and pulmonary embolus once each, cardiac arrhythmia in 3 patients, and other pulmonary problems in 15.

## POSTOPERATIVE HOSPITAL MORTALITY RATES

A postoperative mortality rate of 2–5% or lower for pancreatoduodenectomy has now been achieved in numerous centers (Table 55.4), even though the operation has been extended in magnitude, offered selectively to patients in their eighth decade of life, and performed for more extensive disease. Over 100 consecutive resections (for multiple disease) have now been achieved in several centers without an intervening postoperative death (29, 43, 63). In most studies, pancreatoduodenectomy for chronic pancreatitis has resulted in a low mortality rate. Thus, Gall (65) reported 289 pancreatic resections of various types for chronic pancreatitis with three deaths, a mortality rate of 1%. As surgeons have learned to prevent or anticipate early hemodynamic complications, death within 30 days of operation is no longer an adequate yardstick. Approximately half of postoperative deaths now occur after 30 days, resulting from pancreatic anastomotic leakage, infection, hepatic failure, and other complications. Although the reduction in mortality is due to multiple factors, perhaps the greatest advance in the treatment of pancreatic cancer in the last half of the 20th century is the emergence of specialized centers of excellence for the study and treatment of this disease.

## FOLLOW-UP CARE

At the time of hospital discharge, the author leaves the T tube in situ. If the patient is to receive postoperative radiotherapy, the T tube is left in place until after the therapy is completed, with the thought that it might prevent fibrotic stenosis of the irradiated choledochojejunostomy. Although the need for prolonged biliary intubation is not proved, benign stricture of the biliary anastomosis has not been a problem. Each patient is taught to irrigate the T tube daily with an ounce or more of sterile saline. The tube is left open to a drainage bag during the night and is often clamped during the day, until the serum bilirubin level returns to normal. The pancreatic catheter is removed after the sixth week, when the patient is seen in follow-up.

Adjuvant therapy seems essential to continued improvement in long-term survival after resection of exocrine pancreatic cancer. Consultation is routinely sought from colleagues in radiotherapy and chemotherapy, even after "curative resection" (see Chapter 60). Depending on how far away the patient lives, follow-up is initially frequent. This is primarily to evaluate the patient's nutrition, to monitor the jejunostomy feeding often continued as a dietary supplement, and to participate in adjuvant therapy, which appears advisable in patients with exocrine pancreatic cancer. Pancreatoduodenectomy places a major responsibility on the surgeon for follow-up. The patient with pancreatic cancer may not continue to prosper and will lean on the surgeon for help, including moral support. For most patients, *an acceptable quality of life seems to require the maintenance of hope.* Although the family is fully informed about the patient's prognosis and the patient is told that the prognosis is not good, unless the patient asks directly for specific statistics, the author attempts to maintain continuing hope, advises the patient to live month by month, year by year, and assures his continuing support.

Clinical follow-up is requested at 3-month intervals, more frequently for patients living nearby. Emphasis is placed on weight maintenance, which is monitored regularly; the patient maintains a daily log during periods of nutritional instability. Nutritional supplements, including elemental diets such as Vitale or Vivonex as well as nonelemental supplements such as Ensure or Carnation Instant Breakfast, are accepted to varying extents by individual patients; they are preferably taken by mouth, by jejunostomy tube if required. Pancreatic enzyme supplements are prescribed liberally.

During the first year, a postoperative serum CA19-9 assay is obtained 2–3 weeks after operation and then at intervals of 3 months (as is the serum bilirubin level) in the 90% of patients who are positive for one of the Lewis blood types. In patients whose CA19-9 level was elevated prior to operation and in whom the CA19-9 fell to within a normal range after operation, the prognosis has been relatively good. Conversely, among patients whose elevated CA19-9 level prior to operation did not drop to within the normal range after resection, the prognosis has not been so good, as the persistent elevation reflects a residual burden of tumor and predicts a shorter survival (8, 9). A secondary rise in the CA19-9 level is usually the earliest indication of recurrent pancreatic cancer. This is recognized before changes in the CT scan can be detected. CT scan of the abdomen is obtained at 3- to 4-month intervals for the first year, but its interpretation is difficult after pancreatoduodenectomy; visualization of the liver for metastases is its most important value (66).

Secondary elevation in the CA19-9 level of patients with a good nutritional status has led the author to evaluate secondary laparotomy. In five patients, local recurrence of the cancer in the bed of the resected pancreas, in the liver, or in the pancreatic remnant led to secondary resections, including completion pancreatectomy. A secondary drop in the CA19-9 level followed. In these few carefully selected patients, operation was well tolerated, but no patient survived 18 months following the secondary resection. Although secondary resection of recurrent exocrine carcinoma of the pancreas has not yet been demonstrated of value, this is in sharp distinction to patients with metastatic or recurrent neuroendocrine carcinomas of the pancreas, some of whom have been clinically free of disease following secondary resection of hepatic metastasis for prolonged periods.

Recurrent epigastric pain or pain perceived in the back at the level of T9-L1, pain that becomes increasingly constant, described by the patient as boring, often worse at night, heralds recurrent cancer. In these patients, celiac ganglia blockade, first with a local anesthetic, then with alcohol, done percutaneously under CT guidance, is often helpful (Chapter 64). Relief of pain,

**TABLE 55.4. Postoperative Mortality Rate: Whipple Resection—Multiple Diseases (Selected Reports)**

| First Author and Year of Report | No. of Resections | Hospital Mortality % Deaths |
|---|---|---|
| Wade (54) (collected) (U.S. Veterans) (1994) | 251 | 7.7[a] |
| Baumel (40) (collected) (French Assoc) 1994 | 555 | 8.0[a] |
| Siedeck (55) 1985 | 112 | 1.8 |
| Braasch (26) 1986 | 71 | 2.8 |
| Grace (56) 1986 | 74 | 4 |
| Gall (14) 1988 | 36 | 2.3 |
| Trede 1990 | | |
| (1985–1989) | 107 | 0 |
| (1972–1989) | 313 | 1.9 |
| Pellegrini (57) 1989 | 51 | 2 |
| Lygidakis (58) 1989 | 78 | 3.8 |
| Fernandez-del Castillo (59) 1990 | 135 | 1.5 |
| Miedema (30) 1992 | 279 | 3.6 |
| Keck (60) 1992 | 76 | 1.3 |
| Cameron (43) 1993 | | |
| 1988–1991 | 145 | 0 |
| 1969–1986 | 108 | 12.5 |
| Hanyu (17) 1993 | Overall 224 | 5.3 |
| Extended resections | 167 | 3 |
| Rothmund (46) 1994 | 30 | 3 |
| Kingsnorth (51) 1994 | 54 | 0 |
| Ihse (61) 1994 (1985–1994) | 70 | 5 |
| Allema (16) 1995 (1983–1992) | 146 | 4.7 |
| Yeo (62) 1995 | 201 | 5 |
| Fernandez-del Castillo (63) 1995 | 142 | 0 |
| Howard (64) 1997 (1954–1996) | 208 | 2.4 |

[a]30-day mortality rate.

**TABLE 55.5. Exocrine Pancreatic Carcinoma: Survival after Pancreatoduodenectomy (Selected Reports)**

| Author | Number of Resections | 5-Year Survival |
|---|---|---|
| Baumel et al. (40) 1984 (collected) (1982–1988) | 555 | 15%[a] |
| Wade et al. (54) 1994 (collected) (1987–1991) | 327 | 12%[a] |
| Kümmerle and Rückert (15) 1984 | 107 | 8.4% |
| Trede (29) 1990 | 77 | 14% |
| | 130 | 24%[a] |
| Hanyu et al. (17) 1993 (1968–1990) | 167[b] | 8-10% |
| Willett et al. (68) 1993 | 72 | 13%[a] |
| Nitecki et al. (67) 1995 | 174 | 6.8%[a] |
| Yeo et al. (62) 1995 (1969–1994) | 74 | 15% |
| | 201 | 21%[a] |
| Allema et al. (16) 1995 (1983–1992) | 67 | 14%[a] |
| Ihse et al. (47) 1996 | 36 | 7.4% |
| Howard (64) 1997 (1954–1995) | 120 | 7.5% |

[a]Kaplan-Meier estimates.
[b]Extended resection of lymph nodes and veins.

when so achieved, seldom lasts beyond a month or two. Although secondary injection may be offered, patients often refuse. Successful nerve blockade permits a better lifestyle than does reliance on narcotics. The patient is more alert, is less constipated, and has a better appetite than one who is dependent on narcotics.

## SURVIVAL AFTER PANCREATODUODENECTOMY FOR EXOCRINE PANCREATIC CANCER

Five-year postresection survival today approximates 5–15% (Table 55.5). It may be higher, but published statistics are difficult to evaluate because most current reports are based on Kaplan-Meier estimates, some including peripancreatic cancers. Other reports are based on retrospective identification, with exclusion of "palliative" resections that may have been considered "curative" at the time of operation, only to be categorized as "palliative" after postoperative review of the extent of cancer. Some authors designate as palliative all operations in which the cancer has been "peeled off" the portal or superior mesenteric veins; others do not. Some resect the portal vein "for cure," others "for palliation," while some consider it a contraindication to resection of the pancreas. Some authors exclude operative deaths in calculating 5-year survival rates; others do not. Several authors have limited *exploration* and resection to patients with smaller cancers or to those without preoperative indications of peripancreatic extension. Thus, Yeo et al. (62) indicate a 15% 5-year survival rate among 74 patients after an actual 5-year follow-up but a 21% 5-year actuarial estimate of survival among 201 patients resected. Trede et al. (29) observed approximately a 14% 5-year survival among 77 patients followed for 5 years but a 24% 5-year actuarial survival among 130 patients resected. The time spans were not the same in the actual and actuarial follow-up periods, so interpretation of significance is uncertain.

Kümmerle and Rückert (15), with a resectability rate of 22%, reported 9 patients who were alive 5–16 years after resection among 107 undergoing a Whipple resection. Hanyu et al. (17) extended the lymph node dissection and the frequency of portal vein resection and increased their resectability rate to 53%, while retaining a 5-year survival of 8–10%. The prognostic implications of operative findings are analyzed in Chapters 50 and 51, but it is obvious from the above reports that positive resectional margins, positive lymph node metastases, aneuploidy, and, perhaps, large size and poor differentiation of tumor have a deleterious effect on survival. It is also evident that many patients who survive for 5 years subsequently die of recurrent cancer. *Ten-year survivors remain rare.*

Thus, although 5-year estimates of survival are being noted as 20% or higher among *selected groups*, the title of a report by Nitecki, Sarr, Colley, and van Heerden (67) remains pertinent: "Long-term survival after resection for ductal adenocarcinoma of the pancreas. Is it really improving?" Sometimes, the higher survival rate seems to reflect exclusion of an increasing number of patients for laparotomy who might be technically resectable (53). Although such exclusion may prove warranted, the resulting higher survival rate may not reflect overall progress.

## PALLIATIVE RESECTION

As indicated above, others have performed resection "for cure" but after reviewing the retroperitoneal and transected margins have designated many of their operations as "noncurative" and therefore palliative. Vanhooser and Organ (69), reviewing the experience at the University of Oklahoma in the period 1980–1986, noted no 5-year survivors among patients undergoing pancreatoduodenectomy for pancreatic cancer and, therefore, considered the procedure palliative. Their patients with stage 1 and 2 cancers that were resected lived longer and were more comfortable than those with stage 3 and 4 cancers who were bypassed for palliation. They recommended using the Whipple procedure more aggressively to afford better and longer palliation in the hands of experienced surgeons. Resection of tumors that they were describing as palliative, others referred to as "curative." Watanapa and Williamson in 1992 (12) raised the possibility of palliative resection in young patients with limited but incurable disease, a suggestion previously proposed by Forest and Longmire (36).

The author concurs with this approach (70).

The high incidence of postresection recurrence of exocrine pancreatic cancer indicates that in most of our patients with that disease, micrometastases exist after "curative resection." Although our current research frontiers are earlier diagnosis and improved adjuvant therapy, resection remains the essential element. We have learned to perform it safely, and the lessons learned from the Whipple resection for pancreatic cancer permit long-term cure and normal lifestyle for many patients with other pancreatic and peripancreatic diseases, both benign and malignant.

## REFERENCES

1. Sauvé L. Des pancreatectomies et specialement de la pancreatectomie cephalique. Rev Chir 1908;37:113–152.
2. Berns WC. Over Maagresectie. Ned Tijdschr Geneeskd 1881;21:310–318.

3. Kausch W. Die resektion des mittleren duodenums—eine typische operation. Varlaüzige mitterlung. Zentralbl Chir 1909;39:1350.
4. Kausch W. Das carcinoma des papilla duodeni und seine radikale entfornung. Beitr Klin Chir 1912;78:439–486.
5. Whipple AO, Parsons WB, Mullins CR. Treatment of carcinoma of the ampulla of Vater. Ann Surg 1935;102:763–779.
6. Whipple AO. A historical sketch of the pancreas. In: Howard JM, Jordan GL Jr, eds. Surgical diseases of the pancreas. Philadelphia: JB Lippincott, 1960.
7. Malesci A, Montorsi M, Mariani A, et al. Clinical utility of the serum CA19-9 test for diagnosing pancreatic carcinoma in symptomatic patients: a prospective study. Pancreas 1992;7:497–502.
8. Glenn J, Steinberg WM, Kurtzman SH, et al. Evaluation of the utility of a radioimmunoassay for serum CA 19-9 levels in patients before and after treatment of carcinoma of the pancreas. J Clin Oncol 1988;6:462–468.
9. Tian F, Appert HE, Myles JL, Howard JM. Prognostic value of serum CA19-9 levels in pancreatic adenocarcinoma. Ann Surg 1992; 215:350–355.
10. Fernandez-del Castillo C, Warshaw AL. Peritoneal metastases in pancreatic carcinoma. Hepatogastroenterology 1993;40: 430–432.
11. Lei S, Kini J, Kim K, Howard JM. Pancreatic cancer. Cytologic study of peritoneal washings. Arch Surg 1994;129:639–642.
12. Watanapa P, Williamson RCN. Surgical palliation for pancreatic cancer: developments during the past two decades. Br J Surg 1992;79:8–20.
13. Ashton SJ, Longmire WP Jr. Pancreaticoduodenal resection. Twenty three years' experience. Arch Surg 1973;106:813–817.
14. Gall FP, Köckerling F. The problems of radical surgery in pancreatic cancer and its implications for a combined-treatment approach. Recent Results Cancer Res 1988;110:79–86.
15. Kümmerle F, Rückert K. Surgical treatment of pancreatic cancer. World J Surg 1984;8:889–894.
16. Allema JH, Reinders, ME, van Gulik TM, et al. Prognostic factors for survival after pancreaticoduodenectomy for patients with carcinoma of the pancreatic head region. Cancer 1995;75:2069–2076.
17. Hanyu F, Suzuki M, Imaizuma T. Whipple operation for pancreatic carcinoma: Japanese experience. In: Beger HG, Büchler M, Malfertheiner P, eds. Standards in pancreatic surgery. Berlin: Springer-Verlag, 1993:646–653.
18. Hubbard TB Jr. Carcinoma of the head of the pancreas: resection of the portal vein and portacaval shunt. Ann Surg 1958;147: 935–944.
19. Tsuchiya R, Eto T, Tsunoda T. Radical resection of pancreatic and periampullary neoplasms: pancreatoduodenectomy. In: Braasch JW, Tompkins RK, eds. Surgical disease of the biliary tract and pancreas. Multidisciplinary management. St. Louis: Mosby, 1994.
20. Howard JM. Pancreatojejunostomy: leakage is a preventable complication of the Whipple resection. J Am Coll Surg, in press.
21. Tsunoda T, Terada M, Eto T, Tsuchiya R, et al. A study on postoperative mortality and morbidity after pancreatoduodenectomy. Acta Med Nagasaki 1990;35:175–180.
22. Tian F, Appert HA, Howard JM. The disintegration of absorbable suture materials on exposure to human digestive juices: an update. Am Surg 1994;60:287–291.
23. Traverso LW, Longmire WP Jr. Preservation of the pylorus in pancreaticoduodenectomy. Surg Gynecol Obstet 1978;146:959–962.
24. Kozuscheck W, Reith HB, Waleczek H, et al. A comparison of long term results of the standard Whipple procedure and the pylorus preserving pancreatoduodenectomy. J Am Coll Surg 1994;178: 443–453.
25. Sharp KW, Ross CB, Halter SA, et al. Pancreatoduodenectomy with pyloric preservation for carcinoma of the pancreas: a cautionary note. Surgery 1989;105:645–653.
26. Braasch JW, Rossi RL, Watkins E Jr, et al. Pyloric and gastric preserving resection. Experience with 87 patients. Ann Surg 1986;204:411–418.
27. Takada T. Pylorus-preserving pancreatoduodenectomy: technique and indications. Hepatogastroenterology 1993;40:422–425.
28. Van Berge Henegouwen MI, Allema JH, Van Gulik TM. Delayed hemorrhage after pancreatic and biliary surgery. Br J Surg 1995;82:1527–1531.
29. Trede M, Schwall G, Saeger HD. Survival after pancreatoduodenectomy: 118 consecutive resections without an operative mortality. Ann Surg 1990;211:447–458.
30. Miedema BW, Sarr MG, Van Heerden JA, et al. Complications following pancreaticoduodenectomy. Current management. Arch Surg 1992;127:945–949.
31. Gall FP, Muhe E, Gebhardt C. Results of partial and total pancreaticoduodenectomy in 117 patients with chronic pancreatitis. World J Surg 1981;5:269.
32. Johnson CD. Pancreaticogastrostomy after resection of the pancreatic head. In: Beger HG, Buchler M, Malfertheiner P, eds. Standards in pancreatic surgery. Berlin: Springer-Verlag, 1993: 663–681.
33. Cattell RB. A technique for pancreatoduodenal resection. Surg Clin North Am 1948;28:761–775.
34. Warren K. Discussion of paper. Greene BS, Loubeau JM, Peoples JD, Elliott DW. Are pancreatoenteric anastomoses improved by mucosa to mucosa sutures? Am J Surg 1991;161:45–49.
35. Walsh DB, Eckhauser FE, Cronenwett J, Turcotte JG, Lindenauer SM. Adenocarcinoma of the ampulla of Vater, diagnosis and treatment. Ann Surg 1982;195:152–157.
36. Forest JF, Longmire WP Jr. Carcinoma of the pancreas and the periampullary region. A study of 279 patients. Ann Surg 1979;89: 129–138.
37. Büchler M, Friess H, Klempa I, et al. Role of octreotide in the prevention of postoperative complications following pancreatic resection. Am J Surg 1992;163:125–131.
38. Bassi C, Falconi M, Lombardi D, et al. Prophylaxis of complications after pancreatic surgery. Results of a multicenter trial in Italy. Italian Study Group. Digestion 1994;55(suppl):41–47.
39. Johnson CD. Personal communication.
40. Baumel H, Huguier M, Manderscheild JC, et al. Results of resection for cancer of the exocrine pancreas: a study from the French Association of Surgery. Br J Surg 1994;31:102–107.
41. Trede M, Schwall G. The complications of pancreatectomy. Ann Surg 1988;207:39–47.
42. Greer RJ, Brennan MF. Prognostic indicators for survival after resection of pancreatic adenocarcinoma. Am J Surg 1993;165: 68–73.
43. Cameron JL, Pitt HA, Yeo CJ, et al. One hundred and forty five consecutive pancreatoduodenectomies without mortality. Ann Surg 1993;217:430–438.
44. Yeo CJ, Barry MK, Sauter PK, et al. Erythromycin accelerates gastric emptying after pancreaticoduodenectomy. Ann Surg 1993;218:229–237.
45. Williamson RCN, Bliouras N, Cooper MJ, Davies ER. Gastric emptying and enterogastric reflux after conservative and conventional pancreaticoduodenectomy. Surgery 1993;114(1):82–86.
46. Rothmund M, Weinel RJ, Wagner PK. 54 consecutive duodenopancreatectomies without fatality. Dtsch Med Wochenschr 1994; 119(13):445–450.
47. Ihse I, Anderson H, Andrén Sandberg Ä. Total pancreatectomy for cancer of the pancreas; is it appropriate? World J Surg 1996;20: 288–294.
48. Itani KMF, Coleman RE, Ajurai OE, Meyers W. Pylorus preserving pancreaticoduodenectomy: a clinical and physiologic appraisal. Ann Surg 1986;204:655–664.
49. Ozenc A, Ozdemir A, Bozoklu S. Pylorus preserving pancreaticoduodenectomy. Acta Chir Belg 1993;93(4):140–144.
50. Olah A, Bojdan-Rajcs S, Pardan G, Matrai T. Delayed gastric emptying as a frequent complication of pylorus preserving pancreatoduodenectomy. Orv Hetil 1993;134(34):1857–1860.
51. Kingsnorth AN, Berg JD, Gray MR. A novel reconstructive technique for pylorus preserving pancreatoduodenectomy: avoidance of early postoperative gastric stasis. Ann R Coll Surg Engl 1993;75(1):38–42.
52. Zhao Y, Cai L, Zhong S, Zhu Y. 65 cases of pylorus preserving pancreatoduodenectomy: experience and problems. Chin Med Sci J 1994;9(3):171–175.
53. Heise JW, Becker H, Borchard F, Roher HD. Risks of radical treatment in pylorus preserving duodenopancreatectomy in ductal carcinoma. Chirurg 1994;65(9):780–784.
54. Wade TP, Radford DM, Virgo KS, et al. Complications and outcomes in the treatment of pancreatic adenocarcinoma in the United States veteran. J Am Coll Surg 1994;179:38–48.

55. Siedek M, Birtel F, Mitrenga I. Pankreasganganastomose und pankreatojejunoplicatio nach rechtsresektion. Langenbecks Arch Chir 1985;366:610.
56. Grace PA, Pitt HA, Longmire WP. Pancreatoduodenectomy with pylorus preservation for adenocarcinoma of the head of the pancreas. Br J Surg 1986;73:647–650.
57. Pellegrini CA, Heck CF, Raper S, Way LW. An analysis of the reduced mortality and morbidity rates after pancreatico-duodenectomy. Arch Surg 1989;124:778–781.
58. Lygidakis NJ, van der Hyde MN, Houthoff HJ, et al. Resectional surgical procedures for carcinoma of the head of the pancreas. Surg Gynecol Obstet 1989;168:157–167.
59. Fernandez del Castillo C, Warshaw AL. Diagnosis and preoperative evaluation of pancreatic cancer, with implications for management. Gastrointest Clin North Am 1990;19:915–933.
60. Keck H, Steffen R, Neuhaus P. Protection of pancreatic and biliary anastomosis after partial duodenopancreatectomy by external drainage. Surg Gynecol Obstet 1992;174:329–331.
61. Ihse I, Axelson J, Al-Sharoz K, Andrén-Sandberg A. Surgery of periampullary cancer. Dig Surg 1994;11:402–407.
62. Yeo CJ, Cameron JL, Lillemoe KD, et al. Pancreaticoduodenectomy for cancer of the head of the pancreas. 201 patients. Ann Surg 1995;221:721–733.
63. Fernandez del Castillo C, Rattner DW, Warshaw AL. Standards for pancreatic resection in the 1990's. Arch Surg 1995;130:295–300.
64. Howard, personal experience.
65. Gall FP. Chronische Pankreatitis Chirurgesche Therapy durch reseklonsverfahren del Castillo. Langenbecks Arch Surg 1987;372:363–368.
66. Coombs RJ, Zeiss J, Howard JM, et al. CT of the abdomen after the Whipple procedure: value in depicting postoperative anatomy, surgical complications and tumor recurrence. AJR 1990;154:1011–1014.
67. Nitecki SS, Sarr MG, Colby TV, van Heerden JA. Long term survival after resection for ductal adenocarcinoma of the pancreas. Is it really improving? Ann Surg 1995;221:59–66.
68. Willett CG, Lewandrowski K, Warshaw AL, et al. Resection margins in carcinoma of the head of the pancreas. Implications for radiation therapy. Ann Surg 1993;217:144–148.
69. Vanhooser R, Organ CH Jr. Is the Whipple procedure a better palliative option for pancreatic cancer? J Natl Med Assoc 1991;83:405–408.
70. Howard JM. Pancreatoduodenectomy (Whipple resection) with resection of hepatic metastases for carcinoma of the exocrine pancreas. (Letter to the Editor). Accepted for publication Archives of Surgery.

# 56

# *Extended Lymphadenectomy in Pancreatic Resection for Cancer*

Itsuo Miyazaki and Takukazu Nagakawa

Pancreatoduodenectomy (PD) was originated by Whipple (1) in 1935 and has been widely used as a radical operative procedure for carcinoma of the pancreatic head region. The mortality rate of this operation has been significantly reduced as a consequence of technical refinements and the introduction of advanced methods for pre- and postoperative management including percutaneous transhepatic cholangeal drainage (PTCD), endoscopic nasobiliary drainage (ENBD), and total parenteral nutrition. In contrast, the long-term results still remain extremely poor compared with those of carcinoma of other digestive organs (2–14). Efforts have been directed at early diagnosis (15), which enables operative intervention while the lesion is still resectable, and at achieving a cure by means of extended lymphadenectomy combined with resection of the portal vein and adjacent organs (16–18) or even total pancreatectomy (11, 12).

Extended surgery has been performed for pancreatic cancer since 1973 to improve surgical results, based on evaluation of resected and autopsy specimens. The translateral retroperitoneal approach (TRA) was developed as an extended procedure in 1976 (17, 18). In this technique, adequate lymphadenectomy requires wide dissection of the retroperitoneal nodes from the adrenal glands to the iliac bifurcation. The extent of the pancreatectomy depends upon the site of the cancer. For cancers localized to the pancreatic head, the organ is transected to the left of the celiac artery. This is performed in combination with resection of the portal vein and the retropancreatic tissues, including the nerve plexuses of the trunks of the celiac axis and the superior mesenteric artery. For cancers not localized to the head, a total pancreatectomy together with resection of the portal vein and the retropancreatic tissues is performed.

This approach has been used in 58 patients with carcinoma of the head of the pancreas. Of these, 10 patients survived for 5 or more years. This chapter describes the technique, with particular emphasis on the dissection of the retroperitoneum and the region around the superior mesenteric artery. The significance of the operation and associated problems are also discussed.

## TECHNIQUE OF RETROPERITONEAL DISSECTION FOLLOWED BY TRANSLATERAL RETROPERITONEAL APPROACH (TRA)

### Skin Incision

The abdomen is opened through a chevron incision in the epigastric region.

### Retroperitoneal Dissection (Fig. 56.1)

Using electrocautery, the retroperitoneum is entered by incising the peritoneum at the lower margin of the liver, carrying the incision inferiorly and about 3 cm laterally along the right side of the duodenum. The incision is extended further along the right margin of the ascending colon to the cecum, and the duodenocolic ligament is divided. The duodenum is mobilized and elevated along with the pancreas, ascending colon, and transverse colon, thus allowing full access to the retroperitoneum.

The right kidney is first exposed at the lateral aspect of the duodenum, and the fatty tissue attached to it is removed. The right renal artery and vein then become visible. The dissection then proceeds to the left, exposing the inferior vena cava. Care should be taken not to damage the suprarenal vein. Once the inferior vena cava is fully exposed, the dissection is directed inferiorly to remove the soft tissue and lymph nodes along the vena cava. During this maneuver, the testicular or ovarian vein is ligated and divided. Care should be taken not to injure the right ureter. Dissection of the retroperitoneum is carried as far as the bifurcation of the common iliac artery. At this point, dissection proceeds superiorly, exposing the abdominal aorta. Small-caliber vessels of the inferior vena cava and from the abdominal aorta are ligated and divided. The lymph nodes around both renal arteries, particularly the right renal artery, are dissected carefully by retracting the vessels with vascular tapes (Fig. 56.2). Particular attention should be paid to the dissection around the root of the inferior mesenteric artery and the left ureter. The exposure of the abdominal aorta is carried as far as the root of the superior mesenteric artery. The field of dissection is shifted to the retroperitoneum in the vicinity of the foramen of Winslow, exposing the inferior vena cava and left renal vein. Next, the fatty tissue and lymphatics around the left side of the abdominal aorta are ligated to prevent excessive postoperative lymphorrhea.

**Treatment of the Transverse Mesocolon, Dissection of the Hepatoduodenal Ligament, Cholecystectomy, and Gastrectomy.** The greater omentum is divided at its attachment to the transverse colon, and the transverse mesocolon is divided using electrocautery 3 cm distal to its attachment to the pancreas. The middle colic artery and vein are ligated and divided. It is advisable in the subsequent procedure to keep several centimeters of the superior mesenteric vein free distally (Fig. 56.3).

Attention now shifts to the hepatoduodenal ligament. The gastroduodenal artery is ligated and divided at its root, the lesser omentum is divided along the lower margin of the liver, and the stomach is resected. Total gastrectomy is performed in conjunction with total pancreatectomy. Subtotal gastrectomy is performed with proximal PD.

**Dissection around the Celiac Artery and Left Upper Quadrant of the Retroperitoneum, and Division of the Pancreas.** Keeping the stomach elevated toward the right, the lymph nodes around the root of the celiac axis are removed en bloc with the ganglia and nerve plexus. The pancreas is divided along the line of the celiac axis, and the portal and splenic veins are dissected as in a standard PD. The dissection is directed toward the left border of the abdominal aorta. The lymph nodes

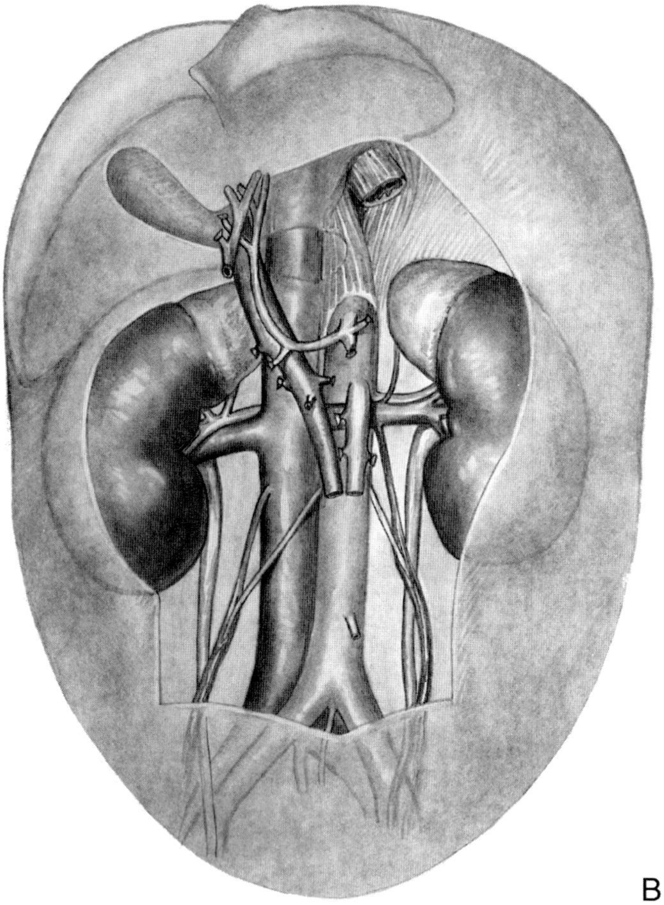

A

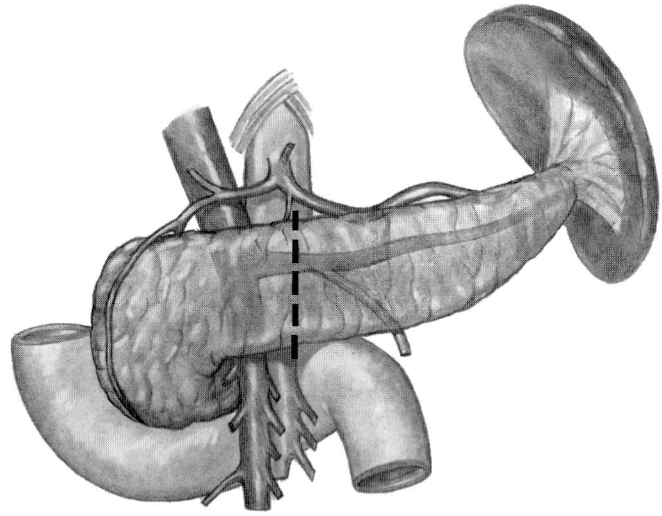

B

**FIG. 56.1.** Resection of pancreatic cancer. **A.** Area of retroperitoneal dissection. **B.** Line of incision of the pancreas.

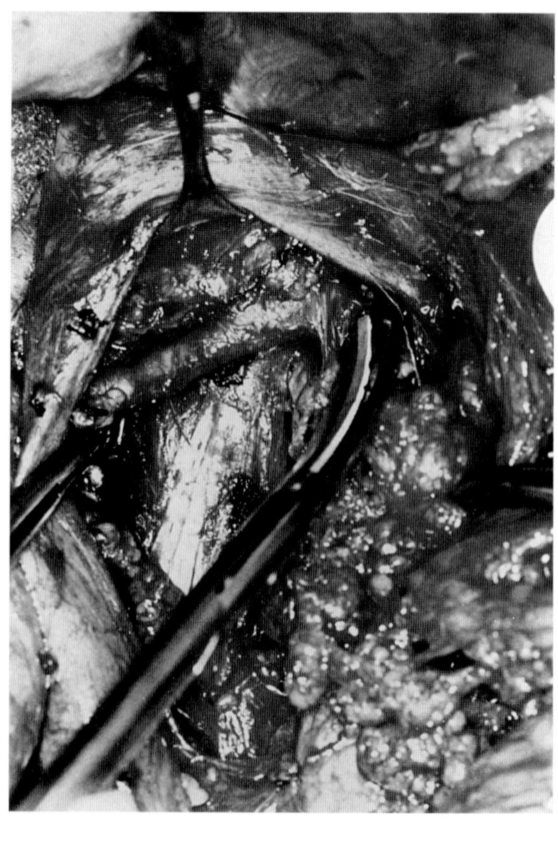

**FIG. 56.2.** Dissection around the right renal artery. The left renal vein is retracted, and the right renal artery is exposed.

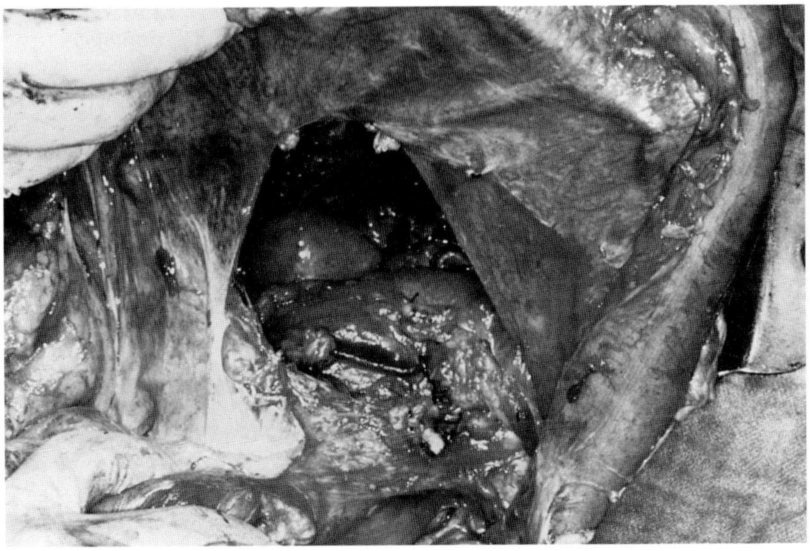

**FIG. 56.3.** Division of the transverse mesocolon. The mesocolon is divided by electrocautery 3 cm distant from the attachment of the pancreas. The middle colic artery and vein are ligated and divided.

around the left renal artery are dissected at this time (Fig. 56.4). This establishes a connection inferiorly with the site of the initial dissection. The splenic artery is ligated and divided in a total pancreatectomy. This maneuver exposes the common hepatic artery.

**Dissection around the Superior Mesenteric Artery.** The jejunum is transected 10–20 cm from the ligament of Treitz. The jejunal crus, which had been divided, is lifted upward from the opening of the above-mentioned incision. The jejunal crus and pancreas are pulled downward and to the right, and the superior mesenteric vein is pulled to the left with a hook. This maneuver exposes the superior mesenteric artery and its nerve plexus. The nerve plexus can be separated from the vessels easily using Kelly hemostats (Fig. 56.5). However, the operator must take care not to avulse any small vessels arising from the superior mesenteric artery (Fig. 56.6). Using scissors, the nerve plexus is dissected away from the superior mesenteric artery and is then divided between ligatures. At this point all retroperitoneal soft tissues and ganglia can be removed en bloc together with the pancreas (Fig. 56.7). A thin layer of nerve plexus around the superior mesenteric artery and the left ganglion at the root of the celiac axis may be preserved.

**Combined Resection of the Portal Vein.** When resection of the portal vein is required, the procedures described above for handling it are not used. Once the retroperitoneum has been dissected, the portal vein can be divided at the upper and lower margins of the pancreas and removed with the organ. An end-to-end anastomosis of the portal vein can be performed easily using 5-0 prolene sutures.

**Reconstruction of Digestive Organs.** The Imanaga (19), Child (20), and Whipple (1) methods have been described as techniques of reconstruction of the digestive tract after PD. Each method has advantages and drawbacks. Recently, the Imanaga method, which has been called a physiologic reconstruction, has been reexamined in an effort to preserve digestive and absorptive function.

The pancreaticojejunostomy is the most important aspect of the reconstruction of the digestive tract after PD. There are several techniques for pancreatojejunostomy. We have used a variety of these since 1973. At present, anastomosis between the pancreatic duct and the jejunum is used, regardless of the size of the duct.

Treatment of the incised end of the pancreas is described first. Suturing and contraction like a fish mouth are not used.

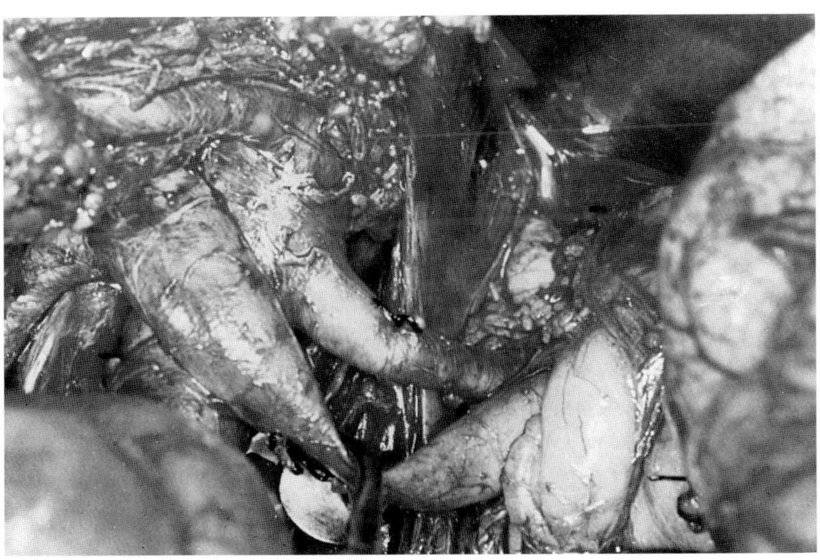

**FIG. 56.4.** Dissection at the left border of the abdominal aorta. The left renal vein is retracted downward, and the left renal artery is exposed from its origin. The origin of the celiac axis and the diaphragmatic crus are visible.

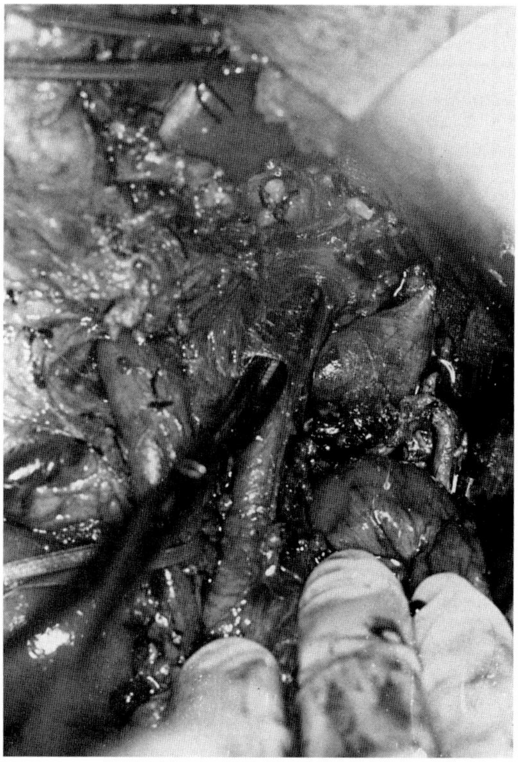

**FIG. 56.5.** Dissection around the superior mesenteric artery. Technique for approaching the superior mesenteric artery. Kelly hemostats are used to strip the nerve tissue from around the artery.

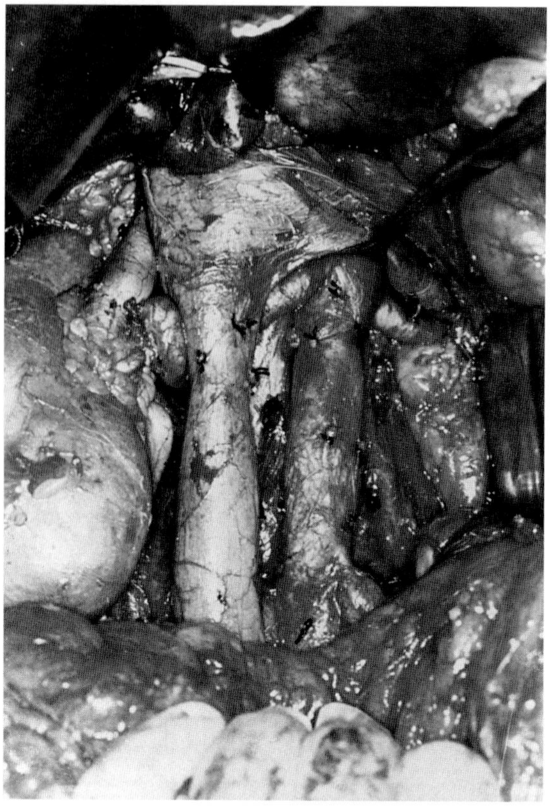

**FIG. 56.7.** Appearance of the retroperitoneum following completion of the dissection. The abdominal aorta and inferior vena cava have been completely skeletonized. Both renal arteries and veins are exposed.

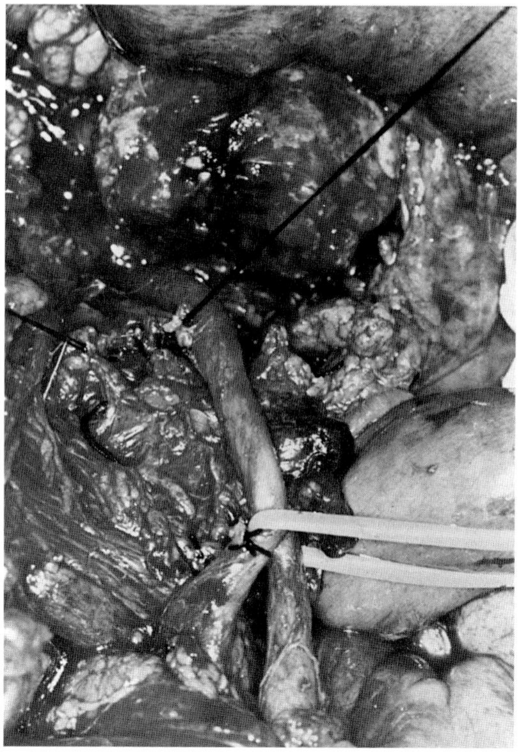

**FIG. 56.6.** Dissection around the superior mesenteric artery. The inferior pancreatoduodenal artery is ligated and divided. The superior mesenteric artery is exposed.

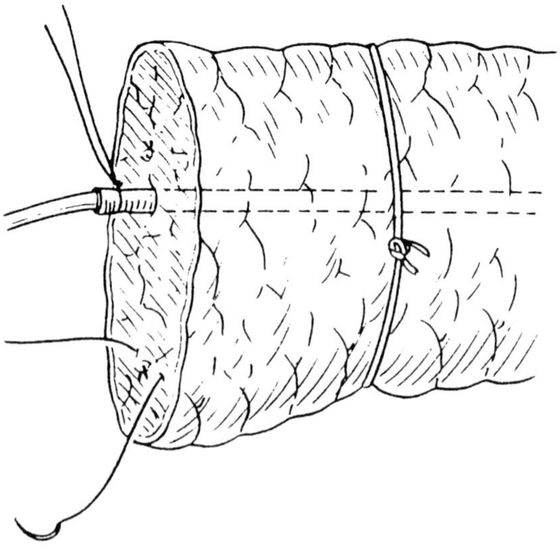

**FIG. 56.8.** Hemostasis is performed by suture ligature of approximately three or more vessels. A tube is inserted and temporarily fixed within the pancreatic duct. The tube has a localized bulge within its intrapancreatic portion to help stabilize its position within the duct. Note the temporary tourniquet around the pancreas.

Hemostasis at the incised end of the pancreas is obtained using 4-0 Maxon suture ligatures in the pancreatic parenchyma (Fig. 56.8). Hemorrhage is always localized and controlled.

An incision is made in the pancreas along a predetermined line. The cranial (resected) side of the pancreas is ligated with a 2-0 silk suture to control its bleeding. The caudal side is temporarily encircled with an atraumatic tourniquet to prevent hemorrhage from the incised end (Fig. 56.8). Alternatively, an assistant may compress the pancreatic parenchyma on the caudal side to prevent hemorrhage from its transected end. We use the latter technique because it permits selective identification of the sites of hemorrhage. In any case, the pancreatic duct should be identified and exposed so that damage to its wall can be avoided. After the pancreatic duct is transected, a no. 4 or 6 pancreatic "duct-tube" with a "bulge" or "bulb" in its intraductal portion is inserted into the cut end (Fig. 56.8). The bulge, or localized area of enlargement, of the tube helps stabilize the tube within the duct.

A small opening is made in the jejunum at the planned site of the anastomosis. If the duct is large, the posterior wall of the pancreatic duct, and of the jejunum are approximated with 5–10 interrupted 6-0 Maxon sutures. If the duct is small, these sutures may sometimes incorporate a limited thickness of adjacent pancreatic parenchyma. The opposite end of the pancreatic duct-tube is then inserted into the jejunum, and the tube is secured with one absorbable suture that attaches the tube to the adjacent wall of the pancreatojejunostomy (Fig. 56.9). The site surrounding the anastomosis is reinforced with interrupted 3-0 or 4-0 absorbable Maxon sutures. The anterior wall is anastomosed in a similar manner.

The capsule and adjacent parenchyma of the pancreas are then sutured to the seromuscular layer of the jejunum by use of a row of interrupted 4-0 nylon sutures that encircle the pancreas as shown in Figure 56.10.

This technique is relatively easy to perform. We have been able to perform this anastomosis on pancreatic ducts with a 1-mm diameter.

The techniques of choledochojejunostomy and gastrojejunostomy are not described here.

**Abdominal Drainage.** In an attempt to prevent the fatal complications of pancreatic leakage, we developed a new method of intraabdominal drainage that involves continuous suction.

The catheter within the pancreatic duct, which crosses the pancreatojejunostomy, is brought through the anterior wall or through the blind end of the Roux-Y segment of jejunum (Figs. 56.10, 56.11) to the abdominal wall. A second decompressive catheter, lying within the lumen of this Roux segment of jejunum, is exteriorized similarly (Fig. 56.11). Immediately after operation, continuous suction is applied to these catheters.

Next, two 18-French double-lumen sump drains are positioned beside the pancreaticoenterostomy and in the left upper quadrant, respectively. Two Penrose drains and a Duple or Faicon tube (Faicon Tube, Fuji Systems Co., Tokyo, Japan) are also inserted near the pancreaticojejunostomy for passive drainage. Immediately after operation, continuous suction is also applied to the sump drains. A common thoracic pump is used for suction, set at a pressure of –20 cm $H_20$. When the sump tube does not function effectively, it should be changed along the Duple drain and its position immediately checked with a plain abdominal roentgenogram.

Amylase concentrations and bacterial cultures of the sump drainage should be examined regularly to detect early dehiscence of the pancreaticojejunostomy. The sump tube should be removed when it drains less than 50 mL in a 24-hour period, provided that the amylase concentration in its drainage has normalized.

**Preoperative Management.** Preoperatively, PTCD or ENBD are used to relieve jaundice. Nutritional support by intravenous hyperalimentation (IVH) is administered routinely in patients with obstructive jaundice. Carbohydrates are given as sugars in amounts of 1000–1800 Kcal/day. Insulin is administered immediately and as needed to keep the blood sugar concentration below 300 mg/dL. Protein is supplied with amino acid preparations, Plasmanate, and plasma. Vitamin preparations and lipids are also administered.

Immediately before surgery, patients should have serum bilirubin concentrations equal to or below 5 mg/dL and a serum protein concentration above 7.0 g/dL.

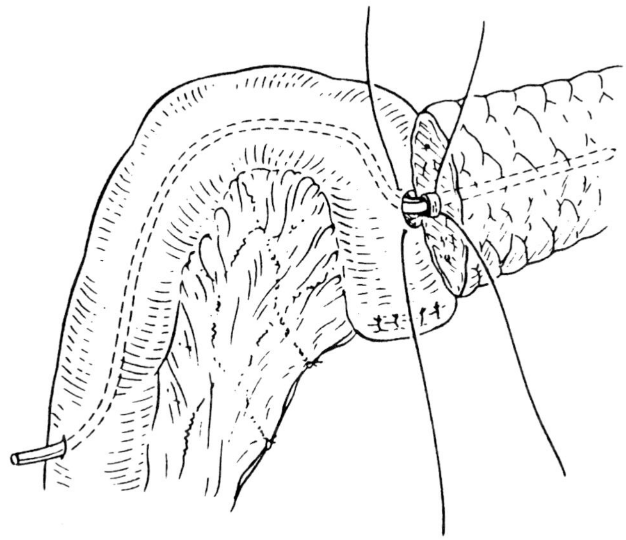

**FIG. 56.9.** The posterior and the anterior walls of the pancreatic duct and the jejunum are sutured with 8–10 6-0 Maxon sutures. (The pancreatic duct has been transected flush with the pancreas.)

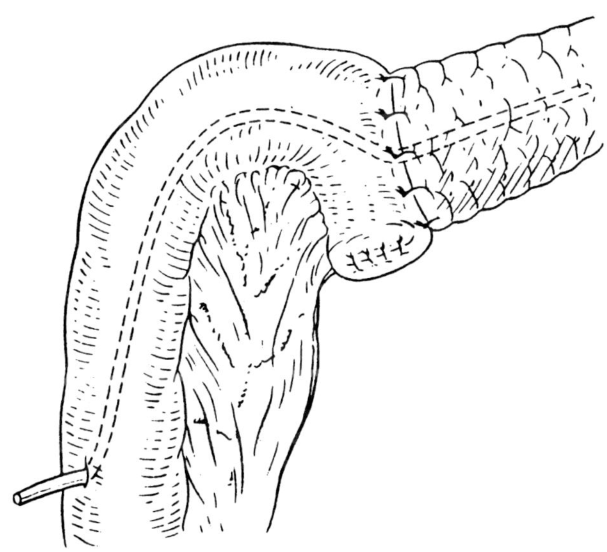

**FIG. 56.10.** After the tissues surrounding the anastomosis are reinforced with three or four 4-0 Maxon (slowly absorbable) sutures, the circumference of the pancreas and the adjacent jejunum are sutured with interrupted 4-0 nonabsorbable nylon sutures. The end of the pancreatic catheter is exteriorized to the abdominal wall.

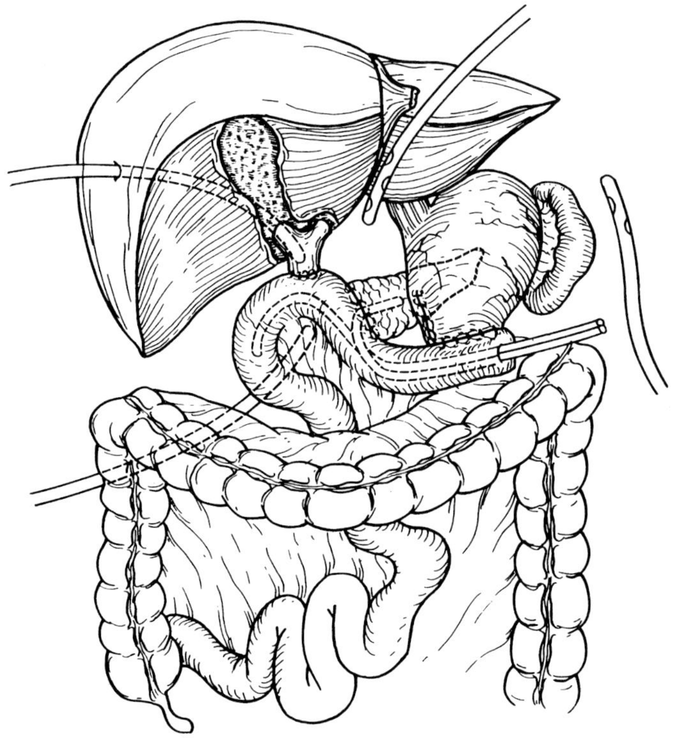

**FIG. 56.11.** Abdominal drainage. Imanaga's method of reconstruction is shown. Two intraluminal catheters and two sump drains are placed on continuous suction.

**Postoperative Management.** The operation usually takes 7–10 hours, with transfusion requirements ranging from 1000 to 3000 mL. Tremendous losses of lymph result from complete peripancreatic lymphadenectomy. Unless supplemented, serum protein levels can fall to 5.0 mg/dL or lower on the first postoperative day.

Patients requiring respiratory support are managed using an endotracheal tube and Servo-type respirator. The oxygen and carbon dioxide tensions are monitored for 24–48 hours.

The principal component of the fluids infused immediately after the operation is sugar. Hypertonic carbohydrate solutions are not used in the first 3 days. Regular insulin (1 U/10 g sugar) is given to patients undergoing resection of the head of the pancreas. After radical pancreatectomy, the dose is doubled (1 U/5 g sugar). Additional supplements of insulin are used to keep the serum glucose concentration between 200 and 300 mg/dL. As a source of protein, 5–10 units of fresh frozen plasma (200 mL each) are administered daily. Neither amino acids nor lipids are given for the first 3 days. Sodium intake is limited during the early postoperative period. The serum chemistries are monitored for hypernatremia and hypokalemia.

At the beginning of the diuretic phase, hypertonic glucose (15–30%), supplying at least 1000 Kcal, is given daily along with insulin and 5 U of fresh frozen plasma or Plasmanate. IVH is continued until oral feedings are started.

With the initiation of oral feeding, diarrhea often results. A large dose of digestive enzymes, as well as loperamide HCl, tincture of opium (3.0 mL/day, given orally in three divided doses 10 minutes before meals) is routinely administered. The concentration of carbohydrate is elevated to 30%, and water intake is restricted. Amino acids and lipids are administered, and IVH is maintained for approximately 3 weeks.

**Long-Term Postoperative Nutritional Management.** Oral feedings of an elemental diet (ED) are increased, as tolerated, limiting the total volume to 3 packs per day. Patients undergoing resection of the head of the pancreas remain on an ED for 6 weeks; those undergoing total pancreatectomy are continued for at least 3 months.

Strict follow-up of patients is necessary after discharge from the hospital. Patients undergoing resection of the head of the pancreas required hospitalization for nutritional support on average twice in the 1st year (for 2 weeks), once or twice in the following year, and rarely in the 3rd. Patients gradually become independent of the tincture of opium and the ED. However, the nutritional status must be carefully followed, even after the 3rd year (Fig. 56.12).

**Surgical Results.** The elements of extended radical pancreatectomy by the TRA include complete excision of the lymph nodes and nerve plexuses of the trunks of both the celiac axis and superior mesenteric artery.

Since 1973, 216 patients with pancreatic cancer have undergone surgical exploration, 147 of whom had cancer of the head of the pancreas. Patients with cystadenocarcinoma, islet cell carcinoma, and carcinoma of the distal bile duct and papilla of Vater were not included in this study. Of those with cancer of the head of the pancreas, there were 101 men and 46 women whose ages at the time of operation ranged from 31 to 82 years (mean, 60.9 years). Resection was performed in 72 patients (49%), including 58 patients (39.5%) undergoing curative resection based on macroscopic criteria and 39 patients (26.5%) undergoing curative resection based on microscopic criteria. In all but seven patients, the TRA facilitated an adequate lymphadenectomy.

**Operative Deaths and Postoperative Complications.** Among the 58 patients who underwent macroscopically curative resections, there were 4 (6.9%) perioperative deaths due to peritonitis or intraperitoneal hemorrhage. Another three patients died within 60 days because of sepsis or hepatorenal failure. Major postoperative complications included wound infection, postoperative hemorrhage, pneumonia, and hepatic and renal insufficiency. The overall incidence of complications in this group was 37.2%.

**Long-Term Survival.** Using the Kaplan-Meier method (throughout), survival was calculated for the 58 patients who underwent a macroscopically curative resection (Fig. 56.13).

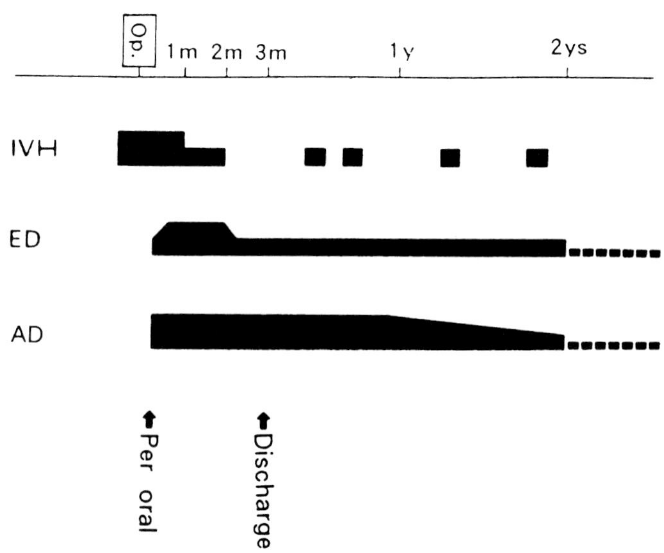


**FIG. 56.12.** Schema of postoperative management after pancreatoduodenectomy. *Op.*, operation; *IVH*, intravenous hyperalimentation; *ED*, elemental diet; *AD*, antidiarrheal medication; *m*, month; *y*, year.

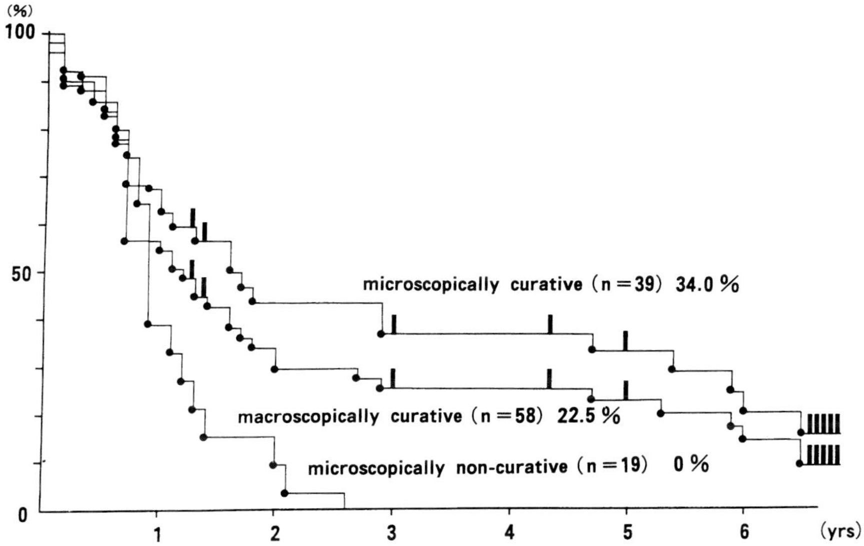


**FIG. 56.13.** Survival rate according to the type of "curative resection" for carcinoma of the head of the pancreas (Kaplan-Meier method). Percentages are given for the 5-year survival rate.

There were 14 3-year survivors and 10 5-year survivors in this group. The overall 5-year survival rate was 22.5% in this macroscopically cured group and 34% in the microscopically cured group. The overall median survival period was 13 months in the macroscopically cured group and 19 months in the microscopically cured group. Late postoperative complications including diarrhea and nutritional disturbances were observed in most patients.

**Prognosis According to Stage of Disease.** The prognoses, related to the spread of the cancer, were calculated on the basis of the 34 patients who survived a microscopically curative resection.

Tumor size was classified as $t_1$, <2.0 cm in diameter; $t_2a$, 2.1–3.0 cm in diameter; $t_2b$, 3.1–4.0 cm in diameter; $t_3$, 4.1–6.0 cm in diameter; or $t_4$, >6.1 cm in diameter. The local extent of disease was evaluated as $s_0$, anterior capsule of the pancreas not invaded; $s_1$, slightly invaded; or $s_2$, invasion of the capsule. The designations $rp_0$, $rp_1$, and $rp_2$ were similarly used depending on whether the retropancreatic tissue had been invaded. Invasion of the portal vein was classified as $pv_0$, no invasion; $pv_1$, invasion to the adventitia or media; or $pv_2$, invasion to the intima or the internal lumen. Involvement of the surgical margin of resection was categorized as $ew_0$, no invasion; $ew_1$, invasion within 5 mm of the surgical margin; or $ew_2$, positive invasion. The surgical margin referred to all margins, most frequently to retroperitoneal invasion. Lymph node metastases were classified as $n_0$, no nodal metastasis; $n_1$, metastasis to group 1 nodes (nos. 6, 81, 8p, $12a_2$, $12p_2$, 13 ab, 14 bcd, 17 ab, above and $n_2$), metastasis to group 2 nodes (nos. 9, 11, 12al, 12pl, 12bl, 12c, 14a, 15, $16a_1$, and $16b_2$). S stages and stages I to IV were used according to the general rules published by the Japan Pancreas Society (21) and outlined in the legend to Figure 56.14.

The generalized Wilcoxon test was used for statistical analysis, and differences were considered significant if the probability was less than .05.

There was no correlation between tumor size and prognosis. There was no 5-year survivor among the patients with $s_2$ disease ($n = 3$); the 5-year survival of patients with $s_0$ disease ($n = 25$) was 43.6% ($p < .05$). There were 5-year survivors in all three retroperitoneal invasion groups ($rp_0$, $rp_1$, or $rp_2$). The survival was significantly better in the $rp_0$ group than in the $rp_1$ or $rp_2$ groups ($p < .05$). Four patients with retroperitoneal invasion survived more than 3 years. There were no 5-year survivors among the patients with positive invasion to the intima or the

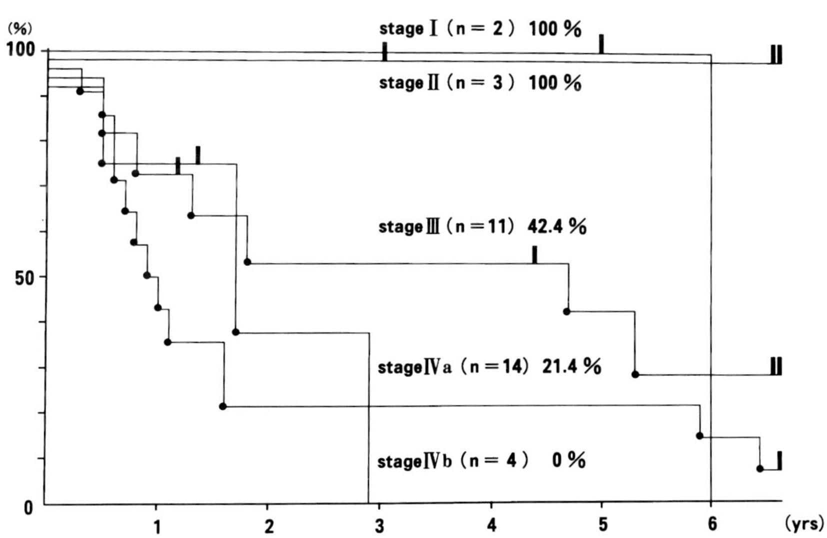


**FIG. 56.14.** Survival rate according to cancer stage. (Kaplan-Meier method). The survival rate was significantly better in patients with stage I and stage II disease than in those with stage IVb disease ($p < .0005$). Percentages are given for the 5-year survival rate. Stage I, $t_1$, $s_0$, $rp_0$, $pv_0$, and $n_0$; stage II, $s_0$, $rp_0$, $pv_0$, and $n_1$; stage III, $s_1$, $rp_1$, or $n_2$; stage IVa, $n_2$; stage IVa, $n_2$ and $s_2$, $rp_2$, $pv_2$; stage IVb, others.

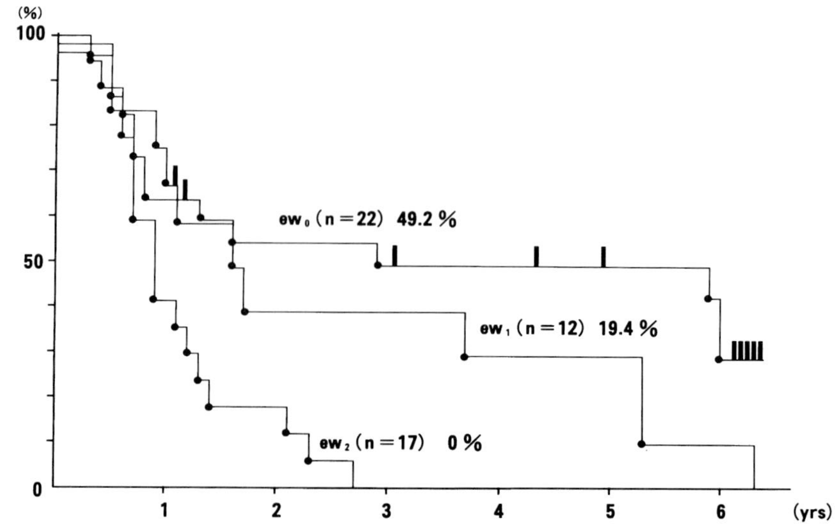


**FIG. 56.15.** Survival rate according to invasion of or near the excisional margin (Kaplan-Meier). Survival was significantly better in patients with $ew_0$ than in those with $ew_2$ ($p < .05$). Percentages are given for the 5-year survival rate. $Ew_0$, negative invasion; $ew_1$, invasion within 5 mm from the surgical margin; $ew_2$, positive invasion; *ew* refers to invasion of any surgical margin, especially the posterior (retroperitoneal) surface.

internal lumen of the portal vein, but there was no statistically significant difference in survival between these groups. The lymph nodes were positive in 22 patients. All patients with $n_2$ disease were dead within 3 years. Patients with $n_0$ disease had a 5-year survival of 76.9%. There was a significant difference in survival between the patients with $n_0$, $n_1$, and $n_2$ disease ($p<.05$). In all patients with metastases to the periaortic lymph nodes, the nodes around the superior mesenteric artery were involved. There were two patients with a single metastasis to the periaortic lymph nodes who lived for more than 2 years. All patients with stage IVb disease died within 3 years (Fig. 56.14). Three patients with stage IVa disease survived more than 5 years. Survival was significantly better in patients with stage I and II disease than in those with stage IVb disease. All patients with microscopic evidence of cancer at the resection margin were dead within 3 years. Of those with a negative margin, a 5-year survival rate of 49.2% was noted. Cancer at the resection margin was statistically correlated with survival ($p < .05$) (Fig. 56.15).

## PROBLEMS WITH EN BLOC REMOVAL

The resection rate for pancreatic carcinoma is increased when advanced techniques such as en bloc removal of the portal vein are used. At the same time, the mortality of extensive operations for pancreatic cancer can be reduced by using ancillary techniques such as percutaneous transhepatic biliary drainage and perioperative nutritional support (22). Despite these approaches, however, the 5-year survival rate after resection is still disappointing, reported to range from 2.3 to 14.3% for cancer of the head of the pancreas (2–14). Because of disappointing long-term survival rates following radical surgery for pancreatic cancer, some authors have suggested that bypass alone should be used as the procedure of choice (23–25).

Our extended radical pancreatectomy is designed to achieve complete resection of the local extent of cancer cells plus wide dissection of the metastatic lymph nodes. Combined resection of the portal vein and the nerve plexuses around the trunks of the celiac axis and the superior mesenteric artery are performed as part of the effort to remove the local extent of disease. Such procedures may be associated with a high postoperative mortality rate (11, 26, 27). Although we lost seven patients (9.7%) within 60 days of the operation, five of the deaths occurred in the earlier years of this series. We have not lost a patient immediately after the operation in the last 5 years. The recent postoperative mortality rate is less than 5%.

**Postoperative Nutritional Disturbance.** The most serious nutritional disturbance was postoperative diarrhea. This results from excision of the sympathetic nerves to the small intestine and can be affected by the method of reconstruction. We have previously investigated this problem clinically and experimentally and found that the degree of disturbance is related to the extent of nerve dissection (22).

Furthermore, reconstruction by the Imanaga method (19), in which the stomach, pancreas, and bile duct are reconstructed in that order, was associated with a more favorable outcome than the Child reconstruction (20). Since this disorder is caused by complete excision of lymph vessels and nerve plexuses, dissection that leaves a thin layer of the nerve plexus around the superior mesenteric artery is recommended in patients with stage I disease. This thin layer does not contain distinct lymph nodes (28) (Fig. 56.16).

Severe malabsorption after PD, particularly after an extended PD has been reported (21). Partial or complete loss of pancreatic and duodenal function after an extended resection and incomplete compensatory adjustments of the residual pancreas and small bowel may contribute to malabsorption. Alternatively, complete resection of the peripancreatic lymph nodes, including the nodes around the base of the superior mesenteric artery, may interrupt lymphatic flow and result in malabsorption.

Triolein fecal excretion rates have been used to demonstrate that malabsorption is more severe after an extended PD than after a standard PD. The pancreatic maldigestive ratio (PMDR) is designed to measure the lack of absorption secondary to pancreatic function by subtracting the intestinal malabsorption factor (d-xylose) from the total malabsorption (urinary excretion of orally administered *p*-aminobenzoic acid [PABA]). The PMDR is higher after extended PD and semiextended PD than after standard PD. This would be predicted, as more pancreatic tissue is resected in the first two methods. Due to diarrhea and malabsorption, the urinary excretion of d-xylose was decreased in the extended PD group. Thus, absorption as assessed by three indicators was greatly impaired by extended PD (Fig. 56.17).

A long-term follow-up study (28a) has shown that fecal excretion of triolein, *d*-xylose urinary excretion, and PMDR returned to normal less than 1 year after standard PD and returned to near-normal within 1 year of semiextended PD. After extended PD, the delay in recovery was more pronounced.

Intravenous injection of 5 g of sugar resulted in decreased potassium levels in 3 of 5 patients treated by extended PD and 2 of 4 patients treated by conventional PD. No significant differences were noted between the two methods.

Reconstructions after PD are classified into two major types according to the location of the gastrojejunostomy. Cattell's (29) method and Imanaga's (19) method (PDIII) allow food to enter the bowel proximal to the pancreaticojejunostomy. The methods (PDII) of Whipple (1) and Child (19), however, in which food enters the gastrointestinal tract distal to the pancreaticojejunostomy, have been widely used to protect the pancreatic anastomosis from disruption.

The differences between the two groups with regard to safety have become less important with the widespread use of early postoperative total parenteral nutrition. We have shown experimentally (30) that following extensive lymph node resection with PD, postoperative digestive and absorptive functions are better preserved by Imanaga's technique (19) (PDIII) than by Child's techniques (20) (PDII). As a result, we have used PDIII clinically since 1983.

The postoperative recovery of digestive and absorptive functions after PDIII has been more favorable than after PDII, as demonstrated by the 5-g *d*-xylose test and the PFD test for urinary *d*-xylose excretion. When the effect of malabsorption of *d*-xylose was excluded from the urinary PABA recovery rate referring to PMDR, no differences in pancreatic exocrine function were observed between the two methods. The favorable results after PDIII are thought to be due to the characteristic way that food passes through the upper jejunum. No marked differences were noted between the two methods following the standard PD. However, since postoperative maldigestion and malabsorption are frequently severe after the extended resection, PDIII, which is associated with better absorption, is recommended.

**Curative Surgery.** Among the 58 patients who underwent macroscopically curative resection, only 39 (67.2%) were microscopically cured (Table 56.1). This was due to retropancreatic invasion, noted microscopically, in numerous patients.

We studied histologically the direction of the retropancreatic invasion toward the superior mesenteric artery, the portal vein, and the inferior vena cava in 21 patients undergoing resection of the head of the pancreas for carcinoma (30). The pattern was reconstructed three-dimensionally by complete serial sectioning in four patients. Retropancreatic invasion of the cancer was detected histologically as spreading toward the superior mesenteric artery, the portal vein, and the inferior vena cava in 17 (81%), 12 (57%), and 16 (76%) patients, respectively. The distances between the histologic carcinoma margin and the pancreatic surface, and the histologic carcinoma margin and the macroscopic tumor margin, were measured in the direction of each vessel. The mean distance of histologic spread, including lymphatic and perineural spread, (carcinoma margin) toward the blood vessels was 3.2 mm (range, 0–13.2 mm) in the direction of the superior mesenteric artery, 0.5 mm (range, 0–2.0 mm) in the direction of the portal vein, and 2.1 mm (range, 0–4.8 mm) in the direction of the inferior vena cava. Three-dimensional reconstruction revealed that the pattern of retropancreatic invasion was composed mainly of neural invasion in the direction of the superior mesenteric artery (Fig. 56.18). Cancer invasion with desmoplasia occurred mainly in the directions of the portal vein and the inferior vena cava.

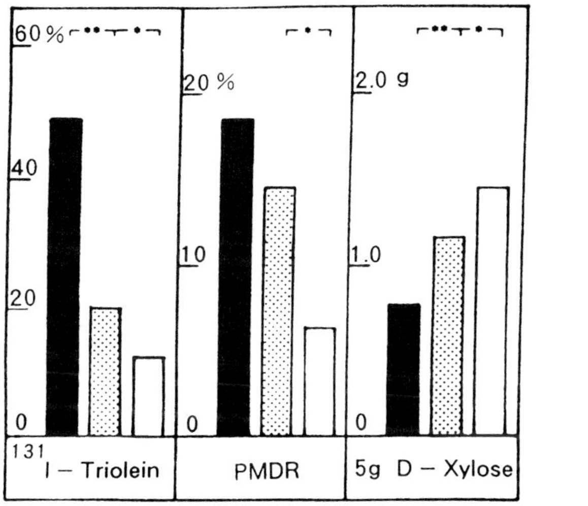


**FIG. 56.17.** Postoperative digestive (triolein excretion) and absorptive (xylose excretion) functions according to operative procedures. *PMDR*, pancreatic maldigestive ratio. ▮, extended pancreatoduodenectomy (PD); ▯, semioxtended resection; ▯, standard PD. *, $p < .05$; **$p < .01$.

The concept of neural invasion is widely accepted in the literature on pancreatic carcinoma. In retroperitoneal dissection of cancer of the head of the pancreas, we emphasized the importance of recognition of neural invasion of the cancer (17, 18, 31–36). The precise mechanisms by which cancer cells invade and progress along the nerves have not been clarified.

The extrapancreatic nerve plexus was divided into two portions on the basis of Yoshioka's study (37): the first portion is distributed from the right celiac ganglia to the upper median

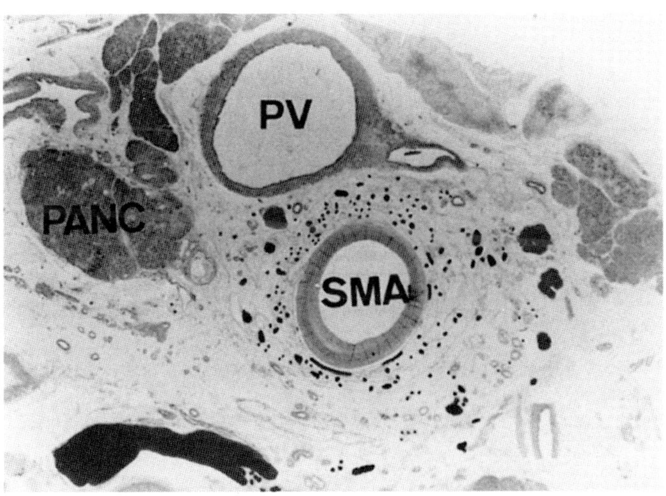


**FIG. 56.16.** Magnified view of the surgical specimen (hematoxylin & eosin stain), showing the position of the pancreas, superior mesenteric artery, and portal vein in the retroperitoneum. *PANC*, pancreas; *PV*, portal vein; *SMA*, superior mesenteric artery.

**TABLE 56.1. Correlation between Retropancreatic Invasion and Cancer Cells at the Surgical Margin**

| Retroperitoneal Invasion[a] | Total Number of Patients | Histologic Invasion of Surgical Margin[b] | | |
|---|---|---|---|---|
| | | $ew_0$ | $ew_1$ | $ew_2$ |
| $rp_0$ | 10 | 10 | | |
| $rp_1$ | 9 | 5 | 3 | 1 |
| $rp_2$ | 39 | 12 | 9 | 18 |

[a] $rp_0$, no invasion of the retropancreatic tissue; $rp_1$, slight invasion of the retropancreatic tissue; $rp_2$, invasion of the retropancreatic tissue.

[b] The surgical margin refers predominantly to the retropancreatic margin of resection. $ew_0$, no invasion of the surgical margin; $ew_1$, invasion within 5 mm of the surgical margin; $ew_2$, positive invasion of the surgical margin.

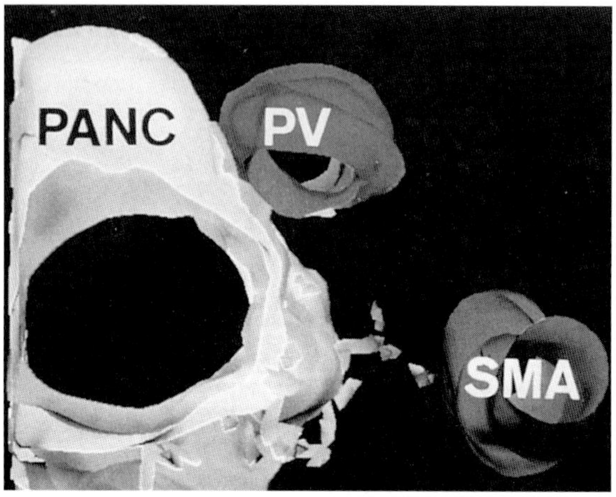


**FIG. 56.18.** Three-dimensional computer-reconstructed image of tumor invasion around the superior mesenteric artery. The tumor cells extend by neural invasion *(green)* and by venous invasion *(light blue)* around the superior mesenteric artery. The most advanced point of stromal invasion consists of neural invasion. The tumor cells extend toward the portal vein, with desmoplastic infiltration of cancer *(purple)*. *PANC*, pancreas. *PV*, portal vein. *SMA*, superior mesenteric artery. See color insert.

margin of the uncinate process, and the second portion extends from the superior mesenteric artery to the median margin of the uncinate process (Fig. 56.19).

Thirty-four patients who underwent resection of cancer of the pancreatic head had specimens examined clinicopathologically to identify neural invasion of the extrapancreatic nerve plexuses. Invasion of the retropancreatic tissue by cancer was seen in 29 (85%) of the 34 patients; neural invasion of the extrapancreatic nerve plexus was seen in 21 (72%) of the 29 with retropancreatic invasion. The incidence of invasion of the second portion of the nerve plexus of the pancreatic head was 67%. Assessment of the relationship between tumor size and invasion into the retropancreatic tissues revealed that the incidence of invasion of the retropancreatic region was high, regardless of $t_1$ tumor size. It is particularly important to note that even two patients with $t_1$ tumors had retropancreatic disease. The degree of neural invasion tended to increase as invasion of the lymph vessels became more marked. Observation of serial sections revealed continuity of the neural invasion to the nerve plexuses (Fig. 56.20). From these findings, we conclude that neural invasion proceeds along peripheral pancreatic nerve branches to the extrapancreatic nerves. The continuity of spread along the nerves is not only from the primary cancer but also from the microscopic positive margins of the spreading cancer. En bloc resection of the retropancreatic tissue involving the nerve plexuses and fatty tissue is necessary in the surgical treatment of cancer of the pancreatic head.

Invasion of the extrapancreatic nerve plexuses was correlated with invasion of the surgical margin of resection (Table 56.2). This shows that extensive dissection of the extrapancreatic nerve plexuses is necessary for a microscopically curative resection for cancer of the head of the pancreas. Although our procedures are similar to those reported by Fortner (16), our 5-year survival rate was higher. The two procedures may differ with respect to the completeness of retroperitoneal dissection, in particular in the dissection of the nerve plexus around the superior mesenteric artery.

**Lymph Node Involvement.** The nomenclature of the major lymph nodes was defined (Figs. 56.1 and 56.2) according to the classification of the general rules for pancreatic cancer and the proposal of the Japan Society for Cancer Therapy (38) (Fig. 56.21) or our own classification of paraaortic lymph nodes (Fig. 56.22).

According to The Japanese Pancreas Society's guidelines for cancer of the pancreas (21), the extent of dissection of area no. 16 is restricted to the paraaortic area ranging from the origin of the celiac artery (upper margin) to the origin of the inferior mesenteric artery (lower margin). However, this description of the area does not include the concept of depth. To more clearly define the anatomic spread of the tumor, we have defined the extent of disease in the cranial and caudal directions (the extent according to the aforementioned guidelines) as lying in a longitudinal plane viewed anteriorly, while the extent in the ventral to dorsal directions lies in a cross-sectional plane.

The incidence of lymph node metastases in cancer of the head of the pancreas is high. Even in resectable disease, Cubilla et al. (39) observed nodal metastases in 19 of 22 patients undergoing PD. Nakao et al. (40) have reported a similar incidence of nodal metastases.

Metastases to the lymph nodes were present in 33 of the 42 patients (78.6%) in our series. The average number of involved lymph nodes in the examined specimens in patients with metastatic disease was 6 (8.1%). The sites of metastasis were areas no. 6, 8, 9, 11, 12, 13, 14, 16, 17, and 18. The prevalence of metastases to area no. 13 was the highest, followed by areas no. 17 and 14. There were 7 patients (16.7%) with metastases to paraaortic area no. 16 (Fig. 56.23).

There was a single nodal metastasis in area no. 16 in 4 patients. Multiple paraaortic nodes were involved in the other 3 patients, with 3, 6, and 9 nodes involved in 1 patient each, respectively. In patients harboring paraaortic nodal metastases, the average number of diseased lymph nodes was 3.1. The average incidence of lymph nodes involved in area no. 16 was 3.2% of those examined. The extent of lymphatic metastasis in area no. 16 increased with the number of involved lymph nodes.

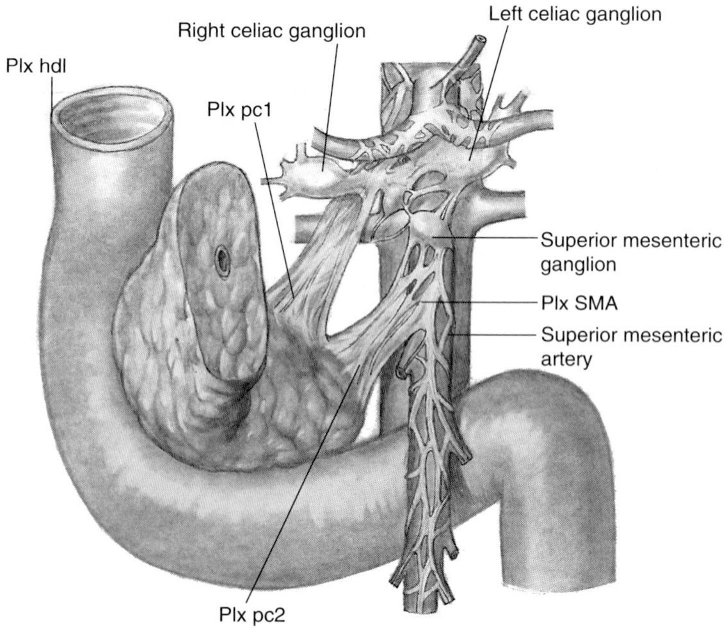


**FIG. 56.19.** Nerve plexuses around the uncinate process and head of the pancreas. *Plx hdl*, nerve plexus of the hepatoduodenal ligament; *Plx pc1*, first region of the nerve plexus of the pancreatic head; *Plx pc2*, second region of the nerve plexus of the pancreatic head; *Plx SMA*, superior mesenteric nerve plexus; *SMA*, superior mesenteric artery.

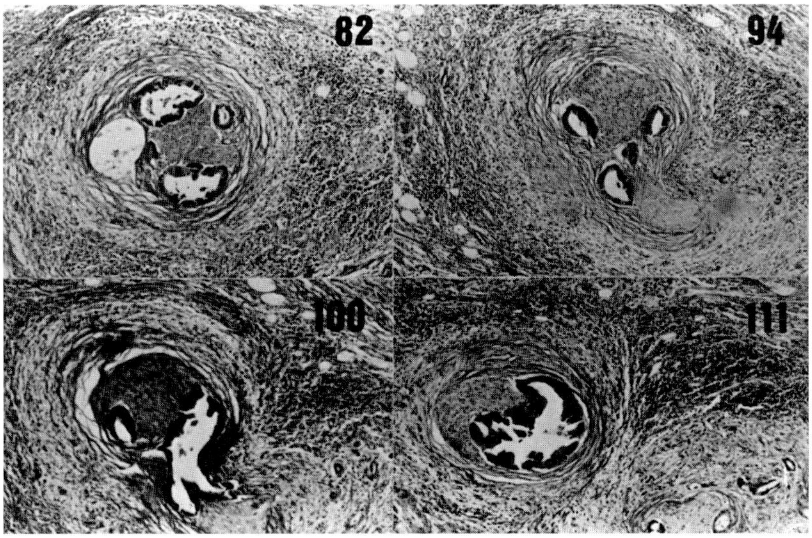


**FIG. 56.20.** Neural invasion and spread in the nerve plexus of the hepatoduodenal ligament (Plx hdl). Cancer cells have spread along the branches of the bifurcated nerve fascicles (×200). The numbers indicate the respective number of the serial sections studied along the course of the nerve. Low numbers represent sections nearer the pancreas. Four different sections are shown in this figure. *Arrows* show cancer cells.

From an anterior view in area no. 16, the incidence of metastases to segment b2 was the highest among those with positive paraaortic nodes (85.5%, 6 of 7 cases), followed by segment b1 (42.9%, 3 of 7 cases). In the transectional view, the incidence of "inter" segment involvement was the highest (71.4%, 5 of 7 cases), followed by the Aor-pre segment (57.1%, 4 of 7 cases) (Fig. 56.22).

Pathways of lymphatic metastasis from the pancreatic head to area no. 16 have been studied by Evans and Ochsner (41), Nagai (42), and Deki and Sato (43). From these studies, it seems that there is a close correlation between area no. 16 and area no. 14 and that the main pathway of metastasis from the pancreatic head to area no. 16 seems to be through area no. 14 (44–46) (Fig. 56.24).

**Combined Resection of the Portal Vein.** The safety of en bloc resection of the portal vein is reasonably well established (47), although the necessity for routine removal of the portal vein is not clear. The invasion of the portal vein observed in our patients suggests that a resection that does not include the periportal tissues would leave cancer cells in the operative field. However, patients with invasion into the intima or the internal lumen of the portal vein did not exhibit long-term survival despite combined resection.

Combined resection of the superior mesenteric artery has been reported by Fortner (16). We also tried this procedure, but the surgical results were poor. This problem should be resolved in the near future.

**TABLE 56.2. Site of Invasion and Spread to the Extrapancreatic Nerve Plexuses: Nerve Plexuses of the Hepatoduodenal Ligament**

| Site of Invasion of Nerve Plexus[a] | Number of Patients with Invasion |
|---|---|
| Plx. hdl. | 2 |
| Plx. pcI | 2 |
| Plx. pcII | 11 |
| Plx. pcI and II | 3 |
| Others | 3 |

[a]Plx. hdl., nerve plexus within the hepato-duodenal ligament; Plx. pcI, first portion of the nerve plexus of the pancreatic head; Plx. pcII, second portion of the nerve plexus of the pancreatic head. See Figure 56.19 for anatomic correlation.

## TOTAL PANCREATECTOMY

It is important to consider the argument of those who maintain that cancer of the pancreas is multifocal (48) and that total pancreatectomy is the only way to deal with this problem. Although there was direct invasion of the neck of the pancreas in 2 of our patients, no multifocal disease was found in the 12 patients who underwent total pancreatectomy. Moreover, we have evaluated autopsy specimens from 68 patients and have been unable to confirm a high rate of multifocal disease. Of the 12 patients who underwent total pancreatectomy, only 1 survived more than 5 years. Consequently, we now depend upon histologic examination of the tissues at the margin of the resection specimen to determine the need for total pancreatectomy. The role of total pancreatectomy for carcinoma of the head of the pancreas may be limited.

## PYLORUS-PRESERVING PANCREATODUODENECTOMY (PPPD)

PPPD (49) has been used recently in the operative treatment of carcinomas in the region of the pancreatic head. Our investigations have shown that PPPD is not proper for resection of pancreatic cancer with invasion of the anterior capsule of the pancreas. Although complete dissection is possible using PPPD, we have not yet performed PPPD for pancreatic cancer except for early-stage disease.

## RESECTION OF CARCINOMA OF THE BODY AND TAIL OF THE PANCREAS

Among the 53 patients with carcinomas of the body and tail of the pancreas, 30 underwent resection. Of these 30 operations, only 3 (5.7%) were macroscopically curative, and only 2 (3.8%) were microscopically curative. The long-term survival rate was very low. We have performed extended resection for carcinoma of the body and tail of the pancreas for the last 5 years. This includes extended retroperitoneal dissection as previously described and a combined resection of the common hepatic artery and the celiac artery (Appleby's operation)(50). Among the six patients in whom this approach was used, two

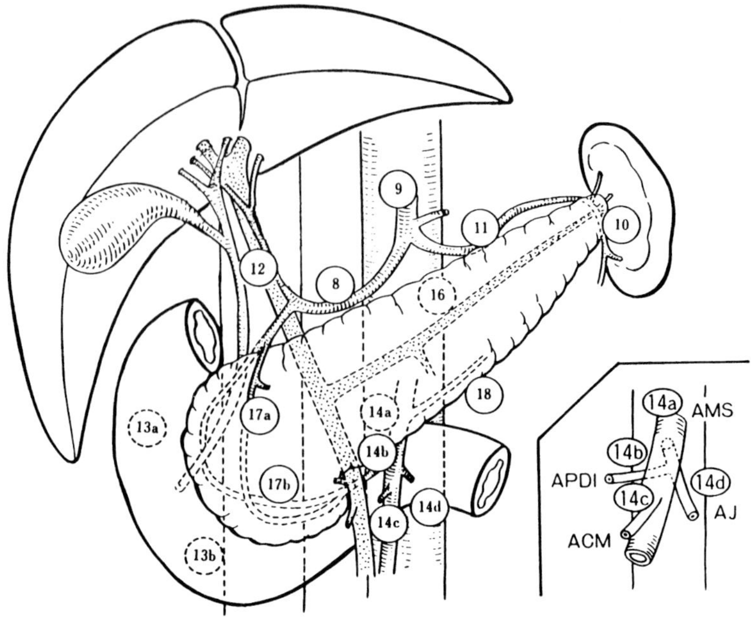


**FIG. 56.21.** Classification of regional lymph nodes of the pancreas. *Inset,* subdivision of area 14. *AMS,* superior mesenteric artery; *AJ,* jejunal artery; *APD1,* inferior pancreaticoduodenal artery; *ACM,* middle colic artery. The *dotted circles* represent retroperitoneal locations.

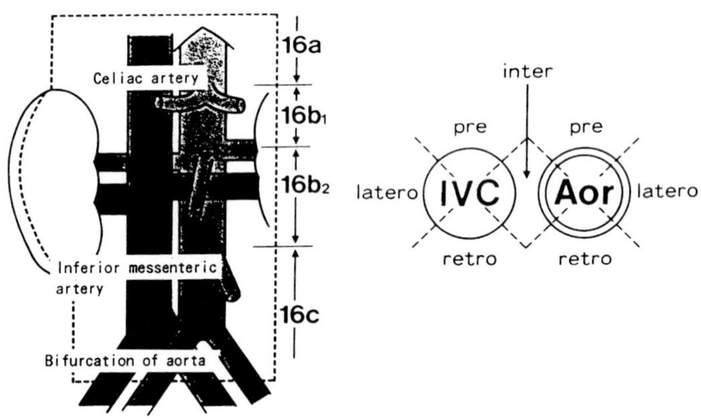


**FIG. 56.22.** Classification of lymph nodes of area no. 16. *A,* frontal (anterior) classification; *b,* transectional segment. *IVC,* inferior vena cava; *Aor,* abdominal aorta.

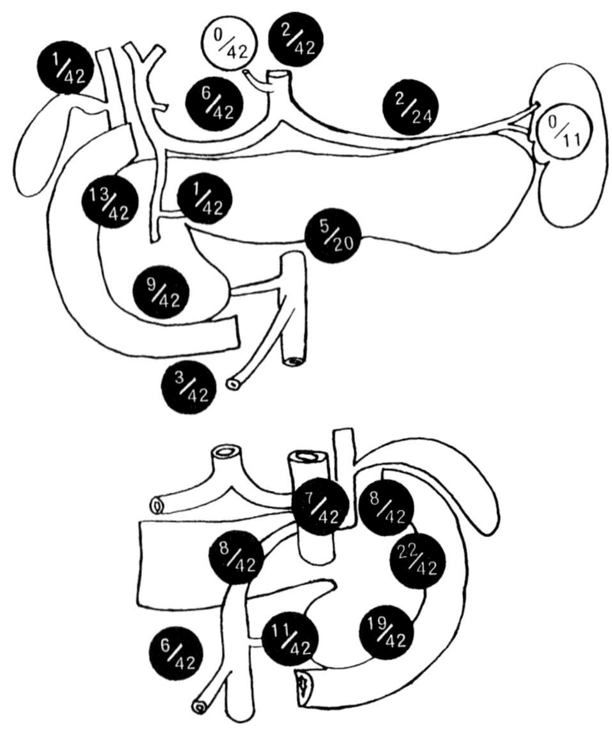


**FIG. 56.23.** Distribution of lymph node involvement in carcinoma of the head of the pancreas. The number beside each circle in which the metastatic rate is shown indicates the lymph node area shown in Figure 56.21. Positive metastatic nodes were present in 33 of 42 patients (78.6%). The average number of positive lymph nodes per patient was 6.1 (8.1%). The incidence of metastases in each nodal area is shown; for example, at area no. 12, nodes were positive in 12 patients (21.4%); 8 in 12b, 0 in 12a, and 1 in 12c. Not all lymph node areas depicted in Figure 56.21 are shown. The *lower drawing* represents the posterior surface of the head of the pancreas, duodenum, and superior mesenteric artery. The pattern shown suggests that metastases to area 16 may occur through area 14. Metastases in each lymph node are shown. No. 6, 1/42 (2.4%); no. 7, 0; no. 8, 6/42 (14.3%); no. 9, 2/42 (4.8%); no. 10, 0; no. 11, 2/24 (8.3%); no. 12, 9/42 (21.4%) -a, 0; b, 8 (19.0%); c, 0; d, 1 (2.4%); 13, 29/42 (69.0%) -a, 22 (52.4%); b, 19 (45.2%); 14, 16/42 (38.1%) -a, 8 (19.0%); b, 11 (26.2%); c, 3 (7.1%); d, 6 (14.3%); 15, 0; 16, 7/42 (6.7%); 17, 17/42 (40.5%) -a, 13 (31.0%); b, 9 (21.4%); 18, 5/20 (25.0%).

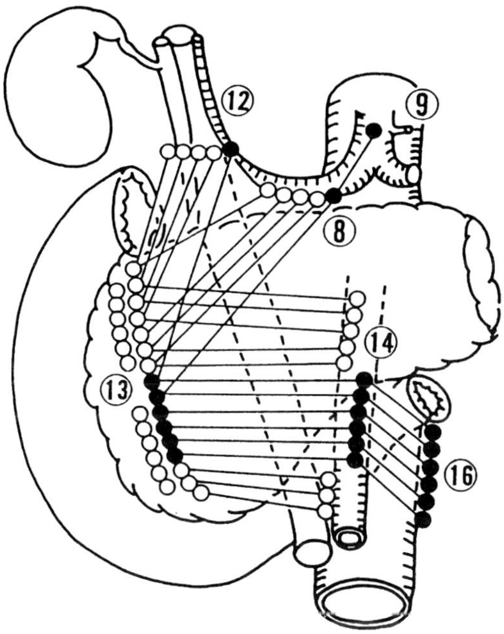


**FIG. 56.24.** Correlation of lymph nodes in 28 patients with area no. 13 lymph node metastases. *Closed circles* indicate patients who also had paraaortic lymph node metastasis. Each circle represents a single patient. Twelve of the 28 patients had metastases only to the group 13 nodes; 16 patients had lymph nodal involvement beyond this regional nodal group.

patients were alive for 3 or more years. These results suggest that such a procedure might be indicated in the treatment of this disease.

## REFERENCES


1. Whipple AO, Parson WB, Mullins CR. Treatment of the carcinoma of ampulla of Vater. Ann Surg 1935;102:763–779.
2. Nagakawa T, Konishi I, Ueno K, Ohta T, Akiyama T, et al. The results and problems of extensive radical surgery for carcinoma of the head of the pancreas. Jpn J Surg 1991;21:262–267.
3. Warren KW, Christophi C, Armendariz R, Basu S. Current trends in the diagnosis and treatment of carcinoma of the pancreas. Am J Surg 1983;145:813–818.
4. Crist DW, Sitzmann JV, Cameron JC. Improved hospital morbidity, mortality, and survival after the Whipple procedure. Am J Surg 1987;206:358–365.
5. Sato T, Saito Y, Noto T, Matsuno S. Follow-up studies of radical resection for pancreaticoduodenal cancer. Ann Surg 1977;186: 581–588.
6. Tsuchiya R, Tomioka T, Izaawa K, Noda T, Yamamoto K, et al. Collective review of small carcinomas of the pancreas. Ann Surg 1986;283:77–80.
7. Nakase A, Matsumoto Y, Uchida K, Honjo I. Surgical treatment of cancer of the pancreas and the periampullary region: cumulative results in 57 institutions in Japan. Ann Surg 1977;185:52–57.
8. Fortner JG. Surgical principles for pancreatic cancer. Regional total and subtotal pancreatectomy. Cancer 1981;47:1712–1718.
9. Nix GA, Schmitz PI, Wilson JH, van Blankenstein M, Groeneveld CF, Hofwijk R. Carcinoma of the head of the pancreas. Gastroenterology 1984;87:37–43.
10. Bjorck S, Svensson JO, Macpherson S, Edlund Y. Cancer of the head of the pancreas and choldeochoduodenal junction: a clinical study of 88 Whipple resections. Acta Chir Scand 1981; 148:353–359.
11. Connoly JR, Dawson PJ, Michelassi F, Moosa AR, Lowenstein F. Survival in 1001 patients with carcinoma of the pancreas. Ann Surg 1987;206:366–373.
12. Moossa AR, Scott M, Lavelle-Jones M. The place of total and extended pancreatectomy in pancreatic cancer. World J Surg 1984;8:895–899.
13. Lygidakis NJ, Hyde MN, Houtoff JH, Schipper ME, Huibregste K, et al. Resectional surgical procedures for carcinoma of the head of the pancreas. Surg Gynecol Obstet 1989;168:157–165.
14. Nagakawa T, Konishi I, Ueno K, Ohta T, Akiyama T, et al. Surgical treatment of pancreatic cancer: the Japanese experience. International J Pancreatol 1991;9:135–143.
15. Takagi K. Early diagnosis of pancreatic cancer (in Japanese). J Japn Med Assoc 1983;90:181–196.
16. Fortner JG. Regional resection of cancer of the pancreas. A new surgical approach. Surgery 1973;73:307–320.
17. Nagakawa T, Konishi K, Kurachi M, Miyazaki I. Retroperitoneal dissection for pancreatic carcinoma: translateral retroperitoneal approach (in Japanese). Igaku no Ayumi 1979;111:324–339.
18. Nagakawa T, Kurachi M, Knoishi K, Miyazaki I. Translateral retroperitoneal approach in radical surgery for pancreatic carcinoma. Jpn J Surg 1982;12:229–233.
19. Imanaga H. A new method of pancreaticoduodenectomy designed to preserve liver and pancreatic function. Surgery 1960;47:577–586.
20. Child CG. Pancreaticojejunostomy and other problems associated with the surgical management of carcinoma involving the head of the pancreas. Ann Surg 1994;119:845–855.
21. The Japan Pancreas Society. Classification of pancreatic carcinoma. Tokyo: Kanehara, 1996.
22. Nagakawa T, Yoshimitsu Y, Suzaki Y, Takeda T, Sanada H, et al. Postoperative digestive function and nutritional management after pancreaticoduodenectomy. Jpn J Bil-Panc Physiol 1993;9: 96–103.
23. Lea MS, Stahlgren LH. Is resection appropriate for adenocarcinoma of the pancreas: a cost-benefit analysis. Am J Surg 1987;154:651–654.
24. Crile G Jr. The advantages of by-pass operation over radical pancreatoduodenectomy in the treatment of pancreatic carcinoma. Surg Gynecol Obstet 1970;130:1049–1053.
25. Hertzberg J. Pancreatoduodenal resection and by-pass operation in patients with carcinoma of the head of the pancreas, ampulla, and distal end of the common duct. Acta Chir Scand 1974;140:523–527.
26. Manabe T, Ohshio G, Baba N, Miyashita T, Asano N, et al. Radical pancreatectomy for ductal cell carcinoma of the head of the pancreas. Cancer 1989;64:1132–1137.
27. Longmire WP Jr. Cancer of the pancreas: palliative operation, Whipple procedure, or total pancreatectomy. World J Surg 1984;8:872–879.
28. Nagakawa T, Mori K, Kayahara M, Ohta T, Ueno K, et al. Three-dimensional studies on the structure of the tissue surrounding the superior mesenteric arteyr. Int J Pancreatol 1994;15: 129–138.
28a. Nagakawa T, Yoshimitu Y, Suzaki Y. Assessment of postoperative digestive function after pancreatico-duodenectomy: a comparison of reconstruction techniques. Hepatogastroenterology 1996;43:1218–1224.
29. Cattell RB. Resection of the pancreas. Surg Clin North Am 1943;23:753–766.
30. Yagi M. Experimental study on reconstruction method and digestive function after pancreatoduodenectomy (in Japanese). Jpn J Gastroenterol Surg 1983;16:1699–1708.
31. Nagakawa T, Takeda T, Ohta T, Kayahara M, Knoishi I, et al. Pathological study of retropancreatic invasion of carcinoma of the pancreas. Cancer Res, in press.
32. Miyazaki I, Bandoh H, Asakura S, Nakagawa T, Hohkoh T, et al. The terms of radical operation for pancreatic cancer (in Japanese). Geka 1969;31:1251–1255.
33. Nagakawa T, Knoishi I, Higashino Y, Ueno K, Ohta T, et al. The spread and prognosis of carcinoma in the region of the pancreatic head. Jpn J Surg 1989;19:510–518.
34. Nagakawa T, Kayahara M, Ueno K, Ohta T, Konishi I, et al. A clinicopathologic study on neural invasion in cancer of the pancreatic head. Cancer 1992;69:930–935.
35. Nagakawa T, Kayahara M, Ohta T, Ueno K, Konishi I, Miyazaki I. Patterns of neural and plexus invasion of human pancreatic cancer and experimental cancer. Int J Pancreatol 1991;10: 113–119.

36. Kayahara M, Nagakawa T, Knoishi I, Ueno K, Ohta T, Miyazaki I. Clinicopathological study of pancreatic carcinoma with particular reference to the invasion of the extrapancreatic neural plexus. Int J Pancreatol 1991;10:105–111.
37. Yoshioka H, Wakabayashi T. Pancreatic nerve plexus (in Japanese). Operation 1957;11:849–857.
38. Japan Society for Cancer Therapy, General rules for reporting clinical oncology (JSCT general rules) (in Japanese). Tokyo: Kanehara, 1991.
39. Cubilla AL, Fortner JG, Fitzgerald PJ. Lymph node involvement in carcinoma of the head of the pancreas area. Cancer 1978;41:880–887.
40. Nakao A, Takeda N, Kasuga T. Significance of dissection of paraaortic lymph nodes in pancreatic cancer (in Japanese). Jpn J Surg Assoc 1990;21:23–26.
41. Evans BP, Ochsner A. The gross anatomy of the lymphatics of the human pancreas. Surgery 1954;36:177–191.
42. Nagai H. Involvement of paraaortic lymph nodes by pancreatic cancer and its lymphatic flow. Jpn J Surg 1987;88:308–317.
43. Deki H, Sato T. An anatomic study of the peripancreatic lymphatic. Surg Radiol Anat 1988;10:121–135.
44. Nagakawa T, Kobayashi H, Ueno K, Ohta T, Kayahara M, Miyazai I. Clinical study of lymphatic flow ot the paraaortic lymph nodes in carcinoma of the head of the pancreas. Cancer 1994;73:1155–1162.
45. Nagakawa T, Kobayashi H, Ueno K, Ohta T, Kayahara M, et al. The pattern of lymph node involvement in carcinoma of the head of the pancreas. Int J Pancreatol 1993;13:15–22.
46. Kayahara M, Nagakawa T, Kobayashi H, Mori K, Nakano T, et al. Lymphatic flow in carcinoma of the head of the pancreas. Cancer 1992;70:2061.
47. Nakao A, Nonami T, Harada A, Kasuga T, Takagi H. Portal vein resection is a new antithrombogenic catheter. Surgery 1990;108: 913–918.
48. Van Heerden JA. Pancreatic resection for carcinoma of the pancreas: Whipple versus total pancreatectomy—an institutional perspective. World J Surg 1984;8:880–888.
49. Traverso LW, Longmire WP Jr. Preservation of the pylorus in pancreaticoduodenectomy. Surg Gynecol Obstet 1978;146: 959–962.
50. Appleby LH. The celiac axis in the expansion of the operation for gastric carcinoma. Cancer 1953;6:704–707.

# 57

# Total Pancreatectomy

A. R. Moossa and Ingemar Ihse

***The feasibility of an operation is not an indication for its performance***
Lord Cohen of Birkenhead

In many ways, the development, evolution, and subsequent abandonment of total pancreatectomy parallels closely the earlier historic fate of total gastrectomy. The complete extirpation of both organs was at first thought to be incompatible with life. As time passed, the second quarter of this century witnessed major pioneering scientific and technical advances in all branches of surgery and in other clinical disciplines. Total resection of both organs became commonplace, but such radical operations were reserved for very advanced tumors with high mortality and morbidity. The operations were next performed more widely for various benign and malignant conditions with gradually decreasing operative risks. By the early 1970s, our understanding of the resulting derangements in upper gastrointestinal physiology and in metabolic processes combined with multiple advances in anesthesia, blood banking, and intensive care monitoring, have led to a more realistic, conservative, and selective approach to radical operations on both organs.

As early as 1908, Sauve reviewed the literature on major pancreatic resection (1). He quoted Mayo Robson who, in 1901, credited the first near-total pancreatectomy to Billroth in 1884. The exact extent of the resection and the end result were never documented. Frank in 1900 also performed an extensive pancreatectomy for pancreatic cancer, preserving only a minute rim of the gland with the duodenum. The patient succumbed 6 months later from recurrent cancer (1). The first authenticated total pancreatectomy was performed by Rockey, but the patient died 2 weeks postoperatively from a disruption of the ligated common bile duct (2). The first long-term survivor after total pancreatectomy is attributed to Priestly et al., who performed the operation for insulinoma in 1942 and reported it in 1944 (3). The patient eventually survived for 29 years (4). This report was the impetus for the performance of total pancreatectomy for various benign and malignant disorders as discussed below.

Four years following the publication of Priestley et al., Gaston reviewed 16 reported cases of total pancreatectomy and added another (5); 11 had been performed for cancer, with 3 survivals, and 6 for benign disease, with 3 deaths. The difficulties of differentiating chronic pancreatitis from cancer were emphasized in 1952 (6), and by 1966, more than 150 successful total pancreatectomies were reported in the literature. Refinement in the technical aspects of the operation continues to this day.

In 1966, Warren recommended the procedure exclusively for patients with end-stage chronic pancreatitis who have disabling symptoms, complete destruction of the glandular parenchyma and multiple areas of ductal obstruction. Six of his patients were closely followed, and good results were reported in five (7). ReMine emphasized in 1970 the disadvantages of total pancreatic extirpation late in the course of chronic pancreatitis when rehabilitation from alcoholism and drug addiction is nearly impossible. His Mayo Clinic series of 36 total pancreatectomies included only 3 patients with benign disease. All three did poorly, two dying within 1 year from hypoglycemia and the third dying 8 years later from massive upper gastrointestinal bleeding (8).

By 1978, Braasch was able to find only 53 instances of total pancreatectomy performed for chronic pancreatitis and added the Lahey Clinic series of 26 patients. There was no operative mortality in his series, but early and late morbidity as well as late deaths were appreciable. There were 12 late deaths, and all patients had difficulty with blood sugar control. Pain relief was considered good, but 3 of the 14 surviving patients were still taking narcotic drugs (9).

In current practice in the 1990s, both the absolute and relative indications for total pancreatectomy are few and have been relegated to special circumstances, depending on the clinical situation and the surgeon's philosophy and personal bias. Total pancreatectomy, as discussed in this chapter, implies excision en bloc of the whole gland, duodenum, distal bile duct, including the gallbladder and cystic duct, distal stomach, spleen, and greater omentum. Depending on the indication, regional lymphadenectomy, soft tissue excision, and skeletonization of the major vessels can also be performed. Technical modifications include pyloric preservation, duodenal preservation, and splenic preservation.

## TOTAL PANCREATECTOMY FOR MALIGNANT TUMORS OF THE PANCREAS

In 1954, Ross was the first to make a strong plea for total pancreatectomy for cancer of the head of the pancreas on the basis of the multicentricity of the tumor (10). By 1958, Milton Porter, from Whipple's institution, had become the major advocate of the operation (11). Two years later, Howard and Jordan published a collective series of total pancreatectomies performed at various institutions by a large number of surgeons and reported a mortality of 37% (12). The impact of this review was such that total pancreatectomy was discarded as an option for nearly a decade; even though, in 1966, Collins et al. emphasized the rationale for total pancreatectomy as the ideal treatment for cancer in the head of the pancreas (13).

The advantages of total pancreatectomy over the Whipple operation for ductal adenocarcinoma of the head of the pancreas are largely theoretic, but nonetheless rational, in spite of the fact that they have not been subjected to statistical validation. The arguments for (pros) and against (cons) total pancreatectomy can be summarized under the following six headings.

#### Multicentricity of Pancreatic Cancer?

***Pros.*** It is reasonable to assume that all ducts within the gland are exposed to the same carcinogenic stimuli. The bulk of experimental, clinical, and pathologic evidence substantiates the theory that cancer of the pancreas, like cancer in many other organs, is potentially multifocal in origin. Careful histologic evaluation of the entire gland following its removal, has revealed multicentric and/or multifocal carcinoma in 16 to 37% of cases (14). Ductal epithelial hyperplasia has been identified in 41% of 141 pancreatic cancer specimens. In four of them, papillary hyperplasia, carcinoma in situ, and invasive carcinoma were found together in the same gland. These data must be compared with the results of routine autopsy examination of 150 pancreatic specimens in which only 9% were found to have ductal hyperplasia (15). Ihse et al. found tumor cells far from the main lesion in 16% of a series of 58 patients with ductal pancreatic cancer in the head of the gland (16). Van Heerden et al. claimed "unequivocal multicentricity" in 29 of 89 patients (33%) (17). Brooks et al. demonstrated tumor foci in the body and tail, free-floating tumor cells in the main pancreatic duct, or tumor extension along the bile duct in 76% of 48 patients with cancer of the pancreatic head (18). Evidence of multicentricity has also been presented by Pliam and ReMine (19).

***Cons.*** In a pain-staking study of 37 total pancreatectomy specimens, Kloppel et al. did not find any real multicentric foci outside the tumor, although there was continuous tumor growth throughout the whole pancreatic duct in two patients (20). Similarly, Motojima et al., using a polymerase chain reaction technique, found multiple mutations in the K-*ras* gene in only 3 of 53 patients with pancreatic cancer, giving strong evidence that multicentric disease exists but at a much lower rate than previously reported (21). Thus, since multicentricity seems to be much less common than previously anticipated, it can no longer be advanced as a strong argument for total pancreatectomy for cancer of the pancreatic head. In addition, it must also be admitted that the natural history and rate of progression of these histologic, dysplastic changes seen in the body and tail of the gland are totally unknown; hence, it is impossible to predict how long it will take for these microscopic changes to evolve into a frankly invasive cancer.

#### More Extensive Lymphadenectomy When the Total Gland is Removed?

***Pros.*** The average number of nodes removed after total pancreatectomy, as reported by Fortner et al., was 48, compared with 28 after a Whipple resection (22).

***Cons.*** It has lately been shown that it is possible to achieve an extensive regional lymphadenectomy, soft-tissue excision, and skeletonization of the vessels, and even partial excision of the portal vein–superior mesenteric vein (PV-SMV) axis, by doing a partial pancreatoduodenectomy of the Whipple type (23, 24). This is currently being practiced more and more at various centers.

#### Decreased Risk of Tumor Growth at the Resection Margin?

***Pros.*** A reason for choosing total pancreatectomy is the risk of leaving tumor tissue at the pancreatic transection margin when a classical Whipple resection is performed. The theoretic possibility of cancer spread by direct extension, intraductal seeding, and lymphatic permeation, therefore, has to be considered. Malignant changes have been demonstrated grossly or histologically at the line of transection of the gland after a partial pancreatectomy of the Whipple type. A positive pancreatic margin is estimated to occur in 14 to 20% (25, 26). In a recent retrospective survey, Willett et al. reported tumor extension to the pancreatic resection margin in 14 of 72 patients who underwent a standard Whipple procedure for cancer of the pancreatic head (26). Malignant viable cells are often present in the obstructed ductal system and, if the gland is transected, may be the source of seeding for local recurrence. Subtle forms of multicentricity or spread are not always readily appreciated at operation, since they can be grossly invisible and impalpable. The average surgical pathologist may have difficulty in providing a frozen-section histologic answer on the surgical margins intraoperatively. Operative indecision and confusion over the exact site of pancreatic transection as well as other time-consuming diagnostic maneuvers are totally eliminated by a total pancreatectomy.

***Cons.*** The true risk of a positive resection margin at the site of glandular transection is probably much smaller than is feared on theoretic grounds. Recently, Trede reported that of 259 Whipple resections, only 3 instances were found to have unexpected tumor growth at the line of resection in spite of routine frozen-section examination of the pancreatic margin (27). Further, local recurrence postoperatively seems to be more frequent in the peripancreatic tissues than in the pancreatic margin itself, as ascertained by autopsy studies. An acceptable alternative to total pancreatectomy is a subtotal resection removing all but 5 to 7 cm of the pancreatic tail, thereby reducing the risk of tumor extension to the resection margin (16).

#### Decrease of Complications Emanating from the Pancreatic Remnant?

***Pros.*** The severity and frequency of complications are anticipated to decrease with performance of a total pancreatectomy, since the need for a pancreatojejunal anastomosis is eliminated. This abolishes the risk of postoperative pancreatitis and the likelihood of pancreatojejunal anastomotic leakage, which can lead to postoperative morbidity and mortality. As far as can be ascertained from the literature, the cause of death in about 40% of patients who underwent a Whipple resection in the 1960s and early 1970s was related to problems with the pancreatojejunal anastomosis (28).

***Cons.*** However, pancreatojejunal anastomosis is no longer the true Achilles' heel of the operation. Our technical ability to avoid complications of a pancreatojejunal anastomosis has improved substantially over the last 10 to 15 years. In addition, a minor pancreatojejunal leak can easily be managed conservatively by a combination of percutaneous drainage by interventional radiology, antibiotics, Sandostatin, and TPN or jejunal feeding. The mortality rate of pancreatojejunal fistula is very low indeed, and it is highly unusual to have to reoperate on a patient and excise the pancreatic remnant. The risk of postoperative pancreatitis is now so low that many publications do not mention it. Warren et al. reported four cases of pancreatitis after 348 Whipple resections (1%) (29); Neoptolemos et al. had one case in 24 consecutive patients (30); and Trede et al. report 1 case in 233 (5%) (28).

#### Postoperative Diabetes Mellitus?

***Pros.*** The fear of inducing diabetes mellitus by total pancreatectomy is somewhat irrational, since at least 30% of all patients with pancreatic cancer are already diabetic at presentation, and another 40 to 50% have an abnormal glucose tolerance curve, as defined by the American Diabetic Association age-adjustment criteria (31).

Irrespective of the technique of pancreatojejunal anastomosis performed, there is a high incidence of both exocrine and endocrine pancreatic insufficiency following the Whipple procedure. The exocrine benefit of any remaining pancreatic tissue after a Whipple operation is often transient, variable, and doubtful, since many pancreatojejunostomies stenose after a variable period. Thus, preservation of the endocrine and exocrine function of the pancreatic remnant does not, by itself, justify leaving some pancreatic tissue behind.

***Cons.*** Total pancreatic extirpation ensures both exocrine and endocrine insufficiency in 100% of cases. While the malabsorption of fat can be controlled by ingestion of enzyme supplements, the diabetes mellitus is sometimes difficult to manage. Andren-Sanberg and Ihse reported 2 patients in a series of 86 who succumbed from hypoglycemia, one while still in the hospital, the other 2 weeks after discharge (32). Grace et al. had one fatality from hypoglycemia among 22 totally pancreatectomized patients (33). Moossa et al. admit to one death from accidental insulin overdose several years after total pancreatectomy (34).

### Is the End Result of Total Pancreatectomy Superior to that of the Whipple Operation for Cancer of the Head of the Pancreas?

***Pros.*** In selected hands, total pancreatectomy produced better survival than the Whipple operation in the 1970s and early 1980s. Brooks, Manabe, Moossa, Moreno-Gonzales, ReMine, all advocated total pancreatectomy in the 1970s as a superior operation (18, 19, 35, 36). Admittedly, their patients were carefully selected on the basis of both functional status and tumor stage. The disparity in reported results from other centers has been largely due to two factors: *(a)* many surgeons abandoned total pancreatectomy after a few early anecdotal adverse experiences with poor results, and *(b)* the operation was reserved for advanced cancers.

Brooks and Culebras pointed out that the results of total pancreatectomy are best when the operation is reserved for stage I and II cancers of the head of the gland (18). The reported increased risk of stomal ulceration after total pancreatectomy is now only of historic interest with the advent of excellent measures, including $H_2$-receptor antagonists and proton pump inhibitors, for controlling gastric acid secretion.

Added to all the above arguments is the admitted prejudice of many surgeons against removing only part of an organ harboring a lethal cancer, since this violates the classical Halstedian surgical oncologic principles.

***Cons.*** Reviews of large retrospective institutional series have failed to demonstrate any survival benefit to total pancreatectomy, compared with the Whipple operation (17). In addition, the results of the Whipple operation have consistently improved over the past two decades, which has abolished many of the indications to extirpate the entire gland (27). If microscopic residual disease is suspected on the basis of pathologic examination of the resected Whipple specimen, as is exhibited by histologic extrapancreatic invasion or nodal invasion, postoperative adjuvant radiotherapy with 5-fluorouracil as a radiosensitizer can be administered and is usually beneficial (37).

## RECOMMENDATIONS FOR CANCER OF THE HEAD OF THE PANCREAS

A rational and sensible compromise in the 1990s is to advocate the following guidelines.

The Whipple resection is the first option for cancer of the head of the gland and periampullary region. To ensure a safe pancreatic margin, the gland should be transected routinely well to the left of its neck, into the proximal body. If tumor extension is suspected at this level of transection, a further 3 to 4 cm of the pancreatic body can be additionally excised. This concept of some pancreatic tissue is attractive, since it decreases the exquisite insulin sensitivity seen in many totally pancreatectomized patients.

Total pancreatectomy is reserved for specific instances such as

1. When the patient is a long-standing insulin-requiring diabetic
2. When there is obvious tumor growth along the main pancreatic duct
3. When the pancreatic remnant is soft and friable and does not hold sutures
4. When a postoperative pancreatojejunal leak cannot be controlled in the early postoperative period

## TOTAL PANCREATECTOMY FOR OTHER TUMORS OF THE PANCREAS

One is rarely called upon to resect a cancer in the body and tail of the pancreas, since ductal adenocarcinoma is usually too advanced at the time of diagnosis. However, if a palliative resection can be used to obtain an exact tissue diagnosis and to palliate the patient, a distal pancreatectomy with splenectomy is usually adequate.

Cystadenoma, cystadenocarcinoma, sarcoma, and apudoma, are all usually confined to one area of the gland and can, in most instances, be dealt with by a partial pancreatectomy. However occasionally, when hyperinsulinism has not been controlled by a distal pancreatectomy and when no discrete tumor can be identified at operation or in the pathologic specimen, a total pancreatectomy is required. In rare instances, a giant cystadenocarcinoma or sarcoma occupies the entire gland and is so extensive that its complete resection can only be achieved by a total pancreatoduodenectomy

### Selection of the Patient and Tumor

As total pancreatectomy is a major operation, a careful evaluation of the patient's general condition is essential. Chronologic age does not seem to matter, but the functional status of the patient and the presence or absence of comorbid factors provides an indication of the operative risk. Careful assessment of cardiopulmonary function and renal function are important. Preoperative correction of blood and fluid deficiencies is highly advisable. Administration of vitamin K is essential for all jaundiced patients. We believe in a 2-day bowel preparation consisting of a clear liquid diet, laxatives, enemas, and/or nonabsorbable oral antibiotics. We routinely administer prophylactic systemic, broad-spectrum antibiotics in the perioperative period.

There is uniform agreement that total pancreatectomy, if used, should be restricted to pancreatic cancer that is potentially curable. This implies that there must be no obvious detectable spread outside the immediate region of the gland. We do not knowingly perform total pancreatectomy for palliation, although this is what we may achieve in many instances. Invasion of the duodenum or distal common bile duct does not seem to influence the prognosis. The presence of a positive regional node per se is not an absolute criterion of unresectability, provided that it falls within the field of resection. Minor invasion of the portal vein and/or superior mesenteric vein can be dealt with by excising a short segment of the vein with end-to-end anastomosis, provided it helps to achieve soft-tissue and nodal clearance. We routinely attempt to perform a regional lymphadenectomy, excision of soft-tissue in the retroperitoneum, and skeletonization of the major vessels. Major arterial excision with reconstruction is no longer recommended, since it does not improve survival and carries a prohibitive postoperative mortality and morbidity.

### Immediate Postoperative Care

Following major pancreatic resection, the patient is transferred to the surgical intensive care unit where experienced nursing and sophisticated monitoring techniques are available. The patient may require respiratory assistance for the first 12 to 24 hours. In the immediate (3–4 days) postoperative period, the patient's blood sugar is checked every 3 to 4 hours, and small doses of regular insulin (2–10 units) are given intravenously as boluses. Alternatively, a continuous intravenous infusion of insulin adequate to maintain the blood sugar between 100 and 200 mg/100 mL can be given. During this early postoperative period when fluid shifts are in a prominent phase and absorption is unpredictable, subcutaneous or intramuscular administration should be discouraged.

### Postoperative Complications

Hemorrhage is still the most common intraoperative and postoperative complication encountered with total pancreatectomy, although the incidence is now well under 5% in our hands. Meticulous preoperative preparation and adequate replacement of blood and clotting factors during the operation are essential. All vessels must be carefully ligated. All vascular areas must be checked for hemostasis before the gastrojejunal and hepaticojejunal anastomosis is performed.

In spite of these precautions, blood may ooze at a fairly alarming rate from the drainage sites during the first 24 hours. Reoperation is mandatory if there is reason to suspect a major bleeding site or when clot accumulation in the abdomen causes distention or tamponade, and/or when a consumption coagulopathy is recognized. In the last situation, one never finds a discrete bleeding point at reoperation. The clots are gently evacuated, and the whole abdomen is irrigated prior to reclosure with drainage.

Gastrointestinal bleeding and intraabdominal sepsis are also well-recognized complications. Other events that may also be fatal include multiorgan failure, mesenteric thrombosis, uremia, liver failure, myocardial infarction, cerebrovascular accident, congestive heart failure, and pulmonary embolism.

Biliary-enteric disruption and leakage from the gastrojejunostomy are very rare and should not occur; they are largely preventable by careful and proper construction of both anastomoses. Other complications that are usually nonfatal include pneumonitis, gastric retention, paralytic ileus, bowel obstruction, wound infection, wound dehiscence, cardiac arrhythmias, fecal fistula, and gastrojejunocolic fistula.

The frequency of postoperative complications varies between different reported series, probably because different populations have different comorbid factors, and possibly because all complications are not always recorded or reported. Thus, it is difficult to compare complication rates between different institutions. In their first published series on total pancreatectomy, Ihse et al. recognized postoperative complications in 46% of 65 patients (38). Edis et al., from the Mayo Clinic, reported a frequency of 55% in their 38 patients (39). Launois et al. recently presented a series of 47 patients who underwent total pancreatectomy with a complication rate of 53% (40). On the other hand, Brooks et al. reported that 27% of their 48 patients suffered postoperative complications (14). Another factor that makes evaluation of the literature difficult is that very often a given patient has more than one complication. This is not always made clear in the reports.

### Operative Mortality of Total Pancreatectomy for Pancreatic Cancer

In 1953, Cattell and Pyrtek collected 33 cases of total pancreatoduodenectomy and reported operative mortalities of 43.5% for malignant disease and 20% for benign disease (41). By 1968, Warren et al. reviewed 6 patients who underwent total pancreatectomy for cancer during the period 1942–1965, inclusive (42). One died in the postoperative period and the others were dead within 1 year, with a mean survival of 8 months. This led Warren to conclude that "such results make it unlikely that this operation is justified for ductal carcinoma of the pancreas, except in the most unusual circumstances. It probably should be reserved for massive cystadenocarcinomas on large islet cell tumors."

The operative mortality following total pancreatectomy for cancer in an early published series was an average of 23% in a total of 293 operations (43). This is almost identical to the 22% in the collective series by Connolly et al. based on 762 Whipple procedures and the 22% reported by Gudjonsson et al. for 1162 resected patients (44, 45). However, these reports are largely of historic interest. As reported lately from several centers, emphasizing a decreased operative mortality for Whipple resection, there has also been a simultaneous dramatic decrease of hospital mortality after total pancreatectomy. In recent years, the operative mortality after total pancreatectomy is in the region of 1 to 2% in experienced hands.

### Long-Term Survival

In a recent patient series comprising 240 totally pancreatectomized patients, the 5-year survival averaged 5% (16). This is comparable to the cumulative experience after pancreatoduodenectomy as reported by Connolly et al. (44). These authors found 27 5-year survivors among 455 patients with cancer of the head of the pancreas, an average 5-year survival of 6%. Again, these data reflect the results of large institutional series analyzing patients with all stages of cancer and involving numerous surgeons with different experience and expertise.

Recently, improved 5-year survival has been reported following Whipple pancreatoduodenectomy, with or without extended lymph node dissection (23–25, 27, 33, 35, 36). Similar data, however, have not yet been reported for total pancreatectomy, but in a carefully selected series of patients, this senior author has a 5-year survival of 21%. In institutions where both operations have been practiced, no statistical difference in survival has been found between the two operations. It is highly unlikely that a prospective randomized study could ever be organized to answer this question, but we have to conclude that long-term survival in pancreatic cancer is not totally dependent on whether a Whipple operation or total pancreatectomy is done, but depends on such other factors as the stage of the tumor, the biologic behavior of the tumor, the surgeon's experience and expertise with the operation, and the functional status of the patient.

## THE PLACE OF TOTAL PANCREATECTOMY IN THE TREATMENT OF CHRONIC PANCREATITIS

As discussed above, in the late 1970s and early 1980s, American surgeons were appropriately cautious and rather timid about advocating total pancreatectomy for chronic pancreatitis. However, European schools, especially in Germany, gained a wider experience in the surgical management of chronic pancreatitis, largely because an increased incidence of disease resulted from changing socioeconomic conditions and increasing alcoholism. In 1981, Gall and his team from Erlangen reported a series of 63 total pancreatectomies performed between 1972 and 1977 (46). Most of their cases were due to chronic alcoholism. Their operative mortality was high (21%) compared with that of Whipple's pancreatoduodenectomy (8%) at that time. Their morbidity was also high; 75% of their patients had problems controlling their blood sugar. Their late mortality was 19%, compared with the 20% late mortality of pancreatoduodenectomy for the same disease.

The wide range in the postoperative mortality from total pancreatectomy in different centers across the world is easily explained by differences in selection criteria. However, the late morbidity and high mortality found in the Lahey Clinic, the Erlangen, and the Chicago experiences confirmed many fears that were voiced in earlier reports (9, 46, 47).

Strumm and Spiro, in 1980, looked carefully at the natural history of chronic pancreatitis and emphasized that the nonoperative treatment of chronic alcoholic pancreatitis is also associated with a late mortality of at least 30% (48). This suggests that the complications of the disease, the psychosocial personality of the patient, and the devastations induced by alcoholism and drug addiction are themselves associated with a poor outcome. The questions remain whether an operation is ever indicated to improve this outcome and whether it is justified for such a high-risk group of patients with a disease that is histologically benign but has a clinically malignant outcome. Currently, in the era of managed care and cost-containment, several health care organizations now give chronic alcoholic pancreatitis a low priority. Many believe that the cost of surgical intervention or even medical care is difficult to justify in a period of diminishing resources (49).

In theory, total pancreatectomy, which ensures the complete ablation of pancreatic tissues, is the only logical operation for chronic pancreatitis. However, because of the multiple medical and psychosocial problems associated with the disease and the metabolic derangements induced by the operation, total pancreatectomy is likely to be the operation of last resort. The operation can only be justified in selected individuals who fulfill strict criteria as described below. In addition, the operation should be performed by a surgeon experienced with the disease and in pancreatic surgery who also has a team interested in managing these complicated patients for a long time. It has been rightly said that total pancreatectomy for chronic pancreatitis fails for four major reasons:

1. The operation is performed too early. The patient still has residual pancreatic exocrine and endocrine function that has to be sacrificed. Conversion of a dependent alcoholic drug addict into an insulin-requiring diabetic is likely to be fatal.
2. The operation is performed too late, when the patient is already a fully entrenched drug addict and a dependent alcoholic.
3. The patient does not have the resources—financial, intellectual, family, backup, etc.—to aid in rehabilitation.
4. The surgeon does not have a substantial interest and expertise in the problem.

Thus, the indications for total pancreatectomy in chronic pancreatitis include:

1. Failure of a Puestow-like procedure or a partial pancreatectomy or pancreatoduodenectomy to control pain
2. Total destruction of the gland without any substantial ductal dilatation
3. Suspicion of cancer in a background of end-stage chronic pancreatitis

Careful assessment and selection of each individual patient is paramount. We believe that total pancreatectomy should rarely, if ever, be performed in patients who have neither overt endocrine nor exocrine insufficiency. Patients must have truly failed all attempts at conservative therapy, including percutaneous celiac nerve blocks to control pain. They must be willing to undergo a program of rehabilitation from alcoholism and narcotic drug addiction. This rehabilitation must be planned and started at least a few weeks prior to operation, to see if they can be compliant or not. All resources, including Alcoholics Anonymous, psychotherapy, and family members, can be usefully involved in the rehabilitation program. Full psychologic assessment is often necessary. The social background, including level of education and understanding and the environment to which they will return must be assessed. Patients must have ready access to adequate medical support. They must not have many comorbid factors such as major impairment of cardiovascular, pulmonary, or renal function. Total pancreatectomy for chronic pancreatitis should never be performed in the absence of pain or suspicion of cancer (50).

### Technical Aspects

Any major resection for chronic pancreatitis is likely to be technically challenging for the surgeon and hazardous for the patient. Chronic or recurrent pancreatic or peripancreatic inflammation results in the fibrotic pancreatic parenchyma being embedded in a cementlike retroperitoneum, which makes delineation of tissue planes and dissection very tedious and time consuming. Involvement of adjacent structures creates further technical problems. These include biliary obstruction, duodenal occlusion, splenic vein occlusion leading to left-sided portal hypertension and splenomegaly, portal vein–superior mesenteric vein (PV-SMV) occlusion leading to more generalized portal hypertension, and pseudoaneurysms of the foregut or midgut vessels. Thus, the surgeon must be aware of where the hazards and the pitfalls are.

1. Intraoperative hemorrhage is the biggest single danger during the operation. The vessels are often embedded in the peripancreatic inflammatory tissue, which renders them vulnerable. In addition, distinct periadventitial planes are often obliterated. Control of bleeding and avoidance of major vessel tears are of paramount importance. The major veins can then be especially troublesome. Unroofing the neck of the pancreas from an adherent PV-SMV axis can be a slow, arduous, and dangerous task. Bleeding from the veins can be aggravated by coexistence of portal hypertension and the development of retroperitoneal collaterals.
2. In the setting of advanced chronic pancreatitis, splenic preservation is rarely desirable or possible. It should never be done in the presence of left-sided portal hypertension.
3. If a pylorus-preserving pancreatoduodenectomy is envisaged, the gastroduodenal artery and the right gastric artery should be preserved.
4. If a duodenum-preserving pancreatoduodenectomy is planned, a Kocher maneuver should not be performed early in the course of the dissection. Preservation of the duodenum should not be attempted when there is evidence of duodenal and/or distal common bile ductal occlusion.

Thus, in our opinion, total pancreatectomy should be confined to end-stage chronic pancreatitis with *(a)* the highly selected patient who can be rehabilitated; *(b)* the surgeon who has interest, experience, skill, and expertise with these potentially difficult operations; and *(c)* specialized centers that have the resources to manage these patients.

## LONG-TERM MANAGEMENT OF THE TOTALLY PANCREATECTOMIZED PATIENT

Long-term management of the totally pancreatectomized patient is best performed by keeping it simple and by educating the patient, the relatives, and the primary physician about the resulting metabolic derangements. It must be understood that *hypo*glycemia is the danger, and the patient must never miss meals. Totally pancreatectomized patients are often exquisitely sensitive to insulin. An occasional *hyper*glycemia or glycosuria is totally acceptable. Patients must be instructed to eat frequent small meals regularly. The diet must have a low-fat content and a high-carbohydrate and high-protein content. Patients must take regular enzyme supplements with each meal and check their blood sugar or urine fractionals at least twice daily. They should use a combination of regular and long-acting insulin, given as one injection in the morning; some patients will need an additional injection of a low-dose of regular insulin toward the end of the day. Patients must carry sugar at all times and must be instructed to take sugar if any untoward symptom such as dizziness, confusion, drowsiness, sweatiness, tachycardia, or weakness, develops. It is sometimes useful to allow patients to have one or two hypoglycemic attacks while in-hospital, so they can see that these symptoms are alleviated by taking adequate sugar. These principles and warnings must be reiterated to patients and relatives at each clinic visit.

## CONCLUSIONS

Total pancreatectomy for malignant disease of the gland or for end-stage chronic pancreatitis, is not a universal panacea. Critical evaluation of the published literature shows that for both benign and malignant disorders, there has been (quite rightly) a tendency to allocate patients to treatment groups on the basis of multiple factors, such as age and fitness of the patient, stage of disease, and the surgeon's personal preference. The small number of patients who are operated on with malignant disease that is still at a curative stage and of chronic pancreatitis patients who can still be rehabilitated makes further interpretation difficult. Statistical analysis of large retrospective series of noncomparable and sometimes incomprehensible data is not always helpful in the management of the individual patient but is often offered to give validity to some preconceived thesis.

Irrespective of the surgeon's bias, total pancreatectomy for benign or malignant disease has a small but definite place in highly selected patients, with careful attention to details in the preoperative preparation, the technical performance of the operation, and the postoperative management of the patient.

## REFERENCES


1. Sauve L. Des pancreatectomies et specialement de la pancreatectomie cephalique. Rev Chir 1908;37:113–152.
2. Rockey EW. Total pancreatectomy for carcinoma: a case report. Ann Surg 1943;118:603–611.
3. Priestley JT, Comfort MW, Radcliffe J Jr. Total pancreatectomy for hyperinsulinism due to islet cell adenoma. Survival and cure at 16 months after operation. Ann Surg 1944;119:211–221.
4. Van Heerden JA. The first total pancreatectomy. Ann Surg 1986;207:39–47.
5. Gaston EA. Total pancreatectomy. N Engl J Med 1948;238:345–354.
6. Gourevitch A, Whitfield AGW. Total pancreatectomy. Br J Surg 1952;40:104–107.
7. Warren KW, Poulantzas JK, Kune GA. Life after total pancreatectomy for pancreatitis; Ann Surg 1966;164:830–834.
8. ReMine WH, Priestley JT, Judd ES, et al. Total pancreatectomy. Ann Surg 1970;172:595–604.
9. Braasch JW, Vito L, Nugent FW. Total pancreatectomy for end-stage pancreatitis. Ann Surg 1978;188:317–322.
10. Ross DE. Cancer of the pancreas: a plea for total pancreatectomy. Am J Surg 1954;87:20–33.
11. Porter MR. Carcinoma of the pancreaticoduodenal area: resectability and choice of procedure. Ann Surg 1958;148:711–724.
12. Howard JM, Jordan GL Jr. Surgical diseases of the pancreas. Philadelphia: JB Lippincott, 1960.
13. Collins JJ, Craighead JE, Brookes J. The rationale for total pancreatectomy for carcinoma of the pancreatic head. N Engl J Med 1966;274:599–602.
14. Brooks JR, Brooks DC, Levine JD. Total pancreatectomy for ductal cell carcinoma of the pancreas—an update. Ann Surg 1989;209:405–410.
15. Sommers SC, Murphy SA, Warren S. Pancreatic duct hyperplasia and cancer. Gastroenterology 1954;27:629–632.
16. Ihse I, Andren-Sandberg A, Anderson R, et al. The role of total pancreatectomy in pancreatic cancer. J Hepatopancreatobiliary Surg 1994;1:546–551.
17. Van Heerden JA, McIlrath DC, Ilstrup M, et al. Total pancreatectomy for ductal adenocarcinoma of the pancreas: an update. World J Surg 1988;12:658–662.
18. Brooks JR, Culebras JM. Cancer of the pancreas: palliative operation, Whipple procedure or total pancreatectomy? Am J Surg 1996;186:416–420.
19. Pliam MB, ReMine WH. Further evaluation of total pancreatectomy. Arch Surg 1975;110:506–511.
20. Kloppel G, Lohse T, Bosselt K, et al. Ductal adenocarcinoma of the head of the pancreas: incidence of tumor involvement beyond the Whipple resection line: histologic and immunocytochemical analysis of 37 total pancreatectomy specimens. Pancreas 1983;2:170–175.
21. Motojima K, Urano R, Nagata Y, et al. Detection of point mutations in the Kirsten-ras oncogene provides evidence for the multicentricity of pancreatic carcinoma. Ann Surg 1993;217:138–143.
22. Fortner JG, Kimn DK, Cubilla A, et al. Regional pancreatectomy—en bloc pancreatic, portal vein, and lymph node resection. Ann Surg 1997;186:42–49.
23. Ishikawa O, Ohhigash H, Sasaki Y, et al. Practical usefulness of lymphatic and connective tissue clearance for carcinoma of the pancreatic head. Ann Surg 1988;208:215–220.
24. Ishikawa O, Ohhigashi H, Imaoka S, et al. Operative indications for external pancreatectomy for locally advanced pancreas cancer involving the portal vein. Ann Surg 1992;215:231–236.
25. Cameron JL, Crist DW, Sitzman JW, et al. Factors influencing survival after pancreaticoduodenectomy for pancreatic cancer. Ann Surg 1991;161:120–125.
26. Willett CG, Lewandrowski K, Warshaw AL, et al. Resection margins in carcinoma of the head of the pancreas: implications for radiation therapy. Ann Surg 1993;217:144–148.
27. Trede M. The surgical options. In: Trede M, Carter DC, eds. Surgery of the pancreas. Edinburgh: Churchill Livingstone, 1993:433–442.
28. Trede M, Schwall G. The complications of pancreatectomy. Ann Surg 1988;207:39–47.
29. Warren KW, Choe DS, Plaza J, et al. Regrets of resection for periampullary cancer. Ann Surg 1975;181:534–540.
30. Neoptolemos JP, Talbott IC, Carr-Locke DL, et al. Treatment and outcome in 52 consecutive cases of ampullary carcinoma. Br J Surg 1987;74:954–961.
31. Schwartz SS, Zeidler A, Moossa AR, et al. A prospective study of glucose tolerance insulin, C-peptide and glucagon responses in patients with pancreatic carcinoma. Dig Dis 1978;23:1107–1114.
32. Andren-Sandberg A, Ihse I. Factors influencing survival after total pancreatectomy in patients with pancreatic cancer. Ann Surg 1983;198:605–610.
33. Grace A, Pitt HA, Tompkins RK, et al. Decreased mortality and morbidity after pancreatoduodenectomy. Am J Surg 1986;151:141–149.
34. Moossa AR, Scott MH, Lavelle-Jones M. The place of total and extended total pancreatectomy in pancreatic cancer. World J Surg 1984;8:895–899.
35. Manabe T, Oshio G, Baba N, et al. Radical pancreatectomy for ductal cell adenocarcinoma of the head of the pancreas. Cancer 1984;64:113–117.
36. Moossa AR. Tumors of the pancreas. In: Moossa AR, Schimpff SC, Robson MC, eds. Comprehensive textbook of oncology. 2nd ed. Baltimore: Williams & Wilkins, 1991:958–988.
37. Kalser MH, Allenberg S. Pancreatic cancer: adjuvant combined radiation and chemotherapy following pancreatoduodenal resection. GITSG randomized study. Arch Surg 1988;120:899–903.
38. Ihse I, Lilja P, Arnesjo B, et al. Total pancreatectomy for cancer: an appraisal of 66 cases. Ann Surg 1977;186:675–680.
39. Edis AJ, Kiernan PD, Taylor WF. Attempted curative resection of ductal carcinoma of the pancreas. Review of Mayo Clinic experience 1951–1975. Mayo Clin Proc 1980;55:531–536.
40. Launois B, Franei J, Bardazoglou E, et al. Total pancreatectomy for ductal adenocarcinoma of the pancreas with special reference to resection of the portal vein and multicentric cancer. World J Surg 1993;17:122–127.
41. Cattell RB, Pyrtek LJ. An appraisal of pancreatoduodenal resection: a follow-up study of 61 cases. Ann Surg 1949;129:840–845.
42. Warren KW, Braasch JW, Thum CR. Current problems in surgery—

diagnosis and surgical treatment of disorders of the pancreas. Chicago: Year Book Medical Publishers, 1968.
43. Cooperman AM, Herter FP, Marboe CA. Pancreatoduodenal resection and total pancreatectomy—an institutional review. Surgery 1981;90:702–712.
44. Connolly MM, Dawson PJ, Michelassi F, et al. Survival in 1001 patients with carcinoma of the pancreas. Ann Surg 1987;206: 366–373.
45. Gudjonsson B, Livstone EM, Spiro HM. Cancer of the pancreas: diagnostic accuracy and survival statistics. Cancer 1978;42:2494–2506.
46. Gall FP, Muhe E, Gebhart C. Results of partial and total pancreatectomy for chronic pancreatitis. Ann Surg 1981;194: 313–318.
47. Prinz RA, Greenlee HB. Pancreatic duct drainage in 100 patients with chronic pancreatitis. Ann Surg 1981;194:313–318.
48. Strum WB, Spiro HW. Chronic pancreatitis. Ann Intern Med 1971;74:264–277.
49. McBride G. Oregon revises health care priorities. Br Med J 1991;302:549.
50. Moossa AR. Surgical treatment of chronic pancreatitis—an overview. Br J Surg 1987;74:661–667.

# 58

# *Resection of the Distal Pancreas*

Henry A. Pitt and Isto H. Nordback

Adenocarcinoma of the pancreas occurs less frequently in the body and tail than in the head, neck, and uncinate. In most series, only approximately one-third of cancers of the pancreas arise in the body and tail (Table 58.1). Because tumors of the body and tail do not obstruct the bile duct and present with jaundice, diagnosis is delayed. As a result, the interval from onset of symptoms until diagnosis is prolonged. Therefore, tumors of the body and tail are, on average, twice as large at the time of diagnosis as are those malignancies that arise in the head and neck of the pancreas. Since most body and tail tumors are more advanced when they do present, the likelihood that resection will be possible is quite low. Nevertheless, if the diagnosis is made when the tumor is localized and not encasing the celiac axis, the superior mesenteric artery, or the portal vein, resection should be undertaken. This chapter reviews the presentation, diagnosis, staging, preoperative preparation, surgical procedures, postoperative complications, and outcome of patients with cancer in the body and tail of the pancreas.

## PRESENTATION

As with adenocarcinoma in the head of the pancreas, patients with cancer in the body and tail have a median age in the sixties (1–6). Similarly, carcinoma of the body and tail of the pancreas occurs with relatively equal distribution in men and women. However, abdominal and/or back pain is the presenting symptom in the vast majority of these patients (Table 58.2). Weight loss is also experienced by most of these patients. Approximately one-third of patients with body or tail cancers will have gastrointestinal symptoms such as nausea, anorexia, early satiety, or steatorrhea. A recent onset of diabetes mellitus or an episode of pancreatitis in an elderly patient without gallstones should raise suspicion of this diagnosis. Unfortunately, the median duration of symptoms before diagnosis is 6 months (2).

Only rarely does a tumor that arises in the body or tail of the pancreas extend far enough into the neck or head to obstruct the bile duct and cause jaundice. These extensive tumors usually encase one or more mesenteric vessels or metastasize to the liver or peritoneum and, therefore, are rarely resectable. Although a moderate percentage of these tumors occlude the splenic vein, causing left-sided portal hypertension and gastric varices, gastrointestinal bleeding is rarely a problem. Most patients have a normal physical examination. A small percentage of patients have a bruit, tenderness, an epigastric mass, or ascites.

## DIAGNOSIS

Laboratory tests also are usually normal. As mentioned above, liver function tests are rarely abnormal in these patients except when a large percentage of the liver is invaded by metastases. Mild anemia and hypoalbuminemia may be found, but the serum amylase and lipase values are usually normal. The search continues for a serum tumor marker that will be sensitive and specific enough to be useful for screening. Many carbohydrate surface antigens, oncofetal antigens, enzymes, and enzyme inhibitors as well as oncogenes have been tested. However, to date, none can accurately differentiate pancreatic cancer from other cancers or benign diseases of the pancreas.

Among the available tumor markers, CA 19-9 has been studied most extensively (7–10). Although the sensitivity and specificity of this test are not sufficient to screen asymptomatic patients, CA 19-9 should be measured in patients with unexplained epigastric or back pain, pancreatitis, or new diabetes (7). While moderate elevations (below 200) are not diagnostic, CA 19-9 levels above 200 strongly suggest pancreatic cancer (8, 9). In addition, preoperative levels may predict resectability and outcome. Moreover, a fall to a normal level after resection indicates a better prognosis, while a subsequent rise may predict recurrence many months before tumor becomes apparent clinically or on scans. Thus, CA 19-9 does have some utility in diagnosis but is more valuable for follow-up and monitoring treatment.

Noninvasive radiologic options for detecting a mass in the body or tail of the pancreas include ultrasound (US), computerized tomography (CT), or magnetic resonance imaging (MRI). US is least expensive and does not involve radiation, but complete visualization of the pancreas is not always possible because of overlying gas. In addition, the ability of US to determine resectability accurately is limited. Endoscopic ultrasound improves the accuracy of this modality but requires sedation and endoscopy and has not been proven to provide advantages over newer CT techniques. In recent years, CT has become the diagnostic test of choice for detecting a mass in the body or tail of the pancreas (Table 58.3). Moreover, with newer spiral techniques, dilation of the distal pancreatic duct, involvement of mesenteric vessels, and detection of liver metastases have become routine with spiral CT (Fig. 58.1).

Until recently, MRI has not provided any advantage over CT in the diagnosis or staging of patients with pancreatic cancer (11). Whether magnetic resonance cholangiopancreatography (MRCP) will become more accurate or cost-effective than other available tests has yet to be determined. Endoscopic retrograde cholangiopancreatography (ERCP) does not need to be performed routinely in these patients. However, the presence of an occluded pancreatic duct in a patient with pain and an equivocal mass on CT scan may confirm the diagnosis (Fig. 58.2). Cytologic examination of cells from a stricture will establish the diagnosis, and elevated carcinoembryonic antigen (CEA) in pancreatic juice can also be used to differentiate chronic pancreatitis from cancer (12). On the other hand, measurement of CA 19-9 in pancreatic juice does not make this differentiation (13).

**TABLE 58.1. Comparison of Pancreatic Cancers by Site of Origin**

| | Head and Neck | Body and Tail |
|---|---|---|
| Frequency | Two-thirds | One-third |
| Presentation | Jaundice | Pain |
| | Pain | Weight loss |
| Size | 3–5 cm | 6–10 cm |
| Resectable | 15–25% | 8–12% |

## STAGING

If the CT scan demonstrates ascites, paracenteses should be performed, and the fluid should be sent for cytologic examination. The presence of malignant cells rules out the possibility of resection for cure. Similarly, the presence of liver lesions on CT is an indication for CT- or US-directed fine-needle aspiration (FNA) of an easily accessible liver mass. The presence of adenocarcinoma in the liver in a patient with a mass in the body or tail of the pancreas documents metastatic disease and precludes prolonged survival and the need for exploration.

In some patients without ascites or liver metastases, the extent of the tumor on CT documents vascular encasement. In these patients, FNA of the tumor should be performed to establish the diagnosis. However, involvement of the splenic artery distant from the celiac axis or the splenic vein at a distance from the portal vein does not prevent resection. On the other hand, involvement of the common hepatic artery or celiac axis or occlusion of the portal vein with multiple collaterals in the region eliminates the possibility of resection (14). Resection may still be possible in up to one-third of patients when the portal vein appears to be encased but not occluded. Therefore, when the CT scan is equivocal, angiography may help to decide whether to explore a patient or help with the focus of that exploration (Fig. 58.3). Again, whether endoscopic ultrasound is as accurate as newer spiral CT techniques in staging these patients has yet to be determined (15).

The role of laparoscopy in the staging of patients with pancreatic cancer in the body and tail also remains controversial. Laparoscopy has the advantage of detecting very small peritoneal and liver metastases that are not seen with CT scanning (16). The addition of US to laparoscopy also improves the ability to detect vascular encasement. However, accurate assessment of encasement of the celiac axis, the superior mesenteric artery, or the portal vein may be difficult even at the time of open exploration because of associated pancreatitis and a desmoid reaction. Thus, laparoscopy may be a reasonable step when CT suggests vascular encasement. If metastatic disease is detected, laparotomy can be avoided. However, if no metastases are found, laparotomy may still be required in a relatively young, healthy patient to determine whether the tumor can be resected.

**TABLE 58.2. Presentation of Carcinoma in the Body and Tail of the Pancreas**

| Symptom | Frequency |
|---|---|
| Abdominal pain | 85–90% |
| Weight loss | 50–60% |
| Nausea/vomiting | 15–20% |
| Diarrhea | 5–10% |
| Jaundice | 2–4% |
| Gastrointestinal bleeding | 2–4% |

Adapted from Nordback IH, Hruban RH, Boitnott JK, Pitt HA, Cameron JL. Carcinoma of the body and tail of the pancreas. Am J Surg 1992; 164:26–31.

In 90–95% of patients with adenocarcinoma of the body or tail of the pancreas, the tumor is unresectable because of local spread (30–40%) or distant metastases (50–65%). As outlined above, these tumors metastasize most frequently to the perito-

**TABLE 58.3. Changing Trends in the Diagnosis of Cancer of the Body/Tail of the Pancreas**

| | 1970s | 1980s |
|---|---|---|
| Computerized tomography | 61% | 99%[a] |
| Ultrasound | 68% | 66% |
| Upper gastrointestinal series | 83% | 57%[a] |
| Esophagogastroduodenoscopy | 37% | 57%[b] |
| ERCP | 17% | 33%[b] |
| Barium enema | 57% | 18%[a] |
| Angiography | 20% | 17% |
| Magnetic resonance imaging | 0% | 7% |

Adapted from Nordback IH, Hruban RH, Boitnott JK, Pitt HA, Cameron JL. Carcinoma of the body and tail of the pancreas. Am J Surg 1992; 164:26–31.

[a] $p < .01$ vs. 1970s.

[b] $p < .05$ vs. 1970s.

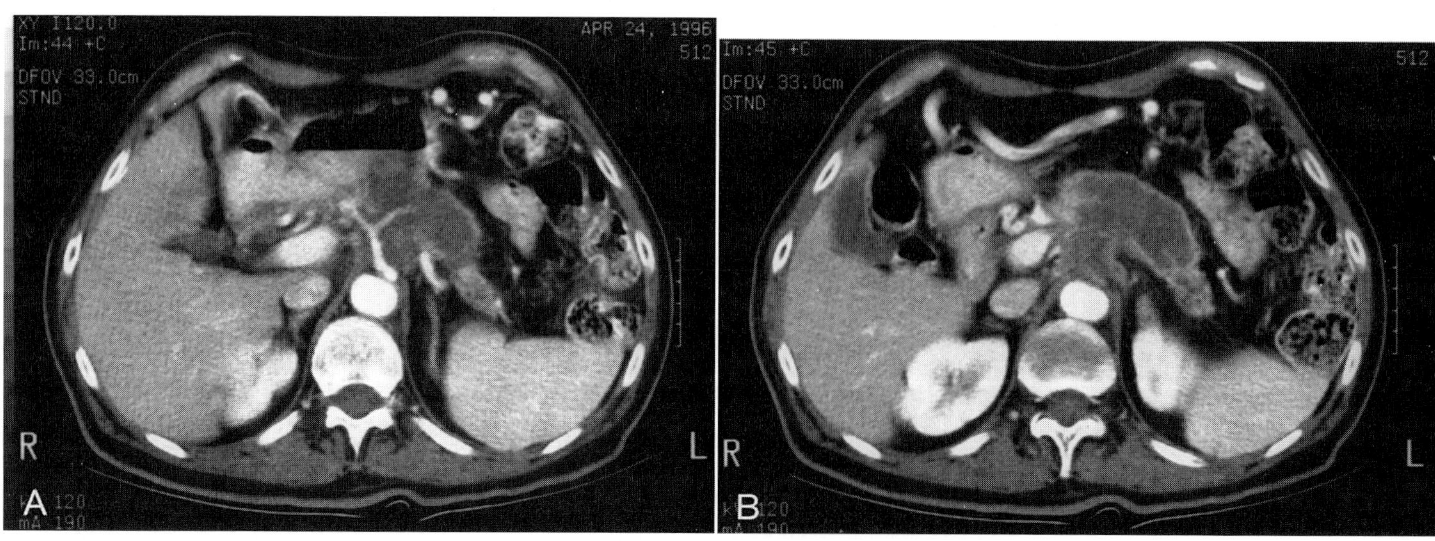


**FIG. 58.1.** **A.** CT scan demonstrating extensive tumor of the body and tail of the pancreas encasing the celiac axis. **B.** CT scan in the same patient. Note the dilated gastroepiploic vein anteriorly, indicating splenic vein occlusion.

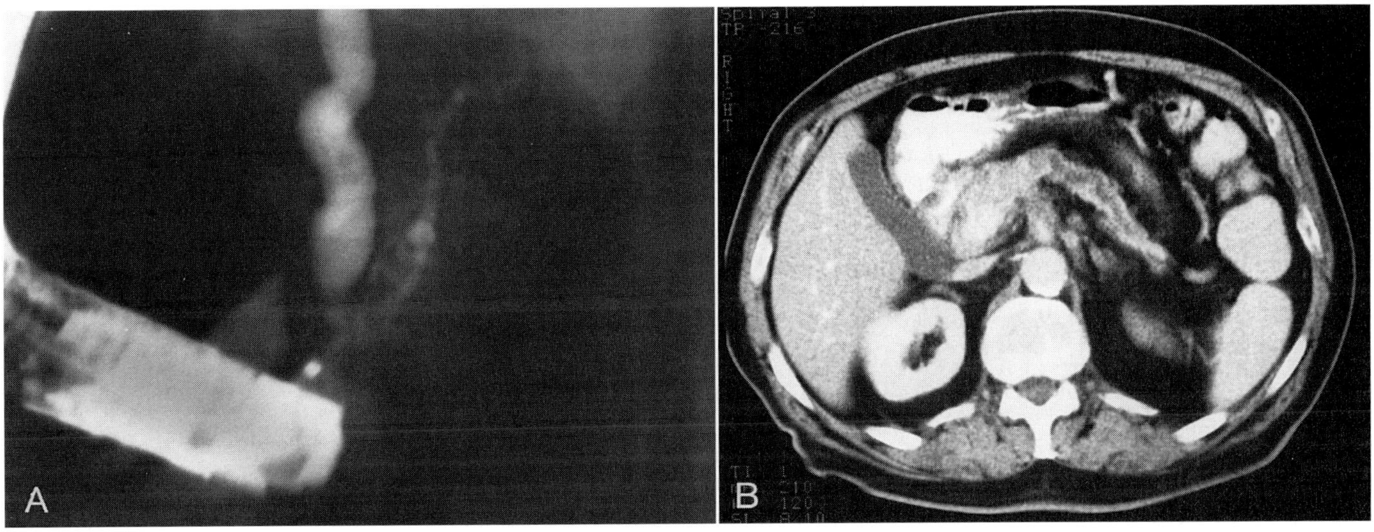


**FIG. 58.2.** **A.** ERCP demonstrates an obstructed pancreatic duct and a normal common bile duct. **B.** CT scan in the same patient does not demonstrate a mass but does show a dilated pancreatic duct in the distal gland and tumor encasing the superior mesenteric artery (SMA).

neum or liver. Any suspicious lesions on chest x-ray should also be investigated further with chest CT and, if a lesion is suspicious for a metastasis, by directed needle biopsy. However, this circumstance is unusual compared with peritoneal or liver involvement. In the 8–12% of patients in whom the tumor seems to be localized to the pancreas without vascular encasement, open exploration is indicated.

## PREOPERATIVE PREPARATION

Tumors in the body and tail of the pancreas that invade adjacent organs are rarely resectable. However, among 26 patients resected at the Mayo Clinic from 1963 to 1987, 11 required concomitant resection of the stomach or colon (2). While resection of an unobstructed stomach requires no special preparation, a mechanical bowel preparation should be performed if colonic resection is anticipated. In this situation, prophylactic use of a systemic antibiotic with anaerobic coverage also would be indicated. However, in most patients with a mass in the body or tail of the pancreas, the operation will be a clean procedure without transection of the gastrointestinal tract. In this circumstance, a first-generation cephalosporin is all that is required for prophylaxis. A single preoperative dose or 24 hours of perioperative coverage should be adequate. The routine use of octreotide to prevent a pancreatic fistula also can be debated. Prospective, randomized trials suggest that complications occur less frequently when octreotide is used (17, 18). However, the risk of a postoperative fistula is greatest when the gland is normal and soft or when the proximal pancreatic duct is strictured. Thus, an argument can be made to reserve prophylactic octreotide for these high-risk situations.

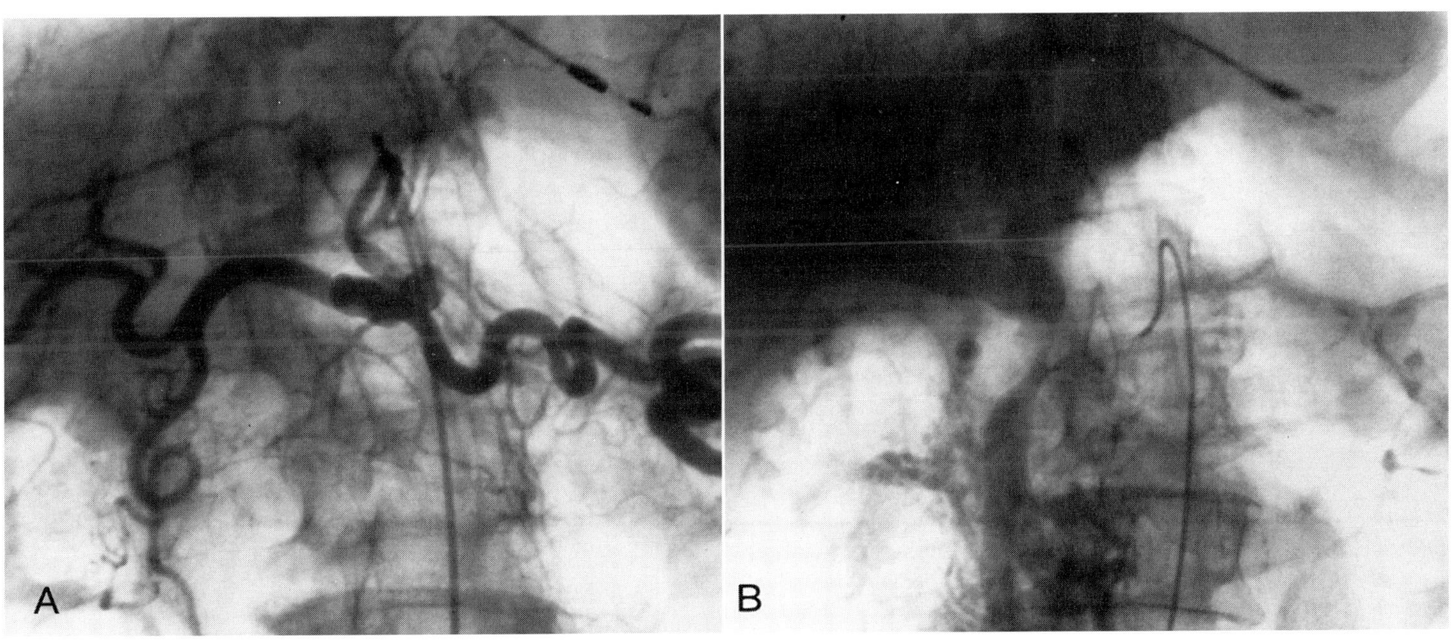


**FIG. 58.3.** **A.** Celiac angiogram demonstrates subtle encasement of splenic artery near its origin from the celiac axis. **B.** Venous phase of SMA injection in the same patient demonstrates severe superior mesenteric vein stenosis.

## SURGICAL TECHNIQUES

In comparing 41 patients managed primarily in the 1970s with 72 patients treated from 1983 to 1989, Nordbach and his associates at Johns Hopkins found substantial changes in practice patterns (Table 58.4). In the 1970s, approximately two-thirds of patients were explored; 15% required a gastric or biliary bypass procedure, and only 5% were resected. In the 1980s, fewer than half the patients required exploration; 17% still needed a bypass procedure, and the percentage resected increased to 10%. When exploration is indicated, the following operative plan should be undertaken.

Under general anesthesia, a midline or left subcostal incision is performed. The entire abdomen is explored to search for metastatic disease. As part of this process, the lesser sac is opened above and below the stomach. The right gastroepiploic artery is preserved, as is the blood supply to the omentum. This local exploration is important because small metastatic deposits are sometimes found on the dorsal serosal surface of the stomach or other peritoneal surfaces of the lesser sac when no tumor spread has occurred elsewhere in the abdomen. Another area to explore carefully is the ligament of Treitz. Tumors in the body of the pancreas may invade the fourth portion of the duodenum at the ligament, which precludes resection without a total pancreatectomy.

If no metastatic disease or duodenal invasion is encountered, the next step is to determine whether vascular encasement will preclude resection. Determining the relationship between the tumor and the celiac axis and its branches is usually undertaken first. Involvement of lymph nodes around the celiac axis does not prevent resection but does diminish the likelihood of long-term survival (5, 6). Encasement of the celiac axis or common hepatic artery makes the tumor unresectable. Encasement of the splenic artery near the spleen is not a problem, but involvement of the splenic artery at its origin from the celiac axis will sometimes make resection with a negative margin impossible. Mobilization of the caudal surface of the body of the pancreas from the retroperitoneum will be necessary to evaluate the relationship between the tumor and the superior mesenteric artery. Establishment of a plane between the neck of the pancreas and the portal vein also will be necessary to perform a resection. Intraoperative ultrasound may help to determine the relationship between the tumor and these vessels. If encasement is encountered in this process, resection should not be undertaken.

If resection is not possible, an alcohol splanchnicectomy should be performed (19). This simple procedure, in which 25 mL of 50% alcohol is injected on either side of the celiac axis, has been shown to reduce or prevent progression of pain for months after the procedure. If the tumor invades the duodenum at the ligament of Treitz, a gastrojejunostomy should be performed. This procedure is most likely to be of benefit when performed retrocolically to the posterior wall of the stomach in an isoperistaltic fashion (20). When the anastomosis is completed, the surrounding stomach is tacked to the transverse mesocolon, creating a dependent funnel that empties easily.

**TABLE 58.4. Changing Trends in the Management of Cancer of the Body/Tail of the Pancreas**

| | 1970s | 1980s |
|---|---|---|
| No operation | 32% | 53%[a] |
| Exploratory laparotomy | 49% | 21%[b] |
| Palliative bypass | 15% | 17% |
| Pancreatic resection | 5% | 10% |

Adapted from Nordback IH, Hruban RH, Boitnott JK, Pitt HA, Cameron JL. Carcinoma of the body and tail of the pancreas. Am J Surg 1992; 164:26–31.
[a] $p < .05$ vs. 1970s.
[b] $p < .01$ vs. 1970s.

As mentioned above, tumors of the body and tail of the pancreas rarely cause obstructive jaundice. However, if the tumor is close to the bile duct and localized but unresectable, a prophylactic biliary bypass should be considered. In general, the results of choledochojejunostomy have been better than those of cholecystojejunostomy. However, with a normal biliary tree, a prophylactic cholecystojejunostomy may be a reasonable compromise as long as the cystic duct enters the common duct at some distance from the tumor. The other situation in which cholecystojejunostomy may be indicated is when the portal vein is occluded and multiple venous collaterals surround the common duct.

If the tumor is localized and not encasing major vessels, resection is indicated. Although the spleen can frequently be preserved when performing a distal pancreatectomy for benign disease, splenic preservation is not indicated when the resection is performed for cancer. Therefore, the splenic artery should be ligated early in the procedure. The short gastric vessels also are divided, and the splenocolic ligament is taken down. Mobilization of the spleen from the retroperitoneum facilitates dissection of the tail of the pancreas from the retroperitoneum (Fig. 58.4). Once fully mobilized, the splenic vein can be divided near its junction with the portal vein. The inferior mesenteric vein can usually be preserved but, if necessary, can be divided without any additional morbidity. The neck of the pancreas is then divided, and the margin is frozen to determine tumor involvement. If tumor is present at the margin, a further resection of the pancreatic neck should be undertaken if possible.

Gentle probing of the proximal duct should be performed to document patency. This step is not necessary if an ERCP was performed preoperatively. Closure of the duct and the pancreatic capsule is then undertaken. If the neck of the pancreas is normal, division and closure of the pancreas can be safely done with a stapler. However, a closed suction drain is routinely left near the closed stump of the pancreas. If proximal obstruction is a problem, a Roux-en-Y pancreatojejunostomy can be performed to prevent a pancreatic fistula. However, this additional procedure is rarely indicated when the distal pancreatectomy is done for cancer and is infrequently indicated in patients with chronic pancreatitis. No data are available to support an extensive retroperitoneal lymph node dissection. However, a substantial number of regional lymph nodes are usually included with the specimen by the time the celiac axis has been dissected and the spleen has been resected.

## POSTOPERATIVE COMPLICATIONS

In reports from specialized centers, morbidity from distal pancreatectomy for pancreatic cancer has been quite acceptable (1, 2, 4, 5). The mortality in 82 patients reported from four institutions was zero (Table 58.5). In comparison, data from the University Hospitals Consortium, a group of 30 academic medical centers, have demonstrated that morbidity is related to surgical volume. Analysis of 1-year data from this group demonstrated that one death occurred among 30 patients (3%). On the other hand, 11 deaths occurred among 128 distal resections (9%) reported by the French Association of Surgery (6). In this large series, hemorrhage was the most common complication (6%) followed by a pancreatic fistula (3%). A similarly low rate of pancreatic fistula following distal pancreatectomy also has been reported by others (2, 5).

The best data on late complications come from the French Association of Surgery survey (6). In this report, diabetes occurred in 11% of resected patients compared with only 2% of bypassed patients and 1% of patients undergoing exploratory laparotomy ($p < .01$). Steatorrhea developed in 5% of those

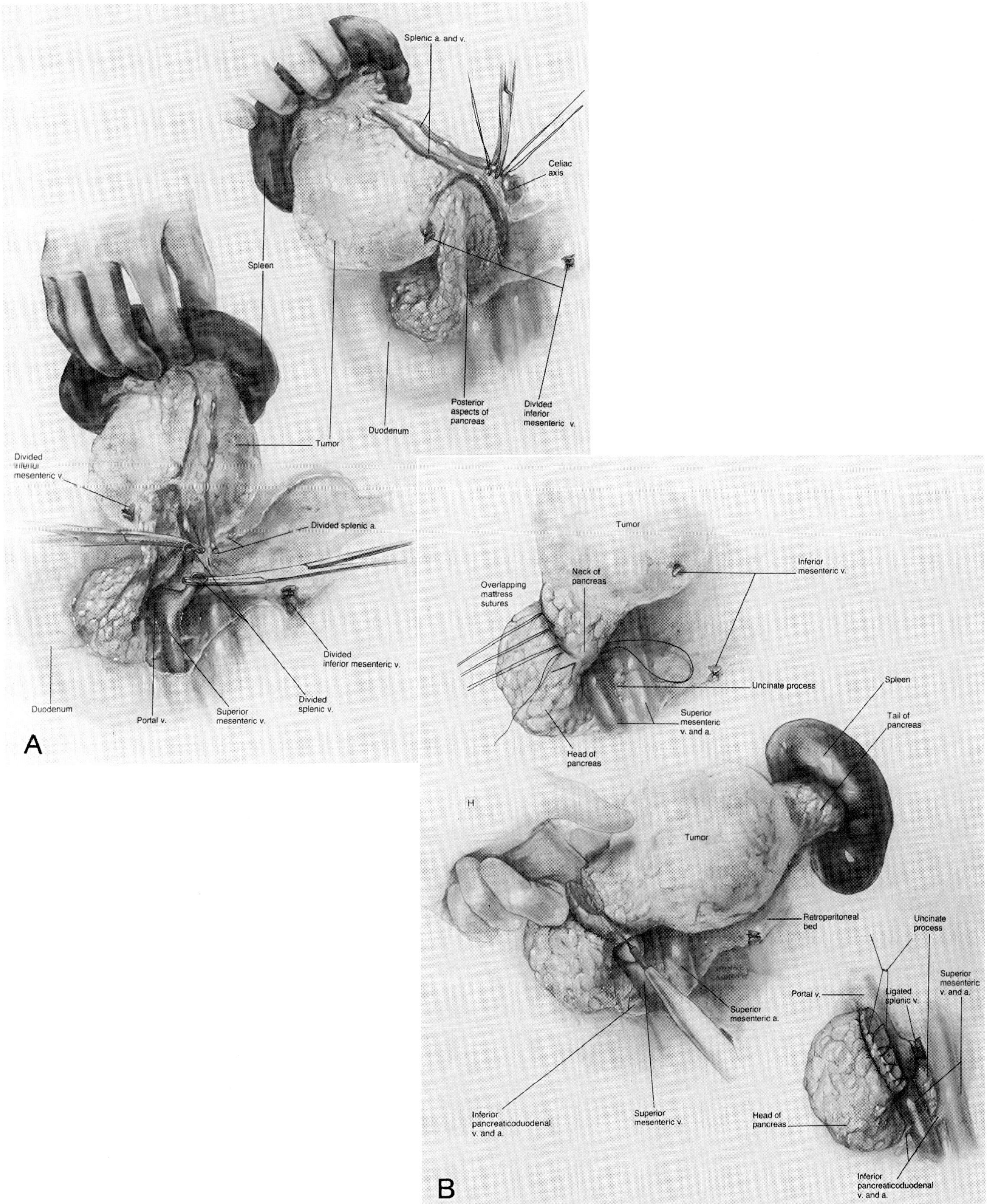


**FIG. 58.4.** **A.** Mobilization of the tail of the pancreas and division of the splenic vein. **B.** Division and oversewing of the pancreatic neck. (Reprinted with permission from Cameron JL. Atlas of surgery. Philadelphia: BC Decker, 1990:433–435.)

**TABLE 58.5. Outcome of Surgery for Carcinoma of the Body/Tail of the Pancreas**

| | | | Resected | | | Survival | |
|---|---|---|---|---|---|---|---|
| Year | Institution | Patients (*N*) | (*N*) | (%) | Operative Mortality | Median (months) | 5-Year |
| 1992 | Johns Hopkins (1) | 113 | 9 | 8% | 0% | 7 | 11% |
| 1992 | Mayo Clinic (2) | NA[a] | 26 | NA | 0% | 10 | 8% |
| 1993 | Univ of Heidelberg (4) | 105 | 13 | 12% | 0% | 13 | 8%[b] |
| 1996 | Memorial (5) | 331 | 34 | 10% | 0% | 12 | 14% |
| 1996 | French Association (6) | NA | 128[c] | NA | 9% | 5 | 1% |

[a]NA, not available.
[b]Estimated.
[c]Includes 28% with metastatic disease.

resected, compared with only 2% of bypassed or exploratory laparotomy patients ($p < .02$). On the other hand, late jaundice was no more common among resected patients (9%) than among bypassed (5%) or explored (6%) patients. Similarly, late bowel obstruction was a problem in only 5% of patients regardless of their initial management.

## OUTCOME

Cancer of the pancreas occurs less frequently in the distal gland and, on average, presents with more advanced disease. Therefore, cancer in the distal pancreas is less frequently resectable for cure. In series from The Johns Hopkins Hospital (1), the University of Heidelberg (4), and the Memorial Sloan-Kettering Cancer Center (5) the resectability rate varied from 8 to 12% (Table 58.5). As with cancer in the head of the pancreas, resection clearly improves long-term survival (1, 4, 5). The median survival for patients who are inoperable or unresectable is less than 6 months, and these patients rarely survive more than 1 year (1, 4). On the other hand, median survival increases to 7–13 months with resection (Table 58.5, Fig. 58.5). Recent data suggest that 5-year survivals of 8–14% can be achieved after resection.

As with cancer in the head of the pancreas, factors such as tumor size, lymph node involvement, surgical margins, and histologic differentiation all affect long-term outcome (5). In the Memorial series, the five patients with tumors less than 2 cm in diameter survived significantly longer ($p < .01$) than the 29 patients with larger tumors. Similarly, the 16 patients with negative lymph nodes lived significantly longer ($p < .05$) than the 18 with positive nodes. In addition, the 23 patients with negative microscopic margins lived longer ($p < .01$) than the 11 with the positive margins. Moreover, the 19 patients with well or moderately differentiated tumors survived significantly longer ($p = .02$) than the 15 patients with poorly differentiated tumors. A multivariate analysis of the French Association series confirmed that tumor size and lymph node involvement were independent predictors of survival (6). This analysis also suggested that involvement of adjacent organs diminished the chance for long-term survival.

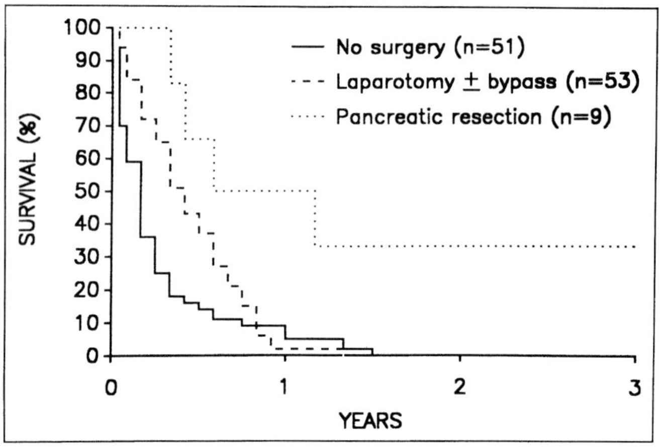


**FIG. 58.5.** Actuarial survival of patients undergoing no surgery, laparotomy with or without bypass procedure(s), or pancreatic resection at Johns Hopkins. (Reprinted with permission from Nordback IH, Hruban RH, Boitnott JK, Pitt HA, Cameron JL. Carcinoma of the body and tail of the pancreas. Am J Surg 1992;164:26–31.)

Data on the role of the adjuvant radiation or chemotherapy after resection for carcinoma of the body or tail of the pancreas is limited. Among 113 patients managed at Johns Hopkins from 1972 to 1989, 52 (46%) received some form of adjuvant therapy (1). Fifteen patients (13%) received chemotherapy alone, 15 (13%) received radiotherapy alone, and only 22 (19%) had chemoradiation. However, with only nine resected patients, no conclusions could be drawn regarding the potential benefit for radiation. Similarly, at the Mayo Clinic, only 7 of 26 resected patients received chemotherapy or radiation. Each of these seven patients experienced recurrent disease, and three had local recurrence as a component of treatment failure.

## CONCLUSIONS

Adenocarcinoma of the body and tail of the pancreas usually presents with epigastric, left upper quadrant, and/or back pain. These body and tail lesions are less common than their counterparts in the head of the pancreas, and they present as larger, more advanced tumors. Spiral CT scans will usually detect a mass, a dilated duct in the tail of the pancreas, vascular involvement, and (if present) liver metastases. A CA 19-9 level above 200 may confirm the suspicion of pancreatic cancer in equivocal cases. Fine-needle aspiration of liver metastases or the pancreas will usually confirm the diagnosis and avoid the need for laparotomy in patients with unresectable tumors. Laparoscopy also may be employed to detect small liver or peritoneal metastases not seen on CT scan. With these newer modalities for diagnosis and staging, the percentage of patients who require laparotomy for diagnosis has diminished substantially in recent years.

Approximately 10% of adenocarcinomas in the body and tail of the pancreas are resectable. In recent series, morbidity and mortality of surgery have been acceptably low at specialized centers. Resection improves survival, which also is influenced by tumor size, lymph node status, tumor presence at resection margin, and degree of differentiation. No good data is available to know whether adjuvant chemoradiation improves survival after distal resection. However, recent information suggests that survival is improved when adjuvant therapy is given after pancreatoduodenectomy (22). Therefore, postoperative chemoradiation after distal resection for adenocarcinoma of the pancreas may be expected to provide a modest improvement in long-term survival. Nevertheless, better methods to establish the diagnosis earlier as well as more effective adjuvant therapies are key to improving the outlook for these patients.

## REFERENCES


1. Nordback IH, Hruban RH, Boitnott JK, Pitt HA, Cameron JL. Carcinoma of the body and tail of the pancreas. Am J Surg 1992;164:26–31.
2. Dalton RR, Sarr MG, van Heerden JA, Colby TV. Carcinoma of the body and tail of the pancreas: is curative resection justified? Surgery 1992;111:489–494.
3. Edge SB, Schmieg RE Jr, Rosenlof LK, Wilhelm MC. Pancreas cancer resection outcome in American University centers in 1989–1990. Cancer 1993;71:3502–3508.
4. Johnson CD, Schwall G, Flectenmacher J, Trede M. Resection for adenocarcinoma of the body and tail of the pancreas. Br J Surg 1993;80:1177–1179.
5. Brennan MF, Moccia RD, Klimstra D. Management of adenocarcinoma of the body and tail of the pancreas. Ann Surg 1996;223:506–512.
6. Fabre JM, Houry S, Manddrscheid JC, Huguier M, Baumel H. Surgery for left-sided pancreatic cancer. Br J Surg 1996;83:1065–1070.
7. Satake K, Takeuchi T, Homma T, Ozaki H. CA 19-9 as a screening and diagnostic tool in symptomatic patients: the Japanese experience. Pancreas 1994;9:703–706.
8. Forsmark CE, Lambiase L, Vogel SB. Diagnosis of pancreatic cancer and prediction of unresectability using the tumor associated antigen CA 19-9Pancreas 1994;9:731–734.
9. Tian F, Appert HE, Myles J, Howard JM. Prognostic value of serum CA 19-9 levels in pancreatic adenocarcinomas. Ann Surg 1992;215:350–355.
10. Sperti C, Pasquali C, Catalini S. CA 19-9 as a prognostic index after resection for pancreatic cancer. J Surg Oncol 1993;52: 137–141.
11. Pitt HA. Classification, diagnosis, staging and preoperative preparation of pancreatic and periampullary neoplasms. In: Braasch JW, Tompkins RK, eds. Surgical disease of the biliary tract and pancreas. Philadelphia: Mosby-Year Book, 1994: 514–527.
12. Matsumoto S, Harada H, Tanaka J, et al. Evaluation of cytology and tumor markers of pure pancreatic juice for the diagnosis of pancreatic cancer at early stages. Pancreas 1994;9:741–747.
13. Gentiloni N, Caradonna P, Costamagna G, et al. Pancreatic juice 90K and serum CA 19-9 combined determination can discriminate between pancreatic cancer and chronic pancreatitis. Am J Gastroenterol 1995;90:1069–1072.
14. Dooley WC, Cameron JL, Pitt HA, Lillemoe KD, Yeo CJ, Vendrux AC. Is preoperative angiography useful in patients with periampullary tumors? Ann Surg 1990;211:649–655.
15. Palazzo L, Roseau G, Goyet B, et al. Endoscopic ultrasonography in the diagnosis and staging of pancreatic adenocarcinoma. Endoscopy 1993;25:143–150.
16. Warshaw AL, Zhuo-yun G, Wittenberg J, Wiltman AC. Preoperative staging and assessment of resectability of pancreatic cancer. Arch Surg 1990;125:230–233.
17. Buchler M, Friess H, Klempa I, et al. Role of octreotide in the prevention of postoperative complications. Am J Surg 1992;163: 125–131.
18. Montsori M, Zago M, Mosca F, et al. Efficiency of octreotide in the prevention of pancreatic fistulas after elective pancreatic surgery: a prospective, randomized clinical trial. Surgery 1995;117: 26–31.
19. Lillemoe KD, Cameron JL, Kaufman HS, Yeo CJ, Pitt HA, Sauter PK. Chemical splanchnicectomy in patients with unresectable pancreatic cancer: a prospective randomized trial. Ann Surg 1993; 217:447–457.
20. Lillemoe KD, Sauter PK, Pitt HA, Yeo CJ, Cameron JL. Current status of surgical palliation of periampullary carcinoma. Surg Gynocol Obstet 1993;176:1–10.
21. Cameron JL. Atlas of surgery. Philadelphia: BC Decker, 1990: 433–435.
22. Yeo CJ, Cameron JL, Lillemoe KD, et al. Pancreaticoduodenectomy for cancer of the head of the pancreas: 201 patients. Ann Surg 1995;221:721–733.

# 59

# Radiotherapy

Ralph R. Dobelbower and Joyce A. Battle

The three traditional modalities for the treatment of cancer are surgery, radiation therapy, and chemotherapy. In spite of major advances in the application of the first two of these modalities in recent decades, the ultimate prognosis for the patient diagnosed with pancreatic cancer remains grim, indeed. According to data from the 1991 National Cancer Data Base, the overall 5-year survival rate for patients with pancreatic cancer is only 3–5%, regardless of the type of treatment: surgery, radiation, chemotherapy, or various combinations thereof (1). This is likely due, at least in part, to the circumstance that the disease is far advanced (AJCC stage IV) in over 50% of patients at the time of diagnosis (1). Clearly, this presents a great opportunity for improvements in early diagnosis as well as effective treatments for this dread disease.

## HISTORIC ASPECTS

The history of the development and implementation of radiation therapy techniques for cancer of the pancreas is an interesting story that has been reviewed in a prior edition of this textbook (2) and elsewhere (3–15). The basic principles of radiation therapy (physics, radiobiology, etc.) as they apply to cancer of the pancreas have also been recently reviewed (4, 16, 17).

This chapter focuses on clinical developments in the field of radiation therapy for cancer of the pancreas that have been reported since the publication of the last edition of this textbook, roughly one decade ago.

## RECENT DEVELOPMENTS

The study of the use of radiation therapy for pancreatic cancer has proceeded at a steady pace over the last decade, with over 100 reports appearing in the English language scientific literature. Most efforts have been directed toward the clinical investigation of specialized radiation modalities, specifically brachytherapy and intraoperative electron beam radiation therapy (IOEBRT). Of course the use of radiation therapy as an adjuvant to resection continues to be of interest, as does the combination of radiation therapy with chemotherapy—principally 5-fluorouracil (5-FU)—for both resectable and unresectable disease. In the past, adjuvant irradiation for cancer of the pancreas has generally been administered in the postoperative setting, after recovery from the effects of surgery. In the recent decade there has been considerable interest in preoperative and (especially) intraoperative irradiation as an adjunct to resection. New radiation techniques, such as 3-dimensional (3-D) noncoplanar external-beam arrangements, infusional brachytherapy, and intraluminal brachytherapy have been reported for use in unresectable pancreatic cancers. The issue of prophylactic hepatic irradiation has been addressed as well. There has also been a modicum of interest in radiation fractionation studies, the combination of radiation therapy with hyperthermia, and the delivery of radiation dose via radiolabeled antibodies.

### Intraoperative Radiation Therapy

The term intraoperative radiation therapy connotes the application of a radiation beam directly to a tumor or tumor bed through a surgical incision (18). With few exceptions, this is accomplished with a beam of high-energy electrons. Electron beams have the advantageous property of delivering a relatively uniform radiation dose to a given depth in tissue while sparing the deeper tissues from radiation. IOEBRT has been applied to unresectable cancers of the pancreas as well as to the tumor bed after resection. Cancer of the pancreas is the disease entity to which IOEBRT has been applied most frequently to date. External-beam radiation therapy has been used in addition to IOEBRT in almost every clinical trial to date. Adjuvant chemotherapy (principally 5-FU) has been very frequently used as well.

In its early years, IOEBRT was felt to hold great promise in the management of cancer of the pancreas. Clinical experience with this modality has documented its usefulness but has generally failed to demonstrate the spectacular survival results once hoped for.

**IOEBRT for Unresectable Pancreatic Cancer.** Unresectable cancer of the pancreas presents a management challenge for the clinical oncologist. Patients with this condition often suffer severe, progressive, unrelenting pain. They are at risk of neoplastic obstruction of the upper gastrointestinal tract as well as the biliary outflow tract. The dose of radiation that may be delivered by external-beam therapy is limited by the surrounding radiosensitive normal tissues such as the stomach, liver, small bowel, kidneys, and spleen. With IOEBRT, one can deliver extraordinarily large single doses of radiation directly to a pancreatic tumor mass with minimal dose to the surrounding normal tissues and organs. Of course, this can be combined with conventional doses of external-beam radiation. The advantages are obvious.

***Feasibility.*** The feasibility of IOEBRT for unresectable pancreatic carcinoma has been widely tested and confirmed (19–51). Most clinical trials have combined IOEBRT with 40–60 Gy external-beam radiation therapy and and various doses of 5-FU. The IOEBRT doses range from 15 to 35 Gy.

The addition of IOEBRT to exploratory/palliative surgery in patients with unresectable pancreatic cancer does not appreciably increase morbidity or mortality (21–23). In three prospective studies of IOERBT conducted by the Radiation Therapy Oncology Group (RTOG), 227 patients were studied. Of these, 129 received IOEBRT, while 98 had disease too far advanced to benefit from IOEBRT and hence underwent palliative surgical procedures only. The wound infection rate in the IOEBRT group was 6%, compared with 2% in the non-IOEBRT group, not a statistically significant difference (21). Two of 51 fully analyzable patients on RTOG-8505 (a prospective study of the use of IOEBRT in the treatment of unresectable pancreatic cancer) developed late major morbidity leading to death: one, a duodenal hemorrhage; the other, biliary obstruction. Major postoperative complications were observed in 12% of patients, but this was not judged to be excessive (20, 22).

***IOEBRT plus External-Beam Therapy.*** Some pilot studies suggest a survival benefit for patients with unresectable pancreatic cancer treated with a combination of IOEBRT and external-beam radiation therapy (9, 10, 34–36, 39, 42, 47); however, many other pilot studies and at least one cooperative group prospective study (20, 22) fail to demonstrate any survival advantage of IOEBRT over conventional radiation therapy for this disease situation.

***Local Control.*** Local control of unresectable pancreatic cancer can be exceedingly difficult to assess accurately; nevertheless, the team of clinical investigators at Mayo Clinic reported achieving local control of cancer in 21 of 27 (78%) patients treated with 50–54 Gy preoperative external-beam radiation therapy ± concomitant bolus 5-FU followed by 20 Gy IOEBRT. The actuarial 2- and 5-year survival rates of patients so treated were 27% and 7%, respectively, significantly ($p$ = .001) better than the 6% and 0% 2- and 5-year actuarial survival rates observed in 56 patients who were previously treated with IOEBRT and postoperative external-beam radiation therapy at the same institution (24). This suggests that the use of preoperative external beam therapy may permit improved patient selection for IOEBRT.

***Palliation.*** Gratifying relief of pain is a common thread that runs through most reports of IOEBRT for unresectable pancreatic cancer (5). Kawamura and associates, for example, observed pain relief in 95% of patients with unresectable disease who had pain (37, 46). Fossati and associates found relief of severe pain in 85% of patients within 12 days of IOEBRT (44, 49). The pain relief was complete in 64% of patients and partial (>50%) in 21% (44).

**IOEBRT for Resectable Pancreatic Cancer.** Even after successful surgical resection of part or all of the pancreas, 3-year survival is the exception rather than the rule for patients with cancer of the pancreas (1). Local recurrence is still the most common type of failure after resection for pancreas cancer (52). The ability of IOEBRT to deliver high radiation doses to the pancreatic resection bed directly through the operative wound makes its use both logical and attractive.

The use of IOEBRT as an adjuvant to surgical resection for pancreatic cancer has now been studied at multiple centers around the world (7, 12, 18, 33–67). Some investigators have studied the use of IOEBRT alone as an adjuvant to resection (37, 41–43, 46, 48–50, 53, 54, 56–58, 61, 64–67); however, in most instances the adjuvant IOEBRT has been combined with external-beam radiation therapy and often with chemotherapy (usually 5-FU) in various regimens. Many investigators have observed that the addition of IOEBRT reduces the incidence of local recurrence; however, there is no convincing evidence that it improves survival.

The Milan experience (52) is illustrative: In a group of 90 patients undergoing resection for pancreatic cancer, 12.5–20 Gy IOEBRT was added for 43 patients; the remaining 47 patients were treated with resection alone. The stage of disease and the extent of tumor clearance were similar in the two groups. Operative mortality and overall early postoperative complication rates (about 2% and 23%, respectively) were nearly identical in the two groups. The local recurrence rate was reduced from 56% to 27% by the addition of IOEBRT ($p$ < .01). The median survival time for the IOEBRT group was increased to 13 months, compared with 8 months for the resection alone group (not statistically significant).

***Preresection IOEBRT.*** Clinical investigators at the University of Innsbruck (53, 57) investigated the use of 15–20 Gy IOEBRT immediately prior to resection in an attempt to decrease any dissemination of viable tumor cells that might occur during necessary manipulation of the tumor and/or the pancreas during resection. A group of 38 patients so treated showed no improvement in survival time attributable to the IOEBRT. The perioperative mortality/morbidity rate (5.6%) was not perceptibly different from their prior experience with resection alone.

***"Sandwich" IOEBRT.*** At the University of Tsukuba, IOEBRT has been employed both before resection (10 Gy) and after resection (10 Gy with a smaller field) in the same patient to take advantage of the putative benefits of both preresection and postresection IOEBRT (50). The number of reported cases is too small to draw any inferences.

## External-Beam Radiation Therapy

External beam radiation therapy may be applied with palliative intent or curative (definitive) intent, although the radiation doses and treatment techniques may differ. External-beam therapy may be given alone or in combination with chemotherapy or other radiation sensitizers. It may be used with or without chemotherapy as an adjuvant to surgical resection.

**External Beam Therapy for Unresectable Pancreatic Cancer.** Standard palliative care for the patient suffering from unresectable cancer of the pancreas often is based primarily upon external-beam radiation therapy. The use of computed tomography (CT), radiation therapy simulators, high-energy radiation beams, and sophisticated computerized radiation treatment planning systems now facilitates the delivery of high radiation doses to unresectable pancreatic cancers. These tools are now widely available for use in the community practice of radiation therapy. In Fort Meyers, for example, 86 patients with unresectable pancreatic cancer were treated in a community hospital setting primarily with radiation therapy; 62 also received chemotherapy (68). The overall probability of survival was 39% at 1 year and 23% at 2 years. The patients who received chemotherapy had a significantly ($p$ = .018) better survival rate (44 vs. 25%) at 1 year.

***Radiation Dose.*** The Louisville experience confirms that total radiation dose is important. Of 77 patients treated with radiation therapy for pancreatic cancer, 35 had localized disease and were treated for cure (69), with 5 receiving less than 40 Gy. The mean survival time of this group of patients was only 5.6 months. Thirty patients received 40 Gy or more and experienced a mean survival time of 14.7 months. Of these 30 patients, 24 received 50 Gy or more and survived an average of 15.4 months; 17 received 60 Gy or more and survived 15.7 months on average. Some palliation of symptoms was achieved in 57% of all patients.

***Split-Course Irradiation.*** Most studies of external-beam radiation therapy for unresectable pancreatic cancer have used daily radiation doses of 1.8–2.0 Gy. Split-course regimens have been in vogue for decades. In the Netherlands, a split-course regimen was combined with intravenous 5-FU (375 mg/m$^2$/day) on the first 4 days of each course of irradiation (70). There was no mortality among 40 patients. Morbidity was moderate. The median survival time was 9 months. Six patients survived 3 years and three patients survived 5 years.

Flickinger et al. (71) used a split-course protocol to manage the radiation therapy for 95 patients with biopsy-proven adenocarcinoma of the pancreas. The radiation schedule consisted of 2 courses of 25 Gy given in 10 treatments, each followed by a 3- to 4-week rest period. Depending on the individual patient's condition and clinical response, a final boost dose of 10 Gy was given in five additional treatment sessions. Of the 55 patients with localized cancers, 25 also received chemotherapy (5-FU or a three-drug combination of 5-FU, mitomycin C, and doxorubicin [FAM]). The median survival times of those patients with localized disease who received doses of 25, 50, and 60 Gy were 3, 7, and 12 months, respectively. These clinical data suggest that preplanned reevaulations during split-course radiation programs may be effective in selecting patients for aggressive external-beam therapy. Similar concepts could well be applied to multimodal treatment regimens for cancer of the pancreas.

***Chemoradiation Studies.*** Most adjuvant chemotherapy regimens have used 5-FU alone or in combination with various other agents. Bruckner et al. (72) treated 20 patients with inoperable locally advanced pancreatic cancer using split-radiation courses of 20 Gy each followed by an additional 14 Gy, separated by 2-week intervals. Simultaneous 5-FU was given intravenously (1 g/m$^2$/day, days 1–5) along with streptozocin (300–500 mg/m$^2$/day, days 1, 2, and 3) and cisplatin (100 mg/m$^2$ on day 3 of every 4-week radiotherapy cycle). The primary tumor, as documented by CT scans, disappeared completely in seven patients. Only three patients had regrowth of tumor in the radiotherapy field.

Ardalan et al. (73) explored the combination of *N*-phosphonacetyl-L-aspartic acid (PALA) and escalating doses of 5-FU with external-beam radiation therapy, 1.8 Gy/day over 6.5 weeks. They found this to be an active regimen, with 250 mg/m$^2$ of PALA given as an intravenous bolus followed 24 hours later by 5-FU, which was given by 24-hour infusion every week. The maximum tolerable dose of 5-FU was 1300 mg/m$^2$. Two patients at this dose level (10 patients in the entire study were evaluable) had a complete response. The median survival time was 12.5 months. Four patients survived more than 1 year.

***Dose Fractionation.*** Relatively few studies have explored the use of daily radiation doses outside the narrow range of 1.8 to 2.0 Gy. The Gastrointestinal Tumor Study Group (GITSG) treated 18 patients with unresectable localized pancreas cancers with a combination of hyperfractionated radiation therapy (1.2 Gy twice daily, 4–6 hours apart, 50.4 Gy total dose) and chemotherapy with streptozocin, mitomycin C, and 5-FU (SMF) (74). During the first and last 3 days of radiation treatment, 5-FU was given at 350 mg/m$^2$. The SMF began on day 53 of the protocol. One patient died of total liver failure 3 months following initiation of treatment. The overall severe toxicity rate was 67%, higher than that in previous combined modality studies. The median survival time was 35 weeks; the 1-year survival rate, 39%. The longest-surviving patient died at 68 months.

Combined chemoradiation therapy was used with hypofractionated radiation in Israel (75). A group of 92 patients was studied: 66 (group 1) with biliary obstruction underwent surgical biliary bypass; 26 (group 2) underwent exploratory laparotomy only. Thirty patients in group 1 and 10 in group 2 received synchronous therapy consisting of 10 intravenous administrations of 5-FU (750 mg/m$^2$) over 8 hours, followed 8 hours later by 4 Gy external-beam radiation therapy. This was repeated every 4 days. Those patients in group 1 who received synchronous therapy had a mean survival time of 13.5 months, compared with 8.9 months for those who did not ($p < .01$). Patients in group 2 who received synchronous therapy had a mean survival time of 5.4 months, compared with 2.7 months for those who did not ($p < .01$). Some 29 of 37 patients (78.4%) with abdominal pain were pain free at the completion of treatment.

***Three-Dimensional Treatment Planning.*** Recent advances in the administration of external-beam radiation treatment include 3-D approaches to radiation dose delivery. In an attempt to minimize the radiation dose to the kidneys, radiation oncologists at the University of Michigan developed a "nonaxial" treatment field orientation, with the anterior radiation beam entering the patient's abdomen from an inferior oblique direction (76). For 14 consecutive patients with pancreatic cancers they carried out radiation treatment planning for both conventional 3- and 4-field arrangements as well as "nonaxial" field arrangements. Comparing the resulting radiation dose distributions with the aid of dose-volume histograms, they showed that the "nonaxial" plan was superior to the standard conventional plan in every case. All patients were treated with the "nonaxial" field arrangements. Gastrointestinal toxicity was not increased, nor was the daily radiation treatment significantly more complex.

Investigators in Chicago also found improved radiation dose distributions with the use of 4 and 6 oblique noncoplanar fields (77). They reduced the radiation dose to the kidneys and/or small bowel with the use of the oblique fields, compared with the dose with conventional 3- and 4-field arrangements.

An even more elegant use of 3-D radiation treatment planning was conceived at the Cleveland Clinic where multiple (as many as 8) noncoplanar fields were used to irradiate pancreas tumors (78, 79). These investigators treated 35 patients to doses of 60 Gy and higher and report excellent patient tolerance (80).

**External-Beam Therapy for Resectable Pancreatic Cancer.** The primary cause of tumor recurrence after resection of pancreatic cancer appears to be residual locoregional subclinical disease (81). Of 72 patients undergoing resection of the head of the pancreas for cancer at the Massachusetts General Hospital (MGH), 37 (51%) were found, by retrospective study, to have tumor extension to the surgical margins (82). The most commonly involved margin was the peripancreatic soft tissue (27 cases), followed by the pancreatic transection line (14 cases) and the bile duct transection line (4 cases). The implications for local adjuvant therapies are obvious.

In a retrospective analysis of 2401 pancreas cancer patients treated in 88 Illinois hospitals (83), it was concluded that the use of multiple treatment modalities warrants further study in organized trials, although the improvement in 3-year patient survival time with combined modality therapy did not achieve statistical significance ($p = .16$). Swedish investigators Andren-Sandberg and Hafstrom (84) voice the opinion that although the overall results of curatively intended surgery for cancer of the exocrine pancreas are slowly improving, adjuvant therapies showing definite impact on long-term survival are lacking. On the other hand, German reviewers Feitkau and Sauer (85) conclude that radiochemotherapy does possibly prolong survival.

***Postoperative Adjuvant Irradiation.*** The current standard of adjuvant therapy for resectable pancreatic cancer includes conventional postoperative radiation therapy. The largest single-institution experience with pancreaticoduodenectomy for cancer of the head of the pancreas reported to date (86) comes from Johns Hopkins, where there were 11 5-year survivors in a group of 201 patients. Univariate analysis showed that the use of postoperative radiotherapy and chemotherapy was one of the factors significantly favoring long-term patient survival. Cameron (87) concludes that adjuvant therapy is effective and should be used routinely.

In an analysis of 29 patients who were treated with postoperative radiation therapy (27 also received adjuvant 5-FU), investigators at the Mayo Clinic found that both median and long-term survival time were twice those of patients treated with surgery alone at the same institution (88). They observed minimal acute toxicity and acceptably low levels of chronic toxicity attributable to the postoperative adjuvant therapies. They noted that 59% of cancer relapses occurred in the liver and/or the peritoneum. They concluded that future improvements in survival can be achieved only by reducing the incidence of liver and peritoneal metastases. Noting similar clinical patterns of failure, investigators at the M. D. Anderson Cancer Center (55) suggested clinical trials of hepatic and whole abdominal chemoradiation. Toxicity data from the RTOG trial of wide-field radiation therapy combined with chemotherapy for unresectable pancreas cancer (89) indicate that such studies in resectable disease, where more long-term survival is to be expected, should be conducted with extreme care because of the potential hazards of hepatic toxicity.

A team of French investigators treated 14 consecutive patients with postoperative radiation alone, without the use of chemotherapy (90). Using a 4-field arrangement of 23-MV photons, they delivered a dose of 54 Gy to the resection bed after resection of pancreatic cancer. Acute toxicities consisted mainly of weight loss (median, 2 kg). Two patients had grade 2 diarrhea, two had grade 2 gastritis. Late effects were minimal and observed in only two patients. The median disease-free survival time was 12 months; the median overall survival time was 23 months. These results are comparable to those of the GITSG adjuvant study that used both 5-FU and split-course radiation therapy, described in detail in the last edition of this textbook (2). Perhaps the use of chemotherapy as a radiosensitizer in this clinical situation is not as necessary as current conventional wisdom indicates.

***Preoperative Adjuvant Irradiation.*** In general terms, whenever postoperative radiation therapy is of value, preoperative (neoadjuvant) radiation therapy may be even more effective. The rationale for, and relative benefits of, this approach are detailed elsewhere (17, 91). The decade since the most recent edition of this textbook has witnessed a surge of interest in preresection chemoradiotherapy in cases of potentially or borderline resectable pancreatic cancer.

Data from the M. D. Anderson Cancer Center (55, 92) have demonstrated the safety of aggressive preoperative chemoradiation and resection (plus IOEBRT). A group of 28 patients was treated with preoperative chemoradiation (5-FU, 300 mg/m$^2$/day and 50.4 Gy). Gastrointestinal toxicity forced hospitalization of 9 patients. Of 23 patients who underwent laparotomy after restaging (5 were found to have metastatic disease), 17 were able to undergo pancreaticoduodenectomy (3 patients had locally unresectable cancers, and 3 others had previously unsuspected intraabdominal metastases). Perioperative complications were observed in three patients. There was one perioperative death from myocardial infarction. The authors noted that this approach avoids resection in patients with rapidly progressive disease and allows radiation therapy to be delivered to well-oxygenated cells before surgical devascularization.

The group at the Fox Chase Cancer Center hypothesized that delivering adjuvant chemoradiotherapy preoperatively might enhance local control of the cancer and patient tolerance for the surgery. They treated 34 patients with localized pancreatic cancer with 5-FU (1000 mg/m$^2$ on days 2–5 and 29–32) and mitomycin-C (10 mg/m$^2$ on day 2) in conjunction with 50.4 Gy external-beam radiation therapy in a preoperative setting (93–95). Nine patients did not have surgery: 1 refused, 1 died of cholangitis, and 7 were found to have distant metastases (5 patients) or unresectable local cancer (2 patients) after radiation therapy. Of the 25 patients who underwent celiotomy, 11 were found to have liver (8 patients) or peritoneal (three) metastases, and 3 had palliative pancreatectomies (2 had concomitant resection of liver metastases, and 1 with hepatic artery and portal vein replacement). The remaining 11 patients (44% of the cohort with surgery, 32% of all patients) had resections with curative intent. Of these, 4 had lesions deemed unresectable at prior celiotomy. One patient developed respiratory failure and another died postoperatively. The median disease-free survival time was 27 months; the median overall survival time was 45 months. The projected 5-year survival rate was 40%. Clearly, this type of approach seems to warrant further clinical investigation. Such studies are ongoing at MGH (82) and elsewhere.

## Brachytherapy

Brachytherapy literally means short-distance therapy (as opposed to teletherapy, therapy from a distance). This radiotherapeutic technique consists of placing radioactive sources in, on, or very near the tissues to be treated. The radioactive sources may be in the form of seeds, tubes, needles, ribbons, or liquids (such as colloidal suspensions). A variety of radioisotopes has been used for brachytherapy. Some of the isotopes that have been more commonly used for pancreatic cancer brachytherapy applications include radium-226 ($^{226}$Ra), radon-222 ($^{222}$Rn), gold-198 ($^{198}$Au), iridium-192 ($^{192}$Ir), iodine-125 ($^{125}$I), palladium-103 ($^{103}$Pd), and phosphorus-32 ($^{32}$P).

In the management of pancreatic cancers, brachytherapy has been applied interstitially (between the tissues), intraluminally (within the pancreatic or biliary ducts), and appositionally (close to or actually touching the tumor). Earlier applications were appositional, but the most common procedures in recent decades have been interstitial brachytherapy (IBT) and intraluminal brachytherapy (ILBT). For pancreatic cancer, brachytherapy has seldom been used in the adjuvant setting. It has been used almost exclusively in unresectable cancer.

**Interstitial Brachytherapy (IBT).** IBT (implantation of radioisotopes directly into tumors) is a method of delivering very high radiation doses to deeply situated pancreatic cancers without overdosing the critical surrounding organs. When combined with external-beam radiation therapy and systemic cytotoxic chemotherapy, it appears to offer the best (currently known) potential for local control of unresectable pancreatic cancer (6, 31, 96, 97), but it is a risky procedure that has failed to substantially improve patient survival beyond that achieved with less toxic external-beam radiation therapy, with or without 5-FU (96).

In Rome, Montemaggi et al. (15) treated seven patients with locally unresectable pancreatic cancer with a 60–100 Gy matched peripheral dose (MPD) by $^{125}$I IBT. One patient died postoperatively of a pulmonary embolus. Four of the remaining six patients received 10.5–30 Gy via external-beam radiation therapy late in the course of the disease because of local tumor progression. One patient developed a pancreaticocutaneous fistula; another developed exacerbation of preexisting diabetes mellitus. The median patient survival time from the date of IBT was 7 months (range, 0–21 months). A group from Valhalla's New York Medical College (98) also called attention to the hazards of pancreaticobiliary fistula and obstructive jaundice complicating $^{125}$I IBT for pancreatic cancer. For the reader with an interest in the brachytherapy of pancreatic cancer, the Montemaggi report (15) contains a comprehensive review of pertinent clinical studies.

At the Medical College of Virginia, data were compared from *(a)* 11 patients with unresectable pancreas cancers treated by $^{125}$I IBT and external-beam radiation therapy, *(b)* 8 patients who received external-beam radiation therapy alone, and *(c)* 23 patients who underwent radical surgical resection (99). Median survival times were 8, 5, and 7.5 months, respectively. Locoregional control of cancer was achieved in 73, 25, and 48% of patients, respectively. Likewise, complete, lasting pain palliation was achieved in 80, 25, and 65% of patients in these respective groups. In spite of surgical unresectability, IBT plus external-beam therapy appears to give results similar to those with radical resection.

Some of the best IBT results in pancreatic cancer have been reported from Thomas Jefferson University (97), where a local control rate of 71% was observed in a group of 81 patients with localized but unresectable pancreas cancers. They were treated with 120-Gy MPD via $^{125}$I IBT plus 50–55 Gy external-beam therapy plus 5-FU and mitomycin-C, with or without CCNU (lomustine) systemic chemotherapy. The early morbidity rate was 34%; the late complication rate was 32%. The median survival time was 12 months, and the 2- and 5-year survival rates were 21 and 7%, respectively—not significantly improved over results reported from the same institution previously using external-beam therapy with or without chemotherapy (96).

Investigators at the University of Copenhagen described a

method of implanting $^{125}I$ seeds into the pancreas percutaneously under ultrasonic guidance (100). They reported that the procedure had been used in 19 patients; 12 had further external-beam irradiation. Clinical improvement was either lacking or slight and short-lived. The median survival time after seed implantation was only 140 days (range, 7–401 days). They concluded that this procedure cannot be recommended for the treatment of the patient with unresectable pancreatic cancer.

High-dose $^{192}Ir$ IBT by use of flexible catheters has been accomplished at some centers (101); however, in spite of excellent palliative results without severe side effects, it has yet to be shown to be superior to more conventional techniques.

**Intraluminal Brachytherapy (ILBT).** ILBT for pancreatic cancer involves the temporary insertion of radioactive sources—usually seeds or wires—into the common bile duct and/or the ducts of Wirsung and Santorini. This can be accomplished via catheters placed percutaneously transhepatically or via surgically placed biliary stents, such as T tubes. A less invasive method involves the use of nasobiliary or nasopancreatic catheters that are positioned endoscopically. The radioisotopes best-suited for this type of procedure appear to be $^{125}I$, $^{192}Ir$, and $^{103}Pd$. Of course the biliary or pancreatic duct stents themselves provide significant palliation of obstructive symptoms, but ILBT is effective in preventing or relieving tumorous obstruction of the stent (102). Endoluminal ultrasound can be very helpful in correct positioning of the radioactive sources (103).

At the Universita Cattolica del Sacro Cuore in Rome, Montemaggi's group treated 31 patients with unresectable cancers to doses of 20–50 Gy by use of ILBT. This was supplemented by external-beam radiation therapy plus 5-FU in some cases. Of the 31 patients, 13 had pancreatic cancers (18 had biliary cancers). No direct treatment-related acute toxicity was observed. Three patients developed late gastrointestinal bleeding. Jaundice was relieved in all patients, pain in 85%. Local control of cancer was reported in 46% of pancreas cancer patients. The 1-year survival rate for patients with unresectable pancreatic cancer was 80%. The median survival time was 21 months (14, 104). (For a comparative review of the use of ILBT, see Montemaggi's second report [14]).

**Infusional Interstitial Brachytherapy.** Infusional brachytherapy techniques using radioactive $^{32}P$ have been developed by Order et al. (105). For this procedure, a liquid suspension of radioactive $^{32}P$ particles is injected directly into the tumor through a fine needle positioned with CT guidance. In some patients, a portion of the radioactive material is "secreted" into the duodenum; in others, some of the radioactive liquid is "shunted" to the liver. Apparently, very high local tumor doses can be achieved in this fashion. In an initial group of 16 patients, Order's team was able to deliver tumor doses of 230–5000 Gy without significant toxicity. The median survival time will be in excess of 12 months. The efficacy of this novel type of brachytherapy in combination with conventional external-beam radiation therapy plus systemic 5-FU is being tested at five cooperating U.S. centers using a prospective phase II protocol.

## Hyperthermia

Heat treatment (hyperthermia) has been used as a sole modality for cancer treatment, but it is much more effective when combined with radiation therapy as a biologic response modifier (17, 106). Temperatures of 41–49°C are necessary to achieve the desired effect. Establishing, measuring, and maintaining such temperature gradients in the pancreas are not simple tasks. Techniques that have been used to heat the pancreas preferentially include interstitial radiofrequency capacitive heating (107–109), ultrasonic heating (110), and microwave heating (111). In most cases, the hyperthermia has been combined with external-beam radiation therapy, IOEBRT, and chemotherapy. All of the series reported to date are small (<20 patients). Although the morbidity and mortality rates seem to be significant (however, not entirely unacceptable), no clear benefit has been demonstrated in either patient survival or local tumor control. There is still a great need for technologic development to facilitate further clinical study of this therapeutic modality for cancer of the pancreas (110, 112).

## Immunotherapy

Although the decade since the last edition of this textbook has seen major advances in tumor imaging by techniques involving the use of antibody fragments and simple direct labeling with radioisotopes, the use of radiolabeled antibodies for cancer therapy in general (and for treatment of pancreatic cancer in particular) has been a more difficult and less successful endeavor, primarily because the immunologic technologies currently available cannot deliver adequate radiation doses (113).

## Radiotherapy of Less Common Pancreas Tumors

**Cystadenocarcinoma.** Cystadenocarcinoma of the pancreas is generally considered to be unresponsive to radiotherapy and/or chemotherapy; however, clinical investigators at Cedars-Sinai Medical Center in Los Angeles reported two cases of laparotomy-proven unresectable cystadenocarcinoma that showed marked shrinkage of tumor and reduction of carcinoembryonic antigen (CEA) levels after intravenous 5-FU (1000 mg/m$^2$/24 hr × 5 days × 2) and 40 Gy external-beam radiation therapy (111). At reexploration, both lesions had become completely resectable, with histologically clear margins and negative lymph nodes.

**Neuroendocrine Tumors.** For a review of the use of radiation therapy in the management of pancreatic neuroendocrine tumors, see Kimmig's summary of the reported experience (115).

**Islet Cell Tumors.** Four groups of clinical investigators have reported beneficial effects of radiation therapy in the management of nine patients with advanced malignant islet cell tumors. These data have been summarized by Torrisi et al. (116). Although a variety of treatment techniques (external beam, intraoperative, and brachytherapy) was used, clinical improvement was observed in every case. While most tumors recurred, the palliation lasted as long as 6 years. Reduction in tumor size, complete relief of pain, and palliation of diarrhea were seen.

**Lymphoma.** Lymphoma confined to or involving the pancreas is uncommon, but this diagnosis does not carry the dismal prognosis of ordinary pancreatic malignancy. With chemotherapy and external-beam radiation therapy given in conventional fashion, as many as 40% of such patients will survive 3 years free of disease (117). Myles et al. (118) have suggested that there may be an association between malignant lymphoma and pancreatic adenocarcinoma. If a patient with malignant lymphoma develops a pancreatic mass, the lesion should be investigated to rule out the presence of a second neoplasm, as the treatment may be much different than that for lymphoma.

**Pancreatoblastoma.** To our knowledge, there is only one case report of the use of external-beam radiation therapy in the management of infantile pancreatic carcinoma (pancreatoblastoma) (119). A 3-year-old girl was treated with 46.2 Gy in 28 fractions over 7 weeks for a second recurrence of pancreatoblastoma after surgery. Multiple biopsies performed at the time of reexploration 6 weeks later showed no residual tumor. The patient was disease free 2 years following radiotherapy.

**Solid and Papillary Tumors.** A single case report of an 18-year-old woman with a solid and papillary tumor of the pancreas treated with 40 Gy external-beam radiation therapy (split course) suggests that these neoplasms may be radiosensitive (120). Her lesion was too large to resect safely. Serial posttreatment CT scans documented tumor regression. She was symptom free 3 years after radiation therapy.

**Tumors Metastatic to the Pancreas.** Metastases to the pancreas are uncommon, but they can be highly symptomatic. In many instances, modest doses of conventional external-beam radiation therapy can provide significant symptom palliation. However, metastatic lesions in the pancreas, particularly from primary breast cancer, can present a histologic picture that is difficult to differentiate from primary adenocarcinoma of the pancreas (121). Histopathologic comparison of specimens from the primary lesion with those from the pancreatic lesion is the most reliable method to establish the correct diagnosis. The long-term prognosis for the patient with a pancreatic metastasis from a primary breast cancer may be much more favorable than that for the patient with a primary pancreatic cancer, given appropriate treatment for either entity; so the distinction is more than academic.

## REFERENCES

1. Niederhuber JE, Brennan MF, Menck HR. The national cancer data base report on pancreatic cancer. Cancer 1995;76(9): 1671–1677.
2. Dobelbower RR, Milligan AJ. Radiotherapeutic approaches to treatment of pancreatic cancer. In: Howard JM, Jordan GL Jr, Reeber HA, eds. Surgical diseases of the pancreas. Philadelphia: Lea & Febiger, 1987:734–747.
3. Dobelbower RR. The radiotherapy of pancreatic cancer. Semin Oncol 1979;6(3):378–389.
4. Dobelbower RR. Therapy by irradiation. In: Go VLW, Gardner FP, Lebenthal E, DiMagno EP, Scheele GA, eds. The exocrine pancreas: biology, pathobiology, and diseases. New York: Raven Press, 1986:699–711.
5. Dobelbower RR, Bronn DG. Radiotherapy in the treatment of pancreatic cancer. In: Neoptolemos JP, ed. Balliere's clinical gastroenterology 4(4): Cancer of the pancreas. London: Balliere-Tindall, 1990:969–983.
6. Merrick HW, Dobelbower RR. Aggressive therapy for cancer of the pancreas: does it help? In: Steinberg WM, ed. Gastroenterology clinics of North America 19(4): Disorders of the pancreas. Philadelphia: WB Saunders, 1990:935–962.
7. Douglass HO. Current approaches to multimodality management of advanced pancreatic cancer. Hepatogastroenterology 1993:40(5):433–442.
8. Trodella L, Caiazza A, Fusco V, Valentini V. Combined treatment in pancreatic carcinoma: review of the literature. Rays 1991; 16(1):76–81.
9. Abe M, Shibamoto Y, Ono K, Takahashi M. Intraoperative radiation therapy for carcinoma of the stomach and pancreas. Front Radiat Ther Oncol 1991;25:258–269,330–333.
10. Merrick HW III, Dobelbower RR Jr, Konski AA. Intraoperative radiation therapy for pancreatic, biliary and gastric carcinoma: the US experience. Front Radiat Ther Oncol 1991;25:246–257.
11. Harter KW, Dritschillo A. Cancer of the pancreas: are chemotherapy and radiation appropriate? Oncology 1989;3(6):27–30,31,35,37.
12. Heijmans HJ, Hoekstra HJ, Mehta DM. Is adjuvant intra-operative radiotherapy (IORT) for resectable and unresectable carcinoma of the pancreas worthwhile? Hepatogastroenterology 1989;36(6):474–477.
13. Dobelbower RR, Montemaggi P. Brachytherapy for pancreatic cancer: a review. Hepatogastroenterology, 1996;43:333–337.
14. Montemaggi P, Morganti AG, Dobelbower RR, Brizi G, Smaniotto D, et al. Role of intraluminal brachytherapy (ILBT) for extrahepatic bile duct *(EHBD)* and pancreas *(PC)* cancers: is it just for palliation? Radiology 1996;199:861–866.
15. Montemaggi P, Dobelbower R, Crucitti F, Caracciolo F, Morganti AG, Smaniotto D, Luzi S, Cellini N. Interstitial brachytherapy for pancreatic cancer: report of seven cases treated with $^{125}$I and a review of the literature. Int J Radiat Oncol Biol Phys 1991;21: 451–457.
16. Bagne FR, Dobelbower RR, Milligan AJ. Radiation therapy in cancer management: history and basic principles. In: Moossa AR, Schimpff SC, Robson MC, eds. Comprehensive textbook of oncology. Baltimore: Williams & Wilkins, 1991:477–485.
17. Dobelbower RR. Principles and practical aspects of radiation therapy. In: Skeel RT, Lachant NA, eds. Handbook of cancer chemotherapy. Boston: Little, Brown & Co, 1995:52–70.
18. Dobelbower RR Jr, Abe M, eds. Intraoperative radiation therapy. Boca Raton, FL: CRC Press, 1989.
19. Mohiuddin M, Regine WF, Stevens J, Rosato F, Barbot D, et al. Combined intraoperative radiation and perioperative chemotherapy for unresectable cancers of the pancreas. J Clin Oncol 1995;13(11):2764–2768.
20. Tepper JE, Noyes D, Krall JM, Sause WT, Wolkov HB, et al. Intraoperative radiation therapy of pancreatic carcinoma: a report of RTOG 8505. In: Abe M, Takahashi M, eds. Intraoperative radiation therapy. Tokyo: Pergamon Press, 1991:231–233.
21. Noyes RD, Weiss SM, Krall JM, Sause WT, Owens JR, et al. Surgical complications of intraoperative radiotherapy: the Radiation Therapy Oncology Group experience. J Surg Oncol 1992;50(4): 209–215.
22. Tepper JE, Noyes D, Krall JM, Sause WT, Wolkov HB, et al. Intraoperative radiation therapy of pancreatic carcinoma: a report of RTOG-8505. Int J Radiat Oncol Biol Phys 1991;21(5): 1145–1149.
23. Seo Y, Hata K, Wada S, Wakasugi H, Furusawa M. Intraoperative and external beam irradiation for unresectable pancreatic cancer. In: Abe M, Takahashi M, eds. Intraoperative radiation therapy. Tokyo: Pergamon Press, 1991:251–253.
24. Garton GR, Gunderson LL, Nagorney DM, Donohue JH, Martin JK, et al. High dose preoperative external beam and intraoperative irradiation for locally advanced pancreatic cancer. Int J Radiat Oncol Biol Phys 1993;27(5):1153–1157.
25. Willich N, Denecke H, Grab J. Advantageous palliative effects and dose-related complications of IORT in nonresectable pancreatic cancer. In: Abe M, Takahashi M, eds. Intraoperative radiation therapy. Tokyo: Pergamon Press, 1991:257–259.
26. Zhong YB, Pan RQ, Wang JY, Liu PF, Qin LL, et al. Intraoperative radiotherapy for pancreatic carcinoma. In: Abe M, Takahashi M, eds. Intraoperative radiation therapy. Tokyo: Pergamon Press, 1991:268–269.
27. Willich N, Kramling H-J, Rube C. Study on IORT of 44 patients with unresectable carcinoma of the pancreas. In: Schildberg FW, Willich N, Kramling HJ, eds. Intraoperative radiation therapy. Essen: Verlag Die Blaue Eule, 1993:311–314.
28. Kimura Y, Kobari M, Akaishi S, Matsuno S. Clinical advantage in radiation therapy for unresectable adenocarcinoma of the pancreas. In: Abe M, Takahashi M, eds. Intraoperative radiation therapy. Tokyo: Pergamon Press, 1991:278–279.
29. Yamaue H, Tanimura H, Aoki Y, Iwashashi M, Tani M, et al. Clinical and immunological evaluation of intraoperative radiation therapy for patients with unresectable pancreatic cancer. J Surg Oncol 1992;49(1):10–15.
30. Kishi K, Shirai S, Yamada R, Tsuji K, Yamaui H, Tanamura H. Effect of single session intraoperative radiotherapy for advanced pancreatic cancer. In: Abe M, Takahashi M, eds. Intraoperative radiation therapy. Tokyo: Pergamon Press, 1991:272–273.
31. Mohiuddin M, Regine W, Rosato F, Barbot D, Schuricht A, et al. A comparison of intraoperative radiation therapy (IORT) and $^{125}$I implantation for cancer of the pancreas. In: Schildberg FW, Willich N, Kramling HJ, eds. Intraoperative radiation therapy. Essen: Verlag Die Blaue Eule, 1993:315–323.
32. Yasukawa H, Kojima Y, Kimura T, Katayama K, Note M, et al. Radiotherapy-centered multimodal treatment for unresectable pancreatic cancer. In: Abe M, Takahashi M, eds. Intraoperative radiation therapy. Tokyo: Pergamon Press, 1991:288–289.
33. Rich TA, Evans DB, Levin B. Current status of IORT in the treatment of pancreatic cancer. In: Schildberg FW, Willich N, Kramling HJ, eds. Intraoperative radiation therapy. Essen: Verlag Die Blaue Eule, 1993:273–277.
34. Dobelbower RR Jr, Konski AA, Kamen C, Merrick HW III. Intraoperative electron beam radiation therapy (IOEBRT) for cancer of the pancreas. In: Abe M, Takahashi M, eds. Intraoperative radiation therapy. Tokyo: Pergamon Press, 1991:234–236.
35. Abe M, Shibamoto Y, Nishimura Y. Intraoperative radiotherapy for pancreatic cancer in Japan: multi-institutional and Kyoto University experiences. In: Schildberg FW, Willich N, Kramling HJ, eds. Intraoperative radiation therapy. Essen: Verlag Die Blaue Eule, 1993:278–281.
36. Gilly FN, Gerard JP, Braillon G, Romestaing P, Berard P, et al. Intraoperative radiation therapy (IORT) for resectable and

unresectable pancreatic carcinoma. In: Abe M, Takahashi M, eds. Intraoperative radiation therapy. Tokyo: Pergamon Press, 1991:244–245.
37. Kawamura M, Kataoka M, Fugii T, Itoh H, Ishine M, et al. Electron beam intraoperative radiation therapy (EBIORT) for localized pancreatic carcinoma. Int J Radiat Oncol Biol Phys 1992;23(4): 751–757.
38. Manabe T, Shibamoto Y, Ono K, Sasai K, Baba N, et al. Combined modality treatment for cancer of the pancreas: intraoperative and external radiotherapies. In: Abe M, Takahashi M, eds. Intraoperative radiation therapy. Tokyo: Pergamon Press, 1991:246–248.
39. Dobelbower RR, Konski AA, Merrick HW. Intraoperative electron beam radiation therapy (IOEBRT) and postoperative precision external beam radiation therapy (PEBERT) for adenocarcinoma of the pancreas: a report of 60 cases. In: Schildberg FW, Willich N, Kramling HJ, eds. Intraoperative radiation therapy. Essen: Verlag Die Blaue Eule, 1993:301–308.
40. Gilly FN, Gerard JP, Braillon G, Romestaing PM, Rocher FP, et al. IORT and surgery for resectable and unresectable pancreatic adenocarcinoma: a series of 48 patients treated according to the Lyon intraoperative system. In: Schildberg FW, Willich N, Kramling HJ, eds. Intraoperative radiation therapy. Essen: Verlag Die Blaue Eule, 1993:309–311.
41. Sakamoto J, Yasue M, Morimoto T, Morita K. Intraoperative radiation therapy for advanced carcinoma of the pancreas. In: Abe M, Takahashi M, eds. Intraoperative radiation therapy. Tokyo: Pergamon Press, 1991:254–256.
42. Dobelbower RR Jr, Konski AA, Merrick HW III, Bronn DG, Schifeling D, Kamen C. Intraoperative electron beam radiation therapy (IOEBRT) for carcinoma of the exocrine pancreas. Int J Radiat Oncol Biol Phys 1991;20(1):113–119.
43. Ebe K, Nishikawa E, Suda H, Honma Y, Nakada T, et al. Intraoperative radiation therapy for carcinoma of the pancreas. In: Abe M, Takahashi M, eds. Intraoperative radiation therapy. Tokyo: Pergamon Press, 1991:270–271.
44. Fossati V, Zerbi A, Cattaneo GM, Parolini D, Reni M, et al. Combination or not of IORT with external radiotherapy (ERT) and chemotherapy (CHT) in pancreatic carcinoma. In: Schildberg FW, Willich N, Kramling HJ, eds. Intraoperative radiation therapy. Essen: Verlag Die Blaue Eule, 1993:297–300.
45. Sasai K, Shibamoto Y, Manabe T, Baba N, Takahashi M, et al. External beam and intraoperative radiation therapy for pancreatic cancer. In: Abe M, Takahashi M, eds. Intraoperative radiation therapy. Tokyo: Pergamon Press, 1991:274–275.
46. Kawamura M, Kataoka M, Tanada M, Takashima S, Inoue K, et al. Electron beam intraoperative radiation therapy (EBIORT) for pancreatic carcinoma. In: Abe M, Takahashi M, eds. Intraoperative radiation therapy. Tokyo: Pergamon Press, 1991:276–277.
47. Gilly FN, Romestaing PJ, Braillon GG, Sayag AC, Sentenac IJ, et al. Experience of three years with intra-operative radiation therapy using the Lyon intra-operative device. Int Surg 1990; 75(2):84–88.
48. Ikeda H, Matayoshi Y, Murayama S, Inoue T, Kozuka T, Monden M. Intraoperative radiation therapy for the patients with locally advanced pancreatic carcinoma. In: Abe M, Takahashi M, eds. Intraoperative radiation therapy. Tokyo: Pergamon Press, 1991: 280–281.
49. Fossati V, Cattaneo GB, Zerbi A, Galli L, Bordogna G, et al. The role of intraoperative therapy by electron beam and combination of adjuvant chemotherapy and external radiotherapy in carcinoma of the pancreas. Tumori 1995;81(1):23–31.
50. Ohara K, Tatsuzaki H, Sugahara S, Yoshida T, Todoriki T, et al. IORT for pancreatic cancer with special reference to pre- and post-resection IORT. In: Abe M, Takahashi M, eds. Intraoperative radiation therapy. Tokyo: Pergamon Press, 1991:282–283.
51. Yamaue H, Tanimura H, Tsunoda T, Iwahashi M, Tani M, et al. Effects of intraoperative radiotherapy on immunological parameters in patients with pancreatic cancer. In: Abe M, Takahashi M, eds. Intraoperative radiation therapy. Tokyo: Pergamon Press, 1991:292–293.
52. Zerbi A, Fossati V, Parolini D, Carlucci M, Bordogna G, et al. Intraoperative radiation therapy adjuvant to resection in the treatment of pancreatic cancer. Cancer 1994;73(12):2930–2935.
53. Glaser K, Bodner E, Klingler A. Adjuvant intraoperative radiation therapy (IORT) of pancreatic cancer during radical resection. In: Schildberg FW, Willich N, Kramling HJ, eds. Intraoperative radiation therapy. Essen: Verlag Die Blaue Eule, 1993:282–286.
54. Hiraoka T, Tashiro S, Kamimoto I, Kanemitsu K, Saitoh N, et al. Combination of intraoperative radiation with resection for cancer of the pancreas. In: Abe M, Takahashi M, eds. Intraoperative radiation therapy. Tokyo: Pergamon Press, 1991:239–241.
55. Rich TA, Evans DB, Curley SA, Ajani JA. Adjuvant radiotherapy and chemotherapy for biliary and pancreatic cancer. Ann Oncol 1994;5(suppl)3:75–80.
56. Grab J, Kramling H-J, Willich N, Schildberg FW. IORT in the treatment of resectable pancreatic carcinoma. In: Schildberg FW, Willich N, Kramling HJ, eds. Intraoperative radiation therapy. Essen: Verlag Die Blaue Eule, 1993:287–290.
57. Glaser K, Bodner J, Tshmelitsh J. Adjuvant IORT during duodenopancreatectomy. In: Abe M, Takahashi M, eds. Intraoperative radiation therapy. Tokyo: Pergamon Press, 1991:237–238.
58. Gotoh M, Sakon M, Kanai Y, Umeshita K, Ikeda H, Mori T. Intraoperative irradiation in resected carcinoma of the pancreas and portal vein. Arch Surg 1992;127(10):1213–1215.
59. Doglietto GB, Bossola M, Belantone R, Ratto C, Valentini V, et al. Intraoperative and external beam radiation therapy for resectable carcinoma of the head of the pancreas. In: Schildberg FW, Willich N, Kramling HJ, eds. Intraoperative radiation therapy. Essen: Verlag Die Blaue Eule, 1993:291–293.
60. Hanyu F, Hatori T, Imaizumi T, Suzuki M, Nakasako T, et al. Intraoperative radiotherapy for patients with carcinoma of the head of the pancreas. In: Abe M, Takahashi M, eds. Intraoperative radiation therapy. Tokyo: Pergamon Press, 1991:242–243.
61. Gotoh M, Monden M, Sakon M, Kanai T, Umeshita K, et al. Control of subclinical disease by intraoperative radiotherapy after radical resection of pancreatic cancer. In: Schildberg FW, Willich N, Kramling HJ, eds. Intraoperative radiation therapy. Essen: Verlag Die Blaue Eule, 1993:294–296.
62. Manabe T, Baba N, Ono K, Sasai K, Takuhashi M, et al. Radical pancreatectomy with intraoperative radiation therapy for pancreatic head cancer. In: Abe M, Takahashi M, eds. Intraoperative radiation therapy. Tokyo: Pergamon Press, 1991:249–250.
63. Ozaki H, Kinoshita T, Kosuge T, Egawa S, Kishi K. Effectiveness of multimodality treatment for resectable pancreatic cancer. Int J Pancreatol 1990;7(1–3):195–200.
64. Zerbi A, Fossati V, Carlucci M, Staudacher C, Volerrani F, Di Carlo V. Intraoperative radiation therapy adjuvant to pancreatoduodenectomy with neoprene injection into the pancreatic stump. In: Schildberg FW, Willich N, Kramling HJ, eds. Intraoperative radiation therapy. Essen: Verlag Die Blaue Eule, 1993: 324–327.
65. Schildberg FW, Grab J, Willich N, Pratschke E. Experience with intraoperative radiotherapy in resectable pancreatic cancer. In: Abe M, Takahashi M, eds. Intraoperative radiation therapy. Tokyo: Pergamon Press, 1991:284–285.
66. Hiraoka T, Uchino R, Kanemitsu K, Toyonaga M, Saitoh N, et al. Combination of intraoperative radiation with resection of cancer of the pancreas. Int J Pancreatol 1990;7(1–3);201–207.
67. Gotoh M, Monden M, Sakon M, Kanai T, Umeshita K, et al. Venous bypass and intraoperative radiotherapy in cases of combined resection of the pancreas and the portal vein for patients bearing pancreatic cancer. In: Abe M, Takahashi M, eds. Intraoperative radiation therapy. Tokyo: Pergamon Press, 1991: 294–295.
68. Blitzer PH, Katin MJ, Rubenstein JH, Harwin WN, Raymond MG, et al. Radiation and chemotherapy. Treatment of localized pancreatic carcinoma. J Fla Med Assoc 1994;81(6):403–407.
69. Tisdale BA, Paris KJ, Lindberg RD, Jose B, Spanos WJ Jr. Radiation therapy for pancreatic cancer: a retrospective study of the University of Louisville experience. South Med J 1995;88(7): 741–744.
70. Treurniet-Donker AD, van Mierlo MJ, van Putten WL. Localized unresectable pancreatic cancer. Int J Radiat Oncol Biol Phys 1990;18(1):59–62.
71. Flickinger JC, Jawalekar K, Deutsch M, Webster J. Split course radiation therapy for adenocarcinoma of the pancreas. Int J Radiat Oncol Phys 1988;15:359–364.
72. Bruckner HW, Kalnicki S, Dalton J, Schwartz GK, Chesser MR, et al. Combined modality therapy increasing local control of pancreatic cancer. Cancer Invest 1993;11(3):241–246.

73. Ardalan B, Ucar A, Reddy R, Livingstone AS, Markoe A, et al. Phase I trial of *N*-phosphonacetyl-L-aspartic acid and high dose 5-fluorouracil administered concomitantly with radiation therapy for unresectable localized adenocarcinoma of the pancreas. Cancer 1994;74(7):1869–1873.
74. Seydel HG, Stablein DM, Leichman LP, Kinzie JJ, Thomas PRM. Hyperfractionated radiation and chemotherapy for unresectable localized adenocarcinoma of the pancreas: the Gastrointestinal Tumor Study Group experience. Cancer 1990;67: 1478–1482.
75. Kahn PJ, Skornick Y, Inbar M, Kaplan O, Chaichik S, Rozin R. Surgical palliation combined with synchronous therapy in pancreatic carcinoma. Eur J Surg Oncol 1990;16(1):7–11.
76. Robertson JM, Marsh L, Ten Haken RK, Lawrence TS. The clinical application of a non-axial treatment plan for pancreatic and biliary malignancies. Radiother Oncol 1992;24:198–200.
77. Chu JC, Solin LJ, Hwang CC, Kessler H, Hanks GE. Three-dimensional dosimetric comparison of radiation therapy treatment planning for the pancreas. Med Dosimetry 1992;17(4): 199–203.
78. Schell MC, Cheng S, Tefft M, Fine R, Higgins PD. Conformal radiation therapy of pancreatic carcinoma (Abstract). Int J Radiat Oncol Biol Phys 1991;21(suppl 1):1078.
79. Higgens PD, Sohn PW, Fine RM, Schell MC. Three-dimensional conformal pancreas treatment: comparison of four- to six-field techniques. Int J Radiat Oncol Biol Phys 1995;31(3):605–609.
80. Fine R. Personal communication. January 1994.
81. Abrams RA, Grochow LB. Adjuvant therapy with chemotherapy and radiation therapy in the management of carcinoma of the pancreatic head. Surg Clin North Am 1995;75(5):925–938.
82. Willett CG, Lewandrowski K, Warshaw AL, Efird J, Compton CC. Resection margins in carcinoma of the head of the pancreas. Implications for radiation therapy. Ann Surg 1993;217:144–148.
83. Sener SF, Fremgen A, Imperato JP, Sylvester J, Chmiel JS. Pancreatic cancer in Illinois. A report by 88 hospitals on 2,401 patients diagnosed 1978–84. Am Surg 1991;57(8):490–495.
84. Andren-Sandberg A, Hafstrom A. Curatively intended surgery for exocrine pancreas cancer. Gastroenterologist 1994;2(1):20–26.
85. Feitkau R, Sauer R. Future prospects of radiotherapy in pancreatic cancer. Eur J Surg Oncol 1991;17(2):201–210.
86. Yeo CJ, Cameron JL, Lillemoe KD, Stitzman JV, Hruban RH, et al. Pancreaticoduodenectomy for cancer of the head of the pancreas. 201 cases. Ann Surg 1995;221(6):721–733.
87. Cameron H. The current management of carcinoma of the head of the pancreas. Annu Rev Med 1995;46:361–370.
88. Foo ML, Gunderson LL, Nagorney DM, McIlraith DC, van Heerden JA, et al. Patterns of failure in grossly resected pancreatic ductal adenocarcinoma treated with adjuvant irradiation +/- 5-fluorouracil. Int J Radiat Oncol Biol Phys 1993; 26(3):483–489.
89. Komaki R, Wadler S, Peters T, et al. High dose local irradiation plus prophylactic hepatic irradiation and chemotherapy for inoperable adenocarcinoma of the pancreas: a preliminary report of a multi-institutional trial (Radiation Therapy Oncology Group protocol 8801). Cancer 1992;69(11):2807–2812.
90. Bosset JF, Pavy JJ, Gillet M, Mantion G, Pelissier E, Schraub S. Conventional external radiation alone as adjuvant treatment in resectable pancreatic cancer: results of a prospective study. Radiother Oncol 1992;24(3):191–194.
91. Dobelbower RR, Konski AA. Radiation therapy in cancer management: clinical considerations. In: Moossa AR, Schimpff SC, Robson MC, eds. Comprehensive textbook of oncology. Baltimore: Williams & Wilkins, 1991:486–492.
92. Evans DB, Rich TA, Byrd DR, Cleary KR, Connelly JH, et al. Preoperative chemoradiation and pancreaticoduodenectomy for adenocarcinoma of the pancreas. Arch Surg 1992; 127(11):1335–1339.
93. Hoffman JP, Weese JL, Solin LJ, Agarwal P, Engstrom P, et al. A single institution experience with preoperative chemoradiotherapy (CTRT) for stage I-III pancreatic adenocarcinoma. Am Surg 1993;59(11):772–781.
94. Yeung RS, Weese JL, Hoffman JP, Solin JP, Paul AE, et al. Neoadjuvant chemoradiation in pancreatic and duodenal carcinoma. A phase II study. Cancer 1993;72(7):2124–2133.
95. Hoffman JP, Weese JL, Solin LJ, Engstrom P, Agarwal P, et al. A pilot study of preoperative chemoradiation for patients with localized adenocarcinoma of the pancreas. Am J Surg 1995; 169(1):71–77.
96. Dobelbower RR, Wagner SM, Fadell RJ, Howard JA, DiDio LA. Pancreatic cancer. In: Dobelbower RR, ed. Gastrointestinal cancer: radiation therapy. Hamburg: Springer-Verlag, 1990: 115–148.
97. Mohiuddin M, Rosato F, Barbot D, Schuricht A, Biermann W, Cantor R. Long-term results of combined modality treatment with I-125 implantation for carcinoma of the pancreas. Int J Radiat Oncol Biol Phys 1992;23(2):305–311.
98. Lebobvics E, Mittleman A, Del Guercio LR, Hilaris B, Moorthy C, et al. Pancreaticobiliary fistula and obstructive jaundice complicating $^{125}$I interstitial implants for pancreatic cancer: endoscopic diagnosis and management. Gastrointest Endosc 1990; 36(6):610–611.
99. Goertz SR, Ali MM, Parker GA. Local management of pancreatic carcinoma: iodine-125 implantation. Clin Oncol (R Coll Radiol) 1990;2(1):22–26.
100. Joyce F, Burcharth F, Holm HH, Stroyer I. Ultrasonically guided percutaneous implantation of iodine-125 seeds in pancreatic carcinoma. Int J Radiat Oncol Biol Phys 1990;19(4):1049–1052.
101. Warszawski N, Pfreundner L, Bratengeier K, Bohndorf W, Feustel H. Combined isodose curves of high-dose rate interstitial brachytherapy with external-beam radiation therapy in pancreatic carcinoma. Strahlenther Onkol 1992;168(9):552–557.
102. Glaser M, Laurence BH, Cameron FG, Relief of tumorous obstruction of a metal biliary stent with palliative intraluminal iridium-192 therapy. Gastrointestinal Endoscopy 1992;38(4): 496–498.
103. Minsky B, Botet J, Gerdes H, Lightdale C. Ultrasound directed extrahepatic bile duct intraluminal brachytherapy. Int J Radiat Oncol Biol Phys 1992;23(1):165–167.
104. Montemaggi P, Costamagna G, Dobelbower RR, Cellini N, Morganti AG, et al. Intraluminal brachytherapy in the treatment of pancreas and bile duct carcinoma. Int J Radiat Oncol Biol Phys 1995;32(2):437–443.
105. Order SE, Siegel JA, Lustig RA, Principato R, Zeiger LS, et al. Infusional brachytherapy in the treatment of non-resectable pancreatic cancer: a new radiation modality (preliminary report of the phase I study). Antibody Immunoconj Radiopharm 1994;7(1):11–27.
106. Kapp D S. Hyperthermia. In: Moossa AR, Schimpff SC, Robson MC, eds. Comprehensive textbook of oncology. Baltimore: Williams & Wilkins, 1991:653–659.
107. U R, Sugahara T. The use of hyperthermia in cancer treatment. An analysis of clinical investigations on deep seated malignant tumor control with a radiofrequency capacitive hyperthermia system (Thermotron RF-8). Adv Exp Med Biol 1990;267:79–94.
108. Goldson AL, Ashayeri E. Update on intraoperative interstitial hyperthermia (IOIBT) and intraoperative radiotherapy (IORT) for pancreatic cancer at Howard University. In: Abe M, Takahashi M, eds. Intraoperative radiation therapy. Tokyo: Pergamon Press, 1991:260–262.
109. Yamashita T, Nakazawa M, Sekiguchi K, Uchida I, Hori M, Nishi M. Intraoperative radio therapy (IOR) and intraoperative hyperthermia (IOH) for unresectable pancreatic cancer. In: Abe M, Takahashi M, eds. Intraoperative radiation therapy. Tokyo: Pergamon Press, 1991:286–287.
110. Colacchio TA, Couglin C, Taylor J, Douple E, Ryan T, Crichlow RT. Intraoperative radiation therapy and hyperthermia. Morbidity and mortality from this combined treatment modality for unresectable intra-abdominal malignancies. Arch Surg 1990; 125(3):370–375.
111. Endow M, Suzuki H, Nakashima Y, Nagashima K, Miyamoto K, Ishikawa T. Seven pancreatic patients with cancer receiving multimodal treatment with intraoperative irradiation and hyperthermochemotherapy. In: Abe M, Takahashi M, eds. Intraoperative radiation therapy. Tokyo: Pergamon Press, 1991:290–291.
112. Kojima Y, Kimura T, Yasukawa H, Katayama K, Note M, et al. Radiotherapy-centered multimodal treatment of unresectable pancreatic carcinoma. Int Surg 1991;76(2):87–90.
113. Goldenberg DM. Imaging and therapy of gastrointestinal cancers with radiolabeled antibodies. Am J Gastroenterol 1991; 86(10):1392–1403.

114. Wood D, Silberman AW, Heifitz L, Mesmic L, Shabot MM. Cystadenocarcinoma of the pancreas: neo-adjuvant therapy and CEA monitoring. J Surg Oncol 1990;43(1):56–60.
115. Kimmig BN. Radiotherapy for gastroenteropancreatic neuroendocrine tumors. Ann NY Acad Sci 1994;733:488–495.
116. Torrisi JR, Treat J, Zeman R, Dritschilo A. Radiotherapy in the management of pancreatic islet cell tumors. Cancer 1987;60: 1226–1231.
117. Hart MJ, White TT, Brown PC, Freeny PC. Potentially curable masses in the pancreas. Am J Surg 1987;154:134–136.
118. Myles JL, Howard JM, Kim K, Dobelbower RR. Association of malignant lymphoma with pancreatic adenocarcinoma: a clinicopathologic study of three patients. Pancreas 1991;6(2): 249–252.
119. Griffin BR, Wisbeck WM, Schaller RT, Benjamin DR. Radiotherapy for locally recurrent infantile pancreatic carcinoma (pancreatoblastoma). Cancer 1987;60:1734–1736.
120. Fried P, Cooper J, Balthazar E, Fazzini E, Newall J. A role for radiotherapy in the treatment of solid and papillary neoplasms of the pancreas. Cancer 1985;56:2783–2785.
121. Whitington R, Moylan D, Dobelbower RR, Kramer S. Pancreatic tumours in patients with previous malignancy. Clin Radiol 1982;33:297–299.

# 60

# *Adjuvant Therapy*

Richard H. Bell, Jr.

## DEFINITION OF ADJUVANT THERAPY

Surgical removal of pancreatic cancer currently is the only therapy shown to result in cure. In this context, adjuvant therapy is defined as therapy added to surgery in an attempt to increase the likelihood of complete cancer eradication and long-term survival. Typically, radiation therapy and chemotherapy have been employed in combination as adjuvant modalities in pancreatic cancer, although some adjuvant programs have used radiation or chemotherapy alone in addition to surgery. Radiation therapy in pancreatic cancer is used to enhance local control of the tumor. Radiation therapy complements surgical excision because surgery is effective at removing bulk disease but potentially ineffective near the margins of invasion, whereas radiation therapy is effective in killing small numbers of well-oxygenated cells near the tumor periphery, but less effective in treating the central, relatively hypoxic portions of bulky tumor. In the adjuvant setting, chemotherapy is employed both for its radiation-sensitizing effects and to treat micrometastatic disease. Adjuvant therapy may be used prior to surgical resection (neoadjuvant therapy), at the same time as surgery (intraoperative radiation therapy), following surgical excision of the tumor, or in combinations of the above (e.g., preoperative external-beam radiotherapy and chemotherapy combined with intraoperative radiation therapy and postoperative chemotherapy). The possible timing of adjuvant therapy in relation to surgery is depicted in Figure 60.1.

## RATIONALE FOR ADJUVANT THERAPY IN PANCREATIC CANCER

### Adjuvant Therapy to Control Local Recurrence

Approximately 80–90% of patients with apparently resectable pancreatic cancer who undergo what appears to be a curative resection develop recurrent cancer. As a result, the 5-year cure rate in this group of patients is only 10–25% (1). In examining the pattern of tumor recurrence following apparently complete resection, Tepper et al. (2) reviewed the course of 31 patients who had apparently curative surgery for carcinoma of the pancreas (none of whom received additional therapy) and found that 50% developed a local recurrence in a follow-up period of 5 years. Griffin et al. (3), in analyzing 36 patients with a median follow-up of 51 months after tumor resection, found that 27% developed an isolated local recurrence. Local recurrence was a component of failure in 70% of patients relapsing after operation. Kayahara et al. (4) reviewed the records of 45 patients who had undergone macroscopically curative resection for carcinoma of the pancreas, of whom 30 ultimately developed recurrent cancer; 25 of the 30 patients (83%) failed in the retroperitoneal area, either exclusively or in association with distant metastases. In a revealing study, Guthoff et al. (5) intensively followed 24 patients, after Whipple resection for ductal carcinoma, with tumor markers and imaging studies every 4–8 weeks; 20 patients developed recurrence within 8 months. In all but two of these patients, the first site of recurrence was local—in the retroperitoneal soft tissue posterior to the portal vein, near the superior mesenteric artery.

Locoregional failure following removal of carcinoma of the head of the pancreas is probably due to at least two factors. First is the high incidence of tumor extension to the retroperitoneum at the time of surgery. In reviewing the operative and pathologic findings in 163 patients who underwent resection for carcinoma of the head of the pancreas, Tsuchiya et al. (6) found that the incidence of invasion into the retroperitoneal soft tissues ranged from 22% in T1 tumors to 56% in T3/T4 tumors. Willett et al. (7) reviewed the pathology and clinical course of 72 patients who had undergone resection of carcinoma of the head of the pancreas to identify the frequency of tumor involvement at the standard surgical resection margins (stomach, duodenum, pancreatic neck, and bile duct) as well as the peripancreatic soft tissue margin. Of the 72 patients undergoing resection, 37 (51%) had microscopic tumor extension to at least one margin. The most commonly involved margin was the peripancreatic soft tissue (27 patients), where the ability to achieve tumor-free margins is hampered by the proximity of the uncinate process of the head of the pancreas to the superior mesenteric artery and vein. There were no 5-year survivors in the group of patients with positive margins, whereas 5-year survival and local control in 35 patients with negative resection margins were 22% and 43%, respectively. This study suggested that preoperative radiation therapy might shrink tumors sufficiently to reduce the incidence of positive margins and that intraoperative radiotherapy might be of benefit by killing tumor cells at positive resection margins.

The second factor favoring a high incidence of locoregional recurrence following pancreaticoduodenectomy is the frequent presence of lymph node metastases, which may or may not be adequately excised as part of the primary operation. The overall incidence of lymph node metastases at the time of resection of pancreatic carcinoma is approximately 60% (8). The incidence of lymph node metastases is 30% even in patients with primary tumors 2 cm or smaller (9). In reviewing the pathologic findings in lymph nodes removed during pancreatic resection with radical lymphadenectomy, the Japan Pancreatic Cancer Registry (10) and Cubilla and Fitzgerald (11) showed that the nodes most frequently involved with metastatic deposits, as expected, are those in immediate proximity to the pancreatic head. On the other hand, a significant number of microscopic metastases occur to regional nodes that are not ordinarily removed in the course of standard pancreaticoduodenectomy. These include nodal groups along the superior mesenteric artery, nodes along the common hepatic artery, nodes in the area of the celiac plexus,

| | PREOPERATIVE PERIOD | RESECTION | POSTOPERATIVE PERIOD |
|---|---|---|---|
| POSTOPERATIVE ONLY | | | WBRT, 5-FU |
| INTRAOPERATIVE ONLY | | IORT | |
| PREOPERATIVE ("NEOADJUVANT) ONLY | EBRT, 5-FU | | |
| COMBINED | EBRT, 5-FU | IORT BOOST | 5-FU |

**FIG. 60.1.** Four possible schemata for the delivery of adjuvant therapy for carcinoma of the pancreas. In all cases, surgical resection of the tumor is assumed. *EBRT,* external-beam radiation therapy; *IORT,* intraoperative radiation therapy; *5-FU,* 5-fluorouracil.

paraaortic nodes behind the pancreas, and nodes along the superior and inferior borders of the body of the pancreas.

In Japan, the realization that nodal metastases are often present outside the bounds of traditional pancreaticoduodenectomy has led to the general adoption of an extended pancreatectomy, which includes a radical upper abdominal lymphadenectomy. In the United States, this procedure has not been widely accepted, and it is possible that the same objective (elimination of occult regional lymph node metastases) can be accomplished by pre- or postoperative radiation therapy, without an increase in the scope of the operation. The possibility that radiation therapy is effective in sterilizing regional lymph node beds is suggested by one study of the pathologic findings in patients explored after preoperative radiotherapy (12). Of 13 patients undergoing resection for pancreatic cancer after preoperative radiation therapy, only 2 (15%) demonstrated lymph node metastases in the operative specimen. On the other hand, another study (13) found no difference in the incidence of lymph node involvement in the resected specimens of patients undergoing preoperative irradiation and nonrandomized historic control patients from the same institution who received no radiation. In rectal cancer, where there has been a longer experience with adjuvant therapy, several studies suggest that preoperative irradiation may have the effect of sterilizing regional lymph nodes (14).

### Adjuvant Therapy for Downstaging

Although tumor resection offers the possibility of cure with pancreatic cancer, most patients present with disease that is too extensive to allow safe removal of all gross tumor. In a consecutive series of 213 patients evaluated by dynamic computed tomography (CT) scan (15), resection was precluded by metastases, local peripancreatic extension, or contiguous organ invasion in all but 25 patients. Common local barriers to resection were invasion/encasement of the portal/superior mesenteric/splenic vein complex (79% of patients) or involvement of the celiac, splenic, hepatic, or superior mesenteric arteries (60% of patients). If a preoperative adjuvant program could significantly shrink tumor volume, it is possible that some patients with advanced local disease could become candidates for resection.

### Adjuvant Therapy for Prevention of Distant Metastases

Autopsy studies demonstrate that nearly all patients who die of pancreatic cancer have distant metastases (16). In patients who have undergone resection of their primary tumor, distant metastases ultimately occur in approximately 80% (3, 4). The most common site of distant metastases is the liver (60% of patients). Peritoneal carcinomatosis is also relatively common (40%). Pulmonary or other extraabdominal metastases occur in about 20% of patients. Presumably, many patients with otherwise apparently resectable pancreatic cancer have distant micrometastases, not yet clinically apparent, which could be targeted by adjuvant therapy while the tumor burden is small. Possible forms of adjuvant therapy that may be useful in this regard include systemic chemotherapy or immunotherapy, as well as regional strategies targeted at the high-risk organs (hepatic perfusion with chemotherapeutic agents, whole liver irradiation). Thus far, the use of adjuvant therapies in pancreatic cancer has focused primarily on the prevention of locoregional recurrence, and experience with adjuvant therapy to prevent distant metastases is relatively limited; the results of the few existing trials are discussed below. As our ability to control locoregional disease improves, however, the need for effective systemic strategies will become increasingly important.

## TIMING AND RESULTS OF ADJUVANT THERAPY IN PANCREATIC CANCER

In the following discussion of the results of adjuvant therapy in pancreatic cancer, the various existing trials are grouped into postoperative, intraoperative, and preoperative interventions in an attempt to bring some order to the various studies that have been reported. Grouping the trials in this way also emphasizes the fact that preoperative (neoadjuvant) therapy differs from postoperative therapy in that there is the possibility of downstaging in addition to prevention of recurrence, whereas postoperative therapy is designed purely for prophylaxis of recurrent disease. On the other hand, grouping the trials in this fashion overlooks the fact that adjuvant programs increasingly combine preoperative, intraoperative, and postoperative therapy, so that the distinctions are somewhat artificial.

### Postoperative Adjuvant Therapy

The first, and in retrospect the most influential, prospective trial of adjuvant therapy for resectable pancreatic cancer was initiated by the Gastrointestinal Tumor Study Group (GITSG) in 1973. The target study population consisted of patients who had undergone an apparently curative resection of histologically confirmed adenocarcinoma of the pancreas. Patients with periampullary tumors, islet cell tumors, and cystadenocarcinoma were excluded. The margins of resection of the surgical specimen were required to be free of disease, with no evidence of distant metastases. Patients meeting these criteria were randomized to receive either radiation therapy and 5-fluorouracil (5-FU) or follow-up and evaluation but no adjuvant therapy. In the treated group, postoperative external-beam radiation was started 4–13 weeks postoperatively and given as a split course of 40 Gy with a 2-week rest period between two courses of 20 Gy each. The treatment field included all of the remaining pancreas as well as the major upper abdominal lymph node–bearing areas. 5-FU was administered as an intravenous bolus of 500 mg/m$^2$ body surface area. It was given on three consecutive days at the beginning of each 20-Gy radiation course and then continued on a once-weekly basis for 2 years or until recurrence was noted.

Accrual into this trial was extremely slow. After 8 years, during which time a total of 43 patients had been entered, it became apparent that there was a survival difference in the treated and nontreated groups. The study was halted, and the results reported (17). At that point, the enrolled patients had been followed for a median of 5.5 years. Median survival was 11 months in the control group and 20 months in the treated group, a statistically significant difference. Disease-free survival was also significantly extended in patients treated with radiation and 5-FU. The maximum separation of the survival curves was at 2 years postoperatively, at which time 42% of the treated group were still alive as opposed to 15% of the control group (Fig. 60.2).

Because the number of patients treated with radiation and chemotherapy in this trial was small, the GITSG reopened the treatment arm of the original study to recruit a new cohort of patients, all of whom received 40 Gy radiation and 5-FU as in the first trial. An additional 30 patients were accrued. In this confirmatory trial (18), the results were quite similar to the treated group in the original study—median survival was 18 months, and 2-year survival, 46%. In both the randomized and

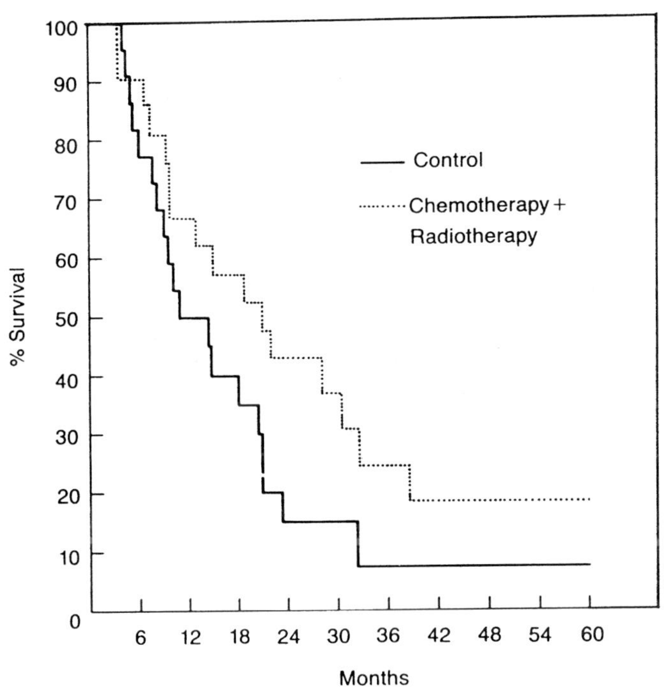


**FIG. 60.2.** Survival comparison of 21 patients who received postoperative external beam radiotherapy and 5-FU after apparently curative pancreatic resection with 22 patients randomized to observation only following resection. Survival was greater in the treated than in the control group at all intervals of follow-up (*p* = .03). (Reproduced with permission from Kalser MH, Ellenberg SS. Pancreatic cancer. Adjuvant combined radiation and chemotherapy following curative resection. Arch Surg 1985;120: 899–903.)

the confirmatory trials, toxicity from the adjuvant regimen was quite tolerable. There was an 18% incidence of severe leukopenia, with leukocyte counts between 1200 and 1900 per mL; 6% of patients experienced mucositis and diarrhea. There were no life-threatening toxic reactions or deaths attributed to adjuvant therapy.

In 1990, Douglass and Stablein (19) reported long-term follow-up data from the original randomized GITSG trial. At that point, median time on study was 11 years. Carcinoma had recurred in 95% of the control group but only 67% of the group receiving radiation and 5-FU; 19% of the treated patients survived 10 years in contrast to none of the control patients.

Since the publication of the GITSG trials, the use of postoperative radiation and 5-FU following resection for pancreatic carcinoma has been adopted as relatively routine therapy in the United States. Subsequent reported experiences from nonrandomized trials have generally supported the GITSG findings. In 78 patients treated at Johns Hopkins since 1991, for example, 2-year survival for patients who received 5-FU/radiation was 35%, compared with 0% in patients not receiving adjuvant therapy following tumor resection (8).

Studies in adjuvant therapy of rectal carcinoma suggest that continuous infusion of 5-FU during radiation therapy is more efficacious than the bolus therapy used in the GITSG trials (20). A phase I trial of protracted 5-FU infusion in combination with radiation therapy was recently reported in patients with pancreatic or biliary cancer (21). In this study, 25 patients with unresectable, residual, or recurrent cancer were treated with a total external radiation dose of 59.4 Gy using conventional fractionation of 1.9 Gy daily. 5-FU began within the first 24 hours of radiation and was administered continuously. The maximum tolerated dose of 5-FU in this setting was found to be 250 mg/m$^2$/day. At this dose range, toxicity was generally mild and self-limited. No episodes of severe mucositis were observed. The most severe hematologic toxicity was grade II. Most patients experienced nausea, but none required placement of feeding tubes or lost more than 10% of pretreatment weight. Most currently ongoing adjuvant trials in pancreatic cancer use continuous infusion rather than bolus 5-FU.

It is possible that multidrug chemotherapy regimens will prove more effective than 5-FU alone in postoperative adjuvant trials. Based on experience with carcinoma of the colon, one group of investigators has added leucovorin to the postoperative 5-FU/radiation regimen (22), although no results of this therapy have yet been reported. Bruckner et al. (23) reported the use of 54 Gy of radiation therapy and a multidrug regimen (5-FU, streptozotocin, and cisplatin) in patients with advanced pancreatic cancer. Although toxicity was significant, all patients completed treatment. This regimen has not yet been evaluated in the adjuvant setting.

Bakkevold et al. (24) evaluated a multidrug chemotherapy postoperative adjuvant regimen without radiation. Some 61 radically resected patients with carcinoma of the pancreas or papilla of Vater were randomized to receive either *(a)* combination chemotherapy with 5-FU (500mg/m$^2$), doxorubicin (40 mg/m$^2$), and mitomycin C (6mg/m$^2$) once every 3 weeks for six cycles or *(b)* no adjuvant therapy. Toxicity appeared to be more significant than in the GITSG radiation/5-FU trial; only 13 of 24 patients who started chemotherapy were able to complete the prescribed six courses. Five patients developed sepsis during chemotherapy; one patient died as a result. The chemotherapy group overall, however, enjoyed a significantly increased median survival—23 months, versus 11 months in the control group. On the other hand, there was no statistically significant advantage in 5-year survival. Thus, the results in terms of survival were quite similar to those of the original GITSG randomized trial using 5-FU/radiation; toxicity of the combination chemotherapy approach without radiation seemed more significant.

**Postoperative Therapy Targeted to the Liver.** Ishikawa et al. (25) reported the use of a 28-day combined portal vein and hepatic arterial infusion of 5-FU in the adjuvant setting following pancreatic resection. At the time of tumor removal, a catheter was placed in a portal venous branch, and a catheter attached to an infusion port was placed into the hepatic artery through the gastroduodenal artery. Immediately following surgery, 125 mg/day of 5-FU was infused into each catheter, and the infusion continued for 1 month. Twenty-one patients were treated. There was no liver dysfunction, hematologic toxicity, or catheter-related morbidity. Compared with historic controls treated with no adjuvant therapy or with systemic 5-FU, the patients treated with the double hepatic infusion of 5-FU demonstrated a significant increase in survival and a marked decrease in death from hepatic metastases. In colorectal cancer, a 7-day postoperative portal venous infusion of 5-FU has not been shown to prolong survival (26). However, the results reported by Ishikawa are intriguing and deserve further evaluation.

An alternative approach to the prevention of hepatic metastases is prophylactic hepatic radiation. The efficacy and toxicity of this approach are not well documented in the adjuvant setting. In 16 patients with unresectable carcinoma of the pancreas, one study (27) reported the use of external-beam irradiation to the pancreas plus prophylactic hepatic irradiation and intermittent bolus 5-FU. Treatment to the liver was begun 4 weeks after commencing pancreatic irradiation. The total dose delivered to the liver was 23.4 Gy in 13 fractions over 2.5 weeks. The entire liver was encompassed within the radiation field. 5-FU was delivered on 3 days at the start of hepatic irradiation. Toxicity was reported to be relatively mild (transient elevations of liver enzymes were noted). Only one patient suffered a major complication during radiotherapy. Survival data revealed an improvement over previous studies (GITSG) that did not include hepatic radiation. Only four patients (25%) developed liver metastases during the period of follow-up. A similar but larger study of 81 patients reported by the Radiation Therapy Oncology Group (28) showed a 31% liver failure rate for patients treated with chemoradiation prophylaxis to the liver, a lower rate of hepatic metastasis than in trials not including hepatic irradiation. In this study, which used continuous infusion 5-FU, toxicity was significant. Approximately half of the patients treated experienced severe or life-threatening toxicity, and two patients died of complications of therapy.

There are no mature data about using whole hepatic irradiation as part of the adjuvant regimen after apparently curative resection for carcinoma of the pancreas, although one group is currently evaluating a combination of postoperative 5-FU/leucovorin, irradiation to the pancreas bed and lymph nodes, and 27 GY of whole hepatic radiation (22).

### Intraoperative Adjuvant Radiation

Intraoperative radiation therapy (IORT) in the adjuvant setting is designed to prevent locoregional recurrence after apparently complete tumor resection. IORT allows the delivery of relatively large radiation doses to the tumor bed after resection, but minimizes the risk of radiation injury to surrounding normal structures. IORT is delivered via high-energy electron beams from a linear accelerator. Radiation doses used for adjuvant IORT in pancreatic cancer have ranged from 10 to 30 Gy delivered over a period of approximately 20 minutes. Radiation is delivered after tumor resection but prior to the performance of the reconstructive anastomoses to the bile duct, pancreas, and stomach. Some institutions have built IORT suites in the operating room. In other institutions, the anesthetized patient must be transported from the operating room to a separate radiation facility.

Radiation is delivered through cylinders ranging in diameter from about 5 to 12 cm. In each case, a treatment cylinder of the appropriate shape and size is chosen to conform to the field to be radiated. One end of the cylinder is placed in direct contact with the operative bed, and the other end is attached to the accelerator through a gantry mechanism. The treatment cylinder acts as both a radiation shield and a retractor, preventing surrounding tissues from inadvertently entering the radiation field (Fig. 60.3). During the delivery of radiation, the patient's condition is monitored by the anesthesiologist from an adjacent shielded suite by use of telemetry.

Hiraoka et al. (29) reported 14 patients who received 30 Gy of IORT following extended pancreatectomy for ductal carcinoma. IORT was given over an extended field from the diaphragm to the inferior mesenteric artery. No other adjuvant treatment was given. There were no apparent complications attributable to IORT. Five-year actuarial survival was 33%, an improvement over that of historic control patients undergoing either standard or extended operation without IORT. Local control of tumor appeared to have been achieved in autopsied patients who underwent extended pancreatectomy plus IORT.

In a large single-institution experience, Evans et al. (30) reported 41 patients who underwent IORT in conjunction with pancreaticoduodenectomy for periampullary carcinomas. Twenty-four patients also received preoperative external-beam radiotherapy and 5-FU; 8 other patients received postoperative external-beam therapy and 5-FU. A relatively wide retroperitoneal lymph node and soft tissue dissection was performed in all patients. The retroperitoneal margin near the superior mesenteric artery was examined by frozen section in all patients, and the dose of IORT based on those findings: 10 Gy for negative margins, 15 Gy when microscopically positive, and 20 Gy when grossly positive. The IORT field encompassed the resection bed from the transected bile duct above to the right kidney laterally and to the pancreatic remnant medially. The cut margins of the bile duct and pancreas were, however, excluded from the field. IORT fields ranged from 5 to 10 cm in diameter. Operative mortality was 2%, and 13 patients (32%) experienced some type of postoperative complication, similar to figures reported for pancreaticoduodenectomy alone. There were no complications directly attributable to IORT, although a relatively high incidence of abscesses and wound infections may have been related to possible breaks in sterile technique during positioning for IORT.

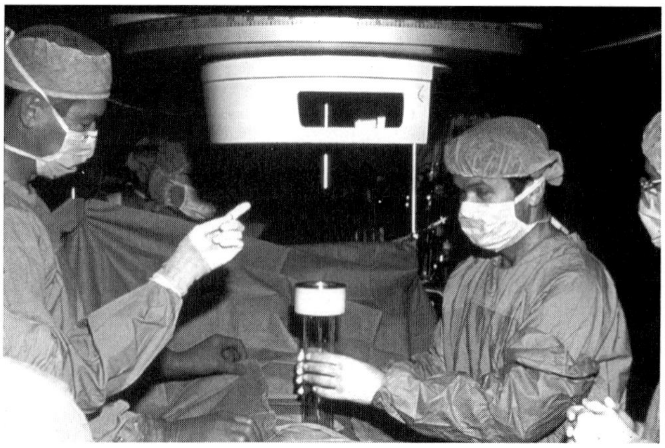

**FIG. 60.3.** Intraoperative radiotherapy for carcinoma of the pancreas. The cone that retracts adjacent viscera and protects them from radiation injury has been placed through the abdominal wound. The gantry unit attached to the linear accelerator will be lowered to engage the cone. (Photograph courtesy of Dr. Kenneth Russell, Department of Radiation Oncology, University of Washington School of Medicine.)

Okamoto et al. (31) studied 11 patients who received IORT with apparently curative resection for pancreatic carcinoma; 10 patients also received postoperative external-beam radiotherapy. An extended retroperitoneal dissection was performed with pancreatectomy. IORT doses ranged from 18 to 30 Gy over a field 6–8 cm in diameter. Median survival in this group of patients was 39 months; 45% survived 5 years. These survival figures were not statistically different from those of a historic control group of patients treated by radical surgery alone. However, resection with IORT appeared to confer a survival advantage over resection alone in the subset of patients with positive lymph nodes. Autopsies were performed on nine patients who died following curative resection and IORT. Four of nine demonstrated recurrence within the irradiated field. In three of these cases, local recurrence occurred along with distant metastases. Five patients who showed no evidence of recurrence within the irradiated field died of distant metastasis.

Zerbi et al. (32) studied 43 patients who underwent IORT in conjunction with resection for carcinoma of the pancreas. Radiation doses ranged from 12.5 to 20 Gy to treatment fields of 6–10 cm. No other adjuvant therapy was given. The results of treatment were compared with those of 47 patients who underwent resection without IORT during the same time period. Although patients were not randomized, the two groups appeared comparable in cancer extent. Operative blood loss and postoperative hospital stay were similar in the two groups. IORT, which required transporting the patients, added an average of 70 minutes to operative time. There was no significant difference in operative mortality or morbidity. Median survival and long-term survival did not differ between the two groups of patients. Local recurrence developed in significantly fewer (27%) patients treated with surgery plus IORT than in patients treated with surgery alone (56%), suggesting that IORT improves local control but fails to enhance long-term survival.

Only one randomized trial of IORT in the adjuvant setting has been reported (33). After apparently curative resection of stage II or higher pancreatic cancer, patients were randomized to treatment with either 20 Gy IORT or 45–55 Gy EBRT. No adjuvant chemotherapy was used. In follow-up, 60% of patients failed locally or regionally. There was no difference in the efficacies of IORT and of EBRT, but the number of evaluable patients was very small.

### Preoperative Adjuvant Therapy

In recent years, there has been increasing interest in preoperative chemoradiation for apparently resectable pancreatic cancer (Fig. 60.4). The development of endoscopic stents for the palliation of jaundice has allowed time to deliver radiation and chemotherapy prior to attempted surgical resection. Preoperative radiation therapy is potentially attractive in pancreatic cancer because of the possibility of treating the periphery of the tumor and decreasing the incidence of positive resection margins. Preoperative radiation therapy might also reduce the implantability of tumor cells shed into the peritoneal cavity or bloodstream during the manipulation of surgery, thus reducing the risk of distant recurrence. Preoperative radiation also has the advantage of avoiding delays in radiation therapy, which often occur when radiation is given in the postoperative setting because patients experience postsurgical complications that delay treatment.

Preoperative chemoradiotherapy has the particular attraction of possibly converting some patients with nonresectable or marginally resectable cancer to candidates for resection, a possibility suggested by the first report of neoadjuvant therapy in pancreatic cancer (34), in which 16 patients were treated with external-beam radiotherapy who had been deemed at operation to have surgically unresectable or borderline resectable pancreatic cancer. Following completion of 40–50 Gy radiotherapy, 11 of these patients were reexplored, and 6 were able to have their tumor resected. The study demonstrated that radiation therapy prior to surgical resection was feasible and suggested the possibility that tumors might be downstaged by preoperative RT. However, subsequent studies (see below) have shown that

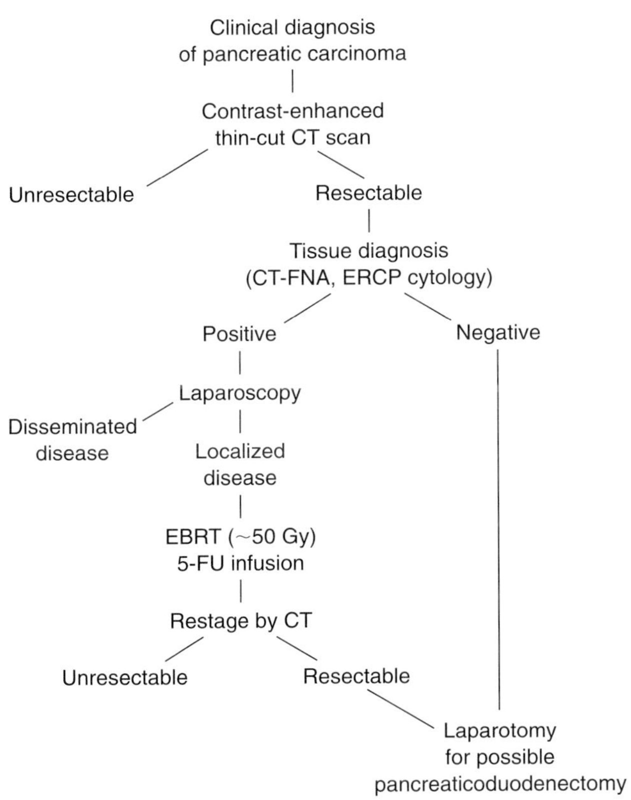


**FIG. 60.4.** Scheme for preoperative adjuvant therapy of pancreatic cancer. Patients with clinical symptoms and signs suggesting pancreatic carcinoma are initially evaluated by CT scan. Those with an apparently resectable tumor in whom a tissue diagnosis can be made by CT-guided biopsy or cytology undergo staging laparoscopy and peritoneal washings. Those who still have evidence of localized resectable disease are treated with external beam radiation therapy and continuous infusion 5-FU. Following completion of chemoradiotherapy, patients are restaged by CT. Those who still have evidence of localized resectable disease undergo laparotomy for possible tumor resection. Patients who have clinical and radiologic signs of pancreatic carcinoma but in whom a tissue diagnosis cannot be made are not candidates for neoadjuvant therapy and should proceed directly to laparotomy. *EBRT,* external-beam radiation therapy; *5-FU,* 5-fluorouracil; *CT,* computerized tomography; 9FNA, fine-needle aspiration; *ERCP,* endoscopic retrograde cholangiopancreatography.

although occasional tumor downsizing occurs after preoperative therapy (Fig. 60.5), preoperative chemoradiation does not result in consistent reduction in tumor size. Thus far, there has not been significant success in converting unresectable to resectable tumors, although this is theoretically possible if adjuvant regimens improve.

Coia et al. (12) recently reported the results of a trial of neoadjuvant therapy begun in 1986 at the Fox Chase Cancer Center in Philadelphia involving 31 patients with documented stage I, II, or III adenocarcinoma of the pancreas or duodenum. Initially, the program enrolled only patients thought to have locally unresectable disease, but after the treatment of the first 16 patients, patients with resectable tumors were also eligible for the trial. Eleven patients had what was believed to be unresectable cancer on prior laparotomy. Staging prior to initiating radiation included abdominal CT scanning, chest x-ray or chest CT, and occasionally arteriography. Total parenteral nutrition (TPN) was instituted in patients with significant malnutrition. Preoperative chemoradiation consisted of 50.4 Gy over 6 weeks, with two courses of infusional 5-FU (weeks 1 and 5) and a single bolus of mitomycin C on day 2. Radiotherapy was initially given to the tumor and a 2- to 3-cm margin to a dose of 39.6 Gy. An additional 10.8 Gy was then delivered to a coned-down field with a 1- to 2-cm margin around the tumor. Radiation fields included lymph nodes in the portal and celiac regions. Surgery was scheduled 4–6 weeks after the completion of radiation therapy if there was no evidence of local progression to unresectability or distant metastases.

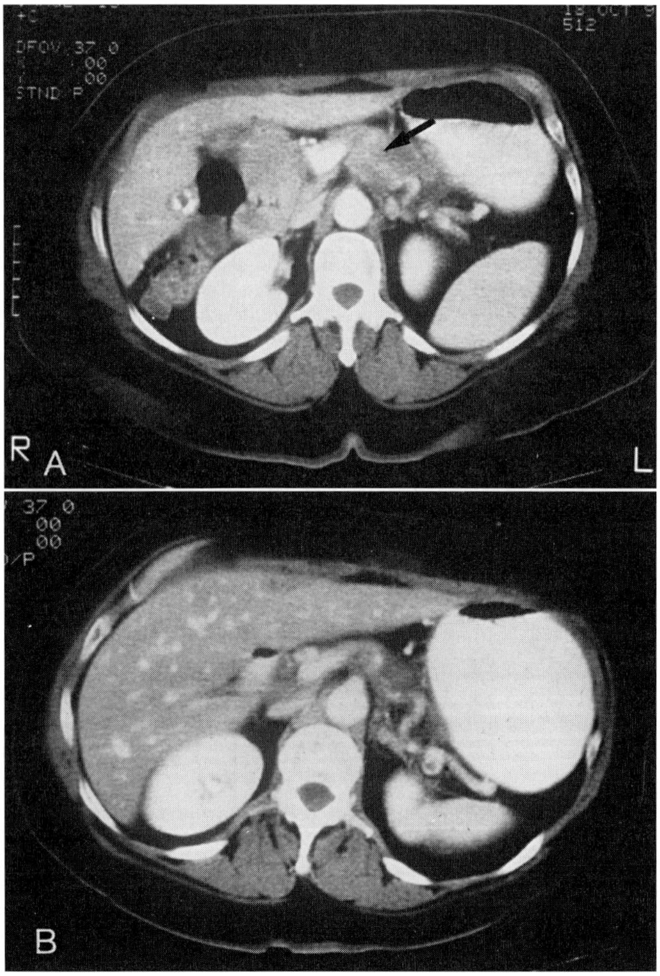


**FIG. 60.5.** Substantial tumor reduction in response to preoperative neoadjuvant therapy in a 68 year old woman. **A.** Initial CT scan demonstrating adenocarcinoma of the body of pancreas *(arrow)*, which was confirmed by fine-needle aspiration cytology. **B.** CT following treatment with 45 Gy external-beam radiation, 5-FU, and interferon-$\alpha$, demonstrating approximately 75% reduction in tumor size. The carcinoma was removed by distal pancreatectomy. Margins of resection and lymph nodes were negative for tumor.

Grade 3 or 4 toxicity of chemoradiation occurred in 8 of 31 patients (26%). Seven patients had to have radiation interrupted for more than 3 days. One patient died of sepsis in the first week of therapy. However, 29 of 31 patients completed the course of 50.4 Gy. There was little evidence of tumor shrinkage by radiologic criteria. One patient had a more than 50% reduction in tumor size; all others had stable local disease. Three patients were found to have developed liver metastases when restaged prior to laparotomy. No patient with superior mesenteric artery (SMA) involvement or portal vein occlusion was converted to resectable status. Of the total of 31 patients, 22 patients underwent exploration, and 17 underwent resection. Of 10 patients initially deemed completely resectable, 7 underwent resection. Of 21 patients initially deemed locally unresectable, 10 were able to undergo resection. Operative mortality was 12%. Following preoperative radiation, all resected patients with pancreatic cancer had negative margins in the surgical specimen, and 11 of 13 patients had no evidence of residual nodal involvement. For the 13 patients with pancreatic cancer who underwent resection, 3-year survival was 43%. This group included 10 patients initially deemed unresectable. Only one patient undergoing preoperative chemoradiation followed by pancreatectomy developed a locoregional recurrence.

A similar experience with preoperative chemoradiation has been reported by Rich and Evans from the M. D. Anderson Cancer Center (35). Some 28 patients were judged to have resectable pancreatic carcinoma by contrast-enhanced thin-cut CT. All patients had the diagnosis confirmed by CT-guided fine-needle aspiration (FNA). Patients with major arterial encasement or venous occlusion were excluded. Chemoradiation consisted of 5-FU at doses of 250–300 mg/m$^2$/day given 5 days per week during external-beam radiation. Total doses of radiation were 50.4–55.0 Gy over 5.0–5.5 weeks. Grade 3 toxicity occurred in 21% of patients, and grade 4 in 32%. This degree of toxicity exceeded that in the Fox Chase trial cited above, probably because of the continuous treatment with 5-FU throughout the period of radiation. At the conclusion of radiation treatment, all patients were restaged; 23 underwent laparotomy, and 17 were able to undergo a potentially curative resection. There was one postoperative death (4%). Pathologic examination of the resected specimens revealed evidence of tumor cell injury in all patients. Four patients had fewer than 10% of viable-appearing tumor cells remaining. However, none of the 17 patients achieved a complete pathologic response.

Ishikawa and his associates from Osaka have treated 23 patients with apparently resectable carcinoma of the head of the pancreas with 50 Gy of preoperative external-beam irradiation over 5 weeks (13). At the time of restaging prior to laparotomy, there was a mean reduction in tumor diameter of approximately 20%. No patients in this study were found to have developed distant metastases or progression while awaiting laparotomy. Following a 3- to 6-week rest period after radiation, laparotomy was performed with the intention of performing pancreaticoduodenectomy with extended lymphadenectomy; 17 of 23 (74%) patients were able to undergo resection of the tumor at laparotomy. Perioperative complications were no higher than in a group of 31 concurrent (but nonrandomized) patients operated upon without preoperative irradiation. Long-term survival in patients undergoing preoperative radiation was not improved over that of the nonradiated group of patients. Irradiated patients, however, exhibited a significant reduction in the rate of locoregional recurrence.

Jessup et al. (36) attempted to improve resectability and survival in 16 patients with locally advanced pancreatic cancer with preoperative radiation and 5-FU. Twelve of the 16 patients had been deemed unresectable at previous laparotomy. Four others had radiologic evidence of encasement of major mesenteric vessels. Preoperative chemoradiation consisted of at least 45 Gy of external-beam radiation in combination with a daily infusion of 5-FU (225 mg/m$^2$/day) throughout radiation therapy. Performance status of the protocol patients worsened from a mean ECOG score of 1.2 before therapy to 2.1 after neoadjuvant therapy. As in Ishikawa's experience above, radiologic evaluation at restaging showed a mean 20% reduction in tumor size after completing chemoradiation. Ten of the 16 patients were ultimately explored; only 2 were able to undergo successful resection. The remainder of the patients demonstrated either persistent advanced local disease or peritoneal implants undetected by preoperative imaging.

## PROBLEMS WITH ADJUVANT THERAPY FOR PANCREATIC CANCER

The randomized trial of postoperative chemoradiation following curative resection of pancreatic cancer performed by the Gastrointestinal Tumor Study Group (17) made it clear that chemoradiation in the adjuvant setting is effective in prolonging survival. Nevertheless, most patients who undergo resection continue to succumb to recurrent disease. Adjuvant chemoradiation therapy appears to decrease the incidence of locoregional recurrence to about 20–30% of patients, but there is still no firm evidence that adjuvant protocols prevent the development of disseminated disease. Adjuvant therapy may prolong time to recurrence and shift the site of first recurrence to distant sites such as the liver or peritoneal surface (37). Whether adjuvant therapy will ultimately result in many more long-term cures following resection of pancreatic cancer remains problematic. Modalities to prevent hepatic metastases, such as infusional chemotherapy and whole liver irradiation, have as yet to be rigorously evaluated. Therapies to deal with metastases beyond the liver and with peritoneal recurrence have not yet been developed. Although higher-dose chemotherapy and multidrug chemotherapy could conceivably address these issues, toxicity will increase with these sorts of regimens and may exceed the potential benefit.

For adjuvant therapy to make an even greater impact on the overall patient population with pancreatic cancer, the development of preoperative regimens that substantially downstage locally advanced tumors would be an important breakthrough. As indicated above, the degree of reduction in tumor size achieved with current protocols is modest; no patients achieve complete pathologic remission, and few patients are converted from the locally unresectable to the resectable category. To achieve improved downstaging will be difficult, since doses of radiation therapy now being used are near the maximally tolerated levels. Currently, attempts to increase the biologic activity of the radiation by hyperfractionated delivery schedules (38) are under way at some institutions, but there are no data yet on the use of hyperfractionation in the adjuvant setting. The development of new drug regimens that are additive to radiation above and beyond the effect of 5-FU would be an important possible breakthrough in neoadjuvant therapy, but the spectre of toxicity may restrain developments in this area, particularly since pancreatic cancer patients with advanced disease often have poor functional performance and limited ability to withstand the complications of chemotherapy.

## CONCLUSIONS

Adjuvant therapy for pancreatic cancer by use of radiation therapy and 5-FU prolongs survival. 5-FU and external-beam radiotherapy should be considered standard therapy following successful resection of a pancreatic adenocarcinoma. At this point, it is difficult to say whether preoperative chemoradiation offers any significant advantage over the same therapy in the postoperative setting. Intraoperative radiation (IORT), although theoretically attractive, has not yet been convincingly demonstrated to have any advantage over conventional external-beam therapy.

For the present, patients who undergo resection of a ductal carcinoma of the pancreas should receive postoperative radiation therapy to the tumor bed of approximately 54 Gy with continuous infusion of 5-FU during radiation treatment. Continued trials of IORT and neoadjuvant therapy will be needed to demonstrate their value. Improvements in neoadjuvant therapy potentially have the greatest dividend, since preoperative therapy holds out the possibility of both preventing recurrence after surgery as well as making more patients eligible for surgical resection by downstaging locally advanced tumors.

## REFERENCES

1. Bell RH. Neoplasms of the exocrine pancreas. In: Bell RH, Rikkers LF, Mulholland MW, eds. Digestive tract surgery. A text and atlas. Philadelphia: Lippincott-Raven, 1996:849–878.
2. Tepper JE, Nardi GL, Suit HD. Carcinoma of the pancreas. Review of MGH experience from 1963 to 1973.Analysis of surgical failure and implications for radiation therapy. Cancer 1976;37:1519–1524.
3. Griffin JF, Smalley SR, Jewell W. Patterns of failure after curative resection of pancreatic carcinoma. Cancer 1990;66:56–61.
4. Kayahara M, Nagakawa T, Ueno K, Ohta T, Takeda T, Miyazaki I. An evaluation of radical resection for pancreatic cancer based on the mode of recurrence as determined by autopsy and diagnostic imaging. Cancer 1993;72:2118–2123.
5. Guthoff A, Rothe B, Klapdor R, Kloppel G, Greten H. Site of recurrence after resection for pancreatic carcinoma (Abstract). Dig Dis Sci 1987;32:1168.
6. Tsuchiya R, Oribe T, Noda T. Size of the tumor and other factors influencing prognosis of carcinoma of the head of the pancreas. Am J Gastroenterol 1985;80:459–462.
7. Willett CG, Lewandrowski K, Warshaw AL, Efird J, Compton CC. Resection margins in carcinoma of the head of the pancreas. Implications for radiation therapy. Ann Surg 1993;217:144–148.
8. Yeo CJ, Cameron JL, Lillemoe KD, et al. Pancreaticoduodenectomy for cancer of the head of the pancreas. 201 patients. Ann Surg 1995;221:721–733.
9. Tsuchiya R, Noda T, Harada N, et al. Collective review of small carcinomas of the pancreas. Ann Surg 1986;203:77–81.
10. Ozaki H. Modern surgical treatment of pancreatic cancer. Int J Pancreatol 1994;16:121–129.
11. Cubilla AL, Fitzgerald PJ. Surgical pathology aspects of cancer of the ampulla-head of pancreas region. In: Fitzgerald PJ, Morrison AB, eds. The pancreas. Baltimore: Williams & Wilkins, 1980:67–81.
12. Coia L, Hoffman J, Scher R, et al. Preoperative chemoradiation for adenocarcinoma of the pancreas and duodenum. Int J Radiat Biol Phys 1994;30:161–167.
13. Ishikawa O, Ohigashi H, Imaoka S, et al. Is the long-term survival rate improved by preoperative irradiation prior to Whipple's procedure for adenocarcinoma of the pancreatic head? Arch Surg 1994;129:1075–1080.
14. Horn A, Morild I, Dahl O. Tumour shrinkage and down staging after preoperative radiation of rectal adenocarcinomas. Radiother Oncol 1990;18:19–28.
15. Freeny PC, Traverso LW, Ryan JA. Diagnosis and staging of pancreatic carcinoma with dynamic computed tomography. Am J Surg 1993;165:600–606.
16. Bell RH. Exocrine pancreatic neoplasms. In: Greenfield LJ, Mul-

holland MW, Oldham KT, Zelenock GB, eds. Surgery: scientific principles and practice. Philadelphia: JB Lippincott, 1993: 816–833.

17. Kalser MH, Ellenberg SS. Pancreatic cancer. Adjuvant combined radiation and chemotherapy following curative resection. Arch Surg 1985;120:899–903.
18. Gastrointestinal Tumor Study Group. Further evidence of effective adjuvant combined radiation and chemotherapy following curative resection of pancreatic cancer. Cancer 1987;59:2006–2010.
19. Douglass HO Jr, Stablein DM. Ten-year follow-up of first generation surgical adjuvant studies of the Gastrointestinal Tumor Study Group. In: Salmon SE, ed. Adjuvant therapy of cancer VI. Philadelphia: WB Saunders, 1990:405–415.
20. O'Connell MJ, Martenson JA, Wieand HS, et al. Improving adjuvant therapy for rectal cancer by combining protracted infusion fluorouracil with radiation therapy after curative surgery. N Engl J Med 1994;331:502–507.
21. Whittington R, Neuberg D, Tester WJ, Benson AB III, Haller DG. Protracted intravenous fluorouracil infusion with radiation therapy in the management of localized pancreaticobiliary carcinoma: a phase I Eastern Cooperative Oncology Group trial. J Clin Oncol 1995;13:227–232.
22. Abrams RA, Grochow LB. Adjuvant therapy with chemotherapy and radiation therapy in the management of carcinoma of the pancreatic head. Surg Clin North Am 1995;75:925–938.
23. Bruckner HW, Kalnicki S, Dalton J, et al. Survival after combined modality therapy for pancreatic cancer. J Clin Gastroenterol 1993;16:199–203.
24. Bakkevold KE, Arnesjo B, Dahl O, Kambestad B. Adjuvant combination chemotherapy (AMF) following radical resection of carcinoma of the pancreas and papilla of Vater—results of a controlled, prospective, randomised multicentre study. Eur J Cancer 1993;29A:698–703.
25. Ishikawa O, Ohigashi H, Sasaki Y, et al. Liver perfusion chemotherapy via both the hepatic artery and portal vein to prevent hepatic metastasis after extended pancreatectomy for adenocarcinoma of the pancreas. Am J Surg 1994;168:361–364.
26. Beart RW Jr, Moertel CG, Wieand HS, et al. Adjuvant therapy for resectable colorectal carcinoma with fluorouracil administered by portal vein infusion. Arch Surg 1990;125:897–901.
27. Komaki R, Hansen R, Cox JD, Wilson JF. Phase I-II study of prophylactic hepatic irradiation with local irradiation and systemic chemotherapy for adenocarcinoma of the pancreas. Int J Radiat Oncol Biol Phys 1988;15:1447–1452.
28. Komaki R, Wadler S, Peters T, et al. High-dose local irradiation plus prophylactic hepatic irradiation and chemotherapy for inoperable adenocarcinoma of the pancreas. A preliminary report of a multi-institutional trial (Radiation Therapy Oncology Group protocol 8801). Cancer 1992;69:2807–2812.
29. Hiraoka T, Uchino R, Kanemitsu K, et al. Combination of intraoperative radiation with resection of cancer of the pancreas. Int J Pancreatol 1990;7:201–207.
30. Evans DB, Termuhlen PM, Byrd DR, Ames FC, Ochran TG, Rich TA. Intraoperative radiation therapy following pancreaticoduodenectomy. Ann Surg 1993;218:54–60.
31. Okamoto A, Tsuruta K, Isawa T, Kamisawa T, Tanaka Y, Onodera T. Intraoperative radiation therapy for pancreatic carcinoma. Int J Pancreatol 1994;16:157–164.
32. Zerbi A, Fossati V, Parolini D, et al. Intraoperative radiation therapy adjuvant to resection in the treatment of pancreatic cancer. Cancer 1994;73:2930–2935.
33. Johnstone PA, Sindelar WF. Patterns of disease recurrence following definitive therapy of adenocarcinoma of the pancreas using surgery and adjuvant radiotherapy: correlations of a clinical trial. Int J Radiat Oncol Biol Phys 1993;27:831–834.
34. Pilepich MV, Miller HH. Preoperative irradiation in carcinoma of the pancreas. Cancer 1980;46:1945–1949.
35. Rich TA, Evans DB. Preoperative combined modality therapy for pancreatic cancer. World J Surg 1995;19:264–269.
36. Jessup JM, Steele G Jr, Mayer RJ, et al. Neoadjuvant therapy for unresectable pancreatic adenocarcinoma. Arch Surg 1993;128: 559–564.
37. Foo ML, Gunderson LL, Nagorney DM, et al. Patterns of failure in grossly resected pancreatic ductal adenocarcinoma treated with adjuvant irradiation ± 5 fluorouracil. Int J Radiat Oncol Biol Phys 1993;26:483–489.
38. Seydel HG, Stablein DM, Leichman LP, Kinzie JJ, Thomas PRM. Hyperfractionated radiation and chemotherapy for unresectable localized adenocarcinoma of the pancreas. The Gastrointestinal Tumor Study Group experience. Cancer 1990;65: 1478–1482.

# 61

# Treatment Using Combined Modalities

Takehisa Hiraoka and Keiichiro Kanemitsu

Despite general advancement in diagnostic, surgical, and anesthetic techniques and in general supportive care, the overall survival of patients with pancreatic cancer remains dismal. Attempts at extending traditional surgical procedures have not produced a discernible benefit, and even following extended surgery, a high proportion of patients have local recurrence and hepatic metastases at autopsy. Therefore, treatment modalities combined with resection have been introduced to improve the prognosis of pancreatic cancer. Since 1969, we have used intraoperative operative radiation therapy (IORT) for patients with unresectable pancreatic cancer, and since 1976, we have combined IORT with resection of the pancreas. The results of our approach of combined therapy for pancreatic cancer are presented below.

## TREATMENT COMBINED WITH IORT

### General Aspects

Pancreatic cancer was regarded as a radioresistant tumor. This notion has been challenged, and now this tumor is thought to be moderately radioresponsive, similar to adenocarcinomas of the rectum, prostate, and breast. The role of radiation therapy in the management of pancreatic malignancy has expanded dramatically. Pancreatic cancer, however, is surrounded by radiosensitive organs, such as the stomach, small intestine, liver, kidney, and spinal cord. If direct irradiation can be applied to advanced pancreatic cancer while sparing the normal tissues as much as possible, some clinical benefits can be expected. Normal tissues may be excluded from the irradiated area by operative displacement from the beam path or by protection with shielding materials positioned at surgery. The rationale for the use of IORT is to maximize the dose of radiation delivered to neoplastic tissues and to minimize the radiation dose to normal tissues that surround the neoplastic area (Fig. 61.1).

The prognosis for patients with resectable pancreatic cancer has consistently been poor; at best, resection offers a modest prolongation of life or temporary palliation of symptoms. The results of total pancreatectomy and regional pancreatectomy, including resection and reconstruction of the portal vein and/or superior mesenteric artery, have not been shown to be superior to less extensive procedures in terms of either operative mortality or morbidity or in terms of long-term survival (1–5).

One reason is local recurrence in the soft tissue around the celiac axis, mesenteric vessels, and aorta as found by autopsy. This suggests that cancer cells in lymphatics, lymph nodes, soft tissue, and nerve plexuses around the pancreas are not completely removed by the surgical procedure alone. To overcome this problem, it is reasonable to apply IORT to the tumor bed following resection for pancreatic cancer. IORT delivers a large single dose of radiation directly to the bed of the resected tumor. Manipulations to protect normal tissues at the time of IORT may permit high tumoricidal doses of radiation to abdominal malignancies that otherwise might not be possible by conventional radiotherapy techniques.

### Historic Background of IORT

In 1907, IORT was first described by Beck (6) for a patient with advanced pyloric cancer; 2 years later, he reported seven patients with unresectable gastric cancers and one with colon cancer in whom he pulled the tumor into the abdominal wounds to irradiate them directly (7). In 1915, Finsterer (8) reported the clinical results of patients with unresectable carcinoma who were treated in a similar fashion. These techniques may be classified as IORT in the broad sense that radiotherapy was performed during surgical procedures. The practice of IORT at that time, however, differed markedly from current methods; the purpose then was to deliver a dose to deep-seated tumors with the low-energy radiation beams then available.

Current IORT was introduced by Abe et al. (9) using a megavoltage machine in 1964. The advent of megavoltage radiotherapy made it possible to deliver a sufficient dose to any location in the body, significantly improving the cure rate of malignant disease. They defined IORT as a treatment modality in which resectable lesions are removed surgically and the remaining cancer cells are sterilized by irradiation during a surgical procedure. The authors reported that IORT is best performed with an electron beam, since a specific beam energy can be chosen to produce the desired depth of tissue penetration. There is a sharp falloff of radiation dose with increasing depth in tissue, which avoids exposure of normal tissues beneath the tumors. Some patients who underwent noncurative surgery with incomplete resection for gastric cancer were cured by intraoperative electron-beam irradiation to the unresectable tumor remnant.

IORT for unresectable pancreatic cancer was introduced by Umegaki in 1963 (10) and by Abe in 1964 (9). We applied IORT for unresectable pancreatic cancer in 1969 (11) and first introduced IORT combined with resection for pancreatic cancer in 1976 (12).

### Electron-Beam IORT Technique

**IORT for Unresectable Cancer.** Under general anesthesia, the pancreatic tumor is exposed, and a needle or incisional biopsy is performed to obtain histologic confirmation of the diagnosis. The extent of the tumor and its local spread are defined. This requires taking down the gastrocolic omentum, reflecting the stomach superiorly, and performing a Kocher maneuver. When the tumor is situated at the head or body of the pancreas, gastrectomy by the Billroth II method may be needed to facilitate adequate exposure of the tumor, as well as to reroute the alimentary tract. Biliary diversion procedures are also done if

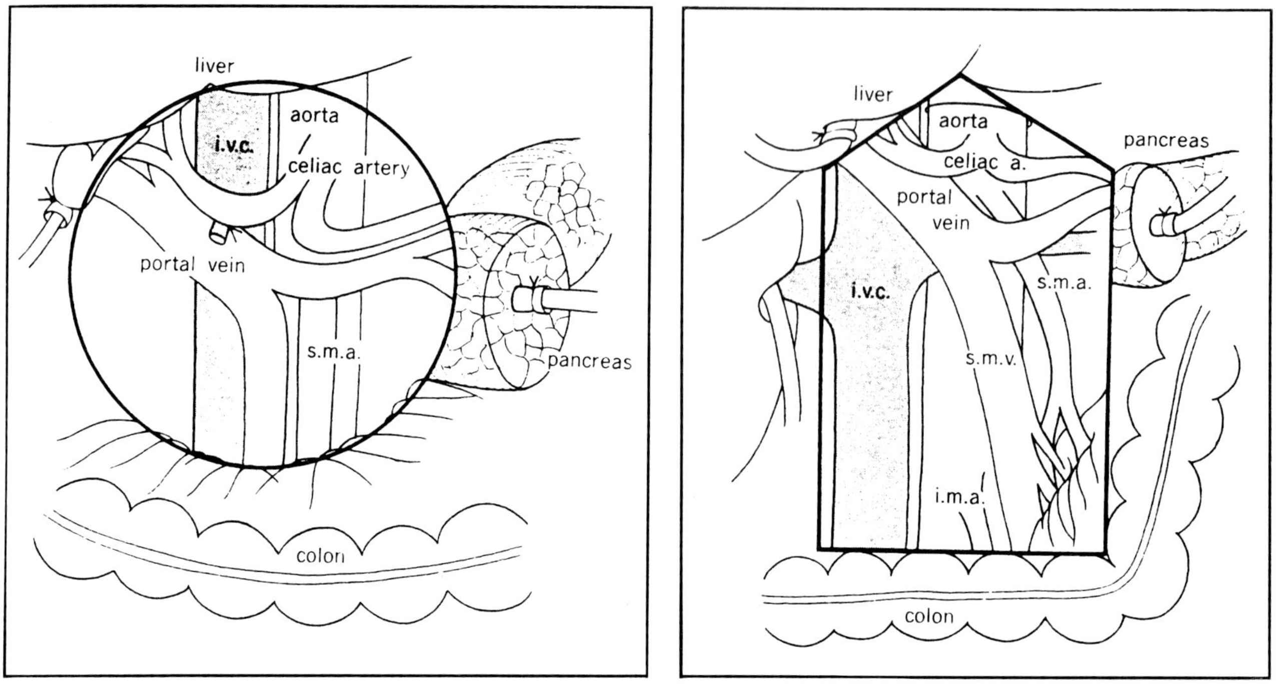


**FIG. 61.1.** Radiation field of extended IORT combined with conventional surgery *(left side)* and extended surgery *(right side)*. The circle *(left side)* and pentagon *(right side)* indicate the borders of the radiation field.

necessary. In our clinic, patients in the operating room are transferred to a radiation room. Remote physiologic monitoring is carried out during irradiation. The electron beam is delivered from a linear accelerator in our institute. After the adjacent normal tissues and organs are displaced outside the planned radiation field, an applicator from the linear accelerator is placed on the surface of the lesions. The energy of the electron beam is selected on the basis of the thickness of the tumor. We use the energy range from 10 to 18 meV and a radiation dose range of 25–40 Gy (10).

### IORT Combined with Resection

***IORT combined with conventional resection.*** Resection of the pancreatic lesion and dissection of the lymph nodes around the celiac axis and superior mesenteric artery are performed. A dose of 30 Gy of 8-meV electrons from a linear accelerator is administered to the operative field, including the celiac axis and superior mesenteric artery, using a 6- to 8-cm circular applicator in our series (11, 12).

***IORT combined with extended resection.*** A dose of 30 Gy of 9–12 meV electrons is administered to the operative field, including the paraaortic area from the diaphragm above to the inferior mesenteric artery below, using a special applicator. To expand the IORT portal, we use a special applicator that we can vary in size depending on the patient's body size to irradiate around the aorta from the diaphragm above to the inferior mesenteric artery below. This applicator is metallic and pentagonal, 6 cm wide by 10–18 cm long (11, 12). The field to be irradiated can be confirmed by observation through the window at the side of the adaptor of the applicator. The pancreatic remnant and the bile duct are kept outside the irradiation field. The electron beam can be sharply focused and concentrated within a depth of approximately 5 cm from the surface, thus minimizing unnecessary exposure to adjacent normal tissues. A sterilizing, cancericidal dose is administered to the target volume with sharp limitation. Patients are anesthetized with either epidural anesthesia or endotracheal anesthesia with nitrous oxide and oxygen.

### IORT for Unresectable Pancreatic Cancer

From 1966 to 1986, 30 patients were treated with IORT for unresectable cancer of the pancreas in our institute. Of the 30 patients, 18 underwent a surgical bypass procedure with IORT. The selection criteria for inclusion in this study were *(a)* biopsy-proven adenocarcinoma of the pancreas, *(b)* a localized unresectable tumor that could be included in a high-dose intraoperative "boost" field, *(c)* no distant metastatic disease (except to the liver), and *(d)* no contraindications to surgical exploration.

The postoperative survival time of these 30 patients ranged from 1 to 15.4 months. The mean survival of all the patients was $4.8 \pm 3.4$ months. In spite of palliative benefits, the survival time of patients treated with IORT was not longer than that of patients without IORT. The survival results of patients with liver metastases were especially poor.

The most obvious merit of IORT in cancer of the pancreas was the alleviation of pain; 80% of patients with pain experienced relief within 4 weeks of irradiation. A decrease in tumor size was found in 85% of the patients who were evaluated by palpation, CT, and/or autopsy. Radiation-related complications were found in 4 of the 30 patients.

Postmortem examinations were performed on 11 of the 30 patients. The tumor in 9 of the 11 patients had become smaller than before irradiation. In all 11 patients, microscopic examination showed the cancer was completely replaced by connective tissue in wide areas of the central portions of the tumor, to which a dose of 30 Gy had been administered. However, there were a few recognizable tumor cells in the superficial and deep portions of the tumor. The extent of damage to the tumor cells caused by the irradiation corresponded well with the distribution of the radiation dose. In one patient, in whom a fistula developed 23 days after IORT, massive radiation necrosis was followed by abscess formation sharply delimited from the nonirradiated area.

IORT on normal tissue at the periphery of the irradiated area usually caused destruction and marked atrophy of the glandular cells in pancreatic parenchyma. Interstitial fibrosis was seen, and glandular tissue was replaced by connective tissue. The islet tissue remained normal in the irradiated field. Fibrous thickening of the walls of arteries in the irradiated field resulted in luminal narrowing of the blood vessels. No remarkable changes were detected in the neighboring organs, such as the liver, kidney, stomach, or aorta, except for the jejunum irradiated accidentally in one patient.

In our series with IORT for unresectable pancreatic cancer, survival was not prolonged, but palliative effects, such as relief of pain, decrease in tumor size, and improvement in the general condition were obtained. Such palliative effects are reported in a collective review by Abe (13).

Tepper et al. (14) reported a multiinstitutional study of IORT (20 Gy) plus external-beam radiation therapy (50.4 Gy) for patients with locally unresectable, nonmetastatic pancreatic cancer. Chemotherapy with 5-fluorouracil (5-FU) (500 mg/m$^2$/day) was combined on the first 3 days of the external-beam treatment. Eighty-six patients were registered, and 51 of them were analyzable. Median survival time was 9 months, with an 18-month actuarial survival rate of 9%. Local control could not be adequately evaluated. Major postoperative complications occurred in 12% of patients. This study did not demonstrate any advantages of IORT over conventional therapy for this disease.

Autopsy of patients who underwent IORT for unresectable pancreatic cancer in our series showed remarkable local anticancer effects. In the central portion of the tumor, subjected to the peak absorbed dose of 25–40 Gy with 10- to 18-meV electrons, cancerous tissues were almost completely replaced by connective tissues. This may indicate that the dose of 30 Gy is suitable as a cancericidal dose.

## Combined Treatment with Conventional Surgery and IORT

IORT has been combined with pancreatic resection at the Kumamoto University Medical School since 1976 (15). From 1966 to 1981, 34 patients with adenocarcinoma of the pancreas underwent conventional resection; 15 of the 34 were combined with IORT. The 34 patients were divided into two groups as follows.

***Group 1.*** From 1966 to 1975, inclusive, 19 patients had a conventional resection, defined as a pancreatectomy or distal pancreatectomy with dissection of the primary group of lymph nodes draining the pancreas. Eleven of the 19 had macroscopic tumor clearance. The 19 patients included 2 classified as stage I; 4, stage II; 10, stage III; and 3, stage IV, according to the classification of the Union Internationale Contre le Cancer (UICC) (16).

***Group 2.*** From 1976 to 1981, inclusive, 15 patients had a conventional resection combined with IORT. Nine of the 15 had macroscopic tumor clearance. Of the 15 patients, 2 were classified as stage II; 10, stage III; and 3, stage IV. Following resection, a dose of 30 Gy of 8-meV electrons from a linear accelerator was administered to the operative field, including the celiac axis and superior mesenteric artery, using a 6- to 8-cm circular applicator (Fig. 61.1).

There was no significant difference in the survival rates between the 19 patients who had conventional resection alone and the 15 patients in whom it was combined with IORT. These patients died within 2.1 years after the operation. There were no other postoperative complications that could be attributed to IORT.

Autopsies were performed in seven patients. In autopsies of four patients who had had conventional pancreaticoduodenectomy alone, all four showed local recurrence at the origin of the superior mesenteric artery, at the celiac axis, and around the aorta. One of the patients also had recurrence in the pancreatic remnant, and three also had liver metastases. In autopsies of three patients who had had conventional pancreaticoduodenectomy combined with conventional IORT, each showed no local recurrence in the radiated area but showed local recurrence around the aorta surrounding the radiation field and liver metastases. Two of the three patients also had involvement of lymph nodes in the mesentery of the jejunum. The remaining patient also had recurrence in the pancreatic remnant.

Sindelar (17) performed a prospective randomized trial comparing IORT with conventional treatment in resectable carcinomas of the pancreas. The experimental group received pancreatectomy with intraoperative electron-beam irradiation (8–14 meV) delivered at a dose of 20 Gy to the resection bed and to regional nodal basins or to areas of potential contiguous tumor spread. The conventional therapy group received pancreatectomy followed by conventional external-beam irradiation (50 Gy in 175–200 cGy/day fractions) after recovery from surgery.

Twenty-six patients with resectable carcinomas of the pancreas were randomized, 13 receiving IORT and 13 receiving conventional therapy. More patients with early-stage disease were included in the control group than in the IORT group, and more advanced-stage patients were entered into the IORT group than into the conventional-treatment group. No statistically significant differences have developed between the IORT and standard therapy groups with respect to overall survival, disease-free interval, and local disease control. If operative deaths are excluded, then IORT appears to prolong overall survival (IORT group, median survival, 18 months; control group, median survival, 10 months), disease-free interval (IORT median, 11 months; control median, 8 months), and local disease control (IORT median, 18 months, control median, 9 months). Survival and local tumor control have been enhanced in advanced-stage patients who have been treated with pancreatectomy and IORT, compared with patients who have been treated with pancreatectomy and conventional external-beam radiation therapy (EBRT).

As the first step, we applied IORT to the celiac axis and mesenteric region following pancreatoduodenectomy, but no remarkable prolongation of survival in patients with pancreatic cancer resulted from this combined therapy, in spite of the local effects of IOR (15). We found that in-field local recurrences developed rarely in the areas where IORT was administered, but recurrences developed surrounding the radiation field. This represents a significant step forward in designing treatment strategies for pancreatic cancer. As a next step, we expanded the IORT portal from the 6- to 8-cm circular applicator used initially to a larger radiation field, encompassing the area from the diaphragm to the level of the inferior mesenteric artery. A special variable applicator was made to irradiate around such areas depending on the body size.

## Combined Treatment with Extended Resection and IORT

As the next step, we have been using IORT combined with extended resection since 1984. From 1982 to 1995, 39 patients with adenocarcinoma of the pancreas of duct cell origin underwent extended resection in our institute. Thirty of the 39 were combined with IORT. The 39 patients were divided into two groups as follows.

***Group 1.*** In 1982 and 1983, nine patients underwent an extended radical resection. This involved pancreatectomy with almost complete resection en bloc of the lymph nodes around the porta hepatis, the celiac axis, the origin of the superior mesenteric artery, and the aorta extending from the diaphragm above to the inferior mesenteric artery below. The inferior vena cava

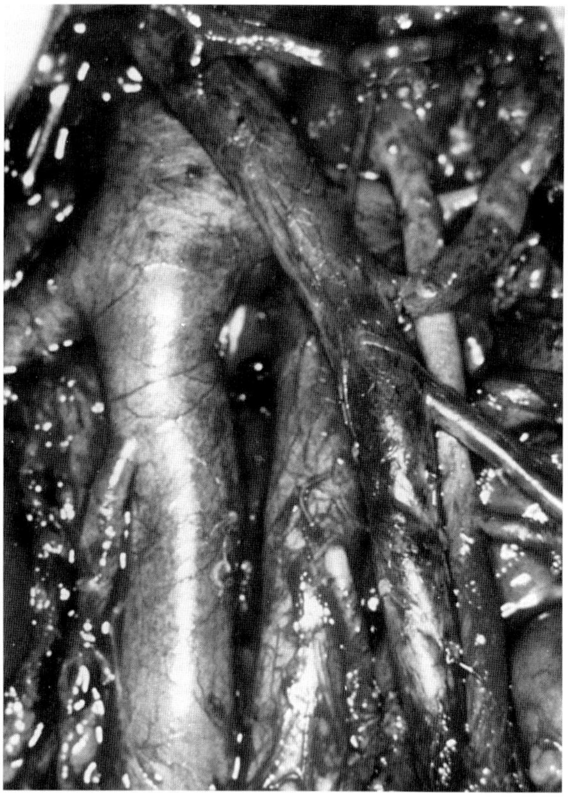

**FIG. 61.2.** The extent of dissection in extended radical resection of the pancreas. The inferior vena cava, aorta, mesenteric artery, and celiac axis are routinely skeletonized.

and aorta were also skeletonized, with all tissue removed en bloc (Fig. 61.2). Six underwent total pancreatectomy; two, pancreaticoduodenectomy; and one, distal pancreatectomy. The pancreatic segment of the portal vein was removed in five of the nine patients. One of the five with resection of the portal vein also underwent resection and reconstruction of the hepatic artery. All nine patients had macroscopic tumor clearance, but two of the nine had histologically incomplete tumor clearance.

***Group 2.*** From 1984 to 1995, inclusive, 30 patients underwent extended radical resection with IORT; 22 underwent pancreaticoduodenectomy; 2, total pancreatectomy; and 6, distal pancreatectomy. The pancreatic segment of the portal vein was removed in 11 of the 30 patients. One of the 11 with resection of the portal vein underwent resection of the common hepatic artery. Twenty-six of the 30 had macroscopic tumor clearance, but 5 of the 26 had histologically incomplete tumor clearance. Following extended resection, a dose of 30 Gy of 9- to 12-meV electrons was administered to the operative field, including the paraaortic area from the diaphragm above to the inferior mesenteric artery below (Fig. 61.1), using a special applicator (11).

The pancreatic cancers were staged in accordance with the UICC classification. The tumor staging and macroscopic tumor clearance of the patients in each of the two groups are summarized in Table 61.1. At the present time, only seven patients who had extended radical resection combined with IORT are still alive from 1 month to 11 years and 7 months postoperatively.

The cumulative survival rates of all patients in the two groups who had extended radical resection are shown in Figure 61.3. Nine patients with extended radical resection alone died within 3.2 years after the operation. The survival rate improved when extended radical resection was combined with IORT. The 5-year survival rate was 18.5% in all 30 cases, but this improvement was not significant. The 5-year survival rate of 23 patients who had complete macroscopic clearance of all tumor in combination with IORT, excluding 3 patients who died at the hospital, was 24.9% (Fig. 61.4). Of these 23 patients, 5 had histologically incomplete tumor clearance. The 5-year survival rates of 14 patients who had complete microscopic clearance of all tumor and 5 patients who had incomplete microscopic tumor clearance were 31.7% and 11.1%, respectively. One of two with stage I tumor is still alive more than 10 years after the operation. The other patient classified stage I died of liver metastases. Four of five patients with stage II tumor died within 3 years after the operation. Two of these four died of liver metastases. The 5-year survival rate of 17 patients with stage III tumor was 22.3%. Three with stage IV tumor died within 1 year (Fig. 61.5). According to the degree of involvement of lymph nodes in the TNM classification of the UICC, the 5-year survival rates of six patients of pN0 and 18 patients of pN1 were 25.0 and 22.3%, respectively. Three patients of pM1 (LYM) died within 1 year (Fig. 61.6). Four patients survived more than 5 years; three were stage III, and one, stage I. Three of these four had lymph node involvement. One of the four underwent macroscopic complete tumor clearance, but microscopically incomplete tumor clearance.

Eighteen patients who had extended combined surgical and radiation therapy died of tumor recurrence within 8 years and 2 months after the operation. Eleven of the 18 patients died of liver metastases, 4 died with carcinomatosis peritonei, 1 died from ileal perforation associated with metastases, 1 died of recurrent tumor in the remnant pancreas, and the remaining patient died with pleural carcinomatosis (Table 61.2).

In autopsies of seven persons in group 2 (Table 61.3), five had no evidence of any local recurrence in the radiation field, but peritoneal tumor seedings were found in two patients and liver metastases in one. The other two patients showed no evidence of any recurrence at autopsy. These two patients died of sepsis associated with severe nutritional disturbance. Two who had incomplete tumor clearance showed no local recurrence.

The remaining two patients had autopsies 8 months and 5.1 years following extended resection and IORT, respectively. Both had cancer of the body of the pancreas. Local microscopic recurrence was found within the radiation field around the aorta just above the left renal artery in one patient, and recurrence was found around the aorta from the level of the celiac axis to the level of the common iliac artery in the other. Microscopically there were sporadic cancer cells and cancer cell clumps in connective tissues, in perineural spaces, and in a small lymph node. On the other hand, the autopsies of two patients who underwent extended total pancreatectomy alone showed extensive macroscopic local recurrence around the celiac axis, the superior mesenteric artery, and the aorta from the diaphragm to the inferior mesenteric artery in one patient, and recurrence at the mesentery of the jejunum in the other.

**TABLE 61.1. Patients with Extended Resection for Pancreatic Cancer**

| | | Tumor Stage | | | | Macroscopic Tumor Clearance | |
|---|---|---|---|---|---|---|---|
| | | I | II | III | IV | Complete | Incomplete |
| Extended resection (1982–1983) | $n = 9$ | 0 | 4 | 5 | 0 | 9 | 0 |
| Extended resection + IORT (1984–1995) | $n = 30$ | 3 | 5 | 19 | 4 | 26 | 4 |

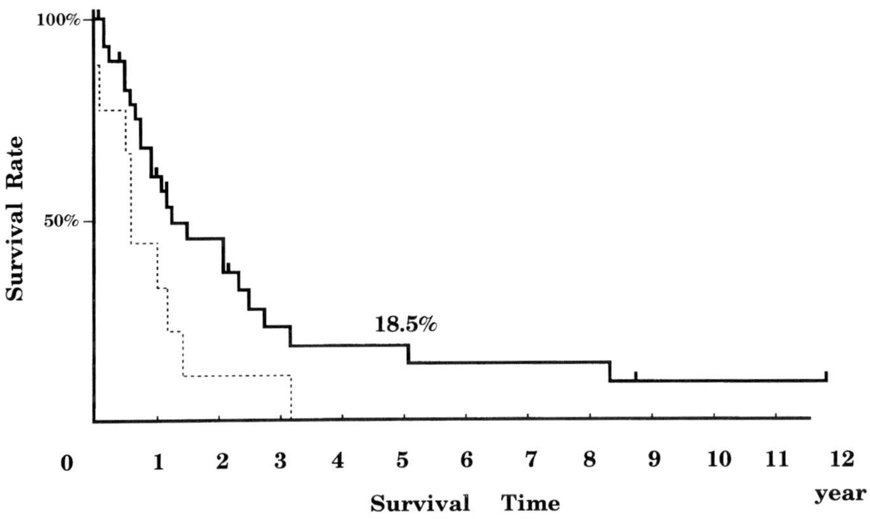


**FIG. 61.3.** Cumulative survival rates of patients who had extended resection for cancer of the pancreas, either alone ($n$ = 9; *small hatched line*) or in combination with IORT ($n$ = 30; *thick line*), including operation-related deaths ($n$ = 3) and noncuratively resected patients ($n$ = 9).

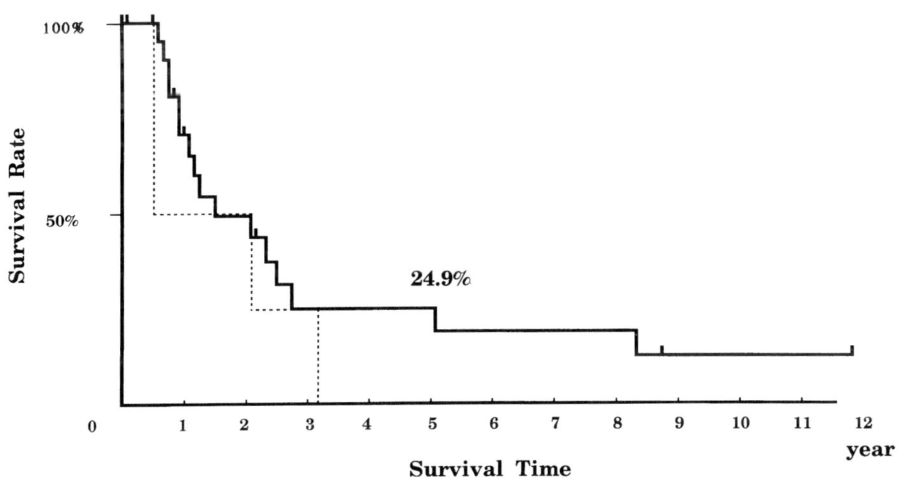


**FIG. 61.4.** Cumulative survival rates of patients who had extended resection for cancer of the pancreas according to whether there was incomplete macroscopic tumor clearance ($n$ = 4: stage II, 2; III, 1; IV, 1. *small hatched line*) or complete macroscopic tumor clearance ($n$ = 23: stage I, 2; II, 3; III, 17; IV, 2. *thick line*), excluding 3 patients who died of operation-related complications.

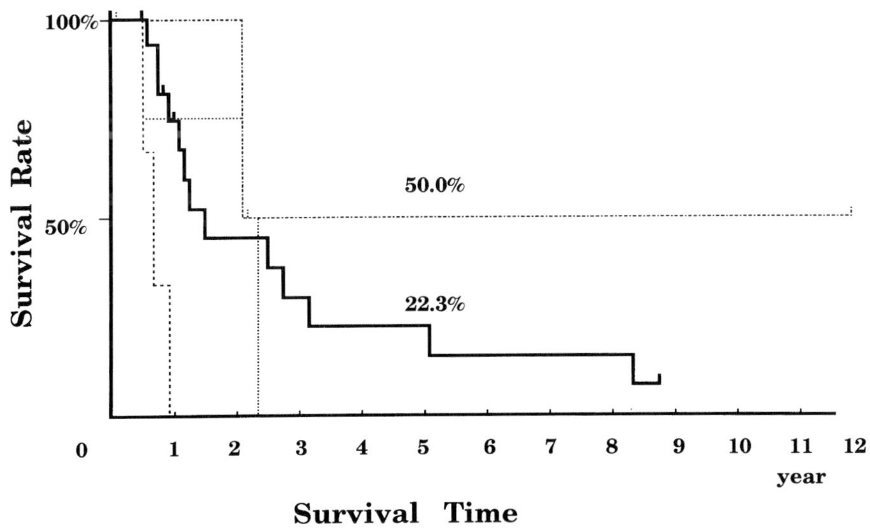


**FIG. 61.5.** Cumulative survival rate of patients who had extended resection for cancer of the pancreas according to the UICC stage of the tumor, excluding operation-related deaths (stage I, 2. *chain line;* II, 5. *small hatched line;* III, 17. *thick line;* IV, 3. *big hatched line*).

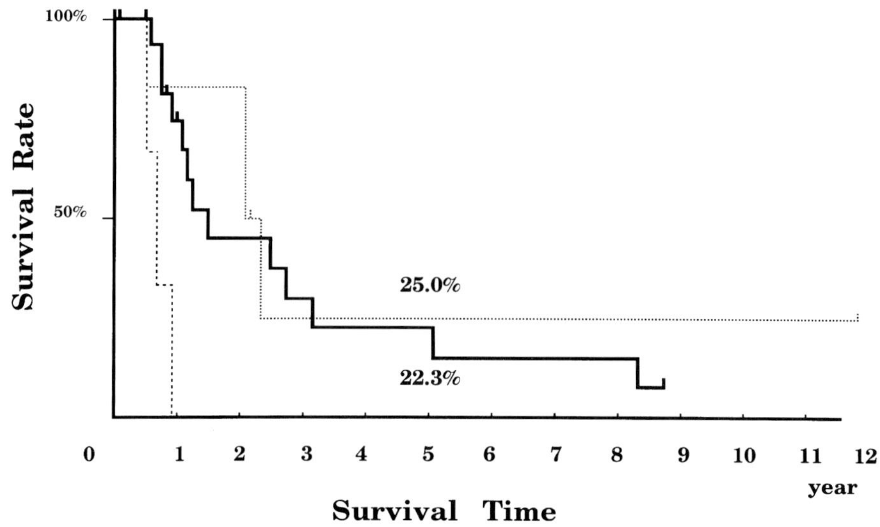


**FIG. 61.6.** Cumulative survival rate of patients who had extended resection for cancer of the pancreas according to the UICC classification of lymph node involvement, excluding operation-related deaths. (NO, 6. *small hatched line;* N1, 18. *thick line;* M1 (LYM), 3. *big hatched line*).

Sindelar (18) tried combining IORT in 11 of 20 patients with regional pancreatectomy for far-advanced cancer. In this trial, he reported that the IORT group did not have any long-term survival benefit compared with external radiation therapy. However, the local recurrence rate 1-year postoperatively was lower in the IORT group. Manabe et al. (19) noted a modest improvement in the survival rate and local recurrence rate in patients given IORT with a dose of 25–30 Gy with 6–10 meV combined with extended resection, but it was not significant. Hanyu et al. (20) did not find any benefit from IORT with a dose of 25 Gy with 9–15 meV in resected pancreatic cancer. Our results are better than those of some authors (18–20) but not as good as those of other authors (5, 21–24). Extended radical surgery and expansion of the IORT portal seems to result in improved local control. Improvements in local control, however, do not translate into increased survival because of the high incidence of subsequent liver and peritoneal failures. Our combined therapy will not benefit patients with stage II and IV tumors. In fact, these patients died of distant metastases (mainly hepatic metastases).

Results of combined therapy with resection and radiation are affected by differences in IORT technique, tumor stage, and degree and extent of dissection of lymph nodes in the resection. The tumor must be reduced as much as possible with resection to achieve the best effect with radiation therapy. The combination of extended surgery and extended IORT may be the best approach for local control of pancreatic cancer. Further study with a large population is required to clarify the clinical significance of such combined therapy.

No early radiation-related complications were noted postoperatively in patients who underwent IORT; nevertheless, when radiation is given over such an extended field, consideration should be given to the low tolerance of other structures, especially the ureter (maximum dose, 30 Gy) (25).

Judging from autopsy findings and causes of death in patients with extended resections combined with IORT, local recurrence of the tumor cannot be completely controlled; however, the incidence of local recurrence is decreased with this extended combined therapy. Moreover, autopsy of two patients who underwent our combined therapy only found local microscopic recurrence enclosed by thick, firm connective tissues. These findings will not directly cause death. In our series of patients with combined therapy, the cause of death of those with tumor recurrence was almost always due to metastasis via vessels.

## CONCLUSION

Further studies, including a prospective randomized trial, will be required to establish the role of these combined approaches fully. At present, we believe it is important to perform an extended pancreatectomy with extended IORT on well-selected patients for possible cure of pancreatic cancer. This extended approach is indicated for patients with advanced local cancer but may not be needed for patients with a tumor at an early stage. Extended pancreatectomy combined with IORT is the most effective treatment for local disease control at present. Enhanced local control induced by this combined therapy, however, has only

**TABLE 61.2. Results of 30 Patients Treated by Extended Resection Combined with IORT**

| | | |
|---|---|---|
| 30 Patients | 23 Dead | 3 Hospital deaths |
| | | 2 Other diseases |
| | | 18 Recurrences (site) |
| | | 11 Liver |
| | | 4 Peritoneum |
| | | 1 Ileum and liver |
| | | 1 Pleura and lung |
| | | 1 Remnant pancreas |
| | 7 Alive | |

**TABLE 61.3. Autopsy Findings of Patients with Extended Operation plus IORT**

| Local Recurrence | Other Recurrence Site |
|---|---|
| Negative: 5 | |
| Curative resection: 3 | 2: None (died of sepsis) |
| Noncurative resection: 2 | 1: Liver metastasis |
| | 2: Peritoneal seeding |
| Positive: 2 | 1: Liver metastasis |
| Curative resection: 2 | 1: Left adrenal gland, lung pleura |

limited impact on overall survival, because of systemic disease progression, especially hepatic metastases. Therefore, as a next step, anticancer treatment of metastases to the liver will become very important for the cure of pancreatic cancer.

## REFERENCES


1. Fortner JG. Regional pancreatectomy for cancer of the pancreas, ampulla, and other related sites, tumor staging and results. Ann Surg 1984;199:418–425.
2. Longmire WP Jr. Cancer of the pancreas: palliative operation, Whipple procedure, or total pancreatectomy. World J Surg 1984;8:872–879.
3. Moosa AR, Scott MH, Lavell-Jones M. The place of total and extended total pancreatectomy in pancreatic cancer. World J Surg 1984;8:895–899.
4. Van Heerden JA. Pancreatic resection for carcinoma of the pancreas: Whipple versus total pancreatectomy—an institutional perspective. World J Surg 1984;8:880–888.
5. Brooks JR, Brooks DC, Levine JD. Total pancreatectomy for ductal cell carcinoma of the pancreas. An update. Ann Surg 1989;209:405–410.
6. Beck C. Uber Kombinationasbehandlung bei bösartigen Neubildungen. Klin Wochenshr (Berlin) 1907;44:1335–1338.
7. Beck C. On external Roentgen treatment of internal structures (eventration treatment). NY Med J 1909;89:621–622.
8. Finsterer H. Zur Therapie inoperabler Magen und Darmkarzinome mit Freilegung und nachfolgender Röntgenbestrahlung. Strahlentherapie 1915;6:205–213.
9. Abe M, Fukuda M, Yamano K, Matsuda S, Handa H. Intraoperative irradiation in abdominal and cerebral tumours. Acta Radiol 1971;10:408–416.
10. Umegaki Y, Hamada M, Mitsukuri S, Nakano M, Karakawa J, et al. Clinical experience of high energy radiation therapy (in Japanese). J Jpn Radiol Assoc 1964;24:875–876.
11. Hiraoka T, Nakamura I, Tashiro S, Miyauchi Y. Intraoperative radiation therapy for pancreatic cancer in Japan. In: Dobelbower RR Jr, Abe M, eds. Intraoperative radiation therapy. Boca Raton, Florida: CRC Press, 1989:181–193.
12. Hiraoka T, Watanabe E, Mochinaga M, Tashiro S, Miyauchi Y, et al. Intraoperative irradiation combined with radical resection for cancer of the head of the pancreas. World J Surg 1984;8:766–771.
13. Abe M, Takahashi M. Intraoperative radiotherapy: the Japanese experience. Int J Radiat Oncol Biol Phys 1981;7:863–868.
14. Tepper JE, Noyes D, Krall JM, Sause WT, Wolkov HB, et al. Intraoperative radiation therapy of pancreatic carcinoma: a report of PTOG-8505. Int J Radiat Oncol Biol Phys 1991;21:1145–1149.
15. Hiraoka T, Uchino R, Kanemitsu K, Toyonaga N, Saitoh N, et al. Combination of intraoperative radiation with resection for cancer of the pancreas. Int J Pancreatol 1990;7:201–207.
16. Hermanek P, Sobin LH. UICC: TNM classification of malignant tumors. 4th ed. Berlin: Springer-Verlag, 1987:65–67.
17. Sindelar WF. Intraoperative radiotherapy in carcinoma of the stomach and pancreas. Recent Results Cancer Res 1988;110:226–243.
18. Sindelar WF. Clinical experience with regional pancreatectomy for adenocarcinoma of the pancreas. Arch Surg 1989;24:127–132.
19. Manabe T, Sibamoto Y, Ono K, Sasai K, Baba N, et al. Combined modality treatment for cancer of the pancreas: intraoperative and external radiotherapies. In: Abe M, Takahashi M, eds. Intraoperative radiation therapy. New York: Pergamon Press, 1991:246–248.
20. Hanyu F, Hatori T, Imaizumi T, Suzuki M, Nakasako T, et al. Intraoperative radiation therapy for patients with carcinoma of the head of the pancreas. In: Abe M, Takahashi M, eds. Intraoperative radiation therapy. New York: Pergamon Press, 1991:242–243.
21. Michelassi F, Erroi F, Dawson PJ, Pietrabissa A, Noda S, et al. Experience with 647 consecutive tumors of the duodenum, ampulla, head of the pancreas, and distal common bile duct. Ann Surg 1989;210:544–556.
22. Ishikawa O, Ohigashi H, Sasaki Y, Kabuto T, Fukuda I, et al. Practical usefulness of lymphatic and connective tissue clearance for the carcinoma of the pancreas head. Ann Surg 1988;208:215–220.
23. Trede M, Schwall G, Saeger HD. Survival after pancreatoduodenectomy: 118 consecutive resections without an operative mortality. Ann Surg 1990;211:447–458.
24. Cameron JL, Crist DW, Sitzmann JV, Hruban RH, Boitnott JK, et al. Factor influencing survival after pancreatoduodenectomy for pancreatic cancer. Ann J Surg 1991;161:120–125.
25. Sindelar SF, Tepper J, Travis EL, Terill R. Tolerance of retroperitoneal structure to intraoperative radiation. Ann Surg 1982;196:601–608.

# 62

# *Hormonal Therapy and Immunotherapy*

Åke Andrén-Sandberg and Pia Lena Bäckman

If recognized early, pancreatic adenocarcinoma can be removed surgically. However, only in a minority of the patients does surgery lead to definitive cure. Therefore other options are eagerly looked for, one of them being hormonal treatment.

The pancreas is not primarily regarded as a target organ for sex hormones, but a number of observations have suggested a reassessment of this opinion. For example, a role for sex hormones in pancreatic cancer development is suggested by epidemiologic data. Exocrine pancreatic cancer is significantly more common in younger men than in younger women. The male to female sex ratio in most countries is between 1.25 and 1.75 to 1.00, but it decreases with increasing age. In Sweden it is 1.75:1.00 below the age of 50 years, but there is no difference beyond the age of 70 years (1, 2). Moreover, in one study, prior oophorectomy appeared to be significantly more common in women with pancreatic cancer than in controls (3).

The gut hormones cholecystokinin (CCK) and gastrin are phylogenetically and structurally related. Under normal conditions, postprandial CCK stimulates the secretion of the exocrine pancreas. Long-term endogenously induced hypercholecystokininemia in rats not only induces hypertrophy of the exocrine pancreas, but also causes pancreatic hyperplastic nodule formation (4). Gastrin has been reported to stimulate growth of several human pancreatic cancer cell lines (5), and an increased incidence of pancreatic neoplasias has been found in patients with pernicious anemia, who are known to have raised levels of gastrin in serum (6).

Hormonal treatment is in routine clinical use for prostatic (7), breast (8, 9), endometrial, and ovarian carcinomas (10) and has also brought about some success in renal carcinoma (11). It has been suggested that hormonal treatment may also be of value in pancreatic cancer (12–14). Even if the benefit were small, such an approach would be of significance given the overall prevalence of the disease and the relatively poor results achieved with current treatment. The sex hormones and peptides of the cholecystokinin and the gastrin families are to date the most studied hormones in pancreatic cancer research.

## INFLUENCE OF ESTROGENS ON THE EXOCRINE PANCREAS

More than 30 years ago, Ullberg and Bengtsson (15) reported increased accumulation of radiolabeled estrogen in the exocrine pancreas. Labeled estradiol or estriol has also been found to be selectively retained in the pancreas of male dogs, rats, and baboons in addition to other organs including the kidney, prostate, testis, muscle, and thyroid (16, 17). Such selective concentration in the pancreas was unaffected by testosterone or cortisol. Using autoradiography, Sandberg and Rosenthal (18) confirmed that the estrogen was predominantly localized in the cytoplasm of the acinar cells. Moreover, normal human pancreatic tissue has been shown to be capable of converting both estrone and estrone sulfate into the biologically active estrogen 17-ß-estradiol at a rate comparable with that of an established estrogen target tissue, such as breast cancer (19).

Boctor et al. reported (20) that the accumulation of zymogen granules, which occurred after adrenalectomy in male rats, was reversed by giving 17-ß-estradiol. A putative receptor for 17-ß-estradiol, distinct from the uterine receptor, was also identified. Evidence that this receptor was restricted to the exocrine pancreas was based on experiments using streptozotocin, which selectively destroys islet cells but does not affect the estrogen receptors (19).

The binding of steroid hormone to pancreatic acinar tissue requires the presence of a coligand (21), one possible candidate being somatostatin (22). This hormone, however, also inhibits the translocation of proteins into the endoplasmic reticulum, which might explain how somatostatin reduces exocrine secretion.

Estrogens appear to be necessary for the synthesis of pancreatic digestive enzymes. Following adrenalectomy in male rats and adrenalectomy and oophorectomy in female rats, there is a marked depletion of zymogen granules in the acinar cells. Treatment with either triamcinolone or estradiol reverses this effect, while there is no influence by testosterone (23). Moreover, estrogen administration results in decreased secretion of zinc and bicarbonate in pancreatic juice, whereas amylase and lipase are increased. In pancreatic tissue, triglycerides and total lipids are increased by estrogens (24, 25).

In contrast to the effects on pancreatic enzyme synthesis, estrogens appear to have an inhibitory effect on pancreatic growth. Lhoste et al. (26) showed that the pancreatic weight of normal male rats was 35% higher than that of normal females, even when corrected for body weight. Guo and Singh (27) demonstrated that chronic treatment of guinea pigs with estradiol resulted in a significant reduction in pancreatic weight and an amylase content comparable to that in castrated control animals, without an associated change in body weight. The pancreatic weight loss with estradiol treatment was primarily due to reduced pancreatic growth in terms of cell numbers, as the DNA content per unit pancreatic weight was identical between treated and control groups.

In contradistinction to estrogens, some other male and female sex hormones appear to have a trophic effect on the pancreas. Orchidectomy in male rats was found to decrease pancreatic weight, which was reversed by testosterone administration (26). Beaudoin et al. (28) reported that dexamethasone replacement therapy in castrated and adrenalectomized rats partially restored the level of pancreatic amylase, while estradiol had no effect on the amylase content and was associated with the presence of unusual "halo" granules. While some have shown that glucocorticoids produce a significant increase in pancreatic weight, total

DNA, RNA, and protein content in the rat (29, 30), others have shown that corticosteroids produce a decrease in pancreatic weight, protein, DNA content (23, 31), and cell proliferation (31, 32) in the same species. There are also several reports on the influence of estrogens on lipid metabolism and its secondary morphologic and biochemical changes in the pancreas, causing acute pancreatitis (33–35).

Guo and Singh (27) have shown increased release of amylase by CCK in oophorectomized guinea-pigs treated with estradiol. Although the total amount of amylase released was less in the latter because of a reduction in the amount of acinar tissue, the proportional release of amylase was significantly greater. This appeared to be due to specific up-regulation of the pancreatic CCK receptors, as the receptor density for vasoactive intestinal polypeptide (VIP) was unaltered. That the estrogenic effect on the CCK receptor was organ specific was suggested by the finding of normal receptor density for both CCK and VIP in the gallbladder.

The mechanism by which estradiol mediates its multiple effects on pancreatic growth and enzyme production and release remains uncertain. At least some of these effects, however, may be due to a direct interaction of estradiol with estradiol-binding protein observed in the rat pancreas (18, 20, 36).

## STEROID RECEPTORS

When Jensen and Jacobson (37) first described in 1962 that $^3$H-estrogen was accumulated and retained in target tissue (e.g., breast cancer) but not in control tissue (e.g., diaphragm muscle), they assumed the presence of specific estrogen-binding molecules ("estrogen receptors"). Steroid receptors, including the receptor for estradiol, are located in the nucleus. Estrogen receptors (ER) belong to a large family of hormone-dependent DNA-binding proteins with a "zinc-finger" motif, a family including receptors for other steroids, thyroid hormone, retinoic acid, vitamin $D_3$, and some "orphan receptors" whose ligands have yet to be identified (38). The hormones, at least estradiol, cross the cell membrane, probably by diffusion, and are bound to the receptor; the complex can then bind to specific sites on the chromosome.

The estrogen receptor gene consists of more than 140 kilobases of genomic DNA divided into eight translated exons. The interaction of estradiol with the steroid-binding domain of the receptor leads to strong binding of the receptor to the estrogen-response elements of target genes. This binding is brought about by the zinc fingers of the receptor, resulting in a range of transcription events that produce several types of mRNA. The resulting translations induce the production of progesterone receptor and a variety of other proteins and peptides (39). These estrogen-regulated agents include c-fos, classical growth factors such as transforming growth factor (TGF)-α, insulin-like growth factors (IGFs) I and II, acid and basic fibroblast growth factors (FGFs), and epidermal growth factor–like protein, which when secreted can activate membrane receptors on the same cells. Also influenced by the estrogen level are proteases such as plasminogen activator and precursors of cathepsins, which stimulate cell proliferation as well as enhance invasiveness by breaking down the extracellular matrix. The extent to which these growth factors are involved in pancreatic cancer is currently debated (40).

Currently much research worldwide focuses on the steroid receptor homologies similar to those of the viral oncogene v-*erb* A and its cellular equivalent c-*erb* A. This has inevitably raised questions as to the oncogenic potential of steroid receptors, particular as c-*erb* A has been found to be a thyroid hormone receptor (41). Since the DNA-binding domains of this receptor family are similar, there is the possibility of interaction (either competitive or synergistic) between their respective ligands at the DNA level (38). Two different types of ERs have been defined, and it has been proposed that ER type II is of special interest for estrogen-induced proliferation (42, 43).

Although much of the work relating to steroids has inevitably centered on the breast, there is increasing attention on the effect of steroid hormones on the structure and function of the exocrine pancreas (23, 28, 44). There are sex-steroid biosynthetic enzymes in pancreatic tissue (16, 28), and the demonstration of testosterone biotransformation by the isolated perfused pancreas (45) strongly suggests the participation of androgens in pancreatic function. Specific sex-steroid-binding sites have been demonstrated in the pancreas of dogs (17, 46), rats (18, 20, 47, 48), hamsters (36), and humans (49, 50). Various effects of other steroid hormones on the exocrine pancreatic functions have also been reported (17, 27, 29, 51–54).

## ESTROGEN RECEPTORS AND ESTROGEN-BINDING PROTEINS IN THE EXOCRINE PANCREAS

ERs have been identified in pancreatic adenocarcinoma as well as in the healthy pancreas of humans (55–57). That such receptors may be important was suggested by the finding of progesterone receptors in human pancreatic tissue (58), since these require activated ERs for their expression (59). However, there are also reports of an absence of ERs (60–63) in both normal and cancerous exocrine pancreas investigated by immunoassay and immunohistochemistry, even though almost one-fourth of the normal specimens showed an increased level of progesterone receptors. In one study, no progesterone receptors were found in pancreatic cancer, and the authors suggested that progesterone receptors found in healthy pancreatic tissue may be situated on the endocrine and not the exocrine cells (60).

There is little doubt that there are several proteins with estrogen affinity in the pancreas, but their biologic function is mainly unknown. Estrogen-binding protein has been separated from the nuclear and microsomal fractions of the rat pancreas and characterized by Boctor et al. (20). This protein has a sedimentation constant of 4S and binds estradiol with a high binding capacity (about $1 \times 10^3$ fmol estradiol/mg pancreatic tissue) and a low affinity (dissociation constant, $K_d > 1$ nM). This estrogen-binding protein has a distinctly lower affinity, but a capacity approximately a thousand times higher than that of the ER. An estrogen-binding protein has been identified in healthy pancreatic tissue of several species, including man, and also in human pancreatic cancer (29, 47, 56). This protein has not been found in other tumors nor in normal tissues other than the pancreas. Proteins of a similar size, binding steroids with a lower capacity but a higher affinity ($K_d < 1$ nM) are, however, also characteristically present in uterine, prostatic, and breast tissue (64, 65). Estrogen-binding protein from the pancreas (unlike that from the uterus) requires a coligand for maximum binding. The physiologic action of pancreatic estrogen-binding protein may also be different, since it does not appear to translocate estradiol to the nucleus and may be involved in acinar cell secretion (31). The fact that these proteins do not have an antigen structure identifiable by anti-ER or anti-PgR monoclonal antibodies might question the existence of biologically active ER or PgR in normal or neoplastic tissue, given that the detection levels for the monoclonal antibodies used are relevant also for the pancreas. This issue remains to be settled.

Estramustine, a nornitrogen mustard derivative of estradiol, is a cytotoxic agent used for treating advanced prostatic cancer. Of particular interest is that an estramustine-binding protein has also been found in human pancreatic tissue. This protein binds estramustine and its metabolite estromustine but not estradiol or tamoxifen (12, 66). Estramustine is bound with an affinity 20 times that with which estrogen-binding protein binds estradiol. This estramustine-binding protein has not been identified in other malignancies, including breast and renal cancers, malignant melanoma, and, surprisingly, prostatic cancer (where there is another estramustine-binding protein described). Moreover, Björk et al. (67) found that estramustine phosphate, estramustine, and estromustine were bound with a relatively high affinity ($K_d$ = 10 nM) to protein-binding sites (24–30 kDa) constituting 0.02–0.03% of total protein in the rat pancreas. Similar binding sites were present in the human pancreatic cancers examined but absent in the only histopathologically normal pancreas examined so far.

## INFLUENCE OF ESTROGENS ON EXPERIMENTAL PANCREATIC CANCER

Strong suggestions of a role for estrogen in promoting pancreatic cancer come from studies both in vivo and in vitro. Lacaine et al. (68) reported that the in vivo growth of a grafted hamster ductular pancreatic cancer cell line that binds 17-ß-estradiol and dihydrotestosterone was significantly reduced in estrogen-treated animals. Estradiol treatment is highly effective in a dose-dependent manner in inhibiting the development and growth of preneoplastic pancreatic lesions in rats treated with azaserine, which induces acinar, but not ductular, pancreatic cancer (69).

The possible hormone sensitivity of the pancreas is further indicated by the presence of several sex-steroid biosynthetic enzymes in normal and malignant tissue. Estrone sulfate, which is quantitatively the most important estrogen in nonpregnant individuals, is converted into the biologically active 17-ß-estradiol by human pancreatic homogenates in vitro. Also, the enzymes 5-α-reductase (which converts testosterone to the more potent androgen 5-dihydrotestosterone) and aromatase (which converts Δ-4-androstenedione to estrone and testosterone to estradiol) have been found in human pancreatic cancer tissue (70).

In a series of in vitro experiments, Benz et al. (71) compared the steroid responsiveness of four human and one rodent pancreatic tumor cell line with that of an ER-positive breast cancer cell line. They found that all four human pancreatic tumor cell lines contained measurable levels of specific estradiol-binding sites, with a $K_d$ that ranged from 1 to 9 nM, which contrasted with the higher affinity found in the breast cancer cell lines, with a $K_d$ < 1 nM. Growth of one of the pancreatic tumor cell lines was stimulated by about 40% following exposure to nanomolar concentrations of estradiol. Moreover, both glucocorticoids and androgen also stimulated the proliferation of the pancreatic tumor cell lines by as much as 30%. Growth of the other pancreatic tumor lines was inhibited to varying degrees following exposure to micromolar concentrations of estrogen, antiestrogen, antiandrogen, progesterone, and inhibitors of steroid-metabolizing enzymes but with little relationship to the ER content of the tumors. In general, progesterone was slightly more growth inhibiting to these pancreatic tumor lines than the other endocrine agents, including tamoxifen. An inhibitor of 5-α-reductase with minimal affinity for androgen receptors inhibited the growth of the pancreatic tumor cell lines to less than 40% of controls, whereas a potent androgen receptor antagonist with no direct influence on 5-α-reductase inhibited growth of two cell lines but not the others. This suggests that the steroid-dependent growth-inhibitory mechanisms of some pancreatic cancers might involve both receptor antagonism and direct inhibition of steroidal oxidoreductases.

In 1982 Benz et al. (72), using the ER-expressing human pancreatic cancer cell line COLO-357, found that the binding of estradiol to the receptor could be inhibited with diethylstilbestrol. When cytotoxic concentrations of 5-fluorouracil were combined with estradiol, progesterone, or tamoxifen, there was a fivefold increase in cytotoxicity. On the other hand, randomized addition of aminoglutethimide, an inhibitor of the aromatase enzyme, did not add to the survival of patients with advanced pancreatic carcinoma treated with FAM (5-fluorouracil, adriamycin, and mitomycin) (73).

## INFLUENCE OF ANDROGENS ON EXOCRINE PANCREATIC CANCER

An androgen receptor has also been identified in the rat pancreas (74) and is present in human healthy and malignant pancreatic tissue (75). Exogenous testosterone also localizes selectively in the pancreas (17). In the rat, a transcriptional activity of the androgen receptor gene in the pancreas has been found, which seemed to be modulated by the androgenic milieu in the tissue, similar to that reported for the classical androgen-responsive organs (76). Adequate characterization of these receptors is still not complete. There are, however, also reports of an absence of androgen receptors in both normal and cancerous pancreas (60).

Hayashi and Katayama (77) found that growth of aminoquinolone-induced pancreatic tumors was increased by injections of testosterone propionate in female and male rats following bilateral oophorectomy and orchidectomy, respectively. On the other hand, oophorectomy alone gave a decreased incidence of pancreatic tumors. Similarly, Lhoste et al. (26) reported that 4 months after azaserine administration, preneoplastic atypical acinar cell foci and nodules were smaller and less numerous in female and castrated male rats than in intact males. Although testosterone treatment partly reversed the effect of orchidectomy, no high-affinity androgen receptors were detected. Orchidectomized rats with azaserine-induced pancreatic tumors developed fewer and smaller atypical acinar cell nodules, which was partially reversed with testosterone treatment (78). Greenway et al. (79) reported that testosterone stimulated the growth of human pancreatic cancer xenografts in nude mice, while growth was inhibited by cyproterone acetate and an antiandrogen.

In human studies Sperti et al. (80) and Greenway et al. (81, 82) reported significantly lower serum concentrations of total testosterone in patients with pancreatic cancer than in patients with other types of gastrointestinal cancers or with benign pancreatic diseases. There were no differences between free testosterone and androstenedione levels in pancreatic cancer patients and other cancer patients (80). Since normal or low levels of follicle-stimulating hormone (FSH) and luteinizing hormone (LH) were also found in association with the low total testosterone levels, it was assumed that there might be a dysfunction of the hypothalamic-hypophyseal feedback mechanism (83, 84), but this was subsequently contradicted by the finding of similar levels of FSH and LH in patients with chronic pancreatitis (85).

Robles-Diaz et al. (86) found a low ratio of serum testosterone to 5-α-dihydrotestosterone in comparison with patients with other gastrointestinal malignancies and chronic pancreatitis, and high androstenedione levels (87). They attributed this to an increased testosterone uptake by the tumor and increased 5-α-reductase activity in pancreatic tumor tissue.

The role of androgens and androgen receptors in human pancreatic cancer still remains unclear. An alternative explanation for the reported findings relating to serum testosterone is that they are secondary to cancer cachexia rather than a primary cancer effect (88), as total serum testosterone levels correlate significantly with poor nutritional status (80, 89). The impaired hepatic function and diabetes that might be associated with pancreatic cancer have also been suggested as a possible explanation for the low testosterone concentration (89).

## TAMOXIFEN AND PANCREATIC CANCER

In 1982 Wilking et al. (90) described the distribution of radioactively labeled tamoxifen—considered to be a competitive inhibitor of estrogens on the ERs—given intravenously to oophorectomized mice. Rather low amounts of uptake were found in normal estrogen target tissues, such as breast and uterus, but high concentrations of tamoxifen were detected in the lungs, adrenals, and pancreas. This observation coupled with the in vitro effects of tamoxifen in pancreatic cancer cells might suggest a benefit for tamoxifen in vivo. However, tamoxifen had no effect on the growth of human pancreatic cancer xenographs in nude mice (79). That study also found no effect of the synthetic nonsteroidal estrogen stilbestrol. A situation analogous to that of breast cancer may pertain, in which hormone manipulation with antiestrogens is more likely to be effective if the pancreatic cancer expresses ERs. Thus, in a recent study of xenografted human pancreatic cancer cell lines in nude mice, growth was significantly reduced by somatostatin given alone or as a combined regimen with tamoxifen (91). Also the DNA, RNA, and protein content in the tumors was reduced. In one of the cell lines, tamoxifen was effective. These data were supported by a nonrandomized human series of 12 patients treated with a low dose of a synthetic somatostatin, octreotide, combined with tamoxifen, who showed a longer survival than expected, 12 months (92).

A few phase II clinical trials of tamoxifen treatment in patients with advanced pancreatic cancer have been published. In a small study, Theve et al. (93) found a median survival of 9 months in patients with unresectable and histologically proven adenocarcinoma given tamoxifen 20 mg a day. In three of the men, survival extended to 22 months. The overall survival was significantly better than that of a historic control group surviving in median only 3 months. Tönnesen and Kamp-Jensen (94) similarly reported a median survival of 7 months in patients treated with tamoxifen 10 mg daily. However, Crowson et al. (95) failed to demonstrate any effect by tamoxifen. Based on serial computerized tomography studies, the mean interval for disease progression was 3 months (range, 1–8 months) in this study. A loading dose of 160 mg tamoxifen was given followed by 40 mg once daily. Only one of the patients survived more than 6 months.

Wong et al. (96) treated 24 pancreatic cancer patients with tamoxifen 20 mg daily, with a median survival of 7 months. In men, the median survival was 4 months; in women (all of whom were postmenopausal), 10 months. Six of these women survived for more than 1 year, and three survived for more than 2 years.

There are also some phase III studies of tamoxifen treatment in pancreatic cancer. In the prospective controlled trial reported by Keating et al. (97), 108 patients with pancreatic adenocarcinoma were randomly allocated to receive daily tamoxifen 20 mg, cyproterone acetate 100 mg, or no active treatment. The median survival of those receiving tamoxifen was 5 months, compared with 4 months for the cyproterone acetate group. There was no survival benefit for either of these groups compared with the control group, which had a median survival of 3 months. A regression analysis of 12 clinical and biochemical features showed, not surprisingly, that for the entire group of patients, survival was significantly longer in younger patients, those undergoing surgical bypass, and those with better performance status. Adjustment for the distribution of these prognostic variables confirmed the lack of benefit of different treatments.

In a Norwegian multicenter study of 173 patients with pancreatic cancer and cancer of the papilla of Vater, a randomization was done between 30 mg tamoxifen daily or placebo (98). Treatment was continued until death or 10 months after accrual into the trial. The median survival in the tamoxifen group was 115 days, compared with 122 days in the placebo group. Although there was no difference in survival between men and women, a retrospective analysis of women with stage III cancer showed that the median survival was 195 days in the treatment group, compared with 45 days in the control group, which is a significant difference. Three women (7%) were still alive after 2.5 years in the treatment group, and none in the control group; no men survived after this time. The findings in the Norwegian study in women with stage III cancer might be conceived as supporting the view of Wong et al. (96) that tamoxifen is beneficial in postmenopausal women. The final answer to the question of whether tamoxifen is of benefit in postmenopausal women with pancreatic cancer requires further phase III trials.

## CHOLECYSTOKININ AND EXOCRINE PANCREATIC CANCER

The influence of CCK on exocrine pancreatic cancer has been studied extensively during recent years. Only a few aspects that might be of importance for the carcinogenic process are discussed here.

An increase in the size and weight of the pancreas in response to CCK administration was described as early as in 1967 (99). A number of later studies have shown that administration of all forms of cholecystokinins—CCK-8, CCK-33, and the CCK analogue cerulein—induces exocrine pancreatic hypertrophy and hyperplasia in rats (100–103). A trophic effect of CCK-8 and cerulein on the pancreas has also been found in hamsters (104, 105) and mice (106, 107). The trophic effect of exogenous CCK seems to be mediated by the CCK-A receptor (108–110), since it can be mimicked by CCK-A receptor agonists (109, 111) and blocked by CCK-A receptor antagonists (112).

Studies with CCK receptor binding, hybridization with radiolabeled cDNA probes, or reverse transcription–polymerase chain reaction, have shown that CCK-A receptors also are present in rat pancreatic putative preneoplastic lesions and cancer tissue induced by azaserine (113–115), rat pancreatic cancer cell lines (116–119), pancreatic carcinomas in transgenic mice (120), hamster pancreatic cancer (121), and human pancreatic cancer cell lines and tumors (122–125). Also, CCK-B receptors have been found in rat pancreas (108), a rat pancreatic cancer cell line (126, 127), experimentally induced rat pancreatic carcinomas (123, 128), and human pancreatic carcinomas and cancer cell lines (119, 120, 129). However, neither CCK-A nor -B receptors have been found uniformly in investigations of pancreatic cancer (130).

Pancreatic cancer has been connected etiologically to diet; for example, intake of fat (3). Thus, there may be an association between pancreatic cancer and dietary fat, inducing the release of CCK and thereby affecting the acinar target cells. However, whether ductal cells—probably the origin of the cancerigenic process—are also affected is not that evident.

Another way to stimulate the exocrine pancreas endogenously is by the feed-back mechanism exerted by intraduodenal trypsin. Presence of trypsin in the duodenum seems to be the main negative feedback stimulus to CCK release (131, 132). Feeding rats and hamsters with protease inhibitors such as raw soya bean flour or camostate induces endogenous hypercholecystokininemia leading to pancreatic hypertrophy. This trophic effect can be abolished or markedly reduced by administration of a CCK-A receptor antagonist (133, 134). Transposing the orifice of the pancreaticobiliary ducts distally into the small intestine frees proximal jejunal and duodenal CCK-secreting cells from the negative feedback. In rats and hamsters, such pancreaticobiliary diversion (PBD) causes a persistent rise in the CCK concentrations in plasma, leading to pancreatic hyperplasia and hypertrophy (135–138). This pancreaticotrophic response can also be abolished by administration of a CCK-A receptor antagonist, indicating that the trophic effect of PBD is mediated by CCK acting through the CCK-A receptor (112, 139).

Exogenously infused CCK-8 or cerulein (109, 140, 141) as well as hypercholecystokininemia endogenously induced by oral trypsin inhibitor administration (142), feeding rats raw soya flour (143, 144), fat promotion (141), PBD (4, 110, 138, 145, 146), and partial gastrectomy (147) has promoted the development of atypical acinar cell foci, which are regarded as preneoplastic lesions (148–152). CCK has also been shown to stimulate growth of human pancreatic carcinoma cell lines (153). Unfortunately, there are few studies on the effects of CCK and its analogues on the growth of carcinoma xenografts. A stimulating effect was found in a hamster ductal carcinoma transplanted to hamsters (154) and in a human pancreatic carcinoma transplanted to nude mice (155). However, inhibition of carcinogenesis by CCK has also been reported in experimental pancreatic cancer (156–158), and in one study no effect of cerulein was found (159). There are also reports of resistance against TGF-α and EGF in preneoplastic pancreatic lesions of azaserine-treated rats if treated by the CCK-analogue cerulein, indicating that CCK acts independently of these growth factors (160).

Studies on the effect of exogenous CCK or feeding with protease inhibitors in the hamster nitrosamine model, which leads to development of ductal pancreatic neoplasia (161), show conflicting results, ranging from promotion (105, 140, 162) or no effect (133, 159, 163, 164) to inhibition (164–168).

The hypothesis that CCK antagonists would be useful as antitumor drugs has been tested in animal studies, but experiments using CCK antagonists in vivo to study the effect on pancreatic cancer have given conflicting results. Devazepide infusion, blocking the CCK-A receptor, did not inhibit tumor initiation in the hamster model (133, 169), but it inhibited tumor growth in human pancreatic cancer transplants in nude mice (155) and decreased tumor size in rats (148). There are several reports of CCK antagonists inhibiting experimental carcinogenesis induced by azaserine (141, 170), anthracene (171), pancreaticobiliary diversion (172), and xenografted cancers (173–175). A clinical trial of devazepide in patients with advanced pancreatic cancer failed to demonstrate any impact on tumor progression, pain, or nutrition, and several patients experienced toxic reactions, even at a lower dosage than that used in animal studies (176). The lack of clinical effects of devazepide may have several explanations: first, human pancreatic cancer is of ductal origin, and CCK seems to influence acinar cells preferably; second, in most studies, devazepide has been given continuously in those with negative results but intermittently in those with positive results. During continuous administration of devazepide, there could be up-regulation of the CCK-A receptor, as an effect on cell proliferation was seen as early as 36 hours (177).

A comprehensive review on the role of cholecystokinin in pancreatic cancer was recently published (178).

## GASTRIN AND EXOCRINE PANCREATIC CANCER

Whether gastrin exerts a trophic effect on the exocrine pancreas or not has long been a matter of controversy (179). However, in one study in mice, administration of gastrin-17 resulted in an increase in the volume, the mean nuclear diameter, and the volume of nucleoli of acinar cells (180). Administration of pentagastrin has repeatedly been reported to induce growth of the exocrine pancreas in rats (181–185), an effect even found in hypophysectomized rats (181). Gastrin-17 also augments pancreatic enzyme secretion at doses that are below the maximum for gastric acid secretion in the human (181, 186, 187). On the other hand, some studies in different rodents have shown that neither potent inhibition of acid secretion, leading to hypergastrinemia (188–190), nor gastrin-17 infusion (191) caused pancreatic hypertrophy in rats. There was a significant increase in pancreatic weight and secretory volume in rats with endogenous hypergastrinemia induced by transposing the gastric antrum to the colon (192); however, this may be an effect of other changes in the levels of gastrointestinal hormones induced by the surgery. In rats, antrectomy, which leads to hypogastrinemia, has been shown to induce atrophy of the exocrine pancreas. This hypotrophic effect of antrectomy was prevented by treatment with pentagastrin, indicating that endogenous gastrin (which in some respects differs physiologically from pentagastrin) could play a role in the regulation of growth of the pancreas in rats (193). In the hamster, fundectomy, leading to hypergastrinemia, induced pancreatic exocrine tissue hyperplasia and hypertrophy, whereas antrectomy led to retardation of pancreatic growth (194). The effects of fundectomy, which last about half of the life span in rats caused pancreatic hyperplasia and hypertrophy, as well as development of acidophilic atypical acinar cell foci (195) and enhancement of the development of precancerous pancreatic changes after azaserine treatment (196). However, Håkansson and coworkers suggested that the increase in pancreatic weight and DNA content after fundectomy and gastrectomy cannot be explained by means of only gastrin or CCK, as there are other, complex hormonal interactions after these unphysiologic operations (197).

If gastrin and its analogues exert any effects on the exocrine pancreas, they are probably mediated through CCK receptors. Cholecystokinin-B receptors and gastrin receptors are thought to be the same and are present in rat pancreas (108). A recent study showed that a CCK-B, but not a CCK-A, receptor antagonist significantly reduced the enhancement of DNA synthesis in the pancreas caused by pentagastrin treatment in fasted rats, indicating that the effect of pentagastrin may be mediated by CCK-B receptors but not CCK-A, receptors (198). Whether this is only a quantitative difference due to different affinities or a qualitative difference is presently not known.

Besides stimulating pancreatic growth, gastrin-17 and pentagastrin also stimulate growth of a rat pancreatic carcinoma cell line (126, 199) and several human pancreatic cancer cell lines (200). Another study showed that split gastrojejunostomy, which leads to hypergastrinemia as well as hypercholecystokininemia, enhanced azaserine-induced pancreatic carcinogenesis in the rat (201). However, the growth of two human pancreatic cancer cell lines was unaffected by gastrin-17 or its antagonist, although it could be enhanced by epidermal growth factor (202). The influence of gastrin on pancreatic cancer needs to be studied further, with special reference to interaction of gastrin with other gastrointestinal hormones.

## CONCLUSIONS

At present there are no data confirming a role for estrogens, androgens, or their antagonists in clinical treatment of exocrine pancreatic cancer; neither are there data supporting the use of cholecystokinin, gastrin, or their antagonists. However, there is strong evidence for an influence of these hormones not only on nonmalignant pancreatic tissue, but also on carcinogenesis and perhaps on the growth of established pancreatic cancers. These observations make further studies on these mechanisms worthwhile, with the aim of finding new, combined strategies for treatment of pancreatic cancer in an adjuvant, and perhaps also a palliative, setting.

## REFERENCES

1. Andrén-Sandberg Å. Demographics of exocrine pancreatic cancer with special reference to age, sex, and time trends. Int J Pancreatol 1993;16:214–216.
2. Bäckman PL, Barlow L, Andrén-Sandberg Å. Decreasing incidence of exocrine pancreatic cancer in Sweden. Int J Pancreatol 1995;18:289–290.

3. Lin RS, Kessler JI. A multifactorial model for pancreatic cancer. JAMA 1981;245:147–152.
4. Stace NE, Palmer TJ, Vaja S, Dowling RH. Long-term pancreaticobiliary diversion stimulates hyperplastic and adenomatous nodules in the rat pancreas: a new model for spontaneous tumor formation. Gut 1987;28(S1):265–268.
5. Smith JP, Fantaskey AP, Liu GZ, Zagon IS. Identification of gastrin as a growth peptide in human pancreatic cancer. Am J Physiol 1995;268:R135–141.
6. Borch K, Kullman E, Ledin T, Ihse I. Increased incidence of pancreatic neoplasia in pernicious anemia. World J Surg 1988;12:866–870.
7. McConnell J. Physiologic basis for endocrine therapy for prostatic cancer. Urol Clin North Am 1991;18:1–13.
8. Early Breast Cancer Trialists Collaborative Group. Systemic treatment of early breast cancer by hormonal, cytotoxic, or immune therapy. 133 randomised trials involving 31,000 recurrences and 24,000 deaths among 75,000 women. Lancet 1992;339:1–15,71–85.
9. Clark G, Wenger CR, Beardslee S, et al. How to integrate steroid hormone receptor, flow cytometric, and other prognostic information in regard to primary breast cancer. Cancer 1993; 71:2157–2162.
10. Kaupilla A. Protestin therapy of endometrial, breast and ovarian carcinoma. A review of clinical observations. Acta Obstet Gynecol Scand 1984;63:4414–50.
11. Romics I, Russel C, Bach D. Experience with hormone receptors in renal cancer. Int Urol Nephrol 1990;22:507–512.
12. Andrén-Sandberg Å. Estrogens and pancreatic cancer. Some recent aspects. Scand J Gastroenterol 1986;21:129–133.
13. Andrén-Sandberg Å. Progress in estrogen receptors and estrogen-binding proteins in pancreatic cancer. Organ System Newsl 1986;2(3):12–13.
14. Greenway BA. Carcinoma of the exocrine pancreas: a sex hormone responsive tumour? Br J Surg 1987;74:441–442.
15. Ullberg S, Bengtsson G. Autoradiographic studies with natural oestrogens. Acta Endocrinol 1963;43:75–86.
16. Mendoza-Hernández G, López-Solache I, Rendón JL, Dìaz-Sánchez V, Díaz-Zagoya JC. 17-ß-Hydroxysteroid dehydrogenase activity in canine pancreas. Biochem Biophys Res Commun 1988;152:376–382.
17. Sandberg AA, Rosenthal HE. Steroid receptors in exocrine glands: the pancreas and prostate. J Steroid Biochem 1979;11: 293–299.
18. Sandberg AA, Rosenthal HE. Estrogen receptors in the pancreas. J Steroid Biochem 1974;5:969–975.
19. Fernstad R, Pousette Å, Carlström K. Metabolism of estrone sulphate by normal human pancreatic tissue in vitro. Scand J Gastroenterol 1987;22:644–648.
20. Boctor AM, Band P, Grossman A. Analysis of binding of ($^3$H)estradiol to the cytosol fraction of rat pancreas: comparison with sites in the cytosol of uterus. Endocrinology 1983;113:453–462.
21. Boctor AM, Band P, Grossman A. Requirement for an accessory factor for binding of ($^3$H)estradiol to protein in the cytosol fraction of rat pancreas. Proc Natl Acad Sci USA 1981;78:5648–5651.
22. Band R, Richardson SB, Boctor AM, Grossman A. Somatostatin enhance binding of ($^3$H)estradiol to a cytosolic protein in rat pancreas. Possible role of oligopeptide coligands in secretions. J Biol Chem 1983;258:7284–7287.
23. Grossman A, Boctor AM, Band P, Lane B. Role of steroids in secreting-modulating effect of triamcinolone and estradiol on protein synthesis and secretion from the rat exocrine pancreas. J Steroid Biochem 1983;19:1069–1081.
24. Tiscornia OM, Cresta MA, de Lehman ES, Behlardi G, Dreiling DA. Estrogen effects on exocrine pancreatic secretion in menopausal women: a hypothesis for menopause-induced chronic pancreatitis. Mount Sinai J Med 1986;53:356–360.
25. Tiscornia OM, Cresta MA, de Lehman ES, Celener D, Dreiling DA. Effects of sex and age on pancreatic secretion. Int J Pancreatol 1986;1:95–118.
26. Lhoste EF, Roebuch BD, Stern JE, Longnecker DS. Effect of orchidectomy and testosterone on the early stages of azaserine-induced pancreatic carcinogenesis in the rat. Pancreas 1987;2:38–43.
27. Guo YS, Singh P. Effects of estradiol on pancreatic amylase and cholecystokinin binding in ovariectomized guinea pigs. J Steroid Biochem 1989;33:459–464.
28. Beaudoin AR, Grodin G, St-Jean P, Vachereau A, Cabana C, Grossman A. Steroids and the secretory function of the exocrine pancreas. Endocrinology 1986;119:1195–2106.
29. Morisset J, Jolicoeur L. Effect of hydrocortison on pancreatic growth in rats. Am J Physiol 1980;239:G95–98.
30. Werlin SL, Stefanick J. Effects of hydrocortison and cholecystokinin-octapeptide on neonatal rat pancreas. J Pediatr Gastroenterol 1982;1:591–595.
31. Leung YK, Jirapinyo P, Lebenthal E, Lee PC. Effect of hydrocortisone on the maturation of cholecystokinin (CCK) binding and CCK stimulated amylase release in pancreatic acini of neonatal rats. Pancreas 1987;2:73–78.
32. Rall L, Pictel R, Githens S, Rutter WJ. Glucocorticoids modulate the in vitro development of the embryonic rat pancreas. J Cell Biol 1977;75:398–409.
33. Greenberger NJ, Hatch FT, Drummey GD, Isselbacher KJ. Pancreatitis in hyperlipedemia. A study of serum lipid alterations in 25 patients with acute pancreatitis. Medicine (Baltimore) 1966;45:161–174.
34. Glueck CJ, Scheel D, Fishback J, Steiner P. Estrogen-induced pancreatitis in patients with previously covert familial type V hyperlipo-proteinemia. Metabolism 1972;21:657–666.
35. Davidoff F, Tischler S, Rosoff C. Marked hyperlipedemia and pancreatitis associated with oral contraceptive therapy. N Engl J Med 1973;289:552–555.
36. Saydjari R, Singh P, Affini B, Townsend DM, Thompson JC. The isolation and characterization of estrogen binding proteins in the pancreas of male and female hamsters. J Steroid Biochem 1988;29:41–45.
37. Jensen EV, Jacobson HI. Basic guides to the mechanism of estrogen action. Recent Prog Horm Res 1962;18:387–414.
38. Parker MG. Structure and functions of estrogen receptors. Vitam Horm Adv Res Appl 1996;51:267–287.
39. Rochefort H, Capony F, Augereau P, et al. The estrogen-regulated 52K-cathepsin-D in breast cancer: from biology to clinical applications. Int J Rad Appl Instrum (B) 1987;14:377–384.
40. Lemoine NR, Hall PA. Models of pancreatic cancer. In: Lemoine NR, Wright NA, eds. The molecular pathology of cancer. New York: Cold Spring Harbor Laboratory Press, 1993:135–155.
41. Sap J, Munoz A, Damm K, Goldberg Y, Ghysdael J, et al. The c-erb-A protein is a high-affinity receptor for thyroid hormone. Nature 1986;324:635–640.
42. Markaverich BM, Roberts RR, Alejandro MA, Clark JH. An endogenous inhibitor of $^3$H-estradiol binding to nuclear type II estrogen binding sites in normal and malignant tissues. Cancer Res 1984;44:1575–1579.
43. Markaverich BM, Roberts RR, Alejandro MA, Clark JH. The effect of low dose continuous exposure to estradiol on the estrogen receptor (type I) and nuclear type II sites. Endocrinology 1984;114:814–820.
44. Grossman A, Boctor AM, Lane B. Dependence of pancreatic integrity on adrenal and ovarian secretions. Endocrinology 1969;85:956–959.
45. Fernández-del Castillo C, Díaz-Sánchez V, et al. Testosterone biotransformation by the isolated perfused canine pancreas. Pancreas 1991;6:104–111.
46. Singh P, Owlia A, Townsend CM, Thompson JC. Estradiol and progesterone receptors in the stomach and pancreas of dogs. Can J Physiol Pharmacol 1986;64:469–473.
47. Rosenthal HE, Sandberg AA. Estrogen binding proteins in rat pancreas. J Steroid Biochem 1978;9:1133–1139.
48. Sing P, Townsend CM, Thompson JC. Presence of estradiol binding proteins in gastrointestinal tissues of male rats. Endocrinol 1986;119:1648–1653.
49. Pousette Å, Carlström K, Sköldefors H, Wilking N, Theve NO. Purification and partial characterization of a 17-ß-estradiol-binding macromolecule in the human pancreas. Cancer Res 1982;42:633–637.
50. Pousette Å, Fernstad R, Theve NO, Sköldefors H, Carlström K. Further characterization of the estrogen binding macromolecule in human pancreas. J Steroid Biochem 1985;23:115–119.
51. Logsdon CD, Williams JA. Pancreatic acini in short-term culture

regulation by EGF, carbachol, insulin, and corticosterone. Am J Physiol 1983;244:G675–682.
52. Logsdon CD, Mössner J, Williams JA, Goldfine ID. Glucocorticoids increase amylase mRNA levels, secretory organelles, and secretion in pancreatic AR42J cells. J Cell Biol 1985;100:1200–1208.
53. Gullo L, Priori P, Labo G. Influence of adrenal cortex on exocrine pancreatic function. Gastroenterology 1982;83:92–96.
54. Singh P, Guo YS, DeBouno JF, Owlia A. Effect of estradiol on amylase release from pancreatic acini of ovariectomized guinea pigs. Endocrinology 1987;120:192–194.
55. Greenway B, Iqbal MJ, Johansson PJ, Williams R. Oestrogen receptor protein in malignant and fetal pancreas. Br Med J 1981;283:751–755.
56. Andrén-Sandberg Å, Borg Å, Dawiskiba S, Ihse I, Fernö M. Estrogen receptors and estrogen binding protein in pancreatic cancer (Abstract). Digestion 1982;25:12.
57. Petersen A, Lea A, Bakkewold K, Arnesjö B. Progress in pancreatic oestrogen receptors. Eur J Surg Oncol 1986;12:321–324.
58. Corbishley TP, Iqbal MJ, Johnson PJ, Williams R. Progesterone receptors in malignant and foetal pancreatic tissue. IRCS Med Sci 1984;12:575–583.
59. McGuire WL. Hormone receptor: their role in predicting prognosis and response to endocrine therapy. Semin Oncol 1978;5:428–451.
60. Taragona EM, Pons MD, Gonzales G, Boix L, Marco V, Marco C. Is exocrine pancreatic cancer a hormone-dependent tumor? A study of the existence of sex hormone receptors in normal and neoplastic pancreas. Hepatogastroenterology 1991;38:165–169.
61. Taylor OM, Teasdeale J, Cowen PN, McMahon MJ, Benson EA. Oestrogen receptors in exocrine pancreatic carcinoma. Digestion 1988;42:118–125.
62. Taylor OM, Harrisson J, Cowen PN, McMahon MJ, Benson EA. Are there oestrogen receptors in pancreatic carcinoma? Br J Surg 1989;76:638–640.
63. Seitz G, Pollow K, Hinkeldey K, Schouder G, Wernet N. Immunohistochemical estrogen demonstration in pancreas, pancreatic carcinomas and other gastrointestinal carcinomas. Verh Dtsch Ges Pathol 1987;71:140–143.
64. Clark JH, Hardin JW, Uchurch S, Eriksson H. Heterogeneity of estrogen binding sites in the cytosol of the rat uterus. J Biol Chem 1978;253:7630–7634.
65. Panko WB, Watson CS, Clark JH. The presence of a second, specific estrogen binding site in human breast cancer. J Steroid Biochem 1981;14:1311–1316.
66. Björk P, Jönsson U, Andrén-Sandberg Å. Binding sites for the cytotoxic metabolites of estramustine phosphate (Estracyt) in rat and human pancreas that are distinct from pancreatic estrogen binding protein. Pancreas 1990;6:77–89.
67. Björk P, Andrén-Sandberg Å. Distribution of estramustine-binding protein (EMBP) in pancreas from male and female rats and the effect of hormonal withdrawal on its expression. In: Björk P. Expression of estramustine-binding protein (EMBP) in normal and neoplastic tissues. Biochemical characterization and study of hormonal influence on its expression (Dissertation). Lund, Sweden: Department of Oncology, Lund University, 1991.
68. Lacaine F, Houry S, Clough K, Lointier P, Huguier M. Is pancreatic tumor growth inhibited by sex steroid hormones? An experimental study in hamster. Dig Dis Sci 1986;31:S68–70.
69. Sumi C, Longnecker DS, Roebuck BD, Brinck-Johnsen T. Inhibitory effects of estrogen and castration on the early stage of pancreatic carcinogenesis in Fischer rats treated with azaserine. Cancer Res 1989;49:2332–2336.
70. Iqbal MJ, Greenway BA, Wilkinson ML, Johnson PJ, Wiliams R. Sex-steroid enzymes aromatase and 5-$\alpha$-reductase in the pancreas: a comparison of normal adult, foetal and malignant tissue. Clin Sci 1983;65:71–75.
71. Benz C, Hollander C, Miller B. Endocrine-responsive pancreatic carcinoma: steroid binding and cytotoxicity studies in human tumor cell lines. Cancer Res 1986;46:2276–2281.
72. Benz C, Lehmn C, Lee S. Steroid sensitivity and modulation of 5-fluorouracil toxicity in a human pancreatic carcinoma (Abstract). 8th annual meeting of the European Society for Medical Oncology, Nice, December 10–13, 1982. Berlin: Springer-Verlag, 1983:3.
73. Lipton A, Harvey HA, Santen RJ, et al. FAM chemotherapy +/- aminoglutethimide in the treatment of pancreatic carcinoma. Eur J Surg Oncol 1990;16:12–14.
74. Pousette Å. Demonstration of an androgen receptor in rat pancreas. Biochem J 1976;157:229–232.
75. Corbishley TP, Iqbal MJ, Wilkinson ML, Williams R. Androgen receptor in human normal and malignant pancreatic tissue and cell lines. Cancer 1986;57:1992–1995.
76. Díaz-Sánchez V, Morimoto S, Morales A, Robles-Díaz G, Cerbón M. Androgen receptor in the rat pancreas: genetic expression and steroid regulation. Pancreas 1995;11:241–245.
77. Hayashi Y, Katayama H. Promoting effect of testosterone propionate on experimental exocrine pancreatic tumors by 4-hydroxyaminoquinoline-1-oxide in rats. Toxicol Lett 1981;9:349–354.
78. Meijers M, Visser CJT, Klijn JG, et al. Effects of orchidectomy, alone or in combination with testosterone, and cyproterone acetate on exocrine pancreatic carcinogenesis in rats and hamsters. Int J Pancreatol 1992;11:137–146.
79. Greenway B, Duke D, Pym B, Iqbal MJ, Johnson PJ, Williams R. The control of human pancreatic adenocarcinoma xenografts in nude mice by hormone therapy. Br J Surg 1982;69:595–597.
80. Sperti C, Bonadimani B, Cuolo P, et al. Androgen profile in patients with pancreatic carcinoma. Ital J Gastroenterol 1992;24:328–331.
81. Greenway B, Iqbal MJ, Johnson PJ, Williams R. Serum sex-steroid concentration in patients with pancreatic carcinoma. Br J Surg 1982;69:293–296.
82. Greenway B, Iqbal MJ, Johnson PJ, Williams R. Low serum testosterone concentrations in patients with carcinoma of the pancreas. Br Med J 1983;286:93–95.
83. Militello C, Sperti C, Foresta C. Plasma levels of testosterone and hypophyseal gonadotropins in men affected by pancreatic cancer (Abstract). Digestion 1984;30:122.
84. Shearer MG, Taggart D, Gray C, Imrie CW. Useful differentiation between pancreatic carcinoma and chronic pancreatitis by testosterone assay (Abstract). Digestion 1984;30:106.
85. Pasquali C, Marra S, Scandellari C, Pedrazzoli P. Testosterone and hypophyseal gonadotropin plasma levels in men affected by pancreatic cancer (Abstract). Ital J Gastroenterol 1985;17:56.
86. Robles-Díaz G, Díaz V, Ornelas R, Mendez JP, Wolpert E. Testosterone:dihydrotestosterone ratio, a new tumor marker in pancreatic cancer. Dig Dis Sci 1986;31:S68–70.
87. Fernández-del-Castillo C, Robles-Díaz G, Díaz-Sánchez V, Altamirano A. Pancreatic cancer and androgen metabolism: high androstenedione and low testosterone serum levels. Pancreas 1990;5:515–518.
88. Todd BD. Pancreatic carcinoma and low serum testosterone: a correlation secondary to cancer cachexia? Eur J Surg Oncol 1988;14:199–202.
89. McColl KE. Low serum testosterone concentrations in carcinoma of the pancreas. Br Med J (Clin Res Ed) 1983;286:641–642.
90. Wilking N, Appelgren LE, Carlström K, Pousette Å, Theve NO. The distribution and metabolism of $^{14}C$-labeled tamoxifen in spayed female mice. Acta Pharmacol Toxicol 1982;50:161–168.
91. Poston GJ, Townsend CM, Rajaraman S, Thompson JC, Singh P. Effect of somatostatin and tamoxifen on the growth of human pancreatic cancers in nude mice. Pancreas 1990;5:151–157.
92. Rosenberg L, Barkun AN, Denis MH, Pollak M. Low dose octreotide and tamoxifen in the treatment of adenocarcinoma of the pancreas. Cancer 1995;75:23–28.
93. Theve NO, Pousette Å, Carlström K. Adenocarcinoma of the pancreas—a hormone sensitive tumor? A preliminary report on Nolvadex treatment. Clin Oncol 1983;9:193–197.
94. Tönnesen K, Kamp-Jensen M. Antiestrogen therapy in pancreatic carcinoma: a preliminary report. Eur J Surg Oncol 1986;12:69–70.
95. Crowson MC, Dorrell A, Rolfe EB, Fieldling JW. A phase II study to evaluate tamoxifen in pancreatic adenocarcinoma. Eur J Surg Oncol 1986;12:335–336.
96. Wong A, Chan A, Arthur K. Tamoxifen therapy in unresectable

adenocarcinoma of the pancreas. Cancer Treat Rep 1987;71: 749–750.
97. Keating JJ, Johnson PJ, Cochran AMG. A prospective randomized controlled trial of tamoxifen and cyproterone acetate in pancreatic carcinoma. Br J Cancer 1989;60:789–792.
98. Bakkevold KE, Pettersen A, Arnesjö B, Espehaug B. Tamoxifen therapy in unresectable adenocarcinoma of the pancreas and the papilla of Vater. Br J Surg 1990;77:725–730.
99. Rothman SS, Wells H. Enhancement of pancreatic enzyme secretion by pancreozymin. Am J Physiol 1967;213:215–218.
100. Ihse I, Arnesjö B, Lundquist I. Effects on exocrine and endocrine rat pancreas of long-term administration of CCK-PZ (cholecystokinin-pankreazymin) on synthetic octa-peptide-CCK-PZ. Scand J Gastroenterol 1976;11:529–535.
101. Solomon TE. Regulation of exocrine pancreatic cell proliferation and enzyme synthesis. In: Johnson LR, ed. Physiology of the gastrointestinal tract: New York: Raven, 1981:873–892.
102. Fölsch UR. Regulation of pancreatic growth. Clin Gastroenterol 1984;13:679–699.
103. Johnson LR. Trophic effects of gut peptides. In: Makhlouf GM, ed. Handbook of physiology. Section 6: The gastrointestinal system. Vol II: Neural and endocrine biology. Bethesda: American Physiological Society, 1989:291–310.
104. Pfeiffer CJ, Chernenko GA, Kohli Y, Barrowman JA. Trophic effects of cholecystokinin octopeptide on the pancreas of the Syrian hamster. Can J Physiol Pharmacol 1982;60:358–362.
105. Satake K, Mukai R, Kato Y, Umeyama K. Effects of cerulein on the normal pancreas and on experimental pancreatic carcinoma in the Syrian golden hamster. Pancreas 1986;1:246–253.
106. Niderau C, Liddle RA, Williams JA, Grendell JH. Pancreatic growth: interaction of exogenous cholecystokinin, a protease inhibitor, and a cholecystokinin receptor antagonist in mice. Gut 1987;28(suppl 1):63–69.
107. Gasslander T, Smeds S, Blomqvist L, Ihse I. Proliferative response of different exocrine pancreatic cell types to hormonal stimuli. I. Effects of long-term cerulein administration. Scand J Gastroenterol 1990;25:1103–1110.
108. Monstein HJ, Nylander AG, Salehi A, Chen D, Lundquist I, Håkansson R. Cholecystokinin-A and cholecystokinin-B/gastrin receptor mRNA expression in the gastrointestinal tract and pancreas of the rat and man. A polymerase chain reaction study. Scand J Gastroenterol 1996;31:383–390.
109. Povoski SP, Zhou W, Longnecker DS, Roebuck BD, Bell RH. Stimulation of growth of azaserine-induced putative preneoplastic lesions in rat pancreas is mediated specifically by way of cholecystokinin-A receptors. Cancer Res 1993;53:3925–3929.
110. Watanapa P, Flaks B, Oztas H, Deprez PH, Calam J, Williamsson RCN. Inhibitory effect of a cholecystokinin antagonist on pancreatic carcinogenesis after pancreatobiliary diversion. Br J Cancer 1993;67:663–667.
111. Dawra R, Saluja A, Lerch MM, Saluja M, Logdson C, Steer M. Stimulation of pancreatic growth by cholecystokinin is mediated by high affinity receptors on rat pancreatic acinar cells. Biochem Biophys Res Commun 1993;193:814–820.
112. Axelson J, Håkansson R, Ihse I, Lilja I, Rehfeld JF, Sundler F. Effects of endogenous and exogenous cholecystokinin and infusion with the cholecystokinin antagonist L-364,718 on pancreatic and gastrointestinal growth. Scand J Gastroenterol 1990;25: 471–480.
113. Bell RH, Kuhlmann ET, Jensen RT, Longnecker DS. Overexpression of cholecystokinin receptors in azaserine-induced neoplasms of the rat pancreas. Cancer Res 1992;52:3295–3299.
114. Zhou WG, Povoski SP, Longnecker DS, Bell RH. Novel expression of gastrin (cholecystokinin-B) receptors in azaserine-induced rat pancreatic carcinoma—receptor determination and characterization. Cancer Res 1992;52:6905–6911.
115. Povoski SP, Zhou WG, Longnecker DS, Roebuck BD, Bell RH. Stimulation of growth of azaserine-induced putative preneoplastic lesions in rat pancreas is mediated specifically by way of cholecystokinin-A receptors. Cancer Res 1993;53:3925–3929.
116. Logsdon CD. Glucocorticoids increase cholecystokinin receptors and amylase secretion in pancreatic acinar AR42J cells. J Biol Chem 1986;261:2096–2101.
117. Zhou WG, Povoski SP, Bell RH. Overexpression of messenger RNA for cholecystokinin-A receptor and novel expression of messenger RNA for gastrin (cholecystokinin-B) receptor in azaserine-induced rat pancreatic carcinoma. Carcinogenesis 1993;14: 2189–2192.
118. Smith JP, Kramer S, Solomon TE. CCK stimulates growth of six human pancreatic cancer cell lines in serum free medium. Regul Pept 1991;32:341–349.
119. Zhou WG, Povoski SP, Tsuei BJ, Bell RH. Gene expression of the cholecystokinin-A receptor and the cholecystokinin-B (gastrin) receptor in human pancreatic carcinomas. Gastroenterology 1994;106:A331–333.
120. Povoski SP, Zhou WG, Longnecker DS, Bell RH. Novel expression of gastrin (CCK-B) receptors in pancreatic carcinomas and dysplastic pancreas from transgenic mice. Am J Surg 1994;167: 120–127.
121. Singh P, Townsend CM, Upp J, Lridjani A, Thompson JC. Characterization of cholecystokinin receptors (CCK-R) in normal and cancerous human pancreas. Fed Proc 1986;45: 291–292.
122. Upp JR, Singh P, Townsend CM, Thompson JC. Predicting response to endocrine therapy in human pancreatic cancer with cholecystokinin receptors. Gastroenterology 1987;46:1677–1679.
123. Shivaram S, Crist KA, Chadhuri B, Mucci SJ, Chadhuri PK. Effect of CCK receptor antagonist on growth of pancreatic adenocarcinoma. J Surg Res 1992;53:234–237.
124. Singh P, Townsend CM, Poston GJ, Reubin JC. Specific binding of cholecystokinin, estradiol and somatostatin to human pancreatic cancer xenografts, J Steroid Biochem Mol Biol 1991;39: 759–767.
125. Smith JP, Liu GZ, Soundararajan V, Mclaughlin PJ, Zagon IS. Identification and characterization of CCK-B/gastrin receptors in human pancreatic cell lines. Am J Physiol 1994;266:R277–283.
126. Scemama JL, Fourmy D, Zahidi A, Pradayrol L, Susini C, Ribet A. Characterization of gastrin receptors on a rat pancreatic acinar cell line (AR42J). A possible model for studying gastrin mediated cell growth and proliferation. Gut 1987;28(S1):233–236.
127. Seva C, DeVries L, Scemama JL, et al. Gastrin modulates growth of a rat acinar pancreatic cell line: receptor analysis and signal transduction. Digestion 1990;46(suppl 2):166–169.
128. Povoski SP, Zhou WG, Longnecker DS, Bell RH. Temporal expression of the gastrin (CCK-B) receptor during azaserine-induced pancreatic carcinogenesis. Pancreas 1993;8:615–621.
129. de Weerth A, von Schrenck T, Mirau S, Raedler A, Greten H, Kalthoff H. Human pancreatic cancer cell lines express the CCK-B/gastrin receptor. Gastroenterology 1994;106;A289–291.
130. Adrian TE, Permert J, Wang Q, et al. Is CCK involved in pancreatic ductal cell cancer? 10th international symposium on gastrointestinal hormones. Santa Barbara, California, 1994.
131. Ihse I, Lilja P, Lundquist I. Trypsin as a regulator of pancreatic secretion in the rat. Scand J Gastroenterol 1979;13:873–880.
132. Liddle RA, Goldfine ID, Williams JA. Bioassay of plasma cholecystokinin in rats: effects of food, trypsin inhibitor, and alcohol. Gastroenterology 1984;87:542–549.
133. Herrington MK, Permert J, Kazakoff KR, et al. Effects of raw soya diet and cholecystokinin receptor blockade on pancreatic growth and tumor initiation in the hamster. Cancer Lett 1994; 82:7–16.
134. Wisner JR, McLaughlin RE, Rich KA, Ozawa S, Renner IG. Effects of L-364,718, a new cholecystokinin receptor antagonist, on camostate-induced growth of the rat pancreas. Gastroenterology 1988;94:109–113.
135. Miazza BM, Turberg Y, Guillaume P, Hahne W, Chayvialle JA, Loizeau E. Mechanism of pancreatic growth induced by pancreatico-biliary diversion in the rat. Scand J Gastroenterol 1985;20(suppl 112):75–83.
136. Dowling RH, Hosomi M, Stace NH, et al. Hormones and polyamines in intestinal and pancreatic adaptation. Scand J Gastroenterol 1985;20(suppl 112):84–95.
137. Gasslander T, Chu M, Smeds S, Ihse I. Proliferative response of different exocrine pancreatic cells after surgical pancreatico-biliary diversion in the rat. Scand J Gastroenterol 1991;26: 399–404.
138. Chu M, Borch K, Lilja I, Blomqvist L, Rehfeld JF, Ihse I. Endogenous hypercholecystokininemia model in the hamster: trophic effect on the exocrine pancreas. Pancreas 1992;7:220–225.

139. Gasslander T, Axelson J, Håkanson R, Ihse I, Lilja I, Rehfeld JF. Cholecystokinin is responsible for growth of the pancreas after pancreaticobiliary diversion in rats. Scand J Gastroenterol 1990;25:1060–1065.
140. Howatson AG, Carter DC. Pancreatic carcinogenesis—enhancement by cholecystokinin in the hamster-nitrosamine model. Br J Cancer 1985;51:107–114.
141. Appel MJ, Meijers M, van Garderen-Hoetmer A, et al. Role of cholecystokinin in dietary fat-promoted azaserine-induced pancreatic carcinogenesis in rats. Br J Cancer 1992;66:46–50.
142. Lhoste EF, Roebuck BD, Longnecker DS. Stimulation of the growth of azaserine-induced nodules in the rat pancreas by dietary camostate (FOY 305). Carcinogenesis 1988;9:901–909.
143. McGuinness EE, Morgan RGH, Levison DA, Frape DL, Hopewood D, Wormsley KG. The effects of long-term feeding of soya flour on the rat pancreas. Scand J Gastroenterol 1980;15: 497–502.
144. Roebuck BD, Baumgartner KJ, Thron CD. Characterization of two populations of pancreatic AACF induced by azaserine in the rat. Lab Invest 1987;50:141–146.
145. Miazza BM, Widgren S, Chayvialle JA, Nicolet T, Loizeau E. Exocrine pancreatic nodules after long-term pancreaticobiliary diversion in rats. An effect of raised CCK plasma concentrations. Gut 1987;28(S1):269–273.
146. Stewart ID, Flaks B, Watanapa P, Davies PW, Williamsson RCN. Pancreaticobiliary diversion enhance experimental pancreatic carcinogenesis. Br J Cancer 1991;63:63–66.
147. Watanapa P, Flaks B, Oztas H, Deprez PH, Calam J, Williamsson RCN. Enhancing effect of partial gastrectomy on pancreatic carcinogenesis. Br J Cancer 1992;65:383–387.
148. Douglas BR, Woutersen RA, Jansen JBMJ, Rovati LC. Influence of cholecystokinin antagonist on the effects of cholecystokinin and bombesin on azaserine-induced lesions in rat pancreas. Gastroenterology 1989;96:462–469.
149. Lhoste EF, Longnecker DS. Effect of bombesin and caerulein on early stages of carcinogenesis induced by azaserine in the rat pancreas. Cancer Res 1987;47:3273–3277.
150. Douglas BR, Woutersen RA, Jansen JBMJ, Rovati LC. Influence of cholecystokinin antagonist on the effects of cholecystokinin and bombesin on azaserine-induced lesions in rat pancreas. Gastroenterology 1989;96:462–469.
151. Douglas BR, Johnson LR. Effects of gastrointestinal hormones on pancreatic growth. Cancer 1981;47:1640–1645.
152. Smith JP, Solomon TE, Bagheri S, Kramer S. Cholecystokinin stimulates growth of human pancreatic adenocarcinoma SW-1990. Dig Dis Sci 1990;35:1377–1384.
153. Smith JP, Kramer ST, Solomon TE. CCK stimulates growth of six human pancreatic cancer cell lines in serum-free medium. Regul Pept 1991;32:341–349.
154. Townsend CD, Franklin RB, Wilson LC, Glass EJ, Thompson JC. Stimulation of pancreatic cancer growth by caerulein and secretin. Surg Forum 1981;32:228–229.
155. Smith JP, Kramer S, Bagheri S. Effect of a high-fat diet and L 364,718 on growth of human pancreatic cancer. Dig Dis Sci 1990;35:726–732.
156. Johnson FE, LaRegina MC, Martin SA, Bashiti HM. Cholecystokinin inhibits pancreatic and hepatic carcinogenesis. Cancer Detect Prev 1983;6:389–402.
157. Pour PM, Lawson T, Helgeson S, Donelly T, Stepan K. Effect of cholecystokinin on pancreatic carcinogenesis in the hamster model. Carcinogenesis 1988;9:597–601.
158. Karsenty L, Hajri A, Aprahamian M, Garaud JC, Doffoél M, Damgé C. Inhibition of growth of a transplanted rat pancreatic acinar carcinoma with CCK-8. Pancreas 1993;8:204–211.
159. Andrén-Sandberg Å, Dawiskiba S, Ihse I. Studies on the effect of cerulein administration on experimental pancreatic carcinogenesis. Scand J Gastroenterol 1984;19:122–128.
160. Visser CJ, Woutersen RA, Bruggink AH, et al. Transforming growth factor-alpha and epidermal growth factor expression in the exocrine pancreas of azaserine-treated rats: modulation by cholecystokinin or a low fat, high fiber (caloric restricted) diet. Carcinogenesis 1995;16:2075–2082.
161. Pour PM, Runge RG, Birt D, et al. Current knowledge of pancreatic carcinogenesis in the hamster and its relevance to the human disease. Cancer 1981;47:1573–1587.
162. Meijers M, Roverts WG, Lamers CBHW, Jansen JBMJ, Rovati LC, Woutersen RA. Modulation of development of (pre)neoplastic lesions in hamster pancreas by cholecystokinin, bombesin and camostate: effect of the cholecystokinin receptor antagonist CR-1409. Digestion 1989;43:162.
163. Meijers M, van Garderen-Hoetmer A, Lamers CRHW, Rovati LC, Jansen JBMJ, Woutersen RA. Role of cholecystokinin in the development of BOP-induced pancreatic lesions in hamsters. Carcinogenesis 1990;11:2223–2226.
164. Pour PM, Lawson T, Helgeson S, Donnely T, Stepan K. Effect of cholecystokinin on pancreatic carcinogenesis in the hamster model. Carcinogenesis 1988;9:597–601.
165. Johnson FE, LaRegina MC, Martin SA, Bashiti HM. Cholecystokinin inhibits pancreatic and hepatic carcinogenesis. Cancer Detect Prev 1983;6:389–402.
166. Liener IE, Hasdai´A. The effect of long-term feeding of raw soyflour on the pancreas of the mouse and hamster. Adv Exp Med Biol 1986;199:189–197.
167. Meijers M, van Garderen-Hoetmer A, Lamers CRHW, Rovati LC, Jansen JBMJ, Woutersen RA. Effects of the synthetic trypsin inhibitor camostate on the development of *N*-nitrosobis(2-oxopropyl)amine-induced pancreatic lesions in hamsters. Cancer Lett 1991;60:205–211.
168. Takahashi M, Imaida K, Furukawa F, Hayshi Y. Inhibitory effect of soybean trypsin inhibitor during initiation and promotion phases of *N*-nitrobis(2-oxopropyl)amine-induced hamster pancreatic carcinogenesis. Prog Clin Biol Res 1991;369:145–154.
169. Herrington MK, Permert J, Kazakoff KR, et al. Effects of high fat diet and cholecystokinin receptor blockade on pancreatic growth and tumor initiation in the hamster. Carcinogenesis 1993;14:1021–1026.
170. Meijers M, Appel MJ, van Garderen-Hoetmer A, et al. Effects of cholecystokinin and bombesin on development of azaserine-induced pancreatic tumours in rats: modulation by the the cholecystokinin receptor antagonist lorglumide. Carcinogenesis 1992;13:1525–1528.
171. Sperti C, Militello C, Rovati L, et al. Effect of cholecystokinin analogue caerulein and cholecystokinin antagonist lorglumide on pancreatic carcinogenesis in the rat. J Surg Oncol 1994;57: 11–16.
172. Watanapa P, Flaks B, Oztas H, Deprez PH, Calam J, Williamson RC. Inhibitory effect of a cholecystokinin antagonist on pancreatic carcinogenesis after pancreatobiliary diversion. Br J Cancer 1993;67:663–667.
173. Nio Y, Tsubono M, Morimoto H, et al. Loxiglumide (CR1505), a cholecystokinin antagonist, specifically inhibits the growth of human pancreatic cancer lines xenografted into nude mice. Cancer 1993;72:3599–3606.
174. Morimoto H, Nio Y, Tsubono M, et al. Inhibitory effect of a cholecystokinin antagonist, loxiglumide (CR-1505), on the growth of freshly separated and xenografted human pancreatic cancer. J Surg Oncol 1993;53:47–53.
175. Shivaram S, Crist KA, Chaudhuri B, Mucci SJ, Chaudhuri PK. Effect of CCK receptor antagonist on growth of pancreatic adenocarcinoma. J Surg Res 1992;53:234–237.
176. Abbruzzese JL, Gholson CF, Daugherty K, et al. A pilot clinical trial of the cholecystokinin receptor antagonist MK-329 in patients with advanced pancreatic cancer. Pancreas 1992;7: 165–171.
177. Ohlsson B, Axelson J, Sternby B, Rehfeld JF, Ihse I. Time-course of pancreatic changes following stimulation or inhibition of the CCK-A receptor. Int J Pancreatol 1995;18:59–66.
178. Herrington MK, Adrian TE. On the role of cholecystokinin in pancreatic cancer. Int J Pancreatol 1995;17:121–138.
179. Håkansson R, Blom H, Carlson E, Larsson H, Ryberg B, Sundler F. Hypergastrinemia produces trophic effects in stomach but not in pancreas and intestines. Regul Pept 1986;13:225–233.
180. Balas D, Senegas-Balas F, Pradayrol L, Vayssette J, Bertrand C, Ribet A. Long-term comparative effect of cholecystokinin and gastrin on mouse stomach, antrum, intestine, and exocrine pancreas. Am J Anat 1985;174:27–43.
181. Mayston PD, Barrowman JA. Influence of chronic administration of pentagastrin on the pancreas in hypophysectomized rats. Gastroenterology 1973;64:391–399.
182. Petersen H, Solomon T, Grossman M. Effect of chronic penta-

gastrin, cholecystokinin, and secretin on pancreas of rats. Am J Physiol 1978;234:E286–293.
183. Majumdar APN, Goltermann N. Chronic administration of pentagastrin. Digestion 1979;19:144–147.
184. Dembinski AB, Johnson LR. Stimulation of pancreatic growth by secretin, caerulein, and pentagastrin. Endocrinology 1980;106:323–328.
185. Solomon TE, Morisset J, Wood JG, Bussjaeger LJ. Additive interaction of pentagastrin and secretin on pancreatic growth in rats. Gastroenterology 1987;92:429–435.
186. Valenzuela JE, Walsh JH, Isenberg JI. Effect of gastrin on pancreatic enzyme secretion and gallbladder emptying in man. Gastroenterology 1976;71:409–411.
187. Mayston PD, Barrowman JA. Influence of chronic administration of pentagastrin on the rat pancreas. Q J Exp Physiol 1971;56:113–122.
188. Håkansson R, Axelson J, Ekman R, Sundler F. Hypergastrinemia evoked by omeprazole stimulates growth of gastric mucosa but not pancreas or intestines in hamster, guinea pig and chicken. Regul Pept 1988;23:105–115.
189. Oscarson J, Håkansson R, Liedberg G, Lundqvist G, Sundler F, Thorell J. Variated serum gastrin concentration: trophic effects on the gastrointestinal tract of the rat. Acta Physiol Scand 1979;suppl 475:3–27.
190. Niderau C, Niderau M, Klonowski H, Luthen R, Ferrell LD. Effect of hypergastrinemia and blockade of gastrin-receptors on pancreatic growth in the mouse. Hepatogastroenterology 1995;42:423–431.
191. Ryberg B, Axelson R, Håkanson R, Sundler F, Mattsson H. Trophic effects of continuous infusion of (Leu$^{15}$)-gastrin-17 in the rat. Gastroenterology 1990;98:33–38.
192. Reber HA, Johnson F, Deveney K, Montgomery C, Way LW. Trophic effects of gastrin on the exocrine pancreas in rats. J Surg Res 1977;22:554–560.
193. Dembinski AB, Johnson LR. Growth of pancreas and gastrointestinal mucosa in antrectomized and gastrin-treated rats. Endocrinology 1979;105:769–773.
194. Chu M, Rehfeld JF, Borch K. Effects of gastric fundectomy and antrectomy on the exocrine pancreas in the hamster. Int J Pancreatol 1992;12:139–144.
195. Chu M, Franzén L, Sullivan S, Wingren S, Rehfeld JF, Borch K. Pancreatic hypertrophy with acinar cell nodules after long-term fundectomy in the rat. Gut 1993;34:988–993.
196. Chu M, Franzén L, Sullivan S, Rehfeld JF, Ihse I, Borch K. Effects of pancreaticobiliary diversion and gastric fundectomy on azaserine-induced pancreatic carcinogenesis in the rat. Pancreas 1991;8:330–337.
197. Chen D, Nylander AG, Norlén P, Håkansson R. Gastrin does not stimulate growth of the rat pancreas. Scand J Gastroenterol 1996;31:404–410.
198. Konturek SJ, Dembinski A, Warzecha Z, et al. Antagonism of receptors for bombesin, gastrin and cholecystokinin in pancreatic secretion and growth. Digestion 1991;48:89–97.
199. Seva C, Scemama JL, Bastié MJ, Pradayrol L, Vaysse N. Lorglumide and loxiglumide inhibit gastrin-stimulated DNA synthesis in a rat tumoral acinar pancreatic cell line (A42J). Cancer Res 1990;50:5829–5833.
200. Smith JP, Fantaskey AP, Liu GZ, Zagon IS. Identification of gastrin as a growth peptide in human pancreatic cancer. Am J Physiol 1995;268:R135–141.
201. Watanapa P, Flaks B, Oztas H, Deprez PH, Calam J, Williamsson RCN. Duodenogastric reflux enhances growth and carcinogenesis in the rat pancreas. Br J Surg 1992;79:791–794.
202. Robertson JFR, Watson SA, Hardcastle JD. Effect of gastrointestinal hormones and synthetic analogues on the growth of pancreatic cancer. Int J Cancer 1995;63:69–75.

# 63

# *Palliative Biliary and Gastroenteric Bypasses*

Toshiyuki Mori and Yutaka Atomi

Modern imaging modalities have made it possible to diagnose pancreatic cancer in earlier stages and more accurately. Even with these sophisticated imaging modalities and advanced surgical techniques, only about 20% of patients have disease potentially curable by resection (1). Most, therefore, require some form of palliation. Patients with pancreatic cancer require surgical palliation for jaundice, duodenal obstruction, and pain. The goal of surgical palliation is to improve the quality of life of patients whose life expectancy does not exceed several months. Surgical palliation, thus, should meet several requirements. First, the surgical mortality and morbidity rates should be low, as a prolonged hospital stay would compromise the quality of life. Second, the palliation should relieve the symptom as long as possible, one hopes until the patient's death. Third, it should not be accompanied by tubes or bags that might require irrigation or replacement since these devices would be a nuisance to the patient and compromise the life quality (2, 3).

## JAUNDICE

Obstructive jaundice is present at the time of diagnosis in up to 90% of patients with carcinoma of the head of the pancreas (4). The primary cause of obstructive jaundice is stenosis or obstruction of the intrapancreatic portion of the common bile duct because of invasion or compression of the tumor (4, 5). It is less likely in patients with carcinoma of the body or tail of the pancreas because of the greater distance of the tumor from the common bile duct (6). As disease progresses, lymph node involvement in the porta hepatis may compress the common bile duct, resulting in obstructive jaundice (7). Another cause of jaundice is metastasis to the liver. Obstructive jaundice occurs in about 70% of patients with pancreatic cancer at some time during the course of the disease.

Biliary bypasses for the relief of obstructive jaundice should be performed in most patients when pancreatic cancer obstructs the bile ducts, for several reasons. First, relief of the obstruction leads to longer survival by diminishing the serious complications of coagulopathy and metabolic disturbances. Sarr and Cameron in their review reported that over 8000 patients who underwent a biliary bypass procedure had a mean survival of 5.44 months, compared with 3.5 months for those who underwent laparotomy alone (8). Although this study was retrospective and patients who underwent biliary bypass were generally better operative risks than those who did not and probably would have lived longer anyway, it is reasonable to believe that biliary bypass improves survival. Second, longstanding obstructive jaundice may result in progressive hepatic failure. Cholangitis may also occur in the presence of biliary obstruction. Although less frequent than when choledocholithiasis is the cause of the jaundice, cholangitis is seen in about 10% of patients, sometimes becoming life threatening. Third, pruritus occurs in at least one-quarter of these patients and may be a severe and intractable symptom. Moreover, psychologic benefit to the patient would be another aim of biliary bypass procedures, since the continued presence of obstructive jaundice may serve to remind the patient that the disease persists.

Although most clinicians believe that biliary bypass procedures effectively relieve jaundice, few objective data are available to prove it. Howard et al. noted that jaundice requires from 4 to 8 weeks for complete resolution, but the frequency with which jaundice cleared completely was not discussed (9). Buckwalter et al. observed that jaundice decreased in 77% of 128 patients who underwent biliary bypass. Only 45% of them experienced a measurable decrease in serum bilirubin (10). Pellegrini et al. found that only 67% of patients with malignant obstruction of the bile duct from a variety of causes (pancreatic cancer, bile duct and other periampullary cancers) had a return of the bilirubin concentration to normal when the obstruction was relieved (11). In patients with normal liver function and extrahepatic biliary obstruction, the bilirubin concentration in plasma fell an average of 8% of the preoperative value per day when the obstruction was relieved; however, in patients with extensive hepatic metastases, in those with high preoperative bilirubin concentrations (>15 mg/dL), and in those obstructed for longer than 1 month, the serum bilirubin concentration may never return to normal.

## CHOICE OF PROCEDURE

Several procedures have been used to bypass obstruction of the common bile duct by pancreatic tumors. Discussion about the merit of each is concerned mostly with the choices between the gallbladder and the common bile duct for the biliary anastomosis. The most common procedures are cholecystojejunostomy and choledochojejunostomy. Cholecysto- or choledochoduodenostomy, cholecystogastrostomy, and external drainage of the common bile duct by T tube or of the gallbladder by cholecytostomy tube have also been used.

### Cholecystojejunostomy and Choledochojejunostomy

Cholecystojejunostomy and choledochojejunostomy are equally effective in relieving malignant biliary obstruction. In a collected series of 2493 patients, cholecystoenteric bypasses ($n$ = 237) in comparison with choledochoenteric bypasses ($n$ = 1770) were associated with higher postoperative mortality (20 vs. 14%), lower long-term morbidity (26 vs. 35%), and a lower survival rate (means, 3.2 vs. 5.2 months) (9).

Much has been written about the relative merits of loop vs. Roux-en-Y cholecystojejunostomy and choledochojejunostomy. Although Roux-en-Y anastomoses are preferred in situations in which long-term survival is expected (e.g., biliary diversions for benign disease), they are unnecessary in malignant obstruction.

Anastomoses to a loop jejunum can be done more quickly, and since these patients rarely survive longer than 1 year, cholangitis is unusual. It is also unnecessary to perform a jejunojejunostomy to divert food from the gallbladder or the bile duct.

When performing a cholecystojejunostomy, one must make sure that the gallbladder is in continuity with the obstructed bile duct through a patent cystic duct (9). At operation, it is frequently possible to ascertain cystic duct patency by inspection, and the cystic duct can be seen to enter the common bile duct well away from the tumor. If there is any question about cystic duct patency, an operative cholangiography should be obtained. This can be done easily by inserting a needle into the unopened gallbladder, aspirating bile, and injecting contrast material. In about 10% of patients, the cystic duct runs for some distance along the side of the common bile duct and eventually joins it close to the duodenum. In that case, the tumor may encroach upon the cystic duct and obstruct it in a short time postoperatively. In the young, fit patient in whom a more lengthy survival is anticipated, a diverting enteroenterostomy is added to reduce the risk of intestinal obstruction caused by tumor extension encroaching and invading the biliary-junostomy area. Most surgeons prefer to perform a cholecystojejunostomy if the anatomic arrangement allows it, because it can be done quickly and easily. When the gallbladder is not present or is chronically inflamed and packed with stones, or if it is so close to the tumor that later obstruction is a concern, the common bile duct should be used for decompression. Either an end-to-end or side-to-side anastomosis of the common bile duct to the jejunum is satisfactory. The gallbladder probably should be removed when the common duct is used for the anastomosis.

The more complex Roux-en-Y jejunostomy, designed to minimize reflux of intestinal content into the biliary tree and to reduce cholangitis (12, 13), is time consuming and probably of little benefit to patients with an overall short survival.

### Cholecystoduodenostomy and Choledochoduodenostomy

Cholecystoduodenostomy and choledochoduodenostomy have been used less frequently than bypass procedures to the jejunum, but substantial experience has been accumulated. In a collection of published series, choledochoduodenostomy ($n$ = 1159) and choledochojejunostomy ($n$ = 611) had similar rates of postoperative mortality (14 vs. 13%), morbidity (26 vs. 27%), and incidence of recurrent jaundice (8 vs. 7%) and similar median survival times (5.4 vs. 5.0 months). The operative mortality rate for choledochoduodenostomy was higher than that for cholecystoduodenostomy (22 vs. 11.7%), but this difference may not be significant (14). Although Stuart et al. preferred a cholecystojejunostomy when the gallbladder could be used for biliary bypass, they favored the use of choledochoduodenostomy rather than choledochojejunostomy when it could not. They reported 48 patients with an operative mortality rate of 10% and no deaths directly related to the choledochoduodenal anastomosis. There were seven complications (14.6%) that were related to the anastomosis: six bile fistulas, and one episode of cholangitis. Of the 48 patients, 23% subsequently developed duodenal obstruction, and jaundice recurred in 10.4% as the tumor progressed (15). It is this latter problem that concerns many surgeons. The editors prefer to avoid the duodenum for biliary-enteric anastomoses in all patients with malignant periampullary disease. The proximity of the tumor to the anastomosis and its unpredictable tendency to invade and reobstruct the bile duct support such a view. Anastomoses to the jejunum can be performed safely and easily in most instances, and reobstruction is less likely.

Cholecystogastrostomy is not recommended for several reasons. It may cause bile gastritis. Reflux of food and gastric juice into the gallbladder may lead to inflammatory changes in it in the occasional patient who survives longer than usual. Hypersecretion of gastric acid may occur because the normal inhibition of antral gastrin release may be interfered with (9). Finally, it is easier to anastomose the thin-walled gallbladder to the small intestine than to the thick-walled stomach. Thus, although it provides effective decompression, cholecystogastrostomy is done infrequently because it may create other problems and there are usually simpler alternatives.

External drainage of the common duct or gallbladder via tube is not desirable because patients must spend the rest of their lives with a tube and biliary drainage bag in place. In the frail elderly patient, in whom laparotomy is to be avoided, however, percutaneous internal/external or endoprosthetic techniques are the procedures of choice (16). There is no clear leader with regard to any of these methods (17). The final choice often depends on the local expertise available. The mean survival of patients undergoing percutaneous (8 months) or endoprosthesis (6 months) biliary decompression is acceptable, particularly as the radiologist and endoscopist are often at the end of the line when dealing with very ill or very frail patients (18).

## DUODENAL OBSTRUCTION

Although nausea and vomiting are part of the initial symptom complex in half to one-third of patients with pancreatic cancer, duodenal obstruction by the tumor is responsible for these symptoms in only about 5%. Some would argue that routine gastroenterostomy is unnecessary, lengthening the operative procedure and giving increased mortality related to a second anastomosis. They restrict its use to patients with large tumors threatening early mechanical duodenal obstruction. Nevertheless, in a collected series of 900 patients who underwent biliary bypass only (i.e., no evidence existed of duodenal obstruction), 22.9% subsequently developed duodenal obstruction as early as 1 month later (9). In this series, the addition of gastrojejunostomy to biliary bypass did not increase the operative morbidity or mortality rate (17 vs. 18%). Richards and Sosin have shown that up to one-third of patients undergoing palliative biliary tract bypass alone will eventually require reoperation for duodenal obstruction, and of those who do not undergo gastroenterostomy, 10 to 20% will die with symptoms of duodenal obstruction (19). Many surgeons believe that a gastrojejunostomy should be performed prophylactically along with biliary bypass in all patients in whom survival is likely to exceed a few weeks. Because duodenal obstruction is found infrequently in the absence of biliary obstruction, it is unusual to have gastrojejunostomy performed as the only procedure. The diagnosis of duodenal obstruction usually can be made preoperatively by upper gastrointestinal roentgenogram and esophagogastroscopy. These studies may reveal duodenal compression or deformity. Frequently, evidence exists of duodenal or antral compression at operation as well.

An antecolic loop gastrojejunostomy should be placed distal to the cholecysto(docho)jejunostomy, because a retrocolic gastrojejunostomy may become obstructed by tumor in the base of the transverse mesocolon. Nevertheless, occasionally the anatomy requires that a retrocolic anastomosis be done. Concern about stomal ulceration and bleeding after gastrojejunostomy, leads a few surgeons to advocate truncal vagotomy to prevent this complication (20); but because it occurs rarely, it probably should be done only in patients with preexisting duodenal ulcer disease. An alternative approach is the use of $H_2$-antagonist therapy to suppress gastric acid secretion. Especially in patients in whom duodenal obstruction is not yet complete, some surgeons perform jejunojejunostomy close to the gastrojejunal anastomosis, because of concern that food in the afferent limb might regurgitate back into the stomach. The efficacy of the procedure has not been proven.

Although gastrojejunostomy usually bypasses the obstruction effectively, some patients are still unable to tolerate an oral diet, and the stomach does not empty well. Mechanical causes must be ruled out by upper gastrointestinal roentgenogram and endoscopy, and parenteral nutrition should be begun early while these diagnostic procedures are performed. In some patients, the return of gastric motility may be hastened by giving metoclopramide (10–30 mg 4 times a day), but occasionally nothing helps. This is particularly frustrating for both the physician and patient, since the inability to eat prolongs hospitalization and seriously compromises the quality of palliation. In such cases, gastroparesis may be a result of autonomic nerve involvement by tumor. No effective treatment for this is known.

## PANCREATIC PAIN

Anterior abdominal and back pain can be the most incapacitating and distressing symptom of pancreatic cancer, and it is often most severe in association with body and tail lesions. Bypass surgery does nothing to relieve this discomfort (21, 22), which is caused by the retroperitoneal extension of the tumor and involvement of the celiac plexus. Various approaches to surgical neurotomy have been tried, but overall, the results have been disappointing, providing only transient symptomatic relief (23, 24). Chemical splanchnicectomy by injecting 5% phenol or 50% alcohol around the celiac axis, as introduced by Bridenbaugh et al. (25), is far more effective. Intraoperative chemical splanchnicectomy is associated with 80% relief of pancreatic cancer pain, which in most instances is permanent (26). In frail patients, percutaneous chemical splanchnicectomy may be performed under computed tomography or ultrasonography guidance. Distal pancreaticojejunostomy has been used occasionally to provide relief from pain believed to be due to obstruction of the pancreatic duct (27). The limited success achieved with this approach together with the fear of complication related to a pancreatic anastomotic leak has discouraged its widespread adoption. For the relief of pancreatic pain, radiotherapy is reported to be more effective than other, surgical treatments (14).

## LAPAROSCOPIC APPROACH

Laparoscopy is a useful tool both for staging and for palliative procedures (28). Staging of pancreatic cancer still represents a challenge for surgeons, and the presence of peritoneal dissemination or small hepatic metastasis (<2 cm) is a frequent surprise at laparotomy and forces the surgeon to use a palliative procedure (29). Since palliative procedures such as bilioenteric and gastroenteric bypasses can be performed with recent techniques of laparoscopic surgery (30, 31), it may be reasonable to use laparoscopy to judge the resectability of the tumors and to perform palliative procedures with laparoscopic surgery in those with unresectable tumors. This approach can avoid the unnecessary laparotomy and may achieve rapid palliation with minimum morbidity (32). Patients with advanced pancreatic cancer and a limited life expectancy may benefit greatly from the shortened hospital stay and convalescence this manner of treatment offers.

## REFERENCES


1. Livingston EH, Welton ML, Reber HA. Surgical treatment of pancreatic cancer. The United States experience. Int J Pancreatol 1991;9:153–157.
2. Shumate CR, Baron TH. Palliative procedures for pancreatic cancer: when and which one? South Med J 1996;89:27–32.
3. Lillemoe KD, Barnes SA. Surgical palliation of unresectable pancreatic carcinoma. Surg Clin North Am 1995;75:935–968.
4. Warren KW, Braasch JW, Thum CW. Diagnosis and surgical treatment of carcinoma of the pancreas. Curr Probl Surg 1968;June:3–70.
5. Howard JM, Jordan GL Jr. Cancer of the pancreas. Curr Probl Cancer 1977;2:5–52.
6. Die Goyanes A, Pack GT, Bowden L. Cancer of the body and tail of the pancreas. Rev Surg 1971;28(3):153.
7. Anderson A, Bergdhal L. Carcinoma of the pancreas. Am Surg 1976;42:173–177.
8. Sarr MG, Cameron JL. Surgical management of unresectable carcinoma of the pancreas. Surgery 1982;91:123–133.
9. Howard JM, Jordan GL Jr, Reber HA. Surgical diseases of the pancreas. Philadelphia: Lea & Febiger, 1987.
10. Buckwalter JA, Lawton RL, Tidrick RT. Bypass operation for neoplastic biliary tract obstruction. Am J Surg 1965;109:100.
11. Pellegrini CA, Thomas MJ, Way LW. Bilirubin and alkaline phosphatase values before and after surgery for biliary obstruction. Am J Surg 1982;143:67.
12. Musgrove JE, Grindlay JM, Karlson AG. Intestinal-biliary reflux after anastomosis of common duct to duodenum or jejunum. Arch Surg 1952;92:579–584.
13. Diamond D, Fisher B. Pancreatic cancer. Surg Clin North Am 1975;55:363–376.
14. Huguier M, Baumel H. Manderscheid JC, et al. Surgical palliation for unresected cancer of the exocrine pancreas. Eur J Surg Oncol 1993;19(4):342–347.
15. Stuart M, Keo T, Hermann RE, et al. Palliation of malignant obstruction of the common bile duct by side to side choledochoduodenostomy. Am J Surg 1971;121:505.
16. Klempa I, Arnold W. Palliative surgical and endoscopic therapy of malignant bile duct occlusion. Chirurg 1994;65(10):836–848.
17. Cotton PB. Endoscopic method for relief of malignant obstructive jaundice. World J Surg 1984;8:854–861.
18. Leung JW, Emery R, Cotton PB, et al. Management of malignant obstructive jaundice at the Middlesex Hospital. Br J Surg 1983;74:584–586.
19. Richards AB, Sosin H. Cancer of the pancreas. The value of radical and palliative surgery. Ann Surg 1973;177:325.
20. Vijayanagar R, Tolins SH. Evaluation of palliative operations for carcinoma of the head of the pancreas: a ten year study. Mt Sinai J Med (NY) 1970;37:115.
21. Elmslie RG, Slavotinek AM. Surgical objectives in unresected cancer of the head of the pancreas. Br J Surg 1972;59:508–511.
22. Flanigan DP, Kraft RO. Continuing experience with palliative chemical splanchnicectomy. Arch Surg 1978;113:509–511.
23. Ray BS, Console AD. The relief of pain in chronic (calcareous) pancreatitis by sympathectomy. Surg Gynecol Obstet 1949; 89:1–7.
24. Yoshioka M, Wakabayashi T. Therapeutic neurotomy on head of pancreas for relief of pain due to chronic pancreatitis. Arch Surg 1958;76:546–549.
25. Bridenbaugh LD, Moore DC, Campbell DD. Management of upper abdominal cancer pain: treatment with celiac plexus block with alcohol. JAMA 1964;190:377–381.
26. Sharp KW, Stevens EJ. Improving palliation in pancreatic cancer: intraoperative celiac plexus block for pain relief. South Med J 1991;84(4):469–471.
27. Aplakis A, Dussault J, Knight M, et al. Relief of pain from pancreatic cancer. Ann R Coll Surg Engl 1977;59:401–403.
28. Cuschieri A. Laparoscopy for pancreatic cancer: does it benefit the patient? Eur J Surg Oncol 1988;14(1):41–44.
29. Meduri F, Diana F, Merenda R, et al. Implication of laparoscopy and peritoneal cytology in the staging of early pancreatic cancer. Zentralbl Pathol 1994;140(3):243–246.
30. Shimi S, Banting S, Cuschieri A. Laparoscopy in the management of pancreatic cancer: endoscopic cholecystojejunostomy for advanced disease. Br J Surg 1992;79(4):317–319.
31. Cuschieri A. Laparoscopic surgery of the pancreas. J R Coll Surg Edinb 1994;39(3):178–184.
32. Mouiel J, Katkhouda N, White S, et al. Endolaparoscopic palliation of pancreatic cancer. Surg Laparosc Endosc 1992;2(3): 241–243.

# 64

# *Treatment of Pancreatic Cancer Pain*

Keith D. Lillemoe

Pancreatic cancer is the fifth leading cause of cancer death in the United States, with more than 28,000 people dying from this disease each year. Unfortunately, despite substantial progress in the last two decades in diagnosis and management, it remains a disease with a grim prognosis. Most tumors are not resectable for cure at the time of presentation, and only 20% of affected patients survive 1 year after diagnosis. Since cure is unlikely for most patients, palliation of symptoms—obstructive jaundice, duodenal obstruction, and pain—is of primary importance.

Results of surgical palliation of pancreatic cancer have improved substantially in recent years. Furthermore, nonoperative methods can effectively relieve obstructive jaundice in patients deemed inoperable because of either the extent of their disease or their general medical condition. Yet, perhaps the most disturbing and incapacitating symptom of pancreatic cancer, pain, is often poorly managed and can remain a major problem for many patients until death. This chapter describes recent advances in our understanding of pancreatic cancer pain and outlines current treatment of this problem.

## INCIDENCE AND PREVALENCE OF PAIN IN PANCREATIC CANCER

Pancreatic cancer has long been regarded as one of the most painful forms of malignancy. Compared with patients with other cancers, such as lung, prostate, or uterine/cervix, the proportion of patients with pancreatic cancer who have pain of moderate-to-severe intensity is high (1). In 1989, Saltzburg and Foley reviewed 19 studies evaluating the incidence and various features of pain in over 2200 patients with pancreatic cancer (2). Most of these studies were retrospective and published prior to 1970. These authors found that pain was present at diagnosis in 50–97% of patients, with most studies noting an incidence of 80% or more. Pain occurred at some point in the course of the disease in up to 89% of patients in those studies in which pain prevalence was specifically evaluated.

Pain can develop from pancreatic cancer arising in any part of the gland. The incidence of pain at diagnosis in patients with cancer originating in the head of the pancreas ranged from 49 to 93%. Over 70% of patients with tumors originating in the body or tail have pain at the time of diagnosis. The corresponding figures for pain at any time during the course of the disease were 68 and 98%, respectively.

More recently, perhaps because of greater awareness of the diagnosis, the percentage of patients with pancreatic cancer presenting with substantial pain has decreased. Prospective analysis from the Memorial Sloan Kettering Cancer Center demonstrated that 40% of patients with pancreatic cancer reported no pain at the time of referral, and another 30% had only minimal complaints of pain (3). Moderate-to-severe pain was present in only 30% of patients, with only 10% of patients in the latter category. Similarly, prospective data collected from the Johns Hopkins Hospital has also demonstrated that only 20% of patients reported clinically relevant pain, as assessed by a visual analogue scale (4).

## PATHOPHYSIOLOGY OF PAIN

The pathogenesis of pain associated with pancreatic cancer can be classified into two general categories. The first mechanism is obstruction of either the biliary or pancreatic ducts and is associated with dilation of these structures. Pathologic changes of chronic pancreatitis are usually seen in the gland distal to the obstructing lesion. This pain is generally located in the upper abdomen and is exacerbated by oral intake. Often during the early stages of the disease, this pain is poorly characterized because of its vague, nonspecific nature. In many patients, investigation for peptic ulcer disease, gallstones, or other benign gastrointestinal conditions may markedly delay the diagnosis. Pain associated with pancreatic cancer arising in the head of the gland arises primarily in the epigastrium and the right upper quadrant. Pain from cancer of the body or tail may also involve the upper abdomen but more frequently will occur in the back and involve the lumbar, thoracic, and iliac regions. Regardless of the site of the pancreatic involvement by the tumor, abdominal pain can radiate directly through to the back. Most patients describe the pain from pancreatic cancer as a constant dull ache. Superimposed paroxysms of colicky pain are also common. Typically, the pain with tumors in the body and the tail is most severe when the patient is supine. This pain often wakes the patient at night and is relieved by sitting forward.

The second mechanism of pain from pancreatic cancer comes from retroperitoneal nerve invasion. Neural invasion by pancreatic cancer can be demonstrated in most patients undergoing pancreatic resection. It is likely that most patients with unresectable cancer will have progressive nerve involvement as their disease advances. Pain due to retroperitoneal nerve involvement is usually constant and is often relieved by sitting forward.

## MANAGEMENT OF PANCREATIC CANCER PAIN

### Pharmacologic Approaches

Analgesic drugs are the cornerstone of the pharmacologic management of pain due to pancreatic cancer. The classes of drugs that can be used include nonnarcotic analgesics, narcotic analgesics, and adjuvant medications. Aspirin, acetaminophen, and nonsteroidal antiinflammatory agents are nonnarcotic analgesics that can be used for pain of mild intensity. Furthermore, combining these agents with narcotic analgesics can enhance pain control while lessening the dose of narcotics. A wide range of narcotic analgesics is available, from weaker agents such as codeine, oxycodone, and propoxyphene to stronger agents such as morphine, hydromorphone, and methadone. In addition to different potencies, these agents vary with respect to efficacy and the degree and type of side effects.

Each patient's pain management should be individualized, based on the intensity of pain and the side effects of the pharmacologic regimen. Patients should be counseled concerning the role of narcotics early in the course of their disease so that they feel comfortable using these agents. This approach minimizes their concern about side effects and dependence. Standard oral pain medication management should begin with an adequate trial of the agent with the lowest potency that provides pain relief. Patients with more severe pain should generally receive narcotic pain medications on a regular schedule at fixed time intervals, not on an as-needed basis. The goal of this fixed administration is to maintain a plateau of analgesia without breakthrough periods of pain and its associated anxiety. Sustained-release oral morphine preparations (MS Contin) appear to be well-suited for this technique. The provision of "rescue" or "breakthrough" medications for periods of pain in the interval between medication dosages is also appropriate.

Side effects of potent narcotics are well known and often provide the greatest limitation to their use. Constipation is the most frequent uncomfortable side effect. Measures should be instituted at the onset of an opiate regimen to ensure maintenance of a regular bowel pattern. Central nervous system side effects include an often desired euphoria, excessive sedation, drowsiness, and confusion. The effects are frequently noted at the initiation of therapy but usually clear in 3–5 days. Nausea and vomiting can be annoying side effects that can usually be prevented or treated effectively. Respiratory depression, perhaps the most feared side effect of potent opiates, accounts for much of the hesitancy to provide adequate dosing of these agents. It is extremely uncommon, however, in patients who are not narcotic naive. Finally, tolerance, physical dependence, and addiction can occur with all potent opiates. The earliest sign of tolerance is the patient's complaint that the duration and/or degree of analgesia have decreased. Although cross-tolerance among opiates can occur, it is often incomplete; therefore, alternate opiates can often be used at equianalgesic doses. Concern for physical dependence or addiction is often cited as a primary factor for underdosing of opiates in patients with cancer pain. In reality, opiate addiction with appropriate medical use rarely, if ever, occurs. Furthermore, in the dying cancer patient, addiction should not be considered a reason for withholding increased doses of opiates.

The dose-limiting side effects of narcotics can be minimized by using various adjuvant drugs. Phenothiazines with their antiemetic properties may be useful in patients with nausea and vomiting, whether it is disease or medication related. These agents are available for oral, rectal, or parenteral administration. Antidepressants such as amitriptyline, imipramine, and doxepin can be used to elevate mood, increase sedation, and ensure sleep. Amphetamines can be used to potentiate the analgesic activity of opiates while antagonizing their sedative effects, elevating mood, and increasing activity.

Overall, standard therapy with oral opiates and adjuvant drugs can be successful in up to 85–90% of patients with pancreatic cancer pain. In the near terminal state, progressive pain can also interfere with the ability to take oral medications. This problem can be overcome by other routes of narcotic delivery. Most opiates are now available as rectal suppositories with an efficacy nearly equal to that of oral administration. The potent, lipid-soluble opiate fentanyl can also be administered transdermally using a skin patch. Recently, patient-controlled analgesic techniques have been offered to ambulatory patients with cancer. Intravenous and subcutaneous continuous infusions of opiates with patient-directed boluses, as needed, can be valuable in minimizing the fluctuations in blood levels, toxicity, and analgesia seen with intermittent-dosing schedules. Opiates can also be administered in the epidural, subarachnoid, or intraventricular spaces to minimize systemic toxicity and side effects. All such administration techniques require catheter access and sophisticated and carefully monitored delivery systems. Although these highly technical methods for opiate administration can offer certain advantages in selected patients, no substantial evidence supports their overall superiority to standard oral dosing. Such technology is definitely associated with an increase in the overall cost of cancer pain management.

### Anesthetic Approaches

Most pancreatic cancer pain is transmitted centrally via the celiac plexus. Interruption of the nociceptive input at the level of the celiac plexus or the splanchnic nerves from which it forms is therefore a potentially effective means of controlling visceral pancreatic pain and serves as a basis for celiac plexus block and other related techniques. The celiac plexus, the largest sympathetic nervous system plexus in the body, contains no somatic fibers. It enervates most of the upper abdominal viscera, including the stomach, liver, pancreas, spleen, kidneys, omentum, small and large bowel, abdominal aorta, and mesentery, as well as the ovaries, uterine fundus, and spermatic cord. It is composed of visceral afferent and efferent fibers from T-5 through T-12 sympathetic ganglia. The parasympathetic vagus fibers contribute to the plexus to a minor extent, with the right posterior vagus contributing most of these fibers. The plexus itself is a dense network of fibers derived from the right and left celiac ganglia and a few above-mentioned vagal fibers. The ganglia are located close to the aorta at the level of the origin of the celiac artery.

Percutaneous celiac block can be done via either fluoroscopic or computed tomographic guidance. In most techniques, a test injection with short-acting local anesthetic is performed prior to injection of a permanent neurolytic solution, most commonly 50% alcohol. The procedure can usually be performed on an outpatient basis, with a short period of observation with intravenous fluid administration following the procedure.

The results of percutaneous celiac plexus block have been cited as good to excellent in up to 80–90% of patients, but correlations of pain site, extent of disease, and previous therapies have not been made (5–7). Similarly, quantitative pain assessment and serial evaluations have often not been reported. A review of the English literature over the last 25 years found 15 series reporting the use of celiac plexus block for pancreatic cancer in 480 patients (7). Although this report appeared to show that pain control was achieved in 70–95% of patients, major deficiencies were present in each study.

When properly performed, celiac plexus block has minimal complications. Orthostatic hypotension is a consequence of splanchnic vasodilation secondary to sympathetic blockade. Although it occurs almost universally, orthostatic hypotension is primarily a problem in the older patient in whom compensation by extrasplanchnic vasoconstriction occurs over 2–3 days. The effect of splanchnic vasodilation can be minimized by crystalloid administration at the time of the procedure. Other rare complications include chest and leg pain attributed to neuritis and even rare cases of motor weakness or paralysis. In addition, inadvertent puncture of an adjacent organ such as kidneys, lungs, blood vessels, or upper abdominal viscera may occur. Finally, increased bowel motility may result from the relative excess of parasympathetic tone as a consequence of sympathetic blockade. In some patients, a diminution of nausea and vomiting may also be noted.

A second regional analgesic technique involves the administration of opiates or anesthetic agents into the subarachnoid or epidural space. This technique is an extension of the popular anesthetic technique and can now be provided not only for hospitalized patients but also for outpatients. In most cases, the catheter is tunneled subcutaneously, with the patient controlling the administration of the drug by a programable pump system. The technique offers the advantages of less systemic opiate effects but may still have the associated complications of respiratory depression, nausea and vomiting, pruritus, urinary retention, tolerance, and catheter-related problems. Fortunately, this technique is rarely necessary in patients with pancreatic cancer.

### Antitumor Approaches

A number of series have reported the impact of external-beam radiation on pain in patients with pancreatic cancer. Symptomatic improvement has been described in one-third to three-quarters of patients (8–10). Unfortunately, many of these reports did not use quantitative measures of pain assessment nor did they perform serial assessment of pain relief at regular intervals. In one of the few studies in which the issue of pain management was specifically addressed, only 31% of patients were able to discontinue pain medications for an unspecified amount of time after completion of radiation therapy (10). Moreover, pain relief from radiation may not occur until several weeks after initiation of therapy, leaving patients with substantial pain for much of their very limited life expectancy. Currently, no series has provided a randomized comparison of the use of radiation therapy versus treatment with oral medications for pain control in patients with unresectable pancreatic cancer. Most current regimens for treatment of unresectable pancreatic cancer combine external-beam radiation with 5-fluorouracil as a radiosensitizer. There is no evidence to support any single agent or combination therapy for either objective tumor response or pain control in patients with pancreatic cancer.

### Surgical Approaches

The surgical options for the management of pancreatic cancer include resection (if appropriate, based on the extent of tumor) and surgical palliation for obstruction of the biliary tree or gastrointestinal tract. Pancreatic resection in which all gross tumor is removed offers not only relief of symptoms, including pain, but also offers the chance of long-term survival. Palliative resection, in which gross and/or microscopic tumor is left behind, has recently been demonstrated to offer some survival advantage; however, the long-term effect on quality of life and, specifically, pain control has not been well defined (11).

Conventional palliation of pancreatic cancer includes biliary bypass and, in most cases, a gastrojejunostomy. Biliary bypass will relieve that component of the patient's pain which is due to biliary obstruction. Gastric outlet obstruction is seldom a cause of pain but can cause early satiety, nausea, and vomiting. There is no role for surgical bypass of an obstructed pancreatic duct due to pancreatic cancer. Nonoperative management of obstructive jaundice can also be accomplished by the placement of percutaneous transhepatic or endoscopic stents. As with surgical bypass, these procedures are likely to relieve the pain due to biliary obstruction. Although attempts at endoscopic placement of pancreatic duct stents for pancreatic cancer have been reported, in general, these techniques have not shown a major long-term benefit in the relief of pain.

**Intraoperative Chemical Splanchnicectomy.** Chemical splanchnicectomy, employing principles of neurolysis of the celiac ganglia as in percutaneous celiac block, can also be performed at laparotomy for unresectable pancreatic cancer. Chemical splanchnicectomy for unresectable pancreatic cancer was first described by Copping et al. in 1969 (12). In the 1978 update of their experience with the technique including 41 patients, 88% of patients with pain due to pancreatic cancer experienced relief of pain postoperatively (13). Most of these patients underwent palliative biliary and gastrointestinal bypass at the same operation. These results were compared with those of a group of historic controls in which only 21% of patients had pain control after similar palliative procedures. There were no reported complications of chemical splanchnicectomy. Since that time, the procedure has been advocated by many surgeons, with anecdotal reports appearing in the literature, describing successful control of pain in most patients (14, 15).

Intraoperative chemical splanchnicectomy can be performed as part of any surgical procedure performed for palliation of pancreatic cancer. Patients should undergo appropriate preoperative assessment and preparation prior to their planned resection or palliative procedure. After determining at laparotomy that the patient's tumor is unresectable, intraoperative chemical splanchnicectomy can be performed. The procedure is indicated whether the patient has severe pain or is pain free at the time of surgery. The technique is applicable whether the cancer arises in the head, body, or tail of the gland. There would not appear to be a need for chemical splanchnicectomy following pancreaticoduodenectomy or distal pancreatectomy if resection is completed with grossly clear margins. In the unusual situation in which resection is completed but gross tumor is left at the margins, chemical splanchnicectomy may be performed in the hope of treating and/or preventing future pain due to retroperitoneal invasion by the remaining tumor. Laparotomy is not indicated if its sole purpose is to perform intraoperative chemical splanchnicectomy. This is especially true in patients who are otherwise not candidates for surgical exploration or palliation because of extent of disease, age, or medical disability. The availability of percutaneous celiac block has eliminated the need for this procedure in almost all patients.

***Technique.*** Intraoperative chemical splanchnicectomy can be performed through either an upper midline or bilateral subcostal incision. After determining that the patient is unresectable and having completed a biliary bypass and/or gastrojejunostomy as indicated, chemical splanchnicectomy is carried out. A 50% alcohol solution should be prepared in a sterile fashion by dilution of absolute alcohol with sterile injectable saline. A 20-mL syringe with either a 20- or 22-gauge spinal needle is used for the injection.

The lesser omentum is incised so that the celiac axis can be palpated as it arises from the aorta. A palpable thrill due to the high blood flow through the celiac axis is usually apparent. The spinal needle is then advanced on each side of the aorta at the level of the celiac axis (Fig. 64.1), and 20 mL of 50% alcohol solution is injected on both sides of the aorta. Prior to and during the injection, the syringe should be aspirated to ensure that neither the vena cava, aorta, nor adjacent lumbar vessels has been cannulated. After completion of both injections, the sites are inspected for hemostasis. If minor bleeding is observed, the area is simply packed and compressed for a short time. The anesthesiologist should be notified at the time of injection, because some hypotension may occur with adequate sympathetic block. This situation can be managed by intraoperative administration of crystalloid solution.

The addition of intraoperative chemical splanchnicectomy should not alter postoperative management of the patient undergoing laparotomy and a palliative procedure for unresectable pancreatic cancer. When only a biopsy for tissue diagnosis and a chemical splanchnicectomy are performed, the patient can resume oral intake as tolerated and be discharged as soon as possible after the procedure. During the first attempts at postoperative ambulation, the patient should be observed for any evidence of orthostatic hypotension. This effect, if noted at all, is seldom long lasting.

***Results.*** In 1993, a prospective, randomized, placebo-controlled study of chemical splanchnicectomy was completed (4). In this study, pre- and postoperative pain was assessed by use of questionnaires including a visual analogue scale. The two groups were similar with respect to age, sex, location and stage of tumor, operation performed, use of postoperative chemo- and

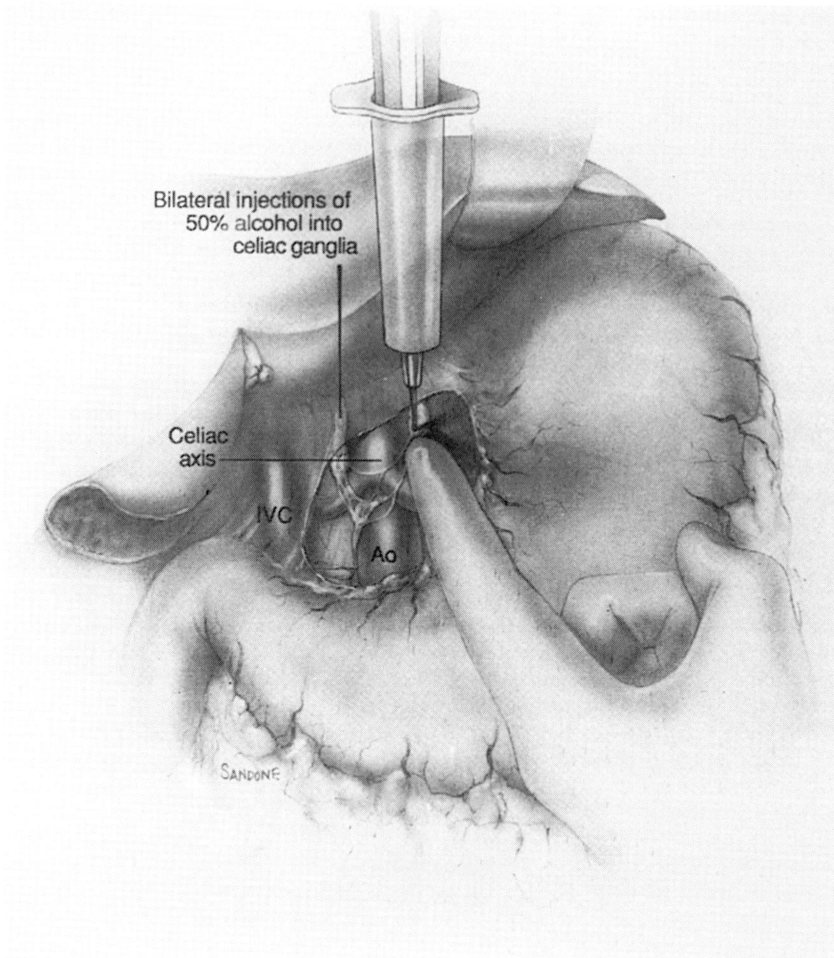


**FIG. 64.1.** Chemical splanchnicectomy was performed using a syringe and a 20- or 22-gauge spinal needle. Solution (20 mL) was injected on each side of the aorta *(Ao)* at the level of the *celiac axis* (*IVC,* inferior vena cava). (From Lillemoe KD, et al. Chemical splanchnicectomy in patients with unresectable pancreatic cancer. Ann Surg 1993;70;730–732.)

radiation therapy, and initial assessment scores for pain, mood, and disability. There was no difference between the patients receiving chemical splanchnicectomy and the control group with respect to perioperative morbidity, mortality, length of nasogastric drainage, days until oral intake, or postoperative length of stay. Mean postoperative pain scores at all assessment points for all randomized patients were significantly lower following chemical splanchnicectomy with alcohol than those of control patients. The subgroup of patients with preexisting pain had a statistically significant decrease in postoperative pain scores, compared with control patients (Fig. 64.2). Some 70% of patients with preexisting pain receiving alcohol decreased their narcotic requirement, compared with none of the placebo patients. Patients receiving alcohol experienced a mean of 3.3 pain-free months, compared with 0.8 pain-free months for the control patients. Unfortunately, pain did recur before death in 65% of the patients who received an alcohol block.

Patients with no preexisting pain also showed a statistically significant decrease in mean postoperative pain scores compared with the placebo controls. The average number of months without substantial pain was 7.2 months in the alcohol group and only 3.0 months in the placebo group. Only 46% of patients receiving alcohol block ever required major doses of narcotic pain medications, compared with 60% of the placebo patients. Finally, before death, 56% of patients receiving alcohol splanchnicectomy never reported having severe pain, compared with only 34% of patients in the placebo group.

An unexpected finding in this study was a highly significant increase in survival among patients with severe preoperative pain who underwent chemical splanchnicectomy, compared with similar patients in the control group (Fig. 64.3). These two subgroups were analyzed with respect to age, tumor location, tumor stage, operation performed, the use of chemo- and radiation therapy, baseline mood, and disability. No significant difference was apparent in any of these comparisons, suggesting that adequate pain control may improve patient survival with this disease.

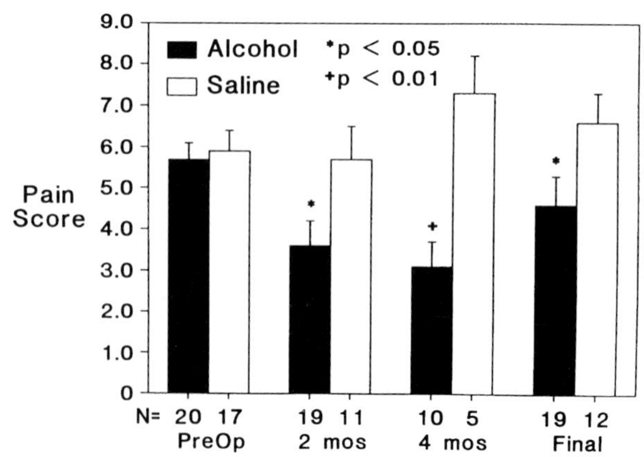


**FIG. 64.2.** Mean pain scores measured at the preoperative, 2- and 4-month, and final assessments for all patients with substantial preoperative pain surviving at each point. (From Lillemoe KD, et al. Chemical splanchnicectomy in patients with unresectable pancreatic cancer. Ann Surg 1993;70;730–732.)

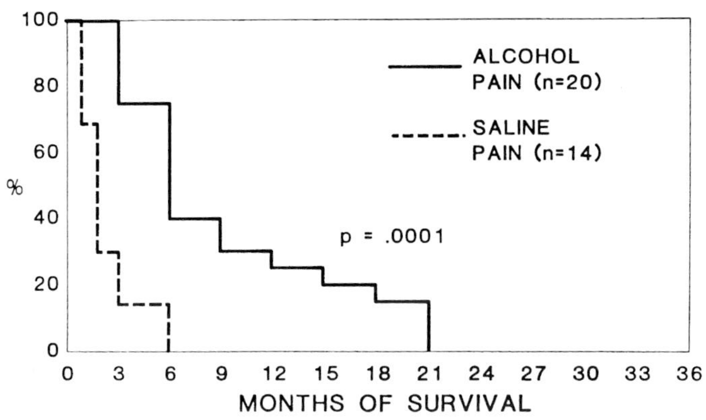


**FIG. 64.3.** Kaplan-Meier survival curves determined from the time of hospital discharge for patients with significant preoperative pain. (From Lillemoe KD, et al. Chemical splanchnicectomy in patients with unresectable pancreatic cancer. Ann Surg 1993;70:730–732.)

**Thoracoscopic Pancreatic Denervation.** The recent advances in laparoscopic and thoracoscopic surgery have led to the technical description of thoracoscopic pancreatic denervation performed via the left chest (16). This technique appears to be most applicable in patients in whom percutaneous celiac block cannot be performed. Patients requiring thoracoscopy must be suitable candidates for general anesthesia, but there is no other special preparation. The procedure provides adequate pain control via a minimally invasive technique. Laparotomy and the associated postoperative pain are avoided.

***Operative technique.*** Thoracoscopic pancreatic denervation is performed through the left chest, with the patient placed on the operating room table in the right lateral decubitus position. A double-lumen endotracheal tube allows the left lung to be deflated, which facilitates visualization. The arm is elevated on a sling to a 90° angle to the chest wall, and the table is tilted posteriorly to about 15°. A 1-cm incision is made in the fourth intercostal space and anterior axillary line. After single-lung (right) ventilation, an 11-mm thoracoscopic cannula is inserted, and the thoracoscope is introduced. Three additional 11-mm cannulas are placed in the sixth intercostal space in the anterior axillary line and through the seventh and ninth spaces in the posterior axillary line of the left chest. The sympathetic chain is identified coursing over the ribs 2 cm posterior and lateral to the aorta (Fig. 64.4). The upper end of the sympathetic chain is noted, and the stellate ganglion is identified. The greater splanchnic nerve (T5-T9) and lesser splanchnic nerve (T10-T11) are identified. The parietal pleura is incised and dissected superiorly and inferiorly. Each nerve should be doubly clipped and divided.

To add a vagotomy to the procedure, a semiflexible dilator or a flexible endoscope is inserted into the distal esophagus to facilitate its identification. The left lung is retracted anteriorly and cephalad away from the esophagus using an atraumatic fanlike instrument. It may be necessary to divide the inferior pulmonary ligament to adequately retract the lung away from the distal third of the esophagus. The pleura overlying the esophagus is opened with either blunt or sharp dissection, and

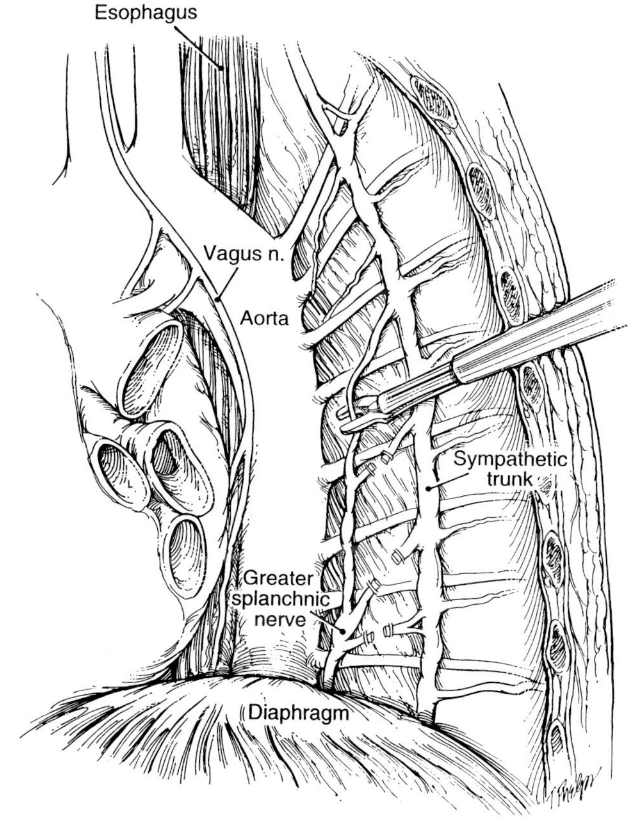


**FIG. 64.4.** The sympathetic chain is identified coursing over the ribs 2 cm posterior and lateral to the aorta. The upper end of the sympathetic chain is noted, and the stellate ganglion is identified. The greater splanchnic nerve (T5-9) and lesser splanchnic (T10-11) are identified.

the esophagus is identified. The left vagus nerve (anterior) is easily visualized over the anterior surface of the esophagus and is dissected free from the underlying muscle fibers. The structure is then doubly clipped and divided. Access to the right (posterior) vagus nerve usually requires complete mobilization of the esophagus, and the dilator or endoscope should be withdrawn to a point above this area. After identification of the posterior vagus, it can be doubly clipped and divided. A small (28–32 Fr) chest tube is inserted through a lower cannula incision.

Following thoracoscopic pancreatic denervation, the chest tube can be removed on the first or second postoperative day and the patient discharged shortly thereafter. No prospective randomized trials have been performed to evaluate thoracoscopic pancreatic denervation. A number of authors, however, have reported significant pain control following this procedure, with minimal perioperative morbidity (16). Gastric emptying problems following vagotomy have not been reported as yet.

## CONCLUSION

Pain associated with pancreatic cancer remains an important clinical problem. With greater recognition and earlier diagnosis, the percentage of patients with pancreatic cancer presenting with substantial pain may be lower than in past decades. Patients with unresectable disease, however, are still likely to develop pain problems before death. Although the rare patient may be extremely difficult to manage, the armamentarium of currently available techniques should provide suitable alternatives for almost all patients with this disease. In patients not considered surgical candidates, the use of narcotic analgesics with adjuvant agents administered orally will usually provide good pain control. If pain relief is ineffective or side effects of these agents become too disabling, percutaneous chemical splanchnicectomy should be performed at an early stage to allow the patient maximal benefit prior to death.

In patients found to have unresectable pancreatic cancer during exploration or undergoing an operative biliary or gastric bypass, intraoperative chemical splanchnicectomy with 50% alcohol offers excellent, albeit not permanent, control of pain. The technique adds very little time and morbidity to the procedure and should be considered as a part of surgical palliation in patients undergoing operation for unresectable pancreatic cancer.

## REFERENCES


1. Greenwald HP, Bonica JJ, Bergner M. The prevalence of pain in four cancers. Cancer 1987;60:2563–2569.
2. Saltzburg D, Foley KJ. Management of pain in pancreatic cancer. Surg Clin North Am 1989;69:629–649.
3. Hudis C, Kelsen D, Niedzwiecki D, Banks W, Portenoy R, Foley K. Pain is not a prominent symptom in most patients with early pancreas cancer. Proc Am Soc Clin Oncol 1991;10:326.
4. Lillemoe KD, Cameron JL, Kaufman HS, Yeo CJ, Pitt HA, Sauter PK. Chemical splanchnicectomy in patients with unresectable pancreatic cancer: a prospective randomized trial. Ann Surg 1993; 217:447–457.
5. Leung J, Bowen-Wright M, Avelig W, Shorvon PJ, Cotton PB. Celiac plexus block for pain in pancreatic cancer and chronic pancreatitis. Br J Surg 1983;70:730–732.
6. Brown DL, Bulley CK, Quiel EL. Neurolytic celiac plexus block for pancreatic cancer pain. Anesth Analg 1987;66:869–873.
7. Lebovits A, Lefkowitz M. Pain management of pancreatic carcinoma: a review. Pain 1989;36:1–11.
8. Haslam JB, Cavanaugh PJ, Stroup SL. Radiation therapy in the treatment of irresectable adenocarcinoma of the pancreas. Cancer 1973;32:1341–1345.
9. Whittington R, Dobelower RR, Mohiuddin M, Rosato FE, Weiss SM. Radiotherapy of unresectable pancreatic carcinoma: a six-year experience with 104 patients. Int J Radiat Oncol Biol Phys 1981;7:1639–1644.
10. Gastrointestinal Tumor Study Group. Radiation therapy combined with adriamycin or 5-fluororacil for the treatment of locally unresectable pancreatic cancer. Cancer 1985;56:2563–2568.
11. Lillemoe KD, Cameron JL, Yeo CJ, et al. Pancreaticoduodenectomy: does it have a role in the palliation of pancreatic cancer? Ann Surg 1996;223:718–728.
12. Copping J, Willix R, Kraft R. Palliative chemical splanchnicectomy. Arch Surg 1969;98:418–420.
13. Flanigan DP, Kraft RO. Continuing experience with palliative chemical splanchnicectomy. Arch Surg 1978;113:509–511.
14. Gardner AM, Solomon G. Relief of pain of unresectable carcinoma of the pancreas by chemical splanchnicectomy during laparotomy. Ann R Coll Surg 1984;66:409–411.
15. Sharp KW, Stevens EJ. Improving palliation in pancreatic cancer: intraoperative celiac plexus block for pain relief. South Med J 1991;84:469–471.
16. Worsey J, Ferson PF, Keenen RJ, Julian TB, Landreneau RJ. Thoracoscopic pancreatic denervation for pain control in irresectable pancreatic cancer. Br J Surg 1993;80:1051–1052.

# 65

# Connective Tissue Tumors

Jan Axelson, Sigmund Dawiskiba, Måns Åkerman, and Ingemar Ihse

In chronic pancreatitis and in pancreatic cancer, secondary changes are found in the pancreatic neural tissue (peripheral nerves). Fibrosis is a prominent feature of both. However, primary tumors of the pancreatic mesenchymal tissue (fibrous, adipose, vascular) are rare, as are tumors originating from muscle and neural tissue. Tumors arising from such structures are referred to as soft tissue tumors. They are a heterogenous group of tumors comprising benign, borderline, and malignant (sarcoma) entities. In addition to lesions with known origin, described previously, there are a number of soft tissue tumors, benign as well as malignant, with unknown or debated histogenesis. Table 65.1 shows retroperitoneal soft tissue tumors in adults diagnosed at Lund University Hospital between 1979 and 1995.

Soft tissue sarcomas account for less than 1% of all malignancies in adults, which underlines the rarity of such pancreatic tumors (1). They are generally described in case reports or in studies comprising tumors from multiple sites. In a report of 647 periampullary tumors, seven sarcomas (1.1%) were found, all of which originated from the duodenum (2). Table 65.2 summarizes cases of soft tissue tumors of the pancreas reported between 1948 and 1995.

## ETIOLOGY

The etiology of soft tissue tumors is largely unknown. A genetic predisposition has been proved in the so-called Li-Fraumeni syndrome, which implies a familial occurrence of carcinomas and soft tissue sarcomas and is caused by an inborn mutation in the suppressor oncogene P53. Increased incidence of soft tissue sarcoma has also been reported in patients with different kinds of hereditary diseases (3, 4). Exposure to herbicides as a cause of soft tissue sarcoma is debated (5, 6), whereas thorium dioxide and vinyl chloride have been proved to cause sarcoma, especially angiosarcoma (7). The risk of Kaposi sarcoma is increased by immunosuppression (8, 9). Radiotherapy may induce soft tissue sarcoma, especially angiosarcoma (10). The aforementioned factors, however, represent an etiology in only a minority of the sarcomas or soft tissue tumors. We have not found any reports on specific etiologic suggestions for any of the soft tissue tumors described in the pancreas (Table 65.2).

## CLINICAL FEATURES AND DIAGNOSTIC METHODS

The sarcomas found in the pancreas have in common a similar biologic behavior and clinical presentation; often situated in the head of the gland, they may also involve the whole organ. Depending on the localization within the pancreas, soft tissue tumors may grow to a considerable size before a mass is noted by the patient or symptoms occur (e.g., due to obstruction of nearby hollow viscera). In later stages, weight loss and general malaise are the main clinical features, which are not different from what is seen in patients with adenocarcinoma.

Ultrasonography and computerized tomography (CT) can disclose small pancreatic tumors, but cannot differentiate between tumors of different origin (12, 13). With the increasing use of these diagnostic procedures, a higher incidence of asymptomatic tumors could have been expected. However, this opinion is not supported by the current literature reports.

Fine-needle aspiration cytology (FNAC) has many advantages and is currently used in the diagnosis of trunk and extremity sarcomas in many centers, but transabdominal fine-needle aspiration is controversial because of the proposed risk of seeding of malignant cells intraabdominally (see Chapter 10). The recommended method for microscopic diagnosis of suspected sarcoma of the pancreas is intraoperative fine-needle aspiration or surgical biopsy.

Specific blood tests or markers are not available to distinguish sarcomatous tumors from adenocarcinoma, although CA 19-9 and CA 50 are sometimes used to identify the latter. Due to the origin of tumors from connective tissue, they generally do not express p53 and Ki-*ras* mutations nor the most common tumor markers (11). Chromogranin A is a usable tool to exclude an endocrine origin.

## CLASSIFICATION, GRADING, AND STAGING

Several attempts have been made to classify the soft tissue tumors. Early classifications were mainly descriptive and predominantly based on morphologic criteria. In 1969, the World Health Organization (WHO) proposed a classification based on clinical findings and histologic typing. It was strongly stressed that close cooperation between clinicians and pathologists was important for establishing a reliable diagnosis. With the use of adjunctive diagnostic methods such as electron microscopy, immunohistochemistry, and cytogenetic analysis, the recognition of different histotypes has improved as has the accuracy of diagnosis. For an updated classification of the soft tissue tumors based on current histogenetic criteria, the reader is referred to the textbooks of Enzinger and Weiss (14), Meis-Kindblom and Enzinger (15), and the WHO international histologic classification (16).

Grading and staging are important for accurate planning of therapy and for prognostic evaluation. Histologic malignancy grading is based on the combined assessment of different histologic parameters. Presently, no grading systems have been accepted worldwide. In all major systems, the degree of differentiation, cellularity, cellular pleomorphism, mitotic activity, and the presence of necrosis are important parameters. Other proposed prognostic criteria are the mode of growth (expansive or infiltrating), the presence of vascular invasion, and the

**TABLE 65.1. Retroperitoneal Soft Tissue Tumors in Adults—University Hospital, Lund 1979–1995**

| Benign | *(N)* | Malignant | *(N)* |
|---|---|---|---|
| Fibrosis | 8 | Sarcoma NOS | 6 |
| Neurolemoma | 5 | Leiomyosarcoma | 4 |
| Lipoma | 3 | Liposarcoma | 4 |
| Hemangiopericytoma | 2 | Hemangiopericytoma malignant | 1 |
| Ganglioneuroma | 1 | | |
| Leiomyoma | 1 | Malignant fibrous histiocytoma | 1 |
| Lymphangioma | 1 | | |
| | | MPNST[a] | 1 |
| | | Rhabdomyosarcoma | 1 |
| | | Synovial sarcoma | 1 |
| Total | 21 | Total | 19 |

[a]Malignant peripheral nerve sheath tumor.

DNA ploidy status. Most systems use a 3 or 4 grade scale, in which grades 1 and 2 correspond to low-grade malignancy and grades 3 and 4 to high-grade malignant sarcomas. In some other systems, each parameter is graded in 0–2 or 3 points, and the sum of points determines the degree of malignancy.

Staging provides information on the state of the disease at the time of histologic diagnosis. Several staging systems are in use; common parameters are the location, size, and extension of the sarcoma and the presence of lymph node or other metastases. Commonly used staging system are the American Joint Committee for Cancer staging system (17) and the Enneking system (18).

## MORPHOLOGIC FEATURES OF FREQUENTLY OCCURRING PANCREAS SARCOMAS

The typical cell of leiomyosarcoma is elongated with abundant cytoplasm. The nucleus, which usually is centrally located, is typically blunt ended or "cigar shaped" and may be truncated. The cells are arranged in fascicles of varying size, and in low-grade malignant tumors the fascicles intersect each other at right angles (Fig. 65.1*A*). The cellular pattern of leiomyosarcoma, however, may vary considerably. In high-grade malignant tumors, the cellular pleomorphism is pronounced and multinucleated tumor giant cells are common; in the epithelioid leiomyosarcomas, the cells are epithelial-like, sometimes with vacuolated cytoplasm, features that might cause confusion with carcinomas. In the cytologic examination of fine-needle aspirates the cellular features are much like those in histologic sections, while the tissue pattern is often more difficult to appreciate (Fig. 65.1*B*).

The microscopic characteristics of liposarcoma are demonstrated in Figure 65.2, *A–D*. Histologically, these tumors may show considerable variation in pattern and cellular appearance, but the identification of more or less atypical lipoblasts is important for the diagnosis. In the most common subtype—the myxoid liposarcoma—the presence of a myxoid matrix and a plexiform capillary network are other diagnostic signs. For the cytologic examination, the comments given above for leiomyosarcoma are valid.

For detailed information on the microscopic appearance of other soft tissue tumors that may occur in the pancreas, see reference 14.

## TREATMENT

Benign soft tissue tumors of the pancreas are mainly treated with resection, ranging from simple excision to pancreaticoduodenectomy, depending on the size of the tumor. Although resection harbors a good possibility for cure, the morbidity and mortality risks related to the larger operations must be considered.

After the establishment of the diagnosis of a malignant soft tissue tumor, the surgical procedure includes the same judgments pre- and perioperatively as those for the more common pancreatic adenocarcinoma. However, connective tissue tumors of the pancreas may reach a larger size than pancreatic adenocarcinoma and still be resectable without local or distant metastases. The histopathologic grading is important not only for prognosis but also for therapeutic decisions. The aim of surgical treatment must be to perform a radical resection, regardless of a subtotal or total pancreatectomy with removal of adjacent structures. Local resections may sometimes seem feasible, but one should bear in mind that such procedures in general have a high local recurrence rate, which is followed by dissemination of the disease. Macroscopically, these tumors are often thought to be encapsulated. Microscopically, only a pseudocapsule of compressed tumor cells are found. Thus a nonradical resection confined to "the encapsulation" only gives unnecessary spillage of tumor cells in the operative field. To choose the proper surgical procedure, preoperative assessment with CT, using intravenous contrast, is advisable. It may give valuable information on tumor invasion or dislocation of major vessels as well as of extrapancreatic spread. Transabdominal ultrasonography and a chest x-ray should also be included in the preoperative assessment. However, the final decision on what procedure to use is done by the surgeon at operation. The surgeon doing a diagnostic laparotomy in these patients should also be prepared to continue with a major pancreatic procedure.

The survival rate for patients with periampullary soft tissue tumors was found to depend not only on the histologic diagnosis of a nonadenocarcinoma with localization to the ampullary duodenum, but also on the curative intention of surgery (2). All patients treated for a soft tissue sarcoma and with a reported survival of 5 years or more were operated on with a subtotal or total pancreatectomy irrespective of the histologic origin of the tumor: unspecified sarcoma (12–14), fibrosarcoma (17, 19), liposarcoma (21), rhabdosarcoma (26), and neuroblastoma (36).

Adjunctive intraoperative and postoperative radiation therapy may possibly, as shown for sarcomas of other locations (3, 43), increase the curative potential of the surgical procedure. However, radiotherapy alone is generally without effect. Whether chemotherapy is useful is not known. There are ongoing trials with chemotherapy for soft tissue sarcomas of other locations

**TABLE 65.2. Primary Soft Tissue Tumors of the Pancreas: Summary of Case Reports in the Literature 1966–1995**

| Benign | *(N)* | Malignant | *(N)* |
|---|---|---|---|
| Lymphangioma | 36 | Leiomyosarcoma | 17 |
| Lipomatosis | 12 | Malignant fibrous histiocytoma | 10 |
| Hemangioma | 6 | | |
| Neurolemoma | 4 | Fibrosarcoma | 7 |
| Leiomyoma | 2 | Sarcoma NOS | 6 |
| Lipoma | 2 | Liposarcoma | 3 |
| Hemangiopericytoma | 1 | MPNST[a] | 2 |
| Neurofibroma | 1 | Hemangiopericytoma malignant | 1 |
| | | Neurofibrosarcoma | 1 |
| | | Rhabdomyosarcoma | 1 |
| Total | 64 | Total | 48 |

[a]Malignant peripheral nerve sheath tumor.

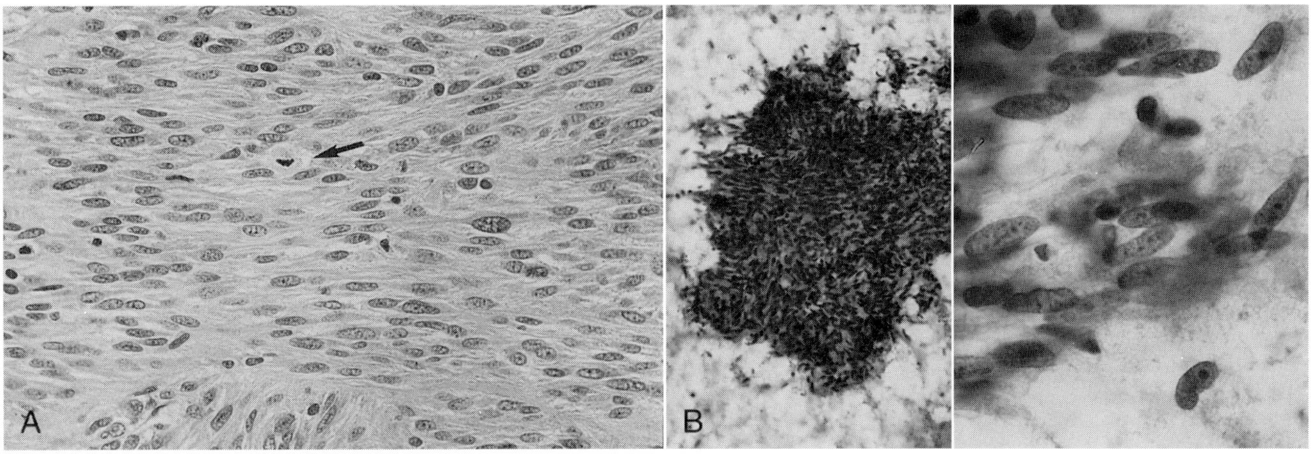

**FIG. 65.1. A.** Leiomyosarcoma, histologic section. A cellular tumor composed of bundles of spindly hyperchromatic, pleomorphic tumor cells and fibrovascular stroma. Numerous mitotic figures *(arrow)*. **B.** Leiomyosarcoma, fine-needle aspirate (metastasis of the same tumor). Tumor tissue fragment with a few isolated tumor cells *(left)*. Tumor cells are orderly arranged in parallel rows, often with ill-preserved cytoplasm. The nuclei are different sized, ovoid or elongated with blunt ends. Between nuclei there is often a red intercellular substance *(right)*. (*A, B,* hematoxylin-erythrosin. *A,* ×50; *B, left* ×25, *right* ×100). See color insert.

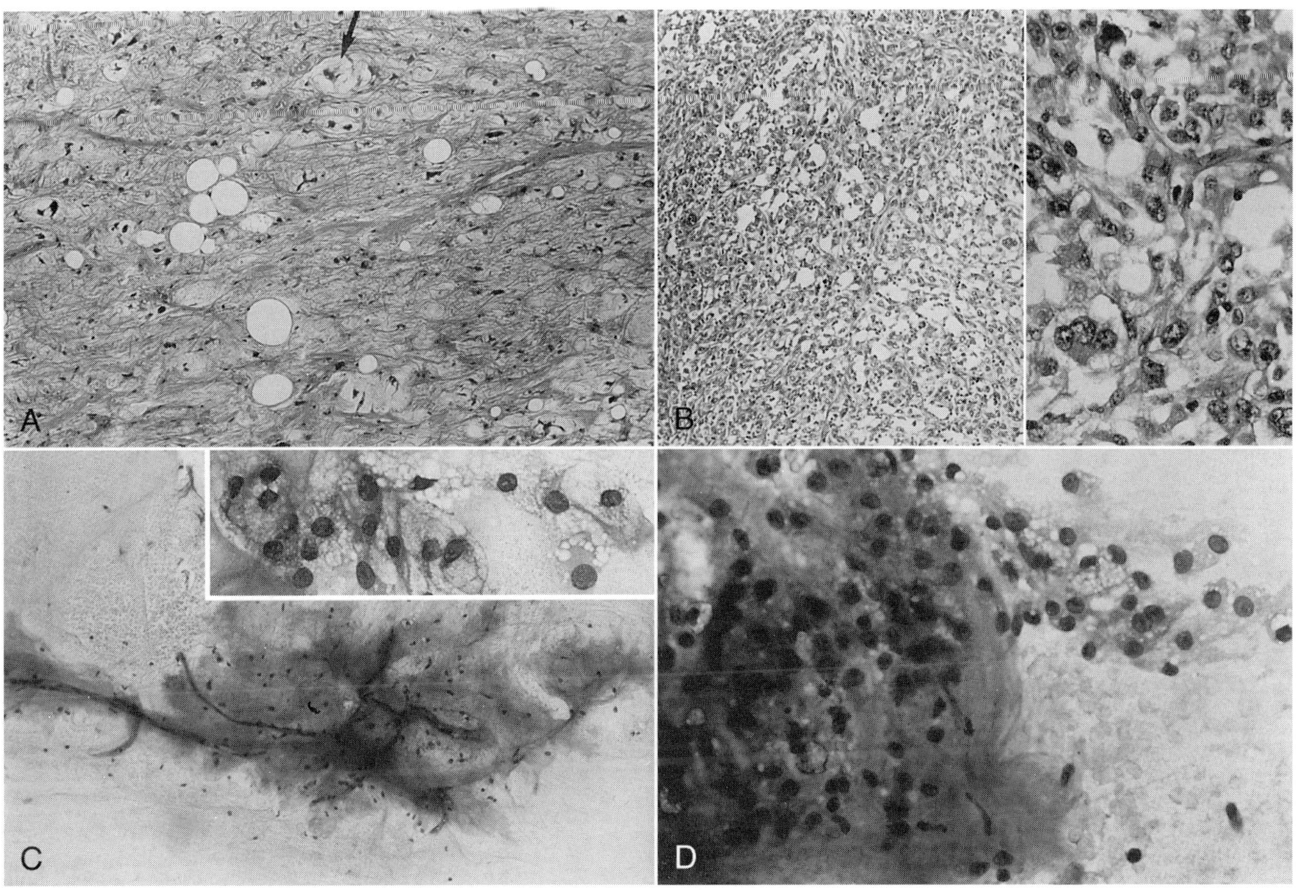

**FIG. 65.2. A.** Histologic section of a primary well-differentiated liposarcoma. It is composed of numerous multivacuolated lipoblasts *(arrow)* in the background of a fine capillary network, sclerosed stroma, and a few normal fat cells. **B.** Section of recurrent dedifferentiated liposarcoma. There are a large number of highly pleomorphic atypical mesenchymal cells, ranging from slender and plump spindle cells to bizarre vacuolated lipoblasts *(left)*. Multinucleated giant cells and atypical mitoses occur *(right)*. **C.** Fine-needle aspirate of myxoid liposarcoma shows fatty tissue fragment with myxoid background substance and branching capillaries. Multivacuolated lipoblasts with scalloped nuclei are present *(insert)*. **D.** Cytologic smear of poorly differentiated round cell liposarcoma (another area of the same tumor) shows a number of dispersed tumor cells with rounded atypical nuclei and some multivacuolated lipoblasts in the myxoid background. (*A, B,* hematoxylin-erythrosin; *C, D, May-Grünwald-Giemsa; A,* ×50; *B, left* ×25, *right* ×100; *C,* ×25, *insert* ×100; *D,* ×100). See color insert.

(44). The treatment of soft tissue tumors in the pancreas has to be based on multidisciplinary cooperation, including surgeons, pathologists, radiotherapists, and oncologists, to individualize and optimize management of the patient.

## SUMMARY

The treatment of soft tissue tumors of the pancreas is primarily surgical. Radical resection gives the only documented chance for cure. Contrary to adenocarcinomas of the pancreas, large tumor size does not preclude resection. Although the role of radiotherapy and chemotherapy is unsettled, management of patients with soft tissue tumors requires teamwork by surgeons, pathologists, radiotherapists, and oncologists.

## REFERENCES

1. Surgical lesions of the pancreas. Arch Surg 1941;42:819–838.
2. Michelassi F, Erroi F, Dawson PJ, et al. Experience with 647 consecutive tumours of the duodenum, ampulla, head of the pancreas, and distal common bile duct. Ann Surg 1989;210: 544–554.
3. Haggitt RC, Reid BJ. Hereditary gastrointestinal polyposis syndromes. Am J Surg Pathol 1986;10:871–887.
4. Malkin D, Li F, Strong L, et al. Germline p53 mutations in a familial syndrome of breast cancer, sarcomas, and other neoplasms. Science 1990;250:1233–1238.
5. Greenwald P, Kovasznay B, Collins DN, et al. Sarcomas of soft tissue after Vietnam service. JNCI 1984;73:1107–1109.
6. Hardell L, Sandstrom A. Case control study: soft tissue sarcoma and exposure to phenoxyacetic acids or chlorophenols. Br J Cancer 1979;39:711–717.
7. Evans DM, Williams WJ, Jung IT. Angiosarcoma and hepatocellular carcinoma in vinyl chloride workers. Histopathology 1983;7: 377–388.
8. Giraldo G, Beth E, Buonaquaro FM. Kaposi's sarcoma, a natural model of interrelationship between viruses, immunologic response, genetics, and oncogenesis. Antibiot Chemother 1984; 32:1–11.
9. Klepp O, Dahl O, Stenwig J. Association of Kaposi's sarcoma and prior immunosuppression therapy: 5 year material of Kaposi's sarcoma in Norway. Cancer 1978:42:2626–2630.
10. Laskin WB, Silverman TA, Enzinger FM. Postradiation of soft tissue sarcomas: an analysis of 53 cases. Cancer 1988;62:2330–2340.
11. Gatteschi B, Saccomanno S, Bartoli FG, et al. Mixed pleomorphic osteoclast-like tumor of the pancreas. Int J Pancreatol 1995;18: 169–175.
12. Russ PD. Leiomyosarcoma of the pancreatic bed detected on CT scans. AJR 1993;161:210–213.
13. Laverdiere JT, van Sonnenberg E, Strum WB, et al. Pleomorphic pancreatic sarcoma mimicking pseudocyst: CT appearance. AJR 1992;158:87–89.
14. Enzinger FM, Weiss SW. Soft tissue tumors. 3rd ed. New York: CV Mosby, 1995.
15. Meis-Kindblom J, Enzinger FM. Color atlas of soft tissue tumors. New York: CV Mosby, 1995.
16. Weiss SW. Histologic typing of soft tissue tumors. 2nd ed. In collaboration with LH Sobin and pathologists in 9 countries. Berlin: Springer-Verlag, 1994.
17. Russel WO, Cohen J, Enzinger FM, et al. A clinical and pathological staging system for soft tissue sarcomas. Cancer 1977;40:1562–1570.
18. Enneking WF. Musculoskeletal tumor surgery. New York: Churchill Livingstone, 1983.
19. Moore GE, Ure B. One-stage pancreatoduodenectomy with resection of the superior mesenteric vein. Surgery 1954;35: 734–742.
20. Piorkowski RJ, et al. Pancreatic and periampullary carcinoma—experience with 200 patients over a 12 year period. Am J Surg 1982;143:189–193.
21. Neibling HA. Primary sarcoma of the pancreas. Am Surg 1968; 34:690–693.
22. Brooke WS, Maxwell JG. Primary sarcoma of the pancreas. Am J Surg 1966;112:657–661.
23. Elliott TE, Albertazzi VJ, Danto LA. Pancreatic liposarcoma: case report with review of retroperitoneal liposarcomas. Cancer 1980;45:1720–1723.
24. ReMine WH. The surgical management of malignant lesions of the pancreas. Jpn J Surg 1979;9:271–278.
25. Ross DE. Cancer of the pancreas with two case reports of five years survival. Am J Surg 1957;93:990–994.
26. Lindberg RD, Martin RG, Romsdahl MM, et al. Conservative surgery and postoperative radiotherapy in 300 adults with soft tissue sarcomas. Cancer 1981;47:2391–2395.
27. Keus RB, Rutgers EJT, Ho GH, et al. Limb-sparing therapy of extremity soft tissue sarcomas: treatment outcome and longterm functional results. Eur J Cancer 1994;30A:1459–1463.
28. Issels R. Soft tissue sarcomas—what is currently being done? Eur J Surg Oncol 1995;21:469–477.

# 66

# *Pancreatic Lymphoma*

Lee Jenkins and Richard Prinz

A mass in the head of the pancreas raises the spectre of neoplasia. Most pancreatic masses are malignant, and the vast majority of these are adenocarcinomas. The prognosis of adenocarcinoma of the pancreas has been relatively bleak, although advances have been made in recent years. Because of the poor prognosis of ductal carcinoma of the pancreas, a defeatist attitude can be engendered when a physician encounters a patient with a mass in the pancreas. A fatalistic approach to the diagnosis and treatment of pancreatic masses ill serves those patients who have more favorable lesions. Lymphoma is an excellent example of the importance of recognizing that not all masses in the pancreas are adenocarcinomas. With appropriate therapy, pancreatic lymphoma is associated with a reasonably good outcome. Without treatment, its prognosis parallels that of untreated adenocarcinoma of the pancreas. It is therefore imperative to evaluate all patients with pancreatic masses to ensure that an accurate diagnosis is made and optimal therapy is administered. This chapter reviews the clinical presentation, methods of diagnosis, characterization of tumor type, and treatment of pancreatic lymphoma.

## BACKGROUND

Lymphoma is a malignant neoplasm that originates from the B or T lymphocytes. It usually presents as nontender lymphadenopathy involving one or more lymph node basins, but it can involve virtually any organ of the body. The lymphadenopathy may be asymptomatic or may be accompanied by systemic findings including fever, night sweats, weight loss, and pruritus. When present, these symptoms connote a poorer prognosis (1). With involvement of extranodal tissue, site-specific symptoms can ensue including bone, back, and abdominal pain. Gastrointestinal (GI) tract involvement can be accompanied by nausea, vomiting, anorexia, early satiety, and upper GI hemorrhage. Jaundice occurs in 1.3% of patients with lymphoma, from involvement of the pancreas and extrahepatic biliary tree (2).

Lymphomas are divided into Hodgkin's disease, characterized by the presence of Reed-Sternberg cells, and the non-Hodgkin's lymphomas (NHLs). Hodgkin's disease is subclassified into four subtypes under the Rye system—lymphocyte predominant, mixed cellular, lymphocyte depleted, and nodular sclerosing. Characteristically, Hodgkin's disease involves contiguous lymph node basins. Most patients present with stage I or IIa disease under the Ann Arbor staging system (Table 66.1), and involvement of extranodal tissue is uncommon.

No single classification system exists for NHL. The Rappaport system proposed in 1966 was somewhat successful in estimating prognosis, and because of this usefulness, it was the most commonly used system in the 1980s. The principal defining characteristics under the Rappaport system are cell type (histiocytic, lymphocytic, lymphoblastic, etc.) and growth pattern within the individual lymph nodes (nodular vs. diffuse). With the development of immunohistochemical staining techniques, further differentiation of NHLs became possible, and the Rappaport system has been supplanted by the World Health Organization's working formulation proposed in 1982. This system adds cellular grade—low, intermediate, and high—as a third factor for categorization. Unlike Hodgkin's disease, NHLs frequently involve noncontiguous lymph node basins and extranodal tissue and are often disseminated at the time of diagnosis. Jones et al. (3) examined 405 cases of NHL and found that 39% of patients presented with stage IV disease, including 16% with GI involvement at the time of diagnosis. When considering only patients with diffuse subtypes of NHL, 43% presented with stage IV disease, and GI involvement was present in 22–39%. Rudders et al. (4) found 39 (10%) primary extranodal lymphomas among 380 patients with NHL. Although one-third were of GI tract origin, no patient in their series had primary pancreatic lymphoma.

## PRESENTATION

Pancreatic involvement in Hodgkin's lymphoma is rare, but it is not uncommon in non-Hodgkin's lymphoma. This is particularly true of the diffuse histiocytic subtype of NHL, in which up to 29% of patients are found to have pancreatic involvement at autopsy (5). Lymphoma initially presenting as a pancreatic mass is less common, occurring in 0.7–2.2% of patients with NHL (6, 7). Less than 5% of pancreatic masses are found to be lymphomas, with reported series ranging from 0.16 to 4.9% (3, 7–9). When lymphoma predominantly involves the pancreas, the resulting symptoms are due primarily to the location and size of the mass rather than its lymphomatous nature. As such, its presentation is similar to that of pancreatic adenocarcinoma. The most common symptoms reported with pancreatic lymphoma are abdominal pain (56–86%), nausea and vomiting (33–71%), weight loss (42–77%), anorexia (42–77%), and jaundice (36–57%) (7, 10–13). Relatively few patients present with systemic symptoms typically associated with lymphoma, such as a history of fever or night sweats (0–22%) or pruritus (0–17%) (7, 10–13). Additional symptoms related to the position of the mass and its bulky nature have been described. Webb et al. (7) found symptoms of gastric outlet obstruction in three of nine patients (33%). Hart et al. (12) reported that 2 of 14 patients (14%) in their series had evidence of upper GI hemorrhage, and 1 patient (7%) had new-onset diabetes. Mansour et al. (10) also found new-onset diabetes in 1 of 12 patients (8%), while only 1 patient had evidence of upper GI bleeding (8%). Freed et al. (14) reported a patient with acute pancreatitis and pancreatic abscess formation secondary to lymphomatous involvement of the pancreas. In patients with pancreatitis and no evidence of the commonly associated risk factors of alcohol abuse and/or biliary

**TABLE 66.1. Ann Arbor Staging System for Lymphoma**

| | |
|---|---|
| Stage I | Disease restricted to one lymph node–bearing area |
| Stage II | Two or more areas of nodal involvement on one side of the diaphragm |
| Stage III | Lymphatic involvement on both sides of the diaphragm |
| Stage IV | Liver, bone marrow, or other extensive, extranodal disease present |
| Substage E | Localized extranodal disease present |
| Symptom status | |
| a | Absence of fevers, night sweats, or weight loss |
| b | Unexplained fevers above 38°C, night sweats, loss of more than 10% of body weight in the preceding 6 months |

tract disease, clinicians should remember that lymphoma and other pancreatic malignancies can present in this fashion. This is particularly true if the patient has a mass lesion in the pancreatic head.

## DIAGNOSIS

Several factors may suggest the diagnosis of lymphoma in a patient with a pancreatic mass. These include a prior history of lymphoma; a history of immunosuppression or immune system compromise; a palpable abdominal mass, palpable peripheral lymphadenopathy, and/or chylous ascites; and a short duration of symptoms. A past history of lymphoma suggests the possibility of recurrent disease as the etiology of the pancreatic mass. Immunodeficiency has been demonstrated to be a risk factor for lymphoma (15). Furthermore, immunodeficiency-related lymphomas, including AIDS-associated malignant lymphoma and organ transplantation–related lymphoma, are typically (80–90%) high-grade, B-cell varieties of NHL (15). They are frequently related to Epstein-Barr virus infection and involve extranodal tissue in 75–90% of patients. The GI tract is involved in 26% of these patients (15–17). Palpable peripheral lymphadenopathy and a palpable abdominal mass are frequent findings in patients with pancreatic lymphoma, occurring in 33% (7, 10, 18) and 33–57%, respectively (7, 10–13). Abdominal involvement in lymphoma is the most common cause of chylous ascites in the adult population (19, 20). Therefore, the presence of chylous ascites in the setting of a mass in the head of the pancreas is highly suggestive of pancreatic lymphoma. A palpable abdominal mass, peripheral lymphadenopathy, and chylous ascites are very uncommon findings in pancreatic adenocarcinoma. Mansour et al. (10) noted that a long history of symptoms is suggestive of lymphoma. Most other authors have found that patients with pancreatic lymphoma usually present with symptoms they have had for 6 weeks or less (2, 7, 11, 14, 18).

Tuchek et al. (11) reported that patients with pancreatic lymphoma are older than the typical patient with pancreatic adenocarcinoma, with a mean age at diagnosis of 68 years. Crist et al., in a series of adenocarcinomas of the pancreas, reported a mean age of 58 years (21). However, other authors, including Hart et al. (12), Brown et al. (13), Boddie et al. (2), and Young et al. (18), have reported that the age profiles of their patients were more similar to those with pancreatic adenocarcinoma; the mean ages were 59 years (Hart et al. and Brown et al.), 38 years (Boddie et al.), and 54 years (Young et al.). Because of the relative rarity of pancreatic lymphoma, each series involves only a small number of patients. Sampling error is therefore likely, making comparisons of this sort very difficult.

Most patients with pancreatic involvement in lymphoma have laboratory evidence of biliary obstruction. Hyperbilirubinemia occurs in 36–57% of patients (7, 10–13). An elevated alkaline phosphatase level is found in 33–89% (7, 11) of patients, and hepatic transaminases are also elevated in 57–78% (7, 11). However, lymphomatous lesions in the pancreatic head can become quite large prior to the development of jaundice. Those that occur in the body and tail of the pancreas, like adenocarcinomas occurring in these locations, may not be accompanied by any biochemical abnormalities. Elevation of the white blood cell count is an infrequent finding, occurring in 0–8% of patients (11).

Computed tomography (CT) is currently the most useful imaging test for evaluating pancreatic masses. Findings on CT that suggest lymphoma include the presence of a homogeneous pancreatic mass larger than 10 cm, retroperitoneal adenopathy, and/or direct invasion of retroperitoneal structures (Fig. 66.1*A*) (22, 23). In a review of 100 consecutive patients with pancreatic adenocarcinoma, Ward et al. (24) found that 60% were 4–6 cm and that no tumors were larger than 10 cm. Most lymphomas that have been evaluated with CT have been larger than 6 cm. Tuchek et al. (11) reported three of seven lymphoma patients with masses 10 cm or larger, with five of seven being 6 cm or larger. Webb et al. (7) found that the pancreatic lymphomas had a median mass size of 7 cm, with eight of nine patients having masses 6 cm or larger. Mansour et al. (10) found that 4 of their 12 patients had masses larger than 10 cm. Several case reports have also described masses that were 8 cm or larger (14, 18, 25–29).

Prayer et al. (23) compared the CT findings in 10 patients with histologically confirmed pancreatic lymphoma with CTs from 50 patients with histologically confirmed nonlymphomatous pancreatic masses. They found that 50% of the lymphomas were larger than 10 cm and the remaining 50% were 5–10 cm. In comparison, 76% of the nonlymphomatous masses were less than 5 cm, and none were larger than 10 cm. Additionally, lymphomas were more likely to appear homogeneous (100 vs. 28%), to involve retroperitoneal lymph nodes (70 vs. 58%), and to invade retroperitoneal structures (90 vs. 22%). Involvement of lymph nodes below the renal veins was particularly suggestive of lymphoma. Although only 30% of the patients with lymphoma had lymphadenopathy below the renal veins, this was significantly more common than the 2% involvement seen with nonlymphomatous masses.

Although they are not routinely needed in the evaluation of pancreatic masses, findings from several other studies can suggest lymphoma. Barium swallow may demonstrate distortion of the duodenal c-loop or duodenal obstruction (10). Endoscopic retrograde cholangiopancreatography may demonstrate normal pancreatic ductal anatomy with external duct compression or even a cutoff sign (10, 11, 30). Lymphoma appears on mesenteric angiography as a hypovascular mass that displaces the large pancreatic and small intrapancreatic arteries (Fig. 66.1*B*) (31). This is in contrast to adenocarcinoma and cystadenocarcinoma of the pancreas, which typically appear as hypervascular masses with little associated mass effect. As endoscopic ultrasound (EUS) becomes more widely available as an adjunct in the preoperative assessment of pancreatic masses, it may be useful in demonstrating retroperitoneal and peripancreatic lymphadenopathy suggesting pancreatic lymphoma (32).

The key to proper management of pancreatic lymphoma is correct tissue diagnosis. If the clinical picture is consistent with pancreatic lymphoma, it is desirable to confirm the diagnosis without performing an exploratory laparotomy. In a patient with accessible peripheral lymphadenopathy, this can be best

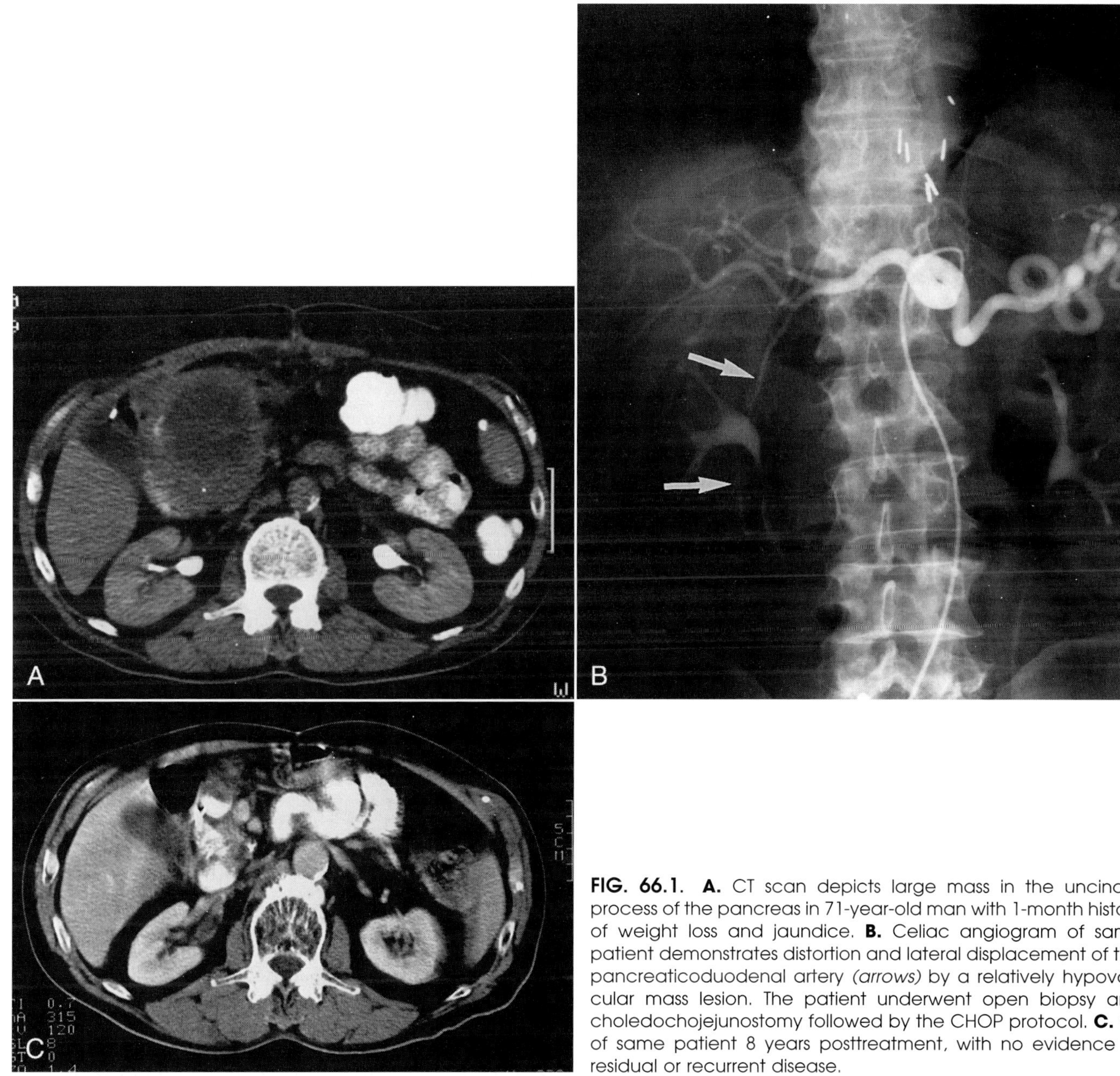


**FIG. 66.1.** **A.** CT scan depicts large mass in the uncinate process of the pancreas in 71-year-old man with 1-month history of weight loss and jaundice. **B.** Celiac angiogram of same patient demonstrates distortion and lateral displacement of the pancreaticoduodenal artery *(arrows)* by a relatively hypovascular mass lesion. The patient underwent open biopsy and choledochojejunostomy followed by the CHOP protocol. **C.** CT of same patient 8 years posttreatment, with no evidence of residual or recurrent disease.

achieved with an excisional lymph node biopsy. In the absence of peripheral lymphadenopathy, options include bone marrow biopsy, CT- or ultrasound-guided percutaneous biopsy of the pancreatic mass, or laparoscopic pancreatic needle biopsy. Of these options, CT-guided biopsy appears to be the best first alternative in patients with suspected pancreatic lymphoma. Webb et al. (7) reported correct diagnosis in four of four attempted CT-guided percutaneous biopsies. Fine-needle aspiration (FNA) of the pancreas for suspected carcinoma has been reported to have sensitivity rates of 76–87% and specificity rates approaching 100% (33–35). Additionally, with the advent of improved cytologic techniques, including immunohistochemical staining, previously reported difficulties in differentiating lymphoma from anaplastic carcinoma (26) present less of a problem (36, 37).

Other authors have had less success with percutaneous biopsy. Tuchek et al. (11) had no correct diagnoses among five patients who underwent CT-guided percutaneous pancreatic biopsy. Mansour et al. (10) had two nondiagnostic samples and two misdiagnoses as adenocarcinoma among four percutaneous biopsies performed on patients in their series. Fine-needle biopsy was also attempted in the patient reported by Shtamler et al. (28); a nondiagnostic sample was obtained, and the patient developed severe intraperitoneal hemorrhage requiring emergent operation. Clearly a team consisting of a skilled invasive radiologist and an experienced cytopathologist is needed if optimal results are to be obtained with percutaneous needle biopsy of a suspected pancreatic lymphoma.

Less than 50% of patients with NHL will have bone marrow involvement at the time of their initial presentation, and this limits the diagnostic yield of bone marrow biopsy. Mansour et al. (10) performed bone marrow biopsy in all 12 of their patients with pancreatic lymphoma but found no positive specimens.

Recently, laparoscopy has been advocated as a means of prelaparotomy staging of pancreatic cancer (38, 39). Laparoscopy, by detecting unsuspected peritoneal seeding and liver metastases, may allow the patient to avoid the morbidity of a full laparotomy. It can also be used for biopsy of suspected pancreatic lymphomas. The principal advantage of CT-guided FNA in the setting of suspected pancreatic lymphoma is that it avoids the use of general anesthesia, which is usually required with laparoscopic needle biopsy.

Tuchek et al. (11) and Hart et al. (12) have argued that exploratory laparotomy is necessary in patients with pancreatic lymphoma, citing the need for appropriate staging of the lymphoma and for obtaining sufficient tissue for subclassification. Conversely, Webb et al. (7) state that exploratory laparotomy is not required for appropriate management of pancreatic lymphoma if the diagnosis can be confirmed by other means. They point out that recommended therapy for pancreatic involvement with lymphoma consists of systemic chemotherapy alone, without radiation therapy. This therapeutic approach eliminates the need for more precise staging than that obtained by CT scanning of the abdomen and CT-directed biopsy. They further state that there is little reason to subclassify the lymphoma precisely, as most are high grade, and therefore aggressive chemotherapy is appropriate in all patients. The gain associated with further staging and subclassification afforded by exploratory laparotomy is marginal and probably does not outweigh the risk of surgery. In their series, Tuchek et al. (11) had one mortality, secondary to pulmonary embolism, among the six patients who underwent exploratory laparotomy—a 17% mortality rate.

Our approach is to perform laparotomy only when CT-guided biopsy is not diagnostic or when there is an associated condition requiring laparotomy, such as gastric outlet obstruction. We do not advise routine biopsy of all pancreatic masses but use it selectively when we have a high index of suspicion that the mass is a lymphoma.

## HISTOLOGY

Hodgkin's disease rarely presents with primary pancreatic involvement. Apparently, only two patients have been reported in the literature. The first, a 28-year-old white male reported by Boddie et al. (2), was diagnosed with stage IIb, mixed-cellular Hodgkin's disease. He was initially treated with ionizing radiation, 3800 rads in a mantle distribution. Two recurrences were treated with radiation therapy and MOPP chemotherapy. He subsequently developed jaundice and was found on exploration to have Hodgkin's involvement of the porta hepatis and peripancreatic tissue. The histology at that time was lymphocyte depleted. He became septic secondary to leakage from his choledochojejunostomy and died 2 months postoperatively. The second patient was a 68-year-old woman reported by Benning et al. (40). She had primary pancreatic Hodgkin's disease at the time of initial diagnosis.

The remaining patients reported in the literature have all had NHLs. Under the Rappaport system of classification, diffuse histiocytic lymphoma is the most common histologic type found in the pancreas, accounting for two-thirds of cases (7, 11–13, 25). The equivalent classes under the WHO working formulation would be either intermediate-grade diffuse, large cell or high-grade large cell, immunoblastic (41). Mixed histiocytic and lymphocytic (0–22%), poorly differentiated lymphocytic (10–18%), and well-differentiated lymphocytic (0–8%) were the next most commonly observed histologic types (7, 12, 13, 25). Rarely reported histologic types include Burkitt's lymphoma (25), T-cell lymphoma (12), and undifferentiated non-Burkitt's lymphoma (2, 12).

## TREATMENT

In the early 1980s, Coltman et al. (42) demonstrated that high-grade NHLs could be cured with combination chemotherapy using the CHOP (cyclophosphamide, hydroxydaunorubicin, oncovin, and prednisone) regimen. Complete response rates with this regimen were 40–55%, with 30–35% long-term survivors (1). Subsequent studies have added additional agents to the CHOP regimen. Combinations used include CAMEL (cyclophosphamide, adriamycin, VP-16, methotrexate, and leucovorin rescue), MACOP-B (methotrexate, adriamycin, cyclophosphamide, vincristine, prednisone, and bleomycin), and ProMACE-MOPP (alternating cycles of *(a)* prednisone, methotrexate, adriamycin, cyclophosphamide, and VP-16 and *(b)* prednisone, nitrogen mustard, oncovin, and procarbazine). In trials directly comparing CHOP with these subsequent regimens, no additional benefit was observed with the newer-generation drugs (43). However, increased morbidity and mortality did occur with their use. Combination chemotherapy with CHOP therefore remains the best available treatment for patients with advanced-stage intermediate- and high-grade NHL. Current recommendations for the CHOP regimen are at least six 21-day cycles consisting of cyclophosphamide 750 mg/m$^2$, doxorubicin 50 mg/m$^2$, and oncovin 1.4 mg/m$^2$ administered intravenously on day 1. On days 1–5, 100 mg of prednisone is taken orally. Treatment is typically continued for two cycles beyond remission.

AIDS-associated lymphoma is extremely resistant to chemotherapy, with complete remission occurring in only 20–28% of patients treated with standard protocols (15). More aggressive chemotherapeutic regimens have fared no better and have resulted in unacceptably high rates of morbidity and mortality (up to 78%) secondary to opportunistic infection (15). Currently under investigation as potential treatments are interferon-$\alpha$, interleukin-2, antiidiotype antibody therapy, and immunotoxin therapy. At present, these agents show no proven benefit over CHOP used alone. Their ultimate role in lymphoma may be in the treatment of low-grade lymphomas, which have a more indolent course but respond poorly to chemotherapeutic intervention (1).

The patient with lymphoma involving the pancreas usually requires treatment of obstructive jaundice, so that hepatic function can be normalized before treatment with cytotoxic chemotherapeutic agents begins. Alternatives for managing biliary obstruction include noncytotoxic chemotherapy, ionizing radiation, endoscopic stenting, and surgical biliary bypass. Boddie et al. (2) used ionizing radiation in five patients to relieve biliary obstruction. Daily doses of 180–400 rads were used, with total doses below 2000 rads. They reported dramatic responses, with resolution of jaundice within 2 weeks of onset of therapy. However, all five of their patients died within 6 months of treatment, which prevented investigation of long-term results and complications. Webb et al. (7) have suggested that potential long-term complications from this approach could include biliary stricture, duodenal stricture, and duodenal ulceration.

Webb et al. at Johns Hopkins University (7) used noncytotoxic chemotherapy to treat obstructive jaundice in three patients. Jaundice resolved in all three within 2 weeks of initiating therapy. The regimen consisted of cyclophosphamide 1000 mg/m$^2$ and prednisone 100 mg/m$^2$ orally for 5 days. After resolution of jaundice, one of the combined chemotherapy regimens was started. Tuchek et al. (11) found that more effective and more rapid relief of biliary obstruction was provided by operative bypass than by chemotherapy for jaundiced patients. Hart et al. (12) also used operative bypass and endoscopic stenting in their jaundiced patients, with good results. All approaches should result in rapid resolution of jaundice, allowing early initiation of definitive chemotherapy. Given the higher potential for morbidity using ionizing radiation and operative decompression, we favor chemotherapeutic treatment of biliary obstruction as first-line therapy in patients with histologically confirmed lymphoma. We reserve endoscopic and operative decompression for refractory cases and those who require operative intervention for other reasons (e.g., gastric outlet obstruction).

## PROGNOSIS

Pancreatic lymphoma is often quite responsive to chemotherapy, and a good long-term prognosis can be expected. Tuchek et al. (11) reported a mean survival of 6.3 years among three patients treated with combination chemotherapy, including one patient alive at 8 years, without evidence of disease. Among four untreated patients, mean survival was 5 months, with a maximum survival of 8 months. Mansour et al. (10) reported 4 long-term survivors in their series of 12 patients, including disease-free survivors who were alive at 3 and 7 years. Webb et al. (7) reported a 66% complete response rate, with patients alive with no evidence of disease at 14, 21, 31, 37, 69, and 95 months posttreatment. Hart et al. (12) reported 6 of 14 patients alive and disease free an average of 32 months posttreatment. These results certainly indicate that an aggressive approach to the diagnosis and treatment of pancreatic lymphoma is warranted.

## SUMMARY

Pancreatic involvement in lymphoma is not uncommon in NHLs, and obstructive jaundice can occur in up to 1.3% of patients with NHL. A diagnosis of pancreatic involvement with lymphoma in a patient with a pancreatic mass is suggested by a history of lymphoma or immunocompromise or the presence of a palpable abdominal mass, peripheral lymphadenopathy, or chylous ascites. CT scanning typically demonstrates a mass lesion of the pancreas that is larger than 6 cm, associated with retroperitoneal lymphadenopathy. When suspected preoperatively, pancreatic lymphoma can be diagnosed by peripheral lymph node biopsy or CT-guided needle biopsy, thus avoiding laparotomy. Treatment consists of combination chemotherapy (CHOP). Obstructive jaundice must be rectified before this regimen can be instituted. Approximately 50% of patients will have a complete response to therapy, with one-third being cured.

## REFERENCES


1. Foon KA, Fisher RI. Lymphomas. In: Beutler E, Lichtman MA, Coller BS, Kipps TJ, eds. Williams' hematology. 5th ed. New York: McGraw-Hill, 1995:1076–1096.
2. Boddie AW Jr, Eisenberg BL, Mullins JD, Schlichtemeier AL. The diagnosis and treatment of obstructive jaundice secondary to malignant lymphoma: a problem in multidisciplinary management. J Surg Oncol 1980; 14:111–123.
3. Jones SE, Fuks Z, Bull M, Kadin ME, Dorfman RF, et al. Non-Hodgkin's lymphomas IV. Clinicopathologic correlation in 405 cases. Cancer 1973;31:806–823.
4. Rudders RA, Ross ME, DeLellis RA. Primary extranodal lymphoma. Cancer 1978;42:406–416.
5. Rosenberg SA, Diamond HD, Jaslowitz B, Craver LF. Lymphosarcoma: a review of 1269 cases. Medicine 1961;61:31–84.
6. Goffinet DR, Warnke R, Dunnick NR, Castellino R, Glatstein E, et al. Clinical and surgical (laparotomy) evaluation of patients with non-Hodgkin's lymphomas. Cancer Treat Rep 1977;61:981–992.
7. Webb TH, Lillemoe KD, Pitt HA, Jones RJ, Cameron JL. Pancreatic lymphoma: is surgery mandatory for diagnosis and treatment? Ann Surg 1989;209:25–30.
8. Reed K, Vose PC, Jarstfer BS. Pancreatic cancer. Am J Surg 1979;138:929–932.
9. Baylor SM, Berg JW. Cross-classification of survival characteristics of 5000 cases of pancreatic cancer. J Surg Oncol 1973;5: 335–358.
10. Mansour GMI, Cucchiaro G, Niotis MT, Fetter BF, Moore J, et al. Surgical management of pancreatic lymphoma. Arch Surg 1989;124:1287–1289.
11. Tuchek JM, De Jong SA, Pickleman J. Diagnosis, surgical intervention, and prognosis of primary pancreatic lymphoma. Am Surg 1993;59:513–518.
12. Hart MJ, White TT, Brown PC, Freeny PC. Potentially curable masses in the pancreas. Am J Surg 1987;154:134–136.
13. Brown PC, Hart MJ, White TT. Pancreatic lymphoma, diagnosis and management. Int J Pancreat 1987;2:93–100.
14. Freed JS, Dreiling DA, Reiner MA. Non-Hodgkin's lymphoma of the pancreas producing acute pancreatitis and pancreatic abscess. Mt Sinai J Med 1983;50:424–427.
15. Levine AM. Aids-associated malignant lymphoma. Med Clin North Am 1992;76(1):253–268.
16. Kaplan LD, Abrams DI, Feigal E, McGrath M, Kahn J, et al. AIDS-associated non-Hodgkin's lymphoma in San Francisco. JAMA 1989;261:719–724.
17. Ziegler JL, Beckstead JA, Volberding PA, Abrams DI, Levine AM, et al. Non-Hodgkin's lymphoma in 90 homosexual men. N Engl J Med 1984;311:565–569.
18. Young IF, Roberts-Thomson IC, Sullivan JR. Histiocytic lymphoma presenting with extrahepatic biliary obstruction: a report of three cases. Aust NZ J Surg 1981;51:181–183.
19. Fischer MG, Kabakow B. Lymphoma of the pancreas. Mt Sinai J Med 1987;54:423–426.
20. Press OW, Press NO, Kaufman SD. Evaluation and management of chylous ascites. Ann Intern Med 1982;96:358–364.
21. Crist DW, Sitzmann JV, Cameron JL. Improved hospital morbidity, mortality, and survival after the Whipple procedure. Ann Surg 1987;206:358–365.
22. Friedman AC, Edmonds PR. Rare pancreatic malignancies. Radiol Clin North Am 1989;27:177–190.
23. Prayer L, Schurawitzki H, Mallek R, Mostbeck G. CT in pancreatic involvement of non-Hodgkin lymphoma. Acta Radiol 1992;33: 123–127.
24. Ward EM, Stephens DH, Sheedy PF. Computer tomographic characteristics of pancreatic carcinoma: an analysis of 100 cases. Radiographics 1983;3:547–563.
25. Cappell MS, Yao F, Cho KC, Axiotis CA. Lymphoma predominantly involving the pancreas. Dig Dis Sci 1989;34(6):942–947.
26. Ackerman NB, Aust JC, Bredenberg CE, Hanson VA, Rogers LS. Problems in differentiating between pancreatic lymphoma and anaplastic carcinoma and their management. Ann Surg 1976; 184:705–708.
27. Teefey SA, Stephens DH, Sheedy PF II. CT appearance of primary pancreatic lymphoma. Gastrointest Radiol 1986;11:41–43.
28. Shtamler B, Bickel A, Manor E, Shahar MB, Kuten A, Suprun H. Primary lymphoma of the head of the pancreas. J Surg Oncol 1988;38:48–51.
29. Case records of the Massachusetts General Hospital (case 11-1985). N Engl J Med 1985;312:706–711.
30. Borrowdale R, Strong RW. Primary lymphoma of the pancreas. Aust NZ J Surg 1994;64:444–446.
31. Neiman HL, Goldstein HM, Silverman PJ, Bookstein JJ. Angiographic features of peripancreatic malignant lymphoma. Radiology 1975;115:589–592.
32. Rosch T, Braig C, Gain T, Feuerbach S, Siewert JR, et al. Staging of pancreatic and ampullary carcinoma by endoscopic ultrasonography. Gastroenterology 1992;102:188–199.
33. Al-Kaisi N, Siegler EE. Fine needle aspiration cytology of the pancreas. Acta Cytol 1989;33(2):145–152.
34. Pinto MM, Avila NA, Criscuolo EM. Fine needle aspiration of the pancreas. Acta Cytol 1988;32:39–42.
35. Pilotti S, Rilke F, Claren R, Milella M, Lombardi L. Conclusive diagnosis of hepatic and pancreatic malignancies by fine needle aspiration. Acta Cytol 1988;32:27–37.
36. Imam A, Taylor CR. Application of immunohistochemical methods in the diagnosis of malignant disease. Cancer Invest 1985;3: 339–359.

37. Picker LJ, Weiss LM, Medeiros LJ, Wood GS, Warnke RA. Immunophenotypic criteria for the diagnosis of non-Hodgkin's lymphoma. Am J Pathol 1987;128:181–201.
38. John TG, Greig JD, Carter DC, Garden OJ. Carcinoma of the pancreatic head and periampullary region: tumor staging with laparoscopy and laparoscopic ultrasonography. Ann Surg 1995; 221:156–164.
39. Warshaw AL, Tepper JE, Shipley WU. Laparoscopy in the staging and planning of therapy for pancreatic cancer. Am J Surg 1986;151:76–80.
40. Benning TL, Silverman JF, Berns LA, Geisinger KR. Fine needle aspiration of metastatic and hematologic malignancies clinically mimicking pancreatic carcinoma. Acta Cytol 1992;36:471–476.
41. Banks PM. Pathology of malignant lymphomas. In: Beutler E, Lichtman MA, Coller BS, Kipps TJ, eds. Williams' hematology. 5th ed. New York: McGraw-Hill, 1995:1049–1057.
42. Coltman CA Jr, Dahlberg S, Jones SE, Miller TP, Dana BW, et al. CHOP is curative in thirty percent of patients with diffuse large cell lymphoma: a twelve year Southwest Oncology Group follow-up. Proc Am Soc Clin Oncol 1986;5:197.
43. Fisher RI, Gaynor ER, Dahlberg S, Oken MM, Grogan TM, et al. Comparison of a standard regimen (CHOP) with three intensive chemotherapy regimens for advanced non-Hodgkins lymphoma. N Engl J Med 1993;328:1002–1006.

# 67

# *Metastases to the Pancreas*

Daniel J. Deziel

Metastatic tumors to the pancreas are not infrequent, but they are an uncommon cause of clinically relevant symptoms. With few exceptions, they are associated with metastatic disease at other, extrapancreatic sites. When secondary pancreatic tumors are diagnosed prior to death, the patient is often at an advanced stage of disease. For these reasons, while of interest to pancreatic surgeons, the topic has received relatively little attention in the literature.

Current diagnostic modalities have increased the antemortem recognition of metastases to the pancreas. Formerly, the diagnosis depended on progression of clinical symptoms or subsequent laparotomy or autopsy. The use of serum tumor markers and improved imaging systems for surveillance of patients following treatment of primary malignancies has allowed earlier and more accurate detection of metastatic lesions. The availability of percutaneous fine-needle aspiration has made it further possible to differentiate some cases of secondary pancreatic tumors from primary malignancies. The overall necessity for treatment specifically aimed at metastatic lesions in the pancreas remains limited. However, surgical intervention may be warranted in selected situations for palliation of tumor-related complications or as an attempt to prolong disease-free survival, depending upon the specifics of tumor biology and the extent of disease.

## PATHOLOGY

Metastases to the pancreas have been observed in 3–12% of autopsy cases with malignant disease (1–4). The frequency of metastatic tumors in the pancreas varies in comparison to primary pancreatic malignancy according to the population studied. Berge and Lundberg examined a well-defined population in which 62.6% of individuals who died in Malmö, Sweden, were autopsied (2). Of 16,294 total necropsies, 7,246 individuals had malignant tumors; among these there were 297 with primary pancreatic cancers and 187 with metastatic tumors to the pancreas. Cubilla and Fitzgerald, on the other hand, found metastatic pancreatic involvement more often than primary cancer in a cancer center–based series (3). Of 2587 consecutive autopsies at Memorial Hospital in New York, there were 261 individuals with metastases to the pancreas and 63 with primary pancreatic neoplasms. Similarly, Abrams et al. documented 32 cases of primary pancreatic cancer and 116 cases of metastases to the pancreas in a series of 1000 consecutive autopsies on individuals with epithelial malignancies (4). In the clinical experience from the Mayo Clinic, metastases accounted for only 2% of pancreatic tumors requiring operation (5).

The lung is the most common site of primary tumors that metastasize to the pancreas. In combined autopsy series of 734 patients (Table 67.1), the origin of pancreatic metastases in order of frequency included lung (174), breast (100), melanoma (89), stomach (68), colon or rectum (43), kidney (29), and ovary (29). A somewhat different relative frequency has been observed in smaller clinical series: renal neoplasms have accounted for a greater proportion of pancreatic metastases, while malignant melanoma has been seen less often (Table 67.2). This difference may be explained by the observation that pancreatic metastases from renal cancer are more often symptomatic than those from melanoma (7).

Although all malignant neoplasms can potentially spread to the pancreas, most metastatic lesions are of epithelial origin. This review specifically excludes pancreatic involvement with lymphoma or systemic hematologic malignancy. Occasionally the pancreas may be involved by various metastatic sarcomas including leiomyosarcoma, chondrosarcoma, osteogenic sarcoma, Ewing's sarcoma, lymphosarcoma, neurofibrosarcoma, and angiosarcoma (1, 3, 8–13). Other cell types that have rarely metastasized to the pancreas include meningioma, medulloblastoma, neuroblastoma, cystosarcoma phyllodes, and cutaneous Merkel cell tumors (3, 10, 14–18).

Certain malignancies have a greater predilection toward pancreatic spread. For example, the prevalence of pancreatic involvement at necropsy has been reported to be 5% in colon cancer (4), 8–12% in carcinoma of the lung (4, 19, 20), 11–19% in breast cancer (4, 21–23), and nearly 40% in melanoma (24, 25). In bronchogenic carcinoma, the incidence of metastases to the pancreas is related to the histologic type of the primary tumor: squamous 3.5%, adenocarcinoma 5%, anaplastic 14%, and "oat cell" or small cell cancer 23–40% (19, 20, 26). A variant of lobular carcinoma of the breast with signet ring features has been described as having a predilection for gastrointestinal metastases. Among four patients with this cell type metastasizing to the gastrointestinal tract, all had serosal pancreatic involvement as well (27).

Metastases may reach the pancreas by any of the recognized routes of tumor dissemination. Hematogenous spread is considered the most frequent. The intraparenchymal location of multiple tumor deposits in a pattern that does not correspond to the anatomic arrangement of peripancreatic lymph nodes supports this premise (10). Blood-borne spread is also evidenced by the typical presence of concurrent metastases at multiple extrapancreatic and extraabdominal sites.

The pancreas may be secondarily involved by metastases spread via the lymphatic system in the form of focal intraglandular lesions or by direct extension of peripancreatic lymph nodes that contain metastatic tumor. The lymphatic route has been considered a likely mode of metastases for colon cancers because the pattern of lymphatic drainage follows the mesocolic vessels to the root of the mesocolon overlying the gland (28). Lymphogenous spread of renal cancers may occur by retrograde lymph flow when tumor infiltrates retroperitoneal lymphatics (29).

**TABLE 67.1. Origin of Pancreatic Metastases in Autopsy Series**[a]

| Reference | Total Number | Primary Site[b] | | | | | | |
|---|---|---|---|---|---|---|---|---|
| | | Lung | Breast | Melanoma | Stomach | Colorectal | Kidney | Ovary |
| Abrams (4) | 116 | 16 | 23 | NA | 28 | 6 | 2 | 10 |
| Berge (2) | 189 | 64 | 11 | 34 | 12 | 11 | 7 | 5 |
| Cubilla (3) | 261 | 49 | 51 | 23 | 19 | 25 | 7 | 13 |
| Havig (6) | 26 | 9 | 0 | 0 | 9 | 0 | 0 | 1 |
| Willis (1) | | | | | | | | |
| Personal series | 15 | 2 | 3 | 1 | 0 | 1 | 1 | 0 |
| Literature | 127 | 34 | 12 | 31 | NA | NA | 12 | NA |
| Total | 734 | 174 | 100 | 89 | 68 | 43 | 29 | 29 |

[a]Excludes lymphoma and hematologic malignancy.
[b]Other primary tumors less frequently seen include soft tissue sarcomas, esophagus, prostate, uterine cervix, liver, thyroid, biliary tract, small intestine, head and neck, salivary gland, bladder, ureter/renal pelvis, testes, adrenal gland, vulva, and skin.

Pulmonary lesions may reach subdiaphragmatic sites via lymphatic communications to the upper abdominal viscera (30). Willis noted that gastric carcinoma could involve the pancreas by lymphatic permeation without gross tumor formation, although he found no evidence of such spread in a series of 500 autopsies for malignant disease (1).

Pancreatic invasion can occur by direct extension of tumors originating in adjacent anatomic structures. Typical primary tumor sites capable of this include the stomach, the transverse colon and colonic flexures, the upper retroperitoneal soft tissues, the kidneys, and any peripancreatic lymph nodes. The sources referenced in this chapter have generally made an effort to differentiate discontinuous pancreatic involvement from contiguous invasion, but this distinction may not always be possible. Willis documented 18 cases of contiguous invasion and 15 cases of hematogenous metastases to the pancreas among 500 autopsies for malignancy (1). Gastric carcinoma was responsible for 13 of the cases of direct invasion. Cubilla and Fitzgerald also found that the stomach was the most common site for primary tumors with direct extension to the pancreas, accounting for 6 of 16 cases among their 2587 autopsies (3). Other primary sites included the colon, duodenum, ovary, gastroesophageal junction, gallbladder, and retroperitoneum.

The histologic pattern of metastases to the pancreas typically demonstrates involvement of the pancreatic lobules. Normal acinar tissue is destroyed and replaced by malignant cells that also invade and widen the interlobular septa (9, 30). A variable degree of inflammatory infiltrate, fibrosis, and necrosis may be present. Intraductal tumor deposits and ductular ectasia with microscopic ductal disruption may also occur (1, 30, 31). The islets of Langerhans are usually preserved by both secondary and primary pancreatic tumors (1, 30). In fact, hyperplasia and hypertrophy of the islets may be present at tumor margins.

The gross patterns of metastatic involvement of the pancreas that have been observed are influenced by the method of detection. Autopsy studies have provided scarce detail regarding glandular morphology. Willis noted that metastatic tumors were usually well-defined nodules, more often multiple than single, and seldom large (1). Clinical reports more often describe solitary larger lesions, which have been selected either because they exceed some clinical threshold for diagnosis (i.e., size, symptoms) or because of a particular treatment rendered (i.e., resection). In patients from five combined series, pancreatic involvement was described as solitary in 50, multiple in 24, and diffuse in 7 (5, 7, 9, 10, 32). Tumors that appear solitary on imaging studies may histologically be composed of multiple small tumor foci (9).

The fact that many reported metastases to the pancreas have been large likely reflects limitations of diagnostic imaging. In the Mayo Clinic experience, only 1 of 27 patients had a tumor under 2 cm (5). Tumor size was 2–5 cm in 8 patients and exceeded 5 cm in 18 patients. Similarly, Boudghène et al. found that 11 of 18

**TABLE 67.2. Origin of Pancreatic Metastases in Clinical Series**[a]

| Reference | Total Number | Primary Site[b] | | | | | |
|---|---|---|---|---|---|---|---|
| | | Lung | Kidney | Breast | Colorectal | Melanoma | Liver |
| Benning (18) | 10 | 4 | 0 | 0 | 0 | 0 | 1 |
| Biset (32) | 7 | 2 | 3 | 0 | 0 | 0 | 0 |
| Boudghène (7) | 24 | 9 | 6 | 1 | 0 | 4 | 0 |
| Carson (17) | 11 | 4 | 1 | 1 | 1 | 0 | 1 |
| Muranka (9) | 30 | 10 | 1 | 5 | 2 | 2 | 3 |
| Opocher (47) | 13 | 1 | 6 | 1 | 0 | 0 | 2 |
| Roland (5) | 27 | 5 | 3 | 3 | 6 | 2 | 0 |
| Rumancik (10) | 7 | 0 | 2 | 2 | 0 | 1 | 0 |
| Swenson (48) | 12 | 3 | 0 | 0 | 3 | 0 | 1 |
| Wernecke (8) | 7 | 2 | 0 | 0 | 2 | 0 | 0 |
| Whittington (42) | 4 | 1 | 1 | 2 | 0 | 0 | 0 |
| Total | 152 | 41 | 23 | 15 | 14 | 9 | 8 |

[a]Excludes lymphoma and hematologic malignancy.
[b]Other primary tumors less frequently seen include stomach, esophagus, soft tissue sarcomas, ovary, biliary tract, uterine cervix, prostate, uterus, skin, duodenum, salivary gland, and testes.

tumors examined by ultrasound and 16 of 29 tumors examined by computed tomography were larger than 2 cm (7). In contradistinction, Wernecke et al. observed that in 6 of 7 patients with ultrasonographically imaged metastases to the pancreas, the lesions were under 2 cm (8). One-half to two-thirds of clinically diagnosed metastases to the pancreas have been located in the head of the gland (5, 10, 17, 28). Presumably, tumors at this site are more likely to cause symptomatic biliary or duodenal obstruction.

Both necropsy and clinical reports agree that the vast majority of patients with metastases to the pancreas have metastatic disease elsewhere. In Berge and Lundberg's comprehensive autopsy series, the pancreas was never the sole site of metastases from any primary tumor (2). Moreover, disease was usually widespread. The number of organs involved in individuals with metastases to the pancreas was distributed as follows: 2 sites (5), 3 sites (7), 4 sites (16), 5 sites (26), and 6 or more sites (135).

## CLINICAL PRESENTATION

The frequency of metastases to the pancreas exceeds the rate of clinical detection. Most secondary pancreatic tumors do not cause organ dysfunction or specific symptoms. Since they are usually diagnosed in patients with advanced malignancy, any direct consequences of the pancreatic lesions may be obscured by manifestations of disease elsewhere. In one review of 222 patients presenting for radiation treatment for unusual metastases, pancreatic involvement was not mentioned (33).

Patients diagnosed with metastases to the pancreas are usually in the 6th or 7th decade of life. Gender distribution corresponds to that of the primary tumor. Jaundice and abdominal pain are the most frequent symptoms of secondary pancreatic tumors (Table 67.3). Other presenting symptoms include weight loss, abdominal mass, gastrointestinal hemorrhage, duodenal obstruction, and inferior vena cava obstruction. Symptoms of exocrine or endocrine insufficiency may occur but are unusual. Gastrointestinal bleeding may be from direct tumor invasion or associated gastritis. Metastatic renal cell cancers are typically hypervascular and have a tendency to present with gastrointestinal hemorrhage (29).

Acute pancreatitis is an unusual but well-recognized manifestation of secondary pancreatic tumors (30, 31, 34–41). Mechanical obstruction of the pancreatic duct by tumor is a plausible initiating event. On histologic examination, intraductal tumor deposits, ductal dilation, and duct rupture can be demonstrated (30, 31, 34). Other possible mechanisms of tumor-induced acute pancreatitis include vascular compromise and tumor necrosis. Acute pancreatitis may occur as the initial manifestation of the primary tumor or later in the course of the disease. Small cell carcinoma of the lung is the primary tumor most frequently associated with metastases-induced acute pancreatitis. Autopsy studies have revealed focal acute

**TABLE 67.3. Clinical Symptoms in 89 Patients with Metastases to the Pancreas**

| Symptom | Number of Patients |
|---|---|
| Asymptomatic | 29 |
| Jaundice | 21 |
| Abdominal or back pain | 19 |
| Weight loss | 7 |
| Abdominal mass | 7 |
| Gastrointestinal bleeding | 5 |
| Intestinal obstruction | 4 |
| Acute pancreatitis | 3 |
| IVC obstruction | 1 |

Data from references 5, 8, 9, 10, 17, 28, 32, and 42.

pancreatitis and fat necrosis in nearly all patients with pancreatic metastases from bronchogenic small cell cancer (26). In some cases, massive necrosis and hemorrhagic pancreatitis have been found.

## DIAGNOSIS

Metastases to the pancreas may be discovered incidentally or during a directed investigation of clinical symptoms. Clinical detection of many lesions is limited by their small size and absence of symptoms. Asymptomatic tumors are often identified when a computed tomographic scan or ultrasound is done for staging or follow-up or when evaluation is prompted by elevated serum tumor markers.

The possibility of metastatic disease should be considered for any pancreatic mass, particularly if the patient has had a previous malignancy. An accurate and well-communicated history is, therefore, of paramount importance. Although metastases to the pancreas may occasionally be the first manifestation of malignancy, most patients have a known primary site (17, 18). The previous tumor may have been chronologically remote from the metachronous pancreatic lesion. This information also may not be consistently communicated to the radiologist or pathologist. Thus, metastatic tumors can be misinterpreted as primary pancreatic malignancies. Whittington et al. found that 12 of 110 patients referred for radiation treatment of primary pancreatic tumors had a previous nonpancreatic malignancy (42). Upon further investigation, five of these patients were found to have metastases to the pancreas. Differentiating secondary from primary pancreatic malignancies has apparent therapeutic implications.

The time interval between the diagnosis of a primary tumor and metastases to the pancreas varies. The apparent disease-free interval is influenced by the type of tumor. Pancreatic metastases from lung cancers tend to be diagnosed early, with a mean interval of 1.5 years (7). Metastatic breast cancer is also usually diagnosed within the first few years, although intervals as long as 18 years have been reported (10, 42–44). Discovery of pancreatic metastases from colon cancer ranges from 6 months to 14 years, with a mean of 32 months (28). A longer average interval of 6 years is more characteristic of melanoma and renal cell cancer; occasionally these tumors have not presented for more than 20 years after the diagnosis of the primary tumor (7, 29, 45, 46).

Imaging by ultrasound or computed tomographic (CT) scan may demonstrate a focal mass or masses (Fig. 67.1), an abnormal contour or enlargement of the gland, and dilation of the pancreatic duct or common bile duct in cases of metastases to the pancreas (7–10, 28, 32). Metastases to the liver or elsewhere outside the pancreas may also be detected. The radiologic features of secondary pancreatic tumors in general are not distinguishable from those of primary neoplasms. The presence of multiple lesions suggests a secondary process, especially in a patient with a history of malignant disease. Additionally, findings of a large mass in the head of the gland without bile duct dilation and preservation of the retropancreatic fat regardless of tumor size may be more indicative of metastatic disease than of a primary pancreatic tumor (7).

On ultrasonography, metastatic lesions are usually solid, regular nodules that are hypoechoic compared with the normal pancreatic parenchyma (7, 8, 32). Some lesions may have a heterogeneous or hyperechoic pattern if fatty or vascular. Rarely, secondary tumors may appear cystic. Experience with endoscopic ultrasonography and metastases to the pancreas has not been widely reported.

Metastatic masses detected by CT scans tend to demonstrate lower attenuation than the surrounding parenchyma (7, 9, 10, 28, 32). Diffuse pancreatic involvement may have an isodense or

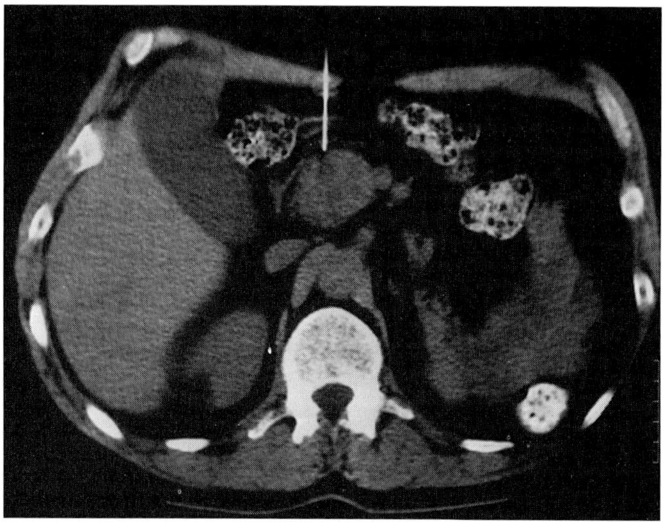

**FIG. 67.1.** CT scan shows a percutaneous biopsy of a mass in the head of the pancreas that was found to be metastatic renal cell carcinoma.

homogeneous attenuation. Smaller lesions that have CT attenuation similar to that of the surrounding parenchyma are not likely to be detected unless they produce an abnormal bulge in the contour of the gland. Ultrasound may sometimes demonstrate the smaller lesions if their acoustic impedance varies sufficiently from that of normal parenchyma (8). On the other hand, dynamic contrast-enhanced CT may detect small lesions not seen by ultrasound and may be better suited to the identification of small lesions in the tail of the gland (32).

Hypervascular tumors may demonstrate intense enhancement in the arterial phase of dynamic CT pancreatography. This most typically occurs with renal cell cancer but may be seen with metastatic breast cancer as well (7, 10, 32). Duplex sonography and angiography (Fig. 67.2) will also demonstrate hypervascular tumors. Demonstration of a hypervascular tumor is more suggestive of a metastatic lesion than of a primary pancreatic malignancy (29, 47).

There are few published descriptions of endoscopic pancreatography in secondary pancreatic tumors. Occlusion and stenosis of the main pancreatic duct are the most common findings, but these do not differentiate metastases from primary tumors or even from benign conditions such as chronic pancreatitis (48). Intraductal filling defects and multiple short asymmetric stenoses of the main pancreatic duct have been noted in metastatic tumors (37, 49).

Percutaneous fine-needle aspiration of pancreatic masses may be useful in diagnosing metastatic tumors. Such biopsies can be performed under ultrasound or CT guidance using a 22-gauge needle. Benning et al. diagnosed secondary pancreatic tumors in 19 patients (9 lymphomas, 10 epithelial malignancies) in a series of 304 pancreatic fine-needle aspirations (18). Thirteen of these patients had a history of prior malignancy. Carson et al. found metastatic malignancy in 13 of 117 pancreatic fine-needle aspirations (17). The fact that 9 of these patients had a prior malignancy again emphasizes the importance of interpreting pathologic material in the appropriate clinical context.

Specific cytologic features may help differentiate primary and secondary tumors. Since most primary pancreatic malignancies are adenocarcinomas, any nonglandular cytomorphology suggests a possible secondary neoplasm. When cellular differentiation is glandular, other cytologic characteristics may indicate a renal, prostatic, or hepatocellular source (17).

## TREATMENT

The treatment of metastases to the pancreas depends on the nature of the primary tumor, the extent of disease, and the presence of organ-specific symptoms or complications. Since most pancreatic metastases are clinically not apparent, no specific therapy is rendered. When pancreatic metastases are known, malignancy is often widespread and the patient's condition poor. Management in this situation is therefore supportive or directed at the systemic disease in general. Survival after the diagnosis of metastases to the pancreas is usually measured in weeks or months. Roland and van Heerden noted a mean survival of 8.7 months following diagnosis of metastases to the pancreas (5). Twenty of 27 patients in their series died within 1 year, and the longest survival time was 26 months.

Pancreas-related conditions that require therapy include pain, exocrine or endocrine insufficiency, obstruction of the biliary or gastrointestinal tracts, gastrointestinal bleeding, and metastases-induced acute pancreatitis. For patients with advanced malignancy and a limited life expectancy, these conditions are treated by nonoperative modalities (pharmacologic, endoscopic, percutaneous) to the extent possible, as long as these approaches offer a reasonable likelihood of relief.

Complications of metastases to the pancreas may prompt operative intervention for palliative intent in patients with a reasonable survival expectancy. Indications for surgery include gastrointestinal bleeding, gastrointestinal obstruction, biliary

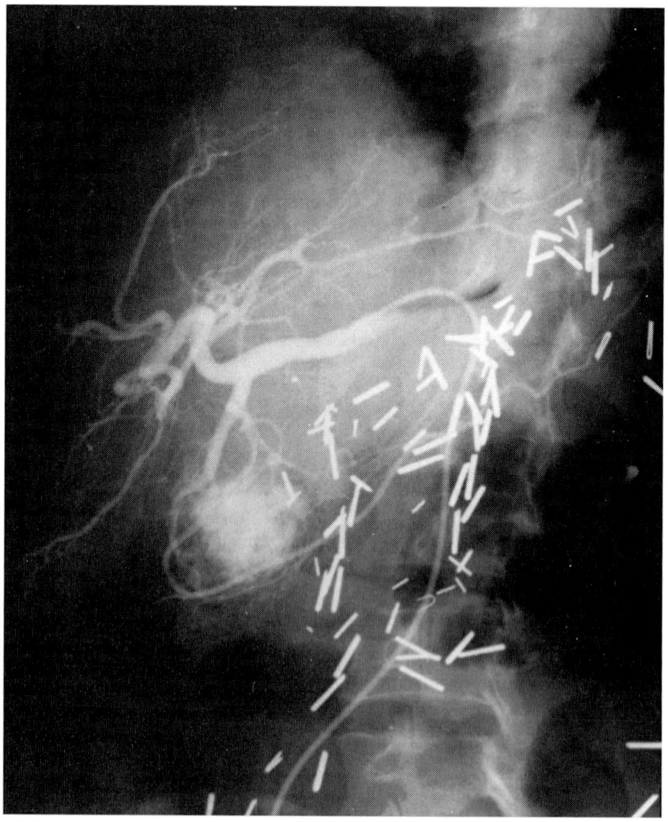

**FIG. 67.2.** Oblique view of an arterial phase angiogram demonstrates hypervascular mass in the head of the pancreas. This was a solitary metastasis from bilateral renal cell cancer. Clips are from previous left radical and right partial nephrectomy. Pancreaticoduodenectomy was subsequently performed. (From Saxon A, Gottesman J, Doolas A. Bilateral hypernephroma with solitary pancreatic metastasis. J Surg Oncol 1980;13:317–322, with permission.).

obstruction, and treatment of complications of pancreatitis such as secondary infection or symptomatic pancreatic pseudocyst. Palliative surgical bypass has been advocated for patients with biliary obstruction and pancreatic metastases as long as diffuse liver metastases are not present (50).

The management of metastases-induced acute pancreatitis merits special consideration. This is a rare consequence of metastatic disease that has most frequently been described with small cell cancer of the lung (30, 31, 34–41). Acute pancreatitis may be the initial manifestation of the malignant process. The diagnosis of metastases as the cause of acute pancreatitis has usually been presumptive, based on clinical and biochemical evidence of acute pancreatitis in a patient with confirmed malignancy from another site and the absence of other usual causes of acute pancreatitis. The pancreatic pathology has been confirmed with subsequent laparotomy or autopsy. The pancreatitis may be severe with evidence of necrosis, sepsis, hemorrhage, and pseudocyst formation. Survival has typically been poor; most patients are dead within a few weeks.

The primary therapeutic decision is whether patients with metastases-induced acute pancreatitis should be given systemic chemotherapy, particularly in metastatic small cell cancer, which can respond to multidrug regimens. It has been suggested that treatment of patients with this condition be based on the severity of the pancreatitis. Conventional supportive management is appropriate for patients with severe pancreatitis who have an extremely poor prognosis and are unlikely to tolerate cytotoxic therapy. For patients with less severe pancreatitis on the basis of standard stratification criteria, chemotherapy has been associated with rapid clinical improvement of pancreatitis and survival of 4–6 months (34–36).

Most patients with metastases to the pancreas have been treated without pancreatic resection. Occasionally, resection has been undertaken for patients with apparent solitary metastases, particularly if there has been a relatively long disease-free interval. Among 27 patients with metastases to the pancreas reviewed at the Mayo Clinic, there were five resections performed, including two distal pancreatectomies, two total pancreatectomies, and one tumor debulking (5). Most reports concerning pancreatic resections for metastatic tumors deal with renal cell carcinoma (29, 45, 46, 51–53). Although the incidence of apparent solitary metastases at any site from renal cell cancer is only 1–3%, resection has been associated with 5-year survivals of 35–50% (54, 55). Stankard and Karl reviewed 16 cases of surgical resection for metastatic renal cell cancer to the pancreas (51). Procedures consisted of 7 pancreaticoduodenectomies, 5 total pancreatectomies, 1 subtotal pancreatectomy, and 3 distal pancreatectomies; there were two postoperative deaths. Two patients died after 6 months and 15 months, respectively, whereas 12 patients were alive with follow-up times ranging from 1–28 months. One patient later had a thyroidectomy for additional metastases. In one study of solitary metastases from renal cell cancer, 10 of 19 patients developed further metastatic lesions at intervals ranging from 3 to 39 months after treatment of the apparent solitary lesion (54). No patients with pancreatic metastases were included in this review, however.

Two reports describe long-term survival after pancreatic resection for metastatic breast cancer. In both patients the diagnosis was not suspected at the time of operation, and resection was done for a presumed primary pancreatic tumor. Azzarelli et al. performed pancreaticoduodenectomy on a 49-year-old woman for metastatic infiltrating lobular carcinoma 4 years after radical mastectomy for a 3.5-cm tumor with one positive axillary lymph node (43). She was subsequently irradiated for castration and was reported well and free of disease 6 years after pancreatic resection. Mehta et al. performed pancreaticoduodenectomy on a 33-year-old woman for metastatic infiltrating ductal cancer of the breast 3 years after modified radical mastectomy for a T-2 N0 M0 lesion (44). Multidrug chemotherapy and tamoxifen were given following pancreatectomy, and the patient was disease free 27 months later. Additionally, an unusual patient with a distal pancreatectomy for an apparent solitary metastases of cystosarcoma phyllodes of the breast has been reported (16).

Roland and van Heerden reported one patient alive 27 months after distal pancreatectomy for metastatic colon cancer (5). The patient was receiving chemotherapy for hepatic metastases apparently present at the time of pancreatectomy. Pancreaticoduodenectomy has also been performed for melanoma metastatic to the pancreas (56, 57). One patient was reported disease free 16 months after resection, while another patient was found to have melanoma of the nasal cavity 1 year following pancreatectomy. Whether the pancreatic melanoma was primary or metastatic in this patient is uncertain.

## SUMMARY

Autopsy studies demonstrate that metastases to the pancreas are not uncommon. The most frequent primary sites are lung, breast, cutaneous melanoma, stomach, colon, kidney, and ovary. Metastases to the pancreas are usually part of a pattern of widespread malignancy and are seldom associated with organ-specific symptoms. Occasionally, operative intervention may be indicated for treatment of tumor-related biliary or gastrointestinal obstruction, hemorrhage, or complications of metastases-induced acute pancreatitis. Resection is appropriate for good-risk patients with apparent solitary metastases, particularly if there has been a relatively long disease-free interval.

## REFERENCES

1. Willis RA. The spread of tumours in the human body. 3rd ed. London: Butterworth, 1973:216.
2. Berge T, Lundberg S. Cancer in Malmö 1958–1969: an autopsy study. Acta Pathol Microbiol Scand (Suppl) (A) 1977;260.
3. Cubilla AL, Fitzgerald PJ. Tumors of the exocrine pancreas. In: Atlas of tumor pathology, series 2, fascicle 19, 1984. Washington, DC: Armed Forces Institute of Pathology, 1984.
4. Abrams HL, Spiro R, Goldstein N. Metastases in carcinoma: analysis of 1000 autopsied cases. Cancer 1950;3:74–85.
5. Roland CF, van Heerden JA. Nonpancreatic primary tumors with metastasis to the pancreas. Surg Gynecol Obstet 1989;168: 345–347.
6. Havig O. Some autopsy findings in malignant pancreatic lesions. Scand J Gastroenterol 1975;10(suppl 34):23–24.
7. Boudghène FP, Deslandes PM, LeBlanche AF, Bigot JMR. US and CT imaging features of intrapancreatic metastases. J Comput Assist Tomogr 1994;18:905–910.
8. Wernecke K, Peters PE, Galanski M. Pancreatic metastases: US evaluation. Radiology 1986;160:399–402.
9. Muranaka T, Teshima K, Honda H. Nanjo T, Hanada K, Oshiumi Y. Computed tomography and histologic appearance of pancreatic metastases from distant sources. Acta Radiol 1989;30: 615–619.
10. Rumancik WM, Megibow AJ, Bosniak MA, Hilton S. Metastatic disease to the pancreas: evaluation by computed tomography. J Comput Assist Tomogr 1984;8:829–834.
11. Waga S, Matsushima M, Ando K, Morii S. Intracranial chondrosarcoma with extracranial metastases: a case report. J Neurosurg 1972;36:790–794.
12. Mikhail MGS, Lim KB. Dedifferentiated chondrosarcoma metastasizing to the pancreas in pregnancy. Acta Obstet Gynecol Scand 1989;68:467–468.
13. Rao NG, Krishnaswami S, Cherian G, Krishnaswami H. Sarcoma of the pulmonary artery with metastases to pancreas and adrenal glands. Chest 1974;66:459–462.
14. Tanabe S, Soeda S, Mukai T, Oki S, Yun K, Miyahara S. A case report of pancreatic metastasis of an intracranial angioblastic menin-

gioma (hemangiopericytoma) and a review of metastatic tumor to the pancreas. J Surg Oncol 1984;26:63–68.
15. Krouwer HGJ, Vollmerhausen J, White J, Prados MD. Desmoplastic medulloblastoma metastatic to the pancreas: case report. Neurosurgery 1991;29:612–616.
16. Wolfson P, Rybak BJ, Kim U. Cystosarcoma phyllodes metastatic to the pancreas. Am J Gastroenterol 1978;70:184–187.
17. Carson HJ, Green LK, Castelli MJ, Reyes CV, Prinz RA, Gattuso P. Utilization of fine-needle aspiration biopsy in the diagnosis of metastatic tumors to the pancreas. Diagn Cytopathol 1995; 12:8–13.
18. Benning TL, Silverman JF, Berns LA, Geisinger KR. Fine needle aspiration of metastatic and hematologic malignancies clinically mimicking pancreatic carcinoma. Acta Cytol 1992;36:471–476.
19. Line DH, Deeley TJ. The necropsy findings in carcinoma of the bronchus. Br J Dis Chest 1971;65:238–242.
20. Berge T, Toremalm NG. Bronchial cancer—a clinical and pathological study. Scand J Resp Dis 1975;56:109–119.
21. Lee YN. Breast carcinoma: pattern of metastasis at autopsy. J Surg Oncol 1983;23:175–180.
22. de la Monte SM, Hutchins GM, Moore GW. Endocrine organ metastases from breast carcinoma. Am J Pathol 1984;114:131–136.
23. Cifuentes N, Pickren JW. Metastases from carcinoma of mammary gland: an autopsy study. J Surg Oncol 1979;11:193–205.
24. de la Monte SM, Moore GW, Hutchins GM. Patterned distribution of metastases from malignant melanoma in humans. Cancer Res 1983;43:3427–3433.
25. Patel JK, Didolkar MS, Pickren JW, Moore RH. Metastatic pattern of malignant melanoma. A study of 216 autopsy cases. Am J Surg 1978;135:807–810.
26. Matthews MJ. Morphology of lung cancer. Semin Oncol 1974;1: 175–181.
27. Merino MJ, Livolsi VA. Signet ring carcinoma of the female breast: a clinicopathologic analysis of 24 cases. Cancer 1981;48:1830–1837.
28. Charnsangavej C, Whitley NO. Metastases to the pancreas and peripancreatic lymph nodes from carcinoma of the right side of the colon: CT findings in 12 patients. AJR 1993;160:49–52.
29. Strijk, SP. Pancreatic metastases of renal cell carcinoma: report of two cases. Gastrointest Radiol 1989;14:123–126.
30. Levine M, Danovitch SH. Metastatic carcinoma to the pancreas: another cause for acute pancreatitis. Am J Gastroenterol 1973;60:290–294.
31. Niccolini DG, Graham JH, Banks PA. Tumor-induced acute pancreatitis. Gastroenterology 1976;71:142–145.
32. Biset JM, Laurent F, de Verbizier G, Houang B, Constantes G, Drouillard J. Ultrasound and computed tomographic findings in pancreatic metastases. Eur J Radiol 1991;12:41–44.
33. Brady LW, O'Neill EA, Farber SH. Unusual sites of metastases. Semin Oncol 1977;4:59–64.
34. Yeung K, Haidak DJ, Brown JA, Anderson D. Metastasis-induced acute pancreatitis in small cell bronchogenic carcinoma. Arch Intern Med 1979;139:552–554.
35. Stewart KC, Dickout WJ, Urschel JD. Metastasis-induced acute pancreatitis as the initial manifestation of bronchogenic carcinoma. Chest 1993;104:98–100.
36. Chowhan NM, Madajewicz S. Management of metastases-induced acute pancreatitis in small cell carcinoma of the lung. Cancer 1990;65:1445–1448.
37. Noseda A, Gangji D, Cremer M. Acute pancreatitis as presenting symptom and sole manifestation of small cell lung carcinoma. Dig Dis Sci 1987;32:327–331.
38. Gutman M, Inbar M, Klausner JM. Metastases-induced acute pancreatitis: a rare presentation of cancer. Eur J Surg Oncol 1993;19(3):302–304.
39. Hall M, Bundred NJ, Hall AW. Oat cell carcinoma of the bronchus and acute pancreatitis. Eur J Surg Oncol 1987;13:371–372.
40. MacLennan AC, MacLeod IA. Case report: small cell carcinoma induced acute pancreatitis. Br J Radiol 1993;66:161–162.
41. McLatchie GR, Imrie CW. Acute pancreatitis associated with tumor metastasis in the pancreas. Digestion 1981;21:13–17.
42. Whittington R, Moylan DJ, Dobelbower RR, Kramer S. Pancreatic tumours in patients with previous malignancy. Clin Radiol 1982; 33:297–299.
43. Azzarelli A. Clemente C, Quagliuolo V, Baticci F. A case of pancreatoduodenectomy as resolutive treatment for a solitary metastasis of breast cancer. Tumori 1982;68:331–335.
44. Mehta SA, Jagannath P, Krishnamurthy SC, De Souza LJ. Isolated pancreatic metastasis from locally controlled breast cancer: a case report. Indian J Cancer 1991;28:48–50.
45. Temellini F, Bavosi M, Lamarra M, Quagliarini P, Giuliani F. Pancreatic metastasis 25 years after nephrectomy for renal cancer. Tumori 1989;75:503–504.
46. Rypens F, Van Gansbeke D, Lambilliotte JP, Van Regemorter G, Verhest A, Struyven J. Pancreatic metastasis from renal cell carcinoma. Br J Radiol 1992;65:547–548.
47. Opocher E, Galeotti F, Spina GP, Battaglia G, Hernandez C. La diagnosi dei tumori secondari del pancreas: analisi di 13 casi. Minerva Med 1982;73:577–581.
48. Swenson T, Osnes M, Serck-Hanssen A. Endoscopic retrograde cholangio-pancreatography in primary and secondary tumours of the pancreas. Br J Radiol 1980;53:760–764.
49. Oda K, Itoh J, Hachisuka K, Yamaguchi A, et al. Value of computer image analysis in improving ERCP images in metastatic tumor of the pancreas. AJR 1993;161:885–886.
50. Pappo I, Feigin E, Uziely B, Amir G. Biliary and pancreatic metastases of breast carcinoma: is surgical palliation indicated? J Surg Oncol 1991;46:211–214.
51. Stankard CE, Karl RC. The treatment of isolated pancreatic metastases from renal cell carcinoma: a surgical review. Am J Gastroenterol 1992;87:1658–1660.
52. Saxon A, Gottesman J, Doolas A. Bilateral hypernephroma with solitary pancreatic metastasis. J Surg Oncol 1980;13: 317–322.
53. Guttman FM, Ross M, Lachance C. Pancreatic metastasis of renal cell carcinoma treated by total pancreatectomy. Arch Surg 1972;105:782–784.
54. Tolia BM, Whitmore WF. Solitary metastasis from renal cell carcinoma. J Urol 1975;114:836–838.
55. Klugo RC, Detmers M, Stiles RE, Talley RW, Cerny JC. Aggressive versus conservative management of stage IV renal cell carcinoma. J Urol 1977;118:244–246.
56. Rutter JE, De Graaf PW, Kooyman CD, Van Leeuwen MS, Obertoop H. Malignant melanoma of the pancreas: primary tumour or unknown primary? Case report. Eur J Surg 1994;160: 119–120.
57. Karakousis CP, Velez A, Driscoll DL, Takita H. Metastasectomy in malignant melanoma. Surgery 1994;115(3):295–302.

SECTION XII

ADJACENT TUMORS REQUIRING PANCREATIC RESECTION

# 68

# Carcinoma and Other Tumors of the Ampulla of Vater

Charles J. Yeo and John L. Cameron

## ETIOLOGY AND PATHOLOGY

The ampulla of Vater is a compact anatomic site, typically located in the more distal aspect of the second portion of the duodenum, and representing the interface between the duodenum, pancreas, extrahepatic biliary tree, and the pancreatic ductal systems. The ampulla of Vater is the area of the small bowel (duodenum, jejunum and ileum) with the highest incidence of neoplastic transformation and malignancy, presumably because of the local production of carcinogens and promoters through the combined interaction of the many components of bile, duodenal content, and pancreatic exocrine secretions. A number of different neoplasms have been identified at the ampulla of Vater (Table 68.1).

Adenocarcinoma of the ampulla of Vater accounts for less than 10% of all cases of periampullary carcinoma (considered to be cancers of the head of the pancreas, distal common bile duct, peri-Vaterian duodenum, and ampulla). However, if one considers only the subgroup of surgically resectable periampullary malignancies, ampullary adenocarcinoma can be the final pathologic diagnosis in up to 25% of patients who undergo resection. Adenocarcinoma is by far the most common malignant ampullary neoplasm. Ampullary adenocarcinoma is believed to originate from the mucosal cells of the ampulla through the process of malignant transformation. Benign ampullary adenomas undergo dysplastic degeneration, with subsequent progression to adenocarcinoma (1), in similar fashion to the adenoma-carcinoma sequence that is so well known for colon cancer.

The frequency of K-*ras* oncogene mutations in ampullary carcinomas appears to differ from that in pancreatic adenocarcinoma. Oncogenes encode proteins that, when overexpressed or activated by mutation, possess transforming properties. K-*ras* is the most widely studied oncogene in pancreatic adenocarcinoma, with activating point mutations of K-*ras* (using allele-specific oligonucleotides or direct sequencing methods) found in 80–90% of patients with pancreatic cancer (2). In contrast, ampullary adenocarcinoma has been reported to have a 13% incidence of K-*ras* mutations (3), a frequency more similar to bile duct carcinoma (cholangiocarcinoma) than that of pancreatic adenocarcinoma. One can speculate that the carcinogenic process may be similar, therefore, between ampullary adenocarcinoma and bile duct carcinoma as compared with pancreatic carcinoma.

Ampullary adenoma is a rare neoplasm. First reported by Calzavara in 1895 (4), the incidence in autopsy studies varies between 0.04% and 0.62%, with most lesions being asymptomatic (5). Ampullary adenoma affects both sexes equally and is typically seen after the 5th decade of life. Histologically, ampullary adenomas appear as glandular proliferations arising from the intestinal-type epithelium of the ampulla. The incidence of residual adenoma at the edge of a true ampullary carcinoma varies between 20 and 80%. Ampullary adenoma has been associated with the familial adenomatous polyposis (FAP) syndrome (7), as well as with polycystic kidney disease, an autosomal dominant trait (8).

Other benign tumors of the ampulla of Vater include leiomyoma, lipoma, lymphangioma, and hemangioma, as well as neuroendocrine tumors (carcinoid tumors). Ampullary carcinoids are associated with von Recklinghausen's disease (neurofibromatosis) (9, 10).

Metastatic carcinoma to the ampulla of Vater is extremely uncommon (Table 68.1). Rare cases have been reported of melanoma, lymphoma, and renal cell carcinoma metastasizing to the region of the ampulla (11, 12). The ampulla can also be locally invaded by other primary malignancies, most commonly by tumors of the duodenum, pancreas, or bile duct. The focus of the remainder of this chapter is on ampullary adenocarcinoma, with reference to other lesions as appropriate.

## DIAGNOSIS

### Clinical Presentation

The mean age of patients with ampullary adenocarcinoma approximates 60 years, with no gender predilection. Jaundice, the most common presenting symptom, is exhibited in approximately 80% of patients at the time of diagnosis (13). Nonspecific gastrointestinal symptoms such as dyspepsia, malaise, and anorexia typically occur in 15–30% of patients. Roughly one-half of all patients complain of pruritus. Occasionally, the jaundice and pruritus of ampullary adenocarcinoma may be intermittent, apparently related to repeated necrosis and sloughing of the obstructing tumor mass, which allows temporary resolution of the symptoms. Hematemesis or melena is rare, although a microcytic anemia due to occult gastrointestinal (GI) bleeding from neoplastic ulceration may be seen in up to one-third of all patients.

Typical findings on physical examination include, in descending order, scleral or cutaneous icterus, cutaneous evidence of pruritus, hepatomegaly, Hemoccult-positive stool, and occasionally a palpable gallbladder.

Two infrequent modes of presentation merit description. First, ampullary adenoma or adenocarcinoma may primarily obstruct the pancreatic duct, causing hyperamylasemia and symptoms of pancreatitis. Second, patients may complain of gray stools, which occur as the result of GI tract blood loss (melena) in combination with an acholic stool.

### Laboratory Tests

Nearly all patients have abnormalities of serum liver function tests. Both the alkaline phosphatase and γ-glutamyl transferase, sensitive markers of cholestasis, are abnormal in most patients.

**TABLE 68.1. Tumors of the Ampulla of Vater**

| |
|---|
| Primary tumors |
| Adenocarcinoma |
| Adenoma |
| Neuroendocrine tumor (carcinoid) |
| Leiomyoma (GIST)[a] |
| Lipoma |
| Lymphangioma |
| Hemangioma |
| Metastatic tumors |
| Melanoma |
| Lymphoma |
| Renal cell carcinoma |
| Local invasion from other primary tumors |
| Duodenal cancer |
| Pancreatic cancer |
| Bile duct cancer |
| Colon cancer |
| Gastric cancer |
| Gallbladder cancer |

[a]GIST, gastrointestinal stromal tumor.

Elevations of serum bilirubin and amino transferases are also found in most patients. Approximately one-third of patients may have evidence of a microcytic, hypochromic anemia due to chronic GI blood loss from the surface of the neoplasm. Hyperamylasemia and hyperlipasemia, presumably related to pancreatic ductal obstruction, are found in a minority of patients. In patients with longstanding jaundice, the prothrombin time may be prolonged, resulting from cholestasis-induced malabsorption of fat-soluble vitamins, most notably vitamin K.

## Endoscopy

Fiberoptic upper GI endoscopy is a highly useful diagnostic procedure in most cases of presumed ampullary carcinoma. Using a standard side-viewing upper endoscope, the ampulla can be visualized (Fig. 68.1), evaluated, subjected to biopsy, and cannulated for cholangiography, pancreatography, or biliary decompression. The endoscopic appearance of ampullary cancer can vary widely. Ampullary adenomas may also be seen, varying in appearance from a nearly normal ampulla to a greatly distorted ampulla with an exophytic lesion of a papillary or sessile nature. Some ampullary abnormalities may appear polypoid and pedunculated, while other lesions may appear infiltrating and ulcerated, with a broad base. Biopsy specimens and brushings obtained via the upper endoscope may allow pathologic or cytologic diagnosis. A normal biopsy specimen does not exclude invasive carcinoma, because of possible sampling error. Biopsy specimens can demonstrate adenomatous tissue but underestimate the extent of dysplasia or invasive carcinoma.

Endoscopic ultrasonography (Fig. 68.2) has been reported to be reliable and accurate in assisting in the diagnosis and staging of ampullary carcinoma (14, 15). In a prospective study by Rosch et al., endoscopic ultrasonography was compared with transabdominal ultrasonography, computed tomography (CT), and angiography in 60 consecutive patients with either ampullary or pancreatic cancer. Endoscopic ultrasonography was superior to both abdominal ultrasonography and CT in determining tumor size and presence of lymph node metastases. Further, involvement of the portal venous system was correctly assessed by endoscopic ultrasonography in 95% of cases, whereas angiography (85%), CT (75%), and abdominal ultrasonography (55%) were less sensitive. These authors concluded that endoscopic ultrasonography was the most effective single imaging procedure for local tumor staging in pancreatic and ampullary carcinoma. However, this imaging modality is extremely dependent upon the experience of the endoscopic ultrasonographer both in performing the procedure and in interpreting the images. Further, endoscopic ultrasonography cannot accurately image the liver for hepatic metastases, an aspect of the evaluation that is mandatory for complete tumor staging.

## Radiographic Imaging

Transabdominal ultrasonography is used by some physicians to evaluate patients with abdominal pain or suspected extrahepatic biliary obstruction. This simple, noninvasive test is particularly useful for the presence of gallstones within the gallbladder, in evaluating for choledocholithiasis, and in diagnosing extrahepatic and intrahepatic biliary dilation. In patients with ampullary neoplasms, visualization of the primary ampullary tumor mass is rare. Transabdominal ultrasonography alone cannot accurately analyze the size of the primary tumor, extent of the primary tumor, or extent of peritumor lymph node metastases.

In most patients being evaluated with the suspicion of

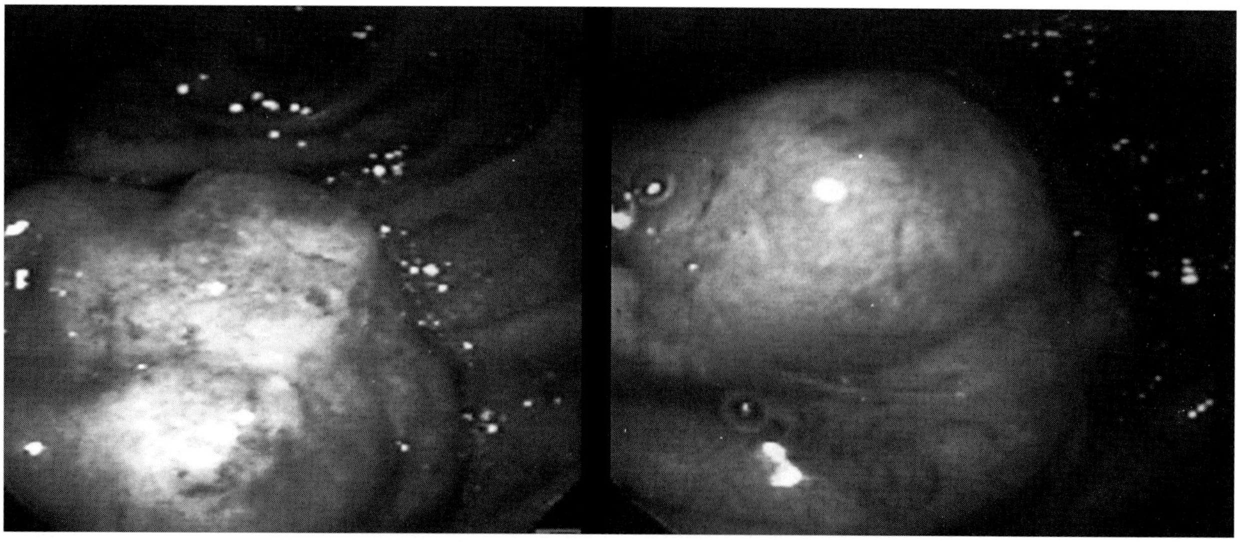

**FIG. 68.1.** Two endoscopic photographic images of the same exophytic, bulging ampullary mass, which proved to be an ampullary adenocarcinoma.

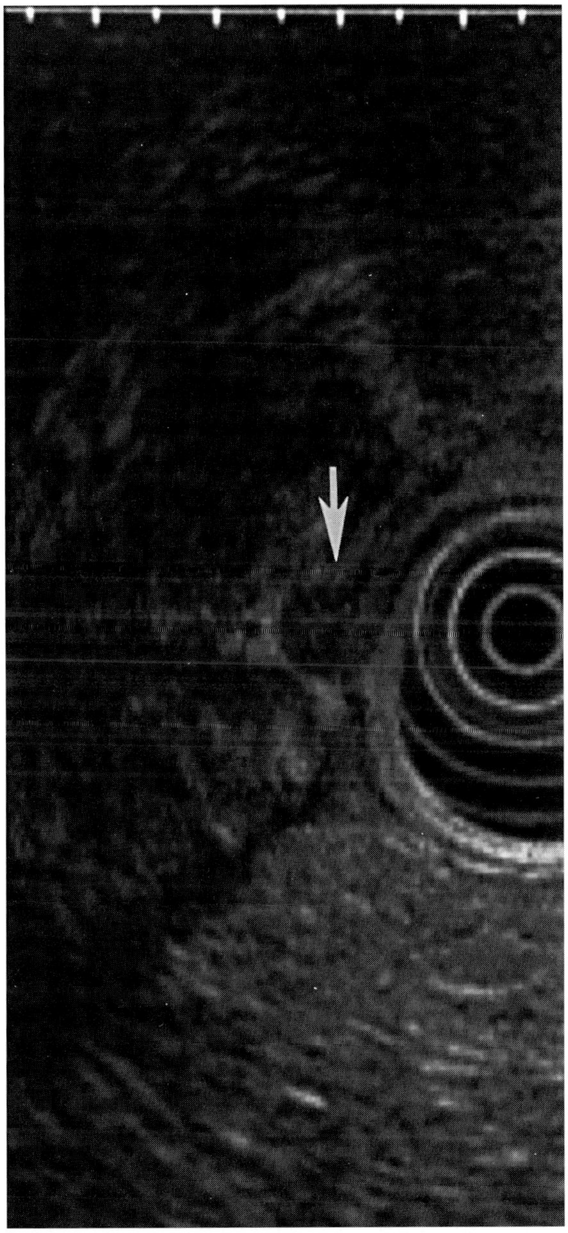

**FIG. 68.2.** An image from an endoscopic ultrasound study revealing a discrete ampullary abnormality *(arrow)* consistent with an ampullary adenocarcinoma.

ampullary carcinoma, the most useful noninvasive imaging modality is CT of the abdomen, using both intravenous and oral contrast (Figs. 68.3 and 68.4). Such a contrast-enhanced dynamic CT scan provides better information than transabdominal ultrasonography. The CT images can demonstrate biliary and pancreatic ductal dilation and a mass lesion at the ampulla and can also provide information regarding the hepatic parenchyma and the presence or absence of hepatic metastases. CT is clearly superior to transabdominal ultrasound in its ability to demonstrate the extent of local disease, encasement of the superior mesenteric or portal venous vessels, and regional lymphadenopathy.

Upper GI barium studies or hypotonic duodenography were used in the past to evaluate the second portion of the duodenum for mucosal abnormalities. Currently neither modality is commonly used because of their low sensitivity and inability to

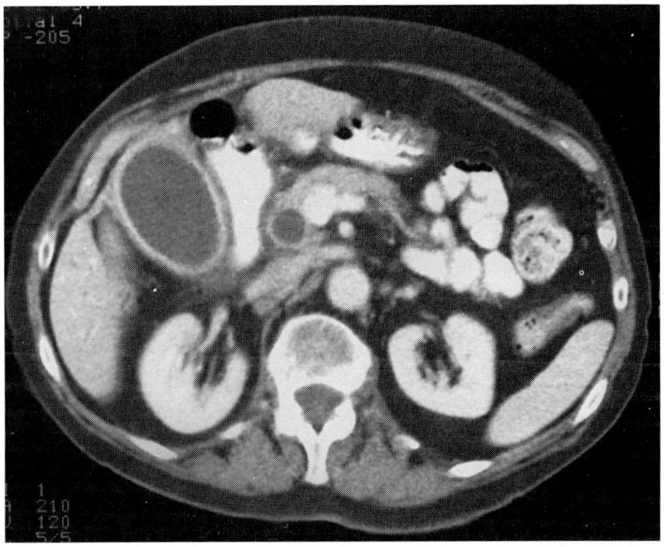

**FIG. 68.3.** An abnormal CT scan with both intravenous and oral contrast in a patient with a 9-mm ampullary adenocarcinoma. There is evidence of dilated intrahepatic ducts, a distended gallbladder, and a dilated distal common bile duct in the head of the pancreas.

provide a tissue diagnosis. Upper endoscopy has largely supplanted the use of both upper GI barium studies and hypotonic duodenography in the evaluation of periampullary abnormalities.

In most patients with ampullary carcinoma, mesenteric angiography is not needed. Most patients with ampullary carcinoma have small tumors, well away from the superior mesenteric vein and portal vein, with CT scan findings that fail to suggest evidence of tumor involvement of any major mesenteric or portal venous structure. Patients with unusually large ampullary carcinomas or with CT scans suggesting possible vessel encasement or occlusion can be further staged by mesenteric angiography.

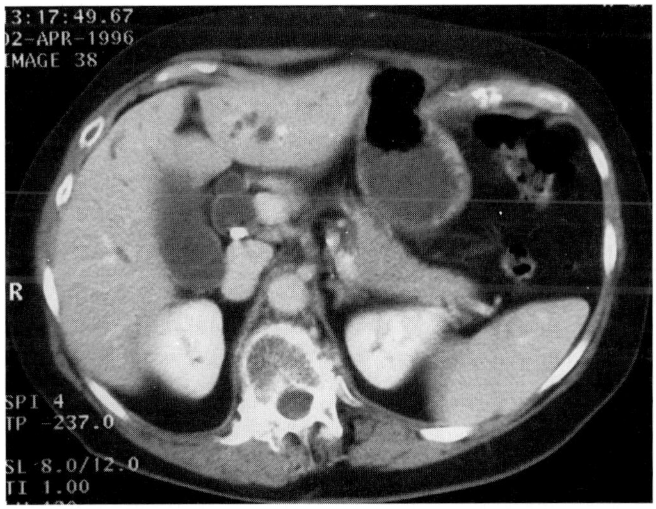

**FIG. 68.4.** An abdominal CT scan in a patient with an ampullary adenocarcinoma. Dilated bile ducts are visible within the hepatic parenchyma. The gallbladder appears distended. The extrahepatic biliary tree is dilated, with a recently placed (but nonfunctional) biliary endoprosthesis seen in the dorsalmost aspect of the biliary tree.

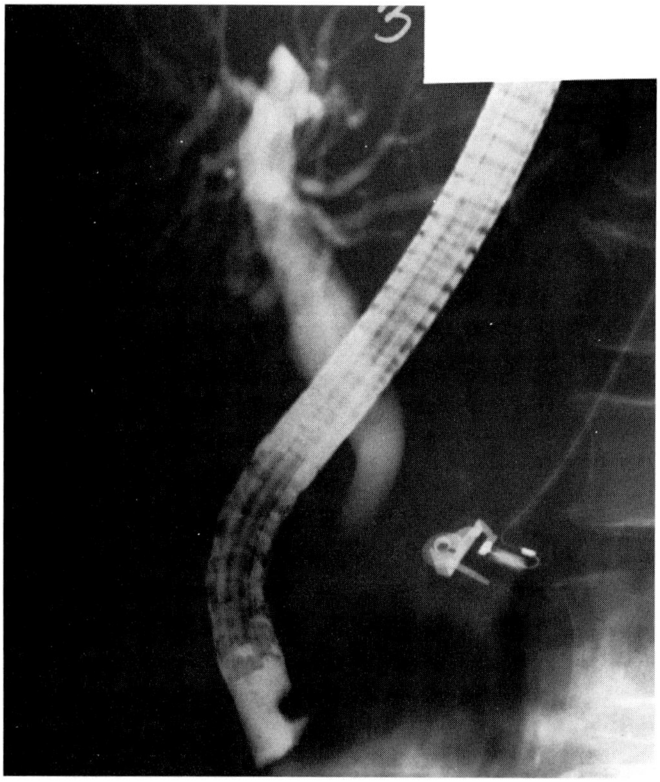


**FIG. 68.5.** An ERCP in the same patient as in Figure 68.3. The extrahepatic and intrahepatic biliary tree are dilated down to the level of the ampulla. At endoscopy, a visible neoplastic abnormality was present at the ampulla.

Another potential benefit of angiography, demonstrating major arterial anomalies (such as replaced right hepatic artery originating from the superior mesenteric artery (SMA) or proximal celiac artery stenosis), has been cited as a reason for performing routine angiography prior to resection. Currently, we do *not* use angiography routinely in the evaluation of ampullary cancer; rather, we use it selectively in patients with large bulky tumors, those with abnormal CT scans, or those with notable systemic atherosclerotic disease, which may be accompanied by celiac or superior mesenteric artery stenosis.

Cholangiography can be performed via either the endoscopic or percutaneous transhepatic approach. The route chosen depends upon the local expertise, the presence or absence of coagulopathy, the apparent level of extrahepatic bile duct obstruction, and the upper GI tract anatomy. In most cases of ampullary carcinoma, cholangiography demonstrates a combination of proximal dilation of the entire extrahepatic biliary tree with an obstructing irregular filling defect at the most distal common bile duct (Fig. 68.5). Overall, the sensitivity and specificity of both cholangiographic approaches are similar. Both approaches also allow placement of indwelling biliary stents for preoperative or palliative drainage of the biliary tree. The advantages of endoscopic cholangiography in cases of ampullary carcinoma include *(a)* luminal access for biopsy confirmation of malignancy; *(b)* direct visualization of the ampulla; *(c)* the ability to treat definitively and safely such alternative diagnoses as choledocholithiasis or sphincter of Oddi dysfunction; *(d)* better patient tolerance because of the avoidance of a percutaneous puncture and an indwelling catheter; and *(e)* the ability to perform a pancreatogram and demonstrate a normal pancreatic duct, which virtually excludes ductal carcinoma of the pancreas.

Percutaneous transhepatic cholangiography is generally best reserved for lesions that obstruct the more proximal biliary tree and may be necessary when a tumor extends proximally to involve the bifurcation of the hepatic duct or when endoscopic cholangiography cannot be performed for technical reasons. In selected cases, percutaneous transhepatic cholangiography with placement of an indwelling percutaneous transhepatic catheter may benefit the surgeon by allowing use of the percutaneous transhepatic catheter during and following either local resection or pancreaticoduodenectomy, helping to locate the ampulla intraoperatively and obviating the need for an intraoperatively placed T tube.

## MANAGEMENT

### Staging

The primary staging system for ampullary carcinoma currently in use is the TNM system (Table 68.2). Ampullary carcinoma is classified according to the extent of tumor invasion, tumor size, presence of lymph node metastases, and presence of distant metastases.

A suggested plan for evaluation and treatment of patients with ampullary tumors is shown in Figure 68.6. Patients who are good operative risks without evidence of distant metastases should undergo surgical exploration. When preoperative evaluation reveals distant metastases, or when a patient is not an operative candidate because of serious medical problems, then nonoperative palliation with a biliary endoprosthesis combined with palliative chemoradiation therapy should be considered.

### Operative Resection

#### Local Excision

In 1899, Halsted reported the first successful local excision of an ampullary carcinoma, reimplanting the pancreatic and bile ducts into the duodenal wall (16). Local resection of ampullary tumors has been advocated for patients with benign adenomas, rare patients with ampullary endocrine tumors, and highly selected patients with ampullary carcinoma (17–19).

Local resection is an uncommonly performed procedure, as evidenced by the report of Asbun et al. (19), who reported 14 patients undergoing ampullary resection over a 16-year period at the Lahey Clinic. Of these 14 patients, 2 were converted to pancreaticoduodenectomy at the first operative procedure, and 2 underwent pancreaticoduodenectomy 5 days and 8 months following ampullectomy. A recent report by Rattner et al. (18)

**TABLE 68.2. TNM Staging of Ampullary Carcinoma**

Tumor
- $T_1$ = Tumor limited to ampulla of Vater
- $T_2$ = Tumor invades duodenal wall
- $T_3$ = Tumor invades ≤2 cm into pancreas
- $T_4$ = Tumor invades >2 cm into pancreas and/or into adjacent organs

Nodes
- $N_0$ = No regional lymph node metastases
- $N_1$ = Regional lymph node metastases

Metastases
- $M_0$ = No distant metastases
- $M_1$ = Distant metastases

| Stages | T | N | M |
|---|---|---|---|
| Stage I | $T_1$ | $N_0$ | $M_0$ |
| Stage II | $T_2$-$T_3$ | $N_0$ | $M_0$ |
| Stage III | $T_1$-$T_3$ | $N_1$ | $M_0$ |
| Stage IV | $T_4$ | any N | $M_0$ |
| | any T | any N | $M_1$ |

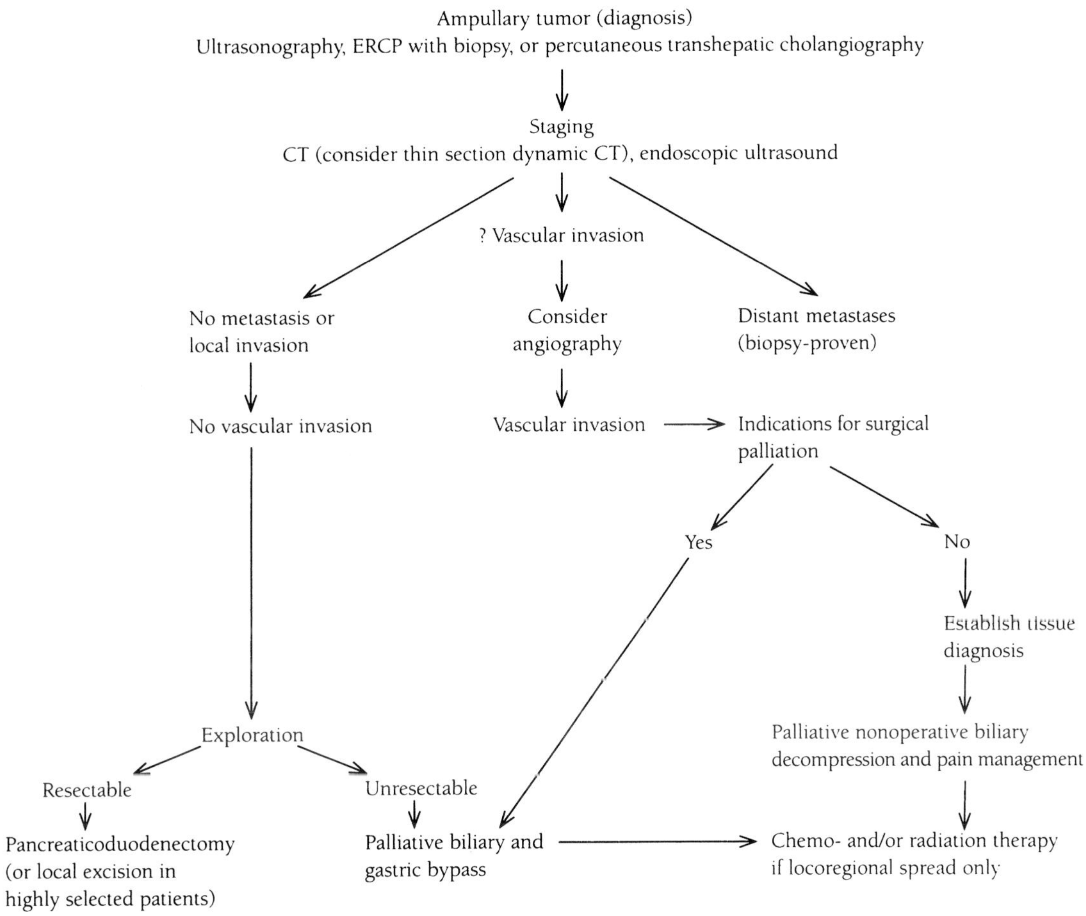


**FIG. 68.6.** Management of patients with ampullary carcinoma. (From Oishi AJ, Murr MM, Petersen BT, Sarr MG. Ampullary carcinoma. In: Pitt HA, Carr-Locke DL, Ferrucci JT, eds. Hepatobiliary and pancreatic disease: the team approach to management. Boston: Little, Brown & Co, 1995:467.)

compares 14 patients who underwent ampullectomy with 12 patients undergoing pancreaticoduodenectomy for ampullary neoplasms. As expected, the length of hospital stay was shorter, and the postoperative complication rate was lower for those undergoing local resection. Survival data cannot be compared because the two groups did not have comparable pathology.

In general, local resection of ampullary neoplasms appears appropriate for benign adenomas with or without dysplasia (generally 3 cm or smaller in diameter), for selected ampullary neuroendocrine tumors, and in highly selected patients with $T_1$ ampullary adenocarcinomas that are pathologically ultimately stage I. The technique of local resection is depicted in Figure 68.7. There is some suggestion that a satisfactory local resection for $T_1$ ampullary adenocarcinomas should have a 1-cm duodenal mucosal margin. Following successful local resection, it is recommended that patients undergo annual upper GI endoscopy for an unspecified period of time, to detect evidence of local recurrence or the development of new lesions.

**Pancreaticoduodenectomy.** A report in 1935 by Whipple et al. described a two-stage pancreaticoduodenal resection in three patients with ampullary carcinoma (20). In 1941, Trimble et al. reported on a one-stage pancreaticoduodenectomy in patients with carcinoma of the ampulla of Vater, leading toward the modern era of pancreaticoduodenal resection for these tumors (21). In the 1940s, 1950s, and 1960s, acceptance of pancreaticoduodenectomy as a viable resectional procedure for ampullary and other periampullary tumors was difficult because of high operative complication rates and operative mortality rates approaching 25%. However, in recent years, advances in pre- and postoperative care, surgical technique, and anesthesia have all contributed to a decrease in the morbidity rates (which now approximate 30–40%) and a dramatic fall in the mortality rate to less than 3% in experienced centers (22, 23). Pancreaticoduodenectomy today is the curative procedure of choice for the vast majority of patients with localized ampullary carcinoma.

The operation is typically begun with an upper midline or limited right subcostal incision. The entire abdominal cavity is examined for evidence of peritoneal or hepatic metastases, and evidence of unresectability is diligently sought. If no evidence of adenocarcinoma is found outside the intended resection zone, then the incision is extended, and resection is begun. Typically, the duodenum and pancreatic head are widely elevated in the ventral direction, being lifted off of the vena cava and aorta with a generous Kocher maneuver. In most cases of ampullary carcinoma, a small tumor mass will be palpated at the site of the ampulla, and there will be no evidence of extraampullary disease. In addition, the remainder of the pancreas will typically be normal and soft, and there will be no evidence of nodal metastases within the celiac axis or in the hepatoduodenal ligament. A detailed description of pancreaticoduodenectomy is beyond the scope of this chapter.

Our preference for resection in cases of ampullary carcinoma is to use the pylorus-preserving modification of pancreaticoduodenectomy with its advantages of diminished operative time, theoretically more physiologic postoperative GI function, retention of the entire stomach as a reservoir, and reduced

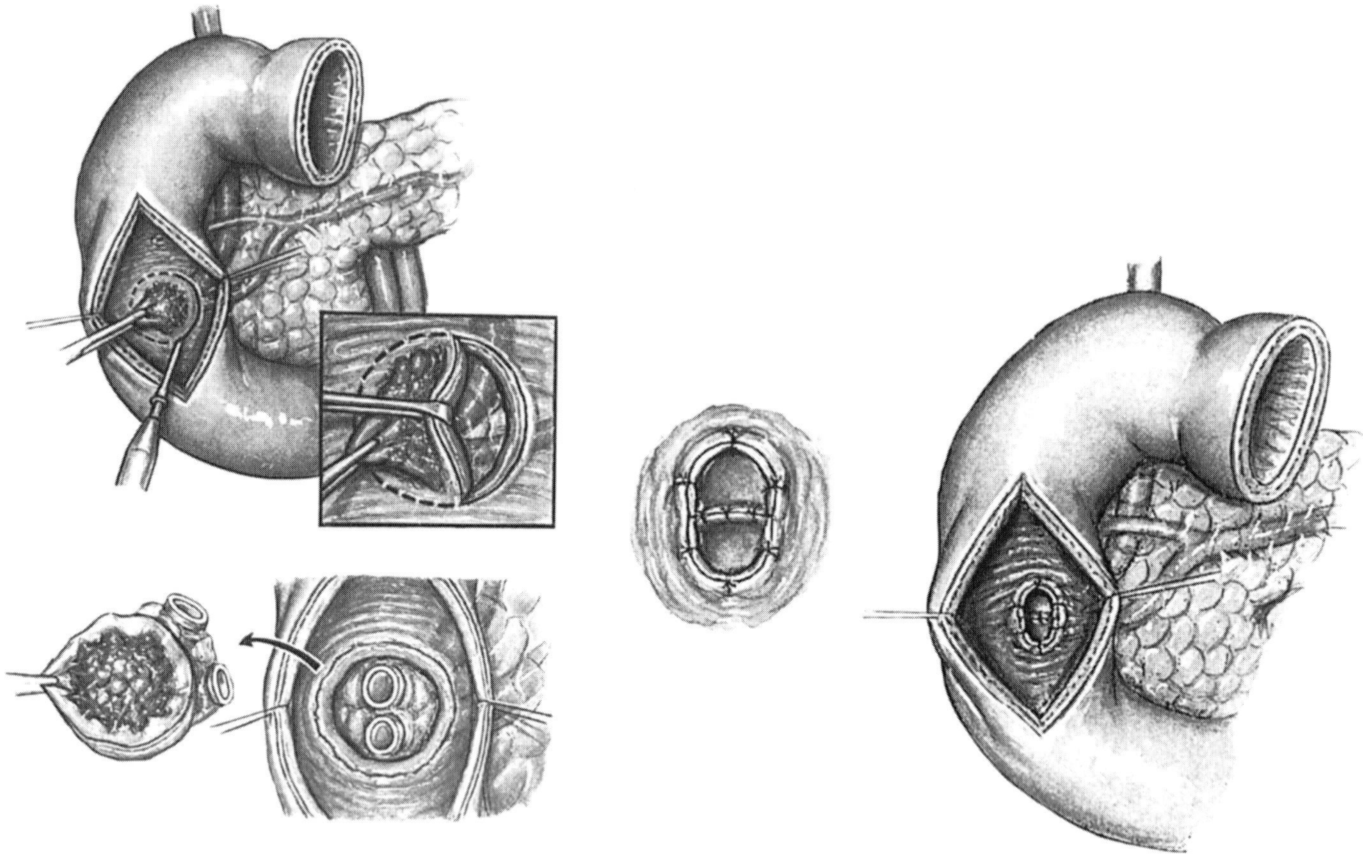

**FIG. 68.7.** Technique of local resection of an ampullary neoplasm. *Left,* A wide excision is performed including a portion of the duodenal wall and the periampullary portions of the pancreatic and common bile ducts. Injection of the submucosal area with 1:100,000 epinephrine solution can help define the correct plane of dissection. *Right,* The pancreatic and common bile ducts are sutured together to form a common septum. The adjacent duodenal wall is then sutured to the pancreatic and common bile ducts. (From Asbun HJ, Rossi RL, Munson JL. Local resection for ampullary tumors: is there a place for it? Arch Surg 1993;128:515–520.)

anastomotic ulceration at the duodenojejunostomy. The type of pancreatic-enteric anastomosis performed varies—either a pancreaticojejunostomy or pancreaticogastrostomy. While the rates of pancreatic fistula formation were equivalent when these two methods of pancreatic reconstruction were studied in prospective, randomized fashion (24), pancreaticogastrostomy may be beneficial in patients with large soft pancreatic remnants that are not easily invaginated into a small-caliber jejunum. We use erythromycin as prophylaxis against the occurrence of delayed gastric emptying, a common and troublesome complication occurring in 20–30% of patients following any form of pancreaticoduodenectomy (25).

## Operative Palliation

In patients who are ultimately determined to have ampullary carcinoma, and whose preoperative staging studies such as abdominal CT scan and/or endoscopic ultrasound and/or angiography reveal no evidence of unresectability, the resectability rate is in excess of 85%. In a minority of patients, surgical exploration will reveal unanticipated metastatic tumor outside the resection specimen or vascular involvement that precludes curative resection. In this situation, a palliative operative procedure is appropriate (26). Decompression of the biliary tree is typically performed as a biliary-enteric anastomosis. We prefer to perform this as a Roux-en-Y hepaticojejunostomy, using a defunctionalized jejunal limb and performing a cholecystectomy. A gastrojejunostomy is performed in patients with compromise of the duodenal lumen or symptoms of gastric outlet obstruction. We prefer to perform the gastrojejunostomy in a retrocolic isoperistaltic fashion. The patient is subsequently placed on long-term $H_2$-receptor antagonists or omeprazole to reduce gastric acid secretion, thereby preventing the occurrence of marginal ulceration. In patients without obvious compromise of the duodenal lumen and without symptoms of gastric outlet obstruction, the decision to perform a prophylactic gastrojejunostomy remains unsettled. In our experience, adding a gastrojejunostomy to a biliary enteric bypass has been safe, and the data suggest that a prophylactic gastrojejunostomy averts the need for reoperation for subsequent duodenal obstruction in approximately one in six patients with periampullary cancer in whom a gastrojejunostomy has not been performed.

The final issue in patients undergoing operative palliation deals with pain relief and pain management. A prospective, randomized trial by Lillemoe et al. (27) showed a significant reduction of pain, with an associated reduction of narcotic analgesic use, in patients with pancreatic and periampullary cancer who underwent intraoperative periaortic celiac ganglion block using 50% alcohol. This study showed no increase in morbidity related to the block, and patients with preoperative pain who underwent the intraoperative alcohol block had better survival than those in the placebo saline control group. While no similar studies compare the efficacy of chemical splanchnicectomy for the relief of pain in patients with ampullary carcinoma, it is reasonable to expect similar results. Thus, this simple and straightforward intraoperative chemical splanchnicectomy should be considered in patients with unresectable ampullary adenocarcinoma.

### Nonoperative Palliation

Most patients with the diagnosis of ampullary carcinoma have localized disease and are candidates for operative therapy. In patients who are not candidates for abdominal exploration because of major medical illness, or in those patients who are found to have unresectable disease on the basis of preoperative staging studies (most typically biopsy-proven hepatic metastases), nonoperative palliation is appropriate. The two approaches to palliate jaundice involve endoscopic or percutaneous techniques. Placement of a biliary endoprosthesis through the ampullary region to provide biliary decompression is a standard approach to the palliation of jaundice. Using either the older plastic endoprostheses or the newer metallic ones, this method allows internal drainage of the bile into the duodenum and avoids the placement of an external apparatus. Endoscopic placement is preferred by many over a percutaneous route because it avoids transhepatic puncture and the attendant risk of hemorrhage, hemobilia, and bile leak. Most reserve percutaneous transhepatic placement of a biliary drainage catheter for situations in which biliary decompression cannot be established endoscopically.

Patients initially treated nonoperatively via biliary decompression who later develop duodenal obstruction can undergo laparotomy for gastrojejunostomy in selected cases. In those who are not candidates for surgical exploration, there are some newer techniques on the horizon that may allow endoscopic laser therapy of an obstructing duodenal lesion and safe placement of an endoluminal stent. At the current time, these techniques remain experimental.

Patients with abdominal, epigastric, and back pain related to unresectable adenocarcinoma of the ampulla may benefit from narcotic analgesics given either orally or topically. Selected patients may benefit from percutaneous chemical splanchnicectomy using 50% alcohol, typically injected paraspinally under fluoroscopic control.

Several randomized studies have compared complication rates and survival rates in patients undergoing nonoperative biliary decompression with those of patients who have surgical bypass for relief of malignant biliary obstruction. These studies have generally involved patients with unresectable periampullary neoplasms, including pancreatic, bile duct, duodenal, and ampullary tumors. In general, nonoperative palliation has been associated with fewer procedure-related complications, a shorter initial period of hospitalization, but an increased need for follow-up intervention for occlusion of the biliary endoprosthesis from biliary sludge and debris, resulting in the recurrence of jaundice or cholangitis. Recent trials with self-expanding metal stents have demonstrated improved patency and some improvement in the incidence of recurrent jaundice and cholangitis.

### Chemotherapy and Radiotherapy

Unfortunately, data are not available to provide unqualified support for the use of chemotherapy and radiation therapy in the adjuvant setting in patients who have undergone resection of ampullary carcinoma via pancreaticoduodenectomy. Combined-modality therapy using 5-fluorouracil-based chemotherapy with external-beam radiation improves survival in patients with resected adenocarcinoma of the head of the pancreas (28–30). It is tempting to extrapolate these results to ampullary carcinoma, although no large studies provide good supportive data. Additionally, limited data suggest that postoperative adjuvant combination chemotherapy alone (using fluorouracil, doxorubicin, and mitomycin C) delays tumor recurrence in patients with ampullary adenocarcinoma (31), but more data are necessary.

In patients with unresectable ampullary adenocarcinoma, there are limited data concerning the use of palliative chemotherapy and/or radiotherapy. Most studies in this setting include groups of unresectable patients with all four periampullary tumors; therefore, results for ampullary adenocarcinoma alone are not available. There is no consensus regarding the use of palliative chemo- or radiotherapy in such patients.

## RESULTS

The overall 5-year survival rates for patients with ampullary adenocarcinoma undergoing pancreaticoduodenectomy approximate 30–50%. Factors that favor long-term survival include confinement of the tumor to the ampulla or duodenum ($T_1$ or $T_2$ lesions), the absence of regional nodal metastases ($N_0$ lesions), and the absence of positive resection margins. In patients who undergo operative palliation without resection, the 5-year survival rates approach 0, with a median survival of approximately 6–12 months. Survival data for patients who undergo local excision of ampullary carcinoma are largely not available, because most published series are small and include a mixture of patients with benign ampullary adenomas and ampullary adenomas with carcinoma in situ, as well as true ampullary adenocarcinoma.

## CONCLUSIONS

Ampullary tumors, although uncommon, can be the most rewarding of all the periampullary tumors to manage. Patients typically present with jaundice and pruritus, often with some evidence of GI blood loss. The jaundice and pruritus may be intermittent, related to intermittent obstruction of the ampulla, associated with tumor sloughing and necrosis. Occasional patients may present initially with pancreatitis. The diagnostic workup involves routine serum laboratory determinations as well as abdominal CT scanning and endoscopy. An endoscopic biopsy of an abnormal ampulla may provide pathologic verification of the diagnosis, and endoscopic ultrasound may provide information regarding the depth of tumor penetration. In most patients with ampullary adenocarcinoma, pancreaticoduodenectomy is the operation of choice. Local excision may be performed in carefully selected patients with benign ampullary pathology. For patients who are poor operative risks or who have evidence of distant metastatic disease, nonoperative palliative methods exist. While the benefits of radiotherapy and chemotherapy remain unproven in patients with ampullary adenocarcinoma, increasing evidence in patients with pancreatic carcinoma suggests that these modalities may be useful, particularly in the adjuvant setting in patients who have undergone resection. Overall 5-year survival rates in patients with resected ampullary adenocarcinoma approximate 40% and are largely determined by the status of resected lymph nodes and resection margins.

## REFERENCES

1. Gouma DJ, Obertop H, Vismans J, Willebrand D, Soeters PB. Progression of a benign epithelial ampullary tumor to adenocarcinoma. Surgery 1987;101:501–504.
2. DiGuiseppe JA, Yeo CJ, Hruban RH. Molecular biology and the diagnosis and treatment of adenocarcinoma of the pancreas. Adv Anat Pathol 1996;3:139–155.
3. Motojima K, Tsunoda T, Kanematsu T, Nagata Y, Urano T, Shiku H. Distinguishing pancreatic carcinoma from other periampullary carcinomas by analysis of mutations in the Kirsten-ras oncogene. Ann Surg 1991;214:657–662.
4. Calzavara C. Ueber adenome des uerdaungskanales. Virchows Arch Pathol Anat Physiol 1895;141:221.

5. Baggenstoss AH. Major duodenal papilla: variation of pathology interest and lesions of the mucosa. Arch Pathol 1938;26:853–868.
6. Yamaguchi K, Enjoji M. Carcinoma of the ampulla of Vater. A clinicopathologic study and pathologic staging in 109 cases of carcinoma and 5 cases of adenoma. Cancer 1987;59: 506–515.
7. Spigelman AD, Williams CB, Talbot IC, Domizio P, Phillips RKS. Upper gastrointestinal cancer in patients with familial adenomatous polyposis. Lancet 1989;2:783–785.
8. Norton ID, Pokorny CS, Painter DM, Johnson JR, Perkins KW. Fraternal sisters with adult polycystic kidney disease and adenoma of the ampulla of Vater. Gastroenterology 1995;109:2007–2010.
9. Klein A, Clemens J, Cameron JL. Periampullary neoplasms in von Recklinghausen's disease. Surgery 1989;106:815–819.
10. Hough DR, Chan A, Davidson H. Von Recklinghausen's disease associated with gastrointestinal carcinoid tumors. Cancer 1983; 51:2206–2208.
11. Venu RP, Geenen JE. Diagnosis and treatment of diseases of the papilla. Clin Gastroenterol 1986;15:439–456.
12. Leslie KA, Tsao JI, Rossi RL, Braasch JW. Metastatic renal cell carcinoma to ampulla of Vater: an unusual lesion amenable to surgical resection. Surgery 1996;119:349–351.
13. Walsh DB, Eckhauser FE, Cronenwett JL, Turcotte JC, Lindenauer SM. Adenocarcinoma of the ampulla of Vater. Diagnosis and treatment. Ann Surg 1982;195:152–157.
14. Tio TL, Mulder CJJ, Eggink WF. Endosonography in staging early carcinoma of the ampulla of Vater. Gastroenterology 1992;102: 1392–1395.
15. Rosch T, Braig C, Gain T, et al. Staging of pancreatic and ampullary carcinoma by endoscopic ultrasonography. Comparison with conventional sonography, computed tomography, and angiography. Gastroenterology 1992;102:188–199.
16. Halsted WS. Contributions to the surgery of the bile passages, especially of the common bile duct. Boston Med Surg J 1899; 141:645–654.
17. Gertsch P, Matthews JB, Lerut J, Baer HU, Blumgart LH. The technique of papilloduodenectomy. Surg Gynecol Obstet 1990; 170:254–256.
18. Rattner DW, Fernandez-del Castillo C, Brugge WR, Warshaw AL. Defining the criteria for local resection of ampullary neoplasms. Arch Surg 1996;131:366–371.
19. Asbun HJ, Rossi RL, Munson JL. Local resection for ampullary tumors. Is there a place for it? Arch Surg 1993;128:515–520.
20. Whipple AO, Parsons WB, Mullins CR. Treatment of carcinoma of the ampulla of Vater. Ann Surg 1935;102:763–779.
21. Trimble IR, Parsons JW, Sherman CP. A one stage operation for the cure of carcinoma of the ampulla of Vater and the head of the pancreas. Surg Gynecol Obstet 1941;73:711–722.
22. Cameron JL, Pitt HA, Yeo CJ, Lillemoe KD, Kaufman HS, Coleman J. One hundred and forty-five consecutive pancreaticoduodenectomies without mortality. Ann Surg 1993;217:430–438.
23. Yeo CJ. Management of complications following pancreaticoduodenectomy. Surg Clin North Am 1995;75:913–924.
24. Yeo CJ, Cameron JL, Maher MM, et al. A prospective randomized trial of pancreaticogastrostomy versus pancreaticojejunostomy after pancreaticoduodenectomy. Ann Surg 1995;222: 580–592.
25. Yeo CJ, Barry MK, Sauter PK, et al. Erythromycin accelerates gastric emptying following pancreaticoduodenectomy: a prospective, randomized placebo controlled trial. Ann Surg 1993; 218:229–238.
26. Lillemoe KD, Sauter PK, Pitt HA, Yeo CJ, Cameron JL. Current status of surgical palliation of periampullary carcinoma. Surg Gynecol Obstet 1993;176:1–10.
27. Lillemoe KD, Cameron JL, Kaufman HS, Yeo CJ, Pitt HA, Sauter PK. Chemical splanchnicectomy in patients with unresectable pancreatic cancer: a prospective randomized trial. Ann Surg 1993; 217:447–457.
28. Kalser MH, Ellenberg SS. Pancreatic cancer. Adjuvant combined radiation and chemotherapy following curative resection. Arch Surg 1985;120:899–903.
29. Gastrointestinal Tumor Study Group. Further evidence of effective adjuvant combined radiation and chemotherapy following curative resection of pancreatic cancer. Cancer 1987;59:2006–2010.
30. Yeo CJ, Cameron JL, Lillemoe KD, et al. Pancreaticoduodenectomy for cancer of the head of the pancreas: 201 patients. Ann Surg 1995;221:721–733.
31. Bakkevold KE, Arnesjo B, Dahl O, Kambestad B. Adjuvant combination chemotherapy (AMF) following radical resection of the pancreas and papilla of Vater—results of a controlled, prospective, randomized multicentre study. Eur J Cancer 1993; 29A:698–703.

# 69

# *Distal Bile Duct Tumors*

Constantine V. Godellas, Yuman Fong, Murray F. Brennan, and Leslie H. Blumgart

Tumors of the bile duct may occur at any level throughout the biliary tree. The common sites are at the confluence of the hepatic ducts or in the mid and low bile duct. The latter are less common than those in the area of the confluence and are more readily managed by established surgical techniques. That lesions in the mid and low common bile duct are less frequently encountered than those above the level of the cystic duct is attested to by the experience of Tompkins and colleagues (1), who recorded a total of 95 tumors: 47 high in the bile duct and the remainder below the cystic duct level. Similarly, experience at the Lahey Clinic over a 13-year period (1965–1978) revealed that 83 of 109 patients had tumors in the proximal bile duct, 13% in the distal bile duct and 11% in the mid bile duct (2). At Hammersmith Hospital, London, 15 distal cholangiocarcinomata were treated over a 5-year period during which 94 proximal lesions were encountered (3).

Both primary benign and malignant tumors are encountered, but metastatic cancer is also rarely encountered (Table 69.1). In addition, a number of benign conditions may present as tumor-like masses or as strictures of the low bile duct and may mimic malignancy in their clinical behavior.

### Prevalence

Benign biliary tumors are clinical rarities that have been the subject of infrequent case reports in the past, usually combined with a review of the literature. Benign bile duct tumors have been reported in 0.1% of all biliary tract operations and constitute only 6% of all extrahepatic bile duct neoplasms (4). To date, only some 200 cases of benign bile duct tumor have been reported in the English literature. As a further measure of their infrequent occurrence, only two operations for benign extrahepatic tumors were performed during a total experience of 4200 biliary tract operations at the Charity Hospital in New Orleans (5).

The incidence of malignant bile duct tumors in large autopsy series varies from 0.01 to 0.2%, and they may constitute about 2% of all cancers found at autopsy (6, 7). While still relatively rare, 4500 new cases per annum may be expected in the United States, an incidence similar to that of carcinoma of the tongue. Of these, we estimate that approximately 2000 cases will involve the distal bile duct.

While there is some evidence that the incidence of the disease is increasing, the advent of new diagnostic methods applicable in obstructive jaundice has led to the preoperative discovery of many more of these lesions almost certainly misdiagnosed in the past. Most of these cancers are found in the proximal biliary ductal system in the region of the hepatic bifurcation. Distal common bile duct cancers make up less than half of these tumors.

Most cancers occur in the 50- to 70-year-old age group, and males are slightly more commonly affected than females. In a recent 10-year review from Memorial Sloan-Kettering Cancer Center, distal bile duct cancers were 1/13th as common as pancreatic ductal carcinoma and represented only 5% of all periampullary cancers (8).

## BENIGN TUMORS AND PSEUDOTUMORS

### Clinical Presentation and Diagnosis

Patients with benign biliary tract tumors and often those with inflammatory masses masquerading as neoplasms almost invariably present with clinical manifestations of jaundice. The onset of icterus may be insidious or intermittent with few other symptoms, or it may be sudden and associated with colicky epigastric pain referred to the back or shoulder, nausea, and vomiting. There is seldom any significant weight loss. As these tumors are relatively slow-growing, some of the clinical symptoms may be intermittent or gradually progressive over an extended period of time only to culminate with obstructive jaundice. There are no clinical symptoms that can assist the physician in differentiating a benign biliary tract tumor from the other more common causes of biliary tract obstruction.

Physical findings are likewise nonspecific: liver enlargement, a palpable gallbladder, tenderness to palpation in the right hypochondrium, and jaundice. Because of the lack of characteristic symptoms and physical findings, benign biliary tumors are often not diagnosed preoperatively.

Reports since the early 1970s have emphasized the usefulness of percutaneous transhepatic cholangiography (PTC) and, more recently, endoscopic retrograde cholangiopancreatography (ERCP) in establishing a preoperative diagnosis of extrahepatic obstruction and in distinguishing between calculus and tumor as a cause (9, 10). Jain et al. (11) in their report of a patient with granular cell myoblastoma, suggested that an eccentric, short stenosis might be associated with a benign biliary tumor. However, obstructive changes identical to those seen in malignant neoplasms are not uncommon and indeed may be produced by inflammatory masses (12, 13). While PTC and ERCP will not distinguish between a benign tumor and a malignant one, adequate visualization of the ductal system provides vital information concerning tumor location, extension, and size, as well as the status of the intrahepatic ductal system. However, unless cytologic specimens obtained by brushings of the biliary tree at ERCP suggest malignancy, there is no preoperative diagnostic study capable of reliably distinguishing benign from malignant tumorous obstruction of the biliary ducts.

Caution is required regarding the use of PTC in the diagnosis of biliary tract obstruction. Although it is highly accurate in predicting tumorous involvement of the biliary tree, there are recorded instances of a tumor suggested to be at the confluence of the hepatic ducts found later to be in the periampullary region. Such misinterpretation at PTC is almost always due to poor radiologic technique and, in particular, failure to place the

**TABLE 69.1. Tumors Involving the Distal Common Bile Duct**

| |
|---|
| Benign |
| Papillomatous polyp |
| Adenomatous polyp |
| Multiple biliary papillomatosis |
| Biliary cystadenoma |
| Granular cell myoblastoma |
| Neural tumors |
| Leiomyoma |
| Pseudotumors |
| Heterotopic tissue |
| Malignant |
| Adenocarcinoma |
| Neuroendocrine tumors |
| Cystadenocarcinoma |
| Malignant fibrous histiocytoma |
| Rhabdomyosarcoma/leiomyosarcoma |
| Metastatic tumors |
| Lymphoma |

patient in an upright position; late films should be repeated at an interval of up to 3 hours. This allows complete mixing of contrast material with stagnant and often viscous bile. Failure to demonstrate dilated intrahepatic ducts does not preclude a diagnosis of partial obstruction of the biliary tract but should at least lead to questioning and stimulate further studies.

### Papilloma and Adenoma

The most common variety of benign tumor of the extrahepatic biliary tree is that arising from the glandular epithelium lining the ducts. Roughly two-thirds of reported benign neoplasms fall into the category of polyps, adenomatous papilloma, or adenoma. There is a slight female predominance in the incidence of these lesions (1.3:1), and the average age at diagnosis is 58 years. Leriche (14) reported a massive papillomatous tumor weighing 750 g arising from the common bile duct of a 4-year-old child. Most are found either in the ampulla or in close proximity to the Vaterian system (47%); the common bile duct (27%) is the second most frequent site.

Chu, in his classic review of benign biliary neoplasms, found that 26 of 30 cases studied were either papillomas or adenomas (15). Later, Dowdy et al. (16) observed that 36 of the 43 cases they reviewed were similarly classified. Since 1962, 53 additional patients have been added to the English literature (17–25). Presently, we have traced a total of 115 patients reported with either benign polyps, adenoma, or cystadenoma.

The onset of symptoms may vary from a few weeks to 35 years. Jaundice, a presenting symptom in over 90% of patients (26) occurs intermittently in approximately 40% of patients. Most patients complain of right upper-quadrant pain associated with jaundice. Wright (27) reported a patient with relapsing pancreatitis who was cured by excision of a common bile duct polyp that had prolapsed into the ampulla of Vater. Gallstones or biliary calculi are reported in only 20% of patients found to have benign extrahepatic ductal tumors. Cattell and Pyrtek (28) suggest that recurrence of symptomatology following cholecystectomy should suggest the possibility of a tumor in the ampullary area rather than biliary dyskinesia. A benign adenomatous tumor should be included on the differential list in all secondary operations of the biliary tree performed for obstruction. These lesions, generally soft and difficult to palpate, present little or no resistance to exploring ductal probes and are thus difficult to detect at the operating table. They are more frequently detected by intraoperative cholangiography, ultrasonography, or choledochoscopy. Misinterpretation of cholangiographic images followed by insertion of an endoscopic stent can dislodge these tumors and make subsequent operative detection impossible. Alternatively, we have seen lesions developing in the lower common bile duct near the ampulla actually protrude through the papilla and be visible endoscopically. In contrast, malignant lesions developing in the ampullary area tend to be infiltrative, are usually large, firm, and more likely to be ulcerated. Presenting symptoms related to bleeding in association with benign adenomatous polyps of the bile ducts are exceedingly rare, although Teter (29) recorded a death due to massive hemorrhage secondary to such a lesion.

Kozuka et al. (30) suggested that most polypoid or papillary cancers of the extrahepatic duct arise from preexisting adenomas. In a review of 43 carcinomas of the extrahepatic tree, Kozuka identified an adenomatous residue in 9 (21.4%). Certainly others have suggested that suprapapillary ductal papillomatous lesions may be precancerous. Gouma et al. (22) reported a case of intrahepatic bile duct papillomata associated with changes of nuclear atypia and reviewed the literature suggesting that it is reasonable to regard these lesions as of low-grade malignant potential. The rarity of benign lesions of the extrahepatic bile ducts makes substantiation of this theory difficult. Although the etiology of bile duct adenomas is uncertain, these lesions have been produced experimentally by performing a choledochopancreatostomy in puppies, a model for anomalous choledochopancreatic ductal junction. After several years, mucosal hyperplasia was observed in 100% of the dogs, with almost one-half having bile duct adenomas (31).

**Treatment.** In 1962, Dowdy et al. (16) reviewed the literature and detailed the operative procedures for 37 patients with papillomas or adenomas. They reported that four of the five recognized tumor recurrences were in patients who had had local tumor excision as primary therapy. Since then, 37 additional patients have been reported for whom both operative procedure and follow-up data are available. Fifteen patients underwent local excision, presumably including the stalk and/or base of the polyp, two of whom had recurrences that necessitated reoperation. Fourteen patients with lesions in or near the ampulla had local excision by way of transduodenal papillotomy without recorded tumor recurrence. In three additional patients, curettage of a polypoid tumor was accomplished without recurrence. One patient had local resection of the duct, and one had local resection of the duct wall without recurrence. Three patients had a Whipple resection for a low-lying tumor initially thought to be malignant.

Based upon these reports and our own experience, it appears that the choice of operative procedure while somewhat dependent on the patients age, medical condition, and location of the tumor, should include total resection of the lesion. Pancreaticoduodenectomy may be necessary. However, lesions arising in the ampulla can be successfully managed by wide local excision embracing the entire ampullary apparatus as described by Gertsch et al. (32). Endoscopic snaring has been suggested, but we do not recommend this approach.

### Multiple Biliary Papillomatosis

Multiple biliary papillomatosis presenting as diffuse intrahepatic and extrahepatic biliary papillomata is extremely rare; most cases involve predominantly the common and intrahepatic bile ducts, although presentation with mid and distal biliary tumors also occurs. There may be a prolonged history of partial and intermittent obstruction of the bile duct by fragments of the villous tumor. In some patients, however, the only symptom has been abdominal pain. The history may be prolonged and be associated with anemia as a result of bleeding. Concomitant cholelithiasis and choledocholithiasis have been reported.

Tompkins et al. (33) have emphasized the value of intraoperative endoscopy in the evaluation of the biliary tree for multiple lesions. Certainly proximal endoscopy is indicated if there is a papillary tumor in the region of the low bile duct.

## Other Tumors and Pseudotumors

While most benign tumors of the low bile duct are adenomas, a number of other benign conditions can present as distal biliary obstruction and should be considered in the differential diagnosis. Distal bile duct obstruction due to pancreatitis can be a source of confusion, but in such instances, a typical history and pancreatic ductal changes at ERCP are extremely valuable. Demonstration of chronic pancreatitis on a pancreatogram should evoke careful consideration of pancreatitis as the reason for biliary obstruction. Gallstones impacted distally at the ampulla of Vater can occasionally be confusing but are usually easily differentiated from tumor at endoscopy.

**Biliary Cystadenoma.** Although most biliary cystadenomas occur in the intrahepatic biliary system, approximately 15% are found in the extrahepatic biliary tree, and another 15% occur in both the liver and extrahepatic biliary system. While these lesions may progress to cystadenocarcinoma in the liver, there is only one report of this occurring in the extrahepatic biliary system (34). Complete excision is curative.

**Granular Cell Myoblastoma.** Granular cell myoblastoma is a very rare benign tumor of uncertain etiology occasionally encountered in the extrahepatic biliary tree. Indeed, the lesion constitutes less than 10% of all benign tumors of the extrahepatic biliary tree (35). While reported in anatomic locations as varied as the pituitary and appendix, the lesions are most commonly encountered in the tongue, breast, and subcutaneous tissues, with less than 1% of granular cell myoblastomas occurring in the extrahepatic biliary tree (35–36). Black women are predominantly affected, and 15% have multicentric lesions (37).

Coggins (38) first described a granular cell myoblastoma arising from the common bile duct near the ampulla of Vater. Since Coggin's initial autopsy report, 47 additional patients have been reported with this lesion: 30 had lesions arising in the hepatic or common duct, most commonly the lower common bile duct, and 15 were reported in the cystic duct (10, 39–52). The average age of patients with this tumor is 34.5 years.

Multiple tumors within the extrahepatic biliary tree have been reported in five patients (10, 45, 48, 52, 53). Synchronous tumors have been noted in four patients with bile duct lesions: a separate gastric tumor, three patients with skin lesions, and one with multiple simultaneous lesions in the gallbladder and cystic duct (47, 55, 56). Clinical symptoms associated with granular cell myoblastoma arising in extrahepatic biliary ducts tend to be those of painless jaundice, while a presentation consistent with cholecystitis is more commonly associated with lesions involving the cystic duct. Other described symptoms include anorexia, weight loss, nausea, and vomiting. Granular cell myoblastoma might be included in the differential diagnosis of obstructive jaundice in a black female, especially if she has a tumor nodule in the tongue, breast, or subcutaneous tissue. However, this clinical presentation would be extraordinarily rare.

Most tumors have been described as firm to palpation, localized, confined to the wall of the common bile duct or cystic duct, and generally less than 3 cm in diameter. The mucosa overlying the tumor has generally been intact and histologically normal. On cut section, granular cell myoblastoma is yellowish white; microscopically it consists of fibrous tissue diffusely infiltrated by elongated large polygonal cells or cells containing small, dark nuclei and an abundant eosinophilic granular cytoplasm. The cytoplasmic granules are markedly positive with the periodic acid-Schiff reaction. Frozen-section diagnosis is adequate for delineating these lesions. While this tumor usually does not metastasize, local recurrence may occur, especially if excision is incomplete.

The histogenesis is uncertain and is marked by controversy. The tumor was initially termed granular cell myoblastoma because it was thought to be derived from "myoid cells." Indeed, characteristics of the cells in tissue culture suggest a myogenic origin (57). More recently, other cellular origins have been proposed. Studies have suggested that perineural fibroblasts, histiocytes, Schwann cells, primitive mesenchymal cells, or even multiple cell lines may serve as the origin of this tumor.

***Treatment.*** Treatment should consist of total excision of the bile duct segment containing the lesion, with reconstruction by Roux-en-Y choledochojejunostomy or hepaticojejunostomy for lesions arising in the common hepatic duct (58). Chandrasoma and Fitzgibbons (59) and Manstein et al. (58) have reported successful management of lesions occurring in the intrapancreatic duct by pancreaticoduodenectomy. There is one documented local recurrence and an additional patient who required a second operation because of an incomplete local resection (35, 58).

**Neural Tumors.** The incidence of neural tumors appears to be lower than expected when one considers the abundant network of neural tissue that normally surrounds the extrahepatic bile ducts. In 1955, Oden (60) reported a neurinoma in a 40-year-old woman who presented with jaundice and mild epigastric discomfort. At operation, a cystic tumor was found displacing the common bile duct medially. The cyst was extirpated, but the wall contiguous to the common bile duct was left in situ. Several common duct stones were also removed. She was asymptomatic 18 months later.

Von Recklinghausen's neurofibromatosis is well recognized to produce gastrointestinal symptoms. Although bleeding, perforation, and obstruction due to intussusception, volvulus, or stenosis have been reported, only one instance of obstructive jaundice secondary to visceral neurofibromatosis is recorded in the literature. Curry and Gray (61) reported finding, at autopsy, a submucosal nodular tumor (25-mm diameter) protruding into the duodenum around the ampullary opening.

While paragangliomata commonly arise in the adrenal gland as pheochromocytoma, extraadrenal lesions are occasionally found in the neck, the mediastinum, and around the aorta. Paragangliomas have also been observed in the gallbladder, gastrointestinal tract, and genitourinary tract. Sarma et al. (62) recorded a case in the extrahepatic biliary tree.

**Leiomyoma.** Leiomyomas are the most common benign tumors of the esophagus, stomach, and small intestine; in the extrahepatic biliary tree they are among the least common. The scanty presence of muscle fibers in the normal common bile duct probably accounts for the fact that only five such lesions have been reported. Each of these patients presented with progressive jaundice, itching, nausea, vomiting, and weight loss. The first patient reported had a tumor confined to the intrapancreatic segment of the common bile duct, which was locally excised along with some of the overlying pancreatic tissue and ligation of the duct of Santorini. The proximal bile duct was anastomosed to the jejunum. This patient was reported well 3 years following surgery (63). Kune and Polgar (64) reported a 49-year-old male treated by pancreaticoduodenectomy for a 4-cm tumor in the intrapancreatic segment of the common bile duct, which was assumed to be a pancreatic carcinoma at surgery. Microscopically, the lesion was observed to arise from the bile duct wall. The patient was well 28 months after operation. The third patient died of septicemia following ERCP demonstration of a tumor obstructing the lower part of the common bile duct, seemingly as a result of external compression. Autopsy examination revealed an angioleiomyoma of the common bile duct. The mucosa overlying the tumor was observed to be intact (65). A fourth recorded leiomyoma occurred at the ampulla of Vater (66). Recently, Mandeville and Stawski (67) reported a fifth patient in whom a leiomyoma of the hepatic duct bifurcation was treated.

**Pseudotumors.** Nonmalignant lesions that may cause obstruction of the extrahepatic biliary ductal system and may closely resemble neoplasms at investigation and even at laparotomy occur frequently enough to be seriously considered in the differential diagnosis of any lesion suspected to be a bile duct tumor (13, 68–69). Lesions should not be assumed to be neoplastic without histologic proof, and certainly a presumed diagnosis of neoplasm should not be the signal for incomplete drainage procedures carried out surgically, percutaneously, or endoscopically. Such maneuvers are inevitably followed by infection, necessitate repeat drainage procedures, and compromise effective surgery.

Stamatakis et al. (12) reported a benign inflammatory mass of the common bile duct in a 13-year-old girl who presented with obstructive jaundice and abdominal pain. PTC demonstrated complete obstruction of the common hepatic duct with intraluminal shouldering, suggesting a tumor. At operation, a 3-cm spherical mass was found to be closely applied to the porta hepatis, necessitating excision of the confluence, common hepatic duct, and common bile duct, with reconstruction by Roux-en-Y hepaticojejunostomy. Pathologic examination demonstrated nearly complete obstruction of the common hepatic and common bile ducts by an encapsulated yellowish brown mass. Microscopically, the encased bile duct exhibited loss of muscular coat, loss of ductal epithelium, and replacement by collagenous fibrous tissue. Scattered throughout the fibrous tissue were foci of acute inflammatory cells. The authors concluded that the mass represented an excessive inflammatory reaction to some local chemical or infective irritant and further speculated that the lesion might represent a form of localized sclerosing cholangitis. Similar cases have been reported by Haith et al., Golematis et al., and Heuser and Polk (70–72).

Standfield et al. (73) reported an interesting group of 12 patients with localized strictures of the extrahepatic biliary system. None had a history of trauma, gallbladder stones, or antecedent diseases generally associated with sclerosing cholangitis. All were found to have histologic evidence of chronic inflammation, fibrosis, and epithelial ulceration. The authors believed this entity was distinct from sclerosing cholangitis in that the mucosa remained intact in that disease. Similarly, Hadjis et al. (13) described 8 of 104 patients at the Hammersmith Hospital, London, submitted to surgery with a clinical diagnosis of malignant obstruction at the confluence of the bile ducts, who had benign disease. The benign nature of the lesion was not certain in six of these patients, even at laparotomy. Comprehensive investigation had failed to give an accurate preoperative diagnosis, although biliary obstruction was accurately shown in all patients, and preoperative assessment using cholangiographic and angiographic data indicated that all were potentially resectable. Microscopic examination of the biopsy specimens taken from the bile ducts of these patients showed an extensive increase of fibrous tissue in all sections. Sections of associated lymph nodes and of the gallbladder were unremarkable. No vascular changes were identified. In particular, no specimen showed evidence of dysplastic, neoplastic, or preneoplastic cytologic change. We have encountered two such cases in the intrapancreatic bile duct.

The diagnostic difficulty is compounded in that cholangiocarcinoma has been described in association with, or as a complication of, primary sclerosing cholangitis. In the presence of a localized bile duct stricture, it is impossible to make a definitive diagnosis without specific biopsy or cytology.

**Heterotopic Tissue.** Symptomatic heterotopic tissue arising in the biliary tree is an exceedingly rare finding. In 1967, Whittaker et al. (74) first observed heterotopic gastric mucosa in a cystic duct that had obstructed the gallbladder. Welling et al. (75) later recorded a similar mucosal mass obstructing the common bile duct at the level of the cystic duct. More recently, Kalman et al. (76) reported a 1-cm papillary tumor arising in the common hepatic duct, which on microscopic examination demonstrated gastric fundal mucosa replacing the full thickness of the bile duct wall.

Heterotopic gastric mucosa occurring at the ampulla of Vater was observed to be the basis for biliary tract obstruction by Blundell et al. (77). Although occurrence elsewhere in the gastrointestinal tract is well documented, this appears to be the first documented ampullary obstruction secondary to heterotopic gastric mucosa.

Kalman et al. cite two hypotheses for the etiology of heterotopia (76). First, they suggest metaplasia with heterotopic differentiation. Several authors have described metaplastic gastric replacement of the gallbladder mucosa in cases of chronic cholecystitis. Usually the metaplastic glands resemble pyloric and Brunner's glands, while specialized chief and parietal cells are absent. A second, and perhaps more tenable, theory is based on the observation that embryologically, the epithelial lining of the foregut and the parenchyma of the liver and pancreas arise from the same primitive endoderm (see above). Kalman states that because of the "common origin of these structures lined by multipotential cells capable of differentiation along several cell lines, it is not unreasonable to conclude that the heterotopic gastric replacement may have resulted from congenitally replaced tissue."

Heterotopic pancreatic tissue has been observed to occur from the stomach to the ileum, as well as in the omentum, spleen, gallbladder, and common bile duct. Seven cases have been reported in which heterotopic pancreatic tissue was found in the common bile duct or ampulla of Vater (78–81).

## MALIGNANT TUMORS

The paucity of published data on distal bile duct cancers is a direct reflection of the rarity of this entity. Between October, 1983, and October, 1994, we collected prospective data on 1978 periampullary cancers seen at the Memorial Sloan-Kettering Cancer Center. This database of periampullary cancer indicates that distal bile duct cancer is 1/13th as common as pancreatic ductal carcinoma and represents only 5% of all cancers in this region. Since approximately 24,000 cases of pancreatic ductal carcinoma are found in the United States each year (82), fewer than 2000 cases of distal bile duct cancer would be expected. Thus it is not surprising that few previous reports devoted to this entity have been published. Most data on this cancer have been part of reports of either periampullary cancers (83–86) or of all bile duct cancers (1, 2, 87) (Table 69.2). These data indicate that distal bile duct cancer represents approximately 5–10% of all periampullary cancers and 20% of all bile duct cancers.

The overwhelming majority of bile duct cancers are adenocarcinomas. Most occur as slow-growing lesions, and while lymphatic metastases occur in approximately one-third of patients, blood-borne metastases are unusual. The tumors spread by local invasion involving neural, perineural, and lymphatic tissues. There is also a well-described subepithelial spread of these cancers, which is important in defining tumor-free margins at resection.

Less common primary distal bile duct tumors include neuroendocrine tumors, encompassing carcinoid tumors, cystadenocarcinoma, and malignant fibrous histiocytoma (Table 69.1). Rhabdomyosarcoma, predominantly seen in infants, has also been identified (88). In addition to these rare primary tumors of the distal bile duct, metastatic malignant melanoma as well as metastatic tumors from renal cell cancer, oat cell cancer of the lung, breast carcinoma, ovarian carcinoma, and colonic carcinoma may occur in the periampullary region and lead to distal

**TABLE 69.2. Studies of Distal Bile Duct Cancer**

| Author | Years | Institutions *(n)* | Total *(n)* | Resected *(n)* | Operative Mortality (%) | Med Survival (months) | Survival 3-year (%) | Survival 5-year (%) |
|---|---|---|---|---|---|---|---|---|
| Warren, 1975 | 30 | 1 | — | 47 | 21 | — | 32 | 25 |
| Nakase, 1975 | 25 | 57 | 309 | 161 | 22 | 17 | 8 | 5 |
| Tompkins, 1981 | 25 | 1 | 18 | 12 | 8 | 18 | 28 | 28 |
| Alexander, 1983 | 13 | 1 | 14 | 14 | 21 | 16 | 20 | 18 |
| Lerut, 1983 | 15 | 1 | — | 5 | — | 11 | 0 | 0 |
| Tarazi, 1986 | 35 | 1 | — | 11 | 0 | — | — | 17 |
| Nagourney, 1994 | 10 | 1 | 39 | 22 | — | 24 | 40 | 40 |
| Fong, 1996 | 10 | 1 | 104 | 45 | 4 | 33 | 46 | 27 |

common bile duct obstruction. Lymphoma, which usually occurs in the pancreatic head, may also cause distal bile duct obstruction.

## Presentation and Evaluation

The clinical presentation of distal bile duct cancer is very similar to that of pancreatic adenocarcinoma or higher bile duct tumors, with jaundice, pruritus, and weight loss the predominant presenting symptoms. In a recent review of 104 distal bile duct cancers (8), jaundice was the most common presenting symptom, occurring in 75% of all patients. Jaundice is usually steadily progressive; however, on occasion, jaundice may be intermittent, particularly if the bile duct cancer is of the papillary variety. Weight loss is also common, occurring in one-third. Pruritus or pain was reported in one-quarter of patients at presentation. The presentation of distal bile duct cancer is therefore similar to that of any condition that causes bile duct obstruction. Distal bile duct cancer can usually be distinguished from choledocholithiasis by preoperative sonography or ERCP. However, distinguishing it from other periampullary cancers by preoperative or even operative evaluations is often difficult.

Evaluation of patients with distal bile duct cancers usually begins like that of all patients with distal bile duct obstruction. The history should evaluate the pattern of biliary obstruction. Any history consistent with past cholelithiasis, cholecysticitis, or pancreatitis should be sought, as well as any symptoms of exocrine or endocrine pancreatic insufficiency. Physical examination should include a search for distended gallbladder and signs of portal hypertension. Initial imaging studies should include sonography and/or computed tomography. If these studies demonstrate extrahepatic bile duct dilation, no signs of biliary stones, and a mass localized to the head of the pancreas, periampullary tumor should be strongly suspected. Baring definitive signs of unresectable tumor, such as encasement of celiac, superior mesenteric, or portal vessels, surgical intervention should be planned. If no mass is noted, ERCP can be useful in demonstrating a malignant stricture. Cytologic evaluation of specimens obtained by brush biopsy during ERCP may also allow definitive diagnosis prior to therapeutic intervention. PTC, a useful test in the evaluation of *high* bile duct obstruction, is usually not necessary for diagnosis of malignant obstruction low in the bile duct. Staging laparoscopy with endoscopic ultrasound may provide further evaluation of intrabdominal spread and resectability.

## Natural History

In our recent report of 104 distal bile duct cancers, the median survival of the 59 patients who were not resected with curative intent was 7 months, with no patient in this group surviving to 2 years (8). These data echo those of previous reports (1–2, 83–87) demonstrating that patients who do not undergo resection with curative intent usually succumb to their cancer within 6 months. Death is related to local tumor spread and associated biliary or portal venous obstruction leading to liver failure or biliary sepsis. Since multiple series have reported 5-year survivors (1–2, 8, 83, 85–87) after potentially curative resections, surgical excision is the treatment of choice.

## Surgical Resection

The mainstay of treatment for distal bile duct cancer is resection, usually consisting of a pancreaticoduodenectomy. Patients with truly localized, very early cancers may be treated with wide local duct excision. This usually represents a minority of cases, however. Of a series of 45 resected distal bile duct cancers, only 6 were treated by local duct excision (8). Most patients require a pancreaticoduodenectomy for extirpation of tumor. In the not-too-distant past, this operation was associated with an operative mortality of over 20%. With the dismal prognosis associated with periampullary lesions, most of which were pancreatic adenocarcinomas, some felt that pancreaticoduodenectomy was not justified (89). Over the last 2 decades, the safety of pancreaticoduodenectomy has steadily improved. In major centers, this operation can now be performed with a perioperative mortality of less than 5% (90–94). In our recent series of distal bile duct cancers, the perioperative mortality for 45 resected patients was 4% (8); median hospital stay was 17 days (range, 1–82) for resected patients; and complications occurred in 17 of the resected patients (38%). The most common complications were intraabdominal abscess and pancreatic fistulae.

## Long-Term Survival and Predictors of Outcome

Surgical resection can clearly result in long-term survival and cure. In the resected patients, median survival can be expected to be between 16 and 33 months, with 5-year survival expected in up to 27% of patients (Table 69.2). In comparison, patients offered no surgical therapy or subjected to only diagnostic laparotomy had a median survival of 6–7 months. Patients palliated by surgical bypass had a longer median survival (10 months) but were still unlikely to be alive 2 years after diagnosis (8). Major predictors of long-term outcome are resectability and nodal status. Parameters that do not correlate with long-term outcome include gender, age, preoperative stenting, preoperative bilirubin level, and tumor grade (8).

As stated above, distal biliary obstruction may be produced by any of the tumors of the periampullary region, including pancreatic ductal adenocarcinoma, ampullary carcinoma, duodenal carcinoma, and distal bile duct carcinoma. Though both clinical presentation and therapy are very similar for these four tumors, outcome after resection may be very different. Recent publications from our institution are summarized to compare the long-term survival for each of these entities (8, 93, 95, 97–98) (Fig. 69.1). After curative resection of pancreatic adenocarcinoma, 5-year survival is expected to be less than 15% (91, 92, 96), while 5-year survival for ampullary carcinoma is

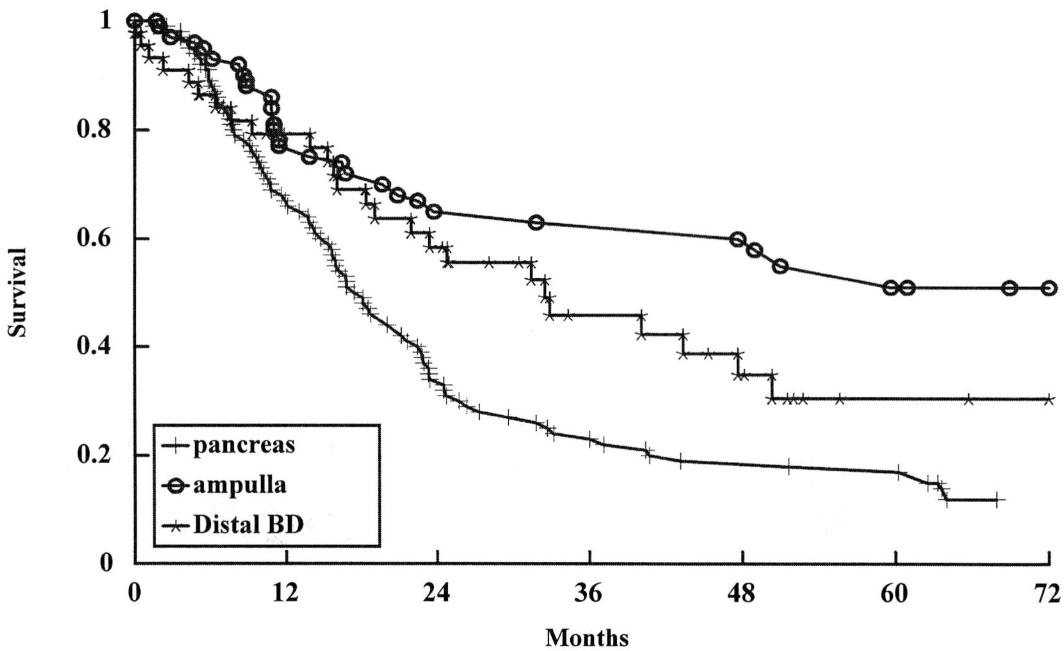


**FIG. 69.1.** Comparison of survival of patients after resection of pancreatic cancer, ampullary cancer, or distal bile duct cancer. (Data for pancreatic cancer are from Geer RJ, Brennan MF. Prognostic indicators for survival after resection of pancreatic adenocarcinoma. Am J Surg 1993;165:68–73; data for ampullary cancer from Matory YL, Gaynor J, Brennan MF. Carcinoma of the ampulla of Vater. Surg Gynecol Obstet 1993;177:366–370; and data for distal bile duct cancer from Fong YF, Blumgart LH, Lin E, et al. Outcome of treatment for distal bile duct cancer. Br J Surg 1996;83:1712–1715.)

more likely to approach 50% (83–86). The results for distal bile duct cancer are intermediate, with 5-year survival of approximately 30%.

## Palliation

Palliation for unresectable distal bile duct cancer is mainly directed at biliary obstruction and gastric outlet obstruction. For the latter, surgical gastrojejunal bypass is indicated, except for patients with far-advanced disease, for which an endoscopically placed gastrostomy may be the best option. For biliary obstruction, both nonsurgical and surgical means of relieving the obstruction exist. The decision to decompress the distal bile duct obstruction is the same as for any malignancy and depends on the clinical condition of the patient, associated medical problems, and the expertise of the particular institution.

Prior to the advent of endoscopic biliary intubation techniques, surgical biliary enteric bypass was the standard of care for obstructive jaundice produced by unresectable tumors of the periampullary region. The advantages of surgical bypass include complete relief of the obstruction, prolonged patency, and low incidence of cholangitis. The risks of general anesthesia, the recovery associated with the surgical procedure, and the short survival associated with unresectable malignancies of this region have prompted a greater enthusiasm for endoscopic stenting for malignant distal biliary obstruction. Clear indications for surgical bypass are *(a)* failure at endoscopic stenting, *(b)* gastric outlet obstruction preventing endoscopic access and requiring simultaneous gastroenteric bypass, and *(c)* obstructed patients explored for resection of tumor but found to be unresectable. Recent advances in laparoscopic techniques also allow laparoscopic biliary bypasses to be performed. Laparoscopic bypasses have been suggested to have less risk and shorter hospital stays than bypasses performed by the traditional open techniques. A prospective clinical trial comparing endoscopic stenting with laparoscopic bypass using hospital stay, morbidity, and long-term patency as outcome parameters is sorely needed.

The only indication for emergent biliary decompression and the only indication for preoperative biliary decompression prior to an exploration for potential resection of tumor is cholangitis. Usually, low bile duct obstruction can be decompressed endoscopically. However, when patients have associated gastric outlet obstruction or other technical factors not allowing access to, or cannulation of, the papilla, or if a skilled endoscopist is not available, percutaneous drainage may be necessary.

In contrast to high bile duct tumors, where biliary drainage should never be undertaken for jaundice without itching or cholangitis, in the distal duct we feel that jaundice alone constitutes adequate indication for drainage. The reason for this more liberal policy regarding the distal duct is the relative risk of life-threatening biliary sepsis at each site. For high bile duct cancers, the tumors often grow to involve second- and third-order intrahepatic ducts, and excluded segments of liver are not uncommon. Therefore, biliary sepsis often occurs after instrumentation insolvable by further instrumentation. Drainage is much simpler for distal bile duct tumors, and dealing with infection in the biliary tract is more straightforward.

Nonsurgical drainage should be performed for patients with malignant lesions demonstrated to be clearly unresectable by preoperative imaging and with no gastric outlet obstruction. Biliary drainage is maintained by either plastic or metallic endoprostheses. A detailed discussion of endoprostheses is beyond the scope of this chapter and the reader is referred to standard texts. Briefly, the advantages of plastic stents include the ease of placement and exchange of these stents and the low cost. Disadvantages include the possibility of migration of the stent and the high likelihood that they will become occluded and require exchange every 2–3 months. Metallic expandable stents offer a lesser chance of migration and longer patency but suffer from expense and the fact that they are essentially not removable or exchangeable. Our bias is to use plastic stents, accepting the need to replace them every 2–3 months.

### Chemotherapy and Radiotherapy

Because of the rarity of distal bile duct cancers, there are no trials examining chemotherapy or radiotherapy for this disease entity. Clinical practice of these palliative anticancer therapies is based on the few available data for pancreatic cancer extrapolated to distal bile duct cancer. 5-fluorouracil (5-FU) is the chemotherapy most often used in patients with primary, locally unresectable, metastatic, or recurrent low bile duct cancers. There is certainly no study demonstrating a benefit for postoperative adjuvant chemotherapy after complete resection of tumor. Radiotherapy has also been advocated for patients with locally unresectable, metastatic, or recurrent disease, again based on data extrapolated from pancreatic or high bile duct cancers. Our practice is to use no chemotherapy or radiotherapy in the adjuvant setting. Combined external-beam radiation with 5-FU chemotherapy is offered to patients with locally advanced and unresectable disease. As with other sites, intraluminal radiation therapy has been used, with limited efficacy in very small numbers of patients.

## REFERENCES


1. Tompkins RK, Thomas D, Wile A, et al. Prognostic factors in bile duct carcinoma. Analysis of 96 cases. Ann Surg 1981;194:447–456.
2. Alexander F, Rossi RL, O'Bryan M, et al. Biliary carcinoma. A review of 109 cases. Am J Surg 1984;147:503–509.
3. Soreide O, Kelley CJ, Czerniak A, et al. Clinical spectrum and diagnostic strategies in non-calculous lower bile duct obstruction. Dig Surg 1986;2(4):209–221.
4. Burhans R, Meyer RT. Benign neoplasms of the extrahepatic biliary ducts. Am Surg 1971;37:161–166.
5. Farris KB, Faust BF. Granular cell tumors of the biliary ducts. Arch Pathol Lab Med 1979;103:510–512.
6. Kirschbaum JD, Kozoll DC. Carcinoma of the gallbladder and extrahepatic bile ducts. Surg Gynecol Obstet 1941;73:740–754.
7. Kuwayti K, Baggenstoss AH, Stauffer MH, et al. Carcinoma of the major intrahepatic and the extrahepatic bile ducts exclusive of the papilla of Vater. Surg Gynecol Obstet 1957;104:357–366.
8. Fong YF, Blumgart LH, Lin E, et al. Outcome of treatment for distal bile duct cancer. Br J Surg 1996;83:1712–1715.
9. Hossack KF, Herron JJ. Benign tumors of the common bile duct: report of a case and review of the literature. Aust NZ J Surg 1972;42:22–26.
10. Kittredge RD, Baer JW. Percutaneous transhepatic cholangiography: problems in interpretation. AJR 1975;125:35–46.
11. Jain KM, Hastings OM, Rickert RR, et al. Granular cell tumor of the common bile duct. Am J Gastroenterol 1979;71:401–407.
12. Stamatakis JD, Howard ER, Williams R. Benign inflammatory tumour of the common bile duct. Br J Surg 1979;66:257–258.
13. Hadjis NS, Collier NA, Blumgart LH. Malignant masquerade at the hilum of the liver. Br J Surg 1985;72:659–661.
14. Leriche R. Volomineuse tumeur papillomateuse du choledoque chez un enfant. Lyon Chir 1934;31:598–602.
15. Chu PT. Benign neoplasms of the extrahepatic bile ducts. Arch Pathol 1950;50:84–87
16. Dowdy GS, Olin WG, Shelton EL, et al. Benign tumors of the extrahepatic bile ducts: report of three cases and review of the literature. Arch Surg 1962;85:503–513.
17. Bahuth JJ, Winkley JH. Benign tumor of the common bile duct. Calif Med 1966;104:307–309.
18. Short WF, Nedwich A, Levy HA, et al. Biliary cystadenoma. Arch Surg 1971;102:78–80.
19. Sull WJ, Brown HW. Benign extrahepatic biliary tumor associated with acute diverticulitis. Int Surg 1972;57:330–333.
20. Archie JP JR, Murray HM Jr. Benign polypoid adenoma of the ampulla of Vater. Treatment by double sphincteroplasty. Arch Surg 1978;113:180–181.
21. Lukes PJ, Nilson AE, Rolny P, et al. Premalignant lesions of the papilla of Vater and the common bile duct. Acta Chir Scand 1979;145:545–548.
22. Gouma DJ, Mutum SS, Benjamin IS, et al. Intrahepatic biliay papillomatosis. Br J Surg 1984;71:72–74.
23. Van Steenbergen W, Povette E, Marchal G, et al. Cystadenoma of the common bile duct demonstrated by endoscopic retrograde cholangiography: an uncommon cause of extrahepatic obstruction. Am J Gastroenterol 1984;79:466–470.
24. Thomsen P, Vasehus Modsen P, Moesgaard F, et al. Biliary cystadenoma of the common bile duct with secondary biliary cirrhosis. Acta Med Scand 1984;216:327–330.
25. Byrne DJ, Walker Ma, Pringle R, et al. Extrahepatic biliary cystadenoma: report of a case and review of the literature. J R Coll Surg Edinb 1989;34:223–224.
26. McIntyre JA, Pay-Zen C. Adenoma of the common bile duct causing obstructive jaundice. Can J Surg 168;11:215–218.
27. Wright RB. Relapsing pancreatitis: report of a case with unusual features. Br J Surg 1958;45–394–395.
28. Cattell RB, Pyrtek LJ. Premalignant lesions of the ampulla of Vater. Surg Gynecol Obstet 1950;90:21–30.
29. Teter LF. Massive hemorrhage from benign adenoma of the biliary duct causing death. J Mich Med Soc 1954;53:62–63.
30. Kozuka S, Tsubone M, Hachisuka K. Evolution of carcinoma in the extrahepatic bile ducts. Cancer 1984;54:65–72.
31. Miyano T, Tadaaki T, Suzuki F, et al. Adenoma and stone formation of the biliary tract in puppies that had choledochopancreatic anastomosis. J Pediatr Surg 1989;24:539–542.
32. Gertsch P, Thomas P, Baer H, et al. Multiple tumors of the biliary tract. Am J Surg 1990;159:386–388.
33. Tompkins RK, Johnson J, Storm FK, et al. Operative endoscopy in the management of biliary tract neoplasms. Am J Surg 1976;132: 174–182
34. O'Shea JS, Shah D, Cooperman AM. Biliary cystadenocarcinoma of extrahepatic duct origin arising in previously benign cystadenoma. Am J Gastroenterol 1987;82(12):1307–1310.
35. Dursi JF, Hirschl S, Gomez R, et al. Granular cell myoblastoma of the common bile duct: report of a case and review of the literature. Rev Surg 1975;32:305–310.
36. Paskin DL, Hull JD, Cookson PJ. Granular cell myoblastoma: a comprehensive review of 15-years experience. Ann Surg 1972; 175:501–504.
37. Vance SF, Hudson RP. Granular cell myoblastoma. Am J Clin Pathol 1969;52:208–211.
38. Coggins RP. Granular-cell myoblastoma of common bile duct—report of a case with autopsy findings. Arch Pathol 1952;54: 398–402.
39. Duncan JT, Wilson H. Benign tumor of the common bile duct. Ann Surg 1957;145:271–274.
40. Whitmore JT, Whitley JP, LaVerde P, ,,et al. Granular cell myoblastoma of the common bile duct. Am J Dig Dis 1969;14:516–520.
41. Abt AB, Feinberg E, Kunitz S. Granular cell myoblastoma of the extrahepatic biliary tract. Mt Sinai J Med (NY) 1971;38:456–461.
42. Savage A, Devitt P. Granular cell myoblastoma of the biliary tree. Postgrad Med J 1977;53:574–577.
43. Zvargulis JE, Keating JP, Askin FB, et al. Granular cell myoblastoma. Am J Dis Child 1978;132:68–70.
44. Dewar J, Dooley JS, Lindsay I, et al. Granular cell myoblastoma of the common bile duct treated by biliary drainage and surgery. Gut 1981;22:70–76.
45. Aisner SC, Khanega S, Ramirez O. Multiple granular cell tumors of the gallbladder and biliary tree: report of a case. Arch Pathol Lab Med 1982;106:470–471.
46. Balart LA, Hines C, Mitchell W. Granular cell schwannoma of the extrahepatic biliary system. Am J Gastroenterol 1983;78: 297–300.
47. Orenstein HH, Brenner LH, Nay HR. Granular cell myoblastoma of the extrahepatic biliary system. Am J Surg 1984;147:827–831.
48. Cheslyn-Curtis S, Russell RCG, Rode J, et al. Granular cell tumors of the common bile duct. Postgrad Med J 1986;62:961–963.
49. Kienzle HF, Bahr R, Stolte M, et al. Granularzell tumor des ductus choledochus. Dtsch Med Wochenschr 1986;111:197.
50. Butterly LF, Shapiro RH, LaMuraglia GM, et al. Biliary granular cell tumor: a little-known curable bile duct neoplasm of young people. Surgery 1988;103:328–334.

51. Eisen RN, Kirby WM, O'Quinn JL. Granular cell tumor of the biliary tree. A report of two cases and a review of the literature. Am J Surg Pathol 1991;15:460–465.
52. Sanchez JA, Nauta RJ. Resection of granular cell tumor at the hepatic confluence. A precarious location for benign tumor. Am Surg 1991;56:446–450.
53. Mauro MA, Jaques PF. Granular cell tumors of the esophagus and common bile duct. J Can Assoc Radiol 1981;32: 254–256.
54. LiVolsi VA, Perzin KH, Badder EM, et al. Granular cell tumors of the biliary tract. Arch Pathol 1973; 95:13–17.
55. Whisnant JD, Bennett SE, Huffman SR, et al. Case report: common bile duct obstruction by granular cell tumor (schwannoma). Dig Dis 1974;19:471–476.
56. Assor D. Granular cell myoblastoma involving the common bile duct. Am J Surg 1969;137:673–675.
57. Murray MR. Cultural characteristics of three granular cell myoblastomas. Cancer 1951;4:857–865.
58. Manstein ME, McBrearty FX, Pellechia PE, et al. Granular cell tumor of the common bile duct. Dig Dis Sci 1981;26:938–942.
59. Chandrasoma P, Fitzgibbons P. Granular cell tumor of the intrapancreatic common bile duct. Cancer 1984;53:2178–2128.
60. Oden B. Neurinoma of the common bile duct. Acta Chir Scand 1955;108:393–397.
61. Curry B, Gray N. Visceral neurofibromatosis. Br J Surg 1972;59: 494–496.
62. Sarma DP, Rodriguez FH, Hoffman EO. Paraganglioma of the hepatic duct. J South Med Assoc 1980;73:1677–1678.
63. Archambault H, Archambault R. Leiomyoma of the common bile duct. Arch Surg 1952;64:531–534.
64. Kune GA, Polgar V. Leiomyoma of the common bile duct causing obstructive jaundice. Med J Aust 1976;1:698–699.
65. Ponka A, Laasonen L, Strengell-Usanov L. Angioleiomyoma of the common bile duct. Acta Med Scand 1983;213:407–410.
66. Fernandez JMC, Gonzales-Bueno CM. Leiomyoma of the ampulla of Vater. Rev Esp Enferm Apar Dig 1974;47:165–172.
67. Mandeville GA, Stawski WS. Obstructing leiomyoma of the common bile duct bifurcation simulating a Klatskin tumor. Am Surg 1991;57:676–678.
68. Smadja C, Bowley NB, Benjamin IS, et al. Idiopathic localised bile duct strictures: relationship to primary sclerosing cholangitis. Am J Surg 1983;146:404–408.
69. Verbeek PCM, Van Leeuwen DJ, DeWit LT, et al. Benign fibrosing disease at the hepatic confluence mimicking Klatskin tumors. Surgery 1992;112:866–871.
70. Haith EE, Kepes JJ, Holder TM. Inflammatory pseudotumor involving the common bile duct of a six-year-old boy: successful pancreatico-duodenectomy. Surgery 1954;56:436–441.
71. Golematis B, Giannopoulos A, Papachristou DN, et al. Sclerosing cholangitis of the bifurcation of the common hepatic duct. Mt Sinai J Med (NY) 1982;49:38–40.
72. Heuser LS, Polk HC Jr. Proximal hepatic duct lesion. Surg Rounds 1983:48–52.
73. Standfield NJ, Salisbury JR, Howard ER. Benign non-traumatic inflammatory strictures of the extrahepatic biliary system. Br J Surg 1980;76:849–852.
74. Whittaker LD, Lynn HB, Dockerty MB, et al. Heterotopic gastric mucosa in the wall of the cystic duct: report of a case. Surgery 1967;62:382–385.
75. Welling RE, Krause RJ, Alamin K. Heterotopic gastric mucosa in the common bile duct. Arch Surg 1970;101:626–627.
76. Kalman PG, Stone RM, Philips MJ. Heterotopic gastric tissue of the bile duct. Surgery 1981;89:384–386.
77. Blundell CR, Kanun CS, Earnest DL. Biliary obstruction by heterotopic gastric mucosa at the ampulla of Vater. Am J Gastroenterol 1982;77:111–114.
78. Barbosa JJ, Dockerty M, Waugh J. Pancreatic heterotopia. Surg Gynecol Obstet 1946;82:527–547.
79. Weber C, Zito P, Becker S. Heterotopic pancreas: an unusual cause of obstruction of the common bile duct. Am J Gastroenterol 1968;49:153–159.
80. Sabini A, Baden J, Norman J, et al. Heterotopic pancreatic tissue in the common bile duct or ampulla of Vater. Am Surg 1970;36: 662–666.
81. Laughlin E, Keown M, Jackson J, et al. Heterotopic pancreas obstructing the ampulla of Vater. Arch Surg 1983;118:979–980.
82. Wingo PA, Tong T, Bolden S. Cancer statistics, 1995. CA 1995 45:8–30.
83. Warren KW, Choe DS, Plaza J, et al. Results of radical resection for periampullary cancer. Ann Surg 1975;181:534–540.
84. Nakase A, Matsumoto Y, Uchida K, et al. Surgical treatment of cancer of the pancreas and the periampullary region: cumulative results in 57 institutions in Japan. Ann Surg 1977;185: 52–57.
85. Lerut JP, Gianello PR, Oile JB, et al. Pancreaticoduodenal resection. Surgical experience and evaluation of risk factors in 103 patients. Ann Surg 1984;199:432–437.
86. Tarazi RY, Hermann RE, Vogt DP, et al. Results of surgical treatment of periampullary tumors: a thirty-five year experience. Surgery 1986;100:716–723.
87. Nagorney DM, Donohue JH, Farnell MB, et al. Outcomes after curative resections of cholangiocarcinoma. Arch Surg 1993;128: 871–879.
88. Albores-Saavedra J, Henson DE. Tumors of the gallbladder and extrahepatic ducts. In: Hartman WH, ed. Atlas of tumor pathology, second series, fascicle 22. Washington DC: Armed Forces Institute of Pathology, 1986.
89. Crile GJ. The advantages of bypass operations over radical pancreaticoduodenectomy in the treatment of pancreatic cancer. Surg Gynecol Obstet 1970;130:1049–1053.
90. Cameron JL, Pitt Ha, Yeo CJ, et al. One hundred and forty-five consecutive pancreaticoduodenectomies without mortality. Ann Surg 1993;217:430–435.
91. Pellegrini CA, Heck CF, Raper S, et al. An analysis of the reduced morbidity and mortality rates after pancreaticoduodenectomy. Arch Surg 1989;124:778–781.
92. Trede M, Schwall G, Saeger HD. Survival after pancreaticoduodenectomy. 118 consecutive resections without an operative mortality. Ann Surg 1990;211:447–458.
93. Geer RJ, Brennan MF. Prognostic indicators for survival after resection of pancreatic adenocarcinoma. Am J Surg 1993;165: 68–73.
94. Lieberman MD, Kilburn H, Lindsey M. et al. Relation of perioperative deaths to hospital volume among patients undergoing pancreatic resection for malignancy. Ann Surg 1995;222(5): 638–645.
95. Matory YL, Gaynor J, Brennan MF. Carcinoma of the ampulla of Vater. Surg Gynecol Obstet 1993;177:366–370.
96. Carey LC. Pancreaticoduodenectomy. Am J Surg 1992;164: 153–162.
97. Conlon KC, Klimstra DS, Brennan MF. Long-term survival after curative resection for pancreatic ductal adenocarcinoma. Ann Surg 1996;223:273–279.
98. Harrison LE, Klimstra DS, Brennan MF. Isolated portal vein involvement in pancreatic adenocarcinoma. A contraindication for resection. Ann Surg 1996;224(3):342–347.

# 70

# Benign and Malignant Tumors of the Duodenum

Kenneth A. Leslie and John W. Braasch

Tumors of the duodenum, like tumors of other portions of the gastrointestinal tract, are made up of a wide variety of histologic types (Table 70.1), but they differ from colonic and gastric tumors in that duodenal tumors are rare. Benign and malignant lesions occur with about equal frequency. As an index of their rarity, the most common malignant neoplasm, adenocarcinoma, is found in only 0.035% of autopsies, and it makes up only 0.35% of all gastrointestinal cancers (1).

The classification of duodenal tumors is similar to that of tumors in other areas of the small intestine. However, the frequency of individual tumors differs, depending on their location—duodenal, jejunal, or ileal (Table 70.2) (2, 3). Adenocarcinomas are more common in the duodenum, and lymphomas are more common in the jejunum and ileum. When these differences are adjusted for mucosal surface areas of the three small intestinal divisions, these differences are more striking. Leiomyosarcomas may also be more common in the duodenum. The duodenum has a considerably higher concentration of neuroendocrine cells than the rest of the small intestine, which explains the high incidence of gastrinomas in the wall of the duodenum (4, 5).

Before the last 2 decades, the diagnosis of duodenal tumors was difficult and relied on barium contrast studies. With refined endoscopic instruments, their recognition has become much more definitive, although the third and fourth portions of the duodenum are difficult to inspect endoscopically. Endoscopic biopsies can be misleading because of sampling errors, especially with villous tumors. Early diagnosis by endoscopy in patients with upper abdominal pain, melena, anemia, jaundice, nausea and vomiting, or weight loss requires a high index of suspicion for endoscopic evaluation. It is indicated in patients with Peutz-Jeghers and familial or nonfamilial polyposis syndromes and in familial multiple endocrine neoplasia syndromes, because the duodenum can harbor malignant polyps or functioning tumors.

The location and anatomic relationships of the duodenum cause problems with resection of the whole or its parts. The second part of the duodenum is pierced by the common bile duct and the ducts of Santorini and Wirsung, which limit sleeve resections and often require reimplantation of these ducts. Lymph node excision and wide resections require a Whipple-type procedure, and the closeness of the great veins means that medial-posterior margins tend to be limited, even when pancreatoduodenectomy is performed. For lesions of the third and fourth portions of the duodenum, which are covered anteriorly by the transverse colon and its mesentery and the mesenteric arteries and veins, direct access can be gained only by the relatively unknown Cattell maneuver (6).

## VILLOUS TUMORS

The most common benign tumor of the duodenum is the villous tumor, which is rare. The largest series (7) reported 47 cases. First described by Perry (8) in 1893, it was first resected by Halsted (7) in 1899. These tumors are found most commonly in the ampullary region (see Chapter 68) but occur in all parts of the duodenum as well.

Most patients with villous tumors have vague nonspecific symptoms of nausea, fatigue, or vague upper abdominal pain on presentation, but others note jaundice or anemia, depending on the location relative to the ampulla of Vater or the tendency to bleed. About one-fifth are asymptomatic (9).

Their most important characteristic is their malignant potential, and a cancer is found in 33–63% of resected tumors (9–16). Preoperative endoscopic biopsy of these lesions is associated with a sensitivity for diagnosing malignancy of only 52% (9), which is the basic problem of their treatment. Attempts at defining characteristics that predict malignancy have been controversial. In one report (12), tumors smaller than 4 cm in diameter were at low risk for malignant change, whereas other authors (9, 11, 15) found no relationship of size to malignancy. In one study (12), age over 50 years and location in the distal duodenum indicated a greater chance of malignancy. It is understandable that the presence of jaundice is a malignant predictor (9). Endoscopic ultrasonography (17) and computed tomography (18) are of uncertain predictive value and rely on demonstrating appreciable invasion of the duodenal wall.

The appropriate therapy for patients with villous tumors is controversial. Some authors (9, 13, 14, 16) advocate aggressive surgical management for all tumors in good-risk patients because of the high incidence of carcinoma. Other authors (11, 12) favor a more conservative approach, with endoscopic resection for benign lesions and aggressive management for those with malignant change. The problem with local endoscopic biopsy and resection is that the whole lesion needs to be examined, and parts can be missed or lost with this method of removal. The problem with open excision and frozen section examination at the time of surgery is that frozen section can have a false-negative rate of 35% (9). After local or endoscopic resection, the recurrence rate in one report (10) was 28%. Other authors (13) reported a recurrence rate of 17% but noted that invasive carcinoma did not

**TABLE 70.1. Tumors of the Duodenum**

| |
|---|
| Benign |
| Adenoma |
| Villous polyp |
| Adenomatous polyp |
| Mesenchymal |
| Leiomyoma |
| Lipoma |
| Hemangioma |
| Neurofibroma |
| Hamartoma (Peutz-Jeghers) |
| Pancreatic (rest) |
| Brunner's gland hyperplasia |
| Neuroendocrinoma |
| Gastrinoma |
| Others |
| Malignant |
| Adenocarcinoma |
| Villous adenocarcinoma |
| Mesenchymal |
| Leiomyosarcoma |
| Lymphoma |
| Neuroendocrinoma |
| Gastrinoma |
| Carcinoid |
| Others |
| Metastatic carcinoma |

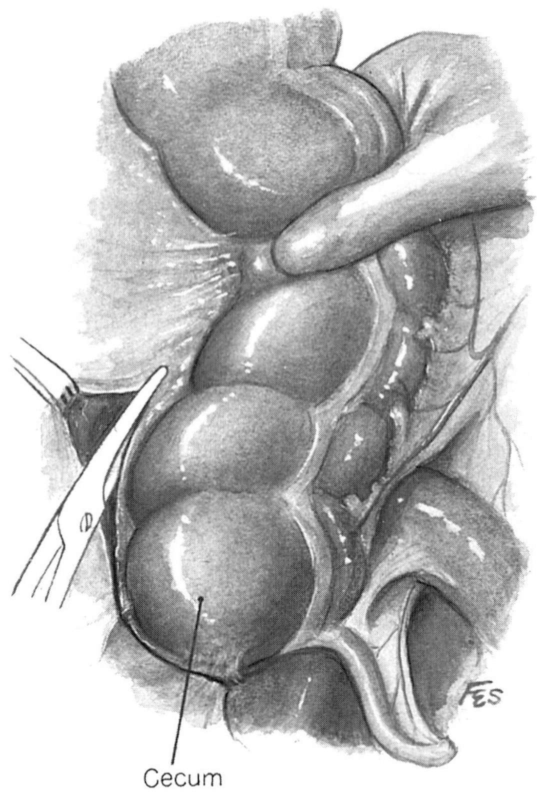


**FIG. 70.1.** The area to be elevated to gain exposure to the retroperitoneal duodenum is shown. (From Cattell RB, Braasch JW. A technique for the exposure of the third and fourth portions of the duodenum. Surg Gynecol Obstet 1960;111:378–379. By permission of Surgery, Gynecology and Obstetrics, now known as the Journal of the American College of Surgeons.)

develop in the long term in any patient with recurrence (including carcinoma in situ). For this reason, they advised local resection for benign lesions, with close endoscopic surveillance in long-term follow-up. For extensive villous tumors, total or near total duodenectomy with preservation of the pancreatic head has been carried out. Reimplantation of the bile and pancreatic ducts is necessary. Five patients have been reported (16) who did well with this approach.

For villous tumors with malignant change showing invasion, major resection of surrounding tissue with node removal is the treatment of choice. For tumors near the pancreatic head, a Whipple type of operation should be performed. For tumors in the fourth or distal third portion of the duodenum, sleeve resection with removal of adjacent nodes is advised.

The polyposis syndromes are associated with a high incidence of duodenal polyps, which are at risk for malignancy and need aggressive surgical resection. In patients with familial polyposis coli, duodenal carcinoma is the most frequent extracolonic malignancy, found in 2–12% of patients (10, 20). In most series of villous tumors, 20% are in patients with polyposis syndromes. The mean time to occurrence of a villous tumor or adenocarcinoma of the duodenum in patients after colectomy is 17 years (10).

**TABLE 70.2. Occurrence of Small Bowel Tumors Related to Portions of the Small Intestine**

| | Duodenum | Jejunum | Ileum |
|---|---|---|---|
| Adenocarcinoma | 131 | 119 | 52 |
| Lymphoma | 7 | 69 | 106 |
| Carcinoid | 13 | 21 | 233 |
| Pancreatic rest | 31 | 4 | 1[a] |
| Adenoma | 53 | 55 | 55 |

Adapted from Mason R. Tumors of the duodenum and small intestine. In: Sabiston DC Jr, ed. Textbook of surgery. 14th ed. Philadelphia: WB Saunders, 1991:803.
[a]In Meckel's diverticulum.

## MISCELLANEOUS BENIGN TUMORS

For other benign tumors, local excision, either endoscopically or at open operation, should be accomplished for identification purposes. In the course of resection, protection of the ampulla of Vater and orifice of Santorini is essential. Full-thickness excisions on the lateral wall are reasonably easy, provided an extensive Kocher maneuver has been performed.

## MALIGNANT TUMORS

### Adenocarcinoma

Adenocarcinoma, although a rarity, is the most common malignancy of the duodenum, representing 0.35% of gastrointestinal tract malignancies. Four major reports (1, 21–23) of this lesion described 140 cases. Adenocarcinoma of the small intestine is more common in the first and second portions of the duodenum. In one series (22), a preexisting villous adenoma was noted in one-half of the patients. The most common presenting symptoms and signs are pain, anemia, nausea and vomiting, jaundice, and weight loss.

Pancreatoduodenectomy is the procedure of choice for lesions of the proximal duodenum and includes the proximal third portion of the duodenum. For lesions of the distal duodenum, access is afforded by the Cattell maneuver (Figs. 70.1, 70.2, and 70.3) (6) by elevating the mesenteric small bowel and right colon with their blood supply. This permits direct inspection and manipulation of this retroperitoneal structure. Segmental resection of the involved duodenum with or without resection of the body of the pancreas may then be curative. Although experience is not extensive, resection of the body of the pancreas does not add to survival.

The 5-year survival rate after pancreatoduodenectomy for duodenal adenocarcinoma has ranged from 40 to 62% (1, 21–23). Only one study (21) reported results at 6, 10, 16, 45, 84, 88, and 150 months after resection of distal lesions and found no evidence of disease in seven patients.

Reports on the use of adjuvant therapy are few and involve few patients. In one report (24), preoperative radiotherapy, 5-fluorouracil, and mitomycin were found to facilitate resection and were associated with downstaging of disease.

## Gastrinoma

Perhaps most patients with Zollinger-Ellison syndrome have a gastrinoma of the duodenum as the source of the hypergastrinemia (4, 5, 25). This is not too surprising in view of the fact that the duodenum contains many neuroendocrine cells. In multiple endocrine neoplasia type I, both the duodenal wall and pancreas often contain gastrinomas.

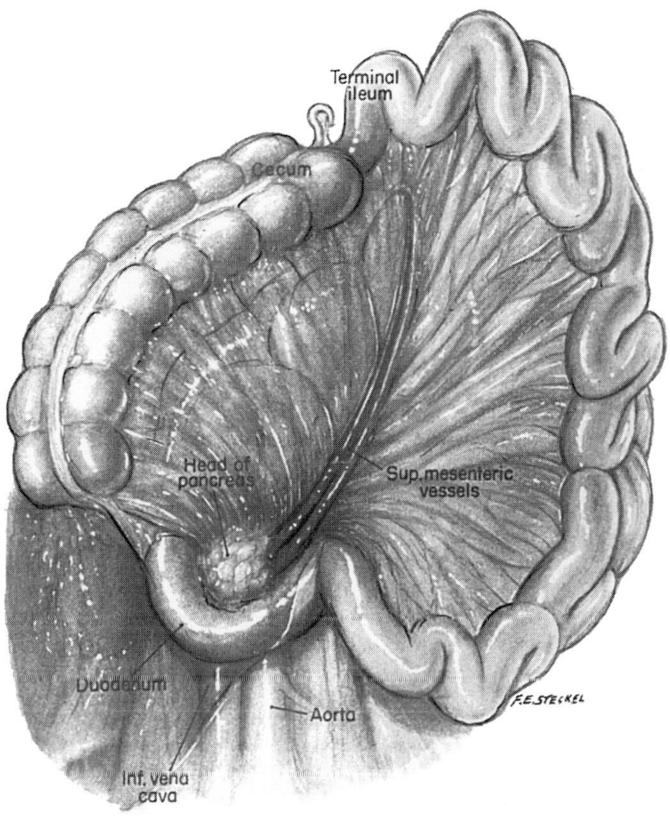


**FIG. 70.3.** Exposure of the retroperitoneal duodenum gained after elevation of the right colon and superior mesenteric artery and vein with the small bowel mesentery.

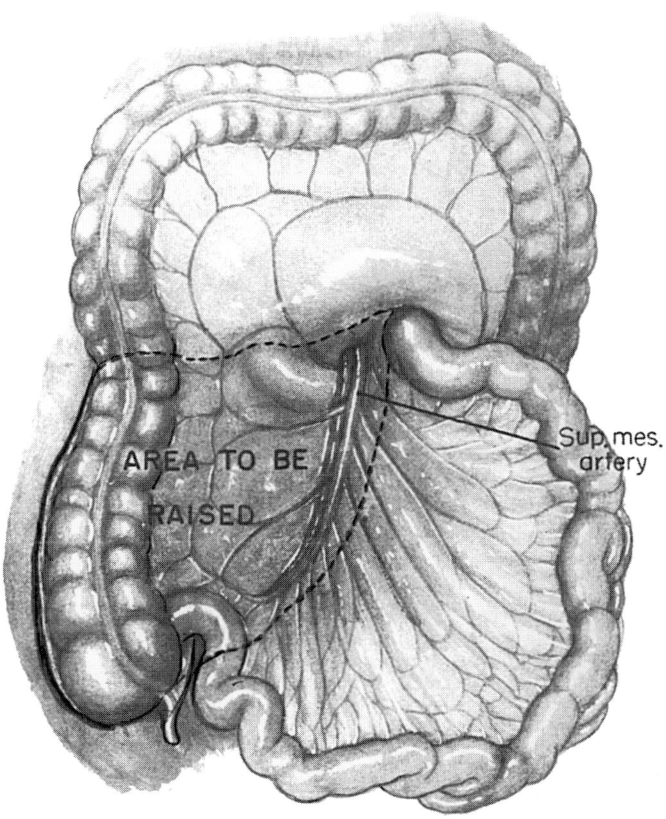


**FIG. 70.2.** The elevation of the right colon and its blood supply is begun. (From Cattell RB, Braasch JW. A technique for the exposure of the third and fourth portions of the duodenum. Surg Gynecol Obstet 1960;111:378–379. By permission of Surgery, Gynecology and Obstetrics, now known as the Journal of the American College of Surgeons.)

Because many duodenal gastrinomas are less than 8–10 mm in diameter, it is necessary to perform duodenotomy for inspection and bimanual palpation to locate the tumors, which may be multiple and in all parts of the duodenum (25). The use of endoscopic transillumination at operation or intraoperative ultrasonography does not increase identification (25).

Once located, they and other possible gastrinomas in the pancreas should be excised along with nodes in the duodenal pancreatic triangle. Because duodenal gastrinomas might be slower growing than those in the pancreas (5), the use of pancreatoduodenectomy in their treatment is controversial; however, resection of liver metastases is reasonable.

## Other Malignant Lesions

Leiomyosarcoma is the most common duodenal sarcoma. Radical resection is the treatment of choice and is followed by long-term survival when the patient has an early lesion.

Lymphoma of the duodenum is rare. Pure bowel involvement is exceedingly uncommon. Treatment can be by resection and radiation or just radiation, which is associated with a risk of perforation (26).

## REFERENCES

1. Rotman N, Pezet D, Fagniez PL, Cherqui D, Celicout B, Lointier P. Adenocarcinoma of the duodenum: factors influencing survival. Br J Surg 1994;81:83–85.
2. Cooper MJ, Williamson RC. Enteric adenoma and adenocarcinoma. World J Surg 1985;9:914–920.

3. Mason GR. Tumors of the duodenum and small intestine. In: Sabiston DC Jr, ed. Textbook of surgery. 14th ed. Philadelphia: WB Saunders, 1991:802–807.
4. Thompson NW, Pasieka J, Fukuuchi A. Duodenal gastrinomas, duodenotomy, and duodenal exploration in the surgical management of Zollinger-Ellison syndrome. World J Surg 1993;17: 455–462.
5. Modlin IM, Lawton GP. Duodenal gastrinoma: the solution to the pancreatic paradox (Editorial). J Clin Gastroenterol 1994;19: 184–188.
6. Cattell RB, Braasch JW. A technique for the exposure of the third and fourth portions of the duodenum. Surg Gynecol Obstet 1960;111:378–379.
7. Halsted WS. Contributions to the surgery of the bile passages, especially of the common bile duct. Boston Med Surg J 1899; 141:645–649.
8. Perry EC. Papilloma of duodenum. Trans Pathol Soc 1893;44:84.
9. Pezet D, Rotman N, Slim K, Boudet MJ, Chipponi J, Fagniez PL. Villous tumors of the duodenum: a retrospective study of 47 cases by the French Associations for Surgical Research. J Am Coll Surg 1995;180:541–544.
10. Galandiuk S, Hermann RE, Jagelman DG, Fazio VW, Sivak MV. Villous tumors of the duodenum. Ann Surg 1988;207:234–239.
11. Bjork KJ, Davis CJ, Nagorney DM, Mucha P. Duodenal villous tumors. Arch Surg 1990;125:961–965.
12. Kutin ND, Ranson JH, Gouge TH, Localio SA. Villous tumors of the duodenum. Ann Surg 1975;181:164–168.
13. Ryan DP, Schapiro RH, Warshaw AL. Villous tumors of the duodenum. Ann Surg 1986;203:301–306.
14. Celik C, Venditti JA Jr, Satchidanand S, Freier DT. Villous tumors of the duodenum and ampulla of Vater. J Surg Oncol 1986;33: 268–272.
15. Komorowski RA, Cohen EB. Villous tumors of the duodenum: a clinicopathologic study. Cancer 1981;47:1377–1386.
16. Chappuis CW, Divincenti FC, Cohn I Jr. Villous tumors of the duodenum. Ann Surg 1989;209:593–599.
17. Tio TL, Sie LH, Verbeek PC, Dé Wit LT, Tytgat GN. Endosonography in diagnosing and staging duodenal villous adenoma. Gut 1992;33:567–568.
18. Kazerooni EA, Quint LE, Francis IR. Duodenal neoplasms: predictive value of CT for determining malignancy and tumor resectability. Am J Roentgenol 1992;159:303–309.
19. Chung RS, Church JM, van Stolk R. Pancreas-sparing duodenectomy: indications, surgical technique, and results. Surgery 1995; 117:254–259.
20. Penna C, Phillips RK, Tiret E, Spigelman AD. Surgical polypectomy of duodenal adenomas in familial adenomatous polyposis: experience of two European centres. Br J Surg 1993;80: 1027–1029.
21. Lowell JA, Rossi RL, Munson JL, Braasch JW. Primary adenocarcinoma of third and fourth portions of duodenum: favorable prognosis after resection. Arch Surg 1992;127:557–560.
22. Scott-Coombes DM, Williamson RC. Surgical treatment of primary duodenal carcinoma: a personal series. Br J Surg 1994;81:1472–1474.
23. Delcore R, Thomas JH, Forster J, Hermreck AS. Improving resectability and survival in patients with primary duodenal carcinoma. Am J Surg 1993;166:626–631.
24. Yeung RS, Weese JL, Hoffman JP, Solin LJ, Paul AR, et al. Neoadjuvant chemoradiation in pancreatic and duodenal carcinoma. Cancer 1993;72:2124–2133.
25. Sugg SL, Norton JA, Fraker DL, Metz DC, Pisegna JR, et al. A prospective study of intraoperative methods to diagnose and resect duodenal gastrinomas. Ann Surg 1993;218:138–144.
26. Muchmore JH, Haddad CG, Goldwag S. Primary non-Hodgkin's lymphoma of the duodenum. Am Surg 1994;60:924–928.

SECTION XIII

TRUE CYSTS AND CYSTIC TUMORS OF THE PANCREAS

# 71

# *True Cysts and Related Disorders*

Louis T. Merriam and Raymond J. Joehl

True nonneoplastic pancreatic cysts are uncommon compared with other cystic diseases of the pancreas. The paucity of case reports and reviews in the adult and pediatric literature reflects the rarity with which physicians encounter these lesions and emphasizes that the true prevalence, clinical characteristics, and natural history of these benign lesions is poorly understood. The fact that most of these cysts cause few if any clinical symptoms has deemphasized much of their clinical importance. However, as true pancreatic cysts resemble both pseudocysts and mucinous cystic neoplasms in radiographic and gross appearance, a working knowledge of the clinical and biologic characteristics of these apparently innocuous lesions is vital. In addition, true pancreatic cysts are found in a number of other clinical disorders and congenital syndromes. Proper recognition, diagnosis, and understanding of this association play an important role in treating patients with this condition appropriately. Finally, cysts that arise in extrapancreatic locations mimic all types of pancreatic cysts. These may be true, parasitic, or inflammatory cysts, and, as their origin is not within the pancreas itself, are considered separately.

## TRUE PANCREATIC CYSTS

A variety of terminologies have been suggested to describe these lesions and the various clinical syndromes in which they occur (1, 2). In general, three types of true cysts of the pancreas can be described: *(a)* primary pancreatic cysts, *(b)* pancreatic cysts associated with hereditary disorders and other congenital syndromes, and *(c)* miscellaneous true cysts of the pancreas. Although the pathogenesis, morphology, and clinical presentation may differ among the various types, the presence of a fibrous capsule with an epithelial lining is common to all true cysts. Many neoplastic cysts possess a variable epithelial lining, both benign and malignant, and are considered to be true cysts. This chapter focuses on nonneoplastic and parasitic cysts of the pancreas.

### Primary Pancreatic Cysts

Primary pancreatic cysts are true, nonneoplastic cysts that arise from within the pancreatic parenchyma (1). Histologically, these lesions are fluid-filled, simple cysts possessing a low cuboidal, nonmucinous epithelium (Fig. 71.1). Most clinicians believe they originate as the result of errors in pancreatic development in utero, when anomalous sequestration of small segments of ductal elements leads to formation of fluid-filled microscopic and macroscopic cysts within the pancreatic parenchyma (3). This notion has led to the term *congenital pancreatic cyst,* a term often used in the literature to include the variety of true cysts that presumably develop before birth. Support for this concept is present in the literature, because histologically confirmed cysts have been found at a variety of ages, from neonates well into adulthood.

Most primary pancreatic cysts have been described in children less than 10 years of age (3, 4). There is considerable heterogeneity among the gross and radiographic appearance, size, and location of these lesions. They are usually less than 10 cm in diameter, are more often unilocular than multilocular, and tend to arise as solitary lesions with no specific intrapancreatic location (4, 5). Although these lesions have been reported to cause a variety of symptoms from gastric outlet and biliary obstruction to pancreatitis, which are described primarily in the pediatric population, the vast majority remain asymptomatic throughout life (3, 4, 6). Most first present during a laparotomy or radiologic evaluation that is being performed for a disorder unrelated to the pancreatic cyst.

Diagnosis and treatment of primary cysts of the pancreas depend on the age of the patient and the clinical presentation. The unilocular gross and radiologic appearance of these lesions (Figs. 71.2 and 71.3) often causes physicians to confuse them with pancreatic pseudocysts or mucinous cystadenoma or cystadenocarcinoma. In adults, therefore, a complete history including prior symptoms and presence of acute or chronic pancreatitis is critical. Patients with pseudocysts usually have a history of acute pancreatitis and/or prior pseudocyst. However, the distinction between primary cysts and mucinous cystadenoma/carcinoma is more difficult, particularly because these neoplastic cysts present asymptomatically in many cases. In this setting, most surgeons advocate complete cyst excision with pancreatectomy to avoid missing neoplastic disease. This technique not only provides the best chance of adequate resection margins in the presence of neoplastic disease, but also reduces the risk of pancreatic leak associated with isolated intrapancreatic cystectomy. Large cysts or those that elicit substantial inflammation may involve surrounding tissues and vasculature, making dissection difficult. Uncommonly, resection of adjacent organs may be necessary (Fig. 71.4). Therefore, appropriate preoperative planning and preparation of the patient is mandatory. In the rare event that the cyst is located extrinsic to the pancreatic parenchyma, simple cystectomy can be safely performed. Recent advances in computed tomography (CT)-guided aspiration and analysis of cyst fluid for amylase, cytology, and tumor markers provide another means of noninvasively distinguishing neoplastic from benign disease. Presence of neoplastic cells and elevated levels of fluid viscosity, CEA, and CA125 have been associated with mucinous cystic neoplasms (7) and, in their absence, may allow observation of lesions in patients thought to have primary cysts. This diagnostic option may be of particular value in older patients and those who are at high operative risk.

In children, cystic neoplasms and pseudocysts are extremely uncommon. After appropriate evaluation for the presence of other disorders associated with pancreatic cysts, patients with asymptomatic unilocular cysts can most often be observed. Several reports of antenatal diagnosis of pancreatic cysts have

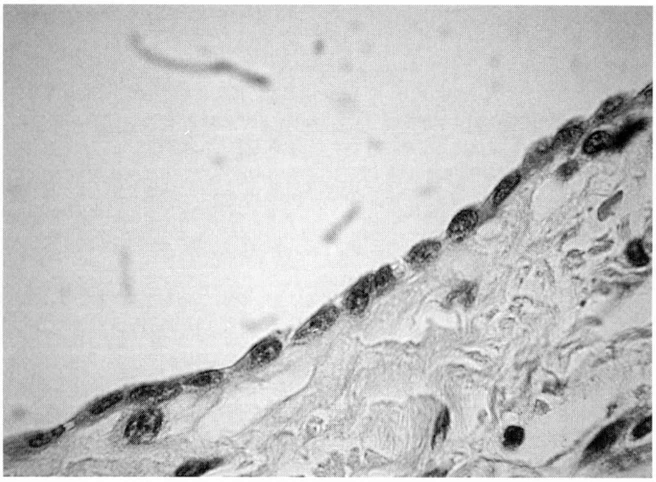

**FIG. 71.1.** Photomicrograph (400× original magnification) of the simple, nonmucinous low cuboidal epithelium of a true pancreatic cyst. See color insert.

been documented in the literature (6). These are unusual occurrences, and clinical relevance is more often placed on the possibility of associated congenital abnormalities or syndromes than on the indications for surgical excision.

### Hereditary Disorders and Congenital Syndromes Associated with True Pancreatic Cysts

A number of inherited diseases are associated with simple, cuboidal epithelium-lined cysts of the pancreas. The most common of these are von Hippel-Lindau, autosomal dominant polycystic kidney disease, polycystic liver disease, polycystic disease of the pancreas, and cystic fibrosis. Pancreatic cysts associated with these diseases are usually asymptomatic; thus, patients seldom require an operation. However, identification of simple pancreatic cysts in any patient without a history of inherited disease should prompt a thorough evaluation.

The von Hippel-Lindau syndrome (HLS) is autosomally inherited and characterized most commonly by retinal angiomatosis, central nervous system hemangioblastomas, pheochromocytoma, renal cysts, renal cancer, papillary cystadenoma of the epididymis, and cystic lesions of the pancreas. The incidence of pancreatic cysts in HLS is highly variable among affected kindreds, ranging from 0 to 90% (8, 9). Most cystic lesions in HLS are fluid-filled, simple, cuboidal epithelium-lined cysts or microcytic serous cystadenomas (8). Although cystic islet cell tumors have been described in these patients, they are rare and, usually, are identified by a substantial solid component on CT scan (9). The extent of cystic involvement varies from the isolated true cyst to polycystic change of the entire pancreas. Although important complications (e.g., biliary obstruction and acute pancreatitis) have been described, the vast majority of these cysts are asymptomatic or cause only mild clinical symptoms (10). Diagnostic evaluation of patients with HLS and pancreatic cysts includes CT, magnetic resonance imaging (MRI), or abdominal ultrasonography. Although studies specifically evaluating the accuracy of these different imaging techniques are lacking, the best imaging study is probably ultrasonography because of the ease in performing initial and follow-up examinations, as well as lower cost than CT and MRI. Treatment of true pancreatic cysts in HLS is observation, unless patients have symptoms requiring intervention. Because mucinous cystadenoma and cystadenocarcinoma have not been described in these patients, confusion surrounding recognition of potentially malignant mucinous cystic lesions is not a serious concern.

Autosomal dominant polycystic kidney disease (ADPK) accounts for approximately 8% of dialysis patients in the United States and represents the most common type of polycystic kidney disease (11). Patients typically present with palpable abdominal masses, pain, other urinary symptoms, and gradually decreasing renal dysfunction in adulthood. Patients with ADPK often have associated cysts in other organs, most commonly in the liver (up to 43% of patients). Associated cysts of the pancreas are less common and are present in up to 9% of ADPK patients (11–13). Similarly, polycystic disease of the liver can have associated true cysts of the pancreas. Polycystic liver disease is a developmental disorder similar to polycystic kidney disease with an incidence of 8 per 11,245 autopsies (14). Pancreatic cysts in these disorders are almost always asymptomatic and usually require no further evaluation or treatment after initial diagnosis.

Isolated polycystic pancreas has been described. However, this condition is exceedingly rare (1). Characterized by multiple, usually unilocular cysts throughout the pancreas, this disorder may simply represent multiple primary cysts and not a true congenital syndrome. The paucity of cases make in-depth investigation into this question difficult. As with the other hereditary lesions described above, these cysts are usually asymptomatic and, therefore, require no specific treatment.

Cystic fibrosis (CF), an autosomal recessive disorder estimated to occur in 1:2000 live births, represents the most common, lethal, genetic defect of the white population (15). Disturbances in mucus and electrolyte secretion in patients with CF result in marked exocrine dysfunction affecting multiple organ systems, particularly the lungs and gastrointestinal tract. Pancreatic manifestations of CF were among those recognized in the original descriptions of the disease and, since then, have been

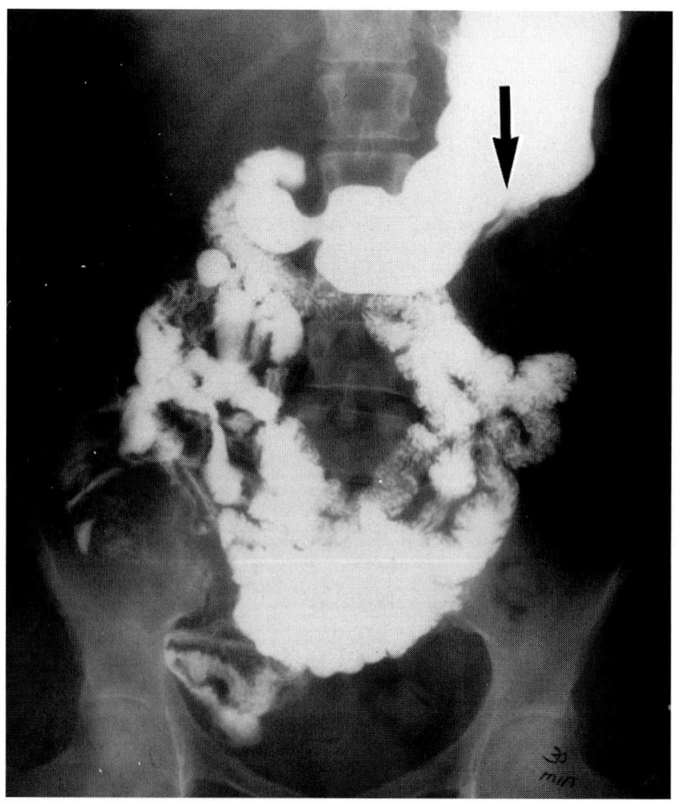

**FIG. 71.2.** Upper gastrointestinal contrast x-ray of a 45-year-old woman who presented with several days of abdominal pain and a palpable mass in the left flank. *Arrow* indicates large pancreatic cyst indenting greater curvature of stomach.

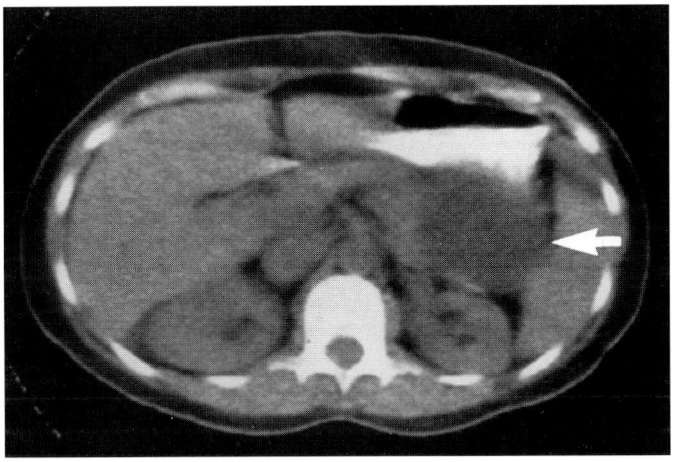

**FIG. 71.3.** Abdominal CT scan of the same patient as Figure 71.2. Unilocular, fluid-filled, cystic mass in the tail of the pancreas is contiguous with the posterior stomach wall.

extensively studied. Inspissated secretions, ductal obstruction, and dilation lead to progressive acinar atrophy, fibrosis, and cystic degeneration. Although pancreatic dysfunction is present in 85–95% of patients, the severity of pancreatic pathology varies considerably (16, 17). The pancreas may contain a variable number of true, epithelium-lined microscopic and small macroscopic cysts, depending on the stage of disease. Macroscopic cysts larger than 1 cm in diameter are uncommon, and those measuring more than 5 cm are exceedingly rare (17–19). Pancreatic cysts in cystic fibrosis do not require detailed evaluation or treatment.

A variety of congenital syndromes have been described that are associated with cystic disease of the pancreas. Most, if not all, of these cysts are of little surgical concern and are more important for their contribution to phenotypic expression of rare and incompletely understood multiple congenital abnormalities. Many of these lesions are found as part of a constellation of developmental abnormalities that are often incompatible with life. Antenatal diagnosis using ultrasonography has enabled early diagnosis of some lesions that, in combination with other anomalies, can serve as a guide to diagnosis and perinatal prognosis. Examples include asphyxiating thoracic dysplasia, short-rib polydactyly syndrome, renal-pancreatic-hepatic dysplasia sequence and the oral-facial-digital syndrome type I (20–22).

### Miscellaneous True Cysts

**Lymphoepithelial Cysts.** Lymphoepithelial cysts are very uncommon pancreatic cysts, with 10 cases reported to date (23–25). These lesions are true cysts lined with a stratified squamous epithelial lining, filled with serous fluid, and surrounded by lymphoid tissue with germinal centers. The origin of these unusual cysts is uncertain, but current theories suggest either development of squamous metaplasia in areas of obstructed pancreatic ducts with subsequent inflammation and involvement of surrounding lymph node(s), abnormal cystic degeneration of ectopic pancreas within peripancreatic lymph nodes, or the formation of cysts in misplaced branchial cleft tissue that took place during development (25). The clinically important concepts regarding these cysts are similar to those reviewed for simple pancreatic cysts. The clinical presentation varies from lesions found incidentally to patients with abdominal pain and a palpable mass (23–27). The small experience with these lesions precludes an assessment of their true natural history. Treatment adheres to the principles adopted for simple cysts, particularly because these lesions appear similar radiographically.

**Splenic Epidermoid Cysts.** Splenic epidermoid cysts are squamous epithelium-lined true cysts originating from aberrant ectodermal and entodermal epithelium within the spleen. Brief mention here is warranted as these lesions have been described to occur within the pancreas (five cases reported) and may appear similar to true cysts described previously (24). How these cysts arise within the pancreas is uncertain yet may involve the development of abnormal pancreatic ductal epithelium in an intrapancreatic accessory spleen. Treatment options are the same as for simple pancreatic cysts.

**Enterogenous Cysts.** Enterogenous or duplication cysts are foregut-derived true cysts originating from errors in embryologic development. Starting during the 4th week of embryogenesis, the primitive forgut gives rise to the pharynx, tracheobronchial tree, and upper GI tract, including the stomach, duodenum, liver, pancreas, and biliary tree. Enterogenous cysts, although considered rare, have been described in virtually all of these anatomic locations (28, 29). Pancreatic enterogenous cysts are extremely uncommon, with only four reported cases in the literature (30, 31). Histopathologic characteristics include either a ciliated, simple, and/or pseudostriated or gastric epithelium-lined cyst surrounded by an abundance of smooth muscle and connective tissue. Pancreatic and other enterogenous cysts exhibit a variety of contents, ranging from clear serous fluid to milky white or brown mucoid material (31). The secretory nature of the epithelium causes intraluminal fluid accumulation, with expansion of cyst volume and formation of a complex cystic mass. Over time, continued enlargement leads to expansion within the pancreas and into neighboring organs. Although the natural history and true incidence of asymptomatic lesions has not been studied, patients described in the literature have all presented with symptoms of an abdominal mass and pain due to either tumor mass effect or pancreatitis (28, 32). Options for treatment in these patients are primarily surgical resection of the entire cyst. Internal or external drainage procedures are associated with considerable morbidity. The high rate of chronic draining fistula in patients having drainage procedures indicates that this ap-

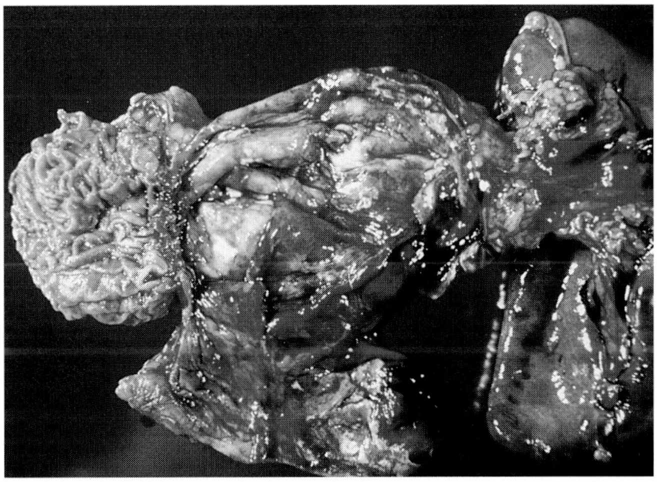

**FIG. 71.4.** Gross photograph of surgically excised specimen from patient in Figures 71.2 and 71.3, containing an 8-cm pancreatic cyst. Gastric resection (stomach at *left side* of specimen) and splenectomy (spleen at *right side*) were required because of the possibility of malignancy, the degree of adherence to adjacent viscera, and pericystic inflammation. Histopathologically, this was a primary pancreatic cyst (Fig. 71.1). See color insert.

proach is a temporary treatment option for patients with major comorbidities who are unable to have immediate surgery or those with infected cysts prior to definitive surgical resection.

## PARASITIC AND EXTRAPANCREATIC CYSTS

### Hydatid Cysts

Although the most common site of hydatid cysts is the liver, multiple anatomic sites including the lungs, brain, bone, kidneys, heart, and pancreas have been described. Unilocular hydatid cysts of the pancreas are rare, with an incidence of 0.25% in a series of patients surgically treated for symptomatic echinococcal disease (33). The true incidence of extrapancreatic hydatid cysts is not known. These cysts are typically fluid filled and may show multiple internal septae with calcifications located peripherally in the wall of the cyst. Daughter cysts with developing scolices arise within the center and gradually enlarge, producing a sandlike sediment within the cyst. These lesions are highly variable in growth rate, some taking years to reach 10 cm or more. Differential diagnosis includes other cystic lesions of the pancreas and is aided by the patient's travel history, clinical presentation, presence of eosinophilia, and cyst appearance on CT or ultrasound. Percutaneous aspiration is often helpful in identifying scolices; however, it is considered undesirable because of possible postaspiration leakage, spillage of daughter cysts, and the subsequent risk of anaphylaxis.

Two-thirds of symptoms in patients with hydatid disease are due to hepatic involvement, usually from cyst rupture, secondary bacterial infection, or tumor mass impinging on the biliary system or neighboring organs (34). Although rare events, pancreatic hydatid cysts cause a variety of symptoms, including biliary obstruction, acute pancreatitis, and pancreatic abscess (35–37). Symptoms require prompt treatment and, as with liver hydatid cysts, are most effectively relieved by surgical excision. Medical management with antiparasitic agents such as albendazole and mebendazole are generally ineffective and should not be used as a primary treatment with unruptured cysts. New therapeutic approaches using ultrasound-guided percutaneous cyst drainage followed by infusion with scolicidal agents (such as 95% ethanol) have had promising results in patients with hepatic cysts (38). However, as experience is small and studies have not been performed in patients with pancreatic cysts, the recommended treatment in these patients remains surgical excision. Meticulous care must be taken in dissection and removal of hydatid cysts, as rupture releases numerous daughter cysts, which may cause anaphylaxis as well as extensive intraabdominal encystation.

### Extrapancreatic Cysts

Extrapancreatic cystic lesions arising in the vicinity of the pancreas present with clinical symptoms and radiographic signs as pancreatic cysts. Although uncommon entities in themselves, cystic lesions of the spleen, adrenals, mesentery, omentum, and retroperitoneum and small bowel duplication cysts have all been described and may appear on imaging studies to originate within the pancreas (1). With refinements in CT scanning and ultrasonography, identifying the anatomic origin of these lesions has become less puzzling. However, persistent dilemmas in diagnosis, inability to exclude neoplastic disease, and the presence of symptoms often demand surgical excision and definitive histologic evaluation in these patients.

### Splenic Cysts

Cystic lesions of the spleen are uncommon; three-quarters of them are pseudocysts that arise secondary to splenic trauma (39). Primary splenic cysts, which include true, congenital, neoplastic, and parasitic cysts, comprise the remainder of lesions. Presenting symptoms in these patients are usually vague or absent. Rarely, they may be large enough to cause splenic rupture, hemorrhage, infection, or compression of adjacent organs. Most occur as solitary, unilocular lesions, and if not confined within the splenic parenchyma, they can be mistaken for pancreatic cysts. Differential diagnosis in these situations includes mucinous cystic neoplasm; therefore, cyst removal is mandatory. The splenic origin of these lesions is usually determined at the time of operation, and surgical removal can be achieved with partial or total splenectomy. In an asymptomatic patient with a definite diagnosis of nonneoplastic or parasitic splenic cyst, simple observation is warranted.

### Adrenal Cysts

Because of their location, adrenal cysts may mimic cysts arising in the pancreas. Their rarity (an incidence of 0.06–0.18% at autopsy (40)) precludes an extensive study of their natural history. They are usually asymptomatic. However, hemorrhage into the cyst, infection, or compression of neighboring organs are reported to precipitate symptoms. Adrenal cysts are almost always unilateral and show no predilection for either side. They vary considerably in size at presentation and can be uni- or multilocular. Etiologies include pseudocysts, parasitic cysts, and a variety of true, epithelium-lined cysts (40). Indications for surgical excision include presence of symptoms, abnormal secretory function, parasitic infestation, or appearance suggesting malignancy. Malignant adrenal cysts are rare; however, distinguishing them from benign lesions can be difficult. A complex mass with heterogenous composition by CT or ultrasound suggests malignancy; definitive diagnosis relies on tissue analysis. Therefore, many of these lesions require surgical removal, as the definitive diagnosis is often uncertain preoperatively. If a cyst appears intrapancreatic in origin, excision is usually indicated to rule out neoplastic disease.

### Mesenteric, Omental, and Retroperitoneal Cysts

Mesenteric, omental, and retroperitoneal cysts are discussed together, as they all are likely to develop from a common, congenital origin. The pathogenesis is uncertain, but most believe they originate from sequestration or obstruction of lymphatic vessels, leading to the term *lymphangiomatous cysts* (41, 42). Others believe that cysts develop secondary to errors in fusion of mesenteric leaves during embryologic development or as a result of trauma, chronic inflammation, or lymphadenopathy; lymphatic obstruction leads to cyst development over time. Whatever the pathogenesis, these lesions can be large and compress intraabdominal organs, which may cause symptoms. Although uncommon, these lesions have been reviewed in both the pediatric and adult literature (41–45). Although most surgeons will see patients with these lesions who are symptomatic, requiring excision for relief, the preoperative diagnosis is correct in less than 25% of cases (45). Depending on the location, the differential diagnosis can be extensive, including ovarian, renal, splenic, duplication, and pancreatic cysts. Most patients are evaluated with CT or ultrasound, which usually assists in decreasing the diagnostic possibilities. As with extrapancreatic cysts, discussed above, they appear similar to mucinous neoplasms and, thus, require surgical excision, even in the absence of symptoms (46).

### Enterogenous Cysts

Enterogenous, or duplication, cysts, in addition to arising within the pancreas, arise from stomach and small bowel and may appear to originate within the pancreas. Persistent secretion within the cyst may lead to expansion and encroachment onto neighboring organs, including the pancreas. Symptomatic and indeterminate lesions mandate resection for definitive histologic diagnosis.

## REFERENCES


1. Yeo CJ, Sarr MG. Cystic and pseudocystic diseases of the pancreas. Curr Probl Surg 1994;31:167–243.
2. Howard JM. Cystic neoplasms and true cysts of the pancreas. Surg Clin North Am 1989;69:651–655.
3. Auringer ST, Ulmer JL, Sumner TE, Turner CS. Congenital cyst of the pancreas. J Pediatr Surg 1993;28:1570–1571.
4. Mao CM, Greenwood S, Wagner S, Howard JM. Solitary true cyst of the pancreas in an adult. Int J Pancreatol 1992;12:181–186.
5. Ross PR, Hamrick-Turner JE, Chiechi MV, Ros LH, Gallego P, Burton SS. Cystic masses of the pancreas. Radiographics 1992;12: 673–686.
6. Shieh C, Eng HL, Huang S, Chuang J. Case report: congenital pancreatic cyst presenting as acute pancreatitis in an adolescent. J Pediatr Gastroenterol Nutr 1994;18:490–493.
7. Lewandrowski KB, Southern JF, Pins MR, Compton CC, Warshaw AL. Cyst fluid analysis in the differential diagnosis of pancreatic cysts. Ann Surg 1993;217:41–47.
8. Neumann HPH, Dinkel E, Brambs H, Wimmer B, Friedburg H, et al. Pancreatic lesions in the von Hippel-Lindau syndrome. Gastroenterology 1991;101:465–471.
9. Choyke PL, Glenn GM, Walther MM, Patronas NJ, Linehan WM, Zbar B. von Hippel-Lindau disease: genetic, clinical and imaging features. Radiology 1995;194:629–642.
10. Deboever G, Dewulf P, Maertens J. Common bile duct obstruction due to pancreatic involvement in the von Hippel-Lindau syndrome. Am J Gastroenterol 1992;87:1966.
11. Delaney VB, Adler S, Bruns FJ, Licinia M, Segel DP, Fraley DS. Autosomal dominant polycystic kidney disease: prevention, complications and prognosis. Am J Kidney Dis 1985;5:104–111.
12. Hatfield PM, Pfister RC. Adult polycystic disease of the kidneys (Potter type 3). JAMA 1972;222:1527–1531.
13. Milutinovic J, Schabel SI, Ainsworth SK. Autosomal dominant polycystic kidney disease with liver and pancreatic involvement in early childhood. Am J Kidney Dis 1989;4:340–344.
14. Brown RAP. Polycystic disease of the kidneys and intracranial aneurysms. Glasgow Med J 1951;32:332.
15. Oppenheimer EH, Esterly JR. Pathology of cystic fibrosis. Review of the literature and comparison with 146 autopsy cases. Perspect Pediatr Pathol 1975;2:241–247.
16. Park RW, Grand RJ. Gastrointestinal manifestations of cystic fibrosis: a review. Gastroenterology 1981;81:1143–1161.
17. Liu P, Daneman A, Stringer DA, Durie PR. Pancreatic cysts and calcification in cystic fibrosis. J Can Assoc Radiol 1986;37:279–282.
18. Hernanz-Schulman M, Teele RL, Perez-Atayde A, Zollars L, Livine J, et al. Pancreatic cystosis in cystic fibrosis. Radiology 1986;158: 629–631.
19. Churchill RJ, Cunningham DG, Henkin RE, Reynes CJ. Macroscopic cysts of the pancreas in cystic fibrosis demonstrated by multiple radiological modalities. JAMA 1981;245:72–74.
20. Carles D, Serville F, Dubecq JP, Gonnet JM. Renal, pancreatic and hepatic dysplasia sequence. Eur J Pediatr 1988;147:431–432.
21. Kennedy SM, Hashida Y, Malatack J. Polycystic kidneys, pancreatic cysts and cystadenomatous bile ducts in the oral-facial-digital syndrome type I. Arch Pathol Lab Med 1991;115: 519–523.
22. Bronstein M, Reichler A, Borochowitz Z, Bejar J, Drugan A. Early prenatal diagnosis of polycystic pancreas with narrow thorax and short limb dwarfism. Am J Med Genet 1994;49:6–9.
23. Koga H, Takayasu K, Mukai K, Muramatsu Y, Mizuguchi Y, et al. CT of lymphoepithelial cysts of the pancreas. J Comp Assist Tomogr 1995;19:221–224.
24. Morohoshi T, Hamamoto T, Kunimura T, Yoshida E, Kanda M, et al. Epidermoid cyst derived from an accessory spleen in the pancreas. A case report. J Soc Pathol 1991;41:916–921.
25. Fitko R, Kampmeier PA, Batti FH, Benjoya RA, Rao SM. Lymphoepithelial cyst of the pancreas with sebaceous differentiation. Int J Pancreat 1994;15:145–147.
26. Truong LD, Rangdaeng S, Jordan PH. Lymphoepithelial cyst of the pancreas. Am J Surg Pathol 1987;11:899–903.
27. Mockli GC, Stein RM. Cystic lymphoepithelial lesion of the pancreas. Arch Pathol Lab Med 1990;114:885–887.
28. Pilcher CS, Bradley EL, Majmudar B. Enterogenous cyst of the pancreas. Am J Gastroenterol 1982;77:576–577.
29. Moore KL. The developing human. Philadelphia: WB Saunders, 1973.
30. Kohzaki S, Fududa T, Fujimota T, Hiara K, Matsungaga N, et al. Case report: ciliated foregut cyst of the pancreas mimicking teratomatous tumour. Br J Radiol 1994;67:601–604.
31. Pins MR, Compton CC, Southern JF, et al. Ciliated enteric duplication cyst presenting as a pancreatic cystic neoplasm: report of a case with cyst fluid analysis. Clin Chem 1992;38:1501–1503.
32. Lyon DC. Recurrent pancreatitis caused by peptic ulceration in an intrapancreatic gastric reduplication cyst. Br J Clin Pract 1969;23:425.
33. Kattan TB. Hydatid cysts in the pancreas. Br Med J 1975;27: 729–730.
34. Thompson RCA. The biology of echinococcus and hydatid disease. London: George Allen & Unwin, 1986.
35. Lemmer ER, Krige JEJ, Price SK, Girdwood AH. Hydatid cyst in the head of the pancreas with obstructive jaundice. J Clin Gastroenterol 1995;20:136–138.
36. Mathai V, Banerjee Jesudason SR, Muthusami JC, Kuruvilla R, Idikula J, Sada P. Chronic pancreatitis caused by intraductal hydatid cysts of the pancreas. Br J Surg 1994;81:1029.
37. Papadimitriou J. Pancreatic abscess due to infected hydatid cyst. Surg 1987;102:880–882.
38. Filice C, Pirola F, Brunetti E, Duchetti S, Strosselli M, Foglieni CS. A new therapeutic approach for hydatid liver cysts. Gastroenterology 1990;98:1366–1368.
39. Dawes LG, Malangoni MA. Cystic masses of the spleen. Am Surg 1986;52:333–335.
40. Sroujieh AS, Farah GR, Haddad MJ, Abu-Khalaf MM. Adrenal cysts: diagnosis and management. Br J Urol 1990;65:570–575.
41. Bliss DP, Coffin CM, Bower RJ, Stockmann PT, Ternberg JL. Mesenteric cysts in children. Surgery 1994;115:571–577.
42. Stoupis S, Ros PR, Abbitt PL, Burton SS, Gauger J. Bubbles in the belly: imaging of cystic mesenteric or omental masses. Radiography 1994;14:729–737.
43. Hebra A, Brown MF, Mcgeehin KM, Ross AJ. Mesenteric, omental and retroperitoneal cysts in children. South Med J 1993;86: 174–176.
44. Kurtz RJ, Heimann TM, Beck AR, Holt J. Mesenteric and retroperitoneal cysts. Ann Surg 1986;103:109–112.
45. Vanek VW, Phillips AK. Retroperitoneal, mesenteric and omental cysts. Arch Surg 1984;119:838–842.
46. Burnett JS, Pickleman J. The rationale for surgical treatment of mesenteric and retroperitoneal cysts. Am Surg 1994;60:432–435.

# 72

# *Cystadenoma and Cystadenocarcinomas, Serous Adenomas*

Roland Andersson and Ingemar Ihse

Cystic neoplasms of the pancreas are uncommon lesions, accounting for only 10–15% of all pancreatic cysts and reported to represent about 1% of pancreatic malignancies (1–3). Pancreatic pseudocysts, which constitute the vast majority of pancreatic cysts, are distinguished from true cysts by their fibrous lining and absence of epithelium (4). The true, rare, cystic lesions were described in the beginning of the 19th century (5, 6), and the first malignant pancreatic cystic tumor was reported by Luecke and Klebs in 1867 (7).

By now, the list of differential diagnoses when considering cystic tumors of the pancreas has become quite extensive (8, 9). Among proliferative pancreatic cysts, serous (microcystic; benign) and mucinous (macrocystic, malignant or with a malignant potential) are dealt with in detail in this chapter. The long, though not complete, list of differential diagnoses (Table 72.1), contains some rare conditions, also within proliferative tumors.

Papillary cystic neoplasm of the pancreas is an infrequent tumor in young women, often remaining asymptomatic until presenting as an abdominal mass or by a complication such as rupture, hemorrhage, or infection. This tumor probably originates from the cells of the terminal pancreatic ductule, appears to have a limited malignant potential, and rarely metastasizes. The prognosis is excellent after surgical resection, even after reoperation for recurrence (10–13).

Mucinous ductal ectasia of the pancreas (MDE) is a recently recognized condition, judged a premalignant lesion. It is morphologically characterized by papillary hyperplasia and mucin overproduction along the pancreatic duct, endoscopically seen as mucus extruding from the ampulla of Vater or partial duct obstruction and proximal dilation, clinically resulting in attacks of obstructive pancreatitis (14–17).

The outcome of patients with pancreatic cystic tumors does not (as discussed below) seem to be comparable with the otherwise poor outcome following radical resection of common pancreatic adenocarcinoma in general. The substantially better prognosis in patients with cystic lesions motivates the relatively great interest directed to these rare conditions, as these patients probably constitute a great part of the few with evident or potentially malignant pancreatic tumors that can be offered cure by radical pancreatic resection.

## DEFINITIONS AND HISTOPATHOLOGIC APPEARANCE

*Serous cystadenomas,* or *microcystic adenomas,* consist of collections of cysts, usually up to 2 cm in diameter, possessing a honeycomb-like appearance on cut section, even though occasional macrocystic cystadenomas have been described (18, 19). The cysts are often located in the head of the pancreas and are lined by a single layer of flattened or cuboidal epithelium, separated by fibrous septa. The cytoplasm contains glycogen and no or little mucin, and the cyst fluid is clear. Most serous cystadenomas occur in women in their 6th and 7th decades and are universally considered benign (20), though one case of malignant transformation, metastasizing to the liver and stomach, has been described (21).

*Mucinous (macrocystic) cystic neoplasms* are larger (5 cm or more), though a clear distinction from serous cystadenomas does not exist. Mucinous cystic tumors, usually located in the body or tail of the pancreas, predominate in females in their 4th and 5th decades. The cysts are lined by tall columnar epithelium, often with papillary extrusions, and the cells are rich in mucin but lack glycogen (22). These cysts are often frankly malignant *(mucinous cystadenocarcinoma)* or are otherwise considered premalignant with the potential of malignant transformation *(mucinous cystadenoma)*. Malignant transformation of mucinous cystadenomas has been described, with them recurring after several years as cystadenocarcinomas (22–24).

Histopathologic differentiation between these different cyst types and also with pancreatic pseudocysts is often difficult. Macroscopic appearance (these cysts classically are thin walled and relatively free from surrounding tissues, while pseudocysts tend to be thick walled and adherent), as well as size and location, is not always helpful (25). Except for the areas of serous and mucinous epithelium that are often mixed in mucinous cystic lesions, parts of the epithelial lining of the cysts are often absent, a frequent cause of misdiagnosis (22). Warshaw et al. (14) reported irregularity of the tumor cyst epithelium in 40% of serous cystadenomas and 72% of mucinous tumors, involving an average of 40% (up to a maximum of 98%) of the cyst wall area. Moreover, mucinous cystic tumors frequently have a nonuniform epithelium that contains not only mucinous cells (26). These histopathologic features are other reasons for misdiagnosis. Not infrequently, the cysts are incorrectly classified as pancreatic pseudocysts. An inaccurate judgment of frank malignancy occurs when evaluating diagnostic punctures and frozen section at operation, resulting in concomitant inaccurate surgical treatment (25, 27). The only way to avoid incorrect diagnosis and inaccurate treatment is thus for the pathologist to have the entire cyst wall for complete histologic examination (14, 22).

## DIAGNOSTIC PROCEDURES

In the series by Warshaw et al. (14) on 67 patients with cystic tumors of the pancreas (including 18 serous cystic adenomas, 15 benign mucinous cystic neoplasms, and 27 mucinous cystadenocarcinomas), 39% of patients had no symptoms, a finding supported by other authors (28). In a report on serous cystadenomas alone, Pyke et al. (9) reported that one-third of the cysts (13 of 40) were incidental findings. Most patients with cystic

**TABLE 72.1. Differential Cystic Lesions of the Pancreas**

| |
|---|
| Congenital true cysts |
| Single cysts |
| Polycystic disease of the pancreas without related anomalies |
| Pancreatic macrocysts associated with cystic fibrosis |
| Pancreatic cysts associated with cerebellar tumors and retinal angiomas (von Hippel-Lindau's disease) |
| Pancreatic cysts associated with polycystic disease of the kidneys (Potter type I or II) |
| Enterogenous cysts |
| Dermoid cysts |
| Acquired cysts |
| Pseudocysts, in association with either acute or chronic pancreatitis |
| Parasitic cysts *(Echinococcus, Taenia solium)* |
| Retention cysts |
| Angiomatous cysts |
| Simple or proliferative cysts |
| Proliferative cysts (cystic neoplasms) |
| Serous (microcystic; benign) cystadenoma |
| Mucinous (macrocystic) cystadenoma and cystadenocarcinoma |
| Papillary cystic neoplasm |
| Cystic islet cell tumor |
| Mucinous ductal ectasia |
| Ductal adenocarcinoma with cystic necrosis |
| Teratomatous cysts |
| Cystic choriocarcinoma |
| Neuroendocrine cystic tumors of the pancreas |

neoplasms of the pancreas, however, have symptoms, mainly related to pressure effects of the cyst, including abdominal pain, abdominal mass, nausea, vomiting, and weight loss (9, 28). Less than 10% present with obstruction of the common bile duct, and occasionally, diagnosis is made after admission for abdominal emergencies (e.g., hemorrhage into the neoplasm, or tumor rupture and hemoperitoneum).

The average size of the cysts is often reported to be in the range of 6 to 10 cm. The mean size of symptomatic lesions (7.5 cm) was not found to differ from that of asymptomatic serous cystadenomas (mean size 6 cm) (9).

## Plain Abdominal X-Ray

Plain abdominal x-ray can demonstrate calcification of the capsule and internal septations in up to 10% of microcystic adenomas and mucinous cystic neoplasms (29, 30). Types of cysts may differentiated by the pattern of calcification; microcystic adenomas are reported to exhibit a starburst pattern of calcifications, while the calcifications in mucinous cystic neoplasms are concentric (29). The generalized distribution of pancreatic calcifications in chronic pancreatitis differs from the localized areas of calcification noted in cystic pancreatic neoplasms.

## Ultrasonography

Ultrasonography may readily demonstrate a cystic lesion of the pancreas. Sometimes the ultrasonographic findings allow differentiation of neoplastic cysts with their complex internal architecture and might even distinguish the multiple small cysts of a microcystic adenoma from mucinous cysts with larger cystic cavities and septa (31). However, in practice it is often difficult to differentiate cystic neoplasms from pancreatic pseudocysts by ultrasound, because of the frequent presence of hemorrhage or necrosis within a pseudocyst (30–32) (Table 72.2).

## Computed Tomography

Computed tomography (CT) may be useful for detection of cystic lesions of the pancreas, distinguishing the group of benign microcystic serous adenomas and demonstrating rim calcification, but not reliably differentiating neoplasms from pseudocysts, serous from malignant, or benign from malignant lesions (14). Others have, however, reported that CT may be beneficial in the differentiation against pseudocysts, especially by the use of intravenous contrast to distinguish papillary excrescences and septa in cystic neoplasms from the hemorrhage and necrosis that might occur in a pseudocyst (31, 33). It has also been stated that the CT appearance could suffice to differentiate between serous and mucinous tumors, with mucinous cysts seen as masses with large cystic cavities and thick walls, while microcystic adenomas have a characteristic honeycomb appearance due to fibrous septa seen after intravenous contrast (31, 33). A solid component or irregularity in the cyst does not always reliably indicate a tumor (34, 35). Calcifications are common in cystic neoplasms of the pancreas (36) and a central scar with sunburst calcification has been described as characteristic of serous cystadenomas (31, 37) but has been found more infrequently by others (14). On CT, pancreatic pseudocysts are usually identified by thin, smooth walls and their usually extrapancreatic location; those located in the pancreas and those multilocated or containing debris, bleeding, or occasionally calcifications may be difficult to differentiate from true cystic pancreatic neoplasm (37). It has been postulated that the combination of preoperative CT scan and ERCP may increase diagnostic accuracy (38, 39).

The limited experience with magnetic resonance imaging *(MRI)* has not yet shown this technique to be superior to CT in the diagnosis and characterization of cystic pancreatic neoplasms (36).

Yamaguchi et al. (40) consider structural complexity on ultrasonography or CT, including irregularity in size and shape of the cysts, cyst walls, internal septa, and solid areas, as well as hypervascularity on angiography to provide crucial infor-

**TABLE 72.2. Diagnostic Investigations in Cystic Neoplasms of the Pancreas**

| Investigation | Comment |
|---|---|
| Ultrasonography | Difficulties differentiating cysts and pseudocysts |
| Computed tomography | Difficulties differentiating cysts and pseudocysts |
| Magnetic resonance imaging | Limited experience |
| Endoscopic pancreatography | No communication with the cyst |
| Angiography | Hypervascularity *may* indicate neoplasm |
| Cyst fluid analysis | |
| Cytology | High rate of false negatives |
| Amylase, lipase, elastase | Contradictory results |
| Tumor markers | |
| CEA | High levels in mucinous cysts |
| CA 19-9 | Nondiscriminatory |
| CA 125 | High levels in malignant cysts |
| CA 72-4 | Increase after malignant transformation |
| CA 15-3 | Increase after malignant transformation |
| Viscosity | High in mucinous cysts |

mation in the assessment of the grade of malignancy prior to operation.

### Arteriography

Arteriography may demonstrate hypervascularity, which often indicates a neoplasm, though not its specific type, as opposed to pancreatic pseudocysts that are described as hypovascular on angiography (14, 40, 41). Vascular obstruction and encasement may signal malignancy (42). Microcystic adenomas frequently appear as hypervascular tumors with large feeding vessels and neovascularity, while mucinous cystic neoplasms have hypovascular areas corresponding to the large cystic cavities and increased vascularity localized to the septa and walls (31, 43, 44). Angiographic interpretation is further confused by the fact that a number of cystic neoplasms have also been found to be hypovascular (41, 45).

### Fine-Needle Puncture

Fine-needle puncture and aspiration has been reported helpful in the preoperative diagnosis and differentiation of various cystic pancreatic lesions (14, 23, 46, 47). Analysis of cyst fluid might help in the differentiation of cystic tumors of the pancreas. Serous cystadenomas should be characterized by cyst contents showing no mucin (20), a positive periodic acid-Schiff (PAS) reaction (2), low amylase levels, and no increase in CA 19-9 or carcinoembryogenic antigen (CEA) levels (48). For comparison, pseudocysts in general have increased amylase and elastase-1 levels. Cytologic examination of cyst fluid aspirates may in some instances show mucinous or malignant cells, thus contributing to accurate preoperative diagnosis (14, 46), though the rate of false-negative outcomes is probably high. Amylase content of neoplastic cysts has been described as both low (14) and high (49, 50).

Lewandrowski et al. (51) analyzed cyst fluid from various pancreatic cystic lesions including inflammatory pseudocysts, benign serous tumors, and mucinous neoplasms (some frankly malignant). Analysis included tumor markers (CEA, CA 125, and CA 19-9), amylase content, amylase isoenzymes, relative viscosity, and cytology in 26 pancreatic cysts. The results demonstrated that CEA levels were high in benign and malignant mucinous cysts but low in benign serous cystadenomas and pseudocysts. CA 125 values were high in malignant cysts, low in pseudocysts, and variable in serous cystadenomas and mucinous cystic neoplasms. The combination of high levels of both CEA and CA 125 would thus predict mucinous cystadenocarcinoma. CA 19-9 levels were determined in a limited number of pancreatic cysts, but levels were highly variable and nondiscriminatory, e.g. high levels could be seen in pseudocyst, then probably correlating to elevated serum levels of CA 19-9 in patients with pancreatitis (52). Amylase and lipase content tended to be high in pseudocysts and low in cystic tumors, and amylase isoenzyme further differentiated pseudocysts from cystic tumors. Cyst fluid relative viscosity was high in mucinous cystic tumors and low in serous cystadenomas and pseudocysts. Cytology was of diagnostic value only when malignant cells could be found. Altogether, the combination of viscosity, CEA, CA 125, and cytologic determinations of cyst fluid was considered to distinguish reliably between malignant cystic tumors and potentially premalignant cystic lesions.

Others have also reported the use of tumor markers like CEA and CA 19-9 together with cytologic findings, but the studies are often performed in a limited number of patients, so evaluation of the diagnostic accuracy is difficult (51, 53–55). The addition of cyst fluid analysis of the tumor marker CA 15-3, a mucin glycoprotein antigen present in a variety of adenocarcinomas, has been suggested to be of value in the preoperative diagnosis, as production of CA 15-3 by the tumor seems to occur only after malignant transformation. Thus, CA 15-3 could potentially offer differentiation between benign and malignant mucinous pancreatic cysts (56). Similarly, expression of CA 72-4, the tumor-associated glycoprotein 72 (TAG-72), seen in a variety of gastrointestinal and pancreatic malignancies (57), could be added to the panel of tumor markers for identification of malignant transformation. Alles et al. (58) showed that cyst fluid CA 72-4 determinations distinguished malignant mucinous cystadenocarcinomas from other types of pancreatic cysts.

Overall, it is recommended that mucinous cystic tumors of the pancreas be radically resected because of their malignant potential, if they are not already frankly malignant, which makes the preoperative differentiation between benign and malignant mucinous tumors important, especially in those who for medical reasons are not candidates for surgery (59, 60).

The potential, though probably infrequent, hazards of fine-needle aspiration cytology (FNAC)—primarily the risk of seeding of malignant cells and the development of implantation metastases especially along the needle track, as has been described for FNAC of other pancreatic and liver tumors (61–63)—should be taken into account. The risk of sampling error, lack of characteristic cystic contents, and complications such as pancreatitis should also be considered (9, 64).

### Endoscopic Pancreatography

Endoscopic pancreatography (ERP) did not show communication to the cyst cavity in any of 37 investigated patients with cystic tumors of the pancreas, while stenosis or obstruction indicated cancer (14). Other studies support the lack of communication between the cyst and the pancreatic duct at ERP in pancreatic cystic neoplasms, and also indicate ductal anomalies such as duct occlusion, narrowing, or displacement signal malignancy (38). This is to be compared with the frequent communication with the pancreatic duct demonstrated in pancreatic pseudocysts (65), together with some duct irregularities and calcifications away from the cystic lesion (66, 67). Not all investigators find ERP helpful in the differentiation of cystic tumors from pseudocysts, as even tumors occasionally may communicate with the pancreatic duct (49, 50, 68). Some authors have, however, postulated the superiority of ERCP to CT in obtaining an accurate diagnosis of pancreatic neoplasms (39, 69) and suggest that ERCP may provide a valuable adjunct to the preoperative diagnosis of cystic neoplasms of the pancreas (70–72).

## DIFFICULTIES WITH ACCURATE DIAGNOSIS

Warshaw et al. (14) reported that 37% of cystic tumors of the pancreas (in a total series of 67 patients) were initially misdiagnosed as pseudocysts, similar to results reported by Delcore et al. (25): 43% of patients who had undergone previous surgical exploration with cyst wall biopsies were still misdiagnosed as having pancreatic pseudocysts and thus not accurately treated. In the report by Turnage et al. (41), a correct preoperative diagnosis was reached in only 35% of patients. de Calan et al. (73) found the accuracy of preoperative morphologic investigations, including ultrasonography, CT, angiography, and MRI, to be even lower. In eight patients whose pancreatic cystic neoplasms were misdiagnosed and treated improperly (five drained by anastomosis, one by aspiration, and drainage recommended for the other two), five proved to have malignant disease, and three patients with no metastases at the first operation had metastatic spread at reoperation (27). However, neither tumor size nor previous inaccurate surgical intervention precludes an attempt at curative removal of the pancreatic cyst (74, 75).

The difficulties in obtaining a correct diagnosis without histologic examination of the entire cyst wall must be emphasized. Of course, suspicion should be raised by the presentation of a cystic lesion, especially in women, without a history of pancreatitis or alcoholism, together with abdominal pain, weight loss, or a palpable mass. Pancreatic pseudocysts either spontaneously resolve or collapse after percutaneous, endoscopic, or surgical management (76, 77), while proliferative pancreatic cysts persist.

## SURGICAL TREATMENT AND PROGNOSIS

The historic development of the surgical management of cystic neoplasms of the pancreas includes cyst puncture, marsupialization, and internal drainage and has now reached the generally accepted use of resection and total excision for pancreatic proliferative cystic neoplasms (78). Still, the inability to reliably differentiate between benign serous cystadenomas and malignant cystic neoplasms of the pancreas remains unsolved, exemplified by the fact that 36 of 40 patients (90%) with benign serous cystadenomas were resected in the series by Pyke et al. (9).

Cystadenocarcinomas have been considered highly curable and resectable, in contrast to the common pancreatic adenocarcinoma, with generally good results, and as many as two-thirds of patients with mucinous cystadenocarcinomas have been reported as long-term survivors after surgical resection (28, 59, 79, 80). These promising results are shown, for example, in the report by Delcore et al. (25) of 10 patients with mucinous cystadenocarcinomas treated by resection: 1 died of recurrence after 8 months, and the remaining 9 were without recurrence after a mean of 6 years. Others present results implying two different grades of malignancy and prognosis of mucinous tumors of the pancreas (14). However, the prognosis is poor in disease that is unresectable because of local extension or distant metastases; for example, did death occur at a mean of 4 months in 10 patients with unresectable cystadenocarcinoma (14), and three patients with metastases and unresectable disease died within 9 months (25)?

Drainage procedures are to be discouraged as they withhold the possibility of definite cure and long-term survival by a complete surgical resection for the cystic lesion. Beyond this, surgical drainage may result in persistent fistulas and eventual skin involvement with tumor growth (81).

## CONCLUSIONS

All mucinous cystic neoplasms of the pancreas should be considered potentially malignant, perhaps being dormant for long periods of time until becoming truly invasive cancers. The low operative mortality and decreasing morbidity following pancreatic resections, the generally high rate of cure, and the still unsatisfactory ability to differentiate reliably between different types of pancreatic cystic tumors, motivate an aggressive surgical approach in most cystic tumors of the pancreas, excluding only those reliably identified as benign serous adenomas and those in patients unfit for surgical intervention.

## REFERENCES


1. Becker WF, Welsh RA, Pratt HS. Cystadenoma and cystadenocarcinoma of the pancreas. Ann Surg 1965;161:845–863.
2. Cubilla AL, Fitzgerald PJ. Tumors of the exocrine pancreas. In: Atlas of tumor pathology, 2nd series, fascicle 19. Armed Forces Institute of Pathology 1984;109–110:185–194.
3. Hoover E, Natesha R, Dao A, Adams CZ, Barnwell S. Proliferative pancreatic cysts: pathogenesis and treatment options. Am J Surg 1991;162:274–277.
4. Jordan J, Durh MS. Injury to the pancreas: a cause of effusions into the lesser peritoneal cavity. Br Med J 1892;2:1051.
5. Cruveihler J. Kyste pancreatique. Essai sur l'anatomie pathologoque, T I. 1816:286.
6. Gross SD. Serous cysts of the pancreas. In: Pathological anatomy, vol. II. Boston: Marsh, Capen, Lyon & Webb, 1839:361–362.
7. Luecke A, Klebs E. Beitrage zur Ovariotomie and zur Kentniss der abdominal Gewchwiste. Virchows Arch 1867;XLI:1–14.
8. Howard JM. Cystic neoplasms and true cysts of the pancreas. Surg Clin North Am 1989;69:651–665.
9. Pyke CM, van Heerden JA, Colby TV, Sarr MG, Weaver AL. The spectrum of serous cystadenoma of the pancreas—clinical, pathologic, and surgical aspects. Ann Surg 1992;215:132–139.
10. Compagno J, Oertel JE, Krezmor M. Solid and papillary epithelial neoplasms of the pancreas, probably of small duct origin: a clinicopathologic study of 52 cases. Abstr Lab Invest 1979; 40:12.
11. Sanfey H, Mendelsohn G, Cameron JL. Solid and papillary neoplasm of the pancreas. A potentially curable lesion. Ann Surg 1983;197:272–275.
12. Rustin RE, Broughan TA, Hermann RE, Grundfest-Broniatowski SF, Petras RE, Hart WR. Papillary cystic epithelial neoplasms of the pancreas. A clinical study of four cases. Arch Surg 1986;121:1073–1076.
13. Kaufman SL, Reddick RL, Stiegel M, Wild RE, Thomas CG Jr. Papillary cystic neoplasm of the pancreas: a curable pancreatic tumor. World J Surg 1986;10:851–859.
14. Warshaw AL, Compton CC, Lewandrowski K, Cardenosa G, Mueller PR. Cystic tumors of the pancreas—new clinical, radiologic, and pathologic observations in 67 patients. Ann Surg 1990;212:432–443.
15. Bastid C, Bernard JP, Sarles H, Payan MJ, Sahel J. Mucinous ductal ectasia of the pancreas: a premalignant disease and a cause of obstructive pancreatitis. Pancreas 1991;6:15–22.
16. Warshaw AL. Mucinous cystic tumors and mucinous ductal ectasia of the pancreas. Gastrointest Endosc 1991;37:199–201.
17. Nickl NJ, Lawson JM, Cotton PB. Mucinous pancreatic tumors. ERCP findings. Gastrointest Endosc 1991;37:133–138.
18. Lewandrowski K, Warshaw A, Compton C. Macrocystic serous cystadenoma of the pancreas: a morphologic variant differing from microcystic adenoma. Hum Pathol 1992;23:871–875.
19. Mori K, Takeyama S, Hirosawa H, Watanabe T, Taniya T, et al. A case of macrocystic serous cystadenoma of the pancreas. Int J Pancreatol 1995;17:91–93.
20. Compagno J, Oertel JE. Microcystic adenomas of the pancreas (glycogen rich cystadenomas): a clinicopathologic study of 34 cases. Am J Clin Pathol 1978;69:289–298.
21. George DH, Murphy F, Michalski R, Ulmer BG. Serous cystadenocarcinoma of the pancreas: a new entity? Am J Surg Pathol 1989;13:61–66.
22. Compagno J, Oertel JE. Mucinous cystic neoplasms of the pancreas with overt and latent malignancy (cystadenocarcinoma and cystadenoma): a clinicopathologic study of 41 cases. Am J Surg Pathol 1978;69:573–580.
23. Hodgkinson DJ, ReMine WH, Weiland LH. Pancreatic cystadenoma: a clinicopathologic study of 45 cases. Arch Surg 1978;113:512–519.
24. Yamaguchi K, Enjoji M. Cystic neoplasms of the pancreas. Gastroenterology 1987;92:1934–1943.
25. Delcore R, Thomas JH, Forster J. Characteristics of cystic neoplasms of the pancreas and results of aggressive surgical treatment. Am J Surg 1992;164:437–442.
26. Shorten SD, Hart WR, Petras RE. Microcystic adenomas (serous cystadenomas) of pancreas: a clinical investigation of eight cases with immunohistochemical and ultrastructural studies. Am J Surg Pathol 1986;10:365–372.
27. Warshaw AL, Rutledge PL. Cystic tumors mistaken for pancreatic pseudocysts. Ann Surg 1987;205:393–398.
28. Tarpila E, Borch K, Franze N, Andersson R, Evander A, et al. Cystic neoplasms of the pancreas: a clinicopathological study of 38 cases. Dig Surg 1989;6:138–141.
29. Barbee CL, DeMello FB, Grange TB. Cystadenoma and cystadenocarcinoma of the pancreas. J Surg Oncol 1976;8:1–10.
30. Freeny PC, Weinstein CJ, Taft DA, Allen FA. Cystic neoplasms of the pancreas: new angiographic and ultrasonographic findings. Roentgenology 1978;131:795–802.
31. Friedman AC, Lichenstein JE, Dachman AH. Cystic neoplasms of the pancreas: radiologic-pathologic correlation. Radiology 1983; 149:45–50.
32. Busilacchi P, Rizzatto G, Bazzocchi M, Boltro E, Caridiana F, et al. Pancreatic cystadenocarcinoma: diagnostic problems. Br J Radiol 1982;55:558–561.
33. Itai Y, Moss A, Ohtomo K. Computed tomography of cystad-

enoma and cystadenocarcinoma of the pancreas. Radiology 1982;145:419–425.
34. Itai Y, Ohhashi K, Furui S, Araki T, Muakami Y, et al. Microcystic adenoma of the pancreas: spectrum of computed tomographic findings. J Comput Assist Tomogr 1988;12:797–803.
35. Corbally MT, McAnena OJ, Urmacher C, Herman B, Shiu MH. Pancreatic cystadenoma, a clinicopathologic study. Arch Surg 1989;124:1271–1274.
36. Minami M, Itai Y, Ohtomo K, Yoshida H, Yoshikawa K, Iio M. Cystic neoplasms of the pancreas: comparison of MR imaging with CT. Radiology 1989;171:53–56.
37. Zirinsky K, Abiri M, Baer JW. Computed tomography demonstration of pancreatic microcystic adenoma. Am J Gastroenterol 1984;79:139–142.
38. Pinson CW, Munson JL, Deveney CW. Endoscopic retrograde cholangiopancreatography in the preoperative diagnosis of pancreatic neoplasms associated with cysts. Am J Surg 1990;159: 510–513.
39. Foley WD, Stewart ET, Lawson TL, Geenan J, Loguidice J, et al. Computed tomography, ultrasonography, and endoscopic retrograde cholangiopancreatography in the diagnosis pancreatic disease: a comparative study. Gastrointest Radiol 1980;5:29–35.
40. Yamaguchi K, Hirakata R, Kitamura K. Mucinous cystic neoplasm of the pancreas: estimation of grade of malignancy with imaging techniques and its surgical implications. Acta Chir Scand 1990; 156:553–556.
41. Turnage RH, Eckhauser FE, Vinik AI, Strodel WE, Thompson NW, et al. Diagnostic dilemmas in patients with cystic neoplasms of the pancreas. Int J Pancreatol 1988;3:477–490.
42. Uflacker R, Amaral NM, Lima S, Aakhus T, Pereira E, Kuroda K. Angiography in cystadenoma and cystadenocarcinoma of the pancreas. Acta Radiol (Diagn) 1980;21:189–195.
43. Thompson NW, Eckhauser FE, Vinik AI, Lloyd RV, Fiddian-Green RG, Strodel WE. Cystic neuroendocrine neoplasms of the pancreas and liver. Ann Surg 1984;199:158–164.
44. Pogany AC, Erlan RK Jr, Karan JH, LeQuesne SP, Ring EJ. Cystic insulinoma. AJR 1985;142:951–952.
45. Pressman BD, Asch T, Casarella WJ. Cystadenoma of the pancreas: a reappraisal of angiographic findings. AJR 1973;119: 115–120.
46. Katoh H, Rossi RL, Braasch JW, Munson JL, Shimozawa E, Tanabe T. Cystadenoma and cystadenocarcinoma of the pancreas. Hepatogastroenterology 1989;36:424–430.
47. Gupta RK, AlAnsari AG. Needle aspiration cytology in the diagnosis of mucinous cystadenocarcinoma of the pancreas. Int J Pancreatol 1994;15:149–153.
48. Albores-Saavedra J, Angeles-Angeles A, Nadja M, et al. Mucinous cystadenocarcinoma of the pancreas: morphologic and immunocytochemical observations. Am J Surg Pathol 1987;11: 11–20.
49. Lumsden A, Bradley EL III. Pseudocyst or cystic neoplasm? Differential diagnoses and initial management of cystic pancreatic lesions. Hepatogastroenterology 1989;36:462–466.
50. Sachs JR, Deren JJ, Sohn M, Nusbaum M. Mucinous cystadenoma: pitfalls of differential diagnosis. Am J Gastroenterol 1989;84:811–816.
51. Lewandrowski KB, Southern JF, Pins MR, Compton CC, Warshaw AL. Cyst fluid analysis in the differential diagnosis of pancreatic cysts: a comparison of pseudocysts, serous cystadenomas, mucinous cystic neoplasms, and mucinous cystadenocarcinoma. Ann Surg 1993;217:41–47.
52. Steinberg M, Gelfand R, Anderson KK, Glenn J, Kurtzman SH, et al. Comparison of the sensitivity and specificity of the CA 19-9 and carcinoembryonic antigen assays in detecting cancer of the pancreas. Gastroenterology 186;90:343–349.
53. Tatsua M, Iishi H, Ichii M, Noguchi S, Yamamoto R, et al. Values of carcinoembryonic antigen, elastase 1, and carbohydrate antigen determinant in aspirated pancreatic cystic fluid in the diagnosis of cysts of the pancreas. Cancer 1986;57:1836–1839.
54. Nishida K, Shiga K, Kato K, Kunihiro K, Fujii T, et al. Two cases of pancreatic cystadenocarcinoma with elevated CA 19-9 levels in the cystic fluid in comparison with two cases of pancreatic cystadenoma. Hepatogastroenterology 1989;36:442–445.
55. Pinto M, Meriano F. Diagnosis of cystic pancreatic lesions by cytologic examination and carcinoembryonic antigen and amylase levels of cysts contents. Acta Cytol 1991;35:456–463.
56. Rubin D, Warshaw AL, Southern JF, Pins M, Compton CC, Lewandrowski KB. Expression of CA 15.3 protein in the cyst contents distinguishes benign from malignant pancreatic mucinous cystic neoplasms. Surgery 1994;115:52–55.
57. Kornek G, Depisch D, Rosen H, Temsch EM, Scheithauer W. Comparative analysis of CA 72-4, CA 195 and carcinoembryogenic antigen in patients with gastrointestinal malignancies. J Cancer Res Clin Oncol 1992;118:318–320.
58. Alles AJ, Warshaw AL, Sothern JF, Comptom CC, Lewandrowski KB. Expression of CA 72-4 (TAG-72) in the fluid contents of pancreatic cysts. Ann Surg 1994;219:131–134.
59. Hoover E, Natesha R, Dao A, Adams CZ Jr, Barnwell S. Proliferative pancreatic cysts: pathogenesis and treatment options. Am J Surg 1991;162:274–277.
60. Ferucci JT, Wittenberg J, Mueller PR, Simeone JF, Harbin WP, et al. Diagnosis of abdominal malignancy by radiologic fine-needle aspiration biopsy. AJR 1980;134:323–330.
61. Ihse I, Isaksson G. Pancreatic carcinoma: diagnosis and treatment. Clin Gastroenterol 1984;13:961–984.
62. Andersson R, Andrén-Sandberg Å, Lundstedt C, Tranberg KG. Implantation metastases after percutaneous puncture or biliary drainage of gastrointestinal malignancies. Eur J Surg 1996;162: 551–554.
63. Bergenfeldt M, Genell S, Lindholm K, Ekberg D, Aspelin P. Needle-tract seeding after percutaneous fine-needle biopsy of pancreatic carcinoma. Acta Chir 1988;154:77–79.
64. Jones EC, Suen KC, Grant DR, Chan NH. Fine-needle aspiration cytology of neoplastic cysts of the pancreas. Diagn Cytopathol 1987;3:328–343.
65. O'Connor M, Kolars J, Ansel U, Silvis S, Vennes J. Preoperative endoscopic retrograde cholangiopancreatography in the surgical management of pancreatic pseudocysts. Am J Surg 1986; 151:18–24.
66. Heij HA, Obertop H, van Blankenstein M, Nix GAJJ, Westbroek DL. Comparison of endoscopic retrograde pancreatography with functional and histological changes in chronic pancreatitis. Acta Radiol 1987;28:289–293.
67. Mahlfartheimer P, Buchler M. Correlation of imaging and of function in chronic pancreatitis. Radiol Clin North Am 1989;27: 51–64.
68. Delcenserie R, Dupas JL, Joly JP, Descombes P, Mortier F, Capron JP. Microcystic adenoma of the pancreas demonstrated by endoscopic retrograde pancreatography. Gastrointest Endosc 1988;34:52–54.
69. Dimagno EP, Magalegada JR, Taylor WF, Go VLW. A prospective comparison of current diagnostic tests for pancreatic cancer. N Engl J Med 1977;297:737–742.
70. Herrera L, Glassman CI, Komins JI. Mucinous cystic neoplasms of the pancreas demonstrated by ultrasound and endoscopic retrograde pancreatography. Am J Gastroenterol 1980;73: 512–515.
71. Mannell A, Tim LO. Cystadenoma of the pancreas: report of a case diagnosed by endoscopic retrograde pancreatography. Aust NZ J Surg 1981;51:201–203.
72. Cross MR. Mucinous cystadenoma of the pancreas: endoscopy as an aid to diagnosis. Gastroenterology 1980;79:944–947.
73. de Calan L, Levard H, Hennet, Fingerhut A. Pancreatic cystadenoma and cystadenocarcinoma: diagnostic value of preoperative morphological investigations. Eur J Surg 1995;161:35–40.
74. Taft DA, Freeney PC. Cystic neoplasms of the pancreas. Am J Surg 1981;142:30–35.
75. Corrente RF. Cystadenocarcinoma of the pancreas. Am J Surg 1980;139:265–267.
76. Bradley EL, Clements JL, Gonzalez AC. The natural history of pancreatic pseudocysts: a unified concept of management. Am J Surg 1979;137:135–141.
77. Warshaw AL, Rattner DW. Timing of surgical drainage for pancreatic pseudocyst: clinical and chemical criteria. Ann Surg 1985;202:720–724.
78. Zamora JL. Cystic neoplasms of the pancreas: evolution of a concept. Am J Surg 1985;149:819–823.
79. Hodgkinson DJ, ReMine WH, Weiland LH. A clinicopathologic study of 21 cases of cystadenocarcinoma of pancreatic cystadenocarcinoma. Ann Surg 1978;188:679–684.
80. Kerlin DL, Frey CF, Bodai BI, Twomey PL, Ruebner B. Cystic neoplasms of the pancreas. Surg Gyn Obstet 1987;165:475–478.
81. Campbell JA, Cruickshank AH. Cystadenoma and cystadenocarcinoma of the pancreas. J Clin Pathol 1962;15:432–437.

# 73

# *Papillary Cystic and Solid Tumors*

Mustafa Guvendi and John M. Howard

The papillary cystic and solid tumor of the pancreas (PCSTP) characteristically presents as a dramatic but often unexpected finding on computed tomography (CT) scanning in an adolescent or young female. Symptoms are often minimal. The management of the patient usually proves gratifying to both patient and surgeon, for the results of treatment are excellent.

The tumor was originally described by Frantz (1) in 1959. The nomenclature has been confusing, as the tumor has been described as cystic and/or solid tumor, papillary and/or epithelial cystic and/or solid tumor of the pancreas, on the basis of gross and histologic descriptions by pathologists. The term "papillary cystic and solid tumor of the pancreas," introduced by Kloppel in 1981 (2), is now widely used. In the classification of the World Health Organization, the tumor is classified as a "solid—pseudopapillary tumor" under the group heading of "borderline-tumors of uncertain malignant potential," unless it is obviously malignant, when it is classified as a "solid—pseudopapillary carcinoma."

The following three patients illustrate the presentation, management, and excellent results characteristic of the PCSTP. They are presented within the framework of a review of the world's literature, consisting of a total of 352 patients; an effort was made to exclude duplication (3–111).

## PRESENTATION OF THREE PATIENTS

**Patient 1.** A 32-year-old white female was hospitalized with a history of nausea and mild abdominal and back pain of 3-week's duration. CT scan showed a large, thick-walled, septated cyst in the left half of the pancreas (Fig. 73.1). Endoscopic retrograde cholangiopancreatography (ERCP) revealed complete obstruction of the pancreatic duct in its midportion, and arteriography revealed displacement without invasion of the spleen by an avascular tumor (Fig. 73.2). A large tumor in the tail of the pancreas was resected by distal pancreatectomy and splenectomy (Fig. 73.3, *A-C*). Neither invasion nor metastasis was detected. The cystic tumor measured 13 × 8 × 7 cm, was multilocular, was encapsulated, and contained dark brown fluid (Fig. 73.3*D*). The neoplasm was composed of slightly pleomorphic cells with round to oval nuclei and variable amounts of granular amphophilic neoplasm. It contained organizing hematoma with dense fibrosis and numerous pigment-laden macrophages at the periphery of the neoplasm. Electron microscopy revealed a moderate number of mitochondria and a rough endoplasmic reticulum. No neuroendocrine granules were seen. The patient remains well 4 years after operation. Follow-up consists of clinical examination at 6-month intervals and annual CT scanning of the abdomen.

**Patient 2.** A 21-year-old black female was hospitalized shortly after a motor vehicular accident. A CT scan demonstrated a mass in the tail of the pancreas (Fig. 73.4). Laparotomy revealed the mass, measuring 14 × 10 × 9 cm, in the tail of the pancreas. Distal pancreatectomy was performed, the spleen being preserved. Neither local invasion nor metastasis was found. Six years after operation, the patient is without evidence of disease.

The tumor was large, pale, and solid but soft, with a dense fibrous capsule (Fig. 73.5). The central portion of the tumor was necrotic and hemorrhagic. Histologically, the neoplasm consisted of uniformly round to cuboidal cells arranged in solid sheets and papillary structures separated by delicate vascular stroma (Fig. 73.6). The cells had eosinophilic granular cytoplasm and uniform round nuclei. Electron microscopy demonstrated uniform round epithelial tumor cells, rich in mitochondria. No neurosecretory granules were identified in the tumor cells, and only a few zymogen granules were identified. No ultrastructural evidence of exocrine pancreatic acini or ductal cells was found.

**Patient 3.** A 68-year-old white female was hospitalized with epigastric pain for the past year. CT scan revealed a 13-cm diameter tumor, well localized, in the tail of the pancreas (Fig. 73.7). Distal pancreatectomy with splenectomy included the large cystic mass in the tail of the pancreas. Neither invasion nor metastasis was detected. The cystic tumor contained approximately 100 mL of serosanguinous fluid and had a thick, fibrous wall. One portion of the cyst contained a well-circumscribed 3.5-cm diameter nodule consisting of multiple papillary structures lined by a single layer of cuboidal to columnar cells and supported by a hyaline vascular core. Abnormal mitotic figures were not identified. Electron microscopy revealed tumor cells in sheets and cords, surrounding a prominent fibrovascular stalk. Numerous dense-core neurosecretory granules were apparent in the cytoplasm.

The patient is living without recurrence 5 years after operation, having subsequently undergone resection of a primary carcinoma of the colon, and is currently under treatment for multiple myeloma.

## CHARACTERIZATION OF PCSTP

### Diagnosis

Clinically, the most important feature is that the patient is likely to be a young woman with a large pancreatic tumor. Patient complaints are usually minimal, although nausea, a sense of fullness, or dull pain across the upper abdomen may be noted. The patient or the physician may detect an asymptomatic mass as the first indication of the tumor's presence. Occasionally, obstructive jaundice may be an initial manifestation. By whatever means, recognition of a large pancreatic tumor in a young woman is the most significant lead to its diagnosis. Several radiologists

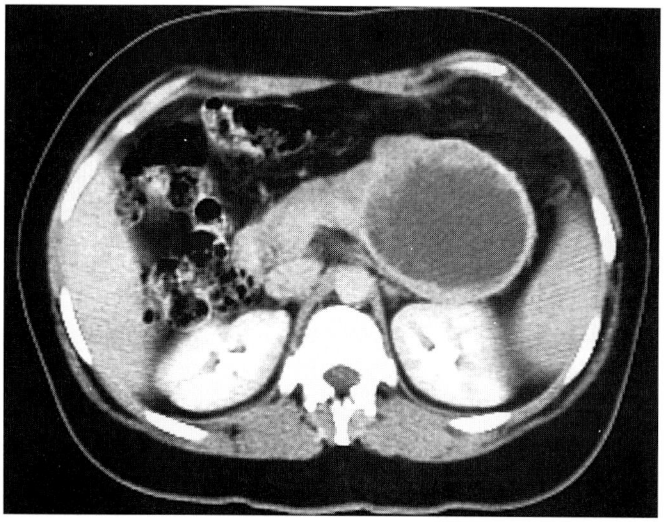

**FIG. 73.1.** CT (patient 1) showing 13-cm diameter papillary cystic and solid tumor in a 32-year-old female.

have commented that the incidence of PCSTP is higher among black people (93, 113), but the writers have not discovered such documentation.

## Special Studies

Although not diagnostic, abdominal films may show displacement of the stomach, duodenum, or transverse colon, depending upon the location of the tumor. Splenomegaly is infrequent, but again, the striking characteristic is a large tumor, usually in a young woman. Barium studies may also show displacement without obstruction of the stomach, duodenum, or transverse colon.

## CT and Ultrasound Scans

CT scans provide the most information of any of the clinical studies, usually showing the tumor to be large and round or, occasionally, bilobar. Characteristically, the tumor is hypodense and well circumscribed, with a definite capsule. Occasionally the capsule is incomplete if the tumor invades the adjacent pancreas. Septation may, or may not, be noted. The presence or absence of calcification is not diagnostic. CT may show solid and cystic components. The fluid component of the cyst has a higher density than water, usually the density is that of hemorrhagic necrotic tissue. Even the solid tumors tend to be hypodense (90). Dynamic studies show the tumor to be hypovascular. Choi et al. (45) emphasized that CT findings include a well-defined round or lobular mass consisting of both cystic and solid components in all instances, although the ratio of cystic to solid elements may vary from tumor to tumor. When the above findings are noted in a young female, and when the CT density numbers of the cystic spaces are higher than that of water, they consider PCSTP to be the primary consideration. They also noted that in one patient with a malignant PCSTP with hepatic and multiple lymph nodal metastases, the CT appearance of the metastases was similar to that of the primary tumor, including well-defined outer margins and mixed solid and cystic components.

Ultrasound with PCSTP (42, 90) provides useful information, although most observers prefer CT scanning.

## Calcification

Although limited areas of calcification of the capsule (92) or of the parenchyma (45) may occur, it is neither characteristic nor diagnostic of this tumor (14, 25). Several authors have described one or more small round areas of calcification, "marblelike" in appearance. Others have noted an "eggshell" (93) appearance or more nondescript (45) areas of calcification. These are best seen on CT scans, although Friedman et al. (26), Strauss et al. (99),

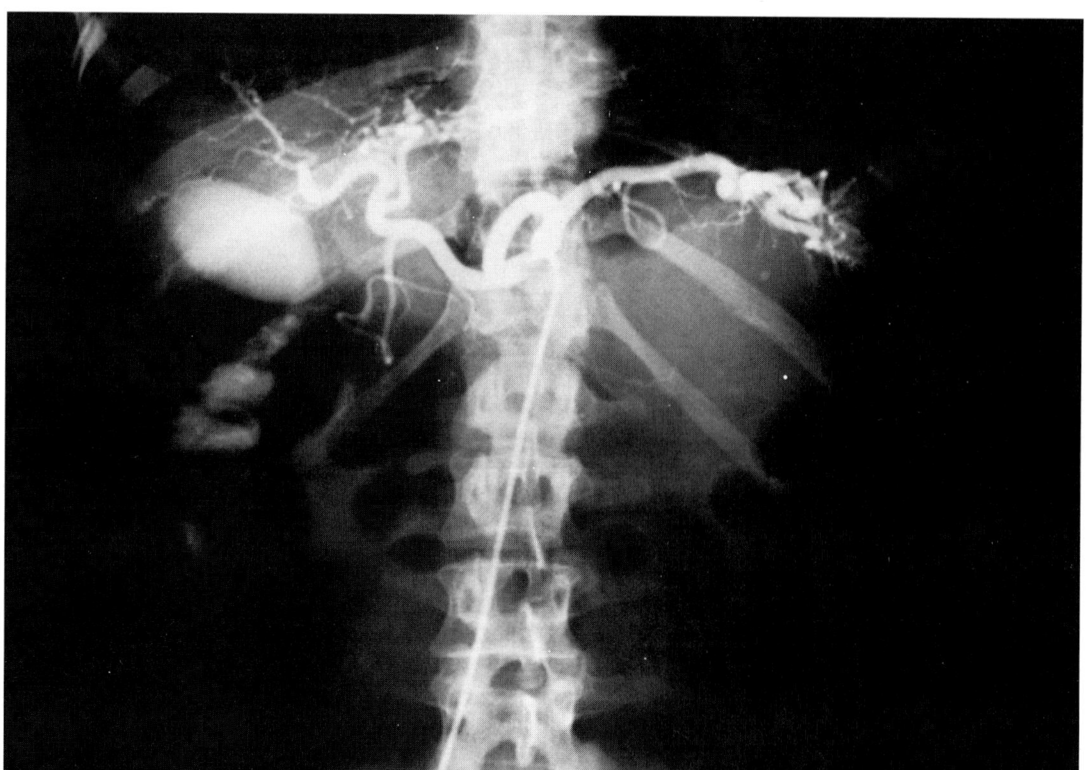

**FIG. 73.2.** Selective celiac arteriogram (patient 1) showing displacement of the splenic artery by the strikingly hypovascular tumor.

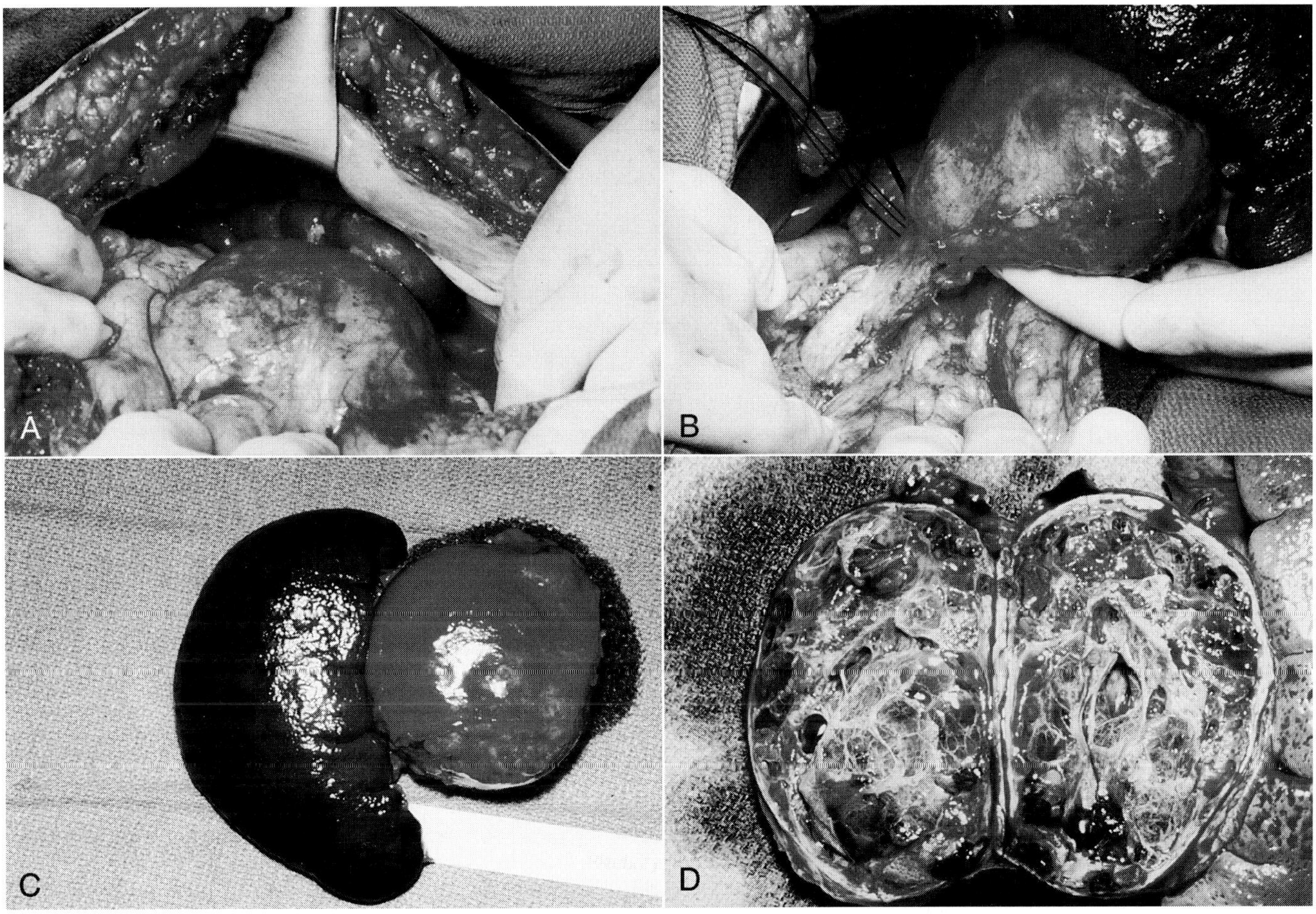


**FIG. 73.3.** Patient 1. **A.** Intraoperative view showing huge pancreatic tumor abutting the spleen. **B.** Intraoperative view demonstrating mobilization of the spleen and tumor of the tail of the pancreas. Note the relatively sharp line of demarcation between the tumor and the body of the pancreas. **C.** Surgical specimen. Not seen is the 2-cm margin of resected pancreas with negative line of transection (frozen section). **D.** Cross-section of fresh tumor. Multiple areas of cystic degeneration. This is the ``cystic or cystic and solid'' form of the tumor. See color insert.

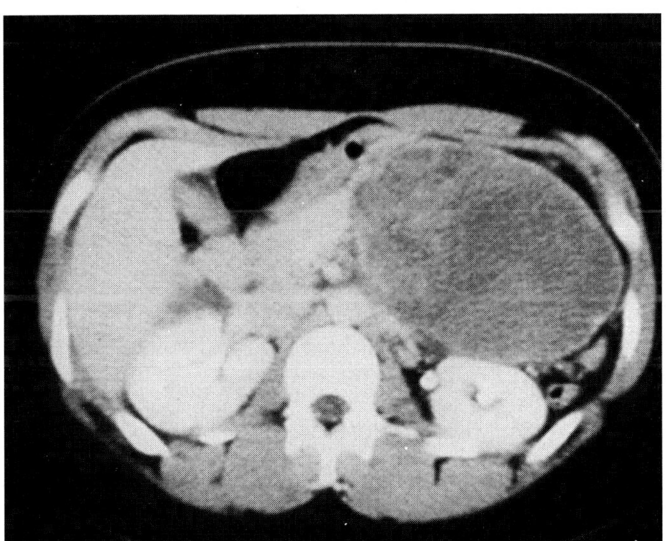

**FIG. 73.4.** CT (patient 2) showing 14-cm diameter tumor of the tail of the pancreas in a 21-year-old female.

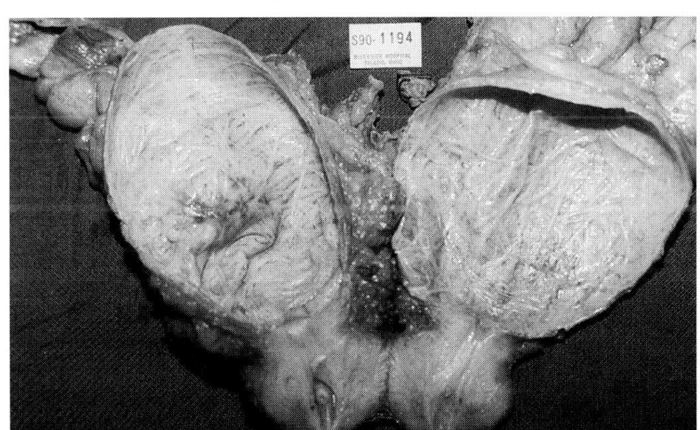


**FIG. 73.5.** Cross-section (patient 2) of the solid form of the tumor. Although largely solid, a central portion of the tumor was hemorrhagic and necrotic.

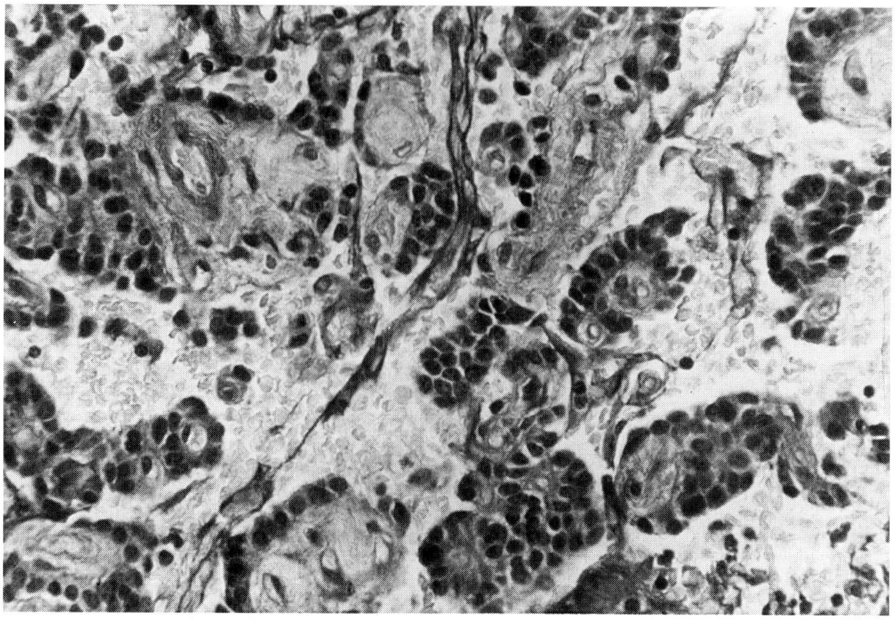

**FIG. 73.6.** Within microcystic spaces, the tumor consisted of uniformly round to cuboidal cells arranged in solid sheets and papillary structures separated by delicate vascular stroma and microcystic spaces (patient 2). (H & E, ×125).

and Matsunou et al. (66) reported calcification on flat plate. Yamaguchi et al. (90) noted a striking calcification of PCSTP on a plain radiograph; CT scanning showed the tumor to have a thick-walled calcified capsule but also discrete "nodules" of parenchymal calcification. Matsunou et al. (66) found an area of calcification and ossification in a tumor in a 44-year-old female.

## Magnetic Resonance Imaging

Although the emerging new techniques with magnetic resonance imaging may demonstrate striking advances in defining this tumor, prior to 1997 its use has made little contribution. Compared with CT scanning, Ohtomo et al. (93) (1992) noted that MRI clearly delineated the solid and cystic components of the tumor as well as its capsule.

## Angiography

With very few exceptions, these tumors are avascular or hypovascular. Large vessels may be displaced and occasionally encased, but seldom occluded. Hypervascularity is quite unusual, and when noted raises the question of the possible diagnosis of an islet cell tumor. Yamaguchi et al. (90) studied nonmetastasizing PCSTPs angiographically, and found 1 to be avascular, 5 hypovascular, 1 mildly hypervascular, and 1 normal.

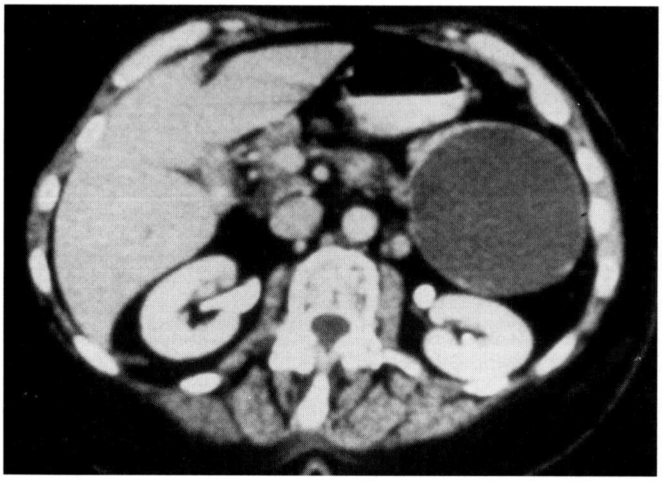

**FIG. 73.7.** CT (patient 3). Papillary cystic and solid tumor, diameter 13 cm, in a 68-year-old female.

## Endoscopic Retrograde Cholangiopancreatography

Pancreatography may show an abrupt obstruction of the main pancreatic duct at the level of the tumor, as in patient 1. The unobstructed duct may sometimes be displaced and occasionally compressed. One report described ductules coursing through the tumor (62), but this is atypical and almost incompatible with the general concept of the tumor. Communication of the duct with the cystic spaces of the tumor is not a feature.

## Tumor Markers

No studies and few observations of serum markers have been made (93). CA 19-9 serum levels have been mentioned. Ohtomo et al. (93) and Yagi et al. (106) noted a slight elevation; Yamanishi et al. (103) found a normal level in individual patients. Similarly, only an occasional mention has been made of the CEA level (111). Neither avenue has been explored, but the limited data do not provide encouraging leads. Several authors (16) have failed to detect CEA in tumor stains.

## Fine-Needle Biopsy

Although its indication has not been clearly defined, fine-needle biopsy and cytologic diagnosis of this tumor are practical, and the cytologic characterization of the cellular aspirate is well established (13, 34, 44, 54, 55, 69, 77, 80, 94, 98, 102, 104, 109). So much of the tumor may consist of blood and necrotic tissue, however, that false-negative findings constitute a continuing possibility (70). Distinction between PCSTP and islet cell tumors is not always possible (73). Greenberg et al. (96) concluded that when used either preoperatively or intraoperatively, cytologic examination is a reliable method of diagnosis. The fact that the histologic features of the tumor may vary from area to area and that the tumor will obviously require laparotomy, together with the inherent danger of tumor spread, bleeding, or infection, has influenced the authors against preoperative biopsy, but others may find its advantages to sometimes outweigh its potential disadvantages.

### Differential Diagnosis

Earlier, cystic tumors of the pancreas were considered either cystadenomas or cystadenocarcinomas. Subsequently, the serous cystadenoma and the malignant or potentially malignant mucinous cystadenoma were identified. In addition, the occasional solid or cystic acinar cell tumor, the cystic islet cell tumor, and the papillary mucinous ectatic tumor were identified—each a separate entity. Short of histologic examination, the various cystic tumors cannot be differentiated from each other with certainty; but because cystic tumors of the pancreas, in general, have a good prognosis following resection, the surgeon should approach them aggressively, anticipating complete removal of the tumor and complete histologic and immunohistochemical study of the entire cyst.

Clinically, the differentiation of PCSTP from other cystic tumors of the pancreas is becoming easier as information accumulates. As indicated, PCSTP is noted predominantly in young women. As stated above, it is well circumscribed, usually large and round or ovoid; it may or may not be septated; it has both cystic areas and solid components; the CT density of the cystic areas is higher than that of water; and it is relatively avascular. No endocrine syndrome is apparent.

The serous cystadenoma, on the contrary, often occurs in older patients and is honeycombed and more vascular. The rare true congenital cyst usually occurs in childhood and lacks a solid component. The cystic islet cell tumor may present with a hormonal syndrome. The mucinous cystadenoma or cystadenocarcinoma may be more difficult to distinguish clinically. It does not usually have the multiplicity of cystic areas seen with PCSTP, and the patient with a mucinous cystadenoma may have an elevated CEA level.

At operation, PCSTP is an encapsulated tumor, usually large, with features that vary relative to the predominance of the cystic component to the solid element. The cystic component, dominant in 95% of these tumors, reflects necrosis and hemorrhage confined within the necrotic spaces. Of 307 cases reviewed, 17 (5.5%) were considered "solid," but they, too, had areas of cystic necrosis (Table 73.1). Unlike most cancers of the pancreas, the benign or malignant PCSTP projects well above the surface of the pancreas.

Histologically, the nonnecrotic portion of the tumor is characterized by papillary projections of solid sheets of epithelial cells, which tend to be round or cuboidal, giving a monomorphic appearance. The cells are slightly eosinophilic, and mitoses are usually infrequent. The areas of necrosis may reveal hemorrhage, hyalinization, and cholesterol granulomas (73). Problems have arisen in the differentiation of PCSTP from the rarer pancreatoblastoma of childhood. The very rare oncocytic tumor is a diagnostic consideration; several authors observed an oncocytic appearance in certain PCSTPs. Table 73.2 (110) summarizes the clinicopathologic features of these three tumors. The acinar cell carcinoma, a very rare aggressive tumor, occurring mainly in adults, might also occasionally be considered in the differential diagnosis.

## NATURAL HISTORY OF THE PCSTP: ORIGIN OF THE TUMOR AND IMMUNOHISTOCHEMICAL AND ELECTRON MICROSCOPIC STUDIES

Because the histogenesis of PCSTP is unknown, there have been extensive attempts to elucidate an islet, acinar, or ductal cell origin or an origin from the embryonic stem cell from which both the endocrine and exocrine pancreatic systems evolve. Electron microscopy has been used because it permits *(a)* identification of neurosecretory granules, pointing toward the hormonal products of islet cells, or *(b)* identification of zymogen granules, implicating the enzyme secretions of the acinar components. Complementing these studies, immunohistochemical techniques permit identification of enolase and/or specific neuroendocrine hormones of islet cells on one hand or identification of the α-1-antitrypsin or α-1-antichymotrypsin of acinar cells on the other. In some studies, the absence of the above findings has been interpreted as evidence of a ductal cell origin. Studies in 234 tumors from the world's literature were reviewed and referenced in the 1995 report by the authors and their colleagues (110). Positive findings have not been consistent from tumor to tumor.

As described by Liu and Potter (112), the islets and acini of the human pancreas appear first during the 3rd month of embryonic development; the islet and acinar cells each arise from a common embryonic stem cell. For many investigators (17, 40, 47, 56, 58, 63, 66, 68, 74, 80, 85, 86, 110), including the writers, the demonstration of subcellular components of both endocrine and exocrine tissue in the tumor supports the concept of the origin of the tumor from these embryonic multipotential stem cells that can differentiate to ductal, acinar, or endocrine components, each of which has been identified by election microscopy or immunohistologic staining in individual tumors. The female sex prevalence for this tumor remains unexplained, although it is perhaps its single most striking characteristic.

### The Patient and the Tumor

The natural history of the tumor is obviously not fully described. Collected data show (Table 73.1) that the tumor usually presents in females: 90.3% of 352 patients. Only 34 tumors, (9.7%) have been found in men. Although the tumor was recognized in a 2-year-old, it has apparently not been described at or before birth. The oldest patient was diagnosed at age 81, but the mean age among 338 patients is 25.3 years. As noted in Table 73.1, the tumors are distributed rather evenly throughout the pancreas. By the time of diagnosis of 307 PCSTPs, 290 (94.5%) were described as cystic or cystic and solid; only 17 tumors (5.5%) were solid in appearance. The tumors are characteristically large; their mean maximal diameter reaches 10.8 cm, with a range of 2.0–25 cm.

The great majority (86%) of PCSTPs behave as benign tumors; 50 tumors, (14% of the total), (45 in females and 4 in males, 1 unspecified) have been malignant (Table 73.1). Twelve malignancies, all in females, were diagnosed before the age of 20 (Table 73.3). Three patients, females aged 10–12 years, presumably prepubertal, were reported with malignancies. Conversely, only four patients were diagnosed with malignancy at age 60 or older, one male and three females (Table 73.3). Of the patients for whom age data for malignancies are available, 12 patients were in their second decade, 14 in the third, 8 in the fourth, 5 in the fifth, 2 in the sixth, 2 in the seventh, and 2 in the eighth. Only four of the patients with malignancies were male (8%), and three were in their fifth to seventh decade. Thus the approximate incidence (8%) of males with malignancies is roughly proportional to their incidence (9.7%) in the overall tumor population. Nevertheless, the younger age of recognition of malignancy in females is of interest: 29 years versus 53 years.

At the time of reporting, only three (7.5%) of the patients with malignancies, all females, had died of their disease; three others died of unrelated causes, one known to have residual cancer. Of the three deaths from cancer, each patient had peritoneal dissemination at the time of diagnosis.

There are few data regarding the growth rate of the tumors. Kingsnorth et al. (79) described the CT identification of a 20-cm tumor in a 14-year-old Chinese girl. No treatment of the mass in the head of the pancreas was permitted. Five years later, she became jaundiced. No change in CT measurement was detected. Resection then revealed invasion of the capsule and the local lymphatics, without recognizable metastases. Professor Kingsnorth reports that the patient remains well 4 years after operation. Yamaguchi et al. (90) noted no change in the CT size and

**TABLE 73.1. The Patient and the Tumor: Clinical Observations**

| | | | |
|---|---|---|---|
| Gender | | | |
| Females | 318 (90.3%) | | |
| Males | 34 (9.7%) | | |
| Total | 352 | | |
| Age | ($n$ = 338) | | |
| Mean | 25.3 years | | |
| Span | 2-81 years | | |
| | Benign | Malignant | |
| Females | 273 (90%) | 45 (92%) | |
| Males | 30 (10%) | 4 (8%) | |
| Total Incidence | 303 (86%) | 49 (14%) | One cancer patient of unstated age |
| Malignancies | | | |
| | Mean Age ($n$ = 45) | Range | |
| Female ($n$ = 45) | 29 years | 10–77 years | |
| Male ($n$ = 4) | 53 years | 43–65 years | |
| Benign Tumors | | | |
| Gender | | | |
| Female ($n$ = 273) | 23.8 years | 2–81 years | |
| Male | 25.4 years | 14–55 years | |
| Tumor Size | | | |
| Maximum diameter ($n$ = 316) | 10.8 cm | (range, 2.0–25 cm) | |
| Site of Tumor | Number | | |
| ($n$ = 278) | | | |
| Head | 94 | | |
| Head and body | 10 | | |
| Body and tail | 58 | | |
| Body | 39 | | |
| Tail | 72 | | |
| Ectopic | 3 | | |
| Multicentric | 1 or 2 | | |
| Total | 278 | | |
| Gross appearance of Tumor ($n$ = 307) | Number | Percentage | |
| Cystic or cystic and solid | 290 | (94.5%) | |
| Solid | 17 | (5.5%) | |

Modified from Mao C, Guvendi M, Domenico DR, Kim K, Thomford NR, Howard JM. Papillary cystic and solid tumors of the pancreas. A pancreatic embryonic tumor? Studies of 3 cases and cumulative review of the world's literature. Surgery 1995; 118:821–828. With permission.

shape of a tumor in a 51-year-old female over a 5-year span. Curative resection was subsequently achieved.

Zinner et al. (63) noted local invasion of adjacent structures (duodenum, splenic vessels, portal vein) in four of six patients, aged 16–24 years, without evidence of metastases; however, a fifth patient with local invasion had an hepatic metastasis. Ohtomo et al. (93) described a 73-year-old female with a history of a mass, apparently in the pancreas, with calcification of the tumor noted on a flat plate 50 years before the diagnosis, at age 73, of a PCSTP with 5 metastases in the right lobe of the liver.

**TABLE 73.2. Differential Diagnosis of PCSTP, Pancreatoblastoma, and Oncocytic Tumors of the Pancreas**

| | PCSTP | Pancreatoblastoma | Oncocytic Tumor |
|---|---|---|---|
| Reported incidence | More frequent 352 cases | Rare<br>Approx. 35 cases | Rare<br>Fewer than 10 cases |
| Age (mean) | 2–81 years (25.3 years) | 3 weeks to 8 years (4.3 years) | 40–73 years (56.8 years) |
| Sex | Females predominate (90%) | Male babies predominate | — |
| α-Fetoprotein level | Normal | Elevated | Normal |
| Malignancy grade | Low | Moderate | Moderate |
| Histologic characteristics | Papillary structures, cystic changes | Organoid structure | Oncocytes |

Modified from Mao C, Guvendi M, Domenico DR, Kim K, Thomford NR, Howard JM. Papillary cystic and solid tumors of the pancreas. A pancreatic embryonic tumor? Studies of 3 cases and cumulative review of the world's literature. Surgery 1995; 118:821–828. With permission.

**TABLE 73.3. Malignant PCSTP**

| Case No. | Reference | Gender | Age | Site | Diameter (cm) | Invasion/Metastases | Treatment/Operation | Follow-up (years, months) |
|---|---|---|---|---|---|---|---|---|
| 1. | Balercia (95) 1995 Zamboni (108) 1993 | F | 23 | H | 12 | Pancreas & vein | Whipple | Alive and well (3,11)[a] |
| 2. | Yamanishi (103) 1995 | F | 77 | T | 7 | Lymph nodes | Distal pancreatectomy, lymph node dissection | Alive and well (5,0) |
| 3. | Sayer (107) 1994 | F | 50–70 | | 5–6 | Metastases to liver | | |
| 4. | Strauss (99) 1993 | F | 15 | B | 15 | Invasion of superior mesenteric vein, initially unresectable | 5-FU and cisplatinum for 6 months then Whipple resection | Alive and well (3,0) |
| 5. | Schneider (100) 1993 | 1 M<br>3 F | | 2 Head<br>2 Tail | | All 4 tumors "curativey" resected | | 1-Alive and well (6,0)<br>1-Alive and well (2,6)<br>1-Died without tumor (3,9)<br>1-Living with breast cancer |
| 6. | Ohtomo (93) 1992 | F | 73 | T | 12.5 | 5 Liver metastases (3 cm diameter) | Distal pancreatectomy, rt hepatic lobectomy | Living with liver metastases (4,8)[a] |
| 7. | Kamei (91) 1991 | F | 45 | T | 9 | Liver metastases 3 years after resection of primary tumor | Primary resection | Living with metastases (3,0) |
| 8. | Nishihara (86) 1993 | F | 21 | BT | 8.5 | Lymph node metastasis | Partial resection | Alive and well (1,1) |
| 9. | Nishihara (86) 1993 | F | 28 | H | 8.5 | Lymph node metastasis; peritoneal dissemination (colon) | Partial resection; secondary resection | Recurrence (10,10);<br>Alive and well (14,5) |
| 10. | Nishihara (86) 1993 | F | 36 | BT | 8.0 | Liver metastasis; peritoneal dissemination | Partial resection | Recurrence (4,9);<br>died of disease (10,11) |
| 11. | Nishihara (86) 1993 | F | 42 | HB | 9.5 | Invasion of vein | N/A | Alive and well (0,3) |
| 12. | Nishihara (86) 1993 | M | 65 | H | 18.0 | Invasion of duedenum and vein | N/A | Alive and well (1,1) |
| 13. | Jeng (84) 1993 | F | 28 | H | 10.0 | Invasion of portal vein | Whipple | Died of unrelated cause (5,6) |
| 14. | Jeng (84) 1993 | F | 19 | H | 15.0 | Invasion of portal vein and superior mesentery artery | Unresectable | Died of unrelated cause (6,11) |
| 15. | Jeng (84) 1993 | F | 22 | HB | 9.0 | Invasion of portal vein | Whipple | Alive and well (3,4) |
| 16. | Kingsnorth (79) 1992 | F | 19 | H | 20.0 | Lymph node metastasis and invasion of duodenum | Whipple | Alive and well (4,0)[a] |
| 17. | Jaksic (78) 1992 | F | 12 | T | 10.0 | Lymph node and peritoneal dissemination (pelvic) | Distal pancreatectomy | Alive and well (5,0) |
| 18. | Jaksic (78) 1992 | F | 10 | T | 14.0 | Invasion | Distal pancreatectomy | Alive and well (5,0) |
| 19. | Stommer (68) 1991 | F | 18 | H | 5.0 | Lymph node metastasis and liver metastasis | Whipple | Alive with liver metastasis (3,0) |
| 20. | Stommer (68) 1991 | F | 20 | T | 8.0 | Invasion of spleen | Distal pancreatectomy | Recurrence (1,0) |
| 21. | Sciafani (71) 1991 | F | 20 | T | 8.0 | Liver metastasis | Unresectable | Alive with tumor (1,10) |
| 22. | Chu (74) 1991 | M | 51 | T | 13.0<br>9.0 | Lesser sac and inguinal "metastasis" | Distal pancreatectomy and tumor resection | Alive (23 days) |
| 23. | Tsunoda (75) 1991 | M | 43 | H | 4.5 | Pancreatic parenchyma and veins invaded | Whipple | Alive (1,10) |
| 24. | Zinner (63) 1990 | F | 33 | H | 15.0 | Liver metastasis | Unresectable | Alive with tumor[a] |
| 25. | Zinner (63) 1990 | F | 24 | BT | 11.0 | Invasion of spleen | Distal pancreatectomy | Alive and well (7.0) |

**TABLE 73.3. Malignant PCSTP—*continued***

| Case No. | Reference | Gender | Age | Site | Diameter (cm) | Invasion/Metastases | Treatment/Operation | Follow-up (years, months) |
|---|---|---|---|---|---|---|---|---|
| 26. | Zinner (63) 1990 | F | 21 | H | 7.0 | Invasion of duodenum | Whipple | Alive and well (12,0) |
| 27. | Zinner (63) 1990 | F | 21 | B | 20.0 | Invasion of portal vein | Distal pancreatectomy | Alive and well (4,0) |
| 28. | Zinner (63) 1990 | F | 16 | H | 12.0 | Invasion portal vein | Total pancreatectomy | Alive and well (7,0) |
| 29. | Matsunou and Konishi (56) 1990 | F | 60 | BT | 7.0 | Liver metastasis and peritoneal dissemination | Distal pancreatectomy | Died of disease (6,0) |
| 30. | Matsunou and Konishi (56) 1990 | F | 47 | BT | 15.0 | Invasion (portal vein, hepatic artery) and peritoneal dissemination | Unresectable | Died of disease (3,11) |
| 31. | Cappellari (55) 1990 | F | 32 | HB | 20.0 | Liver metastasis and peritoneal dissemination | Unresectable | Alive with tumor (4,0) |
| 32. | Hernandez-Maldonodo (51) 1989 | F | 22 | T | 16.0 | Peritoneal dissemination (cul-de-sac) | Distal pancreatectomy | Alive and well (1,0) |
| 33. | Heitz (50) 1989 | F | 21 | T | 6.0 | Invasion of spleen | Distal pancreatectomy | Alive and well (2,0) |
| 34. | Todani (47) 1988 | F | 12 | H | 7.0 | Peritoneal dissemination | Resection | Recurrence (9,2)<br>Alive and well[a] (1,5) |
| 35. | Chol (45) 1988 | N/A | N/A | BT | N/A | Liver metastasis, peritoneal dissemination, invasion | Resection | Alive and well[a] |
| 36. | Stachura (44) 1988 | F | 39 | BT | 14.0 | Retroperitoneal and vascular metastasis | Unresectable | Alive with tumor (4,0)[a] |
| 37. | Matsuda (37) 1987 | F | 42 | H | 8.0 | Invasion of portal vein and liver metastasis | Chemoembolization | Alive with tumor (5,0) |
| 38. | Lieber (39) 1987 | F | 33 | B | 5.0 | Invasion of stomach | Resection | Recurrence (2,0)<br>Alive with tumor (3,0) |
| 39. | Persson (33) 1986 | F | 16 | BT | 8.0 | Invasion of spleen | Distal pancreatectomy | Alive and well (0,6) |
| 40. | Rustin (32) 1986 | F | 31 | T | 9.5 | Liver metastasis | Resection | Alive and well (2,0) |
| 41. | Kaufman (31) 1986 | F | 19 | BT | 10.0 | Subcutaneous tissue | Distal pancreatectomy; marsupialization | Alive and well (5,6) |
| 42. | Warren (23) 1985 | F | 30 | T | 14.0 | Liver metastases | Distal pancreatectomy | Alive and well (1,8) |
| 43. | Fried (24) 1985 | F | 18 | HB | 12.0 | Invasion of portal vein and hepatic artery | Unresectable; radiation therapy | Alive and well (3,0) |
| 44. | Dales (11) 1983 | F | 33 | B | 8.0 | Invasion of portal vein | Total pancreatectomy; radiation therapy | Alive and well[a] |
| 45. | Sanfey (10) 1982 | F | 21 | H | 12.0 | Superior mesenteric artery | Total pancreatectomy | Alive and well (0,7) |
| 46. | Schlosnagle and Campbell (8) 1981 | F | 21 | H | 8.0 | Invasion of duodenum | Whipple | Alive and well[a] |
| 47. | Benjamin and Wright (6) 1980 | F | 16 | T | 11.0 | Omental metastases | Resection | Alive and well (0,2) |

Modified from Mao C, Guvendi M, Domenico DR, Kim K, Thomford NR, Howard JM. Papillary cystic and solid tumors of the pancreas. A pancreatic embryonic tumor? Studies of 3 cases and cumulative review of the world's literature. Surgery 1995; 118:821–828. With permission.

[a]Personal communication.

It has been proposed that growth within a nonexpandable capsule may result in ischemic necrosis of the tumor. However, as pointed out by Mao et al. (110), the extent of necrosis of the tumor is not always proportional to the size of the tumor; a 2-cm diameter tumor may have undergone cystic changes (23), and large tumors sometimes remain essentially solid (24, 44). PCSTP appears at present to be, in most instances, a benign tumor with a tendency to local invasion of the capsule. In an occasional patient with capsular invasion, obvious metastases may develop, and the primary or metastatic tumors may continue to grow. Phillips et al. (92) described focal invasion of the tumor capsule in a 17-year-old female as indicating the tumor's malignant potential. Pettinato et al. (80) studied 20 patients with what appeared to be a benign tumor and found invasion of the capsule in over 60%. Others concurred (4, 8, 9, 15, 47, 87). Kamei et al. (91) noted capsular invasion in a primary tumor associated with hepatic metastases.

The present knowledge of PCSTP is reminiscent of that of islet cell tumors in the 1940s, when Frantz (114) described insulinomas as benign, malignant (with metastases), or histologically malignant but clinically benign. The third group were designated "suspiciously malignant." By definition, in the last group, no metastases were present and the localized tumor showed either invasion of the capsule or blood vessel, local organ invasion, or cellular anaplasia with numerous mitoses. Subsequent follow up of this group of "suspiciously malignant" islet cell tumors showed that metastases seldom, if ever, developed, and the patients remained well after tumor resection. Perhaps, the PCSTP with local invasion or some subset without evidence of metastasis should, for the present, be considered "suspiciously malignant," as our knowledge of the natural history of this tumor evolves. The fact that approximately one of seven (14%) PCSTPs has been malignant at the time of diagnosis leads to the strong suspicion that the others should be considered potentially premalignant (110).

## Malignant Metastasizing Potential

Nishihara et al. (86) studied 3 metastasizing PCSTPs, 2 invasive but nonmetastasizing PCSTPs, and 17 noninvasive PCSTPs; the 5 metastasizing or invasive tumors showed venous invasion. They concluded that venous invasion, nuclear grade, and prominent necrobiotic nests are useful parameters for detecting the malignancy or malignant potential of these tumors. In a related report, they noted that the mitotic rate was considered an important parameter (97) and that the nuclei in tumors that metastasized were significantly larger than in the others, and suggested that nuclear size might also be useful for estimating the tumor's potential for metastasis.

Kamei et al. (91) compared one malignant with two benign PCSTPs and noted the prominent cellular atypia and frequent mitotic figures in the former. In addition, the proliferative activity (P1) was higher in the malignant tumor.

Matsunou et al. (56) studied four solid-type PCSTPs that were invading the adjacent pancreas (in patients aged 39–51 years) and noted pleomorphic atypism in three of them, in contrast to five nonmalignant tumors. None of the invasive tumors had metastasized, nor did any recur within 3–4 years after resection.

## Information from Flow Cytometry

Numerous tumors have been studied by flow cytometry. Pettinato et al. (80) in an intensive study of nonmalignant PCSTP, found eight tumors to be diploid with low-to-moderate proliferative activity, indicated by S-phase fraction values of 7% and 14%. One tumor was hyperdiploid with a DNA index of 1.1. Nishikara et al. (86) found one metastasizing tumor to be aneuploid and eight nonmetastasizing tumors to be diploid. Kamei et al. (91) found two benign tumors to be diploid, with mitotic indices of zero; proliferative indices of 8 and 13, respectively; and a DNA index of 1.0 in each. The third tumor, involving hepatic metastases, was aneuploid, with a mitotic index of 3–4, a proliferative index of 25, and a DNA index of 1.65. Cellular atypia and mitotic figures were prominent in the aneuploid malignant tumor but not in the benign ones.

## Progesterone/Estrogen Receptors

Because of the high female sex dominance in this tumor and the possible younger age of cancer development in females, numerous tumors have been assayed for estrogen and progesterone receptors. Mao et al. (110) reviewed reports of 46 tumors; only 2 were positive for estrogen receptors, and 9 for progesterone receptors. Since that review, Zamboni et al. (95) studied the tumors of 10 patients; each tumor showed progesterone reactivity, and none was estrogen-receptor positive. Eight of the patients were young women, one was a postmenopausal woman, and the tenth was a young boy. In one tumor, two types of cell populations were observed. The more anaplastic invasive-type cell was progesterone negative; the more typical cell was progesterone positive. The authors postulated that a possible pathogenetic role of progesterone in this tumor is independent of the patient's sex and age. Balercia et al. (108) updated this study to 14 patients. Others found one of seven tumors to be estrogen-receptor positive (98). Thus, the existence of sex hormone tumor receptors is currently controversial, and the data do not provide a basis for estimating a potential adjuvant role for Nolvadex therapy.

## Ectopic and Multicentric Tumors

Klöppel et al. (73) reported a 25-year-old male with an asymptomatic mass of 7–8 cm in diameter. A retroperitoneal PCSTP was found beneath the transverse colon and the head of the pancreas. It was not attached to the pancreas or any other organ and was easily removed. The patient was well 24 months following resection. The authors noted ductal structures in the fibrous capsule of the tumor, raising the question of the possible origin of the tumor from "ectopic pancreas."

Earlier, Kim et al. (111) described two ectopic, primary, benign PCSTPs within the liver. The patient, a 41-year-old female had a 30-cm tumor in the right lobe of her liver and a 5.5-cm tumor in the left lobe. The larger tumor had been noted 4 years earlier, but the patient declined treatment. A right hepatic lobectomy and resection of the tumor of the left lobe were subsequently performed. Each was considered a nonmalignant PCSTP. No tumor was found in the pancreas. The patient was well 13 months postresection. Chu et al. (74) described a large PCSTP in the tail of the pancreas along the lesser curvature of the pancreas and in the bilateral inguinal areas. No description of any metastases to the lymph nodes nor to the liver was given. Whether these represented ectopia or metastases is uncertain. Orlando et al. (70) reported a 26-year-old female in her first trimester of pregnancy with obstructive jaundice and a large tumor of the head of the pancreas. The pregnancy was therapeutically terminated. Total pancreatectomy confirmed a 9-cm diameter PCSTP of the head of the pancreas. In addition, a more solid (2.8-cm diameter) PCSTP was found in the tail of the pancreas. The tumors were separate and distinct; each was encapsulated. The patient was well 9 months after resection. As noted above, the earlier report of Kim et al. (111) described two synchronous PCSTPs ectopic in the liver.

## Rupture

Sanchez et al. (62) reported a 13-year-old girl struck in her left side while wrestling at a party. Hemoperitoneum resulted. Hemorrhagic hypotension resulted in emergency resection of a ruptured PCSTP of the tail of the pancreas. She was well 4 years later. Mao et al. (110) (1995) noted that in their collected series, eight (2.7%) patients had undergone rupture of the tumor with resultant hemoperitoneum: two from trauma (39, 62), two from malignancy (68, 71), and four others (15, 47, 51, 84). As they pointed out, rupture is unusual for a slowly growing tumor.

## Treatment

The treatment of PCSTP is resection, and the long-term results are excellent. In the absence of overt malignancy, resection has been curative. Recurrence or metastasis after resection of the "benign" tumor is so rare that it should be reported. The body of information is incomplete, however, suggesting that such patients should be followed closely by clinical and CT examinations for an indefinite period of time.

The limited experience with the treatment of the malignant PCSTP suggests that it too, along with its metastases, deserves an aggressive approach by resection. Resection of invaded vessels, such as the portal vein, should be considered, possibly even in the presence of a resectable metastasis. Ohtomo et al. (93) described resection of the tumor in the tail of the pancreas along with a right hepatic lobectomy in a 73-year-old female. Five metastases, two being 3 cm in diameter, were present in the resected lobe. Ohtomo (personal communication) writes that the patient is living with recurrent hepatic metastases 4 years and 8 months after operation. These represent parameters not yet fully tested. Since few surgeons will have the opportunity to treat a significant series of such patients, information should be pooled as it accumulates.

Resection of most of these tumors is straightforward. Although previously described as tending to occur on the left side of the pancreas, 94 tumors (one-third) have occurred in the head. Resection of the head of the pancreas (Whipple resection) or the left side of the pancreas is performed as with other tumors. Since the tumor may or may not invade the adjacent pancreas or adjacent organs, resection with a 2-cm margin would appear appropriate. For the same reason, in resecting the tail of the pancreas, most surgeons have included splenectomy. Clear margins need to be obtained, with histologic verification during operation. The question has been raised whether radical resection (e.g., pancreatoduodenectomy) for a tumor in the head of the pancreas is justified in children. Published experience does not provide a complete basis for decision. Nevertheless, one in seven PCSTPs is malignant, and of the malignancies, one in four was found in patients below the age of 20 years. In safe hands, complete resection seems essential.

Should regional lymphadenectomy be performed in the absence of recognized nodal involvement? The vast majority of these tumors do not justify prophylactic nodal dissection, as most behave as benign tumors "after resection." Local recurrence following resection has been quite infrequent. Todani et al. (47) described resection of a 7-cm diameter, well-encapsulated tumor in a 12-year-old girl. No invasion or metastasis was found. Nine years later she developed a "fist-sized" recurrence in the transverse mesocolon. Following its resection, she was well, 1 year and 5 months later. In their 1988 review they reported three previous patients with recurrence of tumors that had not originally been considered malignant (12, 18, 115). Kamei, et al. described hepatic metastases 3 years after primary resection. In such cases, recurrence may be related to inadequate local resection or vascular metastasis, rather than metastasis to lymph nodes. Total pancreatectomy, however, would not appear justifiable except under rare and unforeseen circumstances. If the nature of the tumor is not recognized either preoperatively or at operation, a decision about whether to biopsy must be made before resection. In the three cases reported by the writers resection was performed without biopsy. An experienced pancreatic surgeon or pathologist may be able to tentatively diagnose the tumor by gross appearance in the operating room, especially on cross-section. Biopsy prior to resection by an experienced surgeon may not be necessary. However, an immediate histologic study of the resected specimen should be obtained, and if positive for malignancy, a radical resection should be performed. Resection of regional lymph nodes and any involved large vessels should be carefully considered. Because of multiple areas of necrosis in these tumors and because of their potential for malignancy, the entire resected tumor needs careful histologic scrutiny.

No chronic cyst of the pancreas should be drained externally or internally without histologic study of its wall. As with all types of malignant, premalignant, or true congenital cysts of the pancreas, the occasional surgeon has initially failed to recognize the nature of the lesion. Zinner et al. (63) reported a female patient who, at age 19 years, had undergone a drainage procedure for a "pancreatic pseudocyst." Another "pseudocyst" was diagnosed when she was 24. At age 30, she bled into a "pseudocyst." At no time had a biopsy been taken. At age 33 years, the authors found an unresectable PCSTP with a 15-cm mass in the head of the pancreas and multiple metastases to the liver. Kuo et al. (16) reported a 15-cm diameter PCSTP in a 2-year-old female that was biopsied but anastomosed to the jejunum. The patient was living and "well" 34 months later. Sclafani et al. (71) reported a 15-year-old boy who had previously undergone a cytogastrostomy with a presumptive diagnosis of traumatic pseudocyst; however, a biopsy had been taken, which permitted an uneventful resection of the tumor 4 months later.

## Adjuvant Therapy

The tumors are so rare and the results of resection have been so good that few investigators have evaluated adjuvant therapy. Fried et al. (24) described an 18-year-old female who had a PCSTP invading the portal vein, which was considered unresectable. Exploration was followed 4 weeks later by 4000 cGY in 20 fractions over 6 weeks. Two years later, CT scanning revealed marked shrinkage of the tumor without evidence of hepatic metastasis. The patient was living and asymptomatic 3 years after the operation. Cappellari et al. (55) reported a 34-year-old female given 4000 cGY to a PCSTP and its hepatic metastases. Resection was not performed. At age 36, a rupture of the hepatic metastasis led to resection of the metastasis. This was followed by $\alpha$-interferon therapy. The patient felt better 15 months later. Zinner et al. (63) also reported shrinkage of a PCSTP after radiotherapy.

Strauss et al. (99) reported a 15-year-old female with a 15-cm PCSTP, unresectable because of invasion of the superior mesenteric vein. After treatment with *cis*-platinum and 5-fluorouracil for 6 months, reoperation permitted resection of the residual 3.5-cm tumor.

Even if definitive resection seems impossible or if the patient declines therapy, the present available information suggests the possibility of a significant period of life and relative well being, even if no therapy is rendered. Adjuvant therapy, as a clinical investigation under such circumstances, would seem worthwhile.

## Results

When Compagno and Oertal (3) reviewed 52 patients in 1979, they noted that only a single patient was known to have died of metastatic disease. Three patients with malignant PCSTP survived more than 10 years after their first operation; 11 survived more than 5 years (Table 73.3). Of the 50 patients in Table 73.3, 23 had metastases: hepatic and or peritoneal dissemination in 20; lymph nodes in 6; and in 26, the tumor had directly invaded adjacent organs, including the portal or other large vein in 13 and large arteries in 4. Eight patients with metastases or unresectable primary cancers lived more than 5 years, one of whom lived 14 years. Others did well following resection of recurrent cancers.

Although unanticipated recurrence has seldom been reported, accumulated experience is limited, so follow-up for an indefinite period would seem appropriate.

The authors acknowledge an earlier review with their colleagues (110) that provided a basis for this review of worldwide experience. Patient 3 is included by courtesy of Dr. Neil R. Thomford.

## REFERENCES

1. Frantz VK. Tumors of the pancreas. In: Atlas of tumor pathology, sec. VII, fasc. 27 and 28. Washington, DC: Armed Forces Institute of Pathology, 1959.
2. Klöppel G, Morohoshi T, John HD, et al. Solid and cystic acinar cell tumor of the pancreas. Virchows Arch 1981;392:171–183.
3. Compagno J, Oertel JE, Kremzar M. Solid and papillary epithelial neoplasm of the pancreas, probably of small duct origin: a clinicopathologic study of 52 cases. Lab Invest 1979;40:248–249.
4. Borr PJ, Swanson MR. Papillary-cystic neoplasm of the pancreas. Am J Surg Pathol 1979;3(1):69.
5. Cubilla AL, Fitzgerald PJ. Classification of pancreatic cancer (nonendocrine). Mayo Clin Proc 1979;54:449–458.
6. Benjamin E, Wright DH. Adenocarcinoma of the pancreas of childhood: a report of two cases. Histopathology 1980;4:87–104.
7. Alm P, Jonsson PE, Karp W, Lindberg LG, et al. A case of papillary-cystic epithelial neoplasm of the pancreas. Acta Pathol Microbiol Scand 1981;89:125–132.
8. Schlosnagle DC, Campbell WG. The papillary and solid neoplasm of the pancreas: a report of two cases with electron microscopy, one containing neurosecretory granules. Cancer 1981;47:2603–2610.
9. Klöppel G, Morohoshi T, John HD, et al. Solid and cystic acinar cell tumour of the pancreas. Virchows Arch 1981;392:171–183.
10. Sanfey H, Mendelsohn C, Cameron JL. Solid and papillary neoplasm of the pancreas: a potentially curable surgical lesion. Ann Surg 1983;197:272–275.
11. Dales RL, Garcia JC, Davies RS. Papillary-cystic carcinoma of the pancreas J Surg Oncol 1983;22:115–117.
12. Lack EE, Levey R, Cassady, Vawter GF. Tumors of the exocrine pancreas in children and adolescents—a clinical and pathologic study of eight cases. Am J Surg Pathol 1983;7:319–327.
13. Bondeson L, Bondeson AG, Genell S, et al. Aspiration cytology of a rare solid and papillary epithelial neoplasm of the pancreas. Acta Cytol 1984;28:605.
14. Balthazar EJ, Subramanyam BR, Lefleur RS, Barone CM. Solid and papillary epithelial neoplasm of the pancreas. Radiology 1984; 150:39–40.
15. Bombi JA, Milla A, Badal JM, et al. A papillary-cystic neoplasm of the pancreas. Cancer 1984;54:780–784.
16. Kuo TT, Su IJ, Chien CH. Solid and papillary neoplasm of the pancreas: report of three cases from Taiwan. Cancer 1984;54: 1469–1474.
17. Morrison DM, Jewell LD, McCaughey WTE, et al. Papillary cystic tumor of the pancreas. Arch Pathol Lab Med 1984;108:723–727.
18. Cubilla AL, Fitzgerald PJ. Tumors of the exocrine pancreas. In: Atlas of tumor pathology, ser. 2, fasc. 19. Washington, DC: Armed Forces Institute of Pathology, 1984;201–207.
19. Yano H, Komura JI, Tetsuo T, et al. Papillary and solid neoplasm of the pancreas in a child. Jpn J Pediatr Surg 1985;17:1079–1087.
20. Kubo T, Hirose T, Takanashi R, et al. A case of solid and cystic tumor of the pancreas. Jpn J Cancer Clin 1985;31:882–888.
21. Learmouth GM, Price SK, Visser AE, Emms M. Papillary and cystic neoplasm of the pancreas—an acinar cell tumour? Histopathology 1985;9:63–79.
22. Duff P, Greene VP. Pregnancy complicated by solid-papillary epithelial tumor of the pancreas, pulmonary embolism, and pulmonary embolectomy. Am J Obstet Gynecol 1985;152: 80–81.
23. Warren RB. Papillary cystic tumor of the pancreas (Letter). Arch Pathol Lab Med 1985;109:706.
24. Fried P, Cooper J, Balthazar E, et al. A role for radiotherapy in the treatment of solid and papillary neoplasms of the pancreas. Cancer 1985;56:2783–2785.
25. Kim SY, Lim JH, Lee JD. Papillary carcinoma of the pancreas: findings of US and CT. Radiology 1985;154:338.
26. Friedman A, Lichtenstein JE, Fishman EK, et al. Solid and papillary epithelial neoplasm of the pancreas. Radiology 1985;154: 333–337.
27. Murayama T, Kataoka H, Kohno T. An operated case of solid and cystic acinar cell tumor of the pancreas in a 12-year-old boy (in Japanese). Trans Soc Pathol Jpn 1985;74:377–378.
28. Shirayi F, Nakamula S, Takada K, Kina I. Solid and cystic acinar cell tumor of the pancreas: 2 case reports. J Soc Pathol Jpn 1985;74:378.
29. Komorn HJ, Zirkin RM, Nathan LE. Papillary cystic neoplasm of the pancreas: report of two cases of a surgically curable tumor. Surgery 1986;99:110–113.
30. Foote A, Simpson JS, Steward RJ, Wakefield JSJ, et al. Diagnosis of the rare solid and papillary epithelial neoplasm of the pancreas by fine needle aspiration cytology: light and electron microscopic study of a case. Acta Cytol 1986;30:519–522.
31. Kaufman S, Reddick RL, Stiegel M, et al. Papillary cystic neoplasm of the pancreas: a curable pancreatic tumor. World J Surg 1986;10:851–859.
32. Rustin RB, Broughan TA, Hermann RE, et al. Papillary cystic epithelial neoplasms of the pancreas. Arch Surg 1986;121:1073–1076.
33. Persson M, Bisgaard, Nielsen BB, et al. Solid and papillary epithelial neoplasm of the pancreas presenting as a traumatic cyst: case report. Acta Chir Scand 1986;152:223–226.
34. Wrba F, Chott A, Ludvik B, et al. Brief report: solid and cystic tumour of the pancreas; a hormonal-dependent neoplasm? Histopathology 1988,12.330–340.
35. Morohoshi T, Kanda M, Horie A, et al. Immunocytochemical markers of uncommon pancreatic tumors. Cancer 1987;59: 739–747.
36. Kamisawa T, Fukayama M, Koike M, et al. So-called "papillary and cystic neoplasm of the pancreas": an immunohistochemical and ultrastructural study. Acta Pathol Jpn 1987;37:785–794.
37. Matsuda Y, Imai Y, Kawata S, et al. Case report: papillary cystic neoplasm of the pancreas with multiple hepatic metastases: a case report. Gastroenterol Jpn 1987;22:379–384.
38. Farman J, Chen CK, Schulze G, Teitcher J. Solid and papillary epithelial pancreatic neoplasm: an unusual tumor. Gastrointest Radiol 1987;12:31–34.
39. Lieber MR, Lack EE, Roberts JR, et al. Solid and papillary epithelial neoplasm of the pancreas: an ultrastructural and immunocytochemical study of six cases. Am J Surg Pathol 1987;11:85–93.
40. Miettinen M, Partanen S, Fraki O, Kivilaakso E. Papillary cystic tumor of the pancreas. An analysis of cellular differentiation by electron microscopy and immunohistochemistry. Am J Surg Pathol 1987;11:855–865.
41. Ladanyi M, Mulay S, Arseneau J, Bettez P. Estrogen and progesterone receptor determination in the papillary cystic neoplasm of the pancreas. Cancer 1987;60:1604–1611.
42. Sheen IS, Chang-Chien CS, Wu CS. Solid and papillary neoplasm of the pancreas: a report of an unusual pattern of calcification. Am J Gastroenterol 1988;83:789–791.
43. Pezzi CM, Schuerch C, Erlandson RA, Deitrick J. Papillary-cystic neoplasm of the pancreas. J Surg Oncol 1988;37:278–285.
44. Stachura J, Popiela T, Pietron M, et al. Cytology of solid and papillary epithelial neoplasms of the pancreas: a case report. Diagn Cytopathol 1988;4:339–341.
45. Choi BI, Kim KW, Han MC, et al. Solid and papillary epithelial neoplasms of the pancreas: CT findings. Radiology 1988;166: 413–416.
46. Yagihashi S, Sato I, Kaimori M, et al. Papillary and cystic tumor of the pancreas: two cases indistinguishable from islet cell tumor. Cancer 1988;61:1241–1247.
47. Todani T, Shimada K, Watanabe Y, et al. Frantz's tumor: a papillary and cystic tumor of the pancreas in girls. J Pediatr Surg 1988;23:116–121.
48. Hata Y, Sasaki F, Alam S, et al. Solid and cystic tumor of the pancreas in a child: case report and review of the literature. Pediatr Surg Int 1989;4:303–305.
49. Yamaguchi K, Miyagahara T, Tsuneyoshi M. Papillary cystic tumor of the pancreas: an immunohistochemical and ultrastructural study of 14 patients. Jpn J Clin Oncol 1989;19:102–111.
50. Heitz PU, Stolte M, Kloeppel G, et al. Large pancreatic tumor in a young woman. Ultrastruct Pathol 1989;13:589–592.
51. Hernandez-Maldonodo II, Rodreguez-Bigas MA, Gonzalez De Pesanta A, et al. Papillary cystic neoplasm of the pancreas: a

report of a case presenting with carcinomatosis. Am Surg 1989;55:552–559.
52. Carbone A, Ranelletti FO, Rinelli A, et al. Type II estrogen receptors in the papillary cystic tumor of the pancreas. Am J Clin Pathol 1989;92:572–576.
53. Nagai H, Mori T, Wada Y, et al. Solid and cystic tumor of the pancreas (in Japanese). Geka (Surgery) 1989;51:364–373.
54. Jayaram G, Chaturvedi KU, Jindal RK, et al. Papillary cystic neoplasm of the pancreas: report of a case diagnosed by fine needle aspiration cytology. Acta Cytol 1990;34:429–433.
55. Cappellari JO, Geisinger KR, Albertson DA, et al. Malignant papillary cystic tumor of the pancreas. Cancer 1990;66:193–198.
56. Matsunou H, Konishi F. Papillary-cystic neoplasm of the pancreas: a clinicopathologic study concerning the tumor aging and malignancy of nine cases. Cancer 1990;65:283–291.
57. Carter T, Caputo C, O'Hara B. Papillary-cystic tumor of the pancreas: a curable neoplasm. Hosp Physician 1990;26:13–15.
58. Doberstien C, Kirchner R, Gordon L, et al. Cystic neoplasms of the pancreas. Mt Sinai J Med 1990;57:102–105.
59. Kalloo AN, Nauta RJ, Benjamin SB. Solid and papillary epithelial neoplasm of the pancreas: clinical findings of a rare tumor. J Clin Gastroenterol 1990;12:325–328.
60. Katz LBK, Ehya H. Aspiration cytology of papillary cystic neoplasm of the pancreas. Am J Clin Pathol 1990;94:328–333.
61. Von Herbay A, Sieg B, Otto HF. Case report: solid-cystic tumour of the pancreas—an endocrine neoplasm? Virchows Arch (A) 1990;416:535–538.
62. Sanchez JA, Newman KD, Eichelberger MR, Nauta RJ. The papillary-cystic neoplasm of the pancreas. Arch Surg 1990;125: 1502–1505.
63. Zinner MJ, Shurbaji MS, Cameron JL. Solid and papillary epithelial neoplasms of the pancreas. Surgery 1990;108:475–480.
64. Warshaw AL, Compton CC, Lewandrowski K, et al. Cystic tumors of the pancreas: new clinical, radiologic and pathologic observations in 67 patients. Ann Surg 1990;212:432–445.
65. Ohahima A, Yamaguchi K, Koi R, Enjoji M. Incipient papillary cystic tumor of the pancreas. Am J Gastroenterol 1990;85:1437–1438.
66. Matsunou H, Konishi F, Yamamichi N, et al. Solid, infiltrating variety of papillary cystic neoplasm of the pancreas. Cancer 1990;65:2747–2757.
67. Eason JD, Eason JH, George SM, et al. Solid and papillary epithelial neoplasm of the pancreas. South Med J 1991;84:247–249.
68. Stommer P, Kraus J, Stolte M, Giedl J. Solid and cystic pancreatic tumors: clinical, histochemical and electron microscopic features in ten cases. Cancer 1991;67:1635–1641.
69. Mendonca ME, Bivar-Weinholtz J, Soares J. Fine needle aspiration cytology of a solid and papillary epithelial neoplasm of the pancreas. Acta Cytol 1991;35:258–260.
70. Orlando CA, Bowman RL, Loose JH. Multicentric papillary-cystic neoplasm of the pancreas. Arch Pathol Lab Med 1991;115: 958–960.
71. Sclafani LM, Reuter VE, Coit DG, Brennan MF. The malignant nature of papillary and cystic neoplasm of the pancreas. Cancer 1990;68:153–158.
72. Rouquette I, Parent M, Lecomte-Houte M, et al. A papillary and cystic tumor of the pancreas: case report with histological, immunochemical and ultrastructural study (in French). Arch Anat Cytol Pathol 1990;39:38–41.
73. Klöppel G, Maurer R, Hofmann E, et al. Solid-cystic (papillary-cystic) tumours within and outside the pancreas in men; report of two patients. Virchows Arch (A) 1991;418:179–183.
74. Chu HW, Lin W, Chang SM. Malignant papillary cystic tumor of the pancreas: report of a case and review of the literature. China Med J (Taipei) 1991;47:139–144.
75. Tsunoda T, Eto T, Tsurifune T, et al. Solid and cystic tumor of the pancreas in an adult male. Acta Pathol Jpn 1991;41:763–770.
76. Kakihara T, Fukuda T, Nemoto K, et al. Unusual pancreatic tumor resembling solid and cystic tumor with somatostatin production and aberrant crystalloid structures. Acta Pathol Jpn 1991;41: 629–635.
77. Wilson MB, Adams DB, Garen PD, Gansler TS. Aspiration cytologic, ultrastructural and DNA cytometric findings of solid and papillary tumor of the pancreas. Cancer 1992;69:2235–2243.
78. Jaksic T, Yaman M, Thorner P, et al. A 20-year review of pediatric pancreatic tumors. J Pediatr Surg 1992;27:1315–1317.
79. Kingsnorth AN, Galloway SW, Lewis-Jones, et al. Papillary cystic neoplasm of the pancreas: presentation and natural history in two cases. Gut 1992;33:421–423.
80. Pettinato G, Manivel JC, Ravett C, et al. Papillary cystic tumor of the pancreas: a clinicopathologic study of 20 cases with cytologic, immunohistochemical, ultrastructural, and flow cytometric observations, and a review of the literature. Am J Clin Pathol 1992;98:478–488.
81. Munoz NA, Takehara H, Komi N, Hirose T. Papillary and cystic tumor of the pancreas possibly concealed within a pseudocyst. Acta Paediatr Jpn 1992;34:316–323.
82. Tomioka T, Inoue K, Yamamoto T, et al. Solid and cystic tumor of the pancreas occurring without cyst formation in an adult male: case report. Int J Pancreatol 1993;14:195–200.
83. Ward HC, Leake J, Spitz I. Papillary cystic cancer of the pancreas: diagnostic difficulties. J Pediatr Surg 1993;28:89–91.
84. Jeng LBB, Chen MF, Tang RP. Solid and papillary neoplasm of the pancreas: emphasis on surgical treatment. Arch Surg 1993;128: 433–436.
85. Lee WY, Tzeng CC, Jin YT, et al. Papillary cystic tumor of the pancreas: a case indistinguishable from oncocytic carcinoma. Pancreas 1993;8:127–132.
86. Nishihara K, Nagoshi M, Tsuneyoshi M, et al. Papillary cystic tumors of the pancreas: assessment of their malignant potential. Cancer 1993;71:82–92.
87. Hamoudi AB, Misugi K, Grosfeld JL, Reiner CB. Papillary epithelial neoplasm of pancreas in a child: report of a case and electron microscopy. Cancer 1970;26:1126–1133.
88. Ohashi K, Nakajima Y, Hisangaga M, et al. A solid and papillary (solid-cystic) tumor of the pancreas occurring in a 36-year-old man: report of a case. Jpn J Surg 1993;23:551–555.
89. Ebisui S, Kawamoto K, Mitufuju S, et al. A case report of solid and cystic tumor (SCT) of the pancreas and literature review of cases of Japan (in Japanese). Gastroenterol Endosc 1990;32:1692–1701.
90. Yamaguchi K, Hirakata R, Kitamuri K. Papillary cystic neoplasm of the pancreas: radiological and pathological characteristics in 11 cases. Br J Surg 1990;77:1000–1003.
91. Kamei K, Funabiki T, Ochiai M, et al. Three cases of solid and cystic tumors of the pancreas. Analysis comparing the histopathological findings and DNA histograms. Int J Pancreatol 1991;10:269–278.
92. Phillips GWL, Chou ST, Mulhauser J. Papillary and cystic tumour of the pancreas: findings at computed tomography and ultrasound. Br J Radiol 1991;64:367–369.
93. Ohtomo K, Furui S, Onoae M, et al. Solid and papillary neoplasm of the pancreas: MR imaging and pathologic correlation. Radiology 1992;184:567–570.
94. Bapat KC, Pandet AA, Joshi AS, Vora IM. Aspiration cytology of a papillary cystic neoplasm of pancreas: a case report. Indian J Cancer 1992;29:100–103.
95. Zamboni G, Bonetti F, Scarpa A, et al. Expression of progesterone receptors in solid-cystic tumour of the pancreas: a clinicopathological and immunohistochemical study of ten cases (in Japanese). Virchows Arch (A) 1993;32:1692–1701.
96. Greenberg ML, Rennie Y, Grierson JM, et al. Solid and papillary epithelial tumour of the pancreas: cytological case study with ultrastructural and cytometric evaluation. Diagn Cytopathol 1993;541–546.
97. Nishihara K, Tsuneyoshi M. Papillary cystic tumours of the pancreas: an analysis by nuclear morphometry. Virchows Arch (A) 1993;422(3):211–217.
98. Paes de Lima A, Bellotti M, Elsner B, et al. Papillary and cystic tumors of the pancreas. Clinico-pathological cystopathological, immunohistochemical,and nuclear ploidy study (in Spanish). Medicina 1993;53:(6):481–486.
99. Strauss JF, Hirsch VJ, Rubey CN, et al. Resection of a solid and papillary epithelial neoplasm of the pancreas following treatment with *cis*-platinum and 5-fluorouracil: a case report. Med Pediatr Oncol 1993;21(5):365–367.
100. Schneider C, Reck T, Greskotter KR, et al. Cystic pancreatic tumors (in German). Langenbecks Arch Chir 1993;378(5): 281–287.
101. Brandeo C, Urrutia M, Gill del Real de Cano P, et al. Epithelial solid and papillary neoplasms of pancreas. Description of two cases. Rev Med Panama 1994;19:27–36.

102. Lunetta P, Piatti B, Ferrario D, et al. Cystic papillary tumors of the pancreas: 3 new cases (in Italian). Pathologica 1994;86:(2)211–216.
103. Yamanishi M, Miyata M, Kitagawa T, et al. Papillary cystic neoplasm (PCN) of the pancreas with lymph node metastasis: case report of a 77-year-old woman and a review of 198 reported cases. J Hepatobiliarypancreatic Surg 1994;4:413–418.
104. Ryley NG, Baigrie CF, Buley ID. Papillary and solid neoplasm of the pancreas: fine needle aspiration cytology. Cystopathology 1994;5:310–315 (and personal communication).
105. Goldstein J, Benharroch D, Sion-Vardy N, et al. Solid cystic and papillary tumor on the pancreas with oncocytic differentiation. J Surg Oncol 1994;56:63–67.
106. Yagi M, Shiraiwak O, Abiku M, et al. A solid and cystic tumor of the pancreas in a 10-year-old girl: report of a case and review of the literature. Surg Today 1994;24:826–828.
107. Soyer P, Rabenandrasana A, Van Beers B, et al. Cystic tumors of the pancreas: dynamic CT studies. J Comput Assist Tomogr 1994;18(3):420–426.
108. Balercia G, Zamboni G, Bogina G, Mariuzzi GM. Solid-cystic tumor of the pancreas. An extensive ultrastructural study of fourteen cases. J Submicrosc Cytol Pathol 1995;27:331–340.
109. Naresh KN, Borges AM, Chinoy RF, et al. Solid and papillary epithelial neoplasm of the pancreas. Diagnosis by fine needle aspiration cytology in four cases. Acta Cytol 1995;39(3):489–493.
110. Mao C, Guvendi M, Domenico DR, Kim K, Thomford NR, Howard JM. Papillary cystic and solid tumors of the pancreas. A pancreatic embryonic tumor? Studies of 3 cases and cumulative review of the world's literature. Surgery 1995;118:821–828.
111. Kim YI, Kim ST, Lee GK, Choi BI. Papillary cystic tumors of the liver. Cancer 1990;65:2740–2746.
112. Liu HM, Potter EL. Development of the human pancreas. Arch Pathol 1962;74:439–452.
113. Nokes SR, Harter SB, Baker JW, et al. Radiological case of the month. Papillary epithelial neoplasm of the pancreas. J Arkansas Med Soc 1994;91(1):53–54.
114. Frantz VK. Tumors of islet cells with hyperinsulinism: benign, malignant and questionable. Ann Surg 1940;112:161–176.

# 74

# *Mucinous Papillary Cystic Tumors with Ductal Ectasia*

Tomoo Kosuge, Kazuaki Shimada, and Junji Yamamoto

The concept of mucinous papillary cystic tumors with ductal ectasia (MPCT) was developed recently. Ohashi and Takagi first reported a patient with a polypoid cancer inside a markedly dilated main pancreatic duct in 1980 (1). Ohashi et al. collected four similar cases and reported them, using the tentative name mucin-producing cancer of the pancreas, in a Japanese journal (2). With the increasingly widespread use of ultrasonography (US) and computed tomography (CT), an increasing number of patients with dilated pancreatic ducts have been found and treated. Consequently, similar clinical conditions have been found to arise from benign lesions such as adenomas and hypertrophy, and the concept of the disorder was expanded to include various degrees of epithelial atypia. At present, over 100 cases have been reported under various names, such as (intraductal) mucin-[producing or (hyper)secreting] [cancer, adenocarcinoma, tumor, or neoplasm], ductectatic (-type) mucinous cystadenoma and cystadenocarcinoma, intraductal papillary [neoplasm or adenocarcinoma], mucinous [ductal or pancreatic duct] ectasia and papillary adenoma of the pancreas with excessive mucin secretion (2–17) (Table 74.1).

Despite wide recognition of this peculiar pancreatic disorder, its natural history has not yet been established fully. This plus the use of many different names has resulted in some confusion about this pancreatic neoplasm. In this chapter, the authors use a single term, MPCT, to avoid confusion.

## CONCEPT OF THE DISEASE

MPCTs are characterized by hypersecretion of mucin from the atypical epithelial cells of the pancreatic duct, leading to localized or generalized dilatation of the pancreatic duct. A typical endoscopic finding is a wide-open duodenal papilla filled with mucoid material, and pancreatography demonstrates filling defects in the markedly dilated pancreatic duct. These findings reflect accumulation of mucoid material secreted by papillary tumors into the pancreatic duct.

The epithelial cells of the affected pancreatic duct show varying degrees of atypia from hypertrophy to adenocarcinoma, even in a single patient, suggesting step-wise progression of the disease. A common malignancy is intraductal papillary adenocarcinoma with or without minimal infiltration of the pancreatic parenchyma. Tubular adenocarcinoma, which is the most common pancreatic cancer, is rarely observed. In general, the prognosis associated with the malignant variant of MPCT is far better than that with ordinary ductal pancreatic cancer. Although both cancers are of duct cell origin, they should be distinguished clearly.

MPCT has many characteristics in common with classical mucinous cystic neoplasms (cystadenomas and cystadenocarcinomas), such as mucin production, rare incidence, ductal origin, low-grade malignancy, diverse histologic appearance, and good prognosis after surgical resection. However, some differences between them have been noted. MPCTs occur more frequently in males, commonly develop in the head region, and present with abdominal pain due to obstructive pancreatitis; mucinous cystic neoplasms are predominant in females, usually develop in the body and tail region, and present with symptoms attributable to a mass effect. Some authors consider that both disorders are variants of the same basic disease category (9, 18); others insist they are different disease entities (17).

It is convenient in clinical practice to regard MPCTs and mucinous cystic neoplasms as variants of a single family. A common treatment policy can be applied, because their disease courses are similar. Confusion of MPCT with ordinary ductal pancreatic cancer must be avoided both in practice and in carrying out investigations, in view of the considerably different clinical features.

## CLASSIFICATION

In 1986 the pathologists who contributed to Ohashi's reports proposed a classification of the particular pancreatic cancers that were characterized by overproduction of extracellular mucin (18) (Table 74.2). They attempted to integrate malignant MPCT variants with classical mucinous carcinomas and cystadenocarcinomas. Two types of MPCT were considered to be subcategories: lesions involving the main duct were designated intraductal papillary adenocarcinomas, and those developing in the branch ducts were defined as belonging to a ductectatic subtype of cystadenocarcinoma. Since then, the relationship between MPCTs and mucinous cystic neoplasms has been debated and remains to be settled. However, the morphologic classification of MPCT has been generally accepted by Japanese clinicians.

Currently, it is popular to classify MPCT into two groups according to the predominant site of involvement: main duct and branch duct or ductectatic types. Some investigators add another group called the peripheral or megacystic type, which corresponds to the classical mucinous cystic neoplasm.

## DIAGNOSIS

Modern imaging modalities, such as US, computed tomography (CT), and magnetic resonance imaging (MRI), are sensitive for visualizing dilated and cystic pancreatic ducts. In particular, increasingly widespread use of US has contributed to the detection of asymptomatic patients with pancreatic duct dilatation (19–22). Endoscopic retrograde cholangiopancreatography (ERCP) helps to establish a diagnosis, not only by producing a clear pancreatogram, but also by enabling specimen collection for cytology and gene analysis (1, 2, 22, 23). An enlarged duodenal papilla with a wide-open orifice (Fig. 74.1) and

**TABLE 74.1. Various Terms Used to Describe Mucinous Papillary Cystic Neoplasms with Ductal Ectasia**

| |
|---|
| Mucin-producing cancer of the pancreas (2)[a] |
| Ductectatic mucinous cystadenoma and cystadenocarcinoma (3) |
| Intraductal papillary neoplasms (4) |
| Mucinous pancreatic duct ectasia (5) |
| Intraductal mucin-hypersecreting neoplasms (6) |
| Mucin-hypersecreting tumor (7) |
| Mucin-producing tumor (8, 9) |
| Mucinous ductal ectasia (10) |
| Mucin-producing cystic adenocarcinoma (11) |
| Intraductal mucin-producing tumors (12) |
| Papillary adenoma of the pancreas with excessive mucin secretion (13) |
| Intraductal papillary adenocarcinoma (14) |
| Ductectatic-type mucinous cystadenoma and cystadenocarcinoma (15) |
| Mucin-secreting tumors (16) |
| Mucin-producing neoplasms (17) |

[a]Numbers in parentheses correspond to the reference numbers.

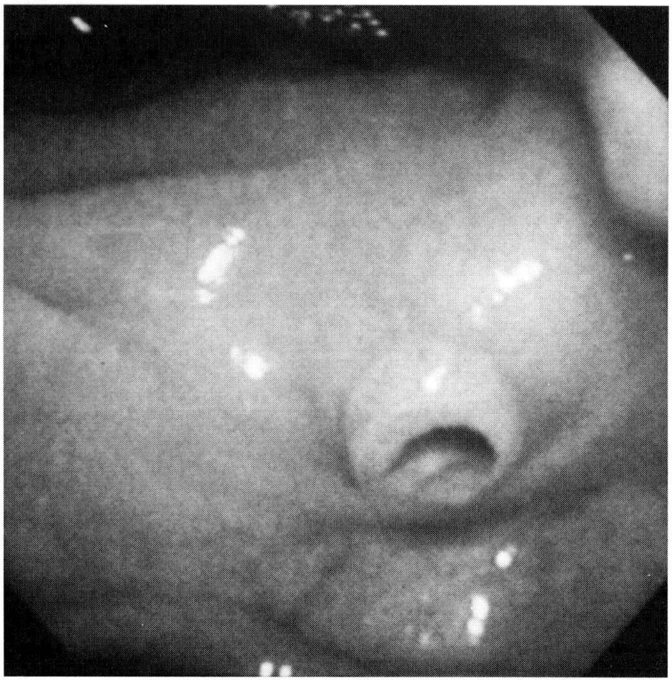

**FIG. 74.1.** Endoscopic view of the duodenal papilla. The orifice was filled with transparent mucin.

dilatation of the main pancreatic duct with filling defects (Fig. 74.2) are diagnostic of MPCT. The presenting finding of the branch duct type is a cystic mass, usually in the uncinate process. A collection of dilated ducts occasionally resembles a mucinous cystic neoplasm or serous cystadenoma. In such cases, associated dilatation of the main duct because of inflow of copious mucin through the communicating branch helps one arrive at the correct diagnosis (Fig. 74.3) (3, 15, 22).

Dilatation of the pancreatic duct and formation of a cystic mass are also common in patients with chronic pancreatitis. Furthermore, hypersecretion of mucin by an MPCT often induces obstructive pancreatitis, resulting in clinical symptoms and laboratory data suggesting pancreatic inflammation. For this reason, many patients have been diagnosed incorrectly as having chronic pancreatitis (11, 13, 22). Understanding the disease and careful examination, particularly looking for hypersecretion of mucin, are mandatory for accurate diagnosis.

Various efforts to improve diagnostic accuracy are in progress, and there is particular interest in differentiating benign and malignant MPCT variants. In addition to conventional measures (24–26), application of new imaging technology is being attempted. Intraductal US with a high-resolution transducer appears to be effective for evaluating small papillary lesions (27). Magnetic resonance–cholangiopancreaticography (28) is expected to facilitate evaluation of the pancreatic duct in a noninvasive manner. The diagnostic value of gene analysis using pancreatic juice is still controversial. Mutations of the K-*ras* gene have been investigated with enthusiasm (29–35). Some investigators suggested they have a strong relationship with malignancy because they found mutations only in patients with carcinomas (29, 30). However, with rapid improvements in detection sensitivity, it became apparent that K-*ras* point mutation was frequently associated with adenoma and hyperplasia (31–34), and currently, it is considered a relatively early event in carcinogenesis. A more intimate relationship between p53 gene mutation to malignancy has been suggested (29, 31), but the diagnostic value remains to be investigated.

**TABLE 74.2. Classification of "Mucin-Producing Cancers" by Katoh and Yanagisawa**

1. Mucinous or muconodular carcinoma
2. Cystadenocarcinoma
   a. Megacystic
   b. Ductectatic
3. Intraductal papillary carcinoma

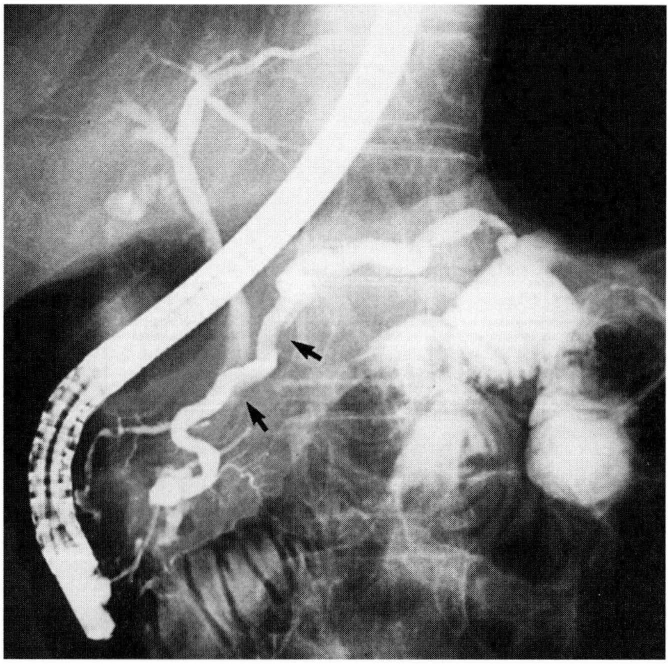

**FIG. 74.2.** ERCP of the main duct–type MPCT. Generalized dilatation of the main pancreatic duct with filling defects *(arrows)*.

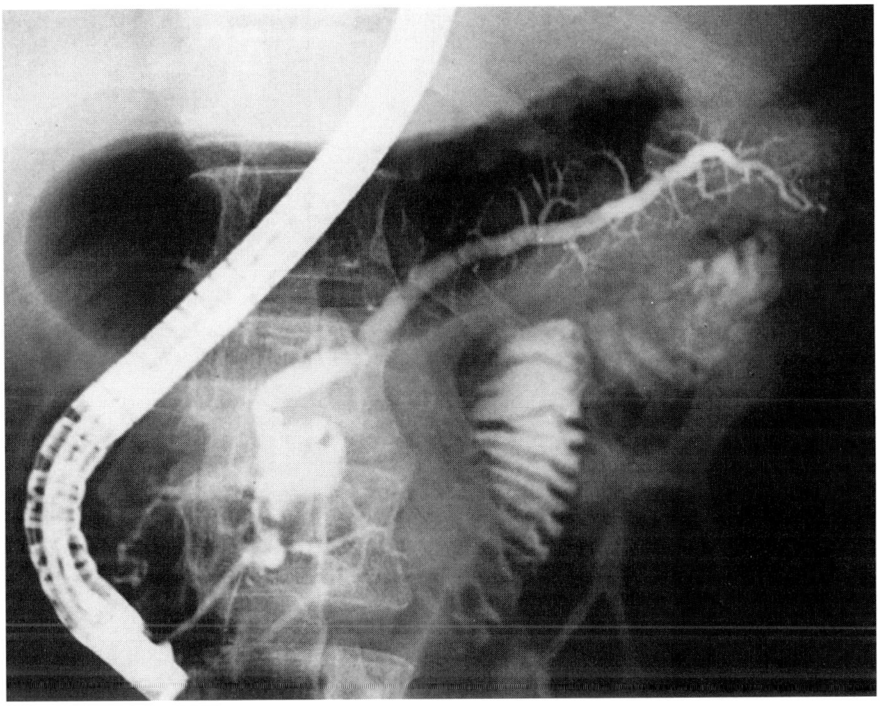

**FIG. 74.3.** ERCP of the branch duct–type MPCT. Cystic dilatation of the branch duct in the uncinate process is visualized. Dilatation of the main duct is also notod.

## TREATMENT

The results of surgical resection for malignant MPCT variants are far better than those with ordinary ductal cancer. Even benign variants are considered precancerous, and consequently, surgical resection is recommended for most patients with MPCTs. Some authors recommend radical resection, including total pancreatectomy. However, performing a really radical procedure including wide retroperitoneal dissection is not justified in view of the relatively low invasiveness of MPCT and relatively high postoperative morbidity. Precise evaluation of the ductal epithelium is important to avoid unnecessary total pancreatectomy. Intraoperative US (Fig. 74.4) and pancreatic ductoscopy are useful to determine the cut line of the pancreas. Our standard procedures are pylorus-preserving pancreatoduodenectomy or distal pancreatectomy depending on the location of the lesion. We do not perform retroperitoneal dissection. We have experienced no postoperative recurrence after resection in 19 patients, including 8 with cancer.

Although surgical resection appears to be the best treatment for most patients with MPCTs, the risks and disadvantages of pancreatic resection should be considered in elderly patients and those with advanced medical problems, in view of the slow progression of the disease. Simple follow-up or palliative treatment may be justified in such cases.

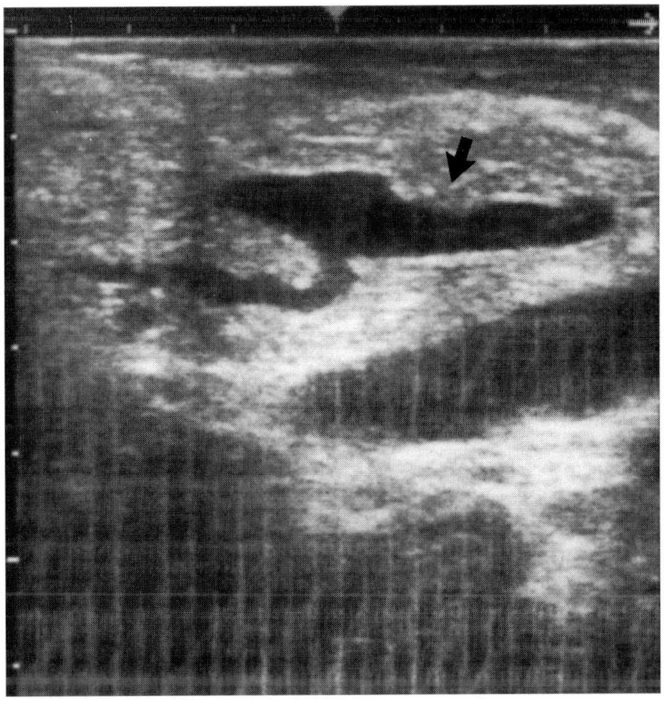

**FIG. 74.4.** Intraoperative US demonstrating a cancerous lesion as a flat elevation in the dilated pancreatic duct *(arrow)*.

## COMMENTS

Japanese investigators predominate in MPCT studies and reports. The apparent rarity of MPCT in western countries may reflect less understanding of the disease concept, although it is possible that geographic and/or racial factors affect the prevalence of MPCT. However, the authors expect that MPCT will prove to be an universal disease and that increasing numbers of patients with this lesion will be found in the future. It is important to understand the common clinical features of MPCTs and classical mucinous cystic neoplasms, but a confusing use of terms should be avoided until a conceptual relationship between the two diseases has been established.

**Acknowledgment**

The authors thank Dr. Hitoshi Kondoh for preparing the photos of ERCP.

## REFERENCES

1. Ohashi K, Takagi K. ERCP and imaging diagnosis of pancreatic cancer (in Japanese). Gastroenterol Endosc 1980;77:1493–1495.

2. Ohashi K, Murakami Y, Maruyama M, et al. Four cases of mucin producing cancer of the pancreas on specific findings of the papilla of Vater (in Japanese). Prog Digest Endosc 1982;20: 348–351.
3. Itai Y, Ohashi K, Nagai H, et al. Ductectatic mucinous cystadenoma and cystadenocarcinoma of the pancreas. Radiology 1986;161:697–700.
4. Morohoshi T, Kanda M, Asanuma K, Klopel G. Intraductal papillary neoplasms of the pancreas: a clinicopathologic study of six patients. Cancer 1989;64:1329–1335.
5. Agostini S, Choux R, Payan MJ, Sastre B, Sahel J, Clement JP. Mucinous pancreatic duct ectasia in the body of the pancreas. Radiology 1989;170:815–816.
6. Rickaert F, Cremer M, Deviere J, et al. Intraductal mucin-hypersecreting neoplasms of the pancreas. A clinicopathologic study of eight patients. Gastroenterology 1991;101:512–519.
7. Yamaguchi K, Tanaka M. Mucin-hypersecreting tumor of the pancreas with mucin extrusion through an enlarged papilla. Am J Gastroenterol 1991;86:835–839.
8. Obara T, Maguchi H, Saitoh Y, et al. Mucin-producing tumor of the pancreas: a unique clinical entity. Am J Gastroenterol 1991;86: 1619–1625.
9. Yamada M, Kozuka S, Yamao K, Nakazawa S, Naitoh Y, Tsukamoto Y. Mucin-producing tumor of the pancreas. Cancer 1991;68:159–168.
10. Bastid C, Bernard P, Sarles H, et al. Mucinous ductal ectasia of the pancreas: a premalignant disease and a cause of obstructive pancreatitis. Pancreas 1991;6:15–22.
11. Kawarada Y, Yano T, Yokoi H, Murayama T, Nakano T, Mizumoto R. Mucin-producing cystic adenocarcinoma of the pancreas, a case report, 7-year follow-up period. Hepatogastroenterology 1992;39:478–480.
12. Kawarada Y, Yano T, Yamamoto T, et al. Intraductal mucin-producing tumors of the pancreas. Am J Gastroenterol 1992;87: 634–638.
13. Obara T, Saitoh Y, Maguchi H, et al. Papillary adenoma of the pancreas with excessive mucin secretion. Pancreas 1992;7: 114–117.
14. Kojima Y, Akiyama T, Saito H, et al. Multifocal intraductal papillary adenocarcinoma of the pancreas: report of a case. Surg Today 1993;23:471–475.
15. Yanagisawa A, Ohashi K, Hori M, et al. Ductectatic-type mucinous cystadenoma and cystadenocarcinoma of the human pancreas: a novel clinicopathological entity. Jpn J Cancer Res 1993;84:474–479.
16. Lichtenstein DR, Carr-Locke DL. Mucin-secreting tumors of the pancreas. Gastrointest Endosc Clin North Am 1995;5:237–258.
17. Shyr YM, Su CH, Tsay SH, Lui WY. Mucin-producing neoplasms of the pancreas. Intraductal papillary and mucinous cystic neoplasms. Ann Surg 1996;223:141–146.
18. Kato Y, Yanagisawa A. Mucin producing carcinoma—concept and classification (in Japanese). Tan To Sui (Biliary tract and pancreas) 1986;7:731–737.
19. Ikeda M, Sato T, Morozumi A, et al. Morphologic changes in the pancreas detected by screening ultrasonography in a mass survey, with special reference to main duct dilatation, cyst formation, and calcification. Pancreas 1994;9:508–512.
20. Soyer P, Rabenandrasana A, Van Beers B, et al. Cystic tumors of the pancreas: dynamic CT studies. J Comput Assist Tomogr 1994;18:420–426.
21. Itoh S, Ishiguchi T, Ishigaki T, Sakuma S, Maruyama K, Senda K. Mucin-producing pancreatic tumor: CT findings and histopathologic correlation. Radiology 1992;183:81–86.
22. Procacci C, Graziani R, Bicego E, et al. Intraductal mucin-producing tumors of the pancreas: imaging findings. Radiology 1996;198:249–257.
23. Nickl NJ, Lawson JM, Cotton PB. Mucinous pancreatic tumors: ERCP findings. Gastrointest Endosc 1991;37:133–138.
24. Yamaguchi K, Ogawa Y, Chijiiwa K, Tanaka M. Mucin-hypersecreting tumors of the pancreas: assessing the grade of malignancy preoperatively. Am J Surg 1996;171:427–431.
25. Uehara H, Nakaizumi A, Iishi H, et al. Cytologic examination of pancreatic juice for differential diagnosis of benign and malignant mucin-producing tumors of the pancreas. Cancer 1994;74: 826–833.
26. Centeno BA, Lewandrowski KB, Warshaw AL, Compton CC, Southern JF. Cyst fluid cytologic analysis in the differential diagnosis of pancreatic cystic lesions. Am J Clin Pathol 1994;101: 483–487.
27. Furukawa T, Tsukamoto Y, Naitoh Y, Mitake M, Hirooka Y, Hayakawa T. Differential diagnosis of pancreatic diseases with an intraductal ultrasound system. Gastrointest Endosc 1994;40: 213–219.
28. Laubenberger J, Buchert M, Schneider B, Blum U, Hennig J, Langer M. Breath-hold projection magnetic resonance-cholangio-pancreaticography (MRCP): a new method for the examination of the bile and pancreatic ducts. Magn Reson Med 1995;33:18–23.
29. Sessa F, Solcia E, Capella C, et al. Intraductal papillary-mucinous tumours represent a distinct group of pancreatic neoplasms: an investigation of tumour cell differentiation and K-ras, p53 and c-erbB-2 abnormalities in 26 patients. Virchows Arch 1994;425: 357–367.
30. Van Laethem JL, Vertongen P, Deviere J, et al. Detection of c-Ki-ras gene codon 12 mutations from pancreatic duct brushings in the diagnosis of pancreatic tumours. Gut 1995;36:781–787.
31. Hoshi T, Imai M, Ogawa K. Frequent K-ras mutations and absence of p53 mutations in mucin-producing tumors of the pancreas. J Surg Oncol 1994;55:84–91.
32. Satoh K, Sawai T, Shimosegawa T, et al. The point mutation of c-Ki-ras at codon 12 in carcinoma of the pancreatic head region and in intraductal mucin-hypersecreting neoplasm of the pancreas. Int J Pancreatol 1993;14:135–143.
33. Yanagisawa A, Kato Y, Ohtake K, et al. c-Ki-ras point mutations in ductectatic-type mucinous cystic neoplasms of the pancreas. Jpn J Cancer Res 1991;82:1057–1060.
34. Yanagisawa A, Ohtake K, Ohashi K, et al. Frequent c-Ki-ras oncogene activation in mucous cell hyperplasias of pancreas suffering from chronic inflammation. Cancer Res 1993;53: 953–956.

SECTION XIV

THE ENDOCRINE PANCREAS

# 75

# *Morphology and Physiology*

Gregory LaValle and Deborah Martinez

The main function of the endocrine pancreas is the maintenance of physiologic levels of glucose within the extracellular fluid compartment and delivery of this metabolic fuel to cells throughout the organism. The main source of glucose is from gastrointestinal (GI) tract absorption; however, it is also produced in the liver by the breakdown of stored glycogen (glycogenolysis) and by the conversion of amino acids and fatty acids (gluconeogenesis). Though most cells in the body can use sources of fuel other than glucose, certain cells such as those in the brain, retina, and germinal epithelium of the gonads can only use glucose for their energy requirements. These specialized cells thus require a consistent amount of glucose best supplied by maintaining a relatively constant concentration of glucose in the surrounding bloodstream. In humans, this level is kept between 70 and 120 mg/dl. Fuel sources other than glucose, such as fatty acids and amino acids, become important sources of energy, especially when carbohydrate stores have been depleted and oral intake of glucose is inadequate. Thus the pancreatic endocrine tissue in the nondiseased state allows the appropriate utilization and storage of glucose. In addition, insulin can also cause deposition of fat within adipocytes, intracellular uptake of amino acids in a variety of cells, and the sparing of intracellular protein, thus making it an important promoter of anabolism.

## DEVELOPMENT

The endocrine pancreas initially develops as single cells randomly dispersed among those cells destined to become the exocrine pancreas. The origin of the stem cell necessary for islet cell formation has been debated. Islet cells do produce tyrosine hydroxylase, which would suggest a cell type of neural crest origin (1). However, they can develop from within the basement membrane of the ductal exocrine tissue and have been demonstrated to arise from endomesodermal tissue in quail-chick chimeras (2), findings that dispute a neural crest origin. The production of insulin from the pancreatic islets for the maintenance of glucose homeostasis begins in the developing embryo, and insulin is measurable in the blood of the fetus. Fetal production of insulin is thought to be important as maternal insulin will not cross the placenta and can occur from the pancreatic B cells as well as the yolk sac and fetal liver (3, 4). Fetal insulin production is not under glucose control until immediately prepartum when acute hypoglycemia occurs. Instead, growth hormone, glucagon, and amino acids, especially arginine, are thought to be important stimuli for insulin production in the fetus (5, 6).

Cells destined to become part of the endocrine pancreas quickly coalesce to form islets, ovoid or spherical collections numbering from several to thousands of cells. These structures are randomly distributed throughout the entire gland and are first observed by the end of the 3rd month of gestation (7). The islet cell mass increases during in utero development and into adulthood. However, the ratio of islet tissue to exocrine pancreatic tissue decreases from birth, when the islets comprise 15% of the pancreatic mass, to adulthood, when they comprise 1–2% of the pancreatic mass and weigh approximately 1 g in total (8). In the adult, the islets receive almost 20% of the pancreatic blood flow despite their relatively small mass (9). In the absence of disease, very little turnover of islet cells is thought to occur.

## ISLET CELL HORMONE AND PEPTIDE PRODUCTION

### B Cell Peptides

**Insulin.** Insulin was the first protein to be structurally defined, by Sanger in 1959 (10). The insulin gene was subsequently cloned and sequenced by Bell (11) and found to be located on the short arm of chromosome 11 (12). The gene contains 3 exons encoding the A and B chains as well as the intervening C-peptide and a signal-peptide sequence (13). Mutations in this gene have uncommonly been reported involving one allele and appear to result in no or only mild clinical diabetes with associated elevated levels of serum insulin or proinsulin levels (14). These mutations are rarely associated with clinically severe diabetes, as the wild-type allele is capable of producing enough native hormone to sustain relatively normal glucose homeostasis.

The pancreas was first reported to be the source of insulin production in 1921 by Banting and Best (15). Insulin production and secretion from the pancreatic islet B cell was proposed several years later, and it is now known that the B cell mass comprises 60–75% of the islet cell mass (16). Insulin is produced initially as a preprohormone with a molecular weight of 11,500. This molecule is cleaved within the rough endoplasmic reticulum (RER) to proinsulin with a molecular weight of 9000, but unlike most prohormones formed in the RER, proinsulin is not glycosylated (17). The proinsulin is further cleaved in the Golgi apparatus to insulin, a 5800-molecular-weight peptide consisting of A and B chains joined by 2 disulfide bonds, and C-peptide, which is thought to provide the support necessary for formation of the proper disulfide bonds between the A and B chains (18). Insulin and C-peptide are stored in secretory granules in equimolar concentrations (19). The stimuli for insulin release are discussed below; however, both insulin and C-peptide are released at the same time. Interestingly, the amino acid structure of insulin is highly conserved, allowing its production from other species for use in treating diabetes in humans; however, the structure of C-peptide varies significantly from species to species (20). The plasma half-life of insulin is approximately 6 minutes, the peptide either binding to its receptor in most tissues of the body and promoting glucose uptake by these tissues or being degraded by insulinase, predominantly in the liver, kidney, and muscle.

**Amyloid.** Islet-amyloid associated polypeptide (IAPP), or amylin, is produced as an 89-amino-acid precursor formed in pancreatic B cells that is cleaved to a 37-amino acid peptide (21). The 37-amino-acid peptide IAPP is sequestered in the same secretory granules that contain insulin and C-peptide, at approximately 10% the concentration of insulin (22). The physiologic function of IAPP has not been established; however, this material has a toxic effect on B cells in vitro, and deposits of this material are demonstrated in the B cells of non-insulin-dependent diabetics (23).

**Pancreastatin.** The 49-amino-acid peptide pancreastatin is produced by the islet B cells and released with insulin. This peptide has a known inhibitory role in insulin secretion as well as glucagon and pancreatic acinar cell secretion in animal models (24). The role of this peptide in human glucose homeostasis is not well defined at present.

### A Cell Peptides

**Glucagon.** Glucagon, a peptide hormone with a molecular weight of 3500, is produced in the alpha or A cells of the pancreatic islets as well as the GI tract (25). Pancreatic A cells make up 15–20% of cells within the islets of the dorsal pancreas but are uncommonly found in islets of the ventral pancreas, in contradistinction to pancreatic-polypeptide-producing F cells, which are the predominant non-B cell in the islets of the ventral pancreas (26). The A cells represent the majority cells in the mantle zone of the islets in the ventral region of the pancreas (see "Architecture," below) and are the first cell type to become distinguishable in the developing pancreas, appearing at the 20-somite stage (27). Glucagon activity results in increased blood glucose levels, thus antagonizing the effects of insulin. The stimuli for glucagon production and effects on target tissue are discussed below.

### D Cell Peptides

**Somatostatin.** Somatostatin is produced in the delta or D cells of the pancreatic islets as well as cells of the GI tract as a 92-amino-acid prosomatostatin (28). This prohormone is processed differently in these two sites: the 14-amino-acid somatostatin is the main product of the pancreatic islet D cells, while the 28-amino-acid somatostatin is the main product of the GI tract D cells (29). D cells make up approximately 5% of cells within the islet (30). In experimental preparations, somatostatin potently inhibits the secretion of insulin and glucagon; however, the role of somatostatin in affecting the physiologic function of the pancreatic islets is somewhat controversial, as blood flow through the larger islets appears to bathe the mantle zone (A, D, and F) cells after having perfused the B cell region (see "Architecture" below) (31). This suggests that its role in islet cell function is perhaps limited to its effect on regional A and PP cells, though somatostatin production from pancreatic islets may be so minor that it is doubtful that A and PP cells are significantly affected. The major role of this hormone may be its effect on inhibiting pancreatic acinar cell function.

**Diazepam-Binding Inhibitor (DBI).** DBI is an 86-amino-acid polypeptide produced in the D cells of human islets. The polypeptide binds to the benzodiazepine recognition site within the γ-aminobutyric acid (GABA)-receptor complex and appears to inhibit insulin secretion in experimental preparations, though its physiologic effect has not been established (32, 33).

### F Cell Peptides

**Pancreatic Polypeptide.** Pancreatic polypeptide is produced in the islet F cells as a 95-amino-acid precursor that is cleaved to form an active 36-amino-acid hormone (34). The F cells comprise approximately 15–20% of cells within the islets of the ventral pancreas but are uncommonly found in the dorsal pancreatic islets. The hormone is released by vagal stimulation and experimentally can suppress insulin secretion as well as pancreatic juice and bile secretion (35); however, its physiologic role in islet cell function and glucose homeostasis is not defined.

## ARCHITECTURE

The arrangement of endocrine cells within the islets is relatively constant. A collection of beta cells is present usually in the center of the islets and is surrounded by a variety of A, D, and F cells, this outer layer 3 to 4 cells in width (36). Each individual islet is supplied by one to five arterioles that penetrate the islet at the periphery (37). However, the direction of blood flow through highly fenestrated capillaries and the sites at which collecting venules form are a matter of some controversy. This controversy has physiologic ramifications because if B cells are perfused prior to cells within the mantle, insulin within the efferent capillaries would then be in a position to exert physiologic effects on the cells of the mantle zone, ultimately affecting the secretion of hormones from these cells. If the blood flow were in the opposite direction, from the mantle to the beta cell zone, the A, D, and F cells would be in a position to exert a significant physiologic effect on the insulin production of B cells. Current evidence appears to support, but not conclusively prove, the former hypothesis (38). In addition, somatostatin produced within the mantle region may be important for acinar cell regulation, and thus an insulo-acinar axis has been proposed in which blood initially perfuses the islet cell mass, the secretion of insulin, glucagon, somatostatin, and pancreatic polypeptide from the islets in turn affecting the exocrine pancreatic function (39). Of the four hormones produced by the endocrine pancreas, somatostatin appears to be the most potent in its effect on the pancreatic acinar cells, by inhibiting acinar cell output.

## PHYSIOLOGY

### Stimuli for Insulin Release

**Metabolic.** Maintenance of serum glucose within a relatively constant range is accomplished by a well-orchestrated release of the aforementioned hormones, in particular insulin and glucagon. Various stimuli for the release of these hormones contribute to this orchestrated release; however, the serum glucose level appears to be the most potent initiating stimulus. Glucose is conducted across the membrane of the B cells by GLUT-2, a glucose transporter protein, whose production and function are not controlled by insulin (40). The GLUT-2 protein allows rapid equilibrium of glucose across the B cell membrane. However, the rate at which glucose is transported across B cell membranes is not related to GLUT-2 function but to the activity of the enzyme glucokinase, which promotes the phosphorylation of the 6 position of glucose to glucose-6-phosphate (41). Other substances known to physiologically enhance the secretion of insulin when present in the extracellular fluid in increased concentrations include amino acids, the most potent of which are arginine and lysine.

**Hormonal.** A question that has been difficult to explain until recently is how, if the serum glucose is kept at constant levels within the blood, does release of insulin occur. The answer appears to be that oral glucose administration stimulates the release of the incretins, polypeptides produced within the mucosa of the GI tract. The incretins include the truncated and amidated form of glucagon-like peptide GLP-1 (GLP-1 [7–36] amide) processed from proglucagon in the intestinal L cells (42) and gastric inhibitory polypeptide (GIP) produced in the K cells of the duodenum and proximal jejunum (43). Cholecystokinin (CCK) is also a candidate, but its physiologic role as an incretin in humans is not established. Though these substances enhance the secretion of insulin from the pancreatic B cells, the mechanism of action of the incretins is not well understood at present.

Following a rise in the serum glucose level, usually above 100 mg/dL, and under the assistance of the incretins, insulin is released from the pancreatic B cells and the plasma level increases 10-fold within 3–5 minutes after the blood glucose rise. There is an initial fall in serum insulin for 10 minutes, then a second rise and plateau for 2–3 hours. The insulin response is terminated within 5 minutes after a fall in the blood glucose to the fasting level.

Other hormones known to directly or indirectly stimulate insulin secretion in experimental models and in humans include the peptide hormones glucagon, growth hormone, gastrin, and secretin, as well as the steroid hormones cortisol, estrogen, and progesterone. It is doubtful that such hormones, with the exception of glucagon, play an influential role in the acute physiologic release of insulin after meals. However, pathologic long-term release of glucagon, growth hormone, and cortisol found in patients with tumors secreting these substances have profound effects on glucose metabolism and can produce diabetes clinically, presumably by antagonizing the effects of insulin in the peripheral tissues.

Hormones known to have an inhibitory effect on insulin secretion in experimental models include somatostatin, pancreatic polypeptide, IAPP, pancreastatin, DBI, peptide YY, galanin, and neuropeptide Y. The physiologic role of these hormones in insulin homeostasis in humans is not completely understood.

**Neural.** Sympathetic, parasympathetic, and sensory nerves innervate the islets. Sympathetic nerve stimulation has complex effects on insulin secretion: stimulation of B cell $\alpha_2$-adrenergic receptors inhibits insulin release, while stimulation of B cell $\beta_2$-adrenergic receptors stimulates insulin release (44). The relative density of $\alpha_2$- and $\beta_2$-receptors on B cells may be the most important determinant of whether sympathetic stimulation causes inhibition or stimulation of insulin release.

By use of immunohistochemistry, the adrenergic nerve terminals have been found to contain neuropeptide Y (NPY) (45) and galanin (46), candidate neurotransmitters that dramatically inhibit insulin secretion in some species. However, the physiologic role of these neurotransmitters on human islet function is not resolved, as marked variations in physiologic effects are observed between species.

Vagal nerve stimulation promotes both insulin and glucagon release (47). However, the pure acetylcholine inhibitor—atropine—does not completely abolish vagally mediated stimulation of insulin or glucagon in some species. In pancreatic islet nerve endings, both vasoactive inhibitory polypeptide (VIP) and gastrin-releasing peptide (GRP) exist, and both are released following vagal stimulation of the islets (48, 49). Both substances are potent stimulators of insulin and glucagon secretion and may mediate in part the effects of vagal stimulation on insulin and glucagon secretion.

It is possible that the observed effects on insulin/glucagon secretion by autonomic stimulation and the neurotransmitters are related to alterations in blood flow to regions of each islet by virtue of the effects of these stimuli on vascular tone (50). Such a mechanism has not been conclusively proven to be physiologically important in humans.

### Insulin Effect

The physiologic result of insulin secretion from the pancreatic B cells is to reduce the blood glucose concentration. This process is initiated with the binding of insulin to its receptor in target cells and is greatest in the liver, muscle, and adipose tissue. Within seconds after binding to its receptor, the target cell membranes become permeable to glucose, allowing rapid entry of glucose as well as amino acids, potassium, and phosphate ions into the cells. The effect of insulin on most tissues, especially liver, muscle, and adipocytes, is to cause a rapid uptake of glucose within the cells which is then phosphorylated by glucokinase. The phosphorylation of glucose retards the movement of glucose out of the cell. In addition, insulin promotes the production of glycogen in the liver and muscle as a source of fuel for these tissues during periods of relative glucose lack, by stimulation of the enzyme glycogen synthase. Following optimum glycogen formation, excess glucose is converted to fatty acids by the stimulation of insulin. These fatty acids are subsequently manufactured into triglycerides and transported via very-low-density lipoproteins from the liver to adipocytes and stored for future energy needs.

Insulin causes transfer of amino acids into cells, those most effectively transferred include valine, leucine, isoleucine, tyrosine, and phenylalanine. In addition, insulin inhibits the rate of gluconeogenesis in the liver, thus sparing the amino acids that can be used as substrates for this process. Finally, insulin inhibits the breakdown of cellular protein and thus is referred to as an anabolic hormone.

### Stimuli for Glucagon Release

Glucagon release is stimulated when blood glucose levels fall below approximately 90 mg/dL. Its major physiologic effects include the breakdown of liver glycogen as well as gluconeogenesis in the liver. An additional stimulus for glucagon release is an elevated serum concentration of amino acids, as occurs after a meal. Interestingly, an elevated serum level of amino acids also exacerbates insulin release. Finally, glucagon release is stimulated by strenuous exercise, thus preventing a potential fall in serum glucose levels. As with insulin release, the physiologic effect of autonomic neural stimuli in the secretion of glucagon in humans is not yet established.

### Glucagon Effect

The main effect of glucagon secreted by the A cells is to increase both glycogenolysis (breakdown of liver glycogen to glucose) and gluconeogenesis (production of new glucose by the liver). The biochemical effects produced by this polypeptide after binding to its cell surface receptor include stimulation of adenyl cyclase in the hepatic cell membrane, production of cyclic adenosine monophosphate (cyclic AMP), and ultimately, stimulation of *phosphorylase a*, promoting the degradation of glycogen to glucose-1-phosphate, which is subsequently dephosphorylated to produce glucose.

## REFERENCES

1. Pearse AGE, Polak JM. Neural crest origin of the endocrine polypeptide (APUD) cells of the gastrointestinal tract and pancreas. Gut 1971;12:783–788.
2. Fontaine J, Le Douarin N. Analysis of endoderm formation in the

avian blastoderm by the use of quail-chick chimeras. The problem of the neuroectodermal origin of the cells of the APUD series. J Embryol Exp Morphol 1977;41:209–222.
3. Adam PA, Teramo K, Raiha N, Gitlin D, Schwartz R. Human fetal insulin metabolism early in gestation. Response to acute elevation of the fetal glucose concentration and placental transfer of human insulin-$^{131}$I. Diabetes 1969;16:409–416.
4. Giddings SJ, Carnaghi LR. Selective expression and developmental regulation of the ancestral rat insulin II gene in fetal liver. Mol Endocrinol 1990;4:1363–1369.
5. Milner RDG, Ashworth MA, Barson AJ. Insulin release from human foetal pancreas in response to glucose, leucine and arginine. J Endocrinol 1972;51:321–327.
6. Formby B, Ullrich A, Coussens L, Walker L, Peterson CM. Growth hormone stimulates insulin gene expression in cultured human fetal pancreatic islets. J Clin Endocrinol Metab 1988;66:1075–1079.
7. Liu HM, Potter EL. Development of the human pancreas. Arch Pathol 1962;74:439–452.
8. Rahier J, Wallon J, Henquin JC. Cell populations in the endocrine pancreas in human neonates and infants. Diabetologica 1981; 20:540–546.
9. Jansson L, Hellerstrom C. A rapid method of visualizing the pancreatic islets for studies of islet capillary blood flow using non-radioactive microspheres. Acta Physiol Scand 1981;113: 371–374.
10. Sanger F. Chemistry of insulin. Science 1959;129:1340–1344.
11. Bell GI, Pictet RL, Rutter WJ, et al. Sequence of the human insulin gene. Nature 1980;284:26–32.
12. Owerbach D. Bell GI, Rutter WJ, et al. The insulin gene is located on the short arm of chromosome 11 in humans. Diabetes 1981;30:267–270.
13. Steiner DF, Chan SJ, Welsh JM, Kwok SCM. Structure and evolution of the insulin gene. Annu Rev Genet 1985;19:463–484.
14. Haneda M, Polonsky KS, Bergenstal RM, et al. Familial hyperinsulinemia due to a structurally abnormal insulin: definition of an emerging new syndrome. N Engl J Med 1984;310:1288–1289.
15. Banting FG, Best CH. The internal secretion of the pancreas. J Lab Clin Med 1922;7:251–266.
16. A proinsulin trafficking and processing in the B-cell. Trends Endocrinol Metab 1990;1:261–265.
17. Patzelt C, Labrecque AD, Duguid JR, et al. Detection and kinetic behavior of preproinsulin in pancreatic islets. Proc Natl Acad Sci USA 1978;75:1260–1264.
18. Rhodes CJ, Halban PA. Newly synthesized proinsulin/insulin and stored insulin are released from pancreatic B cells predominantly via a regulated, rather than a constitutive pathway. J Cell Biol 1987;105:145–153.
19. Docherty K, Steiner DF. Post-translational proteolysis in polypeptide hormone biosynthesis. Annu Rev Physiol 1982;44: 625–638.
20. Dayhoff MO. Atlas of protein sequence and structure, vol 5, suppl 3. Silver Spring, MD: National Biomedical Research Foundation, 1978.
21. Cooper GJS. Amylin compared with calcitonin gene-related peptide: structure, biology and relevance to metabolic disease. Endocr Rev 1994;15:163–201.
22. Kahn SE, D'Alessio DA, Schwartz MW, et al. Evidence of cosecretion of islet amyloid polypeptide and insulin by beta-cells. Diabetes 1990;39:634–638.
23. Clark A. Islet amyloid: an enigma of type 2 diabetes. Diabetes Metab Rev 1992;8:117–132.
24. Sanchez-Margalet V, Lucas M, Goberna R. Pancreastatin: further evidence for its consideration as a regulatory peptide. J Mol Endocrinol 1996;16(1):1–8.
25. Habener JF, Drucker DJ, Mojsov S, et al. Biosynthesis of glucagon. In: Samols E, ed. The endocrine pancreas. New York: Raven Press 1991:125.
26. Dumonteil E, Philippe J. Insulin gene organisation, expression and regulation. Diabetes Metab 1996;22:164–173.
27. Kaung HLC. Growth dynamics of pancreatic islet cell populations during fetal and neonatal development in the rat. Dev Dynamics 1994;200:163–175.
28. Reichlin S. Somatostatin. N Engl J Med 1983;309:1495–1501.
29. Polonsky KS, Shoelson SE, Docherty HM. Plasma somatostatin-28 increases in response to feeding in man. J Clin Invest 1983;71: 1514–1518.
30. Larsson LI. Distribution and morphology of somatostatin cells. Adv Exp Med Biol 1985;188:383–402.
31. Gray PW, Glaister D, Seeburg PH, et al. Cloning and expression of DNA for human diazepam-binding inhibitor, a natural ligand of an allosteric regulatory site of the gamma-aminobutyric acid type A receptor. Proc Natl Acad Sci USA 1986;83:7547–7551.
32. Guidotti A, Forchetti CM, Corda MG, et al. Isolation, characterization, and purification to homogeneity of an endogenous polypeptide with agonistic action on benzodiazepine receptors. Proc Natl Acad Sci USA 1983;80:3531–3535.
33. Sundler F, Bottcher G, Hakanson R, Schwartz TW. Immunocytochemical localization of the icosapeptide fragment of the PP precursor: a marker for "true" PP cells? Regul Pept 1984;8: 217–224.
34. Greenberg GR, McCloy CR, Adrian TE, et al. Inhibition of pancreatic and gallbladder output by pancreatic polypeptide. Lancet 1978;2:1280–1282.
35. Floyd JC, Fajans SS, Pek S, Chance RE. A newly recognized pancreatic polypeptide: plasma levels in health and disease. Recent Prog Horm Res 1977;33:519–570.
36. Orci L. The microanatomy of the islets of Langerhans. Metabolism 1976;25:1303–1313.
37. Brunicardin FC, Tagner J, Bonner-Weir S, Wayland H, Kleinman R, et al. Microcirculation of the islets of Langerhans. Diabetes 1996;45:385–392.
38. Bonner-Weir S. The microcirculation of the islets of Langerhans. In: Samols E, ed. The endocrine pancreas. New York: Raven Press, 1994.
39. Murakami T, Fujita T, Miyake T, Ohtsuka A, Taguchi T, Kikuta A. The insulo-acinar portal and insulo-venous drainage systems in the pancreas of the mouse, dog, monkey, and certain other animals: a scanning electron microscopic study of corrosion casts. Arch Histol Cytol 1993;56:127–147.
40. Elsas LJ, Longo N. Glucose transporters. Annu Rev Med 1992;43: 377–393.
41. Meglasson MD, Matschinsky FM. New perspectives on pancreatic islet glucokinase. Am J Physiol 1984;246(1 pt):E1–13.
42. Goke R, Fehman HC, Goke B. Glucagon-like peptide I (7–36) amide is a new incretin/energastrone candidate. Eur J Clin Invest 1991;21:135–141.
43. Ahren B, Pettersson M, Uvnas-Moberg K, et al. Effects of cholecystokinin (CCK)-8, CCK-33, and gastric inhibitory polypeptide (GIP) on basal and meal-stimulated pancreatic hormone secretion in man. Diabetes Res Clin Pract 1991;13:153–161.
44. Dunning BE, Taborsky GJ Jr. Neural control of islet function by norepinephrine and sympathetic neuropeptides. Adv Exp Med Biol 1991;291:107–127.
45. Waeber G, Hurlimann J, Nicod P, Grouzmann E. Immunolocalization of neuropeptide Y in human pancreatic endocrine tumors. Peptides 1995;16(5):921–926.
46. Ahren B, Rorsman P, Berggren PO. Galanin and the endocrine pancreas. FEBS Letters 1988;229(2):233–237.
47. Ahren B, Karlsson S, Lindskog S. Cholinergic regulation of the endocrine pancreas. In: Aquilonius SM, Gillberg PO, eds. Progress in brain research. Amsterdam: Elsevier Science, 1990:209–218.
48. Holst JJ, Fahrenkrug J, Knuhtsen S, et al. Vasoactive intestinal polypeptide (VIP) in the pig pancreas: role of VIPergic fibers in control of fluid and bicarbonate secretion. Regul Pept 1984;8: 245–259.
49. Knuthsen S, Holst JJ, Baldisscra FGA, et al. Gastrin-releasing peptide in the porcine pancreas. Gastroenterology 1987;92: 1153–1158.
50. Svensson AM, Abdel-Halim SM, Efendic S, et al. Pancreatic and islet blood flow in F1-hybrids on the non-insulin dependent diabetic GK-Wistar rat. Eur J Endocrinol 1994;130:612–616.

# 76

# Imaging Procedures for the Endocrine Pancreas

Donald L. Miller and Peter C. Buetow

The radiologist contributes to the management of patients with pancreatic endocrine tumors by evaluating them for metastases and by localizing tumors. Insulinomas and gastrinomas, often small and elusive, are the only islet cell tumors for which extensive localization efforts are often required. Other islet cell tumors, whether functioning or clinically silent, are usually large enough to be obvious on imaging studies.

Critical evaluation of the various localization procedures used in patients with islet cell tumors is difficult for a number of reasons. Islet cell tumors are uncommon, and relatively few patients with these lesions are seen at most institutions. Findings from a series of 25 patients with breast cancer or colon cancer probably would not be statistically significant and might not be considered reliable, but 25 patients is a large series for insulinomas. Conflicting results are therefore commonly seen when published studies on patients with islet cell tumors are compared.

Because accrual is so slow, there is a tendency to report on patients studied over a long period of time—often 5–10 years or more. However, imaging technologies have evolved so rapidly in the 1980s and 1990s, that results obtained even 5 years ago do not accurately reflect the capabilities of current-generation ultrasound, computed tomography (CT), and magnetic resonance imaging (MRI) units.

Another common approach used to compensate for the rarity of these disorders is to combine the results obtained from patients evaluated at a number of different centers. The problem with multicenter reports is that performance of many radiologic techniques is highly operator dependent, and for all of them, the interpretation of the results depends entirely on the skill and interest of the individual radiologist.

The most reliable results tend to come from centers with the largest numbers of patients, such as the Mayo Clinic and the National Institutes of Health (NIH) in the United States. These series nonetheless reflect the biases and preferences of practitioners at the individual institutions. Further, the results achieved by radiologists at these centers may not be reproducible by radiologists who are less familiar with islet cell tumors. The choice and sequence of localization studies of necessity depends on the preferences of the surgeon and the ability and experience of the radiologists at each institution. There is no single "right way" to evaluate these patients.

## Noninvasive Imaging Studies

Four noninvasive imaging studies are currently in use for localization of primary islet cell tumors and detection of hepatic metastases: ultrasound, CT, MRI, and somatostatin receptor scintigraphy. Ultrasound, CT, and MRI are cross-sectional imaging studies that enable detection of a lesion by directly imaging it. Somatostatin receptor scintigraphy is a functional study that enables identification of lesions on the basis of a functional characteristic (expression of somatostatin receptors) rather than imaging of the lesion itself. Each modality has advantages and disadvantages, and each is described individually.

**Ultrasound.** The effectiveness of ultrasound depends in large part on how close the imaging transducer can be brought to the area of interest. High-frequency (7.5–10 MHz) transducers provide better spatial resolution than lower frequency transducers but cannot penetrate as deeply into tissues. For this reason, conventional (transabdominal) ultrasound has been supplemented with endoscopic ultrasound and intraoperative ultrasound. These two imaging modalities are described below with the other invasive imaging studies.

Large islet cell tumors are easily detected with all imaging modalities, and ultrasound is no exception (Fig. 76.1) (1). There is no characteristic ultrasound appearance, and these tumors may be homogeneous or inhomogeneous. In a series of 12 nonfunctioning islet cell tumors examined with ultrasound, 10 lesions were hypoechoic, 1 was hyperechoic, and 1 was cystic with multiple septations (2). Cystic changes, necrosis, and calcification are all more common in large islet cell tumors than in small ones (3). Cystic islet cell tumors are uncommon but must be included in the differential diagnosis of large cystic (especially multicystic) pancreatic masses (3–9). Cystic or necrotic islet cell tumors are unlikely to be insulinomas (3). Occasionally, cystic islet cell tumors may mimic pancreatic pseudocysts in appearance (8, 10).

Conventional transabdominal ultrasound typically demonstrates small islet cell tumors as round or oval, smoothly marginated areas of decreased echogenicity (Figs. 76.2 and 76.3) (10). When the primary tumor is larger than 2 cm, the sensitivity of ultrasound is 60–65% (11). As with all localization techniques that image lesions directly, the ability of ultrasound to enable localization depends on lesion size. The technique is relatively insensitive for localization of small islet cell tumors. Ultrasound has a reported sensitivity of 25–30% for gastrinomas and 25–75% for insulinomas (10, 12–17). Note, however, that the published literature that indicates a high sensitivity for insulinoma localization is from only two centers, the Mayo Clinic and the University of Mainz (Germany) (18–22). At other institutions, the sensitivity of ultrasound for insulinoma localization is no higher than 25% (15, 23–26).

The technique is more useful for the detection of hepatic metastases (27); which may be either hypoechoic or hyperechoic (Fig. 76.4). In one study of 25 patients with endocrine tumors, 17 of whom had liver metastases, ultrasound was superior to both

The opinions expressed herein are those of the authors and do not necessarily reflect the views of the United States Navy, the United States Army, or the Department of Defense.

CT and MRI (28). Other studies have yielded conflicting results (15, 27, 29), and the mean sensitivity of the technique for detection of hepatic metastases is only 20% (17), but ultrasound remains popular as the initial imaging study for patients with pancreatic endocrine tumors. In part, this is because it is the least expensive noninvasive screening study for hepatic metastases at most institutions. It has the additional advantage of avoiding the admittedly minimal risks associated with the use of ionizing radiation and intravenous contrast material.

**Computed Tomography.** Large islet cell tumors are readily apparent on CT (Fig. 76.1) (2, 30). Certain CT features are highly suggestive of islet cell tumor: unusually large size, intratumoral calcifications, and marked enhancement following the intravenous administration of contrast material (2, 30). In a series of 27 nonfunctioning islet cell tumors, 30% were larger than 10 cm in diameter, 20% contained calcium, and 80% demonstrated contrast enhancement of part or all of the lesion (30). Contrast enhancement differentiates islet cell tumors from pancreatic adenocarcinomas, which virtually never enhance (10). Intratumoral calcification may occasionally mimic the "sunburst" pattern sometimes seen in microcystic adenomas of the pancreas (Fig. 76.1) (31).

Like ultrasound, CT is relatively insensitive for the detection of primary islet cell tumors, with a reported overall sensitivity of 45–70% (the mean sensitivity is about 50%), and reported sensitivities for detection of primary gastrinomas and insulinomas of 30–60% and 30–75%, respectively (10, 13, 16, 17, 32, 33). The sensitivity of the technique is highly dependent on lesion size (16, 34). Diagnoses of endocrine disorders are now made earlier in the course of the disease than in previous years, so that patients now present with smaller tumors, and the sensitivity of standard CT has dropped. Some series now report sensitivities for gastrinoma localization of less than 30% (15, 35, 36). CT should be performed with 5-mm-thick sections through the pancreas during the rapid intravenous infusion of contrast material (dynamic scanning) (35, 37).

If available, a helical CT scanner should be used. This is the newest CT scanner technology. It is likely to yield better results than are possible with conventional CT scanners, for several reasons (32, 38–41). Helical CT permits scanning of the entire pancreas during the period when there is maximal arterial opacification by intravenously injected contrast material, which maximizes the attenuation difference between the hypervascular islet cell tumor and surrounding structures (Fig. 76.5). It also permits imaging of the pancreas with thin sections in a single "breath-hold," minimizing the portion of the pancreas that is not imaged because of patient motion. Finally, the data from the helical CT study can be postprocessed in ways that data from conventional CT cannot, often permitting better visualization of small masses.

Small islet cell tumors are seen on CT as well-defined, round or oval masses. They enhance (become brighter) on CT scans obtained during the intravenous administration of contrast material, but they have equal, higher, or lower attenuation than the surrounding normal pancreas (Fig. 76.6) (1, 10, 42). On occasion, the tumor may be isodense with the surrounding pancreas, and a contour abnormality of the pancreas may be the only indication of its presence (42). In rare cases, small islet cell tumors may not exhibit any contrast enhancement at all (43, 44). CT during the intraarterial infusion of contrast material via the celiac axis has been tried, but in general this technique has not improved the sensitivity of CT (Fig. 76.7) (45). It is occasionally

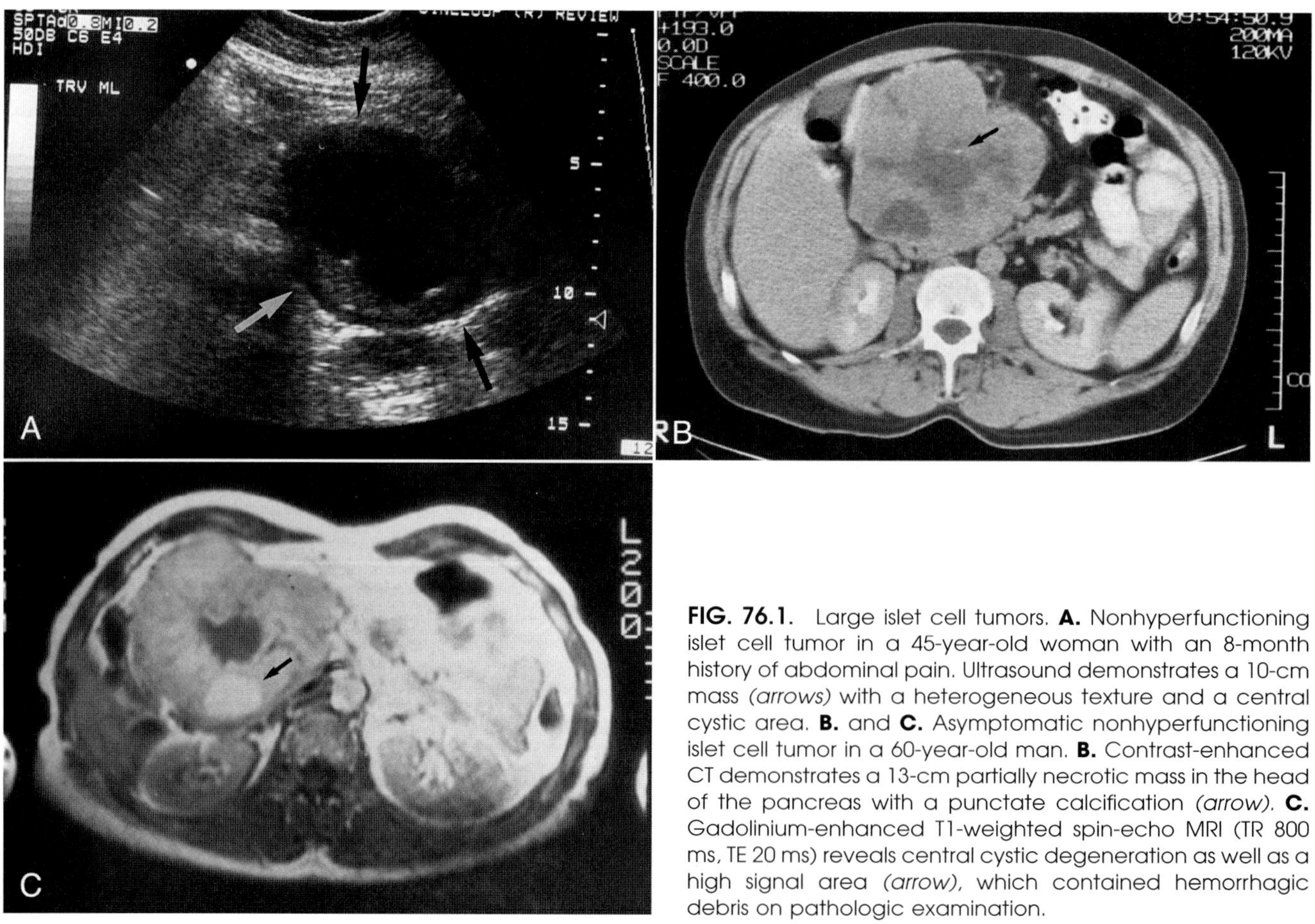


**FIG. 76.1.** Large islet cell tumors. **A.** Nonhyperfunctioning islet cell tumor in a 45-year-old woman with an 8-month history of abdominal pain. Ultrasound demonstrates a 10-cm mass *(arrows)* with a heterogeneous texture and a central cystic area. **B.** and **C.** Asymptomatic nonhyperfunctioning islet cell tumor in a 60-year-old man. **B.** Contrast-enhanced CT demonstrates a 13-cm partially necrotic mass in the head of the pancreas with a punctate calcification *(arrow)*. **C.** Gadolinium-enhanced T1-weighted spin-echo MRI (TR 800 ms, TE 20 ms) reveals central cystic degeneration as well as a high signal area *(arrow)*, which contained hemorrhagic debris on pathologic examination.

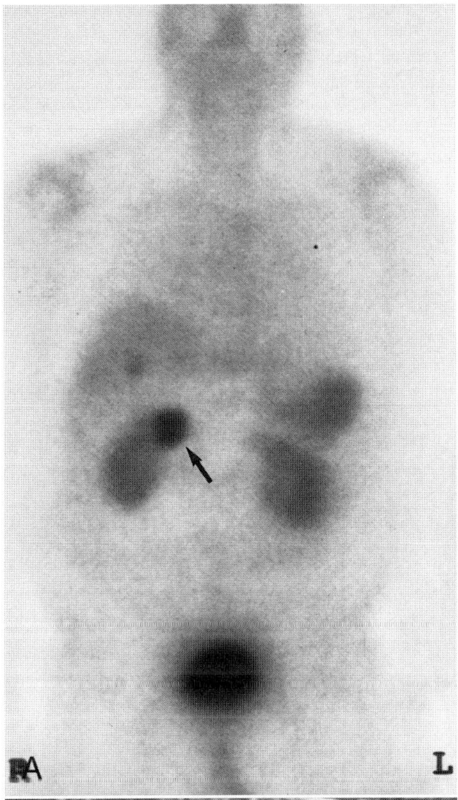


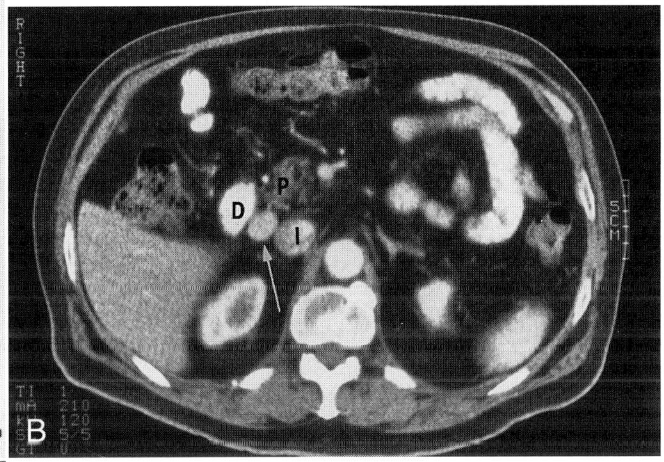


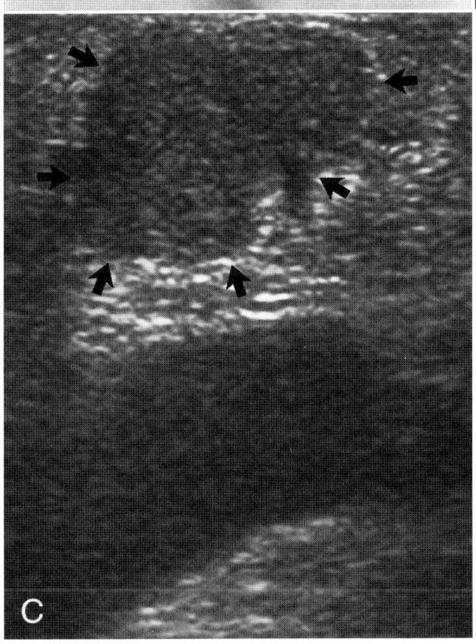


**FIG. 76.2.** Small extrapancreatic gastrinoma. This 69-year-old man with Zollinger-Ellison syndrome presented with upper gastrointestinal bleeding due to peptic ulcer disease. **A.** Planar somatostatin receptor scintigraphy reveals focal increased uptake in the region of the pancreatic head *(arrow)*. Activity in the kidneys, bladder, liver, gallbladder, and stomach is normal. **B.** Contrast-enhanced CT shows the 1.3-cm homogeneously enhancing mass *(arrow)* between the pancreatic head *(P)*, the IVC *(I)*, and the duodenum *(D)*. **C.** Intraoperative ultrasound demonstrates a homogeneous, oval, slightly lobulated, hypoechoic mass *(arrows)* with smooth margins.

helpful for hypovascular tumors (43). Similar images are obtained with helical CT during the arterial phase of contrast enhancement, without the need for arterial catheterization (Fig. 76.5).

Liver metastases from pancreatic endocrine tumors are hypervascular. Since they enhance during the administration of intravenous contrast material, they may become isodense with the normal liver parenchyma on CT (37, 46). Bressler et al. demonstrated that administration of intravenous contrast material during CT scanning could make liver metastases from these tumors invisible on CT (46). However, two other series concluded that CT scans of the liver obtained without the use of intravenous contrast material did not identify significantly more lesions in patients with hypervascular metastases than CT scans obtained with it (47, 48). With helical CT, scanning prior to contrast material administration is unlikely to reveal additional hepatic lesions. Bolus intravenous infusion of contrast material and dynamic scanning through the liver during both arterial and portal phases of hepatic enhancement make it much less likely that metastases will be missed.

Overall, CT is an excellent method for detecting liver metastases, with a sensitivity of 70–85% (29, 42, 49, 50). CT arterial portography may also be used and may further improve the sensitivity of hepatic CT (46, 51, 52).

**Magnetic Resonance Imaging.** Pancreatic endocrine tumors typically have a low signal intensity (dark) on T1-

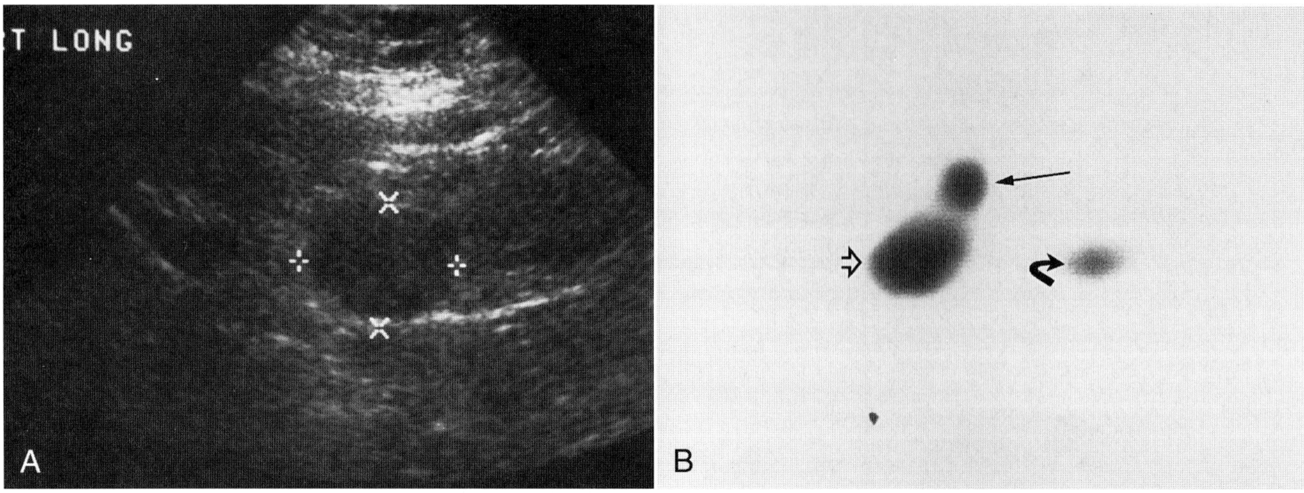


**FIG. 76.3.** Juxtaduodenal gastrinoma in a 65-year-old woman with a 6-year history of peptic ulcer disease. **A.** Transabdominal ultrasound demonstrates a solid 2.6-cm hypoechoic oval mass with smooth borders near the head of the pancreas *(cursors).* **B.** The gastrinoma *(long arrow)* demonstrates focal uptake of indium-111 octreotide on an axial SPECT image from a somatostatin receptor scintigraphy study (*open arrow,* right kidney; *curved arrow,* left kidney).

weighted MR images (Figs. 76.6 and 76.7). They demonstrate high signal intensity (bright) on T2-weighted images (Figs. 76.6 and 76.8), but fluid-filled bowel loops may have a similar appearance. MRI with gadolinium-complex contrast agents is more sensitive for the detection of vascular tumors than is CT with standard intravenous iodinated contrast agents and may therefore permit detection of lesions that cannot be identified on CT (53, 54). On these MR images, pancreatic endocrine tumors may appear very bright (high signal intensity), depending on the pulse sequence used (Fig. 76.8).

MRI of the pancreas has been difficult to perform and to interpret because of inherent motion artifacts caused by respiration, cardiac motion, and peristalsis in adjacent bowel (55). Motion artifacts can be overcome by breath-holding techniques and by the use of fat-suppression pulse sequences (56).

In some small series, insulinomas have been localized with a sensitivity of 100% using T1- and T2-weighted spin-echo pulse sequences (Fig. 76.6) (55). Other, larger series have suggested that it is not a useful modality, except for relatively large primary tumors (13, 15, 57). MRI is likely to become more important for localization of islet cell tumors, but its role is not yet established. When appropriate pulse sequences are used, it is at least as good as CT and ultrasound for the detection of hepatic metastases in patients with pancreatic endocrine tumors (15, 29, 58).

**Somatostatin Receptor Scintigraphy.** Somatostatin receptor scintigraphy was introduced in the late 1980s (59). Iodine-123-Tyr-3-octreotide was initially used as the radiopharmaceutical, but a number of different somatostatin analogues and isotopes have since been developed (59, 60). Currently, indium-111-TPA-*D*-Phe-octreotide (Octreoscan 111, Mallinckrodt Diagnostica, Petten, the Netherlands) is probably the most commonly used agent. Somatostatin receptor scintigraphy is a functional technique in that the lesions are not imaged directly. Theoretically, its sensitivity for the detection of pancreatic endocrine tumors should be independent of tumor size and depend only on tumor expression, cellular concentration, and total number of somatostatin receptors (61). Unfortunately, this means that tumors with a low somatostatin receptor density, whether large or small, will not be imaged (62). There is also

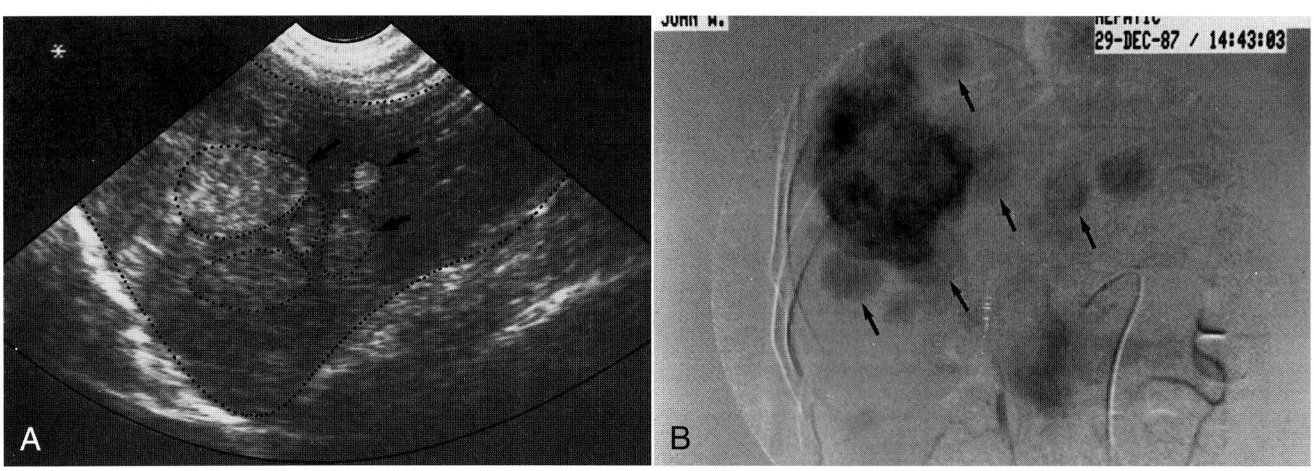


**FIG. 76.4.** Hepatic metastases in a 38-year-old man with metastatic glucagonoma. **A.** Transabdominal ultrasound demonstrates several hyperechoic masses of different sizes *(arrows)* within the liver. **B.** These lesions correspond to the hypervascular masses seen on the late phase of a hepatic arteriogram, several of which are indicated by *arrows.*

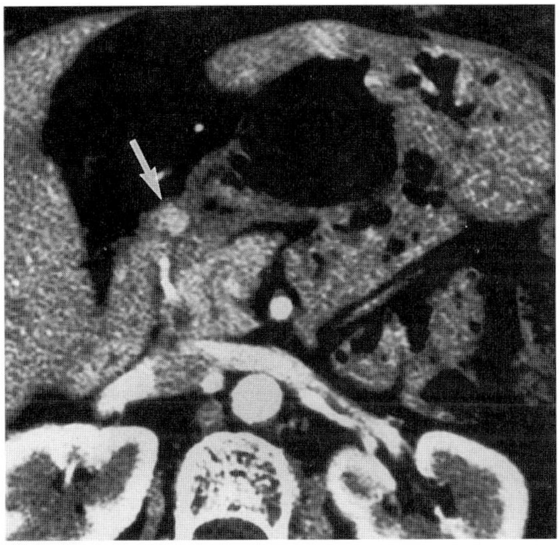

**FIG. 76.5.** Extrapancreatic gastrinoma in a 51-year-old woman with Zollinger-Ellison syndrome. A well-circumscribed area of nodular enhancement *(arrow)* is seen on the late arterial phase of this helical CT. At surgery, a 6-mm juxtaduodenal gastrinoma was identified at this site.

evidence that small tumors are less likely to be detected by somatostatin receptor scintigraphy than by other techniques, such as arteriography (13).

The technique is theoretically applicable to all tumors that express the somatostatin receptor. Most pancreatic endocrine tumors, including gastrinomas, express this receptor, but only 60–70% of insulinomas do (63–65). The sensitivity of somatostatin receptor scintigraphy for primary insulinomas is only 10–50% (66, 67). Insulinomas may be more readily detected with agents directed at vasoactive intestinal peptide receptors, although experience with these agents is currently very limited (68). Alternatively, agents may be directed at other somatostatin receptor subtypes; at least five have been described (59, 64, 66). Octreoscan 111 appears to have particular affinity for the somatostatin-2 subtype (59, 66).

For gastrinomas, sensitivities as high as 75–100% have been reported (66, 67, 69). Sensitivity for duodenal gastrinomas seems to be lower (approximately 50%) (69). The use of both planar and single photon emission computed tomography (SPECT) images is advisable to achieve these high sensitivities (Figs. 76.2 and 76.3). Even with SPECT, scintigraphic images do not provide the same precise anatomic localization as CT and ultrasound, although they may focus attention on an anatomic region (Fig. 76.3). Cross-sectional imaging studies such as ultrasound and CT may complement somatostatin receptor

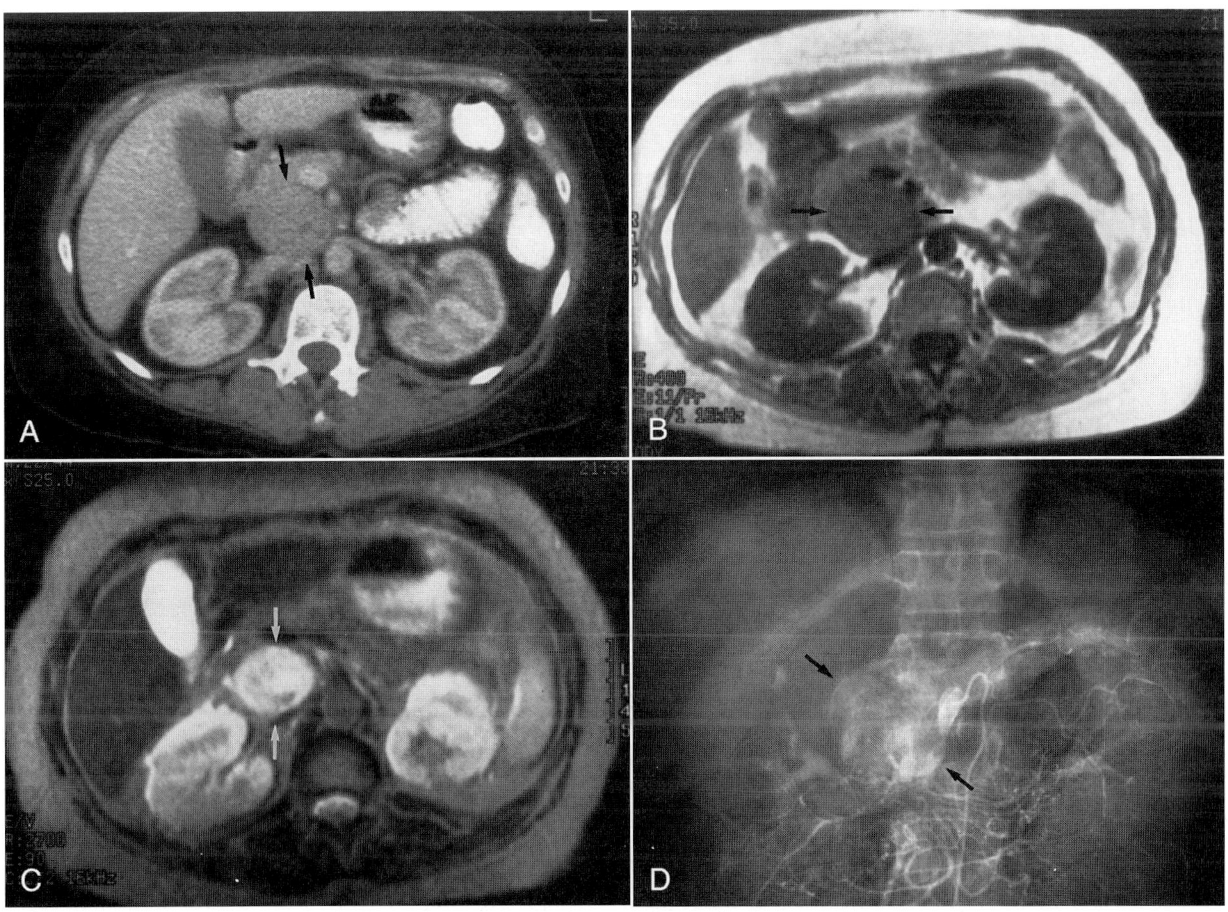


**FIG. 76.6.** Pancreatic head gastrinoma. This 50-year-old man had peptic ulcer disease refractory to medical management. **A.** Contrast-enhanced CT demonstrates a 3.5-cm minimally enhancing mass in the pancreatic head *(arrows)*. The lesion is nearly isodense to the normal pancreatic parenchyma. **B.** A T1-weighted spin-echo (TR 400, TE 11) MR image shows a mass with homogeneous low signal *(arrows)*. **C.** The lesion demonstrates high signal intensity on the T2-weighted (TR 2700, TE 90) spin-echo image *(arrows)*. **D.** During the early capillary phase of a superior mesenteric artery arteriogram, a hypervascular blush is present in the tumor *(arrows)*. A 3.5-cm gastrinoma was subsequently resected from the head of the pancreas.

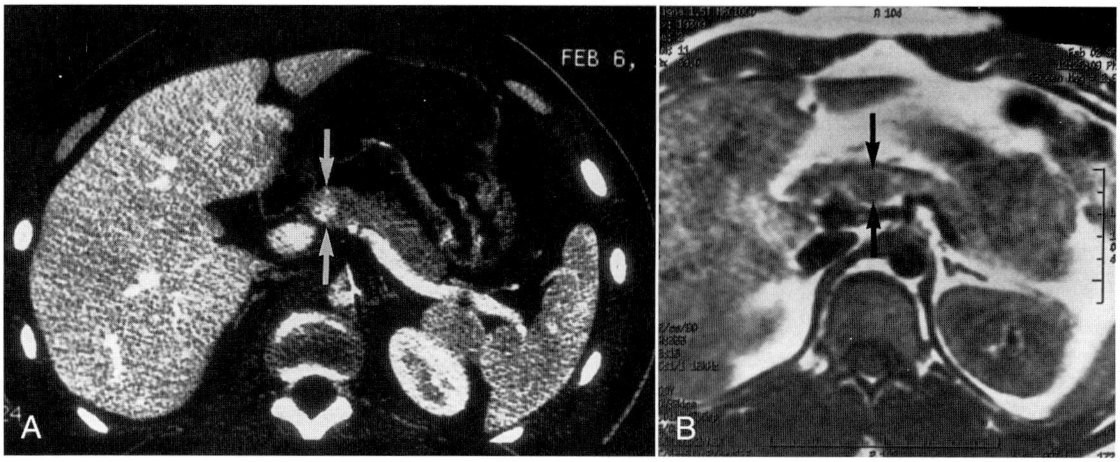

**FIG. 76.7.** Small intrapancreatic insulinoma. This 23-year-old man presented with seizures due to hypoglycemia. **A.** CT during selective arterial injection of contrast material into the celiac axis demonstrates a hypervascular mass in the neck of the pancreas *(arrows)*. **B.** This lesion was identified in retrospect as a focus of low signal intensity on T1-weighted spin-echo (TR 333, TE 16) MR *(arrow)*.

scintigraphy, since scintigraphy permits detection of some tumors missed by cross-sectional studies and vice versa (62, 70). Somatostatin receptor scintigraphy appears to be particularly valuable for the detection of metastatic disease from pancreatic endocrine tumors, especially for detection of metastases outside the liver (61, 63, 66, 71–73). These may be difficult to identify with other imaging modalities.

## Invasive Imaging Procedures

Invasive imaging procedures include endoscopic ultrasound, arteriography, arterial stimulation and venous sampling, portal venous sampling, and intraoperative ultrasound. Endoscopic ultrasound, arteriography, and intraoperative ultrasound are imaging studies that enable direct demonstration of the lesion. Arterial stimulation and venous sampling and portal venous sampling are functional imaging studies that allow determination of the presence of lesions on the basis of detection of elevated hormone levels in samples of venous blood.

**Endoscopic Ultrasound.** With endoscopic ultrasound, the ultrasound transducer may be placed much closer to the pancreas than is possible with conventional ultrasound. A water-filled balloon at the tip of the endoscope acts as an acoustic window for ultrasound beam transmission. The duodenum and pancreatic head are examined with the endoscope in the duodenum, while the remainder of the pancreas is examined through the posterior wall of the stomach. Body habitus and intestinal gas do not hamper visualization of the pancreas, as they do with conventional ultrasound. The technique has no value for the detection of liver metastases.

Small islet cell tumors have a characteristic appearance (Fig. 76.9) (74–76). They are hypoechoic with respect to the pancreas. A central echogenic focus, either regular or irregular, may be present. Echogenic foci may be due to necrosis, hyalinosis, calcification, microcysts, or a disorderly arrangement of tumor cells and stroma (74). A regular echogenic focus has been reported only in benign lesions (74, 75). Small islet cell tumors demonstrate clearly defined, smooth or slightly irregular mar-

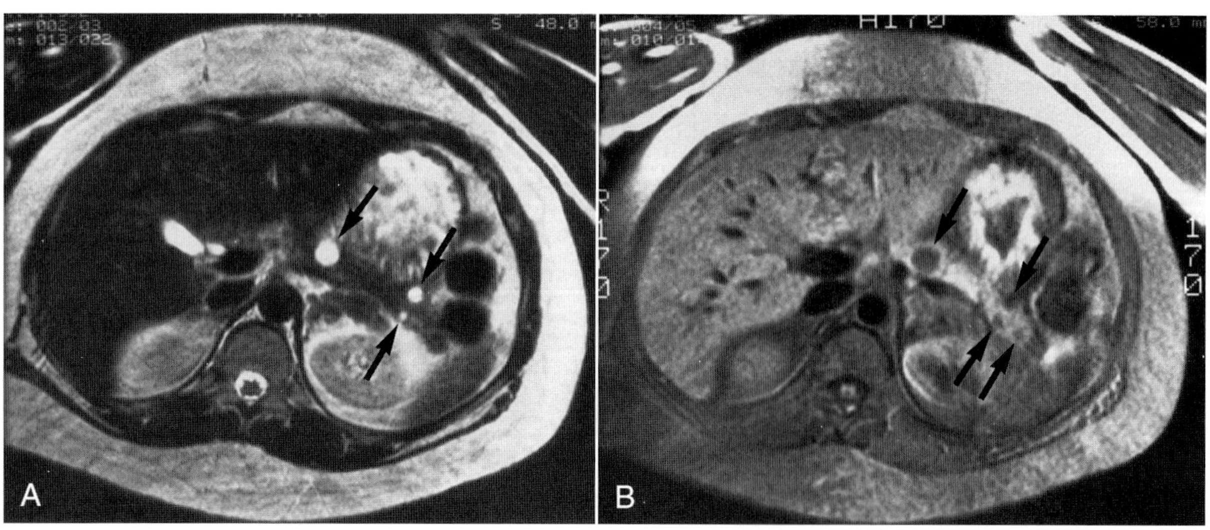

**FIG. 76.8.** Multiple islet cell tumors; 29-year-old woman with multiple endocrine neoplasia syndrome, type 1 (MEN I) and Zollinger-Ellison syndrome. **A.** Several high signal intensity masses are seen within the pancreas on a T2-weighted spin-echo (TR 7000, TE 102) MR image *(arrows)*. **B.** The lesions *(arrows)* demonstrate peripheral enhancement on this fat-saturated T1-weighted spin-echo (TR 500, TE 11) MR image obtained after intravenous administration of a gadolinium-complex contrast agent.

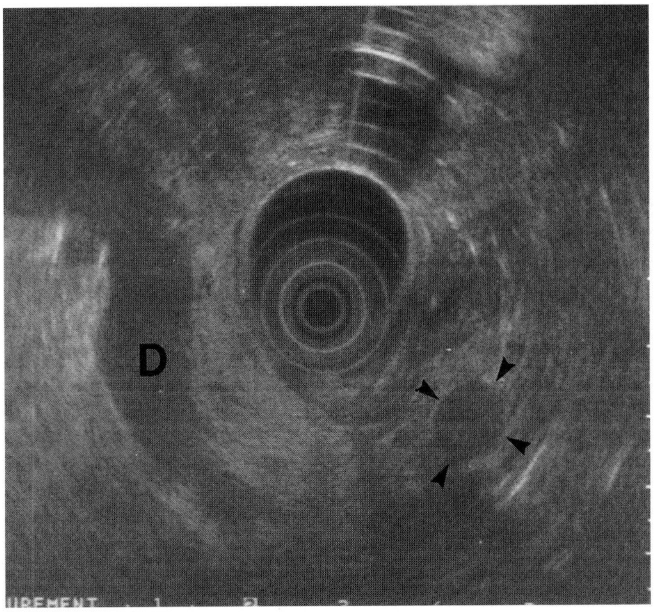


**FIG. 76.9.** Intrapancreatic insulinoma in a 65-year-old man with episodic hypoglycemia, lightheadedness, and agitation. Endoscopic ultrasound demonstrates a smoothly marginated hyperechoic mass *(arrowheads)* within the pancreas. At surgery, this was a 1-cm pancreatic head lesion. The distal common bile duct *(D)* is also clearly visible.

gins. In larger tumors, an irregular tumor margin is a reliable sign of malignancy, but in tumors smaller than 2 cm, partially irregular borders may be seen in benign lesions (74, 75).

Endoscopic ultrasound permits detection of lesions as small as 5 mm in the pancreas and 6 mm in the duodenal wall (77). It is more sensitive than either CT or conventional ultrasound for the detection of primary pancreatic endocrine tumors. In one series, conventional ultrasound and endoscopic ultrasound were compared in 20 patients with pancreatic endocrine tumors. Endoscopic ultrasound permitted detection of all 11 tumors smaller than 2 cm, but conventional ultrasound permitted detection of only 9 (74). In another series of 13 patients with pancreatic endocrine tumors, endoscopic ultrasound permitted localization of the primary tumor in 10 of 13 patients (77%), CT enabled localization in 2 of 13 patients (15%), and arteriography was successful in 2 of 8 patients (25%) (77). Overall, reported sensitivities for localization of intrapancreatic endocrine tumors with endoscopic ultrasound range from 75% to 94% (36, 54, 67, 74, 77–82).

Despite the high spatial resolution and sensitivity of endoscopic ultrasound, some lesions will not be detected. Pedunculated pancreatic tumors as large as 3 cm may be missed (81, 82). The proximal pancreatic tail, especially in the vicinity of the splenic hilum, is not as well visualized as the remainder of the pancreas because it is less closely apposed to the stomach. Tumors in this area of the pancreas are less likely to be detected (13, 78–80). In one series, the sensitivity of the technique for detection of duodenal wall lesions (50%) and lymph node lesions (63%) was lower than for pancreatic lesions (75%) (36). This makes endoscopic ultrasound less helpful for localization of gastrinomas, at least 30% of which are extrapancreatic, than for insulinomas, virtually all of which are intrapancreatic (10, 83, 84). Some authors believe that a negative endoscopic ultrasound examination in a patient with Zollinger-Ellison syndrome suggests that the tumor is extrapancreatic (82).

Endoscopic ultrasound has several disadvantages. First, a special expensive endoscope is required, which cannot be used for routine endoscopy because the optical system is compromised by the incorporation of the ultrasound transducer. Second, intravenous sedation is required, as for all gastrointestinal endoscopy. This entails the additional expense of monitoring equipment, nursing support, and postendoscopy recovery. Third, endoscopy is an invasive procedure that entails risk to the patient, both from the endoscopy and from conscious sedation. Finally, as with all ultrasound procedures, the sensitivity and accuracy of the technique are highly operator dependent.

**Arteriography.** Arteriography, once the mainstay of localization techniques, has been largely supplanted as the initial technique for tumor detection by newer, less invasive modalities. It still remains valuable, however, particularly for localization of gastrinomas and in conjunction with arterial stimulation and venous sampling (discussed below) (10, 34, 85). The smallest lesion that can be visualized by arteriography is about 5 mm, versus at least 7 mm for CT and conventional ultrasound, and 5–6 mm for endoscopic ultrasound (1, 77). Pancreatic endocrine tumors and their metastases appear as foci of homogeneous staining during the capillary phase (Figs. 76.4 and 76.10) (10, 85). Neither neovascularity nor arteriovenous shunting is demonstrable in small lesions, but tumors larger than 2 cm may demonstrate abnormal vessels and prominent draining veins (Fig. 76.6). Rarely, islet cell tumors may be hypovascular (43, 44). Arteriography should include selective superior mesenteric, gastroduodenal, splenic, and dorsal pancreatic arteriograms. Selective hepatic arteriography should be performed as well, to search for liver metastases (Fig. 76.4). Arteriography is capable of demonstrating hypervascular hepatic metastases smaller than 5 mm in diameter (28).

The reported sensitivity of arteriography for localization of primary islet cell tumors has fallen in recent years (10). Older studies report a sensitivity of about 65%, but more recent studies suggest that fewer than half of these tumors are detected arteriographically (35, 86). This is probably due in part to earlier detection and in part to referral bias. On the other hand, the false-positive rate is generally reported as less than 10%. The sensitivity of arteriography for locating primary tumors is superior to that of CT, MRI, or ultrasound when all four modalities are compared in the same patient population (10, 15, 49, 87, 88).

**Arterial Stimulation and Venous Sampling.** Arterial stimulation and venous sampling (ASVS), also known (for gastrinomas) as selective arterial secretin injection, is an adjunct to arteriography performed as part of the arteriographic procedure. It was first described in 1987 by Imamura et al. as a method for gastrinoma localization (89). Via a femoral vein puncture, a catheter is placed with its tip in the right hepatic vein. A secretagogue (secretin is used to stimulate production of gastrin by gastrinomas) is injected through the arterial catheter selectively into an artery that supplies the pancreas or the liver. Secretin stimulates gastrin release from gastrinomas by modulating adenylate cyclase activation (90). Blood samples are drawn from the hepatic vein catheter before and at intervals (typically 30 and 60 seconds or 20, 40, and 60 seconds) after the secretagogue injection. Gastrin concentration in these samples reflects hormone output from the gastrinoma. If the gastrin concentration in the hepatic vein samples increases after secretagogue injection, the tumor must lie in the area supplied by the injected artery (Fig. 76.11).

The technique has been refined (86, 91, 92). Thirty IU of secretin is injected intraarterially into each artery, and a 10-minute interval is allowed between secretin injections (86, 92). Secretagogue injections are made into the gastroduodenal artery, the splenic artery, the superior mesenteric artery, and the hepatic artery. (The hepatic artery injection is used to evaluate the liver for metastases.) An increase in hormone concentration of more than 50% at 30 seconds or more than 100% at 60 seconds after secretagogue injection is a positive response according to criteria developed at the NIH (92). Imamura considers an increase in gastrin of more than 80 pg/mL and more than 20% of the baseline value at 40 seconds postinjection to be a positive result (91, 93). Reported sensitivities range from 77 to 100%, with a false-positive rate near 0% (10, 86, 91, 92). The technique is particularly sensitive for the detection of duodenal gastrinomas. It was positive in all 18 patients with duodenal gastrinomas in the NIH series (92).

Doppman and colleagues have extended ASVS to localization of insulinomas as well as gastrinomas, using calcium as the secretagogue (88, 94, 95). An intravenous infusion of calcium stimulates insulin secretion by insulinomas, and Brunt et al. have shown that rapid calcium infusions are more effective than slow calcium infusions (96). Calcium gluconate, between 0.01 and 0.025 mEq $Ca^{2+}$/kg, depending on the patient's weight, is injected in the same fashion as is used for secretin. Hepatic venous blood is sampled and then assayed for insulin. An increase in insulin concentration within 1 minute of calcium injection of at least 100% of the baseline value is considered a positive result (Fig. 76.12) (88). In a series of 25 patients, the sensitivity of the procedure was 88% for localization of insulinomas, with a 12% incorrect localization rate (88).

The major drawback of ASVS is that the information it provides only serves to demarcate a region (a specific arterial territory) in which the lesion must lie, rather than providing the more precise anatomic location that may be gained from imaging studies. It cannot provide localization information any more precise than this. All that may be concluded from an ASVS study is that the tumor lies in the region of the pancreatic head/proximal duodenum or the body/tail of the pancreas. It is not possible to distinguish between a lesion in the head of the pancreas and one in the duodenum or a peripancreatic lymph node. This is a direct result of the functional nature of the test—the lesion is never imaged, unless by the accompanying arteriographic procedure.

The two advantages of ASVS also result from the functional nature of the procedure. First, sensitivity is independent of lesion size, since lesion detection is based on hormone output alone. Second, the technique permits a tissue- and hormone-specific diagnosis. Only ASVS and portal venous sampling (discussed below) can permit differentiation between a functioning and a nonfunctioning islet cell tumor (17). This information is valuable in patients with multiple endocrine neoplasia. These patients may have multiple pancreatic endocrine tumors, of which only one or two are responsible for the clinical syndrome of hormone excess. The lesion producing the clinical endocrine disorder may not be the largest or most obvious on imaging studies. In rare cases of adult nesidioblastosis, venous sampling–based techniques may be the only modalities capable of demonstrating involvement of the entire pancreas (73, 97, 98).

Precise, accurate timing, both for injection of the secretagogue and for sampling hepatic venous blood, is required if accurate results are to be obtained from ASVS. Nonetheless, the procedure itself is no more difficult than visceral arteriography of the liver and pancreas. It is well within the capabilities of any competent interventional radiologist.

Ko and colleagues have suggested intraarterial injection of methylene blue as a means of locating pancreatic endocrine tumors at surgery (12, 99). On the morning of surgery, a catheter is placed in the artery previously identified by ASVS as supplying the tumor. At laparotomy, 2 mL of methylene blue is rapidly injected through the catheter. In their small series of patients, the entire arterial territory immediately stained blue, but the dye was cleared from normal tissues in about 2 minutes, while the islet cell tumor retained the dye for about 15 minutes.

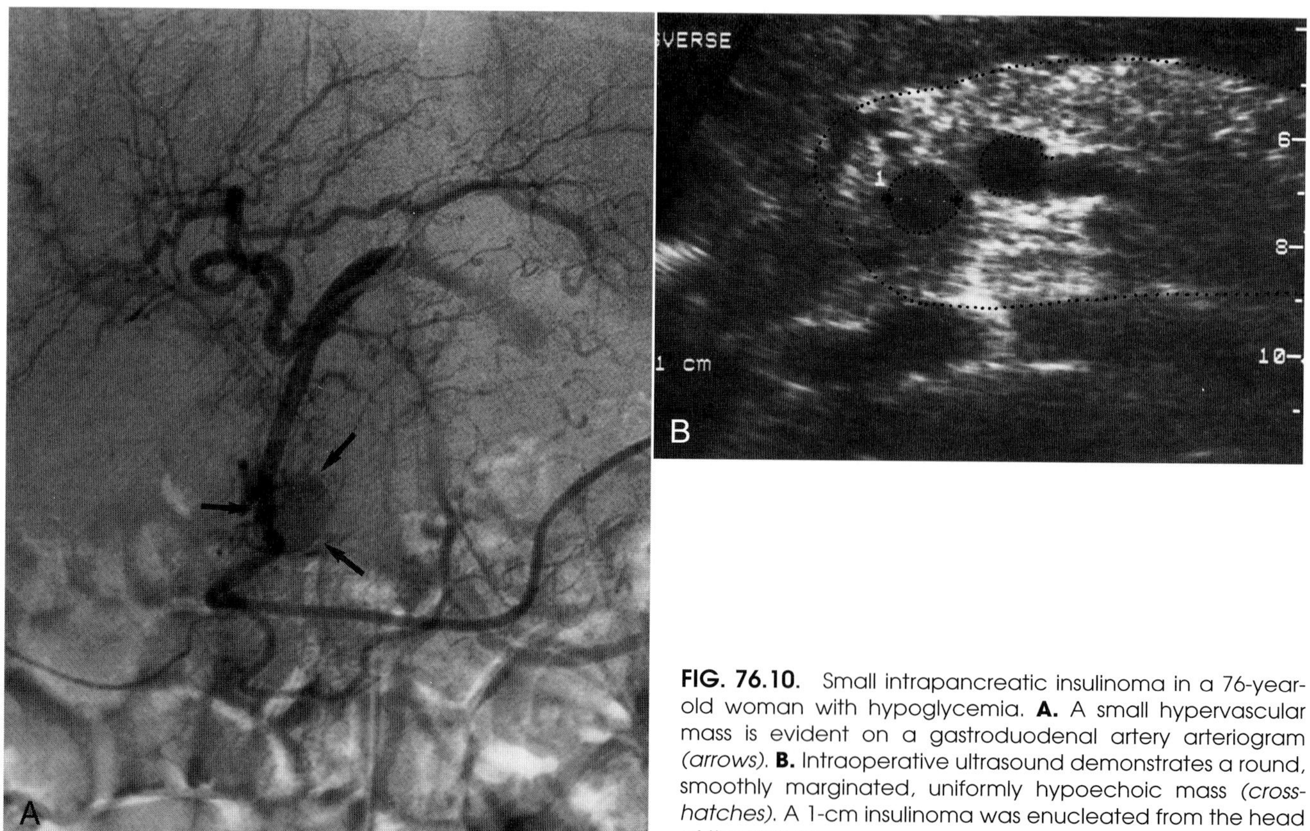


**FIG. 76.10.** Small intrapancreatic insulinoma in a 76-year-old woman with hypoglycemia. **A.** A small hypervascular mass is evident on a gastroduodenal artery arteriogram *(arrows)*. **B.** Intraoperative ultrasound demonstrates a round, smoothly marginated, uniformly hypoechoic mass *(cross-hatches)*. A 1-cm insulinoma was enucleated from the head of the pancreas.

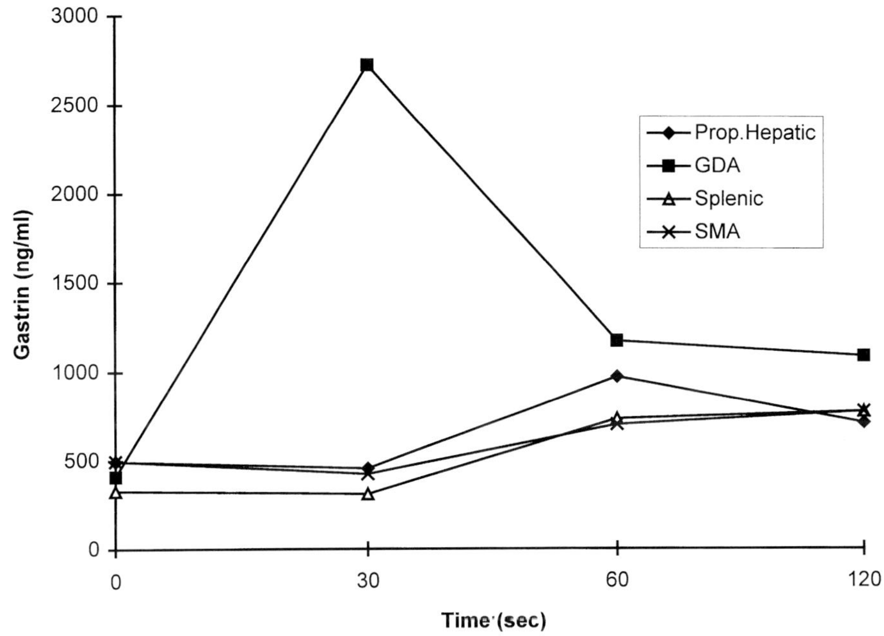


**FIG. 76.11** Results of arterial stimulation and venous sampling in an 86-year-old man with Zollinger-Ellison syndrome. Each line represents gastrin levels in the right hepatic vein after arterial injection of 30 IU of secretin into one of the listed visceral arteries (*Prop. hepatic*, proper hepatic artery; *GDA*, gastroduodenal artery; *Splenic*, splenic artery; *SMA*, superior mesenteric artery). The rapid rise in hepatic vein gastrin levels after stimulation of the gastroduodenal artery with secretin indicates that the tumor lies in the territory supplied by this artery. The gastroduodenal artery arteriogram was negative. At surgery, a 5-mm tumor was removed from the second portion of the duodenum.

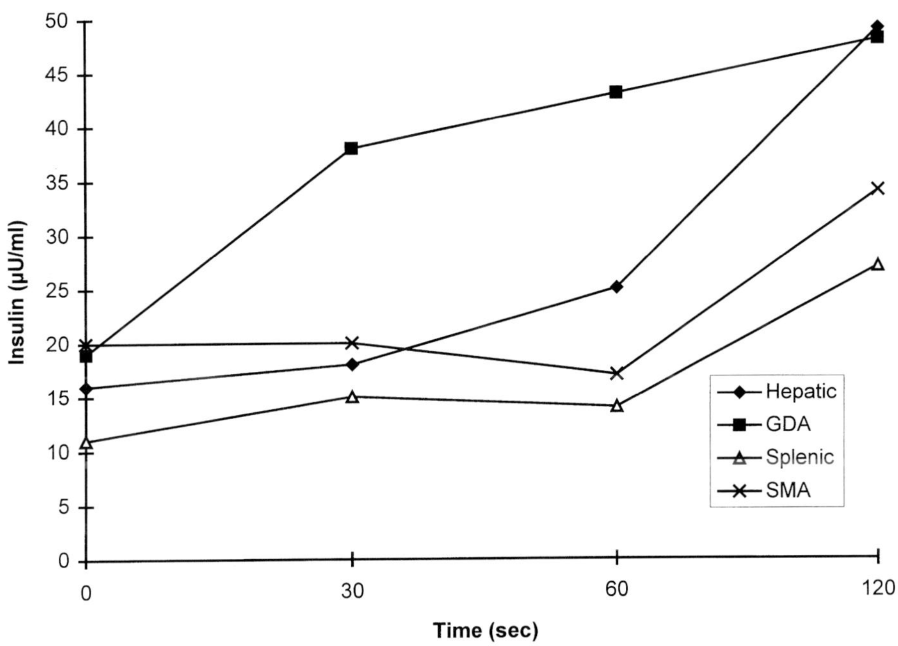


**FIG. 76.12.** Results of arterial stimulation and venous sampling in a 24-year-old man with an insulinoma. Calcium gluconate was used as the secretagogue. (*Hepatic*, proper hepatic artery; *GDA*, gastroduodenal artery; *Splenic*, splenic artery; *SMA*, superior mesenteric artery). Elevations in hepatic vein insulin levels occurring 60 seconds or later after calcium injection are due to systemic recirculation of the secretagogue and have no localizing value. The results of the procedure in this patient indicate that the tumor lies in the arterial territory of the gastroduodenal artery. A hypervascular lesion was identified on the gastroduodenal arteriogram, and a 1.2-cm insulinoma was subsequently resected from the head of the pancreas.

**Portal Venous Sampling.** Portal venous sampling, an older technique than ASVS, requires percutaneous transhepatic catheterization of the portal vein and selective sampling of branches of the portal venous system, including the pancreatic venous arcade (10, 12, 13, 85, 88, 100). The blood samples with the highest concentration of hormone are presumed to come from the veins draining the tumor most directly. The lesion is presumed to lie in the territory drained by these veins. Sampling is sometimes limited to the superior mesenteric, splenic, and portal veins, in part because these are the easiest vessels to catheterize. However, failure to sample the pancreatic venous arcade and the small pancreatic branches of the splenic vein may result in incorrect localization because of streaming of blood flow in the splenic, superior mesenteric, and portal veins (100, 101). As with ASVS, portal venous sampling is a functional localization technique, not an imaging study.

Portal venous sampling is far more difficult technically than ASVS, is riskier, involves greater radiation exposure, and must be performed as a separate procedure from arteriography, which makes it more expensive as well (100). In direct comparisons between portal venous sampling and ASVS in the same groups of patients, ASVS was both more sensitive and more accurate for the detection of gastrinomas (86, 92) and insulinomas (88). For all these reasons, portal venous sampling is now used less frequently than in the past (17).

## INTRAOPERATIVE ULTRASOUND

Intraoperative ultrasound is probably the single most valuable technique for locating pancreatic endocrine tumors, but by its very nature, it cannot be considered a preoperative localizing procedure. It is most accurately thought of as an aid to surgical palpation. Most experienced endocrine surgeons consider intraoperative ultrasound an essential component of surgical exploration of the pancreas in patients with islet cell tumors (12, 16, 102–104).

Since the pancreas is completely exposed and accessible at laparotomy, the entire gland may be examined easily. There is no interference from gas or bone in the sound path. High frequency (7.5 or 10 mHz) transducers are used, providing the highest spatial resolution of any imaging modality. Lesions as small as 3 mm may be detected (10, 13). Islet cell tumors have the same appearance on intraoperative ultrasound as on endoscopic ultrasound (Figs. 76.2, 76.9, and 76.10).

Intraoperative ultrasound is more sensitive for intrapancreatic tumors than for extrapancreatic tumors (105, 106). In one study, the technique had a sensitivity of 93% for intrapancreatic gastrinomas and insulinomas but only 58% for extrapancreatic gastrinomas (105). It is therefore more helpful for localization of insulinomas than for gastrinomas. The sensitivity of intraoperative ultrasound for localization of insulinomas ranges from 75 to 100% in most series, and false-positive results are uncommon (18–20, 26, 105–108). Series comparing intraoperative ultrasound with preoperative imaging methods (CT, ultrasound, arteriography) for localization of insulinomas show it to be the most sensitive examination (18, 20, 26, 107).

Intrapancreatic gastrinomas can be localized by intraoperative ultrasound with the same 90–100% sensitivity obtainable for insulinomas, but the false-positive rate is much higher (26% in a series by Norton et al. (105)). For extrapancreatic gastrinomas, the sensitivity of intraoperative ultrasound is only 50–60%, and the false-positive rate is 28% (105). Ectopic pancreas, scar tissue, and lymph nodes are common causes of false-positive localizations (105). Small, duodenal gastrinomas are infrequently detected. In a study of 35 consecutive patients with suspected duodenal gastrinomas, intraoperative ultrasound had a specificity of 100% but a sensitivity of only 26% for identification of duodenal lesions. All duodenal tumors identified by intraoperative ultrasound were also detected by palpation alone, which had a sensitivity of 67% (109).

In addition to localization of the primary tumor, intraoperative ultrasound also provides valuable information about the anatomic relationships of the tumor to the pancreatic duct and adjacent blood vessels. It may also be used to identify hepatic metastases, especially deeply situated lesions that do not deform the liver capsule and are not easily palpated.

## LOCALIZATION

Radiologic localization procedures are used only after a definite diagnosis of an endocrine disorder. If localization is attempted in the absence of endocrine disease, unacceptably high false-positive rates may be expected. It is not the radiologist's function to establish or confirm the diagnosis, since demonstration of a tumor is not required to diagnose hormone excess.

Preoperative localization efforts are directed to answering two basic questions: has the tumor metastasized to such an extent that surgery is inappropriate? and, for patients in whom surgery is indicated, what is the precise location of the tumor (103)? There is disagreement about how aggressively the answer to the second question should be sought.

For reoperations in patients with gastrinomas or insulinomas, there is general agreement that extensive localization efforts are appropriate. Most surgeons also believe that patients undergoing an initial exploration for gastrinoma, in up to 50% of whom no primary tumor can be identified preoperatively (104), also deserve intensive attempts at localization (12, 13, 16, 17, 34, 73, 103, 104).

There is no consensus, however, on the value of preoperative localization in patients undergoing an initial exploration for insulinoma. In these patients, since the cure rate approaches 100% with the use of intraoperative ultrasound and palpation, some surgeons believe that only one noninvasive imaging modality, usually ultrasound, is needed prior to surgery. It is used only to screen for hepatic metastases. Intraoperative ultrasound is the only imaging technique used to identify the primary tumor (14, 29, 108, 110). Van Heerden, a proponent of this approach, has stated that "extensive preoperative radiologic investigation is neither indicated nor cost effective" in these patients (110).

Other, equally experienced surgeons feel that preoperative localization procedures are essential in patients with insulinomas (12, 13, 19, 111, 112). Some of this variation may be due to the relative expertise of the radiologists at the various institutions, and some is undoubtedly due to differences in surgical philosophy. Certainly, for less experienced surgeons, preoperative localization is likely to contribute significantly to a successful operation. However, the less experienced the radiologist, the less likely it is that these studies will offer anything of value. In particular, false-positive results may cause considerable confusion.

If preoperative localization is performed, what tests should be done? A general algorithm can be suggested, but it is subject to modification depending on the capabilities of the radiologist and surgeon at each individual institution (10, 13, 34). Noninvasive cross-sectional imaging studies (CT, ultrasound, MRI) are usually adequate to evaluate the abdomen for metastatic disease and answer the first question posed above. These studies may also identify the primary tumor and thereby answer the second question, but their likelihood of success for this purpose is lower than for identification of metastatic disease. Ultrasound is the least expensive of these three examinations, but CT is less operator dependent and is probably more sensitive. MRI is the most expensive of the three examinations, and its value for locating primary tumors is not yet established.

CT is the most frequently recommended procedure for initial screening for metastatic disease and for localization, either alone (12, 33, 73, 113), in combination with ultrasound (13, 16, 34) or MRI (17, 103), or with both ultrasound and MRI (104). It should be performed first. If metastases are present, somatostatin receptor scintigraphy may be helpful in further staging the disease and determining whether the tumor expresses somatostatin receptors (17, 73).

Patients who are deemed surgical candidates and in whom cross-sectional imaging studies have not identified a primary tumor, should next undergo either arteriography with ASVS (12, 13, 34, 73, 103, 104, 113) or endoscopic ultrasound (13, 16, 17, 34, 113), depending on the availability of suitable equipment and experienced operators. Somatostatin receptor scintigraphy is helpful for localization of gastrinomas (16, 17, 34, 113). Some authors continue to recommend portal venous sampling as a "last-ditch" localization procedure if all other studies are negative (34, 73, 104). Intraoperative ultrasound is essential during surgery (12, 13, 17, 34, 103, 104).

## CONCLUSION

The wide variety of localization procedures in use at present and the constant development of new techniques underscore the limitations of current methods for preoperative localization of small islet cell tumors. The ideal technique—noninvasive, sensitive, specific, safe, and inexpensive—does not exist. Available methods all have strengths and weaknesses. Since different surgeons have their own personal preferences and many procedures depend for their success on the radiologist's or endoscopist's skill and experience, no one sequence of localization procedures is appropriate for all patients at all times. Just as the patient must rely on the surgeon for the best possible treatment, the surgeon must rely on an experienced radiologist to provide the best possible opportunity for preoperative localization of these often elusive tumors.

## REFERENCES


1. Günther RW, Klose KJ, Rückert K, Beyer J, Kuhn FP, Klotter HJ. Localization of small islet-cell tumors. Preoperative and intraoperative ultrasound, computed tomography, arteriography, digital subtraction angiography, and pancreatic venous sampling. Gastrointest Radiol 1985;10:145–152.
2. Fugazzola C, Procacci C, Bergamo Andreis IA, et al. The contribution of ultrasonography and computed tomography in the diagnosis of nonfunctioning islet cell tumors of the pancreas. Gastrointest Radiol 1990;15:139–144.
3. Buetow PC, Parrino TV, Buck JL, et al. Islet cell tumors of the pancreas: pathologic-imaging correlation among size, necrosis and cysts, calcification, malignant behavior, and functional status. AJR 1995;165:1175–1179.
4. Marrano D, Campione O, Santini D, Piva P, Alberghini M, Casadei R. Cystic insulinoma: a rare islet cell tumour of the pancreas. Eur J Surg 1994;160:519–522.
5. Talamini MA, Pitt HA, Hruban RH, Boitnott JK, Coleman J, Cameron JL. Spectrum of cystic tumors of the pancreas. Am J Surg 1992;163:117–124.
6. Thompson NW, Eckhauser FE, Vinik AI, Lloyd RV, Fiddian-Green RG, Strodel WE. Cystic neuroendocrine neoplasms of the pancreas and liver. Ann Surg 1984;199:158–164.
7. Warshaw AL, Compton CC, Lewandrowski K, Cardenosa G, Mueller PR. Cystic tumors of the pancreas. New clinical, radiologic, and pathologic observations in 67 patients. Ann Surg 1990;212:432–445.
8. Ros PR, Hamrick-Turner JE, Chiechi MV, Ros LH, Gallego P, Burton SS. Cystic masses of the pancreas. Radiographics 1992;12: 673–686.
9. Schwartz RW, Munfakh NA, Zweng TN, Strodel WE, Lee E, Thompson NW. Nonfunctioning cystic neuroendocrine neoplasms of the pancreas. Surgery 1994;115:645–649.
10. Miller DL. Islet cell tumors of the pancreas: diagnosis and localization. In: Freeny PC, Stevenson GW, eds. Margulis and Burhenne's alimentary tract radiology. 5th ed. Hanover: CV Mosby, 1994:1167–1196.
11. Päivänsalo M, Mäkäräinen H, Siniluoto T, Ståhlberg M, Jalovaara P. Ultrasound compared with computed tomography and pancreatic arteriography in the detection of endocrine tumours of the pancreas. Eur J Radiol 1989;9:173–178.
12. Fedorak IJ, Ko TC, Gordon D, Flisak M, Prinz RA. Localization of islet cell tumors of the pancreas: a review of current techniques. Surgery 1993;113:242–249.
13. Hammond PJ, Jackson JA, Bloom SR. Localization of pancreatic endocrine tumours. Clin Endocrinol 1994;40:3–14.
14. Rothmund M. Localization of endocrine pancreatic tumours. Br J Surg 1994;81:164–166.
15. Pisegna JR, Doppman JL, Norton JA, Metz DC, Jensen RT. Prospective comparative study of ability of MR imaging and other imaging modalities to localize tumors in patients with Zollinger-Ellison syndrome. Dig Dis Sci 1993;38:1318–1328.
16. Bonnaud G, Cadiot G, Mignon M, Groupe de Recherches et d'Études du Syndrome de Zollinger-Ellison (GRESZE). Stratégie diagnostique et thérapeutique du syndrome de Zollinger-Ellison. Ann Chir 1994;48:535–546.
17. Orbuch M, Doppman JL, Jensen RT. Localization of pancreatic endocrine tumors. Semin Gastrointest Dis 1995;6:90–101.
18. Grant CS, van Heerden J, Charboneau JW, James EM, Reading CC. Insulinoma: the value of intraoperative ultrasonography. Arch Surg 1988;123:843–848.
19. Böttger TC, Weber W, Beyer J, Junginger T. Value of tumor localization in patients with insulinoma. World J Surg 1990;14: 107–112.
20. Galiber AK, Reading CC, Charboneau JW, et al. Localization of pancreatic insulinoma: comparison of pre- and intraoperative US with CT and angiography. Radiology 1988;166:405–408.
21. Gorman B, Charboneau JW, James EM, et al. Benign pancreatic insulinoma: preoperative and intraoperative sonographic localization. AJR 1986;147:929–934.
22. Böttger T, Weber W, Beyer J, Junginger T. Wertigkeit der Lokalisationsdiagnostik beim Insulinom. Med Klin 1989;84: 415–420.
23. Katz LB, Aufses AH Jr, Rayfield E, Mitty H. Preoperative localization and intraoperative glucose monitoring in the management of patients with pancreatic insulinoma. Surg Gynecol Obstet 1986;163:509–512.
24. Osei K, Falko JM. Clinical features, diagnosis and management of insulinoma in 16 consecutive patients: cost-ineffectiveness of non-invasive imaging modalities. Ohio State Med J 1984;80: 864–869.
25. Proye C, Boissel P. Preoperative imaging versus intraoperative localization of tumors in adult surgical patients with hyperinsulinemia: a multicenter study of 338 patients. World J Surg 1988;12:685–690.
26. Gianello P, Gigot JF, Berthet F, et al. Pre- and intraoperative localization of insulinomas: report of 22 observations. World J Surg 1988;12:389–397.
27. London JF, Shawker TH, Doppman JL, et al. Zollinger-Ellison syndrome: prospective assessment of abdominal US in the localization of gastrinomas. Radiology 1991;178:763–767.
28. Andersson T, Eriksson B, Hemmingsson A, Lindgren PG, Öberg K. Angiography, computed tomography, magnetic resonance imaging and ultrasonography in detection of liver metastases from endocrine gastrointestinal tumours. Acta Radiol 1987;28: 535–539.
29. Wise SR, Johnson J, Sparks J, Carey LC, Ellison EC. Gastrinoma: the predictive value of preoperative localization. Surgery 1989; 106:1087–1093.
30. Eelkema EA, Stephens DH, Ward EM, Sheedy PF II. CT features of nonfunctioning islet cell carcinoma. AJR 1984;143:943–948.
31. Wolf EL, Sprayregen S, Frager D, Rifkin H, Gliedman ML. Calcification in an insulinoma of the pancreas. Am J Gastroenterol 1984;79:559–561.
32. Aspestrand F, Kolmannskog F, Jacobsen M. CT, MR imaging and angiography in pancreatic apudomas. Acta Radiol 1993;34: 468–473.

33. Yeo CJ, Wang BH, Anthone GJ, Cameron JL. Surgical experience with pancreatic islet-cell tumors. Arch Surg 1993;128:1143–1148.
34. King CM, Reznek RH, Dacie JE, Wass JA. Imaging islet cell tumours. Clin Radiol 1994;49:295–303.
35. Doppman JL, Shawker TH, Miller DL. Localization of islet cell tumors. Gastroenterol Clin North Am 1989;18:793–804.
36. Ruszniewski P, Amouyal P, Amouyal G, et al. Localization of gastrinomas by endoscopic ultrasonography in patients with Zollinger-Ellison syndrome. Surgery 1995;117:629–635.
37. Balthazar EJ, Chako AC. Computed tomography of pancreatic masses. Am J Gastroenterol 1990;85:343–349.
38. Heiken JP, Brink JA, Sagel SS. Helical CT: abdominal applications. Radiographics 1994;14:919–924.
39. Zeman RK, Zeiberg AS, Davros WJ, et al. Routine helical CT of the abdomen: image quality considerations. Radiology 1993;189: 395–400.
40. Van Hoe L, Gryspeerdt S, Marchal G, Baert AL, Mertens L. Helical CT for the preoperative localization of islet cell tumors of the pancreas: value of arterial and parenchymal phase images. AJR 1995;165:1437–1439.
41. Winter TC III, Freeny PC, Nghiem HV. Extrapancreatic gastrinoma localization: value of arterial-phase helical CT with water as an oral contrast agent. AJR 1996;166:51–52.
42. Tjon A, Tham RTO, Falke THM, Jansen JBMJ, Lamers CBHW. CT and MR imaging of advanced Zollinger-Ellison syndrome. J Comput Assist Tomogr 1989;13:821–828.
43. Fink IJ, Krudy AG, Shawker TH, Norton JA, Gorden P, Doppman JL. Demonstration of an angiographically hypovascular insulinoma with intraarterial dynamic CT. AJR 1985;144:555–556.
44. Smith TR, Koenigsberg M. Low-density insulinoma on dynamic CT. AJR 1990;155:995–996.
45. Ahlström H, Magnusson A, Grama D, Eriksson B, Öberg K, Lörelius L-E. Preoperative localization of endocrine pancreatic tumours by intra-arterial dynamic computed tomography. Acta Radiol 1990;31:171–175.
46. Bressler EL, Alpern MB, Glazer GM, Francis IR, Ensminger WD. Hypervascular hepatic metastases: CT evaluation. Radiology 1987;162:49–51.
47. Chomyn JJ, Stamm ER, Thickman D. CT of melanoma liver metastases: is the examination without contrast media superfluous? J Comput Assist Tomogr 1992;16:568–571.
48. Patten RM, Byun JY, Freeny PC. CT of hypervascular hepatic tumors: are unenhanced scans necessary for diagnosis? AJR 1993;161:979–984.
49. Frucht H, Doppman JL, Norton JA, et al. Gastrinomas: comparison of MR imaging with CT, angiography, and US. Radiology 1989;171:713–717.
50. Wank SA, Doppman JL, Miller DL, et al. Prospective study of the ability of computed axial tomography to localize gastrinomas in patients with Zollinger-Ellison syndrome. Gastroenterology 1987; 92:905–912.
51. Soyer P, Bluemke DA, Fishman EK. CT during arterial portography for the preoperative evaluation of hepatic tumors: how, when, and why? AJR 1994;163:1325–1331.
52. Little AF, Baron RL, Peterson MS, et al. Optimizing CT portography: a prospective comparison of injection into the splenic versus superior mesenteric artery. Radiology 1994;193:651–655.
53. Semelka RC, Cumming MJ, Shoenut JP, et al. Islet cell tumors: comparison of dynamic contrast-enhanced CT and MR imaging with dynamic gadolinium enhancement and fat suppression. Radiology 1993;186:799–802.
54. Müller MF, Meyenberger C, Bertschinger P, Schaer R, Marincek B. Pancreatic tumors: evaluation with endoscopic US, CT, and MR imaging. Radiology 1994;190:745–751.
55. Pavone P, Mitchell DG, Leonetti F, et al. Pancreatic ß-cell tumors: MRI. J Comput Assist Tomogr 1993;17:403–407.
56. Semelka RC, Ascher SM. MR imaging of the pancreas. Radiology 1993;188:593–602.
57. Carlson B, Johnson CD, Stephens DH, Ward EM, Kvols LK. MRI of pancreatic islet cell carcinoma. J Comput Assist Tomogr 1993; 17:735–740.
58. Larson RE, Semelka RC, Bagley AS, Molina PL, Brown ED, Lee JK. Hypervascular malignant liver lesions: comparison of various MR imaging pulse sequences and dynamic CT. Radiology 1994;192: 393–399.
59. Krenning EP, Kwekkeboom DJ, Bakker WH, et al. Somatostatin receptor scintigraphy with ($^{111}$In-DTPA-*D*-Phe$^1$)- and ($^{123}$I-Tyr$^3$)-octreotide: the Rotterdam experience with more than 1000 patients. Eur J Nucl Med 1993;20:716–731.
60. Ur E, Bomanji J, Mather SJ, et al. Localization of neuroendocrine tumours and insulinomas using radiolabelled somatostatin analogues, $^{123}$I-Tyr$^3$-octreotide and $^{111}$In-pentatreotide. Clin Endocrinol 1993;38:501–506.
61. Kvols LK, Brown ML, O'Connor MK, et al. Evaluation of a radiolabeled somatostatin analog (I-123 octreotide) in the detection and localization of carcinoid and islet cell tumors. Radiology 1993;187:129–133.
62. Scherübl H, Bäder M, Fett U, et al. Somatostatin-receptor imaging of neuroendocrine gastroenteropancreatic tumors. Gastroenterology 1993;105:1705–1709.
63. van Eyck CHJ, Bruining HA, Reubi J-C, et al. Use of isotope-labeled somatostatin analogs for visualization of islet cell tumors. World J Surg 1993;17:444–447.
64. Lamberts SWJ, Krenning EP, Reubi J-C. The role of somatostatin and its analogs in the diagnosis and treatment of tumors. Endocr Rev 1991;12:450–482.
65. Reubi JC, Kvols LK, Waser B, et al. Detection of somatostatin receptors in surgical and percutaneous needle biopsy samples of carcinoids and islet cell carcinomas. Cancer Res 1990;50: 5969–5977.
66. Modlin IM, Cornelius E, Lawton GP. Use of an isotopic somatostatin receptor probe to image gut endocrine tumors. Arch Surg 1995;130:367–374.
67. Zimmer T, Stölzel U, Liehr R-M, et al. Somatostatinrezeptor-Szintigraphie und endoskopischer Ultraschall zur Diagnostik von Insulinomen und Gastrinomen. Dtsch Med Wochenschr 1995; 120:87–93.
68. Virgolini L, Raderer M, Kurtaran A, et al. Vasoactive intestinal peptide-receptor imaging for the localization of intestinal adenocarcinomas and endocrine tumors. N Engl J Med 1994; 331:1116–1121.
69. Krenning EP, Kwekkeboom DJ, Oei HY, et al. Somatostatin receptor scintigraphy in carcinoids, gastrinomas and Cushing's syndrome. Digestion 1994;55(suppl 3):54–59.
70. Weinel RJ, Neuhaus C, Stapp J, et al. Preoperative localization of gastrointestinal endocrine tumors using somatostatin-receptor scintigraphy. Ann Surg 1993;218:640–645.
71. Hammond PJ, Arka A, Peters AM, Bloom SR, Gilbey SG. Localization of metastatic gastroenteropancreatic tumours by somatostatin receptor scintigraphy with ($^{111}$In-DTPA-D-Phe1)-octreotide. Q J Med 1994;87:83–88.
72. Kvols LK. Somatostatin-receptor imaging of human malignancies: a new era in the localization, staging, and treatment of tumors (Editorial). Gastroenterology 1993;105:1909–1911.
73. Perry RR, Vinik AI. Diagnosis and management of functioning islet cell tumors. J Clin Endocrinol Metab 1995;80:2273–2278.
74. Yamada M, Komoto E, Naito Y, Tsukamoto Y, Mitake M. Endoscopic ultrasonography in the diagnosis of pancreatic islet cell tumors. J Ultrasound Med 1991;10:271–276.
75. Hayashi Y, Nakazawa S, Kimoto E, Naito Y, Morita K. Clinicopathologic analysis of endoscopic ultrasonograms in pancreatic mass lesions. Endoscopy 1989;21:121–125.
76. Bolondi L, Li Bassi S, Gaiani S, Campione O, Marrano D, Barbara L. Diagnosis of islet cell tumor by means of endoscopic ultrasonography. J Clin Gastroenterol 1990;12:218–221.
77. Lightdale CJ, Botet JF, Woodruff JM, Brennan MF. Localization of endocrine tumors of the pancreas with endoscopic ultrasonography. Cancer 1991;68:1815–1820.
78. Palazzo L, Roseau G, Salmeron M. Endoscopic ultrasonography in the preoperative localization of pancreatic endocrine tumors. Endoscopy 1992;24(suppl 1):350–353.
79. Rösch T, Lightdale CJ, Botet JF, et al. Localization of pancreatic endocrine tumors by endoscopic ultrasonography. N Engl J Med 1992;326:1721–1726.
80. Glover JR, Shorvon PJ, Lees WR. Endoscopic ultrasound for localisation of islet cell tumours. Gut 1992;33:108–110.
81. Bansal R, Kochman ML, Bude R, et al. Localization of neuroendocrine tumors utilizing linear-array endoscopic ultrasonography. Gastrointest Endosc 1995;42:76–79.
82. Thompson NW, Czako PF, Fritts LL, et al. Role of endoscopic

ultrasonography in the localization of insulinomas and gastrinomas. Surgery 1994;116:1131–1138.
83. Service FJ. Hypoglycemic disorders. N Engl J Med 1995;332: 1144–1152.
84. Howard TJ, Stabile BE, Zinner MJ, Chang S, Bhagavan BS, Passaro E Jr. Anatomic distribution of pancreatic endocrine tumors. Am J Surg 1990;159:258–264.
85. Miller DL. Endocrine angiography and venous sampling. Radiol Clin North Am 1993;31:1051–1067.
86. Doppman JL, Miller DL, Chang R, et al. Gastrinomas: localization by means of selective intraarterial injection of secretin. Radiology 1990;174:25–29.
87. Maton PN, Miller DL, Doppman JL, et al. Role of selective angiography in the management of patients with Zollinger-Ellison syndrome. Gastroenterology 1987;92:913–918.
88. Doppman JL, Chang R, Fraker DL, et al. Localization of insulinomas to regions of the pancreas by intra-arterial stimulation with calcium. Ann Intern Med 1995;123:269–273.
89. Imamura M, Takahashi K, Adachi H, et al. Usefulness of selective arterial secretin injection test for localization of gastrinoma in the Zollinger-Ellison syndrome. Ann Surg 1987;205:230–239.
90. Chiba T, Yamatani T, Yamaguchi A, et al. Mechanism for increase of gastrin release by secretin in Zollinger-Ellison syndrome. Gastroenterology 1989;96:1439–1444.
91. Imamura M, Takahashi K. Use of selective arterial secretin injection test to guide surgery in patients with Zollinger-Ellison syndrome. World J Surg 1993;17:433–438.
92. Thom AK, Norton JA, Doppman JL, Miller DL, Chang R, Jensen RT. Prospective study of the use of intraarterial secretin injection and portal venous sampling to localize duodenal gastrinomas. Surgery 1992;112:1002–1009.
93. Imamura M, Takahashi K, Isobe Y, Hattori Y, Satomura K, Tobe T. Curative resection of multiple gastrinomas aided by selective arterial secretin injection test and intraoperative secretin test. Ann Surg 1989;210:710–718.
94. Doppman JL, Miller DL, Chang R, Shawker TH, Gorden P, Norton JA. Insulinomas: localization with selective intraarterial injection of calcium. Radiology 1991;178:237–241.
95. Doppman JL, Miller DL, Chang R, Gorden P, Eastman RC, Norton JA. Intraarterial stimulation test for detection of insulinomas. World J Surg 1993;17:439–443.
96. Brunt LM, Veldhuis JD, Dilley WG, et al. Stimulation of insulin secretion by a rapid intravenous calcium infusion in patients with ß-cell neoplasms of the pancreas. J Clin Endocrinol Metab 1986;62:210–216.
97. Fajans SS, Vinik AI. Insulin-producing islet cell tumors. Endocrinol Metab Clin North Am 1989;18:45–74.
98. Cho KJ, Vinik AI, Thompson NW, et al. Localization of the source of hyperinsulinism: percutaneous transhepatic portal and pancreatic vein catheterization with hormone assay. AJR 1982;139: 237–245.
99. Ko TC, Flisak M, Prinz RA. Selective intra-arterial methylene blue injection: a novel method of localizing gastrinoma. Gastroenterology 1992;102:1062–1064.
100. Miller DL, Doppman JL, Metz DC, Maton PN, Norton JA, Jensen RT. Zollinger-Ellison syndrome: technique, results, and complications of portal venous sampling. Radiology 1992;182: 235–241.
101. Owens LV, Huth JF, Cance WG. Insulinoma: pitfalls in preoperative localization. Eur J Surg Oncol 1995;21:326–328.
102. Miller DL, Doppman JL. Diagnostic imaging of the adrenal gland. In: Becker KL, ed. Principles and practice of endocrinology and metabolism. 2nd ed. Philadelphia: JB Lippincott, 1995:773–778.
103. Fraker DL, Alexander HR. The surgical approach to endocrine tumors of the pancreas. Semin Gastrointest Dis 1995;6:102–113.
104. Bieligk S, Jaffe BM. Islet cell tumors of the pancreas. Surg Clin North Am 1995;75:1025–1040.
105. Norton JA, Cromack DT, Shawker TH, et al. Intraoperative ultrasonographic localization of islet cell tumors: a prospective comparison to palpation. Ann Surg 1988;207:160–168.
106. Zeiger MA, Shawker TH, Norton JA. Use of intraoperative ultrasonography to localize islet cell tumors. World J Surg 1993;17:448–454.
107. Doherty GM, Doppman JL, Shawker TH, et al. Results of a prospective strategy to diagnose, localize, and resect insulinomas. Surgery 1991;110:989–996.
108. Böttger TC, Junginger T. Is preoperative radiographic localization of islet cell tumors in patients with insulinoma necessary? World J Surg 1993;17:427–432.
109. Sugg SL, Norton JA, Fraker DL, et al. A prospective study of intraoperative methods to diagnose and resect duodenal gastrinomas. Ann Surg 1993;218:138–144.
110. van Heerden JA, Grant CS, Czako PF, Service FJ, Charbonneau JW. Occult functioning insulinomas: which localizing studies are indicated? Surgery 1992;112:1010–1015.
111. Delcore R, Friesen SR. Gastrointestinal neuroendocrine tumors. J Am Coll Surg 1994;178:187–211.
112. Pasieka JL, McLeod MK, Thompson NW, Burney RE. Surgical approach to insulinomas: assessing the need for preoperative localization. Arch Surg 1992;127:442–447.
113. Orloff SL, Debas HT. Advances in the management of patients with Zollinger-Ellison syndrome. Surg Clin North Am 1995;75: 511–524.

# 77

# *Insulinoma and Nesidioblastosis*

Gary R. Peplinski, Michael A. Skinner, and Jeffrey A. Norton

## INSULINOMA

Insulinoma is a neoplasm that arises from the pancreatic insulin-producing beta cells. It is a rare tumor that occurs in approximately 1–6 persons per million population per year (1). Unlike other gastrointestinal endocrine tumors, which are malignant in more than 60% of cases, 90% of insulinomas are benign, solitary growths that occur almost exclusively within the pancreatic parenchyma, with no evidence of local invasion or locoregional lymph node metastases (2). The major cause of morbidity and potential mortality with insulinomas is the hormonal syndrome of hyperinsulinemia and consequent hypoglycemia that is not well controlled long term by medical therapy. The other dilemma in managing this neoplasm is the difficulty in localizing the tumor, which may be as small as 6 mm in diameter and is usually less than 2 cm (3).

Whereas patients with insulinomas commonly died from uncontrolled symptoms and unlocalized tumors only 65 years ago, presently most patients with insulinomas are cured of disease and return to a normal, fully functional lifestyle. Endogenous hyperinsulinism was initially described in 1927, the first syndrome of excessive pancreatic hormone hypersecretion to be identified (1). Roscoe Graham first successfully removed an insulinoma, in Toronto in 1929. Two years later, Evarts Graham in St. Louis successfully resected a 5-mm insulinoma by enucleation, a newly described procedure at the time that remains the operation of choice for benign insulinomas today. In 1935, Whipple proposed a triad of symptoms based on observations in 32 patients: symptoms of hypoglycemia with fasting, a blood glucose level below 50 mg/dL, and relief of symptoms after glucose administration (1). Recognition of this classic triad of symptoms and presently available precise biochemical testing has resulted in accurate diagnosis at an early stage of disease. Refinement of preoperative invasive radiologic means of imaging the tumor and, in cases of nonimageable tumor, regionally localizing the tumor to specific areas of the pancreas based on tumor function, has greatly aided in accurate identification of previously occult tumors and in successful surgical resection. In 1985, the use of intraoperative ultrasound (IOUS) was first reported to localize precisely, at the time of surgery, an occult insulinoma that was not identified by preoperative invasive imaging (4). The use of IOUS has been a major breakthrough in precisely localizing tumors that may not be visualized or palpated by the surgeon and in guiding safe enucleation while avoiding potential morbidity from pancreatic duct or vessel injury (4–6). Ongoing efforts to identify tumors accurately using even less invasive means and newer technology, such as endoscopic ultrasonography (EUS), continue to be evaluated and may further simplify the localization of these small tumors (7–10). Although many techniques in diagnosis and tumor localization have come and gone in an attempt to define the safest and most useful tests as technology advances, the cornerstone of definitive, curative treatment has not changed for almost 70 years—surgery.

### Patient Presentation

Patients with an insulinoma present with symptoms secondary to excessive and physiologically uncontrolled secretion of insulin. Although islet cell tumors, in general, may secrete many hormones and a solitary tumor secreting multiple active peptides may mimic multiple tumors (11), patients usually exhibit symptoms related to only one of these peptides (1).

Patients are usually women (60–75%) with complaints of anxiety, dizziness, obtundation, confusion, unconsciousness, or personality changes (3). These signs and symptoms are due to effects of acute hypoglycemia on the nervous system that typically occur after a period of fasting, commonly during the early morning hours, when glucose reserves are low in the setting of continued endogenous insulin production (3). Seizures may occur in up to 30% (3). Weight gain is reported in 70% of patients, which may be due to either the anabolic effects of excessive insulin production or a learned behavior of frequent eating to avoid symptoms (3). Patients note increased symptoms when food intake is decreased to reduce weight. Patients not uncommonly suffer potentially life-threatening symptoms for several years before the correct diagnosis is considered (3). Many patients have undergone extensive psychiatric evaluation.

### Diagnosis

The major differential diagnosis of hypoglycemia that occurs while fasting is an insulinoma versus factitious hypoglycemia (12). A diagnosis must be substantiated by the standard fasting test with measurement of serum biochemical markers prior to an attempt at tumor localization using radiographic imaging. It is also important to exclude multiple endocrine neoplasia type I syndrome (MEN-1) in all patients with an insulinoma.

**Standard Fasting Test.** Symptomatic patients may initially undergo an overnight fast in an outpatient setting, during which, any symptoms are recorded and the serum glucose and insulin levels can be measured. Development of symptoms along with fasting hypoglycemia strongly suggests an insulinoma. Since management of insulinoma often requires invasive tumor localization tests and surgical resection for cure whereas factitious hypoglycemia is a nonsurgical problem, a 72-hour supervised fast in a hospital setting is necessary to confirm the diagnosis of insulinoma and to exclude factitious hypoglycemia.

The standard fasting test is conducted by placing an intravenous catheter with a heparin lock and allowing the patient to drink only noncaloric beverages (Fig. 77.1). A baseline neurologic examination emphasizing recent memory, calculations, and coordination is done (13). The patient is observed frequently,

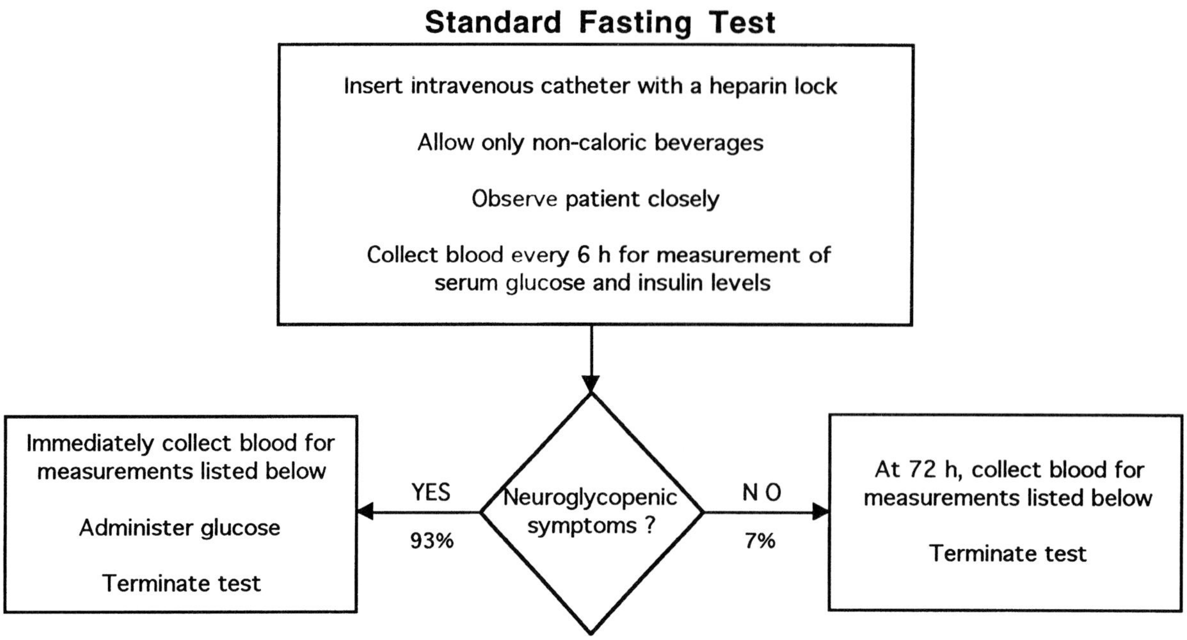


| Blood Test | Normal Range (Fasting) | Result With... Insulinoma | Factitious Hypoglycemia | Test Sensitivity | References |
|---|---|---|---|---|---|
| Glucose | 90-150 mg/dl | < 40 mg/dl | < 40 mg/dl | 99% | 15 |
| Immunoreactive Insulin (IRI) | < 5 μU/ml | > 5 μU/ml | > 10 μU/ml | 100% | 15 |
| C-peptide | < 1.7 ng/ml | > 1.7 ng/ml | < 1.7 ng/ml | 78% | 3, 17, 18 |
| Direct Proinsulin-like Component (PLC) | < 0.2 ng/ml | > 0.2 ng/ml | < 0.2 ng/ml | 85% | 21, 25 |
| PLC/Total IRI | < 25% | > 25% | < 25% | 87% | 15, 21 |

**FIG. 77.1.** Standard fasting test. The diagnosis of endogenous hyperinsulinism is confirmed and factitious hypoglycemia is excluded by the supervised 72-hour fasting test.

and blood is collected every 6 hours for measurement of serum glucose and immunoreactive insulin levels. As the blood glucose level falls below 50 mg/dL, blood samples are collected more frequently (every hour or less), and the patient is observed closely. When neuroglycopenic symptoms appear, blood is collected immediately for determination of serum insulin, glucose, C-peptide, and proinsulin levels, sugar is administered, and the fast is terminated. Few patients with insulinomas remain symptom free for the entire 72 hours, when the test is terminated and the above blood levels are measured. In contrast, approximately 60% of patients with insulinomas develop symptoms in the first 24 hours after fasting begins (1). Some have advocated stimulation tests in which plasma glucose and insulin levels are measured after administration of tolbutamide, calcium, glucagon, or leucine (14). A suppression test involving the administration of porcine or fish insulin, which suppresses human insulin and C-peptide levels in normal subjects but not insulinoma patients, has also been described (1). We do not use these tests in addition to the standard fasting test, and we do not recommend them.

Virtually all patients with insulinoma develop hypoglycemia (blood glucose level <40 mg/dL) during the 72-hour fast, and approximately 93% have neuroglycopenic symptoms (15). Some 16% of patients with insulinoma may develop symptoms with a blood glucose level above 40 mg/dL (3). Virtually all patients have a plasma insulin level that is inappropriately higher than normal (>5 μU/mL) at the time of documented hypoglycemia or symptoms, and the insulin level almost always exceeds 10 μU/mL (3). An elevated insulin level during hypoglycemia is the most definitive diagnostic parameter for insulinoma (15). A ratio of insulin to glucose that is higher than 0.40 may also be useful for diagnosis (16).

Normal insulin secretion requires enzymatic cleavage of a larger single-chain precursor molecule, proinsulin, which results in release of a mature bioactive insulin molecule and an inactive smaller peptide, C-peptide (17–19). Because insulinomas hypersecrete insulin, the C-peptide level is also elevated (>1.7 ng/mL) in most patients (3, 20). Insulinomas also secrete large amounts of uncleaved proinsulin (21, 22), because of incomplete conversion of proinsulin to insulin (23). Prolonged maximal stimulation of insulin secretion in normal subjects does not cause release of proinsulin (24). Patients with tumors that produce large amounts of proinsulin relative to insulin may remain euglycemic and asymptomatic for longer periods during a fast because proinsulin is not biologically active. The proinsulin-like component (PLC) can be measured at the time of hypoglycemia, and this value or the PLC/total immunoreactive insulin percentage is an important confirmatory test for insulinoma (3, 15, 25). In a recent review of 98 patients with pathologically proven insulinoma, 85 patients (87%) had PLC of 25% or more (15). Furthermore, patients with malignant tumors had a higher mean PLC value than patients with benign insulinomas; 17 of 18 (94%) patients with malignant tumors had a PLC above 25%. However, there was considerable overlap between the PLCs of patients with malignant and benign tumors (15).

**Excluding Factitious Hypoglycemia.** Because self-administration of oral hypoglycemic medications or insulin may cause hypoglycemia, "factitious" hypoglycemia is an important differential diagnosis that must be excluded (12). These patients may undergo unnecessary surgery, including pancreatic resection. One may have a high degree of suspicion for factitious hypoglycemia in a patient with diabetic relatives or in a young woman associated with the medical profession, such as a nurse. Sulfonylurea levels in the blood from oral hypoglycemic drugs can be directly measured by gas chromatography and mass spectroscopy. Human antibodies to animal insulin are measurable if the subject is not administering recombinant human insulin. Measurement of blood C-peptide and proinsulin levels further help exclude this diagnosis. Exogenously administered insulin does not contain proinsulin or C-peptide and suppresses their production. Therefore, elevated serum levels of proinsulin or C-peptide during hypoglycemia effectively exclude the diagnosis of factitious hypoglycemia and indicate an endogenous source for the hyperinsulinism. Approximately 13–22% of patients with insulinoma do not have elevated serum proinsulin or C-peptide levels. As a result, a supervised fast prohibiting exogenous hypoglycemic administration remains the "gold standard" for diagnosing insulinoma and excluding factitious hypoglycemia (Fig. 77.1).

**Screening for MEN-1.** About 5–10% of patients with hyperinsulinism have MEN-1. Therefore, careful screening of all patients with insulinoma is necessary to exclude MEN-1 and the possibility of other coexisting conditions associated with this syndrome (26). It is important to recognize patients with this syndrome because multiple pancreatic tumors always exist (27). Other possible manifestations of the syndrome and a family history of endocrine tumors should be sought. Specifically, parathyroid disease is present either concomitant with, or prior to, the diagnosis of an islet cell tumor (26). If the clinical history is equivocal or suspicious for MEN-1, then measurement of serum levels of calcium, prolactin, and pancreatic polypeptide may help confirm or exclude MEN-1. The biochemical parameters measured during the standard fasting test cannot discriminate sporadic insulinoma and MEN-1 (15). Screening of family members for features of MEN-1 is indicated when a patient is suspected of having MEN-1.

Definitive determination of the presence of MEN-1 will soon be possible by genetic testing. The gene believed responsible for MEN-1 is mapped to the long arm of chromosome 11 (28). When the actual gene is cloned, mutational analysis studies may reveal its functional implications, which in turn may enable development of experimental therapeutic strategies aimed at restoring essential gene function or eliminating abnormal gene function.

## Medical Management

In contrast to other syndromes of hormonal excess, which produce distressing symptoms that may be adequately managed by medications such as omeprazole for peptic ulceration in Zollinger-Ellison syndrome, good long-term control of hypoglycemic symptoms by medical management is generally ineffective for patients with insulinoma. As a result, surgery to excise the source of excessive insulin production is the definitive treatment. However, medical management of patients with insulinomas is important during the tumor-localization phase and preoperative period to prevent hypoglycemia, relieve its symptoms, and avoid its life-threatening sequelae. This is accomplished by frequent feedings, including a night feeding. Cornstarch may be added to food to slow absorption. Diazoxide at a dose of 400–600 mg/day inhibits insulin release in approximately 50% of patients with insulinoma (13). Diazoxide should be discontinued 1 week before surgery to avoid intraoperative hypotension. Calcium channel blockers or phenytoin may also suppress insulin production in some cases.

Octreotide is a synthetic, long-acting (half life, >100 min) analogue of the naturally occurring hormone somatostatin. Because octreotide binds to cells expressing somatostatin receptors and activates these receptors, the secretion of many gastrointestinal peptides is inhibited by octreotide. It was initially hoped that this drug would be useful in treating symptoms from excessive hormone production from gastrointestinal endocrine tumors and that radiolabeled octreotide would provide a means of selectively destroying endocrine tumors that express high levels of the somatostatin receptor. Although octreotide may be useful for treating symptoms caused by vipomas and carcinoid tumors (29), it is unpredictable in inhibiting insulin release from insulinomas in adults (30).

In a recent phase II study, 5 of 7 patients with insulinomas treated with octreotide 100–300 μg/day by subcutaneous injection had no hypoglycemic symptoms and normalized blood glucose levels for 0.2 to 54 months (median, 15 months). The other two patients had no evidence of metabolic improvement (31). No significant adverse effects were reported. Similarly, the usefulness of radiolabeled octreotide in imaging insulinomas and in treating metastatic islet cell tumors has been disappointing (32, 33). Therefore, long-term medical management of hypoglycemia in patients with insulinomas generally is reserved for the few patients (<5%) with unlocalized, unresected tumors after thorough preoperative testing and exploratory laparotomy with IOUS or for patients with metastatic, unresectable malignant insulinoma (31). The short-term use of octreotide preoperatively may be beneficial if the patient is not responding well to traditional medical management, and surgery is delayed for tumor localization. The surgeon must know the patient's response to medical management so that the urgency and potential benefits of surgery can be determined (34).

## Preoperative Localization

Once an insulinoma is diagnosed, the goal is to identify, stage, and remove all tumor. Because insulinomas are small and solitary, accurate preoperative tumor localization has traditionally been very important to a successful surgical result (11, 16). Tumor localization may be attempted by use of noninvasive or invasive radiologic imaging techniques. Results of radiologic imaging studies for insulinoma are presented in Table 77.1, and each is discussed in detail below. Noninvasive studies are associated with less morbidity and cost than invasive imaging techniques but identify tumors rarely. Furthermore, despite the sophistication of present noninvasive and invasive radiologic technology, the insulinoma may not be located or, even worse, a

**TABLE 77.1. Localizing Studies for Insulinoma**

| Test | Type | Positive Result | Sensitivity | Usefulness | References |
|---|---|---|---|---|---|
| Transabdominal ultrasonography | Imaging | Sonolucent mass on a uniformly echo-dense background | 0–25% | Useful in nonobese patients | 3, 39, 40, 41 |
| Abdominal CT | Imaging | Pancreatic mass that may brighten with intravenous contrast | 11–40 | May detect primary mass; good for detecting hepatic metastases | 3, 39, 40, 41, 45 |
| Abdominal MRI | Imaging | Pancreatic mass with increased signal intensity on T2 images | 11–43 | Same as for CT | 3, 39, 40 |
| Octreoscan | Functional imaging | Black "hot spot" | 50–80 | Not useful unless tumor binds octreotide; images whole body | 46, 47, 50, 51, 52 |
| Selective arteriography | Imaging | Tumor "blush" upon injection of intraarterial contrast | 40–70 | Useful, but other current tests are better | 40, 41, 45, 54 |
| Portal venous sampling (PVS) | Functional | Increased blood insulin level in veins draining the tumor | 67–100 | Useful to localize tumor to a more specific region of the pancreas | 3, 39, 40, 41, 44, 54 |
| Selective arteriography with calcium stimulation | Functional ±/− imaging | More than 2-fold increase in hepatic vein insulin level 30–60 sec after intraarterial calcium injection | 88 | Useful to regionally localize the tumor and to possibly image the tumor's specific location | 39 |
| Endoscopic ultrasonography (EUS) | Imaging | Sonolucent mass on a uniformly echo-dense background | 70–90 | Useful to avoid other costly invasive preoperative tests if tumor is localized | 7, 8, 9, 10 |
| Intraoperative ultrasonography (IOUS) | Imaging | Sonolucent mass on a uniformly echo-dense background | 75–100 | Very useful to identify nonpalpable tumors, show relationship of vital structures, guide specific enucleation, and find occult insulinomas | 3, 5, 6, 39, 45, 54, 57 |

wrong location may be suggested that misleads the surgeon. The recent advances in ultrasound (namely the development of IOUS and EUS, which are safe and highly effective) make routine use of other preoperative localization studies to obtain as much information as possible about the precise location of the insulinoma prior to surgery questionable (9, 35–38). Currently, the specific tests indicated and the most cost-effective management strategies are being debated.

**Noninvasive Imaging Studies.** Standard transabdominal ultrasonography is the least expensive and least invasive imaging modality for the pancreas. An insulinoma appears sonolucent on a background of "echo-dense" normal pancreas. However, obesity and bowel gas greatly limit the quality of the image. Sensitivity is only 0–25% in most studies (3, 39–42), so this technique has limited utility in localizing insulinomas.

Abdominal computed tomography (CT) may identify pancreatic lesions as small as 1 cm in diameter in a normal pancreas. The addition of intravenous contrast may cause a tumor blush because of increased vascularity of some insulinomas and allow identification of smaller (<1 cm) tumors (43). Oral contrast should also be given to differentiate bowel and define the pancreas more distinctly; cuts of the peripancreatic area 5 mm apart or closer are obtained (44). The sensitivity of CT for insulinomas ranges from only 11 to 40% in most series (3, 39–42, 45). Abdominal magnetic resonance imaging (MRI) may reveal increased signal intensity at the site of an insulinoma on T2-weighted images. The sensitivity of MRI appears to equal that of CT (3, 39, 40). Either imaging modality is, therefore, appropriate to detect hepatic metastases, which may occur in up to 10% of patients with insulinomas, or to detect large (>2 cm) islet cell tumors. Metastases must be identified preoperatively so that the operative approach to resect limited metastases can be planned or, in the case of widespread unresectable metastases, unnecessary surgery can be abandoned. If a tumor is not imaged by CT or MRI, then the incidence of malignancy is virtually zero. Thus, preoperative imaging with abdominal CT or MRI is useful.

Octreoscan is a relatively new imaging modality in which octreotide labeled with a radioactive tracer is given intravenously and binds to tumors with somatostatin receptors, causing the tumor to appear as a "hot spot" on whole-body gamma camera scintigraphy (46). The octreotide scan depends on the ability of a particular tumor to express somatostatin receptors and is considered a functional rather than an anatomic study (47). Because insulinomas do not express high levels of somatostatin receptors consistently, labeled octreotide may not be useful in localizing all insulinomas. If an insulinoma is visualized on an octreotide scan, then the patient is likely to have a favorable symptomatic response to octreotide (48–50). Some 50–80% of insulinomas are imaged by the octreoscan (46, 47, 50–52), and specificity is virtually 100% (51). Many endocrine tumors express large numbers of high-affinity receptors for the hormone vasoactive intestinal polypeptide (VIP). Radioiodinated VIP scanning is a new noninvasive imaging modality for gut tumors, including colorectal adenocarcinomas. This technique localized

4 of 4 insulinomas in one recent study (53). However, experience is presently too limited to make further recommendations.

**Invasive Localizing Procedures.** Because noninvasive imaging studies are poor at detecting small insulinomas, more sensitive invasive tests have been developed to localize the tumor preoperatively. Selective arteriography is more sensitive than noninvasive imaging studies for localizing an insulinoma. Insulinomas are imaged better by arteriography than gastrinomas (44). For this study, the celiac axis is catheterized, and its several tributaries are selectively cannulated and injected with contrast to perfuse different portions of the pancreas parenchyma and liver. Most insulinomas have higher vascularity than the surrounding pancreatic tissue and show up as a "blush" with injection of contrast (Fig. 77.2*A*). Multiple views, including oblique images to evaluate lesions obscured by vessels and bones, may be necessary. Few false-positive results occur. Experienced interventional radiologists are needed for an appropriate study. Several reports indicate that approximately 40–70% of tumors may be identified by this approach (40, 41, 45, 54).

Despite the use of transabdominal US, CT, MRI, and arteriography to image insulinomas, approximately 50% of patients have small (< 2 cm) tumors that are not detected by these imaging tests. These patients routinely require regional localization procedures to localize the insulinoma accurately (3). Regional localization studies rely on the functional activity of the insulinoma (i.e., excessive insulin production) and not on the ability to image the tumor on a radiologic study (i.e. tumor size) to map the tumor to a specific region of the pancreas. However, if imaging studies are negative, whether patients should undergo preoperative regional localization studies or proceed directly to operative exploration is presently controversial. Because insulinomas are often small (<2 cm in diameter) and may not be accurately localized using presently available imaging studies, some have recommended that invasive studies not be done and that the patient undergo abdominal exploration directly, with intraoperative maneuvers to localize the tumor after a diagnosis of insulinoma is made. Increasing experience with IOUS and EUS (discussed below) have greatly increased the operative

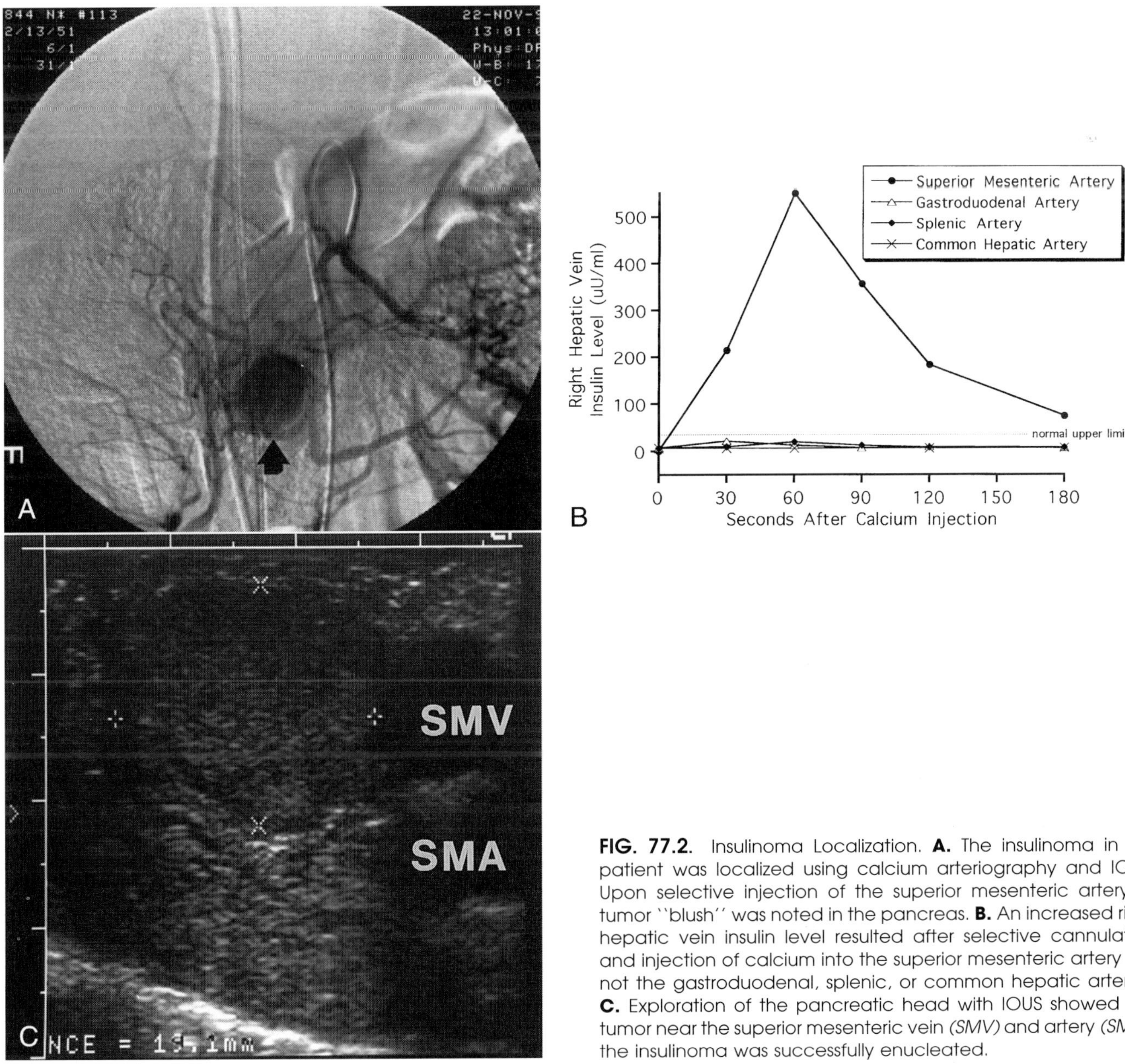


**FIG. 77.2.** Insulinoma Localization. **A.** The insulinoma in this patient was localized using calcium arteriography and IOUS. Upon selective injection of the superior mesenteric artery, a tumor "blush" was noted in the pancreas. **B.** An increased right hepatic vein insulin level resulted after selective cannulation and injection of calcium into the superior mesenteric artery but not the gastroduodenal, splenic, or common hepatic arteries. **C.** Exploration of the pancreatic head with IOUS showed the tumor near the superior mesenteric vein *(SMV)* and artery *(SMA)*; the insulinoma was successfully enucleated.

localization success rate. Proceeding directly to operative exploration may be reasonable for pancreatic endocrine surgeons experienced with these new techniques, especially when sophisticated preoperative radiologic localization studies are not available.

Some endocrine surgeons consider portal venous sampling (PVS) for insulin to be the "gold standard" for localizing insulinomas (9, 16). It may accurately detect tumors as small as 6 mm in diameter. A catheter is placed through the liver percutaneously and positioned in the portal system. More than 20 blood samples are taken from different veins that drain the pancreas and are tested for insulin to localize the insulinoma. Sensitivity ranges from 67 to 100% (3, 39–41, 44, 54), and the false-positive rate is virtually 0%. However, this technique does not localize the tumor precisely, since it only determines whether the portion of the pancreas to the right or left of the superior mesenteric artery (SMA) harbors the insulinoma. Information gained from this test preoperatively can be used to scrutinize the suspicious area of the pancreas more closely at the time of surgery and to resect the appropriate half of the pancreas if a tumor is not positively identified intraoperatively. Besides being costly, an experienced interventional radiologist is needed to pass a catheter through the liver and into the portal circulation. Complications may include hemobilia and hepatic bleeding (55).

The calcium arteriogram appears to be the most sensitive preoperative test for localizing insulinomas and is replacing PVS as the invasive localizing study of choice (39). Arteries that perfuse the pancreatic head (gastroduodenal artery, SMA) and the body/tail (splenic artery) are selectively catheterized, and a small amount of calcium gluconate (0.025 mEq $Ca^{2+}$/kg body weight) is independently injected into each artery. A catheter positioned at the right hepatic vein is used to collect blood for measurement of insulin levels 30–60 seconds after the calcium injection. Calcium stimulates a marked increase in insulin secretion from the insulinoma (Fig. 77.2*B*). A more than twofold increase in the hepatic vein insulin level permits localization of the tumor to the area of the pancreas being perfused by the injected artery. Additionally, injection of contrast may reveal a tumor blush, confirming the location of the insulinoma by imaging the tumor (Fig. 77.2*A*), but this is not a necessary criterion. This test combines the functional advantage of PVS with the more exact localization capability of arteriography. These combined features may be particularly helpful in patients with MEN-1, who always have multiple tumors and may have more than one functional insulinoma. The reported sensitivity of calcium stimulation is 88% (39). In this study, an increase in the hepatic vein insulin level occurred in 25 of 25 patients. Only three patients had false localizations, and all three patients had tumors in the proximal body of the pancreas. There were no major complications (39). The calcium arteriogram is also specific for insulinomas because calcium infusion does not stimulate normal pancreatic beta cells to secrete insulin in patients with factitious hypoglycemia from exogenous insulin administration.

EUS is a new preoperative method to detect pancreatic tumors. An endoscope is passed through the stomach into the duodenum, and a balloon is inflated against the intestinal wall with saline. A 5- to 10-MHz transducer is used to generate an image of the pancreas through the intestinal and stomach walls. Tumors as small as 2–3 mm in diameter can be identified in the pancreatic head by moving the transducer through the duodenum at the junction of the pancreas. The endoscope must be passed well into the third portion of the duodenum to visualize the complete uncinate process adequately (9). Insulinomas in the pancreatic body and tail are imaged by positioning the transducer in the stomach and scanning the posterior wall. In a recent review, transgastric and transduodenal imaging were accomplished in all 10 patients diagnosed with insulinoma who underwent preoperative EUS (9). Seven of 10 (70%) insulinomas were identified, ranging in size from 1.5 to 2.2 cm (mean size, 1.8 cm). Five were located in the pancreatic head/neck region, and two were in the body/tail. Two of three missed tumors occurred in the head. Of the three missed tumors, two were pedunculated, and the other was located in the junction of the head and uncinate process and was not detected, even though it measured 1.2 cm. Because there were no false positives, the authors concluded that in patients with sporadic insulinomas, if the tumor is identified with EUS, then no other preoperative imaging studies are needed, which significantly reduces costs (9). Sensitivity for EUS ranges from 70 to 90% (7–10).

In summary, we recommend that all patients with diagnosed insulinomas initially undergo abdominal CT or MRI to detect potential metastatic disease and to attempt to localize the primary tumor by noninvasive means (Fig. 77.3). Octreoscan may be helpful if an equivocal lesion is identified on CT or MRI. However, a negative octreotide scan does not exclude an insulinoma. If an insulinoma is clearly identified by these studies, then the patient may be taken directly for exploratory laparotomy to evaluate the tumor with IOUS (discussed below) and to resect it. If results of the noninvasive imaging studies are negative, this usually means that the insulinoma is small and that intraoperative localization may be difficult, with a low chance of success if IOUS is not available. Some have advocated EUS as the next localization test because it is very sensitive and may eliminate the costs and morbidity associated with invasive testing (9). However, EUS misses 10–30% of insulinomas (7–10). In cases with an unlocalized insulinoma, the arteriogram with calcium stimulation, which can be performed simply at most hospitals, should be performed preoperatively to increase the chance of localizing the insulinoma. Although up to 12% of insulinomas remain unlocalized by this test, PVS adds little additional information. If the tumor is still not localized by the calcium arteriogram and the diagnosis is certain, then the tumor is considered "occult," and exploratory laparotomy with careful inspection and palpation of the entire pancreas with IOUS is indicated.

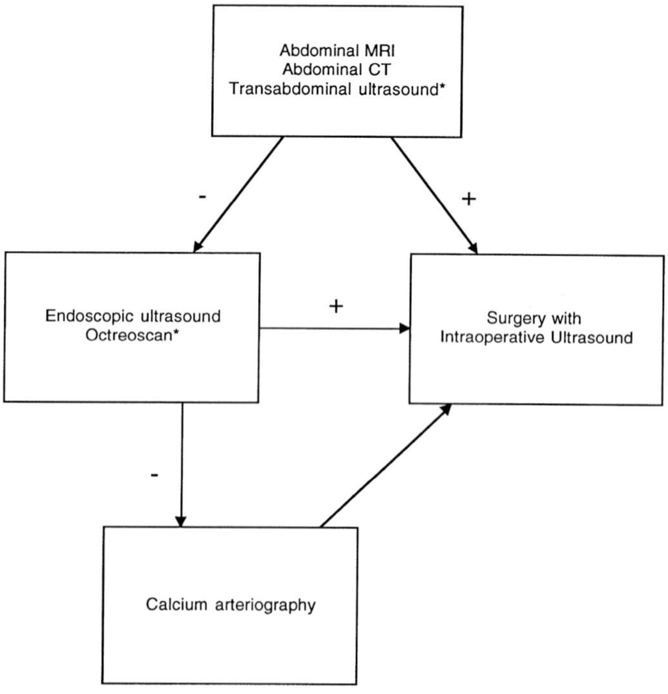


**FIG. 77.3.** Flow chart for the localization of insulinoma. *Only one of the tests listed in each box is necessary for localization.

## Operative Management

Surgery is the main treatment because it is potentially curative for patients with insulinoma. The diagnosis of insulinoma must be firmly established. The goal of surgery is to identify and resect all tumor while preserving as much normal pancreatic tissue as possible. Because insulinomas are small tumors and there is a substantial chance that preoperative localization studies may be negative, precise intraoperative localization is essential. Therefore, experience in this type of surgery is important for a successful, uncomplicated outcome. Accurate localization of the tumor to a specific area of the pancreas using preoperative studies correlates with a high chance of identifying the tumor in the same location at surgery. The likelihood of cure is very good if the area of the pancreas identified as harboring the insulinoma on preoperative studies is resected. Even when preoperative localization studies are inconclusive, adequate mobilization of the pancreas and the use of specific intraoperative maneuvers usually succeed in identifying and resecting the insulinoma.

**Preoperative Preparation.** Patients should be prepared to undergo resection of any portion of the pancreas. A complete bowel preparation is advised in the event bowel resection is required or, rarely, a Whipple pancreaticoduodenectomy is necessary. Each patient should receive pneumococcal vaccination prior to surgery because distal pancreatectomy with splenectomy may be necessary. Treatment of medical conditions is maximized, and an intensive care unit bed is reserved. An antibiotic with broad-spectrum bacterial coverage (such as a second-generation cephalosporin) is given immediately prior to the incision. The prophylactic use of octreotide preoperatively to reduce complications of pancreatic surgery such as fistulas and pseudocysts may be beneficial but is controversial (56).

**Operative Approach.** Adequate exposure of the entire upper abdomen is necessary to expose the entire pancreas and to examine the regional lymph nodes and liver. Prognosis and survival depend on the ability to stage the tumor accurately and completely resect it. A standard midline laparotomy incision or a bilateral subcostal incision is recommended. A fixed upper abdominal retractor greatly facilitates exposure. The entire abdomen is inspected for potential metastases, especially the surface of the liver. Metastatic insulinoma deposits on the liver surface typically appear as firm nodules. IOUS using a 5-MHz transducer may help in identifying deep hepatic metastases. Any suspicious lesions must be either excised, if small and peripheral, or at least have a biopsy done, with immediate frozen-section analysis to exclude tumor.

**Location of Insulinomas.** Virtually all insulinomas are located within the pancreas parenchyma and are uniformly distributed throughout the entire gland (Fig. 77.4) (3). Unlike gastrinomas, insulinomas do not generally occur in extrapancreatic locations such as the duodenal submucosa, and insulinomas do not arise in specific regions, such as the gastrinoma triangle. Tumors that have been found outside the pancreas have occurred in ectopic pancreatic rests. In addition to the primary pancreatic tumor, careful inspection and palpation of the liver and regional lymph nodes is important to exclude metastatic disease, which occurs in 10% of sporadic cases.

**Pancreatic Mobilization.** Because insulinomas are very small and may be found uniformly throughout the entire pancreas, the head, body, and tail of the pancreas must be sufficiently mobilized to permit evaluation of the entire organ. To expose the pancreas adequately, the gastrocolic ligament is divided to open the lesser sac. The hepatic and splenic flexures of the colon are mobilized out of the upper abdomen. An extended Kocher maneuver is required to lift the head of the pancreas out of the retroperitoneum adequately. The head of the pancreas is thick, resulting in poor palpation of tumors that are centrally located. The entire head must be mobilized enough to allow examination of the posterior surface of the pancreatic head and palpation

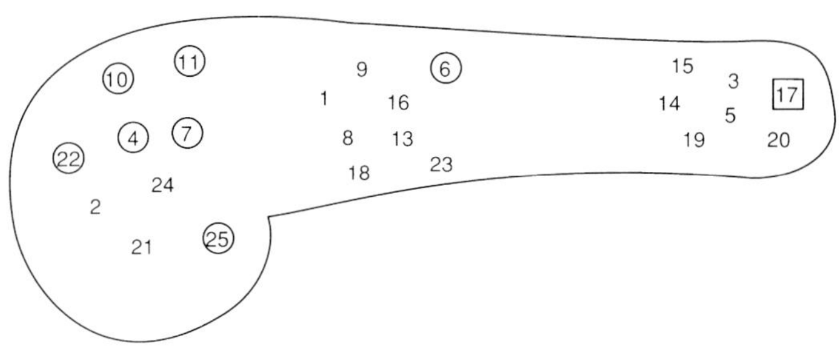

**FIG. 77.4.** Location of benign sporadic insulinomas and mode of intraoperative identification. Each *number* represents the location of the tumor in a separate patient. *Encircled numbers* represent tumors that were not palpable but were found only by ultrasonography. No. 17 *(square)* was found by pathologic study after distal pancreatectomy based on a PVS gradient. Numbers without a circle or square represent tumors that were palpable and could be imaged by IOUS during exploration. (Reprinted with permission from Doherty GM, Doppman JL, Shawker TH, Miller DL, Eastman RC, et al. Results of a prospective strategy to diagnose, localize and resect insulinomas. Surgery 1991;110: 989–997.)

between the thumb and forefinger. Division of attachments at the inferior and posterior border of the pancreas permits evaluation of the posterior body and tail. Meticulous examination of the pancreatic tail may require division of the splenic ligaments to mobilize the spleen completely out of the retroperitoneum. Once the pancreas is fully exposed, the search for the insulinoma begins.

**Intraoperative Maneuvers to Find the Insulinoma.** Precise intraoperative localization of these small tumors is the key to a successful outcome. Intraoperative localization is important because of the inability to localize most (50%) tumors by standard imaging studies preoperatively and the possibility of misinterpretation of data obtained with invasive preoperative localizing studies.

Direct inspection is the first intraoperative localization maneuver. One looks for a brownish red, cherrylike tumor. However, most insulinomas are buried within the pancreatic parenchyma and are not visible.

Careful palpation of the entire pancreas between the thumb and forefinger is the second maneuver that may identify some insulinomas that are not visible. Insulinomas feel hard and nodular compared with the normal pancreas parenchyma. In one study that included patients with insulinomas that could not be found despite intensive noninvasive localization efforts, only 16 of 25 tumors (64%) were identified by standard surgical inspection and palpation (3). Insulinomas in the head of the pancreas are more often missed because the pancreas is thick in this region. Patients with histories of alcoholism have a denser-feeling pancreas, and palpation of the tumor is more difficult. Similarly, previous pancreatic surgery results in a scarred pancreatic parenchyma that may mask the tumor to palpation.

IOUS is the best intraoperative method for localizing the insulinoma and should be considered essential in all cases. IOUS bypasses the obscurity generated by subcutaneous fat and bowel gas and generates an image in direct apposition to the surface of the pancreas. In the study cited above, IOUS identified seven additional patients who did not have palpable tumors (3). To examine the pancreas, a high-resolution near-field real-time transducer is used, usually a 10- or a 7.5-MHz probe with a short focal length and high resolution. The pancreas is covered in a pool of saline to maximize image quality, and the operating room lights are dimmed. Tumors can be identified on the basis of a difference in echogenicity. Insulinomas appear sonolucent on a uniform background of more echo-dense pancreas parenchyma (Fig. 77.2*C*) (5, 6). Having an ultrasonographer in the operating room greatly aids in interpreting ultrasound images. The sensitivity for detecting insulinomas using IOUS is greater than 75% (41, 45, 54, 57) and approaches 100% (3, 39). A distinct, clear margin between the tumor and pancreatic parenchyma is readily identified in benign tumors; malignant insulinomas may have a more irregular or unclear margin suggesting invasion into the pancreatic parenchyma (58). This observation may be an indication for a more radical resection, such as a distal pancreatectomy, rather than the more conventional tumor enucleation. IOUS can also unequivocally identify tumors that are not visualized or are not palpable (3, 58). IOUS is particularly helpful in identifying nonpalpable tumors in the pancreatic head. In conjunction, simultaneous palpation and ultrasonography clarify lesions suspected by either alone (58). Furthermore, by imaging the lesion in longitudinal and transverse planes, IOUS clearly shows the relationship of the tumor to vital structures such as the pancreatic duct or peripancreatic vessels, which may influence the type of resection performed (Fig. 77.2*C*).

Thus, IOUS is a tool to be used by the surgeon as an extension of palpation. IOUS does not replace traditional operative inspection and palpation maneuvers, since tumors that occur in peripancreatic locations (e.g., gastrinomas that arise in the duodenal wall) are not reliably detected with IOUS (58). IOUS allows precise enucleation of the tumor without large incisions into the pancreas and helps avoid complications associated with pancreatic surgery, such as fistulas, pseudocysts, and pancreatitis. Information gained from IOUS can change the course and outcome of the operation for an insulinoma, and we strongly recommend its use.

**Tumor Resection.** Localization of the tumor and delineation of the anatomy surrounding the insulinoma dictates the type of surgery performed, either enucleation or a more formal pancreatic resection. The goal is not to resect pancreas blindly but to remove all hyperfunctioning tissue while preserving normal pancreatic tissue. Insulinomas that occur in the head of the pancreas can usually be enucleated. Similarly, insulinomas arising in the body or tail of the pancreas that are not adjacent to important structures can be enucleated. Enucleation means excision of the entire adenomatous tissue without great margins of normal pancreatic tissue. Because more than 90% of insulinomas are benign, simple tumor enucleation is acceptable for this particular type of islet cell tumor. Evidence of a malignant tumor, such as involved peripancreatic lymph nodes, requires a formal pancreatic resection, not enucleation. Rarely, extremely large tumors in the head that cannot be safely enucleated may require a Whipple pancreaticoduodenectomy, an operation that can be done safely with low mortality and minimal morbidity by experienced surgeons (59). It is important to determine the relationship of the tumor to the pancreatic duct by IOUS prior to tumor excision. If no clear margin of normal pancreatic tissue exists between the insulinoma and the pancreatic duct or major vessels, then a distal or subtotal pancreatectomy is advised. Ductal injury in an attempt to resect a tumor in close proximity to the pancreatic duct results in significantly increased postoperative morbidity (1). Furthermore, adenomatous tissue left behind may cause persistence or recurrence of hypoglycemia. With careful preoperative localization and the availability of IOUS, blind distal pancreatectomy is no longer advocated.

**Postoperative Management.** Closed suction, large-bore drains are placed near the pancreas to empty third-space fluid and to monitor for pancreatic leak postoperatively. Drains are discontinued when the patient tolerates a low-fat diet and drainage is less than 20 mL/day.

In general, morbidity after this type of pancreatic surgery should be below 20%, and mortality should approach 0% (1). Potential complications that are specific to operating on the pancreas include fistula, pseudocyst, pancreatitis, and abscess. Persistent drainage of amylase-rich fluid (>250 mL/day) or increased drainage with eating indicates a pancreatic fistula. An undrained collection of pancreatic fluid results in a pseudocyst. An acute postoperative pseudocyst may be drained percutaneously by interventional radiology. Pancreatic fistulas are treated conservatively with complete bowel rest, total parenteral nutrition, $H_2$-antagonists to decrease emptying of stomach acid and stimulation of pancreatic secretion, and octreotide. Octreotide reduces the amount of drainage (34, 60) and may reduce complications when given both preoperatively and postoperatively (56, 61).

## Outcome

Although the management of patients with an insulinoma may be challenging, virtually all patients with benign, sporadic tumors are cured and have a normal long-term survival (Table 77.2) (62). Proper localization and resection of sporadic insulinomas results in a cure rate above 95% (3, 16, 45, 63). Autonomic and neuroglycopenic symptoms resolve postoperatively, and the fasting morning serum glucose level normalizes (3). Counterregulatory hormonal responses (epinephrine, norepinephrine, glucagon, growth hormone, and cortisol) also normalize after surgery (64). Patients with MEN-1 and insulinomas are usually asymptomatic after surgery but are less commonly cured because of the presence of multiple islet cell tumors, others of which may secrete insulin, and the possibility of malignancy (65, 66). The occurrence of a new insulinoma or the development of metastases may lead to recurrent hyperinsulinism. Surgery can control symptoms and avoid potential life-threatening sequelae associated with the hyperinsulinism from insulinomas even with limited metastases when they can be removed safely with acceptable morbidity and mortality.

## Special Considerations for Insulinoma

**Occult Insulinoma.** An "occult" insulinoma is a tumor unlocalized by nonoperative tests that occurs in a patient with fasting hypoglycemia and hyperinsulinemia. The tumor is bio-

**TABLE 77.2. Insulinoma Tumor Localization and Cure Rate in Selected Recent Studies**

| | | | Tumor Localized | | Patients Cured | |
|---|---|---|---|---|---|---|
| Reference | Year | *n* | *n* | % | *n* | % |
| Doherty GM et al. (3) | 1991 | 25 | 24 | 96 | 24 | 96 |
| Grant CS et al. (45) | 1988 | 36 | 36 | 100 | 35 | 97 |
| Pasieka JL, et al. (16) | 1992 | 45 | 45 | 100 | 45 | 100 |
| Rothmund M, et al. (63) | 1990 | 396 | 394 | 99 | 394 | 99 |
| Totals | | 502 | 499 | 99 | 499 | 99 |

Modified from Norton JA. Neuroendocrine tumors of the pancreas and duodenum. Curr Prob Surg 1994;31:77–164.

chemically proven, but its anatomic site remains unknown. Approximately 10–20% of insulinomas are occult. Each patient should have at least regional localization of the tumor to the right or left of the SMA by calcium arteriography. Exploratory laparotomy is then the last resort to identify the tumor precisely and cure the disease. Surgery should not be performed in these patients unless IOUS is available (3, 58, 67, 68).

In the rare instance in which a tumor remains unlocalized and unresected after thorough exploration with IOUS, the decision whether or not to perform a pancreatectomy depends on the particular patient's response to medical management and the results of the preoperative calcium arteriogram. Pancreatic resection is not indicated if the patient's hypoglycemia can be well controlled with medications, as discussed above. When medical management is unsatisfactory, the only alternative is to perform a pancreatectomy. The type of pancreatectomy to perform depends on the regional localization data from the preoperative tests. For example, if arteriogram with calcium stimulation suggests increased insulin production when the splenic artery is selectively injected, then a distal pancreatectomy is appropriate. A Whipple pancreaticoduodenotomy is indicated when the gastroduodenal or SMA injection is positive on calcium arteriogram, no tumor is palpable or imaged by IOUS, and the hypoglycemia cannot be managed medically.

Blind progressive pancreatic resection has been advocated in the past with intraoperative glucose monitoring for rebound hyperglycemia when the insulinoma is excised (69). However, the reported false-positive and false-negative rates associated with this technique are high, and there is a 33–45% chance that the tumor arises within the pancreatic head and will not be removed using this approach (68). Furthermore, this operative technique may be associated with substantial postoperative morbidity (pancreatitis, fistulas, abscess) and long-term morbidity (exocrine pancreas insufficiency, diabetes mellitus) (70, 71). These factors along with the availability of sensitive, safe localization modalities like IOUS and calcium arteriogram all suggest that blind progressive pancreatectomy should be avoided.

**Malignant Insulinoma.** Malignant insulinoma is very rare and occurs in approximately 5–10% of cases (62, 72). As with other islet cell tumors, no histologic criteria exist to define malignancy. Surgery is the only way to stage the true extent of disease accurately. Histologically proven tumor outside the pancreas, usually in peripancreatic lymph nodes or the liver, definitively fulfills the definition of malignancy. Gross invasion of blood vessels, surrounding pancreas, or adjacent organs may also indicate malignancy (1). IOUS showing indistinct tumor margins may imply local invasion and malignancy (58). If none of these features exist, then the tumor is considered benign. However, because islet cell tumors generally grow slowly, metastases may not become evident until years after the initial primary tumor resection. Large tumors (>5 cm) have an increased risk of being cancerous, but insulinomas rarely attain this size (1). Tumor DNA ploidy and tumoral growth fraction determined by flow cytometry may indicate the biologic behavior of insulinomas (73).

Evaluation of a patient with a malignant insulinoma begins by assessing the extent of disease with imaging studies. CT or MRI may identify disease in the chest and abdomen. The radiolabeled octreotide scan is very useful to identify disease anywhere in the body if the tumor binds this isotope. Specific complaints of bone pain are evaluated with bone scan and x-rays. These preoperative staging studies are important to exclude the few patients who would not benefit from resection, because incomplete resection does not improve the ability to control hypoglycemia. Consequently, subtotal resection is only attempted if most of the tumor can be removed. Approximately 30% of patients with metastatic insulinoma can undergo complete resection of tumor (1).

No prospective, randomized trials exist to guide therapy because of the rarity of malignant insulinoma. Results of treatments for other malignant islet cell tumors may be applicable to malignant insulinomas. Pancreatic neuroendocrine carcinomas have a better prognosis than adenocarcinoma of the exocrine pancreas and are often managed with aggressive surgical resection (74). For example, 30% of patients with gastrinoma present with metastatic disease, and at least one study has demonstrated that aggressive surgical resection of liver metastases improves 5-year survival from 20% in unresected patients to 80% (75).

Although treatment is generally palliative, the only potentially curative therapy for locally advanced tumors and for limited metastases is surgery. Surgery may also be the only therapy that increases survival for patients with limited metastatic disease, because life-threatening symptoms are effectively ameliorated, and tumor growth rate is slow (74, 76). Limited metastases as well as the primary tumor should be resected to debulk tumor enough to eliminate the hormonal syndrome (11, 74, 76). In one study, the median survival was increased from 11 months in patients with metastatic insulinoma who could not undergo resection to 4 years in those in whom tumor debulking was possible (77).

The goal of surgery, then, is to cure the patient, if possible, or at least to palliate. The best opportunity for cure is total resection of all tumor, with negative margins at the initial surgery. Subsequent operations are more difficult and usually of lesser benefit, since new metastases may arise in locations that preclude resection because of difficulty or potential morbidity (72). Approximately 50% of patients with metastatic insulinoma undergoing resection have complete biochemical remission (1). For patients with widespread metastatic disease, medical management with frequent meals, diazoxide, and calcium channel blockers may be attempted to prevent episodes of life-threatening hypoglycemia. If hypoglycemia is poorly controlled by medical management and the patient is medically fit, tumor debulking may control symptoms for prolonged periods, even in the setting of distant metastases (77). Patients may also have obstructive symptoms secondary to the mass effect from the size or location of the tumor or gastrointestinal bleeding from direct tumor invasion into adjacent bowel. These are effectively eliminated by resection of the tumor (74). Pain secondary to neural invasion may be palliated by percutaneous celiac-axis nerve block.

Chemotherapy is not curative but may palliate symptoms. Combination chemotherapy with streptozocin and 5-fluorouracil is the most effective regimen against metastatic insulinoma, producing at least a partial response in 60% of patients (13). Doxorubicin may also be added.

The response to surgery or chemotherapy may be assessed by measuring serum insulin, PLC, and α-human chorionic gonadotropin levels (13). Levels should fall with successful treatment; a rise indicates increasing tumor burden. Disease in more than one lobe of the liver has been treated by hepatic arterial embolization or orthotopic liver transplant.

**Insulinoma and MEN-1.** Insulinoma may occur sporadically or in a familial form in association with MEN-1. MEN-1 is inherited as an autosomal dominant disease, and tumors develop in several endocrine organs. Virtually all patients have four-gland parathyroid hyperplasia, up to 75% develop pancreatic islet cell tumors, and pituitary tumors (usually prolactinomas) occur in less than 50% of patients. Functional pancreatic tumors are most commonly gastrinomas, with insulinomas next most frequent (1). Islet cell tumors of different types may occur simultaneously in a patient with MEN-1. Parathyroidectomy is usually the first operation undertaken in these patients, since most patients have parathyroid pathology concomitant with or preceding the diagnosis of an islet cell tumor. Parathyroidectomy with normalization of the serum calcium level may result in better control of symptoms caused by gastrin hypersecretion (78). Patients may also have thyroid adenomas, adrenocortical tumors, carcinoid tumors, and lipomas (1). Approximately 20% of patients with MEN-1 develop insulinomas, usually multiple and occurring diffusely throughout the pancreas (26). The diagnosis of an insulinoma in a patient with MEN 1 is confirmed by demonstrating fasting hypoglycemia and inappropriate hyperinsulinemia. About 10% of patients with hyperinsulinism have MEN-1; therefore, careful screening of all patients with insulinoma is necessary to exclude this syndrome.

The major difficulty in patients with MEN-1 and hyperinsulinism is the simultaneous occurrence of multiple islet cell tumors within the pancreas (26). The tumors may be small and arise diffusely throughout the pancreas. However, in our experience, insulinomas in MEN-1 patients are usually dominant large tumors (>3 cm) that are readily identifiable on CT scan (65). The objective of therapy for an insulinoma in a patient with MEN-1 is the same as for a sporadic insulinoma, to eliminate the source of the hypersecretion of insulin (11). One must identify the tumor or tumors producing the excessive insulin. Invasive tests such as the calcium arteriogram or PVS usually confirm function of the identified tumor. Other small islet cell tumors may also be identified during the invasive testing, which are usually clinically insignificant (11). However, if no tumor is visualized on noninvasive imaging studies, then the exact tumor or tumors producing excessive insulin may be very difficult to pinpoint. The region of the pancreas containing the insulinoma should be ascertained by calcium arteriography or PVS.

In MEN-1 patients, pancreatic resection is the favored approach, because patients may have multiple tumors (79). If the insulinoma is in the body or tail of the pancreas, a subtotal or distal pancreatectomy is warranted. A tumor in the head of the pancreas that cannot be enucleated should be resected by a Whipple pancreaticoduodenectomy. If multiple tumors are identified in a high-insulin-producing region of the pancreas, then formal resection of that specific area of the pancreas encompassing all the tumors is necessary (i.e., distal pancreatectomy or Whipple procedure).

Successful resection of the tumor or tumors responsible for hyperinsulinism cures most patients of the tumor and hypoglycemia (65). However, some patients with insulinoma and MEN-1 are not cured by surgery and develop either persistent or recurrent hypoglycemia because of a missed insulinoma or metastatic disease from the original tumor (1, 80).

## NESIDIOBLASTOSIS

Neonates and infants may rarely present with hypoglycemic symptoms caused by abnormally high pancreatic insulin production. Unlike older children and adults, neonates and infants do not usually have a single pancreatic adenoma that hypersecretes insulin causing the syndrome (81, 82). A more diffuse primary pancreatic abnormality is responsible. This condition has been called several names, including nesidioblastosis, nesidiodysplasia, congenital hyperinsulinism, and, more recently, islet cell dysmaturation syndrome, or hyperinsulinemic hypoglycemia of infancy. In this chapter, the more common term nesidioblastosis is used.

Nesidioblastosis is a congenital syndrome that occurs in approximately 1 in 50,000 live births (83). Because nesidioblastosis is so rare, it is often a difficult diagnostic and management problem. Onset commonly occurs before 18 months of age. Importantly, the diagnosis of nesidioblastosis in an adult should be critically suspect, because islet cell hyperplasia may be present in the pancreas of patients with insulinomas, and an occult insulinoma can be missed in these cases (1, 84). The existence of adult nesidioblastosis remains controversial (85–89).

### Pathophysiology

The pathophysiology of nesidioblastosis is incompletely understood. Current knowledge suggests that it represents a congenital dysmaturation or malregulation of the neonatal and infant endocrine pancreas, with physiologically uncontrolled hypersecretion of insulin (90–92). This abnormal basal regulation of insulin secretion is inhibited by somatostatin (93). Studies have also suggested that hyperinsulinism may not be the sole disorder. A more generalized disturbance of islet cell function may occur, with dysregulated secretion of other pancreatic hormones such as somatostatin and glucagon (94, 95).

A unifying hypothesis about the cause of the disorder does not exist, and it is debatable whether a true anatomic abnormality exists in the pancreas of neonates or infants with nesidioblastosis. Diffuse and more focal histologic patterns of "nesidiodysplasia" and "beta cell hyperplasia," which are variants of normal adult pancreatic histology, have been described (96, 97). However, careful pathologic analyses have shown that morphologic, immunohistologic, and morphometric features of fetal pancreas remain after birth (98). Histologically, the endocrine pancreas of euglycemic neonates and young infants normally contains poorly organized islets composed of scattered A-cells, B-cells, and somatostatin-producing cells, either singly or in small groups, which occur diffusely throughout the pancreas (91). On pathologic examination, the pancreas from an infant with nesidioblastosis may appear similar to pancreatic tissue from normal children of the same age (99). As a result, the histologic pattern of the pancreas cannot reliably predict the presence of clinical hyperinsulinemic hypoglycemia. Therefore, nesidioblastosis should not be defined anatomically by pancreatic histology, and the terms islet cell dysmaturation syndrome or persistent hyperinsulinemic hypoglycemia of infancy may be more appropriate descriptions.

While most cases of nesidioblastosis occur sporadically, there are rare familial cases of the condition, with an apparent autosomal recessive inheritance pattern (94, 100–102). A single gene that controls islet development or that regulates islet hormone secretion may be involved in initiating the disorder (83). The familial hyperinsulinism gene has been mapped to an 0.8 cM region on chromosome 11p15.1 (103).

### Patient Presentation

Children with hyperinsulinemia usually present with neuroglycopenic symptoms such as lethargy, cyanosis, hypothermia, and seizures (82, 104). Death may occur (105). The severity of the hypoglycemia and corresponding symptoms may be related to the relative amounts of insulin and somatostatin produced by the pancreatic islet cells (106). Since nesidioblastosis is a congenital condition, patients are nearly always younger than 18 months of age. As a result of the meager glucose stores in the neonatal and infant liver, the hypoglycemia may be particularly severe, with extremely low blood glucose levels occurring after only a few hours of fasting (81). Thus, neonates may be diagnosed with nesidioblastosis within the first days of life. However, mild symptoms may go unnoticed initially, especially when frequent feedings are given, and nesidioblastosis may not be diagnosed in these patients until later in infancy when they begin to sleep through the night.

Nesidioblastosis may occur in association with Beckwith-Wiedemann syndrome (omphalocele, macroglossia, gigantism), cerebrohepatorenal syndrome (Bowen-Zellweger syndrome), and in MEN-1 (101, 102, 107, 108). Amniotic fluid levels of glucose, insulin, and C-peptide may allow intrauterine diagnosis of familial nesidioblastosis (109).

### Diagnosis

The differential diagnosis of hypoglycemia in infancy is broad. More common causes include adrenal insufficiency, panhypopituitarism, growth hormone deficiency, and adrenal hyperplasia. These conditions can be excluded by measuring serum levels of cortisol, growth hormone, thyroid-stimulating hormone, and thyroid hormone (81).

As with insulinoma, the hormonal syndrome of hyperinsulinemic hypoglycemia is definitively established by documenting the response to fasting hypoglycemia (110). An inappropriately elevated blood insulin level (>6 μU/mL) that occurs simultaneously with a low blood glucose level (<40 mg/dL) is diagnostic. ß-Hydroxybutyrate blood levels are also significantly decreased in infants with hyperinsulinism (110). The diagnosis of nesidioblastosis as a cause for the hyperinsulinemic hypoglycemia is then one of exclusion. Surreptitious administration of insulin or oral hypoglycemic medication is excluded by closely observing the patient and by measuring blood levels of C-peptide, proinsulin, insulin antibodies, and sulfonylurea (111). With the exclusion of factitious hypoglycemia, a neonate or infant who presents early in life with severe hypoglycemic hyperinsulinemia almost certainly has nesidioblastosis.

Because the surgical managements of nesidioblastosis and insulinoma differ, these two conditions must be differentiated. Age at onset is the most important distinguishing factor. After 18 months of age, nesidioblastosis as a cause for endogenous hyperinsulinemia decreases sharply in frequency, and insulinomas are much more frequent (81). Biochemical tests including blood glucose, immunoreactive insulin, and C-peptide levels do not reliably distinguish hyperinsulinemic hypoglycemia caused by an insulinoma from that attributed to nesidioblastosis (112, 113). Thus, older children with hyperinsulinemic hypoglycemia must be thoroughly evaluated to exclude an insulinoma, which must be localized and resected as for an adult (82). Invasive functional tests, such as selective arteriography with calcium stimulation, may show abnormally high levels of insulin being produced from all areas of the pancreas, which is consistent with nesidioblastosis. However, abnormally high insulin production from a localized area of the pancreas must be regarded as suspicious for insulinoma. Negative preoperative localizing studies do not exclude the diagnosis of insulinoma, since these tumors are commonly less than 2 cm, and up to 12% of patients with insulinomas have unlocalized tumors on preoperative studies (39). An insulinoma may not be definitively excluded until after careful intraoperative exploration of the pancreas using IOUS. Only after an insulinoma has been excluded can the diagnosis of nesidioblastosis be applied.

## Management

The main therapeutic objective is prompt correction of acute hypoglycemia and maintenance of euglycemia to prevent neurologic damage. Long-term therapy depends on the severity of symptoms and the ability of different forms of medical therapy to control them. The effect of medical or surgical therapy long-term has not been well established. No controlled clinical trials have evaluated the safety and efficacy of the different treatment regimens.

**Medical Therapy.** Permanent psychomotor retardation and neurologic dysfunction may result from repeated episodes of hypoglycemia in an infant (82, 104, 114). Therefore, aggressive treatment is advocated initially to correct the hypoglycemia expeditiously and maintain euglycemia.

Infants with severe, symptomatic hypoglycemia are given an immediate intravenous bolus of concentrated glucose (50% dextrose solution) to correct the hypoglycemia. A continuous glucose infusion is usually needed to sustain normal blood glucose levels and to avoid further symptomatic episodes. This may require high rates of glucose infusion (>12–15 mg/kg/min) and early central venous catheter placement (83, 98). Continuous nasogastric tube feedings or frequent oral feedings of a low-protein, high-carbohydrate diet may be instituted in an attempt to withdraw the intravenous glucose infusion (81). Oral cornstarch may be added to slow intestinal transit.

For infants who cannot be weaned from intravenous glucose infusion or who have hypoglycemia while receiving intravenous glucose infusion, the addition of antihypoglycemic medications is indicated. Medical control of hypoglycemia in patients with nesidioblastosis may be more effective than that obtained in those with insulinoma. The drug of choice is diazoxide 8–12 mg/kg administered orally (81). Hypoglycemia can be controlled with diazoxide and a high carbohydrate diet in approximately one-third of patients with nesidioblastosis (Table 77.3) (115, 116). Diazoxide may cause fluid retention with hypertension and edema (83). Thiazide diuretics may be added to decrease these side effects.

In the past, patients unresponsive to diazoxide have traditionally undergone pancreatectomy to control the hypoglycemia. Recent studies with limited follow-up suggest that approximately 19–53% of patients who do not respond to diazoxide may respond to octreotide and avoid surgery (Table 77.3) (115, 116). However, octreotide appears to be most effective after islet cell mass is reduced by pancreatectomy (83). Glucagon has also been added to treatment with octreotide to maintain euglycemia in some patients, but long-acting analogues of glucagon are not available (114, 115).

Octreotide is administered subcutaneously, by repeated injection, or by continuous subcutaneous infusion via a pump (114, 116). Octreotide may cause a prompt fall in blood insulin levels and an elevation of the blood glucose level in patients with nesidioblastosis, including diazoxide-unresponsive patients (117–119). This allows reduction in the rate of glucose infusion and elimination of the intravenous glucose requirement in some patients (116). Early use of octreotide protects cerebral function and may reduce mortality (117). Mild gastrointestinal symptoms that may be experienced at the start of octreotide therapy decrease with more prolonged use. There appear to be no major side effects from more prolonged use of octreotide (116, 120, 121). Administration of octreotide for up to 4.3 years in one study caused some decrease in linear growth and depressed blood levels of insulin-like growth factor 1 and insulin-like growth factor binding protein 3, consistent with suppression of growth hormone by octreotide (115).

Because the hyperinsulinemia associated with nesidioblasto-

**TABLE 77.3. Treatment Required to Control Hypoglycemia in Nesidioblastosis**

| | | | Diazoxide | | Octreotide | | Pancreatectomy | |
|---|---|---|---|---|---|---|---|---|
| Reference | Years | *n* | *n* | % | *n* | % | *n* | % |
| Thornton PS, et al. (115) | 1988–93 | 24 | 8 | 33 | 3 | 13 | 13 | 54 |
| Glaser B, et al. (116) | | | | | | | | |
| Group 1[a] | 1975–86 | 22 | 9 | 41 | — | — | 13 | 59 |
| Group 2[a] | 1986–93 | 18 | 3 | 17 | 8 | 44 | 7 | 39 |
| Totals | | 64 | 20 | 31 | 11 | 17 | 33 | 52 |

[a]Octreotide was not available for group 1 patients.

sis usually improves with time, if patients respond well to octreotide, medical therapy may be the primary and only treatment necessary, and surgery can be avoided (115–117, 120). However, in one study, resistance to treatment with octreotide occurred in 16 of 16 patients, even when doses were increased (115). Long-term treatment with octreotide requires 3–4 daily subcutaneous injections or an implanted subcutaneous pump, multiple daily blood glucose measurements at home, strict diet, and substantial expense (83, 116). Hospitalization is needed for illnesses. Octreotide use may only be appropriate for preoperative preparation and as a trial to avoid surgery for families who can manage the complex treatment regimen (83).

The goal of medical management is to keep blood glucose levels consistently above 60 mg/dL. Gastrostomy may be required for long-term continuous feedings. Some infants improve by 2–6 months of age, while others may require years of medical treatment before therapy can be successfully withdrawn (81, 116). However, patients whose hypoglycemia cannot be controlled with aggressive medical management require surgery.

**Surgery.** Surgery is indicated for infants who do not tolerate medical therapy or who cannot be weaned from intravenous glucose infusions (114, 122). Approximately half of infants with nesidioblastosis require pancreatectomy to control severe hypoglycemia (115, 116). The purpose of surgery is to eliminate the hyperfunctioning insulin-producing tissue so that life-threatening hypoglycemia either does not occur or can be managed with minimal medication and diet modification.

The pancreas is approached so that the entire organ can be appropriately evaluated. A midline incision or a transverse incision above the umbilicus provides good exposure. The bowel and its mesentery are examined for ectopic pancreatic tissue. The gastrocolic ligament is divided to enter the lesser sac. The head of the pancreas is exposed by an extended Kocher maneuver. Adequate exploration of the tail of the pancreas may require mobilization of the spleen from the left upper quadrant. Division of superior and inferior peripancreatic ligaments allows mobilization of the body of the pancreas from the retroperitoneum.

If the patient is over 1 year of age and an insulinoma has not been excluded, then intensive exploration of the pancreas using visualization, palpation, and IOUS is necessary to determine whether an insulinoma is present (3). If a mass consistent with an insulinoma is found, then IOUS-guided enucleation of the mass is indicated. Alternatively, formal pancreatic resection may be necessary if the proximity of the insulinoma to the pancreatic duct or vessels precludes safe enucleation. Blind pancreatectomy is not indicated for an insulinoma (1). If an insulinoma is not identified, then the diagnosis of nesidioblastosis should be entertained. Islet cell hyperplasia can be demonstrated in the pancreas of patients with insulinomas, so biopsy results alone showing a diffuse islet cell disorder in a patient with hyperinsulinism do not exclude the presence of an insulinoma (84).

A near-total pancreatectomy is indicated for nesidioblastosis because this disorder affects the entire pancreas. In general, the spleen can be preserved, decreasing the risk of overwhelming postsplenectomy sepsis (98, 123–125). The pancreatic tail is first mobilized from the splenic hilum, leaving the splenic vessels intact (Fig. 77.5*A*). Pancreatic resection then proceeds toward the duodenum. The splenic artery and vein are carefully separated from the superior aspect of the pancreatic parenchyma and preserved. However, the spleen may be preserved even if the splenic artery is ligated (125). Small vessels penetrating the superior surface of the pancreas are either ligated or cauterized (Fig. 77.5*A*). The pancreas is separated from the superior mesenteric artery and vein. The resection continues toward the duodenum and bile duct. The uncinate process is removed by rotating it anteriorly from behind the duodenum (98). The pancreatic tissue is resected, while carefully preserving the blood supply to the common bile duct and duodenum. A small amount of pancreas is left at the junction of the common bile duct and duodenum. The edge of the pancreas and the pancreatic duct are oversewn (98). Suction drains are left in the vicinity of the oversewn duct.

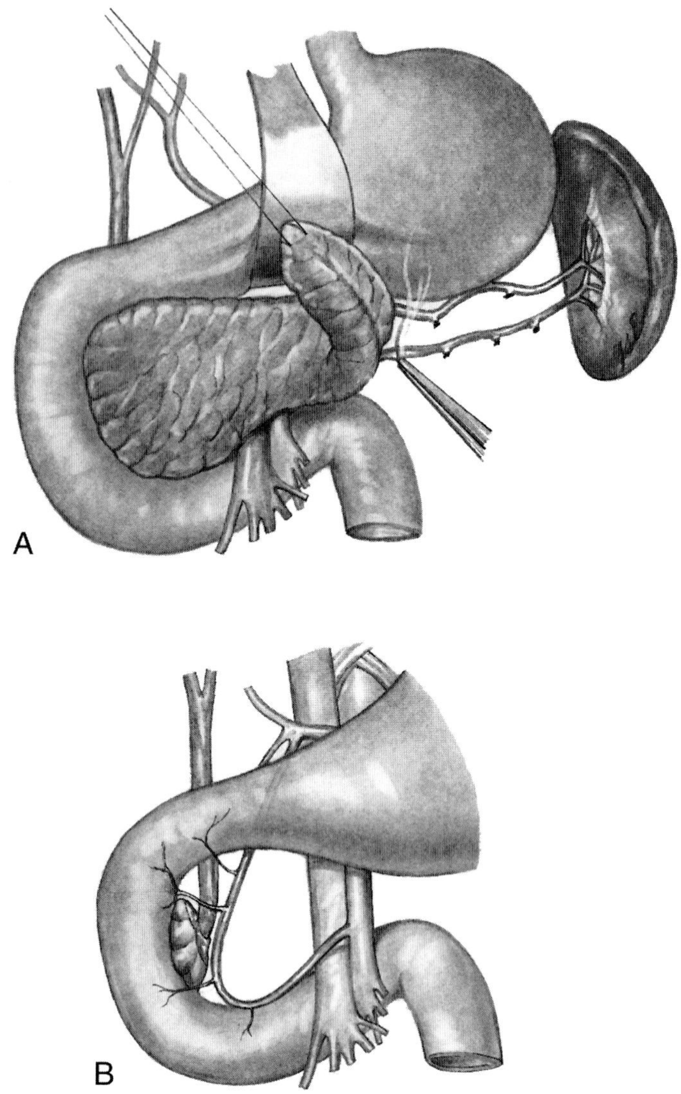

**FIG. 77.5.** Spleen-preserving pancreatectomy for nesidioblastosis. **A.** Mobilization of the pancreas begins at the splenic hilum and proceeds toward the duodenum, while preserving the splenic vessels and ligating or cauterizing vessels that feed directly into the pancreas. **B.** A near-total (95%) pancreatectomy is recommended, leaving a small amount of pancreatic tissue near the junction of the duodenum and common bile duct, which are left well vascularized.

The appropriate amount of pancreas to resect ultimately depends on the severity of the underlying disease in each particular patient. The main objective is to resect enough pancreas so that islet tissue is eliminated and the patient is euglycemic, preferably without medical therapy. It is important to resect enough pancreas at the initial operation, because reoperation may be difficult in a scarred area, especially resecting tissue near the duodenum and bile duct. Near-total pancreatectomy, in which 95% of the pancreas is removed, is recommended (125, 126). Only mild impairment of pancreatic function is demonstrable at 1–2 years after 95% pancreatectomy (127). Preserving some pancreatic tissue is necessary to avoid postoperative diabetes mellitus and exocrine pancreatic insufficiency (127).

## Outcome

Immediately after operation, patients should be euglycemic without concentrated intravenous glucose infusion. Mild hypoglycemia usually responds well to intravenous fluid containing 5% dextrose. As a high-carbohydrate diet is instituted, the blood glucose level is closely monitored to indicate when glucose infusions can be discontinued. After successful pancreatectomy, over half of patients can usually be maintained on frequent feedings of a high-carbohydrate diet alone. The addition of diazoxide or octreotide may be required in a minority of patients to maintain euglycemia postoperatively (115, 120). Persistent, medically untreatable hypoglycemia after partial pancreatic resection is a rare indication for reoperation and resection of more pancreatic tissue (128). Every effort should be made to spare the duodenum and bile duct in these cases.

Although surgery allows effective control of severe hypoglycemia, it does not treat the basic pathogenesis of nesidioblastosis (83). Nesidioblastosis appears to be a lifelong disorder of islet cell malregulation and control of spontaneous hypoglycemia does not correct the primary beta-cell defect. One study found that patients have impaired insulin responses to glucose and are unable to suppress endogenous insulin production for up to 21 years after clinical remission, and a significant proportion develop insulin-requiring diabetes at puberty (129). Whether decreased beta-cell mass after pancreatectomy or beta-cell failure as the natural end-stage of the disease is responsible for the late incidence of diabetes is uncertain (116).

Achieving good long-term control of hypoglycemia, whether by medical or surgical means, remains the prime consideration to prevent damage to the developing neurologic system. Early, aggressive medical therapy and pancreatectomy in patients with medically uncontrolled hypoglycemia results in resolution of the life-threatening symptoms, normal growth, normal neurologic development, and normal psychomotor function (114, 123). Postpancreatectomy diabetes and malabsorption may occur over time, but these conditions are usually easily managed medically (83). Research into the pathophysiologic basis of nesidioblastosis continues, to define new potential treatments for this condition.

## REFERENCES


1. Norton JA. Neuroendocrine tumors of the pancreas and duodenum. Curr Prob Surg 1994;31:77–164.
2. Peplinski GR, Norton JA. Gastrointestinal endocrine cancers and nodal metastases: biological significance and therapeutic implications. Surg Oncol Clin North Am 1996;5:159–171.
3. Doherty GM, Doppman JL, Shawker TH, Miller DL, Eastman RC, et al. Results of a prospective strategy to diagnose, localize and resect insulinomas. Surgery 1991;110:989–997.
4. Norton JA, Sigel B, Baker AR, Ettinghausen SE, Shawker TH, et al. Localization of an occult insulinoma by intraoperative ultrasonography. Surgery 1985;97:381–384.
5. Charboneau WJ, James EM, van Heerden JA, et al. Intraoperative realtime ultrasonographic localization of pancreatic insulinomas. J Ultrasound Med 1983;2:251.
6. Sigel B, Coelho JC, Nyhus LM, Velasco JM, Donahue PE, et al. Detection of pancreatic tumors by ultrasound during surgery. Arch Surg 1982;177:1058–1061.
7. Heyder N. Localization of an insulinoma by ultrasonic endoscopy. N Engl J Med 1985;312:860–861.
8. Glover JR, Shorvon PJ, Lees WR. Endoscopic ultrasound for localization of islet cell tumors. Gut 1992;33:108–110.
9. Thompson NW, Czako PF, Fritts LL, Bude R, Bansal R, et al. Role of endoscopic ultrasonography in the localization of insulinomas and gastrinomas. Surgery 1994;116:1131–1138.
10. Rosch T, Lightdale CJ, Botet JF, Boyce GA, Sivak MV, et al. Localization of pancreatic endocrine tumors by endoscopic ultrasonography. N Engl J Med 1992;326:1721–1726.
11. Debas HT, Mulvihill SJ. Neuroendocrine gut neoplasms: important lessons from uncommon tumors. Arch Surg 1994;129: 965–971.
12. Grunberger G, Weiner JL, Silverman R, Taylor S, Gorden P. Factitious hypoglycemia due to surreptitious administration of insulin: diagnosis, treatment and long-term follow-up. Ann Intern Med 1988;108:252–257.
13. Comi RJ, Gorden P. Hypoglycemic disorders in the adult. In: Becker KL, Kahn CR, eds. Principles and practice of endocrinology and metabolism. 2nd ed. Philadelphia: JB Lippincott, 1995:1342–1351.
14. O'Brien T, O'Brien PC, Service FJ. Insulin surrogates in insulinoma. J Clin Endocrinol Metab 1993;77:448–451.
15. Gorden P, Skarulis MC, Roach P, Comi RJ, Fraker DL, et al. Plasma proinsulin-like component in insulinoma: a 25-year experience. J Clin Endocrinol Metab 1995;80:2884–2887.
16. Pasieka JL, McLeod MK, Thompson NW, Burney RE. Surgical approach to insulinomas: assessing the need for preoperative localization. Arch Surg 1992;127:442–447.
17. Steiner DF, Oyer PE. The biosynthesis of insulin and a probable precursor of insulin by a human islet cell adenoma. Proc Natl Acad Sci USA 1967;57:473–480.
18. Roth J, Gorden P, Pastan I. "Big insulin:" a new component of plasma insulin detected by immunoassay. Proc Natl Acad Sci USA 1968;61:138–145.
19. Conlon JM, Hoog A, Grimelius L. Intracellular degradation of the C-peptide of proinsulin, in a human insulinoma: identification of sites of cleavage and evidence for a role for cathepsin B. Pancreas 1995;10:167–172.
20. Service FJ, O'Brien PC, McMahon MM, Kao PC. C-peptide during the prolonged fast in insulinoma. J Clin Endocrinol Metab 1993;76:655–659.
21. Lazarus NR, Tanese T, Gutman R, Recant L. Synthesis and release of proinsulin and insulin by human insulinoma tissue. J Clin Endocrinol Metab 1970;30:273–281.
22. Monti LD, Sandoli EP, Phan VC, Piatti PM, Costa S, et al. A sensitive and reliable method for assaying true human insulin without interaction with human proinsulin-like molecules. Acta Diabetol 1995;32:57–63.
23. Roth J, Komminoth P, Heitz PU. Topographic abnormalities of proinsulin to insulin conversion in functioning human insulinomas. Comparison of immunoelectron microscopic and clinical data. Am J Pathol 1995;147:489–502.
24. Nauck MA, Siegel EG, Creutzfeldt W. Prolonged maximal stimulation of insulin secretion in healthy subjects does not provoke preferential release of proinsulin. Pancreas 1991;6: 645–652.
25. Kao PC, Taylor RL, Service FJ. Proinsulin by immunochemiluminometric assay for the diagnosis of insulinoma. J Clin Endocrinol Metab 1994;78:1048–1051.
26. Demeure MJ, Klonoff DC, Karam JH, Duh QY, Clark OH. Insulinomas associated with multiple endocrine neoplasia type 1: the need for a different surgical approach. Surgery 1991;110: 998–1004.
27. Thompson NW, Lloyd RV, Nishiyama RH, et al . MEN-1 pancreas: a histological and immunohistochemical study. World J Surg 1984;8:561–574.
28. Nakamura Y, Larsson C, Julier C, Bystrom C, Skogseid B, et al. Localization of the genetic defect in multiple endocrine neoplasia type I within a small region of chromosome II. Am J Hum Genet 1989;44:751–755.
29. Maton PN. Use of octreotide acetate for control of symptoms in patients with islet cell tumors. World J Surg 1993;17:504–510.
30. Arnold R, Frank M, Kajdan U. Management of gastroenteropancreatic endocrine tumors: the place of somatostatin analogues. Digestion 1994;55(suppl 3):107–113.
31. von Eyben FE, Grodum E, Gjessing HJ, Hagen C, Nielsen H. Metabolic remission with octreotide in patients with insulinoma. J Intern Med 1994;235:245–248.
32. Timmer R, Koningsberger JC, Erkelens DW, Thijssen JH, Lips CJ, Koppeschaar HP. No effect of the long-acting somatostatin analogue octreotide in patients with insulinoma. Neth J Med 1991;38:199–203.

33. Arnold R, Neuhaus C, Benning R, Schwerk WB, Trautmann ME, et al. Somatostatin analog sandostatin and inhibition of tumor growth in patients with metastatic endocrine gastroenteropancreatic tumors. World J Surg 1993;17:511–519.
34. Gorden P, Comi RJ, Maton PN, Go VLW. Somatostatin and somatostatin analogue (SMS 201-995) in treatment of hormone-secreting tumors of the pituitary and gastrointestinal tract and non-neoplastic diseases of the gut. Ann Intern Med 1989;110: 35–50.
35. Owens LV, Huth JF, Cance WG. Insulinoma: pitfalls in preoperative localization. Eur J Surg Oncol 1995;21:326–328.
36. Pedrazzoli S, Pasquali C, Alfano D'Andrea A. Surgical treatment of insulinoma. Br J Surg 1994;81:672–676.
37. Bottger TC, Junginger T. Is preoperative radiographic localization of islet cell tumors in patients with insulinoma necessary? World J Surg 1993;17:427–432.
38. Liessi G, Pasquale C, D'Andrea AA, Scandellari C, Pedrazzoli S. MRI in insulinomas: preliminary findings. Eur J Radiol 1992;14: 46–51.
39. Doppman JL, Chang R, Fraker DL, Norton JA, Alexander HR, et al. Localization of insulinomas to regions of the pancreas by intra-arterial stimulation with calcium. Ann Intern Med 1995;123: 269–273.
40. Vinik AI, Delbridge L, Moattari R, Cho K, Thompson N. Transhepatic portal vein catheterization for localization of insulinomas: a ten-year experience. Surgery 1991;109:1–11.
41. Gianello P, Gigot JF, Berthet F, Dardenne AN, Lambotte L, et al. Pre- and intraoperative localization of insulinomas: report of 22 observations. World J Surg 1988;12:389–397.
42. Geoghegan JG, Jackson LE, Lewis MP, Owen ER, Bloom SR, et al. Localization and surgical management of insulinoma. Br J Surg 1994;81:1025–1028.
43. Kurosaki Y, Kuramoto K, Murata S, Itai Y. Improved detection of small insulinomas with intravenous dynamic CT. J Comput Assist Tomogr 1994;18:588–589.
44. Fraker DL, Norton JA. Localization and resection of insulinomas and gastrinomas. JAMA 1988;259:3601–3605.
45. Grant CS, van Heerden J, Charboneau JW, James EM, Reading CC. Insulinoma: the value of intraoperative ultrasonography. Arch Surg 1988;123:843–848.
46. Lamberts SW, Bakker WH, Reubi JC, Krenning EP. Somatostatin receptor imaging in the localization of endocrine tumors. N Engl J Med 1990;323:1246–1249.
47. Lamberts SW, Hofland LJ, van Koetsveld PM, Reubi JC, et al. Parallel in vivo and in vitro detection of functional somatostatin receptors in human endocrine pancreatic tumors: consequences with regard to diagnosis, localization and therapy. J Clin Endocrinol Metab 1990;71:566–574.
48. Nocaudie-Calzada M, Huglo D, Deveaux M, Carnaille B, Proye C, Marchandise X. Iodine-123-Tyr-3-octreotide uptake in pancreatic endocrine tumors and in carcinoids in relation to hormonal inhibition by octreotide. J Nucl Med 1994;35:57–62.
49. Ur E, Bomanji J, Mather SJ, Britton KE, Wass JA, Grossman AB, Besser GM. Localization of neuroendocrine tumours and insulinomas using radiolabelled somatostatin analogues, $^{123}$I-Tyr3-octreotide and $^{111}$In-pentatreotide. Clin Endocrinol 1993;38: 501–506.
50. van Eyck CHJ, Bruining HA, Reubi JC, Bakker WH, Oei HY, et al. Use of isotope-labeled somatostatin analogs for visualization of islet cell tumors. World J Surg 1993;17:444–447.
51. Modlin IM, Cornelius E, Lawton GP. Use of an isotopic somatostatin receptor probe to image gut endocrine tumors. Arch Surg 1995;130:367–373.
52. Ur E, Bomanji J, Mather SJ, Britton KE, Wass JA, et al. Localization of neuroendocrine tumors and insulinomas using radiolabelled somatostatin analogues, 123I-Tyr3-octreotide and 111In-pentatreotide. Clin Endocrinol 1993;38:501–506.
53. Virgolini I, Raderer M, Kurtaran A, Angelberger P, Banyai S, et al. Vasoactive intestinal peptide-receptor imaging for the localization of intestinal adenocarcinomas and endocrine tumors. N Engl J Med 1994;331:1116–1121.
54. Bottger TC, Weber W, Beyer J, Junginger T. Value of tumor localization in patients with insulinoma. World J Surg 1990;14: 107–114.
55. Miller DL, Doppman JL, Metz DC, Maton PN, Norton JA, Jensen RT. Zollinger-Ellison syndrome: technique, results, and complications of portal venous sampling. Radiology 1992;182:235–241.
56. Buchler M, Friess H, Klempa I, Hermanek P, Sulkowski U, et al. Role of octreotide in the prevention of postoperative complications following pancreatic resection. Am J Surg 1992;163:125–131.
57. Angelini L, Bezzi M, Tucci G, Lirici MM, Candiani F, et al. The ultrasonic detection of insulinomas during surgical exploration of the pancreas. World J Surg 1987;11:642–647.
58. Norton JA, Cromack DT, Shawker TH, Doppman JL, Comi R, et al. Intraoperative ultrasonographic localization of islet cell tumors. Ann Surg 1988;207:160–168.
59. Udelsman R, Yeo CJ, Hruban RH, Pitt HA, Niederhuber JE, et al. Pancreaticoduodenectomy for selected pancreatic endocrine tumors. Surg Gynecol Obstet 1993;177:269–278.
60. Heij HA, Bruining HA, Verschoor L. A comparison of the effects of two somatostatin analogues in a patient with an external pancreatic fistula. Pancreas 1986;1:188–190.
61. Lange JR, Steinberg S, Doherty GM, Langstein HN, Shawker T, et al. A randomized prospective trial of postoperative somatostatin analogue in patients with neuroendocrine tumors of the pancreas. Surgery 1992;112:1033–1038.
62. Service FJ, McMahon MM, O'Brien PC, Ballard DJ. Functioning insulinoma—incidence, recurrence, and long-term survival of patients: a 60-year study. Mayo Clin Proc 1991;66:711–719.
63. Rothmund M, Angelini L, Brunt LM, Farndon JR, Geelhoed G, et al. Surgery for benign insulinoma: an international review. World J Surg 1990;14:393–399.
64. Mitrakou A, Fanelli C, Veneman T, Perriello G, Calderone S, et al. Reversibility of unawareness of hypoglycemia in patients with insulinomas. N Engl J Med 1993;329:834–839.
65. Sheppard BC, Norton JA, Doppman JL, Maton PN, Gardner JD, Jensen RT. Management of islet cell tumors in patients with multiple endocrine neoplasia: a prospective study. Surgery 1989;106:1108–1118.
66. Grama D, Skogseid B, Wilander E, Eriksson B, Martensson H, et al. Pancreatic tumors in multiple endocrine neoplasia type 1: clinical presentation and surgical treatment. World J Surg 1992;16:611–618.
67. van Heerden JA, Grant CS, Czako PF, Service FJ, Charboneau JW. Occult functioning insulinomas: which localizing studies are indicated. Surgery 1992;112:1010–1014.
68. Norton JA, Shawker TH, Doppman JL, Miller DL, Fraker DL, et al. Localization and surgical treatment of occult insulinomas. Ann Surg 1990;212:615–620.
69. Katz LB, Aufses AH, Rayfield E, Mitty H. Preoperative localization and intraoperative glucose monitoring in the management of patients with pancreatic insulinoma. Surg Gynecol Obstet 1986;163:509–512.
70. Glickman MH, Hart MJ, White TT. Insulinoma in Seattle: 39 cases in 30 years. 1980;140:119–125.
71. Galbut DL, Markowitz AM. Insulinoma: diagnosis, surgical management and long-term followup. Am J Surg 1980;139:682.
72. Zogakis TG, Norton JA. Palliative operations for patients with unresectable endocrine neoplasia. Surg Clin North Am 1995;75: 525–538.
73. Losada J, Sarria R, Fernandez Val JF, Lopez Ariztegui MA. DNA ploidy and PCNA index in pancreatic lesions producing hyperinsulinemic hypoglycemia. J Surg Oncol 1995;59:14–17.
74. Rothmund M, Stinner B, Arnold R. Endocrine pancreatic carcinoma. Eur J Surg Oncol 1991;17:191–199.
75. Norton JA, Sugarbaker PH, Doppman JL, Wesley RA, Maton PN, et al. Aggressive resection of metastatic disease in selected patients with malignant gastrinoma. Ann Surg 1986;203:352–359.
76. Modlin IM, Lewis JJ, Ahlman H, Bilchik AJ, Kumar RR. Management of unresectable malignant endocrine tumors of the pancreas. Surg Gynecol Obstet 1993;176:507–518.
77. Danforth DN, Gorden P, Brennan MF. Metastatic insulin secreting carcinoma of the pancreas. Clinical course and the role of surgery. Surgery 1984;96:1027–1036.
78. Norton JA, Cornelius MJ, Doppman JL, Maton PN, Gardner JD, Jensen RT. Effect of parathyroidectomy in patients with hyperparathyroidism, Zollinger-Ellison syndrome, and multiple endocrine neoplasia type 1: a prospective study. Surgery 1987;102: 958–966.
79. O'Riordain DS, O'Brien T, van Heerden JA, Service FJ, Grant CS.

Surgical management of insulinoma associated with multiple endocrine neoplasia type I. World J Surg 1994;18:488–493.
80. Rasbach DA, van Heerden JA, Telandar RL, et al. Surgical management of hyperinsulinism in the multiple endocrine neoplasia, type I syndrome. Arch Surg 1985;120:584–589.
81. Glasgow AM. Hypoglycemia of infancy and childhood. In: Becker KL, Kahn CR, eds. Principles and practice of endocrinology and metabolism. 2nd ed. Philadelphia: JB Lippincott, 1995:1360–1368.
82. Bjerke HS, Kelly RE Jr, Geffner ME, Fonkalsrud EW. Surgical management of islet cell dysmaturation syndrome in young children. Surg Gynecol Obstet 1990;171:321–325.
83. Daneman D, Ehrlich RM. The enigma of persistent hyperinsulinemic hypoglycemia of infancy. J Pediatr 1993;123:573–575.
84. Goudswaard WB, Houthoff HJ, Koudstaal J, Zwierstra RP. Nesidioblastosis and endocrine hyperplasia of the pancreas: a secondary phenomenon. Hum Pathol 1986;17:46–54.
85. Walmsley D, Matheson NA, Ewen S, Himsworth RL, Bevan JS. Nesidioblastosis in an elderly patient. Diabetic Med 1995;12: 542–545.
86. Farley DR, van Heerden JA, Myers JL. Adult pancreatic nesidioblastosis: unusual presentations of a rare entity. Arch Surg 1994;129:329–332.
87. Albers N, Lohr M, Bogner U, Loy V, Kloppel G. Nesidioblastosis of the pancreas in an adult with persistent hyperinsulinemic hypoglycemia. Am J Clin Pathol 1989;91:336–340.
88. McHenry C, Newell K, Chejfec G, Barbato A, Lawrence AM, et al. Adult nesidioblastosis: an unusual cause of fasting hypoglycemia. Am Surg 1989;55:366–369.
89. Carlson T, Eckhauser ML, DeBaz B, Khiyami A, Park CH. Nesidioblastosis in an adult: an illustrative case and collective review. Am J Gastroenterol 1987;82:566–571.
90. Gould VE, Memoli VA, Dardi LE, Gould NS. Nesidiodysplasia and nesidioblastosis of infancy: structural and functional correlations with the syndrome of hyperinsulinemic hypoglycemia. Pediatr Pathol 1983;1:7–31.
91. Rahier J, Wallon J, Henquin JC. Cell populations in the endocrine pancreas of human neonates and infants. Diabetologia 1981; 20:540–546.
92. Shermeta DW, Mendelsohn G, Haller JA Jr. Hyperinsulinemic hypoglycemia of the neonate associated with persistent fetal histology and function of the pancreas. Ann Surg 1980;191: 182–186.
93. Hirsch HJ, Loo S, Evans N, Crigler JF, Filler RM, Gabbay KH. Hypoglycemia of infancy and nesidioblastosis: studies with somatostatin. New Engl J Med 1977;296:1323–1326.
94. Schwartz SS, Rich BH, Lucky AW, Straus FH 2d, Gonen B, et al. Familial nesidioblastosis: severe neonatal hypoglycemia in two families. J Pediatr 1979;95:44–53.
95. Shermeta DW, Mendelsohn G. Hyperinsulin hypoglycemia in the neonate: therapeutic choices. J Pediatr Surg 1980;15: 398–399.
96. Goossens A, Gepts W, Saudubray JM, Bonnefont JP, Nihoul-Fekete, et al. Diffuse and focal nesidioblastosis: a clinicopathological study of 24 patients with persistent neonatal hyperinsulinemic hypoglycemia. Am J Surg Pathol 1989;13:766–775.
97. Taguchi T, Suita S, Hirose R. Histological classification of nesidioblastosis: efficacy of immunohistochemical study of neuron-specific enolase. J Pediatr Surg 1991;26:770–774.
98. Warden MJ, German JC, Buckingham BA. The surgical management of hyperinsulinism in infancy due to nesidioblastosis. J Pediatr Surg 1988;23:462–465.
99. Rahier J, Falt K, Muntefering H, Becker K, Gepts W, Falkmer S. The basic structural lesion of persistent neonatal hypoglycaemia with hyperinsulinism: deficiency of pancreatic D cells or hyperactivity of B cells? Diabetologia 1984;26:282–289.
100. Moreno LA, Turck D, Gottrand F, Fabre M, Manouvrier-Hanu S, Farriaux JP. Familial hyperinsulinism with nesidioblastosis of the pancreas: further evidence for autosomal recessive inheritance. Am J Med Genet 1989;34:584–586.
101. Woolf DA, Leonard JV, Trembath RC, Pembrey ME, Grant DB. Nesidioblastosis: evidence for autosomal recessive inheritance. Arch Dis Child 1991;66:529–530.
102. Glaser B, Phillip M, Carmi R, Lieberman E, Landau H. Persistent hyperinsulinemic hypoglycemia of infancy (''nesidioblastosis''): autosomal recessive inheritance in 7 pedigrees. Am J Med Genet 1990;37:511–515.
103. Glaser B, Chiu KC, Liu L, Anker R, Nestorowicz A, et al. Recombinant mapping of the familial hyperinsulinemia gene to an 0.8 cM region on chromosome 11p15.1 and demonstration of a founder effect in Ashkenazi Jews. Hum Mol Genet 1995;4:879–886.
104. Knight J, Garvin PJ, Danis RK, Lewis JE Jr, Willman VL. Nesidioblastosis in children. Arch Surg 1980;115:880–882.
105. Aynsley-Green A, Polak JM, Keeling J, Gough MH, Baum JD. Averted sudden neonatal death due to pancreatic nesidioblastosis. Lancet 1978;1:550–551.
106. Upp JR Jr, Ishizuka J, Lobe TE, Rajaraman S, Townsend CM Jr, Thompson JC. Somatostatin secretion in cultured human islet cells from patients with nesidioblastosis: a compensatory mechanism? J Pediatr Surg 1987;22:1185–1186.
107. Drut R, Jones MC. Congenital pancreatoblastoma in Beckwith-Wiedemann syndrome: an emerging association. Pediatr Pathol 1988;8:331–339.
108. Kloppel G, Willemer S, Stamm B, Hacki WH, Heitz PU. Pancreatic lesions and hormonal profile of pancreatic tumors in multiple endocrine neoplasia type 1: an immunocytochemical study of nine patients. Cancer 1986;57:1824–1832.
109. Bianchi C, Corbella E, Beccaria L, Bolla P, Chiumello G. A case of familial nesidioblastosis: prenatal diagnosis of foetal hyperinsulinism. Acta Paediatr 1992;81:853–855.
110. Stanley CA, Baker L. Hyperinsulinism in infancy: diagnosis by demonstration of abnormal response to fasting hypoglycemia. Pediatrics 1976;57:702–711.
111. Rayman G, Santo M, Salomon F, Almog S, Paradinas FJ, et al. Hyperinsulinaemic hypoglycaemia due to chlorpropamide-induced nesidioblastosis. J Clin Pathol 1984;37:651–654.
112. Amendt P, Kohnert KD, Kunz J. The hyperinsulinaemic hypoglycaemias in infancy: a study of six cases. Eur J Pediatr 1988;148: 107–112.
113. Aynsley-Green A, Jenkins P, Tronier B, Heding LG. Plasma proinsulin and C-peptide concentrations in children with hyperinsulinaemic hypoglycaemia. Acta Paediatr Scand 1984;73: 359–363.
114. Jacobs DG, Haka-Ikse K, Wesson DE, Filler RM, Sherwood G. Growth and development in patients operated on for islet cell dysplasia. J Pediatr Surg 1986;21:1184–1189.
115. Thornton PS, Alter CA, Katz LE, Baker L, Stanley CA. Short- and long-term use of octreotide in the treatment of congenital hyperinsulinism. J Pediatr 1993;123:637–643.
116. Glaser B, Hirsch HJ, Landau H. Persistent hyperinsulinemic hypoglycemia of infancy: long-term octreotide treatment without pancreatectomy. J Pediatr 1993;123:644–650.
117. Tauber MT, Harris AG, Rochiccioli P. Clinical use of the long acting somatostatin analogue octreotide in pediatrics. Eur J Pediatr 1994;153:304–310.
118. Hindmarsh P, Brook CG. Short-term management of nesidioblastosis using the somatostatin analogue SMS 201-995. N Engl J Med 1987;316:221–222.
119. Bruining GJ, Bosschaart AN, Aarsen RS, Lamberts SW, Sauer PJ, Del Pozo E. Normalization of glucose homeostasis by a long-acting somatostatin analogue SMS 201-995 in a newborn with nesidioblastosis. Acta Endocrinol 1986;279:334–339.
120. Wilson DC, Carson DJ, Quinn RJ. Long-term use of somatostatin analogue SMS 201-995 in the treatment of hypoglycaemia due to nesidioblastosis. Acta Paediatr Scand 1988;77:467–470.
121. Delemarre-van de Waal HA, Veldkamp EJ, Schrander-Stumpel CT. Long-term treatment of an infant with nesidioblastosis using somatostatin analogue. N Engl J Med 1987;316:222–223.
122. Harris JP, Ricker AT, Gray RS, Steed RD, Gutai JJ. Reversible hypertrophic cardiomyopathy associated with nesidioblastosis. J Pediatr 1992;120:272–275.
123. Martin LW, Ryckman FC, Sheldon CA. Experience with 95% pancreatectomy and splenic salvage for neonatal nesidioblastosis. Ann Surg 1984;200:355–362.
124. Thomas CG Jr, Underwood LE, Carney CN, Dolcourt JL, Whitt JJ. Neonatal and infantile hypoglycemia due to insulin excess: new aspects of diagnosis and surgical management. Ann Surg 1977;185:505–517.
125. Langer JC, Filler RM, Wesson DE, Sherwood G, Cutz E. Surgical

management of persistent neonatal hypoglycemia due to islet cell dysplasia. J Pediatr Surg 1984;19:786–792.

126. Kramer JL, Bell MJ, DeSchryver K, Bower RJ, Ternberg JL, White NH. Clinical and histological indications for extensive pancreatic resection in nesidioblastosis. Am J Surg 1982;143:116–119.

127. Dunger DB, Burns C, Ghale GK, Muller DP, Spitz L, Grant DB. Pancreatic exocrine and endocrine function after subtotal pancreatectomy for nesidioblastosis. J Pediatr Surg 1988;23: 112–115.

128. Dohrmann P, Mengel W, Splieth J. Total pancreatectomy in a case of nesidioblastosis due to persisting hyperinsulinism following subtotal pancreatectomy. Prog Pediatr Surg 1991;26: 92–95.

129. Leibowitz G, Glaser B, Higazi AA, Salameh M, Cerasi E, Landau H. Hyperinsulinemic hypoglycemia of infancy (nesidioblastosis) in clinical remission: high incidence of diabetes mellitus and persistent beta-cell dysfunction at long-term follow-up. J Clin Endocrinol Metab 1995;80:386–392.

# 78

# Gastrinomas (Zollinger-Ellison Syndrome)

M. Mignon and G. Cadiot

Although rare, Zollinger-Ellison syndrome (ZES) might involve about 0.1% of duodenal ulcer (DU) patients and, according to a Danish epidemiologic study, 1 in 100,000 persons (1). According to epidemiologic data reported by J. A. Norton (2), among both the functioning and nonfunctioning endocrine tumors of the duodenopancreatic area, gastrinomas rank second in terms of incidence per year after insulinomas. Gastrinomas, however, are more prevalent than insulinomas, since gastrinomas are less easily eradicated by surgery.

Since its first description by Zollinger and Ellison in 1955 (3), the diagnostic and therapeutic strategy of ZES has been modified markedly by the advent of powerful gastric antisecretory agents and the recent development of imaging tests, especially endoscopic ultrasonographic (EUS) examination of the duodenopancreatic area and somatostatin receptor scintigraphy (SRS). Both are important components of the strategy aimed at tumor eradication.

Several points are to be emphasized first.

1. Like many ectopic endocrine tumors, gastrinomas are more often malignant (50–60% of cases) than benign and more often multifocal than unifocal. Hepatic metastases are the major cause of death and raise the most difficult therapeutic decisions.
2. Clinically, ZES often presents initially as an isolated simple duodenal ulcer or diarrhea; assessment of gastric acid secretion and serum gastrin both in basal conditions and under secretin are of the greatest importance.
3. Other endocrine involvement and/or familial inheritance must always be investigated; indeed, inclusion of gastrinomas in the context of multiple endocrine neoplasia type 1 syndrome (MEN-1) modifies markedly the usual therapeutic strategy.
4. Once acid overproduction is controlled, the management of the tumor process is the predominant concern in these patients. Although tumor detection has been facilitated by progress in medical imaging techniques, a relatively large number of tumors still escape preoperative detection; thus, in sporadic cases of ZES, explorative laparotomy is usually advocated in the absence of medical contraindications. With such an approach, in our experience, 18–20% of patients with pancreatic gastrinoma and 40–65% of those with extrapancreatic tumors are given a chance of cure.

Whether intraoperative isotopic detection of gastrinomas after $^{111}$In-pentetreotide administration, as assessed currently in our institution, would increase the gastrinoma cure rate remains to be established.

In this chapter, we focus on the diagnostic and therapeutic strategy for the ZES patient according to our personal experience dealing with 240 cases seen in our institution from 1959 to 1995 and partially reported (4–7) together with guidelines proposed by others on this topic (8–11).

## DIAGNOSTIC STRATEGY

According to Zollinger and Ayres (12), the ulcerogenic tumor syndrome has been encountered in patients ranging from 7 to 90 years of age. Development of ulcer symptoms for the first time in the very young or in the elderly should strongly suggest the presence of an ulcerogenic tumor. In contrast to the patient with an ordinary peptic ulcer in whom the age of onset is well below 40 years, the peak of the ulcerogenic syndrome appears to occur in about the 5th decade. The mean age was 47.8 ± 13.2 (SD) for sporadic ZES ($n$ = 127) and 43.8 ± 11.6 for ZES–MEN-1 ($n$ = 45) according to the last reviews of our experience (5). However, careful screening for gastrinoma in MEN-1 families indicated that gastrinomas could be detected at an earlier age (13–15).

According to Zollinger and Ayres (12), there is no clear gender predominance, and nearly 60% of the reported patients are men. In our experience, the male to female ratio was 2.3 for sporadic ZES and 1.8 for MEN-1–ZES (7).

Clinical situations suggesting ZES diagnosis are numerous (Table 78.1). Patients with gastrinoma(s) present mainly with mucosal ulcerations of the upper gastrointestinal tract (UGIT) and diarrhea. Such ulcerative lesions are observed in approximately 85% of cases. One patient in five presents as having a simple chronic duodenal ulcer. Some features, however, suggest the possibility of ZES: female sex, early age, familial peptic ulcer, resistance to medical therapy, *Helicobacter pylori*–negative peptic ulcer or relapsing after successful *H. pylori* eradication, severe peptic ulcer complications, frequent vomiting in the absence of pyloroduodenal stenosis, associated diarrhea, or presence of tumor in the liver. Although not pathognomonic, postoperative peptic recurrence should always suggest the possibility of a previously unrecognized diagnosis of ZES; indeed, 2–10% of these individuals have ZES. Spontaneous or postoperative gastrojejunocolic fistula is rare but highly suggestive of ZES. Multiple peptic ulcers, especially in an atypical site (beyond the duodenal cap down to the duodenojejunal junction or even farther), are rare but highly suggestive of the diagnosis. Isolated esophageal ulcers are seldom observed, but esophagitis of varying degrees is associated with other UGIT ulcerative mucosal lesions in about 45–65% of cases.

Diarrhea, the second main presenting symptom, is important for its frequency and for assessing antisecretory drug efficacy. Diarrhea results from the overwhelming of intestinal and colonic absorptive capacity by excessive secretion from both the stomach and the pancreaticobiliary tracts (16) and maldigestion, particularly of lipids. Alterations in gastrointestinal motility seem to be of minor pathophysiologic importance. Chronic diarrhea is noted in about 65% of cases; it remains isolated or precedes peptic ulcers in about one patient out of five. Frequently, intermittent discharge of bulky loose stools leads to the initial

**TABLE 78.1. Clinical Situations Suggesting Zollinger-Ellison Syndrome (ZES) Diagnosis**

- DU[a] + acid hypersecretion; severe esophagitis related to gastroesophageal reflux
- DU resistant to adequate modern medical therapy
- Postoperative recurrent ulcer
- DU + chronic diarrhea; unexplained chronic diarrhea (steatorrhea)
- DU + primary hyperparathyroidism
- DU + raised serum gastrin to differentiate from antral G cell hyperplasia or hyperfunction
- Liver metastasis ± DU and without primary adenocarcinoma
- Member of a kindred with MEN-1[a] or ZES

[a]DU, duodenal ulcer; MEN-1, multiple endocrine neoplasia type 1.

diagnosis of irritable bowel syndrome. ZES is present in 50% of patients presenting with both steatorrhea and gastroduodenal mucosal ulcerative lesions.

## CURRENT MANAGEMENT STRATEGY IN ZOLLINGER-ELLISON SYNDROME

Once the diagnosis of ZES is considered, the successive steps in management are *(a)* validation of ZES diagnosis; *(b)* control of ZES acid overproduction and symptoms; *(c)* screening for MEN type 1; *(d)* tumor localization; *(e)* decision for laparotomy in case of sporadic ZES and for parathyroidectomy in case of ZES–MEN-1; *(f)* management of hepatic metastases when present; and *(g)* initiation of a surveillance program when all tumor is eradicated.

### Validation of ZES Diagnosis

The definitive diagnosis of ZES depends on histopathologic confirmation. Unfortunately, it is lacking in 20–40% of the reported cases for several reasons: the small size of gastrinomas (early stage of the disease or MEN-1), extrapancreatic location, and difficult location for needle biopsy. Hence the diagnosis of ZES often relies on documenting gastric acid and gastrin overproduction. In patients who have not undergone surgery, a basal acid output (BAO) of 15 mmol/hr or more (17) and/or an acid concentration above 100 mmol/L suggests ZES (18), but considerable overlap exists with DU patients. Demonstration of a definite increase in basal serum gastrin (BSG) concentration in association with increased BAO is a strong indicator of the diagnosis of ZES. Approximately 30% of ZES patients, however, may have fasting BAO and BSG levels in the range of patients with duodenal ulcer or gastroesophageal reflux (19). In these patients, the secretin test is by far the most discriminating test (18).

Secretin is well tolerated and may be used either as an intravenous bolus of 2 clinical units (CU)/kg body weight or as a continuous intravenous infusion of 3 CU/kg body weight/hr. Venous sampling for gastrin radioimmunoassay is performed at 2, 5, 10, 15, and 30 minutes with secretin bolus and at 15, 30, 45, 60, and 75 minutes with continuous infusion. In both cases, it is advisable to obtain two or three gastrin measurements before secretin administration. We measure gastric acid output before and during secretin infusion (four samples of 15 minutes each) to be a valuable addition. We have compared these two techniques for the secretin-provocative test in 9 ZES and 10 DU patients and favor the latter technique (20). As originally described by Isenberg et al. (21), secretin infusion of 3 CU/kg/hr usually induces a marked increase in both serum gastrin and acid output in ZES patients. In DU patients, secretin either has no effect on serum gastrin or causes a slight and transient increase. However, in some DU patients, secretin induces a rather large increase in serum gastrin; this makes it difficult to use gastrin increments for diagnostic purposes either in terms of absolute values or as percentages. By contrast, in these patients, secretin inhibits strongly acid secretion (20).

Table 78.2 indicates the sensitivity of various biologic criteria at specific levels for ZES diagnosis. Values are derived from the study of 80 ZES patients confirmed anatomically (69 without gastrectomy and 11 after previous partial gastrectomy). Threshold values have been established by comparison with 124 nonsurgical DU patients with no pyloric stenosis and 8 DU patients with recurrent ulcer after partial gastrectomy followed at least 5 years (Bichat, unpublished data; 6).

When a diagnosis of ZES is suspected in the case of a postoperative recurrent ulcer, the results of acid and serum gastrin measurements, both baseline and during secretin testing, are sometimes difficult to interpret. Gastric analysis is hampered by difficulties in collecting gastric juice (incomplete collection caused by anastomotic leakage or biliary and/or pancreatic reflux), and serum gastrin may be increased by gastric retention, vagotomy, or residual antral tissue. We have recently suggested criteria of 100% specificity derived from a series of 49 patients with recurrent ulcer after either partial gastrectomy or vagotomy: 28 patients had a histologically confirmed gastrinoma, and 21 had an idiopathic DU before surgery. The respective sensitivities of the threshold values set at 100% specificity for ZES diagnosis are indicated in Table 78.2. The two most discriminating association parameters were secretin acid output and secretin serum gastrin. This combination had no false-negative response. These criteria must be further validated by other investigations in larger groups of both ZES and DU patients.

### Control of Gastric Acid Hypersecretion and ZES Symptoms

Symptoms are almost invariably controlled by use of $H_2$-receptor antagonists and, in the case of failure, $H^+/K^+$-ATPase proton pump inhibitors. Total gastrectomy is no longer necessary to control acid hypersecretion in most patients. Combined total gastrectomy and gastrinoma excision (3) has been drastically reduced in favor of elective tumor removal alone. Total gastrectomy may, however, remain mandatory in symptomatic, medically unresponsive patients who either have negative findings at

**TABLE 78.2. Sensitivity of Various Biologic Criteria at Specific Level for ZES Diagnosis**

| Cutoff Values[a] | Sensitivity (%)[b] |
|---|---|
| BSG ≥ 4.64 N[c] | 61.2 |
| SSG ≥ 3.86 N[c, d] | 70 |
| SSG-BSG ≥ 1.58 N[c, d] | 58.7 |
| • BAO | |
| Without gastrectomy ≥ 37.7 mmol/hr | 47.8 |
| With partial gastrectomy ≥ 14.4 mmol/hr | 18.2 |
| • SAO | |
| Without gastrectomy ≥ 18 mmol/hr[d] | 85.5 |
| With partial gastrectomy ≥ 1.84 mmol/hr[d] | 90.9 |
| • SAO-BAO | |
| Without gastrectomy ≥ 1.41 mmol/hr[d] | 81.6 |
| With partial gastrectomy ≥ 0 mmol/hr[d] | 45.4 |
| • Combined criteria | |
| Without gastrectomy | 97 |
| With partial gastrectomy | 100 |

[a]BSG, basal serum gastrin; SSG, secretin-stimulated serum gastrin; BAO, basal acid output; SAO, secretin-stimulated acid output.
[b]Percentage of patients with gastrinoma above the cutoff point.
[c]Mean of four gastrin determinations expressed as fold upper limit serum gastrin concentration (normal fasting gastrin concentration < 107 pg/mL).
[d]Intravenous infusion of secretin 3 CU/kg for 1 hr.

laparotomy or have a tumor that cannot be safely resected. Proton pump inhibitors (PPIs) are the medical treatment of choice when $H_2$-receptor antagonists have failed because of escape or unwanted side effects. Experience with omeprazole, the first-introduced PPI, and lansoprazole has recently been reviewed by the NIH group (10); PPI doses ranged from 20–360 mg per day. Omeprazole can be administered intravenously in cases of acute presentation and in patients with severe stenosing esophagitis. Pharmacokinetics of intravenous omeprazole in ZES patients and recommendations for proper usage have recently been published; adequate dosage to control acid hypersecretion should be administered every 12 hours (22).

The efficacy of antisecretory drugs is measured by clinical and laboratory criteria. Clinically, diarrhea control and ulcerative mucosal lesion healing should be rapid. However, gastric secretory measurements have the best predictive value—either BAO before the next dose, as advocated by Maton et al. (23), or 24-hour intragastric pH monitoring, as proposed by our group (24). In fact, both methods have advantages. Indications for either one depend upon *(a)* laboratory experience with a given technique; *(b)* type of drug, i.e., its efficacy in reducing both secretory volume and acid concentration and its duration of action; *(c)* the drug regimen; and *(d)* the need for complete control of 24-hour secretion.

Basal acid measurement before the next dose is the method of choice for patients on long-term once- or twice-daily administration of PPIs; it appears reliable and easy to perform and is well tolerated. A BAO below 10 mmol/hr is associated with ulcer healing (10). In patients with previous partial gastrectomy, BAO before the next dosing must be below 5 mmol $H^+$/hr to ensure adequate control, and in patients with severe peptic esophagitis, BAO must be below 1 mmol $H^+$/hr (25).

In contrast, 24-hour intragastric pH monitoring provides the safest technique for monitoring drug efficacy in patients taking antisecretory drugs with a short duration of action, such as $H_2$-receptor antagonists. We correlated 24-hour pH profiles with clinical outcome in ZES patients and showed the predictive value of pH profile types (24). Therapeutic success may be expected when the intragastric pH always exceeds 1 and exceeds 2 and 3.5 for 75% and 50%, respectively, of a 24-hour period.

The risk of developing gastric argyrophil carcinoid tumors is a concern in patients committed to long-term antisecretory treatment, especially in MEN-1–ZES patients. Our group is currently evaluating long-acting somatostatin analogues for these patients, because of their inhibition of acid secretion, gastrin release, and gastrin trophic effects on both fundic parietal and endocrine cell populations.

## Screening for Multiple Endocrine Neoplasia Type 1

MEN-1 syndrome is an autosomal dominant inherited disorder characterized by the development of endocrine cell proliferation (hyperplasia or adenomas), mainly in the parathyroid glands, the endocrine pancreas/duodenum, the anterior pituitary, and the adrenals. In about 60% of patients, the syndrome is familial (26).

Screening for MEN-1 is fundamental in ZES management. Additional endocrinopathies may need specific management and may influence ZES management. Before the availability of PPIs, it was shown that parathyroidectomy reduced hypergastrinemia and improved control of gastric acid hypersecretion (27). Parathyroidectomy should be performed before any attempt at gastrinoma removal. Familial screening should be considered. Management of gastrinoma in MEN-1 patients differs markedly from management of sporadic gastrinoma. Finally, the prognosis of ZES might be different in MEN-1 patients. The MEN-1 screening we offer to patients with ZES and their relatives is summarized in Table 78.3.

ZES occurs as a part of MEN-1 in 10–38% of cases (5, 28–30); in the two largest series, 18% of 185 patients with ZES (28) and 26% of 172 patients seen between 1959 and 1989 in our institution (5), respectively, had MEN-1.

**TABLE 78.3. MEN-1 Screening in ZES Patients**

| |
|---|
| ***Clinical assessment in patients and relatives*** |
| Nephrolithiasis |
| Neuroglycopenia symptoms |
| Signs of diabetes and skin lesions |
| Amenorrhea, galactorrhea |
| Signs of acromegaly, Cushing's syndrome, chiasmatic compression |
| ***Systematic biologic and radiologic screening in patients***[a] |
| *Pancreas* |
| Fasting glucose, insulin, C-peptide |
| Glucagon, VIP, somatostatin |
| *Parathyroids* |
| Basal serum ionized calcium and PTH |
| Oral calcium tolerance test when negative |
| *Pituitary gland* |
| Prolactin, FSH, LH, testosterone in man, estradiol in woman (not done in woman with normal menses) |
| GH, IGF1 |
| Morning cortisol and 24-hour urinary cortisol |
| ACTH |
| MRI (or CT scan) of the pituitary |
| *Adrenal glands* |
| CT scan of the adrenals |
| If positive, serum and urinary K, 24-hr urinary cortisol in basal state and after dexamethasone administration (2 mg per day for 2 days) |
| *Gastric fundus* |
| Endoscopy with systematic fundic mucosal biopsies (Grimelius staining) |

[a]When MEN-1 has been demonstrated in the patient, thymic and bronchial carcinoids should be looked for by chest CT scan in the patient and genetic screening is offered to the relatives. Biologic and radiologic MEN-1 screening and ZES screening is offered to the relatives with positive genetic screening. When genetic screening is impossible, a reduced screening is offered to the asymptomatic relatives (gastrin, calcium, PTH, prolactin).

The *MEN-1* gene has been located on the long arm of chromosome 11 (11q13) (14, 31); it has not yet been cloned. It probably acts as a tumor-suppressor gene, the inactivation of which gives rise to cell proliferation. Familial *MEN-1* genetic screening is available using restriction fragment length polymorphism (RFLP) analysis and markers flanking both sides of the *MEN-1* locus. The DNA from circulating lymphocytes of at least two affected family members and two unaffected family members must be studied to identify the haplotype for the chromosomal region in the family. Accuracy of this genetic testing reaches 99.6%. Until the *MEN-1* gene is cloned, it is not possible to perform genetic testing for *MEN-1* diagnosis in an isolated individual.

The diagnosis of MEN-1 is based on either the presence of MEN-1–related endocrinopathies or secondary islet cell tumors secreting other peptides than gastrin or the presence of ZES- or MEN-1–related endocrinopathies in relatives.

Primary hyperparathyroidism (HPT) is the most frequent MEN-1–related endocrinopathy. The reported prevalence of primary HPT in ZES patients with MEN-1 varies from 50% to almost 100%, but the most recent data suggest that the actual prevalence is 90% or more (5, 28–30, 32). In MEN-1–related HPT, the four glands are pathologic (33, 34). Primary HPT can present several years before or after the diagnosis of ZES is made (13, 15, 29, 32). Normocalcemic primary HPT may exist at the time of the ZES diagnosis (32). Using the oral calcium tolerance test, we recently showed that the usual biologic features of

HPT—both high basal fasting calcium and PTH levels—were lacking in five of eight patients with primary HPT and ZES (32). Since primary HPT is most often the only associated endocrinopathy that would suggest the diagnosis of MEN-1, an oral calcium tolerance test should be considered when typical biologic features of primary HPT are lacking in any patient with ZES (32).

Specific data concerning endocrinopathies other than primary HPT in patients with the ZES are sparse. Pituitary adenomas have been found in 3 (16%) of 19 patients with ZES and MEN-1 (29); 2 were prolactinomas and the other, a basophile adenoma. Cushing's syndrome caused by pituitary production of ACTH has been noted in 19% of patients with ZES and MEN-1 (35). In a series of 10 patients, 2 had a nonfunctioning pituitary adenoma, 3 had adrenal involvement, and 1 had organic hypoglycemia (30). In our experience with 45 MEN-1 patients with ZES, 31% had pituitary involvement, half of whom had increased prolactin serum levels, and 35% had adrenal involvement, 13% of whom had mild hypercortisolism, the other being nonfunctioning (5, 36). Symptomatic insulinomas coexisted with gastrinomas in 13% of our patients with ZES (5). Because of the rarity of a second symptomatic pancreatic endocrine tumor (one insulinoma among 45 patients with ZES) and the high frequency of multiple hormone elevations without any related symptoms, it has been recommended that screening for another pancreatic endocrine tumor syndrome be limited to patients who develop new symptoms after an initial negative screening (37). Severe Cushing's syndrome due to ectopic ACTH secretion by metastases is rarely observed and is independent of MEN-1. Because of the prevalence of sporadic primary HPT in the population, caution must be exercised when a relative of a ZES patient, especially an old one, has isolated primary HPT, particularly when it is due to a single adenoma. Caution must also be exercised when a relative has an isolated adrenal mass (incidentaloma) or an isolated pituitary tumor, for which the respective prevalences could reach 2% with computed tomography (CT) scanning for the former (39) and 10% with magnetic resonance imaging (MRI) for the latter (40) in the general population.

Gastric fundic argyrophil cell carcinoids, composed of enterochromaffin-like cells (ECLomas), are frequently observed in ZES patients with MEN-1 (41, 42). Their prevalence is 29.5% in our experience (7) and 13% in that of the NIH (42). ECLomas are rarely found in sporadic ZES; only three cases have been described (42, 43). Allelic losses at the *MEN-1* locus have been noted in an ECLoma of a patient with ZES and MEN-1, suggesting that these tumors belong to the MEN-1 tumor spectrum (44). However, to our knowledge ECLomas have never been observed in MEN-1 patients without ZES, suggesting that chronic hypergastrinemia is the key factor for their development. Multiple ECLomas might remain one of the very rare indications for total gastrectomy in these patients (41).

## Tumor Localization

Precise localization of all gastrinomas is critical for defining an appropriate therapeutic strategy (18). Great advances in tumor localization have recently occured with the availability of EUS and SRS.

Gastrinomas are mainly located in the "gastrinoma triangle" (45). Primary gastrinomas can also be observed, but less frequently, in the distal duodenum or jejunum and in other parts of the pancreatic gland. Ectopic gastrinomas are rare but hard to localize preoperatively (ovaries, gallbladder). In sporadic ZES, the primary gastrinoma is often single or associated with peripancreatic metastatic lymph nodes (4, 46–49). Primary gastrinomas could be located in lymph nodes, since their resection sometimes led to long-term cure (4, 46–50). Duodenal gastrinomas are increasingly found in recent series (49, 51–53). Recent data suggest that about one-fourth to one-third of the gastrinomas are pancreatic and the others are extrapancreatic, mainly duodenal (49, 50–53). In MEN-1, endocrine tumors are often multiple (5, 7, 18, 46, 47, 51, 54–57). They can be located in both the pancreatic gland and the duodenum. Several types of endocrine tumors may coexist with gastrinomas. It has been suggested that in MEN-1, gastrinomas are preferentially located in the duodenum, the pancreatic endocrine tumors often not being gastrinomas (55), but this has not been confirmed either in our experience (Table 78.4) (5, 57) or in that of the NIH (58–59).

The size of gastrinomas depends on their location. In a recent personal series of patients with sporadic ZES, the median diameter of duodenal gastrinomas was 8 mm (range, 3–15 mm), and the median diameter of tumors in peripancreatic lymph nodes was 16.5 mm (range, 10–30 mm) (53). Data from the NIH show that 77% of the duodenal gastrinomas measured 1 cm or less, whereas 73% of the pancreatic gastrinomas measured 3 cm or more (28).

The ability of imaging modalities to localize primary gastri-

**TABLE 78.4. Nature and Location of Tumors in 45 Patients with MEN-1[a] and ZES**

| | Surgical Patients | | | | | Nonsurgical Patients | | | |
|---|---|---|---|---|---|---|---|---|---|
| | Head | Corpus | Tail | Diffuse | Total | Head | Corpus | Total | Total |
| Pancreatic adenomas | | | | | | | | | |
| Pancreas only | 5 | 2 | 5 | 2 | 14 | | 1[b] | | 15 |
| + duodenal tumor | 1 | | | 1 | 2 | 1[b] | | | 3 |
| + lymph node(s) | 2 | | 3 | | 5 | | | | 5 |
| + lymph node(s) and liver metastases | | | 2 | | 2 | 1[b] | | | 3 |
| + lymph node(s) and duodenal tumor | 1 | | | 2 | 3 | | | | 3 |
| Total | 9 | 2 | 10 | 5 | 26 | | | 3[b] | 29 |
| Duodenal tumors only | | | 3 | | | | | | 3 |
| Liver metastases only | | | | | | | 3[b] | | 3 |
| Lung metastases only | | | | | | | 1[b] | | 1 |
| No tumor | | | 7[c] | | | | 2 | | 9 |

[a]Values indicate the number of patients in each category.
[b]Proven by fine-needle biopsy.
[c]Five of these patients had microscopic lesions at blind distal pancreatectomy.

**TABLE 78.5. Sensitivity and Specificity of Conventional Imaging Techniques[a] in Localizing Gastrinomas**

| | Sensitivity (%) | | Specificity (%) | |
|---|---|---|---|---|
| | Mean | Range | Mean | Range |
| Primary gastrinomas | | | | |
| Ultrasonography | 23 | 21–28 | 92 | |
| CT scan | 50 | 35–59 | 90 | 83–100 |
| MRI | 22 | 20–25 | 100 | |
| Angiography | 68 | 35–68 | 89 | 84–94 |
| Liver metastases | | | | |
| Ultrasonography | 14 | 14–63 | 100 | |
| CT scan | 54 | 35–72 | 99 | 40–100 |
| MRI | 63 | 43–83 | 92 | 88–100 |
| Angiography | 62 | 33–86 | 98 | 96–100 |

Modified from Orbuch M, Doppman JL, Strader DB, Fishbeyn VA, Benya RV, et al. Imaging for pancreatic endocrine tumor localization: recent advances. In: Mignon M, Jensen RT, eds. Endocrine tumors of the pancreas. Recent advances in research and management. Frontiers of gastrointestinal research. Basel: Karger, 1995;23:268–281.
[a]Excluding endoscopic ultrasonography and octreoscanning.

nomas and metastatic gastrinomas to the liver is summarized in Table 78.5. Although noninvasive modalities for tumor localization have high specificity, their sensitivity is often low (59). The sensitivities of ultrasonography (US) and CT scanning are much lower for duodenal gastrinomas than for pancreatic gastrinomas and clearly depend on tumor size (60, 61). The detection rates of US and CT scanning for extrahepatic gastrinomas were 0% for tumors measuring less than 1 cm, 15% and 30%, respectively, for tumors 1–3 cm, and 100% and 95%, respectively, for tumors 3 cm or larger (61–62). US did not detect any duodenal tumor (60), and CT scanning detected only 12% of them in another series (62). Upper digestive endoscopy with biopsy remains a good conventional method to diagnose and localize duodenal gastrinomas; its sensitivity has been set at 40% and 37.5% in two series by our group (53, 63). New MRI technology has proved a real advance in detecting liver metastases (64, 65), with an 83% sensitivity and an 88% specificity (64). One limitation is its inability to differentiate metastases from small hemangiomas (64, 65), which, fortunately, SRS does (66). By contrast, recent improvements in detecting pancreatic endocrine tumors are due to EUS rather than MRI (64, 67). Other techniques such as portal venous sampling of gastrin (59, 68) and angiography with intraarterial injection of secretin with venous sampling of gastrin improve sensitivity to a mean value of 89% for the latter (59, 69, 70). However, these techniques are more invasive and often allow only regional localization of the gastrinomas. A recent study showed that selective intrahepatic arterial secretin stimulation for the detection of liver metastases should be limited to patients whose liver imaging results are ambiguous (71). However, this technique for this indication should be compared with SRS. We almost never use angiography, compared with others (71). Thus, the efficacy of all conventional imaging techniques for the detection of small gastrinomas, mainly duodenal gastrinomas, remains insufficient.

EUS is very useful for detection of endocrine pancreatic tumors (63, 72–76). Its sensitivity (70–94%) is much higher than that of CT scanning (Table 78.6) (63, 72), and its specificity is about 95–100% (63, 72). EUS has detected pancreatic tumors measuring less than 5 mm (72, 76). The sensitivity of EUS for gastrinomas located in lymph nodes is notably lower (62.5%). EUS is also able to detect duodenal gastrinomas: its sensitivity has been 50 and 54%, with excellent specificity in two recent prospective surgical studies (53, 63). EUS precisely localizes tumors, whereas angiography with selective stimulation and venous sampling allows only regional localization (74). However, EUS is a highly observer-dependent technique that demands special expertise of the examiner.

Most endocrine tumors contain a high density of somatostatin receptors that can be detected by scintigraphy using $^{111}$In-DTPA-D-Phe1-octreotide (Octreoscan) (77, 78). SRS is a whole-body noninvasive imaging technique. Nine gastrinomas have been tested in vitro for the presence of somatostatin receptors (77, 79). All nine were positive. In four small series of patients with ZES (10–14 patients), SRS was positive in 90–100% (78, 80–82). In the three largest series of patients (totaling about 150), including our own series of 68 patients, SRS was positive in 69–76% of patients (83–86). In these series, SRS allowed detection of unknown tumors at various sites—liver, bones, mediastinum, lung, duodenopancreatic area—in 35–47% of patients (83). The sensitivity of SRS in detecting liver metastases is almost 100% (66, 84–86). One major advantage of this technique is the detection of liver metastases while the conventional imaging (US, CT, MRI) of the liver is still normal (77, 78, 81, 83–88).

SRS can detect gastrinomas located in the duodenopancreatic area that are not visualized by any other imaging technique, including EUS. In a series of 21 patients with sporadic ZES who did not have pancreatic gastrinomas, SRS was the only technique that showed positive results in the duodenopancreatic area in 32% of the patients (53). Its sensitivity for the detection of pancreatic gastrinomas is probably high (80–100%), but specific data concerning this localization are sparse (80, 82, 83, 85, 87). The sensitivity of SRS for detecting gastrinomas in the duodenum and lymph nodes is probably lower, because of small tumor size. We found it was approximately 58% (53). Differences in the global percentage of positive findings in ZES patients are probably due to the small size of these tumors. However, the combination of EUS and SRS was positive in 90% of our patients with extrapancreatic gastrinomas (53). Therefore, both SRS and EUS should be performed when surgery is contemplated (53, 80). Octreoscan may often alter patient management (84, 86).

However, SRS has several limitations. First, tumors must contain a high density of somatostatin receptors to be visualized. Data are lacking concerning the actual percentage of SR-positive gastrinomas. Second, SRS does not precisely localize tumors in the duodenopancreatic area and sometimes cannot separate tumors located close to each other even by tomography (SPECT) (53, 83). Third, other tumors or tissues are rich in octreotide receptors (78); however, this is not a real limitation in clinical practice. Since activated lymphocytes contain octreotide receptors, SRS should not be performed immediately after surgery or if infection or inflammation is suspected in the studied area. SRS should not be used for a diagnosis of endocrine tumor,

**TABLE 78.6. Comparison of the Sensitivities of Endoscopic Ultrasonography (EUS) and CT Scanning for the Detection of Pancreatic Endocrine Tumors**

| Reference | Patients Studied (*n*) | EUS Sensitivity (%) | CT Scanning Sensitivity (%) |
|---|---|---|---|
| 63 | 22[a] | 75 | 25 |
| 72 | 37 | 82 | 0 |
| 73 | 21 | 79 | 21 |
| 74 | 10[b] | 70 | ND |
| 75 | 17 | 94 | 47 |
| 76 | 19[b] | 89 | 10 |

[a]Gastrinomas.
[b]Insulinomas; other series included various endocrine tumor types.

but because pancreatic adenocarcinomas do not contain somatostatin receptors, a positive SRS is a valid indicator of an endocrine tumor when a pancreatic tumor is visualized by another imaging technique (78). Although bone scintigraphy using a standard technetium tracer is very sensitive for diagnosis of bone metastases, SRS is complementary and has diagnosed bone metastases at an early stage (89).

Extensive evaluation of the extent of gastrinomas in our studies is limited to patients for whom surgery is scheduled. This evaluation includes *(a)* endoscopy, mainly for duodenal gastrinomas; *(b)* CT scanning to identify adrenal abnormalities, liver and lymph node metastases, and large pancreatic tumors; *(c)* EUS for duodenopancreatic tumors or lymph node metastases; and *(d)* SRS for global evaluation of the tumor extent. SRS can also diagnose recurrence early if the primary tumor contains a high density of somatostatin receptors. Despite the improved ability of imaging techniques to localize gastrinomas, a proportion of patients with ZES will still remain who have tumors undetected before surgery (91).

Surgical exploration represents a critical step in the management strategy of sporadic ZES patients. Surgery should be performed by a surgeon experienced in pancreatic endocrine surgery and include the following steps: *(a)* thorough palpation of the liver, pancreas, duodenum, and peripancreatic lymph node areas and *(b)* complete and careful exploration of the entire abdominal cavity, including the peritoneum, ovaries, and tubes in women.

Intraoperative ultrasonography (IUS), duodenal transillumination (DTI) as suggested by the NIH group (11), and perhaps intraoperative radioisotope scanning after $^{111}$In-pentetreotide administration (90) appear to be beneficial technical adjuncts during surgical exploration of ZES patients. Duodenotomy has been advocated by the University of Michigan group (92). According to them, such a maneuver may detect submucosal tumors as small as 1–2 mm in diameter. The efficacy of duodenotomy for tumor localization and excision has been confirmed by Norton et al. (49, 52). Duodenal leak is a potential risk of such surgery.

## Management of the Tumor

**Sporadic ZES Patients.** With the availability of powerful antisecretory agents, tumor excision in patients with ZES has become the predominant concern. There are several reasons for this approach. First, only surgery is capable of definitely curing ZES patients. It avoids continuous administration of powerful antisecretory agents whose long-term safety is still under evaluation and spares the patient the hazardous consequences of long-term hypergastrinemia on fundic and antral endocrine cell proliferation, especially MEN-1–ZES patients. Second, in our experience as in most series in the literature, malignancy is present in 50–60% of cases (18, 93, 97).

Comprehensive reviews of the role of surgery in the management of islet cell tumors have been published by Fraker et al. (93) and by Thompson (with an enthusiastic argument for duodenotomy) (92). In 1986, we reported the results of our management strategy in 144 cases (4), and more recently, we reported 45 cases of MEN-1–ZES patients (7, 97). We present here some guidelines derived from our experience with ZES patient management.

Complete tumor eradication, though desirable, remains rare because gastrinomas are frequently multifocal within the duodenum and pancreas. The rule is to limit tumor excision to *(a)* easily removable gastrinomas located in the body or the tail of the pancreas, *(b)* tumors located near the surface of the pancreas that can be enucleated without risk, and *(c)* extrapancreatic gastrinomas (i.e., tumors in the duodenal and gastric wall, isolated in lymph nodes, in the mesentery, ovaries, tubes, gallbladder, and kidneys).

In the third category, surgery offers an excellent chance of cure in a large proportion of individuals (4, 8). The favorable prognosis of patients with extrapancreatic gastrinomas first noted by Oberhelman (98) has been confirmed by several reports (45, 96–102). The chance of a long-lasting, cure by tumor removal in patients with extrapancreatic gastrinoma may be as high as 65%, compared with only 15–20% in patients with pancreatic gastrinomas (4).

Favorable behavior of duodenal gastrinomas, compared with pancreatic gastrinomas, has been challenged by the NIH group recently, as a result of an 11-year prospective study in 69 patients, including 29 patients with duodenal gastrinomas (49, 103). These authors conclude that duodenal gastrinomas are much more common than previously believed and are more frequently malignant (on the basis of lymph node involvement), and have a chance of cure similar to that of pancreatic tumors. In our experience and that of others (49, 94–103), the possible association of a tumor within the duodenal wall with a gastrinoma located within the pancreas and/or with lymph nodes or hepatic metastases has practical implications: *(a)* it underscores the need for meticulous exploration during surgery of the duodenopancreatic area by an experienced surgeon and *(b)* it mandates close follow-up of patients, including regular clinical evaluation and BAO and serum gastrin determinations, both baseline and (above all) under secretin challenge. Secretin challenge appears to be the best method of assessing and predicting cure in ZES patients after tumor resection (18, 104). Only long-term persistent normalization of the above-mentioned criteria indicates cure.

**MEN-1–ZES Patients.** In contrast to sporadic ZES patients, in whom it appears reasonable to attempt tumor removal in the absence of nonresectable liver involvement, in MEN-1–ZES patients, exploratory laparotomy is seldom indicated (except for symptom-associated endocrine secretion), as a definite cure by surgery is very rare. Parathyroid surgery is often indicated and should take place before any abdominal surgery.

In this clinical setting, the anatomic distribution and tumor morphology differ from those in sporadic cases. Gastrinomas in MEN-1 are usually multiple, disseminated throughout the duodenopancreatic area, small, and often associated with endocrine cell hyperplasia.

Gastric acid secretion parameters and BSG levels are not different from those of sporadic ZES patients; therefore, antisecretory drug management should be the same (5, 57). The prevalence of malignancy is of the same magnitude (Table 78.7) (5, 8, 57), but hepatic metastases seem to follow a more indolent course (5). When the death toll for both categories of ZES is compared (Table 78.7), a tendency favoring the MEN-1–ZES group is noticeable in terms of death related to liver metastases progression. When deaths unrelated to liver metastases are excluded from our evaluation, the survival rate after a median follow-up of 95 months (extremes, 17–278) is 78%, a figure close to the one reported by Weber et al. (28). This may account for a better 15-year survival than that of sporadic ZES patients (63 and 45% for MEN-1–ZES and sporadic ZES, respectively) (Table 78.8) (7).

In patients with hyperparathyroidism, parathyroid surgery should be performed prior to pancreatic surgery, since normalization of blood calcium reduces oversecretion of gastric acid and gastrin (26). Because hyperparathyroidism in MEN-1 patients is usually caused by parathyroid hyperplasia, the acceptable intervention is either removal of three-and-one-half glands or total parathyroidectomy with an implant in the forearm. Subsequent reassessment of acid secretory status and close screening for hyperparathyroidism relapse during follow-up are mandatory.

Opinions diverge about indications for surgical exploration in patients with MEN-1. Opponents of surgical exploration in these patients emphasize *(a)* the multiplicity and diffuse location of

**TABLE 78.7. Main Demographic and Clinical Features of 45 Cases of MEN-1–ZES Compared with 127 Sporadic ZES Cases Followed at Hospital Bichat-Claude Bernard (1959–1989)[a]**

| | MEN-1–ZES (*n* = 45) | Sporadic ZES (*n* = 127) |
|---|---|---|
| % Patients | 26 | 74 |
| Sex ratio, M/F | 1.8 | 2.3 |
| Malignancy % | 47 | 55 |
| Liver metastases | 31 | 30 |
| Other metastases[b] | 16 | 25 |
| Death toll[a, c] | | |
| Total % | 38 | 44 |
| Related to LM % | 12 | 36 |

From Mignon M, Cadiot G, Rigaud D, Ruszniewski PH, Jaïs P, et al. Management of islet cell tumors in patients with multiple endocrine neoplasia type I. In: Mignon M, Jensen RT, eds. Endocrine tumors of the pancreas. Recent advances in research and management. Frontiers of gastrointestinal research. Basel: Karger, 1995;23:342–359.
[a]Median follow-up, 95 months (17–278).
[b]Predominantly lymph nodes.
[c]Death toll related to liver metastases progression tended to be less in ZES–MEN-1 ($p = .11$).

gastrinoma(s) in the pancreas and/or the duodenum as well as their typically small size (8, 57) and *(b)* the extremely limited chance of long-lasting surgical cure in these patients, unless a total pancreatectomy is performed. This drastic procedure is usually rejected by most authorities (8) and can be justified only in exceptional circumstances (105).

Currently, three approaches to the surgical treatment of the tumor process in MEN-1–ZES patients are proposed and being evaluated. The first (106, 107), developed during the past 15 years by Thompson at the University of Michigan, is based on the premise that *(a)* MEN-1 patients with neuroendocrine disease of the pancreas or duodenum can be "cured" of their syndrome providing that the tumor has not metastasized to the liver and that the operation is extensive enough to excise all sites of diseases and *(b)* all gastrinomas have malignant potential whether they are located in the duodenum or pancreas (107). EUS in the hands of this group has replaced the use of THVS for detecting regional secretion of gastrin and thus guiding surgical exploration (108). After a follow-up period of 1–16 years, 11 of 17 patients followed by the Ann Arbor group (106–107) have normal basal serum gastrin levels and are asymptomatic, no longer requiring drug therapy. Whether the routine distal pancreatectomy that is added to the procedure (106) contributes to the apparent success of this strategy by preventing further development of gastrinoma from this area may be questioned. The second strategy (8, 11) recommends an exploratory laparotomy only when a tumor has been clearly identified on preoperative imaging studies. The rationale for this approach is that an imageable tumor may be malignant in 50% of cases (8), and its eradication prevents development of metachronous liver metastases (8).

At surgery, aided by IUS and DTI, gastrinomas are enucleated in the head of the pancreas and in the duodenal wall and usually resected when located in the body and tail of the pancreas (8). Whether the most recent technologic refinements for tumor detection, such as EUS and SRS, by revealing multiple lesions and tumor spread within and outside the abdomen, will alter such aggressive management of the tumor process(es) in MEN-1–ZES is a major area for future study.

Experience gained from our initial aggressive surgical approach (4, 5, 57, 109) indicated that long term, complete cure of MEN-1–ZES is very rare. Actuarial analysis of survival revealed that, for unexplained reasons, at 10 years and thereafter, there was a progressive tendency for better survival in MEN-1 than in sporadic ZES (57) (Table 78.8). We propose close clinical and biologic follow-up of the patient as well as endoscopic and histologic surveillance of the gastric mucosa for argyrophil carcinoid detection. A poor outcome was found when insulinoma was associated with gastrinoma in MEN-1 patients. In our series, this association was found in 6 of 45 gastrinomas in MEN-1 patients (5, 57), and it was a life-threatening condition. We believe that an aggressive approach is indicated in such patients with thorough attempts to locate the tumor, including THVS and urgent and radical surgery. Finally, regarding the very low prevalence of islet cell tumors in general, it is appropriate to initiate a multicenter multinational prospective program for MEN-1 screening in patients and their relatives and for evaluating surgery in MEN-1–ZES patients.

## Management of Secondary Malignancies

Approximately one patient in four has metastases (4, 9, 93). In some, liver involvement is identified only during surgical exploration; in a few others, no primary gastrinoma is found. Although individual patients with long-lasting survival have been observed in most centers caring for ZES patients, commonly less than half of ZES patients with liver metastases survive beyond 5 years (4, 9, 27, 93), and less than 30% beyond 10 years (27); median survival at 5 years ranges from 17 to 53%. In contradistinction to liver metastases, lymph node metastases, although as prevalent, do not seem to influence survival rate in ZES patients, at least in the short term (4, 27, 95).

In sporadic ZES patients, the development of hepatic metastases clearly appears related to the size and location of the primary tumor (27, 93). Patients with hepatic metastases have larger primary tumors than patients without metastases. No such relationship exists between primary tumor size and development of lymph node metastases (28). In the NIH series, 61% of patients harboring tumor(s) larger than 3 cm in diameter, usually in the pancreas, had liver metastases (28). Pancreatic tumors are typically large and are associated with liver metastases in 52% of sporadic cases; 7% of these patients have both lymph node and liver involvement (28). In contrast, duodenal tumors, which are usually small, are associated with liver metastases in only 5% of cases, while they are associated with regional lymph node metastases in the same proportion as in cases of pancreatic primaries (28).

These findings support the anatomic stratification proposed by Howard et al. (96), which separates primaries located on the

**TABLE 78.8. Survival Rate of Patients with MEN-1–ZES Compared with That of Patients with Sporadic ZES[a]**

| | MEN-1–ZES (*n* = 45) | | Sporadic ZES (*n* = 127) | |
|---|---|---|---|---|
| | Patients at Risk | Survival Rate (%) | Patients at Risk | Survival Rate (%) |
| At 5 years | 27 | 67 | 79 | 66 |
| At 10 years | 17 | 63 | 45 | 55 |
| At 15 years | 12 | 63 | 40 | 45 |

[a]Bichat-Claude Bernard ZES series, 1959–1989 (*n* = 172) (5). Two MEN-1–ZES patients were lost for follow-up after 1 and 252 months, respectively. Nine sporadic ZES patients were lost for follow-up after a median follow-up of 56 months; extremes: 2–214 months.

right of the superior mesenteric artery (SMA) within the so-called gastrinoma triangle from those pancreatic tumors to the left of the SMA; in the latter group, liver metastases were much more prevalent (56% of patients), and the actuarial survival was poor (<10% at 10 years).

Clinical experience suggests that the natural history of liver metastases in ZES patients is probably extremely variable from patient to patient. In some patients, growth of individual lesions is also extremely variable (110). Lack of information on the natural history and growth rate of hepatic metastases often makes medical and surgical management of ZES patients with liver involvement difficult; for example, when to start antitumor chemotherapy (111) or whether to propose liver transplantation (112).

Relevant information has been provided recently (110). It appears that hepatic metastases in patients with metastatic gastrinoma grow in three general patterns within a 3- to 6-month observation period: no growth, slow growth, and fast growth. An increase in fasting serum gastrin was the sole significant parameter that separated the three types of growth (110). In our series (112), fast growth seems to correlate with poor patient survival. A study of 35 patients with metastases from endocrine tumors, including 20 cases of ZES, evaluated prognostic factors for survival (112). Among the various elements assessed during an observation period with a median duration of 35 months (range, 5–136 months), only rapid expansion of liver metastases (>25% within 6 months) appeared to be a major prognostic factor. The 5-year survival rate was 52% for enlarging metastases versus 100% for stable metastases. Furthermore, the median interval to death in patients with fast-growing metastases was as brief as 6 (1–24) months (112).

Various therapies for liver metastases have been proposed; surgery is rarely curative, except for some selected cases and in very specialized surgical centers (11, 113). The experience of specialized surgical centers indicates that major hepatic resection is feasible, is safe, and can be repeated. Clinical outcome after hepatic resection demonstrates that this procedure can palliate symptoms and prolong survival in selected patients (113). Partial hepatic resection can be combined with tumor debulking to facilitate the synergistic effect of various other forms of treatment such as chemotherapy, serial arterial embolization, or repeated transient hepatic ischemia.

Vascular occlusive therapy of pancreatic endocrine tumors metastatic to the liver has been updated and reviewed by Arcenas et al. (114). Although it benefits patients with liver metastasis originating from gut carcinoid tumors, its efficacy in gastrinoma patients needs further evaluation (114, 115).

Early experience with systemic chemotherapy found that a combination of streptozotocin (STZ) and 5-fluorouracil (5FU) yielded the best response rates (116). The median duration of remission was 17 months, but there was a trend toward longer survival (26 months) in the STZ-5FU group than in those receiving STZ alone (16.5 months). However, valid interpretation of these results remained uncertain because of the small number of ZES patients included (8 of 84 endocrine pancreatic tumors). Recent prospective studies (117, 118) included 21 and 25 ZES patients, respectively, and measured the response to therapy using both tumor-size regression and survival times. In our trial, STZ-5FU induced *(a)* major and long-lasting tumor size regression (>50% with 55 months duration) in only one case, *(b)* a minor response (25–50% tumor-size regression on CT scans) in three with a transient response, *(c)* stabilization of tumor masses in 28%, and *(d)* liver mass progression in 68% of ZES patients. Actuarial analysis revealed a median survival time of 28 months; 34% of patients were alive at 5 years (118).

Moertel et al. (117) compared STZ + 5FU with chlorozotocin (CZT) and with doxorubicin (DRC) + STZ. Although the combination of STZ + DRC was the most effective, STZ produced frequent and often severe nausea and vomiting and provided a relatively small chance of complete tumor-size regression (18%) and of long-term survival (about 30% of patients were alive at 5 years).

Treatment with a long-acting somatostatin analogue, octreotide acetate, offers the theoretical advantage of acting by inhibiting gastric acid secretion and gastrin release and antagonizing tumor growth. However, clinical use of octreotide is hampered because it cannot be given orally like antisecretory drugs, and its effects on tumor size appear to be modest (111).

There is not yet sufficient experience with interferon (IFN-α) in gastrinoma patients with liver metastases. Interesting results obtained in carcinoid tumors suggested that IFN-α could be worth testing in ZES patients, possibly in association with octreotide (111); however, preliminary data from the NIH group are not encouraging (119).

The advent of liver transplantation raised an interesting therapeutic option for liver metastases from endocrine gut tumors that are slow growing. Makowka et al. from Starzl's group (120) reported the first results from five such patients (one with gastrinoma). Their results appeared encouraging for two glucagonoma patients who remained disease-free 23 and 41 months later. The only gastrinoma patient, who was initially free of extrahepatic metastases, died 8 months later from multiple lung and bone metastases.

A larger French experience with liver transplantation for neuroendocrine liver metastases, extending from 1989 to 1994, has been recently analyzed and published in abstract form (121); the main results are shown in Table 78.9. With the exception of gut carcinoids, the results of liver transplantation for pancreatic endocrine tumors, including gastrinomas, are not encouraging.

In our experience with four ZES patients, the most successful liver transplant was associated with multiple organ removal, including a large pancreatic tumor. The patient survived 26 months after transplantation but developed bone metastases. To identify patients with unrecognized bone metastases, SRS is mandatory before contemplating liver transplantation. SRS is presently the best imaging technique for recognizing distant extraabdominal metastases in these patients—bone, mediastinal, and supraclavicular lymph node metastases would obviously preclude any major surgical procedure.

## Prognosis and Initiation of Surveillance Program

Therapeutic advances have undoubtedly improved the overall survival rate in ZES patients. Greater awareness of the disease and the availability of powerful antisecretory drugs have considerably reduced the number of postoperative deaths and practically eradicated mortality due to peptic ulcer complications.

**TABLE 78.9. French Experience with Liver Transplantation for Metastases from Neuroendocrine Tumors (1989–1994)**

| Actuarial Survival[a] | 1 Year | 2 Years | 5 Years |
|---|---|---|---|
| Carcinoids (*n* = 14) | 78% | 78% | 78% |
| Other NET[b] (*n* = 14) | 28% | 9% | — |

From Le Treut YP, Delpero JR, Houssin D, Cherqui D, Segol P, et al. Que peut-on attendre de la transplantation hépatique (TH) pour métastases des tumeurs neuro-endocrines (NET)? Résultats d'une série multicentrique de 28 cas. Gastroenterol Clin Biol 1995;19:A4.

[a]Postoperative deaths: 21% (4/7 cluster, 3/3 liver-pancreas, 2 early retransplantation).

[b]Gastrinomas, 5; insulinoma, 1; glucagonomas, 3; nonsecreting, 5.

The dramatic refinement of preoperative and intraoperative imaging techniques as well as surgical skill and experience has provided patients with a greater chance of cure. Actuarial estimates of survival up to 20 years among the first 144 patients followed at Bichat Hospital showed that 55 ± 6% of patients survived at 10 years (4). These figures have improved in the last 10 years. A higher survival rate has been observed by the NIH in a group of ZES patients followed for 8 years (28). It is likely that these figures will improve further in the future if *(a)* the suggested stratification of ZES patients into benign and malignant forms is confirmed (28) and *(b)* surgical resection of primary gastrinoma in the sporadic form of the disease is shown to prevent liver metastasis.

For patients in whom laparotomy has been successful, follow-up should include assessing gastric acid secretion and serum gastrin under secretin challenge every 1–2 years. In all other situations, surveillance should cover the following elements at 6- to 12-month intervals: clinical survey, basal serum gastrin levels, and gastrin secretory measurements for drug adjustment, control of tumor growth, and detection of liver metastases. In patients (especially MEN-1–ZES patients) taking long-term, long-acting, gastric antisecretory agents such as PPIs, close survey of gastric endocrine proliferation is mandatory.

The results of an ongoing study in our institution of gastric fundic and antral endocrine cell behavior in 40 ZES patients show that gastrinoma is associated with an enhanced proliferation of fundic endocrine cells, particularly when patients undergo omeprazole therapy. Fundic argyrophil cell densities (namely, of ECL cells) are closely correlated with the serum gastrin level (122) and gastrinoma growth (123). Increased ECL cell proliferation resulted in development of fundic ECLomas in five patients in the MEN-1–ZES group (41), which is consistent with other reports (124). An increase in antral gastrin cell density was noted in patients undergoing long-term antisecretory treatment with omeprazole, apparently because of the extent and duration of hypochlorhydria (123).

## CONCLUSION

A diagnostic and therapeutic strategy for the management of patients with Zollinger-Ellison syndrome has been developed on the basis of our extensive personal experience and the most recent literature. The mainstay of modern ZES management is tumor resection whenever feasible. Diagnosis is centered on gastric acid and gastrin measurements both in basal conditions and with secretin stimulation.

Recognition of other endocrine involvement and familial inheritance is of the utmost importance in distinguishing sporadic ZES patients from those who have MEN-1. Localization of the tumor has been facilitated considerably by recent developments in imaging techniques.

In sporadic ZES, exploratory laparotomy is appropriate, even when preoperative localization of the tumor has failed. Laparotomy will allow detection and resection of gastrinomas in a substantial number of patients. Control of gastric acid secretion is mandatory throughout the workup period. Modern antisecretory agents are efficacious in most cases; total gastrectomy when control of acid hypersecretion has failed is now exceptional. Tumor resection should be attempted in cases of sporadic ZES without unresectable liver involvement. The chance of a definite cure provided by surgical treatment is still difficult to determine precisely. When performed by an experienced surgeon, apparent cure or long-lasting remission seems to be reached in about 50% of cases in the NIH experience.

Indication for surgery is still controversial in MEN-1–ZES patients. We believe that exploratory laparotomy is seldom indicated, as the chance of a definite cure by surgical treatment is low. A national survey of this issue is in progress in France under the aegis of the GRESZE (Groupe de Recherches et D'Etudes sur le Syndrome de Zollinger-Ellison, research group founded by Dr. Michel Mignon). It might alter our present policy if actual prevention of liver metastases by eradication of primaries is confirmed. Parathyroidectomy is often indicated and should take place before any abdominal operation in MEN-1–ZES.

Hepatic metastases remain a major therapeutic problem in ZES patients. Among the various proposed strategies, systemic chemotherapy with STZ and 5FU or DRC has been tried most extensively. Results provide ample justification for continued clinical research into this aspect of the disease.

## REFERENCES


1. Stadil F, Stage JG. The Zollinger-Ellison syndrome. Clin Endocrinol Metabolism 1979;9:433–446.
2. Norton JA. Neuroendocrine tumors of the pancreas and duodenum. Curr Probl Surg 1994;31:81–156.
3. Zollinger RM, Ellison EH. Primary peptic ulceration of the jejunum associated with islet cell tumors of the pancreas. Ann Surg 1955;142:709–728.
4. Mignon M, Ruszniewski P, Haffar S, Rigaud D, René E, Bonfils S. Current approach to the management of tumoral process in patients with gastrinoma. World J Surg 1986;10:703–710.
5. Mignon M, Ruszniewski Ph, Podevin P, Sabbagh L, Cadiot G, et al. Current approach to the management of gastrinoma and insulinoma in adult patients with multiple endocrine neoplasia type I (MEN I). World J Surg 1993;17:489–497.
6. Mignon M, Jaïs P, Cadiot G, Ben Yedder D, Vatier J. Clinical features and advances in biological diagnostic criteria for Zollinger-Ellison syndrome. In: Mignon M, Jensen RT, eds. Endocrine tumors of the pancreas. Recent advances in research and management. Frontiers of gastrointestinal research. Basel: Karger, 1995;23:223–239.
7. Mignon M, Cadiot G, Rigaud D, Ruszniewski P, Jaïs P, et al. Management of islet cell tumors in patients with multiple endocrine neoplasia type I. In: Mignon M, Jensen RT, eds. Endocrine tumors of the pancreas. Recent advances in research and management. Frontiers of gastrointestinal research. Basel: Karger, 1995;23:342–359.
8. Fraker DL, Norton JA. The role of surgery in the management of islet cell tumors. Gastroenterol Clin North Am 1989;4:805–830.
9. Jensen RT, Doppman JL, Gardner JD. Gastrinoma. In: Go VLW, Dimagno E, Gardner JD, et al., eds. The exocrine pancreas: basic and clinical aspects. New York: Raven Press, 1985:727–745.
10. Metz DC, Jensen RT. Advances in gastric antisecretory therapy in Zollinger-Ellison syndrome. In: Mignon M, Jensen RT, eds. Endocrine tumors of the pancreas. Recent advances in research and management. Frontiers of gastrointestinal research. Basel: Karger, 1995;23:240–257.
11. Norton JA. Surgical treatment of islet cell tumors with special emphasis on operative ultrasound. In: Mignon M, Jensen RT, eds. Endocrine tumors of the pancreas. Recent advances in research and management. Frontiers of gastrointestinal research. Basel: Karger, 1995;23:309–332.
12. Zollinger RM, Ayres HP. The Zollinger-Ellison syndrome. In: Nyhus LM, Wastell C, eds. Surgery of the esophagus, stomach and small intestine. 4th ed. Boston: Little, Brown & Co, 1986:491–513.
13. Skogseid B, Eriksson B, Lundqvist G, Lörelius LE, Rastad J, et al. Multiple endocrine neoplasia type I: a ten-year prospective screening study in four kindreds. J Clin Endocrinol Metab 1991;73:281–287.
14. Skogseid B, Öberg K. Genetics of multiple endocrine neoplasia type I. In: Mignon M, Jensen RT, eds. Endocrine tumors of the pancreas. Recent advances in research and management. Frontiers of gastrointestinal research. Basel: Karger, 1995;23:60–69.
15. Benya RV, Metz DC, Venzon DJ, Fishbeyn VA, Strader DB, et al. Zollinger-Ellison syndrome can be the initial endocrine manifestation in patients with multiple endocrine neoplasia type I. Am J Med 1994;97:436–444.

16. Rambaud JC, Matuchansky C. Diarrhoea and digestive endocrine tumours. In: Bonfils S, ed. Endocrine secreting tumours of the gastrointestinal tract. Clin Gastroenterol 1974;3:657–670.
17. Aoyagi T, Summerskill WI IJ. Gastric secretion with ulcerogenic islet cell tumor. Arch Intern Med 1966;117:667–672.
18. Mignon M, Bonfils S. Diagnosis and treatment of Zollinger-Ellison syndrome. In: Piper DW, ed. Peptic ulceration. Baillière's Clin Gastroenterol 1988;2:677–698.
19. Cadiot G, Sékéra E, Mignon M. Gastric secretion in gastroesophageal reflux disease. In: Scarpignato C, Galmiche JP, eds. Functional evaluation in esophageal disease. Frontiers of gastrointestinal research. Basel: Karger, 1994;22:209–222.
20. Mignon M, Rigaud D, Cambray S, Chayvialle JA, Accary JP, et al. A comparative evaluation of secretin bolus and secretin infusion as secretin provocation tests in the Zollinger-Ellison syndrome. Scand J Gastroenterol 1985;20:791–797.
21. Isenberg JI, Walsh JH, Passaro EJR, Moore EW, Grossman I. Unusual effect of secretin on serum gastrin, serum calcium and gastric acid secretion in a patient with suspected Zollinger-Ellison syndrome. Gastroenterology 1972;62:626–631.
22. Vinayek R, Amantea MA, Maton PN, Frucht H, Gardner JD, Jensen RT. Pharmacokinetics of oral and intravenous omeprazole in patients with the Zollinger-Ellison syndrome. Gastroenterology 1991;101:138–147.
23. Maton PN, Gardner JD, Jensen RT. Recent advances in the management of gastric acid hypersecretion in patients with Zollinger-Ellison syndrome. Gastroenterol Clin North Am 1989;18: 847–863.
24. Vallot T, Mignon M, Mazure R, Bonfils S. Evaluation of antisecretory drug therapy of Zollinger-Ellison syndrome (ZES) using 24-hour pH monitoring. Dig Dis Sci 1983;28:577–584.
25. Miller LS, Vinayek R, Frucht H, Gardner JD, Jensen RT, Maton PN. Reflux oesophagitis in patients with Zollinger-Ellison syndrome. Gastroenterology 1990;98:341–346.
26. Lamers CBH, Stadil F, Van Tongeren J. Prevalence of endocrine abnormalities in patients with the Zollinger-Ellison syndrome and in their families. Am J Med 1978;64:607–612.
27. Norton JA, Cornelius MJ, Doppman JL, Maton PN, Gardner JD, Jensen RT. Effect of parathyroidectomy in patients with hyperparathyroidism and Zollinger-Ellison syndrome and multiple endocrine neoplasia type I. Surgery 1987;102:958–966.
28. Weber HC, Venzon DJ, Lin JT, Fishbein VA, Orbuch M, et al. Determinants of metastatic rate and survival in patients with Zollinger-Ellison syndrome: a prospective long-term study. Gastroenterology 1995;108:1637–1649.
29. Melvin WS, Johnson JA, Sparks J, Innes JT, Ellison EC. Long-term prognosis of Zollinger-Ellison syndrome in multiple endocrine neoplasia. Surgery 1993;114:1183–1188.
30. Bardram L, Stage JG. Frequency of endocrine disorders in patients with the Zollinger-Ellison syndrome. Scand J Gastroenterol 1985;20:233–238.
31. Larsson C, Skogseid B, Öberg K, Nakamura Y, Nordenskjöld M. Multiple endocrine neoplasia type I gene maps to chromosome 11 and is lost in insulinoma. Nature 1988;332:85–87.
32. Cadiot G, Houillier P, Allouch A, Paillard M, Mignon M. Oral calcium tolerance test in the early diagnosis of primary hyperparathyroidism and multiple endocrine neoplasia type I in patients with the Zollinger-Ellison syndrome. Gut 1996;39: 273–278.
33. Strewler GJ, Rosenblatt M. Mineral metabolism. In: Felig P, Baxter JD, Frohman LA, eds. Endocrinology and metabolism. New York: McGraw-Hill, 1995:1407–1516.
34. Deftos LJ, Catherwood BD, Bone HG III. Multiglandular endocrine disorders. In: Felig P, Baxter JD, Frohman LA, eds. Endocrinology and metabolism. New York: McGraw-Hill, 1995:1703–1732.
35. Maton PN, Gardner JD, Jensen RT. Cushing's syndrome in patients with the Zollinger-Ellison syndrome. N Engl J Med 1986;315:1–5.
36. Podevin P, Ruszniewski P, Mignon M, Lehy T, Cadiot G, et al. Management of multiple endocrine neoplasia type I (Men I) in Zollinger-Ellison (ZE) syndrome. Gastroenterology 1990;98: A230.
37. Chiang H-CV, O'Dorisio TM, Huang SC, Maton PN, Gardner JD, Jensen RT. Multiple hormone elevations in Zollinger-Ellison syndrome. Prospective study of clinical significance and of the development of a second symptomatic pancreatic endocrine tumor syndrome. Gastroenterology 1990;99:1565–1575.
38. Souquel JC, Sassolas G, Forichon J, Champetler P, Partensky C, Chayvialle JA. Clinical and hormonal effect of a long-acting somatostatin analogue in pancreatic endocrine tumors and in carcinoid syndrome. Cancer 1987;59:1654–1660.
39. Ross NS, Aron D. Hormonal evaluation of the patient with an incidentally discovered adrenal mass. N Engl J Med 1990;323: 1401–1405.
40. Hall WA, Luciano MG, Doppman JL, Patronas NJ, Oldfield EH. Pituitary magnetic resonance imaging in normal human volunteers: occult adenomas in the general population. Ann Intern Med 1994;120:817–820.
41. Lehy T, Cadiot G, Mignon M, Ruszniewski P, Bonfils S. Influence of multiple endocrine neoplasia type I on gastric endocrine cells in patients with the Zollinger-Ellison syndrome. Gut 1992;33:1275–1279.
42. Jensen RT. Gastrinoma as a model for prolonged hypergastrinemia in the human. In: Walsh JH, ed. Gastrin. New York: Raven Press, 1993:373–393.
43. Cadiot G, Vissuzaine C, Potet F, Mignon M. Fundic argyrophil carcinoid tumor in a patient with sporadic type Zollinger-Ellison syndrome. Dig Dis Sci 1995;40:1275–1278.
44. Cadiot G, Laurent-Puig P, Thuille B, Lehy T, Mignon M, Olschwang S. Is the multiple endocrine neoplasia type I gene a suppressor for fundic argyrophil tumors in the Zollinger-Ellison syndrome? Gastroenterology 1993;105:579–582.
45. Stabile BE, Morrow DJ, Passaro E Jr. The gastrinoma triangle: operative implications. Am J Surg 1984;147:25–31.
46. Kaplan EL, Horvath K, Udekwu A, Straus F, Schark C, et al. Gastrinomas: a 42-year experience. World J Surg 1990;14: 365–376.
47. Donow C, Pipeleers-Marichal M, Schröder S, Stamm B, Heitz PU, Klöppel G. Surgical pathology of gastrinoma. Site, size, multicentricity, association with multiple endocrine neoplasia type I and malignancy. Cancer 1991;68:1329–1334.
48. Farley DR, Van Heereden JA, Grant CS, Miller JL, Ilstrup DM. The Zollinger-Ellison syndrome. A collective surgical experience. Ann Surg 1992;215:561–569.
49. Norton JA, Doppman JL, Jensen RT. Curative resection in Zollinger-Ellison syndrome. Results of a 10-year prospective study. Ann Surg 1992;215:8–18.
50. Fraker DL, Norton JA, Alexander R, Venzon DJ, Jensen RT. Surgery in Zollinger-Ellison syndrome alters the natural history of gastrinoma. Ann Surg 1994;220:320–330.
51. Ellison EC. Forty year appraisal of gastrinoma. Back to the future. Ann Surg 1995;222:511–524.
52. Sugg SL, Norton JA, Fraker DL, Metz DC, Pisegna JR, et al. A prospective study of intraoperative methods to diagnose and resect duodenal gastrinomas. Ann Surg 1993;218:138–144.
53. Cadiot G, Lebtahi R, Bonnaud G, Sarda L, Marmuse JP, et al. Detection of extrapancreatic gastrinomas using Octreoscan scintigraphy (SRS): a prospective study. Gastroenterology 1996; 110:A381.
54. Lamers CBHW. Gastrinoma in multiple endocrine neoplasia type I. Acta Oncol 1991;30:489–492.
55. Pipeleers-Marechal M, Somers G, Willems G, Foulis A, Imrie C, et al. Gastrinomas in the duodenum of patients with multiple endocrine neoplasia type I and the Zollinger-Ellison syndrome. N Engl J Med 1990;322:723–727.
56. Norton JA, Jensen RT. Unresolved surgical issues in the management of patients with Zollinger-Ellison syndrome. World J Surg 1991;15:151–159.
57. Ruszniewski P, Podevin P, Cadiot G, Marmuse JP, Mignon M, et al. Clinical, anatomical and evolutive features of patients with Zollinger-Ellison syndrome combined with type I multiple endocrine neoplasia. Pancreas 1993;8:295–304.
58. MacFarlane MP, Fraker DL, Alexander HR, Norton JA, Lubensky I, Jensen RT. Prospective study of surgical resection of duodenal and pancreatic gastrinomas in multiple endocrine neoplasia type I. Surgery 1995;118:973–980.
59. Orbuch M, Doppman JL, Strader DB, Fishbeyn VA, Benya RV, et al. Imaging for pancreatic endocrine tumor localization: recent advances. In: Mignon M, Jensen RT, eds. Endocrine tumors of the

pancreas. Recent advances in research and management. Frontiers of gastrointestinal research. Basel: Karger, 1995;23: 268–281.

60. Miller DL, Norton JA, Jensen RT. Prospective assessment of abdominal ultrasound in patients with Zollinger-Ellison syndrome. Radiology 1991;178:763–767.
61. Wank SA, Doppman JL, Miller DL, Collen MJ, Maton PN, et al. Prospective study of the ability of computerized axial tomography to localize gastrinomas in patients with Zollinger-Ellison syndrome. Gastroenterology 1987;92:905–912.
62. Thom AK, Norton JA, Axiotis CA, Jensen RT. Localization, incidence and malignant potential of duodenal gastrinomas. Surgery 1991;110:1086–1093.
63. Ruszniewski P, Amouyal P, Amouyal G, Grangé JD, Mignon M, et al. Localization of gastrinomas by endoscopic ultrasonography in patients with Zollinger-Ellison syndrome. Surgery 1995;117: 629–635.
64. Pisegna JR, Doppman JL, Norton JA, Metz DC, Jensen RT. Prospective comparative study of ability of MR imaging and other imaging modalities to localize tumors in patients with Zollinger-Ellison syndrome. Dig Dis Sci 1993;38:1318–1328.
65. Berger JF, Laissy JP, Limot O, Henry-Feugeas MC, Cadiot G, et al. Differentiation between multiple liver hemangiomas and liver metastases of gastrinomas: value of enhanced MR examination. J Comput Assist Tomogr 1996;203(3):349–355.
66. Termanini B, Gibril F, Doppman JH, Stewart CA, Sutliff VE, Jensen RT. Somatostatin receptor scintigraphy (SRS), a new method to distinguish hepatic hemangiomas from vascular liver metastases in pancreatic endocrine tumors (PET). Gastroenterology 1996;110:A437.
67. Semelka RC, Cumming MJ, Shoenut JP, Magro CM, Yaffe CS, et al. Islet cell tumors: comparison of dynamic contrast-enhanced CT and MR imaging with dynamic gadolinium enhancement and fat suppression. Radiology 1993;186:799–802.
68. Roche A, Raisonnier A, Gillon-Savouret MC. Pancreatic venous sampling and arteriography in localizing insulinomas and gastrinomas: procedure and results in 55 cases. Radiology 1982; 145:621–627.
69. Imamura M, Takahashi K. Use of selective arterial secretin injection test to guide surgery in patients with Zollinger-Ellison syndrome. World J Surg 1993;17:433–438.
70. Thom AK, Norton JA, Doppman JL, Miller DL, Chang R, Jensen RT. Prospective study of the use of intra-arterial secretin injection and portal venous sampling to localize duodenal gastrinomas. Surgery 1992;112:1002–1009.
71. Gibril F, Doppman JL, Termanini B, Stewart CA, Weber HC, Jensen RT. Is selective intrahepatic arterial secretin stimulation useful in detecting metastatic hepatic gastrinoma? Gastroenterology 1995;108:A357.
72. Rösch T, Lightdale CJ, Botet JF, Boyce GA, Sivak MV Jr, et al. Localization of pancreatic endocrine tumors by endoscopic ultrasonography. N Engl J Med 1992;326:1721–1726.
73. Glover JR, Shorvon PJ, Lees WR. Endoscopic ultrasound for localization of islet cell tumours. Gut 1992;33:108–110.
74. Thompson NW, Czako PF, Fritts LL, Bude R, Bansal R, et al. Role of endoscopic ultrasonography in the localization of insulinomas and gastrinomas. Surgery 1994;116:1131–1138.
75. Zimmer T, Ziegler K, Bäder M, Fett U, Hamm B, et al. Localization of neuroendocrine tumours of the upper gastrointestinal tract. Gut 1994;35:471–475.
76. Ruszniewski P, Amouyal P, Amouyal G, Cadiot G, Mignon M, Bernades P. Endocrine tumors of the pancreas: localization by endoscopic ultrasonography. In: Mignon M, Jensen RT, eds. Endocrine tumors of the pancreas. Recent advances in research and management. Frontiers of gastrointestinal research. Basel: Karger, 1995;23:258–267.
77. Krenning EP, Kwekkboom DJK, Bakker WH, Breeman WAP, Jooij PPM, et al. Somatostatin receptor scintigraphy with (In-111-DTPA-D-Phe(1))- and (I-123-Tyr(3))-octreotide. The Rotterdam experience with more than 1000 patients. Eur J Nucl Med 1993;20:716–731.
78. Krenning EP, Kwekkboom DJK, Pauwels S, Kvols LK, Reubi JC. Somatostatin receptor scintigraphy. In: LM Freeman, ed. Nuclear medicine annual. New York: Raven Press, 1995:1–150.
79. John M, Meyerhof W, Richter D, Waser B, Schaer JC, et al. Positive somatostatin receptor scintigraphy correlates with the presence of somatostatin receptor subtype 2. Gut 1996;38: 33–39.
80. Zimmer T, Liehr RM, Stötzel U, Fett U, Bäder M, et al. Endoscopic ultrasonography (EUS) and somatostatin-receptor-scintigraphy (SRS) for the localization of insulinomas and gastrinomas. Gastroenterology 1994;106:A331.
81. Jamar F, Fiasse R, Leners N, Pauwels S. Somatostatin receptor imaging with indium-111-pentetreotide in gastroenteropancreatic neuroendocrine tumors: safety, efficacy and impact on patient management. J Nucl Med 1995;36:542–549.
82. Ellison EC. Indium-111-pentetreotide scanning versus conventional imaging techniques for the localisation of gastrinoma. Surgery 1195;118:1105–1114.
83. de Kerviler E, Cadiot G, Lebtahi R, Faraggi M, Le Guludec D, et al. Somatostatin receptor scintigraphy in forty-eight patients with the Zollinger-Ellison syndrome. Eur J Nucl Med 1994;21:1191–1197.
84. Gibril F, Reynolds JC, Doppman JL, Chen CC, Termanini B, et al. Does the use of octreoscanning alter management in patients with Zollinger-Ellison syndrome: a prospective study? Gastroenterology 1995;108;A194.
85. Krenning EP, Kwekkeboom DJ, Oei HY, de Jong RJB, Dop FJ, et al. Somatostatin receptor scintigraphy in carcinoids, gastrinomas and Cushing's syndrome. Digestion 1994;55(suppl 3):54–59.
86. Bonnaud G, Cadiot G, Lebtahi R, Sarda L, Le Guludec D, Mignon M. Clinical implications of Octreoscan scintigraphy in 68 patients with the Zollinger-Ellison syndrome (ZES). Gastroenterology 1996;110:A380.
87. Kwekkeboom DJ, Krenning EP, Oei HY, Van Eyck CHJ, Lamberts SWJ. Use of radiolabeled somatostatin to localize islet cell tumors. In: Mignon M, Jensen RT, eds. Endocrine tumors of the pancreas. Recent advances in research and management. Frontiers of gastrointestinal research. Basel: Karger, 1995;23: 298–308.
88. Scherübl H, Bäder M, Fett U, Hamm B, Schmidt-Gayk H, et al. Somatostatin-receptor imaging of neuroendocrine gastroenteropancreatic tumors. Gastroenterology 1993;105:1705–1709.
89. Cadiot G, Lebtahi R, Faraggi M, Le Guludec D, Mignon M. Detection of bone metastases of endocrine tumors: comparison of somatostatin receptor scintigraphy with bone scintigraphy: preliminary results. Gastroenterology 1995;108:A346.
90. Cadiot G, Lebtahi R, Marmuse JP, Le Guludec D, Mignon M. Prospective evaluation of intraoperative isotopic detection of gastrinomas after $^{111}$In-pentetreotide administration: preliminary results in 5 patients. Gastroenterology 1996;110:A381.
91. Gibril F, Fraker DL, Alexander HR, Termanini B, Stewart CA, et al. Does the use of preoperative somatostatin receptor scintigraphy (SRS) have an impact in improving post-operative cure rate in patients undergoing surgery with Zollinger-Ellison syndrome (ZES): a prospective study. Gastroenterology 1996;110:A391.
92. Thompson NW. The surgical treatment of the Zollinger-Ellison syndrome in sporadic and MEN I patients. Acta Chir Austriaca 1992;2:82–87.
93. Fraker DL, Norton JA, Alexander RH, Venzon DJ, Jensen RT. Surgery in Zollinger-Ellison syndrome alters the natural history of gastrinoma. Ann Surg 1994;220:320–330.
94. Ellison EC, Carey LC, Sparks J, O'Dorisio T, Mekhjian HS, et al. Early surgical treatment of gastrinoma. Am J Med 1987;82(suppl 5B):17–24.
95. Stabile BE, Passaro E Jr. Benign and malignant gastrinoma. Am J Surg 1985;49:144–150.
96. Howard TJ, Sawicki MP, Stabile BE, Watt PC, Passaro E Jr. Biologic behavior of sporadic gastrinoma located to the right and left of the superior mesenteric artery. Am J Surg 1993;165:101–106.
97. Mignon MF, Bonfils SJ. Diagnosis and treatment of Zollinger-Ellison syndrome. In: Wastell C, Nyhus LM, Donahue PE, eds. Surgery of the esophagus, stomach and small intestine. 5th ed. Boston: Little, Brown & Co, 1995:631–640.
98. Oberhelman HA. Excisional therapy for ulcerogenic tumors of the duodenum: long-term results. Arch Surg 1972;104:447.
99. Deveney CW, Deveney KS, Way LW. The Zollinger-Ellison syndrome. 23 years later. Ann Surg 1978;188:384–393.
100. Hofman JW, Fox PS, Wilson SD. Duodenal wall tumors and the Zollinger-Ellison syndrome. Arch Surg 1973;107:334–339.

101. Malagelada JF, Edis AJ, Adson MA, Van Heerden JA, Go VLW. Medical and surgical options in the management of patients with gastrinoma. Gastroenterology 1983;84:1524–1532.
102. Thompson JC, Lewis BG, Wiener I, Townsend CM. The role of surgery in the Zollinger-Ellison syndrome. Ann Surg 1983;197: 594–607.
103. Pisegna JR, Norton JA, Metz DC. Duodenal gastrinomas are more common, more malignant and less curable than generally believed. Gastroenterology 1992;102: A286.
104. Fishbeyn VA, Norton JA, Benya RV, Pisegna JR, Metz DC, Jensen RT. Prospective study of the best method to assess and predict cure in patients with Zollinger-Ellison syndrome (ZES) after tumor resection. Gastroenterology 1992;102:A265.
105. Tisell LE, Halman H, Jansson S, Grimelius L. Total pancreatectomy in the MEN I syndrome. Br J Surg 1988;75:154.
106. Thompson NW, Bondeson AG, Bondeson L, Vinik A. The surgical treatment of gastrinoma in MEN I syndrome patients. Surgery 1989;106:1081.
107. Thompson NW. The surgical management of hyperparathyroidism and endocrine disease of the pancreas in the multiple endocrine neoplasia type I patient. J Intern Med 1995;238: 269–280.
108. Carpenter SL, Bansal R, Nostrant TT, Elta GH, Thompson N, Scheiman JM. Accuracy of endoscopic ultrasound in pancreatic neuroendocrine tumor localization. Gastroenterology 1996; 110:A381.
109. Bonfils S, Landor JH, Mignon M, Hervoir P. Results of surgical management in 92 consecutive patients with Zollinger-Ellison syndrome. Ann Surg 1981;194:692–697.
110. Sutliff VE, Doppman JL, Gibril F, Terminini B, Stewart A, Jensen RT. Growth rates of hepatic metastasis in patients with Zollinger-Ellison syndrome (ZES). Gastroenterology 1996;110: A433.
111. Arnold R, Frank M. Systemic chemotherapy for endocrine tumors of the pancreas: recent advances. In: Mignon M, Jensen RT, eds. Endocrine tumors of the pancreas. Recent advances in research and management. Frontiers of gastrointestinal research. Basel: Karger, 1995;23:431–438.
112. Mignon M, Ruszniewski P, Hochlaf S, Sobhani I, Cadiot G, et al. Do endocrine liver metastases have intrinsic evolutive features helping decision making for liver transplantation? Gastroenterology 1991;100:A290.
113. Nagorney DM, Que FG. Cytoreductive hepatic surgery for metastatic gastrointestinal neuroendocrine tumors. In: Mignon M, Jensen RT, eds. Endocrine tumors of the pancreas. Recent advances in research and management. Frontiers of gastrointestinal research. Basel: Karger, 1995;23:416–430.
114. Arcenas AG, Ajani JA, Carrasco HC, Levin B, Wallace S. Vascular occlusive therapy of pancreatic endocrine tumors metastatic to the liver. In: Mignon M, Jensen RT, eds. Endocrine tumors of the pancreas. Recent advances in research and management. Frontiers of gastrointestinal research. Basel: Karger, 1995;23: 439–450.
115. Ruszniewski P, Rougier P, Roche A, Legmann P, Sibert A, et al. Hepatic arterial chemoembolization in patients with liver metastases of endocrine tumors: a prospective phase II study in patients. Cancer 1993;71:2624–2630.
116. Moertel CG, Hanley GA, Johnson LA. Streptozotocin alone compared with streptozotocin alone compared with streptozotocin plus fluorouracil in the treatment of advanced islet cell carcinoma. N Engl J Med 1980;303:1189–1195.
117. Moertel CG, Lefkopoulo M, Lipsitz S, Hahn RG, Klaassen D. Streptozotocin-doxorubicin, streptozotocin-fluorouracil or chlorozotocin in the treatment of advanced islet-cell carcinoma. N Engl J Med 1992;326:519–523.
118. Ruszniewski P, Hochlaf S, Rougier P, Mignon M. Chimiotherapie intraveineuse par streptozotocine et 5 fluoro-uracile des métastases hépatiques du syndrome de Zollinger-Ellison. Etude prospective multicentrique chez 21 patients. Gastroenterol Clin Biol 1991;15:393–398.
119. Pisegna JR, Slimak GG, Doppman JL, Strader DB, Metz DC, et al. An evaluation of human recombinant $\alpha$ interferon in patients with metastatic gastrinoma. Gastroenterology 1993;105:1179–1183.
120. Makowka L, Tijakis AG, Mazzaferro V, Teperman L, Demetris J, et al. Transplantation of the liver for metastatic endocrine tumors of the intestine and pancreas. Surg Gynecol Obstet 1989;168: 107–111.
121. Le Treut YP, Delpero JR, Houssin D, Cherqui D, Segol P, et al. Que peut-on attendre de la transplantation hépatique (TH) pour métastases des tumeurs neuro-endocrines (TNE)? Résultats d'une série multicentrique de 28 cas. Gastroenterol Clin Biol 1995;19:A4.
122. Lehy T, Mignon M, Cadiot G, Elouaer-Blanc L, Ruszniewski P, et al. Gastric endocrine cell behavior in Zollinger-Ellison patients upon long-term antisecretory treatment. Gastroenterology 1989;96: 1029–1040.
123. Cadiot G, Lehy T, Ruszniewski P, Bonfils S, Mignon M. Gastric endocrine cell evolution in patients with Zollinger-Ellison syndrome. Influence of gastrinoma growth and long-term omeprazole treatment. Dig Dis Sci 1993;38:1307–1317.
124. Solcia E, Rindi G, Fiocca L, Villani L, Riva C, Capella C. Endocrine proliferations and carcinoids in hypergastrinemia. In: Walsh JH, ed. Gastrin. New York: Raven Press, 1992:361–372.

# 79

# *Glucagonoma*

Michael S. Sabel and Richard A. Prinz

Neuroendocrine tumors constitute approximately 2% of all gastrointestinal malignancies that are diagnosed each year. While many of these neoplasms are clinically nonfunctioning, others are associated with excess synthesis and secretion of peptides that produce a number of dramatic clinical syndromes. Gastrinomas and insulinomas are the most common functioning islet cell tumors, occurring with an annual incidence of one per million. Glucagon-producing tumors occur less frequently but produce a clinical syndrome that is just as distinctive. The characteristic features of the glucagonoma syndrome are diabetes or abnormal glucose tolerance, a unique rash known as necrotizing migratory erythema, and thromboembolic problems (Table 79.1). Other common findings are weight loss and anemia. Less frequently associated symptoms include gastrointestinal and neurologic disorders. The syndrome is caused by an excess of glucagon produced by pancreatic islet cell tumors that arise from the alpha cells. Advances in biochemistry and molecular biology have rapidly increased our understanding of these neoplasms and of the glucagonoma syndrome. However they continue to present diagnostic and therapeutic challenges.

## HISTORY

Becker et al. are credited with the first description of a patient with a glucagonoma (1). In 1942, they reported a woman with an unusually widespread pruritic rash associated with weakness, an 8-kg weight loss, glossitis, anemia, and an abnormal glucose tolerance test. Iliac vein thrombosis developed, after which she suffered a cardiac arrest and died. An autopsy revealed a large pancreatic islet cell tumor. A similar patient with diabetes, rash, and a pancreatic endocrine tumor was reported by Zhdanov in 1956 (2). The following year, Gossner and Korting induced hyperglycemia in rabbits by injecting an extract of the pancreatic tumor from a patient with the characteristic rash (3). The only thing lacking to confirm the diagnosis of the glucagonoma syndrome in these patients was an elevated circulating glucagon level, which could not be measured at that time.

The development of radioimmunoassay techniques greatly accelerated knowledge and understanding of neuroendocrine tumors. In 1959, Unger et al. reported an assay that could accurately measure circulating and tumor levels of glucagon (4). Four years later, these investigators described four patients with diabetes and islet cell carcinomas who had high levels of immunoreactive glucagon in their tumor extracts. In 1966, McGavran et al. described the first well-diagnosed patient with a glucagonoma (5). In addition to the clinical features of the glucagonoma syndrome, their patient had elevated serum levels of immunoreactive glucagon and an alpha cell tumor of the pancreas that was found at operation. Mallinson et al. described in detail the unique clinical features associated with glucagon-producing alpha cell tumors (6). His nine patients had the characteristic rash, which prompted the diagnosis of glucagonoma syndrome, in addition to weight loss, anemia, and diabetes mellitus. Each of these patients also had hypoaminoacidemia. Four had plasma and tumor glucagon levels measured, all of which were elevated.

## INCIDENCE

Glucagonomas are pancreatic islet cell tumors that arise from the alpha cells. They are rare neoplasms. The incidence is estimated to be one in 20 million to one in 30 million (7); however, the exact incidence is unknown. This is because glucagonomas may be underdiagnosed, since they remain asymptomatic until they grow to a large size, and may be misdiagnosed since the symptoms of excess glucagon can be attributed to other causes. Peak incidence for the glucagonoma syndrome is between the 4th and 6th decade. The mean age at diagnosis is approximately 55 years, but these tumors have been described in patients as young as 19 and as old as 84. So far the syndrome has not been reported in children (7). Speculation on the reason for this is that a certain tumor burden is needed to produce enough glucagon to cause symptoms. The normally slow tumor growth results in late onset of symptoms. Early reports suggested that the tumor occurred predominantly in females. As more patients have been reported, it seems that glucagonomas are only slightly more common in women (58%) than in men (42%). The gender incidence, however, varies between series, and some authors believe there is an equal distribution.

While most glucagonomas present with the clinical manifestations of the glucagonoma syndrome, they can occur in other settings. Using immunohistochemical techniques, Lomsky et al. evaluated the pancreas in 366 autopsies of diabetic patients and found three small glucagonomas, ranging from 3 to 10 mm (8). This would suggest that there is a 0.8% incidence of glucagonomas in patients with diabetes. Rarely, they may be discovered at operation or autopsy in patients without any evidence of the glucagonoma syndrome. They may also be found with computed tomographic (CT) scanning either as an incidental finding or in patients who only have symptoms of an abdominal mass. Glucagonomas may occur in association with other pancreatic islet cell tumors. Patients have been described with glucagonomas combined with gastrinomas, insulinomas, and vipomas (9). Glucagon-producing tumors can also be hereditary and occur as part of the multiple endocrine neoplasia type 1 (MEN-1) syndrome. Patients with a glucagonoma should be screened for other endocrinopathies because of these potential associations.

## TUMOR CHARACTERISTICS

Glucagonomas are usually solitary tumors. They are found almost exclusively in the pancreas, with most being in the body

**TABLE 79.1. Clinical Features of the Glucagonoma Syndrome**

| |
|---|
| Diabetes mellitus or glucose intolerance |
| Dermatitis (NME) |
| Glossitis, cheilitis, vulvovaginitis, nail dystrophy, thinning of hair |
| Weight loss without anorexia |
| Anemia |
| Thromboembolic problems |
| Alterations in mental status (depression, disorientation, nervousness) |
| Neurologic abnormalities (scotomata, optic atrophy) |
| Gastrointestinal disorders (diarrhea, constipation, abdominal pain) |

and tail of the gland. This is consistent with the distribution of A cells in the normal pancreas. However, a neuroendocrine tumor of the duodenum has been reported to produce the glucagonoma syndrome (10), as well as a similar tumor in the kidney (11). Unlike insulinomas, alpha cell tumors are often large, but size varies greatly, ranging from less than 1 cm up to 35 cm. The tumors are usually solid, but they can undergo central necrosis and degenerate. They can then present as a cystic mass.

Approximately 70% of glucagonomas are malignant. Malignancy can only be diagnosed in islet cell tumors by the presence of local invasion or distant metastases. Cellular and other histologic features may be worrisome but are not sufficient criteria to denote malignancy. The presence of metastases does not necessarily correlate with tumor size. Small tumors may metastasize while large tumors may have no evidence of spread. The most common site of metastasis is the liver (50%). The second most common is the peripancreatic lymph nodes. Bony metastases have been identified in several patients. Metastases to the adrenal gland have been described less commonly (9). Direct invasion may occur into the peripancreatic vessels such as the celiac axis, superior mesenteric artery, and splenic and portal veins, and other contiguous structures such as the spleen, stomach, transverse colon, and adrenal gland.

With conventional histology, pancreatic alpha cell tumors do not show any distinctive morphologic features that would distinguish them from other islet cell tumors. They exhibit a variety of cell growth patterns typical of neuroendocrine neoplasms. Cells may be arranged in nests or trabeculae separated by bands of fibrous tissue, or they may have a solid, medullary appearance. Many show a mixed picture, with separate zones of differentiated and anaplastic cells, with the latter types arranged in strands and ribbons. A glandular pattern may also be observed. Extensive fibrosis has been reported in some tumors.

Tumor cells are polygonal or cuboidal. They contain a granular and often abundant cytoplasm with a medium-sized nucleus. Cellular atypia is variable, and malignancy can only be determined by local invasion or metastases. Glucagonoma cells typically show an argyrophilic reaction. As would be expected, glucagonomas contain general markers of neuroendocrine tumors such as neuron-specific enolase, chromogranin, and synaptophysin. Immunofluorescent and immunoperoxidase techniques are needed to demonstrate that these tumors contain large amounts of glucagon, although not uniformly in all cells.

Electron microscopy of glucagonoma cells reveals characteristic dense, round secretory granules, approximately 200 nm in diameter. Immunofluorescent studies indicate these granules contain glucagon. These granules may or may not correspond morphologically to the alpha granules seen in normal islet cells. Sometimes they resemble alpha granules quite closely, but they can appear quite different, particularly in malignant tumors. In general, benign glucagonomas are fully granulated, whereas malignant ones are not. Glucagonoma cells in patients who do not manifest the glucagonoma syndrome may closely resemble normal islet cells (12).

Tumor cells may also contain other islet cell hormones. Pancreatic polypeptide, somatostatin, vasoactive intestinal polypeptide (VIP), insulin, and gastrin can be seen. Metastatic spread of these initially silent cell types can occasionally result in changes in the clinical symptomatology. For instance, the clinical features of a glucagonoma syndrome may change to those of an insulinoma or vice versa. Rarely, glucagonomas may also produce adrenocorticotropic hormone, a parathyroid hormone–like substance, serotonin, and/or melanocyte-stimulating hormone.

Tumor extracts can be assayed for peptide concentrations to enhance the diagnosis. Usually glucagon is found in large amounts, but levels have varied from less than one to several hundred micrograms per gram of wet tissue (13). Tumor content and plasma concentration of glucagon often do not correlate with each other, indicating widely varying rates of hormone synthesis and release. A low concentration of glucagon in a glucagonoma may reflect a high rate of hormone secretion or a low rate of synthesis by the tumor. A gradient in glucagon concentration between the tumor and the normal adjacent pancreas can be demonstrated. Immunoreactive glucagon has also been extracted from metastases.

In addition to variations in glucagon concentration, the molecular forms of the hormone may differ in patients with the glucagonoma syndrome. Four molecular sizes of immunoreactive glucagon-like material have been identified in the plasma of normal subjects. The major component of immunoreactive glucagon circulating in normal subjects has a mass of 3,500 daltons (Da). In addition to this, there is "big" glucagon with a molecular mass of 90,000 Da, proglucagon with a molecular mass of 9,000 Da, and a "small" glucagon of 3,000 Da. In patients with glucagonomas, the major type is not necessarily the 3,500-Da form. It can be any of the other types of glucagon-like molecules. There have not been any molecular forms identified in glucagonoma patients that differ from the four types found normally. There is considerable variation in the quantity of each form found in the plasma of patients with glucagonomas. This variation in molecular species may have pathophysiologic importance. The concentration of immunoreactive glucagon found circulating or in the tumors of these patients has not always correlated well with their clinical or metabolic abnormalities. An explanation could be that the various forms of immunoreactive glucagon may have different biologic potency.

Morphologic changes can be identified in the islet cells of the normal pancreas in the glucagonoma syndrome (14). The chronic excess of glucagon causes a virtual disappearance of A cells. The B cells show a decrease in immunoreactive insulin content and ultrastructural features of enhanced secretion. The content of immunoreactive somatostatin and pancreatic polypeptide (PP) increases substantially. D cells have increased secretory granules, but do not have evidence of increased secretory activity as do the B cells. They often form large clusters in the center of islets, surrounded by B and PP cells.

## CLINICAL FEATURES

### Effects of Glucagon

The symptoms associated with the glucagonoma syndrome are directly or indirectly caused by the excess of circulating glucagon. Glucagon is a straight-chain peptide of 29 amino acids and a molecular weight of 3500. Its amino acid sequence is strikingly similar to that of secretin, VIP, gastric inhibitory polypeptide (GIP), and growth hormone releasing factor (GHRF) (15). After being processed from a preprohormone to the prehormone glicentin and finally to glucagon, it is secreted from the alpha cells, primarily in response to low glucose concentrations. Stress, surgery, infection, strenuous exercise, dietary protein (especially containing the amino acids arginine or alanine), hyperaminoacidemia, starvation or ß-adrenergic stimulation can also stimulate its release from the A cells in the periphery of the islets of Langerhans.

Glucagon is secreted into the hepatic portal circulation and acts primarily on the liver under physiologic conditions (Table 79.2). Glucagon enhances postabsorptive glucose production and increases postabsorptive plasma glucose concentration. It plays a counterregulatory role by promoting glucose recovery from hypoglycemia. Hypoglycemia increases circulating glucagon levels two- to fourfold, whereas hyperglycemia decreases them approximately 50%. The most important action of glucagon is to promote and sustain hepatic glucose output. It binds to specific receptors located on the hepatocyte plasma membrane, activates adenylyl cyclase and increases the intracellular production of cyclic adenosine monophosphate (cAMP). Glucagon is a potent activator of glycogenolysis and gluconeogenesis and increases hepatic glucose production within minutes. This increase is normally transient, as glucagon has a half-life of approximately 6 minutes and a rapid metabolic clearance rate of 600 mL/min. The hepatic extraction of amino acids, especially alanine, is increased. The activities of the gluconeogenic enzymes, pyruvate carboxylase, phosphoenolpyruvate carboxykinase, and fructose 1,6-diphosphatase are increased, while the activities of the glycolytic enzymes phosphofructokinase and pyruvate kinase are decreased.

Another intrahepatic action of glucagon is to direct incoming free fatty acids away from triglyceride synthesis and toward ß-oxidation. Glucagon activates adipose tissue lipase, thereby increasing lipolysis, delivery of free fatty acids to the liver, and ketogenesis. Incoming fatty acids, made abundant through stimulation of lipolysis, are converted into ketone bodies, acetoacetate, and ß-hydroxybutyrate. Although glucagon's ketogenic actions are physiologically relevant, they are easily nullified by rather small amounts of insulin. Other actions of glucagon include stimulation of insulin secretion, inhibition of gastric acid and pancreatic exocrine secretion, relaxation of the smooth muscle of the stomach and duodenum, induction of rapid transit through the small bowel, and increased heart rate and cardiac contractility.

Peptides related immunologically to glucagon are produced in several extrapancreatic tissues such as the brain, salivary glands, and intestine. The gene for proglucagon is expressed not only in the pancreatic A cells, but also in the brain and in the L cells present in the ileal mucosa. The end products of processing, however, are different. The A cells process the proglucagon predominantly to glucagon, glicentin-related pancreatic peptide, and, to a lesser extent, glucagon-like peptide 1 (GLP-1). The intestinal L cells do not form glucagon. Instead they produce large amounts of glucagon-like peptides. GLP-1 is a potent stimulator of insulin release by the pancreatic beta cells. It originates from the intestine to augment insulin release in response to the ingestion of oral nutrients. It also acts as a potent inhibitor of gastric acid secretion (16). While the principal function of glucagon is to regulate carbohydrate, fat, and protein metabolism, it and its related peptides may have more roles. They may act as paracrine agents that communicate with adjacent cells and as neurotransmitters within the nervous system. These less-understood actions may be important in explaining some of the symptoms of the glucagonoma syndrome.

**TABLE 79.2. Systemic Effects of Glucagon**

| |
|---|
| Activates glycogenolysis and gluconeogenesis |
| Inhibits glycolysis |
| Increases β-oxidation of fatty acids |
| Stimulates insulin secretion |
| Inhibits gastric acid secretion |
| Inhibits pancreatic exocrine secretion |
| Relaxes stomach and duodenum smooth muscle |
| Increases transit time through the small bowel |
| Increases heart rate and contractility |

## Diabetes Mellitus

Since the primary function of glucagon is to increase blood sugar, it is not surprising that diabetes mellitus is an almost universal feature of the glucagonoma syndrome. Almost all patients with glucagonomas have either an elevated fasting blood sugar level or an abnormal glucose tolerance test. Since glucagon administration has been shown in animals and man to cause at least transient hyperglycemia, it seems likely that diabetes is a direct result of tumor production of this hormone (9). The diabetes associated with a glucagonoma appears to differ from the usual insulin-dependent disease. It is generally milder, and patients are less prone to ketoacidosis or microvascular complications. It is often well controlled with oral medication and infrequently requires insulin. The mildness of the diabetes is surprising given the very high levels of glucagon found in these patients. There is little correlation between the severity of the diabetes and the level of circulating glucagon or the extent of the tumor.

Elevated insulin levels have often been documented in the glucagonoma syndrome (9). Glucagonomas are slow-growing tumors that usually cause a gradual increase in circulating glucagon levels. Augmented insulin production may be a counterregulating response to the elevated blood sugar that is caused by increased levels of glucagon. This is supported by the pathologic findings of hyperplasia of the pancreatic islet cells, especially the beta cells, after chronic glucagon excess. In rare patients, glucagonomas have even been shown to secrete insulin themselves or to coexist with an insulin-secreting tumor (17).

Other factors may contribute to diabetes in patients with glucagonoma. The pancreas may have a reduced capacity to secrete insulin in response to increased glucose levels. This may be related to the amount of pancreas that has been replaced by tumor or has been removed in surgically treating it. Glucagonomas can produce different molecular types of glucagon. The unequal gluconeogenic potential of these various molecular forms may also explain the poor correlation between hormone levels and the severity of diabetes. Chronic glycogen depletion is another factor that may lessen the severity of diabetes in these patients. Finally, "down-regulation" of either glucagon receptors or hepatic enzymes may occur as glucagon levels gradually rise.

## Rash

The most striking clinical feature of the glucagonoma syndrome is its characteristic rash, known as necrolytic migratory erythema (NME). This is often the most troubling aspect for patients with the syndrome. NME in association with elevated serum glucagon levels is pathognomonic of the glucagonoma syndrome. It is seen in at least 70% of patients (18). The name, which was given by Wilkinson (19), accurately describes both the marked destruction of the epidermis (necrotizing) and the tendency of the rash to heal in one area while developing in others (migratory). Lesions may occur anywhere, but the perineum, buttocks, groin, thighs, distal extremities, and perioral regions are most frequently involved (Fig. 79.1). The rash has a predilection for occurring in areas of friction, such as the intertriginous areas, as well as sites of cutaneous trauma and local irritants such as tight-fitting garments and shoes.

A typical 7- to 14-day cycle occurs in which the lesions undergo several changes. They first appear as red blotches and then become erythematous macules and papules. Superficial

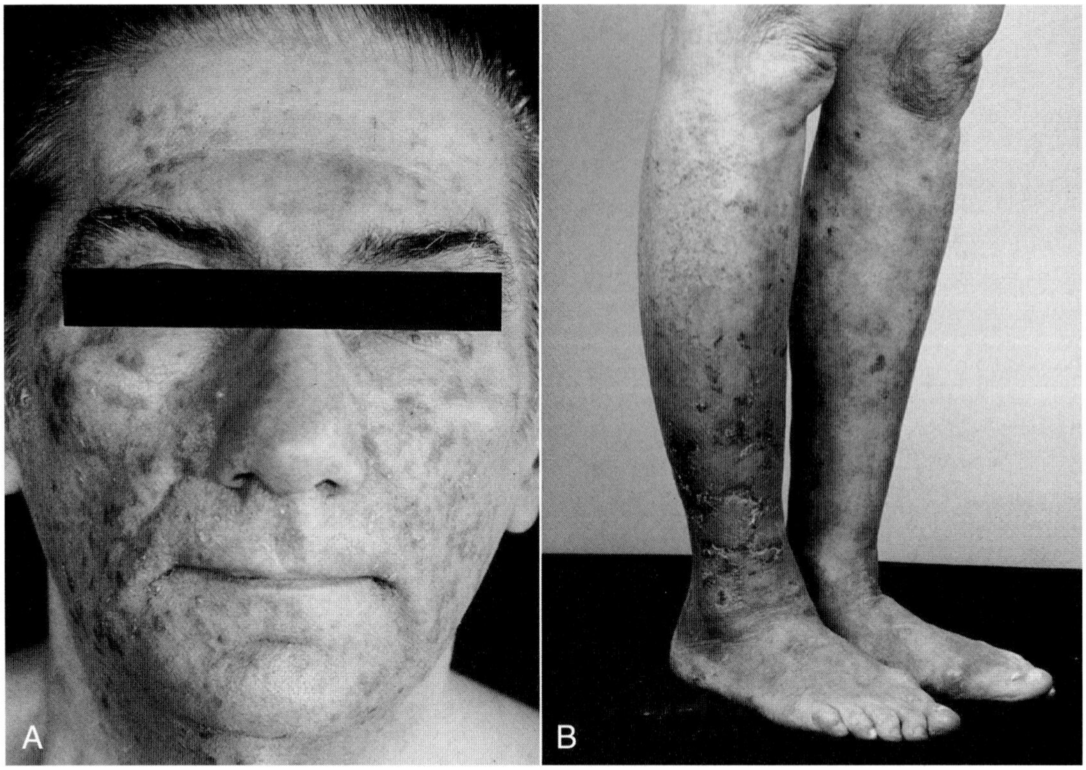

**FIG. 79.1.** Typical appearance of the rash of necrolytic migratory erythema (NME) on the face and legs of a patient with glucagonoma.

scaling develops, resulting in a psoriaform appearance. The rash then begins to resemble a scald as the lesions blister. Central erosions develop in the epidermis overlying the blister, causing oozing and crusting. Neighboring areas may become confluent, and large areas of skin may become involved. As the erythematous margins move peripherally, central healing starts to occur. Healing may be complete without any residual or occur with pigmentation or bronze discoloration marking areas that were previously affected. Stomatitis, angular cheilosis, and painful glossitis with a beefy red tongue often accompany the rash. The finger and toenails can be involved in these dermatologic changes and become dystrophic and brittle.

The rash may be mistaken for many other exanthems, including eczema, psoriasis, pemphigus, pellagra, herpes, zinc deficiency, fatty acid deficiency, and kwashiorkor. Similar eruptions may occasionally be seen with pancreatic cancers, celiac sprue, chronic pancreatitis, ulcerative colitis, jejunal adenocarcinoma, or hepatic cirrhosis (20, 21).

The rash is a cause of substantial morbidity because of its intense pruritus. Secondary infection of the excoriations can occur, and the early clinical signs and symptoms may be dominated by the findings of opportunistic infection by *Staphylococcus aureus* and *Candida* spp. Occasionally, the skin infection may be the presenting symptom. In addition to being difficult to treat, these suprainfections may divert attention away from the true cause, an underlying tumor. Patients have often suffered from NME for many years before the diagnosis is established. Wider knowledge of the characteristic skin changes may lead to earlier recognition of these tumors. However, glucagonomas may occur without skin changes or the skin changes may develop after the tumor is already clinically evident.

Biopsy of a fresh lesion can demonstrate the characteristic histologic picture (Fig. 79.2). The dermis and deeper levels of epidermis are normal, but there is bullous disruption of the superficial epidermis. There is hyperkeratosis, parakeratosis, dyskeratotic cells, papillary dermal angiodysplasia, and cleft formation. Cleavage takes place at the level of the stratum granulosum, with degeneration and necrolysis of these cells. Spongiosis and rarely acantholysis have been described. Fusiform keratinocytes with pyknotic nuclei are found, and a mononuclear inflammatory infiltrate with vascular dilation is often present. Immunofluorescent techniques have not shown any immune complexes in the dermis or epidermis. However, the

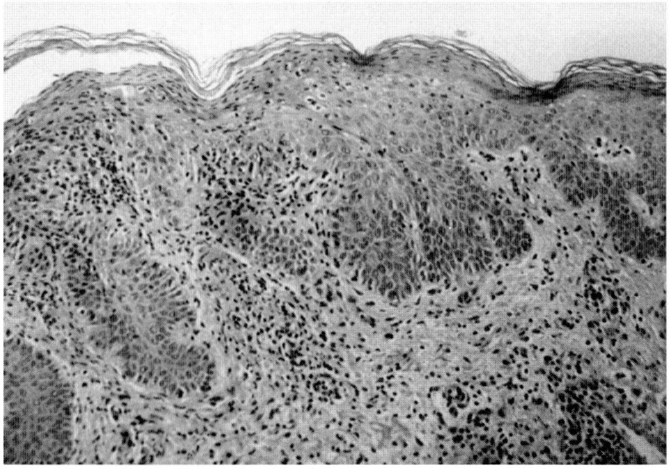

**FIG. 79.2.** The characteristic histologic findings of a chronic NME lesion on skin biopsy. In addition to the marked parakeratosis and psoriaform hyperplasia, there is acantholysis and marked chronic inflammation.

appearance of the rash on histologic examination can be highly variable, and the lack of the classic picture does not rule out NME.

Multiple factors have been implicated as the cause of NME, and several different treatments attempted, including steroids both topically and systemically, antibiotics, irradiation, UV light, nicotinamide, vitamins, methotrexate, hydroxyurea, azathioprine, tar, diiodohydroxyquinlone (Iodoquinol) and dapsone. However, care must be taken in interpreting the results of specific treatments because the rash characteristically waxes and wanes. Improvement, if not shown repeatedly, may be coincidental. A trial of antibiotic therapy may be successful, however, in eradicating opportunistic infections, and topical steroids may provide relief from the pruritus.

Prostaglandins have been implicated because in high concentrations they can cause erythema, increased vascular permeability, and edema. However they do not produce the characteristic skin lesions. Because of similarities with the rash associated with zinc deficiency, Tasman-Jones and Kay postulated that low zinc levels may lead to NME (22). However, investigators have found normal serum zinc levels in these patients. Hair zinc analysis, which is a more accurate assessment of zinc metabolism has also been normal. NME in patients with coexistent zinc deficiency has healed without zinc supplementation, and zinc supplements have not relieved the rash in others.

Another factor that has been implicated in the development of NME is hypoaminoacidemia. Mallinson et al. in 1974 found that amino acid levels were greatly depressed in patients with glucagonomas, and they postulated that amino acid deficiency was the cause of the rash (6). Norton et al. studied a patient with the syndrome whose serum amino acid levels were lower than those seen in starvation (23). The patient's rash disappeared when the serum amino acid levels normalized with parenteral hyperalimentation containing amino acids. On two occasions, the parenteral nutrition was discontinued. Each time the rash reappeared after 2 days and quickly resolved after reinstitution of hyperalimentation. Stacpoole et al. had a similar experience with infusion of amino acids (24). Their patient showed impressive and reproducible improvement in the rash but never had complete resolution. A causal relationship between hypoaminoacidemia and NME remains controversial because restoration of amino acid levels to normal by enteral alimentation has failed to ameliorate the rash in some patients. Furthermore, lower serum amino acid levels can be found in glucagonoma patients without any skin manifestations than those in patients with NME.

The cause of NME remains unclear. The disappearance of the rash in response to surgical excision of the tumor in most patients supports a key role for glucagon. Somatostatin analogue therapy, which decreases circulating glucagon levels, has induced marked improvement in the rash within 48 hours and complete resolution within 1 week (25). When the somatostatin analogue is stopped, the rash usually recurs within 36 hours. Glucagon may not be the only explanation for NME, since resolution of the rash does not always correlate with decreased plasma glucagon levels. In some cases, the rash cleared with octreotide therapy despite plasma glucagon levels either decreasing only mildly or remaining unchanged (26, 27). There may be other hormonally active substances produced by the tumor that are responsible for the rash, or octreotide may have a direct effect on somatostatin receptors on dermal cells. Regardless, the best therapy for the skin lesions is successful tumor treatment with surgery, chemotherapy, or octreotide. Following tumor removal, patients experience almost immediate improvement, with complete clearing of the rash in 7–10 days.

## Weight Loss

Considerable weight loss without anorexia is common in this syndrome and occurs in most patients. As with other malignancies, weight loss can occur from widespread tumor dissemination or from chronic illness. These seem to be the cause in only a minority of patients. Weight loss is often a prominent feature in patients with small, solitary tumors, in whom the tumor burden would not explain such emaciation. The degree of muscle wasting is often out of proportion to the tumor burden. Glucagon is extremely catabolic, and weight loss may reflect a hormonal effect on carbohydrate, protein, and fat metabolism.

## Thrombosis

An increased frequency of thromboembolic disease accompanies glucagon-producing tumors, and these complications may occur in 30–50% of patients. The most plausible explanation for this thrombotic tendency is alteration in factor X levels. Factor X is a vitamin K–dependent serine protease that has a cardinal role in the coagulation process. It converts prothrombin to thrombin after appropriate activation. Although the major source of factor X is the liver, it is also produced by pancreatic alpha cells and is elevated in the glucagonoma syndrome. In these patients, bleeding times and coagulation studies are usually normal when measured.

Deep vein thrombosis and pulmonary emboli are more common in patients with glucagonomas than in patients with other islet cell tumors. Cerebral and renal artery thrombosis can occur. Occlusion of the superior mesenteric artery resulting in small bowel infarction and death has been reported as the initial presentation of an occult pancreatic glucagonoma (28). Because both venous and arterial thrombi and emboli have caused death in some patients, blood clots should be carefully sought and, if found, treated aggressively. It is important to remember this life-threatening problem when evaluating patients with the glucagonoma syndrome for an operation. Careful consideration should be given to prophylactic subcutaneous heparin, intermittent pneumatic calf compression, or other methods of preventing deep venous thrombosis and pulmonary embolus. Aspirin therapy and dipyridamole may also play a role in patients being treated medically for the glucagonoma syndrome.

## Anemia

A normocytic, normochromic anemia is a common finding in the glucagonoma syndrome. Hemoglobin values usually range between 8.5 and 10.5 g/dL, but levels as low as 4 g/dL have been reported (9). The exact cause of the anemia is uncertain. Serum iron, vitamin $B_{12}$, and folate are usually normal, and no reliable response is obtained after treatment with these agents. Bone marrow examination is usually normal. The anemia may be a direct effect of elevated serum glucagon levels. Glucagon has been reported to suppress erythropoiesis in experimental animals (29). Another possibility is that it is secondary to the catabolic state that is induced in these patients. Whatever its cause, the anemia usually responds to successful tumor therapy.

## Hypoaminoacidemia

As mentioned in the discussion of NME, a nearly constant finding in the glucagonoma syndrome is panhypoaminoacidemia. Concentrations of most amino acids are usually depressed to less than 25% of normal, but glucogenic amino acids are affected more than branched-chain amino acids. Plasma hypoaminoacidemia is probably a direct consequence of increased glucagon secretion, and there appears to be some correlation between circulating glucagon levels and amino acid concentrations. Even at physiologic concentrations, glucagon has a pronounced effect on amino acids. It increases intracellular uptake and degradation of amino acids, especially in the liver, and stimulates the conversion of the deaminated carbon skeletons to glucose. A decrease in both total serum protein and serum albumin has been documented in these patients, most likely from this same metabolic pathway. The hypoaminoacidemia may be used to help suggest the diagnosis of glucagonoma. It can be reversed acutely by amino acid infusions or by aggressive dietary supplementation. Surgical extirpation of the glucagonoma or successful chemotherapy provides long-term correction (30, 31).

### Other Characteristics

Alterations in mental status, particularly depression, but also disorientation, insomnia, and nervousness, may accompany the glucagonoma syndrome. It is unclear if these are specific to high glucagon levels or merely the result of a chronic debilitating disease. Neurologic abnormalities, including optic atrophy and reversible scotomata have been found in some patients (30). Various gastrointestinal complaints have also been described. The most common is diarrhea, which may resemble steatorrhea in some patients. This occurs in 15% of patients and may be due to the effect of glucagon on the small bowel mucosa in either reducing absorption or enhancing the net secretion of water and electrolytes. It may also be due to impairment of pancreatic enzyme secretion caused by pancreatic duct obstruction or replacement of the parenchyma by tumor. While weight loss in the glucagonoma syndrome is commonly associated with a normal appetite, some of these patients may have anorexia. Early satiety and constipation are sometimes seen and may be secondary to the smooth muscle–relaxing properties of glucagon. Abdominal pain and nausea and vomiting are less commonly seen. Urinary tract infections occur frequently in women who have perineal involvement with NME. Kidney stones have occasionally been reported.

## DIAGNOSIS

A glucagonoma should be suspected in patients with a rash and evidence of a pancreatic mass. It should also be considered in patients with a chronic unexplained dermatitis that is resistant to therapy. This is especially true if it is accompanied by glucose intolerance and/or thromboembolic phenomena. The possibility of a glucagonoma should be kept in mind in patients with familial MEN type 1 syndrome and their relatives and in asymptomatic patients in whom a pancreatic tumor has been found.

### Glucagon Levels

The diagnosis is made by demonstrating a plasma glucagon concentration that is inappropriately elevated for the level of plasma glucose in patients with the clinical features of this syndrome and/or a pancreatic mass (Table 79.3). Since findings of the glucagonoma syndrome may not appear until the tumor is quite large, plasma glucagon concentrations are usually markedly elevated. When glucagon levels have been measured, patients have almost always had basal glucagon concentrations well over the normal range. Circulating levels have ranged from 300 to 96,000 pg/mL, which is substantially above the normal level of 25–250 pg/mL seen in most assays. For practical purposes, a plasma glucagon concentration above 1000 pg/mL can be considered solid biochemical evidence for a glucagonoma. Although several symptomatic patients with glucagonomas have been found with glucagon concentrations below 1000 pg/mL, most glucagon concentrations of this magnitude have been in asymptomatic patients with small tumors. Rare patients have had glucagon levels above 1000 pg/mL but have had no tumor. These patients have familial hyperglucagonemia, a condition that has been described in two families (13, 31). Involved family members have elevated concentrations of high-molecular-weight immunoreactive glucagon. They have no neoplasm and no clinical signs of the glucagonoma syndrome.

**TABLE 79.3. Laboratory Findings in the Glucagonoma Syndrome**

| |
|---|
| Hyperglycemia |
| Elevated fasting plasma glucagon level |
| Normochromic, normocytic anemia |
| Hypoaminoacidemia |
| Hypoproteinemia |
| Hypocholesterolemia |

**TABLE 79.4. Conditions Associated with Hyperglucagonemia**

| |
|---|
| Prolonged fasting |
| Excessive exercise |
| Severe stress |
| Renal insufficiency |
| Hepatic insufficiency |
| Diabetic ketoacidosis |
| Septicemia |
| Familial hyperglucagonemia |

Glucagon concentrations can be elevated in other disease processes such as hepatic or renal insufficiency and after prolonged fasting and excessive exercise or severe stress (Table 79.4). Elevation can also occur with diabetic ketoacidosis, septicemia, and the use of danazol or oral contraceptives. The plasma glucagon in these conditions rarely exceeds 500 pg/mL. These conditions can usually be excluded by history or the clinical presentation, so the differential diagnosis is not usually a problem.

### Other Diagnostic Tests

An elevated fasting level of immunoreactive glucagon almost always confirms the diagnosis of glucagonoma. In normal subjects, only the 3500-Da form of glucagon should be present in the serum. Detection of the larger 9000-Da peptide in the serum of patients with normal renal function is virtually diagnostic of a glucagonoma (32).

In the rare setting in which a glucagonoma is suspected but the fasting glucagon level is not as dramatically elevated as expected, several other tests may provide additional information (Table 79.5). In healthy people, an oral carbohydrate load increases serum glucose levels and suppresses plasma glucagon levels. A paradoxical rise in circulating glucagon is seen in many patients with a glucagonoma during a glucose tolerance test. Diabetes, cirrhosis, hemosiderosis, and a variety of other conditions can cause the same paradoxical rise. An intravenous infusion of glucose appears to induce the same paradoxical effects (31, 33, 34).

Intravenous secretin can produce a paradoxical increase in glucagon secretion in patients with glucagonoma (35). Just as the rise in circulating gastrin in response to secretin is seen only in patients with gastrinomas, the rise in plasma glucagon is likewise seen only in patients with glucagonomas. Intravenous administration of arginine causes a rise of at least 100 pg/mL in the plasma glucagon level of healthy people (5). The rise is greater in patients with diabetes and is much more prominent in patients with a glucagonoma. After intravenous administration of 30 g of arginine, plasma glucagon levels can rise 100–430% over baseline in glucagonoma patients. The peak is seen between 10 and 30 minutes after infusion (33). Intravenous infusion of tolbutamide suppresses glucagon in healthy people and patients with diabetes. Patients with a glucagonoma usually show a rapid rise in plasma glucagon concentration with intravenous tolbutamide. Calcium and calcitonin infusions induce a biphasic rise in plasma glucagon in patients with glucagonomas. Somatostatin has decreased plasma glucagon levels in patients who have been studied. This finding has therapeutic implications discussed below that are even more important than its diagnostic uses. Unfortunately, there is presently no single reliable provocative test to determine whether moderately elevated glucagon levels are caused by a glucagonoma.

In addition to serum glucagon levels, additional laboratory studies can be obtained to confirm the diagnosis. Since anemia and hypoaminoacidemia are clinical components of the glucagonoma syndrome, a normocytic, normochromic anemia with normal serum $B_{12}$ and folate levels and normal marrow cellularity as well as depressed circulating amino acid levels may help solidify the diagnosis. Relatively low levels of serum cholesterol have been found in several patients with glucagonomas. Decreased dietary intake or the effects of hyperglucagonemia on cholesterol and lipoprotein metabolism are possible, but unproven, explanations. Calcium levels should be checked to rule out concomitant hyperparathyroidism.

## LOCALIZATION

Glucagonomas are less difficult to localize preoperatively than other endocrine tumors of the pancreas because of their size at presentation. Glucagonomas are usually more than 3 cm in diameter and may be larger than 35 cm. These tumors can arise anywhere in the pancreas, but the body and tail of the gland seems to be the most frequent site (36). A review of the anatomic location of glucagonomas showed that 77% of glucagonomas were located to the left of the superior mesenteric artery (37). Approximately half of these were located in the tail and half in the body of the pancreas. It is extremely unlikely to find the tumor outside of the pancreas. There have been only two reports of extrapancreatic tumors; one in the duodenum and one in the kidney.

### Computed Tomography

CT scanning is the technique of choice both to localize the primary glucagonoma and to demonstrate metastatic disease (Fig. 79.3). CT scanning has the obvious advantage of being noninvasive, and successful localization is quite high. As opposed to insulinomas, which are usually relatively small when diagnosed, glucagonomas are usually large enough to be easily detected on CT. Even smaller tumors can be successfully localized with dynamic or spiral scanning.

Glucagonomas as small as 1 cm in diameter can be detected, particularly when the CT scan is equipped with narrow collimation, and dynamic sequencing is performed. Glucagonomas do not have classic diagnostic characteristics on CT to differentiate them from other pancreatic masses. However, tumor calcifications have been noted on CT in some islet cell tumors. Many authors believe that the presence of macroscopic calcifications indicates malignancy. Because glucagonomas are more often malignant than other islet cell tumors, they will more commonly have these calcifications. It may also be helpful to evaluate the fascial planes surrounding the pancreas. Often the extrapancreatic perivascular fat planes and fascial planes in proximity to the tumor are uninvolved. This is opposed to the frequent involvement of such structures in patients with adenocarcinoma of the pancreas, particularly when such tumors are large.

Besides its ability to locate the primary tumor, CT can identify intraabdominal metastases, especially in the liver and peripancreatic lymph nodes. The growth of hepatic metastases and their response to treatment can be followed serially. For these reasons, CT scanning should be the primary radiologic investigation when a glucagonoma is considered.

### Selective Angiography

Selective angiography is also effective in demonstrating glucagonomas. Like other islet cell tumors, they are characteristically highly vascular. Angiographically, they show up with a pronounced tumor "blush." Both primary tumors and metastases are equally well identified because of their vascularity (Fig. 79.4). Selective angiography has identified primary tumors and hepatic metastases that have been missed by CT (38). Some recommend that angiography should be done to augment CT, as it is more sensitive in demonstrating small liver metastases and can also predict major venous involvement by a large tumor involving the head or body of the pancreas. Arteriography has been helpful in demonstrating recurrent disease and metastases after tumor removal. However, the improved technology and widespread use of CT scanning have decreased the importance of angiography.

### Other Localizing Studies

Other modalities have been used to localize glucagonomas. Barium studies are generally not helpful except for large tumors that cause external compression of adjacent viscera. Magnetic resonance imaging (MRI) has been suggested as a sensitive method of detecting the primary tumor and hepatic metastases, but it is uncertain whether it offers any advantages over CT scanning (39). Selective venous sampling can localize glucagonomas by identifying gradients of circulating glucagon levels in caval, portal, and pancreatic venous blood samples (40, 41). However, selective venous sampling is highly invasive and expensive. It requires special expertise to perform and has been associated with morbidity (39). Its use in the localization of glucagonomas is limited.

Endoscopic ultrasound (EUS) of the pancreas allows detailed visualization of the whole gland through the gastric and duodenal walls, with high resolution. Pathologic structures as small as 2–3 mm can be detected by EUS. Rosch et al. studied 37 patients with neuroendocrine tumors of the pancreas from 0.5 to 2.5 cm, including one glucagonoma that was not identified by transabdominal ultrasound and CT scan. EUS was able to localize 32 of the 39 tumors (sensitivity, 82%) (42). No tumor was incorrectly localized. EUS was also able to accurately predict the size within 2 mm. Although EUS is quite accurate for evaluating the pancreas, it does not provide high-resolution images of the liver. EUS must be used with other studies such as CT and scintigraphy so that hepatic metastases can be ruled out.

Somatostatin receptor scintigraphy (SRS) is a new imaging method for localizing and determining the extent of neuroendocrine tumors in the gastrointestinal tract. An indium-labeled somatostatin analogue ([$^{111}$In-DTPA-D-Phe$^{1}$]-octreotide) has been developed for clinical use. Both the binding of this radionuclide to somatostatin receptors and its biologic activity are similar to that of octreotide. Preliminary studies indicate that it

**TABLE 79.5. Effects of Various Stimuli on Glucagon Levels**

| | Effect on Plasma Glucagon Level | |
|---|---|---|
| Stimulus | Normal Subjects | Glucagonoma Patients |
| Oral carbohydrate load | Decrease | Paradoxical increase |
| IV glucose | Decrease | Paradoxical increase |
| Meals with protein, fat, and carbohydrate | Decrease or no effect | Increase |
| IV arginine | Mild increase | Large increase |
| IV tolbutamide | Decrease | Increase |
| IV secretin | Decrease | Increase |

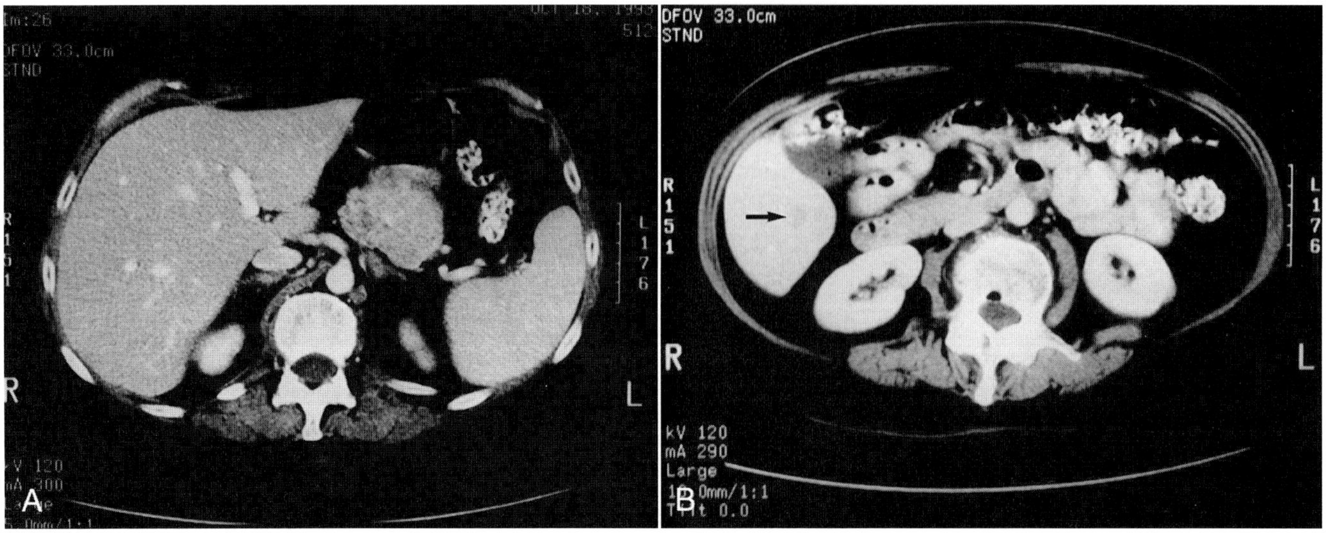


**FIG. 79.3.** CT appearance. **A.** Glucagonoma. **B.** A metastatic lesion in the liver.

is a good radiopharmaceutical for in vivo imaging of somatostatin receptor-positive tumors. A review of the European experience with scintigraphy shows that the overall sensitivity of [$^{111}$In-DTPA-D-Phe$^{1}$]-octreotide scintigraphy for detecting gastroenteropancreatic tumors and their metastases is as high as 80–90%. It is even higher for tumors with a high concentration of somatostatin receptors, such as gastrinomas and glucagonomas. The sensitivity of SRS has been 100% for glucagonomas in several studies (43). Further study is needed to determine its accuracy in identifying metastatic disease.

Positron-emission tomography (PET) is a noninvasive radiologic technique that allows biochemical and metabolic studies of human tumors in vivo. It is a tracer technique, in which bioactive substances, most of them containing carbon, oxygen, nitrogen, or fluoride as natural constituents, are labeled with short-lived positron-emitting radionuclides, that is, $^{11}$C, $^{15}$O, $^{13}$N, and $^{18}$F, with decay times ranging between 2 minutes and 2 hours. Preliminary results with neuroendocrine tumors have been promising, and PET scans may prove beneficial in glucagonoma patients with the labeling of glucagon and its precursors, or somatostatin analogues (44). This very expensive technique is not indicated in all patients.

## TREATMENT

The management of patients with a glucagonoma is directed toward control of the tumor and its hormonally related symptoms. When the tumor is still localized to the pancreas, surgical resection is the optimal treatment because it can completely reverse all clinical manifestations of the syndrome and result in a lasting cure.

### Surgical Therapy

Surgery offers the only chance for cure, but it achieves this goal in only a minority of glucagonoma patients. Greater clinical awareness of these tumors and their clinical features, leading to earlier diagnosis, may improve these results. The prognosis for patients with a glucagonoma is highly variable and depends substantially on the size and metastatic spread of the tumor at the time of diagnosis, as well as the response to treatment, which is not always uniform. There is a dramatic reversal of all clinical features after a curative intervention. Glucagon levels plummet, and improvement in the rash may be noted within 24–48 hours of the operation. The rash resolves within 5–7 days, weight gain begins, and the diabetes, anemia, and hypoproteinemia are reversed. Plasma glucagon levels can be used as a tumor marker after operation to confirm the adequacy of resection and to monitor recurrence at a preclinical stage.

Unfortunately, 75% of glucagonomas are malignant, and 50–60% of patients with the glucagonoma syndrome have metastases at the time of diagnosis. Nevertheless, aggressive surgical resection is indicated because tumor reduction may alleviate the debilitating effects of hyperglucagonemia. Even in

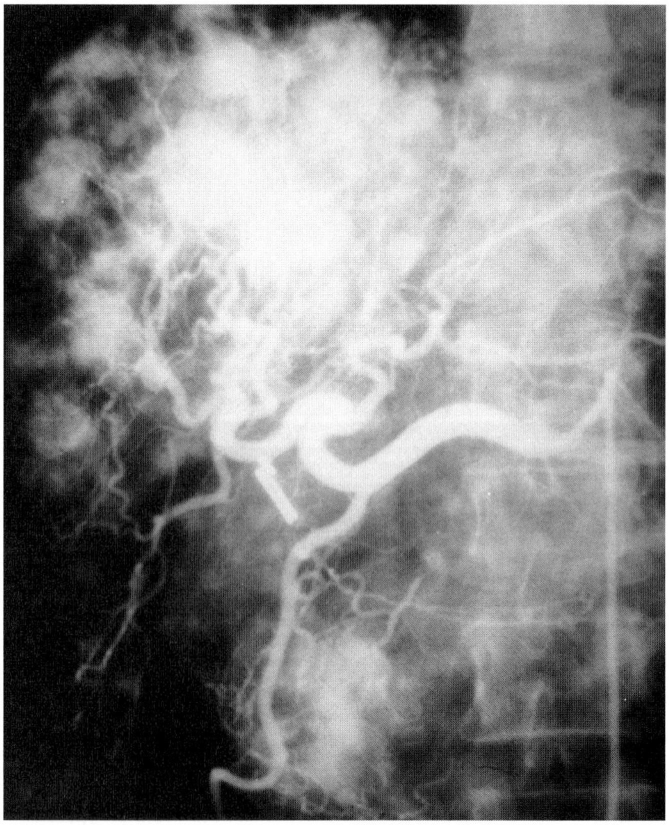

**FIG. 79.4.** Angiogram showing metastatic glucagonoma lesions in the liver.

the face of widespread disease, subtotal removal may provide substantial palliation. Glucagon-producing tumors are slow growing, and hormonal effects may pose a greater danger than the tumor itself. Control of these humoral effects can result in substantial patient benefit. There is also the possibility that the efficacy of other therapeutic modalities can be enhanced by decreasing the tumor burden. As much tumor as safely possible should be removed if curative resection is not possible.

Perioperative management of glucagonoma patients is particularly important. Treatment of a glucagonoma begins with adequate preoperative preparation to control hyperglycemia, improve the rash, and strengthen the patient's nutritional status. In the past, the catabolic effects of glucagon, including severe weight loss, anemia, hypoaminoacidemia, and hypoproteinemia, made these patients poor operative risks. Several options are available to improve their metabolic status before exploration. Oral protein supplementation may be beneficial to reverse the hypoproteinemia and hypoaminoacidemia. Protein solutions administered orally must be used cautiously at first because they may act as a glucagon secretagogue. With severe weight loss, a period of intravenous hyperalimentation can reverse some of the effects of the tumor (23, 45). Hyperalimentation may be even more beneficial to those receiving chemotherapy. The patient's hemoglobin and hematocrit should be checked prior to surgery, and preoperative transfusions should be considered in those with marked anemia. These should also be carefully monitored postoperatively.

Keep in mind that these patients have a predilection for deep venous thrombosis (DVT) and pulmonary embolism. Consideration should be given to aspirin or dipyridamole therapy prior to surgery, even though the efficacy of these agents has not been confirmed in patients with glucagonomas. The patient should have maximum DVT prophylaxis at the time of surgery, including subcutaneous heparin and sequential compression devices. Any thromboembolic complication postoperatively should be aggressively treated with anticoagulation.

The use of somatostatin analogues should also be considered in the preoperative preparation of these patients. Somatostatin and its analogues have been successfully used preoperatively to control the symptoms of hormone excess in patients with endocrine tumors (46, 47). By reducing circulating glucagon levels, octreotide can enhance the nutritional benefit of preoperative intravenous hyperalimentation. It can also reverse the rash and perhaps even decrease the risk of thromboembolic disease.

Hyperglycemia is a normal physiologic response to inhalation and regional anesthesia during laparotomy. Afferent neurogenic stimuli increase the sympathetic outflow and catecholamine release. This stimulates hepatic glycogenolysis and gluconeogenesis. In addition, nitrous oxide/halothane anesthesia alone increases plasma glucagon. Thus, intraoperative and postoperative glucose levels should be monitored. Despite these factors favoring glucose elevation, intraoperative hyperglycemia requiring insulin administration is usually not necessary (48).

An upper abdominal transverse incision is used for a thorough exploration to determine tumor extent. Most of these tumors are malignant and are large and advanced at the time of surgery. Intraoperative ultrasound may be helpful in identifying hepatic metastases or vascular invasion by the primary. A formal pancreatic resection consisting of a distal subtotal pancreatectomy is usually sufficient, since most tumors arise in the body or tail of the pancreas. Enucleation may be considered if the tumor is clearly benign, but this is extremely unusual. As much tumor as possible should be removed, including nodal metastases and lesions in the liver that can be easily and safely wedged out. Formal hepatic resection is indicated if all gross tumor can be excised. Tumor debulking can provide dramatic and rapid improvement in many glucagonoma symptoms. A marked and prolonged decline in serum glucagon is possible with palliative resection, so the hormonal manifestations of this disorder disappear or are ameliorated for many years. Multiple operations aimed at reresecting or debulking recurrent or metastatic disease may also prolong survival (49).

## Chemotherapy

Because glucagonomas are frequently malignant and cannot be completely resected, many patients require chemotherapy. The most commonly used agent has been streptozotocin (STZ), a glucosamine nitrosourea with specific toxicity for islet cells. This has been the basis for most combination chemotherapy regimens in patients with various neuroendocrine tumors. Because of its glucose moiety, increased uptake of this drug occurs in most pancreatic islet cells. Hence it is suitable for glucagonomas. STZ as a single agent has produced a biochemical response (defined as a reduction in hormone levels by at least 50%) in 64% of treated patients and a tumor response (defined as regression of tumor size by at least 50%) in 50% of patients (50). However, most investigators have found a lower response rate than this. STZ must be used with caution because it is nephrotoxic and hepatotoxic and causes severe nausea and vomiting. With the introduction of serotonin blockers, the vomiting can be controlled and is less limiting. Renal dysfunction, the major dose-limiting toxic effect, occurs in 20–75% of patients. Renal, hepatic, and bone marrow function should be closely monitored for toxicity. The response rate can be improved by use of combination chemotherapy, most commonly with 5-fluorouracil (5-FU). The Eastern Cooperative Oncology Group (ECOG) study compared STZ alone with a combination of STZ plus 5-FU in 82 patients with advanced islet cell tumors. Responses were observed in 36% of patients who received STZ alone and 63% of those who received STZ and 5-FU (51). STZ has also been used with in combination with doxorubicin or cyclophosphamide. Unfortunately, none of these combinations has reliably achieved an objective decrease in tumor burden and/or in circulating plasma glucagon levels. Both failure to respond and early relapse have been reported (45, 52).

DTIC (5-{3,3-dimethyl-1-triazeno}imidazole-4-carboxamide) has been reported to be particularly effective in the treatment of glucagonomas. DTIC seems able to induce objective remission in patients failing other drug regimens. It produces less severe gastrointestinal side effects than STZ, but these are still substantial. It causes more bone marrow suppression and more leukopenia and thrombocytopenia. Many studies have found this to be the most effective therapy for advanced disease, and some consider DTIC to be the chemotherapeutic drug of choice for malignant glucagonoma. One must be aware, however, that patients may not respond and that relapses may occur.

Newer chemotherapeutic agents are being investigated as possible treatments for neuroendocrine tumors. Chlorozotocin (CTZ) is structurally similar to STZ. It has less potential for nephrotoxicity and less severe gastrointestinal side effects but increased myelosuppression (53). One advantage of CTZ is that a full dose can be given on a single day every 6–7 weeks, as opposed to STZ which must be given over 5 days every 6 weeks. Another new drug that has been used to treat these types of tumors is ansamitosin (Maytansine). It has generated long-lasting responses in individual cases but has considerable adverse reactions (54).

## Somatostatin Therapy

Patients who are not candidates for curative resection and who have failed to respond to chemotherapy can still be palliated by control of the hormonal manifestations of the glucagonoma syndrome. Somatostatin is a naturally occurring peptide hormone produced in many areas of the body, including the D cells of the islets of Langerhans and mucosa of the gastrointestinal tract. Because it is a potent endogenous inhibitor of peptide release, it has been used to control the hormonal manifestations of neuroendocrine tumors. The clinical usefulness of somatostatin has been limited by its short half-life of less than 4 minutes. Octreotide is a long-acting analogue of somatostatin. Because it has a longer duration of action than naturally occurring somatostatin and because it can be given by subcutaneous injection, octreotide is more suitable for clinical care. It has been used successfully to control hormone secretion and clinical symptomology in patients with glucagonomas, gastrinomas, vipomas, insulinomas, and carcinoid tumors.

Patients can self-administer octreotide at home, using the same subcutaneous injection procedures that diabetics use to administer insulin. Side effects are uncommon and usually mild. Occasionally acute abdominal pain and distension, with or without diarrhea, may occur during the first few days of treatment. Mild steatorrhea and some deterioration in glucose tolerance because of the concomitant inhibition of insulin release may occur with long-term treatment. Also, chronic octreotide administration increases the incidence of small cholesterol gallstones, although these may remain asymptomatic. Surgeons should be cognizant of this side effect and consider removing the gallbladder when operating on patients who are likely to require long-term somatostatin analogue therapy.

Octreotide has been used effectively in patients with glucagonomas. While it does not reliably inhibit tumor growth, it often induces a long-lasting remission of clinical symptoms. The most dramatic improvement is the rapid resolution of disabling NME. The insulin requirements to control diabetes are reduced, and the hemoglobin concentration can normalize with somatostatin analogue therapy. Almost all signs and symptoms are improved in responding patients, including the reversal of neurologic symptoms (18).

These results seem to be secondary to the decrease in plasma glucagon levels. Several studies have documented that somatostatin analogues cause a dramatic decrease in plasma glucagon levels, compared with pretreatment values (Fig. 79.5). However many patients being treated with octreotide do not completely normalize their plasma glucagon levels. This may be misleading because octreotide also inhibits posttranslational conversion of glucagon precursors to bioactive glucagon. Thus, determination of immunoreactive plasma glucagon does not reflect the true suppression of bioactive glucagon. This may explain the occasional discrepancy of a persistently high plasma glucagon despite improvement of clinical symptoms during octreotide therapy (55).

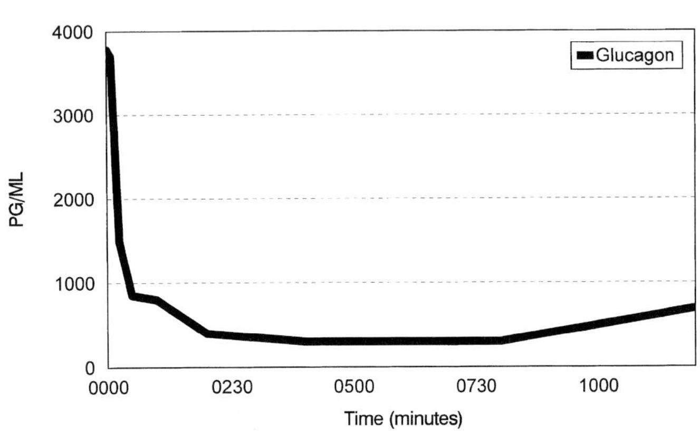


**FIG. 79.5.** Glucagon levels decrease markedly in response to octreotide treatment in a patient with a glucagonoma.

## Hepatic Artery Embolization

Because of the frequency of hepatic metastases, the liver is an important target for locoregional intervention, especially when systemic therapy proves ineffective. Liver metastases of neuroendocrine tumors have a high degree of hypervascularity. Various techniques have been used to interrupt the vascular supply of these liver metastases, including surgical ligation and radiologic embolization of the hepatic arteries. This latter technique has been the most effective method of occluding hepatic vasculature (56). A hepatic arteriogram is performed to assess the arterial anatomy, tumor blood flow, and the patency of the portal vein. The branches of the hepatic artery are selectively catheterized to gain proximity to the vessels supplying the tumor, which are then embolized. The materials used for embolization have been absorbable products, including blood clots, muscle, gelfoam, iodized oil, and collagen; nonabsorbable products, including Ivalon sponge, silicone microspheres, and steel coils; and sclerosing agents such as alcohol. The vascular anatomy, location, and volume of the metastases are all determinants of the extent of vascular occlusion needed. It is important not to occlude the entire vasculature supplying metastases in both lobes of the liver, since fatal liver insufficiency may result.

Contraindications to this form of treatment, as suggested by Carrasco et al., include replacement of more than 50% of the liver, serum LDH above 425 mU/mL, SGOT above 100 mU/mL, and bilirubin above 2 mg/dL (57). Portal vein occlusion, allergy to contrast material, coagulopathy, and substantial extrahepatic disease must also be considered contraindications. The procedure is somewhat toxic. The postembolization syndrome is characterized by liver pain, which can last 3–6 days. It is most severe in the first 36 hours and often requires intravenous narcotics. Nausea and vomiting almost always occur. Patients frequently become febrile, which can last for 72 hours. Other complications include anorexia, hiccups, pleuritic pain, ileus, vascular compromise, gallbladder ischemia, pleural effusions, and pancreatitis. A mortality rate as high as 5% may be anticipated. Hormonal crises due to sudden release of peptides during and after the procedure have decreased dramatically with the pretreatment use of octreotide.

Treatment response can be assessed by the degree of symptomatic improvement, the decrease in the glucagon level, and CT evidence of tumor regression. CT scanning may demonstrate air within the tumor secondary to necrosis. A 50% rate of partial response can be anticipated with the use of vascular occlusion therapy. Improved results can be seen by combining hepatic artery occlusion with the intraarterial infusion of chemotherapeutic agents. Intraarterial chemoembolization involves selective hepatic artery infusions of a chemotherapeutic agent, followed by particulate embolization until blood flow through the feeding arteries to the tumors is blocked. Recent data on chemoembolization using 5-FU in 10 patients with carcinoid tumors revealed a 100% symptomatic improvement with a duration of 22 months. Furthermore, 40% of patients demonstrated significant tumor reduction (58). Similar results have been obtained with chemoembolization using adriamycin (59, 60).

## Interferon Therapy

Interferon-α has been used with some success to treat malignant endocrine tumors, including glucagonomas. Interferon-α stimulates natural killer cell function and increases expression of class I antigens on tumor cells. These immunomodulatory effects may induce autoimmunity against the tumor (61). As the number of tumor cells decrease, they are replaced by fibroblasts. This does not result in any change in tumor size and therefore is not recognized by ultrasound or CT. These changes are nicely demonstrated by PET (62); hence, PET scanning may be an important tool for following patients on interferon treatment. SRS can also be used to demonstrate the fibrosis, since the fibroblasts are unlikely to have these receptors. Reduction in hormone synthesis and release can be noticed early (within days to months) during treatment with interferon-α. A substantial decrease in tumor volume takes a longer time and may not be evident for years. Treatment with interferon-α is not curative, but it can control the disease for extended periods and prolong survival. The mechanism of action is different than that of conventional chemotherapy, and there is no clear correlation between dose and antitumor response. Doses must be titrated individually for each patient for long-term treatment. Adverse reactions include a "flulike" symptom for 3–5 days initially in almost all patients. More severe reactions include fatigue, mild weight loss, and occasional mental depression. These may be difficult to differentiate from similar symptoms that are part of the glucagonoma syndrome. A small percentage of patients may develop anemia, leukopenia, or thrombocytopenia. About one-third of patients may have increased liver enzymes that are mainly dose dependent, and about 20% develop autoimmune reactions.

Interferon-α may not be curative, but it can be combined with other chemotherapeutic agents such as 5-FU to achieve an improved clinical response (63). Increased benefit may also be derived from the combined use of interferon-α and octreotide. Combinations of interferon-α with chemotherapy or octreotide have had additive or synergistic effects in a small number of patients being treated for malignant neuroendocrine tumors (64).

### Other Therapy Possibilities

Scintigraphy with radiolabeled octreotide has demonstrated the expression of a high number of somatostatin receptors on islet cell tumors. The radiotherapeutic potential of radiolabeled octreotide is currently being investigated. Treatment of an inoperable metastatic glucagonoma with peptide receptor radiotherapy has decreased tumor growth and circulating glucagon levels (65). Orthotopic liver transplant has also been used successfully to treat metastatic endocrine tumors, including glucagonomas (66). This option is obviously indicated only when all metastatic tumor can be removed and there is a possibility of cure. Other options that are generally more applicable for treating liver metastases include cryosurgery or percutanous injection of ethanol. Although these modalities offer promise, experience with them is limited, and they must still be considered investigational.

## REFERENCES


1. Becker SW, Kahn D, Rothman S. Cutaneous manifestations of internal malignant tumors. Arch Dermatol Syphilol 1942;45:1069–1080.
2. Zhdanov VC. Diabetes and malignancy of islet cells in pancreas. Arkh Patol (Moskva) 1956;18:92–93.
3. Gossner W, Korting GW. Metastasierendes Inselzellkaszinom vom A-Zell-type bei einem Fall von Pemphigus Folizceus mit Diabetes renalis. Dtsch Med Woschenschr 1960;85:434–440.
4. Unger RH, Eisentraut AM, McCall MS, et al. Glucagon antibodies and their use for immunoassay for glucagon. Proc Soc Exp Biol Med 1959;102:621.
5. McGavran MH, Unger RH, Recant L, Polk HC, Kilo C, Levin ME. A glucagon-secreting alpha cell carcinoma of the pancreas. N Engl J Med 1966;274:1408–1413.
6. Mallinson GN, Bloom SR, Warin AP, Salmon PR, Cox B. A glucagonoma syndrome. Lancet 1974;2:1–5.
7. Delcore R, Friesen SR. Gastrointestinal neuroendocrine tumors. J Am Coll Surg 1994;178:187–211.
8. Lomsky R, Langr F, Vortel V. Demonstration of glucagon in islet cell adenomas of the pancreas by immunofluorescent technic. Am J Clin Pathol 1969;51:245–250.
9. Joyce CD, Prinz RA. The glucagonoma syndrome. Probl Gen Surg 1994;11:1–16.
10. Roggli VL, Judge DM, McGavran MH. Duodenal glucagonoma: a case report. Hum Pathol 1979;19:350–353.
11. Gleeson MH, Bloom SR, Polak JM, et al. Endocrine tumor in kidney affecting small bowel structure, motility and absorptive function. Gut 1971;12:773–782.
12. Bordi C, Ravazzola M, Baetens D, et al. A study of glucagonomas by light and electron microscopy and immunofluorescence. Diabetes 1979;28:925–936.
13. Boden G, Owev OE, Rezvani I, et al. An islet cell carcinoma containing glucagon and insulin. Diabetes 1977;26:128–137.
14. Bani D, Biliotti G, Bani-Sacchi T. Morphological changes in the human endocrine pancreas induced by chronic excess of endogenous glucagon. Virchows Arch (B) 1991;60:199–206.
15. Bromer WW, Sinn LG, Staub A, Behrens OK. The amino acid sequence of glucagon. Diabetes 1957;6:234–238.
16. Wettergren A, Petersen H, Orskov C, et al. Glucagon-like peptide 1 7-36 amide and peptide YY from the L-cell of the ileal mucosa are potent inhibitors of vagally induced gastric acid secretion in man. Scand J Gastroenterol 1994;29:502–505.
17. Lind SE, Weitzman SA. The insidious development of symptomatic secondary hormone syndromes in patients with malignant endocrine tumors. Am J Med Sci 1985;290:107–110.
18. Holmes A, Kilpatrick C, Proietto J, Green MD. Reversal of a neurologic paraneoplastic syndrome with octreotide (Sandostatin) in a patient with glucagonoma. Am J Med 1991;91:434–436.
19. Wilkinson DS. Necrolytic migratory erythema with pancreatic carcinoma. Proc R Soc Med 1971;64:1197–1198.
20. Van der Loos TL, Lambrecht ER, Lambers JCCA. Successful treatment of glucagonoma-related necrolytic migratory erythema with dacarbazine. J Am Acad Dermatol 1987;16:468–472.
21. Goodenberger DM, Lawley TJ, Strober W, et al. Necrolytic migratory erythema without glucagonoma. Arch Dermatol 1979;115:1429–1432.
22. Tasman-Jones C, Kay RG. Zinc deficiency and skin lesions. N Engl J Med 1975;293:830.
23. Norton JA, Hahn CR, Schiebinger R, et al. Amino acid deficiency and the skin rash associated with glucagonoma. Ann Intern Med 1979;91:213–215.
24. Stacpoole PW, Jaspan J, Kasselberg AG, et al. A familial glucagonoma syndrome: genetic, clinical and biochemical features. Am J Med 1981;70:1017–1026.
25. Altimari AF, Bhoopalam N, Prinz RA, et al. Use of a somatostatin analog (SMS201-995) in the glucagonoma syndrome. Surgery 1986;100:989–996.
26. Santangelo WC, Unger RH, Oci L, et al. Somatostatin analog-induced remission of necrolytic migratory erythema without changes in plasma glucagon concentration. Pancreas 1986;1:464–469.
27. Peterson LL, Shaw JC, Acto KM, et al. Glucagonoma syndrome: in vitro evidence that glucagon increases epidermal arachidonic acid. J Am Acad Dermatol 1984;11:468–473.
28. Earl U, Abbott CR. Small bowel infarction associated with pancreatic glucagonoma. Postgrad Med J 1990;66:874–875.
29. Naets JP, Guns M. Inhibitory effect of glucagon on erythropoiesis. Blood 1980;55:997–1002.
30. Prinz RA, Badrinath K, Banerji M, Sparagana M, Dorsch TR, Lawrence AM. Operative and chemotherapeutic management of malignant glucagon-producing tumors. Surgery 1981;90:713–719.
31. Fujita J, Seino Y, Ishida H, et al. A functional study of a case of glucagonoma exhibiting typical glucagonoma syndrome. Cancer 1986;57:860–865.
32. Prinz RA. Glucagonoma syndrome. Surg Rounds 1987;10:63–77.
33. Tiengo A, Fedele D, Marchiori G, et al. Suppression and stimulation mechanisms controlling glucagon secretion in a case of islet cell tumor producing glucagon, insulin and gastrin. Diabetes 1975;25:408–412.
34. Leichter SB. Clinical and metabolic aspects of glucagonoma. 1980;59:100–113.
35. McCarthy D, Jensen R. Zollinger-Ellison syndrome—current issues. In: Cohen S, Soloway R, eds. Hormone producing tumors of the gastrointestinal tract. New York: Churchill Livingstone 1985:25–55.
36. Montenegro-rodas F, Samaan NA. Glucagonoma tumors and syndrome. Curr Probl Cancer 1981;6:1–54.

37. Howard JH, Stabile BE, Zinner MJ, Chang S, Belur BS, Passero E. Anatomic distribution of pancreatic endocrine tumors. Am J Surg 1990;159:258–264.
38. Wawrukiewicz AS, Rosch J, Keller FS, Lieberman DA. Glucagonoma and its angiographic diagnosis. Cardiovasc Intervent Radiol 1982;5:318–324.
39. Bloom SR, Polak JM. Glucagonoma syndrome. Am J Med 1987;82(suppl):25–36.
40. Cho KJ, Wilcox CW, Reuter SR. Glucagon producing islet cell tumor of the pancreas. AJR 1977;145:509–516.
41. Ingemansson S, Holst J, Larsson LI, et al. Localization of glucagonomas by catheterization of the pancreatic veins and with glucagon assay. Surg Gynecol Obstet 1977;145:509–516.
42. Rosch T, Lightdale CJ, Botet JF. Localization of pancreatic endocrine tumors by endoscopic ultrasonography. N Engl J Med 1992;326:1721–1726.
43. Krenning EP, Kwekkeboom DJ, Oei HY, et al. Somatostatin-receptor scintigraphy in gastroenteropancreatic tumors. Ann NY Acad Sci 1994;773:416–424.
44. Eriksson B, Lilja A, Ahlstrom H, et al. Positron-emission tomography as a radiological technique in neuroendocrine gastrointestinal tumors. Ann NY Acad Sci 1994;773:446–452.
45. Marynick SP, Fagadau WR, Duncan LA. Malignant glucagonoma syndrome: response to chemotherapy. Ann Intern Med 1980;93: 453–454.
46. Yoshioka M, Sakazume M, Fukagawa M, et al. A case of the WDHA syndrome: successful preoperative treatment of watery diarrhea with a somatostatin analogue. Jpn J Clin Oncol 1989;19:294–298.
47. Tsai ST, Ekhauser FE, Thompson NW, Strodel WE, Vinik AI. Perioperative use of long-acting somatostatin analog (SMS 201-995) in patients with endocrine tumors of the gastroenteropancreatic axis. Surgery 1986;100:788–795.
48. Boskovski NA, Chapin JW, Becker GL, Edney JA, Sanders WC, Wolpert LA. Anesthesia for glucagonoma resection. J Clin Anesth 1991;3:48–52.
49. Modlin JM, Lewis JJ, Ahlman H, Bilchik AJ, Jumar RR. Management of unresectable malignant endocrine tumors of the pancreas. Surg Gynecol Obstet 1993;176:507–518.
50. Broder LE, Carter SK. Pancreatic islet cell carcinoma: results of therapy with streptozotocin in 52 patients. Ann Intern Med 1973;79:101–107.
51. Moertel C, Hauley J, Johnson L. Streptozotocin alone compared with streptozotocin plus fluorouracil in the treatment of advanced islet cell carcinoma. N Engl J Med 1980;303:1189–1194.
52. Kessinger A, Foley JF, Lemon HM. Therapy of malignant APUD cell tumors. Effectiveness of DTIC. Cancer 1983;51:790–794.
53. Moertel CG, Lefkopoulo M, Lipsitz M. Streptozocin-doxorubicin, streptozocin-fluorouracil or chlorozotocin in the treatment of advanced islet-cell carcinoma. N Engl J Med 1992;326:519–523.
54. Moertel CG. An odyssey in the land of small tumors. J Clin Oncol 1987;5:1503–1522.
55. Jockenhovel F, Lederbogen S, Olbricht T, et al. The long-acting somatostatin analogue octreotide alleviates symptoms by reducing post-translational conversion of preproglucagon to glucagon in a patient with malignant glucagonoma, but does not prevent tumor growth. Clin Invest 1994;72:127–133.
56. Ajani JA, Carrasco CH, Wallace S. Neuroendocrine tumors metastatic to the liver. Ann NY Acad Sci 1994;773:479–487.
57. Carrasco D, Jackson NA. Samaan R, et al. The carcinoid syndrome: palliation by hepatic arterial embolization. Am J Radiol 1986;147:149–154.
58. Hajarizadeh H, Ivancev K, Mueller CR, et al. Effective palliative treatment of metastatic carcinoid tumors with intra-arterial chemotherapy/chemoembolization combined with octreotide acetate. Am J Surg 1992;163:479–483.
59. Perry JL, Stuart K, Stokes KR, Clouse ME. Hepatic arterial chemoembolization for metastatic neuroendocrine tumors. Surgery 1994;116:1116–1117.
60. Urszniewski P, Rougier P, Roche A, et al. Hepatic arterial chemoembolization in patients with liver metastases of endocrine tumors: a prospective phase II study in 24 patients. Cancer 1993;71:2624–2630.
61. Ronnblom LE, Alm GV, Oberg K. Autoimmunity after alpha interferon therapy for malignant carcinoid tumors. Ann Intern Med 1991;115:178–183.
62. Anderson T, Wilander E, Erikson B, Lindgren PG, Oberg K. Effects of interferon on tumor tissue content in liver metastases of carcinoid tumors. Cancer Res 1990;50:3413–3415.
63. Jones DV Jr, Samaan NA, Sellin RV, et al. Metastatic glucagonoma: clinical response to a combination of 5-FU and alpha-interferon. Am J Med 1992;93:348–349.
64. Eriksson B, Oberg K. An update on the medical treatment of malignant endocrine pancreatic tumors. Acta Oncol 1993;32:203–208.
65. Krenning EP, Kooji PPM, Bakker WH, et al. Radiotherapy with a radiolabeled somatostatin analogue, ($^{111}$In-DTPA-D-Phe$^{1}$)-octreotide. Ann NY Acad Sci 1994;773:496–506.
66. Makowka L, Tzakis AG, Mazzaferro V, Teperman L, Demetris AJ, et al. Transplantation of the liver for metastatic endocrine tumors of the intestine and pancreas. Surg Gynecol Obstet 1989;168: 107–111.

# 80

# *The VIPoma Syndrome*

Seth A. Spector, Afaf G. E. Absood, and Dana K. Andersen

The VIPoma syndrome is a gastroenteropancreatic neuroendocrine neoplastic syndrome characterized by watery diarrhea, hypokalemia, and achlorhydria, and was first described in 1958 by Verner and Morrison (1). In 1955, Zollinger and Ellison described an association between islet cell tumors of the pancreas with peptic ulceration. Two years later, Priest and Alexander described the association of diarrhea and a non–beta islet cell tumor as a variant on the Zollinger-Ellison syndrome (2). However, the prominence of hypokalemia and the absence of gastric hypersecretion allowed Verner and Morrison to identify the entity as a separate syndrome in two initial patients studied at Duke University Hospital. Many synonyms were suggested for the syndrome, including "pancreatic cholera" by Matsumoto and colleagues. Marks and associates used the acronym WDHA for watery diarrhea, hypokalemia, and achlorhydria (3). S. I. Said made the definitive association between vasoactive intestinal polypeptide (VIP) and the watery diarrhea syndrome (4).

## VASOACTIVE INTESTINAL POLYPEPTIDE

Vasoactive intestinal polypeptide (VIP) was first discovered in 1970 by Said and Mutt, who isolated the peptide in pure form from the porcine intestine in 1972 (5). It was synthesized and its amino acid sequence was elucidated by the same group in 1973–74 (6, 7).

VIP is a 28-amino-acid polypeptide with a molecular mass of 3326 daltons. Its amino acid sequence demonstrates similarities to secretin, glucagon, peptide histadine isoleucine (PHI), peptide histadine methionine (PHM-27), growth hormone releasing factor (GRF), gastric inhibitory polypeptide (GIP), pituitary adenylate cyclase activating polypeptide (PACAP), helodermin, and helospectin.

VIP is a C-terminal carboxyamidated peptide, cleaved from a large precursor molecule that also generates PHI and PHM and was first thought to be a gastrointestinal hormone. The demonstration of VIP in brain as well as central and peripheral neurons established its identity as a neuropeptide, neurotransmitter, and/or neuromodulator. VIP is a noncholinergic, nonadrenergic transmitter that causes vascular and nonvascular smooth muscle relaxation (8–11). Additional targets of VIP include epithelial cells, secretory acini and ducts, T lymphocytes, myocardium, osteoclasts, and certain neurons and endocrine cells (10). VIP is involved in the regulation of gut function, regional blood flow, cardiovascular dynamics, smooth muscle tone, and the secretion of water, anions, electrolytes, and macromolecules. VIP containing neurons innervate epithelial cells, exocrine glands, smooth muscle, and other neurons. It stimulates pancreatic, intestinal, and gallbladder water and electrolyte secretion as well as pancreatic enzyme secretion and colonic potassium secretion. VIP inhibits absorption of water and electrolytes (sodium, chloride, bicarbonate, and potassium) in the small intestine and colon and also inhibits acid and pepsin secretion in the stomach (Table 80.1, Fig. 80.1).

VIP and related peptides also represent a new class of antiinflammatory agents that elevate plasma cyclic-AMP levels in vivo (12). It inhibits basal and histamine-stimulated proliferation of smooth muscle cells in the human tracheobronchial tree and small cell lung cancer growth in vivo and in vitro (9). VIP stimulates bone resorption and has metabolic effects on liver and adipose tissue (13). It interacts with specific receptors located on the surface of intestinal epithelium (14, 15), colonic epithelium (16), gastric epithelium (17), exocrine pancreas (18), and liver (19). In addition, autoradiographic studies visualize VIP binding sites in almost all layers of the gastrointestinal tract (i.e., mucosa, muscularis mucosa, myenteric plexus and lymph nodes (20)).

VIP receptors are glycoproteins. Activation of VIP receptors is linked to stimulation of adenylate cyclase through stimulatory guanyl (Gs) proteins (21–23). In the digestive tract, VIP receptors have been isolated in an active form from rat liver (24–26), porcine liver (27), rat intestine (23), and human colonic adenocarcinoma cells (21). DNA encoding a VIP receptor protein has been cloned from rat lung.

In the rat small intestine, VIP receptors emerge early during differentiation of epithelial cells from stem cells in the crypt-villus axis (28–29). The epithelial VIP receptor in the intestine is expressed in different phenotypes such as enterocytes (28) and mucus-secreting goblet cells (30). This is consistent with a dual role of VIP in controlling water and electrolyte secretion and mucus output, as evidenced by differentiated clonal cell lines with different phenotypes (28, 30–31). The expression of VIP receptors also extends to cancer cells in the human colon and pancreas (14, 32–34). A study of human colonic adenocarcinoma cells in culture suggests that the expression of VIP receptors may depend on the differentiation of cancer cells (33). VIP may control stimulation of glycogenolysis in colonic cancer cells, which is not shown by normal human adult epithelial cells (35–36).

## VIP AND INTESTINAL SECRETION

VIP inhibits histamine-mediated gastric acid secretion, stimulates intestinal motility, and stimulates intestinal, pancreatic, and biliary secretions. Makhlouf and Said first reported that VIP induced intestinal secretion in dogs, resulting in a dose-dependent increase in fluid secretion when VIP was given intravenously (37). Barbezat reported similar observations in 1973, and numerous other investigators expanded these observations in both in vivo and in vitro models in different animal species (38). The VIPoma syndrome can be mimicked in healthy subjects by prolonged (10-hour) VIP infusion (400 pmol/kg/hr);

**TABLE 80.1. Actions of Vasoactive Intestinal Polypeptide**

| | |
|---|---|
| Cardiovascular system | Vasodilation of peripheral, splanchnic, coronary, extracranial, and cerebral vessels; hypotension; moderate inotropic effect |
| Respiratory system | Bronchodilation; augmented ventilation; pulmonary vasodilation; stimulation of bronchial secretion |
| Digestive systems | |
| Esophagus | Relaxation of lower esophageal sphincter |
| Stomach | Relaxation of fundic smooth muscle; suppression of acid secretion |
| Pancreas, liver | Stimulation of water and bicarbonate secretion (secretin-like action); increased bile flow |
| Gallbladder | Relaxation of isolated smooth muscle; inhibition of contractile effect of CCK |
| Small and large intestine | Inhibition of absorption; stimulation of water and chloride secretion; relaxation of colonic smooth muscle |
| Endocrine function | |
| Pancreas | Release of insulin, glucagon, or somatostatin (depending on experimental conditions) |
| Pituitary-hypothalamus | Stimulation of release of prolactin, growth hormone, and luteinizing hormone; suppression of somatostatin release |
| Adrenal | Adrenocorticotropic hormone–like action (stimulation of steroidogenesis) |
| Kidney | Stimulation of renin release by juxtaglomerular cells |
| Central nervous system | Excitation of cerebral cortical and spinal cord neurons; hyperthermia; stimulation of glycogenolysis and of glucose utilization; hypnogenic and antidipsogenic effects |
| Immune system | Inhibition of mitogen-induced transformation of T lymphocytes; stimulation of immunoglobulin synthesis; inhibition of mast cell histamine release; inhibition of platelet aggregation and secretion |

Adapted from Roczen R, Andersen DK. Gastrointestinal hormones in disease. Probl Gen Surg 1994;11(1):36.

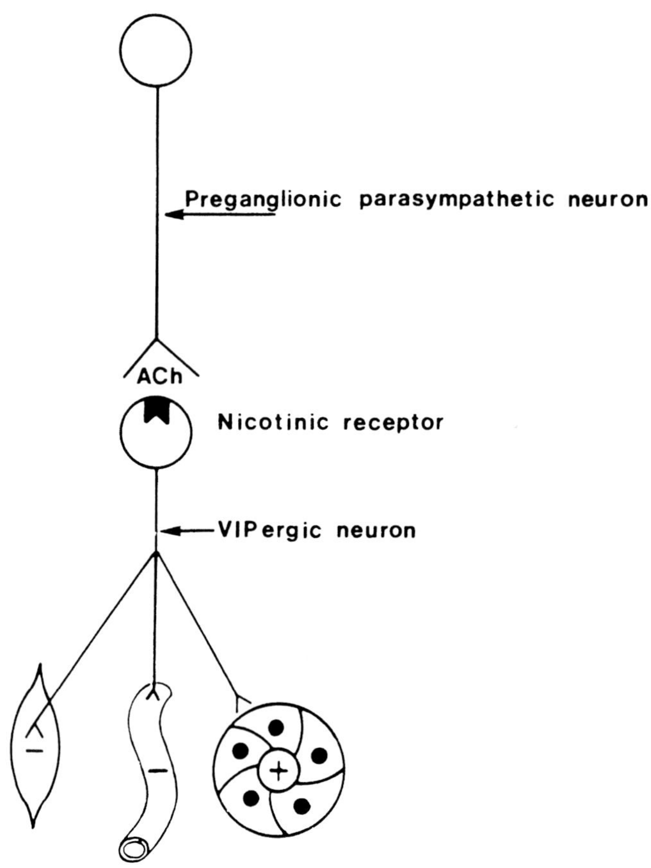


**FIG. 80.1.** Schematic drawing illustrating a working hypothesis on the VIPergic innervation of the digestive tract. Intrinsic *VIPergic neurons* causing relaxation of smooth muscle, vasodilation, and pancreatic bicarbonate secretion are coupled to *preganglionic cholinergic neurons* originating in the central nervous system. The intrinsic VIPergic neurons are also involved in local reflexes. (Adapted from Fahrenkrug J. Physiologic role of VIP in digestion. In: Bloom SR, Polak JM, eds. Gut hormones. 2nd ed. Edinburgh: Churchill Livingstone, 1981:385.)

watery diarrhea (2.4 L/10 hr) and metabolic acidosis develop in all subjects (39–40). Krejs et al. demonstrated active anion secretion in the small intestine in response to VIP (41). Motor and anion secretion in perfused jejunal loops was associated with an increase in the transmucosal potential difference. Chloride and bicarbonate were secreted against an electrochemical gradient, and the secretory effects of VIP were reversed by discontinuation of the infusion (41). When VIP was infused at 500 pmol/kg/hr, a decrease in net absorptive flux in water and electrolytes (sodium, chloride, potassium, and bicarbonate) was noted (Fig. 80.2). In vitro experiments suggest that cyclic-AMP is the second messenger mediating the secretory process induced by VIP (42–43).

## ETIOLOGY OF VIPomas

Since the description of this syndrome in 1958 by Verner and Morrison, the pathophysiology of the disease has been characterized through a variety of clinical and experimental observations. Although calcitonin and prostaglandin $E_2$ ($PGE_2$) have been implicated as tumor products in some patients, the vast majority have an excess of VIP. VIP is produced and released by tumors that arise from the pancreatic islets or from tissue of neural crest origin, such as a neuroblastoma, ganglioneuroma, or ganglioneuroblastoma. Under normal conditions, the low ambient plasma concentrations of VIP probably represent neuronal outflow. Markedly elevated plasma levels of VIP in the VIPoma syndrome lead to intestinal secretion with severe secretory diarrhea, which results in hypovolemia, hypokalemia, and acidosis. VIPoma watery diarrhea is distinguished from diarrhea secondary to a gastrinoma by the presence of low gastric acid secretion. The mechanism of diarrhea is different in the two syndromes, since prevention of acid hypersecretion in gastrinoma patients abolishes the diarrhea (44–45).

Pancreatic VIP-producing tumors associated with the WDHA syndrome have been studied histologically, ultrastructurally, and immunocytochemically. All the tumors contain varying numbers of cells arranged in pseudoglandular structures. The cells show a polar organization, with an apical tuft of microvilli and basal VIP-containing synaptic vesicle-like granules (Fig. 80.3). Based on *(a)* the morphology of the VIPoma cells, which appear to be receptor-associated secretory cells; *(b)* their ability to synthesize and release a peptide that in normal conditions is expressed exclusively by neurons; and *(c)* the

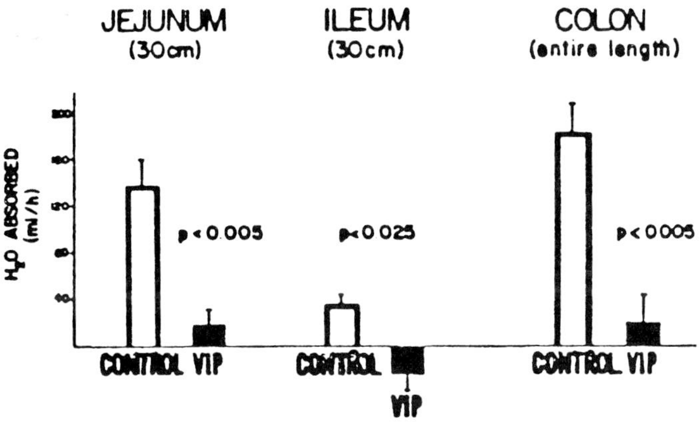


**FIG. 80.2.** Net water movement in the jejunum ($n$ = 6), ileum ($n$ = 10), and colon ($n$ = 8) during control period and VIP infusion. VIP abolished water absorption in all three areas tested. (Adapted from Krejs GJ. Effect of vasoactive intestinal peptide in man. In: Said SI, Mutt V. eds. Vasoactive intestinal peptide and related peptides. Ann NY Acad Sci 1988;527:503.)

absence of VIP-producing endocrine cells in normal pancreas and gastrointestinal mucosa, a hypothesis has been proposed that pancreatic VIPomas are paraneuronal neoplasms, which possibly originate from neuroectodermal elements (46).

## INCIDENCE AND LOCATION

The exact incidence of VIPoma is unknown but is extrapolated to be approximately 1 per 10 million persons. Currently, there are only 201 cases reported in the literature. They occur more frequently in women (65%), and the mean age of patients is 47 years. The tumors have a bimodal distribution that is related to histologic type. In a study of 62 patients, 52 had pancreatic VIPomas, and 10 had extrapancreatic ganglioneuromas. The extrapancreatic sites (adrenal, mediastinal, retroperitoneal) occur predominantly in the pediatric population and demonstrate a less aggressive course, with only a 10% rate of metastasis. Pancreatic VIPomas generally occur singly and average 3 cm or more in diameter at diagnosis. Approximately 75% of tumors are localized to the body and tail of the pancreas, and 40% are malignant. Because of the difficulty in their diagnosis, 30% of these tumors are already metastatic at the time of diagnosis. Up to 5% of VIPoma patients also have the multiple endocrine neoplasia (MEN-I) syndrome (47).

## CLINICAL FEATURES OF VIPoma SYNDROME

Patients present clinically in three typical ways: *(a)* with complaints of voluminous diarrhea; *(b)* with diarrhea, hypokalemic acidosis, and their sequelae; or *(c)* with an abdominal mass. The diarrhea is persistent despite fasting, tends to increase in amount over time, and parallels the increase in tumor burden. This unremitting secretory diarrhea leads to electrolyte disturbances and dehydration that can be life threatening.

The VIPoma syndrome is classically identified by more than 10 episodes of diarrhea per day, with only 30% of patients having less than 3 L of stool per day (39, 48–49). The diarrhea is secretory, and hypermotility does not play a role. The diarrhea is rich in bicarbonate and potassium, the loss of which results in hypokalemia and severe hyperchloremic metabolic acidosis. Potassium is lost in the stool because of a VIP-promoted, cyclic-AMP-mediated secretion of potassium into the intestinal lumen by colonic epithelium. The potassium loss can be in the range of 300 meq/day. Secondary hyperaldosteronism usually accompanies the severe dehydration and adds to the potassium loss. Chloride is reabsorbed in the distal gastrointestinal tract in exchange for bicarbonate, leading to chloride retention and excretion of bicarbonate in the stool. Complete achlorhydria is rare, but hypochlorhydria occurs in 70% of VIPoma patients because of the weak inhibitory effect of VIP on gastric secretion (45). Biopsy of the gastric mucosa reveals normal parietal cell morphology. VIPomas commonly secrete other peptides that may also inhibit gastric acid secretion (50–51).

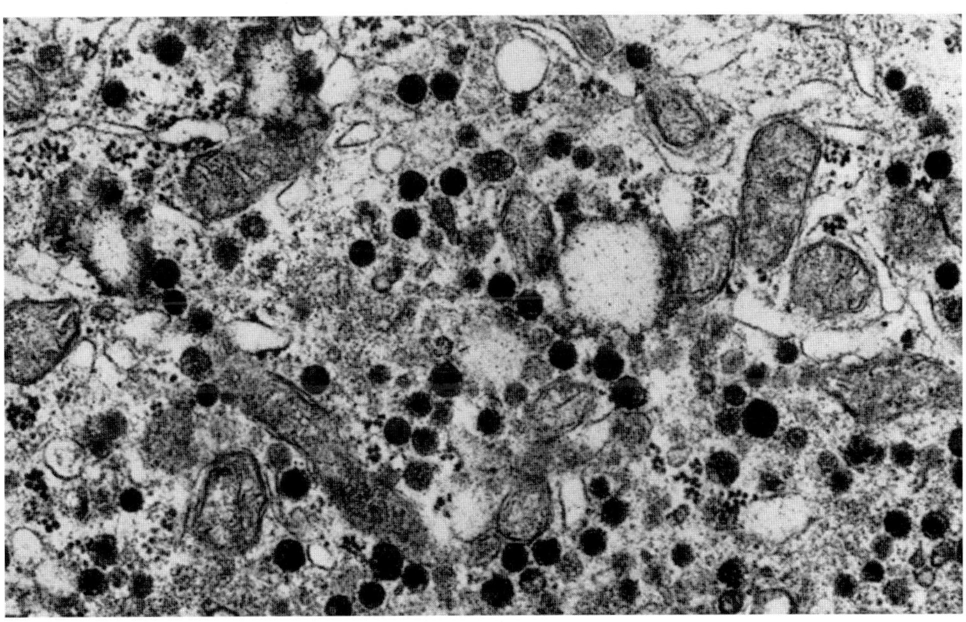

**FIG. 80.3.** Pancreatic diarrheogenic tumor with fairly numerous VIP- and no PP-immunoreactive cells. Note round, thin-haloed secretory granules and a few small clear vesicles. Magnification ×28,000. (Adapted from Solcia E, Capella C, Riva C, Rindi G, Polak JM. The morphology and neuroendocrine profile of pancreatic epithelial VIPomas and extrapancreatic, VIP-producing neurogenic tumors. In: Said SI, Mutt V. eds. Vasoactive intestinal peptide and related peptides. Ann NY Acad Sci 1988;527:512.)

The vasodilatory effects of VIP are probably responsible for the flushing or a rash seen in 20% of patients. The severity is generally dose dependent. In addition, some patients may have episodes of hypotension from severe vasodilation, which may rebound into hypertension once the tumor is removed (52). Hypercalcemia is seen in 50% of patients and is generally due to the osteolytic enhancing effect of VIP and the common coexistence of parathyroid hyperplasia. Parathyroidectomy has been unsuccessful in lowering the calcium level in these circumstances, but VIPoma resection has been universally curative. Glucose intolerance often coexists and can be explained by enhanced hepatic glycogenolysis induced by VIP, probably because of its structural similarity with pancreatic glucagon. Tetany may be seen in patients with pancreatic cholera syndrome and is thought to be due to hypomagnesemia. Other symptoms associated with the VIPoma syndrome include a large gallbladder, generalized myopathy, and excessive lacrimation.

VIP is the major mediator in this syndrome, but like most pancreatic neuroendocrine tumors, many peptides are produced in abnormal quantities. These additional products may counteract each other until one or a few dominate the symptoms (3, 48, 53). These other peptides include pancreatic polypeptide (PP), neurotensin, somatostatin, calcitonin, PHM-27, PHI, helodermin, substance P, neuropeptide Y (NPY), chromogranins A and B, and islet amyloid polypeptide (IAPP) (54–55). NPY and somatostatin-like immunoreactivities have been found in ganglioneuromas, ganglioneuroblastomas, and neuroblastoma (56). The WDHA syndrome has been described with a non-VIP-producing adenoma that was found to secrete $PGE_2$ (57). Family history does not usually play a role in this disease except for patients with the MEN syndrome. The most common causes of death in the untreated VIPoma population are dehydration, hypokalemia, renal failure, or complications associated with the MEN-I syndrome.

## PRIMARY HEPATIC VIPoma

Lundstedt et al. described two cases of neuroendocrine tumors of the liver, positive for VIP, without evidence of a primary tumor outside the liver. One patient had a VIPoma syndrome with diarrhea, hypokalemia, and hypercalcemia. All symptoms were reversed after administration of a somatostatin analogue (octreotide) and arterial liver embolization followed by liver resection. The other patient showed no endocrine symptoms (58). Ayub et al. reported a similar patient with a solitary liver mass and an elevated VIP level. Octreotide acetate administration resulted in prompt cessation of symptoms, and arterial embolization therapy resulted in a temporary response with partial tumor necrosis. Surgical resection of the tumor effected a clinical, biochemical, and radiologic cure over a 20-month follow-up period (59). The mechanism for the development of primary hepatic VIPomas remains unknown.

## THE PEDIATRIC VIPoma SYNDROME

Approximately 10% of VIPomas are found outside the pancreas; they have been found in the adrenals, lungs, mediastinum, retroperitoneum, and the ovaries (Figs. 80.4 and 80.5). Most extrapancreatic tumors are found in the pediatric population and are presumed to be of neural crest origin. Many nonpancreatic tumors secrete catecholamines, and over 30 instances have been described in which diarrhea was the presenting symptom. These patients had high serum levels of VIP, whose origin was traced to ganglioneuromas or neuroblastomas (48). The first description of the WDHA syndrome in a child was by Hawfield and Daisley in 1952. They described the association of a neural crest tumor in a child with intractable diarrhea. At that time it was supposed that these tumors secreted catecholamines that were found in the urine and were thought to cause the diarrhea. However, Stickler and Hallenbeck doubted this theory, and it was later shown that elevated urinary catecholamines were found in children without diarrhea. The chronic diarrhea associated with ganglioneuroblastoma occurs in approximately 10% of cases. The complaints of diarrhea cease after removal of the tumor (60). There have been 54 cases of pediatric VIP-secreting tumors reported to date, including 28 ganglioneuroblastomas, 17 benign ganglioneuromas, 2 pancreatic islet cell tumors, and 1 neurofibroma. The overall survival of children with neuroblastoma is generally poor

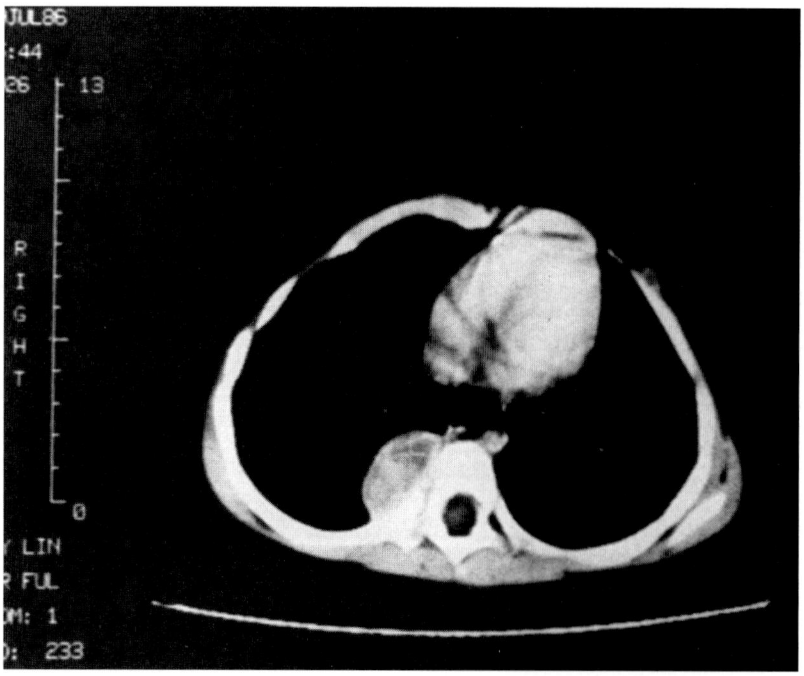


**FIG. 80.4.** Chest computerized tomography of 3-year-old Chinese girl showing the paravertebral soft tissue mass that is secreting VIP. (Adapted from Quak SH, Prabhakaran K, Kwok R, O'Reilly AP. Vasoactive intestinal peptide secreting tumours in children: a case report with literature review. Aust Paediatr J 1988;24:57.)

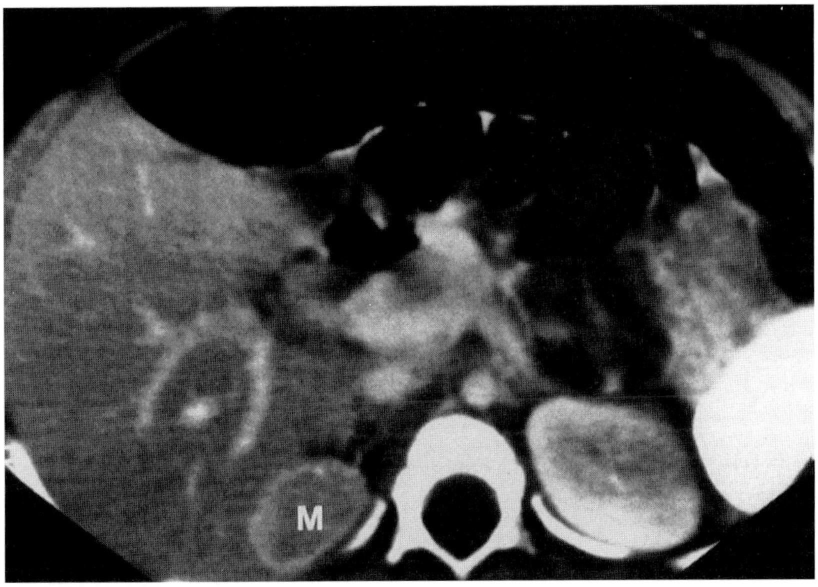


**FIG. 80.5.** A contrast-enhanced CT scan above the upper pole of the right kidney showed a mass *(M)* with an enhancing perimeter. Identified at laparotomy as a ganglioneuroblastoma. (Adapted from Davies RP, Slavotinek JP, Dorney SFA. VIP secreting tumours in infancy: a review of radiological appearances. Pediatr Radiol 1990;20:505.)

(35–40%), whereas the VIP-secreting ganglioneuroblastomas have a survival rate greater than 90% after resection (61).

## DIAGNOSIS AND LOCALIZATION STUDIES

Evidence suggests that the incidence of VIPomas is underreported, and the discovery process may be challenging. The diagnosis requires chemical, hormonal, radiologic, and immunochemical analyses to differentiate this syndrome from the multitude of other secretory diarrheas and to identify the tumor location(s) (Table 80.2).

### Chemical and Biochemical Analysis

The diarrhea must be first evaluated for a secretory nature. This can be confirmed with a trial of fasting for 48–72 hours, which will have no major effect on the diarrhea due to VIPomas. Then, the fecal content of potassium and sodium is determined. The sum of twice the sodium plus the potassium should equal isotonicity in a secretory diarrhea. Additional ingested osmotic agents, such as sorbitol, will result in a diarrheal stool that is low in sodium and potassium. Third, all infectious causes of diarrhea must be excluded.

VIPoma diarrhea usually exceeds 3 L/day, and if less than 750 mL, the diagnosis of VIPoma can be excluded. The stool should be analyzed for mucus, white cells, ova and parasites, fat, and phenolphthalein. A stool pH of 8.0 is also diagnostic, as a result of the bicarbonate loss induced by VIP. Once secretory diarrhea is confirmed and stool examination is negative, serum levels of gastrin, VIP, serotonin, histamine, $PGE_2$, PP, CGA, and urinary 5-HIAA are determined. VIPomas have an increased fasting VIP level, exceeding 190 pg/mL, with a mean 956 (3). An elevated serum VIP concentration with normal levels of gastrin, serotonin, and 5-HIAA strongly suggests a pancreatic VIPoma.

### Radiologic Analysis for Tumor Localization

Once a diagnosis of VIPoma is confirmed, the tumor must be localized. Transabdominal ultrasound is an inexpensive and noninvasive means of evaluating the abdomen for masses but is relatively insensitive for small tumors. Endoscopic ultrasound is helpful in localizing pancreatic tumors and identifying regional adenopathy (62–64) (Fig. 80.6). This method appears to offer the most accurate nonoperative visualization of the pancreas and routinely identifies 2- to 3-mm lesions. Computerized tomographic (CT) scanning is also used to diagnose and localize these neuroendocrine tumors and determine the sites of metastases. Tumors less than 1 cm are difficult to detect by CT scan. The technique visualizes 30% of tumors in the 1- to 3-cm range, however, and 100% of the tumors larger than 3 cm. Magnetic resonance imaging (MRI) and CT scanning are comparable in their applications and sensitivities, although MRI is superior for the detection of metastatic disease. Aspestrand et al. and Grama et al. showed that combinations of angiography and CT are successful in preoperative localization of both primary tumors and metastases (65–66). In 1994, Soyer et al. showed that administration of gadolinium-chelate (gadolinium tetra-azacyclodo-decanetetraacidic acid, Gd-DOATA) enhances the sensitivity of MRI. Twelve patients with pathologically proven metastasis from pancreatic neuroendocrine tumors underwent spin-echo (SE) and dynamic-recalled-echo (DRE) MRI before and after intravenous administration of gadolinium chelate. The DRE images showed marked enhancement of the metastatic deposits (67). Hypervascular tumors such as islet cell carcinoma are easily detected with this technique. Selective venous sampling may also be used to locate a tumor and is helpful when other imaging methods fail to reveal the tumor. VIP levels are measured in the portal, splenic, and mesenteric veins and the vein

**TABLE 80.2. Differential Diagnosis of Secretory Diarrhea**

| |
|---|
| Verner-Morrison syndrome |
| Pseudo-Verner-Morrison syndrome |
| Zollinger-Ellison syndrome |
| Carcinoid syndrome |
| Villous adenoma |
| Medullary carcinoma of the thyroid |
| Celiac disease |
| Infectious or parasitic disease |
| Inflammatory bowel disease |
| Collagen vascular disease |
| Intestinal lymphoma |
| Laxative abuse |

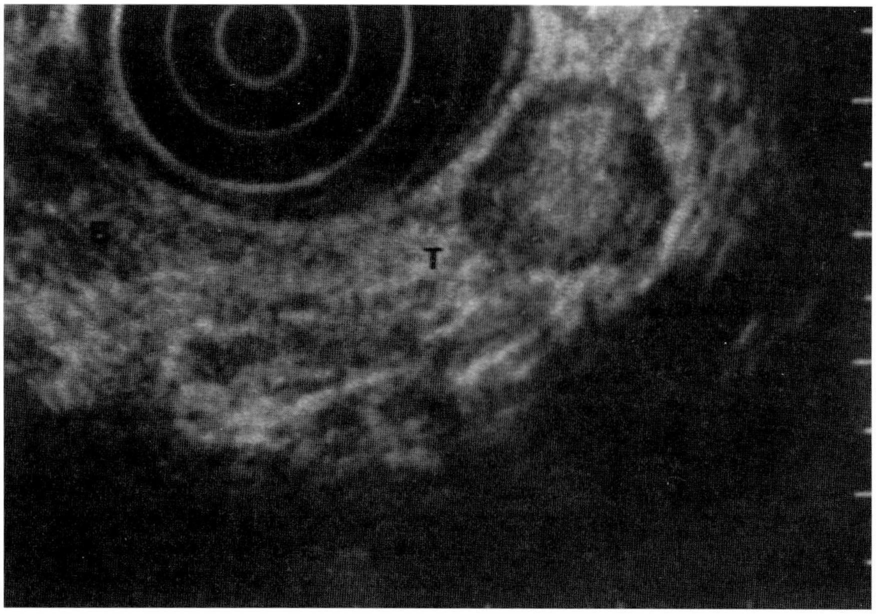


**FIG. 80.6.** Endoscopic ultrasonography of the tumor shows a central echo-rich area but a perimeter that is hypoechoic compared with the rest of the pancreas. *B*, pancreatic body; *T*, pancreatic tail. (Adapted from Rosch T, Lightdale CJ. Localization of pancreatic endocrine tumors by endoscopic ultrasound. N Engl J Med 1992;326(26):1724.)

with the highest level usually drains the area occupied by the tumor.

Radioiodine-labeled octreotide is effective in in vivo imaging of neuroendocrine tumors in the abdomen and is valuable for localizing tumors and metastases preoperatively. Intraoperative localization with the aid of a gamma counter has also been reported (68). $^{111}$In-pentetreotide is a somatostatin analogue that has been used successfully as an agonist for scintigraphic imaging of VIPomas and other gastroenteropancreatic tumors (69–71). The technique is accurate in over 90% of metastatic lesions but is less sensitive for primary pancreatic lesions. Further studies are needed to determine whether this technique will reliably predict treatment responses with long-acting somatostatin analogues (69).

Technetium-99m sestamibi (TC-99m MIBI) imaging was used to visualize a pancreatic VIPoma and parathyroid adenoma in a patient with MEN-I (72). In 1994, Bernay and Sahin demonstrated intestinal uptake of TC-99m methylene diphosphonate in a patient with VIPoma syndrome (73).

In 1994, Virgolini et al. demonstrated the use of $^{123}$I-labeled VIP for localization of gastrointestinal tumors. VIP receptor imaging may have an advantage over octreotide scans for localization of endocrine tumors and intestinal adenocarcinomas because there is less interference due to uptake by the urinary tract. No clinical side effects were noted except for a mild transient drop in blood pressure (Fig. 80.7) (74).

This tumor, as well as other neuroendocrine tumors, is ultimately localized intraoperatively by direct palpation. An aid to this technique is intraoperitive ultrasound (IOUS). The tumor appears as a sonolucent mass with discrete echogenic borders visualized in both the sagittal and transverse planes. IOUS may also help identify adjacent vital structures (75) and deep hepatic metastases and can greatly facilitate the operative management of the patient.

## Immunocytochemistry of Endocrine Tumor Markers

Peptide radioimmunoassay (RIA) has become an important clinical and research tool in understanding the role of peptides in the pathophysiology of gastrointestinal endocrine tumor syndromes. RIA has enhanced our awareness that cooccuring peptide secretion and interaction may modify the clinical expression of these tumors. It has also helped in the development of the rational use of prototype peptides such as VIP, somatostatin (SST), and its long-acting SST analogue, octreotide (76).

Pancreatic VIPomas can produce multiple peptides. The VIPoma syndrome is characterized by elevated levels of VIP and PP (4, 77–80). In vitro, human cultured VIPoma cells release VIP and PP, as well as calcitonin. Patients with VIPoma may have elevated levels of calcitonin, PHI, helodermin, PHM-27, IAPP, chromogranin A (CGA) (201–301), and chromogranin B fragment (314–365) (50, 55, 81–89). Of these additional secretory products, CGA appears to be the most sensitive and useful as a screening tool for an islet cell tumor.

## Immunohistochemistry

VIP-producing tumors overproduce multiple hormones, as shown biochemically and immunohistochemically (50). They are divided histologically into two groups: pancreatic endocrine tumors and neurogenic tumors, including ganglioneuroblastoma, ganglioneuroma, and pheochromocytoma. VIP and PHM-27 have been codetected in the tumors of both groups (Fig. 80.8). Coexpression of VIP and neurotensin was also seen immunohistochemically within some individual VIPoma tumor cells. Immunohistochemical stains of the VIPoma were positive for neuron-specific enolase (NSE), CGA, VIP, neurotensin, and PP (90). Ectopic tumors produce polypeptides other than those normally found in endocrine cells of the adult pancreas. In neurogenic VIPomas, somatostatin, neuropeptide Y (NPY), calcitonin, and substance P (SP) have been reported (91).

In 1993, Kimura et al. demonstrated immunohistochemically that ganglionic tumors were strongly immunoreactive for metenkephalin, SS, NPY, SP, and corticotropin-releasing hormone (CRH). The immunoreactivity was restricted to the cytoplasm of the ganglionic cells and their processes (neurites). A large portion of a VIP-producing ganglioneuroblastoma was composed of ganglionic tumor cells with abundant cytoplasm, large nuclei, and obvious nucleoli; a small portion had neuroblasts and abundant neurites (50).

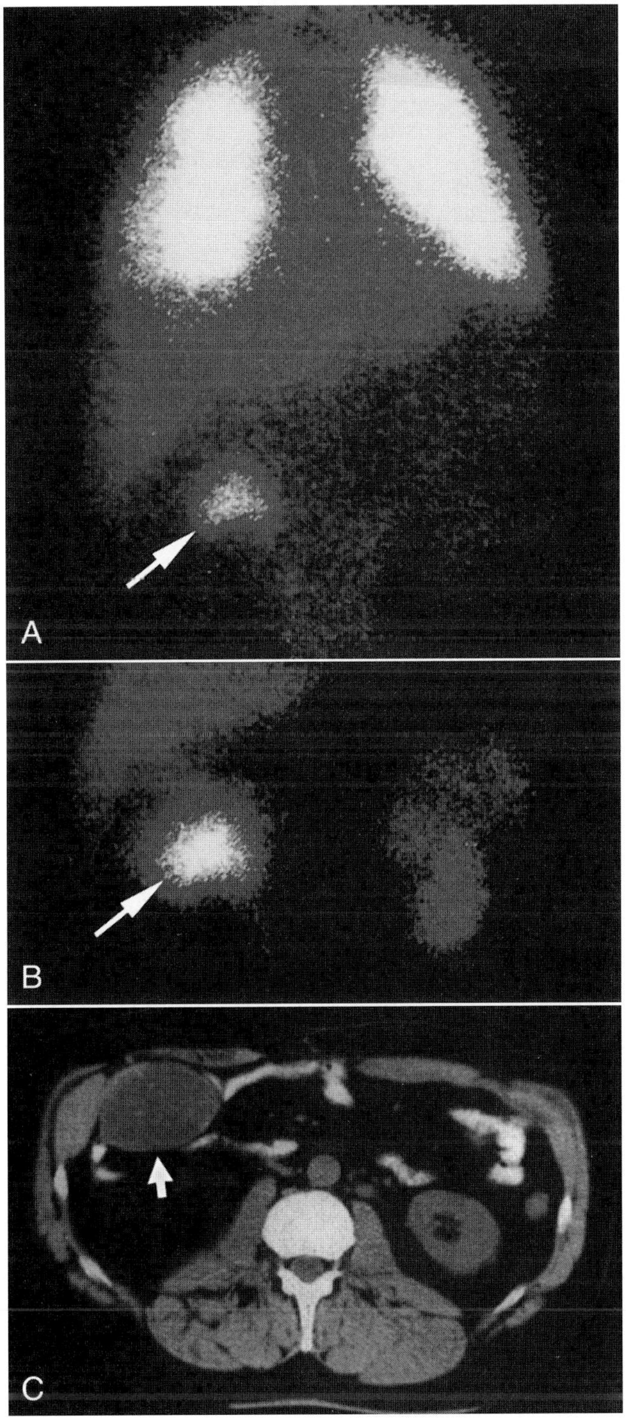


**FIG. 80.7.** Comparison between $^{123}$I-labeled VIP and $^{111}$In-labeled DTPA-D-Phe-octreotide scanning in a man with primary colonic adenocarcinoma. **A.** Anterior image of the tumor 2 hours after the injection of radiolabeled VIP. **B.** Anterior image 6 hours after the injection of $^{111}$In-labeled DTPA-D-Phe-octreotide in the same patient. The interval between the two scans was 3 weeks. **C.** CT scan. In all three panels, the tumor mass is indicated by an *arrow*. (Adapted from Virgolini I, Raderer M, Kunaran A, Angelberger P, Banyai S, et al. Vasoactive intestinal peptide-receptor imaging for the localization of intestinal adenocarcinomas and endocrine tumors. N Engl J Med 1994;27;331(17):1119.) See color insert.

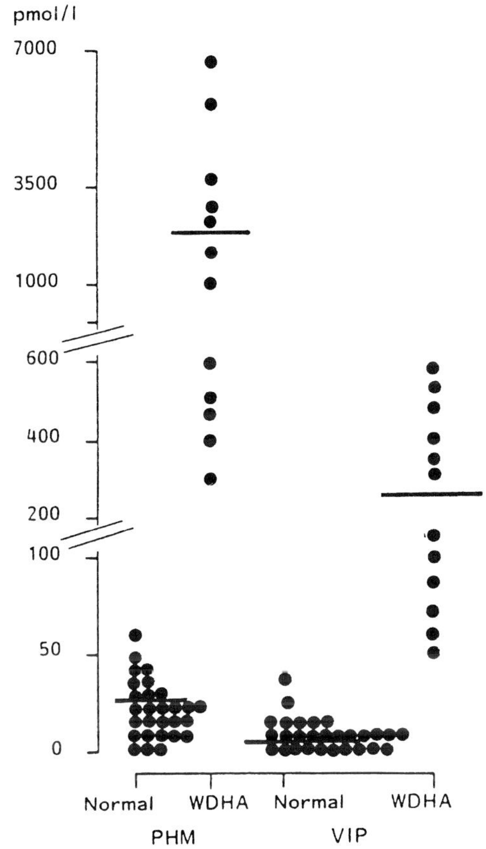


**FIG. 80.8.** Comparison of VIP and PHM plasma levels in normal persons and patients with WDHA. *Horizontal line* represents the median of each group. (Adapted from Bloom SR, Yiangou Y, Polak JM. Vasoactive intestinal peptide secreting tumors: pathophysiological and clinical correlations. In: Said SI, Mutt V. eds. Vasoactive intestinal peptide and related peptides. Ann NY Acad Sci 1988;527:521.)

In 1994, Yasunami et al. investigated the release of VIP and PP from the tumor cells of a VIPoma. They showed that VIPoma cells can be isolated and maintained in vitro and that these cells release VIP and PP simultaneously after stimulation with both carbachol and phorbol-myristate acetate (PMA), a protein kinase activator. The carbachol stimulation was abolished by atropine, which suggests the presence of muscarinic receptors on the cells that mediate VIP and PP release. They also showed that the activation of protein kinase C may play an important role in the stimulus-secretion coupling of these tumor cells. Octreotide directly inhibited the release of VIP and PP after stimulation with carbachol and PMA (81).

Neurotensin, a 13-amino-acid peptide normally present in the brain and gut mucosa, has been found in a small number of pancreatic and nonpancreatic endocrine tumors. Blackburn evaluated 163 patients with a variety of islet cell tumors and found elevated neurotensin levels exclusively in the 56 patients with VIPoma (79). The combined secretion of VIP, neurotensin, calcitonin, and PP has been shown by multiple authors (84, 92–93).

## Provocative Tests

The usefulness of provocative tests in the diagnosis and management of patients with a variety of endocrine neoplasms is well established. Intravenous administration of certain agents may selectively stimulate hormone release from a tumor. In 1985,

Hacki et al. reported dramatic increases in plasma neurotensin levels in response to secretin (75 u/kg) or calcium (15 mg/kg/3 hr) in patients with a pancreatic neuroendocrine tumor (94). In patients with VIPoma, there was a small increase in neurotensin levels in response to secretin and minimal changes after calcium administration (90). Pentagastrin was used intravenously (0.5 μg/kg/5 sec) as a provocative agent in a patient with the VIPoma syndrome. Pentagastrin stimulates the release of VIP and neurotensin over basal levels by 81% and 87%, respectively. After surgery, plasma levels of VIP, neurotensin, and PP were undectectable before and after pentagastrin administration. Provocative agents can be given by selective arterial injection, after which, selective venous sampling is used to locate the tumor. Provocative tests may also aid in postoperative surveillance for tumor recurrence (90).

## TREATMENT

### Preoperative Stabilization

Parallel to the diagnostic process, the primary therapeutic concern should be the stabilization of the patient, with correction of electrolytes, acidosis, and dehydration. The fluid and electrolyte imbalance should be reversed slowly because of its chronic nature. In addition, rapid correction of hypovolemia or hypokalemia can induce other problems with the cardiovascular and renal systems. Because of the combination of hypokalemia and hyperchloremic acidosis, potassium replacement should be in the form of salts other than chloride. In addition, strict intake and output should be recorded. Octreotide acetate (100 μg s.c., t.i.d.) is useful in promptly inhibiting VIP secretion from the tumor and stopping the diarrhea (95) (Fig. 80.9).

### Surgical Therapy

All patients with VIPoma or suspected VIPoma should be evaluated by laparotomy unless metastatic disease is widespread and proven. The availability of octreotide obviates the urgent need for surgery and allows careful localization of the tumor and stabilization of the patient. However, a number of these tumors elude localization efforts and require surgical exploration for definitive recognition and treatment. The retroperitoneum, both adrenal glands, and the pancreas should be meticulously evaluated. The procedure of choice depends on the tumor location: pancreatic head tumors require enucleation or pancreaticoduodenectomy, depending on the size and position of the lesions; body and tail tumors are best managed by distal pancreatectomy. Complete resection of these tumors delivers full symptomatic relief. However, some patients with WDHA have been described in whom no obvious tumor could be identified. Islet cell hyperplasia has been diagnosed by permanent histologic sections in some specimens when no elevated peptide levels have been documented. The entity has been named the pseudo-Verner-Morrison syndrome. For an occult tumor, some authors advocate subtotal pancreatectomy, resecting the pancreas to the left of the superior mesenteric vessels. This treatment is not universally effective (since only 50% of the pancreas is removed), and further resection may be required to control the symptoms. If all apparent tumor cannot be resected or if there is metastatic disease, surgical debulking remains a useful option. Some 75% of malignant VIPomas are metastatic at exploration. A debulking procedure decreases the tumor burden and is symptomatically helpful. If there is recurrence, repeat debulking may be a viable and therapeutic option (53).

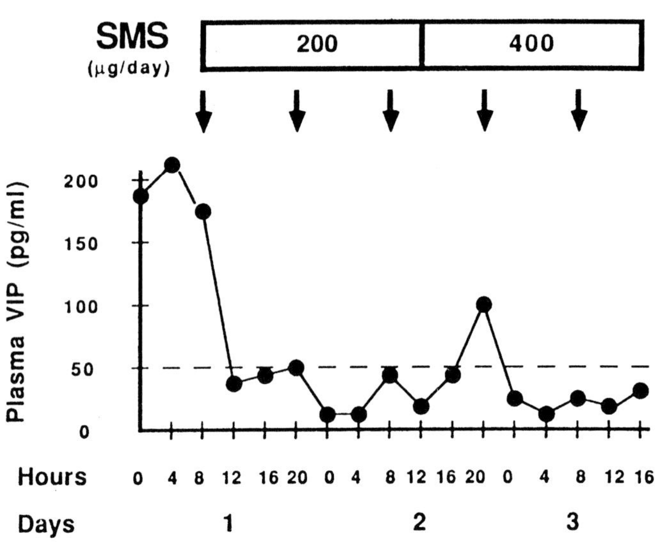


**FIG. 80.9.** Response of VIP levels to treatment with SMS 201-995 in a patient with a metastatic VIPoma. The decline in VIP levels coincides with a disappearance of the diarrhea. (Adapted from Vinik AI, Tsai S, Moattari AR, Cheung P, Eckhauser FE, Cho K. Somatostatin analogue (SMS 201-995) in the management of gastroenteropancreatic tumors and diarrhea syndromes. Symposium on gut endocrinology. Am J Med 1986;81(6B):33.)

### Symptomatic Drug Therapy

The aim of drug therapy is to enhance gastrointestinal absorption or to limit secretion. Corticosteroids, angiotensin, and α-adrenergic agonists promote absorption. On the other hand, indomethacin, opiates, phenothiazines, lithium carbonate, clonidine, metoclopramide, loperamide, trifluoroperazine, adenylate cyclase inhibitors, and calcium channel blockers inhibit secretion into the gastrointestinal tract (48, 51, 96) and may be useful adjuncts or palliative therapies for unresectable or recurrent disease.

### Chemotherapy

There are few well-documented chemotherapeutic agents for the treatment of the VIPoma syndrome. The combination of streptozotocin and 5-fluorouracil (5-FU) was effective in 65% of patients studied in the Eastern Cooperative Oncology Group (97). In 1993, Varkonyi et al. showed that the combination of octreotide and streptozotocin resulted in complete cessation of diarrhea and substantial diminution of tumor mass (98). Once the tumor is maximally debulked, chemotherapy is usually advocated. Chlorozotocin has been compared with streptozotocin and shown to be comparable with diminished nephrotoxic and emetic potentials. Dimethyltriazinoimidazolecarboxaminde (DTIC), human leukocyte interferon, and adriamycin in combination with streptozotocin have been used in small numbers of patients with variable success (51, 96–97, 95, 99). In addition, the combination of human leukocyte interferon and interferon-α, with or without octreotide, is also effective (100–102). Partial responses are seen in 30–60% of patients, although complete responses are rare.

### Peptide Treatment

Somatostatin (or its analogues) is the most promising agent in controlling symptoms and preventing metabolic abnormalities (68). It is capable of inhibiting pathologic secretion in the human intestine secondary to VIP (Fig. 80.10) (89, 103). In 1994, Yasunami et al. demonstrated the direct inhibitory effect of octreotide on VIP and PP release from tumor cells (81). Their observations confirmed that somatostatin and its analogues inhibit mucosal secretion by reducing secretagogue release from endocrine tumors. The natural half-life of somatostatin in the circulation is less than 3 minutes, which makes it unsuitable for

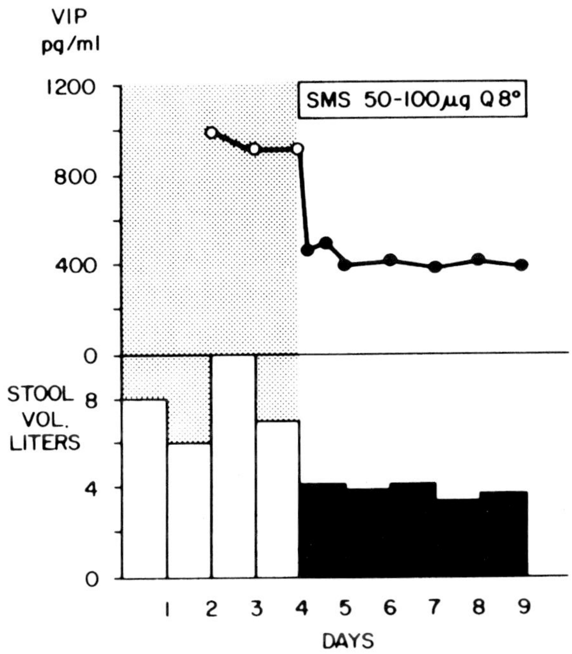


**FIG. 80.10.** Plasma levels of vasoactive intestinal peptide *(VIP)* and stool output before and after treatment with somatostatin analogue *(SMS)* in a patient with VIPoma. (Adapted from Ellison EC, O'Dorisio TM, Benson GD. Modulation of functional gastrointestinal tumors by endogenous and exogenous somatostatin. Am J Surg 1986;151:673.)

outpatient therapy. Octreotide, a long-acting analogue of somatostatin, is a cyclic octapeptide that retains the four amino acids in the biologically active area as well as the cystine bridge of native somatostatin. Subcutaneous injection achieves a peak concentration in 60 minutes with a half life of 70–113 minutes.

The mechanism of action of octreotide and native somatostatin is to interfere with VIP secretion and VIP stimulation of the secretory process at the intestinal epithelial level. In addition, the effects of somatostatin on intestinal motility might slow transit time and thus allow enhanced absorption (104) (Figs. 80.11 and 80.12). VIP also induces intestinal secretion through the cyclic-AMP pathway. Somatostatin may also inhibit the cyclic AMP system and thus antagonize intestinal secretion (105).

Because of the marked interpatient differences in the antidiarrheal effects of octreotide, dose titrations are often necessary. Although all patients have an initial good response, in some the effect is short-lived and requires higher doses. Some patients have recurrence of the diarrhea at higher doses, which may reflect tachyphylaxis. Increasing the dose of octreotide to 1000 μg/24 hours has been reported effective (95). In addition, octreotide has been used effectively for treatment and/or amelioration of metastatic disease (Fig. 80.13).

In 1993, Antonelli et al. demonstrated the effectiveness of octreotide and calcitonin in the VIPoma syndrome and suggested that salmon calcitonin may ameliorate symptomatology and reduce circulating VIP levels in patients with VIPomas (106). In 1994, Marquet et al. showed the effectiveness of sorbin, a 153-amino-acid peptide isolated from porcine intestine, which increases water and ion absorption in the intestine and gallbladder (107). They further showed that a synthetic peptide containing the amidated C-terminus of sorbin had similar activity in increasing duodenal absorption. They compared the effect of two C-terminal derivatives, C20-sorbin and C7-sorbin, with those of metenkephalinamide, NPY, and somatostatin. Sorbin acts as a potent antisecretor and VIP antagonist in rat ileum (107). Another candidate in this class of agents is peptide YY (PYY). In 1992, Okuno et al. demonstrated that PYY enhanced sodium chloride and water absorption in the rat colon in vivo. PYY produced a dose-dependent increase in the net secretion of potassium. In addition, it inhibited the reduction in net absorption of sodium chloride and water evoked by VIP but was without effect on VIP-induced increase in potassium secretion. These findings suggest that PYY enhances sodium chloride and water absorption and is an antagonist to VIP-induced secretion in the colon (108).

Prior to the discovery of somatostatin and octreotide, WDHA patients were treated with glucocorticoids. The initial dose was the equivalent of 60–80 mg of prednisone. These drugs enhance sodium absorption in the small and large intestine and may decrease intestinal secretion by action of the Na/K ATPase (95).

## Immunotherapy

Monoclonal antitumor antibodies have been used for the treatment of various neoplasms, and actual remissions of even metastatic lesions have been reported (109). An efficient proto-

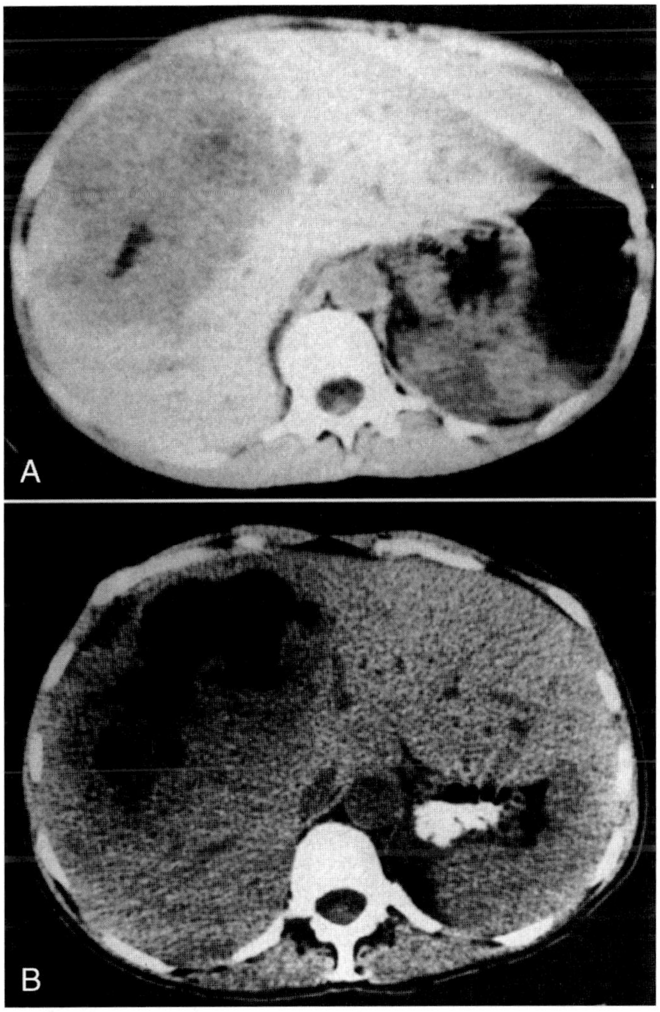


**FIG. 80.11.** VIPoma metastatic to the liver before (**A**) and after (**B**) 6 months of treatment with octreotide. The tumor appears to have undergone infarction. (Adapted from Vinik AI, Tsai S, Moattari AR, Cheung P, Eckhauser FE, Cho K. Somatostatin analogue (SMS 201-995) in the management of gastroenteropancreatic tumors and diarrhea syndromes. Symposium on gut endocrinology. Am J Med 1986;81(6B):32.)

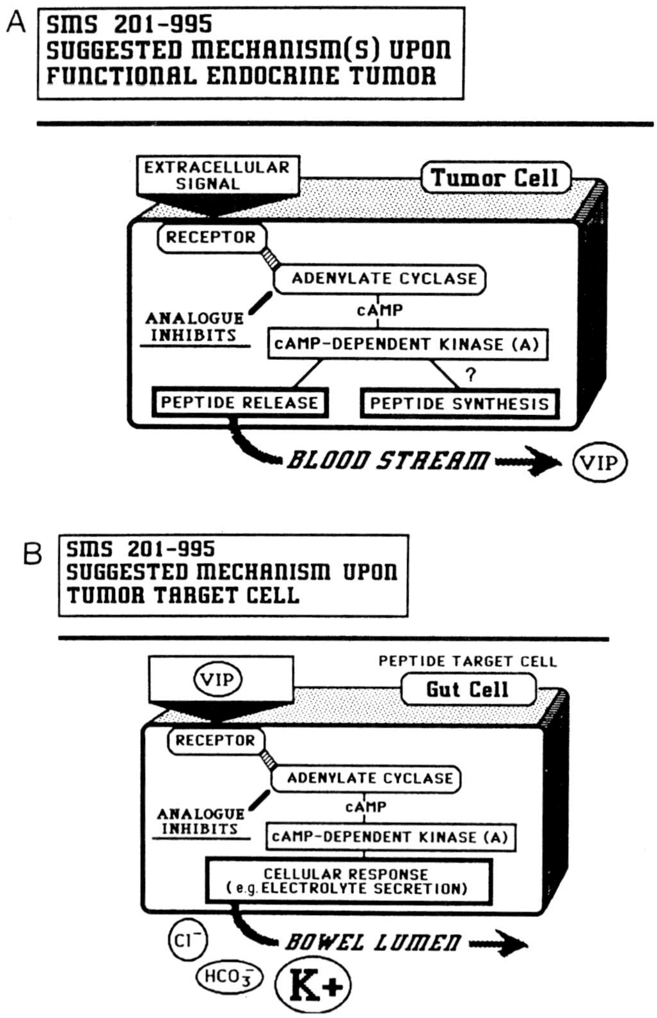


**FIG. 80.12.** *Panel A* demonstrates a hypothetical mechanism whereby the somatostatin analogue SMS 201-995 (and somatostatin) acts on adenylate cyclase to alter the synthesis or release of VIP from a peptide-containing tumor. *Panel B* illustrates a mechanism by which SMS 201-995 may inhibit adenylate cyclase, post–recognition site (VIP receptor), thereby reducing electrolyte secretion by intestinal epithelial cells; inhibition of cAMP stimulation of protein kinase may also occur. (Adapted from O'Dorisio TM, Gaginella TS, Mekhijian HS, Rao B, O'Dorisio MS. Somatostatin and analogues in the treatment of VIPoma. In: Said Si, Mutt V, eds. Vasoactive intestinal peptide and related peptides. Ann NY Acad Sci 1988;527:532.)

col has been established for the generation of monoclonal antibodies recognizing surface structures on endocrine cells (110, 111). In 1994, Juhlin generated murine monoclonal B7 antibody of the IgG2a subtype by immunization with dispersed tumor cells from a pancreatic islet cell carcinoma associated with peritoneal metastases in a therapy-resistant VIPoma syndrome patient. Antibody infusion was accompanied by no apparent adverse reaction (103, 112, 113). Some 100 mg of the antibody was administered into the hepatic artery of a VIPoma patient to obtain high concentrations at the site of the major tumor cell mass. Because murine IgG is rapidly cleared in humans, repeated infusions were administered through an indwelling catheter (112, 114). The treatment with B7 antibody was associated with considerable alteration in diarrhea volume and peripheral hormone excess. These results substantiate that monoclonal antibodies may alleviate symptoms and reduce endocrine tumor mass.

In 1989, Paul described the catalytic hydrolysis in vitro of VIP by IgG immunoglobulin purified from humans (115). The identification of antibodies with high catalytic efficiency that act as site-specific proteases may provide new ways of treating the disease. Iverson and Lerner described an antibody that hydrolyzed a Gly-Phe bond in the presence of a metal cofactor (116). These findings suggest possible future avenues of immunotherapy of the VIPoma syndrome.

### Radiotherapy

In 1992, Tennvall et al. described the modest effectiveness of external radiotherapy of unresectable endocrine pancreatic tumors (117). As is typical of adenocarcinomas, these tumors are relatively radioresistant, and radiotherapy is usually adjunctive rather than primary treatment.

## PROGNOSIS

Most VIPomas (60%) present as benign adenomas, and the survival is very good. Some of these "benign adenomas" may recur, so close surveillance is indicated. VIP levels are an excellent tumor marker for recurrence. Survival of patients with malignancy and/or metastatic disease is disappointing; the average survival is approximately 1 year. The variable response to surgery and therapy underscores the validity of an aggressive approach, and predictions of long-term survival are always estimates at best.

## PSEUDO-VIPoma SYNDROME

According to Krejs, the diagnosis of "pseudo-VIPoma syndrome" may be made in patients with persistent diarrhea for more than 4 weeks, a stool volume above 750 g/24 hr, fecal analysis typical of secretory diarrhea, persistent diarrhea during

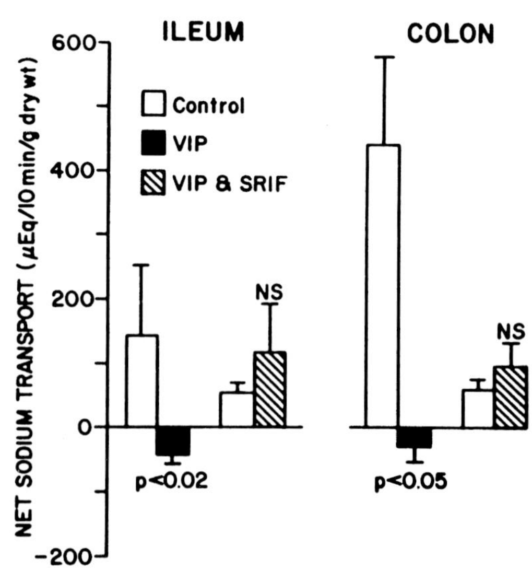


**FIG. 80.13.** Net sodium transport in the rat ileum and colon in response to VIP (14.3 μg/kg/hr i.v.) in the absence and presence of somatostatin (43 μg/kg/hr i.v.). Means ± standard error in 6–8 animals. (Adapted from O'Dorisio TM, Gaginella TS, Mekhijian HS, Rao B, O'Dorisio MS. Somatostatin and analogues in the treatment of VIPoma. In: Said SI, Mutt V. eds. Vasoactive intestinal peptide and related peptides. Ann NY Acad Sci 1988;527:531.)

fasting, no surreptitious laxative or sorbitol ingestion, and no evidence of diseases that are known to cause chronic secretory diarrhea. These patients have normal serum concentrations of VIP, $PGE_2$, and calcitonin (48). The possible etiology of this syndrome has been studied in only a few patients, in whom reduced absorption or increased secretion had been noted (118). By definition, the cause of these abnormalities is unknown. Its severity varies widely, and the prognosis is highly variable. Some patients have severe chronic diarrhea, while others have diarrhea of moderate severity. According to Krejs, some patients benefit from opioid therapy, and one in five benefits from 60–80 mg/day of prednisone. Insertion of a jejunostomy feeding tube for infusion of glucose-containing electrolyte solution may be required in severe cases.

The syndrome of unexplained chronic secretory diarrhea is much more common than the VIPoma syndrome (48). Read et al. suggested the following scheme for the management of patients with pseudo-VIPoma syndrome. First, treatment with nonspecific remedies like opiates should be used for only 6 months. If there is inadequate response to these remedies, abdominal imaging studies or laparotomy should be performed (48). If a tumor is not found at surgery, then "blind" distal pancreatectomy may be considered for those patients whose preoperative plasma concentrations of nonspecific islet cell tumor markers such as pancreastatin were markedly and repeatedly elevated (118). Blind distal pancreatectomy should not be entertained unless careful imaging studies including endoscopic, laparoscopic, and intraoperative ultrasound of the pancreas, liver, and retroperitoneal lymphatics have been unrevealing. The use of somatostatin analogue scintiscans (e.g., Octreoscan) may disclose an extrapancreatic tumor location. This syndrome has been successfully treated with intravenous infusion of native somatostatin and subcutaneous administration of octreotide (119–122). A trial of somatostatin analogue therapy is indicated in virtually all cases.

## REFERENCES


1. Verner JV, Morrison AB. Islet cell tumor and a syndrome of refractory watery diarrhea and hypokalemia. Am J Med 1958;25:374–380.
2. Priest WM, Alexander MK. Islet-cell tumor of the pancreas with peptic ulceration, diarrhea and hypokalemia. Lancet 1957;11: 1145.
3. Mekhjian HS, O'Dorisio TM. VIPoma syndrome. Semin Oncol 1987;14(3):282–291.
4. Said SI. Vasoactive intestinal polypeptide (VIP) as a mediator of the watery diarrhea syndrome. World J Surg 1979;3:559–583.
5. Said SI, Mutt V. Isolation from porcine-intestinal wall of a vasoactive octacosapeptide related to secretin and glucagon. Eur J Biochem 1972;28:199–204.
6. Bodanszky M, Klausent US, Said SI. Biological activities of synthetic peptides corresponding to fragments of the entire sequence of the vasoactive intestinal peptide. Proc Natl Acad Sci USA 1973;70:382–384.
7. Mutt V, Said SI. Structure of the porcine vasoactive intestinal octacosapeptide. The amino-acid sequence. Use of kallikrein in its discrimination. Eur J Biochem 1974;42:581–589.
8. Said SI, Mutt V. Potent peripheral and splanchnic vasodilator peptide from normal gut. Nature 1970b;225:863–864.
9. Said SI. Influence of neuropeptides on airway smooth muscle (Review). Am Rev Respir Dis 1987;136(6 pt 2):S52–S58.
10. Said SI. Vasoactive intestinal peptide (Review). J Endocrinol Invest 1986;9(2):191–200.
11. Absood A, Chen D, Wang Z, Hakanson R. Vascular effects of PACAP: a comparison with VIP. Regul Pept 1992;40:323–329.
12. Absood A, Chen D, Hakanson R. Neuropeptides of the VIP/helodermin/PACAP family elevate plasma cAMP in mice: comparison with a range of other regulatory peptides. Regul Pept 1992;40:311–322.
13. Laburthe M, Karabgi P, Couvineau A, Amiranoff B. Peptide receptors and signal transduction in the digestive tract. Handb Exp Pharmacol 1993;106:133–176.
14. Laburthe M, Rousset M, Boissard C. Vasoactive intestinal peptide (VIP): a potent stimulator of adenosine 3'5' cyclic monophosphate accumulation in gut carcinoma cell lines in culture. Proc Natl Acad Sci USA 1978a;75:2772–2775.
15. Salomon R, Couvineau A, Rouyer-Fessard C. Characterization of a common VIP-PACAP receptor in human small intestinal epithelium. Am J Physiol 1993;264:E294–E300.
16. Broyart JP, Dupont C, Laburthe M, Rosselin G. Characterization of vasoactive intestinal peptide receptors in human colonic epithelial cells. J Clin Endocrinol Metab 1981;52(4):715–721.
17. Gespach C, Cherel Y, Rosselin G. Development of sensitivity to cAMP-inducing hormones in the rat stomach. Am J Physiol 1984;247(3 pt 1):G231–G239.
18. Christophe J, Robberecht P, Cauvin A. Mammalian and lizard helodermin and helodermin-like peptides. New members of the vasoactive intestinal peptide-peptide histidine isoleucine-secretin family. Can Physiol Pharmacol Suppl Gastrointest Hormones 1986;28.
19. Bataille D, Freychet P, Rosselin G. Interaction of glucagon, gut glucagon, vasoactive intestinal polypeptide and secretin with liver and fat cell plasma membranes: binding to specific sites and stimulation of adenylate cyclase. Endocrinology 1974;95: 713–721.
20. Zimmerman RP, Gates TS, Mantyh CR, et al. Vasoactive intestinal polypeptide receptor binding sites in the human gastrointestinal tract: localization by autoradiography. Neuroscience 1989;3. 771–783.
21. El Battari A, Martin JM, Luis J. Solubilization of the active vasoactive intestinal peptide receptor from human colonic adenocarcinoma cells. J Biol Chem 1988;17685–17689.
22. Laburthe M, Couvineau A. Molecular analysis of vasoactive intestinal peptide receptors. A comparison with receptors for VIP-related peptides. Ann NY Acad Sci 1988;527:296–313.
23. Calvo JR, Couvineau A, Guijarro L, Laburthe M. Solubilization and hydrodynamic characterization of guanine nucleotide-sensitive vasoactive intestinal peptide-receptor complexes from rat intestine. Biochemistry 1989;28:1667–1672.
24. Couvineau A, Amiranoff B, Labuthe M. Solubilization of the liver vasoactive intestinal peptide receptor. Hydrodynamic characterization and evidence for an association with a functional GTP regulatory protein. J Biol Chem 1986;261:14482–14489.
25. Couvineau A, Rouyer-Fessar C, Voisin T, Laburthe M. Functional and immunological evidence for stable association of solubilized VIP receptor and Gs protein from rat liver. Eur J Biochem 1990b;187:605–609.
26. Guijarro L, Couvineau A, Calvo JR, Laburthe M. Solubilization of active and stable receptors for vasoactive intestinal peptide from rat liver. Regul Pept 1989;25:37–50.
27. Couvineau A, Voisin T, Guijarro L, Laburthe M. Purification of VIP receptor from porcine liver by a newly designed one-step affinity chromatography. J Biol Chem 1990a:265:13386–13390.
28. Laburthe M, Amiranoff B. Peptide receptors in intestinal epithelium. Sect. 6. In: Makhlouf GM, ed. Handbook of physiology. Bethesda, MD: American Physiology Society, 1989;2:215–243.
29. Voisin T, Rouyer-Fessard C, Laburthe M. Distribution of the common peptide YY neuropeptide Y receptor along rat intestinal vilus-crypt axis. Am J Physiol 1990;258:G753–G759.
30. Laburthe M, Augeron C, Rouyer-Fessard C. Functional VIP receptors in the human mucus-secreting colonic epithelial cell line C1,16E. Am J Physiol 1989;256:G443–G450.
31. Rouyer-Fessard C, Augeron C, Grasset E, Maoret JJ, Laboisse CL, Laburthe M. VIP receptors and control of short circuit current in the human intestinal cell line Cl.19A. Experientia 1989;45(11–12): 1102–1105.
32. Laburthe M, Bataille D, Rousset M. The expression of cell surface receptors for VIP secretin and glucagon in normal and maligant cells of the digestive tract. In: Nicholls P, ed. Membrane proteins. Oxford: Pergamon Press, 1978b:271–290.
33. Laburthe M, Rousset M, Rouyer-Fessard C. Development of vasoactive intestinal peptide-responsive adenylate cyclase during enterocytic differentiation of Caco-2 cells in culture.

Evidence for an increased receptor level. J Biol Chem 1987;262: 10180–10184.
34. Estival A, Mounielou P, Trocheris V. Presence of VIP receptors in a human pancreatic adenocarcinoma cell line, modulation of the cAMP response during cell proliferation. Biochem Biophys Res Commun 1983;111:958–963.
35. Rousset M, Laburthe M, Chevalier G, Boissard C, Rosselin G, Zweibaum A. Vasoactive intestinal peptide (VIP) control of glycogenolysis in the human colon carcinoma cell line HT-29 in culture. FEBS Lett 1981;126(1):38–40.
36. Zweibaum A, Laburthe M, Grasset E, Louvard D. The use of cultured cell lines in studies of intestinal cell differentiation and function. Sect. 6. In: Field M, Frizzel RA, eds. Handbook of physiology. Bethesda, MD: American Physiological Society, 1989–1991;4:223–255.
37. Makhlouf GM, Said SI. The effect of vasoactive intestinal peptide (VIP) on digestive and hormonal function. In: Thompson JC, ed. Gastrointestinal hormones. Austin: University of Texas Press, 1975:599–610.
38. Barbezat GO. Stimulation of intestinal secretion by polypeptide hormones. Scand J Gastroenterol 1973;6:1–21.
39. Kane MG, O'Dorisio TM, Krejs GJ. Production of secretory diarrhea by intravenous infusion of vasoactive intestinal peptide. N Engl J Med 1983;309(24):1482–1485.
40. Krejs GJ. Effect of vasoactive intestinal peptide in man. Ann NY Acad Sci 1988;527:501–507.
41. Krejs GJ, Bakley RM, Reed NW, Forduran JS. Intestinal secretion with choleratoxin in the canine jejunum in vivo. J Clin Invest 1978;61:1337–1345.
42. Schwartz CJ, Kimberg DV, Sheerin HW, Field M, Said SI. Vasoactive intestinal peptide stimulation of adenylate cyclase and active electrolyte secretion in intestinal mucosa. Clin Invest 1974;54:536–544.
43. Racusen LC, Binder HJ. Alteration of large intestinal electrolyte transport by vasoactive intestinal polypeptide in the rat. Gastroenterol 1977;73:790–795.
44. Kraft AR, Tompkins RK, Zollinger R. Recognition and management of the diarrhea syndrome caused by non-beta islet cell tumors of the pancreas. Am J Surg 1970;119:163–170.
45. Verner JV, Morrison AB. Endocrine pancreatic islet disease with diarrhea. Arch Intern Med 1974;133:492–500.
46. Bani Sacchi T, Bani D, Biliotti G. Are pancreatic VIPomas paraneuron neoplasms? A clue to the neuroectodermal origin of these tumors. Pancreas 1992;7:87–97.
47. Delcore R, Friesen SR. Gastrointestinal neuroendocrine tumors. J Am Coll Surg 1994;178:187–211.
48. Krejs GJ. Vipoma syndrome. Am J Med 1987;82(suppl 5B):37–48.
49. Hautefeuille M, Rambaud JC, Ruskone A, Jacquenod P. Diarrhea due to circulating agents. Clin Gastroenterol 1986;15: 312–326.
50. Kimura N, Yamamoto H, Okamoto H, Wakasa H, Nagura H. Multiple-hormone gene expression in ganglioneuroblastoma with watery diarrhea, hypokalemia, and achlorhydria syndrome. Cancer 1993;71:1841–1846.
51. Grier JF. WDHA (watery diarrhea, hypokalemia, achlorhydria) syndrome: clinical features, diagnosis and treatment. South Med J 1995;88(1):22–24.
52. Barraclough MA, Bloom SR. Vipoma of the pancreas. Observations on the diarrhea and circulatory disturbances. Arch Intern Med 1979;139:467–471.
53. Delcore R, Friesen SR. Gastrointestinal neuroendocrine tumors. J Am Coll Surg 1994;178:187–211.
54. Brunt LM, Veldhuis JD, Dilley WG, Farndon JR, Santen RJ, et al. Stimulation of insulin secretion by a rapid intravenous calcium infusion in patients with beta-cell neoplasms of the pancreas. J Clin Endocrinol Metab 1986;62(1):210–216.
55. Stridsberg M, Eriksson B, Lundquist G, Skogeid B, Wilander E, Oberg K. Islet amyloid poplypeptide (IAPP) in patients with neuroendocrine tumors. Regul Pept 1995;55:119–131.
56. Takahashi K, Mouri T, Itoi K, Sone M, Hayashi Y, et al. Neuropeptide Y- and somatostatin-like immunoreactivities in ganglioneuromas, ganglioneuroblastomas and neuroblastoma. Endocrinol Jpn 1989;36(5):627–633.
57. Jaffe BM. Surgery for gut hormone-producing tumors. Am J Surg 1987;82(suppl 5B):68–76.
58. Lundstedt C, Linjawi T, Amin T. Liver VIPoma: report of two cases and literature review. Abdom Imag 1994;19:433–437.
59. Ayub A, Zafar M, Abdulkareem A, Ali MA, Lingawi T, Harbi A. Primary hepatic vipoma. Am J Gastroenterol 1993;88(6): 958–961.
60. Jansen-Goemans A, Englehardt J. Intractable diarrhea in a boy with vasoactive intestinal peptide-producing ganglioneuroblastoma. Pediatrics 1977;59(5):710–716.
61. Rescorla FJ, Vane DW, Fitzgerald JF, West KW, Grosfeld JL. Vasoactive intestinal polypeptide secreting ganglioneuromatosis affecting the entire colon and rectum. J Pediatr Surg 1988;23(7):635–637.
62. Zimmer T, Ziegler K, Liehr RM, Stolzel U, Riecken EO, Wiedenmann B. Endosonography of neuroendocrine tumors of the stomach, duodenum, and pancreas (Review). Ann NY Acad Sci 1994;733: 425–436.
63. Palazzo L, Roseau G, Salmeron M. Endoscopic ultrasonography in the preoperative localization of pancreatic endocrine tumors. Endoscopy 1992;(suppl 1):350–353.
64. Hawes RH, Zaidi S. Endoscopic ultrasonography of the pancreas (Review). Gastrointest Endosc Clin North Am 1995;5(1):61–80.
65. Grama D, Skogseid B, Wilander E, Eriksson B, Martensson H, et al. Pancreatic tumors in multiple endocrine neoplasia type 1: clinical presentation and surgical treatment. World J Surg 1992;16(4):611–619.
66. Aspestrand F, Kolmannskog F, Jacobsen M. CT, MR imaging and angiography in pancreatic apudomas. Acta Radiol 1993;34(5): 468–473.
67. Soyer P, Tidjani K, Laissy JP, Sibert A, Menu Y. Dynamic Gd-DOTA-enhanced MR imaging of hepatic metastases from pancreatic neuroendocrine tumors. Eur J Radiol 1994;18:180–184.
68. Debas HT, Gittes G. Somatostatin analogue therapy in functioning neuroendocrine gut tumors. Digestion 1993;54(suppl 1): 64–71.
69. Nauck C, Ivancevic V, Emrich D, Creutzfeldt W. 111 In-pentetreotride (somatostatin analogue) scintigraphy as an imaging procedure for endocrine gastro-entero-pancreatic tumors. Z Gastroenterol 1994;32:323–327.
70. Scheffold N, Arnold R, Cyran J. Metastasizing pancreatic vipoma. Its diagnosis and therapy with the somatostatin analog octreotide. Dtsche Med Wochenschr 1995;120:1463–1467.
71. Weinel RJ, Neubaus C, Stapp J, Klotter HJ, Trautmann AR, et al. Somatostatin in preoperative therapy and post-operative diagnosis of a patient with Verner Morrison syndrome. Langenbecks Arch Chir 1992;377:345–347.
72. Cesani ER, Walser E, Villanueva-Meyer J. Tc-99m Sestamibi imaging of a pancreatic VIPoma and parathyroid adenoma in a patient with multiple type I endocrine neoplasia. Clin Nucl Med 1994;19(6):532–534.
73. Bernay I, Sahin M. Intestinal uptake of Tc-99m MDP in a patient with vipoma syndrome. Clin Nucl Med 1994;348–349.
74. Virgolini I, Raderer M, Kunaran A, Angelberger P, Banyai S, et al. Vasoactive intestinal peptide-receptor imaging for the localization of intestinal adenocarcinomas and endocrine tumors. N Engl J Med 1994;27;331(17):116–121.
75. King CMP, Reznek JE, Wass JAH. Review imaging islet cell tumours. Clin Radiol 1994;49:295–303.
76. O'Dorisio TM, Mekhjian SH, Ellison EC, O'Dorisio SM, Gaginella TS, Woltering EA. Role of peptide radioimmunoassay in understanding peptide-peptide interactions and clinical expression of gastroenteropancreatic endocrine tumors. Am J Med 1987; 82(suppl 5b):60–67.
77. Said SI. Author's reply re: intractable diarrhea. Gastroenterology 1978;75:153.
78. Said SI. VIP overview. In: Bloom SR, Polak JM, eds. Gut hormones. 2nd ed. Edinburgh: Churchill Livingstone, 1981:379–384.
79. Blackburn AM, Bryant MG, Adrian TE, Bloom SR. Pancreatic tumors produce neurotensin. J Clin Endocrinol Metab 1961;52: 820–822.
80. Lindqvist G, Krause U, Larsson LI. A pancreatic polypeptide-producing tumor associated with the WDHA syndrome. Scand J Gastroenterol 1978;13:715–718.
81. Yasunami Y, Funakoshi A, Ryu S, Shinozaki H, Jimi A, et al. In vitro release of vasoactive intestinal polypeptide and pancreatic polypeptide from human vipoma cells and its inhibition by

somatostatin analogue (SMS 201-995). Surgery 1994;115: 713–717.
82. Gray TK, Bleberdorf FA, Forduran JS. Thyrocalcitonin and the jejunal absorption of calcium, water and electrolytes in normal subjects. J Clin Invest 1973;52:3084–3088.
83. Gray TK, Grannan P, Juan D, Morawski SG, Forduran JS. Ion transport changes during calcitonin-induced intestinal secretion in man. Gastroenterol 1976;71:392–398.
84. Bloom SR, Christofides ND, Delamarter J. Diarrhea in VIPoma patients associated with cosecretion of a second active peptide (peptide histidine isoleucine) explained by single coding gene. Lancet 1983;2:1163–1165.
85. Naruse S, Yasui A, Kishida S. Helodermin: synthesis, existence, and biological actions in mammals. Can J Physiol Pharmacol Gastrointest Hormones 1966;23.
86. Krejs GJ. Gastrointestinal endocrine tumors. Am J Med 1987; 82(suppl 5B):1–3.
87. Woussen-Colle MC, Gourlet P, Vandermeers A, Vandermeers-Piret MD, D'Haens J, et al. Identification of a new chromogranin B fragment (314-365) in endocrine tumors. Peptides 1995;16: 231–236.
88. Woussen-Colle MC, Lingier P, Vertongen P, Vandermeers-Piret MC, Vandermeers A, Robberecht P. Chromogranin A (210-301) is the major form of pancreastatin-like material in human gut extracts and endocrine tumors. Peptides 1994;15:869–874.
89. Krejs GJ. Comparison of the effect of VIP and PHI on water and ion movement in the canine jejunum in vivo. Gastroenterol Clin Biol 1984;8:868.
90. Brunt LM, Mazoujian G, O'Dorisio TM, Wells Jr SA. Stimulation of vasoactive intestinal peptide and neurotensin secretion by pentagastrin in a patient with VIPoma syndrome. Surgery 1994;115:362–369.
91. Viale G, Dell'Orto P, Moro E, Cozzaglio L, Coggi G. Vasoactive intestinal polypeptide-, somatostatin-, and calcitonin-producing adrenal pheochromocytoma associated with the watery diarrhea (WDHH) syndrome. First case report with immunohistochemical findings. Cancer 1985;55(5):1099–1106.
92. Gutniak M, Rosenqvist U, Grimelius L, Lundberg JM, Hokfelt T, et al. Report on a patient with watery diarrhoea syndrome caused by a pancreatic tumour containing neurotensin, enkephalin and calcitonin. Acta Med Scand 1980;208(1–2):95–100.
93. Shulkes A, Chick P, Wong P, Walsh JH. A radioimmunoassay for neurotensin in human plasma. Clin Chim Acta 1982;125(1): 49–58.
94. Hacki WH, Eberle C, Goumoens E, et al. Diagnosis of neurotensin-producing pancreatic tumor by i.v. secretin and calcium provocation tests. Gastroenterology 1985;88:1409.
95. Modlin IM, Lewis JJ, Ahlman H, Bilchik A, Kumar RR. Management of unresectable malignant endocrine tumors of the pancreas. Surg Gynecol Obstet 1993:176:507–518.
96. O'Dorisio TM, Mekhjian HS, Gaginella TS. Medical therapy of vipomas. Endocrinol Metab Clin North Am 1989;18(2):545–556.
97. Moertel CG, Hanley JA, Johnson LA. Streptozocin alone compared with streptozocin plus fluorouracil in the treatment of advanced islet cell carcinoma. N Engl J Med 1980;303:1189–1194.
98. Varkonyi TT, Velosy B, Nagy I, Nemeth J, Lonovics J. Diagnosis of Verner-Morrison syndrome (VDHA) and its treatment with sandostatin and streptozocin. Orv Hetil 1993;134:2599–2602.
99. Juhlin C, Papanicolaou V, Arnberg H, Klareskog L, Lorelius LE, et al. Clinical and biochemical effects in vivo of monoclonal antitumor antibody in Verner-Morrison's syndrome. Cancer 1994;73(5):1346–1352.
100. Eriksson B, Oberg K. An update of the medical treatment of malignant endocrine pancreatic tumors. Acta Oncol 1993;32: 203–208.
101. Grama D, Eriksson B, Martensson H, Cedermark B, Ahren B, et al. Clinical characteristics, treatment and survival in patients with pancreatic tumors causing homonal syndromes. World J Surg 1992;16:632–639.
102. Arnold R, Frank M, Kajdan U. Management of gastroenteropancreatic endocrine tumors: the place of somatostatin analogue. Digestion 1994;55(suppl 3):107–113.
103. Rusone A, Rene E, Chayvialle JA. Effect of somatostatin on diarrhea and on small intestinal water and electrolytic transport in a patient with pancreatic cholera. Dig Dis Sci 1982;27:459–485.
104. Wynick D, Bloom SR. The use of the long-acting somatostatin analog octreotide in the treatment of gut neuroendocrine tumors. J Clin Endocrinol Metab 1991;73(1):1–3.
105. O'Dorisio TM, Gaginella TS, Mekhijian HS, Rao B, O'Dorisio MS. Somatostatin and analogues in the treatment of VIPoma. Ann NY Acad Sci 1988;527:528–535.
106. Antonelli A, Gambuzza C, Bertoni F, Baschieri L. Calcitonin, as SMS 201-995, ameliorates the VIPoma syndrome. J Endocrinol Invest 1993;16(1):57–59.
107. Marquet F, Grishina O, Pansu D, Descroix-Vagne M. Effect of C-terminal derivatives of sorbin on ileal ion transport stimulated by VIP in rats. Gastroenterol Clin Biol 1994;18(8–9):702–707.
108. Okuno M, Nakanishi T, Shinomura Y, Kiyohara T, Ishikawa H, Tarui S. Peptide YY enhances NaCl and water absorption in the rat colon in vivo. Experimentia 1992;48(1):47–50.
109. Catane R, Longo DL. Monoclonal antibodies for cancer therapy (Review). Isr J Med Sci 1988;24(9–10):471–476.
110. Juhlin C, Holmdahl R, Johansson H, Rastad J, Akerstrom G, Klareskog L. Monoclonal antibodies with exclusive reactivity against parathyroid cells and tubule cells of the kidney. Proc Natl Acad Sci USA 1987;84:2990–2994.
111. Juhlin C, Papanicolaou V, Backlin K, Klareskog L, Wilander E, et al. Monoclonal antibodies raised against midgut carcinoid tumor cells. World J Surg 1990;14:386–392.
112. LoBuglio AF, Saleh M, Peterson L, Wheeler R, Carrano R, et al. Phase 1 clinical trial of CO17-1A monoclonal antibody. Hybridoma 1986;5(suppl 1):S117–S123.
113. Sears HF, Herlyn D, Steplewski Z, Koprowski H. Initial trial use of murine monoclonal antibodies as immunotherapeutic agents for gastrointestinal adenocarcinoma. Hybridoma 5(suppl 1): S109–S115.
114. Dillman RO, Shawler DL, Dillman JB, Royston I. Therapy of chronic lymphocytic leukemia and cutaneous T-cell lymphoma with T101 monoclonal antibody. J Clin Oncol 1984;2:881–891.
115. Paul S, Volle DI, Beach CM. Catalytic hydrolysis of vasoactive intestinal polypeptide by human autoantibody. Science 1989; 244:1158–1162.
116. Iverson BL, Lerner RA. Sequence-specific peptide cleavage catalyzed by an antibody. Science 1989;243:1184.
117. Tennvall J, Ljungberg O, Ahren B, Gustavsson A, Nillson LO. Radiotherapy for unresectable endocrine pancreatic carcinomas (Review). Eur J Surg Oncol 1992;18:73–76.
118. Read NW, Read MG, Krejs GJ, Hendler RS, Davis G, Fordtran JS. A report of five patients with large-volume secretory diarrhea but no evidence of endocrine tumor or laxative abuse. Dig Dis Sci 1982;27(3):193–201.
119. Davis GR, Camp RC, Raskin P, Krejs GJ. Effect of somatostatin infusion on jejunal water and electrolyte transport in a patient with secretory diarrhea due to malignant carcinoid syndrome. Gastroenterology 1980;78:346–349.
120. Dharmsathaphorn K, Sherwin RS, Cataland S, Jaffe B, Dobbins J. Somatostatin inhibits diarrhea in the carcinoid syndrome. Ann Intern Med 1980;92:68–69.
121. Santangelo WC, O'Dorisio TM, Kim JG, Severino G, Krejs GJ. Pancreatic cholera syndrome: effect of a synthetic somatostatin analog on intestinal water and ion transport. Ann Intern Med 1985;103:363–367.
122. Maton P, O'Dorisio TM, Howe BA. Effect of a long-acting somatostatin analog (SMS 201-995) in a patient with pancreatic cholera. N Engl J Med 1985;312:17–21.

# 81

# Somatostatinoma

Edgar D. Staren, Louis M. Gianakakis, and Richard A. Prinz

Somatostatin is a cyclic tetradecapeptide that was originally isolated from the hypothalamus of sheep by Brazeau et al. in 1973 (1). At that time, somatostatin was shown to inhibit both the secretion and the action of pituitary growth hormone. It is now known that somatostatin is also produced by the delta cells of the dispersed neuroendocrine cell system (gastroenteropancreatic axis) in man. Delta cells are predominantly located in the pancreatic islets of Langerhans and the fundic/antral regions of the stomach. A lesser number of these cells can be found in the small and large intestine (2, 3).

Somatostatin inhibits the secretion of nearly all gut hormones, including gastrin, secretin, cholecystokinin, vasoactive intestinal peptide, motilin, pancreatic polypeptide, and gastric inhibitory peptide (2, 4). The diffuse location of these somatostatin-producing cells in close proximity to other endocrine cells supports a paracrine activity as well for somatostatin (2, 4). For example, the production of somatostatin by delta cells near the alpha and beta cells of the islets of Langerhans allows paracrine-mediated inhibition of insulin and glucagon release. Thus, somatostatin appears to play a pivotal role as a negative-feedback regulator of peptide hormone–mediated processes in digestion and metabolism. Somatostatin also has a direct inhibitory effect on the motility of the gastrointestinal tract and gallbladder, on pancreatic exocrine and gastric acid secretion, and on the rate of nutrient absorption (i.e., amino acids, carbohydrates, and triglycerides) by the intestine (2–3, 5).

The first patients with a somatostatinoma were reported independently by Ganda et al. and Larsson et al. in 1977 (6, 16). The somatostatinoma "syndrome" was described by Krejs et al. in 1979 (7). Previous reviews have summarized the literature on the somatostatinomas reported between 1977 and 1986 (8, 9). This review incorporates the subsequent 42 patients reported in the English literature from 1987 to 1995, yielding a total of 85 somatostatinomas (15–83).

## DEMOGRAPHICS

There have been 41 males and 42 females reported with somatostatinomas. The gender of 2 individuals was not reported. These patients have an average age of 54 years, with a range of 24–84 years (Table 81.1). The average age of males at the time of diagnosis was 53 years, with a range of 24–79 years. The average age of females at the time of diagnosis was also 53 years, with a range of 28–84 years. The most common location for somatostatinomas was within the pancreas. Among pancreatic somatostatinomas there were 17 males and 24 females, with the gender of two individuals not reported. Extrapancreatic somatostatinomas occurred roughly equally, in 23 males and 19 females.

## CLINICAL SYMPTOMS

The symptoms associated with excessive production of somatostatin are listed in Table 81.2. The classic somatostatinoma syndrome has been characterized by the triad of diabetes, diarrhea/steatorrhea, and gallstones (10). Diarrhea/steatorrhea occurred in 31 (36%) of the 85 patients. Diarrhea results from an increase in the stool osmolarity secondary to malabsorption of fats, sugars, and amino acids. This leads to abnormal liquidity of the stool. Steatorrhea results from decreased pancreatic exocrine secretion and the associated impairment of fat absorption. Excessive somatostatin levels inhibit the release of cholecystokinin, which limits gallbladder contraction as well as the secretion of pancreatic enzymes. Somatostatin also inhibits secretin release, which prevents the pH change necessary for activation of the digestive enzymes in the duodenum. Diarrhea/steatorrhea is uncommon in somatostatinoma patients with low levels of plasma somatostatin-like immunoreactivity (SLI) (5, 11–12).

Weight loss is one of the most common findings and was seen in 33 of the 85 patients (39%). Weight loss may be attributable to malabsorption or possibly to the anorexia that was seen in 10 (12%) patients. Cholelithiasis or a previous cholecystectomy was found in 30 (35%) patients. Somatostatinoma patients are predisposed to gallstone formation as a result of the decrease in gallbladder contractility that accompanies the somatostatin-mediated inhibition of cholecystokinin release (5, 12). Jaundice was observed in 17 (20%) patients. Jaundice may be related to cholelithiasis in some patients, but more often it was due to the tumor directly obstructing bile flow. Abdominal pain was seen in 24 (28%) patients. It can be due to bowel distention from slowed gastrointestinal transit time and malabsorption or from the effects of tumor bulk (12). Nausea/vomiting was seen in 22 (26%) patients and probably results from factors similar to those that account for abdominal pain (5).

Twenty-one (25%) patients with somatostatinomas were diabetic. Diabetes may occur secondary to the direct suppression of insulin release by somatostatin as well as indirectly by suppression of the insulinotropic peptide, gastric inhibitory peptide (GIP). It has been suggested that the substantially higher incidence of diabetes that occurs with pancreatic somatostatinomas is due to their generally higher SLI levels. Tissue destruction by tumor or removal by surgery may lead to diabetes in patients with somatostatinomas. This does not seem to be a likely cause in most patients with diabetes, given the relatively large amount of normal pancreas remaining in them. Generally, diabetes has been relatively mild, with frank ketoacidosis occurring in only three patients. Somatostatinoma patients are thought to have mild diabetes because there is concomitant inhibition of gluca-

**TABLE 81.1. Biographic Data on Patients with a Somatostatinoma**

| Category | Total ($n$ = 85) | ($n$ = 83) Male | Female |
|---|---|---|---|
| Number[a] | 83 | 41 | 42 |
| Age, average | 54 | 53 | 53 |
| Range | 24–84 | 24–79 | 28–84 |

[a]The gender of two patients was not specified.

gon in addition to insulin suppression (5, 12). Somatostatin occurs in various molecular forms: somatostatin 28 and somatostatin 14. The former suppresses insulin activity substantially more than it does glucagon activity. The presence or absence of diabetes in patients with a somatostatinoma may be related to which form predominates.

Less common symptoms observed in these 85 somatostatinoma patients were anorexia in 10 (12%) patients; fatigue in 9 (11%), and anemia in 8 (9%). Interestingly, seven (8%) patients with a duodenal somatostatinoma had neurofibromatosis. The association of duodenal somatostatinomas, neurofibromatosis, and pheochromocytoma has been reported (54). This may be an unusual form of a multiple endocrine neoplasia (MEN) syndrome, since it seems to have a familial relationship. Hypochlorhydria has occurred in some somatostatinoma patients, and this has been viewed as one component of the classic syndrome. It is thought to be due to gastrin inhibition as well as direct suppression of gastric acid secretion by somatostatin. Hypochlorhydria would probably be detected in more patients if specifically sought.

## DIAGNOSTIC EXAMINATIONS

The clinical symptoms of somatostatinomas are generally vague (abdominal pain, diarrhea, etc.). However, somatostatinomas can be relatively large tumors at the time of presentation. In this setting, imaging studies are associated with a high degree of accuracy (Table 81.3). For example, computed tomography (CT) scanning correctly localized the somatostatinoma in 34 of 37 patients with pancreatic tumors (92%). External abdominal ultrasound yielded a positive result in 26 of 30 patients (87%). Angiography correctly identified tumor in 17 of 18 patients (94%). Flexible upper endoscopy was positive in 22 of 26 patients (85%), while endoscopic retrograde cholangiopancreatography (ERCP) was accurate in all 15 patients (100%) in whom it was used. Biopsy and/or fine needle aspiration confirmed the diagnosis in 21 of 25 patients (84%). Because of its ready availability and high degree of accuracy, CT scanning is generally the first imaging study to be used for a clinically suspected somatostatinoma.

Most patients with pancreatic somatostatinomas can have the diagnosis confirmed biochemically by finding elevated plasma levels of somatostatin (normal, <100 pg/mL). When evaluated preoperatively, 34 of 35 (97%) patients had elevated levels of circulating somatostatin. Measurement of plasma SLI may be useful in interpreting otherwise ambiguous symptoms associated with the somatostatinoma syndrome. SLI measurement may also be used to evaluate the success of treatment and to follow patients for possible recurrence. Typically, SLI levels are substantially elevated in patients with pancreatic somatostatinomas but are normal or only slightly elevated with extrapancreatic tumors (13, 14). If baseline plasma SLI levels are not diagnostic, provocative testing may be useful in confirming the diagnosis. Tolbutamide infusion, was used in eight (9%) patients and resulted in substantially increased SLI levels in each. Calcium/pentagastrin stimulation of somatostatin was reported in three patients with normal baseline plasma levels; a 3- to 12-fold rise in plasma concentration of somatostatin was seen in all three. Inhibitory tests using diazoxide have also been used to confirm the diagnosis of a somatostatinoma. Obviously, experience with these tests are limited, and their diagnostic accuracy requires further confirmation.

**TABLE 81.2. Symptoms of Patients with a Somatostatinoma**

| Symptom/Physical Finding | Number of Patients ($n$ = 85) | % |
|---|---|---|
| Weight loss | 33 | 39 |
| Diarrhea/steatorrhea | 31 | 36 |
| Cholelithiasis | 30 | 35 |
| Abdominal pain | 24 | 28 |
| Nausea/vomiting | 22 | 26 |
| Diabetes | 21 | 25 |
| Jaundice | 17 | 20 |
| Anorexia | 10 | 12 |
| Fatigue | 9 | 11 |
| Neurofibromatosis | 9 | 11 |
| Anemia | 8 | 9 |
| Diabetic ketoacidosis | 2 | 2 |

**TABLE 81.3. Accuracy of Diagnostic Tests Performed in 85 Patients with a Somatostatinoma**

| Test[a] | Total | Number Positive | Number Negative |
|---|---|---|---|
| Computed tomography | 37 | 34 | 3 |
| Abdominal ultrasound | 30 | 26 | 4 |
| Endoscopy/EGD[b] | 26 | 22 | 4 |
| Biopsy | 25 | 21 | 4 |
| Upper GI[c] series | 24 | 19 | 5 |
| Angiography | 18 | 17 | 1 |
| ETCP[d] | 15 | 15 | 0 |
| Magnetic resonance imaging | 4 | 3 | 1 |
| PTC[e] | 3 | 3 | 0 |

[a]Tests used for evaluation were not reported in 7 cases.
[b]Esophagogastroduodenoscopy.
[c]Gastrointestinal.
[d]Endoscopic retrograde cholangiopancreatography.
[e]Percutaneous transhepatic cholangiography.

## LOCATION OF PRIMARY TUMOR

Of the 85 reported somatostatinomas, 40 (47%) were found within the pancreas (Table 81.4). The locations of pancreatic somatostatinomas were as follows: 24 were in the head, 8 were in the tail, 3 occupied two-thirds of the organ (body/tail), 2 occupied the whole organ, and 1 did not have its site specified. Of the 45 (53%) extrapancreatic somatostatinomas, 26 were found in the duodenum (second portion), 13 in the ampulla of Vater, 1 in the cystic duct, 1 in the jejunum, 1 in the rectum, and 3 in unspecified locations.

The so-called cardinal symptoms of a somatostatinoma (i.e., mild diabetes, cholelithiasis, diarrhea/steatorrhea) occur almost exclusively with pancreatic rather than extrapancreatic tumors (10). Typically, extrapancreatic somatostatinomas are smaller than their pancreatic counterparts and are characterized by relatively early symptoms of bleeding, jaundice, and abdominal pain resulting from gastrointestinal tract erosion and/or obstruction of the bile duct (47). The somatostatinoma syndrome rarely

**TABLE 81.4. Location of Primary Tumor in Patients with a Somatostatinoma**

| Location | Number of Patients ($n$ = 85) | % |
|---|---|---|
| Duodenum | 26 | 31 |
| Pancreas | 40 | 47 |
| Head | 24 | 28 |
| Tail | 8 | 9 |
| Body/tail | 3 | 4 |
| Whole organ | 2 | 2 |
| Site unknown | 2 | 2 |
| Body | 1 | 1 |
| Ampulla of Vater | 13 | 15 |
| Cystic duct | 1 | 1 |
| Jejunum | 1 | 1 |
| Rectum | 1 | 1 |
| Unknown | 3 | 4 |

occurs with extrapancreatic tumors because they are usually identified and removed before sufficiently high levels of circulating somatostatin are attained.

## SURGERY

Surgical resection is the preferred treatment for patients with somatostatinomas. Unfortunately, the frequent occurrence of metastases at the time of presentation precludes cure for most of these patients. While debulking of tumor has been recommended to palliate symptomatic patients, there are limited data to support the efficacy of this approach in all patients. Surgical judgment is needed to balance the risks and benefits of this form of palliation.

Surgery was performed in 77 of the 85 (91%) patients reported (Table 81.5). As might be expected, given the primary tumor's predilection for the periampullary region, a Whipple resection was the most common procedure, performed in 32 of 85 (38%) patients. Other types of pancreatic resection (i.e., distal, subtotal, or total pancreatectomy) were performed in 17 (20%) patients. Duodenal resection was done in 11 (13%) patients. Tumor removal was performed but the site was not specified in four (5%) patients. Six (7%) patients had laparotomy without tumor resection. In eight patients, no surgical procedure was performed. At the time of operation, 13 (15%) patients had an associated cholecystectomy; 5 (6%) patients had an associated splenic resection either because of tumor spread or for technical reasons.

**TABLE 81.5. Surgical Procedures Performed on Patients with a Somatostinoma**

| Procedure | Number of Patients ($n$ = 85) | % |
|---|---|---|
| Whipple | 32 | 38 |
| Pancreatic resection | 17 | 20 |
| Cholecystectomy | 13 | 15 |
| Tumor resection | | |
| Duodenum | 11 | 13 |
| Not specified | 4 | 5 |
| Laparotomy, tumor not resected | 6 | 7 |
| Splenectomy | 5 | 7 |
| No procedure | 8 | 9 |

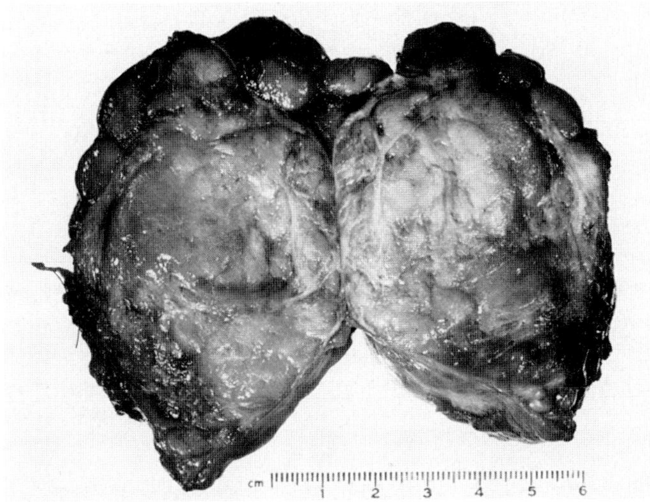


**FIG. 81.1.** An example of a particularly large islet cell tumor locally resected from the pancreas.

## TUMOR CHARACTERISTICS

Somatostatinomas are generally single (90%), moderate-sized, exophytic tumors (Fig. 81.1). The tumor usually presents as a submucosal nodule when located in the intestine. Information on specific tumor size was available in 38 of the patients included in this study. Twenty-three of the 38 patients (61%) had duodenal tumors that ranged from 0.3 to 3.0 cm in diameter. Duodenal tumors larger than 3.0 cm were found in five patients (13%). Five (13%) patients had pancreatic tumors larger than 3.0 cm in diameter, while an equal number (13%) had tumors smaller than 3.0 cm.

On routine histopathologic examination, somatostatinomas appear as well-differentiated neuroendocrine tumors of the islet-cell or carcinoid type (Fig. 81.2). They tend to form solid sheets, cords, or nests of homogeneous-appearing oval or columnar-shaped cells with abundant cytoplasm and small regular nuclei. They may, however, vary from well differentiated to quite undifferentiated tumors. Duodenal somatostatinomas may demonstrate a glandular pattern that can lead to an erroneous diagnosis of adenocarcinoma. Immunohistochemical staining for somatostatin is generally reliable, and a diffusely

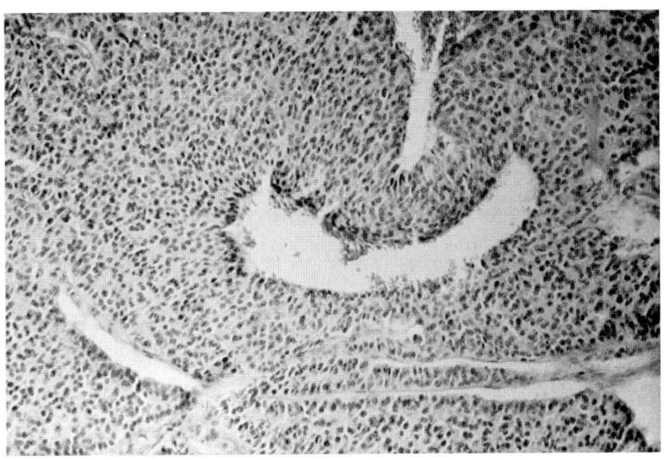

**FIG. 81.2.** Typical histologic appearance of an islet cell carcinoma, showing a solid area, ×50.

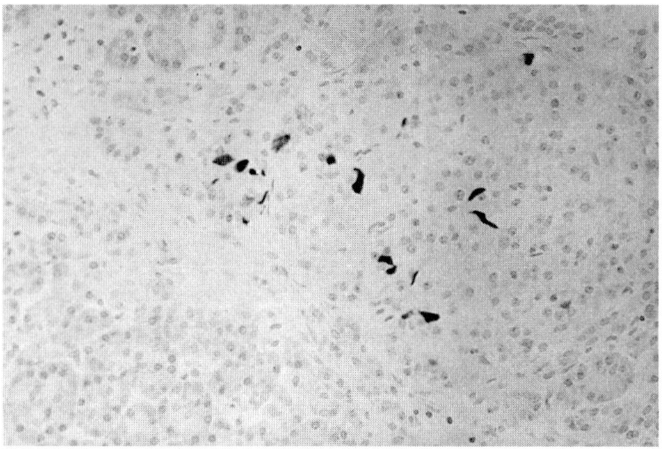

**FIG. 81.3.** Focally intense staining somatostatin-positive cells in this somatostatinoma, ×100.

positive staining pattern is usually seen (Fig. 81.3). Immunohistochemical staining for somatostatin was positive in all 40 tumors in which it was evaluated (Table 81.6). A variety of other hormones may be detected in somatostatinomas including insulin, gastrin, VIP, ACTH, substance P, and others. Ultrastructural evaluation with electron microscopy identifies neurosecretory granules 200–400 nm in size. When present, psammoma bodies strongly suggest an endocrine tumor, particularly a somatostatinoma; they were noted in 23 patients in this series.

Thirty (35%) of the reported patients had no evidence of metastases at the time of diagnosis. In seven patients (8%), the presence or absence of metastases was not specified. Twenty-five patients had metastases to the regional lymph nodes (29%), and 28 patients (33%) had metastases to the liver Fig. 81.4). The other sites of metastases included the duodenum in four patients, bone in three, the spleen in two, and the lung in two. Most somatostatinomas were malignant, and nearly two-thirds of patients had metastases at the time of presentation. The origin of the primary tumor did not seem to influence the biologic aggressiveness of somatostatinomas nor did it appear to influence the predilection for one metastatic site (i.e., liver vs. lymph node) over another.

## CHEMOTHERAPY

Chemotherapy was given to 21 (25%) patients with either metastatic and/or locally advanced disease. The most commonly used chemotherapeutic agents were streptozotocin and/or 5-fluorouracil. They were given alone or in combination to 17 of the 20 patients. Seven of these 20 patients had only chemotherapy, and no surgical intervention was ever performed. The impact of therapy on survival is difficult to evaluate in this small cohort. Twelve patients (60%) given chemotherapy were alive from 1 1/2 to 7 3/4 years after treatment. Ten of the 20 patients had died from 9 months to 3 1/2 years after treatment. Chemotherapy caused tumor regression and symptomatic remission in some patients and is therefore a reasonable consideration in the symptomatic patient with recurrent and/or metastatic disease.

**TABLE 81.6. Immunohistochemical Staining Characteristics of Somatostatinomas (*n* = 54)**

| Category | Number of Patients with Positive Result |
|---|---|
| Somatostatin (tissue) | 42[a] |
| Other peptides | |
| Neuron-specific enolase | 10 |
| Pancreatic polypeptide | 3 |
| Gastrin | 4 |
| Prosomatostatin | 2 |

[a]Ten patients with a positive result were described as "strongly positive."

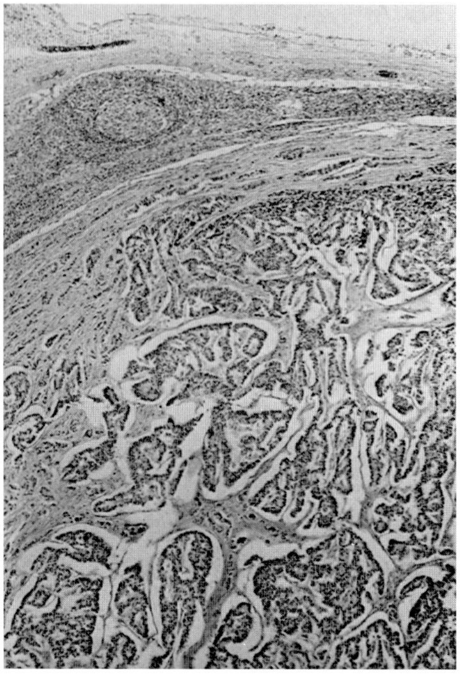

**FIG. 81.4.** An islet cell carcinoma demonstrating obvious regional lymph node involvement, ×16.

## SURVIVAL

As with other islet cell cancers, somatostatinomas may have a rather indolent tumor biology, and long-term survival can occur. Conversely, the highly malignant potential of this tumor warrants aggressive treatment and vigilant follow-up. In this series, survival status was not specified for 18 patients (Table 81.7). Overall, 47 of the 67 (70%) patients for whom length of survival was noted were alive at the time of their report, while 20 (30%) patients were dead. Of the 20 somatostatinoma patients who had died, 9 were known to have persistent or recurrent disease at the time of death. Disease status was unknown in the remaining 10 patients.

## SUMMARY

The somatostatinoma syndrome is characterized by the triad of gallstones, diabetes, and diarrhea/steatorrhea. Less commonly reported symptoms/signs include weight loss and hypochlorhydria. These tumors have a relatively equal gender distribution. The most common age at diagnosis has been in the middle of the 5th decade.

Most somatostatinomas are located within the pancreas (47%). Pancreatic somatostatinomas often exhibit the symptoms typically associated with the syndrome. This is probably related to the fact that pancreatic somatostatinomas are usually associated with high levels of circulating somatostatin. Extrapancreatic tumors most often occur in the duodenum or in the ampulla of

**TABLE 81.7. Survival of Patients with a Somatostatinoma ($n$ = 67)**

| Survival[a] | Alive | NED[b] | Dead | NED[b] |
|---|---|---|---|---|
| Death postoperatively | 0 | — | 5 | — |
| < 6 months | 7 | 5 | 5 | 2 |
| 6 months–1 year | 7 | 4 | 4 | 2 |
| 1–2 years | 15 | 11 | 2 | 1 |
| 2–3 years | 5 | 1 | 2 | 0 |
| 3–4 years | 5 | 2 | 1 | — |
| 4–5 years | 2 | 1 | 1 | 0 |
| > 5 years | 6 | 1 | 0 | — |
| Total | 47 (70%) | | 20 (30%) | |

[a]Survival based on patient status at the time of the case report. Case reports did not specify the survival status of 18 patients.
[b]No evidence of disease.

Vater. Extrapancreatic somatostatinomas frequently do not have the symptomatology associated with the somatostatinoma syndrome but present with bleeding, jaundice, or abdominal pain. This may be secondary to early identification and removal of the tumor before it can produce enough somatostatin to cause the syndrome.

A Whipple resection can be curative if disease is localized to the pancreatic head, but curative surgery is often precluded in these patients by the presence of metastatic disease. Surgical debulking and/or chemotherapy may be indicated to palliate symptomatic patients with metastatic or unresectable disease. Despite the high incidence of malignancy, survival in somatostatinoma patients is generally good. Those patients that died of their disease usually did so within 3 years of their initial presentation.

## REFERENCES


1. Brazeau P, Vale W, Burgus R, et al. Hypothalamic polypeptide that inhibits the secretion of immunoreactive pituitary growth hormone. Science 1973;179:77–79.
2. Krejs GJ. Physiological role of somatostatin in the digestive tract: gastric acid secretion, intestinal absorption, and motility. Scand J Gastroenterol 1986;21(suppl 119):47–53.
3. Schusdziarra V, Schmid R. Physiological and pathophysiological aspects of somatostatin. Scand J Gastroenterol 1986;21(suppl 119):29–41.
4. Lamers CBHW. Clinical and pathophysiological aspects of somatostatin and the gastrointestinal tract. Acta Endocrinol Suppl (Copenh) 1987;286:19–25.
5. Kaplan EL, Michelassi F. Endocrine tumors of the pancreas and their clinical syndromes. Surg Annu 1986;18:181–223.
6. Ganda OP, Weir GC, Soeldner JS, et al. Somatostatinoma: a somatostatin-containing tumor of the pancreas. N Engl J Med 1977;296(17):963–967.
7. Krejs G, Orci L, Conlon M, et al. Somatostatinoma syndrome: biochemical, morphologic, and clinical features. N Engl J Med 1979;301:285.
8. Vinik AI, Strodel WE, Eckhauser FE, Moattari AR, Lloyd R. Somatostatinomas, Pomas, neurotensinomas. Semin Oncol 1987; 14(3):263–281.
9. Harris GJ, Tio F, Cruz AB Jr. Somatostatinoma: a case report and review of the literature. Surg Oncol 1987;36:8–16.
10. Jaffe BM. Surgery for gut hormone-producing tumors. Am J Med 1987;82(5B):68–76.
11. Alam MJ. Chronic refractory diarrhoea: a manifestation of endocrine disorders. Dig Dis 1994,12(1):46–61.
12. Mozell E, Stenzel P, Woltering EA, Rosch J, O'Dorisio TM. Functional endocrine tumors of the pancreas: clinical presentation, diagnosis, and treatment. Curr Probl Surg 1990,27(6):301–386.
13. Delcore R, Friesen SR. Gastrointestinal neuroendocrine tumors. J Am Coll Surg 1994,178(2):187–211.
14. Friesen SR. Update on the diagnosis and treatment of rare neuroendocrine tumors. Surg Clin North Am 1987,67(2):379–393.
15. Kovacs K, Horvath E, Ezrin C, Sepp H, Elkan I. Immunoreactive somatostatin in pancreatic islet-cell carcinoma accompanied by ectopic ACTH syndrome. Lancet 1977;1:1365–1366.
16. Larsson L-I, Holst JJ, Kuhl C, et al. Pancreatic somatostatinoma: clinical features and physiological implications. Lancet 1977;1: 666–668.
17. Alumets J, Ekelund G, Hakanson R, et al. Jejunal endocrine tumor composed of somatostatin and gastrin cells and associated with duodenal ulcer disease. Virchows Arch (A) 1978;378:17–22.
18. Murayama H, Imai T, Kikuchi M, Kamio A. Duodenal carcinoid (apudoma) with psammoma bodies. Cancer 1979;43:1411–1417.
19. Gerlock AJ Jr, Muhletaler CA, Halter S, Goncharenko V. Pancreatic somatostatinoma: histologic, clinical, and angiographic features. Am J Med 1979;133:939–943.
20. Pipeleers D, Somers G, Gepts W, De Nutte N, De Vroede M. Plasma pancreatic hormone levels in a case of somatostatinoma: diagnostic and therapeutic implications. J Clin Endocrinol Metab 1979;49(4):572–579.
21. Kaneko H, Yanaihara N, Ito S, et al. Somatostatinoma of the duodenum. Cancer 1979;44:2273–2279.
22. Marks V, Abolfathi A, Wright J, White WF, Penman E, Wass JAH. Malignant somatostatinoma presenting with hypoglycaemia: clinical and biological studies. In: Andreani D, Lefabvre PJ, Marks V, eds. Hypoglycemia. London: Academic Press, 1979.
23. Asa S, Kovacs K, Killinger D, Marcon N, Platts M. Pancreatic islet cell carcinoma producing gastrin, ACTH, α-endorphin, somatostatin and calcitonin. Am J Gastroenterol 1980;74:30–35.
24. Wright J, Abolfathi A, Penman E, Marks V. Pancreatic somatostatinoma presenting with hypoglycaemia. Clin Endocrinol 1980; 12:603–608.
25. Penman E, Lowry PJ, Wass JAH, et al. Molecular forms of somatostatin in normal subjects and in patients with pancreatic somatostatinoma. Clin Endocrinol 1980;12:611–620.
26. Galmiche JP, Chayvialle JA, Dubois PM, et al. Calcitonin producing pancreatic somatostatinoma. Gastroenterology 1980;78: 1577–1583.
27. Lowery SF, Burt ME, Brennan MF. Glucose turnover and gluconeogenesis in a patient with somatostatinoma. Surgery 1981;89(3): 309–313.
28. Axelrod L, Bush MA, Hirsch HJ, Loo SWH. Malignant somatostatinoma: clinical features and metabolic studies. J Clin Endocrinol 1981;52:886–896.
29. Cantor AM, Rigby CC, Beck PR, Mangion D. Neurofibromatosis, phaeochromocytoma, and somatostatinoma. Br Med J 1982; 285:1618–1619.
30. Shawker TH, Doppman JL, Dunnick NR, McCarthy DM. Ultrasonic investigation of pancreatic islet cell tumors. J Ultrasound Med 1982;1:193–200.
31. Lasson A, Alwmark A, Nobin A, Sundler F. Endocrine tumors of the duodenum: clinical characteristics and hormone content. Ann Surg 1983;197:393–398.
32. Schusdziarra V, Grube D, Seifert H, et al. Somatostatinoma syndrome: clinical, morphological and metabolic features and therapeutic aspects. Klin Wochenschr 1983;61:681–689.
33. Stacpoole PW, Kasselberg AG, Berelowitz M, Chey WY. Somatostatinoma syndrome: does a clinical entity exist? Acta Endocrinol 1983;102:80–87.
34. Kelly TR. Pancreatic somatostatinoma. Am J Surg 1983;146: 671–673.
35. Sakazaki S, Umeyama K, Nakagawa H, et al. Pancreatic somatostatinoma. Am J Surg 1983;146:674–679.
36. Marcial MA, Pinkus GS, Skarin A, Hinrichs HR, Warhol MJ. Ampullary somatostatinoma: psammomatous variant of gastrointestinal carcinoid tumor—an immunohistochemical and ultrastructural study. Report of a case and review of the literature. Am J Clin Pathol 1983;80:755–761.
37. Kaneko H, Toshima M, Kobayashi H, et al. Duodenal somatostatinoma: immunohistopathology and review of the literature. Acta Pathol Jpn 1983;33(1):153–158.
38. Pipeleers D, Couturier E, Gepts W, Reynders J, Somers G. Five cases of somatostatinoma: clinical heterogeneity and diagnostic usefulness of basal and tolbutamide-induced hypersomatostatinemia. J Clin Endocrinol Metab 1983;56:1236–1242.

39. Dayal Y, Doos WG, O'Brien MJ, Nunnemacher G, DeLellis RA, Wolfe HJ. Psammomatous somatostatinoma of the duodenum. Am J Surg Pathol 1983;7(7):653–665.
40. Somers G, Pipeleers-Marichal M, Gepts W, Pipeleers D. A case of duodenal somatostatinoma: diagnostic usefulness of calcium-pentagastrin test. Gastroenterology 1983;85:1192–1198.
41. Nakanome C, Koizumi M, Fujiya H, et al. Somatostatinoma syndrome accompanied by overproduction of pancreatic polypeptide. Tohoku J Exp Med 1984;142:201–210.
42. Griffiths DFR, Jasani B, Newman GR, Williams ED, Williams GT. Glandular duodenal carcinoid—a somatostatin rich tumor with neuroendocrine associations. J Clin Pathol 1984;37:163–169.
43. Goodman ZD, Albores-Saavedra J, Lundblad DM. Somatostatinoma of the cystic duct. Cancer 1984;53:498–502.
44. Jensen SL, Christiansen LA, Oxhole A-M, Holst JJ. Duodenal somatostatinoma. Br J Surg 1984;71(2):159.
45. Roberts L Jr, Dunnick NR, Foster WL Jr, et al. Somatostatinoma of the endocrine pancreas: CT findings. J Comput Assist Tomogr 1984;8(5):1015–1018.
46. Malone MJ, Silverman ML, Braasch JW, Jin GJ, Dayal Y. Early somatostatinoma of the papilla of the duct of Santorini. Arch Surg 1985;120:1381–1383.
47. Shirouzu K, Miyamoto Y, Shiramizu T, Morimatsu M. Somatostatinoma of the pancreas. Acta Pathol Jpn 1985;35(5):1285–1292.
48. Reynolds C, Pratt R, Chan-Yan C, et al. Somatostatinoma—the most recently described pancreatic islet cell tumor. West J Med 1985;142:393–397.
49. Taccagni CC, Carlucci M, Sironi M, Cantaboni A, DiCarlo V. Duodenal somatostatinoma with psammoma bodies: an immunohistochemical and ultrastructural study. Am J Gastroenterol 1986;81(1):33–37.
50. Budmiger H, Buhler H, Hacki W, Stamm B, Streuli R, Ammann R. Comparative diagnostic value of the calcium-pentagastrin test versus the tolbutamide test in a patient with a somatostatinoma. Gastroenterology 1987;92(3):800–804.
51. Stommer PE, Stolte M, Seifert E. Somatostatinoma of Vater's papilla and of the minor papilla. Cancer 1987;60(2):232–235.
52. Jackson JA, Raju BU, Fachnie JD, et al. Malignant somatostatinoma presenting with diabetic ketoacidosis. Clin Endocrinol (Oxf) 1987;26(5):609–621.
53. Griffiths D, Williams G, Williams E. Duodenal carcinoid tumors, pheochromocytoma and neurofibromatosis. Islet cell tumor, pheochromocytoma and the von Hippel-Lindau complex: two distinctive neuroendocrine syndromes. Q J Med 1987;64:769.
54. Kock KF, Sandermann J. A polypoid duodenal somatostatinoma. A case report. Scand J Gastroenterol 1988;23(1):100–102.
55. Willcox PA, Immelman EJ, Barron JL, et al. Pancreatic somatostatinoma: presentation with recurrent episodes of severe hyperglycaemia and ketoacidosis. Q J Med 1988;68(255):559–571.
56. Ranaldi R, Bearzi I, Cinti S, Suraci V. Ampullary somatostatinoma. An immunohistochemical and ultrastructural study. Pathol Res Pract 1988;183(1):8–16.
57. Swinburn BA, Yeong ML, Lane MR, Nicholson GI, Holdaway IM. Neurofibromatosis associated with somatostatinoma: a report of two patients. Clin Endocrinol (Oxf) 1988;28(4):353–359.
58. Levi S, Bjarnason I, Swinson CM, Polak JM, Murray W, Levi AJ. Malignant pancreatic somatostatinoma in a patient with dermatitis herpetiformis and coeliac disease. Digestion 1988; 39(1):1–6.
59. Kusunoki M, Yamamura T, Ichii S, Fujita S, Nakai T, Utsunomiya J. The effects of sodium valproate on plasma somatostatin and insulin in humans. J Clin Endocrinol Metab 1988;67(5):1060–1063.
60. Iguchi H, Kumagai S, Seo IH, Wakasugi H, Hara Y, Abe M. Somatostatin-secreting islet cell tumor (somatostatinoma): suppression of growth hormone (GH) release induced by GH-releasing hormone. J Clin Endocrinol Metab 1988;67(1): 206–210.
61. Davis TM, Bray G, Domin J, Bloom SR. A case of somatostatinoma: responses to food and SMS 201-995 administration. Pancreas 1988;3(6):729–733.
62. Kitagawa M, Hayakawa T, Kondo T, et al. Somatostatinoma of the rectum. Am J Gastroenterol 1989;84(11):1452–1455.
63. Ohtsuki Y, Sonobe H, Mizobuchi T, et al. Duodenal carcinoid (somatostatinoma) combined with von Recklinghausen's disease. A case report and review of the literature. Acta Pathol Jpn 1989;39(2):141–146.
64. Albrecht S, Gardiner GW, Kovacs K, Ilse G, Kaiser U. Duodenal somatostatinoma with psammoma bodies. Arch Pathol Lab Med 1989;113(5):517–520.
65. Anonymous. Case records of the Massachusetts General Hospital. Weekly clinicopathological exercises. Case 15-1989. A 52-year-old man with neurofibromatosis and jaundice. N Engl J Med 1989;320(15):996–1004.
66. Soga J, Suzuki T, Yoshikawa K, Katoh H, Tsuno Y, Muto T. Carcinoid somatostatinoma of the duodenum. Eur J Cancer 1990;26(10): 1107–1108.
67. Konomi K, Chijiiwa K, Katsuta T, Yamaguchi K. Pancreatic somatostatinoma: a case report and review of the literature. J Surg Oncol 1990;43(4):259–265.
68. Soldati T, Del Noce G, Garino M, Farina EC, De Paolis P, Balbo G. Pancreatic somatostatinoma. Panminerva Med 1990;32(3): 141–144.
69. Ohsawa H, Kanatsuka A, Tokuyama Y, et al. Amyloid protein in somatostatinoma differs from human islet amyloid polypeptide. Acta Endocrinol (Copenh) 1991;124:45–53.
70. Farr CM, Price HM, Bezmalinovic Z. Duodenal somatostatinoma with congenital pseudoarthrosis. J Clin Gastroenterol 1991;13(2): 195–197.
71. Yoshida A, Hatanaka S, Ohi Y, Umekita Y, Yoshida H. von Recklinghausen's disease associated with somatostatin-rich duodenal carcinoid (somatostatinoma), medullary thyroid carcinoma and diffuse adrenal medullary hyperplasia. Acta Pathol Jpn 1991;41(11):847–856.
72. Sawady J, Katzin WE, Mendelsohn G, Aron DC. Somatostatin-producing neuroendocrine tumor of the ampulla (ampullary somatostatinoma). Evidence of prosomatostatin production. Am J Clin Pathol 1992;97(3):411–415.
73. Stavri GT, Pritchard GA, Williams EJ, Stamatakis JD. Somatostatinoma of the pancreas with hypercalcaemia. A case report. Eur J Surg Oncol 1992;18(3):298–300.
74. Williams EJ, Ratcliffe WA, Stavri GT, Stamatakis JD. Hypercalcaemia secondary to secretion of parathyroid hormone related protein from a somatostatinoma of the pancreas. Ann Clin Biochem 1992;29(pt 3):354–357.
75. Hagen EC, Houben GM, Nikkels RE, et al. Exocrine pancreatic insufficiency and pancreatic fibrosis due to duodenal somatostatinoma in a patient with neurofibromatosis. Pancreas 1992; 7(1):98–104.
76. Grama D, Eriksson B, Martensson H, et al. Clinical characteristics, treatment and survival in patients with pancreatic tumors causing hormonal syndromes. World J Surg 1992;16(4):632–639.
77. Shaw C, Cormican K, Thim L, et al. Neuropeptide Y and neuropeptide Y 3-36: isolation from human pancreatic endocrine tumours. Regul Pept 1993;45(3):387–394.
78. O'Brien TD, Chejfec G, Prinz RA. Clinical features of duodenal somatostatinomas. Surgery 1993;114:1144–1147.
79. Debas HT, Mulvihill SJ. Neuroendocrine gut neoplasms. Important lessons from uncommon tumors. Arch Surg 1994;129(9):965–971.
80. Tjon A, Tham RT, Jansen JB, Falke TH, Lamers CB. Imaging features of somatostatinoma: MR, CT, US, and angiography. J Comput Assist Tomogr 1994;18(3):427–431.
81. Mao C, Shah A, Hanson DJ, Howard JM. Von Recklinghausen's disease associated with duodenal somatostatinoma: contrast of duodenal versus pancreatic somatostatinomas. J Surg Oncol 1995;59(1):67–73.
82. Anene C, Thompson JS, Saigh J, Badakhsh S, Ecklund RE. Somatostatinoma: atypical presentation of a rare pancreatic tumor. Am J Gastroenterol 1995;90(5):819–821.
83. Dominioni L, Dionigi R, Benevento A, et al. Very late recurrence of a somatostatin cell tumor of the head of the pancreas. Pancreas 1995;10(4):417–419.

# 82

# Cystic and Nonfunctioning Islet Cell Tumors

Alexander R. Miller, Michael G. Sarr, and Jon A. Van Heerden

Islet cell neoplasms of the pancreas, as a whole, constitute a rare clinical entity, with the subset of cystic, nonfunctioning islet cell neoplasms being encountered even less frequently. Despite their rarity, if the clinician does not consider these lesions in the differential diagnosis of pancreatic masses, errors will undoubtedly be made, not only in the diagnostic evaluation, but more importantly, in planning an appropriate therapeutic strategy. This latter concept has direct clinical relevance because this group of pancreatic neoplasms has a uniformly better prognosis than the more common ductal adenocarcinomas of the pancreas. Islet cell neoplasms warrant a much more aggressive surgical approach, even in a setting of advanced local disease. The assumption that a locally advanced pancreatic mass is the more common adenocarcinoma, especially for neoplasms arising in the body and tail of the gland, will deny curative surgery to a major subset of patients. For these reasons, differentiation of islet cell neoplasms from other pancreatic masses is a crucial step in the management of the patient with a presumed pancreatic neoplasm.

## HISTORY/NOMENCLATURE

Neoplasms arising from neuroendocrine tissue within the pancreas were initially described by Nicholls and Fabozzi in the first decade of this century (1, 2). At our institution, recognition of a functioning islet cell neoplasm was reported in 1927 by Wilder et al. (3). These physicians described clearly the clinical manifestations of an islet cell neoplasm producing a systemically active substance, now appreciated as the peptide hormone insulin, from an insulinoma. Since this description, at least 12 distinct types of functional islet cell neoplasms have been recognized by their ability to evoke specific and often pathognomonic clinical syndromes (4).

### Nonfunctioning Islet Cell Neoplasms

Nonfunctioning islet cell neoplasms were originally defined as lesions that do not produce clinical signs or symptoms related to the release of a regulatory peptide hormone. Such a neoplasm was described by Zanetti in 1927 (5). With the advent of radioimmunoassay techniques that allowed direct determinations of serum concentrations of various hormones, nonfunctioning islet cell neoplasms were additionally defined as pancreatic neuroendocrine neoplasms occurring in the absence of both clinical manifestations and increased serum hormone concentrations (6). Depending on the spectrum of peptide hormones assayed, the latter criterion has varied, and no single definition has been accepted universally.

For the following discussion, nonfunctioning islet cell neoplasms are defined as those neoplasms arising from the pancreatic islets that do not produce systemic symptoms related to the release of a regulatory peptide or peptides. Although many of these neoplasms, even in the absence of specific symptoms, will stain immunohistochemically for several peptides, clinically these are nonfunctional islet cell neoplasms. These lesions are referred to as islet cell neoplasms, as opposed to the less discriminating term islet cell "tumors." Their natural history is described, as is their presentation, based on whether they are benign or malignant neoplasms.

### Cystic Islet Cell Neoplasms

Uncertainty regarding diagnosis is enhanced if islet cell neoplasms are found to have a cystic component. The natural history and clinical course of this unusual subgroup can be much different from those of cystadenomas and cystadenocarcinomas of the pancreas and are obviously distinct from postinflammatory cystic disorders of the pancreas (7). Cystic islet cell neoplasms were first recognized by Judd in 1933, and by Thigpen in 1940 (8, 9). Winston later identified cystic features of an islet cell neoplasm in 1965 (10). Subsequently, cystic lesions have been encountered, but only rarely, and continue to be described on a case report basis.

This chapter also describes the epidemiology, clinical presentation, diagnosis, pathophysiology, and therapeutic options in the management of nonfunctional and cystic pancreatic islet cell neoplasms. Though perhaps not as clinically sensational as their functional counterparts, these lesions are worthy of discussion, since appropriate recognition and management will often allow an excellent long-term outcome and avoid unfortunate diagnostic errors.

## EPIDEMIOLOGY

Islet cell neoplasms have been reported to occur in 0.1–1.0 persons per 100,000 population (11). Nonfunctional neoplasms comprise between 15 and 65% of most series, depending on the definition of "nonfunctioning" neoplasm (12–26). Typically, these neoplasms are recognized in patients in their 5th and 6th decades of life, although individuals with multiple endocrine neoplasia type 1 (MEN-1) often develop these lesions, which are frequently multicentric, much earlier in life (27).

There is disagreement in the literature about whether nonfunctioning islet cell neoplasms are being diagnosed more or less frequently than functioning neoplasms. Increased use of newer and more sophisticated imaging modalities has allowed clinically silent intraabdominal masses to be identified incidentally, and many series report an increased incidence of nonfunctioning neoplasms in recent years (16, 22). Conversely, the development of very sensitive immunoassays and immunohistochemical techniques has led to the elucidation of neuroendocrine hormones produced by pancreatic islet cells, thereby allowing previously presumed "nonfunctional" neoplasms to be recognized as expressing peptide hormones that may produce clinically subtle symptoms, such as rare neoplasms releasing pancreatic polypeptide, 7B2, substance P, and neurotensin (22, 28–31). Most recent series have reported that over 50% of clinically nonfunctioning islet cell neoplasms are malignant, as evidenced by local invasion of contiguous organs, lymph node metastases, or distant hematologic metastases (12, 13, 16).

Cystic islet cell neoplasms remain sufficiently rare to be reportable. Approximately 70 cases have been reported to date. Occasionally, these neoplasms are functioning, which may help lead to their recognition, and typically the lesion described is only partially cystic with an associated extrinsic solid component. In our most recent institutional report of 64 patients with islet cell neoplasms, 34 (53%) neoplasms were nonfunctional, and 2 were cystic (24).

## CLINICAL PRESENTATION

Nonfunctioning islet cell neoplasms cause symptoms similar to those with exocrine neoplasms of the pancreas. Generally, the clinical presentation is related to the anatomic location of the lesion. Divergent observations exist about whether the interval from onset of symptoms to diagnosis differs in patients with nonfunctioning neoplasms and those with functional neoplasms. Most reviews, including our own, have not noted any significant difference in the interval to diagnosis between functioning and nonfunctioning neoplasms (24). Several series, however, suggest a longer time to diagnosis in individuals with nonfunctioning neoplasms and have attributed this difference to the more insidious onset of signs and symptoms in this patient group. In contrast to most ductal adenocarcinomas of the pancreas, islet cell neoplasms manifest a different natural history with a slower growth and more gradual development of symptoms related to the mass effect of the primary lesion (32). Many small (≤1 cm) functional islet cell neoplasms can cause systemic symptoms without the development of gastrointestinal or biliary obstruction related to the primary site of origin. Broughan et al. (33) actually observed a significantly shorter median duration of symptoms (6 months) to the time of diagnosis in 21 patients with nonfunctioning neoplasms than in 63 individuals with functioning neoplasms (22 and 36 months for insulinomas and gastrinomas, respectively).

Practically speaking, this interval is clinically unimportant. The critical variable is the duration of the neoplasm before the onset of symptoms or diagnosis. For benign islet cell neoplasms, this interval can often be quite long, as evidenced by functioning benign islet cell neoplasms that have produced a clinical syndrome for months (or years) before the correct diagnosis is reached (14). One would presume that malignant islet cell neoplasms would produce symptoms earlier than the benign lesions, because of a different rate and pattern of growth. The question of whether a benign islet cell neoplasm can undergo malignant transformation remains unanswered, but this phenomenon has been suggested (27).

Most patients with symptoms related to nonfunctional islet cell neoplasms describe a vague spectrum of complaints including nausea, vomiting, and/or abdominal pain; dyspepsia and early satiety may occur with larger neoplasms. Anorexia, malaise, and weight loss are more common with malignant neoplasms. Altered bowel habits such as constipation or steatorrhea may be present but are more common in the setting of ductal adenocarcinoma. As discussed above, these symptoms may have been present for a considerable time prior to diagnosis. Lesions of the head of the pancreas may obstruct the intrapancreatic portion of the common bile duct and cause jaundice, or by "irritating" the intrapancreatic nerves, they may induce back pain, but much less commonly than with ductal adenocarcinomas, which display a distinct predisposition to infiltrate intrapancreatic nerve sheaths (34). Neoplasms arising in the body and tail of the gland present more insidiously, often as a palpable mass. Back pain or upper gut obstructive symptoms related to involvement of the duodenal-jejunal junction may also occur. Gastrointestinal bleeding secondary to direct involvement of the stomach has been reported rarely as a presenting sign of a nonfunctioning islet cell neoplasm (12, 17, 35). It is also not uncommon to identify an islet cell neoplasm inadvertently during abdominal exploration for an unrelated problem; several nonfunctioning and cystic pancreatic islet cell neoplasms have been reported in the setting of elective gastric and biliary surgical procedures for both unrelated and previously unsuspected symptoms (14, 17, 36).

## DIAGNOSIS

Developing a differential diagnosis and determining the correct underlying pathologic entity requires a careful history and physical examination as well as appropriate clinical suspicion. Patients should be questioned about the duration of their symptoms, clinical performance status, family history of similar problems, or the familial occurrence of MEN-1 syndrome. Functional lesions causing hyperglycemia (glucagonoma, somatostatinoma), hypoglycemia and associated psychologic aberrancies (insulinoma), peptic ulcer disease (gastrinoma) or severe diarrhea (gastrinoma, or watery diarrhea, hypokalemia, achlorhydria (WDHA) syndrome), should in large part be ruled out by a careful clinical history. Physical examination should assess the patient's nutritional status, skin color (jaundice), and the presence of any atypical dermatologic conditions such as migratory necrolytic erythema (glucagonoma) and adenopathy (supraclavicular, periumbilical). The abdomen should be palpated for masses. The extremities should be observed for edema or evidence of thrombotic phenomena.

Typically, patients will note many months of symptoms prior to seeking medical attention. Following a precise history and physical examination, the laboratory evaluation should include an analysis of liver enzymes and, when indicated, serum immunoassays for insulin, glucagon, gastrin, somatostatin, or pancreatic polypeptide if a functioning islet cell neoplasm is suspected. On occasion, a serum screen for these peptide hormones may be of therapeutic use at a later stage in determining the need for further therapy in patients with a clinically nonfunctioning islet cell neoplasm or in evaluating prognosis.

A collected summation of previous reviews indicates that the most common symptoms and signs of nonfunctioning islet cell neoplasms include abdominal pain, jaundice, weight loss, and a palpable abdominal mass (12–14, 33, 35, 37, 38). Infrequently, gastrointestinal bleeding secondary to left-sided (sinistral) portal hypertension from splenic vein thrombosis or direct tumor involvement of the stomach has been noted (12, 17, 23, 25, 35). Ten to 15% of lesions were discovered incidentally by radiologic imaging or during operative exploration for other intraabdominal indications.

An important clinical situation involves the differential diagnosis of a solid mass lesion in the pancreas. Several points are relevant and of potential importance for making the diagnosis of nonfunctioning islet cell neoplasms. Because these lesions are so much less common than ductal lesions, a high index of suspicion must be maintained when evaluating a patient with extrahepatic biliary obstruction with a large mass in the head of the pancreas or the individual with a large mass in the body or tail of the gland and systemic symptoms (e.g., weight loss, abdominal pain). The differential diagnosis must include islet cell neoplasms, since the treatment plan and the "aggressiveness" of the surgical approach will vary depending on the cell of origin of the mass. It would be a serious mistake to assume that the lesion necessarily represents the much more common ductal adenocarcinoma and to deny the patient with an unsuspected islet cell neoplasm a potentially curative operation.

The differential diagnosis of cystic lesions of the pancreas is extensive and has been thoroughly reviewed elsewhere (7). Certainly, pancreatic pseudocysts represent the most common cystic entity within the pancreas. Pseudocysts are typically associated with pain and a history of pancreatic inflammation or trauma. However, among the group of "cystic neoplasms of the pancreas," cystic islet cell neoplasms must be considered. Functioning neoplasms can be apparent clinically and evaluated as described above. Nonfunctioning cystic islet cell neoplasms account for 19 of the 26 patients in the most recent 10 reports (24, 36, 39–46). The diagnosis is usually not made until the time of surgical resection. Analysis of cyst fluid has not helped to differentiate these lesions from other cystic neoplasms, but institutional experience is limited.

## Conditions Associated with Islet Cell Neoplasms

One current authority (N. Thompson) has stated that "all patients with MEN I have pancreatic neoplasms" (27). Indeed, such patients have been found to have a high incidence of pancreatic islet cell neoplasms, which are often multiple. Almost all MEN-1 patients develop primary hyperparathyroidism as the initial presentation of their disease. Pancreatic islet cell neoplasms tend to present 1–2 decades after parathyroid pathology develops. Islet cell neoplasms are most commonly functioning, but nonfunctioning neoplasms have been recognized with increasing frequency. Several other disease states, including the von Hippel-Lindau syndrome (47), von Recklinghausen's disease (48), and tuberous sclerosis (49) have also been associated with development of pancreatic islet cell neoplasms. The most recent review from our institution included a total of 64 patients, 6 of whom had MEN-1, and 1 with the von Hippel-Lindau syndrome (24).

## Imaging Techniques

A wide variety of radiologic imaging techniques has been evaluated in the preoperative localization of pancreatic neoplasms. Although real-time (8–10 MHz) transabdominal *ultrasonography* is one of the least costly noninvasive direct imaging techniques available in most hospitals, it is considerably more operator dependent than other imaging modalities such as computerized tomography (CT). Transabdominal ultrasonography has been reported to be 20–70% accurate in identifying the anatomic location of islet cell neoplasms (50). These lesions often demonstrate less echogenicity and a finer parenchymal texture than normal pancreatic tissue (Fig. 82.1); however the ability of ultrasonography to differentiate islet cell neoplasms from the more common pancreatic exocrine neoplasms is unreliable, as it usually is with other imaging techniques as well (50, 51).

Computerized tomography (CT) is currently the "gold standard" for evaluation of pancreatic masses. Over 90% of pancreatic neoplasms 2.5 cm or larger will be localized by use of the more updated CT scanners (Fig. 82.2), particularly when a spiral scanner is used and 4–5 mm sections are obtained through the pancreas. The accuracy and sensitivity of CT in the evaluation of pancreatic masses drop significantly when the lesions are smaller than 2.5 cm (50, 52). Islet cell neoplasms are typically found to be hyperdense after administration of an intravenous contrast agent, relative to normal pancreatic tissue, probably because of their hypervascularity. In contrast, ductal adenocarcinomas of the pancreas are often relatively hypodense (32). Calcification within the mass implies chronicity and suggests the diagnosis of nonfunctional islet cell neoplasm, though this is neither a consistent finding (53) nor one limited exclusively to islet cell neoplasms. CT and ultrasonography may be used in a complementary fashion to stage the lesion by evaluating the liver for metastases, determining the proximity of the pancreatic mass to adjacent organs and mesenteric vessels, and detecting the presence of suspicious lymphadenopathy.

Once imaged, pancreatic masses may safely undergo percutaneous biopsy or fine-needle aspiration if clinically indicated (50, 54). While we do not routinely obtain nor advocate fine-needle aspiration biopsies of clinically resectable pancreatic masses (55), certain situations may warrant obtaining tissue confirmation of the cell of origin *if it will affect or change the proposed treatment*. Since islet cell neoplasms are less aggressive than ductal cancers, obtaining a percutaneous biopsy confirming an islet cell neoplasm may encourage an attempted surgical resection when this approach might not be warranted for a ductal cancer. This is particularly appropriate for large masses in the head of the gland or masses in the body or tail of the gland. We reserve biopsy for patients who would not otherwise undergo surgical exploration.

Magnetic resonance imaging (MRI) has been evaluated in the diagnosis and staging of pancreatic islet cell neoplasms but with disappointing results to date. Because of their hypervascularity, some pancreatic islet cell neoplasms, particularly insulinomas, demonstrate a lower signal intensity on T1 images and a higher intensity using T2-weighted signals than the surrounding normal pancreatic and hepatic parenchyma (51). In contrast, Wise et al. (56) reported that for detecting gastrinomas, which more often do not demonstrate hypervascularity, the sensitivity of MRI was only about 20%, although a specificity of nearly 100% was observed. Additional investigation by Frucht et al. has confirmed these suboptimal results (57). Experience using MRI for nonfunctioning islet cell neoplasms is limited but probably depends on the extent of vascularity of the neoplasm.

Angiography has also been used to localize islet cell neoplasms on the basis of hypervascularity. A persistent blush of contrast agent 4–8 seconds after infusion strongly suggests an islet cell neoplasm as opposed to a ductal cancer (Fig. 82.3) (33, 51, 58). Angiographic localization of functioning islet cell neoplasms by use of selective celiac and/or superior mesenteric arterial injections has been successful in 50–75% of patients, including 6 of 8 nonfunctioning neoplasms described by Broughan et al. (33). When evaluated systematically, the combination of angiography and CT correctly localized 95% of islet cell neoplasms preoperatively. Whether both modalities are needed in all patients is controversial. Usually when CT shows a pancreatic mass presumed to be a nonfunctional islet cell neoplasm, arteriography is not warranted unless there is a question of invasion of a major vascular structure. Even then, many pancreatic surgeons would attempt en bloc resection with vascular reconstruction if appropriate, because of the better prognosis offered by islet cell neoplasms.

Endoscopic retrograde cholangiopancreatography (ERCP) is often used in the evaluation of pancreatic masses, but the information gained is not always useful and does not stage the extent of disease or alter the decision for surgical intervention (55). Findings described include a double duct sign in which both the common bile duct and pancreatic ducts are obstructed, as is more commonly seen with ductal cancers (59). Because islet cell neoplasms do not arise from the epithelium of the pancreatic duct, the main pancreatic duct, instead of being strictured, may be displaced, draped over the mass, or extrinsically narrowed, findings that would be distinctly unusual with ductal adenocarcinoma, which manifests as a circumferential stricture or a complete obstruction. Warshaw and colleagues have described a spectrum of ERCP findings associated with cystic neoplasms that includes pancreatic ductal draping, extrinsic compression, and frank obstruction, all of which may occur with islet cell neoplasms as well (60). Objective information from ERCP regarding the pathologic identity or cell of origin, however, is

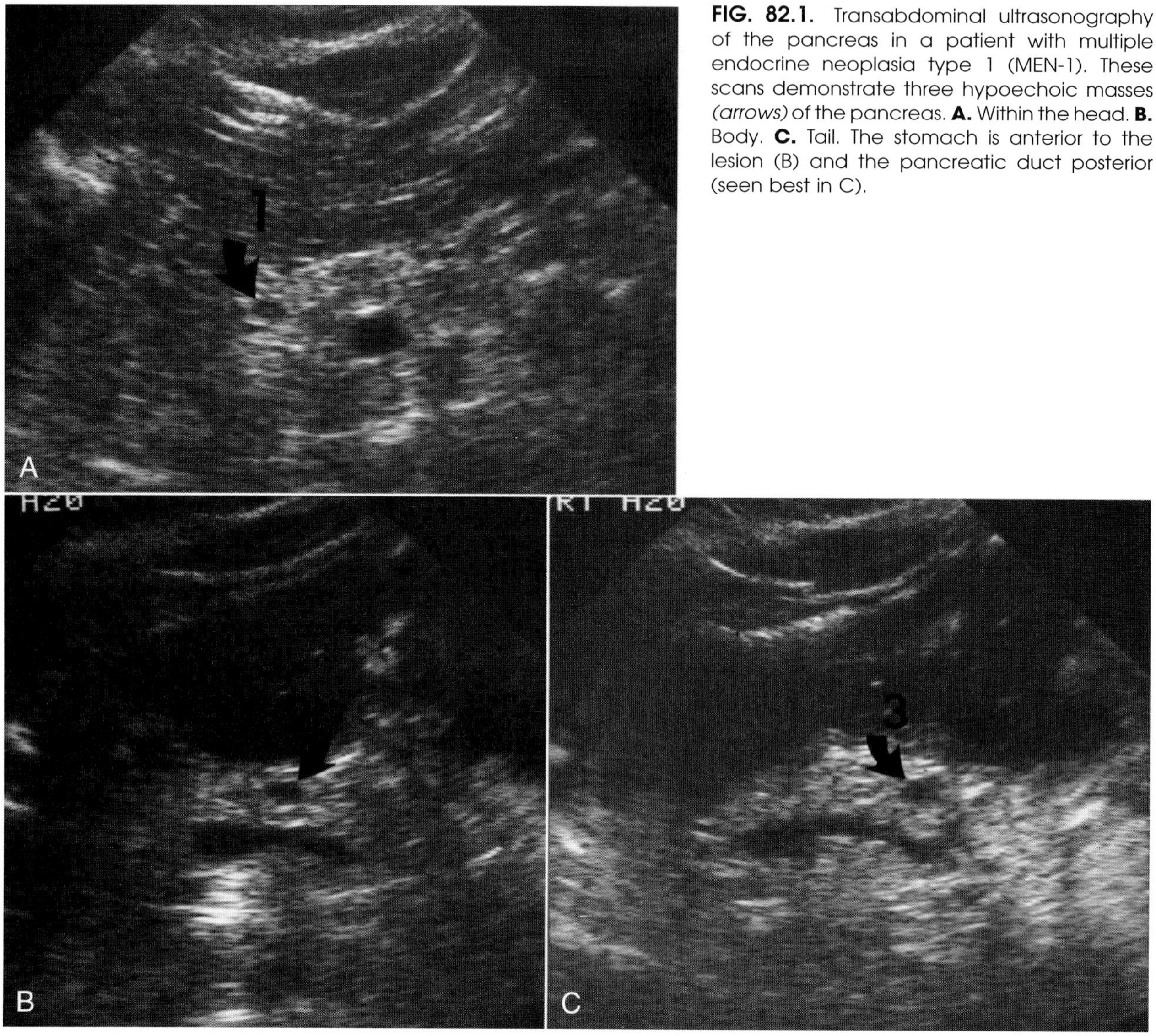


**FIG. 82.1.** Transabdominal ultrasonography of the pancreas in a patient with multiple endocrine neoplasia type 1 (MEN-1). These scans demonstrate three hypoechoic masses *(arrows)* of the pancreas. **A.** Within the head. **B.** Body. **C.** Tail. The stomach is anterior to the lesion (B) and the pancreatic duct posterior (seen best in C).

rarely gained, as blind brushings and biopsies usually miss islet cell neoplasms. If the tissue specimens are negative for malignancy, this information cannot be used to exclude the diagnosis of ductal adenocarcinoma because of the low sensitivity of these techniques.

Endoscopic ultrasonography (EUS) is a newer imaging modality that is gaining in popularity and offers novel and potential applications (61). Glover et al. described 21 patients in whom EUS was evaluated prospectively (62). This modality had a sensitivity of 79%, versus 14% and 21% for transabdominal ultrasonography and CT, respectively (Fig. 82.4). These results were even more impressive because this series involved relatively small neoplasms (0.6–4 cm) not clearly or reliably imaged by other means. Rosch et al. (63) reported a similar improvement in results comparing EUS with transabdominal imaging and angiography; a sensitivity of 82% and specificity of 95% were noted with EUS for neoplasms ranging from 0.5 to 2.5 cm in this multicenter study. EUS is notably inaccurate for imaging lesions in the pancreatic tail near the splenic hilum. This area is considered a relative "blind spot" with EUS.

Ultrasonography may also be used intraoperatively, as discussed below, but it is usually of more use in patients with

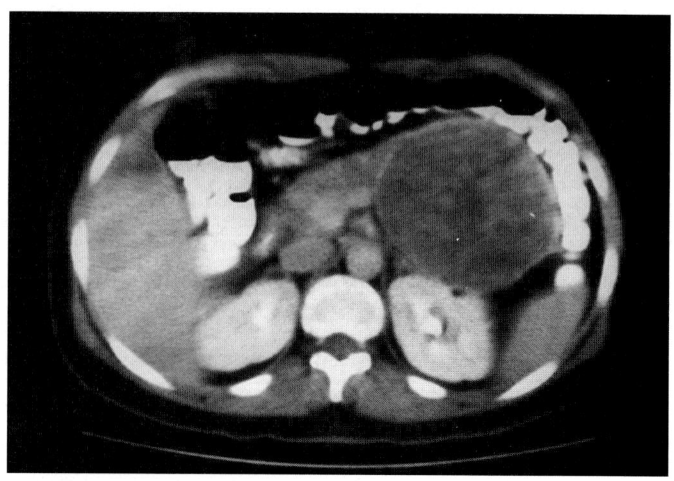

**FIG. 82.2.** CT with intravenous and oral contrast demonstrates a large, partially cystic mass in the tail of the pancreas. The patient underwent complete resection of this neoplasm, and has been without evidence of disease for over 5 years.

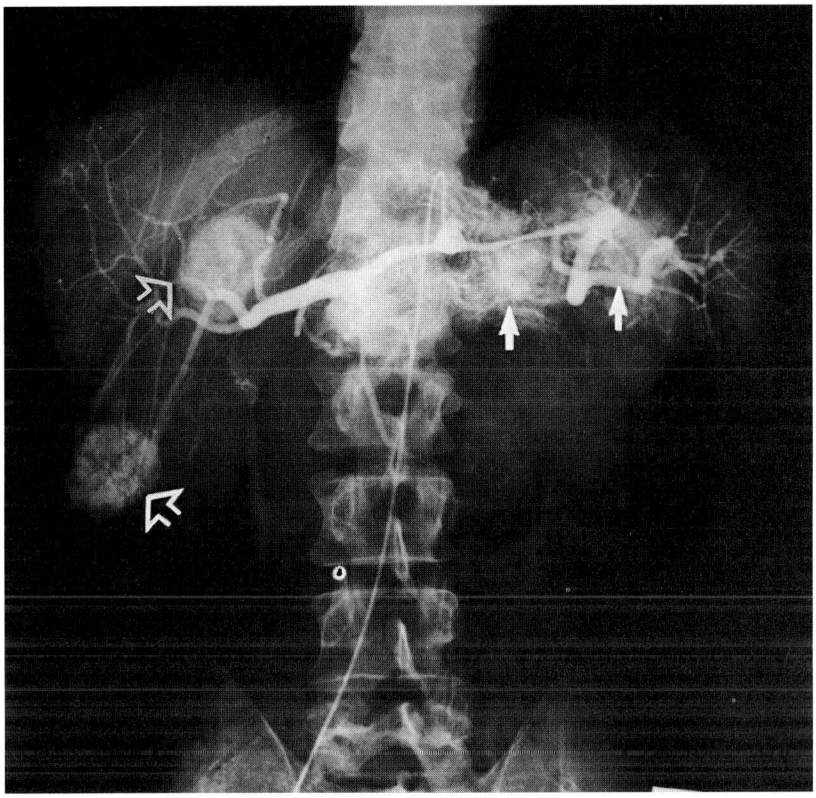

**FIG. 82.3.** A transfemoral mesenteric angiogram with celiac injection demonstrates contrast blushes *(arrows)* involving branches of the splenic and hepatic arteries due to a vascular islet cell carcinoma. The neoplasm encases both the splenic and hepatic arteries. Multiple vascular hepatic metastases are also illustrated.

clinically suspected, functioning islet cell neoplasms (see Chapter 77) (64). In patients with nonfunctioning islet cell neoplasms, one might envision using intraoperative ultrasonography to demonstrate occult hepatic metastases prior to resection or to delineate anatomic relationships between the lesion and the pancreatic duct or mesenteric vessels (Fig. 82.5). Use of intraoperative ultrasonography to screen for multiple islet cell neoplasms would be of little benefit except in patients with the hereditary syndromes predisposing to multicentric islet cell neoplasms (MEN-1, von Hippel-Lindau, von Recklinghausen disease, etc.).

One of the more recently described modalities for localization of otherwise clinically occult neuroendocrine neoplasms involves the radioisotope-labeled somatostatin analogues octreotide and pentatreotide (65–67). A growing experience has been gained with this technique. Even with clinically nonfunctioning islet cell neoplasms, initial reports suggest up to 80% of lesions are visualized. This modality might be of more potential use in patients with a nonfunctioning islet cell neoplasm to detect the presence of distant metastases that might preclude resection.

## PATHOLOGY

Nonfunctioning islet cell neoplasms are usually quite large by the time of diagnosis, ranging from 2 to 15 cm in most series. Their large size is probably due to their presentation by a local mass effect rather than by a systemic syndrome as occurs with functioning islet cell neoplasms or major constitutional symptoms as with ductal carcinomas of the pancreas. Although these neoplasms may arise anywhere in the parenchyma of the gland, most reports have identified a preponderance of lesions in the head region (13, 14). The gross appearance of islet cell neoplasms is a firm, pale white or yellow mass that may be associated with a moderate degree of surrounding fibrosis (Fig. 82.6). Cystic areas within these neoplasms are believed to arise from ischemia, necrosis, and/or degeneration within the mass (40, 68). Rarely an islet cell neoplasm can be a large cystic mass; the cyst walls may be incompletely epithelialized, hyalinized, or partially hemorrhagic, making frozen section histologic determination difficult for the unwary pathologist (36, 41).

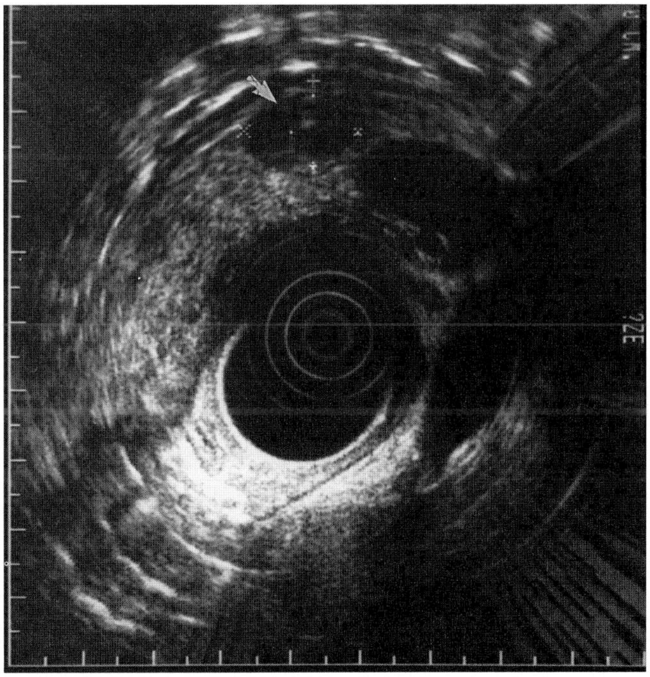

**FIG. 82.4.** An endoscopic ultrasound demonstrates a 1.2 by 1.6 cm hypoechoic islet cell neoplasm *(arrow)* in the neck of the pancreas, adjacent to the pancreatic duct.

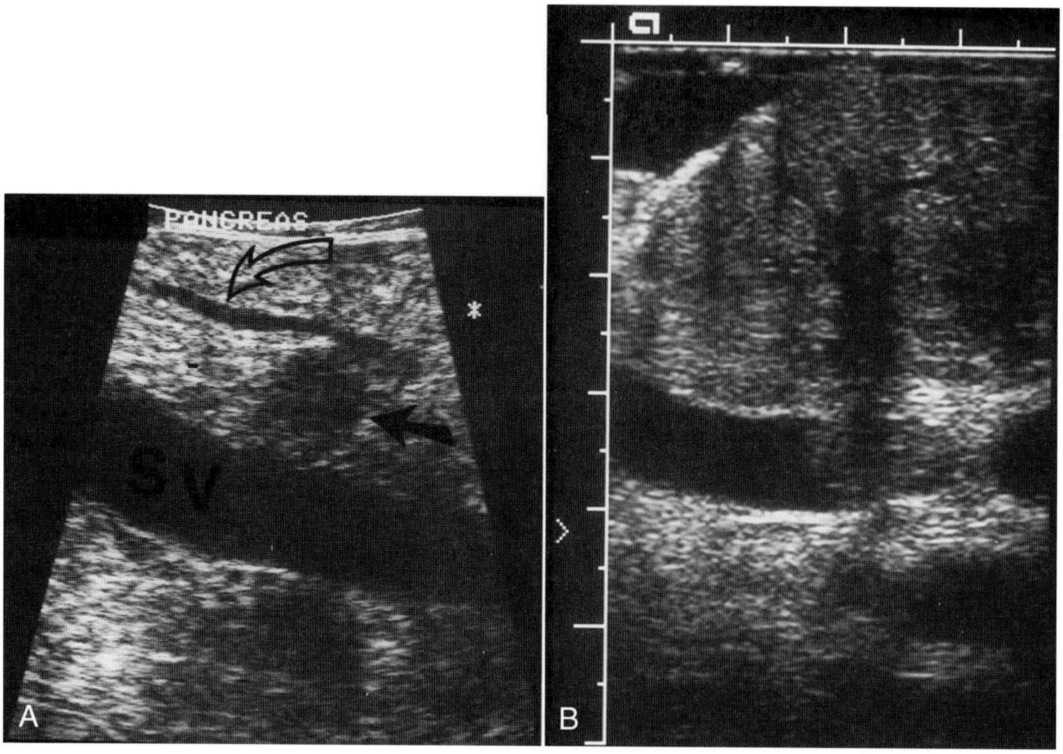


**FIG. 82.5.** **A.** Intraoperative ultrasound of an islet cell neoplasm demonstrates the position of the lesion *(dark arrow)* in the tail of the pancreas between the pancreatic duct *(open arrow)* anteriorly and the splenic vein *(SV)* posteriorly and superiorly. **B.** Intraoperative ultrasound of a large islet cell carcinoma that demonstrates tumor extension into the splenic vein *(arrow)* at the confluence with the superior mesenteric vein *(arrow)*. Complete resection was not possible because of extensive vascular and retroperitoneal involvement of this tumor.

Islet cell neoplasms are neuroendocrine in origin and thus characteristically appear as strands or cords of monotonous-appearing cells of uniform size within a vascular stroma, the so-called starry sky. Mitotic activity is infrequent, even with the obviously invasive islet cell carcinomas (Fig. 82.7). The firm determination of malignancy or benignity is virtually impossible histologically (22). Due to the histologic uncertainty, assignment of a histologic grade is not typically applicable to these cells. Unlike ductal adenocarcinomas, perineural or vascular invasion is rare and is an unreliable predictor of the biologic aggressiveness of islet cell carcinomas, but on occasion, it may be the only criterion by which malignancy can be determined (12). More commonly, the differentiation of an islet cell carcinoma and its benign counterpart is made by the gross findings of direct invasion of adjacent structures or metastatic spread to surrounding lymph nodes or the liver.

### Neuroendocrine Origin

The histologic appearance of islet cell neoplasms on routine hematoxylin and eosin stains is quite suggestive of neuroendocrine cells, but objective confirmation requires further analyses because poorly differentiated adenocarcinomas or lymphomas may have a similar appearance. Transmission electron microscopy will usually reveal dense granules containing secretory products, even in clinically nonfunctional islet cell neoplasms.

Immunohistochemical analysis has proven to be one of the more reliable means of confirming the suspicion of neuroendocrine cell origin. Stains for neural markers such as neuron-specific enolase, synaptophysin, and chromogranin will establish the diagnosis of a neuroendocrine cell and thus of an islet cell neoplasm for masses arising in the pancreas (69). Over 90% of nonfunctioning islet cell neoplasms demonstrate immunohis-

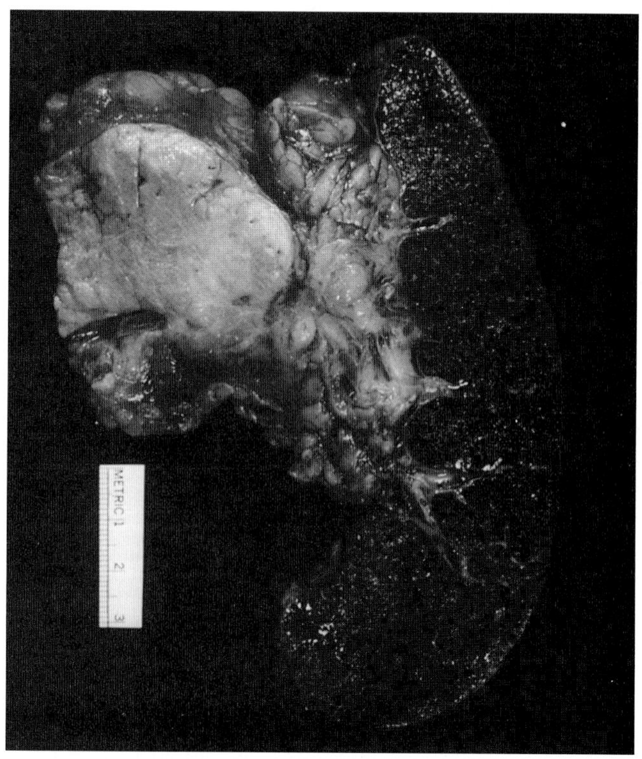

**FIG. 82.6.** Distal pancreatectomy and splenectomy specimen of an islet cell neoplasm arising in the tail of the pancreas. The tumor has a characteristic tan color and firm, scirrhous consistency.

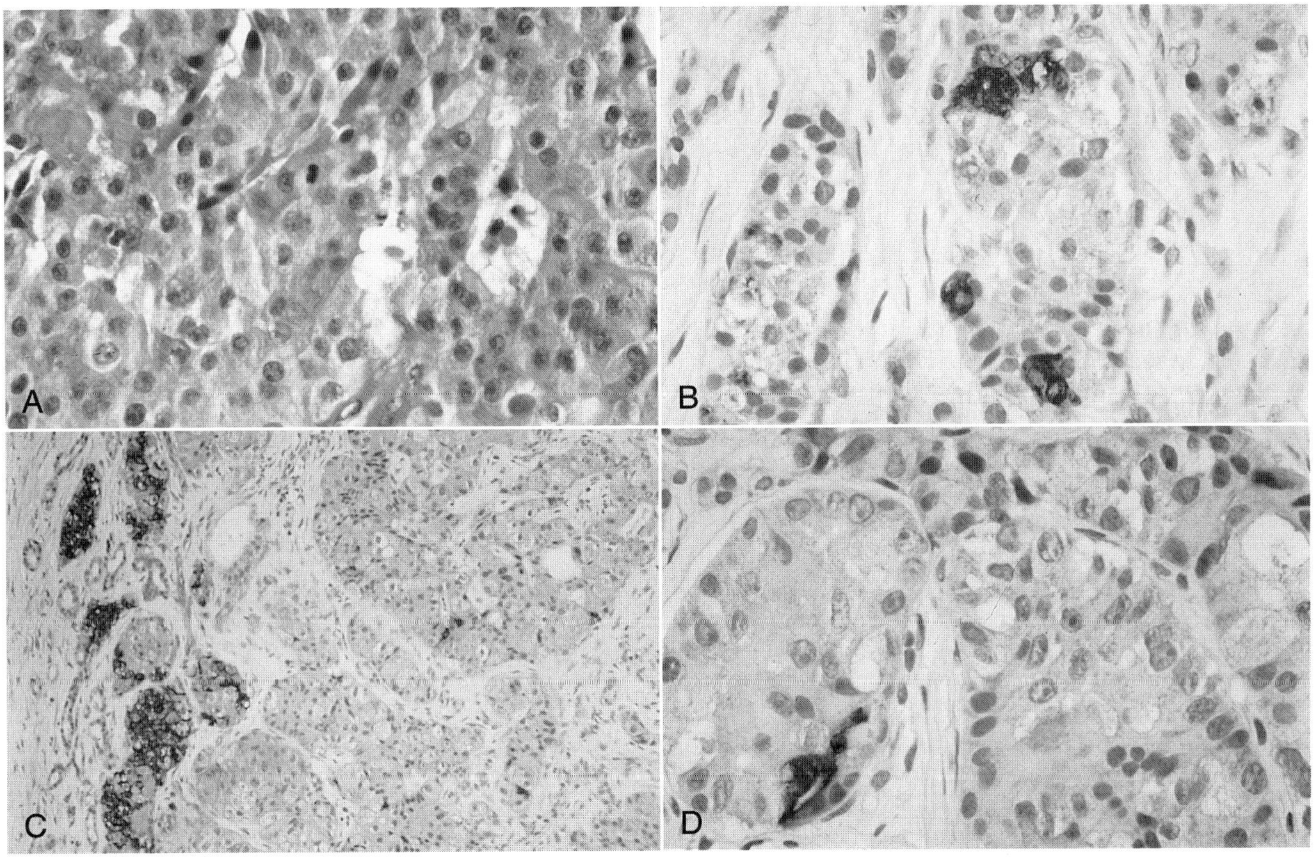


**FIG. 82.7.** Hematoxylin and eosin section of a resected nonfunctional islet cell carcinoma (**A**) in the tail of the pancreas, which demonstrates a monotonous appearing arrangement of islets without significant mitotic activity. The diagnosis of carcinoma was based on gross and microscopic invasion of the splenic vein. The neoplasm stained positively for (**B**) somatostatin, (**C**) insulin, and (**D**) gastrin. See color insert.

tochemical positivity for these relatively specific stains (22). The differential diagnosis of metastatic masses in the lymph nodes or the liver must also include carcinoid tumors, pheochromocytomas, and neoplasms of neural origin.

In addition to neural markers, many clinically "nonfunctional" islet cell neoplasms also stain positively for multiple pancreatic endocrine hormones when investigated immunohistochemically, despite normal serum concentrations of these peptides (Fig. 82.7, *B* to *D*). For instance, Heitz et al. (22) described the immunohistochemical profile of 125 islet cell neoplasms. Of the 30 nonfunctional islet cell neoplasms, 15 stained positive for insulin, 10 for glucagon, 4 for somatostatin, and 23 for pancreatic polypeptide. Indeed, most nonfunctioning islet cell neoplasms have cells that stain positively for multiple pancreatic endocrine hormones. In addition to immunohistochemical techniques, more sensitive molecular tools such as in situ hybridization have been used to recognize messenger RNA for pancreatic endocrine peptides within these neoplasms (70).

## SURGICAL THERAPY

Islet cell neoplasms of the pancreas are slow-growing neoplasms, and a substantial proportion of patients with metastatic disease survive 5 years and longer, even with bulky or widespread metastatic disease. Therefore, in contrast to a more nihilistic approach adopted by some surgeons toward the surgical treatment of ductal adenocarcinoma of the pancreas, especially when metastatic, an aggressive attitude regarding resection, be it curative or palliative, is appropriately held by the surgical community regarding the management of islet cell neoplasms. Most series report that 25–40% of lesions are amenable to curative resection, while nearly 60% of nonfunctioning islet cell neoplasms demonstrate metastatic spread at the time of exploration (13, 15, 24, 32, 71). Of those patients with metastatic or locally unresectable (for cure) disease, many individuals will receive significant palliation by biliary and/or duodenal bypass or by a controlled debulking procedure.

### Curative Resections

A very aggressive operative approach is warranted for islet cell neoplasms, in contrast to ductal adenocarcinomas. Even very large tumors that would be clearly unresectable if of ductal cell origin may prove worthy of resection when known to be of islet cell origin. Islet cell neoplasms tend to be "pushers" rather than "invaders." Whereas ductal adenocarcinomas tend to directly invade adjacent structures such as the duodenum or the portal/superior mesenteric venous confluence, islet cell neoplasms more commonly displace adjacent structures without directly invading them. For instance, Figure 82.8 demonstrates CT *(A)* and angiography (*B* and *C*) of a young woman with a very large nonfunctioning islet cell cancer. Preoperative evaluation showed almost total occlusion of the superior mesenteric vein with the development of very large collateral veins, obviously a process that had been developing for a long time. Despite the size of the lesion and the concern regarding patency of the proximal superior mesenteric vein, the neoplasm proved resectable by a pancreatoduodenectomy and had not invaded but rather extrinsically compressed and functionally obstructed the superior mesenteric vein. Thus, in the absence of known metastatic disease, the size of the primary growth should not necessarily preclude an attempt at curative resection.

The anatomic site of the primary growth will dictate the appropriate type of resection. Unlike insulinomas, which are usually benign and small (<2 cm) and thus often treated by enucleation, nonfunctioning islet cell neoplasms, because of their size and propensity to be malignant, should be managed by a formal pancreatectomy. Rare exceptions might include small neoplasms found incidentally, especially in the head of the pancreas, or small lesions in patients deemed unfit for a major pancreatic resection because of comorbid conditions. All others are best managed by a formal resection.

Nonfunctioning islet cell neoplasms in the body/tail of the gland are best treated by a distal pancreatectomy; while a splenic preserving resection would be technically feasible, the concern for malignancy should argue against this approach. Local involvement of the transverse mesocolon, the stomach, the left adrenal gland, or Gerota's fascia should be removed en bloc. An aggressive attempt at complete resection should be considered even for bulky neoplasms of the proximal body of the pancreas in close proximity to the celiac axis. Unlike for ductal adenocarcinomas in this region, in the absence of distant disease, resection of the celiac axis with reimplantation or revascularization of the common hepatic artery should be considered, albeit rarely.

For neoplasms involving the neck, head, or uncinate process of the pancreas, a pancreatoduodenectomy is warranted (18). While a pylorus-preserving resection remains controversial with ductal adenocarcinomas because of their infiltrative behavior (72), this latter concern does not apply to islet cell neoplasms, and thus, either a pylorus-preserving or classical Whipple-type resection is justified, depending on the surgeon's preference. Nodal metastases outside the usual field of resection (e.g., along hepatoduodenal ligament, common hepatic artery/celiac plexus, or superior mesenteric artery) should not necessarily preclude an attempt at curative resection and can be included with the specimen as a formal node dissection, as routinely performed by other groups for ductal adenocarcinoma (73). However, whether these formal lymphadenectomies should be performed routinely is doubtful and remains controversial, as is the case for ductal

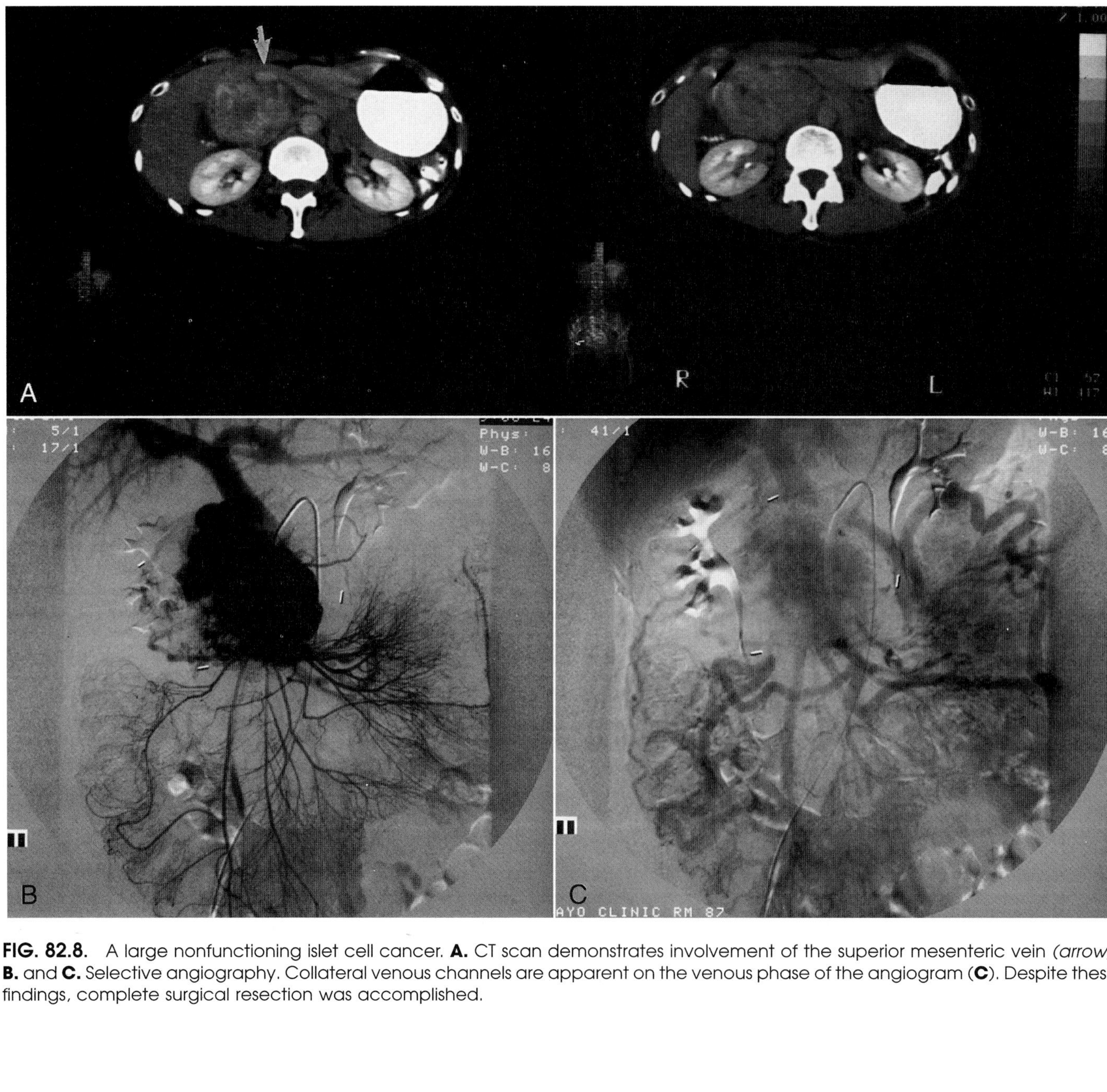


**FIG. 82.8.** A large nonfunctioning islet cell cancer. **A.** CT scan demonstrates involvement of the superior mesenteric vein *(arrow)*. **B.** and **C.** Selective angiography. Collateral venous channels are apparent on the venous phase of the angiogram (**C**). Despite these findings, complete surgical resection was accomplished.

adenocarcinoma (74). The answer to this question will only be provided by a carefully controlled, prospective randomized trial.

### Operative Palliation/Cytoreduction

Physicians and surgeons responsible for the care of patients with metastatic nonfunctioning islet cell neoplasms must not take a nihilistic approach toward their management. Because of their more indolent nature and less aggressive biologic history, consideration should be given to resecting the site of primary origin, even in the presence of distant metastases. Obviously this approach needs to be individualized, but an aggressive approach seems warranted in the good-risk patient, because patients may live for years in apparent harmony with their tumors rather than for several months as with ductal adenocarcinomas. Despite biopsy-proven hepatic metastases, prolonged survival is not unusual. Therefore, the means and extent of "palliation" become an important management consideration.

Islet cell neoplasms can be quite vascular and cause severe gastrointestinal hemorrhage by local invasion of the stomach (with lesions in the body or tail of the gland) or the duodenum (with lesions in the head or neck of the gland). Usually this complication occurs late in the course of the disease, but it can then be difficult, or with time become impossible, to manage. Other local problems related to the mass effect of the primary lesion (pain, gastrointestinal obstruction) may progress and be difficult to palliate later in the course of the disease. Primarily for these reasons, a "palliative" pancreatectomy with a known "noncurative" resection may be considered in selected patients and in experienced centers of expertise (38, 71). This resection involves either a distal pancreatectomy or a pancreatoduodenectomy, depending on the location of the neoplasm. For the more unusual diffuse, nonfunctioning islet cell neoplasms that might require a total pancreatectomy and its attendant metabolic sequelae, the decision becomes more difficult and should be individualized.

For patients with obstructive jaundice secondary to a locally "unresectable" islet cell neoplasm, strong consideration should be given to an operative biliary bypass in contrast to an endoscopically placed biliary endoprosthesis. This operative approach in islet cell neoplasms, as opposed to ductal adenocarcinoma, seems warranted because of the longer expected survival and the well-accepted superiority of operative biliary bypass for long-term control of malignant obstruction of the distal extrahepatic common bile duct. Duodenal bypass via a gastrojejunostomy should also be seriously entertained, again because of the potential for longer-term survival. Prophylactic gastrojejunostomy may be less controversial for these patients than for patients with ductal adenocarcinoma (75).

The concept of "cytoreduction" is less appropriate for the truly nonfunctioning islet cell neoplasms than for metastatic functioning islet cell neoplasms. Debulking or "cytoreduction" is designed to remove as much functioning islet cell carcinoma as possible in an attempt to palliate the systemic effects of the hormone produced, either by decreasing the absolute amount of hormone released or by allowing a more effective chemotherapeutic approach. Because nonfunctioning islet cell neoplasms exert their effect locally by their mass effect, this concept of "cytoreduction" does not truly apply to these neoplasms in the same sense. However, the concept of debulking most of the primary tumor mass, as discussed above, remains a viable therapeutic option when the primary neoplasm causes severe local problems such as bleeding.

Several selected situations require discussion. Although hepatic metastases from islet cell neoplasms are usually multiple and located throughout the liver (and, thereby, preclude curative resection), on rare occasion, the metastatic disease may be anatomically localized and surgically resectable within the liver. Under these circumstances, an attempt at curative resection should be entertained, provided that the site of primary disease can be confidently controlled; reassurance that the hepatic disease is localized should be obtained by the usual methods of preoperative imaging as well as intraoperative ultrasonography. With residual disease outside the liver, hepatic resection is unwarranted because hepatic metastases themselves rarely cause local problems; this approach is unlike the concept of hepatic cytoreduction for functioning islet cell carcinomas (76). Under rare exceptions, selected patients have undergone "cluster" resections with either isolated orthotopic hepatic transplantation (77, 78) or a so-called cluster transplant involving transplantation of a donor liver, duodenum, pancreas, and small bowel (79). This ultraradical approach has yielded controversial results (5-year tumor-free survivals of 64%), bringing into question its appropriate use in the current era of cadaveric organ shortage for recipients with nonmalignant conditions.

### Cystic Islet Cell Neoplasms

Quite often, cystic islet cell neoplasms have been diagnosed mistakenly as pancreatic pseudocysts and treated by internal drainage (41). Principles of management should be followed that pertain to all cystic lesions of the pancreas. When a cystic neoplasm is suspected by the presence of an associated eccentric mass, primary resection should be undertaken under the presumption that this lesion represents a primary pancreatic neoplasm with secondary cystic degeneration. The appropriate management of a presumed pancreatic pseudocyst to be drained internally should almost always warrant a satisfactory biopsy of the wall of the pseudocyst in an attempt to avoid the inappropriate treatment of a cystic neoplasm.

### Multiple Endocrine Neoplasia Type 1

The surgical management of patients with islet cell neoplasms in the setting of the hereditary familial disorder of MEN-1 is controversial. In theory, the entire parenchyma containing islet cell tissue is "at risk." These patients often harbor multicentric neoplasms throughout the gland, functioning and/or nonfunctioning (27). This preneoplastic and overtly neoplastic tendency presents the following difficult dilemma: at the time of operative intervention for a known islet cell neoplasm, should one perform a total pancreatectomy to remove all the tissue at risk (80)? Total pancreatectomy necessitates the certain unavoidable metabolic complications of complete endocrine and exocrine insufficiency, as well as the potential long-term development of hepatic cirrhosis, presumably secondary to loss of the intraportal release of the poorly understood pancreatic trophic factors (81). Total pancreatectomy should be reserved for those patients in whom it is technically necessary to extirpate all overt disease. This clinical situation may be one in which strong consideration is given to enucleation of smaller neoplasms if technically feasible. Most authorities and reviews have suggested that the incidence of malignancy of nonfunctioning islet cell neoplasms in the setting of MEN-1 is not greater than in the setting of sporadic disease (27, 70, 82).

## CHEMOTHERAPY

### Therapeutic

Chemotherapy for nonfunctioning islet cell carcinomas follows many of the same principles used for functioning islet cell carcinomas, with one major exception. For functioning islet cell neoplasms, the somatostatin analogue octreotide has been used primarily to decrease the release of the peptide hormone produced by the neoplasm and to decrease the effect of the peptide on the target organ (e.g., acid release by gastrin from the parietal cell). While there have been rare patients in whom octreotide appears to have had an antineoplastic effect with tumor regression or stabilization, most often octreotide has been used to palliate the effects of excessive production and release of peptide hormones. With nonfunctioning islet cell neoplasms, there is little or no evidence that patients derive symptomatic or survival benefit from the use of octreotide (83, 84).

The primary chemotherapeutic agent used in nonfunctioning islet cell neoplasms is streptozotocin in combination with other cytotoxic agents. Moertel et al. (85) conducted a multicenter trial of chemotherapy for advanced islet cell carcinoma. Streptozotocin in combination with doxorubicin was associated with the greatest tumor response (69%) and longest median survival (2.2 years). Obviously, this regimen and similar protocols are associated with significant toxicity, including vomiting, diarrhea, bone marrow suppression, and renal toxicity.

### Adjuvant/Neoadjuvant Therapy

In contrast to ductal adenocarcinoma of the pancreas in which adjuvant chemoradiation therapy appears to increase survival (86), no such data exist for islet cell neoplasms, probably in part because no single institution has treated enough patients to conduct a definitive study. Concerning neoadjuvant treatment, although it does not appear indicated for clinically resectable islet cell neoplasms, there may be a role, at least in theory, for a course of preoperative (neoadjuvant) chemotherapy in patients with very large masses that demonstrate objective signs of being unresectable on imaging tests. Another possible role is in patients who are explored and found to have locally unresectable disease; one might consider reexploration at a later date if there was marked tumoricidal response. This latter approach is obviously an experimental one that would require special circumstances and mature surgical judgment.

## PROGNOSIS

In sharp contrast to pancreatic exocrine neoplasms, long-term survival is the rule rather than the exception for patients with islet cell neoplasms, often despite the presence of biopsy-proven liver metastases. Most series, including our own most recent review, have not detected a survival difference between functional and nonfunctioning islet cell neoplasms (24). However, the 1986 review of Broughan et al. (33) reported a 10-year survival of 50% for nonfunctioning neoplasms, compared with 68 and 92% for gastrinomas and insulinomas, respectively. The most important predictors of survival are the degree of local and distant spread of the lesion and whether or not the tumor is completely resected. Cystic islet cell neoplasms behave like their solid counterparts in biologic aggressiveness, and the same criteria apply in assessing prognosis and clinical outcome.

Evans et al. (32) divided patients into four groups on the basis of the presence of distant disease and feasibility of resection. Patients without distant metastases in whom a curative resection was performed had a 5-year survival of 72% and a median survival of 6.8 years, whereas individuals with distant metastases who did not undergo resection had a 5-year survival of 38% and a median survival of 3.3 years (32). The recent report of White et al. (13) specifically addressed prognosis in patients with functional versus nonfunctional islet cell carcinomas. Those with nonfunctional neoplasms had a 67% disease-free survival 2 years from the time of diagnosis. These survival data did not differ from those of patients with functioning neoplasms.

## CONCLUSIONS

A variety of reasons explain why many islet cell neoplasms may be clinically silent and thus nonfunctional. Many such neoplasms secrete hormones such as pancreatic polypeptide and neurotensin that cause few or no pathognomonic systemic symptoms, or minute amounts of physiologically functional hormones. The latter may commonly occur, given the fact that the vast majority of these "nonfunctional" islet cell neoplasms contain cells that stain positively for single or multiple pancreatic endocrine hormones. It may also be possible that certain nonfunctioning neoplasms produce an inactive precursor or prohormone (20, 37). Regardless of the reason for their behavior, nonfunctioning pancreatic islet cell neoplasms remain difficult to diagnose yet often allow the host to live in relative harmony with the neoplasm for many years, despite the spread of the lesion. While the standard surgical response is to resect these neoplasms aggressively, long-term survival may occur in patients with unresected lesions. Whether hepatic transplantation for metastatic neuroendocrine malignancies will prove practical and effective is still unknown, because nonfunctioning metastatic lesions usually do not cause life-threatening complications for years after diagnosis.

The very rare cystic islet cell neoplasms, particularly the nonfunctioning subgroup, present an often unique diagnostic dilemma that may not be resolved without operative resection. The key to successful management of cystic pancreatic neoplasms is to maintain a high index of suspicion and not to mistreat these lesions as postinflammatory pseudocysts.

Nonfunctioning and cystic pancreatic islet cell neoplasms, though uncommon entities, must be included in the differential diagnosis of all pancreatic masses, solid and cystic, because of the marked difference in the treatment indicated and the potentially important therapeutic ramifications. It seems clear from the recent literature (87) that major pancreatic resections and complex foregut surgery should be undertaken primarily by individuals and institutions with substantial experience with such cases and a depth of diagnostic and therapeutic capabilities. Referral of such patients to tertiary centers is cost-effective, is associated with reduced patient morbidity, and allows such centers to continue to gain the experience necessary to allow meaningful analysis of therapeutic options involving large patient numbers.

## REFERENCES


1. Nicholls AG. Simple adenoma of the pancreas arising from an island of Langerhans. J Med Res 1902;8:385–395.
2. Fabozzi S. Ueber die Histogenese des primaren Krebes des Pankreas. Beitr Pathol 1903;34:199–214.
3. Wilder RM, Allan FN, Power MH, Robertson HE. Carcinoma of the islets of the pancreas: hyperinsulinism and hypoglycemia. JAMA 1927;89:348–355.
4. van Heerden JA, Thompson GB. Islet cell tumors of the pancreas. In: Trede M, Carter DC, eds. Surgery of the pancreas. London: Churchill Livingstone, 1993:545–561.
5. Zanetti G. Contributo allo studio dei tumori del pancreas. Arch Sci Med 1927;49(35):505–519.
6. Friesen SR. Update on the diagnosis and treatment of rare neuroendocrine tumors. Surg Clin North Am 1987;67:379–393.
7. Yeo CJ, Sarr MG. Cystic and pseudocystic diseases of the pancreas. Curr Probl Surg 1994;31:165–243.
8. Judd ES. Hyperinsulinism, its surgical treatment. JAMA 1933;101: 99–102.
9. Thigpen FM. A pathologic study of cysts of the pancreas (Thesis). Mayo Foundation, Graduate School, University of Minnesota, 1940.
10. Winston JH. Malignant islet cell adenoma in a pancreatic cyst. J Natl Med Assoc 1965;7:203–204.
11. Moldow RE, Connelly RR. Epidemiology of pancreatic cancer in Connecticut. Gastroenterology 1968;55:677–686.
12. Dial PF, Braasch JW, Rossi RL, Lee AK, Jin GL. Management of nonfunctioning islet cell tumors of the pancreas. Surg Clin North Am 1985;65:291–299.
13. White TJ, Edney JA, Thompson JS, Karrer FW, Moor BJ. Is there a prognostic difference between functional and nonfunctional islet cell tumors? Am J Surg 1994;168:627–629.

14. Kent RB III, van Heerden JA, Weiland LH. Nonfunctioning islet cell tumors. Ann Surg 1981;193:185–190.
15. Thompson GB, van Heerden JA, Grant CS, Carney JA, Ilstrup DM. Islet cell carcinomas of the pancreas: a twenty-year experience. Surgery 1988;104:1011–1017.
16. Yeo CJ, Wang BH, Anthone GJ, Cameron JL. Surgical experience with pancreatic islet cell tumors. Arch Surg 1993;128:1143–1148.
17. Debas H, Mulvihill S. Neuroendocrine gut neoplasms. Important lessons from uncommon tumors. Arch Surg 1994;129:965–971.
18. Udelsman R, Yeo CJ, Hruban RH, Pitt HA, Niederhuber JE, et al. Pancreaticoduodenectomy for selected pancreatic endocrine tumors. Surg Gynecol Obstet 1993;177:269–278.
19. Buchanan KD, Johnston CF, O'Hare MM, Ardill JE, Shaw C, et al. Neuroendocrine tumors. A European view. Am J Med 1986;81: 14–22.
20. Kloppel G, Heitz PU. Pancreatic endocrine tumors. Pathol Res Pract 1988;183:155–168.
21. Legaspi A, Brennan MF. Management of islet cell carcinoma. Surgery 1988;104:1018–1023.
22. Heitz PU, Kasper M, Polak JM, Kloppel G. Pancreatic endocrine tumors. Hum Pathol 1982;13:263–271.
23. Broder LE, Carter SK. Pancreatic islet cell carcinoma. Clinical features of 52 patients. Ann Intern Med 1973;79:101–107.
24. Lo CY, van Heerden JA, Thompson GB, Grant CS, Soreide JA, Harmsen WS. Islet cell carcinoma of the pancreas. World J Surg 1996;20:878–884.
25. Kim DG, Chejfec G, Prinz RA. Islet cell carcinoma of the pancreas. Am Surg 1989;55:325–332.
26. Eriksson B, Oberg K, Skogseid B. Neuroendocrine pancreatic tumors. Clinical findings in a prospective study of 84 patients. Acta Oncol 1989:28;373–377.
27. Thompson NW, Lloyd RV, Nishiyama RH, et al. MEN I pancreas: histological and immunohistochemical study. World J Surg 1984; 8:561–574.
28. Feurle GE, Helmstaedter V, Tischbirek K, Carraway R, Forssmann W-G, et al. A multihormonal tumor of the pancreas producing neurotensin. Dig Dis Sci 1981;26:1125–1133.
29. Iguchi H, Yasuda D, Yamada Y, Funakoshi A, Wakasugi H, et al. 7B2, a possible marker for nonfunctioning pancreatic islet cell tumor. Horm Metab Res 1991;23:486–489.
30. Tomita T, Friesen SR, Kimmel JR, Doull V, Pollock HG. Pancreatic polypeptide-secreting islet-cell tumors. Am J Pathol 1983;113: 134–142.
31. Strodel WE, Vomol AO, Lloyd RV, Glaser B, Eckhauser FE, et al. Pancreatic polypeptide-producing tumors. Arch Surg 1984;119: 508–514.
32. Evans DB, Skibber JM, Lee JE, et al. Nonfunctioning islet cell carcinoma of the pancreas. Surgery 1993;114:1175–1182.
33. Broughan TA, Leslie JD, Soto JM, Hermann RE. Pancreatic islet cell tumors. Surgery 1986;99:671–678.
34. Bockman DE, Buchler M, Beger HG. Interaction of pancreatic ductal carcinoma within nerves leads to nerve damage. Gastroenterology 1994;107:219–230.
35. Cheslyn-Curtis S, Sitaram V, Williamson RC. Management of non-functioning neuroendocrine tumours of the pancreas. Br J Surg 1993;80:625–627.
36. Davtyan H, Nieberg R, Reber HA. Pancreatic cystic endocrine neoplasms. Pancreas 1990;5:230–233.
37. Prinz RA, Badrinath K, Chejfec G, Freeark RJ, Greenlee HB. ``Nonfunctioning'' islet cell carcinoma of the pancreas. Am Surg 1983;49:345–349.
38. Eckhauser FE, Cheung PS, Vinik AI, Strodel WE, Lloyd RV, Thompson NW. Nonfunctioning malignant neuroendocrine tumors of the pancreas. Surgery 1986;100:978–988.
39. Schwartz RW, Munfakh NA, Zwqeng TN, Strodel WE, Lee E, Thompson NW. Nonfunctioning cystic neuroendocrine neoplasms of the pancreas. Surgery 1994;115:645–649.
40. Goto M, Nakano I, Sumi K, et al. Cystic insulinoma and nonfunctioning islet cell tumor in multiple endocrine neoplasia type I. Pancreas 1994;9:393–395.
41. Warshaw AL, Comptom CC, Lewandrowski K, Cardenosa G, Mueller PR. Cystic tumors of the pancreas. New clinical, radiologic, and pathologic observations in 67 patients. Ann Surg 1990;212:432–443.
42. Weissman D, Lewandrowski K, Godine J, Centeno B, Warshaw A. Pancreatic cystic islet-cell tumors. Clinical and pathologic features in two cases with cyst fluid analysis. Int J Pancreatol 1994;15:75–79.
43. Iacono C, Serio G, Fugazzola C, et al. Cystic islet cell tumors of the pancreas. A clinico-pathological report of two nonfunctioning cases and review of the literature. Int J Pancreatol 1992;11: 199–208.
44. Dhir V, Mohandas KM, Swaroop VS, et al. Cystic neoplasms of the pancreas: a heterogenous disorder. J Surg Oncol 1992;51; 246–248.
45. Turnage RH, Eckhauser FE, Vinik AI, Strodel WE, Thompson NW, et al. Diagnostic dilemmas in patients with cystic neoplasms of the pancreas. Int J Pancreatol 1988;3:477–489.
46. Thompson NW, Eckhauser FE, Vinik AI, Lloyd RV, Fiddian-Green RG, Strodel WE. Cystic neuroendocrine neoplasms of the pancreas and liver. Ann Surg 1984;199:158–164.
47. Binkovitz LA, Johnson CD, Stephens DH. Islet cell tumors in von Hippel-Lindau disease: increased prevalence and relationship to the multiple endocrine neoplasias. AJR 1990;155:501–505.
48. Swinburn BA, Yeong ML, Lane MR, Nicholson GI, Holdaway IM. Neurofibromatosis associated with somatostatinoma: a report of two patients. Clin Endocrinol 1988;28:353–359.
49. Davoren PM, Epstein MT. Insulinoma complicating tuberous sclerosis. J Neurol Neurosurg Psychiatry 1992;55:1209.
50. Fedorak IJ, Ko TC, Gordon D, Flisak M, Prinz RA. Localization of islet cell tumors of the pancreas: a review of current techniques. Surgery 1993;113:242–249.
51. King CM, Reznek RH, Dacie JE, Wass JA. Imaging islet cell tumours. Clin Radiol 1994;49:295–303.
52. Stark DD, Moss AA, Goldberg HI, Deveney CW, Way L. Computed tomography and nuclear magnetic resonance imaging of pancreatic islet cell tumors. Surgery 1983;94:1024–1027.
53. Eelkema EA, Stephens DH, Ward EM, Sheedy PF II. CT features of nonfunctioning islet cell carcinoma. AJR 1984;143:943–948.
54. Leach SD, Rose JA, Lowy AM, Lee JE, Charnsangavej C, et al. Significance of peritoneal cytology in patients with potentially resectable adenocarcinoma of the pancreatic head. Surgery 1995;118:472–478.
55. Temudom T, Sarr MG, Douglas MG, Farnell MB. Argument against routine percutaneous biopsy, ERCP, or biliary stent in patients with clinically resectable periampullary masses. A surgical perspective. Pancreas 1995;11:283–288.
56. Wise SR, Johnson J, Sparks J, Carey LC, Ellison EC. Gastrinoma: the predictive value of preoperative localization. Surgery 1989;106: 1087–1092.
57. Frucht H, Doppman JL, Norton JA, Miller DL, Dwyer AJ, et al. Gastrinomas: comparison of MR imaging with CT, angiography, and US. Radiology 1989;171:713–717.
58. Fraker D, Norton JA. The role of surgery in the management of islet cell tumors. Gastroenterol Clin North Am 1989;18:805–830.
59. Reber HA. Pancreas. In: Schwartz S, Shives GT, Spencer FC, Husse WC, eds. Principles of surgery. 6th ed. New York: McGraw-Hill, 1994:1421.
60. Gazelle GS, Mueller PR, Raafat N, Halpern EF, Cardenosa G, Warshaw AL. Cystic neoplasms of the pancreas: evaluation with endoscopic retrograde pancreatography. Radiology 1993;188: 633–636.
61. Thompson NW, Czako PF, Fritts LL, Bude R, Bansal R, et al. Role of endoscopic ultrasonography in the localization of insulinomas and gastrinomas. Surgery 1994;116:1131–1138.
62. Glover JR, Shorvon PJ, Lees WR. Endoscopic ultrasound for localisation of islet cell tumours. Gut 1992;33:108–110.
63. Rosch T, Lightdale CJ, Botet JF, et al. Localization of pancreatic endocrine tumors by endoscopic ultrasonography. N Engl J Med 1992;326:1721–1726.
64. Grant CS, van Heerden JA, Charboneau JW, James EW, Reading CC. Insulinoma: the value of intraoperative ultrasonography. Arch Surg 1988;123:843–848.
65. Lamberts SW, Reubi JC, Krenning EP. Validation of somatostatin receptor scintigraphy in the localization of neuroendocrine tumors. Acta Oncol 1993;32:167–170.
66. van Eyck CH, Bruining HA, Reubi JC, Bakker WH, Oei HY, et al. Use of isotope-labeled somatostatin analogs for visualization of islet cell tumors. World J Surg 1993;17:444–447.
67. Jamar F, Fiasse R, Leners N, Pauwels S. Somatostatin receptor

imaging with indium-111-pentatreotide in gastroenteropancreatic neuroendocrine tumors: safety, efficacy and impact on patient management. J Nucl Med 1995;36:542–549.

68. Ros PR, Hamrick-Turner JE, Chiechi MV, Ros LH, Gallego P, Burton SS. Cystic masses of the pancreas. Radiographics 1992;12: 673–686.
69. Lloyd RV, Mervak T, Schmidt K, Warner TFCS, Wilson BS. Immunohistochemical detection of chromogranin and neuron-specific enolase in pancreatic endocrine neoplasms. Am J Surg Pathol 1984;8:607–614.
70. Perkins PL, McLeod MK, Jin L, Fukuuchi A, Cho KJ, et al. Analysis of gastrinomas by immunohistochemistry and in situ hybridization histochemistry. Diagn Mol Pathol 1992;1:155–164.
71. Norton JA. Neuroendocrine tumors of the pancreas and duodenum. Curr Probl Surg 1994;31:77–156.
72. Sharp KW, Ross CB, Halter SA, et al. Pancreaticoduodenectomy with pylorus preservation for carcinoma of the pancreas: a cautionary note. Surgery 1989;105:645–653.
73. Nagakawa T, Konishi I, Ueno K, et al. Surgical treatment of pancreatic cancer: the Japanese experience. Int J Pancreatol 1991;9:135–143.
74. Reber HA, Ashley SW, McFadden D. Curative treatment for pancreatic neoplasms. Radical resection. Surg Clin North Am 1995;75:905–912.
75. Sarr MG, Cameron JL. Surgical palliation of unresectable carcinoma of the pancreas. World J Surg 1984;8:906–918.
76. Que FG, Nagorney DM, Batts KP, Linz LJ, Kvols LK. Hepatic resection for metastatic neuroendocrine carcinomas. Am J Surg 1995;169;36–43.
77. Curtiss SI, Mor E, Schwartz ME, Sung MW, Hytiroglou P, et al. A rational approach to the use of hepatic transplantation in the treatment of metastatic neuroendocrine tumors. J Am Coll Surg 1995;180:184–187.
78. Pichlmayr R, Weimann A, Oldhafer KJ, Schlitt HJ, Klempnauer J, et al. Role of liver transplantation in the treatment of unresectable liver cancer. World J Surg 1995;19:807–813.
79. Alessiani M, Tzakis A, Todo S, Demetris AJ, Fung JJ, Starzl TE. Assessment of five year experience with abdominal organ cluster transplantation. J Am Coll Surg 1995;180:1–9.
80. Tissell LE, Ahlman H, Jansson S, Grimelius L. Total pancreatectomy in the MEN syndrome. Br J Surg 1988;75:154–157.
81. Sarr MG, Behrns KE, van Heerden JA. Total pancreatectomy. An objective analysis of its use in pancreatic cancer. Hepatogastroenterology 1993;40:418–421.
82. Sheppard BC, Norton JA, Doppman JL, Maton PN. Management of islet cell tumors in patients with multiple endocrine neoplasia: a prospective study. Surgery 1989;106:1108–1118.
83. Saltz L, Trochanowski B, Buckley M, Hefferman B, Niedzwiecki D, et al. Octreotide as an antineoplastic agent in the treatment of functional and nonfunctional neuroendocrine tumors. Cancer 1993;72:244–248.
84. Eriksson B, Skogseid B, Lundqvist G, Wide L, Wilander E, Oberg K. Medical treatment and long-term survival in a prospective study of 84 patients with endocrine pancreatic tumors. Cancer 1990; 65:1883–1890.
85. Moertel CG, Lefkopoulo M, Lipsitz S, Hahn RG, Klaassen D. Streptozocin-doxorubicin, streptozocin-fluorouracil, or chlorozotocin in the treatment of advanced islet-cell carcinoma. N Engl J Med 1992;326:519–523.
86. Moertel CG, Frytak S, Hahn RG, et al. Therapy of locally unresectable pancreatic carcinoma: a randomized comparison of high dose (6000 rads) radiation alone, moderate dose radiation (4000 rads + 5-fluorouracil), and high dose radiation + 5-fluorouracil. The Gastrointestinal Tumor Study Group. Cancer 1981;48:1705.
87. Fernandez-del Castillo C, Rattner DW, Warshaw AL. Standards for pancreatic resection in the 1990's. Arch Surg 1995;130; 295–299.

# 83

# Other Rare Tumors of the Endocrine Pancreas

Romano Delcore and Stanley R. Friesen

Tumors of the endocrine pancreas, although frequently reported in the literature, remain extremely rare (1). Nevertheless, with the advent of reliable radioimmunoassays (RIAs), these neoplasms are being recognized with increasing frequency. Endocrine tumors of the pancreas constitute a heterogeneous group that, although closely related in terms of biosynthetic mechanisms, as well as histochemical and ultrastructural features, demonstrate clear-cut differences in morphology, endocrine activity, and prognosis. Even though pancreatic endocrine tumors vary in malignant potential, surgical excision after proper diagnosis and careful localization remains the only curative form of therapy available. Therapeutic strategies for the management of these neoplasms should include the following principles: *(a)* medical control of symptoms in the preoperative phase, *(b)* surgical resection of the primary neoplasm in the absence of metastases or reduction of tumor burden by aggressive surgical debulking when extensive metastases are present, *(c)* medical control of symptoms postoperatively if no tumor can be identified at laparotomy and for patients with unresectable neoplasms, *(d)* control of neoplastic growth by pharmacologic agents, chemotherapy, and tumor embolization or cryotherapy (2). Lymph node metastases should be aggressively resected, and surgical debulking is usually indicated, even when distant metastases are present. The medical treatment of unresectable or residual tumor consists of antisecretory measures, antihormonal therapy, and hormone (i.e., octreotide) or chemotherapeutic (e.g., streptozotocin) inhibition of tumor growth.

Functionally, pancreatic endocrine tumors may be entopic (orthoendocrine), producing abnormal quantities of their inherent native hormone(s); ectopic (paraendocrine), producing substances not expected to derive from those tissues; or nonfunctioning, not associated with a clinically recognizable syndrome caused by the release of peptides into the circulation despite the presence of endocrine cells on histologic examination. The term "ectopic syndrome" was first used by Liddle, who coined the adjective "ectopic" to refer to "any hormone that is produced by a neoplasm which is derived from tissue not normally engaged in the production of the hormone in question" (3). In general, neoplasms producing ectopic hormones are the more malignant, suggesting that they are more profoundly transformed and more aggressive (4).

No single hypothesis explains ectopic hormone production by pancreatic endocrine tumors. Among several suggested theories, the so-called APUD theory of A. G. E. Pearse has attracted the most attention (5). In 1968, Pearse recognized that endocrine cells distributed along the mucosa of the entire gastrointestinal (GI) tract had similar cytochemical and ultrastructural characteristics: these cells contain amines in the cytoplasm, are capable of uptake of amine precursors, and use a decarboxylating enzyme to convert these precursors to amines and/or peptides, which are stored within cytoplasmic secretory granules. He also recognized that this ability for *A*mine *P*recursor *U*ptake and *D*ecarboxylation (APUD) is shared by other cells throughout the body and postulated that these and similar cells throughout the body are all of neuroectodermal origin, implying that they all derive from the same embryonic tissue (neural crest) and constitute a diffuse neuroendocrine system acting in concert with the autonomic nervous system to control the function of all intestinal organs (5). This theory assumes that these cells differentiate from a common progenitor cell and that some metabolic features are retained that can be used to identify this relationship. Numerous neuronal markers are shared by APUD cells (6, 7). Markers found on both gastroenteropancreatic neuroendocrine cells and neurons include neuron specific enolase, a specific acetylcholinesterase, synaptophysin, receptors for tetanus toxoid, protein S-100, and chromogranins A, B, C. However, shared characteristics do not prove a common origin, and this hypothesis has been revised as recent discoveries in cell biology and cytochemistry have shed doubt on some of Pearse's original concepts. The term APUD is now considered inadequate, since several cell types included in the APUD system of cells do not metabolize amines (8). Furthermore, evidence now suggests that some APUD cell types, in particular, the gastroenteropancreatic neuroendocrine cells, are not of neural crest origin but are instead derived from endoderm (9, 10).

Regardless of their exact embryonic derivation, endocrine tumors of the pancreas are of neuroendocrine origin and derive from a primitive stem cell that can differentiate into any one of several adult neuroendocrine secreting cells (11, 12). The primitive stem cell is pluripotent and can synthesize any of the polypeptides and amines normally found in the GI tract. During the maturation process, the primitive stem cell undergoes differentiation that suppresses production of all peptides and amines other than those needed for the normal function of the cell. Neoplasms can arise from each of the four neuroendocrine cell types that normally make up the pancreatic islets of Langerhans. These entopic neoplasms release glucagon from the alpha cells (A-cells) (glucagonomas), insulin from the beta cells (B-cells) (insulinomas), somatostatin from the delta cells (D-cells) (somatostatinomas), and pancreatic polypeptide from the F-cells ($D_2$ or PP-cells) (PPomas). Serotoninomas also arise from the fifth type of neuroendocrine cells present in the normal adult pancreas, the enterochromaffin (EC) cells. Other islet cell neoplasms secrete peptides not normally native to the pancreas. These ectopic neoplasms include the relatively common gastrinomas and VIPomas. In addition, much rarer ectopic neuroendocrine pancreatic neoplasms include ACTHomas, neurotensinomas, parathyrinomas, GRFomas, calcitoninomas, enteroglucagonomas, CCKomas, GIPomas, GRPomas, and IAPPomas. Because the stem cell of origin is pluripotent, pancreatic neuroendocrine neoplasms are frequently of mixed-cell type and secrete several peptides and/or amines simultaneously. One peptide or amine, however, usually predominates and is responsible for the patient's symptoms. Pancreatic neuroendocrine neoplasms are therefore classified and named according to the predominant secretory product or clinical syndrome. Occasionally, however, the clinical presentation is mixed, or the tumor is clinically silent (13).

Nonfunctioning pancreatic islet cell tumors do not produce a well-defined clinical syndrome for one or more of the following reasons (14): *(a)* insufficient peptide production, *(b)* adequate peptide production but insufficient peptide release, *(c)* regulated rather than autonomous peptide secretion, *(d)* concurrent secretion of inhibitory peptides by the tumor, *(e)* production of biologically inactive molecular forms of the peptides, *(f)* production of peptides with little or no clinical effect even at high concentrations, *(g)* production of peptides for which no assays are yet available, *(h)* inadequate clinical investigation of the patient. Most of these neoplasms (70–90%), when adequately studied by careful immunohistochemical tests and ultrastructural analysis, demonstrate characteristics of hormone-producing cells (15, 16). In 1950, a review of 398 reported islet cell tumors revealed a 41% incidence of "nonfunctioning" islet cell neoplasms (17). At that time, any neoplasm not associated with hypoglycemia (i.e., not an insulinoma) was considered nonfunctioning, since assays for other hormones were not yet available. More recent reviews of islet cell tumors have found smaller percentages (15–36%) of nonfunctioning neoplasms (18–22). It is almost certain that as more peptides are identified and patients with "nonfunctioning" pancreatic neuroendocrine neoplasms are routinely studied by the ever-increasing array of assays now available, more of these neoplasms will be identified as "functioning."

## PANCREATIC CORTICOTROPINOMAS (ACTHomas)

Adrenocorticotropic hormone, or corticotropin (ACTH), a well-known polypeptide normally produced by the corticotrope cells of the anterior pituitary gland, promotes growth of the adrenal cortex and stimulates the synthesis of cortisol and other steroid hormones by the adrenal gland. ACTH immunoreactivity has been demonstrated in normal human pancreatic islet cells (23). ACTHomas, also known as corticotropinomas, produce excessive amounts of ectopic ACTH, which overstimulate the adrenal glands. This leads to secondary adrenocortical hyperplasia with hypercortisolemia and causes Cushing's syndrome (the ectopic ACTH syndrome).

Four years before Cushing described the syndrome that now bears his name (24), a patient with an oat cell carcinoma of the bronchus and similar clinical features was reported (25). Not until the 1960s was a clear connection made between Cushing's syndrome and nonpituitary, nonadrenal tumors (26). Since then, many different neoplasms have been found to produce excessive amounts of ACTH and result in the ectopic ACTH syndrome. In four large series that evaluated 812 patients with Cushing's syndrome, ectopic ACTH production was the cause in 9–18% (27–30).

In early reports of ectopic ACTH-producing neoplasms, lung carcinomas predominated; in more recent series, bronchial carcinoids are more common (27). Other less frequent sites of ectopic ACTH-producing tumors are carcinoids of the stomach, appendix, ileum, and ovary; epithelial carcinomas of the thymus; islet cell tumors of the pancreas; medullary carcinoma of the thyroid; and pheochromocytomas (26) and isolated cases of adenocarcinomas of the colon, esophagus, lung, ovary, ileum, and prostate; squamous cell carcinomas of the lung, larynx and cervix; melanoma; and various salivary gland tumors have also been reported (3, 26–28, 31–34) (Table 83.1). However, most neoplasms that produce the ectopic ACTH syndrome belong to one of four histopathologic types: small cell carcinomas of the lung, carcinoid tumors, pancreatic islet cell tumors, and pheochromocytomas (27). Almost all neoplasms that produce ACTH also secrete other hormones (27).

The first pancreatic islet cell neoplasm associated with Cushing's syndrome was reported in 1933 (35). Pancreatic ACTHomas account for 11% (6–25%) of all ectopic neoplasms responsible for Cushing's syndrome (36, 37) (Table 83.1). In a recent prospective study of 42 patients with metastatic pancreatic islet cell neoplasms, 1 patient (2%) had an ACTHoma (38). In

**TABLE 83.1. Types of Neoplasms Causing the Ectopic ACTH Syndrome**

| Type of Neoplasm | Liddle et al., 1969 (3) | Imura et al., 1978 (31) | Davies et al., 1982 (32) | Jex et al., 1985 (26) | Howlett et al., 1986 (28) | Findling et al., 1986 (33) | Doppman et al., 1989 (34) | Wajchenberg et al., 1994 (27) | Total |
|---|---|---|---|---|---|---|---|---|---|
| Lung CA | 52 | 25 | | 5 | 3 | | | 1 | 86 (33%) |
| Misc. CA | 13 | 5 | | 4 | 2 | | | | 24 (9%) |
| Adeno CA, undetermined | 7 | 1 | 4 | | | 4 | 9 | | 25 (10%) |
| Bronchial carcinoid | 5 | 4 | 3 | 7 | 6 | 4 | 11 | 2 | 42 (16%) |
| Thymic carcinoid | 11 | 6 | | 2 | 2 | | 1 | 3 | 25 (10%) |
| Pancreatic islet cell CA | 11 (11%) | 3 (6%) | 1 (10%) | 4 (16%) | 2 (13%) | 1 (10%) | 3 (11%) | 3 (25%) | 28 (11%) |
| Pheochromocytoma | 3 | 1 | 1 | | 1 | | 3 | 3 | 12 (5%) |
| Thyroid medullary CA | 2 | 3 | 1 | 3 | | | | | 9 (4%) |
| GI carcinoid | | 3 | 1 | | | 1 | 1 | | 6 (2%) |
| Total | 104 | 51 | 11 | 25 | 16 | 10 | 28 | 12 | 257 (100%) |

Modified from Wajchenberg BL, Mendonca BB, Liberman B, Pereira MAA, Kirschner MA. Ectopic ACTH syndrome. J Steroid Biochem Mol Biol 1995;53:139–151; and Doppman JL, Nieman L, Miller DL, Pass HI, et al. Ectopic adrenocorticotropic hormone syndrome: localization studies in 28 patients. Radiology 1989;172:115–124.

**TABLE 83.2. Incidence of ACTHomas in Large Series of Pancreatic Neuroendocrine Neoplasms**

| Author (Ref) Year | Pancreatic Neuroendocrine Neoplasms | ACTHomas | Percentage |
|---|---|---|---|
| Broder (39) 1973 | 52 | 2 | 4 |
| Heitz (40) 1979 | 94 | 4 | 4 |
| Kent (19) 1981 | 168 | 2 | 1 |
| Heitz (15) 1982 | 125 | 0 | 0 |
| Durning (41) 1985 | 75 | 4 | 5 |
| Carty (38) 1992 | 42 | 1 | 2 |
| Total | 556 | 13 | 2 |

six large series totaling 556 patients, ACTHomas accounted for 2% of all pancreatic islet cell neoplasms (15, 19, 38–41) (Table 83.2).

In 42 patients reviewed by Clark and Carney, pancreatic ACTHomas were more common in women (27 of 42, 64%) in their 3rd or 4th decade of life (37). The mean age at presentation was 40 years (range, 2–68 years). Three children younger than 16 years of age and four adults over 60 years of age were affected. Two-thirds of patients had symptoms of Cushing's syndrome, including weight gain, acne, hyperpigmentation, hypertension, diabetes mellitus, and hypokalemic alkalosis. Ectopic ACTH secretion was recognized preoperatively as the cause of the syndrome in only six patients. In 18 patients, the pancreatic ACTHomas were diagnosed at laparotomy; of these, 15 had pancreatic tumors, and 3 had metastatic islet cell tumors with an undetected primary lesion. In 10 other patients, the pancreatic ACTHomas were found at autopsy. The remaining 8 patients presented initially with either a gastrinoma (5 patients) or an insulinoma (3 patients) and developed Cushing's syndrome later (37). Histologically, trabecular, acinar, and solid growth patterns were described. Metastases occurred in 37 of 42 patients (88%) (37); 25 of 42 patients (60%) were dead in 2 years or less, and the 5-year survival of 38 patients was 16% (37).

In 17–30% of patients with the Zollinger-Ellison syndrome, the gastrinoma contains both gastrin and ACTH-like immunoreactivity (15, 42, 43). Approximately 5% of patients with the sporadic Zollinger-Ellison syndrome will develop Cushing's syndrome with severe symptoms caused by ectopic ACTH production by their pancreatic neoplasms, usually in the late stages of their disease in the setting of widespread hepatic metastases (44). In contrast, Cushing's disease (ACTH overproduction by a pituitary adenoma), usually mild, occurs in up to 19% of patients with the Zollinger-Ellison syndrome associated with MEN-1 (44). Cushing's syndrome also occurs in about 40% of patients with GRFomas (45, 46). The diagnosis of pancreatic ACTHoma is suggested by a high concentration of circulating ACTH that is not suppressed by high or low doses of oral dexamethasone in a patient with a pancreatic mass. Definitive diagnosis is made by demonstrating neoplastic ACTH production by venous sampling, immunohistochemical staining, or tumor tissue extraction (46).

Pancreatic ACTHomas are aggressive neoplasms that are usually associated with a rapidly progressive clinical course (37). Resection by pancreatoduodenectomy or distal pancreatectomy (depending on tumor location) is the treatment of choice whenever possible. However, metastases occur in 88% of patients, and palliative debulking may be all that can be achieved surgically. Although several adrenal-blocking agents, including aminoglutethimide, metapyrone, and mitotane have been used with varying success in the management of Cushing's syndrome resulting from ectopic ACTH production, these agents are often poorly tolerated and result in severe side effects (47). Octreotide has reduced ACTH secretion from pancreatic ACTHomas and may control their growth; it is the treatment of choice for unresectable or widely metastatic pancreatic ACTHomas (48–50).

The ectopic ACTH syndrome also occurs from excessive ectopic production of corticotropin-releasing hormone (CRH). However, no CRH-producing pancreatic neuroendocrine neoplasm has been reported to date (27).

## PANCREATIC POLYPEPTIDOMAS (PPomas)

PPomas are rare tumors that arise from the PP-secreting cells (also referred to as $D_2$-cells or F-cells) of the GI tract. In mammals, 93% of these cells are located in the pancreas, within the islets of Langerhans and also as occasional single cells scattered in the exocrine parenchyma and lining the pancreatic ducts (51). Within the islets of Langerhans, PP-cells are mainly located in the periphery, wedged between the alpha- and beta-cells and where nerves enter the islets. This may explain the sensitivity of PP-cells to autonomic stimulation and suppression. In the human pancreas, the vast majority of PP-cells are found within a membrane-delineated lobule in the posterior portion of the head of the pancreas, which arises embryonically from the ventral pancreas (52). PP-cells are sparsely located in the human dorsal-derived pancreas, including the anterior portions of the head, as well as the isthmus, body, and tail. Therefore, PPomas are more common in the head of the pancreas but may occur in any area of the pancreas. PP is a 36-amino-acid polypeptide that was independently discovered by Kimmel et al. and Chance et al. in 1972 (53 55). Since then, at least 55 patients with PP-producing tumors have been reported (14, 15, 41, 56–77) (Table 83.3).

The true incidence of PPomas is difficult to assess because many nonfunctioning islet cell neoplasms have not been tested for PP and because PP-producing cells are often found within many other islet cell neoplasms (78). In a recent study of 323 patients with islet cell neoplasms, 12 (3.7%) PPomas were found by immunocytochemistry and determination of elevated circulating PP concentrations (75). Since the study included both pure and combined PPomas, the incidence of pure PP-secreting tumors may be estimated at 1–2% of all islet cell tumors. Pure PPomas, by definition, consist of at least 50% PP-secreting cells, as determined by immunocytochemistry. However, neoplastic PP cells occur frequently in glucagonomas (70%), nonfunctioning islet cell tumors (43%), VIPomas (42%), insulinomas (37%), and gastrinomas (34%) (61). PP cells have also been reported in carcinoid tumors of the rectum and duodenum (66). Similarly, PP hypersecretion is often detectable in many patients with other islet cell neoplasms. VIPomas (74%) are the most likely to present with PP hypersecretion, followed by glucagonomas (58%), somatostatinomas (33%), gastrinomas (31%), and insulinomas (28%) (61). Basal plasma PP concentrations are elevated in 29–50% of patients with the carcinoid syndrome (51, 75).

Detailed information is available for 31 of the 55 patients with PP-producing tumors reported in the literature (14, 15, 41, 56–77) (Table 83.3). PPomas occurred with approximately equal incidence in both sexes (58% women, 42% men). The mean age at presentation was 53 years (range, 20–80 years). Pancreatic PPomas were located in the head of the pancreas in 18 patients (64%), in the body in 3 (11%), and in the tail in 7 (25%). Only three extrapancreatic pure PPomas have been reported: one each in the liver, the stomach, and the ampulla of Vater (64, 66, 71). The mean tumor size was 6.2 cm (range, 0.7–15 cm). In general, PPomas tend to be larger than other functioning islet cell tumors. Histologically, PPomas resemble other gastroenteropancreatic neuroendocrine neoplasms; trabecular, glandular, and medullary cell patterns have been described (79). Benign PPomas are more often trabecular; malignant ones are more

TABLE 83.3. **Clinical Features of PPomas (Modified from references 51 and 61)**

| Case # | Age Sex | Symptoms | Other Findings | Tumor Site | Tumor Size (cm) | Metastases | Operation | Preop Plasma[a] PP (pg/mL) | Tumor PP (ng/g) | Postop Plasma[a] PP (pg/mL) | F/U (years) | Author (Ref) | Year |
|---|---|---|---|---|---|---|---|---|---|---|---|---|---|
| 1 | 45 M | Wt loss<br>Abd pain | DU | Body & tail | 0.7–0.8 | None | DP | | | 2,180 | 5 A | Bordi (56, 57) | 1978 |
| 2 | 41 F | W diarrhea<br>Wt loss | ↓ Gastric acid<br>Acute psychosis | Head | 5.0 | Liver | PD | 197,000 | | 21,000 | 2 D | Lundquist (58, 59) | 1978 |
| 3 | 33 M | None | MEN-1 | Tail | 15 | Liver | DP | 852,000 | 31,220 | 143 | 3.5 D | Friesen (60–63) | 1980 |
| 4 | 29 F | None | MEN-1 | Tail | | None | DP | 3,600 | | nl | 20 A | Friesen (61, 62) | 1980 |
| 5 | 62 M | Abd mass | Heavy drinker | Liver | 14 | LN | HR | | | | A | Warner (64) | 1980 |
| 6 | 55 M | W diarrhea<br>Abd pain | Moderate drinker | Body | 5.0 | None | NR | | | NR | <0.1 D | Hayes (65) | 1980 |
| 7 | 50 M | GI bleeding<br>Diabetes | Heavy drinker | Ampulla of Vater | 2.0 | None | AR | | | nl | 2 A | Ljungberg (66) | 1981 |
| 8 | 58 M | Abd pain<br>Wt loss<br>Diabetes | ↑ Calcitonin | Head & body | | Liver | HAE | 252,000 | | NR | 0.5 D | Manche (41, 67) | 1983 |
| 9 | 26 F | None | MEN-1 | Head | 1.5 | None | NR | 672 | 6,070 | NR | 1.5 UD | Tomita (60, 61) | 1983 |
| 10 | 74 F | None | MEN-1<br>Colon CA | Head | 1.3 | None | NR | 504 | 196,500 | NR | 0.5 UD | Tomita (60) | 1983 |
| 11 | 65 F | Abd mass<br>Diabetes | Cholecystitis<br>Somat | Head | 6.5 | None | PD | 1,000 | 1,340 | | 0.5 A | Nakanome (68) | 1984 |
| 12 | 53 M | Abd pain | GI bleeding | Head | 5.0 | None | PD | 7,520 | | 39 | | Strodel (69) | 1984 |
| 13 | 74 F | W diarrhea<br>Wt loss | | Body | 9.0 | None | SP | 35,100 | | 228 | | Strodel (69) | 1984 |
| 14 | 56 M | Abd pain | | Head | 1.5 | None | PD | 1,870 | | 20 | | Strodel (69) | 1984 |
| 15 | 20 F | Abd pain<br>Wt loss | Jaundice<br>Nausea | Head | 15 | None | PD | 394 | | 15 | 3 A | Strodel (69) | 1984 |
| 16 | 63 F | Wt loss | MEN-1 | Head & tail | 5.0 | None | SP | 1,220 | | 450 | | Strodel (69) | 1984 |
| 17 | 52 M | Abd pain<br>Wt loss | MEN-1 | Head | Multi | None | PD | 2,780 | | 17 | | Strodel (69) | 1984 |
| 18 | 67 M | Wt loss | | Head | Diffuse | Liver | NR | 2,790 | | NR | | Strodel (69) | 1984 |
| 19 | 48 M | Abd pain<br>W diarrhea | GI bleeding | Tail | 4.0 | Liver, LN | Lap | 3,027 | | NR | 2 D | Strodel (69) | 1984 |
| 20 | 57 F | Abd pain<br>Abd mass | ↓ Gastric acid | Head | | Liver, LN | Lap | 126,000 | | NR | 2 A | Nobin (70) | 1984 |

| | | | | | | | | | | | | | |
|---|---|---|---|---|---|---|---|---|---|---|---|---|---|
| 21 | 37 M | Abd pain W diarrhea Wt loss | Heavy drinker DU | Tail | | Liver, LN | NR | 630,000 | | NR | 0.2 D | Nobin (70) | 1984 |
| 22 | 64 F | Abd pain Distention Wt loss Head-aches | Flushing Tachycardia Lacrymation | Stomach | 2.5 | Liver | PG HAE | 298,000 | | nl | >1 yr A | Solt (71) | 1984 |
| 23 | 59 F | Rash | GI bleeding | Head | 10 | Liver | IR | 610 | | 400 | 3 A | Choksi (72) | 1988 |
| 24 | 70 F | Abd pain | | Head | 5.0 | Liver | Bx | nl | | NR | <1 D | Martensson (73) | 1990 |
| 25 | 55 F | Abd pain | | Head | 3.0 | Liver | Bx | 212 | | NR | <1 D | Martensson (73) | 1990 |
| 26 | 55 F | Abd pain | | Head | 3.0 | Liver | Bx | | | NR | <1 D | Martensson (73) | 1990 |
| 27 | 37 M | None | | Head | 2.5 | Liver | PD | 150,000 | | | 4 D | Martensson (73) | 1990 |
| 28 | 59 F | None | | Head | | LN | PD | 30,000 | | | 5 A | Martensson (73) | 1990 |
| 29 | 68 F | None | Hypogly-cemia | Tail | 6.5 | Liver | DP | | 17,600 | | | Tomita (61) | 1991 |
| 30 | 34 F | Abd pain | MEN-1 | Tail | 10 | Liver | DP | | 22,500 | | A | Tomita (61) | 1991 |
| 31 | 80 F | W diarrhea Wt loss Abd pain | | Tail | 16 | Liver | Bx | 2,204 | | NR | A | Uhl (74) | 1992 |
| 32–41 | | Abd pain &/or Abd mass | No hormonal symptoms | | 1–15 | None in 10/10 pts | | 2,520-84,000 | 12,600–176,400 | nl in 5/5 patients studied | 1–10 | Heitz (15) | 1982 |
| 42–53 | | | | | | At least 5 had mets | | 180,058 (31,475–461,114) | | | 3 (1–10) | Adrian & Wynick (75, 76) | 1986/ 1988 |
| 54–55 | | | | | | 1 of 2 | | | | | | Solcia (14, 77) | 1990 |

Modified from Vinik AI, Moattari AR. Treatment of endocrine tumors of the pancreas. Endocrinol Metab Clin North Am 1989;18:483–518, and Tomita T, Friesen SR, Pollack HG, PP-producing tumors (PPomas). In: Dayal Y, ed. Endocrine pathology of the gut and pancreas. Boca Raton, FL: CRC Press, 1991;279–304.

Abbreviations:

| | | | | | |
|---|---|---|---|---|---|
| Wt loss | Weight loss | Bx | Biopsy only | SP | Subtotal pancreatectomy |
| W diarrhea | Watery diarrhea | DP | Distal pancreatectomy | NR | Not resected |
| Abd | Abdominal | PD | Pancreatoduodenectomy | MEN-1 | Multiple endocrine neoplasia type-1 |
| DU | Duodenal ulcer | HR | Hepatic resection | A | Alive |
| Somat | Somatostatinoma | Lap | Exploratory laparotomy only | D | Dead |
| GI | Gastrointestinal | HAE | Hepatic artery embolization | UD | Death unrelated to PPoma |
| Multi | Multiple tumors | AP | Ampullectomy | nl | Normal |
| Preop | Preoperative | IR | Incomplete resection | pos | Positive |
| Postop | Postoperative | CT | Computed tomography scan | neg | Negative |
| Angio | Angiography | ND | Not done | | |

[a]Normal plasma pancreatic polypeptide (PP) concentrations <1000 pg/mL

likely to be medullary (61). The only reliable criteria of malignancy are infiltration into adjacent tissues and/or metastases. Metastases were found in 24 (44%) patients: the liver was involved in 16 patients, lymph nodes in 5, and the site was unspecified in 6. Metastases to lung, brain, and bone have also been reported (63). In general, large PPomas (>5 cm) are likely to be malignant. The incidence of MEN-1 in patients with PPomas is estimated to be between 18–44% (61). In fact, PP determinations have been suggested as a marker for pancreatic neuroendocrine tumors, especially in patients with the MEN-1 syndrome (62, 80–82). Some investigators have suggested that any patient with the MEN-1 syndrome who has a markedly elevated PP level should have the pancreas meticulously evaluated (62, 82). A more recent study questions the use of PP as a marker for sporadic islet cell tumors (83).

Little is known about the physiologic role of PP. Plasma concentrations are known to increase with age, prolonged fasting, exercise, chronic renal failure, chronic pancreatitis, pancreatic carcinoma, and diabetes mellitus. PP inhibits both pancreatic and biliary secretions (80, 84). Its actions appear to be counter to cholecystokinin (CCK) and related to nutrition, especially obesity. This inhibitory action is mediated by an extravagal cholinergic mechanism (85, 86). Eating is followed by a very rapid rise in circulating PP, and this elevation persists for 4–8 hours. The strongest stimulus is protein, followed by fats, and then carbohydrates. Circulating nutrients do not stimulate PP secretion, which shows the importance of the GI tract in mediating signals to the pancreas (51). Plasma PP levels also increase markedly in response to exogenous administration of CCK, secretin, and gastrin-releasing polypeptide (GRP) and to a lesser extent, gastrin and pentagastrin. Physiologic control of PP secretion thus appears to be regulated by intestinal, cephalic, and hormonal phases.

From the known physiologic actions of PP, a PPoma would be expected to be clinically silent, and no characteristic clinical syndrome has been described. However, the clinical picture is complicated by increased PP secretion by other functioning islet cell neoplasms. Watery diarrhea (87), ulcer diathesis (56), jaundice (88), and recently, an erythematous scaly pruritic rash (different from that seen with the glucagonoma syndrome and involving the face, hands, chest, and abdomen) have been reported in patients with increased circulating concentrations of PP (72). Since the hormonal effects of PP are clinically silent, most patients present with an abdominal mass and/or pain from the tumor or its metastases (Table 83.3).

Elevated basal plasma PP concentration, usually more than four times that in age-matched controls, is diagnostic of a PPoma. A fasting plasma level above 300 pmol/L has been reported as diagnostic, regardless of the patient's age (75). Administration of atropine, which reduces PP concentrations in normal individuals but not in patients with PPomas, may assist in the diagnosis of borderline or difficult cases (89). Diagnostic accuracy can also be increased by administration of secretin (51). An exaggerated response of circulating PP to a standard test meal and/or to secretin administration has been used to screen for the genetic trait of MEN-1 and related neoplasms (13, 62). As many as 67% of "nonfunctioning" islet cell neoplasms tested have an exaggerated response to secretin, indicating that many neoplasms previously considered nonfunctioning islet cell tumors may actually be PPomas.

PPomas are usually large and highly vascular; thus computerized tomography is the initial diagnostic test of choice for localization. Although not all patients with an elevated basal plasma PP level have demonstrable tumor, their frequent malignant behavior warrants thorough attempts at localization and even laparotomy to rule out the presence of PPomas (90). Abdominal ultrasonography, computed tomography, and arteriography have all successfully identified tumors in patients with elevated plasma PP levels (69, 73).

Surgical resection is the treatment of choice for PPomas. Small, noninfiltrating, well-circumscribed PPomas can be adequately treated by excision, including the entire capsule and adjacent normal pancreas. Malignant-appearing PPomas should be widely resected by pancreatoduodenectomy or distal pancreatectomy, depending on location. Debulking of large metastatic lesions may be palliative, and clinical responses have been reported with streptozotocin (7, 41). Somatostatin analogue therapy may be useful in patients with unresectable disease (91). Scant data are available on survival, and prognosis depends on tumor size and the extent of metastasis at the time of diagnosis.

## PANCREATIC CARCINOID TUMORS (SEROTONINOMAS)

Neuroendocrine neoplasms of the pancreas that produce serotonin and morphologically resemble carcinoid tumors have been reported but are exceedingly rare (92). The biogenic amine serotonin was first isolated from human serum in 1948 (93) and from enterochromaffin cells in 1952 (94). It was extracted from a carcinoid tumor found at autopsy in 1953 (95), thus implicating its overproduction in the pathogenesis of the carcinoid syndrome (96, 97). Serotonin is normally produced by the enterochromaffin cells of the GI tract, including the pancreas, by hydroxylation and decarboxylation of the essential dietary amino acid tryptophan. Normally only 1–2% of ingested tryptophan is used for serotonin synthesis, but in patients with carcinoid tumors, up to 60% of this amino acid may be diverted for serotonin synthesis at the expense of protein and niacin production. Serotonin is broken down in the liver (by monoamine oxidase) to 5-hydroxyindolacetic acid (5-HIAA), a biologically inactive metabolite that is excreted in the urine. 5-HIAA may be measured in abnormal quantities in the urine of patients with carcinoid tumors, although false-positive results may be caused by drugs and dietary factors. Hepatic metabolism also explains why carcinoid tumors drained by the portal circulation can produce large amounts of serotonin without resulting in the carcinoid syndrome. The carcinoid syndrome is rare (less than 10% of all patients with carcinoid tumors) and occurs only when the humoral output of the neoplasm is released into the systemic circulation and escapes hepatic degradation. This occurs most frequently with hepatic metastases or when the primary is located outside the portal system (e.g., ovarian or bronchial carcinoids). Venous drainage of serotonin directly into the systemic circulation also occurs with extensive retroperitoneal involvement by a pancreatic carcinoid tumor (98).

Carcinoid tumors account for 55–86% of gastroenteropancreatic neuroendocrine neoplasms (1, 99, 100). They were first observed by Lubarsh in 1888 and were later named *karzinoide* ("resembling carcinoma") by Oberndorfer because they were often associated with a benign clinical course even though they appeared to be carcinomas (1). About 89% of carcinoid tumors occur in the GI tract, 10% occur in the lungs (mostly as bronchial carcinoids), and the remainder develop in various other organs such as the larynx, thymus, kidney, ovary, prostate, and skin (101). The histochemical characteristics, biochemical properties, and clinical manifestations of carcinoid tumors vary according to their embryonic origin: thus, they are classified as foregut (bronchus, pancreas, stomach, proximal duodenum), midgut (distal duodenum, jejunum, ileum, appendix, proximal colon, ovary), and hindgut neoplasms (distal colon, rectum) (102). Foregut and hindgut carcinoids exhibit an argyrophil reaction, and all midgut carcinoids show, in addition, an argentaffin reaction. Foregut and hindgut carcinoids are often multihormonal; midgut carcinoids contain a smaller variety of endocrine cells (103). Foregut and midgut carcinoids are associated with the carcinoid syndrome, while hindgut carcinoids seldom, if ever, are. About three-fourths of abdominal carcinoid tumors are of midgut origin. The most frequent location is the appendix

(46%), followed by the small intestine (28%) (usually in the ileum) and the rectum (16%) (101). Pancreatic carcinoids account for less than 2% of abdominal carcinoid tumors (104).

The true incidence of pancreatic carcinoids is unknown but must be very low. Many large series of patients with carcinoid tumors have reported no pancreatic carcinoids. Two major reviews including more than 3000 patients with gastrointestinal carcinoid tumors had no pancreatic carcinoids (101, 105). In another study of 3718 patients with carcinoid tumors, only 2 patients (0.05%) had pancreatic tumors (106). The first pancreatic carcinoid tumor was reported in 1931 (107), and since then, more than 65 cases have been reported (108). Considerable confusion exists because of the histologic similarity of pancreatic carcinoids to pancreatic islet cell tumors, the lack of uniform nomenclature, and the absence of standard diagnostic criteria (92). For example, pancreatic neoplasms that morphologically resemble carcinoid tumors frequently produce multiple peptides. Such neoplasms are usually characterized on the basis of the predominant peptide identified serologically or immunohistochemically. Therefore, minimal serotonin immunoreactivity in a pancreatic neuroendocrine neoplasm that also contains other peptides is not usually considered enough evidence to designate it a pancreatic carcinoid (92). Also, some islet cell neoplasms that were previously considered nonfunctioning in fact do secrete serotonin and should be considered pancreatic carcinoid tumors (109).

The classic carcinoid syndrome is caused by midgut tumors and consists of vasomotor, cardiopulmonary, and GI symptoms. Episodic or continuous cutaneous flushing of the head and torso occurs in 95% of patients. Mild or explosive diarrhea, which does not occur at the time of the flushing episodes, is the second most common symptom (85% of patients), followed by abdominal pain and/or cramping (50%), right heart valvular lesions (50%), and wheezing (6%) (1). Other cutaneous changes include telangiectasia and pellagra dermatosis. Although it was the humoral agent originally identified in carcinoid tumors, hypersecretion of serotonin alone cannot explain all of the manifestations of the carcinoid syndrome. In fact, the substance(s) responsible for the characteristic flushing remains unknown (110, 111). Many other vasoactive substances are produced by foregut carcinoid tumors and by pancreatic carcinoid tumors, including amines (histamine, dopamine, 5-hydroxytryptophan, 5-HIAA), tachykinins (kallikrein, substance P, neuropeptide K), and peptides (PP, ACTH, gastrin, insulin, glucagon, calcitonin, vasoactive intestinal polypeptide [VIP], growth hormone-releasing factor, chromogranins, neurotensin, motilin, and prostaglandins) (112, 113).

Pancreatic carcinoids, like other foregut carcinoids, manifest an atypical carcinoid syndrome, which does not depend upon the presence of hepatic metastases. The interactions of the various substances elaborated by pancreatic carcinoids contribute to the variability of symptoms in the atypical syndrome. In contrast to the classic carcinoid syndrome, the atypical syndrome is characterized clinically by a more livid, severe, and prolonged cutaneous flush. It often has a purplish or violaceous hue rather than the classic pink-red color, and it frequently leaves permanent telangiectasia and hypertrophy of the skin of the face and upper neck. Periorbital edema and lacrimation caused by histamine release are also more pronounced. The patient's face assumes a leonine appearance after repeated episodes (11, 13, 114).

For a pancreatic neuroendocrine neoplasm to be classified as a carcinoid, the following three criteria must be met: *(a)* clinical symptoms and/or biochemical evidence of serotonin production by a pancreatic tumor, *(b)* predominance of serotonin immunoreactivity over that of other secretory products within neoplastic cells, and *(c)* absence of multihormone production (92). The authors of one study found that only 2 of 23 patients met all three criteria for pancreatic carcinoid tumors (11, 115). Another four patients (116–119) fulfilled the first and third criteria but had not been tested for serotonin immunoreactivity (92). A more recent study used somewhat different criteria, namely, a demonstrable pancreatic neuroendocrine tumor and at least one of the following without another dominant hormone being demonstrated: *(a)* elevated serum serotonin or serotonin immunoreactivity in tumor tissue, *(b)* elevated 5-HIAA concentration in the urine, or *(c)* a positive tumor argyrophil and/or argentaffin reaction (108). These authors could identify only 39 patients that met their criteria out of the more than 65 patients with possible pancreatic carcinoids who have been reported (92, 98, 108, 115–142). These authors cited more than 30 other cases previously reported as "pancreatic carcinoid" tumors in which neither silver staining nor production of serotonin or its derivatives was demonstrated (108).

Of the 39 patients that met the authors' criteria, 60% were women. The mean age at presentation was 53 years (range, 23–91 years). Pancreatic carcinoids were located in the head or head and body in 15 patients (43%), in the body in 12 (34%), and in the tail in 8 (23%). Mean tumor size was 4.5 cm (range, 0.5–12 cm). Some 32 patients (82%) had malignant tumors: demonstrated by direct invasion in 13, lymph node metastases in 16, and hepatic or other remote metastases in 22. Only seven patients (18%) had benign tumors (cases #5, 15, 19, 22, 32, 36, 37). Because of the high incidence of malignancy, metastatic disease is often present. Seventeen patients (44%) were surgically resected; 22 patients (56%) were unresectable. Survival data were available for 36 of the 39 patients: 14 patients (39%) died, and 22 were alive at last follow-up. Of the 14 patients, 7 (50%) died within 1 year, 4 (29%) died within 5 years, and 3 (21%) survived for over 5 years. The calculated 5-year survival was 14% (108).

Surgical resection, by pancreatoduodenectomy or distal pancreatectomy, is the treatment of choice for pancreatic carcinoids. In general, metastasis is associated with a poor prognosis, but some patients live several years after demonstrating distant metastases. Therefore, palliative resection (debulking) of metastatic disease is advisable when technically feasible, since it may provide substantial benefit (143). Widespread metastases may require pharmacologic therapy for symptomatic relief of the carcinoid syndrome. The serotonin antagonist ketanserin, as well as octreotide, has proven successful (144, 145). In addition, combination chemotherapy with streptozotocin can produce a beneficial response in as many as 40% of patients with metastatic pancreatic carcinoids (145).

The diagnosis of pancreatic carcinoid is made by demonstrating elevated circulating concentrations of serotonin or by detecting serotonin metabolites such as urinary 5-HIAA. However, pancreatic carcinoids, as other foregut carcinoids, often lack the decarboxylating enzyme (5-hydroxytryptophan decarboxylase) that converts 5-hydroxytryptophan into serotonin. In such patients, serotonin and 5-HIAA determinations in serum and urine may not be diagnostic. In contrast to midgut carcinoids, pancreatic carcinoids often produce elevated serum 5-hydroxytryptophan levels (11). Occasionally, provocative testing with pentagastrin is required for definitive diagnosis (143). Intravenous pentagastrin administration reliably induces flushing, elevations in circulating serotonin concentrations, or both, in patients with carcinoid tumors (144).

## PANCREATIC NEUROTENSINOMAS (NTomas)

Islet cell tumors that secrete neurotensin are exceedingly rare (91). Neurotensin is a 13-amino-acid polypeptide normally produced by the N-cells in the mucosa of the distal jejunum and ileum (146). It is not normally found in the pancreas (147). Neurotensin was first isolated from bovine hypothalamus in 1973 and subsequently from the human GI tract by Caraway et al. (148, 149). Since then, only 35 patients with neurotensin secreting tumors have been reported (41, 76, 150–159) (Table 83.4).

**TABLE 83.4. Clinical Features of Neurotensinomas**

| Case # | Age Sex | Symptoms | Syndrome | Tumor Site | Tumor Size (cm) | Metastases | Operation | Preop Plasma NT (pg/mL) | Tumor NT | Postop Plasma NT (pg/mL) | F/U (years) | Author (Ref) | Year |
|---|---|---|---|---|---|---|---|---|---|---|---|---|---|
| 1 | 65 M | W diarrhea<br>Wt loss<br>Flushing | ↑ Calcitonin<br>↑ Enkephalin<br>Diabetes | Tail | 5.0 | None | DP | 3200 | pos | 24.5 | | Gutniak (150) | 1980 |
| 2 | 48 M | Wt loss | ZES<br>DU | Head | 4.0 | None | E | C 38<br>N 180 | C 250<br>N 164 | C 18<br>N 20 | | Feurle (151) | 1981 |
| 3 | 41 F | W diarrhea, Edema, Vomiting, Pruritis, Flushing, Palpitation | | Head | 4.0 | None | R | High | nl | | | Maier (152) | 1982 |
| 4 | 68 F | None | Bronchial carcinoma | Lung | 8.5 | LN | RP | 200 | 8.5 | 37 | | Wood (153) | 1983 |
| 5 | 49 M | W diarrhea<br>Wt loss | VIPOMA | Tail | | Liver | DP | C 4225 | | nl | <1 A | Bloom (154) | 1983 |
| 6 | 27 F | W diarrhea<br>Wt loss | VIPOMA | Head & tail | 600 g | Liver | DP | C 3700 | | nl | <1 A | Bloom (154) | 1983 |
| 7 | 59 M | W diarrhea | VIPOMS | Head & body | 6.0 | LN | TP | C 225<br>N 1050 | C 168<br>N 1340 | nl | | Shulkes (155) | 1984 |
| 8 | 60 F | | ZES<br>Insulinoma | Pancreas | | Liver | | 310 | 56 | | 6 D | Theodorsson (156, 157) | 1983 |
| 9 | 60 M | W diarrhea | MEN-1<br>↑ Calcitonin<br>WDAH | Pancreas | | Liver | | 175 | | | | Theodorsson (157) | 1983 |

| | | | | | | | | | | | | |
|---|---|---|---|---|---|---|---|---|---|---|---|---|
| 10 | 64 F | Hypoglycemia | ↑ Insulin | Tail | 10 | Liver | | 235 | 58 | 0.9 D | Theodorsson (157) | 1983 |
| 11 | 50 F | W diarrhea<br>Abd pain | WDAH<br>↑ Calcitonin | Body | 8.0 | Liver<br>LN | DP | 315 | 77 | 10 A | Theodorsson (156, 157) | 1983 |
| 12 | ? M | | ZES | Pancreas | | | | 103 | | | Theodorsson (157) | 1983 |
| 13 | ? M | | Glucagonoma<br>↑ Insulin<br>↑ Calcitonin | Pancreas | | | | 921 | | | Theodorsson (157) | 1983 |
| 14 | ? M | Flushing | | Gastric mucosa | | | | 75 | | | Theodorsson (157) | 1983 |
| 15 | ? M | | Carcinoid<br>↑ Serotonin | Ileum | | | | 73 | | | Theodorsson (157) | 1983 |
| 16 | ? M | None | Carcinoid<br>↑ Serotonin | Bronchial carcinoid | | | | 500 | 5200 | | Theodorsson (157) | 1983 |
| 17 | 60 F | Abd pain<br>W diarrhea | | Head | | Liver | NR | | pos | 1.5 D | Durning (41) | 1985 |
| 18–22 | | W diarrhea | VIPOMA | Pancreas | | | | 378 | | | Blackburn (158) | 1981 |
| 23–26 | | | ZES | Pancreas | | | | 4087 (1278–7396) | | | Wynick (76) | 1988 |
| 27–35 | | | ZES | Pancreas | | 3 of 9 patients | | 90–269 | | | Chiang 159 | 1990 |

Modified from Vinik AI, Moattari AR. Treatment of endocrine tumors of the pancreas. Endocrinol Metab Clin North Am 1989;18:483–518.

Abbreviations:

| | | | | | |
|---|---|---|---|---|---|
| W diarrhea | Watery diarrhea | TP | Total pancreatectomy | D | Dead |
| Wt loss | Weight loss | DP | Distal pancreatectomy | pos | Positive |
| Abd pain | Abdominal pain | NR | Not resected | neg | Negative |
| MEN-1 | Multiple endocrine neoplasia type-1 | RP | Right pneumonectomy | ND | Not done |
| C | C-terminal | nl | Normal | | |
| N | N-terminal | A | Alive | | |

In pharmacologic doses, neurotensin induces hypotension, tachycardia, and cyanosis, and stimulates small intestinal secretion (160, 161). It also causes contraction of the ileum and relaxation of both the duodenum and the gastroesophageal sphincter (151, 162). It is normally secreted in response to a meal (163), and high circulating concentrations of neurotensin have been found following duodenal ulcer surgery and jejunoileal bypasses for morbid obesity (164, 165). Neurotensin inhibits the interdigestive myoelectric complex and stimulates insulin release (166). However, the physiologic role of neurotensin remains unknown (167, 168).

As early as 1979, it was noted that some of the non-gastrin-secreting cells in multihormonal gastrinomas showed neurotensin immunoreactivity (169). Neurotensin secretion by a pancreatic tumor was first reported by Blackburn et al. in 1981 (158). In that study, 326 patients with a variety of tumors, including 160 pancreatic neuroendocrine neoplasms, underwent fasting plasma neurotensin determinations; only 6 had increased circulating neurotensin concentrations. All 6 were among the 21 with pancreatic VIPomas associated with the WDHA (watery diarrhea, hypokalemia, achlorhydria) syndrome that were surgically removed during the study (158). In 1981, Feurle described a patient with a high circulating concentration of neurotensin and a pancreatic tumor composed of 79% neurotensin cells. The tumor also secreted gastrin, however, and the patient had the Zollinger-Ellison syndrome (151). In 1983, Bloom described two additional patients with VIPomas and increased circulating neurotensin concentrations (154). Most patients with neurotensin-secreting tumors have had mixed tumors and have presented clinically with either the vipoma syndrome or the Zollinger-Ellison syndrome (Table 83.4).

In 1981, before a pure neurotensin-secreting tumor was identified, it was hypothesized on the basis of the known pharmacologic actions of neurotensin that the neurotensinoma syndrome would include the following features: diabetes, hypotension, vasodilatation, cyanosis, and edema (91). It was also predicted that a pure neurotensinoma would cause net secretion of intestinal fluid and electrolytes, inhibition of gastric acid secretion, infrequent interdigestive myoelectric complexes, and prolonged gastric emptying. So far, the patient reported by Maier et al. (152) (case #3) best exemplifies these predictions (91). Neurotensin and VIP share many biologic actions, including peripheral vasodilatation, hypotension, and the inhibition of both gastric acid production and gastric motility. The clinical symptoms resulting from elevated circulating levels of both peptides may be very similar, and some authors have questioned whether a specific neurotensinoma syndrome actually exists (158).

Recently, 20% of 45 patients with the Zollinger-Ellison syndrome were found to have elevated circulating levels of neurotensin (159). Even though 64% of them had plasma elevations of other peptides, including motilin, PP, and gastrin-releasing peptide, in addition to gastrin and neurotensin, these other elevations were not clinically important in assessing MEN-1 status, extent of disease, or the presence of metastatic disease (159). Furthermore, only one patient developed a secondary clinical syndrome (because of hypersecretion of insulin), yielding a rate of 2 patients/100 patients observed/10 years. Based on these results, the authors concluded that plasma concentrations of additional gastrointestinal peptides should be determined only if new symptoms suggested a secondary clinical syndrome (159).

The true incidence of neurotensinomas remains unknown, but surely some remain undetected because neurotensin is not routinely measured and many of these tumors are mixed. The most common association is with VIP (154, 155, 158), but PP, (151, 159) gastrin, (314, 332) calcitonin, and enkephalin coproduction has also been reported (150). In a study of 20 patients with primary malignant tumors of the liver, all 4 patients with the fibrolamellar variant of hepatocellular carcinoma had elevated circulating neurotensin levels. One other patient, with a nonfibrolamellar hepatic tumor, also had high plasma neurotensin levels. Whether the latter represents an extrapancreatic, primary hepatic neurotensinoma is not clear from the report. The authors concluded that since increased plasma neurotensin levels occur in 100% of patients with the fibrolamellar variant of hepatocellular carcinoma, the test can be used as a marker for this neoplasm (170).

The reported 35 neurotensinomas (41, 76, 150–159) occurred with approximately equal incidence in both sexes (women 53%, men 47%) and presented at the mean age of 54 years (range, 27–68 years) (Table 83.4). Neurotensinomas were usually single large (mean size 6.5 cm, range 4.0–10.0 cm) tumors that were equally distributed between the head, body, and tail of the pancreas. Two extrapancreatic neurotensinomas, both in the lung, have been reported (cases #4 and #16) (153, 157). As with all other gastroenteropancreatic neuroendocrine neoplasms, it is impossible to differentiate malignant from benign neurotensinomas histologically, and demonstration of local invasion and/or metastasis is the only accurate means of diagnosing malignancy. Details regarding metastases are available only in 21 of the 35 reported cases: 12 patients (57%) had metastases to either liver (7 patients) or lymph nodes (5 patients). In three patients the sites of metastases were not specified. Seven patients had normal neurotensin concentrations following resection or excision of the neoplasm.

An elevated circulating concentration of neurotensin suggests the diagnosis of a neurotensin-secreting tumor. Measurement of plasma neurotensin is difficult because the circulating concentration is so low and because of its rapid peripheral degradation; also, biologically inactive N-terminal and C-terminal fragments of neurotensin often cross-react with the assay (151, 155, 171). At present, no provocative or inhibitory tests to confirm the diagnosis of a neurotensinoma are available. Because neurotensinomas are usually large (>3 cm), ultrasound and computed tomography scans are adequate initial localization studies. The efficacy of somatostatin receptor imaging and endoscopic ultrasound for localizing small tumors is not yet clear.

The only curative treatment for neurotensin-secreting tumors is surgical resection. A distal pancreatectomy should be performed for pancreatic body and tail lesions, while pancreatoduodenectomy is the treatment of choice for pancreatic head lesions. If curative resection of all tumor and metastases is not possible, palliative resection of as much primary tumor and metastatic deposits (debulking) as safely possible is probably worthwhile. Continued palliation has been reported after incomplete resection of a further recurrence (172). Streptozotocin alone or in combination with 5-fluorouracil (5-FU) has been used in two patients with good response (154, 157). There are too few neurotensin-secreting tumors for generalization about clinical presentation, prognosis, or results of surgical or chemotherapeutic treatment.

## PANCREATIC PARATHYRINOMAS (PTHomas)

Hypercalcemia is the most common endocrine manifestation of malignant neoplasms, and malignancy is the most common cause of hypercalcemia in hospital practice (173). As early as 1941, it was suggested that nonparathyroid tumors could secrete parathyroid hormone (PTH) (174). Whether the circulating hypercalcemic factor was PTH or a PTH-like substance remained a controversy, exacerbated by cross-reactivity in early PTH RIAs (114). Recently, a PTH-related peptide (PTHrP) was implicated in the pathogenesis of malignant hypercalcemia (175–178). PTHrP is a 141-amino-acid polypeptide (larger than PTH) whose gene is located in a different chromosome than the

PTH gene (176, 179–181). Alternative splicing of the PTHrP gene results in mRNA encoding three related PTHrPs, which have identical sequences for amino acids 1–139 but different C-terminal extensions (182, 183). The biologic activity of PTHrP is attributed to the first 34 amino acids of the N terminus; the physiologic importance of the unique C-terminal sequences, if any, remains unknown (183). The amino acid sequence of PTHrP has striking homology with PTH for amino acids 1–13 but thereafter is unique (183). PTHrP and PTH also bind to the same receptor in bone and kidney (184). PTHrP induces hypercalcemia by mimicking some of the actions of PTH (173).

PTHrP is normally produced by the pancreatic islet cells and was found in 13 of 15 pancreatic neuroendocrine neoplasms tested (185). In fact, PTHrP appears to be ubiquitous in all endocrine tissues, and it normally occurs in the pancreas, brain, hypothalamus, pituitary, thyroid, parathyroid, adrenal, stomach, lactating mammary tissue, and skin (185). PTHrP also has been demonstrated in many neoplasms not associated with hypercalcemia (186). Absence of hypercalcemia in association with PTHrP-producing neoplasms, neuroendocrine or otherwise, may be due to coproduction of counterregulatory substances such as calcitonin or chromagranin (187). The widespread distribution of PTHrP in many different tissues suggests that it may play an important role in the growth, differentiation, or function of numerous cell types, but its physiologic role is unknown (186).

Hypercalcemia associated with pancreatic neuroendocrine tumors is usually caused by primary hyperparathyroidism as part of the MEN-1 syndrome. Paraneoplastic hypercalcemia associated with an islet cell tumor of the pancreas was first reported by O'Neal in 1968 in a patient with the Zollinger-Ellison syndrome (188). Hypercalcemia has also been reported in patients with VIPomas and the WDHA syndrome with low or normal PTH serum concentrations (156, 189–192). Because diarrhea in patients with VIPomas makes evaluation of the hypercalcemia difficult, these patients have been excluded from previous reviews of pancreatic islet cell neoplasms associated with hypercalcemia (173).

Production of a polypeptide with activity like that of PTH by pancreatic neuroendocrine neoplasms results in the so-called ectopic hypercalcemia syndrome (13). The hypercalcemia can be mild or severe with symptoms of lethargy and coma (193). The syndrome is clinically similar to that observed in patients with entopic hyperparathyroidism (i.e., parathyroid neoplasms or parathyroid hyperplasia). It must also be differentiated from paraneoplastic hypercalcemia associated with nonparathyroid and nonendocrine neoplasms, as well as from the hypercalcemia due to nonendocrine carcinomas with bone metastases (194). It is particularly important to distinguish hypercalcemia-inducing neuroendocrine pancreatic neoplasms from exocrine pancreatic adenocarcinomas with paraneoplastic hypercalcemia (14). The hypophosphatemia that accompanies either entopic or ectopic PTH-secreting neoplasms differentiates them from the nonendocrine causes of hypercalcemia with hyperphosphatemia (114).

Historically, the principal problem encountered in the diagnosis of hypercalcemia associated with pancreatic neuroendocrine neoplasms was that the circulating polypeptide demonstrated molecular heterogeneity that was often not recognized by standard RIAs for PTH. In such instances, the hypercalcemia was associated with undetectable concentrations of PTH (195). This hypercalcemic suppression of PTH release from normal parathyroid glands can be applied to the diagnosis of the ectopic neoplasm. For example, pharmacologic reduction of serum calcium concentrations in patients with PTHomas increases the measurable PTH concentration to normal levels, thus confirming normal parathyroid-gland responsiveness (193, 196).

The true incidence of parathyrinomas is difficult to assess because reported cases include both pure and combined parathyrinomas. Hypercalcemia has been seen concurrently in patients with other islet cell neoplasms, most often VIPomas (six patients) (156, 189–192), followed by calcitoninomas (four patients), (156, 197, 198) gastrinomas (two patients), (188, 199) somatostatinomas (one patient) (200), and insulinomas (two patients) (195, 201).

Thirty-three pancreatic neuroendocrine neoplasms associated with hypercalcemia have been reported (21, 156, 173, 184, 188–192, 195–218) (Table 83.5). The pancreatic parathyrinomas occurred with approximately equal incidence in both sexes (51% women, 49% men), and presented at a mean age of 47 years (range, 8–77 years). In 27 patients, the location of the parathyrinoma within the pancreas was noted: 4 (15%) were located in the head of the pancreas, 3 (11%) in the body, 6 (22%) in the body and tail, and 13 (48%) in the tail; in 1 patient (4%), the the entire pancreas was involved. Parathyrinomas are large tumors, with a reported mean tumor size of 9.5 cm (range, 4–18 cm). This is probably an underestimate, since several parathyrinomas were so large that only descriptive terms were used (e.g., "involving the entire pancreas"). Histologically, parathyrinomas resemble other neuroendocrine neoplasms with trabecular, glandular, and medullary cell patterns. Again, the only reliable criteria of malignancy are infiltration into adjacent tissues and/or metastases. Metastases were reported in 25 (76%) of the 33 patients: the liver was involved in all, lymph node metastases were present in 2 patients, and omental metastases were present in 2 patients. Four patients had large, locally invasive, malignant neoplasms without metastases. Only four (cases #1, 3, 12, 20) benign parathyrinomas have been reported (190, 191, 198, 202, 207, 212).

Surgical resection is the treatment of choice for pancreatic parathyrinomas. Because these tumors are almost always malignant (88%), they should be widely resected by pancreatoduodenectomy or distal pancreatectomy, depending on their location. Debulking of large, infiltrating and/or metastatic lesions has provided effective palliation when curative resection was not possible (189, 209, 215). Unresectable or metastatic parathyrinomas often respond favorably to streptozotocin chemotherapy, with prompt and sustained falls in serum calcium concentrations to normal levels (197, 200, 201, 203, 205, 206, 210). Streptozotocin is usually combined with 5-FU (111, 184, 210). Somatostatin analogue therapy also has proven useful in patients with unresectable disease (213–215). Survival can be prolonged even in the presence of liver metastases, and the characteristically slow rate of tumor growth favors aggressive surgical treatment, even when only for palliation (184).

## PANCREATIC GROWTH HORMONE RELEASING FACTOR–PRODUCING TUMORS (GRFomas)

GRFomas are neuroendocrine neoplasms that produce excessive amounts of growth hormone-releasing factor (GRF), also known as somatoliberin or somatocrinin. GRFomas have also been called somatoliberinomas or somatocrininomas (219). GRF, a 44-amino-acid polypeptide structurally similar to VIP, is a potent stimulant of growth hormone release (220). It was first isolated and characterized in 1982 from extracts of pancreatic neuroendocrine neoplasms excised from two acromegalic patients (220–221). Shortly thereafter, it was reported that GRF produced by human pancreatic neuroendocrine neoplasms was identical to that found in the human hypothalamus (222). Hypothalamic GRF was characterized by researchers investigating pancreatic GRFomas (223). Excessive production of GRF by the neoplasm leads to continuous release of growth hormone by the pituitary gland, resulting in acromegaly.

In the 20 years before GRF was characterized, approximately 10 extracranial GRFomas were reported; over 20 cases were reported within the first 5 years after antibodies to GRF made

**TABLE 83.5. Clinical Features of Parathyrinomas**

| Case # | Age Sex | Syndrome | Tumor Site | Tumor Size (cm) | Mets | Operation | Ca (mg/dL) | PTH | Tumor | Postop | Chemo | Autopsy/ Neck Exp | F/U (yr) A/D | Author (Ref) | Year |
|---|---|---|---|---|---|---|---|---|---|---|---|---|---|---|---|
| 1 | 49 F | Hypercalcemia VIPOMA | Tail | 5.5 | Benign | DP | 12.4 | | | nl Ca | None | | 2 A | Matsumoto (190, 202) | 1966 |
| 2 | 48 F | ZES, Cushing's | Tail | | Liver, LN | DP | 11-16 | | Presumptive | ↑Ca | None | NP-A | 2 D | O'Neal (188) | 1968 |
| 3 | 42 F | Hypercalcemia VIPOMA | Tail | 4.5 | Benign | DP | 12.9 | | | nl Ca | None | | 2 A | Lopez (191, 202) | 1970 |
| 4 | 67 M | Hypercalcemia Insulinoma | | | Liver | | 13.9 | ↓ | –PTH | nl Ca after STZ | STZ | NP-A | D | Powel (195, 202) | 1973 |
| 5 | 57 M | Hypercalcemia | Tail | 10 | Liver | Bx | 12-16 | | Presumptive | ↓ Ca after STZ | STZ | NP-E | 3 A | DeWys (203) | 1973 |
| 6 | | Hypercalcemia | Pancreas | | Malig | | | | PTH-LI | | | NP-A | D | Palmeieri (204) | 1974 |
| 7 | 29 M | Hypercalcemia Insulinoma | | | Liver | None | 14.0 | | | nl insulin & Ca after STZ | STZ | | 1.5 A | Laryea (201) | 1974 |
| 8 | 62 M | Hypercalcemia VIPOMA | Tail | 4 | Liver | None | 7 mEq/L | ↑ | Presumptive | | None | NP-A | 2 D | Hirose (192, 202) | 1975 |
| 9 | 8 M | Hypercalcemia | Body & tail | | Liver | SP | 14.4 | nl | Presumptive | ↑ Ca | None | NP-A | 0 D | Friesen (196, 202, 205) | 1975 |
| 10 | 61 F | Hypercalcemia ZES | Pancreas | | Liver | Bx | 13.8–19.4 | nl | | ↓ Ca after STZ | STZ | NP-E | 18 D | Cryer (199, 202, 206) | 1976 |
| 11 | 37 F | CTOMA | Pancreas | | Liver | | nl | ↑ | PTH-LI | ↓ PTH after STZ | STZ | NP-A | D | Deftos (197) | 1976 |
| 12 | 52 F | Hypercalcemia CTOMA | Body & tail | 13 | Benign | DP | 14.8 | nl | Presumptive | nl Calcitonin nl Ca | None | NP-E | 11 A | Heitz (198, 207) | 1981 |
| 13 | 36 M | Hypercalcemia CTOMA VIPOMA | Head | 8 | Liver, oment | PD | 14 | nl | Presumptive | ↑ Calcitonin nl CA | STZ | | 10 A | Oberg (156) | 1981 |
| 14 | 49 F | Hypercalcemia CTOMA VIPOMA | Body | 8 | Liver, oment | | 14.5 | nl | Presumptive | ↓ Calcitonin nl Ca after STZ | STZ | | 7 A | Oberg (156) | 1981 |
| 15 | 44 M | Hypercalcemia | Body & tail | | Liver | DP | 15.3 | | | nl Ca | STZ Adriamycin | | 10 A | Shetty (208, 209) | 1984 |
| 16 | 60 M | Hypercalcemia | Tail | 10 | Liver | Bx | 13.3 | nl | Presumptive | ↓ Ca after STZ | STZ 5FU | | 0.2 A | Rasbach (210) | 1985 |
| 17 | 41 M | Hypercalcemia | Head | 14 | Liver | Bx | 16.8 | | PTH-LI | | None | NP-A | 6.5 D | Arps (211) | 1986 |

| | | | | | | | | | | | | | | | |
|---|---|---|---|---|---|---|---|---|---|---|---|---|---|---|---|
| 18 | 48 M | Hypercalcemia | Head | | Liver | Bx | | ↑ | | | | NP-E | D | Broughan (21) | 1986 |
| 19 | 54 F | Hypercalcemia | Body | | Liver | Bx | | nl | | | | NP-E | D | Broughan (21) | 1986 |
| 20 | 47 F | Hypercalcemia | Body & tail | 9 | None | SP | 16.4 | nl | | n Ca | None | | 2 A | Vair (212) | 1987 |
| 21 | 43 F | Hypercalcemia | | | Malig | | | ↑ | | ↓ Ca after somatos | Chemo Somatos | | 1 | Kvols (213) | 1987 |
| 22 | 54 M | Hypercalcemia VIPOMA | Tail | | Liver | DP | 13.9 | nl | | n CA | Chemo Somatos | | 10 A | Venkatesh (189) | 1989 |
| 23 | 37 F | Hypercalcemia | Tail | 5 | Liver | | 14 | ↓ ↑ | PTHrP | n Ca after Somatos | Somatos | | 0.5 A | Wynick (214) | 1990 |
| 24 | 42 F | Hypercalcemia | Body | Large | Liver | | 19.6 | ↓ ↑ | PTHrP PTHrP | nl Ca after Somatos | Somatos | | 2.5 A | Dodwell (215) | 1990 |
| 25 | 30 F | Hypercalcemia | Tail | 8 | Liver | SP | 14 | nl | PTHrP PTHrP | nl Ca | | | 2 A | Rizzoli (216) | 1990 |
| 26 | 60 F | Hypercalcemia | Head | Large | Liver | Bx | 14.4 | nl | PTHrP | | | NP-A | 1 D | Rizzoli (216) | 1990 |
| 27 | 45 M | Hypercalcemia | Tail | 12 | None | DP | 14.4 | nl | | nl Ca | STZ 5FU | NP-E | 5 A | Breseler (184) | 1991 |
| 28 | 77 F | Hypercalcemia | Tail | Large | Liver | DP | 12 | ↓ ↑ | | nl Ca after STZ | STZ 5FU | | 4.5 A | Mitlak (217) | 1991 |
| 29 | 47 F | Hypercalcemia | Tail | 11 | Liver | DP | 16.6 | | PTHrp PTHrP | nl Ca | | | 3 A | Miraliakbari (218) | 1992 |
| 30 | 30 M | Hypercalcemia Somatostat | Body & tail | Large | Malig | Bx | 17.2 | L | | nl Ca after STZ | STZ | | 1 A | Stavri (200) | 1992 |
| 31 | 41 M | Hypercalcemia | Entire pancreas | 18 | Liver | Bx | 26.4 | nl | PTHrP −PTH | | | | 2.5 D | Mao (173) | 1995 |
| 32 | 43 M | Hypercalcemia | Body & tail | 15 | Liver | DP | 13.6 | ↓ | −PTH +PTHrP | | Chemo Rad Tx | | 10.5 D D | Mao (173) | 1995 |
| 33 | 64 M | Hypercalcemia | Tail | 7 | Liver LN | Bx | 16.4 | nl | −PTH +PTHrP | | | NP-A | 0 D | Mao (173) | 1995 |

Modified from Mao C, Carter P, Schaefer P, Zhu L, et al. Malignant islet cell tumor associated with hypercalcemia. Surgery 1995;117:37–40.

Abbreviations:

| | | | |
|---|---|---|---|
| Oment | Omentum | Malig | Malignant |
| ZES | Zollinger Ellison Syndrome | NP-A | Normal parathyroid gland by autopsy |
| CTOMA | Calcitoninoma | NE-E | Normal parathyroid glands by exploration |
| Somatostat | Somatostatinoma | −PTH | Negative for PTH |
| PTH | Parathyroid hormone | +PTHrP | Positive for PTHrP |
| PTH-LI | PTH-like immunoreactivity | Somatos | Somatostatin |
| PTHrP | PTH-related peptide | | |

RIA and immunohistochemical identification possible (45). GRF is normally produced by cells of the ventromedial and arcuate nuclei of the hypothalamus. Although several investigators detected low levels of GRF immunoreactivity in the pancreas, recent studies showed that this might have resulted from cross-reactivity of the C-terminal-specific anti-GRF serum with the PP molecule (223). The concentration of GRF in normal extracranial tissues, including the pancreas, if any, must be extremely low (45).

As early as 1949, it was suggested that bronchial neuroendocrine neoplasms produced a factor that stimulated adenomatous growth of the pituitary and adrenal glands (224). Subsequently, several patients with acromegaly associated with extrapituitary neuroendocrine neoplasms were reported and the presence of growth hormone-releasing activity in these neoplasms was suggested (45). GRF production has now been demonstrated in a large variety of extracranial neoplasms associated with acromegaly, including pancreatic, pulmonary, intestinal, retroperitoneal, and adrenal neuroendocrine neoplasms. In addition, GRF production has been found in many neoplasms not associated with acromegaly, including pancreatic and jejunal neuroendocrine tumors, medullary carcinoma of the thyroid, small cell carcinoma of the lung, endometrial carcinomas, and neuroendocrine neoplasms of the thymus, appendix, and intestine (45, 225–227). In one study, four of nine pancreatic neuroendocrine neoplasms and three of eight nonpancreatic gastrointestinal neoplasms not associated with acromegaly had GRF immunoreactivity (225). In a more recent study, 6 of 24 pancreatic (25%) and 4 of 35 nonpancreatic (11%) gastrointestinal neuroendocrine neoplasms demonstrated strong GRF immunoreactivity (227). Seven of these 10 neoplasms also had immunoreactivity for a variety of other regulatory peptides and neurotransmitters including gastrin, insulin, glucagon, serotonin, substance P, somatostatin, PP, VIP, and ACTH. Thus, even in the absence of acromegaly, up to 25% of pancreatic neuroendocrine neoplasms may produce GRF. GRF also has been detected in 9 of 18 (50%) VIPomas investigated histochemically (228).

The incidence of GRFomas is unknown. Although the total number of reported patients is still very limited, awareness of the disease has led to increasing recognition (223). While the incidence of GRFomas among patients with acromegaly is less than 1% (229), the markedly different therapeutic approach (i.e., resection of pancreatic GRFoma vs. hypophysectomy) warrants diligent efforts to establish the correct diagnosis (223), and routine measurement of GRF plasma concentration in all patients suffering from acromegaly has been recommended (223, 225, 230). However, fewer than 50 neoplasms secreting ectopic GRF (including the pancreatic GRFomas reviewed here) have been reported (45). Furthermore, of 177 acromegalic patients screened for ectopic GRF production, only 3 (who were already known to have GRFomas) had high circulating GRF concentrations (231).

Of the 23 pancreatic GRFomas reported, 10 had detailed information (45, 219, 220, 225, 227, 231–246) (Table 83.6). GRFomas occurred predominantly in women (80%) and presented at a mean age of 37 years (range, 21–58 years). Extrapancreatic GRFomas have been found most often in the lungs, followed by the extrapancreatic GI tract (421). Histologically, GRFomas resemble other gastroenteropancreatic neuroendocrine neoplasms. Most are composed of trabecular or solid nests and sheets of uniform cells with abundant granular acidophilic cytoplasm (45). Ultrastructurally, GRFoma cells resemble the $D_1$ subtype of PP cells (45). Mean tumor size is 8.0 cm (range, 2–25 cm) and is not related to circulating concentrations of GRF or duration of acromegalic symptoms (45). Tumor size does not seem to correlate with malignancy, since the three largest tumors had neither invasive features nor evidence of metastases. Metastases were found in 3 of 10 patients (30%); the liver was involved in 2 patients and peripancreatic lymph nodes in 1; 2 of these 3 metastatic neoplasms occurred in patients with the Zollinger-Ellison syndrome. In addition, three GRFomas in patients without acromegalic features were malignant; two of these patients also had the Zollinger-Ellison syndrome, and all three had Cushing's syndrome (45). The MEN-1 syndrome was present in 5 of the 10 patients reported in detail (50%). Multiple pancreatic neuroendocrine neoplasms were found in four patients (40%), and all four had features of the MEN-1 syndrome. Thirteen pancreatic GRFomas have been reported in patients without acromegaly (225, 227, 236, 247); most of these 13 patients had associated syndromes including Cushing's syndrome (3 patients), Zollinger-Ellison syndrome (2 patients), insulinoma syndrome (2 patients), and VIPoma syndrome (1 patient).

The clinical presentation of patients with pancreatic GRFomas may include some or all of the following characteristics: *(a)* acromegalic features due to excess GRF and subsequent growth hormone hypersecretion; *(b)* associated features due to hypersecretion of hormones other than GRF; and *(c)* symptoms due to local mass effect of the neoplasm (45). Production of GRF by pancreatic neuroendocrine neoplasms results in the ectopic acromegaly syndrome. The clinical features in these patients are indistinguishable from those of classic acromegaly and include enlargement of the hands and feet, distortion of facial features, skin changes, peripheral nerve entrapments, and headaches (229). Acromegaly is usually insidious, and the onset of symptoms is difficult to assess. The mean duration of symptoms in seven patients with pancreatic GRFomas was 5 years (45). In addition to acromegaly, symptoms associated with hyperparathyroidism (as part of the MEN-1 syndrome), Cushing's syndrome, Zollinger-Ellison syndrome, insulinoma syndrome, and galactorrhea have been noted in patients with pancreatic and extrapancreatic GRFomas (Table 83.6). The diagnosis of a GRFoma is established by the circulating GRF concentration (normal ≤ 10 pg/mL). Classic acromegalics have GRF levels up to 191 pg/mL; the lowest value detected in patients with GRFomas was 299 pg/mL (range, 299–2300 pg/mL). Therefore, circulating concentrations of 300 pg/mL or more in acromegalic patients strongly suggest the presence of a GRFoma (45). There are currently no provocative or inhibitory tests available to confirm the diagnosis of GRFoma (46).

Surgical resection is the treatment of choice for pancreatic GRFomas. Small, noninfiltrating GRFomas have been successfully treated by simple enucleation (243, 247). Any larger, infiltrating, metastatic, or otherwise malignant-appearing GRFoma should be widely resected by pancreatoduodenectomy or distal pancreatectomy, depending on its location. Following complete resection, concentrations of circulating GRF rapidly return to the normal range. Similarly, circulating growth hormone levels rapidly decrease after complete tumor removal, but mild prolonged elevations of growth hormone have been reported, suggesting delayed recovery of the hypothalamohypophyseal axis (45). Octreotide has proven useful in patients with metastatic GRFomas by reducing or normalizing growth hormone concentrations (229, 238, 239). Scant data are available on survival, with follow-up limited to 2 years or less.

A single case of a pancreatic neuroendocrine neoplasm producing excessive amounts of growth hormone in the absence of GRF was reported in a patient with full-blown acromegaly (247). The patient was 60 years old, with a neoplasm 15 cm in diameter in the head of the pancreas. Following enucleation of the tumor, circulating growth hormone levels returned to normal, and all signs and symptoms of acromegaly disappeared rapidly. This is the only well-documented case of an ectopic growth hormone-secreting neoplasm (229).

**TABLE 83.6. Clinical Features of GRFomas**

| Case # | Age Sex | Syndrome | Tumor Site | Tumor Size (cm) | Mets | Operation | GRF <0.1 (ng/mL) | Tumor Immunoreactivity | Preop GH (ng/mL) | Postop GH | Chemo | F/U (years) | Author (Ref) | Year |
|---|---|---|---|---|---|---|---|---|---|---|---|---|---|---|
| 1 | 30 F | Acromegaly | Tail | 10 | None | DP | + Bioactivity | GRF | 14 | <1 | None | 0.7 A | Caplan (219, 232, 233) | 1978 |
| 2 | 21 F | Acromegaly Galactorrhea | Tail | 5 | None | DP | 3.8 | GRF | 95 | nl | None | 0.5 A | Thorner (219, 220, 231, 234, 235) | 1982 |
| 3 | 55 M | Acromegaly HPTH MEN-1 | Head & tail | 25 Multiple | LN | TP | 50 | GRF, PP, ACTH, Somatos, Glucagon | 69 | nl | None | 0.9 A | Barger (236) | 1984 |
| 4 | 25 F | Acromegaly ZES | Tail | | Liver | DP | 5.6 | GRF Gastrin GRP | 488 | nl after somatos | STZ Somatos | 2 A | Wilson (225, 237, 238, 239) | 1984 |
| 5 | 39 F | Acromegaly HPTH | Pancreas | | None | | 0.6 μg/g | | 20.7 | | | | Sano (45) | 1985 |
| 6 | 58 F | Acromegaly HPTH MEN-1 ZES | Pancreas | | Liver | | 2300 | | 25 | nl after somatos | Somatos | | Ch'ng (239, 240) | 1984 |

*Continued on following page*

**TABLE 83.6. Clinical Features of GRFomas—***(continued)*

| Case # | Age Sex | Syndrome | Tumor Site | Tumor Size (cm) | Mets | Operation | GRF <0.1 (ng/mL) | Tumor Immuno-reactiity | Preop GH (ng/mL) | Postop GH | Chemo | F/U (years) | Author (Ref) | Year |
|---|---|---|---|---|---|---|---|---|---|---|---|---|---|---|
| 7 | 54 F | Acromegaly | Head | 10 | None | PD | 1.1 | GRF, NT, PP, VIP, Serotonin | ↑ | nl | None | | Schulte (241, 242) | 1985 |
| 8 | 36 M | Acromegaly HPTH MEN-1 | Tail × 2 | Multiple 4.2 & 2.0 | None | E | 299 | GRF, CT Somatos | 42.4 | nl | None | 1 A | Sano (243) | 1987 |
| 9 | 27 F | Acromegaly MEN-1 | Tail & body | Multiple | None | DP | 0.52 | GRF, PP Gastrin Somatos | 47 | nl | None | 1.5 A | Ramsay (244) | 1988 |
| 10 | 30 F | No Acromegaly Insulinoma MEN-1 ZES | Multiple | 2.3 Multiple | None | SP | 1.28 | GRF Insulin Glucagon Somatos | 32 | nl | None | | Asa (245) | 1978 |
| 11–16 | | No Acromegaly Insulinoma-1 Vipoma-1 | | | | | GRF only 2 | Gastrin-2 Glucagon-4 GRF-6 Insulin-4 PP-3 | ↑ VIP-1 ↑ Seroto-nin-2 | | | | Dayal (227) | 1986 |
| 17–19 | | No Acromegaly Insulinoma-1 | | | | | | | | | | | Bostwick (225) | 1984 |
| 20–23 | | No Acromegaly Cushing's-3 ZES-2 | | | Metastases in all 3 patients | | | | | | | | Sano (246) | 1985 |

Modified from Sano T, Asa SL, Kovacs K. Growth hormone-releasing hormone-producing tumors: clinical, biochemical, and morphological manifestations. Endocrine Rev 1988;9:357–373.

Abbreviations:

| | |
|---|---|
| LN | Lymph nodes |
| nl | Normal |
| DP | Distal pancreatectomy |
| TP | Total pancreatectomy |
| PD | Pancreatoduodenectomy |
| E | Enucleated |
| Somatos | Somatostatin |

## PANCREATIC CALCITONINOMAS (CTomas)

Calcitonin is a polypeptide normally produced by the parafollicular cells (C-cells) of the thyroid gland. It decreases intestinal transit time and increases water and electrolyte secretion in the small intestine. Diarrhea can therefore be expected in patients with hypercalcitoninemia. However, only one-third of patients with medullary carcinoma of the thyroid and excessive circulating calcitonin concentrations have associated diarrhea (248). As early as 1972, elevations of plasma calcitonin were reported in patients with neoplasms other than medullary carcinoma of the thyroid (249–252). Increased circulating calcitonin has been reported in a few patients with pancreatic neuroendocrine tumors but, with two exceptions (cases #9 and 13, Table 83.7), not as the predominant peptide (67, 150, 156, 197, 198, 253–259). Most often, calcitonin has been detected in mixed tumors that also contain VIP. These patients present with the typical WDHA syndrome (156, 253, 254, 258, 259). Calcitonin has also been detected in mixed neoplasms containing primarily somatostatin (255, 257), neurotensin (150), or PP (67, 259).

Only two patients have been reported with what could be considered pure calcitoninomas (156, 198). The first was a 52-year-old female who presented with hypercalcemia and hypercalcitoninemia. Following resection of a pancreatic neuroendocrine neoplasm that demonstrated positive calcitonin immunoreactivity, the hypercalcemia completely disappeared. Her postoperative serum calcitonin concentration remained below 1.7 pg/L after 3 years of follow-up, compared with a preoperative serum level above 10,700 pg/L (198). The second patient was a 49-year-old female who presented with watery diarrhea, hypokalemia, hypercalcemia, hypercalcitoninemia, a neuroendocrine neoplasm of the pancreas, and multiple hepatic metastases. Resection was not performed, and the patient's hypercalcitoninemia slowly decreased following streptozotocin therapy (156). The ectopic production of calcitonin from the pancreatic neoplasm was verified by percutaneous transhepatic catheterization of the portal venous system and by calcitonin immunoreactivity in tumor tissue extracts. The patient had normal serum gastrin, PP, VIP, somatostatin, and PTH concentrations, and the authors suggested that calcitonin secreted by the pancreatic neoplasm was the mediator of the WDHA syndrome (156).

Watery diarrhea has been present in most patients with calcitonin-secreting pancreatic neoplasms. Most of these neoplasms also secreted VIP and PP. The possible interrelationships of VIP, PP, and calcitonin in the pathogenesis of watery diarrhea remain unclear (259). Two patients with watery diarrhea, hypercalcitoninemia, and increased concentrations of both circulating VIP and PP have been reported (259). Octreotide therapy improved the diarrhea and lowered both VIP and PP concentrations but did not alter the serum calcitonin level. The authors speculated that the presence of calcitonin in pancreatic neuroendocrine neoplasms may indicate a clone of cells uniquely unresponsive to octreotide, as is the case with medullary carcinoma of the thyroid (259). Calcitonin, like PP, has been suggested as a possible marker peptide for the diagnosis of pancreatic neuroendocrine malignancies (248).

## PANCREATIC ENTEROGLUCAGONOMAS

Pancreatic glucagon, a 29-amino-acid polypeptide, was first described as a hyperglycemic factor present in a crude extract of bovine pancreas. It was purified and sequenced in 1957 (260). Pancreatic glucagon is produced by the alpha-cells of the islets of Langerhans and belongs to a family of structurally related peptides that includes secretin, VIP, GIP, GRF, and glicentin (261). A heterogeneous group of polypeptides containing glucagon or glucagon-like immunoreactivity, some with more than 29 amino acids in their molecules, have been isolated from the stomach, intestine, and brain (262–263). These polypeptides cross react with nonspecific antiglucagon sera directed toward the N terminus of glucagon but react poorly to specific antiglucagon sera directed toward the C terminus. Of these polypeptides, those isolated from the intestine with molecular structures larger than that of glucagon are collectively referred to as enteroglucagon (261, 263). Enteroglucagon is normally produced by the L-cells of the intestinal mucosa, which are found in highest concentrations in the distal small intestine and colon (261, 263). Enteroglucagon is released into the circulation after a meal, but its biologic actions have not been widely studied (261). An association between intestinal crypt cell production and enteroglucagon has been suggested, since intestinal resection, colonic glucose perfusion, and GRP (bombesin) injection all stimulate intestinal mitotic activity, increase enteroglucagon-cell degranulation, and increase plasma enteroglucagon concentrations (264–267).

In 1971, one patient was reported with a neuroendocrine neoplasm arising in the kidney that appeared to produce enteroglucagon (269). This 44-year-old woman had marked hyperplasia of the intestinal villi, decreased intestinal transit time, and mild fat malabsorption, all of which reversed upon removal of the tumor. The neoplasm demonstrated enteroglucagon-like immunoreactivity (269).

Two pancreatic enteroglucagon-producing neoplasms have been reported (270–272). In both cases, high tissue and plasma concentrations of enteroglucagon were associated with intestinal mucosal hyperplasia and giant intestinal villi. The first was a 45-year-old man with a 6-year history of an itchy bullous rash that had been diagnosed as various different skin conditions, who presented with recurrent diarrhea, weight loss, and diabetes mellitus (270, 271). He had massive hyperglucagonemia, and giant intestinal villi were noted on endoscopy. A 12 × 18 cm neoplasm involving the head and body of the pancreas, the superior mesenteric artery, and the portal vein and extending into the porta hepatis and retroperitoneal space was found at laparotomy. Resection was not performed, and the patient died postoperatively. The tumor reacted only with nonspecific antiglucagon sera directed toward the N terminus of glucagon. This patient had the typical features of the glucagonoma syndrome and also had giant intestinal villi (272).

The second patient was a 41-year-old man who presented with weight loss, diabetes, rash, a glucagon-producing neoplasm of the head of the pancreas, and giant intestinal villi. A 4.5 cm tumor of the head of the pancreas with glucagon-like immunoreactivity and focal, perineural, and vascular invasion but negative lymph nodes was resected by pancreatoduodenectomy. Microscopic examination of the resected proximal jejunum confirmed the marked villous hypertrophy that had been diagnosed preoperatively by CT scanning (272).

## PANCREATIC CHOLECYSTOKININOMAS (CCKomas)

CCK, a 33-amino-acid polypeptide, was first isolated from porcine intestine in 1928 (261). It is not normally found in the pancreas and shares several features in common with gastrin (263). The C-terminal pentapeptide sequences of gastrin and CCK are identical and include the biologically active region for both molecules. The six-amino-acid extensions that immediately follow the pentapeptide sequence are also the same in the human CCK and gastrin precursors. To date, no pure CCK-secreting tumor has been reported (273). However, as early as 1973, a syndrome consisting of diarrhea and severe gastric acid hypersecretion (presumably resulting from the affinity of CCK for the gastrin receptor on the parietal cell) was described in a patient with elevated CCK and normal serum gastrin concentrations (274). Basal pancreatic secretions (volume and bicarbonate output) were increased, but intestinal secretions

**TABLE 83.7. Clinical Features of Calcitoninomas**

| Case # | Age Sex | Symptoms | Syndrome | Tumor Site | Tumor Size (cm) | Mets | Operation | Preop CT (pg/mL)L | Tumor | Postop | Chemo | F/U (years) | Author (Ref) | Year |
|---|---|---|---|---|---|---|---|---|---|---|---|---|---|---|
| 1 | 26 M | W diarrhea Wt loss | VIPOMA | Body & tail | | Liver, LN | SP | | CT 14 ng/g, enteroglu-cagon VIP secretin glucagon serotonin | | STZ 5FU | 0.3 D | Schmitt (253) | 1975 |
| 2 | 37 F | | | Pancreas | | Liver | Bx | CT 24,000 ↑ PTH | PTH, CT | post-STZ, CT 800, PTH 200 | STZ | D | Deftos (197) | 1976 |
| 3 | | W diarrhea | VIPOMA | Pancreas | | Liver | Yes | CT 1710 VIP 312 | VIP, CT | CT 1900 | | | Ram-baud (254) | 1978 |
| 4 | | W diarrhea | VIPOMA | Pancreas | | Liver | Yes | CT 3480 VIP 83 | VIP, CT | CT 1135 | | D | Ram-baud (254) | 1978 |
| 5 | | W diarrhea | VIPOMA | Pancreas | | Liver | No | CT 1740 VIP 227 | VIP, CT | | | D | Ram-baud (254) | 1978 |
| 6 | 70 F | W diarrhea | Somat | Pancreas | 8 | Liver | PD | CT 8700 SOM 9000 | CT 3700 SOM 310,000 | CT 4500 SOM 5700 | | D | Galmiche (1, 225, 256) | 1978 |
| 7 | 52 M | Wt loss | Somat | Head | 5 | Liver | PD | CT 4650 SOM 13,000 | SOM, CT | | STZ 5FU Doxoru-bicin | 8 A | Krejs (257) | 1979 |
| 8 | 65 M | W diarrhea Flushing | NToma | Tail | 5 | None | DP | CT 5000 NT 3200 PP 1400 VIP 250 | NT, CT, En-kephalin | CT 160, NT 24.5, PP 1300, VIP 3.5 | None | 0.2 A | Gutniak (150) | 1980 |
| 9 | 52 F | Hypercal-cemia | CTOMA | Tail | | None | DP | CT 10,700 pmol/L | CT only | CT <1.7 pmol/L | None | 3 A | Heitz (198) | 1981 |

| | | | | | | | | | | | | | | |
|---|---|---|---|---|---|---|---|---|---|---|---|---|---|---|
| 10 | 52 M | W diarrhea | VIPOMA MEN-1 | Tail | Large | None | DP | Ct 480 pmol/L VIP 210 PP 866 | VIP, Gastrin, CT | | STZ | 5 A | Oberg (156) | 1981 |
| 11 | 36 M | W diarrhea Flushing | VIPOMA | Head | 8 | Liver, omentum | PD | CT 830 pmol/L VIP 91 | Gastrin | CT nl VIP 6300 | STZ | 10r A | Oberg (156) | 1981 |
| 12 | 49 F | W diarrhea Hypercalcemia | CTOMA | Body | 8 | Liver, LN | Bx | CT 25,700 | CT, PP | CT 4.6 | STZ | 7 A | OBerg (156) | 1981 |
| 13 | 58 M | Abd pain Constipation | PPOMA | Body & tail | Large | Liver | None | CT 740,000 PP 60,000 | | CT 140,000 PP 50,000 | None | 0.1 A | Manche (67) | 1983 |
| 14 | | W diarrhea | VIPOMA | | | | | | | VIP, PHM, CT | | | Ooi (258) | 1985 |
| 15 | | W diarrhea | VIPOMA | | | | | | VIP, PHM, CT | | | | Ooi (258) | 1985 |
| 16 | | W diarrhea | VIPOMA MEN-1 | | | | | | VIP, PHM, CT | | | | Ooi (258) | 1985 |
| 17 | 63 F | W diarrhea | PPOMA | Body & tail | 7 | Liver | DP | PP 10,000 | VIP, PP, gastrin, CT | PP 149 | | 8 A | McLeod (259) | 1992 |
| 18 | 65 F | W diarrhea Wt loss | VIPOMA | Head | | Liver | Bx | CT 392,700 VIP 209 Serotonin 1043 | VIP, CT | | Octreotide STZ | 3 A | McLeod (259) | 1992 |

Abbreviations:

| | | | |
|---|---|---|---|
| W diarrhea | Watery diarrhea | NTOMA | Neurotensinoma |
| Wt | Weight | CTOMA | Calcitoninoma |
| Bx | Biopsy | PPOMA | Pancreatic polypeptidoma |
| STZ | Streptozotocin | | |

were not. No discrete pancreatic neoplasm was found, but islet cell hyperplasia was present in the resected tail of the pancreas (274).

Recently, two patients with mixed pancreatic CCK-secreting neoplasms have been reported (273, 275). The first was a 57-year-old man who presented with diarrhea, hypokalemia, duodenitis, normal serum gastrin, and a negative secretin-stimulation test for gastrin (275). His symptoms completely resolved following removal of a pancreatic neoplasm and a solitary liver metastasis. Tumor tissue contained substantial amounts of VIP and CCK as well as minute amounts of immunoreactive somatostatin, gastrin, and PP. The second patient was a 68-year-old woman who presented with a perforated postbulbar duodenal ulcer, massive diarrhea, and gastric acid hypersecretion that could not be controlled with high doses of $H_2$ receptor antagonists but was controlled with intravenous native somatostatin (273). Plasma gastrins were repeatedly normal, as was a secretin-stimulation test. She died from respiratory complications, and the autopsy revealed a neuroendocrine neoplasm involving the body and tail of the pancreas. Unfortunately, no immunocytochemical studies were performed (273). A single patient with a mixed extrapancreatic CCK-, VIP-, and bombesin-secreting neoplasm of the ampulla of Vater was recently reported (276).

## PANCREATIC GIPomas

Gastric inhibitory polypeptide (GIP) (also known as glucose-dependent insulinotropic polypeptide) is a 42-amino-acid polypeptide normally produced by the K-cells of the intestinal mucosa. Most of these cells are found in the duodenum and jejunum, but a few K-cells are also present in the ileum and gastric antrum (263). GIP is not found in the normal pancreas (263). GIP was first isolated in 1970 (277), and its correct amino acid sequence was reported in 1981 (278). GIP is an insulinotropic hormone that also inhibits gastric acid secretion and stimulates secretion in the small intestine and mesenteric blood flow (279); however, the physiologic role of GIP remains unclear (263). A single patient with increased plasma GIP concentrations and pancreatic islet cell hyperplasia has been reported (280). This patient had mild chronic watery diarrhea and hypokalemia.

A single pancreatic neoplasm containing GIP (GIPoma) was reported in 1972 (281). The patient was a 41-year-old woman who presented with a 5-month history of severe, intractable, watery diarrhea, hypokalemia, acidosis, hypercalcemia, and a diabetic oral glucose tolerance test. At laparotomy, a 1.5-cm neoplasm in the tail of the pancreas and multiple hepatic metastases were found. The pancreatic neoplasm was resected, and biopsy specimens were obtained from the hepatic metastases. Strong-positive immunofluorescence was seen with GIP antiserum in both the primary neoplasm and the hepatic metastases. Antisera against gastrin, pentagastrin, glucagon, calcitonin, ACTH, insulin, and motilin were negative in both tissues. Postoperatively, the patient received intraarterial hepatic 5-FU infusion, but she died within 4 months from recurrent severe hypokalemic acidosis (281). Since GIP acts as an insulinotropic hormone, increases mesenteric blood flow, and stimulates small-intestinal secretion, high circulating concentrations could have contributed to the clinical findings in this patient (7). However, since GIP cross reacts with VIP, and the VIP content of the tumor was not investigated, this may actually have been a VIPoma that presented with the classic WDHA syndrome. Neurotensinomas and GIPomas are probably best characterized as yet other neoplasms capable of causing the watery diarrhea, hypokalemia, hypochlorhydria, acidosis syndrome (51).

## PANCREATIC BOMBESINOMAS (GRPomas)

GRP, a 27-amino-acid polypeptide, was first isolated from nonantral portions of porcine stomach in 1978 (282, 283). GRP is now known to be the mammalian analogue of bombesin, a peptide with strong GI effects that was first isolated from amphibian skin in 1971 (284). The terms GRP and mammalian bombesin are both used to describe the mammalian polypeptide, and GRPomas are thus also referred to as bombesinomas. GRP and bombesin have amino-acid sequence homology, with close resemblance of the C-terminal sequence. These two peptides also have the same pharmacologic actions, including stimulating release of gastrin and CCK (285, 286). GRP also has widespread excitatory effects on motility and secretion in the mammalian GI tract, which probably result from release of other gastrointestinal peptides. GRP is known to release PP, glucagon, GIP, and somatostatin (287). The release mechanisms and neuronal origin of GRP are consistent with a neurotransmitter function, and although its physiologic role remains unclear, the best documented effect of GRP is gastrin release, in which GRP acts as the noncholinergic mediator of vagally mediated gastrin release (284).

GRP-like immunoreactivity has been demonstrated in various neuroendocrine neoplasms but has not been found in nonneuroendocrine tumors. GRP-like immunoreactivity has been found in medullary thyroid carcinomas (3 of 3), carcinoids of the lung, pancreas, and intestine (22 of 36), paragangliomas (2 of 3), pituitary adenomas (1 of 6), and pulmonary small cell (oat cell) carcinomas with neuroendocrine differentiation (1 of 8) (285). Complete absence of immunoreactivity was observed in 3 pheochromocytomas, 5 Merkel cell tumors, 6 neuroblastomas and 15 nonneuroendocrine tumors (285). In a recent prospective study, elevated plasma concentrations of GRP were detected in 2 of 21 patients (10%) with gastrinomas (159).

A pancreatic GRPoma was reported in 1989 (288). This patient presented with a 20-fold increase in circulating concentrations of GRP-like immunoreactivity and recent-onset type II diabetes, hemorrhagic gastritis, and facial flushing. Peripheral PP, calcitonin, serotonin, carcinoembryonic antigen, and neuron-specific enolase were moderately increased. Fasting gastrin and somatostatin concentrations were normal. Circulating concentrations of GRP-like immunoreactivity were increased further in response to intravenous injection of calcium and pentagastrin. A neoplasm of the head of the pancreas with metastases was found and a biopsy was performed at laparotomy. Immunocytochemistry and electron microscopy confirmed neuroendocrine features. Electron microscopy revealed sparsely granulated neoplastic cells containing small dense granules. The amount of GRP-like immunoreactivity in the neoplastic tissue was 1000 times that of the normal surrounding pancreatic tissue. However, whether the clinical manifestations in this patient were related to the excessive secretion of GRP is unclear. In addition, a neuroendocrine carcinoma of the ampulla of Vater with positive immunoreactivity for GRP, VIP, and CCK has been reported (276).

## PANCREATIC AMYLINOMAS (IAPPomas)

Islet amyloid polypeptide (IAPP), or amylin, is a 37-amino-acid polypeptide that was first identified by purification and chemical characterization of the amyloid component of a human pancreatic insulinoma in 1986 (289, 290). Subsequently, it was isolated from islet amyloid in patients with type II diabetes mellitus (291). IAPP has approximately 50% homology with calcitonin gene-related peptide and is normally located in the pancreatic beta-islet cells where it is stored with insulin in the secretory granules (292). The physiologic role of IAPP is unclear, but it be a regulator of glucose homeostasis (293). It inhibits glycogen synthesis and opposes insulin stimulation of glucose uptake (294). IAPP secretion is regulated by the extracellular glucose level, and circulating levels increase after glucagon stimulation (295, 296). IAPP lowers blood pressure when given intravenously and also may affect calcium homeostasis (297, 298). A role for IAPP in the development of non-insulin-dependent diabetes mellitus (NIDDM) has been suggested, and elevated concentrations of IAPP have been reported in patients with NIDDM (299, 300). A proposed IAPPoma syndrome would thus include symptoms of hyperglycemia, hypocalcemia, and hypotension.

A pancreatic IAPPoma was reported in 1992 (293). The patient was a 50-year-old man who presented with abdominal pain, severe pruritus secondary to obstructive jaundice, flushing, diarrhea, weight loss, night sweats, and hyperglycemia. Three years earlier, a 5 cm neoplasm was found incidentally in the head of the pancreas while he was hospitalized for a hypertensive workup. Pulmonary metastases were identified and biopsy specimens from the pancreatic primary and metastases revealed "carcinoid-like" neoplastic cells. The patient was asymptomatic and received no treatment. Serum gastrin, PP, human chorionic gonadotropin-ß (ß-HCG), insulin, C-peptide, calcitonin, growth hormone, gastrin-releasing polypeptide, VIP, glucagon, and somatostatin levels were all normal. Increased concentrations of serum α-HCG, proinsulin, plasma neuropeptide K, neurotensin, chromagranins A and B, and urinary 5-HIAA were demonstrated along with very high plasma concentrations of IAPP (500 times normal). Ingestion of a mixed meal resulted in a significant rise in IAPP concentration without concomitant release of PP. Recombinant interferon-α improved the patient's symptoms, but his hyperglycemia and high IAPP concentration persisted. He received human leukocyte interferon and later streptozotocin for disease progression, with good clinical response, but the IAPP level was unchanged. He was alive after 5 years of follow-up. In spite of the huge amounts of circulating IAPP-like immunoreactivity, which may have contributed to his altered glucose metabolism, he showed no obvious effects on calcium regulation or systemic blood pressure. More cases are needed before the existence of a distinct IAPPoma syndrome can be established (293).

## REFERENCES


1. Delcore R, Friesen SR. Gastrintestinal neuroendocrine tumors. J Am Coll Surg 1994;178:187–211.
2. Arnold R. Therapeutic strategies of the management of endocrine GEP tumours. Eur J Clin Invest 1990;20:82–90.
3. Liddle GW, Nicholson WE, Island DI, Orth DN, et al. Clinical and laboratory studies of ectopic humoral syndromes. Recent Prog Horm Res 1969;25:283–314.
4. Solcia E, Capella C, Fiocca R, Cornaggia M, Bosi F. The gastroenteropancreatic endocrine system and related tumors. Gastroenterol Clin North Am 1989;18:671–693.
5. Pearse AGE. The cytochemistry and ultrastructure of polypeptide hormone producing cells of the APUD series and the embryologic, physiologic and pathologic implications of the concept. J Histochem Cytochem 1969;17:303–313.
6. Dayal Y. Neuroendocrine cells of the gastrointestinal tract: introduction and historical perspective. In: Dayal Y, ed. Endocrine pathology of the gut and pancreas. Boca Raton, FL: CRC Press, 1991:1–31.
7. Mozell E, Woltering E, Stenzel P, Rosch J, O'Dorisio T. Functional endocrine tumors of the pancreas: clinical presentation, diagnosis, and treatment. Curr Probl Surg 1990;303–386.
8. Kerr DJ, Burt AD, Anderson JR. Tumours of the diffuse system. Eur J Surg Oncol 1987;13:189–195.
9. Delcore R, Friesen SR. Embryologic concepts in the APUD system. Semin Surg Oncol 1993;9:349–361.
10. Debas HT. Clinical significance of gastrointestinal hormones. Adv Surg 1987;21:157–188.
11. Vinik AI, McLeod MK, Fig LM, Shapiro B, Lloyd RV, Cho K. Clinical features, diagnosis, and localization of carcinoid tumors and their management. Gastroenterol Clin North Am 1989;18: 865–896.
12. Vinik AI. A personal historical perspective of the development of the gastrointestinal endocrine system. Endocrinol Metab Clin North Am 1993;22:709–717.
13. Friesen SR. Tumors of the endocrine pancreas. N Engl J Med 1982;306:580–590.
14. Solcia E, Sessa F, Rindi G, Bonato M, Capella C. Pancreatic endocrine tumors: general concepts; nonfunctioning tumors and tumors with uncommon function. In: Y Dayal, ed. Endocrine pathology of the gut and pancreas. Boca Raton, FL: CRC Press, 1991:105–131.
15. Heitz PU, Kasper M, Polak JM, Kloppel G. Pancreatic endocrine tumors: immunocytochemical analysis of 125 tumors. Hum Pathol 1982;13:263.
16. Mukai K, Greider MH, Grotting JC, Rosai J. Retrospective study of 77 pancreatic endocrine tumors using the immunoperoxidase method. Am J Surg Path 1982;6:387–399.
17. Dockray GJ. Physiology of enteric neuropeptides. In: Johnson LR, ed. Physiology of the gastrointestinal tract. New York: Raven Press, 1994:169–209.
18. Somers G. Pancreatic bombesinoma. Eur J Clin Invest 1989; 19:A34.
19. Kent RB, van Heerden JA, Weiland LH. Nonfunctioning islet cell tumors. Ann Surg 1981;193:185–190.
20. Dial PF, Braasch JW, Rossi RL, Lee AK, Jin G. Management of nonfunctioning islet cell tumors of the pancreas. Surg Clin North Am 1985;65:291–299.
21. Broughan TA, Leslie JD, Soto JM, Hermann RE. Pancreatic islet cell tumors. Surg 1986;99:671–678.
22. Kloppel G, Heitz PU. Pancreatic endocrine tumors. Pathol Res Pract 1988;183:155.
23. Larsson LI. Corticotropin-like peptides in central nerves and in endocrine cells of gut and pancreas. Lancet 1977:1321–1323.
24. Cushing H. The basophil adenomas of the pituitary body and their clinical manifestations (pituitary basophilism). Bull Johns Hopkins Hosp 1932;50:137–195.
25. Brown WH. A case of pluriglandular syndrome: diabetes of bearded women. Lancet 1928;28:1022–1023.
26. Jex RK, Van Heerden JA, Carpenter PC, Grant CS. Ectopic ACTH syndrome: diagnostic and therapeutic aspects. Am J Surg 1985;149:227–282.
27. Wajchenberg BL, Mendonca BB, Liberman B, Pereira MAA, Kirschner MA. Ectopic ACTH syndrome. J Steroid Biochem Mol Biol 1995;53:139–151.
28. Howlett TA, Drury PL, Doniach PI, Rees LH, Besser GM. Diagnosis and management of ACTH-dependent Cushing's syndrome: comparison of the features in ectopic and pituitary ACTH production. Clin Endocrinol 1986;24:699–713.
29. Carpenter PC. Diagnostic evaluation of Cushing's syndrome. Endocrinol Metab Clin North Am 1988;17:455–472.
30. Oldfield EH, Doppman JL, Nieman LK, Chrousos GP, et al. Petrosal sinus sampling with and without corticotropin-releasing hormone for the differential diagnosis of Cushing's syndrome. N Engl J Med 1991;325:897–905.
31. Imura H, Nakai Y, Nakao K, Oki S, Matsukura S, Hirata Y. Functioning tumors with special reference to ectopic hormone producing tumors (in Japanese). Tanpakushitsu-Kakusan-Koso 1978;23:641–656.
32. Davies CJ, Joplin GF, Welbourn RB. Surgical management of the ectopic ACTH syndrome. Ann Surg 1982;196:246–258.
33. Findling JW, Tyrrel JB. Occult ectopic secretion of corticotropin. Arch Intern Med 1986;146:929–933.
34. Doppman JL, Nieman L, Miller DL, Pass HI, et al. Ectopic adrenocorticotropic hormone syndrome: localization studies in 28 patients. Radiology 1989;172:115–124.
35. Kepler EJ. Report of four cases. Proceedings of the staff meetings of the Mayo Clinic 1933;8:102–107.
36. Rawlinson DG. Electron microscopy of an ACTH-secreting islet cell carcinoma. Cancer 1973;31:1015–1019.

37. Clark ES, Carney JA. Pancreatic islet cell tumor associated with Cushing's syndrome. Am J Surg Pathol 1984;8:917–924.
38. Carty SE, Jensen RT, Norton JA. Prospective study of aggressive resection of metastatic pancreatic endocrine tumors. Surgery 1992;112:1024–1032.
39. Broder LE, Carter SK. Pancreatic islet cell carcinoma: I. Clinical features of 52 patients. Ann Intern Med 1973;79:101–107.
40. Heitz PU, Kasper M, Polak J, Kloppel G. Pathology of the endocrine pancreas. J Histochem 1979;27:1401–1402.
41. Durning P, Galland RB, Nagorney DM, Welbourn RB. Neuroendocrine tumors of the gut. World J Surg 1985;9:348–360.
42. Larsson LI, Grimelius L, Hakanson R, et al. Mixed endocrine pancreatic tumors producing several peptide hormones. Am J Pathol 1975;79:271–284.
43. Creutzfeldt W, Arnold R, Creutzfeldt TC, Track NS. Pathomorphologic, biochemical and diagnostic aspects of gastrinomas (Zollinger-Ellison syndrome). Hum Pathol 1975;6:47–76.
44. Maton PN, Gardner JD, Jensen RT. Cushing's syndrome in patients with the Zollinger-Ellison syndrome. N Engl J Med 1986;315:1–5.
45. Sano T, Asa SL, Kovacs K. Growth hormone-releasing hormone-producing tumors: clinical, biochemical, and morphological manifestations. Endocrine Rev 1988;9:357–373.
46. Metz DC, Jensen RT. Endocrine tumors of the pancreas. In: Haubrich WS, Schaffner F, Berk JE, eds. Gastroenterology. Philadelphia: WB Saunders, 1995:3002–3034.
47. Loriaux DL, Nieman L. Cushing's syndrome: advances in diagnosis and treatment. Adv Endocrinol Metab 1990;1:223–243.
48. Maton PN. Use of octreotide acetate for control of symptoms in patients with islet cell tumors. World J Surg 1993;17:504–510.
49. Lamberts SWJ, Tilanus HW, Klooswijk AIJ, Bruining HA, et al. Successful treatment with SMS 201-995 of Cushing's syndrome caused by ectopic adrenocorticotropin secretion from a metastatic gastrin-secreting pancreatic islet cell carcinoma. J Clin Endocrinol Metab 1988;67:1080–1083.
50. Ruszniewski P, Girard F, Benamouzig R, Mignon M, Bonfils S. Long acting somatostatin treatment of paraneoplastic Cushing's syndrome in a case of Zollinger Ellison syndrome. Gut 1988;29: 838–842.
51. Vinik AI, Moattari AR. Treatment of endocrine tumors of the pancreas. Endocrinol Metab Clin North Am 1989;18:483–518.
52. Orci L, Malaisse-Lagae F, Baetens D, et al. Pancreatic-polypeptide-rich regions in human pancreas. Lancet 1978;ii: 1200–1202.
53. Kimmel J, Pollack H, Hazelwood R. Isolation and characterization of chicken insulin. Endocrinology 1968;83:1323–1330.
54. Kimmel JR, Hayden LJ, Pollock HG. Isolation and characterization of a new pancreatic polypeptide hormone. J Biol Chem 1975;24:9369–9376.
55. Chance RE, Jones WE. Polypeptides from bovine, ovine, human, and porcine pancreas. United States Patent Office 1974; 842:063.
56. Bordi C, Togni R, Baetens M, et al. Human islet cell tumor storing pancreatic polypeptide. J Clin Endocrinol Metab 1978;56: 215–219.
57. Bordi C, Sivelli R, Lampugnani R, Zanella E, Fajans SS. Horm Metab Res 1985;17:467–470.
58. Lundqvist G, Krause U, Larsson LI, Grimelius L, Schaffalitzky De Muckadell OB, et al. A pancreatic-polypeptide-producing tumour associated with the WDHA syndrome. Scand J Gastroenterol 1978;13:715–718.
59. Larsson L-I, Schwartz T, Lundqvist G, Chance RD, Sundler F, et al. Occurrence of human pancreatic polypeptide in pancreatic endocrine tumors. Am J Pathol 1976;85:675–682.
60. Tomita T, Friesen SR, Kimmel JR, Doull V, Pollock HG. Pancreatic polypeptide-secreting islet-cell tumors: a study of three cases. Am J Pathol 1983;113:134–142.
61. Tomita T, Friesen SR, Pollock HG. PP-producing tumors (PPomas). In: Dayal Y, ed. Endocrine pathology of the gut and pancreas. Boca Raton, FL: CRC Press, 1991:279–304.
62. Friesen SR, Kimmel JR, Tomita T. Pancreatic polypeptide as screening for pancreatic polypeptide apudomas in multiple endocrinopathies. Am J Surg 1980;139:61–72.
63. Tomita T, Friesen SR, Kimmel JR. Pancreatic polypeptide-secreting islet cell tumor: a follow-up report. Cancer 1986;129–133.
64. Warner TF, Seo IS, Madura JA, Polak JM, Pearse AGE. Pancreatic-polypeptide-producing apudoma of the liver. Cancer 1980;46: 1146–1151.
65. Hayes MMM. Report of a pancreatic polypeptide-producing islet-cell tumour of the pancreas causing the watery diarrhoea, hypokalaemia, achlorhydria syndrome in a 55 year old Zimbabwean African male. J Med 1980;9:195–197.
66. Ljungberg O, Jarnerolt G, Rolny P, Wickbon G. Human pancreatic polypeptide immuno-reactivity in an infiltrating tumor of the papilla of Vater with unusual morphology. Virchows Arch A 1981;392:119.
67. Manache A, Wood SM, Adrian TE, Welbourn RB, Bloom SR. Pancreatic polypeptide and calcitonin secretion from a pancreatic tumour—clinical improvement after hepatic artery embolization. Postgrad Med J 1983;59:313–314.
68. Nakanome C, Koizumi M, Fujiya H, Akai H, Toyota T, et al. Somatostatin syndrome accompanied by overproduction of pancreatic polypeptide. Tohoku J Exp Med 1984;142:201–210.
69. Strodel WE, Vinik AI, Lloyd RV, Glaser B, Eckhauser FE, et al. Pancreatic polypeptide-producing tumors: silent lesions of the pancreas? Arch Surg 1984;119:508–514.
70. Nobin A, Berg M, Ericsson M, Ingemansson S, Olsson E, Sundler F. Pancreatic polypeptide-producing tumors: report on two cases. Cancer 1984;53:2688–2691.
71. Solt E, Kadas I, Polak JM, Nemeth A, Bloom SR, et al. A pancreatic-polypeptide-producing tumor of the stomach. Cancer 1984;54:1101–1104.
72. Choksi VA, Sellin RV, Hickey RC, et al. An unusual skin rash associated with a pancreatic polypeptide-producing tumor. Ann Intern Med 1988;108:64.
73. Martensson H, Bottcher G, Sundler F, Nobin A. Localization and peptide content of endocrine pancreatic tumors. Ann Surg 1990;212:607–614.
74. Uhl MD, Diallo G, Cooke AR. Metastatic pancreatic polypeptidoma. Presented at the annual meeting of the American College of Physicians, Kansas Chapter, Overland Park, Sept 11, 1992.
75. Adrian TE, Uttenthal LO, Williams SJ, Bloom SR. Secretion of pancreatic polypeptide in patients with pancreatic endocrine tumors. N Engl J Med 1986;315:287–291.
76. Wynick D, Williams SJ, Bloom SR. Symptomatic secondary hormone syndromes in patients with established malignant pancreatic endocrine tumors. N Engl J Med 1988;319:605–607.
77. Solcia E, Sessa F, Rindi G, Villani L, Riva C, et al. Classification and histogenesis of gastroenteropancreatic endocrine tumours. Eur J Clin Invest 1990;20:S72–S81.
78. Tomita T, Kimmel JR, Friesen SR, Doull V, Pollock HG. Pancreatic polypeptide in islet cell tumors. Cancer 1985;56:1649.
79. Heintz PV. Pancreatic endocrine tumors. In: Kloppel G, Heintz PV, eds. Pancreatic pathology. Edinburgh: Churchill Livingstone, 1984:206–232.
80. O'Dorisio TM, Vinik AI. Pancreatic polypeptide and mixed peptide producing tumors of the gastrointestinal tract. In: Cohen S, Soloway RD, eds. Contemporary issues in gastroenterology. London: Churchill Livingstone, 1985:117–128.
81. Oberg K, Walinder O, Bostrom H, Lundquist G, Wide L. Peptide hormone markers in screening for endocrine tumors in multiple endocrine adenomatosis type 1. Am J Med 1982;73:619–630.
82. Friesen SR, Tomita T, Kimmel JR. Pancreatic polypeptide update: its role in detection of the trait for multiple endocrine adenopathy syndrome type 1 and pancreatic polypeptide-secreting tumors. Surgery 1983;94:1028–1037.
83. Langstein HN, Norton JA, Chiang HCV, et al. The utility of circulating levels of human pancreatic polypeptide as a marker for islet cell tumors. Surgery 1990, 108:1109–1116.
84. Greenburg G, Adrian T, Baron J, et al. Inhibition of pancreas and gallbladder by pancreatic polypeptide. Lancet 1978;2:1280.
85. Glaser B, Floyd JC Jr, Vinik AI, et al. Evidence for extravagal cholinergic dependence of pancreatic polypeptide responses to beef ingestion in man. Clin Res 1979;27:366A.
86. Glaser B, Vinik AI, Sive AA, et al. Plasma human pancreatic polypeptide responses to administered secretion effects of surgical vagotomy, cholinergic blockage and chronic pancreatitis. J Clin Endocrinol Metab 1980;50:1094–1099.
87. Larsson LI, Schwartz T, Lundquist G, et al. Occurrence of human

pancreatic polypeptide in pancreatic endocrine tumors, possible implication in watery diarrhea syndrome. Am J Pathol 1976;85:675–684.
88. Ebeid AM, Dragon R, Brand D, et al. Clinical and pathological consideration on apudomas. Read before the Connecticut Society of American Board Surgeons. New Haven, CT, December 7, 1977.
89. Schwartz TW. Atropine suppression test for pancreatic polypeptide. Lancet 1978;ii:43–44.
90. Gower WR, Fabri PJ. Endocrine neoplasms (non-gastrin) of the pancreas. Semin Surg Oncol 1990;6:98–109.
91. Vinik AL, Strodel WE, Eckhauser FE, et al. Somatostatinomas, PPomas, neurotensinomas. Semin Oncol 1987;14:263–281.
92. Wilson RW, Gal AA, Cohen C, DeRose PB, Millikan WJ. Serotonin immunoreactivity in pancreatic endocrine neoplasms (carcinoid tumors). Mod Pathol 1991;4:727–732.
93. Rapport MM, Green AA, Page IH. Partial purification of the vasoconstrictor in beef serum. J Biol Chem 1948;174:735.
94. Erspamer V, Asero B. Identification of enteramine, the specific hormone of the enterochromaffin cell system, as 5-hydroxytryptamine. Nature 1952;169:800.
95. Lembeck F. 5-Hydroxytryptamine in a carcinoid tumor. Nature 1953;172:910–911.
96. Rosenbaum FF, Santer DG, Claudon DB. Essential telangiectasia, pulmonary stenosis and neoplastic liver disease: a possible new clinical syndrome. J Lab Clin Med 1953;42:941.
97. Thorson A, Bjork G, Bjorkman G, Waldenstrom J. Malignant carcinoid of the small intestine with metastases to the liver, valvular disease of the right heart (pulmonary stenosis and tricuspid regurgitation without septal defect), peripheral vasomotor symptoms, bronchoconstriction and an unusual type of cyanosis. Am Heart J 1954;47:795–817.
98. Haq AU, Yook CR, Hiremath V, Kasimis BS. Carcinoid syndrome in the absence of liver metastasis: a case report and review of literature. Med Pediatr Oncol 1992;20:221–223.
99. Buchanan, KD, Johnston CF, O'Hare MMT, et al. Neuroendocrine tumors—a European view. Am J Med 1986;81:14–22.
100. Watson RGP, Johnston CF, O'Hare MMT, et al. The frequency of gastrointestinal endocrine tumours in a well-defined population—Northern Ireland 1970–1985. Q J Med 1989;267:647–657.
101. Godwin DJ. Carcinoid tumors: an analysis of 2,837 cases. Cancer 1975;36:560–569.
102. Williams ED, Sandler M. The classification of carcinoid tumors. Lancet 1963;1:238–239.
103. Chejfec G, Prinz R, Staren ED, Gould VE. Neuroendocrine tumors of the gastrointestinal tract with and without the carcinoid syndrome. In: Dayal Y, ed. Endocrine pathology gut and pancreas. Boca Raton, FL: CRC Press 1991:134–149.
104. Modlin IM, Lewis JJ, Bilchik AJ, Kumar RR. Management of unresectable malignant endocrine tumors of the pancreas. Surg Gynecol Obstet 1993;176:507–518.
105. MacDonald RA. A study of 356 carcinoids of the gastrointestinal tract: report of four new cases of the carcinoid syndrome. Am J Med 1956;21:867–878.
106. Cheek RC, Wilson H. Carcinoid syndrome. Curr Probl Surg 1970;36:41.
107. Arnett JH, Long CF. A case of congenital stenosis of the pulmonary valve, with late onset of cyanosis: death from carcinoma of the pancreas. Am J Med Sci 1931;182:212–217.
108. Mao C, Attar AE, Domenico DR, Kim K, Howard JM. Carcinoid tumors of the pancreas: status report based on two cases and review of the world's literature. Unpublished.
109. Feldman JM. Carcinoid tumors and the carcinoid syndrome. Curr Probl Surg 1989;831–885.
110. Lucas KJ, Feldman JM. Flushing in the carcinoid syndrome and plasma kallikrein. Cancer 1986;58:2290.
111. Oates JA. The carcinoid syndrome (Editorial). N Engl J Med 1986;315:702.
112. Theodorssom É. Regulatory peptides as tumour markers. Acta Oncol 1989;28:319.
113. Ch'ng JLC, Polak JM, Bloom SR. Miscellaneous tumors of the pancreas. In: Go VLW, Gardner JD, Brooks FP, et al., eds. The exocrine pancreas: biology, pathobiology and diseases. New York: Raven Press, 1986:763–771.
114. Friesen SR. Hormone-producing gastrointestinal tumors. In: Glass GBJ, Sherlock P, eds. Progress in gastroenterology, vol IV. New York: Grune & Stratton, 1983.
115. Ordonez NG, Manning JT, Raymond K. Argentaffin endocrine carcinoma (carcinoid) of the pancreas with concomitant breast metastasis: an immunohistochemical and electron microscopic study. Hum Pathol 1985;16:746–751.
116. Dollinger MR, Ratner LH, Shamoian CH, Blackbourne BD. Carcinoid syndrome associated with pancreatic tumors. Arch Intern Med 1967;120:575–580.
117. Castleman B, McNeely BU. Case records of the Massachusetts General Hospital. N Engl J Med 1967;276:1313–1322.
118. Gordon DL, Lo MC, Schwartz MA. Carcinoid of the pancreas. Am J Med 1971;51:412–415.
119. Patchefsky AS, Gordon G, Harrer WV, Hoch WS. Carcinoid tumor of the pancreas: ultrastructural observations of a lymph node metastasis and comparison with bronchial carcinoid. Cancer 1974;33:1349–1354.
120. Peart WS, Porter KA, Robertson JIS, Sandler M, Baldock E. Carcinoid syndrome due to pancreatic-duct neoplasm secreting 5-hydroxytryptophan and 5-hydroxytryptamine. Lancet 1963:239–242.
121. Van Der Sluys Veer J, Choufoer JC, Querido A, Van Der Heul RO, Hollander CF, Van Rujssel TG. Metastasising islet-cell tumour of the pancreas associated with hypoglycemia and carcinoid syndrome. Lancet 1964:1416–1419.
122. Persaud V, Walrond ER. Carcinoid tumor and cystadenoma of the pancreas. Arch Pathol 1971;92:289–230.
123. Patchefsky AS, Solit R, Phillips LD, Craddock M, Harrer WV, Cohn HF. Hydroxyindole-producing tumors of the pancreas: carcinoid-islet cell tumor and oat cell carcinoma. Ann Intern Med 1972;77:53–61.
124. Gammill SL, Weichert R, Smith SL, Font R, Ingraffia R. Carcinoid-islet cell tumors. Acta Radiol Ther Phys Biol 1973;12:229–240.
125. Greene JF, Doyle WF. Pancreatic islet cell carcinoid: a highly malignant form of carcinoid tumor. J Surg Oncol 1974;6:183–190.
126. Pedinielli L, Quilichini R, Futsch D, Romieu CL, Pujol R, Baldet P. Pancreatic tumours with both endocrine and exocrine components and carcinoid syndrome—report of 2 cases (in French). Chirurgie 1975;101:42–51.
127. Derizhanova IS, Reznikova GL. Clinicoanatomic characteristics of carcinoid tumors of the pancreatoduodenal area (in Russian). Khirurgiia 1981;4:56–59.
128. Wilander E, El-Salhy M, Willen R, Grimelius L. Immunocytochemistry and electron microscopy of an argentaffin endocrine tumour of the pancreas. Virchows Arch 1981;392:263–269.
129. Prinz RA, Bermes EW, Chejfec G, Fareed J, Klich J. A serotonin and ßHCG-producing islet cell carcinoma associated with focal nodular hyperplasia of the liver. J Surg Oncol 1983;24:30–32.
130. Varma JS. Acute chylous ascites with carcinoid of the pancreas. Scott Med J 1985;30:111.
131. Lee C-H, Ching K-N, Lui W-Y, P'eng F-K, Franklin WA, Kaplan L. Carcinoid tumor of the pancreas causing the diarrheogenic syndrome: report of a case combined with multiple endocrine neoplasia, type I. Surgery 1986;99:123–129.
132. Troussier B, Pillon P, Masri B, Grauer JL, Boizel R, et al. Osseous metastasis revealing a carcinoid tumor of the pancreas (in French). Presse Med 1988;17(27):1411.
133. Rowe PH, Taylor PR, Shearer MJ, Owen WJ. Vitamin A deficiency secondary to pancreatic carcinoid. Acta Chir Scand 1988;154: 487–488.
134. Gettenberg G, Zimbalist E, Marini C. Chronic pancreatitis and pseudocyst formation secondary to carcinoid tumor of the pancreas. Gastroenterology 1988;94:1222–1224.
135. Carstens HB, Cressman KF. Malignant oncocytic carcinoid of the pancreas. Ultrastruct Pathol 1989;13:69–75.
136. Kanavaros P, Hoang C, LeBodic MF, Polivka M, Hautefeuille P. Serotonin-producing pancreatic tumour. Histological, ultrastructural and immunohistologic chemical study of a case. Histol Histopathol 1990;5:325–328.
137. Cappellari L, D'Antonio D, Benea M, Felloni M, Zibordi U, Galdoni GP. Una rara localizgazione di tumore carcinoide: il pancreas descrizione di un caso (in Italian). Minerva Chir 1991;46:979–984.
138. Rougier P, Oliveira J, Ducreux M, Theodore C, Kac J, Droz JP. Metastatic carcinoid and islet cell tumours of the pancreas: a phase II trial of the efficacy of combination chemotherapy with

5-fluorouracil, doxorubicin and cisplatin. Eur J Cancer 1991;27: 1380–1382.
139. Deixonne B, Duchene D, Eledjam JJ, Pignodel Ch, Gaujoux A-F, et al. Ec cell (carcinoid) endocrine carcinoma of the pancreas causing chronic diarrhea. J Chir 1991;128:415–418.
140. Nagai E, Yamaguchi K, Hashimoto H, Sakurai T. Carcinoid tumor of the pancreas with obstructive pancreatitis. Am J Gastroenterol 1992;87:361–364.
141. Tadi CH, Soyer PH, Barge J, Amouyal P, Levesque M. Primary carcinoid tumor of the pancreas. J Radiol 1993;74:347–350.
142. Villaneuva A, Perex C, Llauger J. Carcinoid tumors of the pancreas: CT findings. Abdom Imag 1994;19:221–224.
143. Seymour NE, Andersen DK. Pancreatic endocrine tumors: surgical aspects. In: Burns GP, Bank S, eds. Disorders of the pancreas: current issues in diagnosis and management. New York: McGraw-Hill, 1992:460–483.
144. Ahlman H, Dahlstrom A, Gronstad K, et al. The pentagastrin test in the diagnosis of the carcinoid syndrome: blockade of gastrointestinal symptoms by ketanserin. Ann Surg 1985;201: 81–86.
145. Kvols LK, Buck M. Chemotherapy of metastatic carcinoid and islet cell tumors. Am J Med 1987;82:77–83.
146. Polak JM, Sullivan SN, Bloom SR, Buchanan AMJ, Facer P, et al. Specific localization of neurotensin to the N cell in human intestine by radioimmunoassay and immunocytochemistry. Nature 1977;270:183–184.
147. Helmstaedter V, Taugner C, Gearle G, et al. Localization of neurotensin-immunoreactive cells in the small intestine of man and various mammals. Histochemistry 1977;53:35.
148. Carraway R, Leeman SE. The isolation of a new hypotensive peptide, neurotensin, from bovine hypothalami. J Biol Chem 1973;248:6854–6861.
149. Hammer RA, Leeman SE. Neurotensin: properties and actions. In: Bloom SR, Polak JM, eds. Gut hormones. Edinburgh: Churchill Livingstone, 1981;2:290–299.
150. Gutniak M, Rosenqvist U, Grimelius L, et al. Report on a patient with watery diarrhea syndrome caused by a pancreatic tumour containing neurotensin, enkephalin and calcitonin. Acta Med Scand 1980;208:95–100.
151. Feurle GE, Helmstaedter V, Tischbirek K, Carraway R, Forssmann WG, et al. A multihormonal tumor of the pancreas producing neurotensin. Dig Dis Sci 1981;26:1125–1133.
152. Maier W, Schumacher A, Etzrodt H, et al. A neurotensinoma of the head of the pancreas: demonstration by ultrasound and computed tomography. Eur J Radiol 1982;2:125–127.
153. Wood JR, Wood SM, Lee YC, Bloom SR. Neurotensin-secreting carcinoma of the bronchus. Postgrad Med J 1983;59:46–47.
154. Bloom SR, Lee YC, Lacroute JM, Abbass A, Sondag D, et al. Two patients with pancreatic apudomas secreting neurotensin and VIP. Gut 1983;24:448–452.
155. Shulkes A, Boden R, Cook I, Gallagher N, Furness JB. Characterization of a pancreatic tumor containing vasoactive intestinal peptide, neurotensin, and pancreatic polypeptide. J Clin Endocrinol Metab 1984;58:41–48.
156. Oberg K, Loof L, Bostrom H, Grimelius L, Fahrenkrug J, Lundqvist G. Hypersecretion of calcitonin in patients with the Verner-Morrison syndrome. Scand J Gastroenterol 1981;16:135–144.
157. Theodorsson-Norheim E, Oberg K, Rosell S, Bostrom H. Neurotensinlike immunoreactivity in plasma and tumor tissue from patients with endocrine tumors of the pancreas and gut. Gastroenterology 1983;85:881–889.
158. Blackburn AM, Bryant MG, Adrian TD, Bloom SR. Pancreatic tumours produce neurotensin. J Clin Endocrinol Metab 1981;52: 820–822.
159. Chiang HCV, O'Dorisio TM, Huang SC, Maton PN, et al. Multiple hormone elevations in Zollinger-Ellison syndrome. Gastroenterology 1990;99:1565–1575.
160. Andersson S, Rosell S, Hjelmquist U, Chang D, Folkers K. Inhibition of gastric and intestinal motor activity in dogs by (Gln(4))-neurotensin. Acta Physiol Scand 1977;100:231–235.
161. Hammer RA, Leeman SE, Carraway R, Williams RH. Isolation of human intestinal neurotensin. J Biol Chem 1980;255:2476–2480.
162. Rokaeus A, Burcher E, Chang D, Folkers K, Rosell S. Actions of neurotensin and (Gln(4))-neurotensin on isolated tissues. Acta Pharmacol Toxicol 1977;41:141–147.
163. Mashford ML, Nilsson G, Rokaeus A, Rosell S. The effect of food ingestion on circulating neurotensin-like immunoreactivity (NTLI) in the human. Acta Physiol Scand 1978;104:244–246.
164. Besterman MS, Sarson DL, Blackburn AM, Cleary J, Pilkington TRE, Bloom SR. The gut hormone profile in morbid obesity and following jejuno-ilial bypass. Scand J Gastroenterol 1978; 13(Supp 49):15.
165. Blackburn AM, Bloom SR. A radioimmunoassay for neurotensin in human plasma. J Endocrinol 1979;83:175–181.
166. Blackburn AM, Bloom SR, Long RG, Fletcher DR, Christofides ND, et al. Effect of neurotensin on gastric function in man. Lancet 1980:987–989.
167. Blackburn AM, Bloom SR. Neurotensin in man. In: Bloom SR, Polak JM, eds. Gut hormones. Edinburgh: Churchill Livingstone, 1981; 2:290–299.
168. Leeman SE, Carraway RE. Neurotensin: discovery, isolation, characterization, synthesis and possible physiological roles. Ann NY Acad Sci 1982;400:1–16.
169. Sundler F, Alumets J, Hakanson R. Majority and minority cell populations in GEP and bronchial endocrine tumours. Scand J Gastroenterol 1979;14:9–13.
170. Collier NA, Bloom SR, Hodgson HJF, Weinbren K, et al. Neurotensin secretion by fibrolamellar carcinoma of the liver. Lancet 1984:538–540.
171. Carraway RE. Variants of neurotensin. In: Bloom SR, Polak JM, eds. Gut hormones. Edinburgh: Churchill Livingstone, 1981;2: 290–299.
172. Nagorney D, Bloom S, Polak J, et al. Resolution of recurrent Verner-Morrison syndrome by resection of metastatic vipoma. Surgery 1983;93:348.
173. Mao C, Carter P, Schaefer P, Zhu L, et al. Malignant islet cell tumor associated with hypercalcemia. Surgery 1995;117:37–40.
174. Albright F. Case records of the Massachusetts General Hospital no. 27461. N Engl J Med 1941;225:789.
175. Burtis WJ, Wu T, Bunch C, et al. Identification of a novel 17,000-dalton parathyroid hormone-like adrenylate cyclase-stimulating protein from a tumor associated with humoral hypercalcemia of malignancy. J Biol Chem 1987;262:7151–7156.
176. Suva LJ, Winslow GA, Wettenhall REH, et al. A parathyroid hormone-related protein implicated in malignant hypercalcemia: cloning and expression. Science 1987;237:893–896.
177. Strewler GJ, Stern PH, Jacobs JW, et al. Parathyroid hormonelike protein from human renal carcinoma cells: structural and functional homology with parathyroid hormone. J Clin Invest 1987;80:1803–1807.
178. Moseley JM, Kubota M, Diefenbach-Jagger H, et al. Parathyroid hormone-related protein purified from a human lung cancer cell line. Proc Natl Acad Sci USA 1987;84:5048–5052.
179. Mangin M, Webb AC, Dreyer BE, et al. Identification of a cDNA encoding a parathyroid hormone-like peptide from a human tumor associated with humoral hypercalcemia of malignancy. Proc Natl Acad Sci USA 1988;85:597–601.
180. Thiede MA, Strewler GJ, Nissenson RD, Rosenblatt M, Rodan GA. Human renal carcinoma expresses two messages encoding a parathyroid hormone-like peptide: evidence for the alternative splicing of a single-copy gene. Proc Natl Acad Sci USA 1988;85:4605–4609.
181. Broadus AE, Mangin M, Ikeda K, et al. Humoral hypercalcemia of cancer: identification of a novel parathyroid hormone-like peptide. N Engl J Med 1988;319:556–563.
182. Mangin M, Ikeda K, Dreyer BE, Broadus AE. Isolation and characterization of the human parathyroid hormone-like peptide gene. Proc Natl Acad Sci USA 1989;86:2408–2412.
183. Burtis WJ, Brady TG, Orloff JJ, Ersbak JB, et al. Immunochemical characterization of circulating parathyroid hormone-related protein in patients with humoral hypercalcemia of cancer. N Engl J Med 1990;322:1106–1112.
184. Bresler L, Boissel P, Conroy T, Grosdidier J. Pancreatic islet cell carcinoma with hypercalcemia: complete remission 5 years after surgical excision and chemotherapy. Am J Gastroenterol 1991;86:635–638.
185. Asa SL, Henderson J, Goltzman D, Drucker DJ. Parathyroid hormone-like peptide in normal and neoplastic human endocrine tissues. J Clin Endocrinol Metal 1990;71:1112–1118.
186. McAuley P, Asa SL, Chiu B, Henderson J, et al. Parathyroid

hormone-like peptide in normal and neoplastic mesothelial cells. Cancer 1990;66:1975–1979.

187. Deftos LJ, Gaydar AF, Ikeda K, Broadus AE. The parathyroid hormone-related protein associated with malignancy is secreted by neuroendocrine tumors. Mol Endocrinol 1989;3:503–508.
188. O'Neal LW, Kipnis DM, Luse SA, Lacy PE, Jarett L. Secretion of various endocrine substances by ACTH-secreting tumors—gastrin, melanotropin, norepinephrine, serotonin, parathormone, vasopressin glucagon. Cancer 1968;21:1219–1232.
189. Venkatesh S, Vassilopoulou-Sellin R, Samaan NA. Somatostatin analogue: use in the treatment of vipoma with hypercalcemia. Am J Med 1989;87:356–357.
190. Matsumoto KK, Peter JB, Schultze RG, Hakim AA, Franck PT. Watery diarrhea and hypokalemia associated with pancreatic islet cell adenoma. Gastroenterology 1966;50:231–242.
191. Lopes V, Reis DD, Cunha AB. Islet-cell adenoma of the pancreas with reversible watery diarrhea and hypokalemia. Am J Gastroenterol 1970;53:17–35.
192. Hirose S, Kobayashi K, Kijikawa K, Sawabu N, Takeuchi J. A case of watery diarrhea, hypokalemia and hypercalcemia associated with nonulcerogenic islet cell tumor of the pancreas. Am J Gastroenterol 1975;64:382–391.
193. Friesen SR. Endocrine tumors. In: Toledo-Pereyra LH, ed. The pancreas: principles of medical and surgical practice. New York: John Wiley & Sons, 1985:339–357.
194. Friesen SR. Update on the diagnosis and treatment of rare neuroendocrine tumors. Surg Clin North Am 1987;67:379–393.
195. Powell D, Singer FR, Murray TM, Minkin C, Potts JT. Nonparathyroid humoral hypercalcemia in patients with neoplastic diseases. N Engl J Med 1973;289:176–184.
196. Friesen SR, McGuigan JE. Ectopic apudocarcinomas and associated endocrine hyperplasias of the foregut. Ann Surg 1975;182:371–385.
197. Deftos LJ, McMIllan PJ, Sartiano GP, et al. Simultaneous ectopic production of parathyroid hormone and calcitonin. Metabolism 1976;25:543.
198. Heitz PU, Kloppel G, Polak JM, Staub JJ. Ectopic hormone production by endocrine tumors: localization of hormones at the cellular level by immunocytochemistry. Cancer 1981;48:2029.
199. Cryer PE, Kissane JM. Metastatic pancreatic islet cell carcinoma with peptic ulcer disease and hypercalcemia. Am J Med 1977;63:142–151.
200. Stavri GT, Pritchard GA, Williams EJ, Stamatakis JD. Somatostatinoma of the pancreas with hypercalcaemia: a case report. Eur J Surg Oncol 1992;18:298–300.
201. Laryea EA, Brodrick R, Hidvegi R. Hypercalcemia and streptozotocin. Ann Intern Med 1974;80:276.
202. Skrabanek P, McPartlin J, Powell D. Tumor hypercalcemia and "ectopic hyperparathyroidism." Medicine 1980;50:262–282.
203. DeWys WD, Stoll R, Au WY, Salisnjak MM. Effects of streptozotocin on an islet cell carcinoma with hypercalcemia. Am J Med 1973;55:671–676.
204. Palmieri GMA, Nordquist RE, Omen GS. Immunochemical localization of parathyroid hormone in cancer tissue from patients with ectopic hyperparathyroidism. J Clin Invest 1974;53:1726.
205. Friesen SR, Allen MS. Malignant hyperparathyroidism of pancreatic and parathyroid origins. Bull Soc Int Chir 1975;34:439–441.
206. Cryer PE, Hill GJ. Pancreatic islet cell carcinoma with hypercalcemia and hypergastrinemia: response to streptozotocin. Cancer 1976;38:2217–2221.
207. Heitz PU, Harder F, Haas HG, Kloeppel G. Tumor of the pancreas inducing hypercalcemia. Ultrastruct Pathol 1989;13:585–588.
208. Shetty MR. Multiple hormone-producing malignant islet cell tumor: long-term survival with combined treatment. Northwest Community Hosp Med Bull (Arlington Heights, IL 60005) 1984;21:88–93.
209. Shetty MR. Pancreatic islet cell tumors. Surgery 1987;101:380.
210. Rabasch D, Hammond J. Pancreatic islet cell carcinoma with hypercalcemia. Primary hyperparathyroidism or hormonal hypercalcemia of malignancy. Am J Med 1985;78:337.
211. Arps H, Dietel M, Schulz A, et al. Pancreatic endocrine carcinoma with ectopic PTH-production and paraneoplastic hypercalcaemia. Virchows Arch A 1986;408:497–503.
212. Vair D, Boudreau S, Reid E. Pancreatic islet-cell neoplasia, with secretion of a parathormone-like substance and hypercalcemia. Can J Surg 1987;30:108.
213. Kvols LK, Buck M, Moertel CG, et al. Treatment of metastatic islet cell carcinoma with somatostatin analogue (SMS 201-995). Ann Intern Med 1987;107:162–168.
214. Wynick D, Ratcliffe WA, Heath DA, Ball S, Barnard M, Bloom SR. Treatment of a malignant pancreatic endocrine tumour secreting parathyroid hormone related protein. Br Med J 1990;300:1314–1315.
215. Dodwell D, Gurney H, Scarffe H. Treatment of a pancreatic tumour secreting parathyroid hormone related protein. Br Med J 1990;300:1653.
216. Rizzoli R, Sappino AP, Bonjour J-P. Parathyroid hormone-related protein and hypercalcemia in pancreatic neuro-endocrine tumors. Int J Cancer 1990;46:394–398.
217. Mitlak BH, Hutchison JS, Kaufman SD, Nussbaum SR. Parathyroid hormone-related peptide mediates hypercalcemia in an islet cell tumor of the pancreas. Horm Metab Res 1991;23:344–346.
218. Miraliakbari BA, Asa SL, Boudreau SF. Parathyroid hormone-like peptide in pancreatic endocrine carcinoma and adenocarcinoma associated with hypercalcemia. Hum Pathol 1992;23:884–887.
219. Kovacs K, Ryan N, Horvath E, Asa SL, et al. Somatoliberinoma: morphologic characteristics. Arch Pathol Lab Med 1984;108:355–356.
220. Rivier J, Spiess J, Thorner M, Vale W. Characterization of a growth hormone-releasing factor from a human pancreatic islet tumour. Nature 1982;300:276–278.
221. Guillemin R, Brazeau P, Bohlen P, Esch F, Ling N. Growth hormone-releasing factor from a human pancreatic tumor that caused acromegaly. Science 1982;218:585–587.
222. Ling N, Esh F, Bohlen P, Brazeau P, Wehrenberg WB, Guillemin R. Isolation, primary structure, and synthesis of human hypothalamic somatocrinin: growth hormone-releasing factor. Proc Natl Acad Sci USA 1984;81:4302.
223. Frohman LA, Jansson J-O. Growth hormone-releasing hormone. Endocrine Rev 1986;7:223–253.
224. Goldman A. The malignant nature of bronchial adenoma. 1949; J Thorac Surg 18:137.
225. Bostwick DG, Quan R, Hoffman AR, Webber RJ, et al. Growth hormone-releasing factor immunoreactivity in human endocrine tumors. Am J Clin Pathol 1984;117:167–170.
226. Asa SL, Kovacs K, Thorner MO, Leong DA, et al. Immunohistological localization of growth hormone-releasing hormone in human tumors. J Clin Endocrinol Metab 1985;60:423–427.
227. Dayal Y, Lin HD, Tallberg K, Reichlin S. Immunocytochemical demonstration of growth hormone-releasing factor in gastrointestinal and pancreatic endocrine tumors. Am J Clin Pathol 1986;85:13–20.
228. Solcia E, Capella C, Riva C, Rindi G, Polak JM. The morphology and neuroendocrine profile of pancreatic epithelial VIPomas and extrapancreatic VIP-producing neurogenic tumors. Ann NY Acad Sci 1988;527:508.
229. Barkan AL. Acromegaly: diagnosis and therapy. Endocrinol Metab Clin North Am 1989;18:277–310.
230. Melmed S, Rushakoff RJ. Ectopic pituitary and hypothalamic hormone syndromes. Endocrinol Metab Clin 1987;16:805–821.
231. Thorner MO, Frohman LA, Leong DA, Thominet J, et al. Extrahypothalamic growth-hormone-releasing factor (GRF) secretion is a rare cause of acromegaly: plasma GRF levels in 177 acromegalic patients. J Clin Endocrinol Metab 1984;59:846–849.
232. Caplan RH, Koob L, Abellera RM, Poglara Kovacs K, Randall RV. Cure of acromegaly by operative removal of an islet cell tumor of the pancreas. Am J Med 1978;64:874.
233. Frohman LA, Szabo M, Berelowitz M, Stachura ME. Partial purification and characterization of a peptide with growth hormone-releasing activity from extrapituitary tumors in patients with acromegaly. J Clin Invest 1980;65:43–54.
234. Thorner MO, Perryman RL, Cronin MJ, et al. Somatotroph hyperplasia. Successful treatment of acromegaly by removal of a pancreatic islet tumor secreting a growth hormone-releasing factor. J Clin Invest 1982;70:965.
235. Cronin MJ, Rogol AD, Dabney LG, Thorner MO. Selective growth hormone and cyclic AMP stimulating activity is present in a

human pancreatic islet cell tumor. J Clin Endocrinol Metab 1982;55:381–383.
236. Berger G, Trouillas J, Bloch B, Sassolas G, et al. Multihormonal carcinoid tumor of the pancreas. Cancer 1984;54:2097–2108.
237. Wilson DM, Ceda GP, Bostwick DG, Webber RJ. Acromegaly and Zollinger-Ellison syndrome secondary to an islet cell tumor: characterization and quantification of plasma and tumor human growth hormone-releasing factor. J Clin Endocrinol Metab 1984;59:1002–1005.
238. Wilson DM, Hoffman AR. Reduction of pituitary size by the somatostatin analogue SMS 201-995 in a patient with an islet cell tumour secreting growth hormone releasing factor. Acta Endocrinol 1986;113:23–28.
239. Maton PN, Gardner JD, Jensen RT. Use of long-acting somatostatin analog SMS 201-995 in patients with pancreatic islet cell tumors. Dig Dis Sci 1989;34:28S–39S.
240. Ch'ng LJC, Christofides ND, Kraenzlin ME, Keshavarzian A. Growth hormone secretion dynamics in a patient with ectopic growth hormone-releasing factor production. Am J Med 1985; 79:135–138.
241. Schulte HM, Benker G, Windeck R, Olbricht T, Reinwein D. Failure to respond to growth hormone releasing hormone (GHRH) in acromegaly due to a GHRH secreting pancreatic tumor: dynamics of multiple endocrine testing. J Clin Endocrinol Metab 1985;61:585–587.
242. Saeger W, Schulte HM, Kloppel G. Morphology of a GHRH producing pancreatic islet cell tumour causing acromegaly. Virchows Arch 1986;409:547–554.
243. Sano T, Yamasaki R, Saito H, et al. Growth hormone-releasing hormone (GHRH)-secreting pancreatic tumor in a patient with multiple endocrine neoplasia type I. Am J Surg Pathol 1987; 11:810.
244. Ramsay JA, Kovacs K, Asa SL, Pike MJ, Thorner MO. Reversible sellar enlargement due to growth hormone-releasing hormone production by pancreatic endocrine tumors in an acromegalic patient with multiple endocrine neoplasia type I syndrome. Cancer 1988;62:445–450.
245. Asa SL, Singer W, Kovacs K, Horvath E, et al. Pancreatic endocrine tumour producing growth hormone-releasing hormone associated with multiple endocrine neoplasia type I syndrome. Acta Endocrinol 1987;115:331–337.
246. Sano T, Saito H, Yamasaki R, Kimura N, Sasaki A, et al. Immunoreactivity against anti-growth hormone-releasing hormone (GHRH) sera in human pancreas and pancreatic endocrine tumors: evidence of pitfall in immunohistochemical study. Biomed Res 1987;8:407.
247. Melmed S, Ezrin C, Kovacs K, Goodman R, Frohman LA. Acromegaly due to secretion of growth hormone by an ectopic pancreatic islet-cell tumor. N Engl J Med 1985;312:9–17.
248. Krejs GJ. Non-insulin-secreting tumors of the gastroenteropancreatic system. In: Wilson JD, Foster DW, eds. Paraendocrine and neoplastic syndromes. 8th ed. Philadelphia: WB Saunders, 1992:1567–1576.
249. Kaplan EL, Sizemore G, Hill BJ, Peskin GW. Calcitonin in nonthyroid tumors in man. Clin Res 1972;20:724.
250. Coombes RD, Hillyard C, Greenberg PB, MacIntyre I. Plasma-immunoreactive-calcitonin in patients with non-thyroid tumours. Lancet 1974:1080–1083.
251. Sizemore GW, Go VLW, Kaplan EL, Sanzenbacher LJ, Holtermuller KH, Arnaud CD. Relations of calcitonin and gastrin in the Zollinger-Ellison syndrome and medullary carcinoma of the thyroid. N Engl J Med 1973;288:641–644.
252. Abe K, Adachi I, Miyakawa S, et al. Production of calcitonin, adrenocorticotropic hormone, and ß-melanocyte-stimulating hormone in tumors derived from amine precursor uptake and decarboxylation cells. Cancer Res 1977;37:4190.
253. Schmitt MG, Soergel KH, Hensley GT, Chey WY. Watery diarrhea associated with pancreatic islet cell carcinoma. Gastroenterology 1975;69:206–216.
254. Rambaud JC, Nisard A, Modigliani R, Calmette C, et al. Hypercalcitoninemia in vipomas. Lancet 1978:220.
255. Galmiche JP, Chayvialle JA, Dubois PM, Descos DF, et al. Calcitonin-producing pancreatic somatostatinoma. Gastroenterology 1980;78:1577–1583.
256. Galmiche JP, Colin R, DeBois PM, Chavialli JA, Desco P, et al. Calcitonin secretion by a pancreatic somatostatinoma. N Engl J Med 1978;299:1252.
257. Krejs GJ, Orci L, Conlon JM, Ravazzola M, et al. Somatostatinoma syndrome. N Engl J Med 1979;301:285–292.
258. Ooi A, Kameya T, Tsumuraya M, Yamaguchi K, et al. Pancreatic endocrine tumours associated with WDHA syndrome. Virchows Arch 1985;405:311–323.
259. McLeod MK, Vinik AI. Calcitonin immunoreactivity and hypercalcitoninemia in two patients with sporadic, nonfamilial, gastroenteropancreatic neuroendocrine tumors. Surgery 1992;111: 484–488.
260. Bromer WW, Sinn LG, Staub A, Behrens OK. The amino acid sequence of glucagon. Diabetes 1957;6:234–238.
261. Leung YK, Lebenthal E. Gastrointestinal peptides: physiology, ontogeny, and clinical significance. In: Lebenthal E, ed. Human gastrointestinal development. New York: Raven Press, 1989: 41–98.
262. Grimelius L, Capella C, Buffa R, Polak J, Pearse A, Solcia E. Cytochemical and ultrastructural differentiation of enteroglucagon and pancreatic-type glucagon cells of the gastrointestinal tract. Virchows Arch 1976;20:217–228.
263. Walsh JH. Gastrointestinal hormones. In: Johnson LR, ed. Physiology of the gastrointestinal tract. 3rd ed. New York: Raven Press, 1994:1–128.
264. Sagor G, Ghatei M, Al-Mukhtar M, Wright S, Bloom S. Evidence for a humoral mechanism after small intestinal resection. Gastroenterology 1983;84:902–906.
265. Buchan A, Griffiths C, Morris J, Polak J. Enteroglucagon cell hyperfunction in rat small intestine after gut resection. Gastroenterology 1985;88:8–12.
266. Miazza B, Al-Mukhtar M, Salmeron M, Ghatei M, Felce-Dachez M, et al. Hyperenteroglucagonaemia and small intestinal mucosal growth after colonic perfusion of glucose in rats. Gut 1985;26:518–524.
267. Sagor G, Ghatei M, O'Shaughnessy D, Al-Mukhtar M, Wright N, Bloom S. Influence of somatostatin and bombesin on plasma enteroglucagon and cell proliferation after intestinal resection in the rat. Gut 1985;26:89–94.
268. Gleeson MH, Bloom SR, Polak JM, Henry K, Dowling RH. Endocrine tumour in kidney affecting small bowel structure, motility, and absorptive function. Gut 1971;12:773–782.
269. Bloom SR. An enteroglucagon tumour. Gut 1971;13:520–523.
270. Stevens FM, Flannagan J, Buchanan KD, O'Gorman DJ. The first Irish glucagonoma. Ir J Med Sci 1977;146:350.
271. Stevens FM, Flanagan RW, O'Gorman D, Buchanan KD. Glucagonoma syndrome demonstrating giant duodenal villi. Gut 1984;25:784–791.
272. Jones B, Fishman EK, Bayless TM, Siegelman SS. Villous hypertrophy of the small bowel in a patient with glucagonoma. J Comput Assist Tomogr 1983;7:334–337.
273. Debas HT, Mulvihill SJ. Neuroendocrine gut neoplasms: important lessons from uncommon tumors. Arch Surg 1994;129: 965–972.
274. Wilson SD, Soergel K, Go VLW. Diarrhea, gastric hypersecretion, and "cholecystokinin-like" hormone. Lancet 1973:1515–1516.
275. Chayvialle JA, Cuber JC, Partensky C, Berger F, Bernard C. Pseudo-Zollinger Ellison syndrome with pancreatic tumor storing cholecystokinin-like immunoreactivity. Eur Gastroenterol Club 1990;37:260.
276. Sanchez-Sosa S, Angeles AA, Orozco H, Larriva-Sahd J. Neuroendocrine carcinoma of the ampulla of Vater: a case of absence of somatostatin in a vasoactive intestinal polypeptide-, bombesin-, and cholecystokinin-producing tumor. Anat Pathol 1991;95:51–54.
277. Brown JC, Mutt V, Pederson RA. Further purification of a polypeptide demonstrating enterogastrone activity. J Physiol (Lond) 1970;209–257:57–64.
278. Jornvall H, Carlquist M, Kwauk S, Otte SC, McIntosh CHS, et al. Amino acid sequence and heterogeneity of gastric inhibitory polypeptide (GIP). FEBS Lett 1981;123:205–209.
279. Anderson D. Physiological effects of GIP in man. In: Bloom SR, Polak JM, eds. Gut hormones. Edinburgh: Churchill Livingstone, 1981:256–263.

280. Kidd GS, Donowitz M, O'Dorisio T, Cataland S, Newman F. Mild chronic watery diarrhea-hypokalemia syndrome associated with pancreatic islet cell hyperplasia. Am J Med 1979;66: 883–888.
281. Elias E, Bloom S, Welbourn R, et al. Pancreatic cholera due to production of gastric inhibitory polypeptide. Lancet 1972;ii: 791–792.
282. McDonald TJ, Nilsson G, Vagne M, Ghatei M, et al. A gastrin releasing peptide from the porcine non-antral gastric tissue. Gut 1978;19:767–774.
283. McDonald TJ, Jornvall H, Nilsson G, Vagne M, et al. Characterization of a gastrin releasing peptide from porcine non-antral gastric tissue. Biochem Biophys Res Commun 1979;90: 227–233.
284. Anastasi A, Erspamer V, Bucci M. Isolation and structure of bombesin and alytesin, two analogous active peptides from the skin of the European amphibians Bombina and Alytes. Experientia 1971;27:166–167.
285. Bostwick DG, Bensch KG. Gastrin releasing peptide in human neuroendocrine tumours. J Pathol 1985;147:237–244.
286. Varner AA, Modlin IM, Walsh JH. High potency of bombesin for stimulation of human gastrin release and gastric acid secretion. Regul Pept 1981;1:289–296.
287. Dockray GJ. Physiology of enteric neuropeptides. In: Johnson LR, ed. Physiology of the gastrointestinal tract. New York: Raven Press, 1987:41–66.
288. Somers G, Segers O, Marichal M, In't Veld P, Kloppel G. Pancreatic bombesinoma. Eur J Clin Invest 1989;19:A34.
289. Westermark P, Wernstedt C, Wilander E, Sletten K. A novel peptide in the calcitonin gene-related peptide as an amyloid fibril protein in the endocrine pancreas. Biochem Biophys Res Commun 1986;140:827–831.
290. Westermark P, Wernstedt C, Wilander E, Hayden DW, O'Brien TD, Johnson KH. Amyloid fibrils in human insulinoma and islet of Langerhans of the diabetic cat are derived from a neuropeptide-like protein also present in hormonal islet cells. Proc Natl Acad Sci USA 1987;84:3881–3885.
291. Cooper GJ, Willis AC, Clark A, Turner RD, Sim RB, Reid KB. Purification and characterization of a peptide from amyloid-rich pancreas of type 2 diabetic patients. Proc Natl Acad Sci USA 1987;84:8628–8632.
292. Lukinius A, Wilander E, Westermark GT, Engstrom U, Westermark P. Co-localization of islet amyloid polypeptide and insulin in the B cell secretory granules of the human pancreatic islets. Diabetologia 1989;32:240–244.
293. Stridsberg M, Wilander E, Oberg K, Lundqvist G, Eriksson B. Islet amyloid polypeptide-producing pancreatic islet cell tumor: a clinical and biochemical characterization. Scand J Gastroenterol 1992;27:381–387.
294. Leighton B, Cooper GJ. Pancreatic amylin and calcitonin gene-related peptide cause resistance to insulin in skeletal muscle in vitro. Nature 1988;335:632–635.
295. Kanatsuaka A, Makino H. Ohsawa H, et al. Secretion of islet amyloid polypeptide in response to glucose. FEBS Lett 1989;259: 199–201.
296. Van Jaarsveld BC, Hackeng WHL, Nieuwenhus MG, Erkelens DW, Geerdink RA, Lips CJM. Islet-amyloid polypeptide in human plasma. Lancet 1990;1:60.
297. MacIntyre I. Amylinamide, bone conservation and pancreatic B cells. Lancet 1989;2:1026–1027.
298. Brain SD, Wimalwansa S, MacIntyre I, Williams TJ. The demonstration of vasodilator activity of pancreatic amylin amide in the rabbit. Am J Pathol 1990;136:487–490.
299. Cooper GJS, Da AJ, Willis AC, Roberts AN, Reid KBM, Leighton B. Amylin and the amylin gene: structure, function and relationship to islet amyloid and to diabetes mellitus. Biochim Biophys Acta 1989;1014:247–258.
300. Johnson KH, O'Brien TD, Betsholtz C, Westermark P. Islet amyloid polypeptide and diabetes mellitus. N Engl J Med 1989;321: 513–518.

# 84

# *Pancreatic Trauma*

Kimberly K. Nagy and John Barrett

The pancreas is an infrequently injured abdominal organ in both blunt and penetrating trauma. The diagnosis of pancreatic trauma is often difficult. Nevertheless, it is important to recognize it early to minimize complications from this injury. Once the diagnosis is made, the operative treatment is then based upon the location of injury as well as the presence or absence of an associated pancreatic duct injury.

The first report of a pancreatic injury was in 1827, when Travers remarked on the unfavorable prognosis of a pancreatic wound. An abdominal gunshot wound that injured the pancreas among other organs was responsible for President McKinley's death in 1901 (1). In 1957, Hannon and Sprafka performed the first resections for pancreatic trauma (2). Until that time conservative nonoperative treatment was considered appropriate despite the high incidence of pseudocysts and fistulae. They demonstrated that resection was associated with fewer complications than nonoperative therapy, thus changing our approach to the injured pancreas.

Pancreatic trauma is present in less than 5% of all patients who sustain abdominal trauma (3, 4). It occurs slightly more frequently (3–8%) with penetrating abdominal injuries than after blunt abdominal trauma (2–3%) (5–7). Of the patients who sustain penetrating trauma to the pancreas, gunshot wounds occur 4–5 times more frequently than stab wounds (7, 8).

Blunt injuries usually occur when the pancreas is compressed against the underlying lumbar vertebrae (9). The gland may be compressed during deceleration against a steering wheel or an incorrectly placed lap belt during a motor vehicle collision (8, 10). A motorcyclist or bicyclist may strike the epigastrium on the handlebars, resulting in a similar compression injury (10, 11). Even an epigastric blow from a fist may cause a pancreatic injury (11). While the most commonly described injury is compression/transection at the neck of the pancreas from a direct blow, the actual angle of compression may vary, resulting in an injury to the head, body, or tail of the gland (10, 12).

Associated injuries are common, occurring in 90% of all patients who sustain trauma to the pancreas (13). Most (60–85%) patients sustaining blunt pancreatic injury have associated injuries to abdominal organs (5, 7). Virtually all (98–100%) patients who sustain a penetrating pancreatic wound have associated injuries (6, 7).

On average, 2.1–4.3 other abdominal organs are injured in patients with pancreatic trauma (1, 13–15). More abdominal organs are injured by gunshot wounds than by stab wounds or blunt trauma (1). The most common associated injuries after blunt trauma are to the other solid organs, the liver, spleen, and kidney (8, 13). The most common associated injuries following penetrating trauma are to adjacent organs, the liver, stomach, duodenum, and colon (1, 8, 13, 15). The duodenum is injured in 14% of patients sustaining penetrating pancreatic injuries, but only half of these patients have severe injuries to both organs (15). Injuries to major vascular structures occur in 24–30% of penetrating pancreatic injuries (13, 15) and account for much of the mortality of these wounds (14).

## DIAGNOSIS OF PANCREATIC INJURY

It is important to make the diagnosis of pancreatic injury as soon as possible, as a delay can lead to increased complications and mortality (16). Often, the diagnosis is made at the time of laparotomy for associated injuries. Because penetrating wounds almost always injure other organs, these other injuries usually provide the indication for operation. Blunt injuries, on the other hand may be difficult to diagnose, especially if isolated to the retroperitoneum (9). A history of ethanol abuse renders the pancreas more susceptible to blunt trauma (17). Early symptoms of pancreatic injury, if present, consist of mild or moderate epigastric and/or back pain (9, 12). The patient may have mild or vague tenderness in the epigastrium (10, 12). Frequently however, associated skeletal injuries mask symptoms, or associated head injuries render the examination unreliable (5). There may be a transient improvement in abdominal signs and symptoms after 1–2 hours only to worsen again after 6 hours (17). If the diagnosis is not made initially, the examination may progress to peritonitis and hypovolemic shock after 1–2 days (9).

Serum amylase would seem to be a logical initial test to diagnose pancreatic trauma. Unfortunately, serum amylase is a very nonspecific indicator of pancreatic injury. It can be elevated with injuries to other abdominal organs such as the stomach, duodenum, or small intestine (18). It can be elevated with injuries to the head, face, or chest, ethanol intake, or hypotension with decreased renal perfusion (10, 18). Only 34% of patients with penetrating pancreatic injury and 67–78% of patients with blunt pancreatic injury have an elevated serum amylase level (12, 15, 19). In one series, 33% of patients with an elevated serum amylase level had no intraabdominal injury at all (18). Measuring pancreatic isoenzymes may increase the diagnostic yield. The pancreatic isoenzyme, or P-amylase, is derived solely from the pancreas and makes up 35–55% of the total amylase (18, 20). If the P-amylase value is normal, a pancreatic injury may be ruled out. If it is elevated, a pancreatic source is implied, although preexisting pancreatic disease may also elevate the P-amylase (18, 20). Perhaps the most useful role of serum amylase is to follow the patient for the first few days of the hospital course; if the amylase value remains persistently elevated or shows a consistent rise, a pancreatic injury must be strongly considered (7, 10, 21).

Diagnostic peritoneal lavage is an excellent test for diagnosing intraperitoneal injury; however, it will miss an injury that is confined to the retroperitoneum (22). The measurement of amylase in lavage fluid has an extremely low yield that does not justify the extra cost (23). Lavage is still a useful test, as it will diagnose the presence of associated injuries requiring laparotomy (10). Once in the operating room, the surgeon can then make the diagnosis of a pancreatic injury.

Plain radiographs are not helpful in the diagnosis of pancreatic injury. Abdominal radiographs are usually nonspecific but may show a "ground glass" appearance in the upper abdomen secondary to edema late in the hospital course (17). Computed tomography (CT) shows only subtle findings when pancreatic injury is present and may miss up to 40% of acute pancreatic injuries (21, 24). Signs of pancreatic injury on CT include nonspecific edema or thickening of the pancreas, which may be diffuse or localized (12). There may be thickening of the left anterior renal fascia (16). CT gives no information regarding duct integrity and is only useful in a stable patient (12). CT is effective in predicting the presence or absence of injury to the retroperitoneal organs, including the pancreas, following penetrating trauma to the back or flank (25). Ultrasound shows promise as an easily performed test that can be performed in the emergency department, even in an unstable patient. It will show diffuse edema and enlargement of the injured pancreas and may delineate a pancreatic transection (26, 27). Both CT and ultrasound are useful modalities for diagnosis of late complications such as abscess and pseudocyst (10, 24, 27).

Endoscopic retrograde cholangiopancreatography (ERCP) has been proposed as an initial diagnostic test. In one series, it was shown to be both 100% sensitive and specific in patients with blunt abdominal trauma, minimal abdominal pain, and elevated serum amylase (24). Unfortunately, ERCP can only be used in stable patients, may delay treatment of an acutely injured patient, and requires an experienced endoscopist, who may not always be immediately available (12, 22). This is another test that may be better used for the diagnosis of missed injuries and complications (10).

## OPERATIVE MANAGEMENT OF PANCREATIC TRAUMA

Most diagnoses of pancreatic trauma are made at the time of laparotomy for associated injuries (10). The general principles of surgical management of pancreatic injuries are as follows: control hemorrhage, confirm the diagnosis, define the extent of injury, determine if the duct is involved, do selective conservative debridement, and provide adequate drainage for exocrine secretions (8, 15, 28).

The abdomen is explored through a standard midline laparotomy incision. After initial control of hemorrhage and contamination from associated injuries, attention is then turned to the pancreas. Any hematoma, air bubbles, or bile staining over the area of the pancreas requires further evaluation (10, 17, 29). Likewise, any penetrating wound near the pancreas requires close evaluation (17). The anterior, superior, and inferior surfaces of the pancreas are examined by entering the lesser sac through the gastrocolic ligament (Fig. 84.1). The posterior surface of the head of the pancreas is examined by performing an extended Kocher maneuver (17). If the spleen is injured, both it and the pancreas are reflected medially by dividing the lienorenal ligament to examine the posterior surface of the body and tail. If the spleen is intact, this area may be examined by reflecting the pancreas superiorly after incising the retroperitoneal tissue along the inferior border of the pancreas (9, 10). The pancreas should be examined both visually and by manual palpation.

The extent of injury should be defined by location with respect to the superior mesenteric vessels as well as by whether the main pancreatic duct has been injured. Management of pancreatic injury differs depending on whether the injury is proximal (to the right of the vessels) or distal (to the left of the vessels) (Fig. 84.2) (14). The determination of duct injury can be difficult but is an important step toward reducing complications (7, 19). Injury to the duct may be suspected on the basis of direct visualization of an injury, complete transection of the gland, laceration of more than half of the pancreatic parenchyma, a centrally located penetrating wound, or severe maceration of the gland (Fig. 84.3) (30, 31). In a completely transected pancreas, there has obviously been ductal injury; however, the diagnosis is not always so obvious. If the severed end of the duct is identified, it should be ligated to minimize complications (4). Unfortunately, the duct may be obscured by a field of blood, bowel contents, or tissue swelling. In an unstable patient, it should not be sought (3, 22). There is no advantage to reanastomosing a severed duct; this procedure is tedious and time-consuming and has no advantage over duct ligation (10).

Several methods have been described to demonstrate ductal injury radiographically (Fig. 84.4) during laparotomy if the duct itself is not easily seen. A pancreatogram may be obtained by injection of contrast into the distal pancreatic duct after amputation of the tail of the pancreas (32). This procedure is difficult in patients with a normal caliber pancreatic duct and carries the risks of a distal pancreatectomy. Alternatively, a 5 French feeding catheter may be placed retrograde through the ampulla of Vater via a duodenotomy and 2–5 mL of radiopaque dye can be instilled by gravity (Fig. 84.5) (17, 31). The contrast should not be injected too forcefully, as pancreatitis may result. Opening an uninjured duodenum is usually not recommended because it exposes the patient to the risk of a duodenal fistula (19). An ERCP may be performed intraoperatively if an experienced endoscopist is available (6). We have had some success with performance of a cholangiogram, as there is often reflux of contrast into the pancreatic duct. This method will also demonstrate injury to the intrapancreatic portion of the common bile duct (19). With any of these methods, extravasation of contrast indicates a major ductal injury (31).

When the duct cannot be visualized radiographically in a pancreatic wound with a high probability of duct injury, the surgeon should presume that such an injury is present and treat it accordingly by internal drainage or resection (6, 28). If internal drainage or resection is not feasible because of patient instability or associated intestinal injuries, wide external drainage should be performed (19). In any case, one of the most important components of management of pancreatic injuries is associated external drainage to provide for a controlled fistula should one develop (19). If there is an associated vascular injury in proximity to a pancreatic wound, the vascular suture line should be protected from pancreatic secretions by interposing some omentum (8).

When the extent of pancreatic injury has been defined, the next step is determining the appropriate surgical management. The stage of the pancreatic injury will help to determine the operative procedure. Several staging systems have been described (Table 84.1). The most useful system is the Organ Injury Scale developed by the American Association for the Surgery of Trauma (33). This system has five grades (Fig. 84.6). A grade I

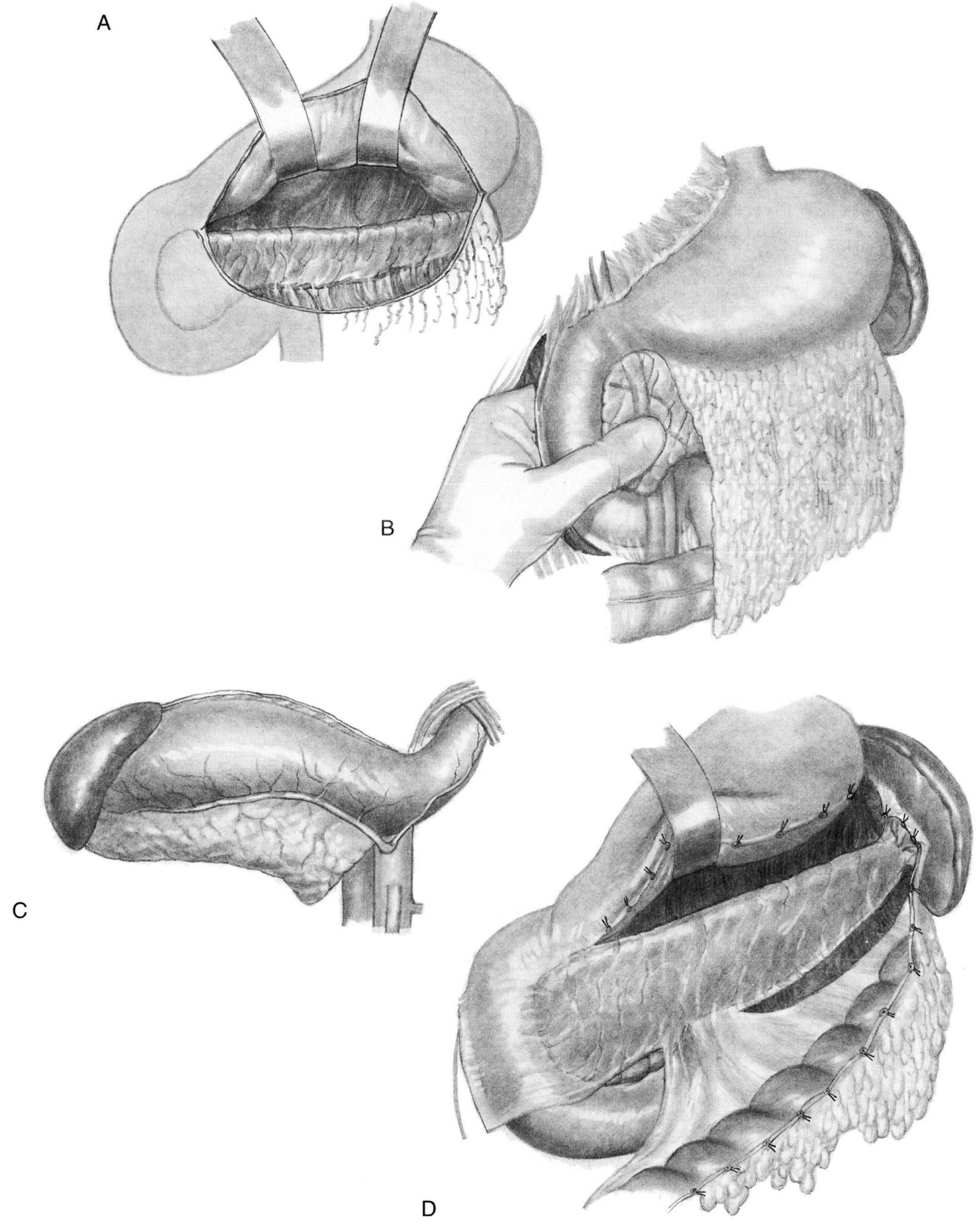


**FIG. 84.1.** Methods of operative exposure of the pancreas. **A.** Division of the gastrocolic ligament to view the anterior surface. **B.** Extended Kocher maneuver. **C.** Reflection of the spleen and pancreas medially after division of the lienorenal ligament. **D.** Reflection of the pancreas superiorly.

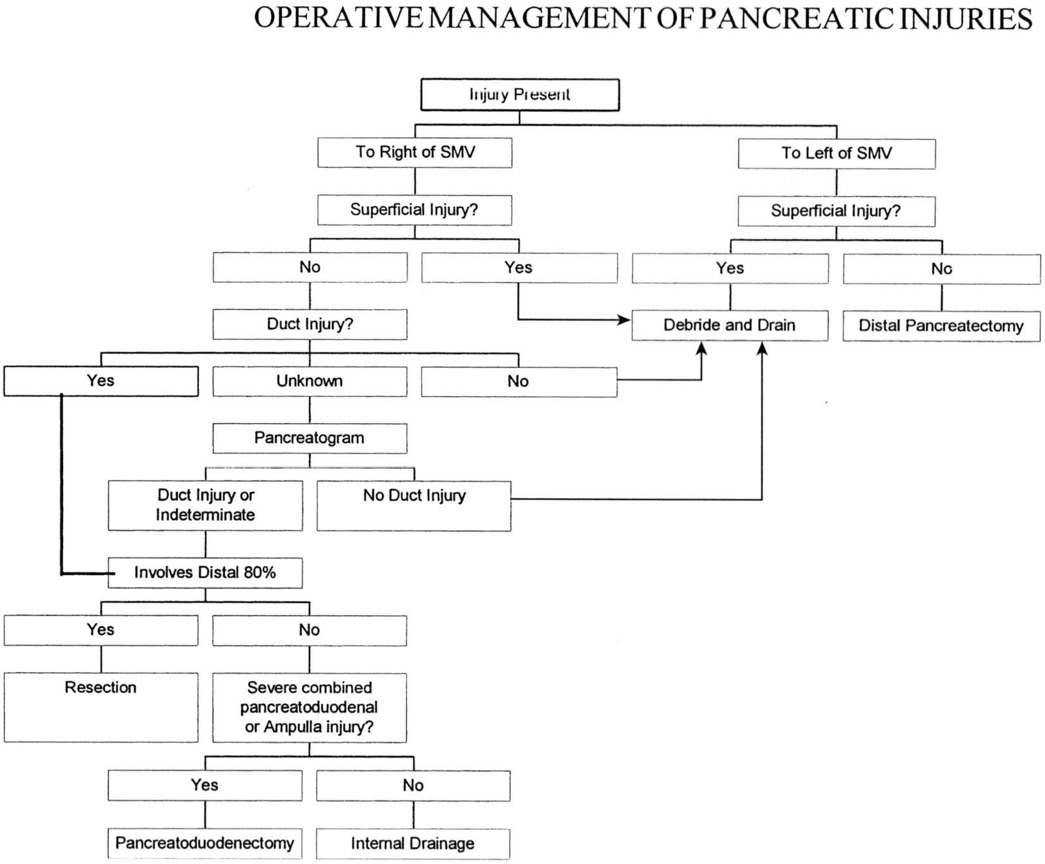


**FIG. 84.2.** Operative management of pancreatic injuries.

pancreatic injury is a minor contusion or superficial laceration anywhere in the gland without associated duct injury. A grade II injury is a major contusion or laceration anywhere in the gland, without duct injury or tissue loss. Grade III injuries involve the distal parenchyma (to the left of the superior mesenteric vein) with a duct injury. Grade IV injuries involve the proximal pancreas and have an associated duct injury. Grade V, the most serious injury, is defined as a massive disruption of the pancreatic head.

## MANAGEMENT OF SPECIFIC PANCREATIC INJURIES

### Superficial Injuries

Grade I and II pancreatic injuries are contusions or superficial lacerations. These injuries make up most (87%) pancreatic injuries seen (8). The only treatment necessary is providing hemostasis and external drainage of pancreatic secretions (15, 17, 29). Drainage is important regardless of how minor the injury appears, as it provides for formation of a controlled fistula and prevents complications such as abscess and pseudocyst (10). Suture repair of the capsule is unnecessary and may increase the rate of pseudocyst formation (10, 17). Active drains appear to have an advantage over passive drains. Stone et al. (8) had a 39% complication rate when Penrose drains were used, compared with a 2% complication rate with sump drains. They feel that passive drains do not adequately prevent accumulation of pancreatic secretions. In a later series, Fabian et al. (34) found that sump drainage was associated with a 21% abscess rate, while closed suction drains had only a 3% rate of abscess formation. They feel that when sump drains are left in place for more than a few days, the tract becomes colonized and bacteria are actually drawn inward. Closed suction drains were equally effective at preventing fluid accumulation. Sump drains tend to be larger and more rigid, which can lead to erosion of adjacent structures (10, 17). At our institution, we prefer to use large-bore closed-suction drains, such as Jackson-Pratt drains.

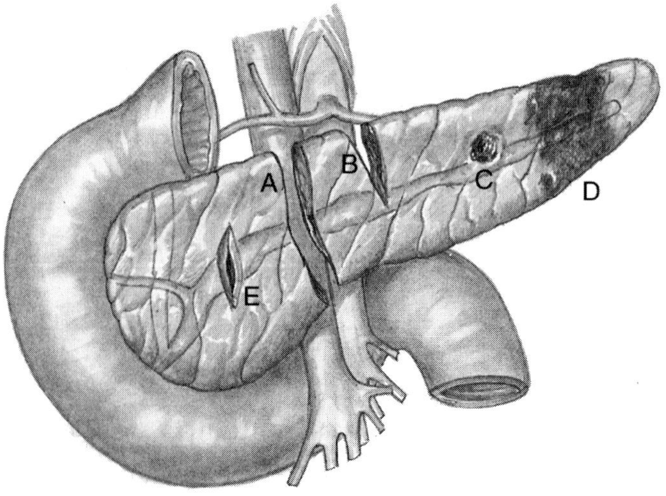


**FIG. 84.3.** Presumptive evidence of duct injury. *A*, Complete transection; *B*, laceration involving over 1/2. of the parenchyma; *C*, centrally located penetrating wound; *D*, severe maceration; *E*, direct visualization of the injured duct.

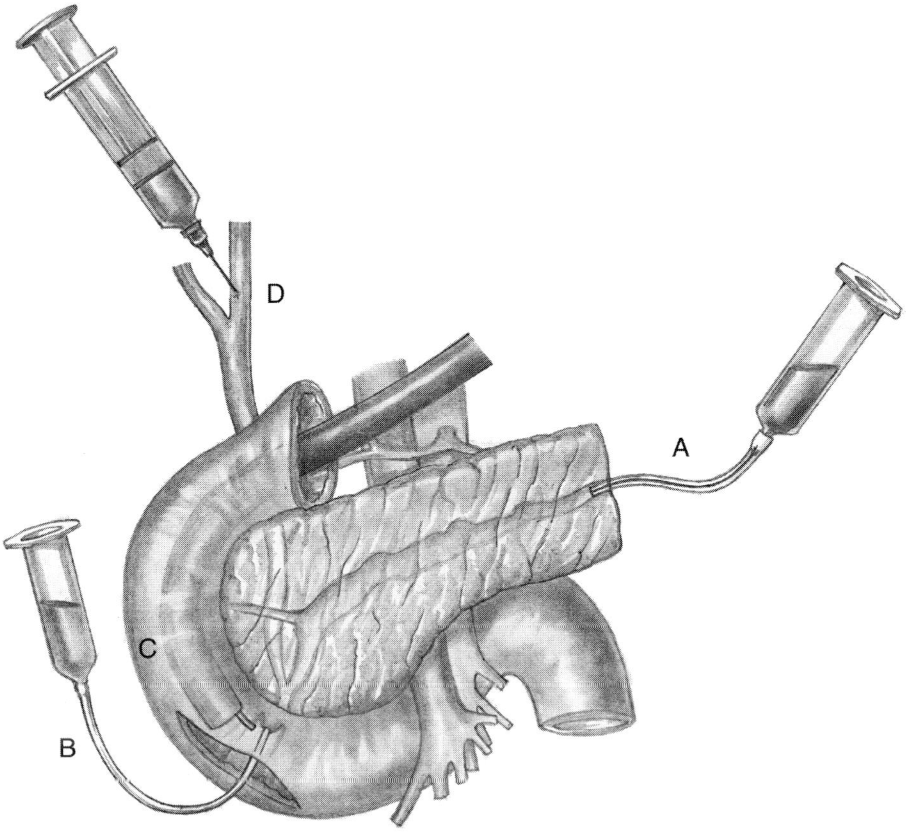


**FIG. 84.4.** Intraoperative radiographic determination of duct injury: *A*, cannulation of distal duct after amputation of the tail; *B*, cannulation of the ampulla of Vater via duodenotomy; *C*, ERCP; *D*, cholangiogram.

### Distal Injuries

Injuries involving the body and tail of the gland make up about 11% of all pancreatic injuries (8). These injuries are best treated with a distal pancreatectomy, as there are more complications related to drainage alone than to resection (19, 29, 30). The spleen is usually removed as well. If the patient has an isolated pancreatic injury or relatively minor associated injuries, the splenic vessels may be dissected away from the distal pancreas, leaving the spleen in situ. Splenic preservation should not be performed in a patient with multiple injuries or hemodynamic instability; the risk of postsplenectomy sepsis is low, and the tedious dissection prolongs the operative time significantly (10, 22). There is also a small risk of splenic vein thrombosis after splenic preservation (10).

If the stump of the pancreatic duct is easily identified, it should be individually ligated; however, there appears to be no increase in complications if it is not ligated (7). The closure of the pancreatic stump may be accomplished by interrupted sutures or stapling (17). Wisner et al. (22) found that nonabsorbable sutures had a higher complication rate than absorbable sutures (58 vs. 31%), although a large multicenter trial showed no difference between suture types and staplers (7). Closure of the pancreatic stump with a TA stapling device (Fig. 84.7) can be accomplished simply and rapidly and includes the duct at the same time (3, 4). Fibrin glue (cryoprecipitate plus a thrombin/calcium mixture) may be applied to the suture line. This has been shown to decrease the rate of fistula formation in distal pancreatectomy performed for nontrauma indications (35). Omentum may be placed over the stump as well. Regardless of the method of closure of the pancreatic stump, the area should be drained externally. In the extremely rare instance in which there is impaired antegrade flow of pancreatic secretions because of associated injury or disease of the proximal duct, the stump may be drained with a Roux-en-Y limb of jejunum (17).

### Proximal Injuries

When a wound involves the head of the pancreas, it is important to determine if the duct is injured as well. If the duct is intact or

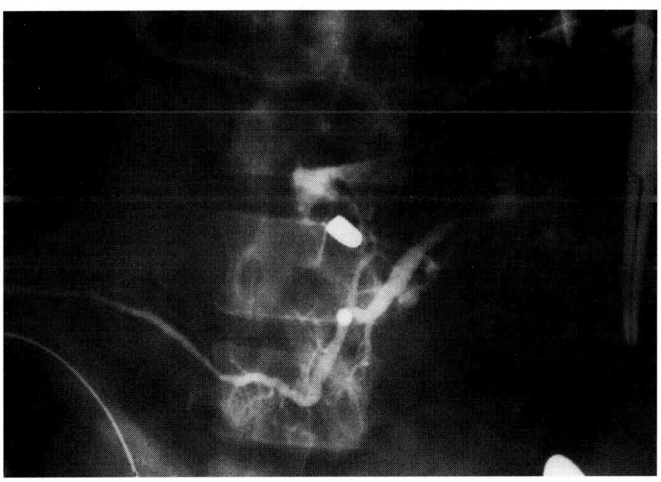

**FIG. 84.5.** Intraoperative pancreatogram performed via duodenotomy; no injury is visualized.

**TABLE 84.1. Comparison of Scoring Systems for Pancreatic Trauma**

| Lucas (17) | Smego et al. (9) | Moore et al. (33) |
|---|---|---|
| I Contusion, peripheral laceration<br>II Distal laceration or transection with duct injury<br>III Proximal laceration or transection with duct injury<br>IV Severe combined pancreatoduodenal injury | I Contusion or hematoma<br>II Minor parenchymal disruption<br>III Major ductal injury<br>IV Severe crush injury | I Superficial laceration or contusion<br>II Major laceration or contusion without duct injury<br>III Distal parenchymal injury with duct involvement<br>IV Proximal parenchymal injury with duct injury<br>V Massive disruption of pancreatic head |

the injury is away from the area of the duct, simple external drainage is all that is necessary (10, 29). If the duct is injured, two alternatives exist. If resection of the gland distal to the injury would leave 20% or more of the pancreas in situ, then an extended distal pancreatectomy may be performed (19). If a resection would involve more than 80% of the pancreas, then internal drainage should be performed to avoid the complication of pancreatic insufficiency (19). Internal drainage is best accomplished with a Roux-en-Y limb of jejunum sewn to pancreatic capsule over the area of injury (Fig. 84.8) (10, 28). This is often a difficult anastomosis and should not be attempted in an unstable patient. In a through and through penetrating wound, it is not necessary to drain both ends of the tract; the opposite wound (usually posterior) is treated with external drainage. This method of internal drainage has the best success, however, if the posterior pancreatic capsule is intact (19). If the patient is unstable or massive destruction makes performance of a pancreatojejunostomy unsafe, wide external drainage may be performed accepting the formation of a pancreatocutaneous fistula (22).

There are few indications for a Whipple procedure following abdominal trauma. These include extensive devitalization of the duodenum and/or pancreatic head (Fig. 84.9), complex injuries

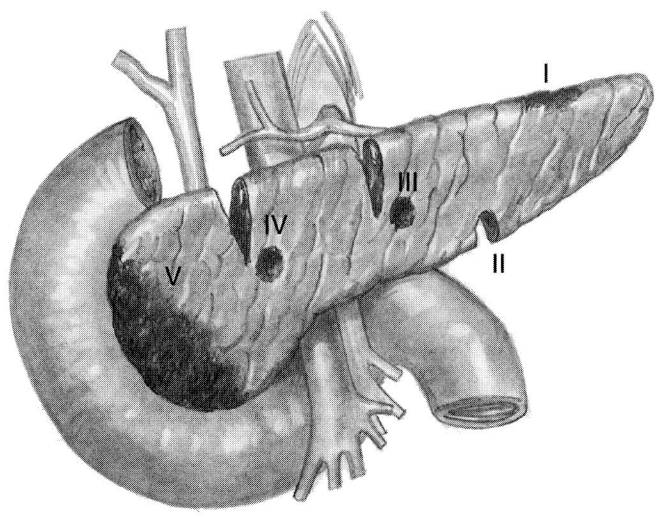


**FIG. 84.6.** Grades of pancreatic injury. A grade I injury is a minor contusion or laceration. A grade II injury is a major contusion or laceration without duct involvement. Grade III injuries contain a duct injury to the left of the superior mesenteric vessels. Grade IV injuries contain a duct injury in the head of the pancreas. Grade V injuries have massive destruction of the pancreatic head.

to both the duodenum and pancreatic head, injury to the ampulla of Vater, and uncontrollable bleeding from the pancreatic head (19, 28, 29). Some authors feel that injuries to the retropancreatic portal vein or the intrapancreatic common bile duct are indications for a Whipple procedure as well (28). In our experience however, the portal vein may be repaired after distal resection of the overlying gland, or in the case of a bile duct injury, a biliary-enteric anastomosis may be performed. Fewer than 3% of patients with a pancreatic injury will require a pancreaticoduodenectomy (10, 13, 19, 36); most combined pancreatic and duodenal injuries may be treated separately (36, 37). The mortality of a pancreaticoduodenectomy for trauma is over 29% and as high as 100% in some series (8, 13, 28, 36). This high mortality is due to the associated vascular injuries in these patients. If a patient is unstable during pancreaticoduodenectomy, the reconstruction may be delayed until after the patient has undergone a period of stabilization (38). Alternatively, the pancreatic duct may be ligated after performance of the gastro- and choledochojejunal anastomoses to avoid breakdown of a pancreatojejunal anastomosis. This duct ligation is associated with a high incidence of fistula formation (50%), pancreatitis (23%), and malabsorption (50%) (39).

Two other methods exist for managing severe combined pancreatic and duodenal injuries if the pancreatic duct is intact: duodenal diverticularization and pyloric exclusion. Duodenal diverticularization consists of antrectomy, gastrojejunostomy, and tube duodenostomy (Fig. 84.10) and diverts gastric drainage away from the injured duodenum (13, 17, 36). Pyloric exclusion is performed by suturing or stapling the pylorus, followed by gastrojejunostomy, and it also diverts gastric drainage away from the site of injury (13, 36). Both procedures are associated with a mortality rate of 12–19% and a pancreatic fistula rate of 12–25% (13).

## POSTOPERATIVE MANAGEMENT OF PANCREATIC TRAUMA

All patients should receive broad-spectrum antibiotic coverage for 24–48 hours following laparotomy (17). Postoperative nutritional support is extremely important. Nutrition may be provided in the form of parenteral alimentation or via a tube jejunostomy (10, 37). Enteral tube feedings distal to the duodenum are cheaper and associated with fewer complications than parenteral nutrition and do not appear to stimulate exocrine pancreatic secretions (10).

Virtually all patients with pancreatic injuries will have external drains in place to minimize complications (14). Regardless of the type of drain, it should be left in for at least a week (29). The drain is usually removed after the output has dropped to less than 30 mL in a 24-hour period and the patient is

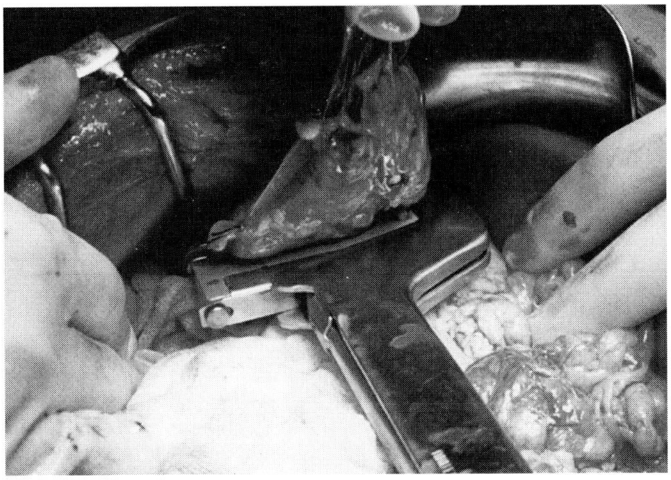

**FIG. 84.7.** Distal pancreatectomy performed with a TA stapling device for a macerated pancreatic tail.

tolerating an oral diet. Persistently high drain outputs should be investigated as possible fistulae by measuring the amylase level in the drainage fluid.

The somatostatin analog octreotide may be useful in reducing the incidence of complications when given prophylactically. It reduced complications from 54% to 32% in a large multicenter trial of patients undergoing elective pancreatic resection (40). In a small retrospective series of pancreatic trauma patients, the incidence of complications related to the pancreas fell from 29% to 0% when octreotide was used prophylactically (41). The usual dose of octreotide in this setting is 50–100 μg subcutaneously three times daily (40, 41).

## OUTCOME OF PANCREATIC TRAUMA

### Natural History

A delay in diagnosis and treatment even as short as 6 hours may increase the complication and mortality rates following pancreatic trauma (16, 22). One series showed a 50% mortality rate in patients whose diagnosis was delayed over 24 hours, and 75% of the survivors developed pancreatic fistulae (17).

Pancreatic injuries may be initially silent. However in a major pancreatic injury, autodigestion of the parenchyma and peripancreatic tissue may occur before a pancreatic transection is recognized hours or days later (21). There may be increasing edema, tissue necrosis, and even erosion into adjacent structures (9). A duct injury if missed, may lead to fistula, abscess, and pseudocyst formation (Fig. 84.11) (10). Later, progressive periductal inflammation and fibrosis may result in chronic pancreatitis, which has been reported up to 21 years following injury (10, 42). This late complication is best treated with distal resection to the left of the area of injury (42). Late complications are most easily diagnosed with a combination of ultrasound, CT, and ERCP (10).

### Morbidity and Mortality

The overall mortality of pancreatic injuries varies from 3 to 24% (7–9, 22). Blunt injuries carry a mortality rate of up to 67% (8, 14, 29, 30), although isolated blunt injuries to the pancreas have a mortality of 3–10% (10). Penetrating wounds to the pancreas carry a mortality rate of 18–22% (3, 19, 29, 30), but this mortality varies widely with the type of weapon involved. Shotgun wounds have the highest mortality at 56–67%, stab wounds have the lowest at 5–8%, and gunshot wounds are intermediate at 11–22% (6, 8, 19). The immediate mortality is usually due to associated injuries, notably hemorrhage from major vascular injuries. Delayed mortality is due to a combination of sepsis from associated hollow viscus injuries and complications from the pancreatic wound itself (3, 14, 22). The pancreatic injury is actually the cause of death in about 3% of patients with pancreatic injuries (19). There is an increase in mortality associated with massive blood requirements and more than four associated organ injuries (19, 30). Mortality is also related to the grade and location of the pancreatic injury, with higher grades and injuries to the pancreatic head having a poorer prognosis (19).

Pancreatic complications are not uncommon after pancreatic trauma. Complication rates range from 25 to 80% (1, 3, 15, 22, 29). Blunt injuries have a higher complication rate than penetrating wounds (29). Complications also vary with the number and type of associated organs injured and the location and severity of the pancreatic wound. There is a higher rate of abscess and fistula formation when the wound involves the head of the pancreas than with an injury in the body or tail (1). Likewise, grade I injuries have a 9% risk of abscess or fistula formation, compared with a 50% risk in grade V injuries (9, 22).

### Hemorrhage

The most serious complication after pancreatic trauma is hemorrhage. This may occur in 5–10% of patients and is the result of incomplete hemostasis of the pancreatic stump, incomplete control of the pancreatoduodenal artery, or erosion of sutures in a nearby vascular anastomosis from pancreatic enzymes (7, 10, 28). Nearly 100% of these patients will require reoperation for control of hemorrhage (10). Protection of a vascular suture line with interposed omentum will minimize the incidence of this complication (8).

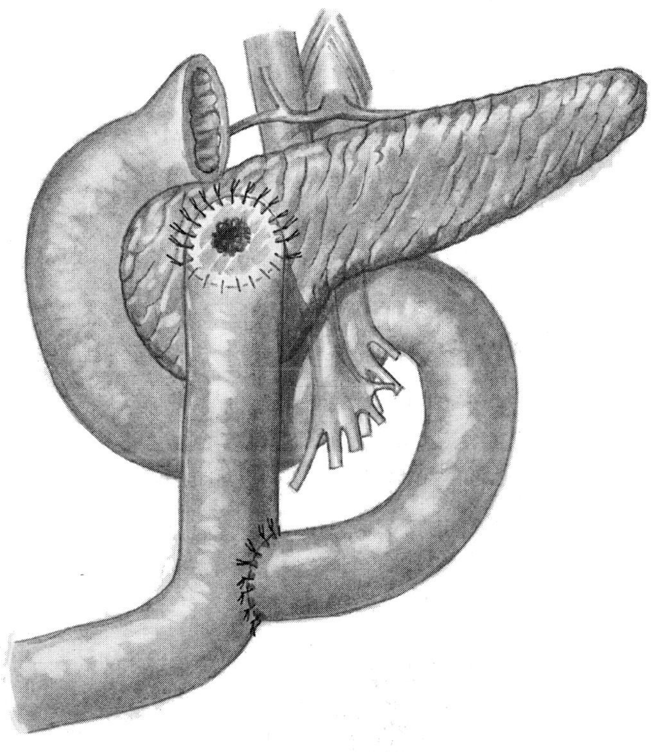

**FIG. 84.8.** Injury to proximal pancreatic duct repaired with a Roux-en-Y pancreatojejunostomy.

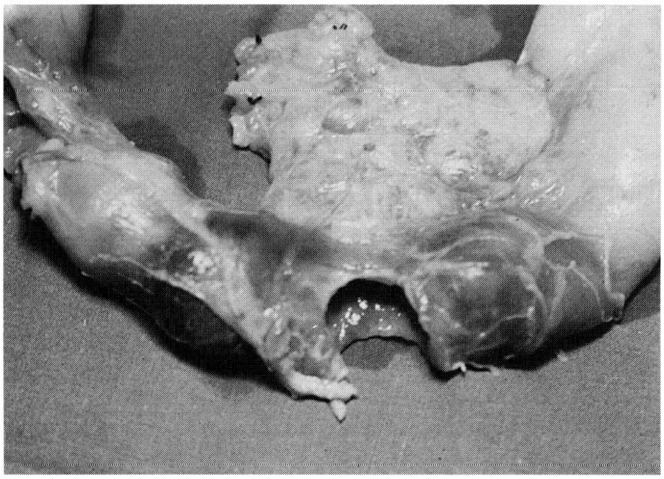

**FIG. 84.9.** Operative specimen after pancreatoduodenectomy for gunshot wound. Note the extensive devitalization of the duodenum and pancreatic head.

### Fistula

Pancreatocutaneous fistulae develop in 6–26% of patients who sustain an injury to the pancreas (6, 7, 10, 36, 43). Different authors have different definitions of what constitutes a fistula,ranging from drainage of over 50 mL of amylase-rich fluid per day for more than 3 days (7) to drainage of over 100 mL of amylase-rich fluid per day for over 7 days (43). The measured amylase in the drainage fluid is markedly higher than the serum amylase (36). The rate of fistula formation is highest after injury to the pancreatic head (10).

Once a pancreatic fistula is diagnosed, the patient is treated supportively. A high-output fistula requires intravenous fluid replacement with normal saline solution. Serum potassium and bicarbonate should be monitored and replaced as needed. If the fistula persists more than a few weeks, zinc and magnesium may also need repletion (10). Most (89%) fistulae close spontaneously within 6–8 weeks, especially if the duct is uninjured or has been drained internally (7, 10, 19, 30, 37). Seventy percent will actually close within 2 weeks (10). Seven to 11% of pancreatic fistulae require reoperation. In this case, a Roux-en-Y limb of jejunum is used to drain the pancreatic secretions internally (10, 17).

### Abscess

An infectious complication will occur in 10–40% of patients with pancreatic trauma (7, 10, 13, 19, 36, 43). This may range in severity from a wound or drain tract infection to an intraabdominal or pancreatic abscess (6, 19). The formation of an intraabdominal abscess correlates with the presence of a hollow viscus injury, particularly of the colon and/or the duodenum (1, 7, 10, 13, 30, 43).

Up to a third of intraabdominal abscesses are pancreatic abscesses (6, 7), which require open surgical debridement and drainage. The remainder are abscesses located elsewhere within the abdomen, most of which (79%) are successfully treated with percutaneous drainage and broad-spectrum antibiotics (7). Unfortunately, the presence of an intraabdominal abscess after pancreatic trauma carries a 20% mortality (10, 19).

### Pancreatic Pseudocyst

A patient treated nonoperatively for a blunt traumatic injury has a 60% chance of developing a pseudocyst (5). If pancreatic injury is diagnosed and treated operatively in a timely manner, the incidence of pseudocyst falls to 2–3% (6, 7, 10). The type of drain used has some effect on pseudocyst formation; passive drains are associated with 7% pseudocyst formation, contrasted with 1% pseudocyst formation after active drainage (8). If the pseudocyst does not resolve spontaneously or develops complications, it will require definitive treatment (7).

### Pancreatitis

Early postoperative pancreatitis occurs in 8–23% of patients who sustain pancreatic trauma (7, 13, 30, 39). It is more likely to occur after pancreatoduodenectomy than with other operative procedures (13, 39). A small percentage of patients (1.2%) actually develop necrotizing pancreatitis (19). The treatment of early posttraumatic pancreatitis is supportive, consisting of nasogastric suction, bowel rest, and nutritional support (10, 17).

Chronic pancreatitis may develop in the patient with unrecognized/untreated duct injury. The patient may present months to years after injury. The diagnosis is made by ERCP demonstration of duct cutoff or stricture. This posttraumatic chronic pancreatitis can be treated with distal pancreatectomy or pancreatojejunostomy (5).

### Pancreatic Insufficiency

Another complication of pancreatic trauma is endocrine and exocrine insufficiency. Endocrine insufficiency may occur in up to 27% of patients undergoing resection of more than 80% of their pancreas and may range from mild glucose intolerance to insulin-dependent diabetes mellitus (7, 19, 43). Symptomatic exocrine insufficiency and malabsorption are rare, even after 80% resection of a normal pancreas (4, 7). Delayed gastric emptying may occur in up to 20% of patients undergoing pancreaticoduodenectomy for trauma (13).

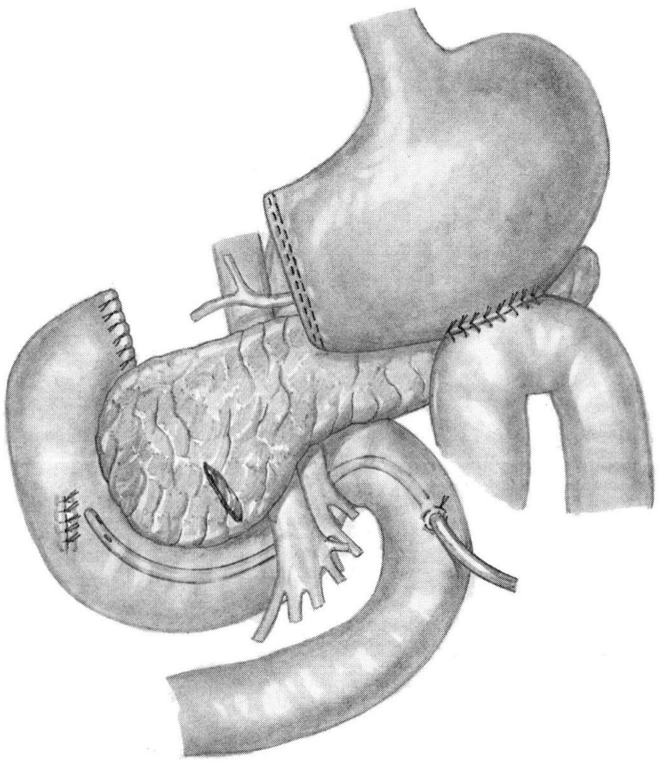

**FIG. 84.10.** Duodenal diverticularization procedure.

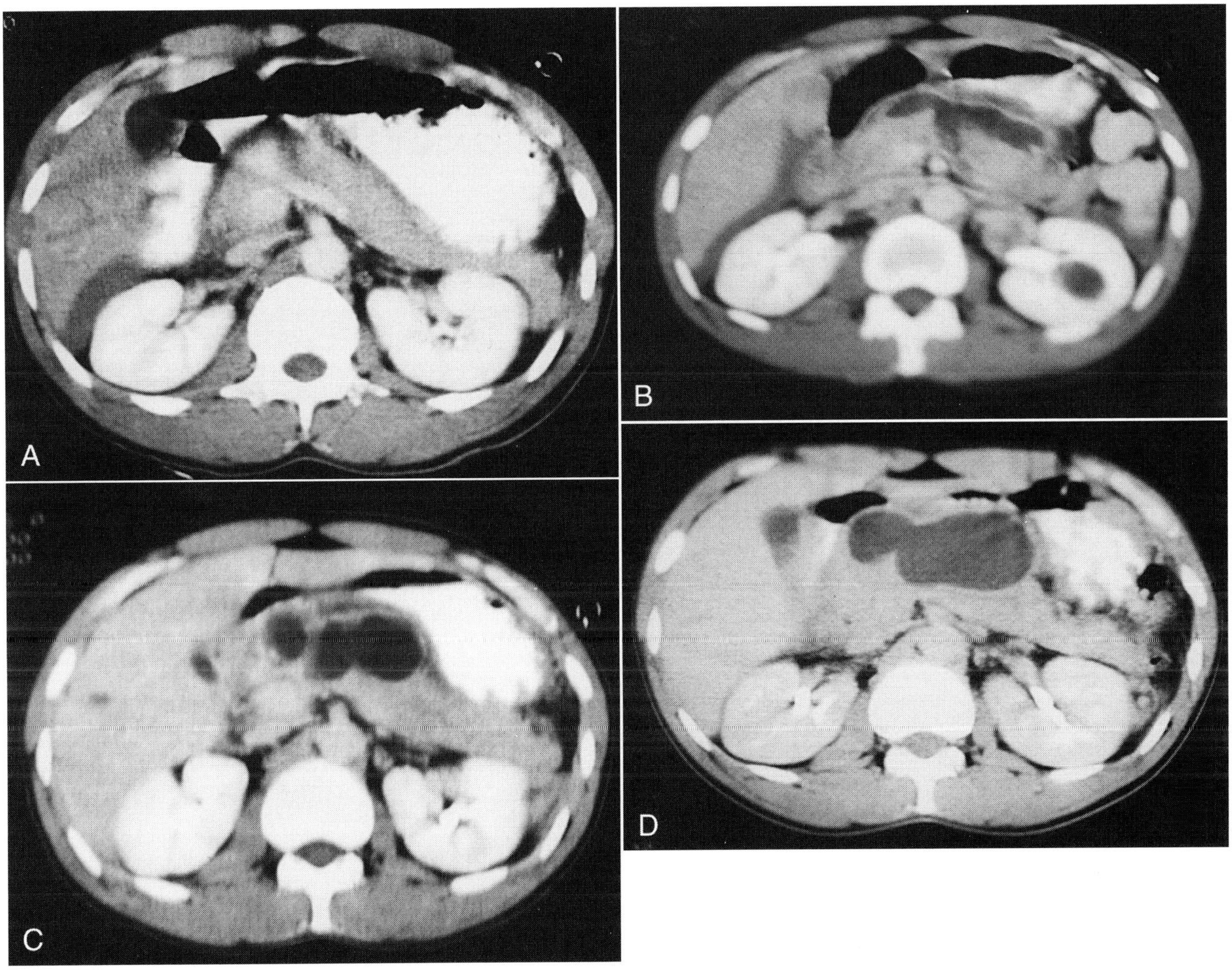


**FIG. 84.11.** CT of untreated pancreatic transection following a blow to the epigastrium. **A.** Initial CT shows a hypodense area in midpancreas. This was not appreciated by the physician initially treating the patient. **B.** Repeat CT 7 days later when the patient returned with abdominal pain. This was treated conservatively. **C.** CT 17 days after injury, when patient was transferred to our hospital. **D.** CT prior to performance of pseudocyst-gastrostomy.

## PANCREATIC TRAUMA IN CHILDREN

Trauma is the leading cause of pancreatitis in children, being responsible for over 50% of cases. Most children with pancreatic trauma are managed nonoperatively. Twenty percent of acute pancreatic injuries in children result in pseudocyst formation. These pseudocysts tend to be large and thin-walled and become acutely symptomatic, requiring earlier treatment than the corresponding adult pseudocysts. Pediatric pseudocysts can be externally drained with a 78–100% success rate. Those that recur may be redrained externally (11).

## SUMMARY

Pancreatic trauma is an infrequent component of abdominal trauma. It is important to diagnose and treat pancreatic wounds in a timely manner to minimize the incidence of complications. The diagnosis is often difficult because of the retroperitoneal location of the pancreas and is frequently made during laparotomy for other indications. Even with early and aggressive operative treatment, there is a high incidence of complications from these injuries.

## REFERENCES


1. Sims EH, Mandal AK, Schlater T, Fleming AW, Lou SMA. Factors affecting outcome in pancreatic trauma. J Trauma 1984;24: 125–128.
2. Hannon DW, Sprafka J. Resection for traumatic pancreatitis. Ann Surg 1957;146:136–138.
3. Andersen DK, Bolman RM, Moylan JA. Management of penetrating pancreatic injuries: subtotal pancreatectomy using the auto suture stapler. J Trauma 1980;20:347–349.
4. Fitzgibbons TJ, Yellin AE, Maruyama MM, Donovan AJ. Management of the transected pancreas following distal pancreatectomy. Surg Gynecol Obstet 1982;154:225–231.
5. Kudsk KA, Temizer D, Ellison EC, Cloutier CT, Buckley DC, Carey LC. Post-traumatic pancreatic sequestrum: recognition and treatment. J Trauma 1986;26:320–324.
6. Laraja RD, Lobbato VJ, Cassaro S, Reddy S. Intraoperative endoscopic retrograde cholangiopancreatography (ERCP) in penetrating trauma of the pancreas. J Trauma 1986;26:1146–1147.
7. Cogbill TH, Moore EE, Morris JA, et al. Distal pancreatectomy for trauma: a multicenter experience. J Trauma 1991;31:1600–1606.
8. Stone HH, Fabian TC, Satiani B, Turkleson ML. Experiences in

the management of pancreatic trauma. J Trauma 1981;21: 257–262.
9. Smego DR, Richardson JD, Flint LM. Determinants of outcome in pancreatic trauma. J Trauma 1985;25:771–776.
10. Wilson RH, Moorehead RJ. Current management of trauma to the pancreas. Br J Surg 1991;78:1196–1202.
11. Warner RL, Othersen HB, Smith CD. Traumatic pancreatitis and pseudocyst in children: current management. J Trauma 1989;29: 597–601.
12. Craig MH, Talton DS, Hauser CJ, Poole GV. Pancreatic injuries from blunt trauma. Am Surg 1995;61:125–128.
13. Oreskovich MR, Carrico CJ. Pancreaticoduodenectomy for trauma: a viable option? Am J Surg 1984;147:618–623.
14. Nowak MM, Baringer DC, Ponsky JL. Pancreatic injuries: effectiveness of debridement and drainage for nontransecting injuries. Am Surg 1986;52:599–602.
15. Sorensen VJ, Obeid FN, Horst HM, Bivins BA. Penetrating pancreatic injuries, 1978–1983 Am Surg 1986;52:354–358.
16. Jeffrey RB, Federle MP, Crass RA. Computed tomography of pancreatic trauma. Radlology 1983;147:491–494.
17. Lucas CE. Diagnosis and treatment of pancreatic and duodenal injury. Surg Clin North Am 1977;57:49–65.
18. Bouwman DL, Weaver DW, Walt AJ. Serum amylase and its isoenzymes: a clarification of their implications in trauma. J Trauma 1984;24:573–578.
19. Jones RC. Management of pancreatic trauma. Am J Surg 1985;150:698–704.
20. Greenlee T, Murphy K, Ram MD. Amylase isoenzymes in the evaluation of trauma patients. Am Surg 1984;50:637–640.
21. Horst HM, Bivins BA. Pancreatic transection: a concept of evolving injury. Arch Surg 1989;124:1093–1095.
22. Wisner DH, Wold RL, Frey CF. Diagnosis and treatment of pancreatic injuries: an analysis of management principles. Arch Surg 1990;125:1109–1113.
23. Alyono D, Perry JF. Value of quantitative cell count and amylase activity of peritoneal lavage fluid. J Trauma 1981;21:345–348.
24. Barkin JS, Ferstenberg RM, Panullo W, Manten HD, Davis RC. Endoscopic retrograde cholangiopancreatography in pancreatic trauma. Gastrointest Endosc 1988;34:102–105.
25. Himmelman RG, Martin M, Gilkey S, Barrett JA. Triple-contrast CT scans in penetrating back and flank trauma. J Trauma 1991;31: 852–855.
26. Kuligowska E, Mueller PR, Simeone JF, Fine C. Ultrasound in upper abdominal trauma. Semin Roentgenol 1984;19:281–295.
27. Van Steenbergen W, Samain H, Pouillon M, et al. Transection of the pancreas demonstrated by ultrasound and computed tomography. Gastrointest Radiol 1987;12:128–130.
28. Lowe RJ, Saletta JD, Moss GS. Pancreatoduodenectomy for penetrating pancreatic trauma. J Trauma 1977;17:732–741.
29. Anane-Sefah J, Norton LW, Eiseman B. Operative choice and technique following pancreatic injury. Arch Surg 1975;110: 161–166.
30. Heitsch RC, Knutson CO, Fulton RL, Jones CE. Delineation of critical factors in the treatment of pancreatic trauma. Surgery 1976;80:523–529.
31. Berni GA, Bandyk DF, Oreskovich MR, Carrico CJ. Role of intraoperative pancreatography in patients with injury to the pancreas. Am J Surg 1982;143:602–605.
32. Gougeon FW, Legros G, Archambault A, Bessette G, Bastien E. Pancreatic trauma: a new diagnostic approach. Am J Surg 1976;132:400–402.
33. Moore EE, Cogbill TH, Malangoni MA, et al. Organ injury scaling, II: pancreas, duodenum, small bowel, colon and rectum. J Trauma 1990;30:1427–1429.
34. Fabian TC, Kudsk KA, Croce MA, et al. Superiority of closed suction drainage for pancreatic trauma: a randomized, prospective study. Ann Surg 1990;211:724–730.
35. Suzuki Y, Kuroda Y, Morita A, et al. Fibrin glue sealing for the prevention of pancreatic fistulas following distal pancreatectomy. Arch Surg 1995;130:952–955.
36. Feliciano DV, Martin TD, Cruse PA, et al. Management of combined pancreatoduodenal injuries. Ann Surg 1987;205: 673–679.
37. Whalen GF, Robbs JV, Baker LW. Injuries of the pancreas and duodenum—results of a conservative approach. S Afr J Surg 1987;25:15–18.
38. Eastlick L, Fogler RJ, Shaftan GW. Pancreaticoduodenectomy for trauma: delayed reconstruction: a case report. J Trauma 1990; 30:503–505.
39. Gentilello LM, Cortes V, Buechter KJ, Gomez GA, Castro M, Zeppa R. Whipple procedure for trauma: is duct ligation a safe alternative to pancreaticojejunostomy? J Trauma 1991;31: 661–668.
40. Büchler M, Friess H, Klempa I, et al. Role of octreotide in the prevention of postoperative complications following pancreatic resection. Am J Surg 1992;163:125–131.
41. Amirata E, Livingston DH, Elcavage J. Octreotide acetate decreases pancreatic complications after pancreatic trauma. Am J Surg 1994;168:345–347.
42. Gholson CF, Sittig K, Favrot D, McDonald JC. Chronic abdominal pain as the initial manifestation of pancreatic injury due to remote blunt trauma of the abdomen. South Med J 1994;87: 902–904.
43. Flynn WJ, Cryer HG, Richardson JD. Reappraisal of pancreatic and duodenal injury management based on injury severity. Arch Surg 1990;125:1539–1541.

# 85

# *Pancreatic Fistula*

Claudio Bassi, Massimo Falconi, and Paolo Pederzoli

Pancreatic fistulas (PFs) are one of the most frequent and feared complications of pancreatic surgery. They may also result from pancreatic trauma, necrotizing acute pancreatitis, abscesses, pseudocysts, and exacerbations of chronic pancreatitis. All these factors can cause destruction of Wirsung's duct or its branches, with consequent leakage of pancreatic juice into the retroperitoneum and/or peritoneum.

If defense processes and serosal reabsorption are not activated, the leakage causes pancreatic ascites or different types of *internal* fistulas such as to the (1) pleural or mediastinal space, (2) bronchi, (3) pericardium, (4) colon, (5) small intestine, (6) portal vein, and (7) bile ducts. Pancreatic ascites and internal fistulas develop within the context of chronic pancreatitis or, less frequently, after surgery (8, 9); *external* PFs are more common in acute pancreatitis or after pancreatic surgery (10).

External PFs are classified as *high-* or *low-output*, depending on their daily output (more or less than 200 mL) (11), and as *pure* or *mixed* with other intestinal fluids. Anatomically, the pancreaticocutaneous connection may be *direct* or *indirect* through a collection or pseudocyst and *simple* or *complex* according to whether the fistulas run straight from the pancreas to the skin or whether they pass via other organs (12). Since there is no universally accepted general classification of PFs, those resulting from acute pancreatitis are hard to categorize in strict nosologic terms; on the basis of the underlying disease, they are often defined as "acute" in contrast to those arising in the course of chronic pancreatitis (9, 10). This terminology seems somewhat misleading, in that adjectives such as "acute" or "chronic" are more useful, indicating the actual length of the fistula formation period.

PFs have not been given a lot of attention in the literature, probably because they were almost always regarded as the unwanted complications of improperly performed surgery. Though it is difficult to quantify them epidemiologically, it is reasonable to believe that their incidence parallels the increasingly widespread practice of pancreatic surgery (12).

Though the advances over the past decade have revolutionized the therapeutic approach to PFs, their basic management is still the one rightly advocated a few years ago (13, 14). Since the condition tends to heal spontaneously, albeit over lengthy time periods, any analysis of the different types of medical or surgical approaches should be based on the actual closure rates achieved as well as on the time and costs involved (12).

## EXTERNAL PANCREATIC FISTULAS

Development of external PFs necessarily entails the disruption of a duct. In acute pancreatitis, such an event may occur spontaneously or, more often, as a result of surgical maneuvers (drainage placement, sequestrectomy, debridement), or radiologically guided drainage procedures (12).

The amount of drainage and discharge appears to depend upon three factors: *(a)* the size of the duct involved, *(b)* the site of the rupture, and *(c)* the functional capability of the sphincter of Oddi. Presumably, the resolution of papillary edema and spasm in the acute phase of the disease is the main mechanism responsible for the rapid spontaneous healing of acute fistulas. This interpretation accounts for the lower tendency of fistulas to heal spontaneously in chronic pancreatitis (owing to the presence of prepapillary fixed intraductal obstacles).

Surgical maneuvers such as extensive debridements and necrosectomies performed on infected necrotic areas or pancreatic abscesses (15–17) may give rise to or uncover a rupture of the ductal system. Drains left in place for lengthy periods may result in pressure erosions. In the acute phase, proteolytic enzyme activity may contribute to the formation of a fistula tract. It is likely that both continuous postoperative lavage techniques (15, 18) and open packing (19) favor persistence of the fistula tract. In this context we feel a need to review the concept of fistulas as complications of procedures that have been important steps forward in terms of reducing mortality due to severe pancreatitis. High-output external PFs requiring specific treatment have an incidence of about 10% in our patients subjected to retroperitoneal drainage and intraperitoneal lavage for necrotizing pancreatitis (15), a figure that appears acceptable in such a severe condition.

### Diagnosis

While there is no generally accepted definition of an external PF, in practice its diagnosis is easy, and in all cases there will be a strong suspicion on the basis of medical history alone. The diagnosis must be considered whenever pancreatic juice emerges from a surgical drain for a period exceeding 2–4 days. If the output is less than 100 mL/day, the fistula will tend to close rapidly and spontaneously with return of gastrointestinal function and progressive improvement in the patient's clinical course. This may occur even in fistulas of higher output (100–700 mL/day), while the likelihood of a rapid, spontaneous closure decreases in the so-called major fistulas (>700 mL/day) (10, 11).

Mixed PFs are obviously not characterized by the presence of crystal-clear or "spring-water" fluid found in the pure forms, but they may present with fluids of different colors, ranging from pale green to dark brown. The pancreatic component in these cases is revealed by skin erosion as a result of activation of the juice by intestinal enterokinase. The clinical suspicion is generally confirmed by finding large amounts of amylase in the drainage with magnitudes being of the order of a few tens of thousands of international units.

Radiology can distinguish between simple and complex fistulas. The diagnostic workup, as regards type and chronologic sequence, is influenced by the particular etiologic factor responsible for formation of the fistula (20). For example, with

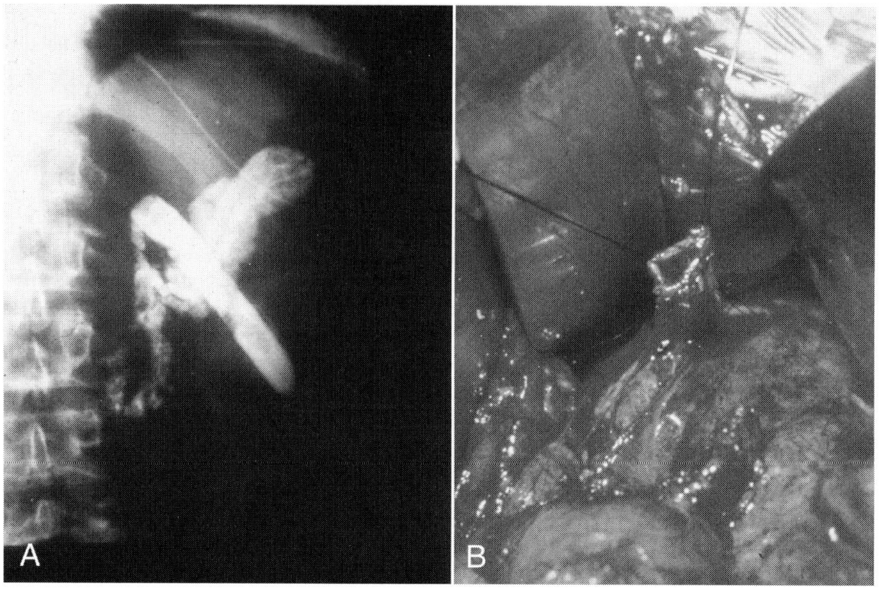


**FIG. 85.1. A.** Fistulography performed through a surgical drain positioned for continuous postoperative drainage and lavage of severe pancreatitis with infected necrosis. The contrast medium displays the Wirsung duct in the body and tail without outlining the head portion, owing to complete rupture of the duct at the level of the head-body transition. This is an absolute impediment to conservative management. **B.** The same patient 4 months after onset of a high-output external fistula. Using the drain as a guide, the fistula tract has organized itself into a fibrous structure that is readily amenable to surgical treatment. The fistula tract, loaded with four stitches, is ready for the construction of a ductojejunostomy using a Roux loop.

*pancreatic trauma*, the serial CT scans necessary to evaluate the patient can document the site and extent of the lesion. Simultaneous CT scan examination and opacification of the fistula tract (CT-fistulography) may demonstrate the presence of collections communicating with the fistula tract or with Wirsung's duct. Since nonopacification of the main duct can be the result of insufficient pressure or insufficient contrast medium with CT fistulography, a conventional fistulography is often needed. Finally, endoscopic retrograde cholangiopancreatography (ERCP) should be obtained whenever the disease persists or deteriorates. ERCP can clarify whether the main duct has been injured, a situation that indicates surgical or endoscopic correction (21, 22).

As stressed above, PF is a well-known complication of pancreatic surgery and many technical and pharmacologic expedients have been suggested for its prevention (23, 24). It is often not possible to determine whether such complications are due to incorrect technique or to the inflammatory process itself.

In the postoperative period, CT is the only diagnostic tool that can detect a possible inflammatory process in the residual parenchyma and which, when used in conjunction with fistulography (CT-fistulography), allows correct staging of the lesion. Unlike posttraumatic fistulas, these fistulas are usually mixed—thus necessitating use of contrast radiography of the digestive tract and/or bile ducts for their complete delineation (20).

ERCP can document lesions arising as a result of left resections, though these generally tend to heal rapidly and spontaneously. Juxtapapillary duct obstructions, which maintain the fistula by impeding outflow, may be relieved with ERCP techniques.

Finally, another factor that may cause external PF formation is surgical or US/CT-guided drainage of complications of necrotizing pancreatitis, such as abscesses and/or pseudocysts. Conventional fistulography can provide basic information about the simple or complex nature of the fistula and its relationship to the ductal system (Fig. 85.1*A*). With complex fistulas, radiologic examination of the gastrointestinal tract is often needed to determine the site and extent of intestinal involvement and to assess the likelihood for spontaneous closure. CT is useful also in pancreatitis because it can detect peripancreatic fluid collections that may be associated with the fistula.

In conclusion, the various other radiologic procedures mentioned play a complementary role to standard fistulography, which remains the examination of choice and is capable, in most cases, of identifying the nature, site, extent, and possible communications of the PF. CT-fistulography is used in the staging of complex fistulas with several branches and when it proves necessary to provide a complete picture of *peripancreatic fluid collections*.

Further techniques are considered in relation to the duration and onset of fistula complications. Cases that show rapid healing do not require investigations in addition to traditional fistulography. In such situations, an excessive use of radiology may even prove counterproductive, by reopening a fistula tract that is on its way to healing.

If the fistula does not heal, an ERCP is advisable to verify the state of patency of the main duct as well as the site of rupture, if any.

### Limitations and Pitfalls of Conservative Management

The availability of potent inhibitors of pancreatic secretion and the refinement of enteral and parenteral nutritional techniques have led some to conclude that all external PFs will ultimately heal. In spite of the enormous progress achieved, in clinical practice there is no clear-cut relationship between the treatment and results obtained. Table 85.1 shows both the elements that hinder (limitations) and those that complicate or jeopardize (pitfalls) definitive healing of external PFs (25, 26). Their presence can be documented clinically and radiologically and must always be assessed before attempting any kind of therapy. For this reason, the following section precedes the discussion on therapy.

An *anatomic discontinuity* that impedes the flow of pancreatic juice into the digestive tract is an obvious obstacle to nonsurgical healing of a fistula. Such a condition may typically occur in acute pancreatitis in a case of complete disruption of Wirsung's duct (Fig. 85.1*A*). In a total of 58 external fistulas resulting from severe pancreatitis, we found 11 patients (18.9%) with complete rupture of Wirsung's duct that required surgical correction.

**Limitations.** A limiting factor may be a *correctable outlet obstruction* such as an intraductal stone or stenosis in chronic pancreatitis. Presence of *infection* is an extremely important factor, since infected fistulas generally tend to have lower healing rates and longer healing times than sterile fistulas (11, 27, 28). Fistula contamination can occur from bacterial colonization by the pathogens responsible for infected pancreatic necrosis or abscess (Fig. 85.2). This situation occurs frequently (roughly

**TABLE 85.1. Management of External Pancreatic Fistulas: Limitations and Pitfalls of Conservative Treatment**

| | | |
|---|---|---|
| Limitations | Absolute | • Pancreaticoenteric anatomic discontinuity (Wirsung rupture) |
| | Relative | • Resolvable outlet obstruction<br>• Descending infection<br>• Negative nitrogen balance |
| Pitfalls | | • Ascending infections (superinfections)<br>• False closure |

90% of the infected patients observed in our series) and is generally caused by gram-negative flora of intestinal origin, i.e. the same organisms that most readily colonize necrotizing pancreatitis (15–19, 29). A descending infection must be detected and adequately treated prior to the use of antisecretory therapy.

Lastly, a *negative nitrogen balance* may hinder healing because of a protein and calorie metabolism imbalance (25, 30).

**Pitfalls.** An important factor that can prevent conservative healing is an *ascending infection.* This clinical situation occurs when originally sterile juice is contaminated with pathogens working their way back up the drainage tract (27). This phenomenon is related to three factors: *(a)* long-standing presence of external drainage; *(b)* reduction in output (spontaneous or due to treatment) with a consequent reduced washout of the fistula tract; and *(c)* lavage maneuvers or radiologic investigations on the tract. The role of skin flora in such infections is clearly demonstrated by the fact that, in our patients, *Staphylococcus* was isolated in only 25% of descending infections (it was never the sole isolate in these cases), compared with 75% in ascending infections (it was the only infecting pathogen in 80% of cases).

The last problem to be considered is related to what we have defined as *false closure* (26, 27). In 15% of the patients we treated with antisecretory drugs, we witnessed a rapid reduction in fistula output culminating in total closure of the fistula, accompanied by the onset of fever and abdominal pain within 12–24 hours. The condition resolves by reopening the fistula tract, either spontaneously or by a simple surgical maneuver. It is always due to a deep-lying collection of pancreatic juice. If the fluid is sterile, failure to absorb it will result in the formation of a pseudocyst within 4 weeks; an abscess will develop if the collection is colonized. The mechanism of false closure may be drug-induced inhibition of pancreatic secretion that allows skin epithelialization in the presence of infected juice. These considerations suggest that antisecretory agents should be used only after sterilization of the PF.

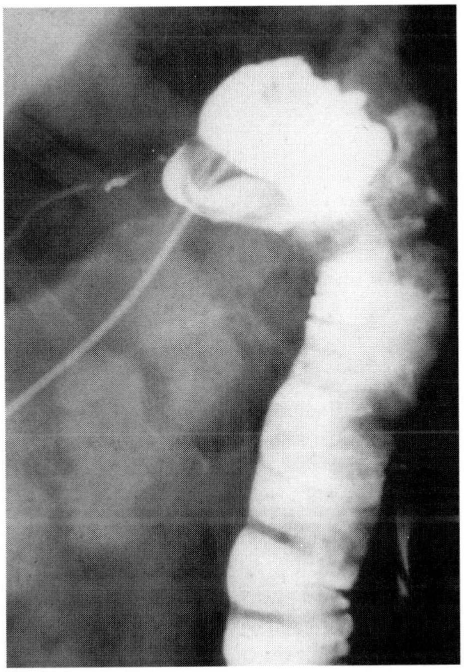

**FIG. 85.2.** Fistulography performed with a drain positioned inside an abscess (infected pseudocyst) of the tail of the pancreas. The contrast medium displays the cystic cavity and, on the left, the main pancreatic duct. The lesions communicate not only with Wirsung's duct but also with the descending colon. Not surprisingly, the pancreatic juice was infected (a descending infection, a relative impediment to conservative management).

## MEDICAL TREATMENT

External PF treatment can be divided into *supportive and specific* treatment.

### Supportive Treatment

Supportive measures allow better clinical management for both the patient and the health care personnel but do not in themselves lead to a reduction in daily fistula output. Though not curative, supportive measures are useful treatments.

*Adequate management of the drains* is a fundamental step to prevent the formation of cavities in which the pancreatic fluid may stagnate and become activated and/or infected. The drain tube should be soft, atraumatic, and easily replaceable. The external orifice of the fistula tends to be irritated and eroded by the local action of activated proteases. *Cutaneous protection* can usually be achieved by use of a sterile bag with adhesive patches.

*Electrolyte imbalance* and *protein-calorie* deficits must be corrected. Since it is difficult to distinguish supportive from specific treatment in this instance, these aspects are discussed below.

Once infection has been documented, specific *antibiotic treatment* is implemented on the basis of antibiotic sensitivity assay. Local administration can be used. In general, the antibiotic is diluted in 50–200 mL of normal saline solution and instilled twice daily into the fistula tract, leaving the drain tube closed for 15–20 min.We advise using the systemic route only when there are signs of sepsis or when there are other concomitant foci of infection.

### Specific Treatment

Specific treatment comprises measures aimed at reducing the fistula output and ultimately achieving complete healing and definitive closure. *Mechanical occlusion of the tract,* which had long been abandoned, has recently been reproposed using fibrin sealant in combination with protease inhibitors (31). To achieve successful results, the procedure must be applied to single tracts that are well consolidated and sterile. Physiologic transduodenal drainage of the pancreatic duct must be present to use mechanical occlusion. The reports in the literature focus mainly on cases resulting from distal surgical resections. This procedure should be used in chronic fistulas that fail to respond to other conservative measures. The application should be neither too early nor too late, when it will not be effective.

*Pancreatic rest* and *inhibition of exocrine secretion* are a sine qua non for achieving fistula closure (12). Numerous pharmacologic agents and regimens have been suggested for this purpose, some of which are now merely of historic interest, while others are still used. The latter comprise parenteral or enteral nutrition (30) and the use of somatostatin compounds. The basic difference between the two is that parenteral nutrition and, to a lesser extent, enteral nutrition are mild inhibitors of pancreatic secretion but excellent calorie-protein reintegrators, while the somatostatin compounds are potent inhibitors of secretion but act only indirectly on the calorie and protein imbalance by reducing the losses. The complementary nature of their actions allows their use in combination (28).

In high-output PFs, *suspension of oral feeding* is mandatory. As a result, alternative forms of nutrition must be used. There are two possibilities: *enteral* and *parenteral nutrition* (30). As regards the former, infusion of elemental formulations into the jejunum evokes a 50–80% pancreatic exocrine response, compared with a standard meal (32). However, these elemental products do not reduce secretion when used in amounts needed to maintain the patient's body weight. The literature does not provide clear data on the specific effects of the various lipid or amino acid compounds used at different gastrointestinal levels (30). Nevertheless, enteral nutrition reduces fistula secretion, acting in particular on the water and bicarbonate components (33). Enteral nutrition has had only limited success is achieving fistula closure.

As far as *parenteral nutrition* is concerned, the available data lead us to conclude that intravenous infusion of glucose (25%) inhibits exocrine secretion (34), infusion of fats stimulates an increase, and amino acids do not produce an inhibitory or a stimulatory effect (35).

Ever since the earliest work by Dudrick et al. (36), *total parenteral nutrition* (TPN) has had an important place among the therapeutic measures adopted for closure of external PFs, and it still remains one of the mainstays of therapy. Its formulation does not require any particular attention except that it needs to be tailored to the individual patient, and some care must be devoted to the lipid component. Fat emulsions, though potentially stimulating exocrine secretion, can be an irreplaceable source of nonprotein calories.

Closure of the fistula tract is obtained in approximately 60% of untreated patients after 2–3 months; this figure rises to approximately 80% in mean periods of 3–4 weeks in patients receiving TPN. The incidence of complications in TPN-treated patients is reduced to half that of controls (from 50 to 25%) (30). TPN management has generally required hospitalization, but care of the central intravenous catheter is now often accomplished in the outpatient setting.

The progressive decline in the use of various drugs that inhibit pancreatic secretion, such as acetazolamide (37), α- and ß-adrenergic agonists (38), atropine (39), calcitonin (40), glucagon (41) and high-dose pancreatic extracts (42), is due to the advent of the *somatostatin compounds* (38). Somatostatin is a tetradecapeptide that has both a paracrine and a direct action on the intestinal mucosa. Its activity is biologically mediated by the presence of specific receptors. It is a powerful inhibitor of exocrine secretion; it can decrease the output of enzymes, bicarbonate, and overall volume after stimulation with secretin and cholecystokinin (CCK) (43). In 1982, this theoretical option was confirmed by two clinical trials in which Di Costanzo et al. (44) and Hild et al. (45) simultaneously reported successful treatment of PFs by combining the hormone with TPN.

In our experience (28) of 45 patients with pure high-output external PFs, 18 were treated with TPN alone, 12 with TPN plus glucagon, 7 with TPN plus calcitonin, and 8 with TPN plus naturally occurring somatostatin at the dose of 250 μg/hr intravenously by continuous infusion. Healing rates were similar between groups, but the TPN plus somatostatin combination was the quickest (6 days vs. 12, 61, and 62, respectively), with a consequent reduction in hospitalization and a saving estimated at the time (1986) to be $2100 per patient.

The short half-life of the naturally occurring hormone means that it has to be administered by continuous intravenous infusion. The introduction of a long-acting synthetic analogue immediately aroused the interest of clinicians. This octapeptide has a half-life of 120 minutes when administered subcutaneously and exerts an action in man comparable to that of the native hormone (46).

In our series of patients treated with octreotide, using a dosage of 0.1 mg three times a day, we found a mean reduction of fistula output of more than 50% as early as treatment day 1, when the drug was used in conjunction with TPN, and healing occurred in more than 80% of patients (25, 38). These data are comparable to figures reported in other studies (47, 48).

Because it can be administered subcutaneously, some investigators have used the drug in outpatients (49–51). We found this approach (0.1 mg, t.i.d.) useful in our experience with 6 patients. So far we have confined such use of home treatment to low-output fistulas.

### Preventive Treatment

In three controlled clinical trials (23, 52, 53), the use of octreotide (0.1 mg t.i.d.) starting at least 1 hour before surgery significantly reduced the incidence of postoperative external PFs in patients undergoing elective pancreatic surgery. Table 85.2 reports our experience in a double-blind, controlled, clinical trial conducted in 252 patients (52). Table 85.3 attempts to summarize current policy for the treatment and prophylaxis of external PFs.

## INTERNAL PANCREATIC FISTULAS

Internal fistulas due to *acute pancreatitis* are a rare occurrence, though they are presumably underdiagnosed (9, 10). Cole (9), in 1992, reviewed the literature on this type of fistula and reported only 31 cases in all. A constant feature is the presence of a pancreatic abscess or infected pancreatic necrosis. The infected juice is activated, and proteolysis of the intestinal structures may account for the fistulization. Cofactors may be the presence of drains with pressure erosions (15, 17) and intestinal ischemia associated with severe pancreatitis. In clinically evident cases, the fistulization is generally associated with a pseudocyst or an abscess.

The presence of a certain amount of fluid in the peritoneal cavity is a frequent event in severe pancreatitis and may be attributed to an inflammatory exudation from the retroperitoneum (15, 17). In a true internal fistula, the activated juice that is present will hinder spontaneous closure and primary and/or subsequent superinfection (10). We have avoided defining these situations of what might be termed "pancreatic peritonitis" as "pancreatic ascites" (1), inasmuch as the latter has to be classified nosologically in the context of chronic pancreatitis (1).

From the point of view of the radiologic diagnosis, US and CT are the first-choice imaging modalities. Radiography of the GI tract and ERCP to display the bile duct and/or pancreatic ducts are performed, depending on the individual case.

It is very difficult to estimate the role of pancreatic rest and inhibition of exocrine secretion in the treatment of internal PFs in acute pancreatitis. In the far more common, clinically less

**TABLE 85.2. External Pancreatic Fistulas Observed in 252 Patients after Pancreatic Surgery**

| | High Risk[a] (%) | Low Risk[b] (%) | Total (%) |
|---|---|---|---|
| Placebo | 20 (69) | 4 (66.7) | 24 (18.5)[c] |
| Octreotide | 9 (31) | 2 (33.3) | 11 (9)[c] |
| Total | 29 (17.9) | 6 (6.7) | 35 (13.9) |

[a] Patients with "soft" pancreas.
[b] Patients with "fibrotic" pancreas.
[c] $P = .03$.

**TABLE 85.3. Conservative Treatment of Pancreatic Fistulas**

| | High output ≥700 mL/day | Medium output >150<700 mL/day | Low output ≤150 mL/day |
|---|---|---|---|
| Prophylaxis | Only in pancreatic surgery: octreotide 100 μg t.i.d. for 1 week perioperatively, starting at least 1 hr prior to surgery | | |
| Specific | | | |
| Mechanical occlusion | ? | ? | ? |
| Nothing by mouth | yes | ? | no |
| TPN | yes | ? | no |
| Somatostatin | yes (naturally occurring or octreotide) | yes (octreotide) | yes (octreotide) |
| Support | | | |
| Adequate drainage | yes | yes | yes |
| Cutaneous protection | yes | yes | yes |
| TPN | yes | ? | no |
| Antibiotics[a] | yes | yes | yes |
| Others[b] | ? | ? | ? |
| Pancreatic extracts | ? | ? | ? |

[a]When pancreatic juice infection is present.
[b]Sphincterotomy plus removal of obstacles, use of endoscopic stents, and sphincter-relaxing drugs.

aggressive situations, medical therapy may promote the resolution of peripancreatic collections that are an expression of internal fistulization phenomena. The more severe forms require surgical treatment, which is necessary because of the concomitant presence of complications such as infected necrosis or abscesses (17, 18).

In contrast to the rarity of internal fistulas in the course of acute pancreatitis, cases associated with *chronic pancreatitis* are being increasingly reported in the literature (2, 9). The most common are *pancreatic ascites* (1) and *pancreatic hydrothorax* (2). The pathogenesis of these pancreatic-mesothelial fistulas is attributable to rupture of the pancreatic duct or of a pseudocyst, with consequent leakage of juice into the abdominal or thoracic cavity (1–4, 9). This theory is supported by findings both by intraoperative pancreatograms and by ERCP, as demonstrated in Figure 85.3. Ascites presumably results from a rupture in the area of the anterior wall of the gland, whereas a posterior leakage should lead to thoracic involvement, by tracking up the loose

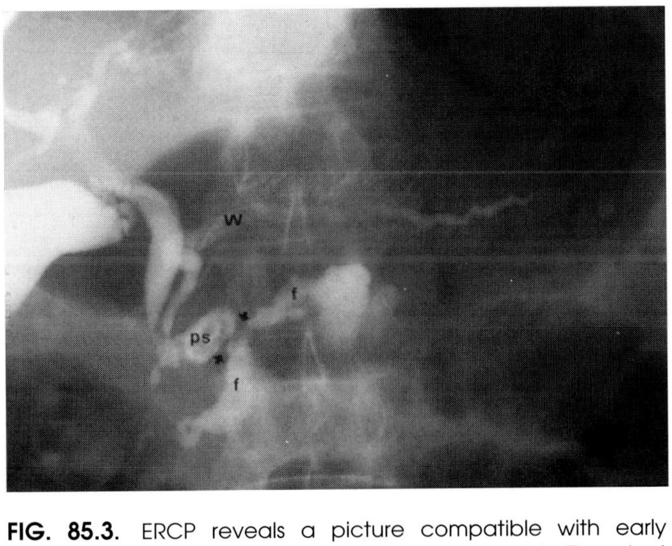


**FIG. 85.3.** ERCP reveals a picture compatible with early chronic pancreatitis in the duct of Wirsung *(w)*. The duct communicates with a pseudocyst *(ps) (arrows)* that leaks *(f)* into the peritoneal cavity, with ensuing ascites.

retroperitoneal tissue and reaching the esophageal and/or aortic hiatus (9). From the mediastinum (2), the leakage can thus reach the pleural space (4) as well as the bronchi (3) and pericardium (4). In view of the amount of fluid present in ascites, the liquid component is unlikely to be solely of pancreatic origin; it seems probable, then, that, in addition to the transudate component, there is also an exudate component originating from a mild peritoneal reactivity. Generally, however, patients complain neither of spontaneous pain nor of tenderness from palpation, because the juice is not activated. This indolent presentation explains the diagnostic difficulty encountered clinically.

In approximately 80% of cases, patients report a history of alcohol abuse and/or chronic pancreatitis (trauma is the most common factor in pediatric cases) with recent onset of progressive abdominal distension, weight loss, malnutrition, diarrhea, and low-grade fever (9). The differential diagnosis also includes cirrhosis, peritoneal carcinomatosis, tuberculous peritonitis, constrictive pericarditis, and Budd-Chiari syndrome.

Thoracic involvement manifests with dyspnea, chest pain, and cough, which, generally speaking, are hardly ever attributed to the underlying pancreatic disease. Clinical suspicion is the first element in reaching the correct diagnosis, which is then confirmed by physicochemical analyses of the fluid. In contrast to cirrhotic ascites, pancreatic ascites has an amylase concentration of the order of several thousand units and an albumin level of about 3 g/dL. The cytologic examination of aspirated fluid must be carefully done, as false-positive cases have been reported. This is probably related to metaplasia of the serosal cells, induced by contact with pancreatic enzymes (9).

The ideal treatment of internal FP in chronic pancreatitis is still a controversial issue. Paracentesis and thoracentesis have only a transient beneficial effect on the symptoms, whereas an adequate supply of calories and protein instituted with enteral or total parenteral nutrition appears to be necessary to improve the patient's general condition, which, as a rule, is substantially compromised.

As with external fistulas, suppression of pancreatic secretion is also a rational goal in internal PFs. A recent review of the experience with octreotide showed healing of 7 of 11 patients treated. In 3 of the 7 healed patients, the drug was used in conjunction with external drainage of the collections (54). Comparable results have been reported with the naturally occurring hormone (55, 56). Based on data reported to date, the role of somatostatin appears to be clearly definable in terms of supportive treatment, whereas further controlled trials are needed to determine the actual value of specific therapy. Though defined empirically, the time limit for evaluating the efficacy of conservative treatment is conventionally set at 3 weeks (9), after which an invasive procedure is advisable, though the period may be shorter if the patient's condition deteriorates.

The surgical strategy first requires identification of the point where the leakage occurs, which usually cannot be visualized directly. In this sense, preoperative ERCP and/or intraoperative contrast injection into the pseudocyst or pancreatic duct may delineate the lesion, thereby serving as a guide for choosing among the technical options available.

Surgical treatment focuses on decompression of the pancreatic ductal system by use of pancreatico-, cysto-, or pancreaticocystojejunostomy with a Roux loop. In the case of pseudocysts of the tail, resection is a good alternative, carrying an acceptable level of risk provided the resection is combined with construction of an anastomosis between jejunum and the residual portion of the pancreas, which in chronic pancreatitis may often have impeded outflow. External drainage of the pseudocyst is not recommended because it is almost certain to produce an external PF. In some cases, however, this option is mandatory, owing to the patient's precarious condition or to the unexpected intraoperative finding of a pseudocyst wall that is not yet mature. The resulting external PF should therefore be treated according to the guidelines outlined previously.

A review of the surgical experience reveals mortality rates ranging from 0 to 14%, with a 12% recurrence rate (23% in patients with medical therapy alone). The choice of surgical or conservative therapy hinges on accurate delineation of the lesion. The right choice of therapy will result in the lowest morbidity and mortality rates (9, 57).

## SURGICAL TREATMENT OF EXTERNAL PANCREATIC FISTULAS

The aim of surgical therapy is to redirect the exocrine pancreatic secretion into the intestinal tract (13, 21, 57). Surgery is indicated in a minority of patients (12.5% in our series). Since pancreatic cachexia resulting from malnutrition caused by major fistulas can be avoided today both by nutritional support and by pharmacologic antisecretory agents, the decision should not be made in haste, as the clinical situation is readily controllable (11, 21).

Before subjecting the patient to surgery, the fistula must be staged, controlled medically, and adequately visualized. The following factors must be identified: *(a)* the nature of the fistula—simple, complex; direct, mediated; communicating/not communicating with Wirsung's duct; *(b)* the point of origin of the fistula, the possible presence of ductal abnormalities and endoscopically treatable obstacles; and *(c)* the adequacy of the drainage. The indications for surgical treatment are summarized in Table 85.4. If there are no contraindications to medical treatment, the individual patient must be carefully assessed, and the choice and type of surgery weighed against the intrinsic possibility of spontaneous healing.

A patient with an external fistula after drainage of a pseudocyst may, for example, be operated on within a short time, once evidence of ductal obstruction not amenable to endoscopic treatment has been found. On the other hand, fistulas resulting from severe necrotic pancreatitis may require much longer waiting periods (at least 6 months from the acute attack) to achieve complete healing of the underlying disease.

Another important factor for the timing of surgery is the simple or complex nature of the fistula (21). While simple fistulas tend not to present problems, complex fistulas are particularly dangerous, because they harbor activated enzymes and are contaminated with microorganisms, which can lead to hemorrhage and sepsis. This situation is typical of pancreatitis involving the residual gland after major resections. If the area is not fully drained, immediate reoperation is mandatory to complete the pancreatectomy and ensure full drainage (8, 58).

**TABLE 85.4. External Pancreatic Fistulas: Surgical Indications**

1. Wirsung rupture with discontinuity between the portion where the fistula arises and the rest of the ductal system (after endoscopic stent failure?)
2. Obstruction of normal pancreaticoduodenal flow not amenable to endoscopic treatment
3. Persistence of the fistula beyond 6 months
4. Recurrent infection caused by an abscess cavity
5. Hemorrhage
6. Pancreatic cachexia

Another situation with a complex external fistula that carries a high mortality rate (60%) is concomitant perforation of a pancreatic abscess in the stomach (59), duodenum (60), or, particularly, the colon (59, 61). In these cases, delay in choosing the surgical option is not advisable, since it is necessary to treat the abscess in conjunction, with a jejunostomy, ileostomy, or colostomy if need be (5, 15, 17).

The surgical options available are *(a)* major pancreatic resections with ligation and/or excision of the fistula tract, *(b)* pancreaticojejunostomy after excision of the fistula tract, and *(c)* ductojejunostomy. The resection approach is reasonable when the fistula tract is in the body or tail. Splenopancreatectomy without jejunal anastomosis, in the experience of Warshaw's group, is indicated in 75% of cases and curative in 90% of fistulas. Recurrences closed spontaneously (21).

When the fistula arises from the head of the pancreas, resection, if performed from left to right, would involve either sacrificing a substantial amount of parenchyma or the high morbidity and mortality risks usually associated with duodenopancreatectomy (23, 24, 58). We believe that such procedures are rarely justified in benign disease and that an anastomosis to a Roux limb of jejunum should be performed in most patients. Pancreatic exocrine secretions can be drained with a Roux-en-Y jejunal onlay directly on the pancreas or on the duct (ductojejunostomy). The first of these options is the more popular of the two (21), because the extensive fibrosis and scar tissue surrounding the fistula tract provides a secure anastomosis. Ductojejunostomy has been abandoned by many surgeons because of the ease of perforating the fistula tract during the difficult dissection. The tract has very poor vascularization. Use of this procedure allows an anastomosis distant from the pancreas, thus avoiding an often long and laborious dissection.

Current medical therapy now controls most clinical situations, so operative intervention can be delayed at least 3–6 months from the date of onset of the fistulas. This permits development and maturation of the fibrous tissue composing the fistula tract around the drain (Fig. 85.1*B*).

For these reasons, we adopted this approach in the last 12 consecutive patients requiring surgical therapy and achieved complete, definitive healing in 11 of them. One additional patient was definitively healed with medical therapy after recurrence 1 month postoperatively.

In conclusion, our surgical preference for both internal and external PFs is for resection only if the origin of the fistula is in the tail. In other situations, one must consider the performing the easiest and safest procedure that will be curative. As a possible alternative to surgery, the use of endoscopic stents has been reported to give promising results, though so far in only a limited number of patients (62).

## REFERENCES


1. Cameron JL, Anderson RP, Zuidema GD. Pancreatic ascites. Surg Gynecol Obstet 1967;125:328–332.
2. Iacono C, Procacci C, Frigo F, Bergami IA, Cesaro G, et al. Thoracic complications of pancreatitis. Pancreas 1988;2:228–236.
3. Govin PR, McMahon SM. Transient expectoration of pancreatic fluids in a patient with pancreaticopleural fistulas. Crit Care Med 1989;17:293–296.
4. Pottmeyer EW, Frey CT, Matsuno S. Pancreaticoploeural fistulas. Arch Surg 1987;122:648–701.
5. Grodinsky C, Ponka JL. The spectrum of colonic involvement in pancreatitis. Dis Colon Rectum 1978;21:66–70.
6. Willis SM, Brewer TG. Pancreatic duct-portal vein fistula. Gastroenterology 1989;97:1025–1027.
7. Miller BM, Traverso LW, Freeny PC. Intrapancreatic communication of bile and pancreatic ducts secondary to pancreatic necrosis. Arch Surg 1988;123:1000–1002.
8. Frey CF. Pancreatic fistulas and tumor of the pancreas. In: Pederzoli P, Bassi C, Vesentini S, eds. Pancreatic fistulas. Heidelberg: Springer-Verlag, 1992:75–90.
9. Cole DJ, Bradley EL III. Internal pancreatic fistulas: classifications, recognition and management. In: Pederzoli P, Bassi C, Vesentini S, eds. Pancreatic fistulas. Heidelberg: Springer-Verlag, 1992: 107–120.
10. Sunderland GT, Imrie CW. Pancreatic fistulas in acute pancreatitis. In: Pederzoli P, Bassi C, Vesentini S, eds. Pancreatic fistulas. Heidelberg: Springer-Verlag, 1992:61–69.
11. Zinner MJ, Beker RR, Cameron JL. Pancreatic cutaneous fistulas. Surg Gynecol Obstet 1974;138:710–712.
12. Pederzoli P, Bassi C. Vesentini S. Pancreatic fistulas. Heidelberg: Springer-Verlag, 1992.
13. Lahey FH, Lium R. Cure of pancreatic fistula by pancreatojejunostomy. Report of a case with review of the literature. Surg Gynecol Obstet 1937;64:78–81.
14. Judd ES, Mattson H, Mahorner HR. Pancreatic cystis: report of 47 cases. Arch Surg 1931;22:838–841.
15. Pederzoli P, Bassi C, Vesentini S, Girelli R, Cavallini G, et al. Retroperitoneal and peritoneal drainage and lavage in the treatment of severe necrotizing pancreatitis. Surg Gynecol Obstet 1990;170:197–203.
16. Bassi C, Vesentini S, Nifosi F, Girelli R, Falconi M, et al. Pancreatic abscess and other pus harboring collections related to pancreatitis: a review of 108 cases. World J Surg 1990;14: 505–512.
17. Pederzoli P, Bassi C, Vesentini S, Iacono C, Nicoli N, et al. Necrosectomy by lavage in the surgical treatment of severe necrotizing pancreatitis. Acta Chir Scand 1990;156:775–780.
18. Beger HG. Surgery in acute pancreatitis. Hepatogastroenterology 1991;38:92–96.
19. Bradley EL III. Management of infected pancreatic necrosis by open drainage. Ann Surg 1987;206:484–487.
20. Pistolesi GF, Procacci C, Residori E, Bicego E, Bertocco M, et al. Radiologic imaging of pancreatic fistulas. In: Pederzoli P, Bassi C, Vesentini S, eds. Pancreatic fistulas. Heidelberg: Springer-Verlag, 1992:10–38.
21. Schmidt J, Rattner DW, Worshaw AL. Surgical treatment of pancreatic fistulas: rationale timing and techniques. In: Pederzoli P, Bassi C, Vesentini S, eds. Pancreatic fistulas. Heidelberg: Springer-Verlag, 1992:176–194.
22. Kellum JM, Holland GF, McNeil P. Traumatic pancreatic cutaneous fistulas: comparison of enteral and parenteral feedings. J Trauma 1988;28:700–704.
23. Büchler M, Friess H, Klempa I, Hermane KP, Sulkowsky U, et al. Role of octreotide in the prevention of postoperative complications following pancreatic resection. Am J Surg 1992;163: 125–131.
24. Bassi C, Falconi M, Lombardi D, Briani G, Vesentini S, et al. Prophylaxis of complications after pancreatic surgery: results of a multicenter trial in Italy. Digestion 1994;55:41–47.
25. Nifosì F, Falconi M, Montresor E, Vesentini S. Limitations of conservative therapy of pancreatic fistulas. In: Pederzoli P, Bassi C, Vesentini S, eds. Pancreatic fistulas. Heidelberg: Springer-Verlag, 1992:155–161.
26. Falconi M, Nifosì F, Lombardi D, Bassi C, Girelli R. Pitfalls in medical treatment. In: Pederzoli P, Bassi C, Vesentini S, eds. Pancreatic fistulas. Heidelberg: Springer-Verlag, 1992:162–166.
27. Bassi C. Microbiological aspects of pancreatic fistulas. In: Pederzoli P, Bassi C, Vesentini S, eds. Pancreatic fistulas. Heidelberg: Springer-Verlag, 1992:121–128.
28. Pederzoli P, Bassi C, Falconi M, Albrigo R, Vantini I, Micciolo R. Conservative treatment of external pancreatic fistulas with parenteral nutrition alone or in combination with continuous intravenous infusion of somatostatin, glucagon or calcitonin. Surg Gynecol Obstet 186;163:428–432.
29. D'Egidio A, Schein M. Surgical strategies in the treatment of pancreatic necrosis and infection. Br J Surg 1991;78:133–137.
30. Vantini I, Scattolini C, Fioretta A. Artificial nutrition in pancreatic fistulas. In: Pederzoli P, Bassi C, Vesentini S, eds. Pancreatic fistulas. Heidelberg: Springer-Verlag, 1992:140–145.
31. Costantino V, Petrin P, Pasquali C, Liessi G, Pedrazzoli S. Use of fibrin sealant in the treatment of pancreatic fistulas. In: Pederzoli P, Bassi C, Vesentini S, eds. Pancreatic fistulas. Heidelberg: Springer-Verlag, 1992:201–210.
32. Vidon N, Hecketswiller P, Butel J. Effect of continuous jejunal perfusion of elemental and complex nutritional solutions on pancreatic enzyme secretion in human subjects. Gut 1978;19: 194–198.
33. Grant JP, Davery-McCrae J, Snyder PJ. Effect of enteral nutrition on human pancreatic secretion. JPEN 187;11:302–304.
34. Zajtchuk R, Amato JC, Shoemaker WC, Baker RJ. The relationship between blood glucose levels and external pancreatic secretion in man. J Trauma 1969;9:629–637.
35. Klein E, Shnebaum S, Ben-Ari A. Effect of total parenteral nutrition on exocrine pancreatic secretion. Am J Gastroenterol 1983;78: 31–36.
36. Dudrick SJ, Wilmore DW, Steiger E, Mackie JA, Fits WT. Spontaneous closure of traumatic pancreaticoduodenal fistulas with total intravenous nutrition. J Trauma 1970;10:542–553.
37. Papastrat LS, Miler JM. Treatment of external pancreatic fistula with Diamox. Am J Dig Dis 1958;3:339–407.
38. Pederzoli P, Falconi M, Bassi C, Benetti L, Briani G. Drugs inhibiting exocrine pancreatic secretion. In: Pederzoli P, Bassi C, Vesentini S, eds. Pancreatic fistulas. Heidelberg: Springer-Verlag, 1992: 146–154.
39. Buzkurt T, Adler G, Koop I, Arnold R. Effect of atropine on intestinal phase of pancreatic secretion in man. Digestion 1988;41: 108–115.
40. Luisetto G, Pilon T, Pederzoli P, Ziliotto D. Treatment of acute edematous pancreatitis and pancreatic fistulas with salmon calcitonin. In Pecile A, ed. Calcitonin 1980 chemistry, physiology, pharmacology and clinical aspect. Proc Int Symp Excerpta Medica, Amsterdam, 1980:336–345.
41. Knight MJ, Condon JR, Smith R. Possible use of glucagon in the treatment of pancreatitis. Br Med J 197;2:440.
42. Garcia-Puges AM, Navarro S, Fernandez-Cruz L, Ros E, Honojosa L, Pera C. Oral pancreatic enzymes accelerate closure of external pancreatic fistulae. Br J Surg 1988;75:924–925.
43. Gullo L, Priori P, Scarpignato C, Baldoni F, Mattioli G, Barbara L. Effect of somatostatin 14 on pure human pancreatic secretion. Dig Dis Sci 1987;32:1065–1070.
44. DiCostanzo J, Cano N, Martin J. Somatostatin in persistent gastrointestinal fistula treated by total parenteral nutrition. Lancet 1982;7:338–339.
45. Hild P, Stoyanov M, Dobroschke J, Aigner K. La somatostatine dans le traitment medical des fistulas du pancreas et de l'intestin grele. Ann Chir 1982;36:193–196.
46. Konturek SJ. Somatostatin and the gastrointestinal secretions. Scand J Gastroenterol 1976;11:1–4.
47. Landsen FT, Adams DB, Anderson MC. Treatment of external pancreatic fistulas with somatostatin. Am Surg 1989;55:695–698.
48. Williams St, Woltering EQ, D'Orisio TM, Fletcher WS. Effect of octreotide acetate on pancreatic exocrine function. Am J Surg 1989;157:459–462.
49. Prinz RA, Pickleman J, Hoffman MD. Treatment of pancreatic cutaneous fistulas with a somatostatin analog. Am J Surg 1987;155:36–42.
50. Prinz RA. Treatment of pancreatic fistulas in outpatients. In: Pederzoli P, Bassi C, Vesentini S, eds. Pancreatic fistulas. Heidelberg: Springer-Verlag, 1992:195–200.

51. Barnes SM, Konty BG, Prinz RA. Somatostatin analog treatment of pancreatic fistulas. Int J Pancreatol 1993;14:181–188.
52. Pererzoli P, Bassi C, Falconi M, Camboni M. Efficacy of octreotide in the prevention of complication of elective pancreatic surgery. Br J Surg 1994;81:265–269.
53. Friess M, Beger HB, Sulkowski U, Becker H, Hofbauer B, et al. Randomized controlled multicentre study of the prevention of complications by octreotide in patients undergoing surgery for chronic pancreatitis. Br J Surg 1995;82:1270–1273.
54. Bassi C, Falconi M, DeSantis L, Caldiron E, Sartori N, Pederzoli P. Role of somatostatin and its analogues in gastrointestinal fistulas, ascites and pancreatic pseudocysts. Dig Surg 1994;11: 451–455.
55. Gilason H, Gronbech JE, Soreide O. Pancreatic ascites: treatment by continuous somatostatin infusion. Am J Gastroenterol 1991; 86:519–521.
56. Pezzilli R, Gullo L, DiStefano M, et al. Treatment of pancreatic ascites with somatostatin. Pancreas 1993;8:120–122.
57. Ihse I, Larsson J, Lindström E. Surgical management of pure pancreatic fistulas. Hepatogastroenterology 1994;41:271–275.
58. Bartoli FG, Arnone GB, Ravera G, Bachi V. Pancreatic fistula and relative mortality in malignant diseases after pancreaticoduodenectomy. Review and statistical meta-analysis regarding 15 years of literature. Anticancer Res 1991;11:1831–1848.
59. Warshaw AL, Mancure AC, Rattner DW. Gastrocutaneous fistulas associated with pancreatic abscess: an aggressive entity. Ann Surg 1989;210:603–606.
60. Doberneck RC. Intestinal fistula complicating necrotizing pancreatitis. Am J Surg 1989;158;581–583.
61. Warshaw AL, Jin G. Treatment of the complications of acute pancreatitis. In: Moody FG, Carey LC, Jones RS, Kelly KA, Nahrwold DL, Skinner DB, eds. Surgical treatment of digestive disease. 1st ed. Chicago: Year Book Medical Publishers, 1986:476–491.
62. Saeed ZA, Ramirez FC, Hepps KS. Endoscopic stent placement for internal and external pancreatic fistulas. Gastroenterology 1993; 105:1213–1217.

# 86

# *Pancreas and Islet Cell Transplantation*

Lawrence P. McChesney, Xavier Martin, and J. M. Dubernard

## PANCREAS TRANSPLANTATION

Diabetes mellitus is a major health problem in all developed countries. In France, a study performed in 1985 revealed the prevalence to be 1 per 200,000 population, with an incidence of 50 new cases of diabetes per million inhabitants per year (1). Similar data from the United States in 1995 reveals a diabetes population of 16 million, with an incidence of 625,000 new cases per year (2). Diabetes can be broken down pathophysiologically into two distinct entities. Type I diabetes mellitus typically occurs during childhood, thus the term juvenile onset diabetes. Though the etiology is yet undetermined, there is a selective immune destruction of the insulin-producing beta cells of the pancreas (3, 4). This results in an insulinopenic state, as can be documented by negligible plasma levels of insulin (5). Type II diabetes mellitus, or adult onset diabetes, accounts for approximately 90% of individuals diagnosed with diabetes and is commonly seen after the fourth decade of life (2). Insulin production in type II is still intact, and plasma levels of insulin are often elevated. The pathophysiologic mechanism in this disease process seems to be the development of insulin resistance (5). Despite the measured elevated insulin levels, individuals with type II diabetes frequently require exogenous insulin to achieve blood glucose control. Therefore, the terminology of insulin-dependent versus non-insulin-dependent does not correlate with the exact pathophysiology of that specific patient's diabetes.

Diabetes is well known because of its secondary complications. Historically these secondary complications were not seen prior to the use of exogenous insulin (6). Individuals with type I diabetes did not survive long enough to develop them. One can view the secondary complications of diabetes as a result of medical treatment of this disease. The goal of most medical therapies for diabetes is to achieve and sustain normoglycemia. Some studies, such as the Diabetes Control and Complications Trial Research Group (DCCT), have shown that prolonged maintenance of near normal blood sugar levels decreases the development of these secondary complications (7). Multiple methods of providing exogenous insulin, such as frequent injections with associated glucose monitoring and use of pumps for continuous infusion have been tried, but none of these techniques have completely aborted the development of degenerative complications.

## INDICATIONS FOR PANCREAS TRANSPLANTATION

### Overview of Indications

When insulin deficiency was identified as the pathophysiologic defect in diabetes, replacing the defective pancreas became a possible treatment for diabetes. The first clinical pancreas transplant for diabetes was performed by Kelly, Lillehei, and Merkel on December 17, 1966. The procedure, performed on a 28-year-old female, combined a segmental pancreas transplant placed in a retroperitoneal iliac position after duct ligation and a concomitant contralateral renal transplant (8, 9). The patient achieved near normal glycemia for a period of days in the absence of exogenous insulin. However, perigraft collections developed, with eventual loss of the graft secondary to rejection. Nevertheless, realization of the concept was achieved despite initial clinical failure.

Currently, pancreas transplantation is indicated only in individuals with at least one major complication of type I diabetes. The International Registry of Pancreas Transplantation reports that 87% of pancreas transplants performed since 1987 were in combination with a kidney transplant (10). Simultaneous pancreas-kidney transplantation (SPK) is performed in individuals with type I diabetes complicated by end-stage renal disease (ESRD). The remaining pancreas transplants were performed as isolated grafts, either after a previously successful kidney transplantation (PAK) (7%) or prior to the onset of ESRD in patients who failed appropriate medical management and thus received a pancreas transplant alone (PTA) (5%) (10, 11).

The overall demographics of patients undergoing pancreas transplantation in the authors respective programs are as follows: patients in Lyon, France, have a mean age of 38 years, duration of diabetes of 25 years, presence of retinopathy in 28%, advanced neuropathy of the lower limbs in 74%, and clinical coronary artery disease in 20%. The Rush program's recipients have a mean age of 34 years, duration of diabetes of 23 years, presence of retinopathy in 80%, advanced neuropathy in 91%, and clinical coronary artery disease in 4%.

### Simultaneous Pancreas Kidney Transplantation (SPK)

Despite the accumulated supporting evidence, an ongoing debate exists regarding the benefits of pancreas transplantation in reversing or halting the secondary complications of diabetes as weighed against the increased risks associated with lifelong immunosuppression. The presence of ESRD in patients with type I diabetes negates this debate. Renal transplantation for ESRD improves quality of life and has an economic advantage over prolonged dialysis (12). For those who choose organ transplantation, lifelong immunosppression is needed, at least for the foreseeable future. However, transplantation of a normal kidney in recipients with unresolved diabetes places this new organ within a persistantly hyperglycemic environment that leads to microangiopathic disease. Simultaneous transplantation of a pancreas restores a euglycemic state that prevents recurrent diabetic nephropathy (13). As a result of newer techniques and better postoperative management, pancreas transplantation does not appear to substantially increase the risks associated with kidney transplantation (14, 15). Survival rates in patients receiving a double graft are not significantly different from those of nondiabetes patients receiving only a kidney graft (16). As is explained below, when simultaneous pancreas-renal transplantation is performed, the kidney allograft frequently serves as a marker for the detection of pancreas rejection and allows superior graft survival rates (17–20).

To achieve the optimal effect of pancreas transplantation, many transplant programs believe that pancreatic-renal transplants should be performed in patients with renal insuffiency, but prior to the institution of dialysis as well as other advanced secondary complications of diabetes. At the center in Lyon, the proportion of dialyzed patients undergoing pancreatic-renal transplantation has dropped from 90% in the late 1980s to 70% presently. However, in the United States, diabetic nephropathy is one of the leading causes of ESRD, accounting for 30–40% of chronic dialysis patients (12). Despite the aggressive application of dialysis, these patients have a substantially decreased survival rate, often noted to be less than 40% at 3 years (21). Transplantation has a life-sparing effect for patients with diabetes already on dialysis. Because of the shortage of usable donor grafts and the number of patients awaiting transplantation, the expansion of predialysis transplantation has been prevented, and many programs feel obligated to transplant the patients on dialysis before nondialysis transplant candidates.

### Pancreas Transplantation after Kidney Transplantation (PAK)

PAK transplantation is applicable in those individuals who did not have access to a program performing pancreas transplantation at the time of their renal transplant or who had previously decided that historic success rates for pancreas transplantation were unsatisfactory. Patients who previously received a living-related/nonrelated renal allograft are also candidates for PAK transplantation. Transplantation of the pancreas after a previous renal transplant is a limited surgical procedure that is performed in a nonuremic patient. Despite this apparent improved candidate, pancreas graft survival in these sequential transplants has been slightly lower than SPK transplant results. The pancreas and renal grafts come from immunologically different donors, and therefore the renal graft cannot be used as a marker for predicting pancreas rejection. Improved graft survival rates are obtained with renal transplant recipients who have the following: *(a)* one or no rejection episodes within the first year, *(b)* a stable immunosuppressive regimen, and *(c)* excellent renal function (22). Some programs have found that using protocol biopsies of the pancreas graft and selecting individuals with good renal function and a stable immunosuppressive regimen has resulted in survival rates between those of the simultaneous pancreas/kidney transplant and those of the isolated pancreas transplant performed prior to renal insufficiency (23).

### Isolated Pancreas Transplantation Alone (PTA)

Another candidate for isolated pancreas transplantation is the nonuremic diabetic patient who has failed aggressive medical management, as documented by secondary diabetes complications. Whether isolated pancreas transplantation for this latter indication does prevent or stabilize the secondary complications of diabetes reliably enough to warrant the present risk of lifelong immunosuppression is debatable. Failure of medical management typically involves complications that are difficult to document objectively, such as frequent unrecognized hypoglycemia, in contrast to more objective data such as deteriorating renal function.

A few centers have substantial experience in performing isolated pancreas transplants in individuals with type I diabetes prior to the onset of ESRD. Ideally, such a transplant could be performed to prevent the ravages of these secondary complications. However, neither the development nor the severity of secondary complications in type I diabetes are predictable in all patients. A reliable method for selecting patients for whom pancreas transplant has a justifiable preventive role has not been found (24–29). The inhibiting factor for PTA is not the operative procedure, but rather the complications of lifelong immunosuppression with its increased incidence of infections, lymphoma, renal impairment, and such. This procedure is currently indicated only in patients with at least one degenerative complication and documented failure of medical management. Sutherland, an advocate for isolated pancreas transplantation in the nonuremic type I diabetes recipient, has shown that the pancreas transplant can reverse and stabilize certain specific secondary complications of diabetes such as neuropathy (30). Despite this preventive effect, enthusiasm for this approach has not increased because of a previously reported 55% 1-year *graft survival* rate. *Patient survival* rates in this same group exceed 90% at 1-year (31).

Newer immunosuppressive agents such as microemulsified cyclosporine A (Neoral), FK506 (Prograf), and mycophenolate mofetil (CellCept) have become available. By combining these agents to obtain more diverse immunosuppression, graft survival rates have significantly improved. The 1-year graft survival rates for technically successful transplants are 77% in PAK transplant and 73% in PTA (31). As graft survival rates improve with decreased complications associated with the newer immunosuppressive agents, then PTA will assume a larger role (32, 33).

## SELECTION AND EVALUATION OF POTENTIAL RECIPIENTS

Pancreas transplantation thus far has only been used in individuals with insulinopenia or type I diabetes but not all patients with this disease will be candidates. Therefore, the differentiation between type I diabetes and type II diabetes is mandatory (Table 86.1). This is easily done by measuring plasma C-peptide levels following adequate stimulation, such as an oral glucose challenge or an injection of glucagon. This stimulated state easily separates the two disease processes (34, 35). Insulin is absent in type I diabetes; therefore, plasma C-peptide levels are negligible. Type II diabetes patients produce insulin, so plasma C-peptide levels are normal or elevated.

Because diabetes produces injury in multiple organ systems, evaluation of the potential pancreas transplant candidate is as inclusive if not more so than any other transplant evaluation (Table 86.2). Baseline data are obtained to evaluate the long-term effects of pancreas transplantation. Because of the variability of secondary complications, the physiologic age of a prospective pancreas transplantation candidate should be used instead of a numerical age restriction. A general evaluation includes a

**TABLE 86.1. Patient Selection Criteria**

1. Documentation of type I diabetes with at least one intractable degenerative complication of diabetes
2. Simultaneous pancreas kidney transplant
   - Presence of end-stage renal disease
   - Prediction of institution of dialysis within 1 year
   - Present renal function <50 mL/min
3. Physiologic age <60 years
4. Absence of irreversible cardiovascular disease
5. Absence of advanced peripheral vascular disease
6. Absence of stroke or unresolved TIA
7. Absence of unresolved malignancy
8. Absence of psychosis
9. Absence of incapacitating neuropathy resulting in a bed-ridden state
10. Absence of incapacitating gastroparesis without reliable enteral access
11. Absence of a history of noncompliance
12. Ability to comprehend consent form

**TABLE 86.2. Pretransplant Evaluation**

1. Laboratory evaluation
   Hemogram, electrolytes, coagulation, liver function, renal function, lipid profile, urinalysis, 24-hr creatinine clearance, and protein, blood group, and screen
2. Immunologic evaluation
   HLA typing, Panel sensitization assay (PRA), CMV IgG, EBV IgG, HIV, hepatitis B virus, hepatitis C virus, RPR, antiislet and antiinsulin antibodies
3. Diabetes exposure
   Glycosylated hemoglobin, stimulated serum C-peptide level
4. Chest x-ray and ultrasound of abdomen (cholelithiasis, etc.)
5. Cardiovascular evaluation
   ECG, thallium Persantine scan, consultation with cardiology, echocardiogram and/or cardiac catheterization, noninvasive vascular studies as indicated
6. Genitourinary evaluation
   Voiding cystourethrogram, cystometrogram as indicated
7. Ophthalmic evaluation including retinograph for comparison
8. Dental evaluation
9. Gynecologic/mammogram evaluation
   Recent PAP smear, if childbearing age: documentation of contraceptive technique, if >50 y/o: recent mammogram
10. Psychologic, social worker, and financial liaison evaluation

search for unsuspected cancers, chronic infections, and other comorbid disease processes. Standard immunologic tests to determine blood group, tissue typing, and presence of antiidiotypic antibodies denoting previous antigen exposure are completed. Serologic markers for hepatitis B and C and human immunodeficiency virus (HIV) and previous exposure to Epstein-Barr virus (EBV) and cytomegalovirus (CMV) are evaluated.

Individuals undergoing pancreas transplant should have the presence and extent of their secondary complications of diabetes carefully documented. Those who are not on dialysis require determination of their glomerular filtration rate (GFR) and proteinuria. If they do not require dialysis at the time of evaluation but do have impaired renal function, institution of cyclosporine- or FK 506–based immunosuppression commonly will reduce their GFR by a mean of 35 mL/min (36, 37). Baseline documentation of the extent of retinopathy is helpful in determining its regression or progression following transplantation. Determining the presence of a neurogenic bladder is important before reinstituting the large urinary output that will follow successful renal transplantation. The most critical aspect of evaluation focuses on the extent of micro- and macrovascular disease. Asymptomatic coronary artery disease is fairly common in patients with diabetes, and the candidate's exercise capacity may be severely limited. Therefore, most patients should have a chemically induced cardiac stress evaluation, i.e., thallium Persantine scan or dobutamine echocardiogram. Abnormalities on either of these evaluations mandates formal coronary angiography. Approximately 4% of patients in the Rush program who underwent these evaluations were found to have coronary artery disease treatable by angioplasty or coronary artery bypass graft.

The macrovascular complications of diabetes frequently manifest as arterial insufficiency of the lower extremities and can result in limb amputation. Sometimes it is difficult to distinguish amputations done for control of osteomyelitis versus those for ischemia and determine their interrelationship. Pancreas and kidney transplants use the iliac vessels for revascularization, so examination of the aortoiliac arterial tree is prudent.

Diabetic neuropathy can be divided into sensory and autonomic neuropathies. Gastroparesis, a complication of autonomic neuropathy, may require insertion of intestinal tubes to maintain nutrition. A neurogenic bladder will complicate the posttransplant course. Somatic neuropathies of diabetes are frequently seen in prospective candidates and can produce an insensate foot, complicated by trophic ulcers. Without aggressive treatment and preventive care, incapacitating complications such as osteomyelitis and Charcot joints may occur.

## VARIATIONS ON PANCREAS TRANSPLANTATION

A segmental graft with ligation of the pancreatic duct was chosen for the first human pancreas transplant (9). In a subsequent series of 13 pancreas transplants performed between 1966 and 1973, 12 used the whole pancreaticoduodenal graft anastomosing the duodenal segment to recipient small bowel for enteric drainage, while one anastomosed the ampulla of Vater to the recipient bowel (38). This initial series of pancreas transplants identified the difficulty in controlling exocrine secretion. Enteric drainage of the secretions evoked frequent anastomotic disruptions and subsequent sepsis. A technique to eliminate acinar drainage was sought. Animal studies performed by Dubernard in the early 1970s led to the technique of intraductal injection of the pancreas allograft (39). Polychloroprene (Neoprene) was found useful because of its property of hardening after injection into the pancreatic duct. Occlusion of the duct by this agent causes atrophy of the exocrine tissue without modifying the function of the islet cells (39). The canines that underwent ductal injection of their pancreata with polychloroprene survived without subsequent development of diabetes.

This technique was first applied to human pancreas transplantation and successfully performed in 1976 (39). Low morbidity has been reported by several centers using this technique (10, 40). Polychloroprene solidifies by flocculation when in contact with an alkaline medium. In practice, this occurs at the level of the pancreatic ductules arising from the acinar cells. Additional substances have been evaluated, such as latex and prolamine (Ethibloc), with similar results. ß-Radioactive substances have been used to destroy the acinar tissue without destroying the islet cells; results have shown a transitory diminution of exocrine secretion without loss of endocrine function. At present, the program in Lyon is evaluating the effect of hematoporphyrin on exocrine secretions after exposure to the red spectrum of light. This application of photodynamic therapy may bring a new technique to the preparation of the pancreas graft.

If the grafts do not undergo intraductal ablation, then acinar drainage can be achieved via an enteric anastomosis to a loop of ileum or a Roux-en-Y limb. Implantation of the whole gland, including a duodenal segment providing enteric drainage into the intestine, was initially complicated by anastomotic breakdown and sepsis that can be associated with the high doses of steroids used for immunosuppression (41). In the early 1980s, clinical application of the immunosuppressant cyclosporine A allowed a reduction in the dose of steroids used for immunosuppression; which resulted in improved wound healing. The ability to reduce steroid usage has resulted in a re-evaluation of the technique of enteric drainage or bladder drainage of the exocrine secretions.

Sollinger et al. described a technique of visceral drainage of acinar secretion by anastomosing the duodenum to the dome of the bladder (42). An advantage of this technique is that it allows collection of amylase as it is secreted in the urine, to monitor the function of the pancreas allograft (42). Collecting the urine and measuring the rate of amylase secretion provides a marker of pancreas function. Reduction of urine amylase has been associated with rejection. Because of the decreased incidence of anastomotic leaks and the ability to monitor urine amylase, bladder drainage of the pancreas graft has been commonly used in the United States and increasingly applied in Europe (10). Alternatively, the duodenal segment can be anastomosed to the bowel for enteric drainage by a direct side-to-side enteric anastomosis or to a prepared Roux-en-Y limb (43, 44). However, no reliable method of monitoring amylase secretion as a marker for rejection has been found with enteric drainage.

The route of venous drainage of the pancreas graft with its high insulin content is another variable in the technique of pancreas transplantation. Physiologic drainage of the beta cell brings insulin through the portal system. Insulin has been identified as a hepatocyte growth factor (45–49). High concentrations of insulin in the liver act as a counterregulatory hormone for gluconeogenesis. Approximately 50–75% of insulin secreted is removed by the first pass through the liver (50).

Presently most pancreas allografts drain into the systemic iliac or caval venous circulation. This allows the pelvic location of the graft to accommodate drainage of acinar secretions into the bladder. Portal drainage with its subsequent physiologic systemic levels of insulin can be achieved by locating the pancreatic allograft in the recipient mesentery. The risk of potential complications is higher than with the systemic drainage techniques described above. Elevated plasma levels of insulin are routinely seen when systemic venous drainage is used. No detrimental long-term effects of these elevated levels of systemic insulin have been found.

The multiple techniques used for pancreas transplantation show that the best technique has yet to be agreed upon. It is difficult to compare the results of various techniques, since their evolution extends over several years with accompanying improvement in many factors other than just technical ones. Prospective trials comparing systemic versus portal venous drainage, segmental versus whole pancreas grafts, and ductal occlusion versus enteric drainage versus bladder drainage may decrease our uncertainty and identify the best technique. Successful transplantation of functioning islet cells could nullify this search. However, the function of grafted islet cells is still confounded by multiple problems, such as a heightened immune response to islet cells, the quantity of islet cells to be transplanted, and the increased number of donors required for such transplants. Resolution of these problems is not expected within the next few years.

## DONOR SELECTION AND PROCUREMENT

### Pancreas Donor Selection and Operation

Criteria that exclude cadaveric pancreas donation are similar to those for other organ transplantation. A donor history of neoplastic disease, other than primary central nervous system tumors, precludes use for transplantation, as does a history of a chronic infectious disease that could be transmitted with the graft, alcoholism, chronic pancreatitis, previous pancreatic surgery and, of course, a history of diabetes. The combination of hypotension and the use of vasopressors is thought to cause ischemic injury to the pancreas, resulting in a poor-quality pancreas allograft. There are no specific biologic markers to determine a suitable pancreas donor. Frequently, direct visualization of the organ by an experienced pancreas transplant surgeon is required. A recent multivariate analysis performed by the University of Minnesota Transplant Program showed association of donor age above 50 years with poor pancreas transplant outcomes. This is due to a decrease in the number of islet cells after this age (51, 52). Marked edema in the pancreas allograft discourages some from transplanting these organs. The Rush program, as others, found that the use of colloids during the resuscitative phase of the donor operation and release of the pancreas from its retroperitoneal attachments commonly reverses this edema, yielding an acceptable allograft.

### Multiorgan Procurement

Organs for transplantation are obtained from brain-dead, heart-beating, normally perfused donors. This maintains normal hemodynamics until the organs are flushed with preservation solution. However, successful pancreas allografts have been recovered from controlled, non-heart-beating donors with rapid flushing and intraabdominal cooling (53). The heart-beating normally perfused cadaveric donor is used as a multiorgan donor, which requires coordination and cooperation between different organ teams (54). Depending upon the hemodynamics and the experience of the team, initial organ dissection can be completed prior to the cessation of blood flow and flushing of the organs. Alternatively, initial arresting of the heart with flushing of the organs allows dissection of the organs in a cool exsanguinous state. Each technique has its own merits.

A generous incision from the jugular notch to the pubis with a median sternotomy is commonly used. Abdominal exploration is carried out to identify unrecognized tumors, infection, or unsuitable organs. The duodenum of the donor is considered contaminated intraluminally; therefore, antibacterial and antifungal agents are instilled into the duodenal lumen by way of a nasogastric tube during the operation. The gastrocolic ligament is divided and carried cephalad, including division of the short gastric vessels. The pancreas is visualized to determine the quality of the organ. A finger is placed through the foramen of Winslow to palpate for a replaced right hepatic artery. The presence of a replaced right hepatic artery originating from the superior mesenteric artery will typically abort whole pancreas procurement, but will allow segmental procurement. An innovative technique includes division of the replaced right hepatic artery at the level of the duodenum, with insertion of the hepatic portion into the stump of the gastroduodenal artery arising from the common hepatic artery. This allows use of both the liver and pancreas for transplantation (Fig. 86.1) (55).

The liver, kidney, and pancreas are initially exposed by mobilizing the right colon, a Cattell maneuver. This allows visualization of the entire inferior vena cava. The posterior peritoneum is dissected further, and the abdominal aorta is exposed. The aorta, proximal to the iliac bifurcation, is then encircled. Next, the triangular ligament of the left lateral segment of the liver is divided, and the supraceliac aorta is dissected and again encircled. These maneuvers provide the exposure needed for rapid cannulation and clamping should hemodynamic instability occur. A generous Kocher maneuver to the level of the superior mesenteric artery (SMA) releases the head of the pancreas from its retroperitoneal attachments. At this time, the middle colic vessels can be divided, and the splenic flexure of the colon taken down to allow the entire colon to be displaced into the pelvis. The spleen is then released from its ligamentous attachments. Using the spleen as a handle to decrease manipulation of the parenchyma of the pancreas, the gland is elevated from its retroperitoneal position. The common bile duct is ligated and divided at the level of the duodenum. The portal vein is then skeletonized so that appropriate sharing of the portal vein between the pancreas and liver can be determined. Following dissection of the liver and pancreas, the kidneys are exposed and the ureters identified.

The arterial supply of the liver is then determined. It is common for the gastroduodenal artery to be ligated and divided at the level of the duodenum. Dissection is then carried along the anterior surface of the common hepatic artery, identifying the branching of the splenic artery and left gastric artery. Division of

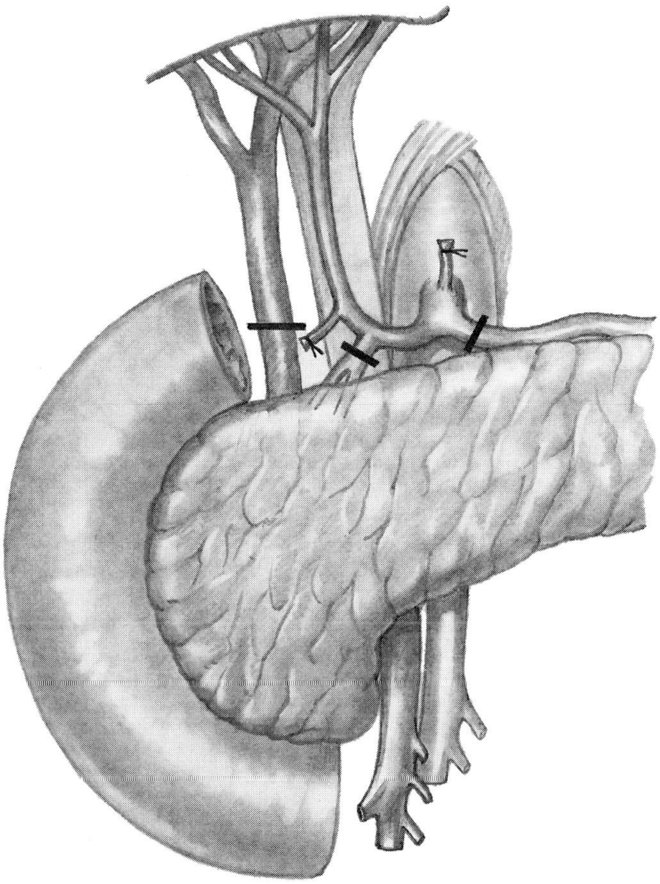

**FIG. 86.1.** General disposition of the main arterial pedicles to the pancreas. At least two of these pedicles are necessary for a total graft. In case of a liver procurement, splenic artery and gastroduodenal artery can be ligated and divided *(black lines)*. Superior mesenteric and splenic arteries will form the two pedicles of the graft.

the semilunar ganglion covering the origin of the celiac trunk provides visualization of the supraceliac aorta.

At completion of the dissection of the varied organs, in coordination with all teams, the infrarenal aorta is cannulated following systemic heparinization. The supraceliac aorta is then clamped, and approximately 3 L of University of Wisconsin solution is infused. Saline slush for topical cooling is applied to all usable organs. Caval exsanguination can be carried out at the pericardium by dividing the right atrium from its suprahepatic caval origin or by cannulation of the infrarenal cava. Direct portal vein flushing is not required. This is achieved by allowing the venous return of the splanchnic vessels with their contents replaced by preservation solution to supplant portal flush. Direct flushing of the liver via the portal vein produces venous hypertension, which exacerbates pancreas edema. If direct portal vein flushing is deemed necessary, one can cannulate the portal vein through the inferior mesenteric vein or a branch of the superior mesenteric vein (SMV) and advance the catheter into the portal vein. Encircling the cannulated hepatic side of the portal vein with a venotomy performed on the pancreas side prevents venous hypertension.

When adequate exsanguination and perfusion of the organs are completed, the liver is removed. Division of the portal vein is done allowing a 1–2 cm length of vein for the pancreas allograft. Division of the arterial tree shared by the liver and pancreas is then done as described above. If the liver team is accustomed to performing a donor common hepatic artery end-to-end anastomosis to the recipient proper hepatic artery, then arterial division can be carried out at the level of the *donor* proper hepatic artery. This allows the celiac and SMA to be taken as an aortic patch for implantation of the pancreas allograft. However, more commonly in the United States, the celiac axis is retained with the liver allograft. In this situation, the splenic artery is divided approximately 0.5 cm at its branching from the celiac axis. It is important not to dissect the splenic artery too far from its branching at the celiac axis. Small branches to the body of the pancreas arise from this section of the splenic artery. Division at the branching of the splenic artery allows the celiac axis to be retained with the liver graft but requires arterial reconstruction of the pancreas graft. The liver is further dissected by taking the diaphragmatic attachments surrounding the suprahepatic cava and dividing the infrahepatic cava at the level of the right renal vein.

With the liver explanted, the duodenum is divided at the level of the pylorus by an automatic stapler. Similarly, the distal portion of the duodenum is divided at the ligament of Treitz. Next, the root of the mesentery is divided, allowing the small bowel to be displaced into the pelvis. It is prudent to divide the left renal vein at its confluence with the vena cava at this point, preventing its injury during renal artery and SMA dissection. The tail and body of the pancreas are then elevated and an aortic patch of the celiac axis and SMA is removed. The renal artery should be identified to prevent injury during the dissection of the SMA. If the celiac axis is to be retained with the liver, then the origin of the SMA is taken at the level of the aorta. The pancreas is lifted from the abdominal cavity and placed in iced University of Wisconsin solution. The kidneys can then undergo their customary dissection and procurement.

### Arterial Reconstruction and Preparation for Implantation

If the celiac axis is retained with the pancreas graft, then reconstruction of the pancreas arterial supply is not needed. However, if the celiac axis is retained with the liver, and the splenic artery is divided at its branching from the celiac axis, then arterial reconstruction is needed for whole pancreas implantation. This can be achieved by anastomosing the divided splenic artery in an end-to-side fashion into the root of the SMA (Fig. 86.2*A*). A more common reconstruction uses the donor iliac artery. Reconstruction is carried out by anastomosing end-to-end the origin of the SMA to the external iliac artery and the divided splenic artery end-to-end to the internal iliac artery (Fig. 86.2*B*). This provides a long arterial graft for its implantation along the recipient arterial tree.

Because of the multiple vessels involved at the root of the mesentery, these vessels are ligated individually to ensure hemostasis after reperfusion of the pancreas. The duodenum is opened and again irrigated with antibacterial and antifungal solutions. The size of the duodenal segment is then reduced to include its second portion. Splenectomy can be carried out at this time or after reperfusion of the pancreas allograft.

Occasionally, while dissecting the donor porta hepatis, there is difficulty identifying arterial structures in situ. If this occurs, then a variation of multiorgan procurement is to remove the liver, pancreas, duodenum, and spleen en bloc. Then the arterial tree and portal vein can be divided in an ice basin in an exsanguinous state.

In segmental pancreas transplantation, the isthmus of the gland is divided at the level of the portal vein. A segment of the portal vein is taken as an extension of the splenic vein, which allows mobility for its venous anastomosis. The splenic artery is divided at its origin from the celiac axis. The pancreas graft splenic artery may be lengthened using a segment of donor iliac artery. If the celiac axis is included with the pancreas allograft, then no further reconstruction is needed.

After all arterial reconstructions are completed, it is common practice to infuse preservation solution through the arterial tree to confirm adequate exsanguination of the graft and to demonstrate arterial communication by the presence of venous flow. This also shows that adequate hemostasis has been achieved by vessel ligation at the root of the mesentery.

### Pancreas Procurement in the Living Donor

Use of living donors for segmental pancreas transplantation has been championed by Sutherland and coworkers at the University of Minnesota (56). Living-related organ donation potentially offers an immunologic advantage over cadaveric transplantation (57, 58). The surgical procedure for living-related pancreas retrieval is similar to segmental pancreas retrieval performed in the cadaver. The spleen is left in place, with its vascular supply and drainage being the short gastric vessels. The splenic artery is divided at its branching from the celiac axis, and the splenic vein is divided at its confluence with the SMV. The pancreas graft is then implanted as a segmental graft. Complications such as splenic infarction and intraabdominal collections have been observed. Additionally, abnormal glucose tolerance has been described in the living-related pancreas *donor* following segmental donation (59, 60).

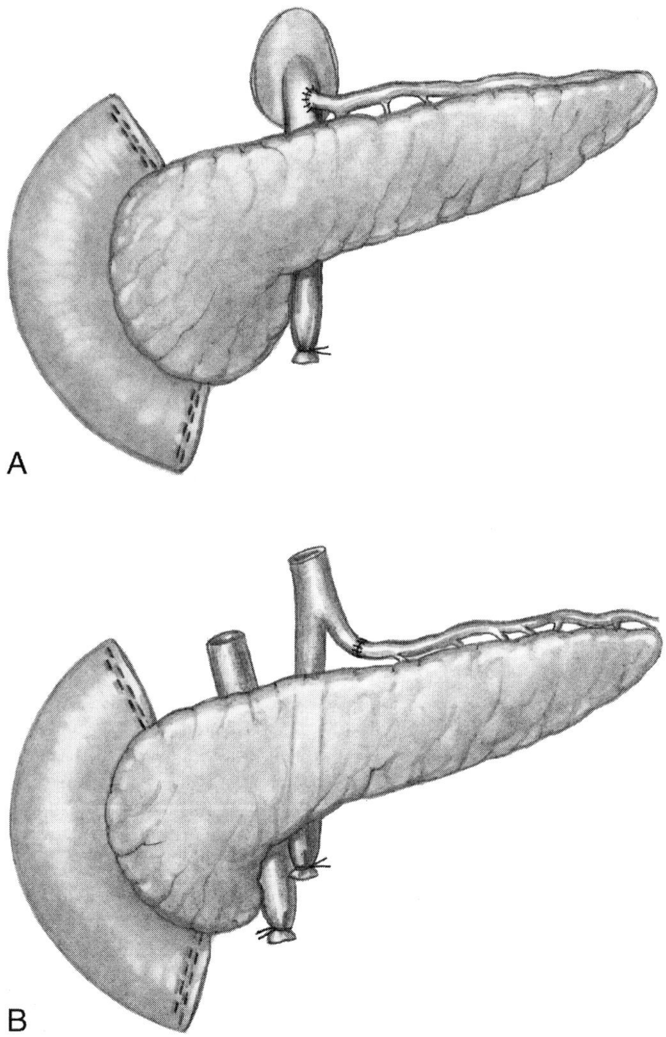

A

B

**FIG. 86.2.** Two types of revascularization of the arteries of a total graft. **A.** Use of the iliac bifurcation for revascularization of splenic and superior mesenteric arteries. **B.** Replantation of the splenic artery on the superior mesenteric artery.

### Pancreas Procurement and Sharing for Two Recipients

Pancreas transplant candidates with previous exposure to human antigens from failed transplants or blood transfusions, historically have a very difficult time obtaining a compatible donor. An exceptional technique is justified when more than one of these recipients is found to be compatible with the same cadaveric donor. Technically the pancreas can be divided to provide two segmental allografts. A total pancreatic duodenal graft is procured as previously described. In the iced basin, the graft is split into segmental grafts as dictated by their vascular supply. The distal segmental graft will be based on the splenic artery and splenic vein. The cephalad graft, consisting of the head of the pancreas and duodenum, is based on the SMA and SMV/portal vein confluence. With arterial and venous reconstruction, two segmental grafts can be fashioned to meet the needs of two highly sensitized recipients.

## OPERATION IN THE RECIPIENT

### Perioperative and Operative Planning

Patients with type I diabetes and ESRD represent the most common recipients of pancreas transplantation. These patients are chronically ill with abnormal metabolism. Initial hospital evaluation confirms absence of an active infection or a recent myocardial event. Despite the patient being NPO in preparation for the operating room, there is still a sustained insulin need. Frequent measurements of blood glucose are required, and the appropriate doses of insulin are administered. Preoperative antibiotics are routinely given. In the operating room, heating blankets and padding are placed, and the recipient is positioned to prevent pressure necrosis or nerve damage by traction.

The incision used for pancreas transplantation depends upon whether enteric drainage or bladder drainage of the pancreas allograft is planned. Since pancreas transplantation is most commonly combined with kidney transplantation, most centers use a midline celiotomy. Some centers favor bilateral iliac incisions with retroperitoneal dissection and allograft placement.

In spite of progress in the control of hypercholesterolemia in patients with diabetes, advanced atheroma of the vessels are commonly encountered. The vessels are frequently calcified and extremely fragile. Thus care must be taken in placing vascular clamps for arterial control. Following reperfusion of the graft, distal arterial patency is confirmed, ensuring that there is no arterial dissection to the involved extremity.

### Intraperitoneal Simultaneous Pancreas Kidney Transplantation

After a midline celiotomy is made down to the pubis, abdominal exploration is performed. Dissection of the iliac vessels is done with great care as previously mentioned. Implantation of the pancreas allograft is usually based on the recipient iliac vessels. The graft is positioned so the duodenal segment abuts the bladder. The recipient iliac vein is mobilized extensively, including division of the internal iliac vein to allow the common and external iliac veins to move anteriorly. This decreases tension on, and subsequent narrowing of, the venous anastomosis, as a result of graft edema. With the posterior aspect of the pancreas allograft facing the midline, an end-to-side portal vein to external iliac vein anastomosis is performed. A segment of donor iliac vein may be used to lengthen the donor portal vein as needed.

The arterial and venous anastomoses are performed at different levels on the iliac vessels. With the extension graft provided by arterial reconstruction of the pancreas allograft, it is possible to place the arterial anastomosis along the recipient proximal external iliac artery. After reperfusion of the pancreas, hemostasis is ensured. If the exocrine secretion of the pancreas is to be drained into the bladder, then an enterotomy is made in the dependent portion of the duodenal segment as well as an opening in the dome of the bladder. A two-layer anastomosis is performed using a hemostatic absorbable mucosal suture followed by a series of interrupted seromuscular sutures. Alternatively, this anastomosis can be done using an EEA stapler through another incision lower on the bladder (61). If splenectomy was not performed prior to implantation, then it is done at this time. If an SPK transplantation is to be performed, the renal allograft is placed in the opposite iliac fossa, and the ureteral anastomosis to the bladder is made on the contralateral side of the bladder (Fig. 86.3).

### Retroperitoneal Simultaneous Pancreas-Kidney Transplantation

If the grafts are to be implanted in the retroperitoneal space, then bilateral iliac incisions are used. The retroperitoneal space is entered, and the peritoneum is swept medially. The iliac vessels are prepared as above. Vascular anastomosis for implantation is the same as intraperitoneal placement. The duodenum-to-bladder anastomosis is completed similarly. Fluid collection with retroperitoneal placement is common; therefore, the peritoneum is opened to allow any peripancreatic fluid collection to be reabsorbed by the peritoneum. Occasionally, the omentum may be long enough to be placed around the pancreas graft through a peritoneal incision. This can help in reabsorption of perigraft fluid. The wound is closed in layers. An iliac incision is made on the contralateral side. The implanted kidney is placed on the exposed iliac vessels and an ureteroneocystostomy is made. Again the wound is closed in layers.

### Pancreas Transplantation with Enteric Drainage of Exocrine Secretions

Following a midline celiotomy, the pancreas allograft is placed in the left gutter, with the duodenal segment oriented superiorly. The previously described vascular anastomoses are carried out, but more proximally along the iliac vessels. A simple side-to-side enteric anastomosis to the duodenal segment is created (62). The site on the ileum for anastomosis should be chosen to prevent subsequent malabsorption diarrhea. Typically, the enteric anastomosis is made 80 cm from the ligament of Treitz. A two-layer anastomosis is done in the usual fashion. Another technique is to create a Roux-en-Y segment of small bowel, producing a defunctionalized enteric anastomosis. The limb of the Roux-en-Y should be approximately 40 cm long. The small bowel mesentery should be reapproximated to prevent internal herniation and subsequent bowel obstruction.

Venous drainage of the pancreas allograft into the iliac system results in systemic hyperinsulinemia (63–65), which some investigators believe may accelerate atherosclerotic vascular disease (66). For this reason, some programs use portal drainage of the pancreas allograft, using the technique of Gaber. Arterial inflow is obtained by tunneling the reconstructed donor iliac arterial graft through the small bowel mesentery for anastomosis to the recipient common iliac artery. The portal vein is then anastomosed to the side of a recipient SMV tributary. Enteric drainage is performed by a Roux-en-Y limb in a side-to-side manner (67, 68).

### Segmental Pancreas Transplantation

Segmental transplantation of the pancreas as developed by Dubernard's team provides a means of eliminating exocrine drainage, which has been a problem in pancreas transplantation. This technique of ablating exocrine secretions with ductal occlusion is simple, with little morbidity (39). A small catheter is

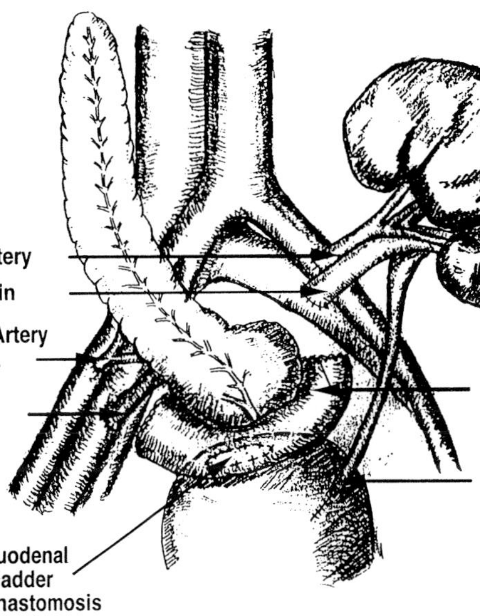


**FIG. 86.3.** Simultaneous pancreas-kidney transplant with bladder drainage.

inserted into the pancreatic duct for approximately 5 cm and secured with a purse-string suture. Two occluding clamps are placed on the neck of the pancreas to prevent reflux of the occluding agent (Fig. 86.4). Approximately 2–5 mL of polychloroprene or a similar substance is injected into the pancreatic duct under low pressure prior to revascularization. Visualization of the occluding substance at the surface of the gland denotes adequate injection.

The segmental pancreas graft can be placed through an iliac incision into a retroperitoneal position or through the previously described midline celiotomy. Both are revascularized using the iliac vessels in proximity. The graft is positioned so the tail of the gland lies in the right lateral gutter, pointing toward the right kidney. Alternatively, the segmental pancreas can be positioned transversely. A small trough is made by mobilizing the anterior aspect of the bladder. This orientation positions the anterior surface of the pancreas adjacent to the anterior abdominal wall. Arterial and venous anastomoses again are placed at separate levels along the iliac vessels. After revascularization of the allograft, hemostasis is achieved, and the graft is positioned to ensure absence of vascular impingement. Commonly, the pancreas allograft secretes a substantial amount of exocrine fluid. If placed in a retroperitoneal location, the peritoneum can be opened and the omentum positioned around the graft to enhance reabsorption of this fluid.

Bladder drainage of the segmental allograft is also possible. The position of the segmental graft is such that the cut surface of the graft abuts the bladder. Arterial and venous vascularization is performed as previously described. An anastomosis between the pancreatic duct and the bladder mucosa is carried out. Additionally, the bladder is sutured to the pancreatic parenchyma to stabilize the anastomosis.

Segmental pancreas transplantation can also be done with intestinal or gastric drainage of the exocrine secretions. Again the revascularization of the pancreas allograft is based on the iliac vessels or the aorta/vena cava. A Roux-en-Y limb of small intestine is anastomosed to the pancreatic duct, with mucosa-to-mucosa apposition. A small Silastic catheter is placed in the duct of Wirsung to provide drainage of the exocrine secretions, to protect the anastomosis. This also allows quantitation of amylase excretion, which can serve as a marker for pancreas

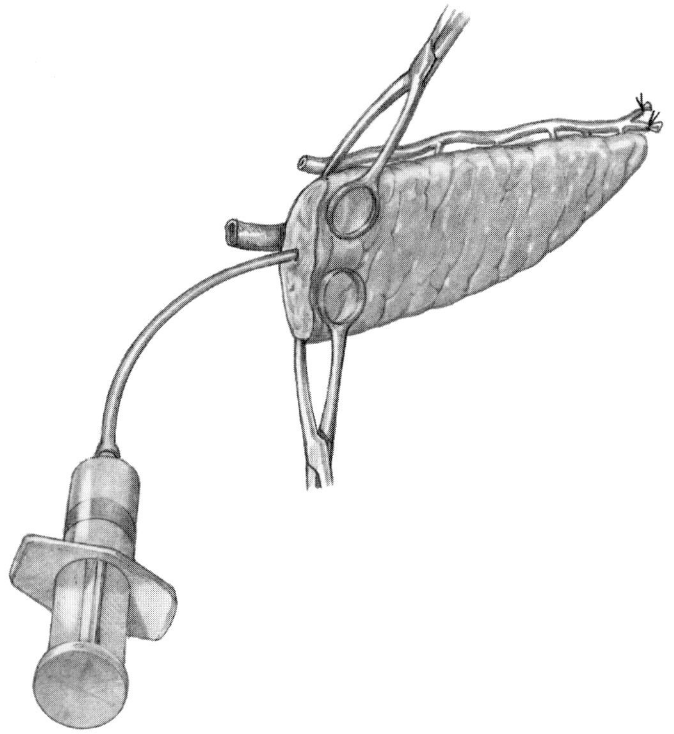

**FIG. 86.4.** Neoprene is injected in the pancreatic duct via a catheter inserted in the duct. Clamps are put on the neck of the pancreas to prevent liquid reflux during injection.

allograft dysfunction. Instead of an intestinal anastomosis, the cut edge of the gland can be anastomosed to the posterior aspect of the stomach. This position allows portal drainage of the pancreas.

### Retransplantation of the Pancreas Allograft

Several second transplants of the pancreas have been performed in the Lyon center. This is always done intraperitoneally. The nonfunctioning pancreas allograft is removed, which may be difficult because of the subsequent fibrosis. The arterial reconstruction of the new pancreas can use the arteriotomy of the failed pancreas, or a new anastomosis can be placed a few centimeters proximally.

## OPERATIVE AND POSTOPERATIVE CARE OF THE PANCREAS TRANSPLANT RECIPIENT

### Surveillance of Postoperative Diabetes

Control of glycemia before, during, and after the pancreas transplant is important. Hyperglycemia may result in excessive stimulation of the pancreas allograft. Continuous insulin infusion is used to achieve normoglycemia. However this requires frequent measurements at 30-minute intervals by a glucometer. The Rush program has seen hypoglycemia after reperfusion of the pancreas, especially if the donor was young, with episodes of hypotension prior to procurement. Glucose is not controlled by an insulin pump because it is costly, requires specially trained staff, and is difficult to adjust with the changing serum glucose levels. Following *whole* pancreas transplantation, insulin requirements decrease dramatically. Most patients no longer require exogenous insulin after the first 1–2 days. Following *segmental* pancreas transplantation, exogenous insulin is needed for a longer time at much higher doses (69, 70).

### Hemodynamic and Renal Monitoring

Patients are frequently extubated at the end of the procedure but are observed in the intensive care unit postoperatively. Routine monitoring of the electrocardiogram, blood pressure, central venous filling pressure, temperature, arterial blood gas, and serum glucose is required. Vascular filling pressures are maintained by use of crystalloid, albumin, and other colloid concentrates as needed. The hematocrit is kept above 20%. Those with a question of cardiac compromise are monitored by Swan-Ganz catheterization. The Lyon center has seen blood pressure instability in 52% of their patients, with episodes of prolonged arterial hypotension (>20 minutes) (71). The Rush program frequently sees hypertension that requires vasodilating therapy. Despite these hemodynamic alterations, acute tubular necrosis is observed in 8% or less of the transplanted kidneys. This has been attributed to the short cold ischemia time associated with combined pancreas kidney transplant.

Patients who have undergone simultaneous pancreas and renal transplantation also require monitoring of urinary output and adjustments of volume status to maintain adequate systemic perfusion. Oliguria, in the face of adequate intravascular volume, suggests vascular compromise of the renal allograft and mandates emergent ultrasonic evaluation of its arterial and venous flow.

### Immunosuppression

Immunosuppressive protocols used in pancreas transplantation are very similar to those of kidney transplantation. The objectives of immunosuppression are to prevent rejection of the allograft, yet maintain an immune system that can respond to infections. Rejection of the allograft has been the weak point of pancreas transplantation. Excluding early graft loss secondary to technical failure and death of the recipient with a functioning transplant, rejection is the most common cause of graft loss (10). Therefore, immunosuppression plays a pivotal role in pancreas transplantation. Most programs, including Lyon and Rush, use quadruple immunosuppression with cyclosporine A (Sandimmune, Neoral) or FK506 (Prograf), azathioprine (Imuran) or mycophenolate mofetil (CellCept), and prednisone. Induction therapy with either polyclonal (ATG) or monoclonal ($OKT_3$) antilymphocyte serum is common. Multiple agents are combined to avoid the toxicities associated with any one agent and to achieve an overall acceptable level of immunosuppression. Frequently, monoclonal antilymphocyte globulin ($OKT_3$) is reserved for the treatment of steroid-resistant rejection (72). The Rush program has used early conversion to oral immunosuppression. The newly developed microemulsified cyclosporine A (Neoral) and FK506 tacrolimus (Prograf) with its increased oral bioavailability have allowed a decrease in antilymphocyte globulin induction therapy (73, 74).

### Anti-thrombotic Therapy

Systemic heparin in low doses of approximately 100 IU/kg/day is used in Lyon, with subsequent conversion to platelet inhibitors during the second postoperative week. The Rush program has avoided the use of heparin. Instead, high-molecular-weight dextran is infused during the first 24 hours, with concomitant administration of low-dose aspirin. Both of these approaches are in response to the historic 6–12% graft thrombosis rate, though there are no reliable studies to prove their effectiveness (75).

## PANCREAS REJECTION

Although the incidence of technical failures in pancreas transplantation is relatively high at 6–12%, rejection represents the most frequent cause of pancreas graft loss after transplantation (76). When grafts lost to technical failure are excluded, graft survival rates differ for SPK transplantation (93%), PAK transplantation (77%), and PTA (73%) (77). These differences have been attributed to the difficulty of diagnosing and successfully treating pancreas allograft rejection. Using both organs from the same donor allows the kidney to act as a biologic marker of pancreas rejection. Diagnosis of rejection is more precise in the kidney allograft than in the pancreas (78). Measurement of serum creatinine to identify dysfunction can often be followed by renal allograft ultrasound and biopsy prior to substantial dysfunction in the pancreas allograft. Successful treatment of rejection in the renal allograft may halt or reverse concomitant pancreas rejection.

In those individuals *not* undergoing a concomitant renal allograft, as in PAK transplant or PTA, other markers of rejection have been sought. The drainage of pancreatic secretions into the bladder allows collection and determination of urinary amylase levels. A drop in urine amylase of 25–50% can act as a marker for pancreas rejection (79, 80). Others have reported success by following serum human anodal trypsinogen levels (81). Still others have favorable results using biopsy of the pancreas or its duodenal segment (82–84). Biopsy of the pancreas can be performed cystoscopically in bladder-drained transplants. Interpretation of the biopsy may be difficult, since reflux pancreatitis can be confused with rejection (85). Segmental duct–injected grafts do not lend themselves to biopsy. The graft becomes atrophic after several weeks, making it a difficult target. Pulse Doppler ultrasonography of the pancreas seems to show promise. Measurement of the resistive index of the intraparenchymal vessels combined with the echogenicity of the parenchyma may be especially helpful in acute allograft rejection (86, 87).

Hyperglycemia is a late finding in pancreas rejection and occurs after approximately 90% or more of the islet cells have been destroyed (88). Percutaneous core biopsy of the pancreas allograft has been avoided for fear of creating a troublesome pancreatic fistula. The Rush program uses fine-needle aspiration (FNA) of the pancreas allograft (89). Comparison studies of FNA and core biopsy of the kidney have shown a good correlation. This has been extended to the pancreas allograft (90, 91). Multiple FNAs of the pancreas allograft under ultrasound guidance have been carried out, obtaining pancreatic acinar tissue and ductal tissue for review. FNA can determine the presence or absence of activated lymphocytes and macrophages consistent with an immunologic inflammatory response. No major complications or morbidity have been seen to date with this technique.

## COMPLICATIONS OF THE PANCREAS TRANSPLANTATION

### Thrombosis

Thrombosis of the pancreas allograft usually occurs early following transplantation. Sudden hyperglycemia with reduction in urine amylase levels is consistent with arterial thrombosis. Duplex Doppler ultrasound or angiography confirms this complication. Graft removal is carried out to prevent subsequent loss of the renal allograft from complications of a retained necrotic pancreas graft.

Most vascular thromboses of the pancreas allograft are venous and occur with an incidence of 6–12% (10). Venous thrombosis is thought to be precipitated because of the high vascular resistance that occurs in the pancreas as a result of tension on the venous anastomosis from graft swelling or intrinsic pancreas venous hypertension postreperfusion. The incidence of venous thrombosis is higher in the segmentally injected graft than in whole pancreas transplantation (70). Venous thrombosis is heralded by the abrupt onset of gross hematuria. The portal vein provides the venous drainage of the transplanted duodenal segment. Thus, acute venous occlusion results in duodenal mucosal congestion and sloughing, with subsequent hematuria. Additionally, swelling of the graft produces local peritoneal inflammation and pain. Recently, immediate thrombectomy following the diagnosis of pancreatic venous thrombosis has been reported to be of benefit (92). Because of the high rate of venous thrombosis, most programs performing pancreas transplantation treat the graft with either anticoagulant or antithrombotic agents. The decrease in the overall incidence of thrombosis in Lyon has been attributed to the use of University of Wisconsin preservation solution and increased monitoring of the hemodynamic parameters postoperatively. Others feel that complete mobilization of the iliac vein decreases narrowing of the venous outflow tract and subsequent thrombosis.

### Arterial Complications

Arterial complications of pancreas transplantation are similar to those of other allografts and other vascular anastomoses. These include anastomotic hemorrhage, hematoma formation, and thrombosis. Meticulous adherence to technique in anastomosis to atherosclerotic iliac arteries is required. Unique to the pancreas allograft is the development of an arterial venous fistula at the ligated root of the transplant mesentery. This complication presents with an asymptomatic bruit or thrill and requires operative correction (93). Pseudoaneurysms and mycotic aneurysms have also been described. Management of these complications may require sacrifice of the graft (94, 95).

A particular manifestation of late arterial stenosis has been seen in the pancreas transplant recipient. Long-term allograft recipients in whom hyperamylasemia occurs associated with hyperglycemia may require reinstitution of insulin as a result of arterial stenosis to the graft. This macrovascular arteriopathy may represent a form of chronic rejection specific to the pancreatic allograft (96).

### Urologic Complications

The recent increase in graft survival has been attributed to bladder drainage techniques used for pancreas transplantation. However, there are urologic complications because of this method. Hematuria occurs commonly following the creation of a bladder-drained pancreas allograft. The mucosa of the duodenal segment is quite friable. Although hematuria is frequent, it is usually self-limited, resolving within a couple of days of onset. No treatment is needed during this phase other than ensuring Foley catheter patency. Patients with hematuria requiring blood transfusions undergo cystoscopy with identification of the bleeding site. Hematuria developing after the first month may represent CMV infection of the duodenal segment or severe cystitis. Differential diagnosis requires cystoscopy. Fulguration may be needed to control a bleeding source. If CMV is confirmed, then a course of ganciclovir is required.

Urinary tract infections occur in up to 50% of individuals with bladder drainage of the allograft. This has been attributed to the alkalinization of the urine from the exocrine drainage, which results in chronic cystitis with bacterial adhesion (97). Although these complications are frequent, they can be reduced with prophylactic antibiotic therapy (98).

Males have more severe complications of bladder drainage, which cause urethritis, urethral strictures, and urethral disruptions. Disruptions commonly present with suprapubic discomfort and scrotal edema (98). The diagnosis is confirmed by a cystogram. Treatment includes cystoscopy and Foley catheter drainage. Previously, urethral disruption was an indication for enteric conversion (99). The Rush program has had two urethral disruptions, neither of which followed instrumentation of the urethra (98). Both patients had a component of meatal stenoses. Neither patient has had a recurrence more than 6 months after urethral dilatation.

Reflux pancreatitis can also be a problem. A neurogenic

bladder is common in diabetes recipients and results in elevated intravesicular pressures. This can almost always be managed with Foley catheter drainage if caught early. However, recurrent pancreatitis warrants conversion to enteric drainage of the pancreas graft (99).

### Anastomotic Leak and Fistula

Pancreatic fistulas occur with an incidence of 50% in segmentally injected pancreas transplants. If a graft is placed in a retroperitoneal location, the fistula exits through the wound. If the fistula output exceeds 300 mL/day, somatostatin analogues have been found useful. There are concerns that somatostatin with its associated effect of decreasing splanchnic blood flow may make the graft more prone to thrombosis as well as altering immunosuppression absorption. Low-volume pancreatic fistulas usually dry up within a few weeks with local care (70, 100). With intraperitoneal segmental grafts, a pancreatic leak may show up as intraabdominal sepsis. However, most low volume fistulas are reabsorbed by the peritoneal cavity and do not cause problems.

Anastomosis of the duodenal segment to the bladder can result in fistula formation with an incidence of 14% (98). This fistula may originate from the duodenal anastomosis to the bladder or from the staple line of the duodenal segment. Patients present with nonlocalized abdominal pain or flank pain. A sensitive method of diagnosis is the technetium voiding cystourethrogram (101, 102). Duodenal bladder anastomotic leaks usually occur within the first 1–2 months postoperatively. Leaks occurring after the second postoperative month frequently involve the duodenal segment staple line. This may represent a manifestation of CMV infection of the duodenal segment. These fistulas can be managed by Foley catheter drainage and appropriate antiviral agents if CMV is the cause.

Because of the frequent complications associated with bladder drainage techniques, enteric conversion is not uncommon. If possible, a wait of 3–6 months between the initial transplant and enteric conversion is recommended (103). Most of the complications for which enteric conversion is considered are self-limited and resolve after this period of time. If enteric conversion is needed, then the duodenum is disconnected from the bladder, and the cystostomy is closed primarily. A Roux-en-Y limb or loop of ileum is anastomosed in a side-to-side fashion with the remaining duodenal segment (103, 104).

As described above, the pancreas-duodenal allograft can be anastomosed primarily to the bowel for enteric drainage. This technique is used less frequently because of a previous anastomotic leakage rate. The increased rate has been attributed to the higher immunosuppression required immediately following transplantation (105, 106). The manifestation of an unrecognized occult leak is sepsis with its associated morbidity and mortality. The Lyon center is convinced that a Roux-en-Y limb is safer and performs the anastomosis with a standard two-layer technique.

### Metabolic Disorders

Hyperkalemic acidosis is frequent following bladder drainage. This has been attributed to the obligatory bicarbonate loss from the duodenal segment and the pancreas. Management is by vigorous hydration and bicarbonate replacement in the form of citrates or salts of bicarbonate. The Rush program has found that limiting the size of the duodenal segment results in decreased bicarbonate loss.

### Other Complications

Candidates for pancreas transplantation have a multitude of metabolic problems and are never considered ideal operative candidates. The most lethal complications following pancreas transplantation are related to the candidate's previous and ongoing cardiovascular disease. In fact, cardiovascular disease represents 50% of the mortalities in the Lyon center and in other groups (106). Cardiovascular complications (angina, myocardial infarction, cardiac insufficiency, arrhythmic disorders, or cardiac arrest) occur in 20% of all patients undergoing pancreas transplants in Lyon. The preexisting hypertension of ESRD is almost universal. Following SPK transplantation, it is not uncommon to have the need for antihypertensive medications reduced or eliminated. This may well represent the reversal of uremia.

Gastroparesis is a common complication of diabetes (108). Many patients require medication to enhance GI motility preoperatively because of this problem. The Rush program has found gastroparesis a limiting factor in early conversion to oral immunosuppressants. To manage this, a transnasal feeding tube is placed at the time of transplantation, providing reliable enteral access in the early postoperative period.

## LONG-TERM RESULTS

### Patient and Graft Survival

Survival rates for both patients and allografts are maintained by the International Pancreas Transplant Registry (IPTR), as well as the United Network of Organ Sharing (UNOS). Over the past 30 years, more than 7500 pancreas transplants have been performed worldwide (77). Inclusive of all implantation techniques used, actuarial patient survival at 1 year is 91% and at 5 years is 80% (20). Again, when all implantation techniques are included, the primary pancreas graft survival rate at 1 year is 75% and at 5 years is 60% (10). Pancreas graft survival rates depend on the drainage technique used. Bladder drainage results in 78% 1-year pancreas graft survival, enteric drainage results in 66% 1-year graft survival, and ductal injection results in 63% 1-year graft survival (10). UNOS and IPTR data reveal that the best pancreas graft survival rates were obtained when SKP transplants were performed and bladder-drainage techniques were used (10, 11). With the elimination of technically unsuccessful grafts, SPK graft survival rates increase to 91% at 1 year and 82% at 5 years (77).

Pancreas transplantation can be done alone or in combination with other organs. In the United States, most pancreas transplants are done in combination with kidney transplants in individuals who are uremic or who will soon require dialysis. UNOS data reveal that in the United States, pancreas allografting is done in combination with kidney transplantation (SPK) 89% of the time, after kidney transplant (PAK) in 7%, and pancreas transplant alone (PTA) in 4% (11). Pancreas graft survival rates differ for SPK and PTA. The 1-year graft survival rate for SPK transplantation is 78%, compared with 60% for PAK and 55% for PTA. Despite the decreased graft survival rates for solitary pancreas transplants, patient survival rates at 1 year are essentially the same, 90–92% (77). The decreased pancreas graft survival rates have inhibited some programs and many third-party payers from performing or paying for pancreas-only transplants (PAK, PTA). However, experienced centers using graft monitoring have reported PAK and PTA graft survival rates at 1 year of 75% or more (109).

### Effects on Secondary Complications of Diabetes

Secondary complications of diabetes are a result of prolonged hyperglycemia with excessive glycosylation of membrane-bound proteins as well as circulating proteins (110–114). The ability to achieve persistent euglycemia and its effects on the secondary complications of diabetes have been approximated by the Diabetes Control and Complications Trial (DCCT) whose results were released in 1993 (7). Using multiple injections of insulin with tight glucose control, microalbuminemia was decreased by 35%, clinical neuropathy by 60%, and major retinopathy by 34–76%. The pancreas allograft is thought to provide a euglycemic state better than intensive insulin therapy does. The negating factor in this formula is the side effects of immunosuppressive medications.

Upon revascularization of the pancreas allograft, there is immediate secretion of insulin and glucagon (115). It is not uncommon to see intraoperative glucose levels plummet, and intensive monitoring is required during this phase. Insulin requirements following whole pancreas transplantation are small compared with those following segmental grafts, reflecting the number of beta cells transplanted with each type of graft. Since most pancreas transplants have their venous drainage into the systemic circulation, this results in elevated systemic insulin levels and delayed postprandial peaks of insulin (116). The Lyon center demonstrated that following an oral glucose load, normoglycemia is achieved only after 180 minutes. This indicates glucose intolerance with delayed insulin secretion compared with normal subjects (117, 118). Despite the theoretical disadvantages of elevated peripheral insulin levels, major complications from systemic drainage of the pancreas allograft have yet to be identified (109).

**Long-Term Metabolic Results.** Maintenance of the euglycemic state has a major impact on the development, stabilization, or progression of the secondary complications of diabetes. A functioning pancreas allograft results in a euglycemic state with normalization of glycosylated hemoglobins (119, 120). Segmental pancreas grafts have maintained normoglycemia for up to 10 years following transplantation despite the persistence of abnormal glucose tolerance test results. Possible explanations for the difference in glucose homeostasis between whole pancreas grafts and segmental grafts is the fibrosis attributed to polychloroprene injection and/or the transplantation of a smaller number of islet cells in the segmental graft. Despite these abnormal glucose tolerance test results with segmental grafts, glycosylated hemoglobin levels remain normal (121).

**Diabetic Retinopathy.** The effect of pancreas transplantation on retinopathy is difficult to interpret because of the advanced state of retinopathy in transplant recipients (122, 123). Some improvement in retinopathy in patients undergoing SPK transplantation has been attributed to the reversal of the uremic state. The Lyon center has studied 38 patients with functioning grafts for a mean of 9 years and compared their retinal status with that of patients who lost their pancreas graft either by rejection or by early thrombosis. No differences were seen in visual acuity, presence of cataracts, or stage of diabetic retinopathy. As was found with the DCCT, stabilization of retinopathy may not be seen in the first few years. Some studies of longer duration (i.e., more than 4 years following pancreas transplantation) have shown stabilization of retinopathy (109, 124, 125). The University of Minnesota program has found stabilization of retinopathy in individuals with a functioning pancreas graft compared with those who lost their pancreas allograft (126). As with other therapies, improvement following pancreas transplantation will not be seen when very advanced retinopathy is present.

**Diabetic Neuropathy.** Diabetic neuropathy is a result of prolonged, uncontrolled glycemia (7). Diabetic neuropathy was studied in 60 patients with a successful pancreas transplant in Lyon. Parameters included clinical findings, sensory motor nerve conduction velocity, and autonomic neuropathy evaluation. Data collected before and after pancreas transplant were compared. The study was carried out for 9 years following transplant. Greater improvement was observed in sensory neuropathy than in autonomic neuropathy. Improvement occurred after 2 years and continued up to 7 years. Such longitudinal data cannot be attributed to the reversal of uremia (127). This improvement in neuropathy has been confirmed by other groups (128–131). Several years of prolonged normoglycemia are required before substantial improvement is seen.

**Diabetic Nephropathy.** Pancreas transplantation prevents the relapse of diabetic nephropathy in the transplanted kidney. The centers in Stockholm and Minneapolis have compared type I diabetes patients who underwent pancreas-kidney transplantation with those who had kidney transplantation alone on a similar immunosuppression regimen (132–134). Biopsies of the transplanted kidneys were obtained to determine the recurrence of diabetic nephropathy. The presence of a successful pancreas transplant prevented the development of microangiopathy in the renal allograft. Isolated pancreas transplant prior to the onset of diabetic nephropathy accounts for a very small portion of the total pancreas transplants performed. However, the University of Minnesota examined this group and found that the nephropathy index of the recipient's native kidney shows a decrease in glomerular volume as well as decreased mesangial volume following successful pancreas transplant (135), despite a subsequent decrease in the overall creatinine clearance (90 ± 21 L/min before vs. 60 ± 14 mL/min after). The decrease in GFR has been attributed to the effect of cyclosporine on the recipients' native kidneys as is commonly seen in extrarenal transplant recipients.

**Quality-of-Life Issues.** Quality-of-life is a major issue affecting individuals with diabetes, especially those who develop ESRD. Improved quality-of-life after successful SPK transplantation with relief from a diabetes- and dialysis-dependent life is profound and has been demonstrated consistently (136–138). Individuals who undergo pancreas transplantation alone because of extreme difficulty with metabolic control or hypoglycemia unawareness realize freedom from exogenous insulin use and from hypoglycemic episodes that have a negative impact on their employment capability (139, 140).

**Recurrence in Diabetes following Transplantation.** Development of type I diabetes is felt to be an autoimmune phenomenon; therefore, an allograft, by definition, does not share the same autoimmune environment. However, in living-related donors sharing identical HLA antigens, histologic relapse of diabetes in the pancreas allograft has been seen under modest immunosuppression (141). Progression of this biologic experiment has resulted in the resumption of insulin therapy 2.5–38 months following transplantation. Histology of the pancreas graft revealed the infiltration of graft islet cells by activated T lymphocytes and macrophages (141).

The most common cause for recurrence of diabetes after pancreas transplantation is allograft loss secondary to acute or chronic rejection. Omitting patients dying with a functioning pancreas graft or losing their graft during the first year, reveals an immunologic loss of the pancreatic allografts of only 8% at 5 years (10).

Temporary recurrence of hyperglycemia has been seen within the first year, not associated with irreversible immunologic injury to the pancreas graft. At the Rush program and in Sweden, temporary return of a hyperglycemic state with elevated C-peptides has been seen, consistent with insulin-resistant type II diabetes (142). Hyperglycemia was reversed by lowering the steroids or administering oral hypoglycemic agents.

## CONCLUSIONS

Pancreas transplantation provides the most stable euglycemic state for patients with type I diabetes. Patient survival rates above 90% approximate the success rates for other more established organ transplants. Graft survival rates, especially when combined with kidney transplantation, approximate that of cadaveric renal transplantation. Improved immunosuppressive medications with decreased side effects combined with an enhanced ability to diagnose rejection in the pancreas allograft, will make pancreas transplantation prior to development of ESRD a clinical reality. Recognition and early treatment of complications minimize mortality and lower morbidity. The ability of pancreas transplantation to normalize the dysmetabolism of patients with type I diabetes shows the advantage of this procedure. Pancreas transplantation prior to the onset of ESRD avoids added years of dialysis with its expense and impact on quality-of-life.

## ISLET CELL TRANSPLANTATION

The defect in type I diabetes is the lack of insulin-secreting beta cells in the pancreas. These islet cells make up approximately 1% of the pancreas. The surgical complications of whole pancreas transplantation are related to the acinar and associated nonislet tissues. The transplantation of beta cells with minimal or no acinar tissue to achieve insulin independence is the primary objective of islet cell transplantation. Although reliable success has been achieved in the rodent, it has not been translated to larger animals or humans, for many reasons. One of the major problems in its clinical application is that islet cell isolation/purification techniques do not yield enough viable cells to achieve insulin independence from a solitary pancreas donor (143–146). There are also unresolved questions regarding the immunologic barriers to transplanted islet cells.

### History

The first attempts at islet cell transplantation were done as autografts. Following total or subtotal pancreatectomy for chronic pancreatitis, the islet cells were isolated and returned to the patient. The removed pancreas was digested, yielding a suspension of both acinar tissue and islet cells. This suspension was infused through the portal vein and engrafted into the native liver. Graft survival was achieved in approximately 30%, with some surviving more than 5 years (147). During this phase, the number of islet cells, or islet cell equivalents (IEQ), required to achieve normoglycemia in an autograft was found to exceed 300,000. A rare complication of hepatic infarction has been attributed to the rapid infusion rate of the nonhomogeneous suspension.

### Human Islet Cell Retrieval/Preparation

The cadaveric pancreas is digested by injecting a buffered salt solution containing collagenase into the ducts of the pancreas. Internal enzymatic digestion produces a slurry of acinar tissue and islet cells; this is described as the isolation phase of the islet cell preparation. This digestant, containing acinar and islet tissue, can be used for transplantation, but most programs purify the islet cells after the isolation phase, which reduces the total number of islet cells. The purification of islet cells is achieved by utilizing the differences in density between acinar and islet cell tissue. Using discontinuous gradient centrifugation, a preparation of more than 90% pure islet cells can be achieved. Ricordi has described an automated technique that combines these phases of islet cell preparation (148). The pancreatic duct is cannulated, and Hank's buffered saline solution containing collagenase is infused. The pancreas is then placed in an agitation chamber and the chamber is perfused with the collagenase-containing solution at 37°C. The cells that separated from the body of the pancreas are collected and washed free of any remaining collagenase. The suspension then undergoes purification using a Ficol gradient in an automated cell separator. A sample of the final preparation is examined and stained with dithizone (DTZ) dye. DZT stains zinc in the insulin granules, which confirms the presence of beta cells. The purified islet cells can be resuspended in an albumin solution and injected into the portal vein or another appropriate engraftment site.

The yield of pancreatic islet cells with this technique is quite variable. Usually two human pancreata are required to obtain the 8000 IEQ/kg needed to achieve normal glycemia using an allograft in patients with type I diabetes (149). The ability to acquire an adequate number of islet cell equivalents from human pancreata also depends upon the quality of the organ undergoing digestion (150). Previously, organs considered inadequate for solid organ transplantation were used for islet cell procurement. However, the factors that result in a poor-quality graft for whole organ transplantation are the same factors that result in low yields of islet cells. Factors involved in high-quality grafts include short preservation times, the use of young donors, prevention of donor hyperglycemia, absence of obesity, and avoidance of pressor agents (151). Therefore, solid organ transplantation and islet cell transplantation compete for the same donor group. Since islet cell transplantation will be applicable to many more individuals with type I diabetes than are presently undergoing whole pancreas transplantation, human sources for pancreatic islet tissue will never meet the potential need. Therefore, xenotransplantation, or transplantation across species, is undergoing intensive laboratory investigation. Xeno islet cells have reversed chemically induced diabetes in the rodent (152–154).

### Islet Cell Transplantation Results

Clinical islet cell allotransplantation has been carried out, but its success rate has been low. This is due not only to the quality and quantity of the islet cells transplanted, but also to the development of subsequent allograft rejection. Transplantation of islet cells from one or more donors exposes the recipient to a multitude of antigens, making subsequent transplantation more difficult. To avoid this antigen sensitization as well as the need for immunosuppression, many investigators are encapsulating islet cells. These capsules are usually made from alginates, which allow glucose and insulin to exchange but limit mediators of rejection from reaching the islet cells (155, 156).

### Clinical Islet Cell Transplantation

Clinical application of islet cell transplantation has been carried out as a solitary graft and in combination with other grafts. Patients undergoing upper abdominal exenteration for cancer that includes a total pancreatectomy have been studied. These individuals undergo liver transplantation and have donor islet cells infused within the portal vein. Approximately 55% of the patients achieved insulin independence until their death from recurrent cancer. One individual has survived 58 months without needing exogenous insulin (157, 158). More recently, simultaneous islet cell and kidney transplant has been done in patients with type I diabetes and ESRD. Serum C-peptide levels were measurable in 60% of the transplant recipients. However, an insulin-independent state was achieved in only 30% for a short period of time (159, 160). Although patients did not achieve long-term insulin independence, the presence of serum C-peptide confirmed islet cell survival. Most clinical attempts at islet cell transplantation have been unable to achieve insulin independence but have noted increased serum C-peptide levels as well as decreased insulin requirements. These studies showed that the number of islet cells should be 8000 IEQ/kg of body weight, preservation times should be less than 8 hours, the implantation site should be the liver, and induction therapy with poly- or monoclonal antilymphocyte antibodies should be used (161–164).

Future improvements in islet cell transplantation will come from several directions (Table 86.3). New agents for immunosuppression as well as immunoalteration of islet cells show promise. The use of transgenic donors, gene transplantation or molecular re-arrangement, can lower islet cell immunogenicity. Intrathymic grafting and the creation of immunotolerant chimerism using donor bone marrow infusion have been successful in animal models. Improvements in cryopreservation of islet cells, with high viability, allow the use of multiple donors to achieve the number of islet cells needed for each recipient. Breakthroughs in the immunology of xenotransplantation will result in an unlimited supply of islet cells for transplantation. These questions are under active investigation and will likely require cooperative

**TABLE 86.3. Future Directions in Islet Cell Transplantation**

Immunomodulation
- Islet cell culture at reduced temperatures
- Donor pretreatment with antilymphocyte antibodies
- Culture of islet cells with antilymphocyte antibodies
- Ultra violet B irradiation of islet cells

Induction of immunologic tolerance
- Donor-specific bone marrow infusion
- Transplant into privileged sites such as intrathymic
- Treatment with anti-CD4 monoclonal antibodies

Fetal islet cells
- Proliferation with growth factors
- Development of a hybrid strain

Immunoisolation techniques
- Alginates for microencapsulation
- Implantable perfusion chambers

Xenotransplantation
- Development of transgenic animals

efforts to achieve clinical relevance similar to that of whole pancreas transplantation for type 1 diabetes.

## REFERENCES

1. Cordonnier D, Halimi S, Benhamou Py. La néphropathie diabétique avant le stade de l'insuffisance rénale. Médicale MSD (Chapitre 1) 1988:9–37.
2. Diabetes Statistics. Prevalence of diabetes in the United States. National Institute of Diabetes and Digestive and Kidney Diseases of the National Institutes of Health (NIH). NIH publ. no. 96-3926. October 1995.
3. Castano L, Eisenbarth GS. Type I diabetes: a chronic autoimmune disease of human, mouse and rat. Annu Rev Immunol 1990;8:647–679.
4. Neurp J, Mandrup-Poulsen T, Molvig J, et al. Mechanism of pancreatic B-cell destruction in type I diabetes. Diabetes Care 1988;11(suppl 1):16–22.
5. Bennett PH. Definition, diagnosis and classification of diabetes mellitus and impaired glucose tolerance. In: Kahn CR, Wein GC, eds. Joslin's diabetes mellitus. Philadelphia: Lea & Febiger, 1994:194–195.
6. Banting FG, Best CH. The internal secretion of the pancreas. J Lab Clin Med 1922;7:257–266.
7. Diabetes Control and Complications Trial Research Group. The effect of intensive treatment of diabetes on the development and progression of long-term complication in insulin-dependent diabetes mellitus. N Engl J Med 1993;329:(14)977–986.
8. Kelly WD, Lillehei RC, Merkel FK, Idezuki Y, Goetz F. Renal and pancreatic allotransplantation in the treatment of diabetic nephropathy in man. In: Advances in transplantation: proceedings of the first international congress of the Transplantation Society. Baltimore: Williams & Wilkins 1968:699–707.
9. Kelly WD, Lillehei RC, Merkel FK. Allotransplantation of the pancreas and duodenum. Diabetic Nephrop Surg 1967;61: 827–837.
10. International Pancreas Transplant Registry. June 1995.
11. Annual report of the United States Scientific Registry of Transplants and Recipients and the Organ Procurement and Transplant Network. 1995:51.
12. Summary statistics on reported ESRD therapy in the US, 1993. USRDS patient database updated from HCFA PMMIS May 1995, quality control filters applied. (Includes only ESRD patients reported through HCFA as receiving renal replacement therapy for ESRD, or approximately 93% of the total number of U.S. ESRD patients.)
13. Bohman SO, Tyden G, Wilezek A. Prevention of kidney graft diabetic nephropathy by pancreas transplantation in man. Diabetes 1985;34:306.
14. Velosa JA, Frohnert PP, Perkins JD, et al. Pancreas transplantation at the Mayo Clinic: patient selection. Mayo Clin Proc 1990;65:475–482.
15. Traeger J, Piatti PM, Monti LD. Indications for combined pancreas and kidney transplantation. In: Dubernard JM, Sutherland DER, ed. International handbook of pancreas transplantation. Boston: Kluwer Academic Publishers, 1989;3:49–57.
16. Lefrançois N, Faure JL, Melandri M, et al. Kidney graft survival in simultaneous kidney pancreas transplantation. Diabetes 1989; 38(suppl):38–39.
17. Sutherland DER, Moudry Munns KD. International Pancreas Transplant Registry report. Transplant Proc 1990;22(4):1605.
18. Florack G. Sutherland DER, Sibley R, et al. Combined kidney and segmental pancreas allotransplantation in dogs. Transplant Proc 1985;17:374–377.
19. Gruessner RWG, Nakhleh R, Tzardis P, et al. Rejection patterns after simultaneous pancreaticoduodenal-kidney transplants in pigs. Transplantation 1994;57(5):756–760.
20. Stratta RJ, Taylor JS, Bynon JA, et al. Patterns of rejection after combined pancreas kidney transplantation. Transplant Proc 1994;26(2):524–525.
21. Friedman EA. Comprehensive care essential to success in diabetic nephropathy. Transplant Proc 1984;16:569.
22. Stratta RJ, Taylor R, Martin G, et al. Experience with protocol biopsies after solitary pancreas transplantation. Transplantation 1995;60;12:1431–1437.
23. Sutherland DER. Indications for pancreas transplantation: a commentary. Clin Transplant 1990;4:242–246.
24. Messent JW, Elliott TG, Hill RD, et al. Prognostic significance of microalbuminuria in insulin-dependent diabetes mellitus: a twenty-three year follow-up study. Kidney Int 1992;41(4): 836–889.
25. Lloyd CE, Becker D, Ellis D, Orchard TJ. Incidence of complications in insulin-dependent diabetes mellitus: a survival analysis. Am J Epidemiol 1996;143(5):431–441.
26. Bender R, Sawicki PT. Effect of intensive treatment in insulin dependent diabetes mellitus with microalbuminuria. Interpretation of study's results is open to criticism (Letter). Br Med J 1996;312(7025):254.
27. Crimi S, Cipolli D, Infantone E, et al. Microalbuminuria and severity of diabetic retinopathy in type 1 diabetic patients: association and relationship with some risk factors. Diabetes Metab 1995;21(6):440–445.
28. Drash AL. The child, the adolescent, and the Diabetes Control and Complications Trial. Diabetes Care 1993;16(11):1515–1516.
29. Chaturvedi N, Fuller JH. Glycosylated hemoglobin and the risk of microalbuminuria in insulin-dependent diabetes mellitus. EURODIAB IDDM Complications Study Group. N Engl J Med 1995;333(14):940–941.
30. Sutherland DER. Effect of pancreas transplantation on secondary complications of diabetes. In: Dubernard JM, Sutherland DER, ed. International handbook of pancreas transplantation. Boston: Kluwer Academic Publishers, 1989;13:257–289.
31. International Pancreas Transplant Registry 1995.
32. Anvessnen RWG. FK506 for induction or rescue therapy after pancreas transplantation: a multicenter analysis. Presented at the XVI international congress of the Transplant Society. Barcelona, August 1996.
33. Bartlett ST, Schweitzer EJ, Johnson LB, et al. Equivalent success of simultaneous pancreas kidney and solitary pancreas transplantation: a prospective trial of tacrolimus immunosuppression with percutaneous biopsy. Annals of Surgery 1996;224(4):40040–40049.
34. Faber OK, Hagen C, Binder C, et al. Kinetics of human connecting peptide in normal and diabetic subjects. J Clin Invest 1988;62:197–203.
35. Gero L, Korany H, Tamas EJ Jr. Residual B-cell function in insulin dependent (type I) and non-insulin dependent (type 2) diabetics. Diabetes Metab 1983;9:183–190.
36. Brennan DC, Stratta RJ, Lowell JA, et al. Cyclosporine challenge in the decision of combined kidney-pancreas versus solitary pancreas transplantation. Transplantation 1994;57(11):1606–1611.
37. Wang YL, Stevens RB, Fioretto P, et al. Correlation of preoperative renal function and identification of risk factors for eventual native renal failure in cyclosporine treated non-uremic diabetes recipients of pancreas transplant alone. Transplant Proc 1993; 25(1):1291–1292.

38. Lillehei RC, Ruix JO, Aquino C, et al. Transplantation of the pancreas. Acta Endocrinol Suppl 1976;205:303–320.
39. Dubernard JM, Traeger J, Neyra P. A new method of preparation of segmental pancreatic grafts for transplantation in trials in dogs and in man. Surgery 1978;84:633–639.
40. Martin X, Lefrancois N, Dawahra M. Pancreas transplantation in the uremic patient: a random trial of pancreas with bladder drainage versus duct obstruction of segmental grafts. Transplant Proc 1993;25:1182–1189.
41. Groth CG, Collste H, Lundgren G, et al. Successful outcome of segmental human pancreatic transplantation with enteric exocrine diversion after modifications in technique. Lancet 1982;1:522–524.
42. Sollinger HW, Cook R, Harps D, et al. Clinical and experimental experience with pancreatico cystostomy for exocrine drainage in pancreas transplants. Transplant Proc 1984;16:749–751.
43. Groth CG, Lundgren G, Arner P, et al. Resection of isolated pancreatic allograft in patients with diabetes. Surg Gynecol Obstet 1976;143:133–140.
44. Tibell A, Brattstrom C, Wadstrom J, et al. Improved results using whole organ pancreatoduodenal transplants with enteric exocrine drainage. Transplant Proc 1994;26(2):412–413.
45. Starzl TE, Watanabe K, Porter KA, Putnam CW. Effects of insulin, glucagon, and insulin/glucagon infusions on liver morphology and cell division after complete portacaval shunt in dogs. Lancet 1976;1(7964):821–825.
46. Starzl TE, Proter KA, Putnam CW. Insulin, glucagon, and the control of hepatic structure, function, and capacity for regeneration. Metabolism 1976;25(11 suppl 1):1429–1434.
47. Starzl TE, Terblanche J. Hepatotrophic substances. Prog Liver Dis 1979;6:135–151.
48. Starzl TE, Francavilla A, Porter KA, Benichou J. The effect upon the liver of evisceration with or without hormone replacement. Surg Gynecol Obstet 1978;146(4):524–532.
49. Starzl TE, Francavilla A, Halgrimson CG, et al. The origin, hormonal nature, and action of hepatotrophic substances in portal venous blood. Surg Gynecol Obstet 1973;127(2): 179–199.
50. Polonsky KS, Jaspan J, Emmanovel D, et al. Difference in the hepatic and renal extraction of insulin and glucogon in the dog: evidence for saturability of insulin metabolism. Acta Endocrinol 1983;102:420–427.
51. Gruessner RWG, Truppmann C, Bynon B, et al. Assessment of donor and recipient risk factors on pancreas transplant outcome. Transplant Proc 1994;26(2):437–438.
52. Pouzdjian V, Gugliuzza K, Fish J. Multivariate analysis of donor risk factors for pancreas allograft failure after simultaneous pancreas-kidney transplantation. Surgery 1994;118(1):73–81.
53. Personal communication. Hoffman R and Sollinger H. University of Wisconsin, Madison, WI, 1994.
54. Sollinger HW, Vernon W, D'Alessandro H, et al. Combined liver and pancreas procurement with Belzer-UW solution. Surgery 1989;106(4):685–691.
55. Thistlethwaite J, Lloyd D, Broelsch C, et al. Whole pancreas and liver procurement from single cadaver organ donor: where should shared vascular structures be divided? Diabetes 1989; 38:232.
56. Sutherland DE, Goetz FC, Najarian JS. Pancreas transplants from related donors. Transplantation 1984;38(6):625–633.
57. Sutherland DER, Gruesser R, Dunn D, et al. Pancreas transplantation from living related donors. Transplant Proc 1994;26; 2:443–445.
58. Gruessner RW, Sutherland DE. Simultaneous kidney and segmental pancreas transplants from living related donors—the first two successful cases. Transplantation 1996;61(8):1265–1268.
59. Kendall DM, Sutherland DE, Goetz FC, et al. Metabolic effect of hemipancreatectomy in donors. Preoperative prediction of postoperative oral glucose tolerance. Diabetes 1989;38(suppl 1):101–103.
60. Seaquist ER, Robertson RP. Effects of hemipancreatectomy on pancreatic alpha and beta cell function in healthy human donors. J Clin Invest 1992;89(6):1761–1766.
61. Douzdjian V, Gugliuzza KK, Fish JC. Handsewn versus staple duodenocystostomy in bladder drained pancreas transplants. Transplant Proc 1995;27;6:3053–3054.
62. Corey RJ, Egidi MF, Shapiro M, et al. Enteric drainage of the pancreas transplants revisited. Transplant Proc 1995;27;6:3048–3049.
63. Blackman JD, Polonsky KS, Japan JB, et al. Insulin secretory profiles and C-peptide clearance kinetics at 6 months and 2 years after kidney-pancreas transplantation. Diabetes 1992; 41(10):1346–1354.
64. O'Meara NM, Sturis J, Blackman JD, Byrne MM, et al. Oscillatory insulin secretion after pancreas transplantation. Diabetes 1993; 42(6):855–861.
65. Diem P, Abid M, Redmon JB, et al. Systemic venous drainage of pancreas allografts as independent cause of hyperinsulinemia in type I diabetic recipients. Diabetes 1990;39(5):534–540.
66. DeFronzo RA, Ferrannini E. Insulin resistance. A multifaceted syndrome responsible for NIDDM, obesity, hypertension, dyslipidemia, and atherosclerotic cardiovascular disease. Diabetes Care 1991;14(3):173–194.
67. Newell KA, Woodle ES, Millis JM. Pancreas transplantation with portal venous drainage and enteric exocrine drainage offers early advantage without compromising safety or allograft function. Transplant Proc 1995;27(6):3002–3003.
68. Gaber AO, Shokouh-Amiri H, Grewal HP, et al. A technique for portal pancreatic transplantation with enteric drainage. Surg Gynecol Obstet 1993;177(4):417–419.
69. Tajra LC, Molina G, Albalate P, Lefrancois N, Brunet M, Martin X. Early postoperative period: study of metabolic profiles after segmental or total pancreas transplantation. Transplant Proc 1994;26,2:478–479.
70. Martin X, Lefrancois N, Dawahra M. Pancreas transplantation in the uremic patient: a random trial of pancreas with bladder drainage versus duct obstruction of segmental grafts. Transplant Proc 1993;25:1182–1189.
71. Mercatello A, Mongin Long D, LefranÇois N. Anesthésie et réanimation de la transplantation pancréatique (Abstract). JEPU 1989:169–199.
72. Lard W. Immunosuppression for pancreas transplantation recipients. In: Dubernard JM, Sutherland DER, ed. International handbook of pancreas transplantation. Boston: Kluwer Academic Publishers, 1989:167–186.
73. Cantarovitch D, Dandal J, Hourmand M. Importance of cyclosporine dosage and blood levels in simultaneous pancreas and kidney transplantation. Transplant Proc 1992;24:890–891.
74. Shapiro ME, Abrams JM, Brown RS, et al. Successful pancreas-renal transplantation without anti T-cell antibody induction. Transplant Proc 1995;27(6):3087–3088.
75. Sutherland DER, Gruessner A. International Pancreas Transplant Registry 1995.
76. Stratta RJ, Taylor RJ, Bynon JS, et al. Patterns of rejection after combined kidney transplantation. Transplant Proc 1994;26;2: 524–525.
77. Sutherland DER, Gruessner RWG. International Pancreas Transplant Registry. Pancreas transplant results in the United States with comparison to non-US data in the international registry. IPTR annual report, 1995.
78. Dubernard JM, Traeger J, Touraine JL, et al. Rejection of human pancreatic allografts. Transplant Proc 1980;12:103–106.
79. Sollinger HW, Cook, Kamps D, et al. Clinical and experimental experience with pancreaticocystostomy of exocrine pancreatic drainage in pancreas transplantation. Transplant Proc 1984;16:749–751.
80. Sollinger HW, Pirsh JD, D'Alessandro AM. Advantages of bladder drainage in pancreas transplantation: a personal view. Clin Transplant 1990;4:32–36.
81. Ploeg RJ, D'Alessandro AM, Groshek M, et al. The efficacy of human anodal trypsinogen for detection of rejection in clinical pancreas transplantation. Transplant Proc 1994;26;2:531–533.
82. Lowell JA, Bynon JS, Nelson N, et al. Improved technique for a transduodenal pancreas transplant biopsy. Transplantation 1994;57(5):752–753.
83. Jones JW, Nakhleh RE, Cassanova D, et al. Cystoscopic transduodenal pancreas transplant biopsy: a new needle. Transplant Proc 1994;26(2):527–528.
84. Klassen DK, Hoehn-Saric EW, Bartlett ST, et al. Isolated pancreas rejection in combined kidney pancreas transplantation. Transplantation 1996;61(6):974–977.

85. Nakhleh RE, Sutherland DER. Pancreas rejection. Significance of histopathologic findings with implications for classification of rejection. Am J Surg Pathol 1992;16(11):1098–1107.
86. Kubota K, Biuing H, Kelter U, et al. Duplex doppler ultrasonography for evaluation pancreatic grafts. Transplant Proc 1990;22: 1–183.
87. Nghiem DD, Ludrosky L, Young JC. Evaluation of pancreatic circulation by duplex color doppler flow sonography. Transplant Proc 1994;26(2):466.
88. Tyden G, Lundgren G, Gunnarson R, et al. Laboratory findings during rejection of segmental pancreatic allografts. Transplant Proc 1984;16:715–717.
89. Egidi MF, Shapiro R, Corey RJ, et al. Fine needle aspiration biopsy in pancreas transplantation. Transplant Proc 1995;27(6):3055–3056.
90. Hayry P, von Willebrand E, Ahonen J, et al. Monitoring of organ allograft rejection by transplant aspiration cytology. Ann Clin Res 1981;13(4–5):264–287.
91. Egidi MF. Fine-needle aspiration biopsy in renal transplantation: a review of cytologic features. Diagn Cytopathol 1990;6(5): 330–335.
92. Fernandez Druz L, Gilavert R, Sabater L. Pancreas graft thrombosis: prompt diagnosis and immediate thrombectomy or retransplantation. Clin Transplant 1993;7:233–234.
93. Lowell JA, Bynon JS, Stratta RJ, et al. Superior mesenteric arterial venous fistulas in vascularized whole organ pancreatic allografts. Surg Gynecol Obstet 1993;177:254–258.
94. Stzakas AG, Carrol PV, Gordon RD, et al. Arterial mycotic aneurysm and rupture. A potentially fatal complication of pancreatic transplantation and diabetes mellitus. Arch Surg 1989;124:660–661.
95. Ciancio G, Burke GW, Viciana AL, et al. Destructive allograft fungal arteritis following simultaneous pancreas kidney transplantation. Transplantation 1996;61:1172–1175.
96. Fakir M, Cardozo M, St. Louis G, et al. Hyperamylasemia associated with pancreatic graft arterial stenosis in combined kidney pancreas transplantation. Transplantation 1992;53;3: 689–691.
97. Smith JL, See WA, Ames SA, et al. Lower urinary tract complications with patients with duodenal cystomies for exocrine drainage of the transplanted pancreas. Transplant Proc 1991;23: 1611–1612.
98. Sollinger HW, Messing EM, Eckhoff DE, et al. Urological complications of 210 consecutive simultaneous pancreas kidney transplants with bladder drainage. Ann Surg 1993;218;4:561–570.
99. Sollinger HW, Sasaki TM, D'Allessandro AM, et al. Indications for enteric conversion after pancreas transplantation with bladder drainage. Surgery 1992;112:842–846.
100. Everett J, Wahoff D, Statz C. Characterization and impact of wound infection after pancreas transplantation. Arch Surg 1994;129(12):1310–1316.
101. Eckhoff DE, Ploeg RJ, Wilson MA, et al. Efficiency off $^{99m}$Tc voiding cystourethrogram for detection of duodenal leaks after pancreas transplantation. Transplant Proc 1994;26(2):462–463.
102. Ozaki C, Stratta R, Taylor R. Surgical complications in solitary pancreas and combined pancreas kidney transplants. Am J Kidney Dis 1992;164:546–551.
103. Sollinger HW, Sasaki TM, D'Alessandro AM, et al. Indications for enteric conversion after pancreas transplantation with bladder drainage. Surgery 1992;112:842–846.
104. Stephanian E, Gruessner RWG, Brayman K, et al. Conversion of exocrine secretions of the bladder to enteric drainage of recipients of whole pancreatoduodenal transplants. Ann Surg 1992;216:663–672.
105. Burke GW, Sutherland DER, Najarian JS, et al. Intra-abdominal fluid collections in pancreas transplant recipients: bladder versus enteric drainage. Transplant Proc 1988;20:87–88.
106. Groth CG. Surgical complications following pancreatic transplantation. In: Groth CG, ed. Pancreatic transplantation. Philadelphia: WB Saunders, 1998:17:219–238.
107. Corey RJ, Nghiem DT, Schanbacher B, et al. Critical analysis or mortality and graft loss following simultaneous pancreatico duodenal transplantation. Transplant Proc 1986;19:2305–2306.
108. Solders G, Tyden G. Improvement of nerve conduction in diabetic neuropathy. A follow up study of 4 years after combined pancreatic and renal transplantation. Diabetes 1992;41:946–951.
109. Stratta RJ, Taylor RJ, Gill IS. Pancreas transplantation: a managed care approach to diabetes. Curr Probl Surg 1996;33(9): 709–816.
110. Nathan DM. Long term complications of diabetes mellitus. N Engl J Med 1993;328:1676–1684.
111. Chase HP, Jackson WE, Hoops SL, et al. Glucose control in renal and retinal complications of insulin dependent diabetes. JAMA 1989;261:1155–1160.
112. Brownle M. Glycosylation and diabetic complications. Diabetes 1994;43:836–841.
113. Bucala R, Cerami A, Vlassara H. Advanced glycosylation end products in diabetic complications. Diabetes Rev 1995;3: 258–268.
114. Strowig SF, Reskan P. Glycemic control and the complications of diabetes. Diabetes Rev 1995;3:237–257.
115. Piatti PM, Traeger J, Dubernard JM, et al. Hormonal evaluation of immediate pancreatic function in simultaneous kidney plus pancreas transplantation during artifical pancreas monitoring. Transplant Proc 1985;17:346–348.
116. Stratta RJ, Taylor RJ, Zorn BH, et al. Combined pancreas kidney transplantation: preliminary results and metabolic effects. Am J Gastroenterol 1991;86:967–703.
117. Secchi A, Dubernard JM, La Rocca E. Endocrinometabolic effects of whole versus segmental pancreas allotransplantation in diabetic patients: a two year follow-up. Transplantation 1991;51:625–629.
118. Diem P, Abid M, Redmon JB, et al. Systemic venous drainage of pancreas allograft as independent cause of hyperinsulinemia in type I diabetes recipients. Diabetes 1990;39:534–540.
119. Katz H, Homan M, Vlosa J, et al. Effects of pancreas transplantation on postprandial glucose metabolism. N Engl J Med 1991;325:1278–1283.
120. Morel P, Goetz FC, Moudry-Muns KC. Long term metabolic control in patients with pancreas transplantation. Ann Intern Med 1991;115:694–699.
121. Morel P, Chau C, Brayman K. Quality of metabolic control at 2 to 12 years after pancreatic transplantation. Transplant Proc 1992;24:835–837.
122. Königsraner A, Miller K, Steurer W, Kieselbach G, Aichbergerc Ö. Does pancreas transplantation influence the course of diabetic retinopathy? Diabetologia 1991;34(suppl 1):86–88.
123. Ulbig M, Kampik A, Thurau S. Longterm follow up of diabetic retinopathy for up to 71 months after combined renal and pancreatic transplantation. Graefes Arch Clin Exp Ophthalmol 1991;229:242–245.
124. Caldara R, Bandello F, Vigano C. Influence of successful pancreatorenal transplantation on diabetic retinopathy. Transplant Proc 1994;26;2:490.
125. Königsrainer A, Miller K, Steuren W. Does pancreas transplant influence the course of diabetic retinopathy. Diabetologia 1991;34(1):586–588.
126. Ramsay RC, Goetz FC, Sutherland DER. Progression of diabetic retinopathy after pancreas transplantation for insulin dependent diabetes. N Engl J Med 1988;318:208–214.
127. Laftavi MRA, Chapuis F, Vial C. Diabetic polyneuropathy: outcome after successful pancreas transplantation 1 to 9 years follow up. Transplant Proc 1995;27,1:1406–1409.
128. Muller-Felber W, Landgraf R, Scheuer R. Diabetic neuropathy 3 years after successful pancreas and kidney transplantation. Diabetes 1993;42:1482–1486.
129. Solders G, Tyden G. Persson A, et al. Improvement in diabetic neuropathy four years after successful pancreatic and renal transplantation. Diabetology 1991;33(1):S125.
130. Boucek P, Bartos V, Vanek Z. Diabetic autonomic neuropathy after pancreas and kidney transplantation. Diabetology 1991; 34(1):S121.
131. Sutherland DER. Effect of pancreatic transplantation on secondary complications of diabetes: review of observations at a single institution. Transplant Proc 1992;24:859–861.
132. Najarian JS, Sutherland DER, Simmons RL. Kidney transplantation for the uremic diabetic patient. Surg Gynecol Obstet 1977;144: 682–688.
133. Cheung AHS, Sutherland DER, Gillingham KJ, et al. Simultaneous

pancreas/kidney transplant vs. kidney transplant alone in diabetic patients. Kidney Int 1992;41:924–929.
134. Bilous RW, Mauer SM, Sutherland DER, et al. The effects of pancreas transplantation on the glomerular structure of renal allografts in patients with insulin-dependent diabetes. N Engl J Med 1989;321(2):80–85.
135. Stratta RJ, Taylor RJ, Ozaki CF, et al. The analysis of benefits and risks of combined pancreas and renal transplantation vs. renal transplantation alone. Surg Gynecol Obstet 1993;177: 163–171.
136. US Renal Data System. USRDS 1992 annual report. Simultaneous kidney pancreas transplantation versus kidney alone: patient survival, kidney graft survival and posttransplant hospitalization. Am J Kidney Dis 1992;20:61–67.
137. Nakache R, Tyden G, Groth CG. Longterm quality of life in diabetic patients after combined pancreas kidney transplantation or kidney transplantation. Transplant Proc 1994;26(2): 510–511.
138. Sutherland DER. Pancreas transplantation: an update. Diabetes Rev 1993;1:152–165.
139. Gross CR, Zehrer CL. Health related quality of life outcomes in pancreas transplant recipients. Clin Transplant 1992;6:165–171.
140. Sibley RK, Sutherland DER. Recurrence of diabetes mellitus in the pancreas graft. In: Groth CG, ed. Pancreas transplantation. Philadelphia: WB Saunders, 1988:339–355.
141. Soulis AK, Farquarson MA, Hardman R. Aberrant expression of class Ii major histocompatibility complex molecules by B cells and hyperexpression of class I major histocompatibility complex molecules by insulin containing islets in type I diabetes. Diabetologia 1987;30:333–343.
142. Wadstrom J, Gannedahl G, Wahlberg J, Frodin L, Tedbrandt A, Berne C. Development of type II diabetes after combined kidney-pancreas transplantation in a patient with type I (insulin-dependent) diabetes. Transplant Proc 1994;26(3):1761–1762.
143. Federlin KF, Bretzel RG. The effect of islet transplantation and complications of experimental diabetes. World J Surg 1984;8: 169–178.
144. Altman JJ, Cugnenc PH, Tessier C. Epiploïc flac: a new site for islet transplantation in man. Horm Metab Res 1990;25:136–137.
145. Scharp DN, Lacy PE, Santagoj U. Results of first nine intraportal islet allografts in type I, insulin dependent diabetic patients. Transplantation 1992;51:76–85.
146. Socci C, Falqui L, Davallia M. Fresh human islet transplantation to replace pancreatic endocrine function in type I diabetic patient. Acta Diabetol 1991;28:151–157.
147. Farney AC, Najarian J, Nakleh RE. Autotransplantation of dispersed pancreatic islet tissue combined with total, or near total pancreatectomy for treatment of chronic pancreatitis. Surgery 1991;110:427–439.
148. Ricordi C, Camello RG, eds. The automated method for islet isolation in pancreas islet cell transplantation. Austin: Landes, 1992.
149. Gores PF, Najarian JS, Stephania NE, et al. Insulin independence in type I diabetes after transplantation of unpurified islet cells from a single donor with 15-deoxyspergualin. Lancet 1993:19.
150. Zeng Y, Torre M, Karrison T. The correlation between donor characteristics and the success of human islet isolation. Transplantation 1994;57:954–958.
151. Gores PF, Gillingham KJ, Dunn DL. Donor hyperglycemia as a minor factor and immunologic variables as major risk: factors for pancreas allograft loss in a multivariate analysis of a single institution's experience. Ann Surg 1992;215:217–230.
152. Ueno M, Nakajima Y, Kanehiro H, Yoshimura A, Nakano H. Immunosuppressive effect in combination therapy of cyclosporine A, FK506 and 15-deoxyspergualin on a pancreatic islet xenotransplantation (in Japanese). Nippon Geka Gakkai Zasshi 1993;94(4):376–382.
153. Iwata H, Takagi T, Amemiya H. Agarose microcapsule applied in islet xenografts (hamster to mouse). Transplant Proc 1992;24 (3):952.
154. Iwata I I, Takagi T, Amemiya I I. Marked prolongation of islet xenograft survival (hamster to mouse) by microencapsulation and administration of 15-deoxyspergualin. Transplant Proc 1992; 24(4):1517–1518.
155. Lim F, Sun AM. Microencapsulated islet cells as bio-artifical endocrine pancreas. Science 1980;908–910.
156. Clayton HA, James RF, London NJ. Islet cell microencapsulation: a review. Acta Diabetol 1993;30(4):181–189.
157. Rilo HLR, Carrol PB, Tzaskis A, et al. Insulin dependence for 58 months following pancreas islet cell transplantation in a patient undergoing upper abdominal exoneration. Transplant Proc 1995;27(6):3164–3165.
158. Rilo HLR, Carrol PB, Shapiro R, et al. Human islet cell transplantation: results of the first 37 patients. Transplant Proc 1995;27(6): 3162–3163.
159. Ricordi C, Tzakis A, Carroli P. Human islet isolation and allotransplantation in 22 consecutive cases. Transplantation 1992;53: 407–414.
160. Warnock GL, Kreteman N, Ryan E. Longterm follow up after transplantation of insulin producing pancreata islets into patients with type I (insulin dependent) diabetes. Diabetologia 1992;35:89–95.
161. Haring BJ, Browstzki CC, Schultz A, et al. Clinical islet cell transplantation registry report accomplishments in the past and future research needs. Cell Transplant 1993;2:269–282.
162. Haring BJ, Geir C, Schultz AO. International Islet Cell Transplant Registry Newsletter 1994;4:1–20.
163. Kneteman N, Alderson D, Scharp D, Lacy P. Longterm angiogenic storage of purified adult human islets of Langerhans. Diabetes 1989;38:386–396.
164. Hayek A, Lopez AD, Beattie G. Factors influencing islet transplantation: number, location and metabolic control. Transplantation 1990;49:224–228.

# Index

* *Italic* page numbers indicate figures; page numbers with *t* indicate tables.

## A

## B

## F



## G

## H

## L



## M

## N



## O



## P

## R

## S



## T

## U



## V